西医经典名著集成

菲兹帕里克皮肤病学

FITZPATRICK'S DERMATOLOGY

9TH EDITION

VOLUME 2

Sewon Kang
Masayuki Amagai
Anna L. Bruckner
Alexander H. Enk
David J. Margolis
Amy J. McMichael
Jeffrey S. Orringer

第9版（双语版）

编译委员会主任委员　陈翔　粟娟

中册

McGraw Hill ｜ 湖南科学技术出版社

CONTENTS

目 录

Volume 1 上 册

PART 1 FOUNDATIONS OF CLINICAL DERMATOLOGY
第一篇 临床皮肤病学基础

1 Fundamentals of Clinical Dermatology: Morphology and Special Clinical Considerations ························ 1
Erin H. Amerson, Susan Burgin, & Kanade Shinkai
第一章 临床皮肤病学基本原理：形态学和特殊的临床考虑

2 Pathology of Skin Lesions ·············· 19
Rosalie Elenitsas & Emily Y. Chu
第二章 皮疹的病理学

3 Epidemiology and Public Health in Dermatology ······················ 42
Junko Takeshita & David J. Margolis
第三章 皮肤病流行病学和公共卫生学

PART 2 STRUCTURE AND FUNCTION OF SKIN
第二篇 皮肤的结构和功能

4 Developmental Biology of the Skin ········ 53
Luis Garza
第四章 皮肤发育生物学

5 Growth and Differentiation of the Epidermis ···· 67
Terry Lechler
第五章 表皮生长和分化

6 Skin Glands: Sebaceous, Eccrine, and Apocrine Glands ······················ 76
Christos C. Zouboulis
第六章 皮肤腺体：皮脂腺、小汗腺和顶泌汗腺

7 Biology of Hair Follicles ················ 96
George Cotsarelis & Vladimir Botchkarev
第七章 毛囊生物学

8 Nail ······························ 114
Krzysztof Kobielak
第八章 甲

9 Cutaneous Vasculature ················ 124
Peter Petzelbauer, Robert Loewe, & Jordan S. Pober
第九章 皮肤血管系统

10 The Immunological Structure of the Skin ···· 139
Georg Stingl & Marie-Charlotte Brüggen
第十章 皮肤免疫系统

11 Cellular Components of the Cutaneous Immune System ···················· 153
Johann E. Gudjonsson & Robert L. Modlin
第十一章 皮肤免疫系统的细胞成分

12 Soluble Mediators of the Cutaneous Immune System ···················· 170
Allen W. Ho & Thomas S. Kupper
第十二章 皮肤免疫系统的可溶性介质

13 Basic Principles of Immunologic Diseases in Skin (Pathophysiology of Immunologic/ Inflammatory Skin Diseases) ············ 204
Keisuke Nagao & Mark C. Udey
第十三章 皮肤免疫性疾病发生的基本原理（免疫性/炎症性皮肤病的病理生理学）

14 Skin Barrier ······················· 219
Akiharu Kubo & Masayuki Amagai
第十四章 皮肤屏障

15 Epidermal and Dermal Adhesion ·········· 246
Leena Bruckner-Tuderman & Aimee S. Payne
第十五章 表皮和真皮的黏附

16 Microbiome of the Skin ················ 268
Heidi H. Kong
第十六章 皮肤微生物组学

1

17 Cutaneous Photobiology ················· 280
Thomas M. Rünger
　第十七章　皮肤光生物学

18 Genetics in Relation to the Skin ············ 305
Etienne C. E. Wang, John A. McGrath, & Angela M. Christiano
　第十八章　皮肤遗传学

19 Carcinogenesis and Skin ·················· 328
Kenneth Y. Tsai & Andrzej A. Dlugosz
　第十九章　癌变与皮肤

20 Pigmentation and Melanocyte Biology ······· 347
Stephen M. Ostrowski & David E. Fisher
　第二十章　色素沉着和黑素细胞生物学

21 Neurobiology of the Skin ·················· 371
Sonja Ständer, Manuel P. Pereira, & Thomas A. Luger
　第二十一章　皮肤神经生物学

PART 3 DERMATITIS
第三篇　皮炎

22 Atopic Dermatitis ························ 383
Eric L. Simpson, Donald Y. M. Leung, Lawrence F. Eichenfield, & Mark Boguniewicz
　第二十二章　特应性皮炎

23 Nummular Eczema, Lichen Simplex Chronicus, and Prurigo Nodularis ··········· 406
Jonathan I. Silverberg
　第二十三章　钱币状湿疹、慢性单纯性苔藓和结节性痒疹

24 Allergic Contact Dermatitis ················ 416
Jake E. Turrentine, Michael P. Sheehan, & Ponciano D. Cruz, Jr.
　第二十四章　变应性接触性皮炎

25 Irritant Dermatitis ······················· 436
Susan T. Nedorost
　第二十五章　刺激性皮炎

26 Seborrheic Dermatitis ···················· 451
Dae Hun Suh
　第二十六章　脂溢性皮炎

27 Occupational Skin Diseases ················ 462
Andy Chern, Casey M. Chern, & Boris D. Lushniak
　第二十七章　职业性皮肤疾病

PART 4 PSORIASIFORM DISORDERS
第四篇　银屑病样皮肤疾病

28 Psoriasis ······························· 483
Johann E. Gudjonsson & James T. Elder
　第二十八章　银屑病

29 Pityriasis Rubra Pilaris ··················· 525
Knut Schäkel
　第二十九章　毛发红糠疹

30 Parapsoriasis and Pityriasis Lichenoides ······ 533
Stefan M. Schieke & Gary S. Wood
　第三十章　副银屑病和苔藓样糠疹

31 Pityriasis Rosea ························· 547
Matthew Clark & Johann E. Gudjonsson
　第三十一章　玫瑰糠疹

PART 5 LICHENOID AND GRANULOMATOUS DISORDERS
第五篇　苔藓样皮炎和肉芽肿性皮炎

32 Lichen Planus ··························· 557
Aaron R. Mangold & Mark R. Pittelkow
　第三十二章　扁平苔藓

33 Lichen Nitidus and Lichen Striatus ·········· 585
Aaron R. Mangold & Mark R. Pittelkow
　第三十三章　光泽苔藓和线状苔藓

34 Granuloma Annulare ····················· 595
Julie S. Prendiville
　第三十四章　环状肉芽肿

35 Sarcoidosis ····························· 603
Richard Marchell
　第三十五章　结节病

PART 6 NEUTROPHILIC, EOSINOPHILIC, AND MAST CELL DISORDERS
第六篇　中性粒细胞、嗜酸性粒细胞、肥大细胞相关性疾病

36 Sweet Syndrome ························· 619
Philip R. Cohen & Razelle Kurzrock
　第三十六章　Sweet综合征

37 Pyoderma Gangrenosum · 638
  Natanel Jourabchi & Gerald S. Lazarus
  第三十七章　坏疽性脓皮病

38 Subcorneal Pustular Dermatosis
  (Sneddon-Wilkinson Disease) · · · · · · · · · · · · · · · 651
  Franz Trautinger & Herbert Hönigsmann
  第三十八章　角层下脓疱病

39 Autoinflammatory Disorders · · · · · · · · · · · · · · · · 656
  Takashi K. Satoh & Lars E. French
  第三十九章　自身炎症性疾病

40 Eosinophilic Diseases · 685
  Hideyuki Ujiie & Hiroshi Shimizu
  第四十章　嗜酸性粒细胞疾病

41 Urticaria and Angioedema · · · · · · · · · · · · · · · · · · 721
  *Michihiro Hide, Shunsuke Takahagi,
  & Takaaki Hiragun*
  第四十一章　荨麻疹和血管性水肿

42 Mastocytosis · 748
  Michael D. Tharp
  第四十二章　肥大细胞增生症

PART 7　REACTIVE ERYTHEMAS
第七篇　反应性红斑

43 Erythema Multiforme · 763
  Jean-Claude Roujeau & Maja Mockenhaupt
  第四十三章　多形红斑

44 Epidermal Necrolysis (Stevens-Johnson
  Syndrome and Toxic Epidermal Necrolysis) · · · · 774
  Maja Mockenhaupt & Jean-Claude Roujeau
  第四十四章　表皮坏死松解症（Stevens-
  　　　　　　Johnson综合征和中毒性表皮
  　　　　　　坏死松解症）

45 Cutaneous Reactions to Drugs · · · · · · · · · · · · · · 791
  Kara Heelan, Cathryn Sibbald, & Neil H. Shear
  第四十五章　药物所致皮肤反应

46 Erythema Annulare Centrifugum and Other
  Figurate Erythemas · 808
  Christine S. Ahn & William W. Huang
  第四十六章　离心性环状红斑和其他形态
  　　　　　　红斑

PART 8　DSORDERS OF CORNIFICATION
第八篇　角化异常性疾病

47 The Ichthyoses · 819
  Keith A. Choate & Leonard M. Milstone
  第四十七章　鱼鳞病

48 Inherited Palmoplantar Keratodermas · · · · · · · · 861
  Liat Samuelov & Eli Sprecher
  第四十八章　遗传性掌跖角化病

49 Keratosis Pilaris and Other Follicular
  Keratotic Disorders · 913
  Anna L. Bruckner
  第四十九章　毛周角化病和其他毛囊性
  　　　　　　角化疾病

50 Acantholytic Disorders of the Skin · · · · · · · · · · · 924
  Alain Hovnanian
  第五十章　棘层松解性皮肤病

51 Porokeratosis · 949
  *Cathal O'Connor, Grainne M. O'Regan,
  & Alan D. Irvine*
  第五十一章　汗孔角化症

PART 9　VESICULOBULLOUS DISORDERS
第九篇　水疱大疱性疾病

52 Pemphigus · 957
  Aimee S. Payne & John R. Stanley
  第五十二章　天疱疮

53 Paraneoplastic Pemphigus · · · · · · · · · · · · · · · · · · 983
  Grant J. Anhalt & Daniel Mimouni
  第五十三章　副肿瘤性天疱疮

54 Bullous Pemphigoid · 994
  Donna A. Culton, Zhi Liu, & Luis A. Diaz
  第五十四章　大疱性类天疱疮

55 Mucous Membrane Pemphigoid · · · · · · · · · · · · 1011
  Kim B. Yancey
  第五十五章　黏膜类天疱疮

56 Epidermolysis Bullosa Acquisita · · · · · · · · · · · · 1023
  David T. Woodley & Mei Chen
  第五十六章　获得性大疱性表皮松解症

57 Intercellular Immunoglobulin (Ig)
  A Dermatosis (IgA Pemphigus) · · · · · · · · · · · · · 1034
  Takashi Hashimoto
  第五十七章　细胞间IgA皮病（IgA天疱
  　　　　　　疮）

58 Linear Immunoglobulin A Dermatosis and
  Chronic Bullous Disease of Childhood · · · · · · · 1046
  *Matilda W. Nicholas, Caroline L. Rao,
  & Russell P. Hall III*
  第五十八章　线状IgA皮病和儿童慢性大
  　　　　　　疱性皮病

59 Dermatitis Herpetiformis · · · · · · · · · · · · · · · · · · 1057
　　Stephen I. Katz
　　第五十九章　疱疹样皮炎

60 Inherited Epidermolysis Bullosa · · · · · · · · · · · 1067
　　M. Peter Marinkovich
　　第六十章　遗传性大疱性表皮松解症

PART 10 AUTOIMMUNE CONNECTIVE TISSUE AND RHEUMATOLOGIC DISORDERS

第十篇　自身免疫结缔组织病和风湿病

61 Lupus Erythematosus · 1093
　　Clayton J. Sontheimer, Melissa I. Costner,
　　& Richard D. Sontheimer
　　第六十一章　红斑狼疮

62 Dermatomyositis · 1118
　　Matthew Lewis & David Fiorentino
　　第六十二章　皮肌炎

63 Systemic Sclerosis · 1144
　　Pia Moinzadeh, Christopher P. Denton,
　　Carol M. Black, & Thomas Krieg
　　第六十三章　系统性硬皮病

64 Morphea and Lichen Sclerosus · · · · · · · · · · · · · 1165
　　Nika Cyrus & Heidi T. Jacobe
　　第六十四章　硬斑病和硬化性萎缩性苔癣

65 Psoriatic Arthritis and Reactive Arthritis · · · · · 1187
　　Ana-Maria Orbai & John A. Flynn
　　第六十五章　银屑病性关节炎和反应性关节炎

66 Rheumatoid Arthritis, Juvenile Idiopathic Arthritis, Adult-Onset Still Disease, and Rheumatic Fever · 1207
　　Warren W. Piette
　　第六十六章　类风湿性关节炎、幼年特发性关节炎、成人Still病和风湿热

67 Scleredema and Scleromyxedema · · · · · · · · · · 1225
　　Roger H. Weenig & Mark R. Pittelkow
　　第六十七章　硬肿症和硬化性黏液水肿

68 Sjögren Syndrome · 1232
　　Akiko Tanikawa
　　第六十八章　干燥综合征

69 Relapsing Polychondritis · · · · · · · · · · · · · · · · · · 1249
　　Camille Francès
　　第六十九章　复发性多软骨炎

PART 11 DERMAL CONNECTIVE TISSUE DISORDERS

第十一篇　真皮结缔组织异常

70 Anetoderma and Other Atrophic Disorders of the Skin · 1255
　　Catherine Maari & Julie Powell
　　第七十章　斑状萎缩和其他萎缩性皮病

71 Acquired Perforating Disorders · · · · · · · · · · · · 1265
　　Garrett T. Desman & Raymond L. Barnhill
　　第七十一章　获得性穿通性皮病

72 Genetic Disorders Affecting Dermal Connective Tissue · 1275
　　Jonathan A. Dyer
　　第七十二章　影响真皮结缔组织的遗传性疾病

PART 12 SUBCUTANEOUS TISSUE DISORDERS

第十二篇　皮下脂肪疾病

73 Panniculitis · 1315
　　Eden Pappo Lake, Sophie M. Worobec,
　　& Iris K. Aronson
　　第七十三章　脂膜炎

74 Lipodystrophy · 1360
　　Abhimanyu Garg
　　第七十四章　脂肪营养不良

Volume 2
中　册

PART 13 MELANOCYTIC DISORDERS

第十三篇　色素细胞性疾病

75 Albinism and Other Genetic Disorders of Pigmentation · 1375
　　Masahiro Hayashi & Tamio Suzuki
　　第七十五章　白化病和其他遗传性色素性疾病

76 Vitiligo · 1397
　　Khaled Ezzedine & John E. Harris
　　第七十六章　白癜风

77 Hypermelanoses · 1419
　　Michelle Rodrigues & Amit G. Pandya
　　第七十七章　色素沉着过度性疾病

PART 14 ACNEIFORM DISORDERS

第十四篇　痤疮样皮肤病

78 Acne Vulgaris · 1461
   Carolyn Goh, Carol Cheng, George Agak,
   Andrea L. Zaenglein, Emmy M. Graber,
   Diane M. Thiboutot, & Jenny Kim
   第七十八章　寻常痤疮

79 Rosacea · 1490
   Martin Steinhoff & Jörg Buddenkotte
   第七十九章　玫瑰痤疮

80 Acne Variants and Acneiform Eruptions · · · · · · 1520
   Andrea L. Zaenglein, Emmy M. Graber,
   & Diane M. Thiboutot
   第八十章　痤疮异型和痤疮样疹

PART 15 DISORDERS OF ECCRINE AND APOCRINE SWEAT GLANDS

第十五篇　汗腺疾病

81 Hyperhidrosis and Anhidrosis · · · · · · · · · · · · 1531
   Anastasia O. Kurta & Dee Anna Glaser
   第八十一章　多汗症和无汗症

82 Bromhidrosis and Chromhidrosis · · · · · · · · · · 1543
   Christos C. Zouboulis
   第八十二章　腋臭和色汗

83 Fox-Fordyce Disease · · · · · · · · · · · · · · · · · · · 1551
   Powell Perng & Inbal Sander
   第八十三章　Fox-Fordyce病

84 Hidradenitis Suppurativa · · · · · · · · · · · · · · · · 1557
   Ginette A. Okoye
   第八十四章　化脓性汗腺炎

PART 16 DISORDERS OF THE HAIR AND NAILS

第十六篇　毛发和甲疾病

85 Androgenetic Alopecia · · · · · · · · · · · · · · · · · · 1575
   Ulrike Blume-Peytavi & Varvara Kanti
   第八十五章　雄激素性脱发

86 Telogen Effluvium · 1588
   Manabu Ohyama
   第八十六章　休止期脱发

87 Alopecia Areata · 1599
   Nina Otberg & Jerry Shapiro
   第八十七章　斑秃

88 Cicatricial Alopecias · 1607
   Nina Otberg & Jerry Shapiro
   第八十八章　瘢痕性脱发

89 Hair Shaft Disorders · 1621
   Leslie Castelo-Soccio & Deepa Patel
   第八十九章　毛干疾病

90 Hirsutism and Hypertrichosis · · · · · · · · · · · · · 1640
   Thusanth Thuraisingam & Amy J. McMichael
   第九十章　多毛和多毛症

91 Nail Disorders · 1655
   Eckart Haneke
   第九十一章　甲疾病

PART 17 DISORDERS DUE TO THE ENVIRONMENT

第十七篇　环境引起的皮肤病

92 Polymorphic Light Eruption · · · · · · · · · · · · · · 1699
   Alexandra Gruber-Wackernagel
   & Peter Wolf
   第九十二章　多形性日光疹

93 Actinic Prurigo · 1716
   Travis Vandergriff
   第九十三章　光化性痒疹

94 Hydroa Vacciniforme · · · · · · · · · · · · · · · · · · · 1723
   Travis Vandergriff
   第九十四章　种痘样水疱病

95 Actinic Dermatitis · 1728
   Robert S. Dawe
   第九十五章　光化性皮炎

96 Solar Urticaria · 1740
   Marcus Maurer, Joachim W. Fluhr, & Karsten Weller
   第九十六章　日光性荨麻疹

97 Phototoxicity and Photoallergy · · · · · · · · · · · · 1747
   Henry W. Lim
   第九十七章　光毒性与光过敏

98 Cold Injuries · 1756
   Ashley N. Millard, Clayton B. Green,
   & Erik J. Stratman
   第九十八章　冻伤

99 Burns · 1769
   Benjamin Levi & Stewart Wang
   第九十九章　烧伤

PART 18 PSYCHOSOCIAL SKIN DISEASE

第十八篇　心理社会性皮肤病

100 Delusional, Obsessive-Compulsive, and Factitious Skin Diseases ·················1783
Mio Nakamura, Josie Howard, & John Y. M. Koo
第一百章　妄想、强迫症和人为皮肤病

101 Drug Abuse ······································1796
Nicholas Frank, Cara Hennings, & Jami L. Miller
第一百零一章　药物滥用

102 Physical Abuse ·································1809
Kelly M. MacArthur & Annie Grossberg
第一百零二章　身体虐待

PART 19 SKIN CHANGES ACROSS THE SPAN OF LIFE

第十九篇　皮肤在人一生中的变化

103 Neonatal Dermatology ·······················1819
Raegan Hunt, Mary Wu Chang, & Kara N. Shah
第一百零三章　新生儿皮肤病学

104 Pediatric and Adolescent Dermatology ······1844
Mary Wu Chang
第一百零四章　儿科和青少年皮肤病学

105 Skin Changes and Diseases in Pregnancy ····1861
Lauren E. Wiznia & Miriam Keltz Pomeranz
第一百零五章　妊娠期的皮肤变化和疾病

106 Skin Aging ······································1877
Michelle L. Kerns, Anna L. Chien, & Sewon Kang
第一百零六章　皮肤老化

107 Caring for LGBT Persons in Dermatology ····1892
Howa Yeung, Matthew D. Mansh,
Suephy C. Chen, & Kenneth A. Katz
第一百零七章　关于LGBT人群的皮肤病学

PART 20 NEOPLASIA

第二十篇　皮肤肿瘤

108 Benign Epithelial Tumors, Hamartomas, and Hyperplasias ····························1901
Jonathan D. Cuda, Sophia Rangwala, & Janis M. Taube
第一百零八章　良性上皮肿瘤、错构瘤和增生性病变

109 Appendage Tumors of the Skin ············1923
Ruth K. Foreman & Lyn McDivitt Duncan
第一百零九章　皮肤附属器肿瘤

110 Epithelial Precancerous Lesions ············1961
Markus V. Heppt, Gabriel Schlager, & Carola Berking
第一百一十章　上皮癌前病变

111 Basal Cell Carcinoma and Basal Cell Nevus Syndrome ····························1989
Jean Y. Tang, Ervin H. Epstein, Jr., & Anthony E. Oro
第一百一十一章　基底细胞癌和基底细胞痣综合征

112 Squamous Cell Carcinoma and Keratoacanthoma ·······························2006
Anke S. Lonsdorf & Eva N. Hadaschik
第一百一十二章　鳞状细胞癌和角化棘皮瘤

113 Merkel Cell Carcinoma ·······················2026
Aubriana McEvoy & Paul Nghiem
第一百一十三章　梅克尔细胞癌

114 Paget's Disease ································2041
Conroy Chow, Isaac M. Neuhaus, & Roy C. Grekin
第一百一十四章　佩吉特病

115 Melanocytic Nevi ·····························2052
Jonathan D. Cuda, Robert F. Moore, & Klaus J. Busam
第一百一十五章　黑素细胞痣

116 Melanoma ······································2090
Jessica C. Hassel & Alexander H. Enk
第一百一十六章　黑色素瘤

117 Histiocytosis ····································2127
Astrid Schmieder, Sergij Goerdt, & Jochen Utikal
第一百一十七章　组织细胞增生症

118 Vascular Tumors ·······························2152
Kelly M. MacArthur & Katherine Püttgen
第一百一十八章　血管性肿瘤

119 Cutaneous Lymphoma ·······················2182
Martine Bagot & Rudolf Stadler
第一百一十九章　皮肤淋巴瘤

120 Cutaneous Pseudolymphoma ···············2219
Werner Kempf, Rudolf Stadler, & Martine Bagot
第一百二十章　皮肤假性淋巴瘤

121 Neoplasias and Hyperplasias of Muscular and Neural Origin ···············2242
Hansgeorg Müller & Heinz Kutzner
第一百二十一章　肌肉和神经源性肿瘤与增生

122 Lipogenic Neoplasms ·················2285
Thomas Mentzel & Thomas Brenn

　　第一百二十二章　脂肪源性肿瘤

PART 21 METABOLIC, GENETIC, AND SYSTEMIC DISEASES

第二十一篇　代谢性、遗传性和全身性疾病

123 Cutaneous Changes in Nutritional Disease ·················2313
Albert C. Yan

　　第一百二十三章　营养性疾病的皮肤改变

124 The Porphyrias ·················2349
Eric W. Gou & Karl E. Anderson

　　第一百二十四章　卟啉病

125 Amyloidosis ·················2374
Peter D. Gorevic & Robert G. Phelps

　　第一百二十五章　淀粉样变性

126 Xanthomas and Lipoprotein Disorders ·······2390
Vasanth Sathiyakumar, Steven R. Jones, & Seth S. Martin

　　第一百二十六章　黄色瘤和脂蛋白紊乱

127 Fabry Disease ·················2410
Atul B. Mehta & Catherine H. Orteu

　　第一百二十七章　Fabry病

128 Calcium and Other Mineral Deposition Disorders ·················2426
Janet A. Fairley & Adam B. Aronson

　　第一百二十八章　钙和其他矿物沉积紊乱

129 Graft-Versus-Host Disease ·················2440
Kathryn J. Martires & Edward W. Cowen

　　第一百二十九章　移植物抗宿主病

130 Hereditary Disorders of Genome Instability and DNA Repair ·················2463
John J. DiGiovanna, Thomas M. Rünger, & Kenneth H. Kraemer

　　第一百三十章　基因组不稳定性和DNA修复障碍的遗传性疾病

131 Ectodermal Dysplasias ·················2494
Elizabeth L. Nieman & Dorothy Katherine Grange

　　第一百三十一章　外胚层发育不良

132 Genetic Immunodeficiency Diseases ·········2517
Ramsay L. Fuleihan & Amy S. Paller

　　第一百三十二章　遗传性免疫缺陷病

133 Skin Manifestations of Internal Organ Disorders ·················2549
Amy K. Forrestel & Robert G. Micheletti

　　第一百三十三章　内脏疾病的皮肤表现

134 Cutaneous Paraneoplastic Syndromes ·······2566
Manasmon Chairatchaneeboon & Ellen J. Kim

　　第一百三十四章　皮肤副肿瘤综合征

135 The Neurofibromatoses ·················2590
Robert Listernick & Joel Charrow

　　第一百三十五章　神经纤维瘤病

136 Tuberous Sclerosis Complex ·················2606
Thomas N. Darling

　　第一百三十六章　结节性硬化症

137 Diabetes and Other Endocrine Diseases ·······2620
April Schachtel & Andrea Kalus

　　第一百三十七章　糖尿病和其他内分泌疾病

Volume 3
下　册

PART 22 VASCULAR DISEASES

第二十二篇　血管性疾病

138 Cutaneous Necrotizing Venulitis ···········2655
Nicholas A. Soter

　　第一百三十八章　皮肤坏死性静脉炎

139 Systemic Necrotizing Arteritis ···········2669
Peter A. Merkel & Paul A. Monach

　　第一百三十九章　系统性坏死性动脉炎

140 Erythema Elevatum Diutinum ···········2694
Theodore J. Alkousakis & Whitney A. High

　　第一百四十章　持久性隆起性红斑

141 Adamantiades–Behçet Disease ···········2701
Christos C. Zouboulis

　　第一百四十一章　白塞病

142 Kawasaki Disease ···········2716
Anne H. Rowley

　　第一百四十二章　川崎病

143 Pigmented Purpuric Dermatoses ···········2728
Alexandra Haden & David H. Peng

　　第一百四十三章　色素性紫癜性皮病

144 Cryoglobulinemia and
Cryofibrinogenemia · 2739
Julio C. Sartori-Valinotti & Mark D. P. Davis

 第一百四十四章 冷球蛋白血症和冷纤维蛋白原血症

145 Raynaud Phenomenon · · · · · · · · · · · · · · · · · · 2755
Drew Kurtzman & Ruth Ann Vleugels

 第一百四十五章 雷诺现象

146 Malignant Atrophic Papulosis
(Degos Disease) · 2774
Dan Lipsker

 第一百四十六章 恶性萎缩性丘疹病

147 Vascular Malformations · · · · · · · · · · · · · · · · · 2782
Laurence M. Boon, Fanny Ballieux, & Miikka Vikkula

 第一百四十七章 血管畸形

148 Cutaneous Changes in Arterial, Venous, and Lymphatic Dysfunction · · · · · · · · · · · · · · · · · · 2817
Sabrina A. Newman

 第一百四十八章 动脉、静脉和淋巴管功能障碍的皮肤表现

149 Wound Healing · 2850
Afsaneh Alavi & Robert S. Kirsner

 第一百四十九章 伤口愈合

PART 23 BACTERIAL DISEASES

第二十三篇　细菌性疾病

150 Superficial Cutaneous Infections and Pyodermas · 2871
Lloyd S. Miller

 第一百五十章 浅部皮肤感染和脓皮病

151 Cellulitis and Erysipelas · · · · · · · · · · · · · · · · · · 2899
David R. Pearson & David J. Margolis

 第一百五十一章 蜂窝织炎和丹毒

152 Gram-Positive Infections Associated with Toxin Production · 2911
Jeffrey B. Travers

 第一百五十二章 产毒素革兰氏阳性细菌感染

153 Necrotizing Fasciitis, Necrotizing Cellulitis, and Myonecrosis · 2924
Avery LaChance & Daniela Kroshinksy

 第一百五十三章 坏死性筋膜炎、坏死性蜂窝组织炎和肌坏死

154 Gram-Negative Coccal and Bacillary Infections · 2937
Breanne Mordorski & Adam J. Friedman

 第一百五十四章 革兰氏阴性球菌和细菌感染

155 The Skin in Infective Endocarditis, Sepsis, Septic Shock, and Disseminated Intravascular Coagulation · · · · · · · · · · · · · · · · · 2971
Joseph C. English III & Misha Rosenbach

 第一百五十五章 感染性心内膜炎、脓毒血症、脓毒性休克和弥散性血管内凝血中的皮肤表现

156 Miscellaneous Bacterial Infections with Cutaneous Manifestations · · · · · · · · · · · · · · · · 2983
Scott A. Norton & Michael A. Cardis

 第一百五十六章 混杂细菌感染引起的皮肤表现

157 Tuberculosis and Infections with Atypical Mycobacteria · 3015
Aisha Sethi

 第一百五十七章 结核和非典型分枝杆菌感染

158 Actinomycosis, Nocardiosis, and Actinomycetoma · 3034
Francisco G. Bravo, Roberto Arenas, & Daniel Asz Sigall

 第一百五十八章 放线菌病、诺卡氏菌病和放线菌瘤

159 Leprosy · 3051
Claudio Guedes Salgado, Arival Cardoso de Brito, Ubirajara Imbiriba Salgado, & John Stewart Spencer

 第一百五十九章 麻风病

PART 24 FUNGAL DISEASES

第二十四篇　真菌性疾病

160 Superficial Fungal Infection · · · · · · · · · · · · · · · 3085
Lauren N. Craddock & Stefan M. Schieke

 第一百六十章 浅部真菌感染

161 Yeast Infections · 3113
Iris Ahronowitz & Kieron Leslie

 第一百六十一章 酵母菌感染

162 Deep Fungal Infections · · · · · · · · · · · · · · · · · · · 3127
Roderick J. Hay

 第一百六十二章 深部真菌感染

PART 25 VIRAL DISEASES

第二十五篇　病毒性疾病

163 Exanthematous Viral Diseases · · · · · · · · · · · · 3151

Vikash S. Oza & Erin F. D. Mathes

　　第一百六十三章　病毒疹性疾病

164　Herpes Simplex ·················3184
Jeffrey I. Cohen

　　第一百六十四章　单纯疱疹

165　Varicella and Herpes Zoster ·············3199
Myron J. Levin, Kenneth E. Schmader, & Michael N. Oxman

　　第一百六十五章　水痘–带状疱疹

166　Poxvirus Infections ···············3230
Ellen S. Haddock & Sheila Fallon Friedlander

　　第一百六十六章　痘病毒感染

167　Human Papillomavirus Infections ·········3261
Jane C. Sterling

　　第一百六十七章　人乳头瘤病毒感染

168　Cutaneous Manifestations of HIV and Human T-Lymphotropic Virus ·········3274
Adam D. Lipworth, Esther E. Freeman, & Arturo P. Saavedra

　　第一百六十八章　HIV和人类嗜T细胞病毒感染的皮肤表现

169　Mosquito-Borne Viral Diseases ···········3303
Edwin J. Asturias & J. David Beckham

　　第一百六十九章　蚊媒病毒性疾病

PART 26 SEXUALLY TRANSMITTED DISEASES

第二十六篇　性传播疾病

170　Syphilis ·····················3315
Susan A. Tuddenham & Jonathan M. Zenilman

　　第一百七十章　梅毒

171　Endemic (Nonvenereal) Treponematoses ·····3345
Francisco G. Bravo, Carolina Talhari, & Khaled Ezzedine

　　第一百七十一章　地方性（非性病性）密螺旋体病

172　Chancroid ···················3360
Stephan Lautenschlager & Norbert H. Brockmeyer

　　第一百七十二章　软下疳

173　Lymphogranuloma Venereum ···········3369
Norbert H. Brockmeyer & Stephan Lautenschlager

　　第一百七十三章　性病性淋巴肉芽肿

174　Granuloma Inguinale ··············3380
Melissa B. Hoffman & Rita O. Pichardo

　　第一百七十四章　腹股沟肉芽肿

175　Gonorrhea, Mycoplasma, and Vaginosis ·····3387
Lindsay C. Strowd, Sean McGregor, & Rita O. Pichardo

　　第一百七十五章　淋病、支原体感染和细菌性阴道病

PART 27 INFESTATIONS, BITES, AND STINGS

第二十七篇　虫媒叮咬和感染性疾病

176　Leishmaniasis and Other Protozoan Infections ···················3405
Esther von Stebut

　　第一百七十六章　利什曼病和其他原虫感染

177　Helminthic Infections ··············3434
Kathryn N. Suh & Jay S. Keystone

　　第一百七十七章　蠕虫感染

178　Scabies, Other Mites, and Pediculosis ·······3458
Chikoti M. Wheat, Craig N. Burkhart, Craig G. Burkhart, & Bernard A. Cohen

　　第一百七十八章　疥疮、其他螨类和虱病

179　Lyme Borreliosis ················3472
Roger Clark & Linden Hu

　　第一百七十九章　莱姆病

180　The Rickettsioses, Ehrlichioses, and Anaplasmoses ···············3492
Maryam Liaqat, Analisa V. Halpern, Justin J. Green, & Warren R. Heymann

　　第一百八十章　立克次体病、埃氏立克次体病和无浆体病

181　Arthropod Bites and Stings ···········3511
Robert A. Schwartz & Christopher J. Steen

　　第一百八十一章　节肢动物咬伤和蜇伤

182　Bites and Stings of Terrestrial and Aquatic Life ··················3526
Camila K. Janniger, Robert A. Schwartz, Jennifer S. Daly, & Mark Jordan Scharf

　　第一百八十二章　陆生和水生生物的叮咬和蜇伤

PART 28 TOPICAL AND SYSTEMIC TREATMENTS

第二十八篇　外用和系统药物治疗

183　Principles of Topical Therapy ··········3553
Mohammed D. Saleem, Howard I. Maibach, & Steven R. Feldman

　　第一百八十三章　外用药物的治疗原则

184 Glucocorticoids ················3573
　　Avrom Caplan, Nicole Fett, & Victoria Werth
　　第一百八十四章　糖皮质激素

185 Retinoids ····················3587
　　Anna L. Chien, Anders Vahlquist,
　　Jean-Hilaire Saurat, John J. Voorhees, & Sewon Kang
　　第一百八十五章　维甲酸类药物

186 Systemic and Topical Antibiotics ······3600
　　Sean C. Condon, Carlos M. Isada,
　　& Kenneth J. Tomecki
　　第一百八十六章　系统使用和外用抗生素

187 Dapsone ····················3617
　　Chee Leok Goh & Jiun Yit Pan
　　第一百八十七章　氨苯砜

188 Antifungals ··················3631
　　Mahmoud Ghannoum, Iman Salem,
　　& Luisa Christensen
　　第一百八十八章　抗真菌药

189 Antihistamines ················3647
　　Michael D. Tharp
　　第一百八十九章　抗组胺药

190 Cytotoxic and Antimetabolic Agents ·····3659
　　Jeremy S. Honaker & Neil J. Korman
　　第一百九十章　细胞毒性和抗代谢药

191 Antiviral Drugs ················3690
　　Zeena Y. Nawas, Quynh-Giao Nguyen,
　　Khaled S. Sanber, & Stephen K. Tyring
　　第一百九十一章　抗病毒药

192 Immunosuppressive and
　　Immunomodulatory Drugs ··········3715
　　Drew Kurtzman, Ruth Ann Vleugels, & Jeffrey Callen
　　第一百九十二章　免疫抑制药和免疫调节药

193 Immunobiologics: Targeted Therapy Against
　　Cytokines, Cytokine Receptors, and Growth
　　Factors in Dermatology ············3730
　　Andrew Johnston, Yoshikazu Takada, & Sam T. Hwang
　　第一百九十三章　免疫生物制剂：皮肤病学中针对细胞因子、细胞因子受体和生长因子的靶向治疗

194 Molecular Targeted Therapies ········3758
　　David Michael Miller, Bobby Y. Reddy, & Hensin Tsao
　　第一百九十四章　分子靶向治疗

195 Antiangiogenic Agents ············3790
　　Adilson da Costa, Michael Y. Bonner,
　　& Jack L. Arbiser
　　第一百九十五章　抗血管生成抑制药

196 Other Topical Medications ··········3810
　　Shawn G. Kwatra & Manisha Loss
　　第一百九十六章　其他外用药

197 Photoprotection ················3824
　　Jin Ho Chung
　　第一百九十七章　光保护剂

PART 29 PHYSICAL TREATMENTS
第二十九篇　物理治疗

198 Phototherapy ·················3837
　　Tarannum Jaleel, Brian P. Pollack, & Craig A. Elmets
　　第一百九十八章　光疗

199 Photochemotherapy and Photodynamic
　　Therapy ····················3867
　　Herbert Hönigsmann, Rolf-Markus Szeimies,
　　& Robert Knobler
　　第一百九十九章　光化学疗法和光动力疗法

200 Radiotherapy ·················3891
　　Roy H. Decker & Lynn D. Wilson
　　第二百章　放疗

PART 30 DERMATOLOGIC SURGERY
第三十篇　皮肤外科

201 Cutaneous Surgical Anatomy ·········3903
　　Arif Aslam & Sumaira Z. Aasi
　　第二百零一章　皮肤外科解剖学

202 Perioperative Considerations in
　　Dermatologic Surgery ·············3913
　　Noah Smith, Kelly B. Cha, & Christopher Bichakjian
　　第二百零二章　皮肤科手术的围手术期注意事项

203 Excisional Surgery and Repair,
　　Flaps, and Grafts ···············3934
　　Adele Haimovic, Jessica M. Sheehan,
　　& Thomas E. Rohrer
　　第二百零三章　肿物切除术和修复、皮瓣和皮片移植

204 Mohs Micrographic Surgery ··········3970
　　Sean R. Christensen & David J. Leffell
　　第二百零四章　莫氏显微外科

205 Nail Surgery ··················3984
　　Robert Baran & Olivier Cogrel
　　第二百零五章　甲部手术

206 Cryosurgery and Electrosurgery ········4002

Justin J. Vujevich & Leonard H. Goldberg

第二百零六章　冷冻疗法和电疗法

PART 31　COSMETIC DERMATOLOGY

第三十一篇　美容皮肤学

207 Cosmeceuticals and Skin Care in Dermatology ························· 4015
Leslie Baumann

第二百零七章　化妆品和皮肤护理

208 Fundamentals of Laser and Light-Based Treatments ················ 4033
Omer Ibrahim & Jeffrey S. Dover

第二百零八章　激光原理和光学治疗

209 Laser Skin Resurfacing: Cosmetic and Medical Applications ················ 4048
Bridget E. McIlwee & Tina S. Alster

第二百零九章　激光皮肤表皮重建：美容和医疗应用

210 Nonablative Laser and Light-Based Therapy: Cosmetic and Medical Indications ··········· 4061
Jeffrey S. Orringer

第二百一十章　非剥脱激光和以光为基础的治疗：美容和医学适应证

211 Noninvasive Body Contouring ············· 4073
Murad Alam

第二百一十一章　无创塑形

212 Treatment of Varicose Veins and Telangiectatic Lower-Extremity Vessels ······· 4088
Daniel P. Friedmann, Vineet Mishra, & Jeffrey T. S. Hsu

第二百一十二章　下肢静脉曲张和毛细血管扩张的治疗

213 Chemical Peels and Dermabrasion ··········· 4113
Gary Monheit & Bailey Tayebi

第二百一十三章　化学剥脱术和磨削术

214 Liposuction Using Tumescent Local Anesthesia ························· 4125
C. William Hanke, Cheryl J. Gustafson, William G. Stebbins, & Aimee L. Leonard

第二百一十四章　局部麻醉下的肿胀吸脂术

215 Soft-Tissue Augmentation ················· 4130
Lisa M. Donofrio & Dana L. Ellis

第二百一十五章　软组织填充术

216 Botulinum Toxin ······················· 4142
Richard G. Glogau

第二百一十六章　肉毒杆菌毒素

217 Hair Transplantation ···················· 4153
Robin H. Unger & Walter P. Unger

第二百一十七章　毛发移植

Melanocytic Disorders

PART 13

第十三篇 色素细胞性疾病

Chapter 75 :: Albinism and Other Genetic Disorders of Pigmentation
:: Masahiro Hayashi & Tamio Suzuki

第七十五章
白化病和其他遗传性色素性疾病

中文导读

本章讲述了与色素生成相关的5种先天性疾病，包括白化病、色素失禁症、斑驳病、Waardenburg综合征和tietz综合征及网状色素异常症。本章对每个疾病分别从临床特征、病因和发病机制、诊断、鉴别诊断、病程、预后和处理等方面来进行详细讨论。

第一节介绍了白化病，分别介绍了两种白化病亚型：综合征型和非综合征型。首先详细阐述了非综合型白化病的临床特征、患病率、各型致病基因的功能及其致病机制、诊断及鉴别、治疗及预后等内容；其次对于综合型白化病的几个亚型包括Hermansky-Pudlak综合征、Chediak-Higashi综合征和Griscelli综合征作了详细介绍。

第二节介绍了色素失禁症，色素失禁症是一种X连锁显性遗传多器官疾病，其特征是从婴儿期到成年期的各种皮肤损伤，伴随有如眼睛、中枢神经系统和肌肉骨骼系统异常等皮肤外症状。重点描述了色素失禁症4个阶段的典型皮肤表现和相应的组织病理表现，并对其致病基因、诊断标准及鉴别、治疗及预后作了说明。

第三节介绍了斑驳病，斑驳病是常染色体显性遗传性疾病，其特征性临床表现即先天性白色额发、分散性色素减退斑和额头三角形的白色斑块，致病基因为KIT及SNAI2基因突变，目前无有效治疗，表皮移植可能有效。

第四节介绍了Waardenburg综合征（WS）和tietz综合征。Waardenburg综合征（WS）是一种罕见遗传病，该疾病的临床特征常表现为先天性色素异常合并感音神经性耳聋，部分患者还伴有面部畸形、先天性巨结肠或严重的神经系统缺陷。根据其临床表现及致病基因、突变位点、遗传方式的不同，可分为不同的亚型。WS的诊断需要满足两个主要标准或一个主要标准和两个次要标准。治疗上并无有效方法。tietz综合征同样表现为先天性色素异常合并感音神经性耳聋，但该疾病的色素减退具有与眼皮肤白化病2型相似的弥漫性色素表型，其致病基因是MITF-Asn210Lys和Arg217del突变。

第五节介绍了网状色素异常症，网状色素异常症是对称性遗传性色素沉着症（DSH）、遗传性泛发性色素沉着症（DUH）、北村网状顶色素沉着症（RAK）和Dowling-Degos病（DDD）的统称。本章总结了它们的临床表现、分型及相应的致病基因、遗传位点和遗传方式（表75-5），并对它们分别进行了阐述。

〔李 吉〕

Albinism is characterized by hypopigmentation of the skin, hair, and eyes, or of eyes only, in the affected individuals. There are 2 albinism subtypes are non-syndromic albinism, with symptoms restricted to impaired melanin biosynthesis (hypopigmentation of skin and hair, and ocular changes such as reduced iris pigment, nystagmus, impaired visual acuity, and foveal hypoplasia), and syndromic albinism, such as Hermansky-Pudlak syndrome, Chediak-Higashi syndrome, and Griscelli syndrome, with various non-pigmentary symptoms, including bleeding diathesis, lung fibrosis, and immunodeficiency. Other congenital disorders involving pigmentation include a wide range of disorders such as piebaldism, Waardenburg syndrome, and reticular pigmentary disorders including dyschromatosis symmetrica hereditaria, dyschromatosis universalis hereditaria, reticulate acropigmentation of Kitamura, and Dowling-Degos disease. This chapter discusses all of the disorders listed above.

- In addition to hypopigmentation, extrapigmentary symptoms in GS1 and GS2 are neurologic abnormalities and hematologic immunodeficiency/abnormalities, respectively. On the other hand, GS3 is restricted to hypopigmentation.
- In some types, hypopigmentation of the skin may gradually improve as the individual grows; the exception is type 1A, where melanin biosynthesis is completely absent.
- Visual disturbances consist of nystagmus, impaired visual acuity, and stereoscopic vision.
- Protection of skin from the sun is required to prevent sunburn and secondary skin change, including solar degeneration and skin cancer.
- Early referral to an ophthalmologist is important to introduce proper ophthalmologic intervention.

OCULOCUTANEOUS ALBINISM

AT-A-GLANCE

- Oculocutaneous albinism is a group of rare genetic disorders with autosomal recessive inheritance, characterized by hypopigmentation of skin, hair, and eyes.
- Seven subtypes and 6 responsible genes (all except for type 5) have been described.

Oculocutaneous albinism (OCA) is a rare genetic condition with autosomal recessive inheritance, and it is characterized by hypopigmentation of skin, hair, and eyes. Currently 7 types of OCA have been identified (Table 75-1), and all of the genes responsible, with the exception of OCA5 (for which the responsible gene has not yet been identified), are associated with melanin biosynthesis or migration of melanocytes/melanocyte precursor cells. The overall prevalence of OCA is estimated at approximately 1:10,000 to 20,000 people; however, the incidence of each type varies depending on geographic region and ethnicity. Some types of albinism are seen more frequently in certain regions as a result of the founder effect.[1]

TABLE 75-1
Ocular Albinism and Oculocutaneous Albinism (Nonsyndromic Albinism)

DISEASE NAME	INHERITANCE	GENES	CHROMOSOMAL LOCATION	OMIM #
OCA1	AR	TYR	11q14.3	203100
OCA2	AR	OCA2	15q12-q13.1	203200
OCA3	AR	TYRP-1	9p23	203290
OCA4	AR	SLC45A2	5p13.2	696574
OCA5	AR	Unknown	4q24	615312
OCA6	AR	SLC24A5	15q21.1	609802
OCA7	AR	C10orf11	10q22.2-q22.3	615179
OA1	X-linked	GPR143	Xp22.3	300500

OA, ocular albinism; OCA, oculocutaneous albinism; OMIM, Online Mendelian Inheritance in Man.

CLINICAL FEATURES

OCULOCUTANEOUS ALBINISM TYPE 1

OCA1 appears to be the most common type of albinism in non-Hispanic white, Chinese, and Japanese patients. OCA1, number 203100 in the Online Mendelian Inheritance in Man (OMIM) system, is divided into 4 subtypes: OCA1A, OCA1B, OCA1 temperature sensitive (TS), and OCA1 minimal pigment (MP).

In OCA1A, the classic tyrosinase-negative OCA, there is a complete inability to synthesize melanin in skin, hair, and eyes, resulting in the characteristic "albino" phenotype (Fig. 75-1A). Affected individuals are born with white hair, white skin, and blue eyes, and there are no changes as they mature. The phenotype is the same in all ethnic groups and at all ages. The hair may develop a slight yellow tint as a consequence of the denaturing of the hair protein from sun exposure and/or shampoo use. The irides are translucent, appear pink early in life, and often turn a gray-blue color with time. No pigmented lesions develop in the skin, although amelanotic nevi can be present. The architecture of skin and hair bulb melanocytes is normal. The melanosomes show a normal melanosomal membrane, and normal internal matrix formation is observed in stage 1 and stage 2 melanosomes.

The phenotype of OCA1B can range from minimal hair pigment to skin and hair pigmentation approaching the normal pigment phenotype. Most individuals with OCA1B have very little or no pigment at birth, and develop varying amounts of melanin in the hair and skin in the first or second decade of life. In some cases, the melanin develops within the first year. The hair color changes to light yellow, light blond, or golden blond at first, as a result of residual pheomelanin synthesis, and eventually can turn dark blond or brown in adolescence and adulthood. The irides can develop light-tan or brown pigment, sometimes limited to the inner third of the iris, and iris pigment can be present on globe transillumination. However, some degree of iris translucency, as demonstrated by slitlamp examination, is usually present. Many individuals with OCA1B will have a tanning ability with sun exposure, although it is more common to burn without tanning. Pigmented lesions (nevi, freckles, and lentigines) develop in the skin of individuals who have developed pigmented hair and skin.

One variation of OCA1B is the temperature-sensitive phenotype (OCA1TS). Certain specific mutations in TYR cause a conformational change of the TYR protein, leading to the production of a thermolabile variant. TYR activity decreases at 37°C (98.6°F) and is retained, at least in part, at approximately 31°C (87.8°F). Pigmentation is found on the extremities where body temperature is relatively low. In this variation, scalp and axillary hair remain white or slightly yellow, but arm and leg hair becomes pigmented. The skin remains white and does not tan. OCA1MP has no eumelanogenesis but is limited to just pheomelanogenesis. Individuals with OCA1MP show white skin and hair and severe visual impairment, resembling OCA1A, but they do develop some freckles.

OCULOCUTANEOUS ALBINISM TYPE 2

OCA2 (OMIM 203200) occurs worldwide, although somewhat more frequently in African, African American, and certain Native American populations. In African and African American individuals, there is a distinct OCA2 phenotype. Hair is yellow at birth and remains so throughout life, although the color may turn darker. The skin is creamy-white at birth and changes little with time. No generalized skin pigment is present, and no tan develops with sun exposure, but pigmented nevi, lentigines, and freckles often develop, as the cutaneous melanocytes in these individuals both remain susceptible to ultraviolet-induced changes early in life and retain some ability to synthesize melanin later. The irides are blue-gray or light tan or brown.

In white and Asian individuals with OCA2, the amount of hair pigment present at birth or developing

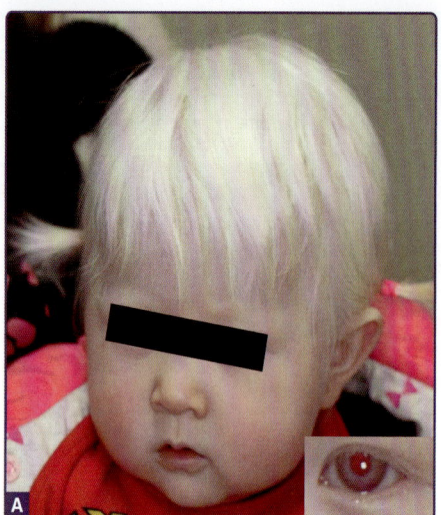
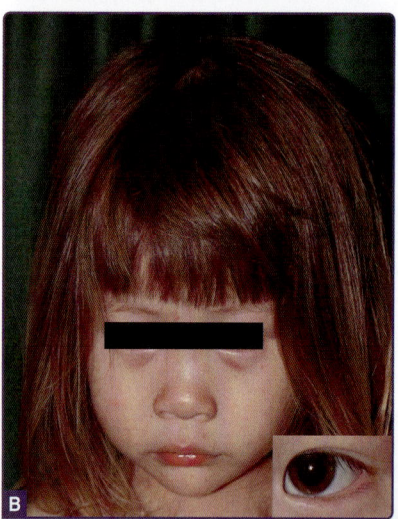
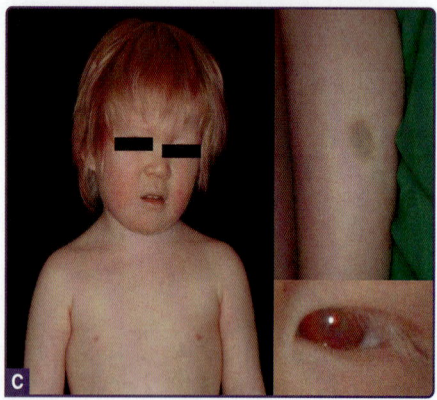

Figure 75-1 Clinical findings of albinism. **A,** OCA1A, 7-month-old boy. He demonstrates complete lack of melanin, and the irides are translucent and reddish. **B,** OCA4, 2-year and 10-month-old girl. Her hair and irides are brown, but the skin is not as pale as for OCA1A. **C,** Hermansky-Pudlak syndrome type 4 (HPS4), 6-year-old girl (reported in Araki Y, Ishii Y, Abe Y, et al[59]). Blonde hair, white skin, and light gray irides with nystagmus are seen. Purpura is also seen on her lower leg.

with time varies from minimal to moderate. The hair can be very lightly pigmented at birth, having a light yellow or blond color, or more pigmented with a definite blond, golden blond, or even red color. The skin is creamy-white and tanning ability varies. The iris color is blue-gray or lightly pigmented, and the amount of translucency correlates with the development of iris pigment. With time, pigmented nevi and lentigines may develop, and freckles are seen in areas with repeated sun exposure. The hair may slowly turn darker through the first 2 or more later decades of life.

OCULOCUTANEOUS ALBINISM TYPE 3

OCA3 (OMIM 203290) is a rare and mild phenotype of OCA. In Africa, distinctive forms of OCA with symptoms different from those of OCA1 and OCA2 have been known, called brown OCA (BOCA) and rufous OCA (ROCA). BOCA and ROCA were stated to be distinguishable based on the color of skin and hair. ROCA is characterized by brick-red, mahogany, or bronze skin color, and the hair color varies from deep mahogany to sandy red; BOCA is characterized by tan or light-brown skin and light-brown hair. Visual disturbances, including nystagmus and impaired visual acuity, tend to be mild or even absent in both BOCA and ROCA.[2] Boissy and associates identified tyrosinase-related protein-1 (*TYRP-1*) as a responsible gene for BOCA in African American males.[3] On the other hand, Manga and associates identified *TYRP-1* as a responsible gene for ROCA by linkage analysis of ROCA families and subsequent DNA sequencing.[2] ROCA and BOCA may be categorized into the same entity by genetic analysis; that is, may share the same responsible gene, *TYRP-1*. The same mutation (c.1103delA, p.K368fs) in *TYRP-1* was reported in both BOCA and ROCA. However, the reason why the phenotypes of BOCA and ROCA differ, although both have the same mutation, is yet to be shown.

The clinical phenotype of OCA3 in non-African individuals, including German, Japanese, and Pakistani patients, has been reported as mild, blond hair, brown eyebrows, dark-brown irides, and lighter skin complexion than those of unaffected parents. There is a possibility that individuals of non-African ethnicity with OCA3 are overlooked, because the effect of diluted pigmentation in OCA3 is mild or even subtle.

OCULOCUTANEOUS ALBINISM TYPE 4

OCA4 (OMIM 696574) is relatively rare in the general population, found in approximately 3% of albino individuals[4]; however, it accounts for 27% of Japanese albinos, and is one of the major types of OCA in Japan.[5] The hypopigmentation of OCA4 varies among individuals (see Fig. 75-1B), similar to OCA2[5] and OCA6,[6] presumably because the responsible genes are found in the same functional entity, ion transporters on melanosomes (see discussions of OCA2 ["Oculocutaneous Albinism type 2" above] and OCA6 ["Oculocutaneous Albinism type 6" below]). The phenotype of OCA4 ranges from light-yellow to brown hair, from blue to red-brown irides with or without nystagmus, and from severe cutaneous hypopigmentation indistinguishable from OCA1A to mild diluted pigmentation with some tanning ability. Furthermore, pigmentation of some individuals tends to recover as individuals mature.[4]

OCULOCUTANEOUS ALBINISM TYPE 5

OCA5 (OMIM 615312) has been reported in 1 consanguineous Pakistani albino family.[7] Individuals with OCA5 display golden-colored hair, white skin, nystagmus, photophobia, foveal hypoplasia, and impaired visual acuity, regardless of their sex and age.[7] No other individual with OCA5 other than this family member has been reported as of this writing.

OCULOCUTANEOUS ALBINISM TYPE 6

OCA6 (OMIM 609802) was initially identified in a Chinese family,[6] although this type has subsequently been reported in several families and in sporadic individuals of Chinese, European, French Guinean, and Middle Eastern origin. The prevalence of OCA6 has been reported as approximately 3% in European albino populations. The phenotype of individuals with OCA6 varies, and is similar to that of individuals with OCA2 and OCA4 (see section "Oculocutaneous Albinism type 2" and "Oculocutaneous Albinism type 4"), ranging from light-brown to platinum blond hair, lighter skin complexion with or without tanning ability, and mild to moderate visual impairment. Some individuals are likely to gain their pigmentation at a later age.[6]

OCULOCUTANEOUS ALBINISM TYPE 7

OCA7 (OMIM 615179) was initially reported in a consanguineous Danish albino family in the Faroe Islands.[8] Recently, more individuals with OCA7 were reported in Iran. Grønskov and associates detailed the phenotype of OCA7, with most of the affected individuals having a light northern European complexion, with a tendency to lighter pigmentation than that of their relatives. Eye symptoms were predominant: nystagmus and iris transillumination were present in all subjects. Extremely sparse pigmentation of the peripheral ocular fundus was seen. Visual impairment in OCA7 is severe, in contrast to relatively mild hypopigmentation of skin and hair.

ETIOLOGY AND PATHOGENESIS

OCA1

OCA1 is caused by loss-of-function of the melanocytic enzyme tyrosinase resulting from mutation of the *TYR* gene.[9] Most individuals with OCA1 are compound heterozygotes with different mutant maternal and paternal alleles. Missense mutations in the *TYR* gene are distributed among distinct regions of the coding sequence, suggesting that the encoded protein has multiple functional domains. Two of the clusters are in the copper-binding regions, with a third near the aminoterminus of the mature protein, in the extramelanosomal domain of tyrosinase shown to require phosphorylation for enzyme activation. Clustering of mutations in discrete regions of the coding sequence is consistent with the importance of these regions either for the melanogenic activity of tyrosinase or for functions related to its maturation and processing.

OCA1A completely lacks TYR activity, whereas OCA1B retains slight TYR activity and may show a unique clinical manifestation, depending on the impact of the mutation. All nonsense and frameshift mutations are associated with a complete loss of tyrosinase activity, presumably because of the resulting production of a truncated protein. Concerning missense mutations, the picture is more complicated. Sets of missense mutations that were associated with OCA1 patients accumulating pigment with age in either OCA1B or OCA1TS patients[10] were shown to have residual enzymatic activity. Hence, it is likely that subsets of *TYR* missense mutations are responsible for the OCA1B and OCA1TS phenotypes as a result of the reduced, rather than absent, tyrosinase activity in their melanocytes.

OCA2

Mutations of the *OCA2 (P)* gene, which maps to chromosome arm 15q, are responsible for OCA2.[11] From the standpoint of melanin synthesis, the defect in OCA2 appears to involve primarily a reduction in eumelanin synthesis, with less effect on pheomelanin synthesis. The predicted structure of the *OCA2* gene, a melanosomal protein, includes 12 transmembrane domains. In sub-Saharan Africa, a single 2.7-kb deletion allele accounts for 60% to 90% of mutant *OCA2* alleles and is associated with a common haplotype, suggesting a common founder.[12] This single mutation is estimated to be associated with 25% to 50% of all mutant *OCA2* alleles in African Americans.[12] Unlike the mutations in *TYR*, the missense mutations described as of this writing in OCA2 do not seem to cluster in any specific region.

Regarding the function of the *OCA2* gene product, it has been shown that melanosomes from P protein–deficient melanocytes have an abnormal pH. Melanosomes in cultured melanocytes derived from wildtype mice are typically acidic, whereas melanosomes from P protein–deficient mice are nonacidic. Hence, it is likely that the P protein regulates the pH of melanosomes, perhaps by functioning as an anion cotransporter in conjunction with a distinct proton pump on the melanosomal membrane. One possibility is that the acidic conditions mediated by the P protein favor the normal biogenesis of melanosomes, including the correct targeting of other melanosomal proteins such as tyrosinase.[13]

OCA3

Mutations in the *TYRP-1* gene result in OCA3. TYRP-1 is implicated in steps downstream from the eumelanogenesis pathway.[14] 5,6-Dihydroxyindole-2-carboxylic acid (DHICA), which is generated from dopachrome by decarboxylation, is oxidized and polymerized by TYRP-1, leading to production of eumelanins. Defective TYRP-1 is unable to oxidize DHICA, hence disrupting eumelanogenesis. In addition, TYRP-1 also has been shown to play a role in stabilizing TYR, indicating that decreased function of TYRP-1 may affect melanogenesis in several ways.

The first described OCA3 mutation was in an African American newborn twin initially classified clinically as having BOCA. Mutation analysis revealed a single-base deletion at codon 368 producing a frameshift and premature stop codon in exon 6, causing a slightly truncated TYRP-1 molecule.[3] This mutation is shared by a substantial proportion of the ROCA population in southern Africa.[2] Additional OCA3-associated *TYRP-1* mutations include a single-base substitution at codon 166, resulting in the alteration of a serine to a premature stop codon in exon 3 and a truncated TYRP-1 molecule,[15] also identified in the ROCA population; and, in a Pakistani kindred, individuals were found to be homozygous for a distinct premature termination mutation.[16] A white male was compound heterozygous for a missense mutation in *TYRP-1* located in the second copper-binding domain, inherited from the patient's mother, and a stop codon, which apparently occurred spontaneously.[17] A Japanese individual with OCA3 harboring a homozygous mutation at c.1100delG (p.G367fsX384), has been reported.[18] The phenotype of this individual was apparently tyrosinase-positive OCA, despite the homozygous frameshift mutation, supporting the idea that the TYRP-1 protein is not the sole rate-limiting factor in melanogenesis. Furthermore, an intriguing p.S166X mutation in *TYRP-1* associated with ROCA[15] was found to modify an OCA2 phenotype to a red-haired variant.[5]

OCA4

SLC45A2, a melanosomal transporter protein, is responsible for OCA4. The function and exact localization of SLC45A2 have not been elucidated, although SLC45A2 is considered to be involved in pH control inside the melanosome, together with OCA2.[19] As melanosome pH influences TYR activity and melanogenesis, disruption of SLC45A2, which controls melanosome pH, would affect melanogenesis. A recent functional study demonstrated that OCA2 and SLC45A2 are also involved in trafficking of melanosomal components, including TYR. Thus, mutations in *SLC45A2* would impair melanin biosynthesis with wide clinical variation depending on the impact of each mutation.[20]

OCA5

Linkage analysis mapped the responsible locus to 4q24; however, subsequent sequence analysis of candidate genes failed to detect the pathologic mutation.[7]

OCA6

SLC24A5 acts as an ion transporter on melanosomal membranes together with OCA2 and SLC45A2.[21] The eumelanin content of hair in individuals with OCA6 is significantly lower than that of unaffected family members (heterozygous carriers). Electron microscopy of skin from individuals with OCA6 revealed fewer mature melanosomes (stage IV), but more immature melanosomes (stages II and III) in both the cell body and dendrites of melanocytes compared with cells from unaffected individuals. This finding suggests that the SLC24A5 protein is required for the maturation of melanosomes or for the production of pigment in mature melanosomes.[6]

OCA7

C10orf11, which is considered a melanocyte differentiation gene, is responsible for OCA7.[8] Immunohistochemistry of skin from human fetuses showed C10orf11-positive cells (melanoblasts) on the dermis, which migrate from the neural crest, while no cells positive for C10orf11 were observed in either fetal or adult retinal pigment epithelium. This finding suggests that C10orf11 is also associated with melanocyte migration.

DIAGNOSIS

Previously OCA was placed into 2 categories, tyrosinase-positive OCA and tyrosinase-negative OCA, based on the finding of dihydroxyphenylalanine (DOPA) staining. However, this method can only distinguish between OCA1A and non-OCA1A subtypes; consequently, it is seldom used. As the phenotypes of different types of OCA show significant overlap, genetic analysis is necessary for definitive diagnosis. Recent advances in genetic analysis enable us to detect additional types of albinism and the genes responsible for these disorders.[6-8] On the other hand, no mutations in known albinism-related genes have been detected in approximately 20% of affected individuals. A genome-wide association study has shown that a single nucleotide polymorphism in the regulatory region upstream of the KIT ligand gene (*KITLG*) is involved in blond hair color in northern European populations,[22] suggesting that genetic alterations in noncoding regions near albinism-related genes also can be associated with the pathogenesis of albinism, as well as mutations in potential albinism genes yet to be identified.

DIFFERENTIAL DIAGNOSIS

The coexistence of systemic symptoms such as bleeding diathesis, interstitial pneumonia, immunodeficiency, and/or neurologic defects is useful in suggesting syndromic OCA. Prader-Willi syndrome and Angelman syndrome, which are characterized by mental retardation, are sometimes accompanied by the symptoms of OCA2 because both conditions are caused by the deletion of chromosome 15q containing the *OCA2* gene. Other congenital or nutritional disorders, including phenylketonuria, histidinemia, homocystinuria, selenium deficiency, copper deficiency, and kwashiorkor, may show hypopigmentation of skin and hair (albinism). These also can be distinguished from OCA by the accompanying symptoms.

CLINICAL COURSE, PROGNOSIS, AND MANAGEMENT

No curative treatment has been found for OCA as of this writing. Early diagnosis is important to allow initiation of appropriate interventions for skin and eye symptoms. For skin, sun protection by wearing of protective clothing and the regular application of sunscreen are essential to prevent sunburn and secondary skin changes, and to decrease the risk of skin cancer in later life. Regular skin checkups for skin cancer are recommended for adult individuals with OCA, especially in cases of severe hypopigmentation. Early referral to an ophthalmologist is mandatory for proper ophthalmologic interventions such as corrective glasses or surgical correction of strabismus and nystagmus. Dark sunglasses may alleviate photophobia. Once pathologic mutations are detected in an affected family member, prenatal diagnosis becomes possible, and diagnosis may be an option for parents and other family members.

The life span of individuals with OCA may be similar to that of unaffected individuals. However, several epidemiologic studies showed that a relatively larger number of albino people is present in the younger age groups.[23] In addition, a retrospective survey of African albinos with skin cancers found that late presentation, mainly attributable to a lack of funding and poor access to health care facilities, led to more-advanced disease status.[24] Lack of preventive resources, including sunscreen, could cause albino people to have more ultraviolet exposure, a major risk factor for skin carcinogenesis.[23] These data may imply that the mortality of people with albinism might be higher than that of people without albinism, although more specific data are required to accurately assess this issue. In terms of public health, albino people have been reported to face social stigma, discrimination, and lower socioeconomic status, particularly in African countries, as a consequence of lack of accurate knowledge and education about albinism.[23]

With the exception of OCA1A, hypopigmentation of skin and hair tends to be alleviated as individuals mature. There are no case-control data regarding whether early ophthalmologic intervention can prevent the progression of visual impairment. However, visual impairment is generally not progressive, and may gradually improve with age. An increased risk for skin cancers, particularly squamous cell carcinoma and basal cell carcinoma, has been reported. The incidence rate of melanoma in individuals with OCA is controversial because of the lack of large population studies; however, it is generally considered that the risk of melanoma is increased in individuals with OCA compared to the risk for unaffected individuals. Melanin is a kind of scavenger that removes free radicals from tissue; thus, decrease or absence of melanin will lead to an increase in the risk of melanoma, squamous cell carcinoma, and basal cell carcinoma.

OCULAR ALBINISM

AT-A-GLANCE

- Ocular albinism is a rare inherited disorder characterized by hypopigmentation of the eyes and visual disturbances.
- The most common type is X-linked ocular albinism (OA), also called OA1, although OA includes heterogeneous conditions accompanied by extraocular symptoms.
- Although hypopigmentation of skin and hair can be seen in some individuals, this is usually mild and not as evident as in the case of oculocutaneous albinism.
- Visual disturbances consist of nystagmus, impaired visual acuity, and stereoscopic vision.
- Early referral to an ophthalmologist is important to introduce proper ophthalmologic intervention.
- Visual acuity is usually stable throughout the life span of an individual, and sometimes improves gradually until adulthood.

Ocular albinism (OA) is a genetic disorder characterized by decreased pigmentation of the eyes and visual disturbances. The most common and recognized form is X-linked OA (also called OA1); however, OA includes heterogeneous conditions accompanied by extraocular symptoms such as sensorineural deafness, sensorineural deafness with autosomal recessive inheritance, and congenital malformation of the maxillary bone. Although hypopigmentation of skin and hair can be seen in some individuals, these manifestations are usually mild and not as visible as those of OCA.

CLINICAL FEATURES

OA1 is characterized by hypopigmentation in the retinal pigment epithelium and iris, nystagmus, photophobia, impaired visual acuity, and foveal hypoplasia. Misrouting of the optic nerve in the chiasm is also observed in visual evoked potential testing. These ophthalmologic findings greatly overlap with those of OCA subtypes. Theoretically, hypopigmentation of skin is not seen in individuals with OA; however, some individuals show mild dilution of the pigmentation in skin and hair compared to unaffected male siblings.

ETIOLOGY AND PATHOGENESIS

The prevalence of OA has been reported as 1:60,000 and 1:50,000 in Danish and U.S. cohorts, respectively. OA1 is caused by a defective G-protein–coupled receptor 143 gene (*GPR143*) located on chromosome Xp.22.2. GPR143 is a melanosome-associated G-protein–coupled receptor involved in melanosome biogenesis during melanocyte differentiation. Electron microscopy of skin melanocytes and retinal pigment epithelium from OA1 patients showed that the number of melanosomes was decreased but their size had increased. GPR143 regulates melanosome size and number via activation of the microphthalmia-associated transcription factor (MITF), a key regulator of melanocyte differentiation.

DIAGNOSIS

OCA can be excluded by the absence of hypopigmentation of skin and hair. In white individuals with pale skin and blond hair, it may be difficult to determine whether the individuals have hypopigmentation of their skin and hair. In such cases, genetic analysis of the *GPR143* and OCA genes may be needed to obtain a definitive diagnosis.

DIFFERENTIAL DIAGNOSIS

OCA can be excluded by the absence of hypopigmentation of skin and hair. There are rare genetic disorders that demonstrate congenital nystagmus, and these also can be distinguished from OA by the absence of hypopigmentation of the iris and retinal pigment epithelium.

CLINICAL COURSE, PROGNOSIS, AND MANAGEMENT

As with the ocular symptoms of OCA, no curative treatment of OA1 exists as of this writing. Early referral to an ophthalmologist is necessary for appropriate intervention. For visual impairment, wearing corrective glasses is necessary, and dark sunglasses may alleviate photophobia. Surgical correction may be preferred for strabismus and nystagmus in some individuals. Regular ophthalmologic examinations should be performed.

OA1 is likely to be a nonprogressive disorder; visual acuity is usually stable throughout the life span of an individual, and sometimes improves gradually until adulthood. Nystagmus also tends to improve as individuals mature, but is unlikely to disappear.

HERMANSKY-PUDLAK SYNDROME

AT-A-GLANCE

- Hermansky-Pudlak syndrome (HPS) is a rare autosomal recessive genetic disorder characterized by hypopigmentation of skin, hair, and eyes accompanied by nonpigmentary symptoms, including bleeding diathesis, caused by platelet storage pool deficiency and accumulation of ceroid in tissues.
- Ten forms of HPS have been identified as of this writing.
- HPS1 and HPS4 are frequently associated with life-threatening symptoms such as interstitial pneumonia or granulomatous colitis mimicking Crohn disease in affected individuals older than age 30 years.
- HPS2 and HPS10 are associated with immunodeficiency and uncontrolled lymphocyte and macrophage activation, leading to subsequent hemophagocytic syndrome.

Hermansky-Pudlak syndrome (HPS) is a rare autosomal recessive disorder characterized by OCA and other nonpigmentary symptoms, such as bleeding diathesis, caused by platelet storage pool deficiency and accumulation of ceroid in tissues.[25] The estimated prevalence of HPS in the general population is 1:500,000 to 1:1,000,000. The region with the highest known prevalence of HPS is Puerto Rico, where approximately 1 in 1800 persons is

TABLE 75-2
Syndromic Oculocutaneous Albinism

DISEASE NAME	INHERITANCE	GENES	CHROMOSOMAL LOCATION	OMIM #
HPS1	AR	HPS1	10q24.2	203300
HPS2	AR	HPS2/AP3B1	5q14.1	608233
HPS3	AR	HPS3	3q24	614072
HPS4	AR	HPS4	22q12.1	614073
HPS5	AR	HPS5	11p15.1	614074
HPS6	AR	HPS6	10q24.32	614075
HPS7	AR	HPS7/DTNBP1	6p22.3	614076
HPS8	AR	HPS8/BLOC1S3	19q13.32	614077
HPS9	AR	HPS9/PLDN	15q21.1	614171
HPS10	AR	HPS10/AP3D1	19p13.3	617050
CHS	AR	LYST	1q42.3	214500
GS1	AR	MYO5A	15q21.2	214450
GS2	AR	RAB27A	15q21.3	607624
GS3	AR	MLPH and MYO5A	2q37.3	609227

AR, autosomal recessive; CHS, Chediak-Higashi syndrome; GS, Griscelli syndrome; HPS, Hermansky-Pudlak syndrome; OMIM, Online Mendelian Inheritance in Man.

affected, and approximately 1 in 22 is a carrier. Almost all of these individuals are type 1 or type 3. Regarding non–Puerto Rican populations, HPS1 is a relatively common type of albinism in Japan and China.[1] HPS is genetically and clinically heterozygous, with 10 types of HPS and their responsible genes reported as of this writing (Table 75-2). By electron microscopy, platelets from individuals with HPS do not contain dense granules, which is a gold standard diagnostic finding.

CLINICAL FEATURES

Patients with HPS show various degrees of hypopigmentation, impaired visual acuity, and bleeding tendency (see Fig. 75-1C). After middle age, it is noteworthy that patients with HPS1 and HPS4 frequently manifest life-threatening symptoms such as interstitial pneumonia, granulomatous colitis mimicking Crohn disease, and, rarely, cardiomyopathy. Because the affected molecular complex is the same in HPS1 and HPS4 (see section "Etiology and Pathogenesis"), the phenotype is identical and cannot be distinguished clinically. HPS3, HPS5, and HPS6 show relatively mild phenotypes lacking pneumonia and colitis. HPS2 and HPS10 are associated with immunodeficiency and uncontrolled lymphocyte and macrophage activation, leading to subsequent hemophagocytic syndrome.

ETIOLOGY AND PATHOGENESIS

HPS is caused by the disruption of lysosomal-related organelles that play important roles in membrane trafficking in many types of cells and organs. The symptoms, including OCA, bleeding diathesis, and deposition of ceroid bodies, are a result of the disruption of membrane trafficking of melanosome-related proteins, platelet-dense granules, and lysosomes. Lysosomal-related organelles are synthesized by several protein complexes that consist of several HPS proteins, including the BLOC (biogenesis of lysosome-related organelles complex) members—BLOC-1, BLOC-2, and BLOC-3, and the adaptor protein (AP) complex—AP-3. Thus, disruption of HPS proteins results in pigmentary and various nonpigmentary symptoms.

BLOC-3 is composed of 2 subunits, HPS1 and HPS4.[26] Analysis of fibroblasts derived from BLOC-3–deficient mice showed altered distribution of late endosomes/lysosomes, suggesting that BLOC-3 may play a role in the proper distribution and motility of organelles, although its pathophysiology in the development of HPS1 and HPS4 remains to be clarified. Depending on where it is expressed, the AP-3 complex has 2 forms, the ubiquitous form and the neuron-specific form.[27] The ubiquitous form plays a role in the efficient trafficking of TYR and OCA2 in melanocytes.[28] The neuron-specific form is necessary for synaptic vesicle formation from endosomes, thus allowing the release of neurotransmitters along developing axons.[29] Although both forms share 3 subunits, AP-3α, AP-3δ, and AP-3μ, the difference between the 2 forms is the presence of AP-3 β3A in the ubiquitous form and the presence of AP-3 β3B in the neuron-specific form. The gene for HPS2 (AP3B1) encodes the β3A subunit. Recently, AP3D1 encoding AP-3δ has been reported to be the gene responsible for HPS10.[27] Clinical symptoms of HPS2 and HPS10 are consistent with these molecular findings, as a defective β3A subunit (HPS2), which is a component of the ubiquitous form but not the neuron-specific form, does not cause neurologic abnormalities, whereas a defective AP-3δ subunit (HPS10) is associated with neurologic symptoms.[27] BLOC-2 is composed of 3 subunits that are responsible for HPS3, HPS5, and HPS6. Melanocytes from individuals with HPS with deficient BLOC-2 showed mislocalization of TYR and TYRP-1, and accumulation of TYR-containing vesicular structures in the cytoplasm. These findings suggest that BLOC-2 is located downstream of BLOC-1 and might play a role in fusion of BLOC-1–dependent transport intermediates with maturing melanosomes.[28] BLOC-1 is a large complex consisting of at least 9 subunits, including HPS7, HPS8, and HPS9. BLOC-1 may play a role in the trafficking of TYR and TYRP-1 in cooperation with AP-1 and AP-3, although the details have not been clarified. BLOC-1–deficient mice show prominent hypopigmentation.[30]

DIAGNOSIS

The clinical diagnosis of HPS is rendered by the lack of platelet dense granules on electron microscopy. Genetic analysis of HPS genes is needed to obtain a definitive diagnosis, because the symptoms of some HPS subtypes (eg, HPS1 and HPS4) are identical—the affected molecular complex is the same—and cannot be distinguished clinically.

DIFFERENTIAL DIAGNOSIS

The differential diagnosis of HPS includes nonsyndromic OCA and Chédiak-Higashi syndrome (CHS). The symptoms of nonsyndromic OCA are restricted to hypopigmentation and visual impairment. CHS is characterized by silvery hair, recurrent pyogenic infection, and subsequent fatal hemophagocytic syndrome, considered the "accelerated phase." Large granules are seen in polymorphonuclear cells from individuals with CHS, which is diagnostic. Immunodeficiency is observed in HPS2 and HPS10.

CLINICAL COURSE, PROGNOSIS, AND MANAGEMENT

For hypopigmentation of skin and visual impairment, early intervention should be introduced (see sections "Intervention and Treatment" in the nonsyndromic OCA and OA above). No curative treatment has been found as of this writing for hypopigmentation. Pirfenidone, corticosteroid, and immunosuppressants have been used to treat pulmonary fibrosis, although the efficacy of these therapies remains controversial. Infliximab and granulocyte colony-stimulating factor are suggested to be effective for colitis and neutropenia/immune deficiency, respectively. Colectomy may be necessary for severe colitis. Hematopoietic stem cell transplantation (HSCT) may be required to prevent the development of hemophagocytic syndrome in individuals with HPS2.

Hypopigmentation of skin and hair tends to be alleviated as individuals mature. Visual impairment is usually nonprogressive. The prognosis of individuals with HPS1, the most common subtype of HPS, can be determined by the interstitial pneumonia.

GRISCELLI SYNDROME

AT-A-GLANCE

- Griscelli syndrome is a rare autosomal recessive genetic disorder characterized by hypopigmentation of skin and hair, with large clumps of pigment in the hair shaft on light microscopy.
- Three forms of Griscelli syndrome (GS) have been identified.
- GS1 and GS2 show extrapigmentary symptoms including neurologic and hematologic abnormalities; GS3 is restricted to hypopigmentation.

Griscelli syndrome (GS) is a rare autosomal recessive genetic disorder characterized by hypopigmentation of skin and hair, with large clumps of pigment in the hair shaft on light microscopy. Three forms of GS have been identified as of this writing (see Table 75-2): GS1 is characterized by hypopigmentation with neurologic abnormalities; GS2 features hypopigmentation accompanied by hematologic immunodeficiency and hematologic abnormalities; GS3 is restricted to hypopigmentation.

CLINICAL FEATURES

GS is characterized by hypopigmentation of skin and silvery hair with large clumps of pigment in the hair shaft. GS1 is associated with severe developmental delay and mental retardation. GS2 is associated with recurrent pyogenic infections and uncontrolled T-cell and macrophage activation leading to hemophagocytic syndrome, the so-called accelerated phase, which can be fatal without immunosuppressive treatment or stem cell bone marrow transplantation. GS3 is restricted to hypopigmentation of skin and hair.

ETIOLOGY AND PATHOGENESIS

The genes responsible for the 3 GS types are *MYO5A* (GS1), *RAB27A* (GS2), and *MLPH* (GS3). They form a complex in melanocytes, connect melanosomes to the actin network, and are involved in melanosome transport at the periphery of melanocytes.[31] MYO5A binds to actin filaments and moves along them like a wheel; MLPH connects RAB27A and MYO5A; and RAB27A connects to melanosomes. Because MYO5A is associated with neurologic development and function,[32] defective MYO5A can cause severe neurologic deterioration. On the other hand, a transcript variant in brain tissue does not contain exon-F of *MYO5A*.[33] Individuals showing hypopigmentation of skin and hair identical to GS3 showed homozygous deletion of *MYO5A* exon-F.[31] RAB27A is also associated with the release of lytic granules from CD8+ T cells. Defective RAB27A causes immunodeficiency and uncontrolled T-cell and macrophage activation leading to fatal hemophagocytic syndrome.[31]

DIAGNOSIS

The presence of large clumps of pigment in the hair shaft is diagnostic for GS, but genetic analysis gives a definitive diagnosis.

DIFFERENTIAL DIAGNOSIS

The differential diagnosis of GS includes nonsyndromic OCA, CHS, and HPS. Nonsyndromic OCA can be excluded based on the presence of nonpigmentary symptoms. GS3 can be distinguished from nonsyndromic OCA by the presence of large clumps of pigment in the hair shaft. Similarly, these observations also can be used to distinguish GS2 from CHS. Peripheral blood smears from individuals with CHS demonstrate giant inclusion bodies in polymorphonuclear neutrophils and some lymphocytes. HPS2 and HPS10 show hypopigmentation together with immunodeficiency, although HPS lacks platelet dense granules on electron microscopy.

CLINICAL COURSE, PROGNOSIS, AND MANAGEMENT

For hypopigmentation of skin and visual impairment, early intervention should be introduced (see "Intervention and Treatment" in the OCA and OA sections above). As of this writing, no curative treatment exists for the neurologic symptoms. However, rehabilitation can alleviate the neurologic symptoms. Stem cell bone marrow transplantation is the only method to cure the hematologic and immunologic abnormalities.

Regarding the prognosis, most patients with GS1 and GS2 reported in the literature died before the age of 10 years. Cağdaş and associates reported healthy 21- and 24-year-old patients with GS3 with only pigmentary dilution.[34]

CHÉDIAK-HIGASHI SYNDROME

AT-A-GLANCE

- Chédiak-Higashi syndrome is a rare genetic disease with autosomal recessive inheritance characterized by reduced pigmentation of skin and eyes, silvery or metallic colored hair, and neurologic and hematologic disorders.
- Approximately 90% of individuals with Chédiak-Higashi syndrome develop lymphoproliferative syndrome, the "accelerated phase" of the disease that tends to be fatal.
- Hematopoietic stem cell transplantation is the only treatment for hematologic and immunologic abnormalities.

CHS is a rare genetic disease with autosomal recessive inheritance characterized by reduced pigmentation of skin and eyes, silvery or metallic colored hair, immunodeficiency, and debilitating neurologic abnormalities. Large granules in polymorphonuclear neutrophils on blood smear are diagnostic, and pigment clumping on the hair shaft is also seen. As of this writing, fewer than 500 cases have been reported. Approximately 90% of individuals with CHS develop lymphoproliferative syndrome, which is known as the "accelerated phase" of the disease and tends to be fatal.

CLINICAL FEATURES

Individuals with CHS show various degrees of hypopigmentation of skin and eyes, silvery or metallic colored hair, and immunodeficiency. Neurologic findings, including low IQ scores, cerebellar ataxia, and peripheral neuropathy, appear in childhood or adolescence and tend to progress gradually. Approximately 90% of individuals with CHS develop lymphoproliferative syndrome, which is called the "accelerated phase" of the disease and tends to be fatal. A case report exists of two brothers with a *LYST* mutation, who showed slowly progressive neurologic symptoms, including spastic paraplegia, cerebral ataxia, and peripheral neuropathy, but lacked hypopigmentation.[35]

ETIOLOGY AND PATHOGENESIS

The gene responsible for CHS is *LYST*, located on 1q42.3, which encodes lysosomal trafficking regulator (LYST), also known as CHS1. Although the biologic function of CHS1 has not been determined, electron microscopy of epidermal melanocytes from an individual with CHS shows the accumulation of large melanosomes on the periphery of the cytoplasm; these melanosomes are not transferred to neighboring keratinocytes. Peroxidase-positive large inclusion bodies are seen in polymorphonuclear neutrophils and occasionally in lymphocytes, which is a characteristic finding in CHS. Neurologic abnormalities may be caused by lysosome dysfunction in neurons and glial cells.[36] Considering these findings, LYST may play roles in vesicle trafficking in various cell types.

DIAGNOSIS

Peroxidase-positive large inclusion bodies are seen in polymorphonuclear neutrophils and, occasionally, in lymphocytes, which is a characteristic finding in CHS. Genetic analysis of CHS1 assists in making a diagnosis of CHS.

DIFFERENTIAL DIAGNOSIS

Differential diagnosis includes diseases showing hypopigmentation of skin, hair, and eyes, and/or immunodeficiency. Nonsyndromic OCA is restricted to hypopigmentation and ocular symptoms, with a lack of immunodeficiency or neurologic abnormalities. Individuals with HPS2 and HPS10 demonstrate neutropenia and immunodeficiency in addition to albinism. Individuals with GS demonstrate symptoms similar to those of CHS; however, GS can be distinguished from CHS by the lack of large inclusion bodies in polymorphonuclear neutrophils. Individuals with HPS also lack dense granules in platelets.

CLINICAL COURSE, PROGNOSIS, AND MANAGEMENT

HSCT is the only treatment for hematologic and immunologic abnormalities. For hypopigmentation of skin and visual impairment, early intervention should be introduced (see "Intervention and Treatment" in the OCA and OA sections). As of this writing, no curative treatment has been established for hypopigmentation.

Most individuals with CHS are required to undergo HSCT; without this treatment, they will die within the early part of their first decade of life. Individuals with mild symptoms or those who do not develop the accelerated phase may survive for a long period of time, although debilitating neurologic abnormalities, such as loss of balance, difficulty with ambulation, and peripheral neuropathy, may appear.[36]

INCONTINENTIA PIGMENTI

AT-A-GLANCE

- Incontinentia pigmenti is a rare genetic multiorgan disorder with X-linked dominant inheritance.
- Various cutaneous lesions are seen from infancy to adulthood, with eye, CNS or musculoskeletal abnormalities.
- Cutaneous lesions usually heal spontaneously with focal hypopigmentation or scarring, but eye and CNS lesions can have serious consequences for the vision and life of patients.

Incontinentia pigmenti (IP) is a rare genetic multiorgan disorder with X-linked dominant inheritance, characterized by various cutaneous lesions from infancy to adulthood, and extracutaneous symptoms such as eye, CNS, and musculoskeletal abnormalities. Skin lesions include erythema, vesicle, hyperkeratotic papule, and hyperpigmentation, and usually heal spontaneously with focal hypopigmentation, scarring, or alopecia. However, eye and CNS lesions can have serious consequences for the vision and life of patients.

CLINICAL FEATURES

Multiple organs including the skin, eye, CNS, and musculoskeletal tissue can be affected in patients with IP. Although cutaneous lesions tend to be self-healing with occasional scarring (Fig. 75-2), they are one of the major diagnostic criteria and a characteristic symptom of IP.

Cutaneous lesions are classified into 4 stages based on clinical findings. Stage I (vesiculobullous stage) is characterized by vesicular/bullous eruptions and erythema distributed in a linear or whorled pattern on

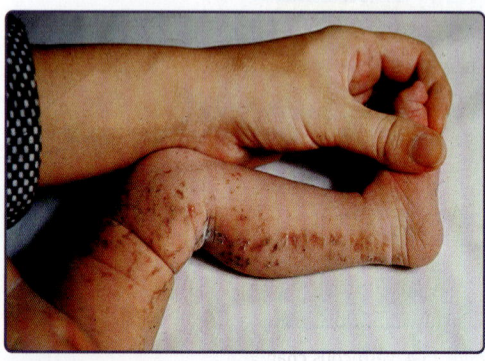

Figure 75-2 Healing vesicle in an infant with incontinentia pigmenti. (Image used with permission from the Graham Library of Wake Forest Department of Dermatology.)

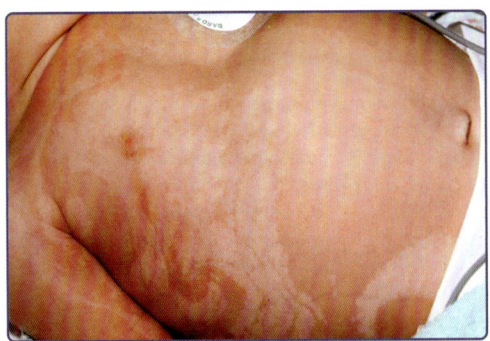

Figure 75-3 Hypopigmented whorls on the abdomen of an infant with incontinentia pigmenti. (Image used with permission from the Graham Library of Wake Forest Department of Dermatology.)

the trunk and extremities (the face is usually spared) that appear within 1 week of birth (Fig. 75-3). The eruption tends to be bilateral but can be unilateral. Eosinophilia is seen in approximately 30% to 60% of the cases, and eosinophilic infiltration in the lesional skin is a characteristic histologic finding. Stage II (verrucous stage) follows stage I, and is characterized by verrucous or lichen planus-like keratotic eruptions on the extremities (Fig. 75-4), particularly the dorsal hand and foot. The distribution of lesions does not necessarily correspond to that of the stage I eruption. The histopathology of stage II eruption shows dyskeratotic keratinocytes, hyperkeratosis, and acanthosis. Stage II lasts for a few months and occasionally, may last up to a few years. The lesions of stage III (hyperpigmentation stage) appear when individuals are 12 to 16 weeks old, and these are characterized by brown to gray-brown pigmentation distributed in whorled or linear patterns, respecting the Blaschko line. Melanophages are prominent in the upper dermis histologically. The pigmentation disappears almost completely by 4 or 5 years of age and may leave focal hypopigmentation, atrophic scar, or alopecia. The eruptions during stages I and II can often be exacerbated by acute viral infection.

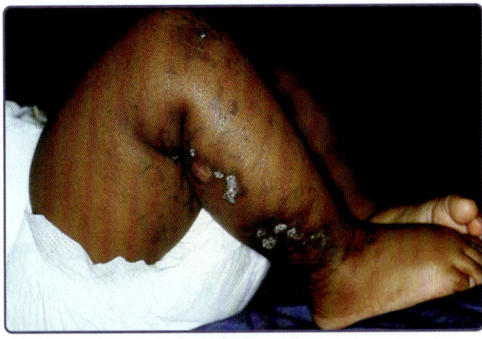

Figure 75-4 Verrucous changes on the leg of deeply pigmented infant with incontinentia pigmenti. (Image used with permission from the Graham Library of Wake Forest Department of Dermatology.)

Several types of eruption may coexist, so each stage may not be clearly determined. Eye abnormalities are seen in 36% to 77% of patients with IP,[37] including both retinal and nonretinal lesions, such as retinal detachment, retinal hemorrhage, strabismus, nystagmus, and uveitis. CNS lesions include seizure, mental retardation, hemiplegia, spasticity, and cerebellar ataxia, some of which can be life-threatening.

ETIOLOGY AND PATHOGENESIS

The responsible gene for IP is *IKBKG* (inhibitor of kappa light polypeptide gene enhancer in B-cells, kinase gamma) located on Xp28. Of patients with IP, 80% harbor an 11.7-kb deletion containing exons 4 to 10 of *IKBKG*, and the function of nuclear factor κB is thereby completely lost. The cells containing aberrant IKBKG are very sensitive to proapoptotic stimuli, and are prone to undergo apoptosis.[37] Abundant eosinophil infiltration is seen in the biopsy from vesicular eruption, and eosinophilia is also observed in 30% to 60% of patients. Jean-Baptiste and associates revealed that the expression of eosinophil-specific chemotactic factor eotaxin in vesicular lesions from IP patients was increased, and keratinocyte expression of eotaxin was induced by the proinflammatory cytokine interleukin-1α in vitro. Overexpression of eotaxin seems to be involved in the eosinophil infiltration and the pathogenesis of IP.[38] The mechanism of eosinophil infiltration can lead to fibrovascular proliferation during the inflammatory process in the eye. The pathogenesis of the CNS lesions in IP has not been determined, although apoptosis and the subsequent inflammatory response caused by the abnormal function of nuclear factor κB seem to be the major events, similar to the pathogenesis of skin lesions.[39]

Because IP is inherited by an X-linked mechanism and a male fetus with aberrant IKBKG is expected to be miscarried, the expected percentage among newborn babies is 33% unaffected females, 33% affected females, and 33% unaffected males. However, more than 100 male patients (6.1% of all IP cases) have been reported. An international IP consortium proposed 3 possible mechanisms for male IP patients. These were less deleterious (hypomorphic) mutations; a 47,XXY karyotype; or somatic mosaicism.[40] Ardelean and Pope reported that the clinicopathologic features of male and female individuals with IP seemed to be similar.[41]

DIAGNOSIS

Landy and Donnai proposed diagnostic criteria for IP in 1993.[42] Their suggestion for a major criterion is cutaneous lesions that occur from infancy to adulthood, while minor criteria include dental, hair, nail, and retinal abnormalities.[37] Mimic and associates suggested the modification that the presence of at least 1 skin lesion should be one of the major criteria, together with CNS abnormalities, multiple miscarriages of male fetuses, and typical skin histologic findings. Genetic analysis of *IKBKG* would also be helpful to render a definitive diagnosis.

DIFFERENTIAL DIAGNOSIS

As the cutaneous symptoms of IP vary depending on the stage and time course, many skin diseases can be the differential diagnosis. At stages I and II, infectious diseases producing similar symptoms include herpes simplex, impetigo, wart, molluscum contagiosum or epidermolysis bullosa. In later stages, the following resemble IP: nonspecific postinflammatory pigmentation, hypomelanosis of Ito, vitiligo, and Naegeli syndrome (although Naegeli syndrome itself is rare).

CLINICAL COURSE, PROGNOSIS, AND MANAGEMENT

Skin lesions of IP tend to be self-healing but may leave scars or hair loss at the affected areas. Secondary infection and strong inflammation may be possible, particularly in the stage I lesions, requiring topical treatment based on the skin condition. Eye and CNS abnormalities can cause serious impacts to the patients including blindness and death. No curative treatment for IP exists as of this writing. Routine regular followup study for extracutaneous lesions including those affecting the eyes and CNS is needed to allow early initiation of appropriate interventions.

PIEBALDISM

AT-A-GLANCE

- Piebaldism is a rare autosomal dominant disease with congenital white patches.
- The patches mainly occur on the forehead, chest, abdomen, and extremities.
- The distribution and shape of white patches remains the same throughout life.
- Usually there are no complications except for skin phenotypes.

Piebaldism is a rare genetic disorder with congenital white patches on the forehead, chest, abdomen, and extremities that result from impairment of melanoblast migration in embryonal development.

CLINICAL FEATURES

Piebaldism is an autosomal dominant disease in which a congenital white forelock, scattered hypopigmented macules, and a triangular-shaped white patch on the forehead are involved (OMIM 172800). The forehead, chest, abdomen, and extremities are typical sites for involvement. White patches are completely depigmented owing to the absence of melanocytes, and often are strikingly symmetrical. Hyperpigmented macules, which are similar to café-au-lait spots, are sometimes involved. A diamond-shaped white forelock is present in 90% of affected individuals. Within depigmented areas, there may be islands of hyperpigmentation, and the margins of lesions are also often hyperpigmented. The distribution of the lesions remains for the entire life of affected individuals. Intrafamilial variability in the degree of lesions is great.

ETIOLOGY AND PATHOGENESIS

Piebaldism is associated with the *KIT* gene.[43] Melanocytes originate from the dorsal portions of the closing neural tube in vertebrate embryos. Progenitor melanoblasts migrate dorsolaterally between the mesodermal and ectodermal layers to reach their final destinations, including the skin. Early melanoblast development requires the presence of stem cell factor (SCF or c-KIT ligand) expressed by epidermal keratinocytes, and its tyrosine kinase transmembrane receptor c-KIT expressed on melanoblasts. Piebaldism results from mutations of *c-KIT* that cause failure of melanoblast migration from the neural crest to the skin.[43] Because the ventral aspect of the body is the area farthest from the dorsally located neural crest, it is more frequently affected than the dorsal aspect.

There is a report that mutation in *SNAI2*, which encodes a zinc finger transcription factor, can cause piebaldism.[44]

DIAGNOSIS

Piebaldism is typically a straightforward clinical diagnosis based on complete depigmentation in chest, abdomen, and extremities, a characteristic white forelock, and a family history. Skin biopsy from the white lesion shows an absence of melanin and melanocytes. The finding of a mutation of *c-KIT* definitely determines the diagnosis as piebaldism.

DIFFERENTIAL DIAGNOSIS

Piebaldism should be distinguished from vitiligo, Vogt-Koyanagi-Harada disease, nevus depigmentosus, hypomelanosis of Ito, tuberous sclerosis, and Waardenburg syndrome.

CLINICAL COURSE, PROGNOSIS, AND MANAGEMENT

The distribution, size, and shape of the lesions will not typically change during life. However, islands of repigmentation, especially in the white patch on the forehead, have been reported to develop in some affected individuals after sun exposure. A patient with typical piebaldism but progressive depigmentation also has been reported.

So far, there are some reports that epidermal transplantation was available, although effective management strategies have not been established yet.

WAARDENBURG SYNDROME AND TIETZ SYNDROME

AT-A-GLANCE

- Waardenburg and Tietz syndromes are rare genetic diseases with congenital pigment disorder plus sensorineural deafness.
- Both mostly have autosomal dominant inheritance.
- White patches are frequently found, but mottled or speckled patterns also are found sometimes.
- Some of the 4 subtypes involve musculoskeletal anomalies, Hirschsprung disease, or severe neurologic defects.
- Tietz syndrome is a kind of variation of Waardenburg syndrome with a diffuse pigmentary phenotype plus severe hearing loss.

WAARDENBURG SYNDROME

Waardenburg syndrome (WS), first reported by Waardenburg in 1951, is a genetic disease consisting of congenital pigment anomalies, including white patches, with sensorineural deafness.[45] According to the clinical manifestations and genetic abnormalities, WS is classified into 4 types (Table 75-3).

CLINICAL FEATURES

Pigment anomalies include both white patches and occasionally occurring mottled or speckled patterns. In patients with WS1, white forelock (hair depigmentation), pigmentary anomalies of the iris (Fig. 75-5), congenital sensorineural deafness, and dystopia canthorum are frequently observed. Depigmented macules or patches, synophrys, broad nasal root, and nose hypoplasia are sometimes accompanying symptoms. In WS3, axial and limb musculoskeletal anomalies are additionally observed. In the case of WS2, the clinical features are similar to those of WS1, except for absence of dystopia canthorum and

TABLE 75-3
Subtypes of Waardenburg Syndrome

DISORDER TYPE	CLINICAL FEATURE	SUBTYPE	OMIM #	RESPONSIBLE GENE	MAPPING	INHERITANCE
WS1	White forelock, heterochromia irides, dystopia canthorum		193500	PAX3	2q35	AD
WS2	Similar to WS1, but no dystopia canthorum	A	193510	MITF	3p14.1-p12.3	AD
		B	600193	?	1p21-p13.3	?
		C	606662	?	8p23	?
		D	608890	SNAI2	8q11	AR
		E	611584	SOX10	22q13	AD
WS3	Similar to WS1, plus axial and limb musculoskeletal anomalies		148820	PAX3	2q35	AD/AR
WS4	Similar to WS1, plus Hirschsprung disease	A	277580	EDNRB	13q22	AD/AR
		B	613265	EDN3	20q13.2-q13.3	AD/AR
		C	613266	SOX10	22q13	AD

AD, autosomal dominant; AR, autosomal recessive; OMIM, Online Mendelian Inheritance in Man; WS, Waardenburg syndrome.

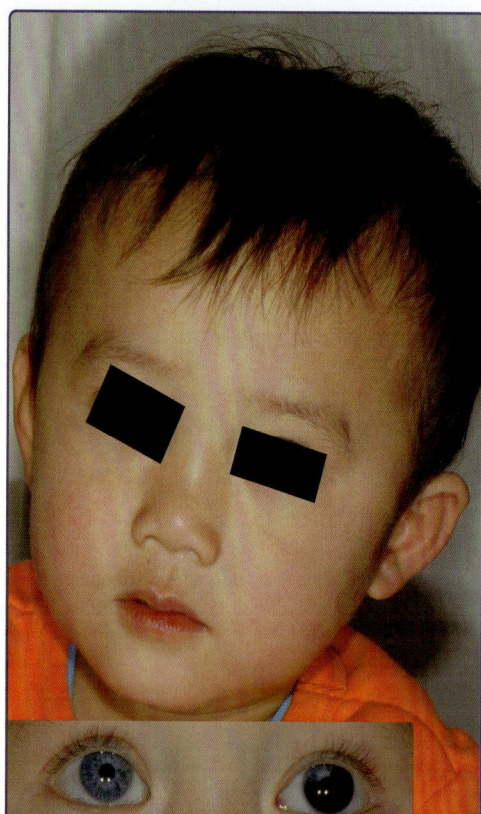

Figure 75-5 Clinical findings of Waardenburg syndrome type 2. Three-year-old boy (reported in Monma F, Hozumi Y, Kawaguchi M, et al[60]). Heterochromia irides are seen, and he showed a frontal white blaze of hair, and leukoderma over his body. Hearing impairment was also reported.

TABLE 75-4

Criteria for Diagnosis of Waardenburg Syndrome[a]

Major Criteria
Characteristic white forelock
Pigmentary anomalies of the iris
Congenital sensorineural deafness
Dystopia canthorum
An affected first-degree relative

Minor Criteria
Depigmented macules or patches
Synophrys
Broad nasal root
Nose hypoplasia
Early graying the hair by age 35 years

[a]Diagnosis requires either 2 major criteria or 1 major and 2 minor criteria.

as responsible genes for another WS2 type.[46] WS4 is also a heterogenic type resulting from mutations in several genes, including the endothelin-B receptor (*EDNRB*), endothelin-3 (*EDN3*), and SOX10 (*SOX10*).[46] Interaction between EDNRB and its ligand EDN3 is essential for the embryologic development of neurons of ganglia in the GI tract, and melanocytes. Mutations in *SOX10* cause myelination deficiency in the central and peripheral nervous systems, and can cause a severe phenotype called PCWH (peripheral demyelinating neuropathy, central dysmyelinating leukodystrophy, Waardenburg syndrome, and Hirschsprung disease).[47]

DIAGNOSIS

Diagnosis requires fulfillment of either 2 major criteria or 1 major and 2 minor criteria (Table 75-4).

CLINICAL COURSE, PROGNOSIS, AND MANAGEMENT

Protection from sunburn is important. In the case of WS4, surgical treatment of the aganglionic segment of bowel is required. Establishing the diagnosis of WS should lead to early detection of hearing loss and appropriate intervention.

TIETZ SYNDROME

Tietz syndrome (OMIM 103500) is caused by specific mutations of *MITF*—Asn210Lys and Arg217del. The hypopigmentation has a diffuse pigmentary phenotype similar to that found in OCA2, not patchy as in WS2. Patients with either mutation present with severe hearing loss. Both mutations are thought to have a dominant-negative effect, resulting in a distinct phenotype, even though mutations exist in the same gene with WS2.[48]

facial abnormalities. WS4 presents with white forelock, isochromatic irides, and the additional feature of Hirschsprung disease (neonatal intestinal obstruction, megacolon).[46]

ETIOLOGY AND PATHOGENESIS

WS1 and WS3 result from loss-of-function mutations in *PAX3*, which encodes a transcription factor regulating expression of MITF. The clinical manifestations observed in WS1 and WS3 can be explained by deregulation of the genes regulated by PAX3, occurring early in embryogenesis in the cells originating from the neural crest. MITF takes a central role in melanogenesis, and also mediates survival of melanocytes via regulation of Bcl2. Defects of MITF cause the pigmentary and hearing symptoms observed in WS1 and WS3.

WS2 is genetically a heterogenic type. Mutations of *MITF* have been found in 89.6% of WS2 cases. *MITF* is a member of the Myc supergene family of transcription factors having a basic helix-loop-helix leucine zipper structure. Two genes, *SNAI2* and *SOX10*, and 2 loci, chromosome 1p and 8p23, have been reported

RETICULATE PIGMENT DISORDERS

AT-A-GLANCE

- The category of reticulate pigment disorders includes dyschromatosis symmetrica hereditaria, dyschromatosis universalis hereditaria, reticulate acropigmentation of Kitamura, and Dowling-Degos disease.
- These 4 diseases can be genetically differentiated.
- All of these are genetic diseases with reticulate pigment phenotype, mostly having autosomal dominant inheritance.
- Some anomalies or complications are sometimes found in addition to skin phenotypes in some of the diseases.

Reticulate pigment disorders involve many diseases. Here, dyschromatosis symmetrica hereditaria (DSH), dyschromatosis universalis hereditaria (DUH), reticulate acropigmentation of Kitamura (RAK), and Dowling-Degos disease (DDD) are included. These are recognized as different diseases, and most of these diseases can be differentiated by genetic analysis.

DYSCHROMATOSIS SYMMETRICA HEREDITARIA

CLINICAL FEATURES

DSH (OMIM 127400) (also called "reticulate acropigmentation of Dohi") is an autosomal dominant disease characterized by a mixture of hyperpigmented and hypopigmented macules distributed on the dorsal aspects of the extremities (Fig. 75-6), and freckle-like macules on the face. The skin lesions usually appear in infancy or early childhood.

Patients with DSH usually have no complications; however, some reports showed that patients with the specific mutation Gly1007Arg in *ADAR1* presented with severe neurologic disorders, such as dystonia, mental deterioration, and brain calcification.[49] So far, this is a unique mutation causing neurologic complications.

ETIOLOGY AND PATHOGENESIS

DSH has been reported mainly in East Asia, although it occurs in families of every ethnic origin worldwide. Histologic and electron microscopic examination has revealed that the number of melanocytes in the hypopigmented areas of patients with DSH is

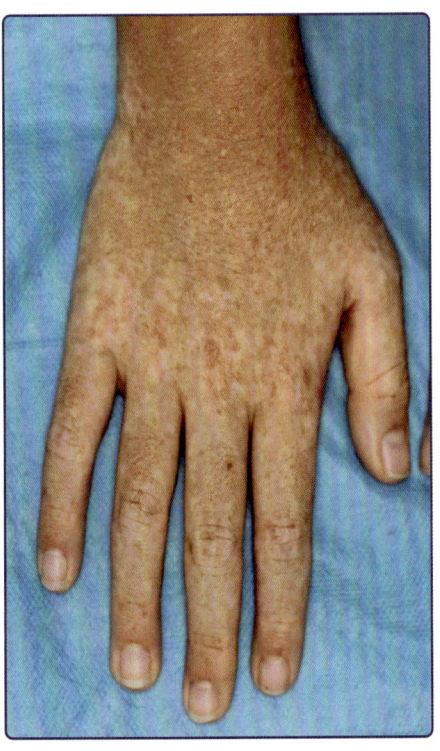 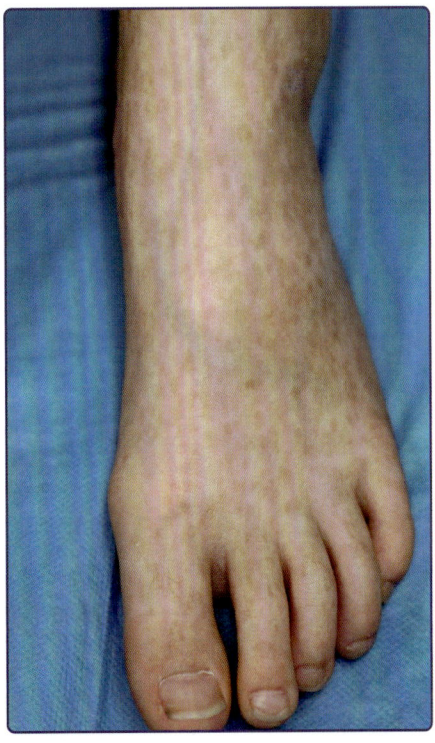

Figure 75-6 Clinical manifestations of dyschromatosis symmetrica hereditaria. Intermingled hyperpigmentation and hypopigmentation of the dorsal aspect of the hand and fingers.

obviously lower than that in normal skin, and that the melanocytes show degenerative vacuolation, indicative of apoptosis.

From linkage analysis and a genome-wide scan, the results indicated that a heterozygous mutation of the RNA-specific adenosine deaminase gene (*ADAR1*) causes DSH.[50] ADAR1 was identified as the first enzyme that converts adenosine to inosine in double-stranded RNA. Previous in vitro studies suggested ADAR1 is involved in several physiologic activities, such as virus inactivation (eg, measles virus, HIV, and hepatitis C virus) and alteration in the properties of the neurotransmitter receptor for L-glutamate (GluR) and serotonin (5-HT2cR) through this A-to-I editing process. Recent studies have revealed that ADAR1 is an important modulator of the innate antiviral response. Haploinsufficiency of ADAR1 causes the phenotypes of DSH, although the mechanisms remain unknown.

DIAGNOSIS

A mixture of hyperpigmented and hypopigmented macules distributed only on the dorsal aspects of the extremities, not on the body, is characteristic of DSH. The frequency of the neurologic complication is very rare. Identification of a pathologic mutation in *ADAR1* makes a definite diagnosis.

DIFFERENTIAL DIAGNOSIS

There are at least 3 diseases showing phenotypes very similar to DSH. One of them is DUH. In DUH, mixtures of hyperpigmented and hypopigmented macules occur all over the body. The other is RAK, which is characterized by "pits" on the palms, and the absence of hypopigmented macules. DDD is another reticulate disease. The DDD phenotype, in which small hyperkeratotic dark-brown papules are found mainly in the flexures, is progressive.

CLINICAL COURSE, PROGNOSIS, AND MANAGEMENT

Skin conditions commonly stop spreading before adolescence and last for life. Transplantation of skin from a normally pigmented area to the white area is a management strategy that has been reported to give good results.

DYSCHROMATOSIS UNIVERSALIS HEREDITARIA

CLINICAL FEATURES

DUH (OMIM 127500) is characterized by asymptomatic hypopigmented and hyperpigmented macules of irregular size and shape in a generalized distribution over the trunk and limbs, and sometimes the face. Skin phenotypes usually appear early in life. Abnormalities of hair and nails have been reported, and DUH may be associated with abnormalities of dermal connective tissue, nerve tissue, or other systemic complications.[51] DUH has been most commonly reported in East Asia, for example, Japan and China, but also has been reported worldwide.

ETIOLOGY AND PATHOGENESIS

Histopathologic examination of a skin lesion showed a pigmented basal layer of the epidermis, pigmentary incontinence in the papillary dermis, and some melanophages and lymphocytes in the upper dermis. These findings indicate that DUH is not a disorder of melanocyte number.

DUH is classified into 3 subtypes. DUH1 (OMIM 127500) is an autosomal dominant disease with linkage to 6q24.2-q25.2. DUH2 (OMIM 612715) is an autosomal recessive disease mapped to chromosome 12q21-q23. DUH3 is caused by heterozygous mutation in the *ABCB6* gene on chromosome 2q35.[51]

DIAGNOSIS

The characteristic phenotype, which is a mixture of hypopigmented and hyperpigmented macules all over the body, can be easily used clinically to diagnose DUH. However, gene analysis is helpful for diagnosis, because subtyping from clinical information is sometimes difficult.

RETICULATE ACROPIGMENTATION OF KITAMURA

CLINICAL FEATURES

RAK (OMIM 615537) is a rare genetic pigmentary disorder that usually shows an autosomal dominant pattern of inheritance with high penetrance, and was first reported worldwide in 1953.[52] RAK is typically characterized by angulate reticulate hyperpigmentation of the dorsum of the extremity (Fig. 75-7A). The palms and soles contain punctate pits (Fig. 75-7B) and breaks in the epidermal rete ridge pattern. Hypopigmented macules are never included in the lesions. The phenotype appears within the first or second decade of life, and continues throughout life. Although RAK has been reported mainly in Japan, considerable numbers of patients have been described from other countries or ethnicities, such as the Middle East, Europe, and Latin America.

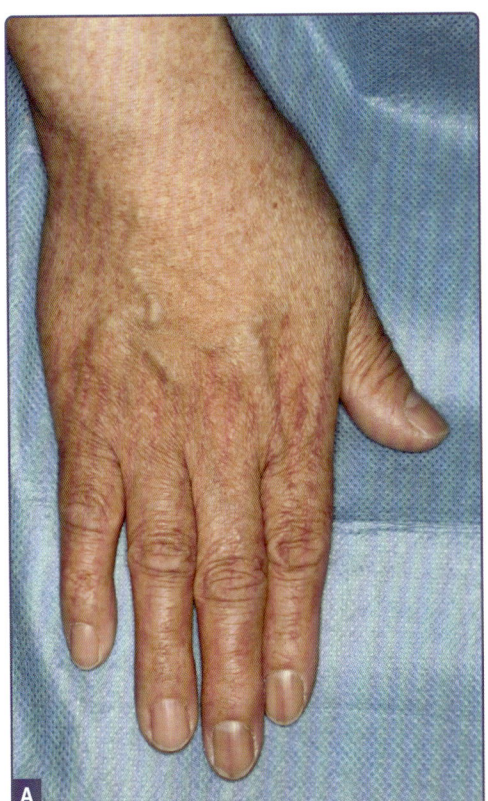

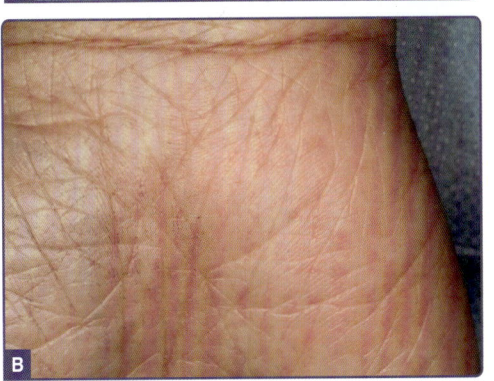

Figure 75-7 Clinical finding of reticulate acropigmentation of Kitamura. **A,** Hyperpigmented macules distributed on the dorsal aspects of the hands. **B,** "Pits" on the palm.

Investigation with electron microscopy showed that the number of melanosomes in the cytoplasm of keratinocytes was obviously increased in hyperpigmented macules, compared with cells from the perilesional skin. A majority of melanosomes observed in the lesion formed melanosome complexes, membrane-bounded vesicles containing several melanosomes. These melanosome complexes were not detected in the perilesional skin. Some melanosome complexes were also observed in melanocytes. Recently, heterozygous mutations in the *ADAM10* gene have been identified as causing RAK.[53]

DIAGNOSIS

The phenotype of reticulate hyperpigmentation on the dorsum of the extremities without hypopigmented macules, plus the punctate pits on the palms and soles, is helpful for the diagnosis of RAK. Identification of a mutation in *ADAM10* can confirm the diagnosis.

DOWLING-DEGOS DISEASE

CLINICAL FEATURES

DDD is an autosomal dominant genodermatosis with reticulate hyperpigmentation that is progressive.[54] Small, hyperkeratotic, dark-brown papules that affect mainly the flexures and great skin folds appear after puberty. Pitted perioral acneiform scars and genital and perianal reticulated pigmented lesions also have been described.[55] Patients usually show no abnormalities of the hair or nails. Histology shows thin branch-like patterns, filiform epithelial downgrowth of epidermal rete ridges, with a concentration of melanin at the tips.

ETIOLOGY AND PATHOGENESIS

ETIOLOGY AND PATHOGENESIS

Histopathologic analyses reported that hyperpigmented macules show hyperkeratosis without parakeratosis, slightly elongated rete ridges, and a small number of inflammatory cells in the upper dermis. In Fontana-Masson staining, the lesion shows hypermelanosis, mainly in the lower epidermis, and absence of obvious IP in the upper dermis. The number of melanocytes is increased in the basal layer of the epidermis.

DDD shows genetic heterogeneity and is classified into 4 types (see Table 75-3). DDD1 is caused by heterozygous mutation in the *KRT5* gene on chromosome 12q13.[56] DDD2 is caused by mutation in the *POFUT1* gene on chromosome 20q11.[57] DDD3 has been mapped to chromosome 17p33.3. DDD4 is caused by mutation in the *POGLUT1* gene on chromosome 3q13.[58] Both of the gene products from POFUT1 and POGLUT1 have been reported to play important roles in the Notch receptor signaling pathway.

DIAGNOSIS

The phenotype of reticulate hyperpigmentation is progressive, and is mainly distributed on

TABLE 75-5
Genetic Heterogeneity of Reticulate Pigment Disorders

DISORDER TYPE	CLINICAL FEATURE	SUBTYPE	OMIM #	RESPONSIBLE GENE	MAPPING	INHERITANCE
DDD	Usually in a flexural distribution, sometimes, generalized distribution	1	179850	KRT5	12q13.13	AD
		2	615327	POFUT1	20q11.21	AD
		3	615674	ND	17q21.3-q22	AD
		4	615696	POGLUT1	3q13.33	AD
DSH	In acral distribution with mixed hyper- and hypopigmentation		127400	ADAR1	1q21	AD
DUH	In generalized distribution over the trunk with mixed hyper- and hypopigmentation	1	127500	ND	6q24.2-q25.2	AD
		2	612715	ND	12q21-q23	ND
		3	615402	ABCB6	2q35	AD
ARK	In an acral distribution		615537	ADAM10	15q21.3	AD

AD, autosomal dominant; AR, autosomal recessive; ND, not determined; OMIM, Online Mendelian Inheritance in Man.

the flexures, although sometimes more generally. Genetic analyses can be helpful for the differential diagnosis, because the responsible genes are different, as shown in Table 75-5.

REFERENCES

1. Ito S, Suzuki T, Inagaki K, et al. High frequency of Hermansky-Pudlak syndrome type 1 (HPS1) among Japanese albinism patients and functional analysis of HPS1 mutant protein. *J Invest Dermatol*. 2005; 125(4):715-720.
2. Manga P, Kromberg JG, Box NF, et al. Rufous oculocutaneous albinism in southern African Blacks is caused by mutations in the TYRP1 gene. *Am J Hum Genet*. 1997;61(5):1095-1101.
3. Boissy RE, Zhao H, Oetting WS, et al. Mutation in and lack of expression of tyrosinase-related protein-1 (TRP-1) in melanocytes from an individual with brown oculocutaneous albinism: a new subtype of albinism classified as "OCA3." *Am J Hum Genet*. 1996;58(6):1145-1156.
4. Rundshagen U, Zuhlke C, Opitz S, et al. Mutations in the MATP gene in five German patients affected by oculocutaneous albinism type 4. *Hum Mutat*. 2004;23(2): 106-110.
5. Inagaki K, Suzuki T, Shimizu H, et al. Oculocutaneous albinism type 4 is one of the most common types of albinism in Japan. *Am J Hum Genet*. 2004;74(3):466-471.
6. Wei AH, Zang DJ, Zhang Z, et al. Exome sequencing identifies SLC24A5 as a candidate gene for nonsyndromic oculocutaneous albinism. *J Invest Dermatol*. 2013;133(7):1834-1840.
7. Kausar T, Bhatti MA, Ali M, et al. OCA5, a novel locus for non-syndromic oculocutaneous albinism, maps to chromosome 4q24. *Clin Genet*. 2013;84(1):91-93.
8. Gronskov K, Dooley CM, Ostergaard E, et al. Mutations in c10orf11, a melanocyte-differentiation gene, cause autosomal-recessive albinism. *Am J Hum Genet*. 2013;92(3):415-421.
9. Spritz RA, Strunk KM, Giebel LB, et al. Detection of mutations in the tyrosinase gene in a patient with type IA oculocutaneous albinism. *N Engl J Med*. 1990; 322(24):1724-1728.
10. King RA, Townsend D, Oetting W, et al. Temperature-sensitive tyrosinase associated with peripheral pigmentation in oculocutaneous albinism. *J Clin Invest*. 1991;87(3):1046-1053.
11. Rinchik EM, Bultman SJ, Horsthemke B, et al. A gene for the mouse pink-eyed dilution locus and for human type II oculocutaneous albinism. *Nature*. 1993;361(6407):72-76.
12. Spritz RA, Fukai K, Holmes SA, et al. Frequent intragenic deletion of the P gene in Tanzanian patients with type II oculocutaneous albinism (OCA2). *Am J Hum Genet*. 1995;56(6):1320-1323.
13. Brilliant M, Gardner J. Melanosomal pH, pink locus protein and their roles in melanogenesis. *J Invest Dermatol*. 2001;117(2):386-387.
14. Hearing VJ. Determination of melanin synthetic pathways. *J Invest Dermatol*. 2011;131(E1):E8-E11.
15. Chiang PW, Fulton AB, Spector E, et al. Synergistic interaction of the OCA2 and OCA3 genes in a family. *Am J Med Genet A*. 2008;146A(18):2427-2430.
16. Kobayashi T, Imokawa G, Bennett DC, et al. Tyrosinase stabilization by Tyrp1 (the brown locus protein). *J Biol Chem*. 1998;273(48):31801-31805.
17. Newton JM, Cohen-Barak O, Hagiwara N, et al. Mutations in the human orthologue of the mouse underwhite gene (uw) underlie a new form of oculocutaneous albinism, OCA4. *Am J Hum Genet*. 2001; 69(5):981-988.
18. Okamura K, Yoshizawa J, Abe Y, et al. Oculocutaneous albinism (OCA) in Japanese patients: five novel mutations. *J Dermatol Sci*. 2014;74(2):173-174.
19. Kondo T, Hearing VJ. Update on the regulation of mammalian melanocyte function and skin pigmentation. *Expert Rev Dermatol*. 2011;6(1):97-108.
20. Inagaki K, Suzuki T, Ito S, et al. Oculocutaneous albinism type 4: six novel mutations in the

membrane-associated transporter protein gene and their phenotypes. *Pigment Cell Res.* 2006;19(5): 451-453.
21. Ito S, Wakamatsu K. Diversity of human hair pigmentation as studied by chemical analysis of eumelanin and pheomelanin. *J Eur Acad Dermatol Venereol.* 2011;25(12):1369-1380.
22. Sulem P, Gudbjartsson DF, Stacey SN, et al. Genetic determinants of hair, eye and skin pigmentation in Europeans. *Nat Genet.* 2007;39(12):1443-1452.
23. Hong ES, Zeeb H, Repacholi MH. Albinism in Africa as a public health issue. *BMC Public Health.* 2006; 6:212.
24. Mabula JB, Chalya PL, McHembe MD, et al. Skin cancers among albinos at a university teaching hospital in Northwestern Tanzania: a retrospective review of 64 cases. *BMC Dermatol.* 2012;12:5.
25. Wei AH, Li W. Hermansky-Pudlak syndrome: pigmentary and non-pigmentary defects and their pathogenesis. *Pigment Cell Melanoma Res.* 2013;26(2): 176-192.
26. Suzuki T, Li W, Zhang Q, et al. Hermansky-Pudlak syndrome is caused by mutations in HPS4, the human homolog of the mouse light-ear gene. *Nat Genet.* 2002;30(3):321-324.
27. Ammann S, Schulz A, Krageloh-Mann I, et al. Mutations in AP3D1 associated with immunodeficiency and seizures define a new type of Hermansky-Pudlak syndrome. *Blood.* 2016;127(8):997-1006.
28. Sitaram A, Marks MS. Mechanisms of protein delivery to melanosomes in pigment cells. *Physiology (Bethesda).* 2012;27(2):85-99.
29. Blumstein J, Faundez V, Nakatsu F, et al. The neuronal form of adaptor protein-3 is required for synaptic vesicle formation from endosomes. *J Neurosci.* 2001;21(20):8034-8042.
30. Dell'Angelica EC. The building BLOC(k)s of lysosomes and related organelles. *Curr Opin Cell Biol.* 2004;16(4):458-464.
31. Ménasché G, Ho CH, Sanal O, et al. Griscelli syndrome restricted to hypopigmentation results from a melanophilin defect (GS3) or a MYO5A F-exon deletion (GS1). *J Clin Invest.* 2003;112(3):450-456.
32. Langford GM, Molyneaux BJ. Myosin V in the brain: mutations lead to neurological defects. *Brain Res Brain Res Rev.* 1998;28(1-2):1-8.
33. Lambert J, Naeyaert JM, Callens T, et al. Human myosin V gene produces different transcripts in a cell type-specific manner. *Biochem Biophys Res Commun.* 1998;252(2):329-333.
34. Cagdas D, Ozgur TT, Asal GT, et al. Griscelli syndrome types 1 and 3: analysis of four new cases and long-term evaluation of previously diagnosed patients. *Eur J Pediatr.* 2012;171(10):1527-1531.
35. Shimazaki H, Honda J, Naoi T, et al. Autosomal-recessive complicated spastic paraplegia with a novel lysosomal trafficking regulator gene mutation. *J Neurol Neurosurg Psychiatry.* 2014;85(9):1024-1028.
36. Tardieu M, Lacroix C, Neven B, et al. Progressive neurologic dysfunctions 20 years after allogeneic bone marrow transplantation for Chediak-Higashi syndrome. *Blood.* 2005;106(1):40-42.
37. Swinney CC, Han DP, Karth PA. Incontinentia Pigmenti: a comprehensive review and update. *Ophthalmic Surg Lasers Imaging Retina.* 2015;46(6):650-657.
38. Jean-Baptiste S, O'Toole EA, Chen M, et al. Expression of eotaxin, an eosinophil-selective chemokine, parallels eosinophil accumulation in the vesiculobullous stage of incontinentia pigmenti. *Clin Exp Immunol.* 2002;127(3):470-478.
39. Minic S, Trpinac D, Obradovic M. Systematic review of central nervous system anomalies in incontinentia pigmenti. *Orphanet J Rare Dis.* 2013;8:25.
40. Kenwrick S, Woffendin H, Jakins T, et al. Survival of male patients with incontinentia pigmenti carrying a lethal mutation can be explained by somatic mosaicism or Klinefelter syndrome. *Am J Hum Genet.* 2001;69(6):1210-1217.
41. Ardelean D, Pope E. Incontinentia pigmenti in boys: a series and review of the literature. *Pediatr Dermatol.* 2006;23(6):523-527.
42. Landy SJ, Donnai D. Incontinentia pigmenti (Bloch-Sulzberger syndrome). *J Med Genet.* 1993;30(1): 53-59.
43. Giebel LB, Spritz RA. Mutation of the KIT (mast/stem cell growth factor receptor) protooncogene in human piebaldism. *Proc Natl Acad Sci U S A.* 1991; 88(19):8696-8699.
44. Sanchez-Martin M, Perez-Losada J, Rodriguez-Garcia A, et al. Deletion of the *SLUG* (*SNAI2*) gene results in human piebaldism. *Am J Med Genet A.* 2003; 122a(2):125-132.
45. Waardenburg PJ. A new syndrome combining developmental anomalies of the eyelids, eyebrows and nose root with pigmentary defects of the iris and head hair and with congenital deafness. *Am J Hum Genet.* 1951;3(3):195-253.
46. Read AP, Newton VE. Waardenburg syndrome. *J Med Genet.* 1997;34(8):656-665.
47. Pingault V, Girard M, Bondurand N, et al. *SOX10* mutations in chronic intestinal pseudo-obstruction suggest a complex physiopathological mechanism. *Hum Genet.* 2002;111(2):198-206.
48. Tassabehji M, Newton VE, Liu XZ, et al. The mutational spectrum in Waardenburg syndrome. *Hum Mol Genet.* 1995;4(11):2131-2137.
49. Kondo T, Suzuki T, Ito S, et al. Dyschromatosis symmetrica hereditaria associated with neurological disorders. *J Dermatol.* 2008;35(10):662-666.
50. Miyamura Y, Suzuki T, Kono M, et al. Mutations of the RNA-specific adenosine deaminase gene (*DSRAD*) are involved in dyschromatosis symmetrica hereditaria. *Am J Hum Genet.* 2003;73(3):693-699.
51. Zhang C, Li D, Zhang J, et al. Mutations in *ABCB6* cause dyschromatosis universalis hereditaria. *J Invest Dermatol.* 2013;133(9):2221-2228.
52. Kitamura K, Akamatsu S, Hirokawa K. A special form of acropigmentation: acropigmentation reticularis [in German]. *Hautarzt.* 1953;4(4):152-156.
53. Kono M, Sugiura K, Suganuma M, et al. Whole-exome sequencing identifies *ADAM10* mutations as a cause of reticulate acropigmentation of Kitamura, a clinical entity distinct from Dowling-Degos disease. *Hum Mol Genet.* 2013;22(17):3524-3533.
54. Dowling GB, Freudenthal W. Acanthosis nigricans. *Proc R Soc Med.* 1938;31(9):1147-1150.
55. Degos R, Ossipowski B. Reticulated pigmentary dermatosis of the folds: relation to acanthosis nigricans [in undetermined language]. *Ann Dermatol Syphiligr (Paris).* 1954;81(2):147-151.
56. Betz RC, Planko L, Eigelshoven S, et al. Loss-of-function mutations in the keratin 5 gene lead to Dowling-Degos disease. *Am J Hum Genet.* 2006;78(3): 510-519.

57. Li M, Cheng R, Liang J, et al. Mutations in POFUT1, encoding protein O-fucosyltransferase 1, cause generalized Dowling-Degos disease. *Am J Hum Genet.* 2013;92(6):895-903.
58. Basmanav FB, Oprisoreanu AM, Pasternack SM, et al. Mutations in *POGLUT1*, encoding protein O-glucosyltransferase 1, cause autosomal-dominant Dowling-Degos disease. *Am J Hum Genet.* 2014;94(1):135-143.
59. Araki Y, Ishii Y, Abe Y, et al. Hermansky-Pudlak syndrome type 4 with a novel mutation. *J Dermatol.* 2014;41(2):186-187.
60. Monma F, Hozumi Y, Kawaguchi M, et al. A novel MITF splice site mutation in a family with Waardenburg syndrome. *J Dermatol Sci.* 2008;52(1):64-66.

Chapter 76 :: Vitiligo
:: Khaled Ezzedine & John E. Harris

第七十六章
白癜风

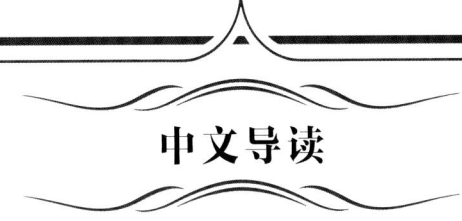

中文导读

白癜风是一种进行性黑素细胞丢失的自身免疫性皮肤病，本章从八个方面全面讲述了白癜风。

第一节讲述了白癜风的定义，描述了白癜风的特征性表现，还讲述了历史上多个古代文明对"白癜风"的描写和记录。

第二节介绍了白癜风的流行病学，世界各地的流行率通常是相似的，估计为0.5%~1%。介绍了白癜风的好发时间、患病率和性别差异，并着重阐述了白癜风对患者生活质量尤其是心理健康的影响。

第三节介绍了白癜风的临床表现，描述了白癜风的典型表现，阐释了反映疾病活动性的临床标志物，介绍了评估和监测白癜风活动的两种量表，讲述了与白癜风重叠发病的自身免疫性疾病的相关情况，尤其提到大多数患者有自身免疫性甲状腺疾病，并介绍了白癜风的并发症，其中较为严重的并发症为Vogt-Koyanagi-Harada综合征（VKHS）和Alezzandrini综合征。

第四节介绍了白癜风的病因和发病机制，白癜风的病因不明，发病机制尚不清楚。介绍并分析了多个看似不相关且相互矛盾的假说，并提出了一个新的假说，同时提出致病的关键细胞及关键细胞因子，最后讨论了白癜风的危险因素。

第五节介绍了白癜风的诊断，通常基于典型临床表现、好发部位、wood灯检测等较容易做出诊断，区分白癜风其节段性变异很重要。如有特定症状，建议酌情检测TSH、全血细胞计数、抗核抗体或其他自身免疫标记物。指出有异常现象时可以行组织学检测，并描述了白癜风的组织学表现和免疫组化特征。

第六节介绍了白癜风的鉴别诊断，非节段型白癜风主要须与炎症性、炎症后、肿瘤性和遗传性（主要是先天性）色素减退相鉴别，将鉴别要点列于表76-1；将节段型白癜风与贫血痣和无色素痣相鉴别，鉴别要点列于表76-1。

第七节介绍了白癜风的临床病程和预后，非节段型白癜风的病程不可预测，倾向于周期性的复发和阶段性的稳定；相反，节段型白癜风起病迅速，但具有自我限制性，病情稳定迅速，疾病发生后一般不再进展。指出有毛发部位治疗效果好，而无毛发部位治疗效果不佳。

第八节介绍了白癜风的治疗，包括外用药、光疗、心理干预治疗、美容治疗、脱色治疗及非传统疗法，治疗方案分别总结在图

76-20和图76-21。本章还总结了白癜风的新治疗进展，包括生物制剂靶向治疗、促进黑素细胞再生、增殖和/或迁移的治疗等。

〔李 吉〕

AT-A-GLANCE

- Vitiligo is a common autoimmune disease of the skin that causes depigmentation through T-cell–mediated destruction of melanocytes.
- Pathogenesis is multifactorial, including genetic predisposition, autoimmunity, and environmental factors.
- Vitiligo can cause significant social stigma, with serious implications for mental health.
- Correlates with increased risk of other autoimmune diseases, but decreased risk of skin cancer.
- Clinical signs of lesional activity include confetti, trichrome, and inflammatory lesions, as well as koebnerization.
- Reversible with treatment, but only in areas with normally pigmented hair.
- Effective treatments include topical and oral immunosuppressants, phototherapy, and chemical depigmenting agents.
- Emerging treatments include targeted immunotherapy and melanocyte-stimulating hormones.

DEFINITION AND HISTORY

Vitiligo, an acquired skin disease of progressive melanocyte loss, is clinically characterized by well-defined milky-white macules that may also include white hairs, or poliosis. The term *vitiligo* initially appears in the first century, although clinical features consistent with vitiligo were described in ancient medical texts during the second millennium before Christ.[1-3] Historically, vitiligo has been confused with leprosy, an infectious disease of the skin that results in ill-defined hypopigmentation. Some texts sought to differentiate the 2 diseases, while others conflated them. As early as 1500 BC, the *Ebers Papyrus* listed 2 diseases that affected skin color—one associated with "swellings," which may have been leprosy, and another that exclusively affected the color, which was likely vitiligo. In the book of "Leviticus" in the *Bible*, also dated between 1500 and 1400 BC, a number of skin diseases could make one "unclean" and required examination by the priest to determine whether isolation was warranted. Skin swelling, lightening, poliosis, and evolution of lesions over time were assessed to make this determination. This protocol may have been designed to distinguish vitiligo from leprosy or other skin diseases. In India, vitiligo was described in the *Atharva Veda* (1400 BC) and the Buddhist *Vinay Pitak* (224 to 544 BC) under the term "Kilas," a Sanskrit word "derived from kil," meaning white.[3-5] Hippocrates (460 to 355 BC) did not discriminate between vitiligo and leprosy. In fact, he included lichenoid eruptions, leprosy, psoriasis, and vitiligo under the same category. Still, today, in geographic areas with high incidence of leprosy, the 2 diseases are often confused.

EPIDEMIOLOGY

PREVALENCE

There have been very few studies conducted in the general population that aim to determine the prevalence of vitiligo. This is a difficult task, because unlike other diseases that cause significant morbidity and mortality, affected patients may not present to a medical facility to be counted. Thus, most estimates of prevalence are based on prospective surveys, retrospective observational studies, and prospective studies in selected populations, which may underestimate or overestimate the prevalence, depending on the approach. The largest epidemiologic study was performed in 1977 in Denmark, on the island of Bornholm, with a calculated prevalence of 0.38%.[6] A study in black people from the French West Indies found it to be similar to established data for white people.[7] However, peaks of prevalence have been reported in subpopulations in India (8.8%) in relationship to chemically induced depigmentation.[8,9] Similarly, higher incidences of vitiligo in Mexico and Japan have been reported.[9] Although the different prevalence rates of vitiligo in various populations could certainly be the result of genetic or environmental differences, one potential reason could be the different social and/or cultural stigmas that influence reporting.[9] In light of these challenges, the prevalence of disease is typically stated to be similar all over the world, estimated at 0.5% to 1%.[10,11]

PATIENT DEMOGRAPHICS

Vitiligo can begin at any age, although it usually starts before the third decade of life with almost half of patients presenting before the age of 20 years, and a third before the age of 12 years.[9,10,12-14] The segmental variant of vitiligo, affecting only 1 side of the body, tends to occur earlier in life.[14] A study in Jordan reported that the prevalence of vitiligo gradually increases with age (0.45% younger than age 1 year; 1% aged 1 to 5 years old, 2.1% aged 5 to 12 years old).[15] Males and females appear to be affected equally, although females may seek treatment more frequently.[10,11]

QUALITY OF LIFE

Vitiligo is frequently dismissed as "cosmetic," however it is often psychologically devastating for patients.[16] Numerous studies show that patients with vitiligo feel stigmatized, have low self-esteem with poor body image, and suffer a considerable psychosocial burden.[17,18] Thus, vitiligo may have a significant impact on quality of life, and patients reportedly have mental impairment similar to psoriasis and atopic dermatitis.[19] Differences in Dermatology Life Quality Index (DLQI) scores have been noted in various cultural groups, which may reflect different social stigmas of having the disease. For example, the mean of Dermatology Life Quality Index scores was 4.95 in a Belgian population, whereas Indian patients experienced a mean of 7.06 in patients with a successful treatment outcome, and 13.12 in those who failed treatment.[20]

CLINICAL FEATURES

PRESENTATION PATTERNS

Typically, vitiligo lesions are asymptomatic, white, nonscaly macules and patches with distinct margins that fluoresce when illuminated by Wood lamp examination. Although a number of patterns have been described, most can be grouped together, except for the segmental variant of vitiligo, which follows a different disease course and experiences a different treatment response. Thus, we will describe these forms separately and highlight differences important to recognize when developing a management plan.

Vitiligo lesions may involve any part of the body, usually with a symmetrical distribution (Figs. 76-1 and 76-2). The disease can start at any site of the body, although the face, as well as acral and genital locations, are often the initial sites. A number of specific clinical patterns have been defined, which include acrofacial, mucosal, generalized, universal, mixed, and rare forms. However, this distinction is not often easy to make, as there is often overlap among these forms, or evolution from one to another. Because many clinicians are familiar with these forms and describe vitiligo accordingly, we briefly describe each one.

Acrofacial vitiligo is reportedly more common in adults and typically involves the hands, feet, and face, particularly the orifices. This form may evolve to typical generalized vitiligo.

Vitiligo universalis is a rare form of widespread disease. It is usually seen in adults, although cases in children have been reported.[14] The form is named "universalis" because it affects a large proportion of the body, frequently defined as greater than 80% of the body surface area. Despite this widespread involvement, hairs may be spared. Classically, vitiligo universalis results from longstanding disease that steadily progresses to nearly complete whitening of the skin.

In *Mucosal vitiligo,* the oral and/or genital mucosae are primarily involved (Fig. 76-3). When strictly limited to the mucosa, the differential diagnosis of lichen sclerosus et atrophicus should be carefully considered (see also section "Differential Diagnosis"). Furthermore, both conditions in the same patients are reported to coexist.[21]

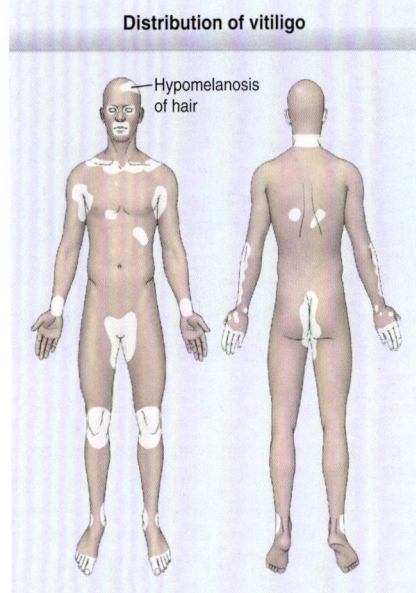

Figure 76-1 Distribution of vitiligo. (From Wolff K, Johnson R, Saavedra AP, et al. *Fitzpatrick's Color Atlas and Synopsis of Clinical Dermatology.* 8th ed. New York, NY: McGraw-Hill; 2017, with permission.)

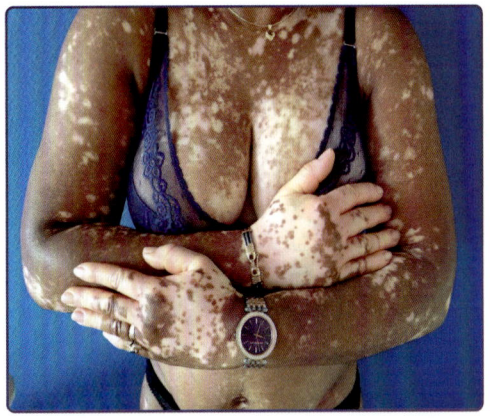

Figure 76-2 Symmetrical patchy depigmentation of vitiligo.

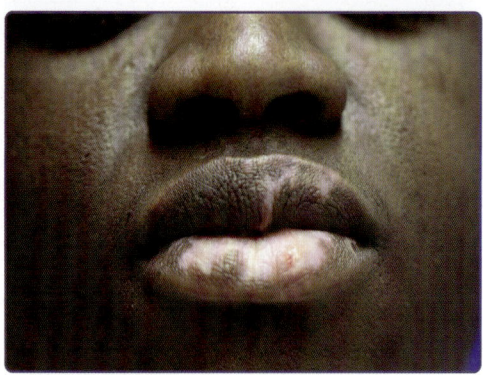

Figure 76-3 Mucosal vitiligo, limited to the lips.

Focal vitiligo consists of small, isolated lesions. In a recent report, long-term followup of 53 cases of focal vitiligo have shown that almost 50% of these cases progress to involve larger areas without any clinical sign that might predict this progression.[22]

The *segmental variant* of vitiligo is seen in 10% to 15% of vitiligo patients who present to the clinic. It is characterized by a unilateral and segmental, or block-shaped, distribution of the lesions (Fig. 76-4). Typically, a single contiguous segment is involved, although 2 or more segments with ipsilateral or contralateral distribution have been described.[23] *Mixed vitiligo* is a rare form of vitiligo that refers to the occurrence of a clear example of segmental vitiligo plus additional macules or patches that do not fit the segment (Fig. 76-5). These additional patches may be remote from the segmental involvement and are bilateral and symmetrical, affecting the contralateral side.[24] In segmental vitiligo, there is frequently early involvement of the follicular melanocyte reservoir, resulting in poliosis.

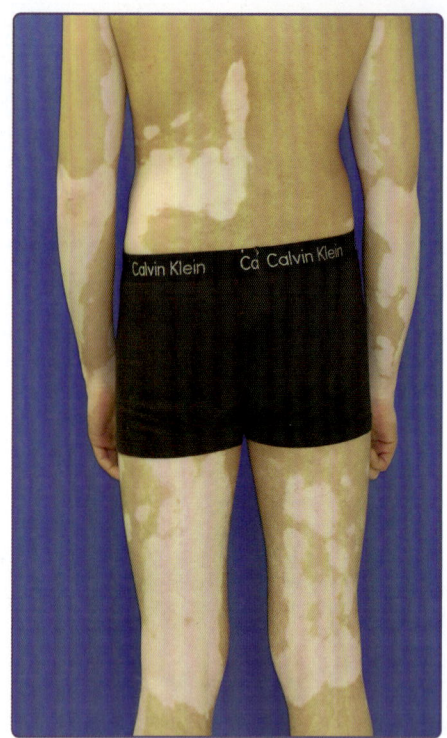

Figure 76-5 Mixed vitiligo, made up of a segmental lesion on the back plus additional bilateral lesions in remote areas.

The disease usually spreads over the segment within 6 to 12 months, and then stabilizes.[25] Although this may initially be difficult to distinguish from focal vitiligo, the rapid progression of segmental disease usually makes it clear within a few weeks to months.

CLINICAL MARKERS OF DISEASE ACTIVITY

In addition to recognized anatomical patterns of vitiligo, there are lesional patterns that indicate disease activity, which are important to recognize when determining the best treatment approach for patients. These patterns include the Koebner phenomenon, trichrome lesions, confetti-like depigmentation, and inflammatory lesions. For example, one study reported that the Koebner phenomenon in vitiligo patients was associated with higher body surface area involvement in vitiligo and poorer response to treatment.[26] Disease activity also has been partially quantified through scoring systems such as the vitiligo disease activity score (VIDA), which relies on patient recall, and the Koebner phenomenon in vitiligo score (K-VSCOR), which is focused on clinical signs.

The *Koebner phenomenon*, also called the isomorphic response, describes the observation that depigmentation occurs readily at the site of skin trauma in patients with active vitiligo. This can be recognized as linear

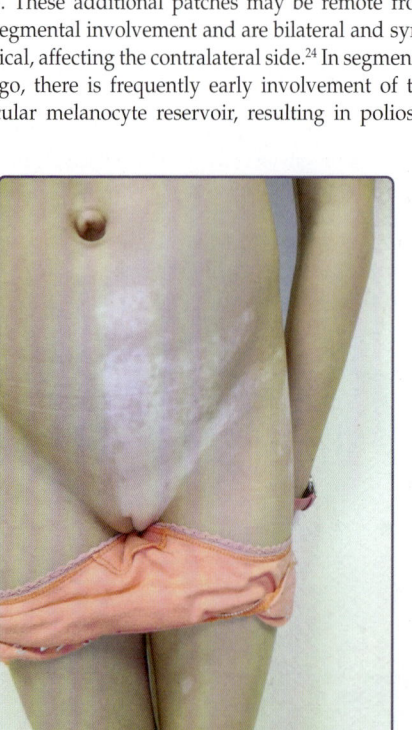

Figure 76-4 Unilateral, block-like depigmentation of the segmental variant of vitiligo.

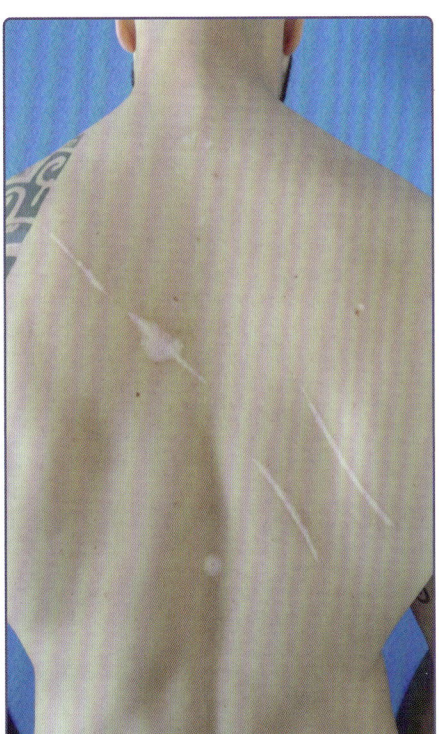

Figure 76-6 Linear depigmentation in locations of skin trauma.

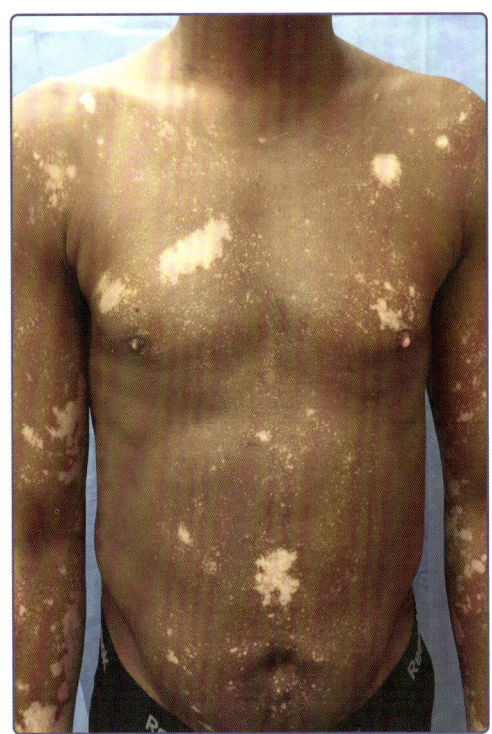

Figure 76-8 Multiple scattered macules of confetti depigmentation in vitiligo.

marks of depigmentation where the skin has been scratched, lacerated, or burned, or nonlinear macules and patches at the site of known skin injury, such as erosions and abrasions (Fig. 76-6).

Trichrome vitiligo is characterized by blurring of lesional borders because of the presence of a hypopigmented zone between the depigmented and normally pigmented border. This results in the appearance of 3 distinct colors: the depigmented skin, normally pigmented skin, and hypopigmented skin (Fig. 76-7). This pattern is associated with active, rapidly spreading vitiligo.[27]

Confetti-like depigmentation consists of multiple small macules of depigmentation clustered together, often at the edge of existing vitiligo lesions (Fig. 76-8). One study used serial photography to demonstrate that these small macules grew and coalesced into larger depigmented areas after just a few weeks, identifying this sign as an important marker of disease activity.[28]

Inflammatory vitiligo is a very rare form of vitiligo characterized by the presence of erythema, scale, and itch at the border of hypopigmented or depigmented lesions (Fig. 76-9). This inflammatory phase is typically transient, lasting just a few weeks to months but rapidly progressing to involve large areas of the body. Early histologic studies in vitiligo were done on

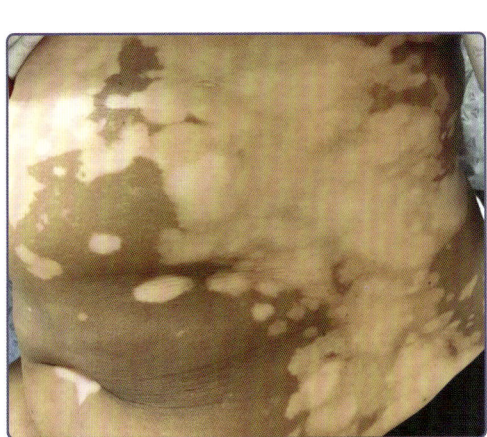

Figure 76-7 Trichrome vitiligo comprised of normal pigmentation, depigmentation, and a zone of hypopigmentation between them.

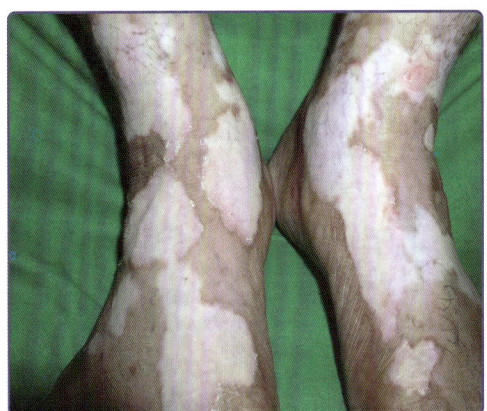

Figure 76-9 Inflammatory vitiligo characterized by erythema and scaling at the margin of the depigmented lesion. (Used with permission from Dr. Shyam Verma.)

inflammatory lesions, where the immune infiltrate could be readily observed.[29]

The *VIDA* score is a 6-point scale that was developed with the aim of assessing and monitoring vitiligo activity.[30] Because this scoring is based on the patient's recollection of disease activity, it may be subject to recall bias. Active vitiligo is defined as the spread of existing lesions or onset of new lesions. The VIDA scores range from +4 (activity lasting 6 weeks or less) to −1 (vitiligo stable for 1 year or more with spontaneous repigmentation). One of the limitations of the VIDA score is that different lesions can have different scores, making it difficult to use in daily practice.

Finally, the *K-VSCOR* uses the Koebner phenomenon and anatomical location of lesions to determine disease activity in vitiligo patients.[31] It is based on the presence or absence of vitiligo lesions at 6 different areas of the body (forehead + scalp areas, eyelids, wrists, genital + belt areas, knees and tibial crests) as well as disease duration. The K-VSCOR ranges from 0 to 56, with 56 corresponding to the highest likelihood of having the Koebner phenomenon, which serves as an indicator of disease activity in the clinic. Further validation is needed to predict the extension of lesions over a longer period of time.

DISEASE ASSOCIATIONS

Vitiligo is an autoimmune disease of the skin that is associated with a number of other autoimmune diseases in other organs through increased incidence of type 1 diabetes, autoimmune thyroiditis, pernicious anemia, Addison disease, lupus, and alopecia areata, in both vitiligo patients and their family members.[32,33] This strongly implicates inherited factors that predispose patients and their family members to a group of autoimmune diseases, and the breadth of diseases found in this overlap suggests that the predisposition is toward autoimmunity in general, rather than specific diseases themselves. Up to 20% of vitiligo patients have at least 1 additional autoimmune disease, and most of these patients (13% to 19%) have autoimmune thyroid disease. This increased risk has prompted some to advocate testing thyroid-stimulating hormone (TSH) in all patients with vitiligo, because the pretest probability of finding a positive result is higher in this patient population. Others suggest, however, that this is unnecessary, because many patients will develop thyroid disease much earlier or later than the onset of vitiligo, and recommend that the presence of symptoms should drive TSH screening.[34]

There has always been some concern that vitiligo patients have a higher risk of skin cancers than the general population because of their loss of pigment in the skin. Although this makes some intuitive sense, the data do not support this hypothesis. Two large studies, one of 1307 participants[35] and another of 10,040 participants,[36] reported that vitiligo patients have close to 3-fold lower risk of developing melanoma, basal cell carcinoma, and squamous cell carcinoma compared to controls. This protection was maintained even when factors like reduced sun exposure and/or increased exposure to phototherapy were factored in. Controls included partners of patients in one study and vascular surgery patients in another. The remarkable agreement between these 2 studies strongly suggests that the data are representative, despite the individual weaknesses of each study. Protection from melanoma is least surprising, as immune surveillance against neoplastic melanocytes should be heightened in vitiligo patients, and because genetic risk alleles for vitiligo are simultaneously protective against melanoma.[37] However, why the incidence of basal cell carcinoma and squamous cell carcinoma are also lower in vitiligo patients is not clear.

DISEASE COMPLICATIONS

Melanocytes are found not only in the epidermis of the skin, but also in the mucous membranes, hair follicles, uveal tract, retinal pigment epithelium, membranous labyrinth of the inner ear, heart, and meninges of the brain. Typically, these sites are spared in vitiligo patients, with the exception of hair follicles, which can be involved when present within lesions. However, some studies report hearing changes in vitiligo patients, with sensorineural hearing loss present with a wide range of prevalence (20% to 60%), depending on the study.[38-40] However, sensorineural hearing loss frequently goes undetected by the patient, and is only observed with formal testing. Ocular abnormalities have been reported in vitiligo patients as well, including pigment changes, scarring, and even uveitis in up to 5% of patients.[41,42] Vogt-Koyanagi-Harada syndrome (VKHS) and Alezzandrini syndrome represent severe, rare forms of vitiligo that affect organs other than the skin. VKHS results in skin depigmentation with prominent poliosis, as well as hearing loss, visual changes, meningitis, and flu-like symptoms. The skin manifestations occur after the systemic ones, so those with classic vitiligo are not known to progress to VKHS.[43] Alezzandrini syndrome has been described in 7 patients, and is characterized by segmental vitiligo (unilateral depigmentation) on the face with poliosis, plus ipsilateral hearing loss and visual changes.[44-46]

ETIOLOGY AND PATHOGENESIS

COMPETING HYPOTHESES AND THE CONVERGENCE THEORY

Vitiligo is an autoimmune disease of the skin in which CD8+ T cells target melanocytes and destroy them, leaving areas without pigment production, which is clinically manifest as white macules and patches. The pathogenesis has been debated for many years, with multiple hypotheses offered as alternative explanations as to what lies at the root of the disease. These alternative hypotheses include cellular stress causing degeneration of melanocytes, chemical toxicity causing melanocyte death, and neural changes that influence melanocytes or their ability to produce melanin. The reason for these alternative explanations were research observations over the years suggesting that much more than simply autoimmune targeting of perfectly normal melanocytes was occurring in vitiligo.

Early clinical observations that other autoimmune diseases occurred frequently in vitiligo patients and their family members hinted, through guilt by association, that vitiligo was itself an autoimmune disease. Additionally, antimelanocyte antibodies appeared to be elevated in vitiligo patients compared to healthy controls, also implicating immune responses in disease pathogenesis. However, others found that melanocytes cultured from vitiligo patients, and thus separated from immune influences, were abnormal—they did not grow well, were susceptible to exogenous oxidative stress, and appeared to have elevated cellular stress. This was manifest by the presence of reactive oxygen species and a dilated endoplasmic reticulum, a marker of activation of the unfolded protein response which is involved in stress responses.[47-52] But histologic studies revealed that CD8+ T cells infiltrated lesional epidermis and were found next to dying melanocytes, strongly supporting T-cell–mediated cytotoxicity as the key event in vitiligo.[29,53] Finally, one group reported that CD8+ T cells isolated from lesional skin of a patient and then coincubated with nonlesional skin from that same patient resulted in melanocyte targeting and death, demonstrating that CD8+ T cells were both necessary and sufficient to cause melanocyte destruction in vitiligo patient skin.[54]

These seemingly unrelated and conflicting observations were later tied together by the convergence theory, which suggested that all of these pathways may synergize to cause vitiligo in patients.[55] Now it appears that melanocytes in vitiligo patients are indeed abnormal and are more sensitive to cellular processes like melanogenesis and energy consumption. This results in the production of reactive oxygen species and activation of the unfolded protein response, which initiate the secretion of signaling intermediates from melanocytes that act as danger signals to alert the innate immune system. Next, innate immune cells activate and recruit adaptive immune CD8+ T cells to the skin, where they find the abnormal melanocytes and kill them. Thus, cellular stress within the melanocyte and autoimmunity work together to cause what we see clinically as vitiligo.[56,57]

Additional studies have now revealed that certain chemicals, typically phenols, induce the cellular stress response in melanocytes by acting as analogs of tyrosine, also a phenol.[56] Thus, these chemicals act as exogenous environmental agents that induce and exacerbate vitiligo by initiating the cellular stress response in otherwise well-compensating melanocytes. Consequently, the "chemical theory" can be incorporated into the inclusive convergence theory as well. Finally, the neural hypothesis was based on the clinical appearance of segmental vitiligo, misinterpreting the unilateral nature of disease for being associated with dermatomes, which is not the case.[58-60] Others reported that catecholamines were increased in the urine of vitiligo patients; however, catecholamines are also secreted by melanocytes, which is a more likely source in vitiligo. Case reports of vitiligo clearing after unilateral nerve injuries suggested nerves as important players in disease pathogenesis, but further observations noted the opposite result as well, eliminating this as strong evidence. The role of emotional stress in worsening vitiligo has been offered as evidence, yet this is common in many diseases that do not appear to be influenced by nerves. Finally, some animals control their pigmentation through innervation (primarily fish), but this has never been observed in mammals. Thus, the "neural hypothesis" remains unsupported by evidence and should be discarded for now.[58]

T CELLS AND CYTOKINES IN AUTOIMMUNITY

As mentioned above, CD8+ T cells play a critical role during the progression of vitiligo, serving as the primary immune effectors that destroy melanocytes. Studies using human tissues and a mouse model of vitiligo have revealed that interferon (IFN)-γ is a key cytokine that drives the disease.[61-64] IFN-γ is secreted by melanocyte-reactive autoimmune CD8+ T cells, and induces the production of CXCL10 and other chemokines from keratinocytes, which promote the further recruitment of additional T cells that progressively destroy more melanocytes as the disease spreads.[64,65] Multiple groups have found that IFN-γ–induced chemokines are elevated in the serum and skin of vitiligo patients, and these may serve as useful biomarkers of disease activity in the future.[64,66-68] In addition, targeting the IFN-γ–chemokine axis during disease may be an effective novel treatment strategy (see section "Emerging Therapies").[69]

THE SEGMENTAL VARIANT OF VITILIGO, A SPECIAL CASE

As mentioned above, segmental vitiligo was initially thought to mirror the distribution of nerves via dermatomes, which led to the "neural hypothesis." Close inspection, however, reveals that segmental vitiligo lesions rarely, if ever, follow dermatomes, and frequently cross these zones in a perpendicular direction.

Depigmented blocks of segmental vitiligo also do not appear to follow blaschkoid lines, especially on the trunk, which are narrow and S-shaped.[59,60] So, the question arises, what defines a segment of vitiligo, and what is the pathogenesis of this variant, considering that immune-mediated disorders do not typically respect the midline? One hypothesis that is gaining acceptance is that segmental vitiligo results from a general autoimmune predisposition combined with melanocytes that have acquired a postzygotic mutation that alters their susceptibility to autoimmune attack, like activation of the cellular stress pathways discussed above. This has the potential to explain (a) why it is unilateral (melanocytes migrate from the neural crest and do not cross the midline), (b) its rapid evolution and stabilization (normal melanocytes create the stable border of the lesion), (c) its resistance to treatments (abnormal melanocytes are unstable and have an impaired ability to repigment the skin), and (d) the successful response to surgical therapies (normal melanocytes transplanted from another region are stable and resistant to autoimmune attack).[70]

RISK FACTORS IN VITILIGO

Similar to other autoimmune diseases, a number of factors influence the risk of developing vitiligo. These include both genetic factors and environmental factors. Vitiligo is more common in family members of affected patients, as 15% to 20% of patients have a family member with the disease, strongly suggesting that genetics influences the risk of getting disease. While the prevalence of vitiligo in the general population is close to 1%, the prevalence in first-degree relatives is 7%, and the prevalence in identical twins of affected individuals is 23%, clearly demonstrating a role for genes in disease. However, the fact that concordance between identical twins is not 100% also clearly demonstrates nongenetic influences in disease, which may represent environmental factors, stochastic influences (those that occur by chance), or both.

Modern genome-wide association studies have identified approximately 50 genetic loci that contribute to the risk of developing vitiligo, clearly demonstrating that it is inherited in a polygenic fashion with a complex interplay among multiple genes that contribute to the total risk. Of these loci, the majority are involved in regulating the immune system, representing key molecules in both innate and adaptive immunity, and thus strongly support the conclusion that disease is immune-mediated. Others appear to influence cellular apoptosis pathways and still others direct melanocyte function, including melanogenesis, supporting a role for the melanocyte in conferring risk for disease. Importantly, those genes involved in melanogenesis also influence the risk of developing melanoma, but in the opposite direction, suggesting that immune responses in vitiligo may be protective against melanoma, and thus may have evolved to protect against the development of this devastating cancer.[37]

In addition to genetic influences, environmental influences are important in vitiligo. The first chemical exposure to be definitively linked to the onset of vitiligo occurred in a group of leather factory workers in 1939. A large proportion of these workers developed depigmentation on their hands and lower arms, and monobenzyl ether of hydroquinone, or monobenzone, was implicated as the cause. Because some of the workers also developed depigmentation at sites remote from the exposure, depigmentation was not simply the result of direct toxicity to the melanocyte, but an exacerbation of the autoimmune destruction.[71] Other chemicals have been similarly implicated since then, including 4-tert-butyl phenol and 4-tert-butylcatechol.[72] An outbreak of vitiligo occurred in Japan in 2013, when a cosmetic company created a new skin lightening cream that resulted in more than 18,000 users getting vitiligo at the site of application and in remote areas.[72] Another study revealed that the use of permanent hair dyes may increase the risk of getting vitiligo by as much as 50%.[73] The common characteristic of implicated chemicals is that they are phenols with a chemical structure that resembles the amino acid tyrosine, also a phenol. Mechanistic studies reveal that these chemicals act as tyrosine analogs, which are taken up by melanocytes instead of tyrosine, interact with tyrosinase, and induce cellular stress pathways that then activate immune inflammation to initiate or exacerbate vitiligo.[56,74-76]

DIAGNOSIS
CLINICAL EXAMINATION

The diagnosis of vitiligo is usually a clinical one, as there is usually no need for additional laboratory or histologic testing to confirm the diagnosis. On physical examination it is important to differentiate vitiligo from its segmental variant, as these 2 forms have different clinical course, prognosis, and treatment responses. Vitiligo is usually characterized by well-defined, symmetrical depigmented lesions that can be distributed on any part of the body, but with a preference for the face (particularly periorificial areas), genitals, and acral areas. Wood lamp examination in a dark room is helpful in differentiating the depigmentation of vitiligo from hypopigmentation seen in other diseases. The disease is also characterized by cycles of flares and stabilization that are unpredictable, which can be distressing for patients. Additional clinical signs that may help with the diagnosis of vitiligo are the presence of multiple halo nevi and poliosis. The presence of repigmentation can be recognized as perifollicular pigmented macules from pigmented hairs at hair-bearing sites (Fig. 76-10) or convex patterns of pigment at lesional borders in glabrous skin (Fig. 76-11). Hair-bearing sites without poliosis repigment easily, whereas glabrous skin and lesions containing mostly white hairs respond poorly.

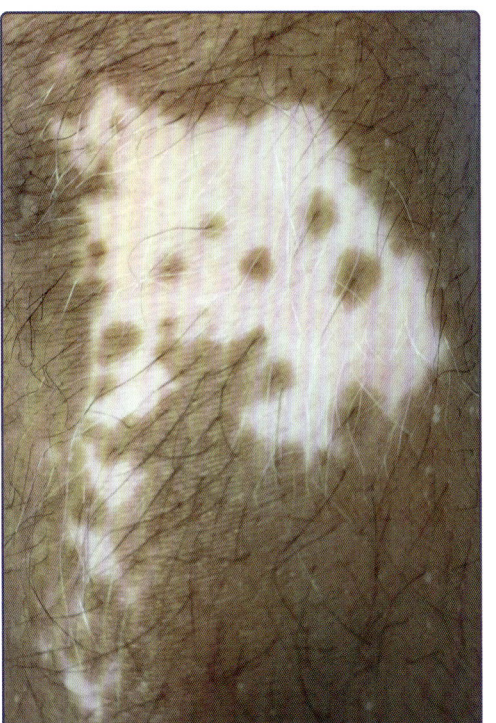

Figure 76-10 Perifollicular repigmentation. Note the lack of repigmentation from white hairs.

In the segmental variant of vitiligo, the lesions are unilateral, typically do not cross the midline, and are organized into block-like patterns, in contrast to the dermatomes of zoster or blaschkoid lines of keratinocyte disorders like segmental Darier disease. These blocks of depigmentation may represent zones of skin that have been affected by postzygotic mutations that create a mosaic distribution of abnormal melanocytes (discussed under section "Segmental Variant Special Case" above).[59,60] The evolution of segmental vitiligo is distinct in that the onset is usually acute with rapid progression over 6 to 12 months before it becomes stable and unchanging for the remaining life of the individual.

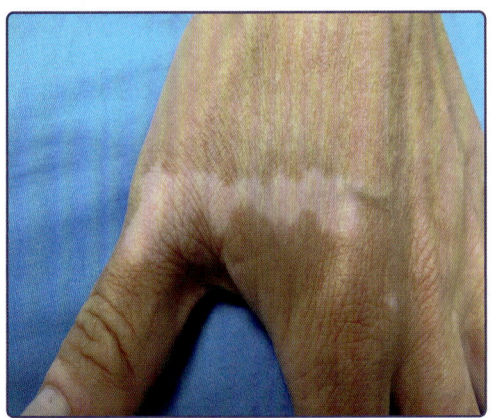

Figure 76-11 Marginal repigmentation in glabrous skin.

LABORATORY TESTING

Because vitiligo is associated with other autoimmune diseases such as thyroid diseases, clinicians should consider laboratory testing for these other diseases when patients' symptoms warrant them. TSH is commonly tested to rule out concomitant Hashimoto thyroiditis, although in the absence of symptoms this testing may not be necessary.[34] Complete blood count and antinuclear antibody testing can be considered in the context of light sensitivity, as phototherapy is a standard in vitiligo treatment. During followup, clinicians should consider testing for other autoimmune markers whenever patients have suggestive signs and symptoms.

HISTOLOGY

When the history and physical examination are consistent with vitiligo, there is usually no need for skin biopsy to confirm the diagnosis. However, when the presentation is unusual, biopsy may help to rule out other disorders of pigment abnormalities that fall within the differential diagnosis (discussed below). When performed, histologic examination and immunohistochemical studies reveal a complete loss of melanocytes within the epidermis,[55] and biopsy near the lesional border during progression may demonstrate an inflammatory infiltrate of CD4+ and CD8+ T cells in an interface pattern, with primarily CD8+ T cells infiltrating the epidermis.[77]

DIFFERENTIAL DIAGNOSIS

The differential diagnosis of vitiligo is broad and is presented concisely in Tables 76-1 and 76-2. In general, inherited hypomelanoses are present at or within a few months after birth, whereas vitiligo is rarely, if ever, present that early. Wood lamp examination helps to differentiate the depigmentation of vitiligo from hypopigmentation of most other diseases. Specifically, vitiligo and its segmental variant have different considerations when thinking about differential diagnoses, because the former is symmetric, often more widespread, and progressive, whereas the latter is focal, unilateral, and stable.

The differential diagnosis of vitiligo includes inflammatory, postinflammatory, neoplastic, and genetic (mostly congenital) disorders of depigmentation. The first helpful step is to determine whether the lesion or lesions are congenital, remembering that in fair skin, lesions may not become apparent until after the first few months of life, often after the first sun exposure. A number of genodermatoses may be initially misdiagnosed as vitiligo, but the most frequent are piebaldism and tuberous sclerosis. In piebaldism, the combination of white forelock, anterior body midline depigmentation,

TABLE 76-1
Differential Diagnoses for Nonsegmental Vitiligo

CONDITION	DISTINGUISHABLE FEATURES
Inherited Hypomelanoses	
Piebaldism (KIT mutation) (Fig. 76-12)	White forelock, anterior body midline depigmentation and bilateral shin depigmentation present at birth (with absence of melanocytes); autosomal dominant
Waardenburg syndrome (PAX3 mutation)	White forelock, white skin macules, hypertelorism, heterochromic or hypoplastic blue irides, deafness, early graying, ± Hirschsprung disease
Tuberous sclerosis (TSC1 and TSC2 mutations) (Fig. 76-13)	Hypomelanotic macules (ash leaf) present within the first years of life; angiofibromas at age 3-4 years; ungual fibromas; cephalic and lumbar (shagreen patch) fibrous plaques; and hypopigmented "confetti" macules appearing in childhood to early adolescence; seizures; autosomal dominant
Ito hypomelanosis	Hypopigmented skin macules and patches along Blaschko lines in a linear pattern, unilateral or bilateral pattern; usually develops within the first 2 years of life; sporadic; chromosomal or genetic mosaicism
Infectious Disorders	
Tinea versicolor (Fig. 76-14)	Well-demarcated finely scaling patches in highly sebaceous areas; yellow-green fluorescence on Wood light
Treponematoses (syphilis and pinta)	Postinflammatory hypopigmented/depigmentated patches) on the neck on trunk, limbs. Positive testing for serologic treponemal infection
Leprosy (tuberculoid/borderline forms) (Fig. 76-15)	Mainly hypopigmented patches; localized anesthesia
Postinflammatory Hypopigmentation	
Discoid lupus erythematosus, scleroderma, lichen sclerosis et atrophicus, psoriasis	History of preexisting condition
Paramalignant Hypomelanoses	
Mycosis fungoides (Fig. 76-16)	Scattered irregular hypopigmented patches on non–sun-exposed areas. Atrophic epidermal surface. Plaque and tumor lesions of mycosis fungoides may be present concurrently. Histology: epidermotropism of atypical lymphocytes
Cutaneous melanoma	Dyschromic lesion combining pigmented areas with depigmentation around or within the tumor
Idiopathic Disorders	
Idiopathic guttate hypomelanosis	Hypopigmented well-circumscribed macules, sharply defined and small in size. Usually localized on photoexposed areas, especially the legs. Very slowly progressive and nonconfluent
Progressive macular hypomelanosis	Nummular, nonscaly hypopigmented spots lesions of the trunk, often confluent. Punctiform red fluorescence on Wood lamp
Postinflammatory pigment loss	History of preceding eruption/injury
Melasma	Hyperpigmented macules and patches, often limited to the face. The contrast between lighter and darker skin may appear hypopigmented; dermoscopy may show capillary network

bilateral shin depigmentation, and large islands of sparing are hallmarks of the disease. Family history will often make the diagnosis of piebaldism straightforward, as it is most often dominantly inherited.

TABLE 76-2
Differential Diagnoses for Segmental Vitiligo

CONDITION	DISTINGUISHABLE FEATURES
Nevus anemicus	Poorly demarcated white macule surrounded by erythema, which disappears with diascopy.
Nevus depigmentosus	Well-delimited hypopigmented macule usually present at birth with irregular, saw-toothed border. Hairs within the lesion generally remain pigmented. The lesion is stable in size but will expand in proportion to growth with age. In fair skin types, parents may note the lesion after first photoexposure of the child

Distinguishing vitiligo from tuberous sclerosis relies on the hypopigmented nature of ash-leaf spots, as well as their stability over time. Of course, the presence of seizures or other cutaneous symptoms that may appear later, such as shagreen patches or angiofibromas, should prompt further investigation for tuberous sclerosis.

If the lesions in question are acquired, the most common differential diagnoses are pityriasis versicolor and postinflammatory hypopigmentation, such as pityriasis alba. Here, a Wood lamp examination is quite helpful, as lesions of vitiligo are depigmented and enhance, while others are hypopigmented and do not. In addition, neoplastic hypomelanoses, in particular hypopigmented mycosis fungoides, should be ruled out. Hypopigmented mycosis fungoides is distributed in sun-protected areas and is hypopigmented, rather than depigmented. Isolated genital involvement should be carefully differentiated from the diagnosis

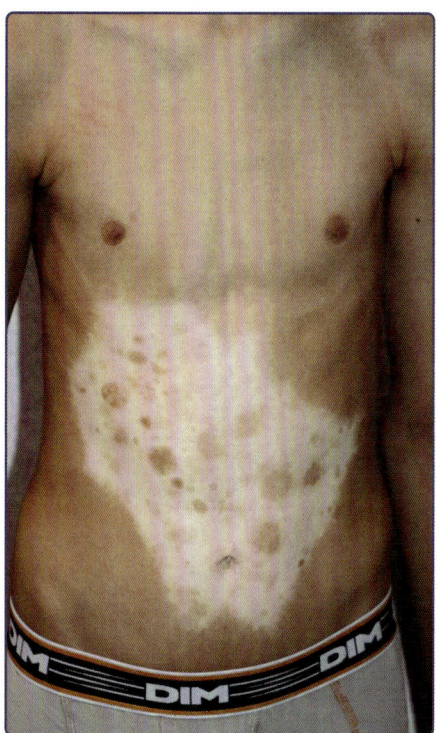

Figure 76-12 Piebaldism. Note large central midline patch of depigmentation with islands of sparing.

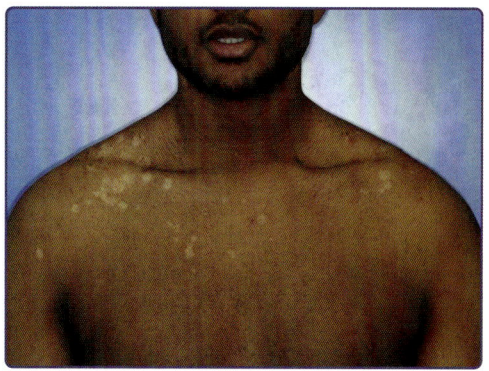

Figure 76-14 Scaly, hypopigmented macules of tinea versicolor.

of lichen sclerosus et atrophicus as this diagnosis can be quite destructive and often is irreversible. Lichen sclerosus is often symptomatic, following a figure-of-eight pattern around the anus and introitus in women, frequently with signs of atrophy and fissuring of the skin. In longstanding cases, it may be accompanied by resorption of normal structures like the labia minora as well as narrowing of the introitus. A complicating factor in the differential diagnosis includes reports of concomitant genital lichen sclerosus and vitiligo. Biopsy can be helpful in difficult cases.

For segmental vitiligo, nevus depigmentosus is the most common consideration in the differential diagnosis. However nevus depigmentosus is usually congenital or recognized within a few months of life and is stable in size, growing only in proportion to the child. In contrast to its name, it is typically hypopigmented rather than depigmented, and the border is frequently jagged rather than smooth, both notable differences from vitiligo. When biopsy is performed, histology displays normal or a slightly decreased number of melanocytes with reduced melanin content, rather than absence of melanocytes. Nevus anemicus is another to condition to rule out and is usually present at birth. Clinically, nevus anemicus corresponds to a poorly demarcated white macule surrounded by erythema, which, contrary to segmental vitiligo, does not

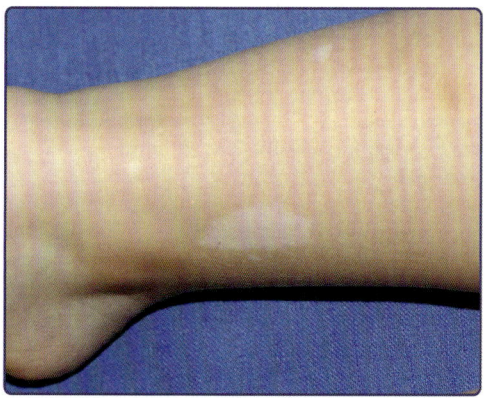

Figure 76-13 Ash-leaf macules in tuberous sclerosis.

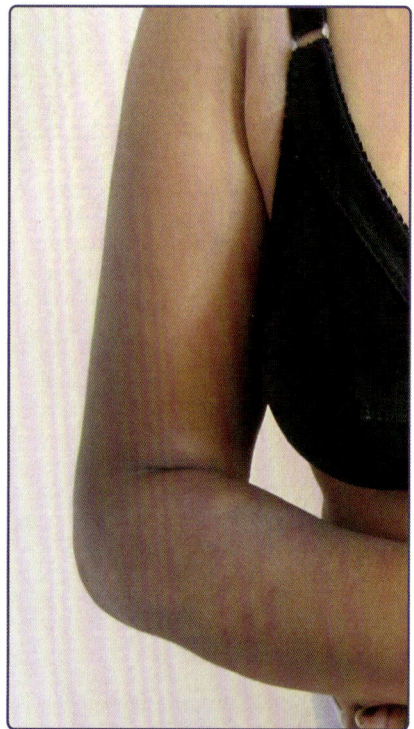

Figure 76-15 Hypopigmented patches of leprosy.

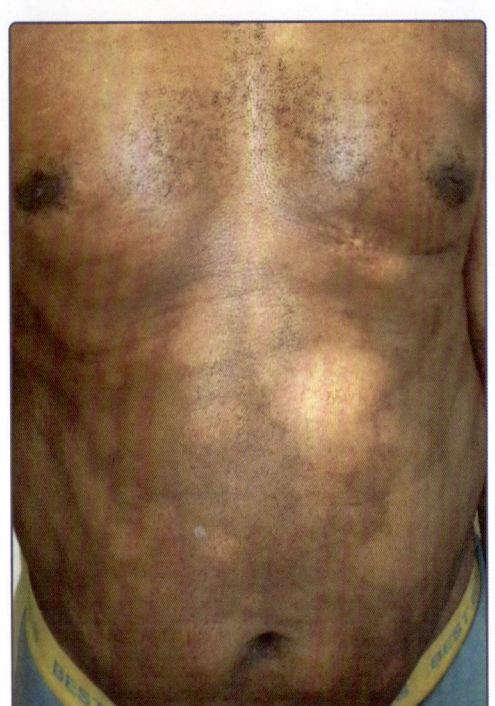

Figure 76-16 Hypopigmented patches of mycosis fungoides.

show accentuation when examined with Wood lamp. It also disappears with diascopy, or other gentle pressure on the skin.

CLINICAL COURSE AND PROGNOSIS

Vitiligo has an unpredictable course with a disposition toward cycles of flares and phases of stability. Early whitening of the hairs is unusual, although this may appear later in the course of the disease. Repigmentation in hair-bearing locations is likely, and may either occur spontaneously, after specific therapeutic intervention, or following sun exposure. However, lesions in glabrous skin are much slower to respond, as they improve from slower marginal repigmentation that is limited to only a few millimeters total, despite long-term treatment. There is some evidence that episodes of stress may trigger disease onset and/or relapse. In contrast, the course of segmental vitiligo is rapid but self-limited, with rapid stabilization and rare progression after this has occurred. The early involvement of hairs makes segmental vitiligo less responsive to treatment, although if caught early good results may be obtained.

MANAGEMENT

When developing a management plan for vitiligo patients, multiple factors should be considered. A thorough examination of patients under natural and Wood lamp light is important to assess the extent of disease. In addition, social and demographic details, family history of the patient, as well as the patient's relevant medical history, should be elicited at the initial consultation. The skin phototype, presence of halo nevi, disease duration and extent, and activity are key items in guiding therapeutic management. Scoring of disease activity by evaluating the probability of Koebner phenomenon also can be considered.[31]

As of this writing most therapies that are effective for vitiligo were developed for other inflammatory skin diseases and are thus used off-label. The management plan for patients with vitiligo will vary according to disease activity and extent. For example, if a patient presents during active progression, combination therapy that includes oral antiinflammatories may be important to halt the progression of disease, as other therapies, such as phototherapy, may take weeks to months to become effective. If the disease is stable, monotherapy is an option as the likelihood of progression while the responses slowly develop is minimal.

TOPICAL THERAPIES

Topical therapies may be used as monotherapy when there is limited surface involvement (less than 5% body surface area); however, they are often used in combination with phototherapy. Two main classes of topical drugs are used in vitiligo: topical steroids and topical calcineurin inhibitors.

The advantages of topical corticosteroids are good efficacy, ease of application, high compliance rate, and low cost. The drawbacks of topical corticosteroids are their side effects, which include skin atrophy, telangiectasia, hypertrichosis, acneiform eruptions, and striae, as well as increased intraocular pressure (exacerbation of glaucoma) when used around the eyes. Typically, ultrapotent formulations are required for reliable efficacy, and most published studies have evaluated the class I steroid clobetasol. They should be applied twice daily and can be used in a discontinuous scheme, such as cycles of 1 week on treatment followed by 1 week off treatment for up to 6 months, to avoid side effects. For childhood vitiligo, a class II potency steroid with a good safety profile, like mometasone, is a good choice. Lower-potency steroids do not have strong evidence to support their use.

Advantages of topical calcineurin inhibitors include their good efficacy and excellent safety profile.[78] They can be used on areas that are not ideal for steroids, such as on the face, neck, intertriginous areas, and on children. Of note, warnings have been placed on the long-term use of topical calcineurin inhibitors in relation to an increased risk of cancer; however, these concerns are based on risks associated with oral dosing of these drugs and have not been observed with topical use. A recent systematic review and meta-analysis concluded that the use of topical steroids and calcineurin inhibitors was unlikely to increase the risk of lymphoma in patients with atopic dermatitis.[79]

Although some concerns about the combining of phototherapy with these drugs promotes skin cancer have been raised, the combination of light therapy with topical calcineurin inhibitors increases their efficacy[80] and there is no clinical data that supports these concerns for increased cancer risk. Thus, clinicians should proceed with these treatments but with caution, and patients should be counseled of these facts when prescribed these therapies, at least until these warnings are removed from the packaging. A recent report tested topical tacrolimus as maintenance therapy in patients who achieved repigmentation through other methods.[81] In this randomized controlled study of 35 patients, more than 90% of those treated with tacrolimus 0.1% only twice weekly maintained their pigmentation without a relapse of their vitiligo, whereas only 60% did so in the placebo group. A small number of studies have compared topical calcineurin inhibitors and topical steroids without significant difference in efficacy between the 2 groups.[82]

PHOTOTHERAPY AND COMBINATION THERAPIES

Because of its efficacy, ease of use, and relatively good safety profile, full-body phototherapy should be considered the first treatment option in patients with more than 5% of the body surface area affected, especially if the disease is rapidly spreading (Fig. 76-17). For those with more limited, focal disease, targeted phototherapy can be considered because of its very high efficacy. However, phototherapy is time-consuming and devices may not be readily accessible to all patients. When this is the case, home phototherapy can be considered, where units are prescribed and purchased for use in the patient's home. Although the strength of home units does not match those in the physician's office, the convenience of getting phototherapy at home often results in excellent responses.[83] Most units require a prescription from a dermatologist, who must provide ongoing codes to enable continued use of the unit after regular in-office assessments. Because some patients with vitiligo have circulating antinuclear antibodies that could sensitize them to light, screening for antinuclear antibodies prior to phototherapy can be considered, particularly if there is a history of sun sensitivity. Overall, the risk-to-benefit profile of all treatments should be considered when developing a management strategy for each patient.

Historically, phototherapy has been administered using different sources, including oral or topical psoralen plus ultraviolet A (PUVA), broadband ultraviolet B, narrowband ultraviolet B (nbUVB), and targeted phototherapy with excimer laser. These are outlined below:

PSORALEN AND ULTRAVIOLET A

PUVA was the first phototherapy treatment reported to be effective for vitiligo; it has since, however, become

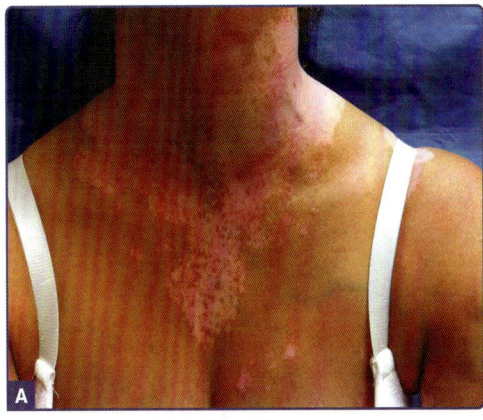
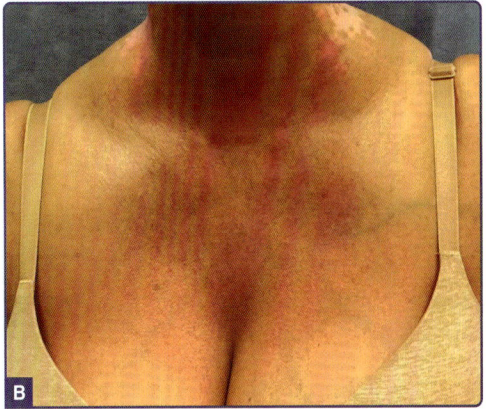

Figure 76-17 Excellent response after about 1 year of narrowband ultraviolet B phototherapy; (**A**) before and (**B**) after therapy.

associated with adverse effects that include nausea, ocular damage, and phototoxic reactions, as well as an increased risk of skin cancer.[84] A 2015 Cochrane review reported that the efficacy of PUVA was inferior to nbUVB in achieving greater than 75% repigmentation in vitiligo patients.[85] In another study, color matching of treated areas with normal skin was inferior in PUVA compared to nbUVB.[86] In addition, nbUVB treatment has fewer short-term (painful erythema) and long-term (epidermal thickening, atrophy, and photocarcinogenesis) adverse reactions than PUVA.[56] Thus, PUVA is no longer first-line therapy for vitiligo, and has been largely replaced by nbUVB. However, PUVA may be considered in patients who fail to repigment with other modalities.[86-88] Like other methods of phototherapy, PUVA is typically administered 2 or 3 times weekly.

NARROWBAND ULTRAVIOLET B

nbUVB has largely replaced other modalities because of its efficacy and better safety profile. It provides 2 particular benefits: (a) repigmentation and (b) stabilization, which is important in those who have active disease. Njoo and colleagues achieved greater than 75% repigmentation in 53% and stabilization in 80%

of children with twice-weekly nbUVB.[89] Increased benefit has been reported with the addition of topical corticosteroids and calcineurin inhibitors. The 2015 Cochrane update for interventions in vitiligo reported that 35 of 96 randomized controlled trials used nbUVB as either monotherapy or in combination with other treatments.[90] nbUVB has potent immunosuppressive effects locally and is able to induce melanocyte differentiation and melanin production.[91]

Treatment with nbUVB should be 2 to 3 times weekly, starting with a dose of 200 millijoules (mJ) with an increase of 10% to 20% increments until reaching the minimal erythema dose, which corresponds to the lowest dose resulting in asymptomatic, visible erythema on depigmented skin that lasts less than 24 hours. A total of 9 to 12 months or more of treatment is required to achieve full repigmentation, with at least 6 months of therapy before determining that the disease is nonresponsive.[86] When used on its own, nbUVB has been reported to induce repigmentation rates ranging from 40% to 100%, depending on the location of the lesion.[89,92-95]

TARGETED ULTRAVIOLET B PHOTOTHERAPY

Targeted UVB phototherapy is achieved using excimer lasers and lamps. They reportedly are equally effective, although excimer lamp induces more erythema.[96] Because of their small treatment size, targeted phototherapy is indicated in patients with limited, focal vitiligo (less than 5% of the body surface area affected with stable disease).[97] Targeted phototherapy is also reportedly the treatment that achieves highest efficacy for segmental vitiligo in its early phase (ie, disease onset of less than 6 months to 1 year). It is also reportedly safe and effective for long-term treatment of pediatric vitiligo patients.[98]

COMBINATION THERAPIES

In the most recent update of the Cochrane review, combination therapies using any type of light were considered the most effective treatment for vitiligo. Even though not necessarily synergistic or even additive, the additional benefit of adding topical therapies when undergoing phototherapy appears to be worthwhile. If large areas are involved, sites that are important to the patient, such as the face and hands, may be selected for adjuvant topical therapy. The combination of oral steroid pulse therapy, such as dexamethasone on weekends or prednisone on alternate days, with light therapy is reportedly helpful in controlling rapidly spreading vitiligo until phototherapy achieves a therapeutic dose.[99]

PSYCHOLOGICAL INTERVENTIONS

The psychological impact of vitiligo includes poor self-perception, low quality of life, poor interpersonal relationships, depression, and anxiety.[100-104] Thus, psychological interventions such as cognitive-behavioral therapy and hypnosis have been shown to improve quality of life, reduce anxiety, improve coping with disease, and even enhance repigmentation in vitiligo.[101,105-107] Importantly, adolescents with vitiligo are uniquely susceptible to social pressure and stigma, and thus should be screened for psychological impairment and referred for management.

COSMETICS

Cosmetic camouflage, especially on visible areas such as the face and the hands, can improve quality of life in patients with vitiligo.[108,109] There are now several water-resistant camouflage dyes and creams that are available with a wide range of color and shades covering all skin types.

DEPIGMENTATION THERAPY

Ever since the observation that monobenzone potently induced and exacerbated vitiligo in exposed individuals, it has been used as a treatment for vitiligo to depigment the skin, removing the remaining pigment and evening out the tone.[110] In fact, it is the only Food and Drug Administration–approved medical therapy for vitiligo. For patients with widespread disease that would be difficult to reverse with the conventional treatments discussed above (many suggest greater than 80% body surface area or significant poliosis), monobenzone can be prescribed as a 20% topical cream to be applied 1 to 2 times daily. It can take 1 to 2 years for complete depigmentation, and it even affects areas remote from the site of application, so it cannot be used for just local depigmentation. Up to 20% of patients develop a contact dermatitis to the cream, which is located only in pigmented skin and may limit treatment. If this occurs, the strength can be decreased to 10%, and concurrent use of topical steroids may limit the reaction. Hair, eyes, and other locations where melanocytes are found are typically spared during depigmentation therapy with monobenzone. Even though this is a drastic and permanent approach to therapy, patients are typically happy with the result. They must be counseled that their skin will be sun-sensitive for the rest of their lives, and sun protection must be strictly followed.

NONTRADITIONAL TREATMENTS

There are numerous nontraditional treatments that have been suggested for vitiligo. Of these, khellin, ginkgo biloba, vitamins and nutritional supplements,

Polypodium leukotomos, topical and systemic phenylalanine, topical calcipotriene, and pseudocatalase cream have been used. Current evidence for their efficacy is weak at best and adding them to a therapeutic strategy should be carefully considered in light of this lack of evidence.

SURGICAL THERAPIES

Surgical therapies for vitiligo can be very successful; however, a key part of surgical therapy is patient selection. Surgery in vitiligo should be reserved for patients with highly stable disease, which has been defined as the absence of new or growing lesions for 1 to 2 years.[111] Segmental vitiligo patients are well suited for this approach because their disease stabilizes quickly, but those who do not have this variant have much-less-successful outcomes.

Several techniques for surgical treatment exist for vitiligo, which can broadly be divided into tissue grafting and cellular grafting. Tissue grafts include thin and ultrathin split-thickness skin grafts, suction blister epidermal grafts, mini punch grafts, and hair follicle grafts. These approaches all use solid-tissue grafts whose size is matched to the donor site in a 1:1 ratio. Alternatively, cellular grafts include noncultured epidermal cell suspension, cultured "pure" melanocytes, cultured epithelial grafts, and autologous noncultured extracted hair follicle suspension. These approaches transplant suspensions of keratinocytes and melanocytes and can cover larger surface areas with up to a 1:10 ratio of donor-to-recipient area.

Each technique has advantages and disadvantages. In general, tissue grafts are easier to perform than cellular grafts, but are limited by the need to harvest tissue in a 1:1 ratio to the donor site. Split-thickness grafting is easy and inexpensive, but frequently results in color mismatch and occasional failure of the graft to take. Punch grafting is easy to perform and inexpensive but should be used in limited areas because of frequent side effects, such as cobblestoning, which describes healing at the recipient site with raised grafts that are visible and palpable, like cobblestones on a path.[112] Blister grafting gives better cosmetic results without cobblestoning, but it is time-consuming and may be more difficult to perform because of handling and placement of the very thin blister roof graft.[113-117]

Because of their improved donor-to-recipient-site ratio, excellent outcomes in percent repigmentation and color match, as well as improved healing, cellular grafts are becoming the first-line in surgical management of stable vitiligo (Fig. 76-18). The most commonly used technique, the melanocyte keratinocyte transplant procedure, creates a suspension of keratinocytes and melanocytes from donor epidermis that is enzymatically digested and mechanically disrupted into a single cell suspension. This technique has been optimized and simplified over the past few years and now requires minimal laboratory support. It is usually conducted in 2 steps. The first consists of shaving an ultrathin skin

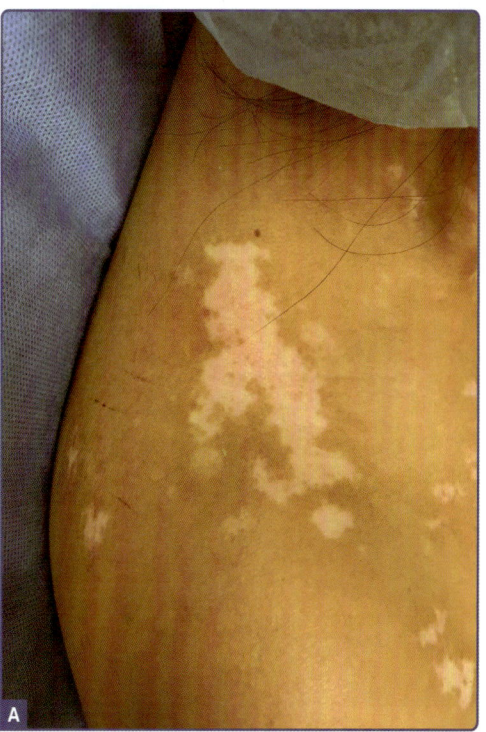 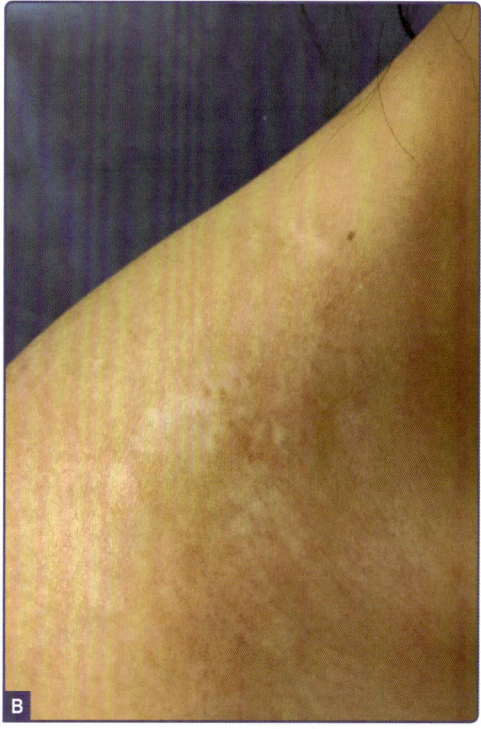

Figure 76-18 Surgical therapy of segmental vitiligo using the melanocyte keratinocyte transplant procedure; (**A**) before and (**B**) after therapy.

donor graft (Fig. 76-19A), which is rinsed and incubated in 0.25% trypsin for 30 minutes at 37°C (98.6°F) before manually removing the epidermis from the dermis, disrupting the epidermis mechanically, and centrifuging the epidermal fragments to create a cellular pellet (Fig. 76-19B, C). This pellet is resuspended in lactated ringers or normal saline in a 1mL syringe. The second step consists of applying this cellular suspension over

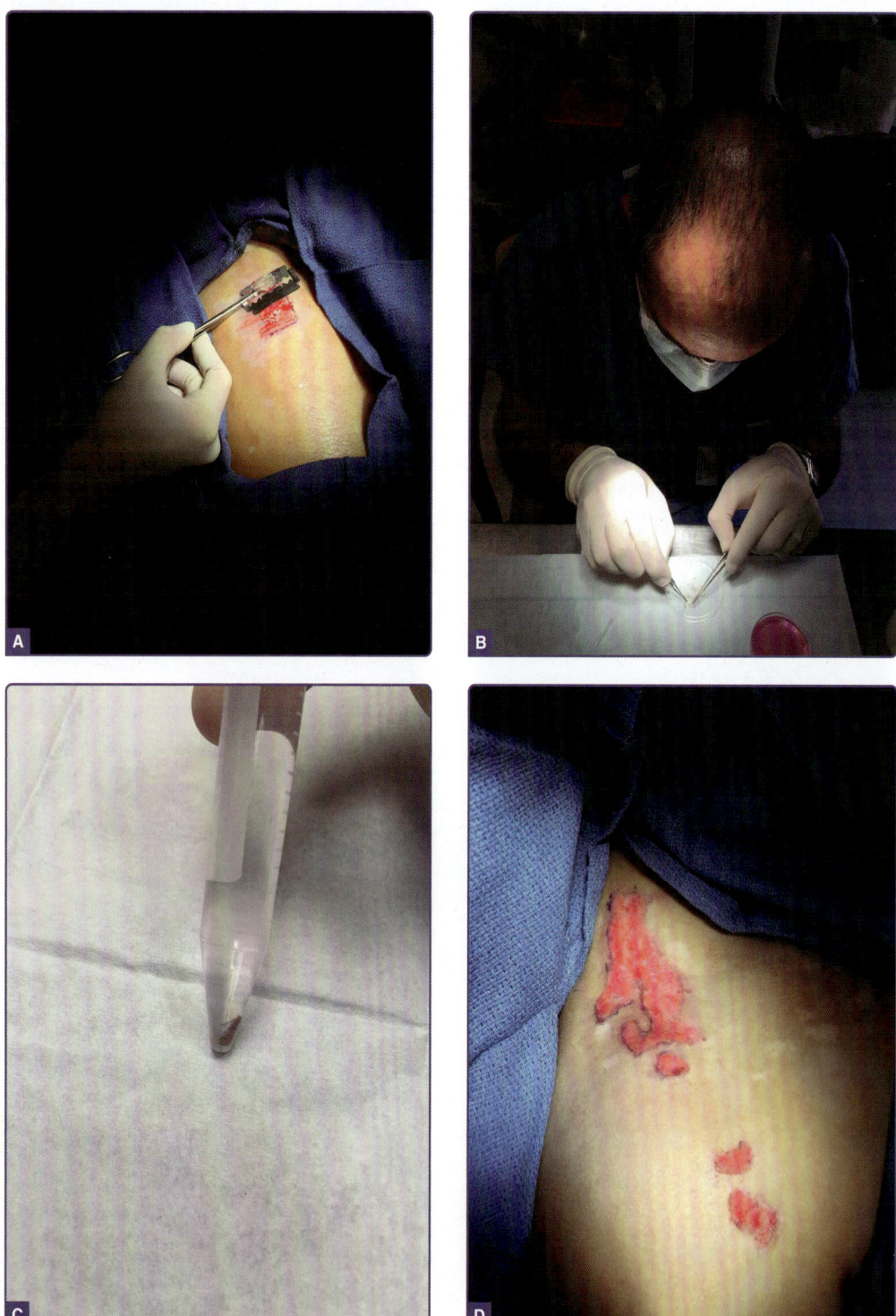

Figure 76-19 Melanocyte keratinocyte transplant procedure. **A,** Harvesting of thin skin graft. **B,** Processing of the skin graft to remove the epidermis and mechanically disrupt it into small pieces. **C,** Pellet of melanocytes and keratinocytes after centrifugation. **D,** Dermabraded skin lesions ready for application of cell suspension.

the recipient site that was previously dermabraded or laser treated to remove the epidermis (Fig. 76-19D). The recipient site is then covered with an appropriate dressing for 4 to 7 days, depending on the treated area.[118,119]

TREATMENT ALGORITHM

We propose 2 treatment algorithms, one for vitiligo (Fig. 76-20) and another for the segmental variant of disease (Fig. 76-21).

EMERGING THERAPIES

As discussed above, vitiligo is driven primarily by the destruction of melanocytes by CD8+ T cells that secrete IFN-γ, which induces chemokines that recruit additional T cells in an ongoing, positive feedback loop. Future targeted therapies are likely to target this and other synergistic cytokine pathways, similar to recent advancements in the treatment of psoriasis. However, psoriasis treatments are ineffective for vitiligo because the interleukin-23–interleukin-17–tumor necrosis factor-α cytokine axis that drives psoriasis is not active in vitiligo.[69]

Examples of future targeted therapies include inhibition of Janus kinases (JAKs), which are required for the signaling of many cytokines, including IFN-γ. In small case studies and series, JAK inhibitors have been reported to promote repigmentation of vitiligo patients, including oral tofacitinib, oral ruxolitinib, and topical ruxolitinib.[120-126] Ongoing clinical trials are currently testing JAK inhibitors as new treatments for patients with vitiligo. In addition, biologics that target other members of the IFN-γ–chemokine signaling axis may be effective, such as antibodies against CXCR3 or its ligands, which have been reported effective in a mouse model of vitiligo.[64,127] Additional cytokine-targeted biologics have been developed for other diseases and may be repurposed for vitiligo.[69] Side effects should be considered for any immunotherapy, which may include increased incidence of infections or decreased tumor surveillance.

Finally, in addition to targeted immunotherapy, treatments that promote melanocyte regeneration, proliferation, and/or migration could also be effective treatments, particularly when combined with immunosuppressive treatments. One example that has been tested in vitiligo patients is afamelanotide, an α-melanocyte–stimulating hormone analog, which, in conjunction with nbUVB, increased the rate and extent of repigmentation in vitiligo patients.[128,129] Side effects of this treatment included nausea, abdominal pain, and darkening of the normal skin of patients, which led to

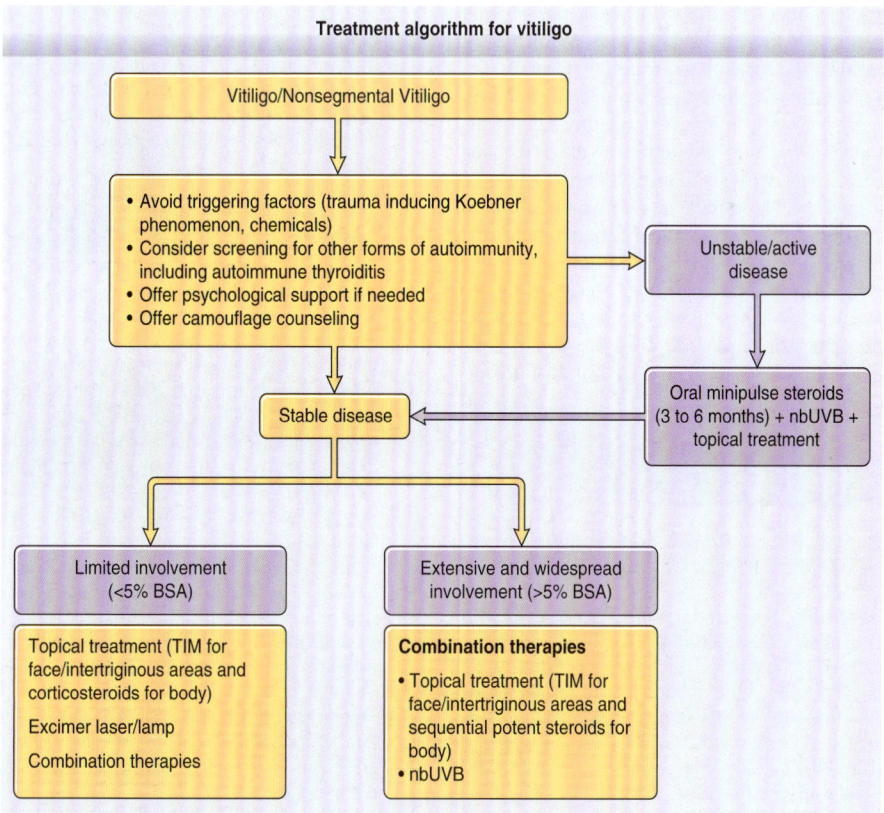

Figure 76-20 Treatment algorithm for vitiligo. BSA, body surface area; nbUVB, narrowband ultraviolet B; TIM, topical immunomodulators.

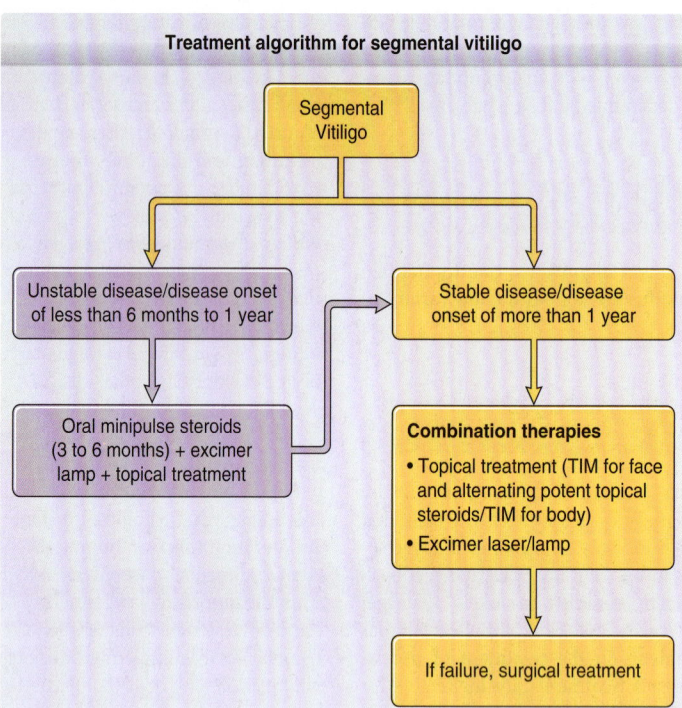

Figure 76-21 Treatment algorithm for segmental vitiligo. TIM, topical immunomodulators.

dissatisfaction and withdrawal of some participants from the study owing to the increased prominence of lesions against the darker background of normal skin.

In summary, recent advances in our understanding of vitiligo have led to the development of new treatment strategies that may have improved efficacy in our treatment of patients with vitiligo. As with any new therapy, safety will have to be monitored and carefully considered when making recommendations for patients suffering with this psychologically, but not physically, debilitating disease. This marks an exciting time for both patients with vitiligo and their caregivers, who are gaining deeper insight into their disease, and may have improved options for management in the near future.

REFERENCES

1. Panda AK. The medico historical perspective of vitiligo (Switra). *Bull Indian Inst Hist Med Hyderabad*. 2005;35(1):41-46.
2. Westerhof W, Njoo MD, Schallreuter KU. Vitiligo [in German]. *Hautarzt*. 1997;48(9):677-693; quiz 693.
3. Goldman L, Moraites RS, Kitzmiller KW. White spots in biblical times. A background for the dermatologist for participation in discussions of current revisions of the bible. *Arch Dermatol*. 1966;93(6):744-753.
4. Donata SR, Kesavan M, Austin SR, et al. Clinical trial of certain ayurveda medicines indicated in vitiligo. *Anc Sci Life*. 1990;4:202-206.
5. Olsson MJ, Juhlin L. Melanocyte transplantation in vitiligo. *Lancet*. 1992;340(8825):981.
6. Howitz J, Brodthagen H, Schwartz M, et al. Prevalence of vitiligo. Epidemiological survey on the Isle of Bornholm, Denmark. *Arch Dermatol*. 1977;113(1):47-52.
7. Boisseau-Garsaud AM, Garsaud P, Calès-Quist D, et al. Epidemiology of vitiligo in the French West Indies (Isle of Martinique). *Int J Dermatol*. 2000;39(1):18-20.
8. Behl PN, Bhatia RK. 400 cases of vitiligo. A clinico-therapeutic analysis. *Indian J Dermatol*. 1972;17(2):51-56.
9. Sehgal VN, Srivastava G. Vitiligo: compendium of clinico-epidemiological features. *Indian J Dermatol Venereol Leprol*. 2007;73(3):149-156.
10. Singh M, Singh G, Kanwar AJ, et al. Clinical pattern of vitiligo in Libya. *Int J Dermatol*. 1985;24(4):233-235.
11. Alikhan A, Felsten LM, Daly M, et al. Vitiligo: a comprehensive overview. Part I. Introduction, epidemiology, quality of life, diagnosis, differential diagnosis, associations, histopathology, etiology, and work-up. *J Am Acad Dermatol*. 2011;65(3):473-491.
12. Das SK, Majumder PP, Chakraborty R, et al. Studies on vitiligo. I. Epidemiological profile in Calcutta, India. *Genet Epidemiol*. 1985;2(1):71-78.
13. Ezzedine K, Diallo A, Léauté-Labrèze C, et al. Pre- vs. post-pubertal onset of vitiligo: multivariate analysis indicates atopic diathesis association in prepubertal onset vitiligo. *Br J Dermatol*. 2012;167(3):490-495.
14. Nicolaidou E, Antoniou C, Miniati A, et al. Childhood- and later-onset vitiligo have diverse epidemiologic and clinical characteristics. *J Am Acad Dermatol*. 2012;66(6):954-958.
15. Al-Refu K. Vitiligo in children: a clinical-epidemiologic study in Jordan. *Pediatr Dermatol*. 2012;29(1):114-115.

16. Ezzedine K, Sheth V, Rodrigues M, et al. Vitiligo is not a cosmetic disease. *J Am Acad Dermatol.* 2015;73(5):883-885.
17. Ongenae K, Dierckxsens L, Brochez L, et al. Quality of life and stigmatization profile in a cohort of vitiligo patients and effect of the use of camouflage. *Dermatology.* 2005;210(4):279-285.
18. Ongenae K, Van Geel N, De Schepper S, et al. Effect of vitiligo on self-reported health-related quality of life. *Br J Dermatol.* 2005;152(6):1165-1172.
19. Linthorst Homan MW, Spuls PI, de Korte J, et al. The burden of vitiligo: patient characteristics associated with quality of life. *J Am Acad Dermatol.* 2009;61(3):411-420.
20. Parsad D, Pandhi R, Dogra S, et al. Dermatology Life Quality Index score in vitiligo and its impact on the treatment outcome. *Br J Dermatol.* 2003;148(2):373-374.
21. Osborne GE, Francis ND, Bunker CB. Synchronous onset of penile lichen sclerosus and vitiligo. *Br J Dermatol.* 2000;143(1):218-219.
22. Lommerts JE, Schilder Y, de Rie MA, et al. Focal vitiligo: long-term follow-up of 52 cases. *J Eur Acad Dermatol Venereol.* 2016;30(9):1550-1554.
23. Ezzedine K, Lim HW, Suzuki T, et al. Revised classification/nomenclature of vitiligo and related issues: the Vitiligo Global Issues Consensus Conference. *Pigment Cell Melanoma Res.* 2012;25(3):E1-E13.
24. Ezzedine K, Gauthier Y, Léauté-Labrèze C, et al. Segmental vitiligo associated with generalized vitiligo (mixed vitiligo): a retrospective case series of 19 patients. *J Am Acad Dermatol.* 2011;65(5):965-971.
25. Mazereeuw-Hautier J, Bezio S, Mahe E, et al. Segmental and nonsegmental childhood vitiligo has distinct clinical characteristics: a prospective observational study. *J Am Acad Dermatol.* 2010;62(6):945-949.
26. van Geel N, Speeckaert R, De Wolf J, et al. Clinical significance of Koebner phenomenon in vitiligo. *Br J Dermatol.* 2012;167(5):1017-1024.
27. Hann SK, Kim YS, Yoo JH, et al. Clinical and histopathologic characteristics of trichrome vitiligo. *J Am Acad Dermatol.* 2000;42(4):589-596.
28. Sosa JJ, Currimbhoy SD, Ukoha U, et al. Confetti-like depigmentation: a potential sign of rapidly progressing vitiligo. *J Am Acad Dermatol.* 2015;73(2):272-275.
29. Le Poole IC, van den Wijngaard RM, Westerhof W, et al. Presence of T cells and macrophages in inflammatory vitiligo skin parallels melanocyte disappearance. *Am J Pathol.* 1996;148(4):1219-1228.
30. Njoo MD, Das PK, Bos JD, et al. Association of the Kobner phenomenon with disease activity and therapeutic responsiveness in vitiligo vulgaris. *Arch Dermatol.* 1999;135(4):407-413.
31. Diallo A, Boniface K, Jouary T, et al. Development and validation of the K-VSCOR for scoring Koebner's phenomenon in vitiligo/non-segmental vitiligo. *Pigment Cell Melanoma Res.* 2013;26(3):402-407.
32. Alkhateeb A, Fain PR, Thody A, et al. Epidemiology of vitiligo and associated autoimmune diseases in Caucasian probands and their families. *Pigment Cell Res.* 2003;16(3):208-214.
33. Gill L, Zarbo A, Isedeh P, et al. Comorbid autoimmune diseases in patients with vitiligo: a cross-sectional study. *J Am Acad Dermatol.* 2016;74(2):295-302.
34. Liu M, Murphy E, Amerson EH. Rethinking screening for thyroid autoimmunity in vitiligo. *J Am Acad Dermatol.* 2016;75(6):1278-1280.
35. Teulings HE, Overkamp M, Ceylan E, et al. Decreased risk of melanoma and nonmelanoma skin cancer in patients with vitiligo: a survey among 1307 patients and their partners. *Br J Dermatol.* 2013;168(1):162-171.
36. Paradisi A, Tabolli S, Didona B, et al. Markedly reduced incidence of melanoma and nonmelanoma skin cancer in a nonconcurrent cohort of 10,040 patients with vitiligo. *J Am Acad Dermatol.* 2014;71(6):1110-1116.
37. Spritz RA. Modern vitiligo genetics sheds new light on an ancient disease. *J Dermatol.* 2013;40(5):310-318.
38. Gopal KV, Rama Rao GR, Kumar YH, et al. Vitiligo: a part of a systemic autoimmune process. *Indian J Dermatol Venereol Leprol.* 2007;73(3):162-165.
39. Akay BN, Bozkir M, Anadolu Y, et al. Epidemiology of vitiligo, associated autoimmune diseases and audiological abnormalities: Ankara study of 80 patients in Turkey. *J Eur Acad Dermatol Venereol.* 2010;24(10):1144-1150.
40. Anbar TS, El-Badry MM, McGrath JA, et al. Most individuals with either segmental or non-segmental vitiligo display evidence of bilateral cochlear dysfunction. *Br J Dermatol.* 2015;172(2):406-411.
41. Albert DM, Wagoner MD, Pruett RC, et al. Vitiligo and disorders of the retinal pigment epithelium. *Br J Ophthalmol.* 1983;67(3):153-156.
42. Wagoner MD, Albert DM, Lerner AB, et al. New observations on vitiligo and ocular disease. *Am J Ophthalmol.* 1983;96(1):16-26.
43. Sakata VM, da Silva FT, Hirata CE, et al. Diagnosis and classification of Vogt-Koyanagi-Harada disease. *Autoimmun Rev.* 2014;13(4-5):550-555.
44. Alezzandrini AA. Unilateral manifestations of tapetoretinal degeneration, vitiligo, poliosis, grey hair and hypoacousia [in French]. *Ophthalmologica.* 1964;147:409-419.
45. Andrade A, Pithon M. Alezzandrini syndrome: report of a sixth clinical case. *Dermatology.* 2011;222(1):8-9.
46. Gupta M, Pande D, Lehl SS, et al. Alezzandrini syndrome. *BMJ Case Rep.* 2011;2011.
47. Schallreuter KU, Moore J, Wood JM, et al. In vivo and in vitro evidence for hydrogen peroxide (H_2O_2) accumulation in the epidermis of patients with vitiligo and its successful removal by a UVB-activated pseudocatalase. *J Investig Dermatol Symp Proc.* 1999;4(1):91-96.
48. Boissy RE, Liu YY, Medrano EE, et al. Structural aberration of the rough endoplasmic reticulum and melanosome compartmentalization in long-term cultures of melanocytes from vitiligo patients. *J Invest Dermatol.* 1991;97(3):395-404.
49. Puri N, Mojamdar M, Ramaiah A. In vitro growth characteristics of melanocytes obtained from adult normal and vitiligo subjects. *J Invest Dermatol.* 1987;88(4):434-438.
50. Puri N, Mojamdar M, Ramaiah A. Growth defects of melanocytes in culture from vitiligo subjects are spontaneously corrected in vivo in repigmenting subjects and can be partially corrected by the addition of fibroblast-derived growth factors in vitro. *Arch Dermatol Res.* 1989;281(3):178-184.
51. Medrano EE, Nordlund JJ. Successful culture of adult human melanocytes obtained from normal and vitiligo donors. *J Invest Dermatol.* 1990;95(4):441-445.
52. Jimbow K, Chen H, Park JS, et al. Increased sensitivity of melanocytes to oxidative stress and abnormal expression of tyrosinase-related protein in vitiligo. *Br J Dermatol.* 2001;144(1):55-65.

53. van den Wijngaard R, Wankowicz-Kalinska A, Le Poole C, et al. Local immune response in skin of generalized vitiligo patients. Destruction of melanocytes is associated with the prominent presence of CLA+ T cells at the perilesional site. *Lab Invest.* 2000; 80(8):1299-1309.
54. van den Boorn JG, Konijnenberg D, Dellemijn TA, et al. Autoimmune destruction of skin melanocytes by perilesional T cells from vitiligo patients. *J Invest Dermatol.* 2009;129(9):2220-2232.
55. Le Poole IC, Das PK, van den Wijngaard RM, et al. Review of the etiopathomechanism of vitiligo: a convergence theory. *Exp Dermatol.* 1993;2(4):145-153.
56. Harris JE. Cellular stress and innate inflammation in organ-specific autoimmunity: lessons learned from vitiligo. *Immunol Rev.* 2016;269(1):11-25.
57. Strassner JP, Harris JE. Understanding mechanisms of autoimmunity through translational research in vitiligo. *Curr Opin Immunol.* 2016;43:81-88.
58. Ortonne J-P, Mosher DB, Fitzpatrick TB. *Vitiligo and Other Hypomelanoses of Hair and Skin.* New York, NY: Plenum Medical; 1983.
59. van Geel N, Speeckaert R, Melsens E, et al. The distribution pattern of segmental vitiligo: clues for somatic mosaicism. *Br J Dermatol.* 2013;168(1):56-64.
60. van Geel N, Mollet I, Brochez L, et al. New insights in segmental vitiligo: case report and review of theories. *Br J Dermatol.* 2012;166(2):240-246.
61. Gregg RK, Nichols L, Chen Y, et al. Mechanisms of spatial and temporal development of autoimmune vitiligo in tyrosinase-specific TCR transgenic mice. *J Immunol.* 2010;184(4):1909-1917.
62. Harris JE, Harris TH, Weninger W, et al. A mouse model of vitiligo with focused epidermal depigmentation requires IFN-gamma for autoreactive CD8(+) T-cell accumulation in the skin. *J Invest Dermatol.* 2012;132(7):1869-1876.
63. Grimes PE, Morris R, Avaniss-Aghajani E, et al. Topical tacrolimus therapy for vitiligo: therapeutic responses and skin messenger RNA expression of proinflammatory cytokines. *J Am Acad Dermatol.* 2004; 51(1):52-61.
64. Rashighi M, Agarwal P, Richmond JM, et al. CXCL10 is critical for the progression and maintenance of depigmentation in a mouse model of vitiligo. *Sci Transl Med.* 2014;6(223):223ra223.
65. Richmond JM, Bangari DS, Essien KI, et al. Keratinocyte-derived chemokines orchestrate T cell positioning in the epidermis during vitiligo and may serve as biomarkers of disease. *J Invest Dermatol.* 2017;137(2):350-358.
66. Wang X, Wang Q, Wu J, et al. Increased expression of CXCR3 and its ligands in vitiligo patients and CXCL10 as a potential clinical marker for vitiligo. *Br J Dermatol.* 2016;174(6):1318-1326.
67. Maouia A, Sormani L, Youssef M, et al. Study of the comparative expression of CXCL9, CXCL10 and IFN-gamma in vitiligo and alopecia areata patients. *Pigment Cell Melanoma Res.* 2017;30(2):259-261.
68. Strassner JP, Rashighi M, Ahmed Refat M, et al. Suction blistering the lesional skin of vitiligo patients reveals useful biomarkers of disease activity. *J Am Acad Dermatol.* 2017;76(5):847-855.e5.
69. Frisoli ML, Harris JE. Vitiligo: mechanistic insights lead to novel treatments. *J Allergy Clin Immunol.* 2017;140(3):654-662.
70. Harris JE. Immunopathogenesis of vitiligo. In: Hamzavi I, Mahmoud BH, Isedeh PN, eds. *Handbook of Vitiligo: Basic Science and Clinical Management.* London, UK: JP Medical Publishers; 2016:21-36.
71. Oliver EA, Schwartz L, Warren LH. Occupational leukoderma. *JAMA.* 1939;113:927-928.
72. Harris JE. Chemical-induced vitiligo. *Dermatol Clin.* 2017;35(2):151-161.
73. Wu S, Li WQ, Cho E, et al. Use of permanent hair dyes and risk of vitiligo in women. *Pigment Cell Melanoma Res.* 2015;28(6):744-746.
74. Kroll TM, Bommiasamy H, Boissy RE, et al. 4-Tertiary butyl phenol exposure sensitizes human melanocytes to dendritic cell-mediated killing: relevance to vitiligo. *J Invest Dermatol.* 2005;124(4):798-806.
75. Toosi S, Orlow SJ, Manga P. Vitiligo-inducing phenols activate the unfolded protein response in melanocytes resulting in upregulation of IL6 and IL8. *J Invest Dermatol.* 2012;132(11):2601-2609.
76. van den Boorn JG, Picavet DI, van Swieten PF, et al. Skin-depigmenting agent monobenzone induces potent T-cell autoimmunity toward pigmented cells by tyrosinase haptenation and melanosome autophagy. *J Invest Dermatol.* 2011;131(6):1240-1251.
77. Faria AR, Tarle RG, Dellatorre G, et al. Vitiligo—part 2—classification, histopathology and treatment. *An Bras Dermatol.* 2014;89(5):784-790.
78. Taieb A, Alomar A, Bohm M, et al. Guidelines for the management of vitiligo: the European Dermatology Forum consensus. *Br J Dermatol.* 2013;168(1):5-19.
79. Legendre L, Barnetche T, Mazereeuw-Hautier J, et al. Risk of lymphoma in patients with atopic dermatitis and the role of topical treatment: A systematic review and meta-analysis. *J Am Acad Dermatol.* 2015;72(6):992-1002.
80. Bae JM, Yoo HJ, Kim H, et al. Combination therapy with 308-nm excimer laser, topical tacrolimus, and short-term systemic corticosteroids for segmental vitiligo: a retrospective study of 159 patients. *J Am Acad Dermatol.* 2015;73(1):76-82.
81. Cavalie M, Ezzedine K, Fontas E, et al. Maintenance therapy of adult vitiligo with 0.1% tacrolimus ointment: a randomized, double blind, placebo-controlled study. *J Invest Dermatol.* 2015;135(4):970-974.
82. Ho N, Pope E, Weinstein M, et al. A double-blind, randomized, placebo-controlled trial of topical tacrolimus 0.1% vs. clobetasol propionate 0.05% in childhood vitiligo. *Br J Dermatol.* 2011;165(3):626-632.
83. Dillon JP, Ford C, Hynan LS, et al. A cross-sectional, comparative study of home vs in-office NB-UVB phototherapy for vitiligo. *Photodermatol Photoimmunol Photomed.* 2017;33(5):282-283.
84. Veith W, Deleo V, Silverberg N. Medical phototherapy in childhood skin diseases. *Minerva Pediatr.* 2011;63(4):327-333.
85. Whitton ME, Pinart M, Batchelor J, et al. Interventions for vitiligo. *Cochrane Database Syst Rev.* 2015;(2):CD003263.
86. Yones SS, Palmer RA, Garibaldinos TM, et al. Randomized double-blind trial of treatment of vitiligo: efficacy of psoralen-UV-A therapy vs narrowband-UV-B therapy. *Arch Dermatol.* 2007;143(5):578-584.
87. Bhatnagar A, Kanwar AJ, Parsad D, et al. Comparison of systemic PUVA and NB-UVB in the treatment of vitiligo: an open prospective study. *J Eur Acad Dermatol Venereol.* 2007;21(5):638-642.
88. Pathak MA, Mosher DB, Fitzpatrick TB. Safety and therapeutic effectiveness of 8-methoxypsoralen, 4,5′,8-trimethylpsoralen, and psoralen in vitiligo. *Natl Cancer Inst Monogr.* 1984;66:165-173.

89. Njoo MD, Bos JD, Westerhof W. Treatment of generalized vitiligo in children with narrow-band (TL-01) UVB radiation therapy. *J Am Acad Dermatol*. 2000; 42(2, pt 1):245-253.
90. Whitton ME, Pinart M, Batchelor J, et al. Interventions for vitiligo. *Cochrane Database Syst Rev*. 2015;2:CD003263.
91. De Francesco V, Stinco G, Laspina S, et al. Immunohistochemical study before and after narrow band (311 nm) UVB treatment in vitiligo. *Eur J Dermatol*. 2008;18(3):292-296.
92. Arca E, Tastan HB, Erbil AH, et al. Narrow-band ultraviolet B as monotherapy and in combination with topical calcipotriol in the treatment of vitiligo. *J Dermatol*. 2006;33(5):338-343.
93. Welsh O, Herz-Ruelas ME, Gomez M, et al. Therapeutic evaluation of UVB-targeted phototherapy in vitiligo that affects less than 10% of the body surface area. *Int J Dermatol*. 2009;48(5):529-534.
94. Kanwar AJ, Dogra S. Narrow-band UVB for the treatment of generalized vitiligo in children. *Clin Exp Dermatol*. 2005;30(4):332-336.
95. Kanwar AJ, Dogra S, Parsad D, et al. Narrow-band UVB for the treatment of vitiligo: an emerging effective and well-tolerated therapy. *Int J Dermatol*. 2005;44(1):57-60.
96. Le Duff F, Fontas E, Giacchero D, et al. 308-nm excimer lamp vs. 308-nm excimer laser for treating vitiligo: a randomized study. *Br J Dermatol*. 2010;163(1):188-192.
97. Ezzedine K, Eleftheriadou V, Whitton M, et al. Vitiligo. *Lancet*. 2015;386(9988):74-84.
98. Koh MJ, Mok ZR, Chong WS. Phototherapy for the treatment of vitiligo in Asian children. *Pediatr Dermatol*. 2015;32(2):192-197.
99. Rath N, Kar HK, Sabhnani S. An open labeled, comparative clinical study on efficacy and tolerability of oral minipulse of steroid (OMP) alone, OMP with PUVA and broad/narrow band UVB phototherapy in progressive vitiligo. *Indian J Dermatol Venereol Leprol*. 2008;74(4):357-360.
100. Gawkrodger DJ, Ormerod AD, Shaw L, et al. Guideline for the diagnosis and management of vitiligo. *Br J Dermatol*. 2008;159(5):1051-1076.
101. Shah R, Hunt J, Webb TL, et al. Starting to develop self-help for social anxiety associated with vitiligo: using clinical significance to measure the potential effectiveness of enhanced psychological self-help. *Br J Dermatol*. 2014;171(2):332-337.
102. Kruger C, Smythe JW, Spencer JD, et al. Significant immediate and long-term improvement in quality of life and disease coping in patients with vitiligo after group climatotherapy at the Dead Sea. *Acta Derm Venereol*. 2011;91(2):152-159.
103. Kossakowska MM, Ciescinska C, Jaszewska J, et al. Control of negative emotions and its implication for illness perception among psoriasis and vitiligo patients. *J Eur Acad Dermatol Venereol*. 2010;24(4):429-433.
104. Picardi A, Abeni D. Can cognitive-behavioral therapy help patients with vitiligo? *Arch Dermatol*. 2001;137(6):786-788.
105. Papadopoulos L, Bor R, Legg C. Coping with the disfiguring effects of vitiligo: a preliminary investigation into the effects of cognitive-behavioural therapy. *Br J Med Psychol*. 1999;72(pt 3):385-396.
106. Papadopoulos L, Bor R, Legg C, et al. Impact of life events on the onset of vitiligo in adults: preliminary evidence for a psychological dimension in aetiology. *Clin Exp Dermatol*. 1998;23(6):243-248.
107. Shenefelt PD. Hypnosis in dermatology. *Arch Dermatol*. 2000;136(3):393-399.
108. Tedeschi A, Dall'Oglio F, Micali G, et al. Corrective camouflage in pediatric dermatology. *Cutis*. 2007; 79(2):110-112.
109. Ramien ML, Ondrejchak S, Gendron R, et al. Quality of life in pediatric patients before and after cosmetic camouflage of visible skin conditions. *J Am Acad Dermatol*. 2014;71(5):935-940.
110. Mosher DB, Parrish JA, Fitzpatrick TB. Monobenzylether of hydroquinone. A retrospective study of treatment of 18 vitiligo patients and a review of the literature. *Br J Dermatol*. 1977;97(6):669-679.
111. Ezzedine K, Lim HW, Suzuki T, et al. Revised classification/nomenclature of vitiligo and related issues: the Vitiligo Global Issues Consensus Conference. *Pigment Cell Melanoma Res*. 2012;25(3): E1-E13.
112. Linthorst Homan MW, Spuls PI, Nieuweboer-Krobotova L, et al. A randomized comparison of excimer laser versus narrow-band ultraviolet B phototherapy after punch grafting in stable vitiligo patients. *J Eur Acad Dermatol Venereol*. 2012;26(6): 690-695.
113. Feetham HJ, Chan JL, Pandya AG. Characterization of clinical response in patients with vitiligo undergoing autologous epidermal punch grafting. *Dermatol Surg*. 2012;38(1):14-19.
114. Gupta S, Ajith C, Kanwar AJ, et al. Surgical pearl: standardized suction syringe for epidermal grafting. *J Am Acad Dermatol*. 2005;52(2):348-350.
115. Agrawal K, Agrawal A. Vitiligo: repigmentation with dermabrasion and thin split-thickness skin graft. *Dermatol Surg*. 1995;21(4):295-300.
116. Malakar S, Malakar RS. Surgical pearl: composite film and graft unit for the recipient area dressing after split-thickness skin grafting in vitiligo. *J Am Acad Dermatol*. 2001;44(5):856-858.
117. Krishnan A, Kar S. Smashed skin grafting or smash grafting-a novel method of vitiligo surgery. *Int J Dermatol*. 2012;51(10):1242-1247.
118. Huggins RH, Henderson MD, Mulekar SV, et al. Melanocyte-keratinocyte transplantation procedure in the treatment of vitiligo: the experience of an academic medical center in the United States. *J Am Acad Dermatol*. 2012;66(5):785-793.
119. Mulekar SV. Melanocyte-keratinocyte cell transplantation for stable vitiligo. *Int J Dermatol*. 2003;42(2):132-136.
120. Craiglow BG, King BA. Tofacitinib citrate for the treatment of vitiligo: a pathogenesis-directed therapy. *JAMA Dermatol*. 2015;151(10):1110-1112.
121. Harris JE, Rashighi M, Nguyen N, et al. Rapid skin repigmentation on oral ruxolitinib in a patient with coexistent vitiligo and alopecia areata (AA). *J Am Acad Dermatol*. 2016;74(2):370-371.
122. Rothstein B, Joshipura D, Saraiya A, et al. Treatment of vitiligo with the topical Janus kinase inhibitor ruxolitinib. *J Am Acad Dermatol*. 2017;76(6): 1054-1060.e1.
123. Liu LY, Strassner JP, Refat MA, et al. Repigmentation in vitiligo using the Janus kinase inhibitor tofacitinib may require concomitant light exposure. *J Am Acad Dermatol*. 2017;77(4):675-682.e1.
124. Kim SR, Heaton H, Liu LY, et al. Rapid repigmentation of vitiligo using tofacitinib plus low-dose,

narrowband UV-B phototherapy. *JAMA Dermatol.* 2018;154(3):370-371.
125. Joshipura D, Plotnikova N, Goldminz A, et al. Importance of light in the treatment of vitiligo with JAK-inhibitors. *J Dermatolog Treat.* 2018;29(1):98-99.
126. Joshipura D, Alomran A, Zancanaro P, et al. Treatment of vitiligo with the topical Janus kinase inhibitor ruxolitinib: a 32-week open label extension study with optional narrow-band ultraviolet B. *J Am Acad Dermatol.* 2018;78(6):1205-1207.e1.
127. Richmond JM, Masterjohn E, Chu R, et al. CXCR3 depleting antibodies prevent and reverse vitiligo in mice. *J Invest Dermatol.* 2017;137(4):982-985.
128. Lim HW, Grimes PE, Agbai O, et al. Afamelanotide and narrowband UV-B phototherapy for the treatment of vitiligo: a randomized multicenter trial. *JAMA Dermatol.* 2015;151(1):42-50.
129. Grimes PE, Hamzavi I, Lebwohl M, et al. The efficacy of afamelanotide and narrowband UV-B phototherapy for repigmentation of vitiligo. *JAMA Dermatol.* 2013;149(1):68-73.

Chapter 77 :: Hypermelanoses
:: Michelle Rodrigues & Amit G. Pandya

第七十七章
色素沉着过度性疾病

中文导读

本章按病因将色素沉着过度性疾病分为先天性色素沉着过度性疾病和获得性色素沉着过度性疾病，分别展开了详细的阐述。

首先介绍了先天性色素沉着过度性疾病，本组疾病的特点在于因基因突变导致色素异常沉着，常发生于出生早期。共介绍了14种色素沉着过度性疾病，分别对每个疾病从临床特征、病因和发病机制、诊断、鉴别诊断、病程、预后和处理等方面来进行详细讨论。

第一节介绍了线状和漩涡状痣样黑素过度沉着病，是一种表现为先天性的沿Blaschko线分布的弥漫性条纹状色素沉着斑的皮肤病。其临床表现以沿Blaschko线分布的泛发条纹状色素沉着斑片为特征，不同表型均可用"色素镶嵌"这一术语来形容。大多数病例是散发的，该疾病的诊断主要依靠典型的临床表现以及组织学改变，常须与色素失禁和表皮痣相鉴别。该疾病随年龄增长可能会逐渐消退。

第二节介绍了色素失禁症，是一种可导致弥漫性线状皮肤色素沉着的X连锁显性遗传病，主要见于女性。病变通常会经历四个阶段（水疱期、疣状期、色素沉着期和色素减退期），在时间上可能有重叠，组织病理学改变对疾病的诊断很重要，该疾病预后良好。

第三节介绍了先天性角化不良（DKC），主要临床表现为皮肤和血液系统病变。本病病因被认为是由端粒维持缺陷引起的，根据致病机制可分为三种亚型。在诊断上认为组织病理学改变缺乏特异性改变，须与Fanconi综合征相鉴别，预后方面常染色体显性遗传的DKC预后比其他DKC好。

第四节介绍了Naegeli-Franceschetti-Jadassohn综合症，是由于常染色体中KRT14基因突变所致外胚层发育异常。该疾病主要临床表现为颈部和腋窝网状色素沉着，指甲、牙齿和出汗异常。其组织学改变为真皮浅层大量黑色素细胞，周边片状表皮色素沉着过度，外分泌腺数量和结构均正常。

第五节介绍了网状色素性皮肤病，首先列举了该病的一系列常见的临床表现，随后提出网状色素性皮肤病是一种罕见的常染色体显性疾病，并描述了该病的组织学改变，为明显的色素失禁、基底细胞液化变性和真皮胶原玻璃样变。

第六节介绍了Dowling-Degos病，是一种罕见的常染色体显性遗传性色素异常性疾病。本病由染色体12q13.13上的KRT5基因突变所致，以网状色素沉着过度和带有痤疮状的口周凹陷和粉刺状的角化丘疹为特征，特征性的病理变化为从表皮和毛囊漏斗部发出的丝状有色素沉着的突出的上皮脚，而黑素细胞没有增加。该疾病必须与黑棘皮病区别开来。疾病进展缓慢，通常从成年早期可见，没有性别偏向。

第七节简单介绍了Galli-Galli病，它被认为是Dowling-Degos病的有棘层松解的一种变异体。

第八节介绍了北村网状色素沉着，描述了疾病的特征性皮损及皮损的临床发展规律，分析了病因及病理生理，提出北村网状色素沉着是由ADAM10基因的突变（15q21.3）所致。本病组织学上可见黑素细胞数量和黑素生成活性均增加，并且存在表皮萎缩。须与Dowling-Degos病、Dohi色素沉着和网状色素性皮病相鉴别。

第九节简单介绍了哈伯综合症，提到患者除了在躯干和腋窝上出现网状色素沉着之外，在躯干还有疣状丘疹样皮损以及明显的光敏性酒渣鼻样面部红斑和毛细血管扩张，最常见于儿童期。

第十到第十三节介绍了太田痣、伊藤痣、蒙古斑、皮肤黑素细胞错构瘤这一组相似的疾病，将其流行病学特点、临床表现、分布、组织学改变、治疗要点及其他相关特点总结归纳于表77-1中。本组疾病各自临床表现展示于图77-2至图77-6中。在该组疾病中，着重介绍了皮肤黑素细胞错构瘤。皮肤黑素细胞错构瘤是由先天因素所导致的以皮肤出现界限分明的色素沉着及着色性斑片为特征的一组疾病，包括Peutz-Jeghers综合征、LEOPARD综合征（着色斑，心电图异常，眼部玻璃体肥大，肺动脉狭窄，生殖器异常，发育迟缓和耳聋）、Carney综合征、Bannayan-Ruvalcaba-Riley综合征和面中部着色斑病。分别就这几个综合作了详细描述。

第十四节介绍了牛奶咖啡斑（CALM），首先描述了牛奶咖啡斑的特点，CALM是界限分明的色素沉着形成的斑片，大小从0.5厘米到更大不等，甚至超过20厘米，通常在出生时出现或出现在生命的头几个月。同时作者提到多发CALM是几种多系统疾病公认的标志物，可见于家族性多发性CALM（Legius综合征）、1型神经纤维瘤病、McCune-Albright综合征、Bloom综合征、Watson综合征和Silver-Russel综合征等。随后就上述几种多系统疾病作了详细阐述。

随后介绍了获得性色素沉着过度性疾病。本节共介绍了17种不同相关因素所导致的获得性色素沉着过度性疾病，并分别从流行病学、临床特征、病因和发病机理、诊断、鉴别诊断、病程、预后和处理等方面来对各疾病进行了详细讨论。

第十五节介绍了内分泌疾病相关的色素沉着，列举了一系列可能引起色素沉着性改变的内分泌系统疾病。作者首先指出在诸如Addison病、Cushing综合征、Nelson综合征、嗜铬细胞瘤、类癌综合征、甲状腺功能亢进症、黑棘皮病和糖尿病等疾病中可能会存在弥漫性、非模式化的色素沉着过度；而在黑棘皮病和成年后皮肤色素异常等情况下可能会出现局限性色素沉着。接下来详细描述了上述疾病中皮肤色素改变的特征，并将特征性的临床表现展示于图77-7至图77-8中。

第十六节介绍了营养性疾病所导致的色素沉着改变。首先提出弥漫性、无规律性的色素变化可继发于营养状况，例如营养不良，维生素B12缺乏，叶酸缺乏或糙皮病。如果纠正营养不足，皮肤变化是可逆的。随后从病因、临床特点及各自代表性的色素沉着改变等方面详细阐述了上述几个营养性疾病。

第十七节介绍了与代谢相关的色素沉着，列举了两种可能导致弥漫性非模式化色素沉着的代谢性疾病：皮肤卟啉病和血色素沉着病。并就这两种疾病的病因、临床特点及皮损特征等作了详细阐述。

第十八节介绍了与肿瘤情况相关的色素沉着，提到肥大细胞疾病和黑素瘤可以导致弥漫性的非模式化的色素沉着，在第四十二章和第一百一十六章也分别有详细讨论。

第十九节介绍了与物理因素相关的色素沉着，主要探讨了紫外线、电离辐射、热辐射、创伤如摩擦性黑变病所导致的获得性色素沉着改变。紫外线、电离和热辐射可能引起受影响的区域发生弥漫性非模式化的色素沉着；而创伤则可能导致慢性摩擦区域的色素沉着过度。

第二十节介绍了与中毒和药物因素相关的色素沉着，从临床表现、病因病理、诊断、预后及治疗五个方面阐述了中毒和药物因素所致的色素沉着性疾病。表77-2中归纳了已被报道可导致色素沉着性疾病的各类常见药物；图77-9至图77-12则展示了毒物及药物因素所致特征性色素沉着改变。

第二十一节介绍了褐黄病，褐黄病可能为先天性疾病或因使用某些药物所致。本章作者主要探讨外源性褐黄病，分别从流行病学、临床表现、病因病理、诊断、鉴别诊断、预后及治疗等方面作出详细阐述。

第二十二节简单介绍了系统性硬皮病伴发的各种色素沉着性改变，在第六十三章有更详细的阐述。

第二十三节介绍了与感染因素相关的色素沉着，主要提到了奇昆古尼亚热，分别从流行病学、临床表现、病因病理、诊断、鉴别诊断、预后及治疗等方面作出详细阐述。

第二十四节介绍了生理性色素沉着，列举了色素分界线（PDLs）、获得性特发性面部色素沉着、眼周色素沉着、黏膜黑素沉着病、纵向黑甲、肢端色素沉着斑等疾病，并从流行病学、临床表现、病因病理、诊断、鉴别诊断、预后及治疗等方面详细描述了上述疾病的特点。图77-13、图77-14和图77-15分别展示了色素分界线、眼周色素沉着及黏膜黑素病的皮损特点。

第二十五节介绍了获得性模式化色素沉着症，提出植物日光性皮炎、博来霉素引起的鞭毛状色素沉着和鞭毛状蘑菇性皮炎都是造成模式化色素沉着的原因，并简述了上述疾病的特点及特征性皮损形态。

第二十六节介绍了火激红斑和色素性痒疹，这两种疾病均以网状色沉为主要临床特点。其中火激红斑是由于经常暴露于热（通常是红外辐射）导致的网状色素沉着，大腿和小腿部位多见。色素性痒疹则多见于躯干。本节分别从上述两类疾病的临床表现、病因病理、诊断、鉴别诊断、预后及治疗等方面进行了详细描述，并在图77-16及图77-17中展示了皮损特点。

第二十七节介绍了以局限性色素增多为代表的一组疾病，包括颧部褐青色痣、贝克痣、牛奶咖啡斑、雀斑、进行性肢端色素沉着病、炎症后色素沉着（PIH）、黄褐斑、部分单侧性雀斑样痣（PUL）、Riehl黑变病。本节分别从流行病学、临床表现、病因病理、诊断、鉴别诊断、预后及治疗等方面详细阐述，并在图77-18及图77-24中展示了各疾病的皮损特点，在表77-3中列举了治疗PIH的外用药物及作用机制。

第二十八节介绍了Cronkhite-Canada综合征和色素性口周红斑这两个非常罕见的色素沉着性疾病。本节分别从流行病学、临床表现、病因病理、诊断、鉴别诊断、预后及治疗等方面作了详细阐述。

第二十九节简单提到了其他能导致色素沉着的疾病，如皮肤淀粉样变、帕西尼-皮耶里尼萎缩皮病、固定型药疹。

第三十节介绍了持久性色素异常性红斑和色素性扁平苔藓这两类特发性发疹性斑状色素沉着症，同样从流行病学、临床表现、病因病理、诊断、鉴别诊断、预后及治疗对上述疾病作了详细阐述。其中图77-25至图77-27展示了持久性色素异常红斑的皮损特点。

第三十一节分别介绍了可导致混合性色素减退和色素沉着的五种疾病，包括遗传性泛发性色素异常症、遗传性对称性色素异常症、多伊网状肢端色素沉着、家族性进行性色素沉着症（Westerhof综合征）伴或不伴色素减退、Vagabond's白斑病。

〔李　吉〕

CONGENITAL HYPERMELANOSIS

LINEAR AND WHORLED NEVOID HYPERMELANOSIS

AT-A-GLANCE

- Congenital diffuse streaky hyperpigmented macules in Blaschko lines.
- Typically seen on the trunk and extremities.
- No preceding inflammation or atrophy.
- Onset in the first few weeks of life.
- May fade with advancing age.

Linear and whorled nevoid hypermelanosis is a congenital condition causing diffuse streaky hyperpigmented macules along the lines of Blaschko.[1]

CLINICAL FEATURES

Linear and whorled nevoid hypermelanosis is characterized by widespread streaky hyperpigmented macules along the lines of Blaschko without preceding inflammation or atrophy in the first few weeks of life. Lesions are typically located on the trunk and limbs and do not cross the midline. Face, palms, soles, eyes, and mucous membranes are spared. Similar cases have been described under different descriptive names (*zosteriform hyperpigmentation*, *zosteriform lentiginous nevus*, *zebra-like hyperpigmentation*). Several cases have been reported with both hyperpigmentation and hypopigmentation. *Pigmentary mosaicism* is a useful term to encompass all these different phenotypes.

Rarely, extracutaneous manifestations, such as developmental and growth retardation, facial and body asymmetry, ventricular septal defects, and pseudohermaphroditism, are observed. The frequency of extracutaneous manifestations is unknown, as these observations have been made in case reports only.

ETIOLOGY AND PATHOGENESIS

Most cases are sporadic but the presence of mosaicism has been confirmed in a few cases (mosaic trisomies 7, 14, 18, and 20, and X-chromosomal mosaicism) by chromosomal analysis.[2]

DIAGNOSIS

In addition to the typical clinical appearance, histologic examination reveals increased pigmentation of the basal layer and prominence or vacuolization of melanocytes. Pigment incontinence is usually absent.

DIFFERENTIAL DIAGNOSIS

Linear and whorled nevoid hypermelanosis should be differentiated from incontinentia pigmenti (IP) and epidermal nevus.

CLINICAL COURSE AND PROGNOSIS

Kalter and colleagues[1] described typical onset in the first few weeks of life with progression during the initial years of life. The pigmentation may fade gradually with advancing age.

INCONTINENTIA PIGMENTI

AT-A-GLANCE

- X-linked dominant disorder resulting from mutation in the *IKBKG* (previously called *NEMO*) gene.
- Lethal in male embryos.
- Four clinical phases commencing at birth: vesicular, verrucous, hyperpigmented, and hypopigmented.
- Congenital diffuse linear hyperpigmented macules in Blaschko lines.

IP, also known as Bloch-Sulzberger syndrome, was first described by Garrod and colleagues in 1906. It is an X-linked disorder primarily seen in females, which results in diffuse linear cutaneous hyperpigmentation.

CLINICAL FEATURES

Lesions usually proceed through 4 cutaneous stages, although the stages may sometimes overlap: (a) vesicular stage (from birth or shortly thereafter), which presents with multiple small and medium-sized vesicles following the lines of Blaschko; (b) verrucous stage (between 2 and 8 weeks of age) consisting of wart-like plaques; (c) hyperpigmented stage (several months of age into adulthood); and (d) hypopigmented stage (from infancy onwards) (Fig. 77-1).

The degree of hyperpigmentation varies among individuals but appears in streaks and whorls along Blaschko lines. Although it can appear on the limbs, it is usually pronounced on the trunk. The hypopigmented

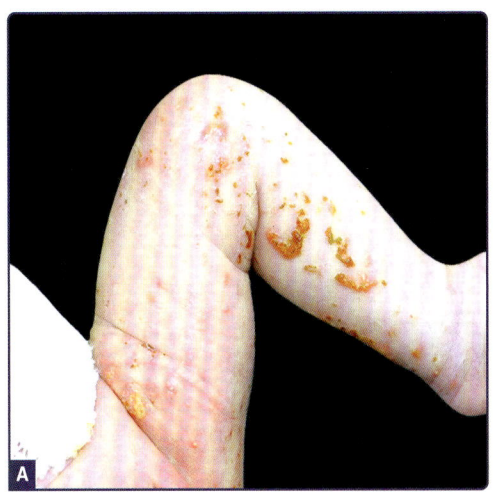

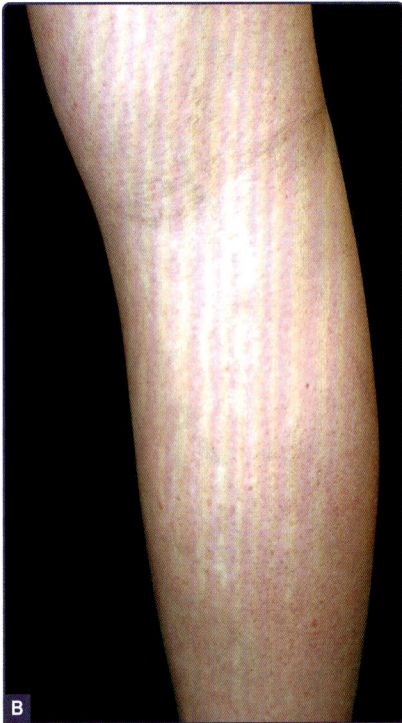

Figure 77-1 Incontinentia pigmenti in a mother and her baby. **A,** Verrucous lesions in a 2-week-old baby. **B,** Hypopigmented atrophic lesions following Blaschko lines.

stage is characterized by linear, atrophic, hairless scars along Blaschko lines.

ETIOLOGY AND PATHOGENESIS

IP is an X-linked, dominantly inherited disorder believed to be embryonically lethal in the majority of males. In most cases, IP is caused by a mutation in the *IKBKG* gene (previously called *NEMO* [nuclear factor κB (NF-κB) essential modulator]) on the X chromosome at Xq28.[3,4] The gene encodes a regulatory component of the IKappaB kinase complex that activates the NF-κB pathway, which is required to protect against tumor necrosis factor-α–induced apoptosis.[5]

In females with IP, inactivation of 1 of the 2 X chromosomes through a process termed *lyonization* occurs during embryogenesis. Epidermal cells expressing the defective *IKBKG* gene give rise to typical skin lesions along the lines of Blaschko, reflecting the embryonic migration path of the affected keratinocytes.

The cutaneous lesions in the vesicular stage represent the population of *IKBKG*-deficient cells that fail to activate NF-κB, leading to apoptosis. The number of *IKBKG*-deficient cells decreases secondary to apoptosis and is replaced by cells expressing the normal allele. Subsequently, the inflammatory and vesicular stage ends. The hyperproliferation in the second stage is likely a result of compensatory proliferation of normal IKBKG keratinocytes. Hyperpigmentation in the third stage results from incontinence of epidermal melanin pigment, which then migrates into the dermis and is engulfed by macrophages.

Extracutaneous manifestations occur in a significant number of patients with IP. Ocular (30% to 70%), CNS (40%), dental, and skeletal anomalies are among the most common.

DIAGNOSIS

Histologically, the number of melanocytes appears to be normal, although a reduced number of melanocytes have been noted. The thin epidermis and absence or reduction of skin appendages in the dermis may contribute to the impression of hypopigmentation.

Histologically, the areas of pigmentation show many melanin-laden melanophages, extensive deposits of melanin in the basal cell layer and dermis. Epidermal basal layer vacuolization and degeneration is also noted.

CLINICAL COURSE AND PROGNOSIS

Usually the hyperpigmentation fades gradually over several years, leaving hypopigmented skin (stage 4), which represents postinflammatory dermal scarring.

MANAGEMENT

A beneficial effect of topical steroids and topical tacrolimus in the vesicular stage has been reported.[6] Hypopigmented and atrophic scarring may be amenable to noncultured epidermal cell grafting.[7]

DYSKERATOSIS CONGENITA

AT-A-GLANCE

- Congenital diffuse reticular hyperpigmentation with nail atrophy and leukoplakia.
- Manifests in the first few years of life.
- Extracutaneous manifestations are bone marrow failure and malignancies.

Dyskeratosis congenital (DKC) or *Zinsser-Cole-Engman syndrome* is characterized by cutaneous and hematologic manifestations.

CLINICAL FEATURES

Reticulate skin pigmentation especially on the neck and chest, nail atrophy in fingernails and toenails, and leukoplakia are seen in those with DKC.

Extracutaneous manifestations include bone marrow failure (in more than 80% of cases) and malignancy in the second and third decades of life.

ETIOLOGY AND PATHOGENESIS

In all cases of DKC, the causative mutations are present in components of the telomerase complex. Rapidly dividing somatic cells express low but detectable levels of telomerase activity that slows telomere shortening occurring with each cycle of DNA replication, which eventually leads to cellular senescence (permanent loss of proliferative capacity). It is now thought that DKC is caused by defective telomere maintenance, which limits the proliferative capacity of hematopoietic and epithelial cells. Increased melanin synthesis occurs in senescent melanocytes, which is likely to account for the pigmentary changes noted in DKC. Critically short telomeres may force cells into "replicative crisis," at which time activation of an alternative "ALT" mechanism for lengthening telomeres in the absence of telomerase may lead to development of malignancies. The role of telomeres in cell biology (cellular aging) was actually first demonstrated through the finding of short telomeres in DKC.[8]

X-linked DKC is caused by mutations in the *DKC1* gene located at Xq28, encoding for dyskerin. Females carrying 1 mutated allele are protected by expression of normal telomerase on the unaffected allele. In autosomal dominant DKC, the majority of cases are caused by mutations in TERC, the RNA component of the telomerase complex. TERT (telomerase reverse transcriptase) is affected much less often in autosomal dominant DKC. In the autosomal recessive form of DKC, mutations in telomerase-associated proteins such as NOP10, NHP2, and TINF2 are involved.[9]

DIAGNOSIS

Skin biopsy of hyperpigmented skin does not demonstrate specific changes. Epidermal atrophy and a chronic inflammatory cell infiltrate with numerous melanophages in the upper dermis are usually observed in histology.

DIFFERENTIAL DIAGNOSIS

DKC may be confused with Fanconi syndrome, which is characterized by short stature, hypoplastic or aplastic thumbs, and a reduced number of carpal bones. The patchy hyperpigmentation of the trunk, neck, groin, and axillary regions in Fanconi syndrome appears earlier than in DKC, that is, in the first few years of life.

CLINICAL COURSE AND PROGNOSIS

The autosomal dominant form has a better prognosis than other forms, possibly because of the presence of an unaffected allele with some preservation of telomerase activity. Usually, the hyperpigmentation fades gradually after several years.

NAEGELI-FRANCESCHETTI-JADASSOHN SYNDROME

AT-A-GLANCE

- Autosomal ectodermal dysplasias.
- Reticulate hyperpigmentation on the neck and axillae.
- Nail, teeth, and sweating abnormalities.

CLINICAL FEATURES

Reticulate hyperpigmentation is most prominent in neck and axillae. Palmoplantar diffuse keratoderma, absence of dermatoglyphs, nail and teeth changes, and heat intolerance owing to diminished or absent sweating are characteristic.[10]

ETIOLOGY AND PATHOGENESIS

The Naegeli-Franceschetti-Jadassohn syndrome and the related dermatopathia pigmentosa reticularis are autosomal dominant ectodermal dysplasias caused by mutations in the *KRT14* gene.[11] The *KRT14* gene codes for keratin 14, which, together with keratin 5, forms intermediate keratin filaments. Keratin 14 is predominantly produced by the keratinocytes in the basal cell layer of the epidermis. Mutations in *KRT14* gene lead to fragility of basal keratinocytes. It plays an important role during ontogenesis of dermatoglyphs and sweat glands.[12]

Dermatopathia pigmentosa reticularis has been distinguished from Naegeli-Franceschetti-Jadassohn syndrome by lifelong persistence of skin hyperpigmentation, partial alopecia, and absence of dental anomalies. Both disorders have been mapped to 17q11.2-q21 and are considered to be allelic.[11]

HISTOLOGY

There are numerous melanophages in the upper dermis, next to a patchy epidermal hyperpigmentation. Eccrine glands histologically appear normal in number and structure.

DERMATOPATHIA PIGMENTOSA RETICULARIS

AT-A-GLANCE

- Autosomal dominant.
- Reticulate hyperpigmentation on the trunk.
- Nail, sweating, and ocular abnormalities with nonscarring alopecia.

CLINICAL FEATURES

Reticulate hyperpigmentation on the trunk, palmoplantar keratoderma with punctiform accentuation, nail and ocular changes, noncicatricial alopecia, ichthyosis, hypohidrosis, widespread hyperkeratotic lesions, ainhum formation, severe periodontal disease, mechanic blister formation, and pigmentation of the oral mucosa are all seen in this condition.[13]

ETIOLOGY AND PATHOGENESIS

Dermatopathia pigmentosa reticularis is a rare autosomal dominant condition.

HISTOLOGY

Histologic examination shows pronounced pigmentary incontinence, liquefaction degeneration of the basal cell layer and hyalinization of dermal collagen.

DOWLING-DEGOS DISEASE

AT-A-GLANCE

- Autosomal dominant.
- Reticulate hyperpigmentation in the flexures with acneiform perioral pits and comedo-like hyperkeratotic papules.

CLINICAL FEATURES

Numerous small symmetrical brown-gray macules usually begin in the groin and axillae in the third or fourth decade of life and then spread to intergluteal and inframammary folds, neck, trunk, and arms. Comedo-like hyperkeratotic follicular papules on the neck and axilla and pitted perioral acneiform scars also appear.[14]

ETIOLOGY AND PATHOGENESIS

This rare autosomal dominant genodermatosis (synonym: *reticular pigmented anomaly of the flexures*) is cause by mutations in the *KRT5* gene on chromosome 12q13.13. Betz and colleagues demonstrated that haploinsufficiency in keratin 5 causes epithelial remodeling, melanosome mistargeting, and altered perinuclear organization of intermediate filaments.[14] Keratin 5 and keratin 14 are 2 proteins that together form a keratin intermediate filament. It is hypothesized that keratin 5 haploinsufficiency causes an excess of keratin 14 that could be responsible for the pathology of Dowling-Degos disease by competing with transport adapters. Keratins could regulate the availability and positioning of AP-3 complexes in keratinocytes or alternatively could regulate the interaction of AP-3–dependent vesicles with motor proteins.

HISTOLOGY

The histology is very characteristic with filiform rete projections from both epidermis and follicular infundibulum with hyperpigmented tips, without an increase of melanocytes. The disorder has to be differentiated from acanthosis nigricans, which has a different histologic appearance.

CLINICAL COURSE AND PROGNOSIS

Progression of the hyperpigmentation is slow and usually is visible from early adult life, without sex predilection.

GALLI-GALLI DISEASE

Patients with Galli-Galli disease show the diagnostic features of Dowling-Degos disease with the additional histopathologic finding of acantholysis in suprabasal epidermal layers. It is regarded as the acantholytic variant of Dowling-Degos disease. Mutations in the keratin 5 gene have been found in some patients.[15]

KITAMURA RETICULAR ACROPIGMENTATION

AT-A-GLANCE

- Autosomal dominant.
- Reticulate hyperpigmentation in the flexures with acneiform perioral pits and comedo-like hyperkeratotic papules.

CLINICAL FEATURES

Kitamura reticular acropigmentation is characterized by angular and sharply demarcated reticulate, freckle-like hyperpigmented macules (but no hypopigmentation as seen in Dohi disorder [see section "Mixed Hypomelanosis and Hypermelanosis"]) beginning on the dorsa of the hands during the first decade of life and subsequently spreading to the rest of the body. The macules are slightly depressed; sometimes palmar pits can be observed. Most cases are from Japan.

ETIOLOGY AND PATHOGENESIS

Mutations in the *ADAM10* gene (15q21.3). *ADAM10* encodes for a zinc metalloprotease, a disintegrin, and a metalloprotease domain containing protein 10, which is involved in the shedding of skin substrates.[16]

HISTOLOGY

There is an increased number of melanocytes and melanogenic activity, and epidermal atrophy is present upon histologic examination.

DIFFERENTIAL DIAGNOSIS

Dowling-Degos disease, acropigmentation of Dohi, and dermatopathia pigmentosa reticularis are all in the differential diagnosis of Kitamura reticular acropigmentation.

HABER SYNDROME

Next to a reticulate pigmentation on trunk and axillae, patients with Haber disease also develop verruciformis papular lesions of the trunk and a distinct photosensitive rosacea-like facial erythema and telangiectasias, most commonly presenting in childhood.[17]

NEVUS OF OTA

AT-A-GLANCE

- Congenital circumscribed tan-brown hyperpigmentation with dermal melanocytosis.
- Unilateral pigmentation in the area of the first and second branches of the trigeminal nerve.
- Of those affected, 60% have scleral involvement.
- Mostly occurs in Asian females.

Nevus of Ota (nevus fuscoceruleus ophthalmomaxillaris) was first described by Ota in 1939.[18] It is characterized by blue-black or gray-brown dermal melanocytic pigmentation on the face.

EPIDEMIOLOGY

Even though nevus of Ota has been described in different skin types, it is most commonly seen in the Asian population with 0.6% of this population affected.[19,20] Onset is usually noted at birth and in females, although it may be noted for the first time in early childhood or puberty.

CLINICAL FEATURES

Unilateral blue-black or gray-brown dermal melanocytic pigmentation is typically seen in areas innervated by the first and second branches of the trigeminal nerve.[21] Nevus of Ota is now subclassified as mild (Type 1), moderate (Type 2), intensive (Type 3), and bilateral (Type 4).

Of those affected, 60% have scleral pigmentation. Other sites of mucosal pigmentation include the conjunctiva and tympanic membrane (oculodermal melanocytosis) (Fig. 77-2).

Malignant melanoma may rarely develop in a nevus of Ota. This necessitates careful followup of the lesion, especially if it occurs in white patients, in whom malignant degeneration seems to be more frequent. Malignant melanocytic tumors in association with nevus of Ota have been shown to arise in the chorioidea, brain, orbit, iris, ciliary body, and optic nerve. In addition, association with ipsilateral glaucoma and intracranial melanocytosis has been described.

ETIOLOGY AND PATHOGENESIS

Various triggers, including infection, trauma, ultraviolet light exposure, and hormonal influences, have been described.

DIAGNOSIS

The diagnosis is usually made clinically but may be confirmed on histology, which reveals evenly spread melanocytes throughout the entire dermis.

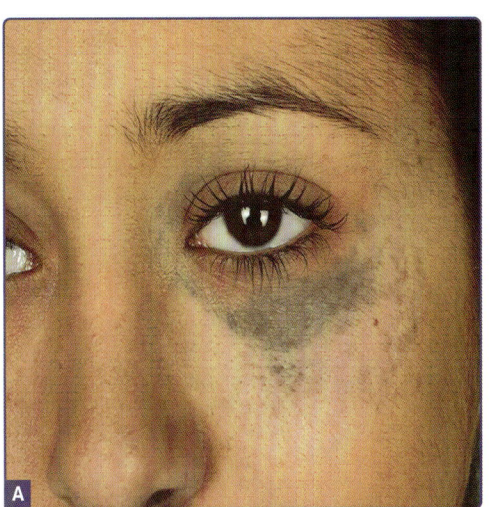

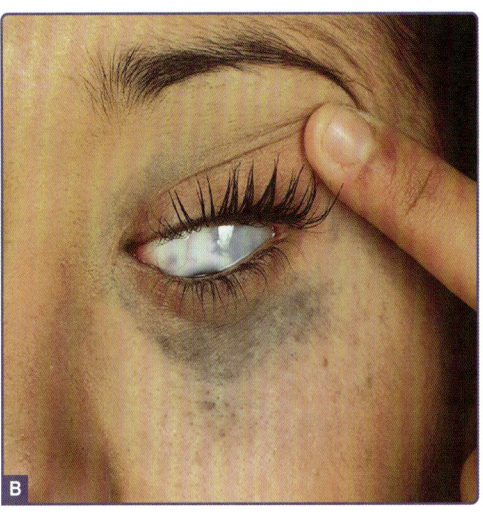

Figure 77-2 Nevus of Ota in a 20-year-old woman. **A,** Hyperpigmentation around the orbit. **B,** The hyperpigmentation extends into the sclera.

DIFFERENTIAL DIAGNOSIS

Bilateral cases should be differentiated from Hori nevus, which is acquired, does not have mucosal involvement, and is less pigmented.

Other dermal melanocytoses include nevus of Ito, Mongolian spots, and dermal melanocyte hamartomas (Table 77-1). Associated vascular malformations have been described in phakomatosis pigmentovascularis (port-wine stain type, Klippel-Trenaunay or Sturge-Weber syndrome).

CLINICAL COURSE AND PROGNOSIS

Nevus of Ota is persistent and does not usually undergo spontaneous regression.

MANAGEMENT

Topical therapies are ineffective in the treatment of this dermal pigmentation. Even though cryotherapy and surgery have been used in the past, they should be avoided because of significant scarring. Laser surgery is the treatment of choice with quality-switched (QS) lasers including quality-switched ruby laser, QS alexandrite laser and QS neodymium:yttrium-aluminum-garnet (Nd:YAG) laser having the most success in the treatment of this condition. Picosecond lasers also have been reported as effective in treating this condition.[22]

NEVUS OF ITO

AT-A-GLANCE

- Congenital circumscribed brown-tan hyperpigmentation with dermal melanocytosis.
- Considered a variant of nevus of Ota.
- Involvement of the acromioclavicular and deltoid region.

Nevus of Ito is a congenital dermal melanocytosis first described by Ito in 1954 as nevus fuscoceruleus acromiodeltoideus.[23] It can be considered as a variant of nevus of Ota.

Clinical, demographic, and histologic characteristics are similar to nevus of Ota and both lesions can occur simultaneously (see Table 77-1 and Fig. 77-3).

MONGOLIAN SPOTS

AT-A-GLANCE

- Congenital circumscribed blue-tinged hyperpigmentation caused by dermal melanocytosis.
- Mainly occurs in persons with skin of color.
- Usually occurs in the sacral region.

EPIDEMIOLOGY

Mongolian spots are more common in the African, Asian, and Hispanic populations and are only rarely seen in whites.[24] They occur in both sexes with a slight male predominance.

TABLE 77-1
Differential Diagnosis and Management of Dermal Melanocytosis

	NEVUS OF OTA	NEVUS OF ITO	MONGOLIAN SPOT	NEVUS OF HORI	DERMAL MELANOCYTE HAMARTOMA
Epidemiology	• Mostly congenital • Sporadic (rare familial cases) • Asian and female predominance	• Mostly congenital • Sporadic (rare familial cases) • Asian and female predominance	• Congenital • Often familial • Asian, African, and Hispanic populations with slight male predominance	• Acquired • Familial or sporadic • Asian and female predominance	• Congenital
Clinical presentation	• Blue to slate-gray mottled macular hyperpigmentation	• Blue to slate-gray mottled macular hyperpigmentation	• Uniform blue to slate-gray macular hyperpigmentation	• Brown-blue progressing to slate-gray mottled macular hyperpigmentation	• Mottled hyperpigmentation with small blue-gray macules in a diffuse pigmented patch
Distribution	• Trigeminal nerve	• Acromioclavicular nerve	• Lower back and sacrum	• Especially malar region of the cheek (also forehead, upper eyelids, temple)	• Dermatomal distribution
Histology	• Spindle-shaped melanocytes diffusely throughout the dermal layers; sometimes more band-like melanocytic proliferation and stromal fibrotic reaction	• Spindle-shaped melanocytes diffusely throughout the dermal layers; sometimes more band-like melanocytic proliferation and stromal fibrotic reaction	• Spindle-shaped melanocytes diffusely throughout the dermal layers	• Dermal melanocytes in the upper and mid dermis	• Dermal melanocytes in the upper two-thirds of the dermis (including subpapillary layer)
Therapy	• Quality-switched laser • Cryotherapy • Surgery	• Quality-switched laser • Cryotherapy • Surgery	• Usually spontaneous regression during childhood	• Quality-switched laser in combination with bleaching cream and chemical peels	• None
Associated features	• Rare malignant transformation	• No associated features of medical concern	• Possible association with inborn errors of metabolism	• No associated features of medical concern	• None

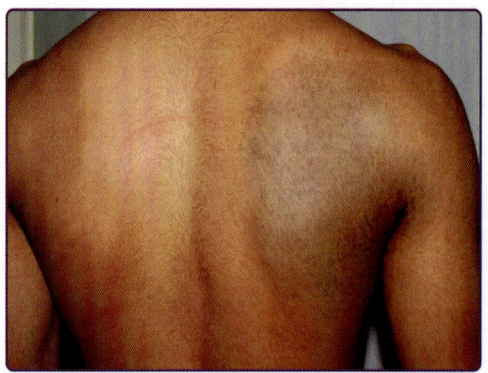

Figure 77-3 Nevus of Ito on the back of a Middle Eastern adolescent.

CLINICAL FEATURES

Well-circumscribed, blue-tinged hyperpigmented macules in the sacral area are most commonly seen (Fig. 77-4). Mongolian spots also can be found in the gluteal and lumbar regions and on the thorax, abdomen, arms, legs, and shoulders.

Several cases are described with extensive Mongolian spots involving large areas of the trunk and extremities that are associated with inborn errors of metabolism, such as lysosomal storage diseases, GM_1-gangliosidosis and mucopolysaccharidosis.[25]

ETIOLOGY AND PATHOGENESIS

Histologically, these macules consist of spindle-shaped melanocytes in the lower dermis that have failed to migrate to the dermal–epidermal junction during fetal life.

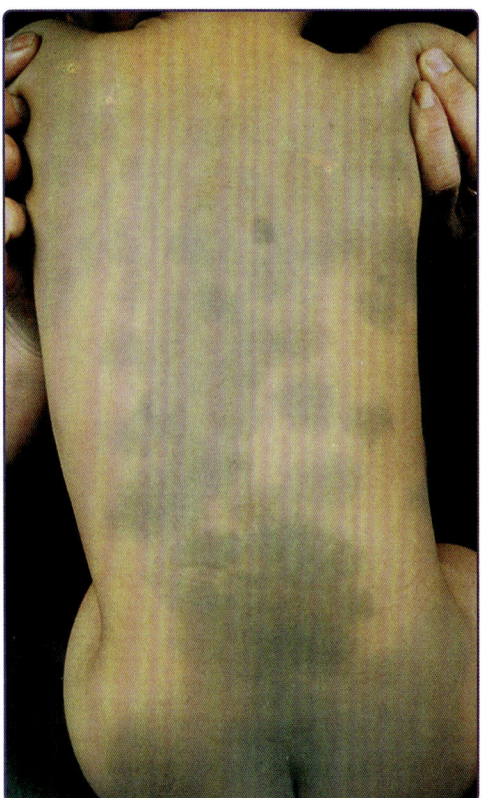

Figure 77-4 Classic Mongolian spots in the lumbosacral region and aberrant or extrasacral Mongolian spots on the back.

DERMAL MELANOCYTE HAMARTOMA

AT-A-GLANCE

- Congenital, circumscribed, blue-tinged hyperpigmentation with dermal melanocytosis.
- Dermatomal patterns have been described.

Dermal melanocyte hamartoma is a distinctive form of congenital dermal melanocytosis, first described by Burkhart and colleagues in 1981.[26] Gray-blue pigmentation, caused by melanocytes residing in the dermis, occurs in a dermatomal pattern.

FAMILIAL LENTIGINOSIS SYNDROMES

AT-A-GLANCE

- Congenital conditions causing well-circumscribed pigmentation with lentiginosis.
- Causes include Peutz-Jeghers syndrome, LEOPARD (lentigines, electrocardiographic abnormalities, ocular hypertelorism, pulmonary stenosis, abnormalities of genitalia, retardation of growth, and deafness) syndrome, Carney complex, Bannayan-Ruvalcaba-Riley syndrome, and centrofacial lentiginosis.

DIAGNOSIS

The diagnosis is usually made clinically, but may be confirmed on histology.

DIFFERENTIAL DIAGNOSIS

Table 77-1 outlines the differential diagnosis and management of Mongolian spots.

CLINICAL COURSE AND PROGNOSIS

In most cases, Mongolian spots spontaneously regress during childhood, but persistence into adulthood has been described.

MANAGEMENT

Spontaneous resolution usually means treatment can be avoided but laser treatment in childhood or adolescence can give favorable results, especially in sacral Mongolian spots.

Familial lentiginosis syndromes are characterized by the presence of lentigines—well-circumscribed brown macules (usually <5 mm in diameter), which have an increased number of melanocytes in the epidermis (epidermal melanocytic hypermelanosis) and an increased incidence of cardiovascular, endocrine, or GI neoplasias. Familial lentiginosis syndromes include Carney complex, Peutz-Jeghers syndrome (PJS), LEOPARD syndrome (lentigines, electrocardiogram conduction defects, ocular hypertelorism, pulmonary stenosis, abnormalities of genitalia, retardation of growth, and sensorineural deafness), arterial dissection and lentiginosis, Laugier-Hunziker syndrome, familial benign lentiginosis, Bannayan-Ruvalcaba-Riley syndrome (BRRS), centrofacial lentiginosis, and segmental and agminated lentiginosis.[27] Genetic loci and gene mutations have been identified for Carney complex, PJS, and BRRS.

PEUTZ-JEGHERS SYNDROME

PJS was first described by Peutz (1921) and Jeghers (1949).[28] It is a rare autosomal dominant genodermatosis with a predisposition for development of malignancies. More than half of all cases of PJS can be attributed to a mutation in STK11 (LKB1) on chromosome 19 (19q13.3),[29] which is thought to act as a tumor-suppressor gene. Close surveillance of PJS patients for malignancies from a young age is warranted.

Mucocutaneous pigmentation and intestinal hamartomatous polyposis are hallmarks of the condition (Fig. 77-5). The pigmentary lesions resemble those of Carney complex, with small hyperpigmented (brown-gray) macules typically appearing in childhood (not present at birth) on the lips and buccal mucosa; however, they may also involve the eyelids, hands, and feet. Quality-switched laser or intense pulsed light can be used to treat the pigmented lesions.

The most common malignancies associated with PJS are GI (small intestine, colorectal, stomach, pancreas), but nongastrointestinal neoplasms, such as breast, cervix, and endocrine tumors (thyroid, testicular, ovarian), have been described.

LEOPARD SYNDROME

LEOPARD syndrome is a rare autosomal dominant condition caused by a heterozygous missense mutation in the *PTPN11* gene, coding for the protein tyrosine phosphatase SHP-2 and situated on chromosome 12 (12q24.1). LEOPARD syndrome is allelic to Noonan syndrome and shares several clinical features with this disorder.[30] The characteristic lentigines usually develop during childhood and in the first months of life (Fig. 77-6). Clinical diagnosis is primarily based on the typical facial features and the presence of hypertrophic cardiomyopathy and/or café-au-lait macules (CALMs). Recently, missense mutations in the *RAF1* gene were found in 2 LEOPARD syndrome patients in whom no *PTPN11* mutations could be discovered.

CARNEY COMPLEX

Carney complex is an autosomal dominant disorder first described by Carney and colleagues in 1985.[31] Clinical components of Carney complex include spotty skin pigmentation, myxomas (heart, skin, breast), endocrine tumors (primary pigmented nodular adrenal disease [Cushing syndrome], testicular large-cell calcifying Sertoli cell tumor [sexual precocity], pituitary adenoma [acromegaly], thyroid tumors, ovarian cysts), and schwannomas.[27] Multiple types of hyperpigmentation, such as lentigines, ephelides, blue nevi, junctional, dermal and compound nevi, and café-au-lait spots, have been described.[32] The typical lesions consist

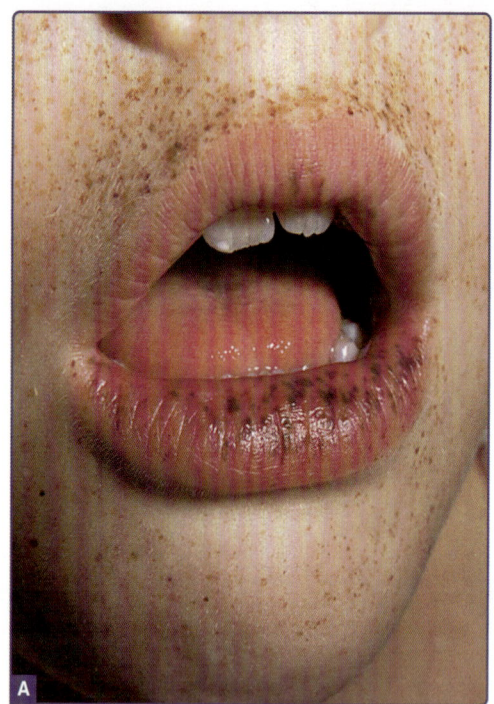
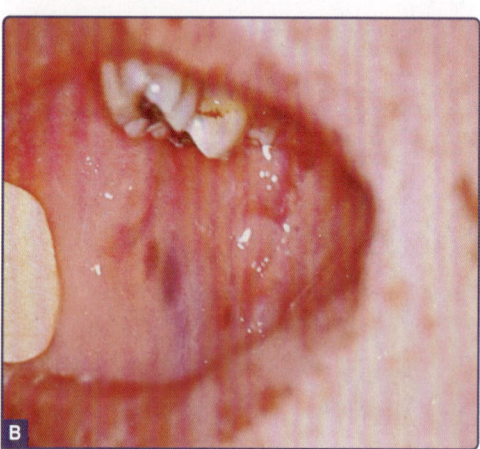

Figure 77-5 Peutz-Jeghers syndrome. **A,** Lentigines, which are dark-brown to gray-blue, appear on the lips, around the mouth, and on the fingers. Lip macules may, over time, disappear. **B,** Macules of the buccal mucosa are blue to blue-black and are pathognomonic; unlike lip lesions, these do not tend to disappear with time.

of spotty centrofacial pigmentation involving the vermilion border of the lips, the lacrimal caruncle, the conjunctival semilunar fold, and sometimes the sclera. Intraoral-pigmented spots are present in a limited number of cases. In at least half of the patients with Carney complex, a mutation in the gene encoding protein kinase A regulatory subunit 1A (PRKAR1A) mapped to 17q22-24 has been identified.[33]

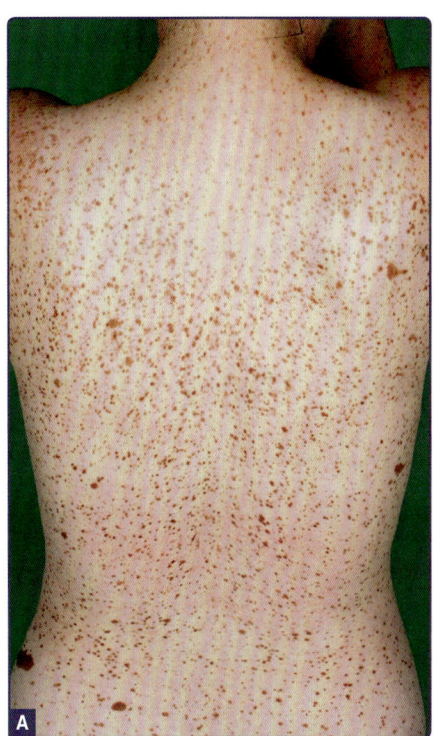

(b) Bannayan-Zonana, and (c) Ruvalcaba-Myhre-Smith syndromes.[34] It is characterized by the classical triad of macrocephaly, genital lentiginosis, and intestinal polyposis. Besides the genital lentiginosis (sometimes presenting as larger CALMs), mucocutaneous manifestations include vascular malformations, lipomatosis, multiple acrochordons, and verrucous facial papules. More than 60% of BRRS patients show germline mutations in the *PTEN* (phosphatase and tensin homolog) gene on chromosome 10q23.3, a gene that is mutated in Cowden syndrome, which displays partial clinical overlap with BRRS[34] Recently, the PTEN hamartoma tumor syndrome, encompassing 4 allelic disorders (Cowden syndrome, BRRS, Proteus syndrome, and Proteus-like syndrome), has been described.[35]

CENTROFACIAL LENTIGINOSIS

A horizontal band of lentigines across the central face is the hallmark of the autosomal dominant centrofacial lentiginosis syndrome. Other associated signs and symptoms include bone abnormalities, endocrine dysfunctions, neural tube defects, and mental retardation.[36]

FAMILIAL CAFÉ-AU-LAIT SYNDROMES

AT-A-GLANCE

- Congenital circumscribed hypermelanosis with café-au-lait macules (CALMs) are seen in conditions like familial multiple CALMs (Legius syndrome), neurofibromatosis Type 1, McCune-Albright syndrome, Bloom syndrome, Watson syndrome, and Silver-Russel syndrome.
- Well circumscribed hypermelanosis with CALMs.

CALMs consist of well-demarcated hyperpigmented patches of skin, varying in size from 0.5 cm to more than 20 cm. They are often present at birth or appear in the first few months of life. Between 0.3% and 18% of all newborns display isolated CALMs.[37] Histologically, isolated CALMs show a normal number of melanocytes but increased epidermal melanin (epidermal melanotic hypermelanosis). Multiple CALMs are well-known markers for several multisystem disorders.

LEGIUS SYNDROME

Legius syndrome is also known as familial multiple CALMs and is autosomal dominant with mutations in the *SPRED1* gene (15q13.2). Multiple CALMs are present and axillary freckling and lipomas may be seen, but no neurofibromas are demonstrated. Macrocephaly and developmental delays are noted but are less severe than what is seen in neurofibromatosis Type 1.[38,39]

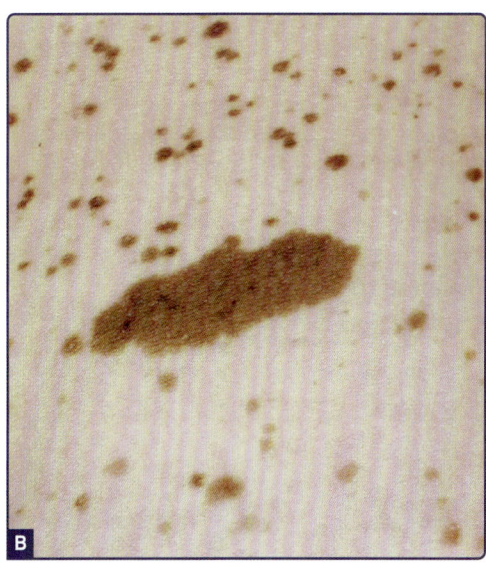

Figure 77-6 LEOPARD (lentigines, electrocardiogram conduction defects, ocular hypertelorism, pulmonary stenosis, abnormalities of genitalia, retardation of growth, and sensorineural deafness) syndrome. **A** and **B,** A 27-year-old woman with LEOPARD syndrome. Note the characteristic widespread lentigines and several café-au-lait macules.

BANNAYAN-RILEY-RUVALCABA SYNDROME

BRRS is a second autosomal dominant hamartomatous polyposis syndrome. This designation replaces 3 previously described entities: (a) Riley-Smith,

NEUROFIBROMATOSIS TYPE 1

Neurofibromatosis Type 1 (NF1) was first recognized by Friedrich von Recklinghausen in 1882 and is also called von Recklinghausen disease (see Chap. 135 for detailed discussions).

NF1 is an autosomal dominant disease caused by a mutation in the *NF1* gene that encodes the neurofibromin protein. The most important neurofibromin function involves downregulation of the Ras signal transduction pathway; consequently, it is considered a tumor-suppressor gene.

NF1 has been considered a neurocristopathy and is characterized by a number of cutaneous and noncutaneous pigment cell-related manifestations such as CALMs, intertriginous freckling, and iris Lisch nodules. (Chap. 135 discusses the clinical diagnostic criteria for NF1.) The presence of 6 or more CALMs larger than 5 mm in greatest diameter in prepubertal individuals or larger than 15 mm after puberty is one of the hallmarks of the disease. NF1-associated CALMs, contrary to isolated CALMs, contain a significantly increased number of melanocytes in the epidermis. Intertriginous freckles, pathognomonic for NF1, also display increased numbers of epidermal melanocytes, which differentiates them from ordinary freckles (ephelides).

MCCUNE-ALBRIGHT SYNDROME

McCune-Albright syndrome was first described by McCune (1936) and Albright (1937) as a triad of poly/monostotic fibrous dysplasia, CALMs, and hyperfunctioning endocrinopathies, including precocious puberty, hyperthyroidism, hypercortisolism, hypersomatotropism, and hypophosphatemic rickets.[40] The CALMs are fewer in number and have more irregular borders than those seen in NF1. They are classically demarcated at the midline. McCune-Albright syndrome is caused by a postzygotic activating mutation of the α subunit of the cyclic adenosine monophosphate–regulating Gs protein. Consequently, a mosaic distribution of McCune-Albright syndrome cells bears the constitutively active adenylate cyclase.

BLOOM SYNDROME

Bloom syndrome is a rare, autosomal recessive, genetic-immunodeficiency-and-cancer-predisposition syndrome. It is characterized by a growth deficiency, unusual facies, CALMs, and a sun sensitivity with telangiectasia and erythema that can result in atrophy and scarring. Neoplasias that occur frequently in Bloom syndrome are acute leukemia, lymphoma, and squamous cell carcinoma.[41] Bloom syndrome is caused by a DNA repair defect, which results in genomic instability, including a high frequency of sister-chromatid exchanges.[42] The causative gene *BLM* has been mapped to 15q26.1 and encodes the BLM RecQ helicase homolog protein, a well-known member of the DNA helicase family, closely related to the helicases that is also defective in Werner syndrome and Rothmund-Thomson syndrome.[43]

WATSON SYNDROME

Watson syndrome is an autosomal dominant condition made up of pulmonary valvular stenosis, CALMs, and lower intelligence, that was first described by Watson in 1967.[44] Later, the clinical phenotype of Watson syndrome was expanded with features overlapping with NF1 (macrocephaly, Lisch nodules, neurofibromas, short stature, intertriginous freckling), and it was shown to be allelic to NF1.[45] Recent studies suggest an overlap of Watson syndrome with neurofibromatosis-Noonan syndrome.

SILVER-RUSSELL SYNDROME

Silver–Russell syndrome (SRS) is a clinically and genetically heterogeneous disorder first described by Silver (1953) and Russell (1954).[46,47] Cardinal features of the disease are low birth weight, short stature resulting from intrauterine and postnatal growth retardation, and a small triangular face. Other associated symptoms include clinodactyly of the fifth finger, relative macrocephaly, and facial, limb, or body asymmetry. CALMs are a variable SRS feature. One or 2 CALMs are present in up to 20% of SRS patients. Many SRS cases are sporadic, but familial cases with different modes of inheritance have been described. Maternal uniparental disomy for chromosome 7 occurs in approximately 10% of patients, and several candidate regions for the SRS gene mutation have been described on this chromosome (7p11.2-p13, 7q31-qter, and 7q21). Other possible gene candidates could be situated on the long arm of chromosome 17 or on chromosome 11p15. Recently, methylation defects in the H19 imprinted domain chromosome 11p15 has been implicated in 35% to 65% of SRS cases.[48]

ACQUIRED HYPERMELANOSIS

ENDOCRINOPATHIES

AT-A-GLANCE

- Diffuse, nonpatterned hyperpigmentation may be seen in conditions like Addison disease, Cushing syndrome, Nelson syndrome, pheochromocytoma, carcinoid syndrome, hyperthyroidism, acanthosis nigricans, and diabetes.

- Circumscribed hyperpigmentation may be seen in conditions like acanthosis nigricans and maturational dyschromia

ADDISON DISEASE

Chapter 137 discusses endocrine diseases in detail.

Addison disease is a clinical syndrome characterized by salt-wasting and diffuse cutaneous hyperpigmentation. In the developed world, Addison disease is usually autoimmune. It is associated with adrenal insufficiency with inadequate secretion of corticosteroid and androgenic hormones, leading to compensatory overproduction of adrenocorticotropic hormone (ACTH) by the pituitary gland.

Hyperpigmentation is the most striking cutaneous sign of patients with chronic Addison disease and is the consequence of ACTH binding to the melanocortin-1 receptor. The hyperpigmentation occurs preferentially on sun-exposed areas (face, neck, hands), sites of trauma, scars, chronic pressure (knees, spine, knuckles, elbows, shoulders), in the palmar creases, nipples, areolae, axillae, perineum, and genitalia.

CUSHING SYNDROME

Chapter 137 discusses endocrine diseases in detail.

Cushing syndrome is characterized by clinical signs and symptoms caused by chronic glucocorticoid excess.

Various degrees of hyperpigmentation can be seen. It is usually most severe in patients with the ectopic ACTH syndrome. Patients present with generalized hyperpigmentation with accentuation in areas of sun exposure, chronic mild trauma, and pressure (shoulders, midriff, waist, elbows, knuckles, spine, knees), and on mucosal surfaces.

NELSON SYNDROME

Nelson syndrome comprises an enlarging pituitary tumor associated with elevated fasting plasma ACTH levels, hyperpigmentation, and neuroophthalmologic symptoms in patients with Cushing disease after bilateral adrenalectomy and inadequate hormonal replacement.[49]

PHEOCHROMOCYTOMA

Pheochromocytoma is a chromaffin cell tumor of the adrenal medulla with associated excessive production of catecholamines. Pallor of the face resulting from vasoconstriction may be observed. In contrast, addisonian-like hyperpigmentation has been reported and is probably caused by ectopic ACTH and melanocyte-stimulating hormone production by the tumor. Pigmentation rapidly fades after surgical treatment.[50]

CARCINOID SYNDROME

Diffuse hyperpigmentation resulting from melanocyte-stimulating hormone–producing tumors, such as gastric or thymic carcinoid tumors, have been described in carcinoid syndrome. Carcinoid syndrome also can be accompanied by a pellagra-like rash occurring on light-exposed skin. The rash is secondary to a tryptophan deficiency, as a large amount of dietary tryptophan is diverted to serotonin by the tumor. Treatment of the underlying tumor is critical in the management of affected patients.

HYPERTHYROIDISM

Chapter 137 discusses endocrine diseases in detail.

Thyrotoxicosis has multiple causes. The most common cause is Graves disease, characterized by circulating antibodies against thyroid-stimulating hormone receptors.

The occurrence of hyperpigmentation in thyrotoxic patients has been estimated to be from 2% to as high as 40% in large series. The increased cutaneous pigmentation can be localized or generalized and is more common in those with dark skin. The distribution of hyperpigmentation is often similar to that in Addison disease with pigment deposition in the creases of the palms and soles. However, in contrast to Addison disease, involvement of the mucous membranes is uncommon and pigmentation of the nipples and genital skin is less striking. Hyperpigmentation associated with thyrotoxicosis is thought to be the result of an increased release of pituitary ACTH, compensating for accelerated cortisol degradation. The response of hyperpigmentation to therapy for the hyperthyroidism is reported to be poor.[51] Autoimmune Graves disease has been reported in association with vitiligo.

DIABETES

Chapter 137 discusses diabetes in detail.

Diabetic dermopathy is characterized by asymptomatic, irregular, light-brown, depressed patches on the anterior lower legs, often after mild trauma or the appearance of bullae. The pathogenesis is unknown.

ACANTHOSIS NIGRICANS

Acanthosis nigricans is characterized by thickened hyperpigmented velvety skin most often noted on the neck, axilla, popliteal and antecubital fossae, and inguinal folds (Fig. 77-7). It has, however, also been

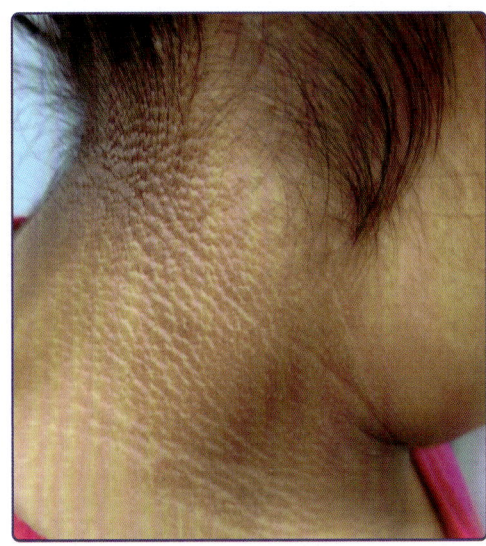

Figure 77-7 Acanthosis nigricans on the neck of a young girl of Filipino origin.

described on the face and should be considered in the differential diagnosis of facial hyperpigmentation. When on the face, acanthosis nigricans presents as poorly demarcated hyperpigmentation with a predilection for the malar region inferior to the zygoma and the nasolabial folds, and has even been described on the supraalar creases.[52] Recognizing this entity is becoming steadily more important as the rates of obesity and non–insulin-dependent diabetes increases. Acanthosis nigricans is discussed in more detail in Chap. 137.

MATURATIONAL DYSCHROMIA

Maturational dyschromia is a recently described entity noted in the African and Indian population in the fourth to fifth decades of life. It presents as dark-brown to black poorly demarcated areas of hyperpigmentation on the lateral forehead, temples, and zygoma. Histologic evaluation of hyperpigmented skin reveals mild to moderate proliferation of melanocytes with some reports of a papillomatous epidermis, suggesting a potential link or continuum with acanthosis nigricans.[53] The etiology is still unclear and further research of this disorder is needed (Fig. 77-8).

NUTRITIONAL CONDITIONS

Chapter 123 discusses nutritional disease in detail. Diffuse, nonpatterned pigmentary changes can be secondary to nutritional conditions such as kwashiorkor, vitamin B_{12} deficiency, folic acid deficiency, or pellagra. The skin changes are reversible if the nutritional deficiency is corrected.

KWASHIORKOR

Kwashiorkor is the result of severe protein malnutrition in the presence of adequate caloric intake. It is a significant cause of death in children between 6 months and 5 years of age in developing countries, and is often associated with GI parasitoses. A child with kwashiorkor ceases to gain weight and becomes irritable and apathic, and develops edema, hepatomegaly, diarrhea, muscle wasting, and photophobia. Cutaneous manifestations are present in most cases. Skin changes usually begin with hypopigmentation of the face. In areas exposed to friction and pressure, such as knees, elbows, and buttocks, hyperkeratoses and scaling in association with hyperpigmentation develop, giving the skin a "flaky paint" appearance. Removing the scale leaves superficial erosions that turn into pale patches. Hair may become hypopigmented. Sometimes there are bands of hypopigmentation along the hair shafts (flag sign), a result of periods of worse malnutrition. Treatment of kwashiorkor consists of replacing protein sources. Changes in skin and hair are reversed by proper nutritional treatment.[54]

Kwashiorkor-like syndrome also has been described in cases of protein loss and malnutrition secondary to bowel disorders such as ulcerative colitis.

VITAMIN B_{12} DEFICIENCY

Cobalamin or vitamin B_{12} deficiency is caused by atrophic gastritis caused by *Helicobacter pylori* infection or an autoimmune process directed against gastric parietal cells, which lead to severe "intrinsic factor" deficiency (pernicious anemia). Blood examination reveals megaloblastic anemia and low levels of vitamin B_{12}. Associated generalized hyperpigmentation of the skin and hypopigmentation/depigmentation or early graying of the hair have been reported. Skin histology shows increased melanin in the basal layer. Electron microscopy reveals a normal complement of melanosomes in melanocytes and surrounding keratinocytes. These findings suggest that an increase in melanin synthesis rather than a defect in melanin transport causes vitamin B_{12} deficiency–associated hyperpigmentation. Supplementation with vitamin B_{12} reverses the hyperpigmentation.

Pernicious anemia is an autoimmune disorder and has been reported in association with vitiligo.[55]

FOLIC ACID DEFICIENCY

Folic acid deficiency associated with megaloblastic anemia has been reported to cause hyperpigmentation of the skin.

PELLAGRA

Pellagra is caused by a deficiency of niacin (vitamin B_3) or its derivatives. The disease is rare and can be caused

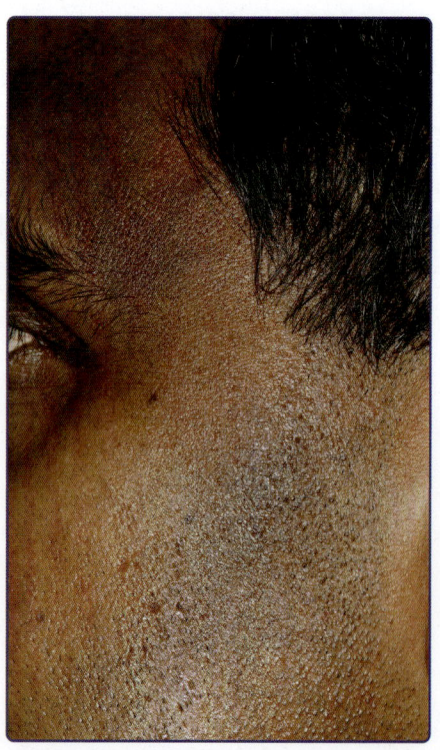

Figure 77-8 Maturational dyschromia on the temple and the lateral zygoma of a middle-aged Indian man.

by chronic alcoholism, certain drugs (isoniazid, anticonvulsants), malabsorption secondary to inflammatory bowel disease, celiac disease, and carcinoid tumors. Pellagra is characterized by the clinical triad of dermatitis, dementia, and diarrhea. The first skin changes are erythema and edema following sun exposure, which fade with a dusky brown–red coloration on face, neck, and dorsal surfaces of the hands, arms, and feet. Later on the lesions become hyperpigmented, hyperkeratotic, and scaly with fissures and crusts ("goose-like"). Niacin supplementation causes a rapid clinical response.[56]

METABOLIC CONDITIONS

AT-A-GLANCE

- Porphyria cutanea tarda and hemochromatosis may cause diffuse nonpatterned hyperpigmentation accentuated in photoexposed sites.

PORPHYRIA CUTANEA TARDA

Chapter 124 discusses the porphyrias in detail.

Porphyria cutanea tarda is a metabolic disorder affecting the synthesis of heme. It is associated with diffuse brown hyperpigmentation, which is accentuated in photoexposed areas. In females, a melasma-like hyperpigmentation of the face may be observed.

HEMOCHROMATOSIS

Hemochromatosis is a disease of iron storage with a heterogeneous genetic basis that results in lowered levels of hepcidin. Approximately 10% of the population has a mutation in the hemochromatosis gene, with a lower prevalence noted in Africans and Asians compared with northern Europeans. This leads to increased intestinal absorption and deposition of iron in the liver, pancreas, and other organs, including the skin.[57] Because hemochromatosis is now usually diagnosed early, hyperpigmentation is less frequently observed. Historically, hemochromatosis was diagnosed at an advanced stage with a classic triad of hyperpigmentation, diabetes mellitus ("bronze diabetes"), and hepatic cirrhosis. Darkening of the skin was present in 70% of the patients because of 2 different mechanisms: (a) hemosiderin deposition causing a diffuse, slate-gray color, and (b) increased epidermal melanin production. The pigmentation is usually generalized, but may be more pronounced in photoexposed areas, genitalia, and scars. Skin bronzing is reversible with phlebotomy, which remains the mainstay of treatment for this condition. Deferoxamine is most commonly used in secondary hemochromatosis.

TUMORAL CONDITIONS

MAST CELL DISORDERS AND MELANOMA

Mast cell disorders and melanoma can lead to diffuse, nonpatterned hyperpigmentation and are discussed in Chaps. 42 and 116, respectively. Diffuse, generalized melanosis associated with advanced metastatic melanoma is a rare, although well-documented, condition. It is characterized by a slate bluish-gray to brown discoloration of the skin. Histology reveals melanin particles and melanin-containing histiocytes and dendritic cells in the dermis and subcutaneous fat. No melanoma cells can be detected in the skin, and there is no increase in epidermal melanin pigment or number of melanocytes. Melanosomes circulating in the blood have been detected, supporting the hypothesis that diffuse melanosis may result from tumor lysis with release of their organelles into the circulation and subsequent deposition in the skin.

PHYSICAL CAUSES

AT-A-GLANCE

- Ultraviolet, ionizing, and thermal radiation may cause diffuse nonpatterned hyperpigmentation in the area(s) affected.
- Trauma may cause localized hyperpigmentation in areas of chronic friction.

ULTRAVIOLET RADIATION AND PIGMENTATION

Chapter 20 discusses pigmentation in detail.

A major acute effect of ultraviolet radiation on normal human skin is tanning.

IONIZING RADIATION

Chapter 200 discusses radiotherapy in detail.

Exposure of skin to ionizing radiation during accidents or after local fractionated radiotherapy can give rise to a cutaneous radiation syndrome characterized by fibrosis, keratosis, telangiectasias, and sharply demarcated lentiginous hyperpigmentation, resembling ultraviolet-induced lentigines (radiation dermatitis). Small hypopigmented macules can be intermingled with zones of hyperpigmentation. Histology reveals altered melanin content in melanocytes and basal keratinocytes. Electron-beam therapy has been reported to induce tan-like transient hyperpigmentation and transverse melanonychia when nails are exposed.[58]

THERMAL RADIATION

In superficial thermal burn injuries, when the melanocyte-bearing basal epidermis has not been destroyed, various degrees of hyperpigmentation result, depending on the patient's skin color and time after the injury. Thermal injury resulting from laser therapy with intense, high-dose visible light also can give rise to hyperpigmentation, especially in dark-skinned patients. Cryotherapy, tissue destruction by application of cold, commonly causes (sometimes permanently) hypopigmentation in combination with peripheral hyperpigmentation in treated skin as a result of melanocyte injury.[59]

FRICTION MELANOSIS

Frictional melanosis in an acquired pigmentary disorder caused by repeated rubbing of the skin, especially over bony prominences. Marked increase in melanin and melanin incontinence is seen histologically.[60] Diffuse hyperpigmentation is noted with some cases revealing mild lichenification.

TOXINS AND MEDICATIONS

AT-A-GLANCE

- Toxins and medications are a common cause of acquired, diffuse, nonpatterned hyperpigmentation.
- Fixed drug eruptions may cause well-demarcated brown-gray mucocutaneous macules.
- Hyperpigmentation may be caused by direct deposition of the drug into the skin, deposition of melanin or melanin-drug complex in the dermis, or nonmelanin pigment produced by the drug.
- Treatment involves cessation of the offending medication, and quality-switched and picosecond lasers.

Hyperpigmentation caused by toxic agents or medication accounts for 10% to 20% of all cases of acquired hyperpigmentation. CNS drugs, antineoplastic agents, antiinfectious drugs, antihypertensive medications, and hormones are most often the responsible agents (Table 77-2).

CLINICAL FEATURES

Clinical features vary with characteristic sites, patterns, and shades of discoloration noted with particular medications and toxins. Bluish-slate gray pigmentation is characteristic of dermal deposition of pigment. Pigmentation associated with melanin accumulation often worsens with sun exposure.

A linear, sometimes flagellate hyperpigmentation can be observed in patients taking bleomycin or zidovudine. A diffuse hyperpigmentation on the palms and soles may be present in patients taking cyclophosphamide or doxorubicin. Diffuse slate-gray pigmentation also may be seen at the site of IV iron infusion (Fig. 77-9). Bleomycin and doxorubicin may produce localized hyperpigmentation around small joints. Estrogen-related hormonal substances and phenytoin-like medication may cause melasma-like pigmentation. Nail unit involvement can be observed with some medications, most frequently chemotherapeutic agents such as cyclophosphamide, zidovudine, psoralens, minocycline, antimalarials, and gold. Mucosal hyperpigmentation has been reported with cyclophosphamide, doxorubicin, zidovudine, minocycline, and some heavy metals.

Amiodarone can produce blue-gray pigmentation in photoexposed areas from accumulation of a lipid-like substance in macrophages. Some of these patients display photosensitivity (Fig. 77-10). Chloroquine may give rise to a yellow-brown to bluish-gray pigmentation on the face, neck, lower extremities, and forearms after several years of intake, a result of deposition of a drug–melanin complex in the dermis. The nail unit and hard palate also may be involved. Exogenous ochronosis has been reported after chronic hydroquinone use (see section "Ochronosis").

Chlorpromazine and related phenothiazines can produce a bluish-gray cutaneous pigmentation that is worse in photoexposed areas with pigmentation of the conjunctivae.

The risk of minocycline-induced pigmentation increases with prolonged therapy at doses above 100 mg daily.[61] Three types of minocycline-induced pigmentation exist: Type 1 consists of blue-gray pigmentation in normal skin and areas of prior inflammation (often on the face) (Fig. 77-11); Type 2 is noted on the lower legs and forearms; and Type 3 is diffuse muddy brown photoexacerbated pigmentation. Pigmentation of the nails, sclerae, oral mucosa, thyroid, bones, and teeth also has been reported.

Argyria patients present with a generalized grayish-blue pigmentation caused by silver ingestion. The nails and the sclerae also may be involved.

Although medication-induced pigmentation usually results in diffuse hyperpigmentation, fixed drug eruptions must be considered when well-demarcated mucocutaneous hyperpigmented macules are the presenting sign (Fig. 77-12). A preceding history of erythema and possible itching with pigmentation as the lesion resolves is classically seen after use of nonsteroidal antiinflammatory medications, certain antibiotics, and drugs containing codeine.

TABLE 77-2
Medications Reported to Cause Hyperpigmentation

TOPICAL TREATMENTS	ANTIINFECTIOUS DRUGS	CNS DRUGS	ANTINEOPLASTIC AGENTS	MISCELLANEOUS
Aminolevulinic acid	Amphotericin B	Amitriptyline	Bevacizumab	Alitretinoin
Carmustine (BCNU)	Ceftriaxone	Carbamazepine	Bleomycin	Amiodarone
Bergamot	Chloroquine	Chlorpromazine	Busulfan	Azathioprine
Bimatoprost	Cidofovir	Citalopram	Capecitabine	Cetirizine
Carteolol	Clofazimine	Clomipramine	Carboplatin	Cevimeline
Chlorhexidine	Dapsone	Clonazepam	Carmustine	Cyclobenzaprine
Hydroquinone	Demeclocycline	Desipramine	Cisplatin	Cyclosporine
Imiquimod	Doxycycline	Diazepam	Cyclophosphamide	Deferoxamine
Latanoprost	Emtricitabine	Donepezil	Dactinomycin	Dicumarol
Nitrogen mustard	Enoxacin	Eletriptan	Daunorubicin	Dinoprostone
Tretinoin	Foscarnet	Fluoxetine	Doxorubicin	Etodolac
Antihypertensive drugs	Ganciclovir	Fluphenazine	Epirubicin	Glatiramer
Acebutolol	Grepafloxacin	Fluvoxamine	Estramustine	Heroin
Betaxolol	Griseofulvin	Haloperidol	Etoposide	Interferon
Bisoprolol	Hydroxychloroquine	Imipramine	Floxuridine	Isotretinoin
Captopril	Indinavir	Kava	Fluorouracil	Ketoprofen
Clonidine	Ketoconazole	Loxapine	Hydroxyurea	Leflunomide
Diltiazem	Linezolid	Mephenytoin	Ifosfamide	Levobupivacaine
Esmolol	Lomefloxacin	Mesoridazine	Irinotecan	Lidocaine
Indapamide	Minocycline	Methamphetamine	Mechlorethamine	Methimazole
Labetalol	Ofloxacin	Molindone	Mercaptopurine	Methoxsalen
Methyldopa	Oxytetracycline	Olanzapine	Methotrexate	Methysergide
Metoprolol	Pyrimethamine	Paroxetine	Mitomycin	Metoclopramide
Minoxidil	Quinacrine	Perphenazine	Mitotane	Niacin
Nisoldipine	Quinine	Phenytoin	Mitoxantrone	Nicotine
Propranolol	Ribavirin	Pimozide	Paclitaxel	Orphenadrine
Spironolactone	Rifabutin	Prochlorperazine	Pentostatin	Pantoprazole
Timolol	Rifapentine	Promazine	Procarbazine	Pentazocine
Heavy metals	Saquinavir	Promethazine	Thiotepa	Phenazopyridine
Arsenic	Sertaconazole	Risperidone	Vinblastine	Phenolphthalein
Bismuth	Smallpox vaccine	Ropinirole	Vincristine	Propylthiouracil
Gold (compounds)	Sparfloxacin	Thioridazine	Vinorelbine	Psoralens
Iron	Sulfadiazine	Thiothixene	Hormones	Quinidine
Lead	Terbinafine	Tiagabine	Chlorotrianisene	Rabeprazole
Mercury	Tetracycline	Tolcapone	Corticosteroids	Riluzole
Silver	Voriconazole	Topiramate	Diethylstilbestrol	Sulfasalazine
	Zidovudine	Trifluoperazine	Estrogens	Tacrolimus
		Venlafaxine	Insulin	Toremifene
		Zaleplon	Leuprolide	Trioxsalen
			Medroxyprogesterone	Vitamin A
			Oral contraceptives	
			Progestins	
			Stanozolol	

ETIOLOGY AND PATHOGENESIS

In the majority of cases of medication-induced hyperpigmentation, the underlying pathogenic mechanism involves one of the following.

1. Deposition of melanin in the dermis, usually in macrophages. Sometimes this melanin is complexed to the drug (drug–pigment complex, eg, hydroxychloroquine). Accumulation of melanin can occur after cutaneous inflammation (postinflammatory) and/or DNA damage (eg, carmustine). This type of hyperpigmentation is often increased by ultraviolet exposure and is usually more pronounced in photoexposed areas.

2. Direct deposition of the medication in the skin (eg, carotene, heavy metals). Sometimes this type of pigmentation is accentuated in photoexposed areas, as ultraviolet light can induce a transformation in the deposited drug, which may then become more visible.

3. Nonmelanin pigments synthesized or produced under the direct or indirect influence of the drug may cause cutaneous pigmentation.

DIAGNOSIS

The diagnosis may be made clinically if the characteristic appearance is seen and a temporal relationship

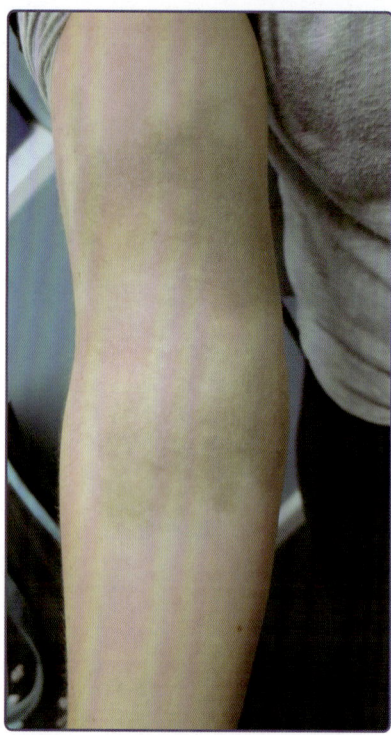

Figure 77-9 Diffuse gray pigmentation secondary to IV iron infusion in the arm of a white woman.

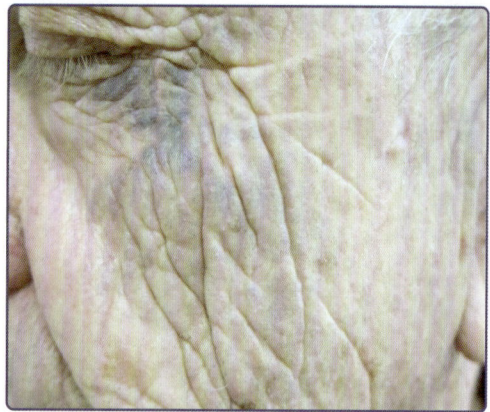

Figure 77-11 Slate-gray minocycline-induced pigmentation on the cheek of a white male.

with exposure to a medication or toxin is noted. A skin biopsy also may be helpful in cases of medication-induced pigmentation.

CLINICAL COURSE AND PROGNOSIS

Ceasing the offending medication is critical, but hyperpigmentation persists in many cases, sometimes for decades, even after discontinuation of the medication.

MANAGEMENT

Sun protection should be advised, especially in forms caused by melanin accumulation. Quality-switched ruby, alexandrite, and Nd:YAG lasers have demonstrated favorable results in some cases (eg, amiodarone and minocycline-induced pigmentation), although multiple treatments spaced over many months is often necessary to achieve clinically notable results. Picosecond lasers have proven efficacious for medication-induced pigmentation in white skin, with fewer treatments over a shorter time frame achieving complete or near complete clearance of the pigmentation.[62]

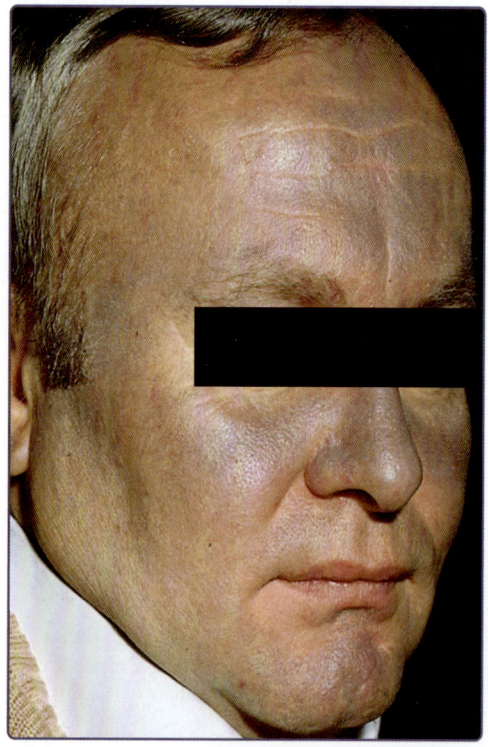

Figure 77-10 Amiodarone hyperpigmentation. This patient exhibits a striking amiodarone-induced, slate-gray pigmentation of the face. The blue color (ceruloderma) is a result of the deposition of a brown pigment in the dermis, contained in macrophages and endothelial cells.

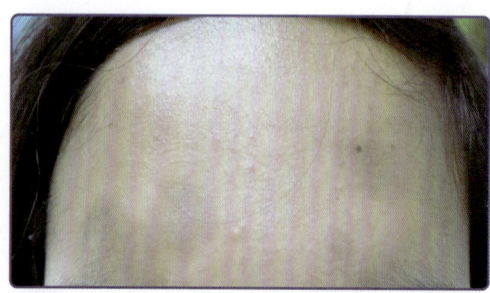

Figure 77-12 Fixed drug eruption on the face secondary to nonsteroidal antiinflammatory medication in a young Sri Lankan girl.

OCHRONOSIS

AT-A-GLANCE

- May be congenital (autosomal recessive) or caused by the use of certain medications.
- Results in asymptomatic diffuse nonpatterned hyperpigmentation.
- More common in persons with skin of color.
- Characteristic histologic appearance is yellow-brown banana-shaped globules in the dermis.

The term *ochronosis* is derived from the Greek word "ochre," which refers to yellow discoloration. Endogenous and exogenous forms of the condition exist.

EXOGENOUS OCHRONOSIS

Epidemiology: Although the majority of ochronosis cases have been reported in darker racial/ethnic groups in Africa, India, Thailand, China, and Singapore, it also has been described in other skin types. The exact worldwide incidence is unknown but assumed to be low.

Clinical Features: Asymptomatic blue-black and gray-black hyperpigmented macules are characteristic and can be found on the face (malar, temples, lower cheeks), posterolateral neck, back, and extensor skin of the extremities. Later stages include progressive hyperpigmented colloid milium ("caviar-like lesions), papulonodular lesions, and areas of scarring.[63]

No systemic involvement is noted with exogenous ochronosis.

Etiology and Pathogenesis: Exogenous ochronosis results from the use of certain medications, which form a homogentisic acid polymer-like substance during their metabolism. It has been most frequently reported in association with hydroquinone, usually at concentrations greater than 4%, and topicals, such as phenol or resorcinol, and quinine, an oral antimalarial.

Exacerbating factors include unprotected ultraviolet light exposure, prolonged application of the offending medication on large surface areas, and use of topical resorcinol, phenol and mercury.

Diagnosis: Although early stages of exogenous ochronosis may appear similar to melasma, dermoscopy may be helpful in differentiating the two. Dark-brown globules and globular-like structures are seen on a diffuse brown background.[64]

Skin biopsy however, remains the gold standard for diagnosis of exogenous ochronosis. Histopathologically, there is a collection of yellowish-brown (ochronotic) banana-shaped globules in the papillary dermis. Homogenous, edematous dermal collagen also may be seen.

Differential Diagnosis: The early stages of ochronosis may be clinically indistinguishable from melasma, especially in Asians.

Clinical Course and Prognosis: Without cessation of the offending agent, exogenous ochronosis is progressive.

Management: Treatment is rarely helpful, but the offending drug should be stopped to prevent progression. Broad-spectrum sunscreen and sun avoidance are important. Topical retinoids, α-hydroxy acids, corticosteroids and physical therapies, such as chemical peels and quality-switched lasers, have all been reported in the treatment of exogenous ochronosis but there has been no universally efficacious treatment documented as of this writing.

The following disorders can be associated with hyperpigmentation and are discussed in their respective chapters: systemic sclerosis (Chap. 63), pinta (Chap. 171), onchocerciasis (Chap. 177), phytophotodermatitis (Chap. 97), and flagellate pigmentation caused by bleomycin (Chap. 45).

SYSTEMIC SCLEROSIS

Chapter 63 discusses systemic sclerosis in greater detail.

AT-A-GLANCE

- Acquired diffuse hyperpigmentation, focal depigmentation over sites of friction, streaky hyperpigmentation, and reticulated pigmentation have all been described.

Different types of abnormal pigmentation have been described in systemic sclerosis. A diffuse, generalized hyperpigmentation similar to Addison's disease but with normal levels of melanocyte-stimulating hormone can be observed in severe systemic sclerosis.

Focal depigmentation with perifollicular hyperpigmentation may occur, especially on sites of friction (eg, shins, elbows, and dorsum of the hands). There can be localized hyperpigmentation and hypopigmentation.

A streaky hyperpigmentation over blood vessels on a background of depigmentation also has been reported. Diffuse reticulated hyperpigmentation accentuated on the trunk has been reported in 1 case.[65]

INFECTIONS

CHIKUNGUNYA

AT-A-GLANCE

- Acquired circumscribed or diffuse hyperpigmentation.
- Caused by a mosquito-borne virus.
- Persistent pigmentation with symptomatic relief being the only treatment option.

Chikungunya is a mosquito-borne virus first described in the 1950s in Tanzania, Africa.

Epidemiology: While first described in Africa, chikungunya has been noted in several dozen other countries in Africa, Asia, Europe, and the Americas. All age groups are affected.[66]

Clinical Features: Pigmentary changes are the most common cutaneous finding. Lentiginous central facial hyperpigmentation, diffuse hyperpigmentation of acrofacial lesions, and flagellate hyperpigmentation have all been described. Striking pigmentation of the nose also has been reported. A case of neonatal hyperpigmentation has been reported in a case of congenital chikungunya.[67]

A maculopapular eruption is noted at the onset of the illness and resolves over 7 to 10 days. Other mucocutaneous manifestations include vesiculobullous lesions, purpuric lesions, aphthous-like ulcers, and exacerbation of other primary dermatoses such as lichen planus and psoriasis.

Systemic symptoms, such as fever, arthralgia, myalgia, and GI upset, are some of the extracutaneous manifestations.

Etiology and Pathogenesis: *Aedes aegypti* (tropics and subtropics) and *Aedes albopictus* (cooler regions of the world) have been implicated in large outbreaks of this mosquito-borne illness.

The mechanism by which cutaneous hyperpigmentation occurs is not understood but various theories exist, including melanocyte phagocytosis of the invading pathogens[68] followed by intraepidermal melanin dispersion or retention triggered by the virus.

Diagnosis: Lymphocytic vasculopathy and increased intraepidermal melanin is noted histologically. Melanophages are also noted and may account for the persistent cutaneous pigmentation.

Differential Diagnosis: Other viral illnesses and mosquito-borne illness fall into the wide differential diagnosis.

Clinical Course and Prognosis: Pigmentation often persists for many months.

Management: Symptom relief is the mainstay of treatment.

OTHER INFECTIONS

Erythematous, scaly papules termed *pintids* develop during the secondary stage of pinta. These initially red lesions can turn brown, slate-blue, black, or grayish.[69]

Chronic papular onchodermatitis is one of the skin manifestations of onchocerciasis. It is characterized by a severely pruritic maculopapular rash with hyperpigmented macules, most often occurring on shoulders, buttocks, and extremities (see Chap. 177).

PHYSIOLOGIC HYPERPIGMENTATION

PIGMENTARY DEMARCATION LINES

AT-A-GLANCE

- More common in persons with skin of color.
- Linear demarcation with opposing hyperpigmentation and hypopigmentation.
- Seen along "embryonic suture lines" in distinct patterns and areas of the face and limbs.
- Can occur on the face, trunk, and limbs.
- Usually become obvious in childhood.

Pigmentary demarcation lines (PDLs) are also known as Voigt or Futcher lines. They are abrupt changes from lighter to darker skin in a linear pattern mostly seen on the limbs, trunk, and face.

Epidemiology: PDLs are most common in persons with skin of color. PDLs often appear in childhood or puberty and persist throughout life.

Clinical Features: PDLs are classified based on location as follows:

- Type A: This is the most common type and involves the lateral aspect of the upper anterior arms (occasionally extending across the pectoral area);
- Type B: Posterior medial lower limb;
- Type C: Vertical hypopigmented line in sternal and parasternal areas;
- Type D: Vertical line in spinal or paraspinal area;

- Type E: Hypopigmented oval areas, streaks, or bands on bilateral aspects of the chest, from the mid-third of clavicle to periareolar skin;
- Type F: V-shaped hyperpigmented line between the malar prominence and the temple;
- Type G: W-shaped hyperpigmented lines between the malar prominence and the temple; and
- Type H: Linear hyperpigmentation from the angle of the mouth to the lateral aspect of the chin.

A pigmentary demarcation line anterior to the ear has not been described in the literature (at the time of this writing) but should now be added as a new pigmentary demarcation line "Type I" (Fig. 77-13).

Etiology and Pathogenesis: The cause of PDLs is unknown. The debate surrounding topography following lines of Blaschko or cutaneous innervation continues. Hormonal and genetic influences have been postulated with onset during pregnancy and variable inheritance patterns noted, including autosomal dominant inheritance patterns in some families.

Diagnosis: The diagnosis can usually be made clinically without need for biopsy.

Clinical Course and Prognosis: PDLs often appear in childhood or puberty and persist throughout life.

Management: Reassurance that these changes are a normal variant is needed. In addition, sun protection may diminish the difference between affected and unaffected skin.

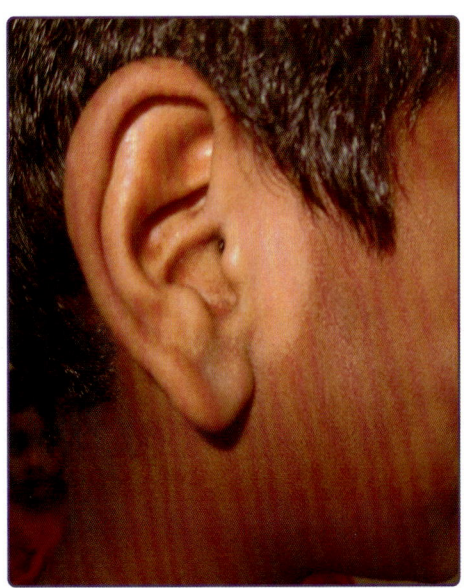

Figure 77-13 Pigmentary demarcation line anterior to the ear in a boy of Sri Lankan descent.

ACQUIRED IDIOPATHIC FACIAL PIGMENTATION

AT-A-GLANCE

- Can be considered as another group of pigmentary demarcation lines.
- More common in persons with skin of color.
- Linear demarcation with opposing hyperpigmentation and hyperpigmentation.
- Predominantly affects periorbital and perioral zones.
- Usually become obvious in adulthood.

Acquired idiopathic facial pigmentation was described recently in the Indian population and can be considered another group of PDLs.[70] The term *acquired idiopathic facial pigmentation* was coined after observing that some types of idiopathic facial pigmentation were nonnevoid, patterned, and bilateral with a dark-brown–gray color located around the eyes, lateral face, and chin.

Epidemiology: Onset is noted in early adulthood with occurrence in males and females in a 1:1 ratio. It often appears in adulthood and persists throughout life.

Clinical Features: Well-demarcated dark-brown–gray macular hyperpigmentation is noted on periorbital, zygomatic, and malar areas, root of the nose, and perioral and mandibular skin. The pigmentation is noted in a similar pattern to other nevoid conditions with patterns reflecting the normal patterns of embryologic spread of pigmentation on face. The absence of symptoms, scale, erythema, and lichenification should help differentiate it from other dermatoses and pigmentary disorders in the area.

Etiology and Pathogenesis: Although the cause is unknown, it is postulated this is a genetic disorder with exacerbation and accentuation resulting from physiologic factors such as ultraviolet light and aging.

Diagnosis: The diagnosis can usually be made clinically without need for biopsy.

Differential Diagnosis: Conditions like melasma and postinflammatory pigmentation may look similar to acquired idiopathic facial pigmentation and should be differentiated clinically and histologically.

Clinical Course and Prognosis: Acquired idiopathic facial pigmentation often appears in adulthood. It darkens with time and persists throughout life.

Management: Sun protection may help diminish the difference between affected and unaffected skin and occasionally topical hydroquinone can subtly lighten excessive pigmentation in the areas affected.

PERIORBITAL PIGMENTATION

> **AT-A-GLANCE**
>
> - Primary dermatoses, such as lichen planus pigmentosus, medication-induced pigmentation, pigmented contact dermatitis, and postinflammatory hyperpigmentation, should be excluded.
> - Familial/racial/constitutional pigmentation is especially common in persons with skin of color.

Periorbital hyperpigmentation is also known as dark circles and is very common in certain racial ethnic types.

Epidemiology: Males and females, mainly with darker-skin types, are commonly affected. Onset is usually noted in young adults.

Clinical Features: Asymptomatic brown-black nonscaly and nonerythematous pigmentation is noted on the upper, lower, or both eyelids. Accentuation of skin creases is noted and visible vessels also may be seen (Fig. 77-14).

Etiology and Pathogenesis: The exact etiology of constitutional pigmentation is yet to be determined.

Diagnosis: A clinical diagnosis is made in most cases. Increased melanin in the basal epidermis and melanophages in the upper dermis are seen histologically in those with constitutional pigmentation.

Differential Diagnosis: Primary dermatoses, like lichen planus pigmentosus, medication-induced pigmentation, and eczema with lichenification, must be excluded.

Clinical Course and Prognosis: Constitutional pigmentation is usually progressive.

Management: Treatment of the underlying dermatosis, if present, is critical. Although topical therapy, peels, lasers, and autologous fat transplants have been reported to be useful, these studies don't often specify the underlying cause of pigmentation, making it difficult to interpret the results.

MUCOSAL MELANOSIS

> **AT-A-GLANCE**
>
> - Physiologic pigmentation in the oral cavity.
> - Macular pigmentation on the gingiva, oral mucosa, lips, and tongue.
> - More common in persons with skin of color.

Mucosal melanosis is common in persons with skin of color and should be differentiated from other causes of pigmentation in the oral cavity.[71]

Epidemiology: The limited literature available on this topic suggests the onset of pigmentation is gradual and likely to occur in middle-aged adults with richly pigmented skin.

Clinical Features: Diffuse and bilateral pigmentation may be noted but localized macular hyperpigmentation may be seen affecting one or more of the following locations: gingiva, buccal mucosa, lips, hard palate, and papillae of the tongue (Fig. 77-15). A study in China concluded that pigmented fungiform papillae

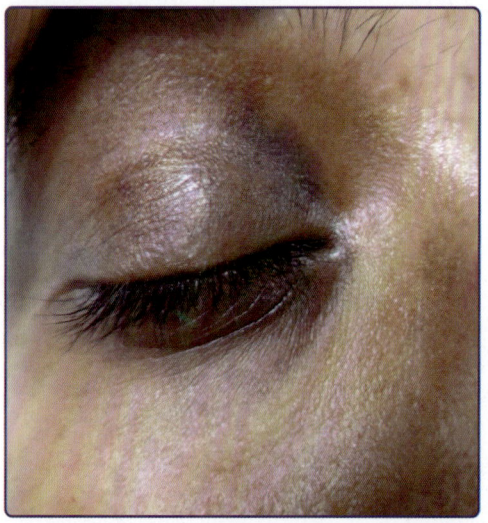

Figure 77-14 Periorbital pigmentation in an Indian lady.

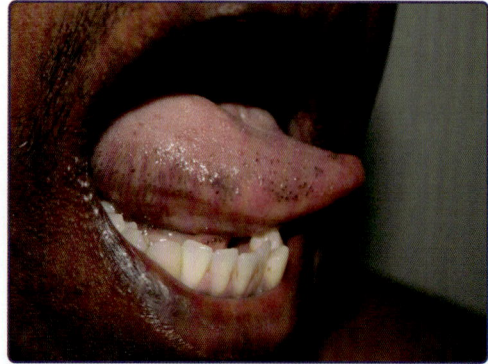

Figure 77-15 Benign pigmentation of the papillae of the tongue in an Indian man.

of the tongue are relatively common in the Chinese population.

Laugier-Hunziker syndrome is an acquired form of hyperpigmentation that presents as longitudinal melanonychia and pigmentation involving the oral mucosa, genitals, perianal region, fingers, and esophagus.

Etiology and Pathogenesis: The cause is unknown.

Diagnosis: The diagnosis can usually be made clinically without need for biopsy but if the diagnosis is in doubt, a biopsy can be helpful. Histologic examination demonstrates basal cell hypermelanosis, increased dermal melanophages, pigment incontinence, and normal melanocytes that in some instances are increased in number.

Differential Diagnosis: Many conditions can cause oral pigmentation. Drug-induced pigmentation, including fixed drug eruption, oral lichen planus, postinflammatory hyperpigmentation, dental amalgam, Addison disease, and malignancy, need to be excluded.

Brown hyperpigmented macules in childhood should prompt investigation for genodermatoses such as Peutz-Jeghers, Bandler, Carney, and Cronkhite-Canada syndromes.

Clinical Course and Prognosis: Mucosal melanosis appears in childhood and persists without consequence throughout life.

Management: Reassurance is the most important component of management. No treatment is required.

LONGITUDINAL MELANONYCHIA

AT-A-GLANCE

- Benign brown-black linear band of pigmentation of the nail plate.
- More common in persons with skin of color.
- Incidence increases with age.

Chapter 91 discusses longitudinal melanonychia in greater detail. Regular, thin hyperpigmented bands on multiple nails is characteristic of benign longitudinal pigmentation seen in darker individuals. Medications, trauma, and nevi in the nail apparatus may also cause longitudinal melanonychia and should be considered in the differential diagnosis. A single band located on the thumb or great toe, should prompt the clinician to diligently look for signs of melanoma clinically and dermoscopically. A biopsy also may be necessary to differentiate benign longitudinal melanonychia from melanoma.

ACRAL HYPERPIGMENTED MACULES

AT-A-GLANCE

- Benign brown well-demarcated macules on palms and soles.
- More common in persons with skin of color.
- Incidence increases with age.

Well-defined brown macules on the palms and soles reveal increased epidermal melanin histologically. Despite the parallel ridge pattern noted on dermoscopy, the number of lesions noted provides a clue to the benign nature of the lesions.[72] It is important to exclude genodermatoses and drug-induced (especially chemotherapy) pigmentation that may present in a similar fashion.

ACQUIRED PATTERNED HYPERMELANOSIS

AT-A-GLANCE

- Phytophotodermatitis, flagellate pigmentation caused by bleomycin, and flagellate mushroom dermatitis are all causes of patterned hyperpigmentation.

PHYTOPHOTODERMATITIS

Contact with plants containing phototoxic agents such as psoralens, with subsequent ultraviolet exposure, may lead to phytophotodermatitis, which is followed by patterned hyperpigmentation.

FLAGELLATE MUSHROOM DERMATITIS

Shiitake mushroom (*Lentinula edodes*) is typically grown and used in Asian cuisine but the Western world now consumes it in large quantities. Oral ingestion of raw or insufficiently cooked shiitake mushrooms is associated with a "flagellate mushroom dermatitis" that appears 12 hours to 5 days after consumption. While most reports have emerged from Japan, cases in Europe, the United States, and Canada also have been described.[73] It is characterized by linear grouped, erythematous, and intensely pruritic papules that resembles bleomycin-induced flagellate dermatitis. A pustular eruption also has been reported. The trunk and limbs are usually involved. The pathogenesis is not yet known, but it is hypothesized that a toxic reaction results from a thermolabile polysaccharide contained within the mushroom.

ERYTHEMA AB IGNE

AT-A-GLANCE

- Acquired diffuse reticulate pigmentation.
- May also have epidermal atrophy, scaling, and hyperpigmentation.
- Caused by chronic exposure to moderate heat.
- Thyroid function should be checked.

Erythema ab igne is caused by frequent exposure to heat, usually infrared radiation, resulting in reticulate hyperpigmentation. Although it may occur anywhere on the body, it is usually localized to the thighs and lower legs.[74]

CLINICAL FEATURES

Tan–red-brown reticulate transient and blanchable erythema is noted acutely (usually about 3 weeks after the heat exposure) but fixed hyperpigmentation may be accompanied by epidermal atrophy, bullous lesions or hyperkeratosis, and scale in chronic cases. Common sites of involvement include the thighs, lower legs, abdomen, and back.

ETIOLOGY AND PATHOGENESIS

Erythema ab igne is caused by chronic exposure to moderate heat. It was seen in the past in people who frequently sat in front of open fires for warmth, but the introduction of central heating has seen a decline in this presentation. Nevertheless, it is seen after local application of heating pads, hot water bottles, or heating blankets (Fig. 77-16). Widespread cases secondary to hot tub bathing in Japan also has been reported.[45] Modern appliances that have been reported to elicit erythema ab igne are furniture with built-in heaters, car heaters, and laptop computers when rested on the thighs or legs.

The reticulate nature of the cutaneous changes is thought to reflect the distribution of blood vessels. The heat is thought to damage superficial blood vessels in the epidermis, which, in turn, results in extravasation of red blood cells and hemosiderin, causing the cutaneous hyperpigmentation.

DIAGNOSIS

The diagnosis is usually made clinically. Thyroid function tests should be considered in patients with symptoms or signs that suggest hypothyroidism.

If a skin biopsy is performed, histologic examination usually reveals vasodilation, extravasation of red blood cells, and deposition of melanin and hemosiderin in the dermis. Dermal edema and lymphohistiocytic dermal infiltration is also noted.[75]

DIFFERENTIAL DIAGNOSIS

Livedo reticularis and its various causes need to be considered, but the history often reveals chronic heat exposure in cases of erythema ab igne.

CLINICAL COURSE AND PROGNOSIS

The pigmentary changes usually resolve when the patient stops using the heat source on the skin, but depending on the chronicity of the exposure, pigmentation may persist for many months. Very rarely squamous cell carcinoma and Merkel cell carcinoma have been reported to arise within chronic lesions of erythema ab igne.

MANAGEMENT

Elimination of the heat source is critical, but topical retinoids and low-fluence quality-switched Nd:YAG laser also have been helpful in some persistent cases.[76]

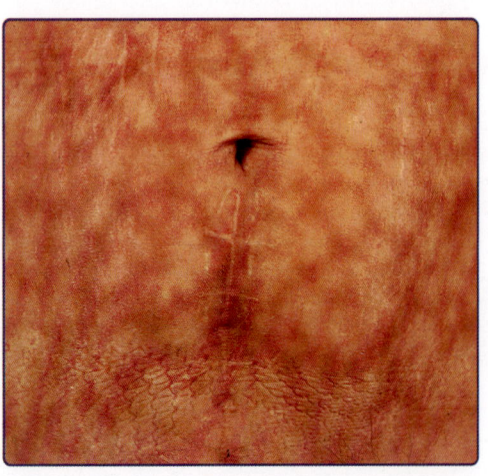

Figure 77-16 Reticular hyperpigmentation (erythema ab igne) on the abdomen resulting from repeated applications of a heating pad over several years.

PRURIGO PIGMENTOSA

AT-A-GLANCE

- Acquired diffuse reticulate pigmentation on the trunk.
- Most common in young females.
- Initial phase of pruritic papules, vesicles, and papulovesicles is followed by asymptomatic hyperpigmentation.
- Tetracyclines and dapsone are helpful for the inflammatory component of the condition.

Prurigo pigmentosa is a rare condition, first described in Japan by Nagashima et al. in 1971.[77] It most commonly affects the trunk and results in reticulated hyperpigmentation.

EPIDEMIOLOGY

While reports as of this writing have largely emerged from Japan, it is becoming increasingly documented in other parts of the world. It is most common in young females in their 20s with a female to male ratio of 4 to 6:1.[78]

CLINICAL FEATURES

Prurigo pigmentosa presents with intensely pruritic symmetrical urticarial, erythematous papules, papulovesicles, and vesicles that evolve into reticulated hyperpigmentation. The lesions develop on the upper back, chest, neck, and lumbosacral region. The papulovesicular lesions heal spontaneously over approximately 1 week, leaving nonpruritic reticular hyperpigmentation in its wake (Fig. 77-17).

No systemic associations have been documented.

ETIOLOGY AND PATHOGENESIS

Environmental and metabolic factors have been suggested as causative agents, but the pathogenesis remains unknown.

DIAGNOSIS

The diagnosis of prurigo pigmentosa requires close clinicopathologic correlation. Histology of early lesions reveals a superficial neutrophilic perivascular and interstitial infiltrate. Later in the disease course, lesions demonstrate lichenoid inflammation with a predominance of lymphocytes. Spongiosis, necrotic keratinocytes, eosinophils, and vesiculation are also noted.[79]

DIFFERENTIAL DIAGNOSIS

Confluent reticulated papillomatosis (no preceding erythematous papules), pigmented contact dermatitis (responds to topical steroids), and Dowling-Degos disease (characteristic histologic findings) are the main differential diagnoses.

CLINICAL COURSE AND PROGNOSIS

The disease has a fluctuating course with exacerbations and recurrences.

MANAGEMENT

The eruption and pruritus respond well to minocycline or doxycycline 100-200 mg daily or dapsone 25 to 100 mg daily. The pigmentation resolves spontaneously.

NEVUS OF HORI

AT-A-GLANCE

- Acquired circumscribed hyperpigmentation in the form of symmetrical pinhead-sized macules on the malar region of the face.
- Noted mainly in Asian populations.
- Often coexists with other pigmentary conditions like melasma and flat seborrheic keratoses.
- Best treated with quality-switched Nd:YAG lasers.

Nevus of Hori was first described in 1984 as acquired bilateral nevus of Ota–like macules (ABNOM) or acquired dermal melanocytosis.[80]

EPIDEMIOLOGY

It is a common condition noted in nearly 1% of the Asian population, particularly the Chinese and Japanese population. It is more common in females and appears in the third to fifth decades of life.

CLINICAL FEATURES

Nevus of Hori consists of blue-brown to slate-gray hyperpigmented macules ranging from pinhead size to a few millimeters in diameter (Fig. 77-18). Lesions are found on the face with predilection for the malar

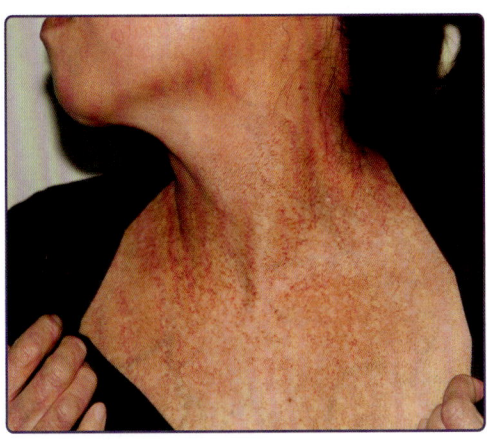

Figure 77-17 Reticulate pigmentation seen in prurigo pigmentosa in a Japanese woman.

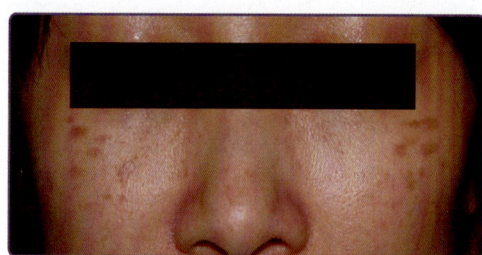

Figure 77-18 Nevus of Hori.

region, although lesions on the temple and nose are not uncommon.

Unlike nevus of Ota, nevus of Hori is bilateral and lacks ocular and mucosal membrane involvement.

ETIOLOGY AND PATHOGENESIS

Hori described 3 possible mechanisms for the pathogenesis of ABNOM: (a) "dropping" of epidermal melanocytes into the dermis, (b) migration of melanocytes from hair bulbs, and (c) reactivation of pre-existing latent or immature dermal melanocytes. The third possibility has been suggested as being the most plausible mechanism with ultraviolet radiation and sex hormones as activating factors.

DIAGNOSIS

The diagnosis may require a biopsy, particularly if other pigmentary disorders, such as melasma, coexist in the affected area. Histology often reveals melanocytosis in the upper and mid dermis.

DIFFERENTIAL DIAGNOSIS

In many cases, ABNOM can occur simultaneously with other pigmentary abnormalities such as melasma, freckles, solar lentigines, and nevus of Ota.

CLINICAL COURSE AND PROGNOSIS

Nevus of Hori is usually gradually progressive.

MANAGEMENT

Although various lasers, such as ablative CO_2, quality-switched 532-nm, quality-switched ruby, and fractional nonablative 2940-nm Erbium:YAG, have been used in isolation or in combination,[81] quality-switched lasers are the most commonly used form of treatment. Obtaining complete clearance is not always possible and multiple treatments are required. Quality-switched and picosecond lasers have demonstrated efficacy in lightening or clearing the lesions, but multiple treatments spaced many months apart are required.[82,83]

NEVUS OF BECKER

AT-A-GLANCE

- Presents with acquired circumscribed hyperpigmentation.
- Most commonly found on the trunk.
- Usually associated with hypertrichosis.
- Treatment with lasers can be attempted but current studies lack statistical significance.

This acquired hyperpigmented epidermal nevus was first described in 1949 (Fig. 77-19) and is also known as Becker hamartoma or Becker melanosis.

EPIDEMIOLOGY

Nevus of Becker appears to be androgen-dependent and is noted in approximately 0.5% of the population, usually becoming more prominent during adolescence. It is said to be more common in males but a newer study revealed equal incidence in male and female children.[84]

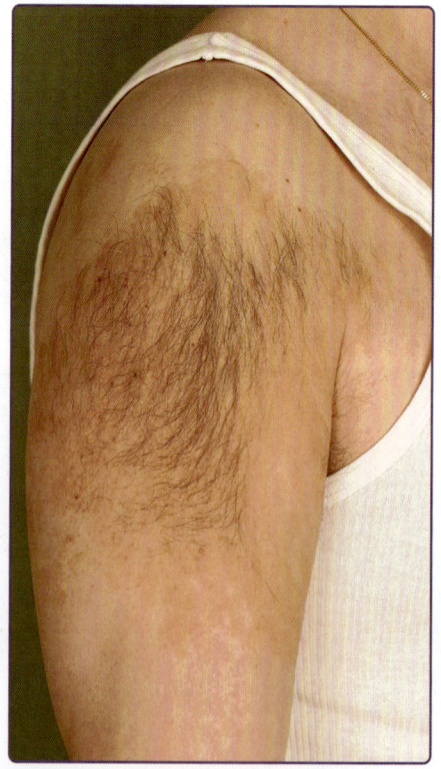

Figure 77-19 Nevus of Becker on the upper arm and shoulder of a young man. Note the typical localization and marked hypertrichosis.

CLINICAL FEATURES

This benign hamartoma may be cosmetically disfiguring and presents with a hyperpigmented macular or speckled area, most commonly in the scapular region, upper arms and chest, although it has been described in any area of the body. Hypertrichosis is common and often develops years after the hyperpigmentation is noted. The hairs are coarse and dark. Becker nevi are often first noted after an episode of intense sun exposure.

Associated anomalies, such as ipsilateral breast hypoplasia, musculoskeletal abnormalities (eg, scoliosis, ipsilateral limb hypoplasia), maxillofacial abnormalities, and additional cutaneous hypoplasias, occur in the rare nevus of Becker syndrome.

ETIOLOGY AND PATHOGENESIS

Nevus of Becker is suggested to follow a paradominant inheritance pattern, which means it (almost) always occurs sporadically. The rare familial cases that have been described (especially in nevus of Becker syndrome) can be explained by a somatic mutation during embryogenesis, resulting in loss of heterozygosity and formation of a mutant cell population. This hypothesis is supported by the identification of chromosomal mosaicism in fibroblasts derived from a Becker nevus.

The exact cause of the hyperpigmentation is unknown.

DIAGNOSIS

Epidermal acanthosis with variable hyperkeratosis and elongation of the rete ridges is noted on histology. Normal numbers of melanocytes, but increased levels of melanin in the basal epidermal layer are demonstrated. In the dermis, the number of arrector pili muscles is increased, making it difficult to differentiate from smooth muscle hamartomas.

DIFFERENTIAL DIAGNOSIS

Congenital hairy nevus, nevus of Ito, and CALMs are all potential differential diagnoses.

CLINICAL COURSE AND PROGNOSIS

Nevus of Becker may appear to darken during pregnancy and in summer. It persists throughout life.

MANAGEMENT

Treatment of nevus of Becker is challenging. If the lesion is small, surgical excision may be appropriate to consider. Although mechanical abrasion, cryotherapy, and argon and CO_2 lasers have been used in the past for larger lesions, the high risk of scarring and dyspigmentation limit their use. Laser hair removal can give the illusion of lightening the lesion. Long-pulsed and picosecond alexandrite laser, as well as quality-switched Nd:YAG, have been cited as useful in some studies, but the current evidence lacks statistical power and has inconsistent findings.[85]

CAFÉ-AU-LAIT MACULES

AT-A-GLANCE

- Acquired circumscribed hyperpigmentation.
- May exist in isolation or as part of a genodermatosis.
- Lasers may be used to lighten spots but relapses are common.

CALMs, also known as café-au-lait spots, may occur spontaneously or as part of a genodermatosis like NF1 and McCune-Albright syndrome.

EPIDEMIOLOGY

Up to one-third of the general population have CALMs. They are more frequent in darker Fitzpatrick skin types, but occur equally in males and females.[86]

CLINICAL FEATURES

Light-brown–tan–dark-brown well-demarcated homogenously hyperpigmented macules or patches can be noted anywhere on the body. The most commonly involved sites are the trunk, buttocks, and lower limbs (Fig. 77-20).

When 6 or more CALMs are noted, investigation for underlying genodermatoses should be commenced.

ETIOLOGY AND PATHOGENESIS

A normal number of melanocytes produce an abnormal amount of melanin.

DIAGNOSIS

Histopathologic examination shows a normal to reduced number of sometimes hypertrophic melanocytes and increased melanin in the basal epidermal layer.

DIFFERENTIAL DIAGNOSIS

Nevus spilus, early nevus of Becker, and congenital nevus are all differential diagnoses.

CLINICAL COURSE AND PROGNOSIS

CALMs persist throughout life.

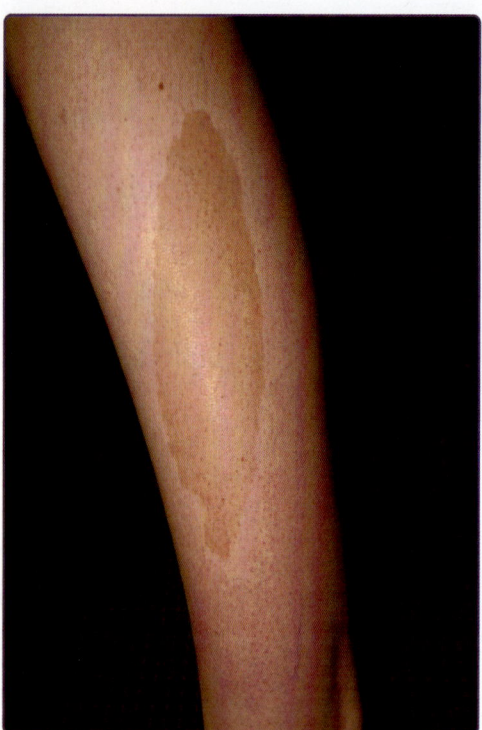

Figure 77-20 Café-au-lait macule on the lower leg of a young girl.

MANAGEMENT

For cosmetic reasons, quality-switched lasers can be used for treatment but relapses are common.

EPHELIDES

AT-A-GLANCE

- Acquired circumscribed hyperpigmentation.
- Autosomal dominant.
- Appear on fair-skinned individuals.

EPIDEMIOLOGY

Ephelides appear in sun-exposed skin of fair-skinned individuals, often those with red or blond hair and Celtic ancestry. Males and females are equally affected.

CLINICAL FEATURES

Ephelides, or freckles, are asymptomatic, small, light-brown macules that appear symmetrically on photo-exposed sites.

ETIOLOGY AND PATHOGENESIS

Ephelides are inherited in an autosomal dominant pattern with a relationship noted to a mutation in the *MCR-1* gene, with carriers demonstrating a significantly increased risk of developing these lesions.[87]

MCR-1 is the receptor for α-melanocyte-stimulating hormone, which activates the melanogenesis pathway via cyclic adenosine monophosphate. Decreased activity of this pathway promotes pheomelanin production.

DIAGNOSIS

Histopathologic examination shows a normal to reduced number of sometimes hypertrophic melanocytes but increased melanin in the basal epidermal layer.

DIFFERENTIAL DIAGNOSIS

Lentigines are the main differential diagnosis. The characteristic appearance in lighter-skin phototypes provides a clue to the diagnosis. The oral mucosa, palms, and soles are spared.

CLINICAL COURSE AND PROGNOSIS

They are more pronounced during spring and summer and fade during the winter. They appear in early childhood and often regress later in life.

MANAGEMENT

Photoprotection is important in those with light skin irrespective of the presence of ephelides but is especially important in individuals who wish to prevent darkening of the lesions. Topical depigmenting agents, such as hydroquinone, retinoids, α-hydroxy acids, and botanicals, may help to lighten pigmentation. Physical therapies, such as cryotherapy, are difficult to perform on very small lesions, so intense pulsed light or quality-switched lasers are preferred, but relapse should be expected.

ACROMELANOSIS PROGRESSIVA

AT-A-GLANCE

- Acquired circumscribed hyperpigmentation in newborns.
- Usually involves acral and perineal areas.
- Spontaneously resolves.

EPIDEMIOLOGY

Very few cases have been described.

CLINICAL FEATURES

Diffuse brown hyperpigmentation is noted in newborns or during the first few weeks of life and is located on acral and or perineal areas. Progression to the trunk, oral mucosal involvement, and seizures were reported in one case.[88]

ETIOLOGY AND PATHOGENESIS

The cause is unknown.

DIAGNOSIS

Acromelanosis progressiva is a clinical diagnosis that becomes apparent over time, as the lesions fade. Histology reveals increased basal epidermal melanocytes.

DIFFERENTIAL DIAGNOSIS

Periungual hyperpigmentation, acropigmentation of Dohi, and reticulate acropigmentation of Kitamura are differential diagnoses to consider.

CLINICAL COURSE AND PROGNOSIS

Spontaneous resolution is noted.

MANAGEMENT

Reassurance is important as treatment is not required.

POSTINFLAMMATORY HYPERPIGMENTATION

AT-A-GLANCE

- Acquired circumscribed hyperpigmentation in sites of prior inflammation or injury.
- More common in persons with skin of color.
- Hydroquinone remains the gold standard treatment.
- Spontaneously resolves over a variable period of time.

Postinflammatory hyperpigmentation (PIH) is a common reactive melanosis caused by numerous preceding inflammatory (eg, acne, lichen planus, psoriasis) and cutaneous insults, such as drug and phototoxic reactions, infections, physical injury or trauma, and allergic reactions.

EPIDEMIOLOGY

PIH is far more common in darker-skin types (Fitzpatrick Types III to VI) and can occur at any age. It is observed in a significant number of individuals of African ancestry who are suffering from acne.[89]

CLINICAL FEATURES

PIH consists of a macular hyperpigmentation at the site of inflammation (Fig. 77-21). A Wood lamp examination can determine the depth of the hyperpigmentation (see section "Melasma"). PIH after epidermal inflammation results in brown discoloration while inflammation in the dermis results in a gray-brown discoloration. The severity of PIH is proportional to the severity of the inflammation and degree of basement membrane disruption.

Discovering the cause of the primary dermatosis should involve examination of the entire skin. Adverse effects on quality of life have been documented, especially in persons with skin of color, and should be addressed.

ETIOLOGY AND PATHOGENESIS

It is thought that inflammatory markers stimulate the melanocytes that drive PIH. Conditions causing epidermal inflammation cause an increase in epidermal keratinocytes, whereas dermal inflammation results in pigment incontinence into the dermis. The melanin is eventually cleared by macrophages.

The cause for increased susceptibility of PIH in persons with skin of color has not been fully elucidated but is thought to relate to the increased amount of melanin in melanosomes.

DIAGNOSIS

Histologic features include pigment incontinence with accumulation of melanophages and increased melanin in epidermal layers.

DIFFERENTIAL DIAGNOSIS

When PIH is widespread on the trunk, it may look similar to urticaria pigmentosa but a positive Darier sign and the history of itching associated with the lesions should help to differentiate PIH from urticaria pigmentosa.

CLINICAL COURSE AND PROGNOSIS

The clinical course is variable and depends on the location of the inflammation or injury. It is more persistent in darker-skin types (Fitzpatrick Types III to VI) and after lichenoid inflammatory processes. Epidermal PIH often has spontaneous but slow fading.

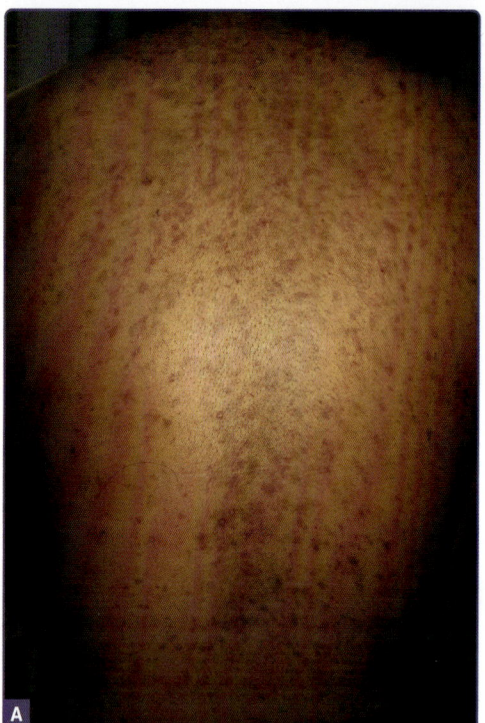

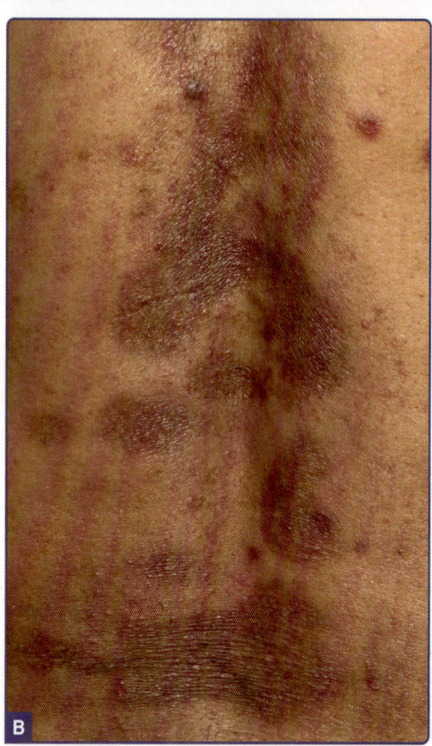

Figure 77-21 **A,** Postinflammatory hyperpigmentation secondary to acne on the back of a young African girl. **B,** Postinflammatory hyperpigmentation secondary to psoriasis on the back of a Chinese man.

MANAGEMENT

Management of PIH remains difficult. It is important, especially when treating patients with skin of color, to treat the primary dermatosis early to prevent PIH.

The importance of photoprotection should not be underestimated. Pretreatment and posttreatment regimens are critical after physical therapies, especially for persons with skin of color, and may include sun protection, hydroquinone, hydroquinone alternatives, or topical corticosteroids.[90]

Topical hydroquinone remains the gold standard treatment for PIH (Table 77-3). A plethora of nonprescription cosmeceuticals containing licorice, soy, niacinamide, and various botanicals are available and numerous prescribed topicals, such as kojic acid, retinoids, and α-hydroxy acids may be used as monotherapy or in combination. Kligman's formula and similar triple-therapy combinations containing hydroquinone, tretinoin, and a topical corticosteroid are also commonly prescribed. Physical therapies, including peels and lasers, should be used with caution given they can induce PIH if used too aggressively. Quality-switched and picosecond lasers have been described in isolation or as part of a broader treatment plan for PIH. Epidermal PIH is more amenable to topical therapy than dermal PIH.

MELASMA

AT-A-GLANCE

- Acquired light-brown to dark-brown poorly circumscribed macules.
- More common in persons with skin of color.
- Malar skin, nose, forehead, and upper lip are commonly involved areas.
- Hydroquinone remains the gold standard treatment.
- Physical and oral therapies also can be used.

TABLE 77-3
Lightening Agents

AGENTS	MECHANISM OF ACTION
Hydroquinone	Tyrosinase inhibitor
Retinoids	Stimulate keratinocyte turnover, reduce melanosome transfer, tyrosinase inhibitor
Arbutin	Tyrosinase inhibitor; inhibits melanosome maturation
Azelaic acid	Tyrosinase inhibitor
Kojic acid	Interacts with copper and inhibits tyrosinase
Tranexamic acid	Plasmin inhibition; antioxidant

Adapted from Chaowattanapanit S, Silpa-archa N, Kohli I, et al. Postinflammatory hyperpigmentation: a comprehensive overview: treatment options and prevention. *J Am Acad Dermatol*. 2017;77(4):607-621.

Melasma is one of the most common disorders of pigmentation and is sometimes referred to as chloasma or the mask of pregnancy.

EPIDEMIOLOGY

Melasma affects millions of people with a reported prevalence ranging from 9% in Hispanic populations in southern United States to 40% in Southeast Asians.[91] It is cited as the most common pigmentary disorder in Indian women. It is mainly seen in premenopausal women, although men and postmenopausal women also may be affected.

CLINICAL FEATURES

Melasma typically presents with diffuse light-brown to dark-brown areas of pigmentation on the central face (Figs. 77-22 and 77-23). The malar and mandibular regions, forehead, chin, and upper lip are most commonly affected—centrofacial (63%: forehead, nose, chin, and upper lip); malar (21%: nose and cheeks); and mandibular (16%: ramus mandibulae) patterns are most common. Melasma spares the periorbital skin as well as the lips, neck, and ears. It may be seen less commonly on the forearms (also known as acquired brachial cutaneous dyschromatosis).

The negative impact on quality of life has been documented repeatedly in the literature; consequently, symptoms of depression and anxiety need to be explored by the treating clinician.

ETIOLOGY AND PATHOGENESIS

The pathogenesis is not completely understood. Biologically active melanocytes, genetic and hormonal influences, and ultraviolet light exposure are known to be important. Specific precipitants, particularly oral contraceptives and estrogen replacement therapy, have been implicated in exacerbating the condition.

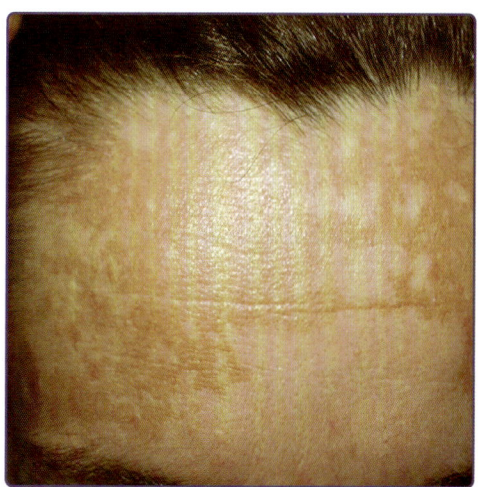

Figure 77-22 Melasma on the forehead of a young woman. Note the well-demarcated brown macules.

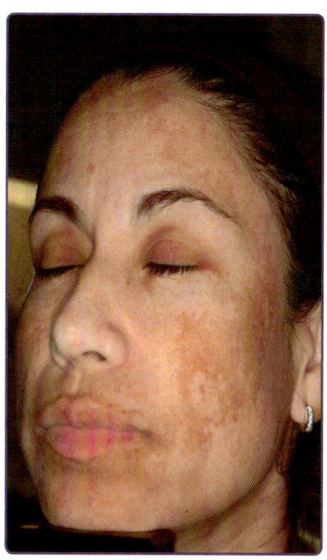

Figure 77-23 Hyperpigmentation of the forehead, cheek, upper lip, and chin caused by melasma in a Latino female.

Recently, visible light in individuals with skin of color and increased vascularity and vascular endothelial growth factor in the epidermis of lesional skin have been implicated in the pathogenesis of melasma.

DIAGNOSIS

A Wood lamp may help differentiate epidermal from dermal and mixed melasma in those with lighter skin types, although even Wood light–enhancing lesions, supposedly signifying epidermal melasma, have dermal melanin.

DIFFERENTIAL DIAGNOSIS

The differential diagnosis may be broad depending on the area affected and the location of the pigment (epidermal, dermal, or mixed). It includes postinflammatory pigmentation, maturational dyschromia, medication-induced pigmentation, lichen planus pigmentosus, and possibly poikiloderma of Civatte.

CLINICAL COURSE AND PROGNOSIS

Despite lightening or resolution with treatment, melasma is a chronic and relapsing condition with exacerbations during pregnancy, sun or visible light exposure, and with certain hormonal treatments.

MANAGEMENT

Managing expectations and counseling on the recurrent and chronic nature of melasma is critical for patient satisfaction. Cessation of any obvious triggers is the first step in management. Photoprotection is central to management and should include sun-avoidance, protective clothing, and regular application of a broad-spectrum sunscreen with a physical blocker. Care should also be taken to protect from visible light in those with Fitzpatrick skin Types IV to VI.

Epidermal pigmentation is known to be more responsive to topical therapy. Even though 4% hydroquinone remains the gold standard, various other topical agents have been used with variable success. Nonprescription creams containing soy, licorice, lignin peroxidase, and niacinamide are just some of the botanicals and vitamins said to help mild epidermal melasma. Preparations containing tretinoin, azelaic acid, and kojic acid are helpful when used for prolonged periods.

Combining topical therapies is a useful strategy for epidermal melasma. Kligman's formula is a popular combination of 5% hydroquinone, 0.1% tretinoin, and a mild topical corticosteroid. Another treatment, commonly referred to as triple-combination therapy, includes 4% hydroquinone, 0.05% tretinoin, and a topical corticosteroid. Both Kligman's formula and triple-combination therapy have been deemed efficacious for epidermal melasma.

Superficial chemical peels have proven efficacious and are useful when used as a treatment adjunct, but the cost and frequency of treatments must be considered. Furthermore, the risk of postinflammatory hyperpigmentation must be considered with appropriate pretreatment and posttreatment care, especially in individuals with skin of color. Laser therapy may be helpful in the treatment of melasma, but can also result in further unwanted hyperpigmentation. Various lasers, including intense pulsed light, erbium:YAG, and nonablative 1550-nm and 1927-nm fractional lasers have all been reported to be effective for melasma but low-fluence quality-switched Nd:YAG laser (also known as laser toning), is the most popular. This treatment modality has proved efficacious and safe when a few treatments are used in carefully selected cases.

Recently, tranexamic acid has been proven to lighten epidermal and dermal melasma. It has been used in topical, intralesional, and oral forms. When used as an adjunct in low doses (500 to 700 mg daily) over a few months, it is efficacious and safe in treatment-resistant cases.[92]

EPIDEMIOLOGY

Usually appears at birth or in childhood.

CLINICAL FEATURES

PUL is characterized by numerous lentigines with sharp margins. Lesions occur in a segmental pattern in the midline in 1 or more dermatomes.[93]

ETIOLOGY AND PATHOGENESIS

Its segmental pattern and presentation, which are accompanied by café-au-lait spots, Lisch nodules, or neurofibromas, suggests that PUL is a variant of mosaic NF1. Genetic studies will help to further elucidate this subject.

DIAGNOSIS

The characteristic history and clinical appearance are often diagnostic.

DIFFERENTIAL DIAGNOSIS

Mosaic NF1.

CLINICAL COURSE AND PROGNOSIS

PUL persists throughout life. No complications have been noted as a result of PUL.

MANAGEMENT

Quality-switched alexandrite and Nd:YAG lasers are reported to be treatment options.

PARTIAL UNILATERAL LENTIGINOSIS

AT-A-GLANCE

- Acquired circumscribed hyperpigmentation.
- Appears at birth or in childhood.
- May be a variant of mosaic neurofibromatosis Type 1.
- Usually within 1 or more dermatomes.

Partial unilateral lentiginosis (PUL) is a rare pigmentary disorder also known as unilateral lentigines, lentiginous mosaicism, zosteriform lentiginous nevus, segmental lentiginosis, and agminated lentiginosis.

RIEHL MELANOSIS

AT-A-GLANCE

- Acquired gray-brown-blue circumscribed reticulate hyperpigmentation.
- Caused by topical contact sensitizers.
- Mostly middle-aged women.
- Located mainly on the face.
- Lasers have been described as a treatment option.

Riehl melanosis, also known as female facial melanosis and pigmented contact dermatitis, was first described in 1917 by Riehl.

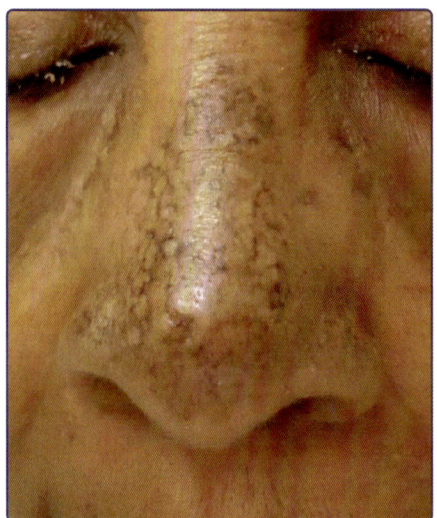

Figure 77-24 Riehl melanosis on the face.

EPIDEMIOLOGY

Riehl melanosis is mostly seen in middle-aged women, especially in darker-skin types, such as Latinos and Asians.

CLINICAL FEATURES

It is characterized by rapid onset of a reticular gray-brown to almost black reticulate hyperpigmentation. The face (especially the forehead, zygomatic area, and temples) and the neck are principally involved, but the hands, forearms, and trunk also may be affected (Fig. 77-24). Inflammatory findings, such as erythema and pruritus, are usually absent although it may be observed in very early stages of the clinical course.

Significant psychological stress may be reported by patients.

ETIOLOGY AND PATHOGENESIS

The pathogenesis is not understood fully understood but the hyperpigmentation has been postulated to be induced by repeated contact with threshold doses of a contact sensitizer such as fragrances, some pigments, and bactericides used in cosmetics and optical whiteners.

DIAGNOSIS

The main histopathologic feature is liquefactive degeneration of the basal layer of the epidermis, resulting in pigment incontinence in the dermis.

DIFFERENTIAL DIAGNOSIS

Poikiloderma of Civatte, erythrose peribuccal pigmentaire of Brocq, erythromelanosis follicularis faciei et colli, and medication-induced pigmentation are all differential diagnoses.

CLINICAL COURSE AND PROGNOSIS

Riehl melanosis is progressive if the contact sensitizer is not avoided. It may take many years to lighten, but no systemic effects are noted.

MANAGEMENT

Unfortunately treatment is challenging. Cessation of the topical sensitizer is critical. Photoprotection and topical depigmenting agents (hydroquinone, α-hydroxy acids, tretinoin) have a limited effect on this dermal pigmentation, with more recent reports describing treatment with lasers and oral tranexamic acid. Intense pulsed-light therapy has been helpful in some cases, but carries the risk of postinflammatory hyperpigmentation. Low-fluence quality-switched Nd:YAG and "laser toning" have demonstrated moderate improvements in Asian skin and have even been used in combination with oral tranexamic acid and hydroquinone.[94]

CRONKHITE-CANADA SYNDROME

AT-A-GLANCE

- Acquired generalized light-brown to dark-brown macules and patches.
- Palms and soles often involved first.
- Onychodystrophy and alopecia are also seen.
- Nutritional supplementation and corticosteroids may help.

Cronkhite-Canada syndrome (CCS) is a very rare condition resulting in cutaneous and GI manifestations.

EPIDEMIOLOGY

Approximately 450 cases are reported in the literature. Adults of Asian (most commonly Japanese) and European extraction are usually affected, starting in the fourth decade of life.

CLINICAL FEATURES

Cronkhite-Canada syndrome initially presents with brown macules and patches noted on the palms and soles. This is followed by generalized pigmentary changes with onychodystrophy and alopecia.[95]

GI symptoms, such as abdominal pain, nausea, diarrhea, and loss of weight, are noted in addition to GI polyposis and occasional malignancies. Complications include, but are not limited to, protein and electrolyte imbalance, anemia, and even portal vein thrombosis and glomerulonephritis.

Cronkhite-Canada syndrome may be associated with other autoimmune conditions like systemic lupus erythematosus and rheumatoid arthritis.

ETIOLOGY AND PATHOGENESIS

An autoimmune process is suspected but the exact etiology remains elusive.

DIAGNOSIS

Clinicopathologic correlation is required to make the diagnosis. Histologic changes include increased epidermal melanin with dermal melanosis. Acanthosis and compact hyperkeratosis of the epidermis are also seen.

DIFFERENTIAL DIAGNOSIS

The differential diagnosis includes other causes of congenital lentigines.

CLINICAL COURSE AND PROGNOSIS

Cronkhite-Canada syndrome is progressive and may cause significant morbidity and mortality because of the systemic manifestations of the condition.

MANAGEMENT

Immunosuppression with corticosteroids and nutritional supplements may be helpful.

ERYTHROSE PERIBUCCAL OF BROCQ

AT-A-GLANCE

- Very rare dermatosis causing diffuse hyperpigmentation, erythema, and folliculocentric skin-colored papules.
- Occurs mainly in women.

Erythrose peribuccal of Brocq is also known as erythrose pigmenta faciei, erythrosis pigmentosa peribuccalis, and melanosis perioralis et peribuccalis.

EPIDEMIOLOGY

Only a few cases, mainly in women, have been reported.

CLINICAL FEATURES

Erythema followed by diffuse light-brown to dark-brown pigmentation in the perioral region affecting the cutaneous upper and lower lip with sparing around the vermilion border is usually seen. In some cases, scale and loss of vellus hairs are noted.

ETIOLOGY AND PATHOGENESIS

The etiology is unknown, although ultraviolet light exposure and fragrances may play a role.

DIAGNOSIS

The diagnosis is usually made clinically. Histologic findings are nonspecific.

DIFFERENTIAL DIAGNOSIS

Melasma and PIH are the main differential diagnoses.

CLINICAL COURSE AND PROGNOSIS

Persistence and progression are the rule.

MANAGEMENT

Photoprotection and avoidance of triggers is recommended.

CUTANEOUS AMYLOIDOSIS

Macular amyloidosis presents as brown to gray-brown macules coalescing to plaques, mainly on the back (see Chap. 125).

ATROPHODERMA OF PASINI-PIERINI

Chap. 70 discusses atrophic disorders of the skin in greater detail. The cutaneous lesions of atrophoderma of Pasini-Pierini can be described as single or multiple gray to violaceous-brown atrophic patches from 1 cm to more than 10 cm in diameter with slight depression and a characteristic "cliff-drop" border.

FIXED DRUG ERUPTION

Fixed drug eruption can cause hyperpigmentation (see earlier in section "Toxins and Medications" and Chap. 45).

ERYTHEMA DYSCHROMICUM PERSTANS

AT-A-GLANCE

- Acquired idiopathic dermal melanosis.
- Blue-gray well-demarcated hyperpigmented macules and plaques.
- Usually intermediate skin types (eg, Hispanic, Asian populations).
- Seen in photoprotected sites.
- Treatment is challenging and may require systemic therapy.

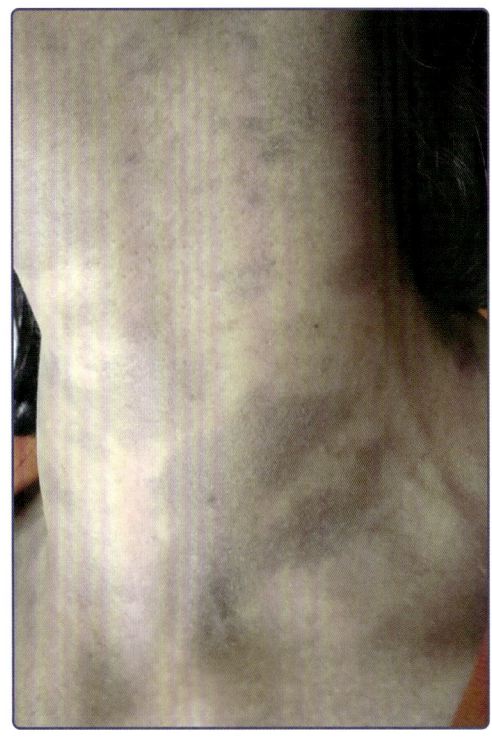

Figure 77-25 Acquired dermal melanosis–erythema dyschromicum perstans/on the neck of a Hispanic woman.

Erythema dyschromicum perstans (EDP), also known as ashy dermatosis, dermatosis cinecienta, and erythema chronicum figuratum melanodermicum, was first described by Ramirez in 1957.[96] Patients with this eruption were labeled as *los cenicientos*, the ashen ones. The terms EDP, lichen planus pigmentosus, and idiopathic eruptive macular pigmentation have been used interchangeably and are often confused in the literature, even though they appear to be distinct clinical entities.

EPIDEMIOLOGY

EDP is mainly observed in females with intermediate skin types (eg, Hispanics and Asians). It is said to be a disease of young adults with most presenting between the second and third decades of life, although a recent review of Korean patients revealed onset in the third and fourth decades of life.

CLINICAL FEATURES

EDP presents with widespread asymptomatic well-demarcated blue-gray macules that are most commonly seen on photoprotected sites (Figs. 77-25 and 77-26). Lesions slowly expand over time and an erythematous border may be seen at the edge of the lesion in the acute stages of the condition. The erythematous border, especially in darker-skin types, may evolve into a hypopigmented border that accentuates the hyperpigmentation.

Mucous membranes are not involved and no extracutaneous manifestations exist.

ETIOLOGY AND PATHOGENESIS

The etiology is unknown although human leukocyte antigen-D related (HLA-DR)–associated susceptibility has been described in a Mexican population.[97]

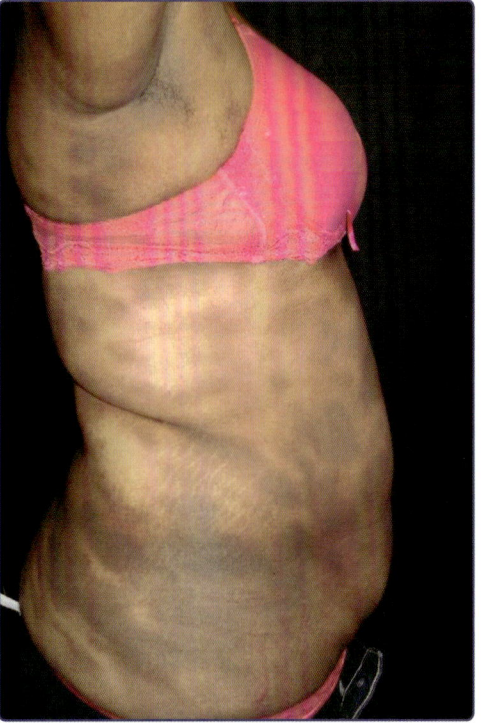

Figure 77-26 Erythema dyschromicum perstans on the trunk. (Used with permission of Juan Carlos Mendez, Department of Dermatology, UANL. Monterrey, México.)

DIAGNOSIS

The diagnosis usually requires clinicopathologic correlation. Histologically, early lesions reveal dermal edema and lichenoid inflammation, basal layer vacuolization and colloid bodies with a perivascular infiltrate. Later, melanin incontinence is noted in the deep dermis along with melanophages.

DIFFERENTIAL DIAGNOSIS

Lichen planus pigmentosus, idiopathic eruptive macular pigmentation, and PIH are the main differential diagnoses. Medication-induced pigmentation must also be excluded.

CLINICAL COURSE AND PROGNOSIS

The condition is chronic and very difficult to treat. There is a slow progression of the lesion over several years, usually without spontaneous regression.

MANAGEMENT

Topical therapies are not helpful for this acquired dermal disorder of pigmentation and improvement with systemic therapy is minimal. An 8- to 12-week course of dapsone 100 mg may lighten pigmentation and clofazimine 100 mg daily has demonstrated improvement in a small study.[98] Unfortunately, even though many other treatments have been evaluated, none have resulted in appreciable lightening. Most recently, laser surgery has been studied by a group in the Netherlands, who concluded fractionated laser was unsuccessful for the treatment of EDP.[99]

LICHEN PLANUS PIGMENTOSUS

AT-A-GLANCE

- Acquired idiopathic dermal melanosis.
- Poorly demarcated brown to gray-brown hyperpigmented macules.
- Usually seen with deeply pigmented skin (eg, South East Asians, Arabic).
- Mostly in photoexposed sites.
- Treatments provide only minimal improvement in pigmentation.

Lichen planus pigmentosus is considered a variant of lichen planus. Lichen planus is discussed in Chap. 32. It is often confused in the literature for EDP and idiopathic eruptive macular pigmentation.

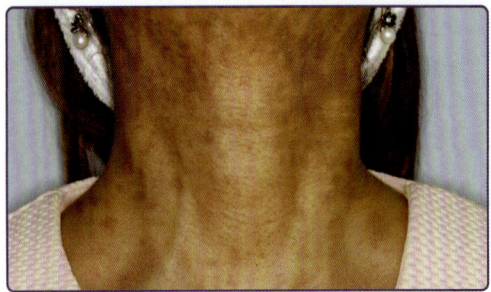

Figure 77-27 Acquired dermal melanosis–erythema dyschromicum perstans/lichen planus pigmentosus on the neck of a Sri Lankan lady.

EPIDEMIOLOGY

Lichen planus pigmentosus is mainly observed in middle-aged (third to fourth decade of life) individuals with more deeply pigmented skin (eg, South Asians, Southeast Asians, and the Arabic population).

CLINICAL FEATURES

Symmetrical brown to gray-brown poorly demarcated macules and patches are seen mainly in photoexposed sites such as the head (forehead and temples) and neck (Fig. 77-27). Lesions also may be seen in skin folds such as the axillae (known as lichen planus pigmentosus–inversus). Lesions may also rarely appear on mucous membranes.

No extracutaneous manifestations exist.

ETIOLOGY AND PATHOGENESIS

The exact etiology is unknown but mustard and amla oils used in cooking and in hair care formulas, respectively, have been listed as possible causes in retrospective studies. Medication-induced pigmentation must also be excluded.

DIAGNOSIS

Biopsy is required and clinicopathologic correlation is critical. Epidermal atrophy, basal layer vacuolation with a perivascular lymphocytic infiltrate, and melanophages in the superficial dermis are noted histologically.

DIFFERENTIAL DIAGNOSIS

EDP, idiopathic eruptive macular pigmentation, and PIH are the main differential diagnoses.

CLINICAL COURSE AND PROGNOSIS

Some cases gradually resolve over many months, but these cases are the exceptions to the rule.

MANAGEMENT

Photoprotection is critical. Topical tacrolimus (0.03% twice daily), topical and systemic corticosteroids, and topical vitamin A may be helpful in lichen planus pigmentosus.[100] Treatment combinations and laser treatments also have been used with variable results. Recently, a prospective study reported low-dose oral isotretinoin (20 mg daily), used over 6 months in conjunction with sunscreen, caused stabilization and decrease in pigmentation, especially when used early in the course of disease.[101]

IDIOPATHIC ERUPTIVE MACULAR HYPERPIGMENTATION

AT-A-GLANCE

- Acquired idiopathic dermal melanosis.
- Well-demarcated brown to gray hyperpigmented macules and plaques.
- Usually smaller lesions than erythema dyschromicum perstans.
- Usually appears in children and adolescents.
- Usually appears on the face, trunk, and proximal extremities.
- Treatments provide only a minimal improvement in pigmentation.

Idiopathic eruptive macular hyperpigmentation is a rare disorder of pigmentation, described initially by Degos and colleagues but first described in English in 1996.[102,103]

EPIDEMIOLOGY

Idiopathic eruptive macular hyperpigmentation is usually seen in children and adolescents.

CLINICAL FEATURES

Idiopathic eruptive macular hyperpigmentation is characterized by an eruption of asymptomatic, well-demarcated, nonscaly, brown macules and plaques (5 mm to several centimeters in diameter) involving the face, neck, trunk, and proximal extremities. No preceding inflammation or erythema is noted.

A subset of patients have been noted to have thickened plaques (epidermal papillomatosis).

No extracutaneous manifestations exist.

ETIOLOGY AND PATHOGENESIS

The etiology is unknown.

DIAGNOSIS

Histopathologically, there is increased melanin in the basal epidermis and melanophages demonstrated in the dermis. The number of mast cells is normal. No basal layer change or lichenoid inflammation is seen.

DIFFERENTIAL DIAGNOSIS

EDP, lichen planus pigmentosus, and PIH are the main differential diagnoses. Drug-induced pigmentation must be excluded.

CLINICAL COURSE AND PROGNOSIS

Lesions spontaneously disappear over several months to years without scarring.

MANAGEMENT

Spontaneous resolution means that in most situations, treatment is not needed. Topical lightening agents like retinoids, α-hydroxy acids, and hydroquinone are possible treatments.

MIXED HYPOMELANOSIS AND HYPERMELANOSIS

AT-A-GLANCE

Causes of mixed hypomelanosis and hypermelanosis include:
- Dyschromatosis hereditaria universalis.
- Dyschromatosis symmetrica hereditaria.
- Reticulate acropigmentation of Dohi.
- Familial progressive hyperpigmentation with (Westerhof syndrome) or without hypopigmentation.
- Vagabond leucoderma.

DYSCHROMATOSIS HEREDITARIA UNIVERSALIS

Dyschromatosis hereditaria universalis is a rare autosomal dominant disorder (mutation in the *ABCB6* gene on chromosome 12q21-q23) that usually presents in infancy or early childhood in Japanese families and is characterized by pinpoint to pea-sized hypopigmented and hyperpigmented macules, distributed in a reticulated pattern over the trunk, abdomen, and limbs, usually sparing the face and palmoplantar surfaces.[104]

RETICULATE ACROPIGMENTATION OF DOHI

Reticulate acropigmentation of Dohi is a localized form of dyschromatosis universalis hereditaria, also called dyschromatosis symmetrica hereditaria. It is characterized by small, symmetric, hyperpigmented and hypopigmented macules on the dorsal hands and feet, and is mainly seen in young children in South American and Asian families.[104]

FAMILIAL PROGRESSIVE HYPERPIGMENTATION WITH (WESTERHOF SYNDROME) OR WITHOUT HYPOPIGMENTATION

Familial progressive hyperpigmentation with or without hypopigmentation is an autosomal dominant condition caused by a heterozygous mutation in the KIT ligand gene (*KITLG*) on chromosome 12q22. It presents at birth or early infancy as diffuse hyperpigmentation and may demonstrate café-au-lait macules and larger hypopigmented ash-leaf macules on the face, neck, trunk, and limbs. The case series of Westerhof syndrome in 1978 described some family members with retarded growth and mental retardation.[105]

VAGABOND LEUKODERMA

Vagabond leukoderma is a condition found in persons living in poor hygienic conditions. Many abuse alcohol, live on an inadequate diet, and are infested with lice and/or scabies. Diffuse light-brown hyperpigmentation is present at the shoulder and waist girdle, and the neck and back are dotted with depigmented macules. The condition improves upon institution of a healthier lifestyle and likely represents a coexistence of many disorders

ACKNOWLEDGMENTS

We would like to acknowledge the contribution of the authors of this chapter in the previous edition: Hilde Lapeere, Barbara Boone, Sofie De Schepper, Evelien Verhaeghe, Mireille Van Gele, Katia Ongenae, Nanja Van Geel, Jo Lambert, and Lieve Brochez.

REFERENCES

1. Kalter DC, Griffiths WA, Atherton DJ. Linear and whorled nevoid hypermelanosis. *J Am Acad Dermatol*. 1988;19:1037-1044.
2. Hartmann A, Hofmann UB, Hoehn H, et al. Postnatal confirmation of prenatally diagnosed trisomy 20 mosaicism in a patient with linear and whorled nevoid hypermelanosis. *Pediatr Dermatol*. 2004;21:636-641.
3. Happle R. A fresh look at incontinentia pigmenti. *Arch Dermatol*. 2003;139:1206-1208.
4. Fusco F, Bardaro T, Fimiani G, et al. Molecular analysis of the genetic defect in a large cohort of IP patients and identification of novel NEMO mutations interfering with NF-kappa B activation. *Hum Mol Genet*. 2004;13:1763-1773.
5. Conte MI, Pescatore A, Paciolla M, et al. Insight into IKBKG/NEMO locus: report of new mutations and complex genomic rearrangements leading to incontinentia pigmenti disease. *Hum Mutat*. 2014;35:165-177.
6. Jessup CJ, Morgan SC, Cohen LM, et al. Incontinentia pigmenti: treatment of IP with topical tacrolimus. *J Drugs Dermatol*. 2009;8:944-946.
7. Schmidt M, Serror K, Chaouat M, et al. Management of hypopigmented scars following burn injuries [in French]. *Ann Chir Plast Esthet*. 2018;63(3):246-254.
8. Vulliamy T, Marrone A, Goldman F, et al. The RNA component of telomerase is mutated in autosomal dominant dyskeratosis congenita. *Nature*. 2001;413:432-435.
9. Walne AJ, Dokal I. Advances in the understanding of dyskeratosis congenita. *Br J Haematol*. 2009;145:164-172.
10. Lugassy J, Itin P, Ishida-Yamamoto A, et al. Naegeli-Franceschetti-Jadassohn syndrome and dermatopathia pigmentosa reticularis: two allelic ectodermal dysplasias caused by dominant mutations in KRT14. *Am J Hum Genet*. 2006;79:724-730.
11. Komaya G. Symmetrische Pigmentanomalie der Extremitaeten. *Arch Derm Syphilol*. 1924;147:389-393.
12. Amyere M, Vogt T, Hoo J, et al. KITLG mutations cause familial progressive hyper- and hypopigmentation. *J Invest Dermatol*. 2011;131:1234-1239.
13. Rycroft RJ, Calnan CD, Allenby CF. Dermatopathia pigmentosa reticularis. *Clin Exp Dermatol*. 1977;2:39-44.
14. Betz RC, Planko L, Eigelshoven S, et al. Loss-of-function mutations in the keratin 5 gene lead to Dowling-Degos disease. *Am J Hum Genet*. 2006;78:510-519.
15. Hanneken S, Rütten A, Pasternack SM, et al. Systematic mutation screening of KRT5 supports the hypothesis that Galli-Galli disease is a variant of Dowling-Degos disease. *Br J Dermatol*. 2010;163:197-200.
16. Kono M, Sugiura K, Suganuma M, et al. Whole exome sequencing identifies ADAM10 mutations as a cause of reticulate acropigmentation of Kitamura, a clinical entity distinct from Dowling-Degos disease. *Hum Mol Genet*. 2013;22:3524-3533.
17. Muller CS, Pfohler C, Tilgen W. Changing a concept–controversy on the confusing spectrum of the reticulate pigmented disorders of the skin. *J Cutan Pathol*. 2009;36:44-48.
18. Ota M. Naevus fusco-caeruleus ophthalmo-maxillaris. *Jpn J Dermatol*. 1939;46:369.
19. Ho SG, Chan HH. The Asian dermatologic patient: review of common pigmentary disorders and cutaneous diseases. *Am J Clin Dermatol*. 2009;10:153-168.
20. Shah VV, Bray FN, Aldahan AS, et al. Lasers and nevus of Ota: a comprehensive review. *Lasers Med Sci*. 2016;31:179-185.
21. Chan HH, Kono T. Nevus of Ota: clinical aspects and management. *Skinmed*. 2003;2:89-96.
22. Forbat E, Al-Niami F. The use of picosecond lasers beyond tattoos. *J Cosmet Laser Ther*. 2016;16:1-3.
23. Ito M. Naevus fusco-caeruleus acromio-deltoides. *Tohoku J Exp Med*. 1954;60:10-12.
24. Leung AK. Mongolian spots in Chinese children. *Int J Dermatol*. 1988;27:106-108.

25. Mimouni-Bloch A, Finezilber Y, Rothschild M, et al. Extensive Mongolian spots and lysosomal storage diseases. *J Pediatr*. 2016;170:333-e1.
26. Burkhart CG, Gohara A. Dermal melanocyte hamartoma. A distinctive new form of dermal melanocytosis. *Arch Dermatol*. 1981;117:102-104.
27. Stratakis CA. Genetics of Carney complex and related familial lentiginoses, and other multiple tumor syndromes. *Front Biosci*. 2000;5:D353-D366.
28. Jeghers H, McKusick V, Katz KH. Generalized intestinal polyposis and melanin spots of the oral mucosa, lips and digits a syndrome of diagnostic significance. *N Engl J Med*. 1949;241:1031-1036.
29. Shah KR, Boland CR, Patel M, et al. Cutaneous manifestations of gastrointestinal disease: part I. *J Am Acad Dermatol*. 2013;68:189.e1-21.
30. Digilio MC, Sarkozy A, de Zorzi A, et al. LEOPARD syndrome: clinical diagnosis in the first year of life. *Am J Med Genet A*. 2006;140:740-746.
31. Carney JA, Gordon H, Carpenter PC, et al. The complex of myxomas, spotty pigmentation, and endocrine overactivity. *Medicine (Baltimore)*. 1985;64:270-283.
32. Mateus C, Palangié A, Franck N, et al. Heterogeneity of skin manifestations in patients with Carney complex. *J Am Acad Dermatol*. 2008;59:801-810.
33. Rothenbuhler A, Stratakis CA. Clinical and molecular genetics of Carney complex. *Best Pract Res Clin Endocrinol Metab*. 2010;24:389-399.
34. Gorlin RJ, Cohen MM Jr, Condon LM, et al. Bannayan-Riley-Ruvalcaba syndrome. *Am J Med Genet*. 1992;44:307-314.
35. Hobert JA, Eng C. PTEN hamartoma tumor syndrome: an overview. *Genet Med*. 2009;11:687-694.
36. Dociu I, Galaction-Nițelea O, Sîrjiță N, et al. Centrofacial lentiginosis. A survey of 40 cases. *Br J Dermatol*. 1976;94:39-43.
37. Alper JC, Holmes LB. The incidence and significance of birthmarks in a cohort of 4,641 newborns. *Pediatr Dermatol*. 1983;1:58-68.
38. Brems H, Chmara M, Sahbatou M, et al. Germline loss-of-function mutations in SPRED1 cause a neurofibromatosis 1-like phenotype. *Nat Genet*. 2007;39:1120-1126.
39. Denayer E, Descheemaeker MJ, Stewart DR, et al. Observations on intelligence and behavior in 15 patients with Legius syndrome. *Am J Med Genet C Semin Med Genet*. 2011;157:123-128.
40. Dumitrescu CE, Collins MT. McCune-Albright syndrome. *Orphanet J Rare Dis*. 2008;3:12.
41. Kaneko H, Kondo N. Clinical features of Bloom syndrome and function of the causative gene, BLM helicase. *Expert Rev Mol Diagn*. 2004;4:393-401.
42. Cheok CF, Bachrati CZ, Chan KL, et al. Roles of the Bloom's syndrome helicase in the maintenance of genome stability. *Biochem Soc Trans*. 2005;33:1456-1459.
43. Ellis NA, German J. Molecular genetics of Bloom's syndrome. *Hum Mol Genet*. 1996;5(spec no):1457-1463.
44. Watson GH. Pulmonary stenosis, cafe-au-lait spots, and dull intelligence. *Arch Dis Child*. 1967;42:303-307.
45. Allanson JE, Upadhyaya M, Watson GH, et al. Watson syndrome: is it a subtype of type 1 neurofibromatosis? *J Med Genet*. 1991;28:752-756.
46. Silver HK, Kiyasu W, George J, et al. Syndrome of congenital hemihypertrophy, shortness of stature and elevated urinary gonadotrophins. *Pediatrics*. 1953;12:386-376.
47. Russel A. A syndrome of intra-uterine dwarfism recognizable at birth with cranio-facial dysostosis, disproportionately short arms, and other anomalies (5 examples). *Proc R Soc Med*. 1954;47:1040-1044.
48. Peñaherrera MS, Weindler S, Van Allen MI, et al. Methylation profiling in individuals with Russel-Silver syndrome. *Am J Med Genet A*. 2010;152A(2):347-355.
49. Pereira MA, Halpern A, Salgado LR, et al. A study of patients with Nelson's syndrome. *Clin Endocrinol (Oxf)*. 1998;49:533-539.
50. Zawar VP, Walvekar R. A pheochromocytoma presenting as generalized pigmentation. *Int J Dermatol*. 2004;43:140-142.
51. Heymann WR. Cutaneous manifestations of thyroid disease. *J Am Acad Dermatol*. 1992;26:885-902.
52. Guffey D, Narahari S, Alinia H. Hyperpigmented plaques of the alar creases: an unusual presentation of acanthosis nigricans. *Pediatr Dermatol*. 2016;33(2):e160-e161.
53. Alexander A. Maturational hyperpigmentation. In: Kelly A, Taylor S, eds. *Dermatology for Skin of Color*. New York, NY: McGraw-Hill Medical; 2009:344.
54. Heilskov S, Rytter MJ, Vestergaard C, et al. Dermatosis in children with oedematous malnutrition (Kwashiorkor): a review of the literature. *J Eur Acad Dermatol Venereol*. 2014;28(8):995-1001.
55. Mori K, Ando I, Kukita A. Generalized hyperpigmentation of the skin due to vitamin B12 deficiency. *J Dermatol*. 2001;28:282-285.
56. Lee LW, Yan AC. Skin manifestations of nutritional deficiency disease in children: modern day contexts. *Int J Dermatol*. 2012;51:1407-1418.
57. Powell LW, Seckington RC, Deugnier Y. Haemochromatosis. *Lancet*. 2016;388(10045):706-716.
58. Quinlan KE, Janiga JJ, Baran R, et al. Transverse melanonychia secondary to total skin electron beam therapy: a report of 3 cases. *J Am Acad Dermatol*. 2005;53:S112-S114.
59. Kelly KM, Svaasand LO, Nelson JS. Further investigation of pigmentary changes after alexandrite laser hair removal in conjunction with cryogen spray cooling. *Dermatol Surg*. 2004;30:581-582.
60. Al-Aboosi M, Abalkhail A, Kasim O, et al. Friction melanosis: a clinical, histologic, and ultrastructural study in Jordanian patients. *Int J Dermatol*. 2004;43(4):261-264.
61. Nisar M, Iyer K, Brodell R, et al. Minocycline-induced hyperpigmentation: a comparison of 3 Q-switched lasers to reverse its effects. *Clin Cosmet Investig Dermatol*. 2013;6:159-162.
62. Rodrigues M, Bekhor P. Treatment of minocycline-induced cutaneous pigmentation with the picosecond alexandrite (755-nm) laser. *Dermatol Surg*. 2015;41(10):1179-1182.
63. Prachi B, Vijay Z, Godse K, et al. Exogenous ochronosis. *Indian J Dermatol*. 2015;60(6):537-543.
64. Romero SA, Pereira PM, Mariano AV, et al. Use of dermoscopy for diagnosis of exogenous ochronosis. *An Bras Dermatol*. 2011;86(suppl 1):S31-S34.
65. Chung, L, Lin J, Furst DE, et al. Systemic and localized scleroderma. *Clin Dermatol*. 2006;24(5):374-392.
66. Gibney KB, Fischer M, Prince HE, et al. Chikungunya fever in the United States: a fifteen year review of cases. *Clin Infect Dis*. 2011;52:e121-e126.
67. Vasani R, Kanhere S, Chaudhari K, et al. Congenital Chikungunya—a cause of neonatal hyperpigmentation. *Pediatr Dermatol*. 2016;33(2):209-212.
68. Gasque P, Jaffar-Bandjee MC. The immunology and inflammatory responses of human melanocytes in infectious diseases. *J Infect*. 2015;71(4):413-421.

69. Engelkens HJ, Niemel PL, van der Sluis JJ, et al. Endemic treponematoses. Part II. Pinta and endemic syphilis. *Int J Dermatol.* 1991;30(4):221-228.
70. Sarma N, Chakraborty S, Bhattacharya SR. Acquired, idiopathic, patterned facial pigmentation (AIPFP) including periorbital pigmentation and pigmentary demarcation lines on face follows the lines of Blaschko on face. *Indian J Dermatol.* 2014;59:41-48.
71. Gondak RO, da Silva-Jorge R, Jorge J, et al. Oral pigmented lesions: clinicopathologic features and review of the literature. *Med Oral Patol Oral Cir Bucal.* 2012;17: e919-e924.
72. Tanioka M. Benign acral lesions showing parallel ridge pattern on dermoscopy. *J Dermatol.* 2011;38:41-44.
73. Netchiporouk E, Pehr K, Ben-Shoshan M, et al. Pustular flagellate dermatitis after consumption of shiitake mushrooms. *JAAD Case Rep.* 2015;1(3):117-119.
74. Takashima S, Iwata H, Sakata M, et al. Widespread erythema ab igne caused by hot bathing. *J Eur Acad Dermatol Venereol.* 2015;29(11):2259-2261.
75. Huynh N, Sarma D, Huerter C. Erythema ab igne: a case report and review of the literature. *Cutis.* 2011; 88:290-292.
76. Cho S, Jung JY, Lee JH. Erythema ab igne successfully treated using 1,064-nm Q-switched neodymium-doped yttrium aluminum garnet laser with low fluence. *Dermatol Surg.* 2011;37:551-553.
77. Nagashima M, Oshiro A, Shimizu N. A peculiar pruriginous dermatosis with gross reticular pigmentation [in Japanese]. *Jap J Dermatol.* 1971;81:78-91.
78. Corley, S, Mauro P. Erythematous papules evolving into reticulated hyperpigmentation on the trunk: a case of prurigo pigmentosa. *JAAD Case Rep.* 2015;1(2):60-62.
79. Boer A, Misago N, Wolter M, et al. Prurigo pigmentosa: a distinctive inflammatory disease of the skin. *Am J Dermatopathol.* 2003;25(2):117-129.
80. Bhat RM, Pinto HP, Dandekeri S, et al. Acquired bilateral nevus of ota-like macules with mucosal involvement: a new variant of Hori's nevus. *Indian J Dermatol.* 2014; 59:293-296.
81. Tian BW. Novel treatment of Hori's nevus: a combination of fractional nonablative 2,940-nm Er:YAG and low fluence 1,066-nm Q-switched ND;YAG laser. *J Cutan Aesthet Surg.* 2015;8(4):227-229.
82. Cho SB, Park SJ, Kim MJ, et al. Treatment of acquired bilateral nevus of Ota-like macules (Hori's nevus) using 1064-nm Q-switched Nd:YAG laser with low fluence. *Int J Dermatol.* 2009;48:1308-1312.
83. Chan JC, Shek SY, Kono T, et al. A retrospective analysis on the management of pigmented lesions using a picosecond 755-nm alexandrite laser in Asians. *Lasers Surg Med.* 2016;48(1):23-29.
84. Patrizi A, Medri M, Raone B, et al. Clinical characteristics of Becker's nevus in children: a report of 118 cases from Italy. *Pediatr Dermatol.* 2012;29:571-574.
85. Momen S, Mallipeddi R, Al-Niami F. The use of lasers in Becker's naevus: an evidence-based review. *J Cosmet Laser Ther.* 2016;18(4):188-192.
86. Shah KN. The diagnostic and clinical significance of café-au-lait macules. *Pediatr Clin North Am.* 2010; 57:1131-1153.
87. Bastiaens M, ter Huurne J, Gruis N, et al. The melanocortin-1-receptor gene is the major freckle gene. *Hum Mol Genet.* 2001;10:1701-1708.
88. Sopena Barona J, Gamo Villegas R, Guerra Tapia A, et al. Acromelanosis [in Spanish]. *An Pediatr (Barc).* 2003;58:277-280.
89. Callender VD, St Surin-Lord S, Davis EC, et al. Postinflammatory hyperpigmentation: etiologic and therapeutic considerations. *Am J Clin Dermatol.* 2011; 12:87-99.
90. Ho SG, Yeung CK, Chan NP, et al. A retrospective analysis of the management of acne post-inflammatory hyperpigmentation using topical treatment, laser treatment, or combination topical and laser treatments in oriental patients. *Lasers Surg Med.* 2011; 43(1):1-7.
91. Rodrigues M, Pandya AG. Melasma: clinical diagnosis and management options. *Australas J Dermatol.* 2015;56(3):151-163.
92. Lee HC, Thng TG, Goh CL. Oral tranexamic acid (TA) in the treatment of melasma: a retrospective analysis. *J Am Acad Dermatol.* 2016;75(2):385-392.
93. Pretel M, Irarrazaval I, Aguado L, et al. Partial unilateral lentiginosis treated with alexandrite Q-switched laser: case report and review of the literature. *J Cosmet Laser Ther.* 2013;15(4):207-209.
94. Kwon HH, Onh J, Suh DH, et al. A pilot study for triple combination therapy with a low-fluence 1064 nm Q-switched Nd:YAG laser, hydroquinone cream and oral tranexamic acid for recalcitrant Riehl's melanosis. *J Dermatolog Treat.* 2016;27:1-5.
95. Kronborg C, Mahar P, Howard A. Cronkhite-Canada syndrome: a rare disease presenting with dermatological and gastrointestinal manifestations. *Australas J Dermatol.* 2016;57(2):e69-e71.
96. Ramirez CO. Los cenisientos: problema clinica. Proceedings of the first Central American Congress of Dermatology. San Salvador, El Salvador; 1957: 122-130.
97. Rodríguez N, Granados J. HLA-DR association with the genetic susceptibility to develop ashy dermatosis in Mexican Mestizo patients. *J Am Acad Dermatol.* 2007;56(4):617-620.
98. Bahadir S, Cobanoglu U, Cimsit G, et al. Erythema dyschromicum perstans: response to dapsone therapy. *Int J Dermatol.* 2004;43:220-222.
99. Kroon MW, Wind BS, Meesters AA, et al. Non-ablative 1550 nm fractional laser therapy not effective for erythema dyschromicum perstans and postinflammatory hyperpigmentation: a pilot study. *J Dermatolog Treat.* 2012;23:339-344.
100. Al-Mutairi N, El-Khalawany M. Clinicopathological characteristics of lichen planus pigmentosus and its response to tacrolimus ointment: an open label, non-randomized, prospective study. *J Eur Acad Dermatol Venereol.* 2010;24:535-540.
101. Muthu SK, Narang T, Saikia UN, et al. Low-dose oral isotretinoin therapy in lichen planus pigmentosus: an open-label non-randomized prospective pilot study. *Int J Dermatol.* 2016;55(9):1048-1054.
102. Degos R, Civatte J, Belaiche S. Idiopathic eruptive macular pigmentation. *Ann Dermatol Venereol.* 1978; 105:177-182.
103. Sanz de Galdeano C, Léauté-Labrèze C, Bioulac-Sage P, et al. Idiopathic eruptive macular pigmentation: report of five patients. *Pediatr Dermatol.* 1996; 13:274-277.
104. Zhang C, Li D, Zhang J, et al. Mutations in ABCB6 cause dyschromatosis universalis hereditaria. *J Invest Dermatol.* 2013;133(9):2221-2228.
105. Westerhof W, Beemer FA, Cormane RH, et al. Hereditary congenital hypopigmented and hyperpigmented macules. *Arch Dermatol.* 1978;114:931-936.

Acneiform Disorders PART 14

第十四篇 痤疮样皮肤病

Chapter 78 :: Acne Vulgaris
:: Carolyn Goh, Carol Cheng, George Agak, Andrea L. Zaenglein, Emmy M. Graber, Diane M. Thiboutot, & Jenny Kim

第七十八章
寻常痤疮

中文导读

寻常痤疮是一种毛囊皮脂腺单元常见的皮肤问题,好发于青少年。本章从流行病学、临床特点、病因和发病机制、诊断、鉴别诊断、临床病程和预后以及治疗这七个方面全面讲述了寻常痤疮。

第一节介绍了寻常痤疮的好发人群和不同年龄阶段的患病人群的性别比例,指出痤疮是全球范围内的十大流行病之一,也是全球疾病负担排名第三的疾病。全球范围内寻常痤疮的发病率在增长,原因不清。

第二节介绍了寻常痤疮的临床特点,将痤疮皮损分为非炎症型皮损(开放性或闭合性粉刺)和炎症型皮损(丘疹、脓疱、结节);痤疮消退后,留下的萎缩性瘢痕根据瘢痕的深度和宽度可以分为冰锥型、厢车型、滚轮样型;同时从心理学角度讲述了痤疮严重损害了患者的心理健康和社交行为,引起抑郁、焦虑、心理压力、社交障碍等,需要及时的心理疏导和干预。

第三节介绍了寻常痤疮的病因和发病机制,指出痤疮的发病机制是多方面的,包括毛囊上皮过度增生、皮脂分泌增多、痤疮丙酸杆菌、炎症和免疫反应等多个关键环节,且这些过程又在激素和免疫的影响下相互作用;还总结了目前较为认可的痤疮发病的病理生理过程:雄激素刺激、亚油酸、IL-1、痤疮丙酸杆菌等因素诱导毛囊上皮过度增生,导致微粉刺形成;雄激素分泌增多,刺激皮脂腺细胞分泌更多的皮脂,痤疮丙酸杆菌分解皮脂为脂质氧化物,释放多种促炎因子，调节和促进痤疮丙酸杆菌的定植，诱导一系列免疫反应和炎症反应；同时微粉刺与角蛋白、皮脂、细菌等继续阻留形成粉刺，持续增大导致破裂，内容物刺激真皮产生一系列的炎症反应；炎症反应的类型决定临床皮损，且在瘢痕化的过程中也起重要作用。

第四节介绍了寻常痤疮一般通过病史和体查即可诊断，提出部分病例需要进一步的检查，尤其是考虑高雄激素血症患者，需要检查血清雄激素水平，如总睾酮、游离睾酮、DHEAS、17-羟孕酮、皮质醇等。

第五节介绍了寻常痤疮需要与毛囊炎、玫瑰痤疮、口周皮炎、面部扁平疣、粟丘疹、药物性痤疮、接触性痤疮等疾病进行鉴别，并将各种不同类型皮损及与之相对应的疾病的鉴别要点，列于表78-1。

第六节介绍了寻常痤疮的临床病程和预后，指出寻常痤疮持续数年可以自行缓解，有些患者可能会延续到35～50岁。家族史、BMI、饮食因素几个方面可以诱发或加重寻常痤疮，导致病程的迁延反复。

第七节介绍了针对痤疮不同皮损和不同严重程度的分级治疗，对其各个病理生理环节联合治疗（表78-2），讲述了常见的外用药和系统药物的种类、剂型、浓度、适应症、不良反应和注意事项（表78-3和表78-4），列举了寻常痤疮各种辅助治疗方法，如粉刺清除术、皮下切开术、皮损内糖皮质激素注射、化学剥脱、光动力、激光、磨削、微针、填充等不同方法的适应症范围、注意事项；同时分析了孕期痤疮治疗时常见的药物及治疗方式的安全性（表78-5）。

〔李　吉〕

AT-A-GLANCE

- Acne vulgaris is a common disorder of the pilosebaceous unit.
- There are four key elements of pathogenesis: (1) follicular epidermal hyperproliferation, (2) sebum production, (3) the presence and activity of *Propionibacterium acnes*, and (4) inflammation and immune response.
- Clinical features include comedones, papules, pustules, and nodules on the face, chest, and back.
- Treatment often includes combinations of oral and topical agents such as antimicrobials, retinoids, and hormonal agents. Laser and light sources are additional treatment options.

INTRODUCTION

Acne vulgaris is a common disorder of the pilosebaceous unit that is seen primarily in adolescents. Most cases of acne present with a pleomorphic array of lesions, consisting of comedones, papules, pustules, and nodules with varying extent and severity. Although the course of acne may be limited in the majority of patients, the sequelae can be lifelong, with scar formation and psychological impairment, especially in young people.

EPIDEMIOLOGY

Acne is one of the top three most common skin diseases, particularly in adolescents and young adults, in whom the prevalence is estimated at 85% (ages 12–25 years).[1,2] Acne has no predilection for ethnicity; thus, it is an important disease worldwide and is considered one of the top 10 most prevalent global diseases.[3-5] It is also considered the third most important disease defined by the global burden of disease.[6] Acne patients report a Dermatology Life Quality Index (DLQI) score of 11.9, considered more detrimental to quality of life than psoriasis (DLQI = 8.8). Thus, acne is not only important for health of a significant number of people in the United States but has an impact globally.

Acne can occur at any age, starting at birth with neonatal acne (presents in the first few weeks of life) and infantile acne (presents between 1 and 12 months) and extending into adulthood. Acne may persist from adolescence into adulthood, or it can have its onset after the adolescent period. The prevalence of acne in adolescents is higher in males, but in adults is higher in females. The prevalence rates in adults have been reported to be as high as 64% in the 20s and 43% in the 30s.[7] After the age of 50 years, 15% of women and 7% of men have been reported to have acne.[8] Because the age of adrenarche appears to be dropping over the years, patients may be presenting with acne at an earlier age.[9] Globally, the incidence of acne vulgaris appears to be rising. The reasons are unclear, although increased exposure to a westernized diet is postulated.[2]

Family history of acne has been reported in 62.9% to 78% of patients.[10,11] Those with family history tend to be male and have an earlier onset of acne, truncal involvement, and scarring.[11] Several twin studies have been done, finding that 81% of acne variation is caused by genetic factors as opposed to 19% environmental factors and that as many as 98% of monozygotic twins both have acne versus 55% of dizygotic twins.[9] The severity of acne may also be genetically determined.[9]

Males tend to have more severe acne, and nodulocystic acne has been reported to be more common in white males than in black males.[6,12] Acne also appears to be more severe in patients with the XYY genotype.[13]

Individual genes responsible for this high heritability remain unclear. Several candidate gene-based studies have identified a few genetic variants associated with acne in *tumor necrosis factor-α* (*TNF-α*), *tumor necrosis factor receptor 2(TNFR2)*,[14] *interleukin-1A (IL1A)*,[15,16] *cytochrome P450, family 17 (CYP17)*,[17] *Toll-like receptor 2(TLR2)*,[14] and *Toll-like receptor 4 (TLR4)*.[18] Genome-wide association studies (GWASs)[19] have also been reported on this common skin condition.

Interestingly, there are two indigenous populations that have been described—one in Papua New Guinea and the other in Paraguay—that do not develop acne.[6] Although this may be genetically determined, environmental factors may also be at play because these groups have not been exposed to a westernized diet.

CLINICAL FEATURES

HISTORY

Most patients with acne vulgaris report a gradual onset of lesions around puberty. Some may develop acne in the years preceding puberty, but others may not develop acne until after puberty. Because of the typical gradual onset, careful history should be obtained from patients describing an abrupt onset of acne to potentially reveal an underlying etiology, such as a medication or an androgen-secreting tumor.

Hyperandrogenism should be considered in a female patient whose acne is severe, in the jawline or lower face distribution, sudden in onset, or associated with hirsutism or irregular menstrual periods. The patient should be asked about the frequency and character of her menstrual periods and whether her acne flares with changes in her menstrual cycle. Flares of acne perimenstrually, however, are common in acne vulgaris, with 56% of adult women reporting worsening of acne before menses.[20] Other signs that may suggest a diagnosis of hyperandrogenism include deepening of the voice, an increase in libido, hirsutism, and acanthosis nigricans.

A complete medication history is also important because some medications can cause an abrupt onset of a monomorphous acneiform eruption. Drug-induced acne may be caused by anabolic steroids, corticosteroids, corticotropin, phenytoin, lithium, isoniazid, vitamin B complexes, halogenated compounds, and certain chemotherapy medications, particularly with epidermal growth factor receptor (EGFR) inhibitors. Furthermore, many patients may be on hormonal therapy, which can exacerbate or induce acne vulgaris. Progestin-only contraceptives, including injectables and intrauterine devices, can exacerbate or induce acne vulgaris.[21] Women approaching or in menopause may be on hormone therapy, including progesterone, and some are treated with dehydroepiandrosterone (DHEA) or testosterone.[22] Men may be on testosterone replacement therapy. Finally, inquiring about supplements is important. In particular, those containing whey protein have been associated with onset or worsening of acne vulgaris.[23]

CUTANEOUS FINDINGS

The primary site of acne is the face and to a lesser degree the back, chest, and shoulders. On the trunk, lesions tend to be concentrated near the midline. Acne vulgaris is characterized by several lesion types: noninflammatory comedones (open or closed) and inflammatory lesions (red papules, pustules, or nodules) (Fig. 78-1). Although one type of lesion may predominate, close inspection usually reveals the presence of several types of lesions. Closed comedones are known as "whiteheads" (Fig. 78-1A), and open comedones are known as "blackheads" (Fig. 78-1B). The open comedo appears as a flat or slightly raised lesion with a central dark-colored follicular impaction of keratin and lipid. It is dark because of oxidation (Fig. 78-2). Closed comedones appear as cream to white, slightly elevated, small papules and do not have a clinically visible orifice (Fig. 78-1A). Stretching, side lighting, or palpation of the skin can be helpful in detecting the lesions.

The inflammatory lesions vary from small erythematous papules to pustules and large, tender, fluctuant nodules (see Figs. 78-1C and 78-1D and Figs. 78-2–78-4). Some of the large nodules were previously called "cysts," and the term *nodulocystic* has been used to describe severe cases of inflammatory acne. True cysts are rarely found in acne; this term should be abandoned and substituted with *severe nodular acne* (see Figs. 78-1D and 78-4). The evolution of an acne lesion is unclear. Although the majority of inflammatory lesions appear to originate from comedones (54%), a significant number of inflammatory (26%) lesions arise from normal uninvolved skin.[24] The mechanisms involved in the evolution of an inflammatory lesion are still unclear, but an inflammatory process is thought to play a role. Whether the lesion appears as a papule, pustule, or nodule depends on the extent and location of the inflammatory infiltrate in the dermis.

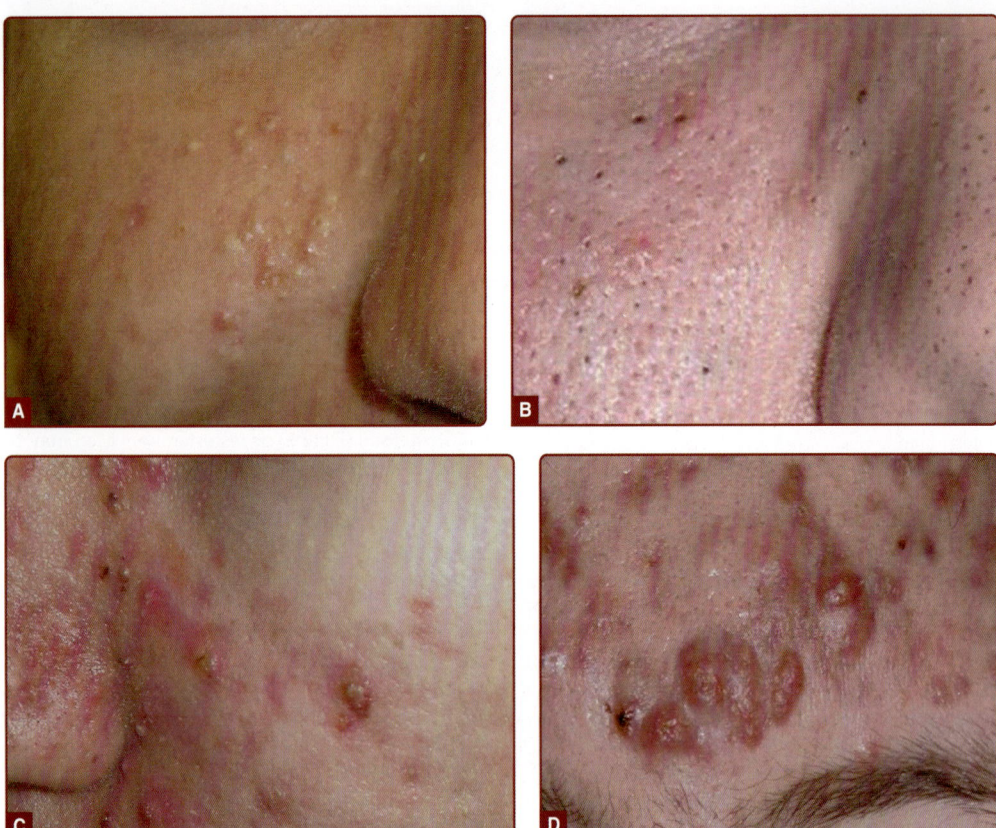

Figure 78-1 Clinicopathologic correlation of acne lesions. **A,** Closed comedone. The follicular infundibulum is distended, filled with keratin and sebum, and the follicular epithelium is attenuated. The follicular ostium is narrow. **B,** Open comedone. Resembles the closed comedone with the exception of a patulous follicular ostium. **C,** Inflammatory papule. Acute and chronic inflammatory cells surround and infiltrate the follicle, which shows infundibular hyperkeratosis. **D,** Nodule. The follicle is filled with acute inflammatory cells. With the rupture of the distended follicle, there is a foreign body granulomatous response.

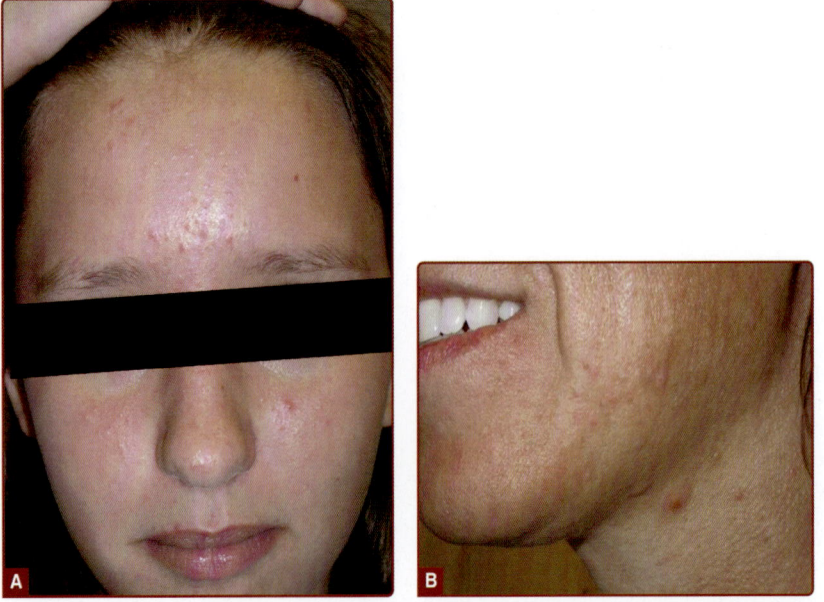

Figure 78-2 Mild acne vulgaris. **A,** A 13-year-old girl with mild acne vulgaris. Scattered comedones or inflammatory lesions (or both) are seen, usually limited to less than half of the face. The T-zone of the face is commonly involved. No nodules are present. **B,** An adult female with primarily inflammatory acne. Note the typical involvement of the jawline.

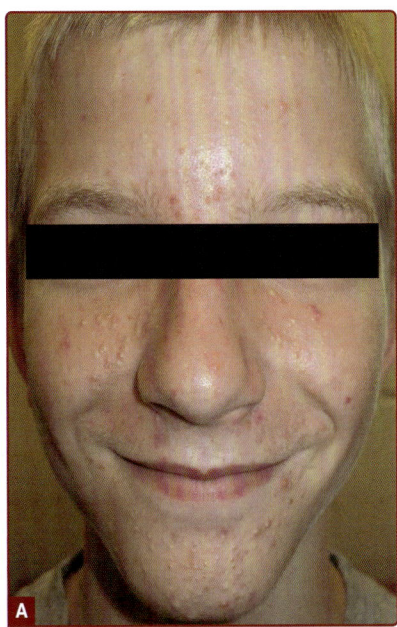 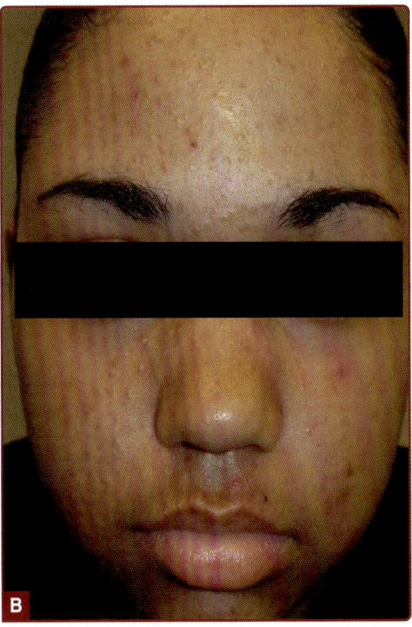

Figure 78-3 Moderate acne vulgaris. **A,** A 15-year-old male patient with moderate acne. Typically, more than half of the face is involved with increasing numbers of lesions, usually a mix of lesions is seen: papules, pustules, and comedones. Infrequent and limited nodules may be present. Chest and back involvement may also be moderately affected. **B,** A 16-year-old female patient with open and deep closed comedones. Scarring and postinflammatory changes are possible sequelae.

NONCUTANEOUS FINDINGS

Acne vulgaris is usually an isolated cutaneous finding. However, it can be part of several syndromes, including those that are associated with hyperandrogenism and inflammatory states (see Chap. 80).

COMPLICATIONS

All types of acne lesions have the potential to resolve with sequelae. Almost all acne lesions leave a transient macular erythema after resolution. In darker skin types, postinflammatory hyperpigmentation may persist for months after resolution of acne lesions. In some individuals, acne lesions may result in permanent scarring. Acne scars can be atrophic or hypertrophic.[25] Atrophic scars can be further categorized based on size and shape: ice pick, boxcar, or rolling[26] (Fig. 78-5). Ice pick scars are narrow, deep scars that are widest at the surface of the skin and taper to a point in the dermis, typically less than 2 mm in diameter. Boxcar scars are wide sharply demarcated scars that do not taper to a point at the base and range in size from 1.5 to 4 mm. Rolling scars are shallow, wide scars (often >4–5 mm) that have an undulating appearance. Perifollicular elastolysis is another type of scar, which typically presents as atrophic soft papules on the upper part of the trunk.[27] Hypertrophic and keloidal scars, in addition to sinus tracts, can also form.

Although not life threatening, acne leads to significant morbidity, including depression, anxiety, and psychosocial stress, and is a major cause of psychosocial and psychological impairment for young people,[28,29] triggering anxiety and mood disorders and affecting self-esteem.[30,31] It is ranked third among chronic skin diseases for causing disability, as measured by equivalent years of "healthy" life lost by virtue of being in states of poor health or disability.[3] Patients experience social isolation and are reluctant to participate in group activities. Unemployment rates are higher among adults with acne than those without. Self-esteem issues are also likely to be the driving force behind higher rates of unemployment in people with acne; however, there is also an existing bias whereby patients with acne are more likely to be passed over by prospective employers.[29] A cross-sectional study found that 14% of students reported "problem acne," which was associated with an increased risk of depressive symptoms as well as suicidal thoughts and attempts.[32,33] One study has estimated the prevalence of suicidal ideation in patients with acne as 7%.[34] In adolescents, two large studies have shown that anxiety, depression, and suicidal ideation are higher in those with self-described "problem acne" or "substantial acne." These findings highlight the importance of appropriate psychiatric screening and referral. Importantly, the impact of acne on patients' lives was often independent of severity, such that some patients with only minimal acne experience psychological and psychosocial distress.[35] Thus, although some consider acne "cosmetic," its impact on one's well-being can be significant.

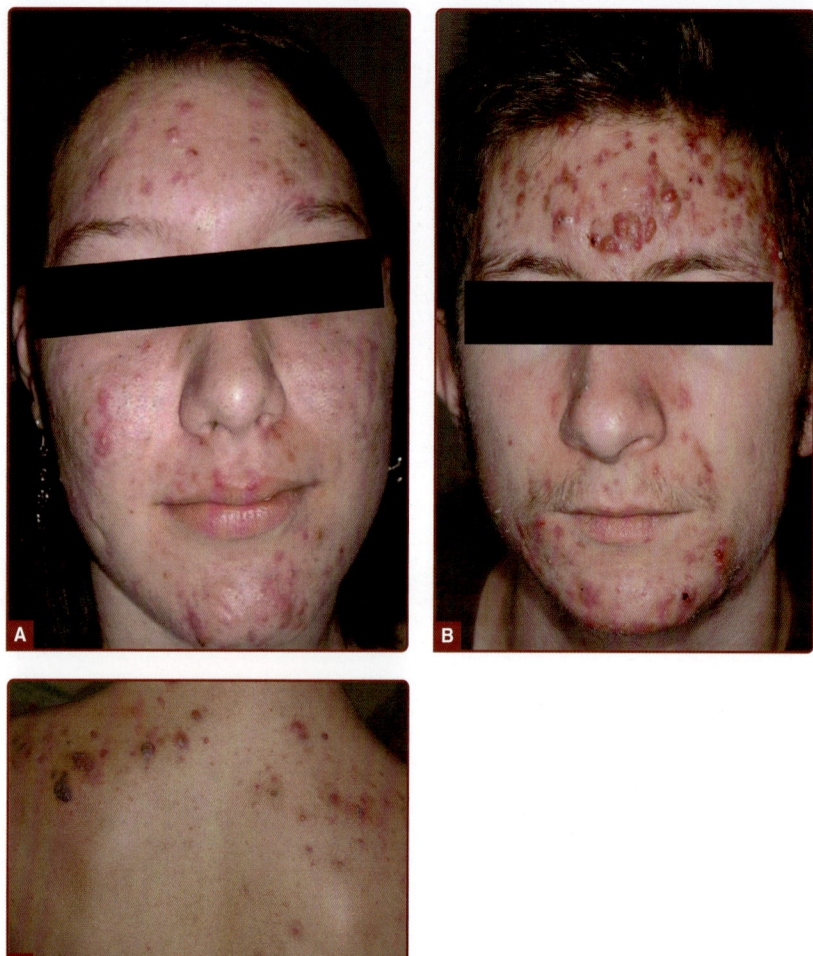

Figure 78-4 Severe acne vulgaris. **A,** A 17-year-old female patient with extensive acne. Numerous pustules and nodular lesions admixed with comedones and smaller papules cover the entire face. **B,** Deep, friable nodules that coalesce into pseudocysts in acne conglobata. **C,** Chest and back involvement can be extensive and severe. Scarring is a common complication in severe acne.

ETIOLOGY AND PATHOGENESIS

Current understanding of acne is that it is a complex and multifactorial inflammatory disease. Recent studies are better defining the cellular and molecular mechanisms involved in acne and the importance of inflammation and the immune response. The pathogenesis of acne is multifaceted, and at least four factors have been identified. These key elements (Fig. 78-6) are (1) follicular epidermal hyperproliferation, (2) sebum production, (3) *Propionibacterium acnes*, and (4) inflammation and immune response. Each of these processes are interrelated and under hormonal and immune influence.

It is thought that all clinical lesions begin with the microcomedo and develop into clinical lesions—comedones, inflammatory lesions, and scarring. Follicular epidermal hyperproliferation results in the formation of a microcomedo. The epithelium of the upper hair follicle, the infundibulum, becomes hyperkeratotic with increased cohesion of the keratinocytes, resulting in the obstruction of the follicular ostium, where keratin, sebum, and bacteria begin to accumulate in the follicle and cause dilation of the upper hair follicle, producing a microcomedo. Exactly what initiates and stimulates the hyperproliferation and increased adhesion of keratinocytes is unknown. Several proposed factors in keratinocyte hyperproliferation include androgen stimulation, decreased linoleic acid, increased IL-1-α activity, and effects of *P. acnes*. Dihydrotestosterone (DHT) is a potent androgen that may play a role in acne. DHT is converted from dehydroepiandrosterone sulfate (DHEA-S) by 17-β hydroxysteroid dehydrogenase (HSD) and 5-α reductase enzymes (Fig. 78-7). Compared with epidermal keratinocytes, follicular keratinocytes have increased 17-β HSD and 5-α reductase, thus enhancing DHT production.[36,37] DHT may stimulate follicular keratinocyte proliferation. Also sup-

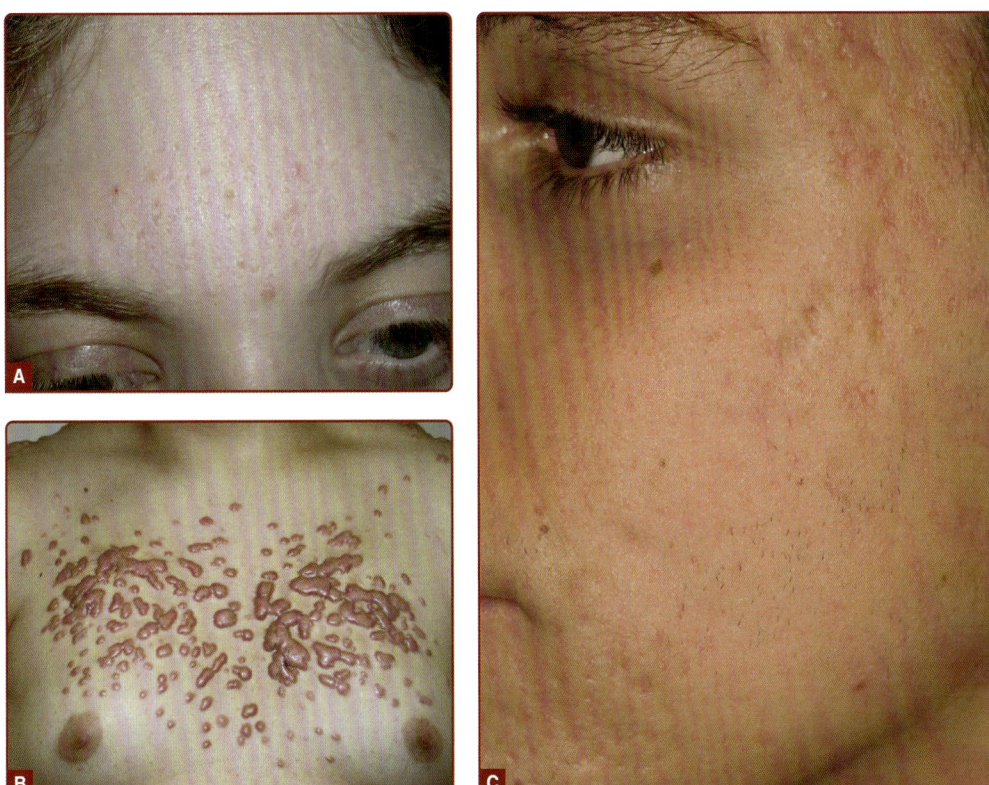

Figure 78-5 Acne vulgaris, scarring. **A,** Honeycomb scarring in a young girl with mild to moderate inflammatory acne. **B,** Extensive keloidal scarring occurring as sequelae of acne fulminans. **C.** Rolling scars.

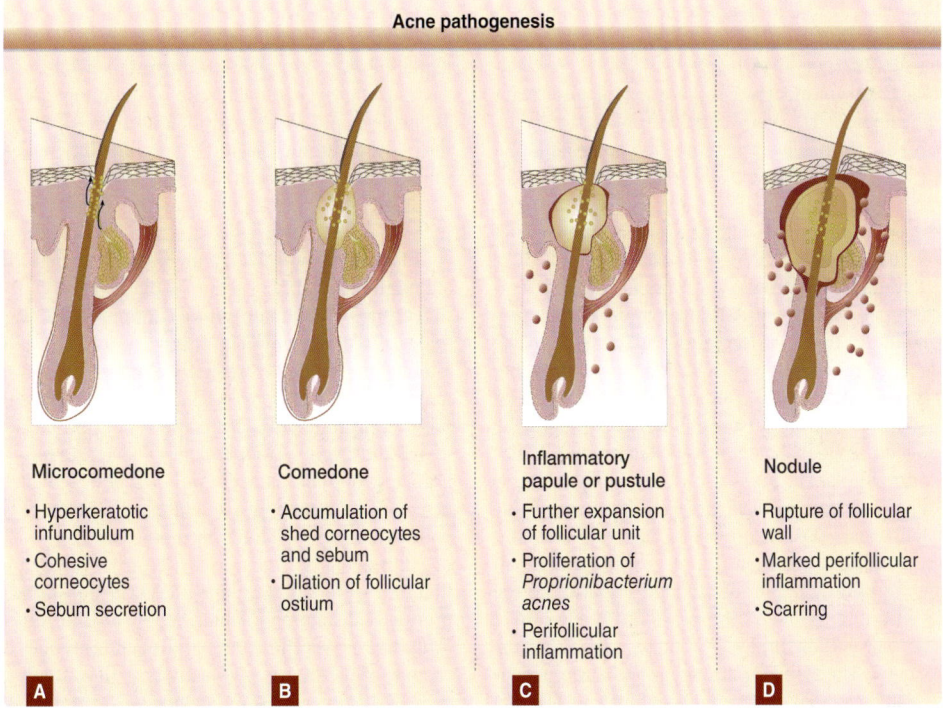

Figure 78-6 **A–D** Acne pathogenesis.

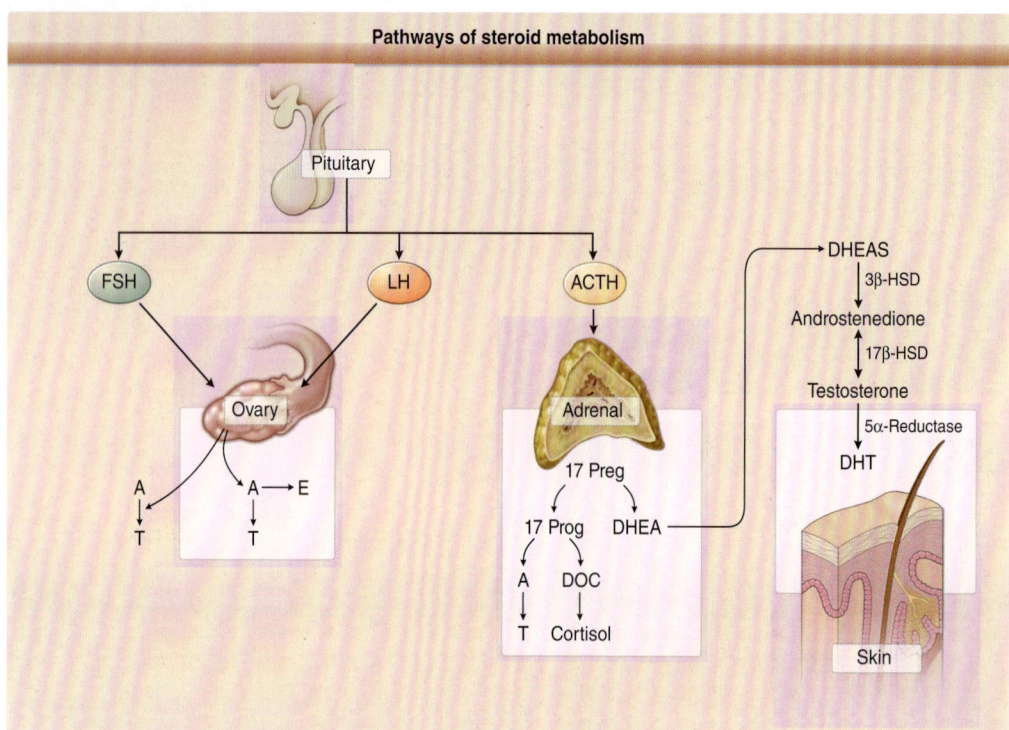

Figure 78-7 Pathways of steroid metabolism. Dehydroepiandrosterone (DHEA) is a weak androgen that is converted to the more potent testosterone by 3β-hydroxysteroid dehydrogenase (HSD) and 17β-HSD. 5-α Reductase then converts testosterone to dihydrotestosterone (DHT), the predominant hormonal effector on the sebaceous gland. The sebaceous gland expresses each of these enzymes. A, androstenedione; ACTH, adrenocorticotropin-stimulating hormone; DHEAS, dehydroepiandrosterone sulfate; DOC, deoxycortisol E, estrogen; FSH, follicle-stimulating hormone; LH, luteinizing hormone; T, testosterone.

porting the role of androgens in acne pathogenesis is the evidence that individuals with complete androgen insensitivity do not develop acne.[38]

Follicular keratinocyte proliferation is also regulated by linoleic acid, an essential fatty acid in the skin. Low levels of linoleic acid induce follicular keratinocyte hyperproliferation and the production of proinflammatory cytokines. The levels of linoleic acid are decreased in individuals with acne and normalize after successful treatment with isotretinoin.[39]

In addition to androgens and linoleic acid, IL-1 α has been shown to contribute to keratinocyte hyperproliferation. IL-1α induces follicular keratinocyte hyperproliferation and microcomedone formation, and IL-1 receptor antagonists inhibit microcomedone formation.[40,41] The initial event that upregulates the production of IL-1α has not been determined. Fibroblast growth factor receptor (FGFR)-2 signaling is also involved in follicular hyperkeratinization. There is a long-established relationship between acne and Apert syndrome, a complex bony malformation syndrome, caused by a gain-of-function mutation in the gene encoding FGFR-2. Mutations in FGFR-2 in a mosaic distribution underlie a nevus comedonicus-like lesion.[42] The FGFR-2 pathway is androgen dependent, and proposed mechanisms in acne include an increased production of IL-1α and 5-α reductase.[43,44]

The second and key feature in the pathogenesis of acne is the production of sebum from the sebaceous gland. Human sebum are composed mainly of triglycerides found ubiquitously and of unique lipids, such as squalene and wax esters not found anywhere else in the body, including the surface of the skin.[45] Increased sebum secretion has been associated with acne. On average, people with acne excrete more sebum than those without acne, and secretion rates have been shown to correlate with the severity of clinical manifestations, although the quality of sebum is the same between the two groups.[46] The main component of sebum, triglycerides, is important in acne pathogenesis. Triglycerides are broken down into free fatty acids by *P. acnes*, normal flora of the pilosebaceous unit. In return, these free fatty acids promote *P. acnes* colonization and induction of inflammation.[47] Lipoperoxides also found in sebum induce proinflammatory cytokines and activate the peroxisome proliferator-activated receptors (PPAR) pathway, resulting in increased sebum.[48,49]

Androgenic hormones activate sebocyte proliferation and differentiation and the induction of sebum production. Similar to their action on the follicular infundibular keratinocytes, androgen hormones bind to and influence sebocyte activity.[50] Those with acne have higher average serum androgen levels (although still within normal range) than unaffected control participants.[51,52] 5-α Reductase, the enzyme responsible for converting testosterone to the potent DHT, has greatest activity in areas of skin prone to acne, face, chest, and back.[44]

The role of estrogen on sebum production is not well defined. The dose of estrogen required to decrease sebum production is greater than the dose required to inhibit ovulation.[53] The mechanisms by which estrogens may work include (1) directly opposing the effects of androgens within the sebaceous gland, (2) inhibiting the production of androgens by gonadal tissue via a negative feedback loop on pituitary gonadotropin release, and (3) regulating genes that suppress sebaceous gland growth or lipid production.[54]

Corticotropin-releasing hormone may also play a role. It is released by the hypothalamus and increased in response to stress. Corticotropin-releasing hormone receptors are present on a vast number of cells, including keratinocytes and sebocytes, and are upregulated in the sebocytes of patients with acne.[55]

The microcomedo continue to expand with densely packed keratin, sebum, and bacteria. Eventually, this distension causes follicular wall rupture. The extrusion of the keratin, sebum, and bacteria into the dermis results in a brisk inflammatory response. The predominant cell type within 24 hours of comedo rupture is the lymphocyte. CD4+ lymphocytes are found around the pilosebaceous unit, and CD8+ cells are found perivascularly. One to two days after comedo rupture, the neutrophil becomes the predominant cell type surrounding the burst microcomedo.[56]

It was originally thought that inflammation follows comedo formation, but there is evidence that dermal inflammation may actually precede comedo formation. Biopsies taken from comedo-free acne-prone skin demonstrate increased dermal inflammation compared with normal skin. Biopsies of newly formed comedos demonstrate even greater inflammation.[57] This may suggest that inflammation actually precedes comedo formation, again emphasizing the interplay between all of the pathogenic factors.

P. acnes is one of the key factors involved in acne pathogenesis. *P. acnes* is a gram-positive, anaerobic, microaerophilic bacterium found in the sebaceous follicle and is the dominant bacterial inhabitant of the human sebaceous gland,[58] accounting for almost 90% of the bacterial 16S transcripts.[59] *P. acnes* is generally believed to play a major role in the pathogenesis of acne vulgaris, in part by eliciting a host inflammatory response.[60] *S. epidermidis* is also present in follicles but is located near the surface, suggesting that it does not contribute to the deeper inflammatory process.[58] There is a significant increase in *P. acnes* colonization at puberty, the time when acne commonly develops, and teenagers with acne can have as many as 100-fold more *P. acnes* bacteria present on their skin than healthy age-matched counterparts.[61] However, there are no consistent data correlating the raw number of *P. acnes* organisms present in a sebaceous follicle and the severity of the acne.[61]

Previously, a shotgun approach to target all *P. acnes* with antibiotics has been used, which has led to significant bacterial resistance in up to 60% clinical isolates, directly correlating with antibiotic treatment failure.[61-63]

The recent association of specific *P. acnes* strains with acne versus healthy skin supports the concept that *P. acnes* is an etiologic agent in the pathogenesis of acne. Certain *P. acnes* strains, as identified by multilocus sequence typing, were found to be associated with acne, designated as type IA_1 or IC strains.[64-67] Acne-associated types were further investigated using full genome sequencing in conjunction with ribotyping.[59,68] Specifically, phylotype IB-1 was associated with acne, as were the ribotype 4 and 5 subgroups of phylotype IA-2. The ribotype 1 subgroup of phylotype IA-2, together with phylotypes IA-1, IB-2, and IB-3, was found evenly distributed in acne patients and individuals with healthy skin. These acne-associated types were present in significant quantity in approximately 30% to 40% of patients but with acne rarely in individuals with healthy skin. Conversely, the phylotype II, ribotype 6 subgroup was found to be 99% associated with healthy skin. Additionally, *P. acnes* isolates belonging to phylotype III were not found in acne lesions but composed approximately 20% of isolates from healthy skin.[64] The genomes of acne-enriched and healthy skin–associated strains were sequenced,[59,68] revealing that the phylotypes associated with acne selectively harbor a plasmid and two chromosomal regions that contain genes possibly involved in pathogenesis, adhesion to epithelial tissues, or induction of human immune response.[59,68] Moreover, the levels of porphyrin production and vitamin B_{12} regulation were recently shown to be different between acne- and health-associated strains, suggesting a potential molecular mechanism for disease-associated strains in acne pathogenesis and for health-associated strains in skin health.[69] Metabolite-mediated interactions between the host and the skin microbiota may also play an essential role in acne development.[70]

Sebocyte differentiation and proinflammatory cytokine and chemokine responses are varied depending on the strain of *P. acnes* predominating within the follicle.[35] Certain strains of *P. acnes* induce a differential host immune response. *P. acnes* ribotypes associated with acne induced distinct T helper 1 (Th1) and Th17 responses, which potentially contribute to inflammation in acne, but *P. acnes* ribotypes associated with health-induced high levels of IL-10, which presumably regulate and inhibit inflammatory responses.[71]

P. acnes directly induces inflammation through various mechanisms. The cell wall of *P. acnes* contains a carbohydrate antigen that stimulates antibody development. Patients with the most severe acne have been shown to have the highest titers of antibodies.[72] The antipropionobacterium antibody enhances the inflammatory response by activating complement initiating a cascade of proinflammatory events.[73] *P. acnes* also facilitates inflammation by eliciting a delayed-type hypersensitivity response and by producing lipases, proteases, hyaluronidases, and chemotactic factors.[72,74] Reactive oxygen species (ROS) and lysosomal enzymes are released by neutrophils and levels may correlate with severity.[75] Additionally, *P. acnes* stimulates host innate responses via secretion of proinflammatory cytokines and chemokines from peripheral blood mononuclear cells (PBMCs) and monocytes[60,76] and inflammatory cytokines and antimicrobial peptides such as human β-defensin-2 (hBD2) from KC[77,78] and sebocytes.[35]

The mechanisms by which *P. acnes* triggers the innate immune response has been studied and includes the activation of pattern recognition receptors (PRRs), which recognize conserved pathogen-associated molecular patterns (PAMPs) and activate specific signaling cascades, resulting in the induction of immune response genes. *P. acnes*–induced secretion of proinflammatory cytokines IL-8, IL-12, and TNF-α in monocytes has been shown to involve TLR2,[60] which is expressed on macrophages surrounding the sebaceous follicles of acne lesions,[60] as well as in the epidermis of inflammatory acne lesions.[79] More recently, *P. acnes* has been shown to induce IL-1β secretion and inflammasome activation via NLRP3 and caspase-1 in monocytes and macrophages,[80,81] as well as sebocytes.[82] Both NLRP3 and caspase-1 colocalize with macrophages in acne lesions,[80] keratinocytes,[77,78] and sebocytes.[35] Although many of the *P. acnes* ligands that trigger these PRRs and pathways are not known, experimental evidence points to a possible role for *P. acnes* peptidoglycan in TLR2 activation[60,76] and a component of peptidoglycan muramyl dipeptide (MDP), which in *P. acnes* is composed of the canonical N-acetylmuramic acid residue linked to the L-alanine D-isoglutamine dipeptide.[83] MDP is a ligand for NOD2,[84,85] a cytoplasmic PRR, and can also activate the inflammasome via NLRP3,[86] hinting at a possible role for NOD2 in *P. acnes*–induced immune activation.

The antimicrobial peptides histone H4 and cathelicidin are also secreted locally in response to *P. acnes*. Histone H4 exerts direct microbial killing, and cathelicidin interacts with components of the innate immune system, such as β defensins and psoriasin, in response to *P. acnes*.[87,88] Another indicator of the role of innate immunity in the pathogenesis of acne is the differentiation of peripheral blood monocytes to CD209+ macrophages and CD1b+ dendritic cells in response to *P. acnes*.[89]

A role for the adaptive immune response has also been suggested based on the detection of CD4+ T cells in the inflammatory infiltrate from early acne lesions,[56] and both Th1 and Th17 responses are prominent in vitro and in vivo at the site of disease.[90-92] Both Th1 and Th17 cells can trigger antimicrobial activity against bacteria, but the lysis of these bacteria can release components that directly activate the innate immune response, resulting in inflammation. Moreover, Th17 characteristically induce the recruitment of neutrophils, which contribute to antibacterial activity but also cause tissue injury. ROS and lysosomal enzymes are also released by neutrophils and levels may correlate with severity.[75,93,94]

The mechanism of acne scarring is not clear, and although scar formation correlates with inflammatory response, there is no direct correlation of severity of disease and development of scar formation can occur in mild to moderate acne.[95]

It has been shown that *P. acnes* induces metalloproteinase (MMP) 1 and 9 and the expression of tissue inhibitors of metalloproteinase (TIMP)-1, the main regulator of MMP-9 and MMP-1. Furthermore, ATRA downregulates MMP and augments TIMP-1, suggesting that one way that ATRA may improve acne scarring is through the modulation of MMP and TIMP expression, shifting from a matrix-degradative phenotype to a matrix-preserving phenotype.

T-cell responses also appear to determine the outcome of scar formation. In nonscarring lesions, initial robust inflammatory response with influx of CD4+ nonspecific response with few memory T cells were shown, which subsided in resolution. In contrast, in scarring lesions, CD4+ T-cell numbers were smaller, although a high proportion were skin-homing memory and effector cells, and inflammation was increased and activated in resolving lesions.[96]

Finally, the impact of diet on acne is an emerging area of interest in the pathogenesis of acne. Recent studies provide evidence that high glycemic load diets may exacerbate acne and dairy ingestion appears to be weakly associated with acne,[97-99] but some studies do not support the role of diet.[100,101] Both are thought to increase insulin-like growth factor (IGF)-1 with possible increase in androgen activity and sebocyte modulation, therefore promoting acne.[97,102] Several studies have reported that molecular interplay of forkhead box transcription factor (Fox)O1 and mammalian target of rapamycin (mTOR)–mediated nutrient signaling are important in acne.[103,104] The roles of omega-3 fatty acids, antioxidants, zinc, vitamin A, and dietary fiber in acne remain to be elucidated. Thus, further randomized controlled studies are needed to have a clear understanding of how diet influences acne.

DIAGNOSIS

The diagnosis of acne vulgaris is typically made by clinical history and physical examination, but in some instances, further workup may be indicated.

LABORATORY TESTING

Laboratory workup may be indicated in patients with acne if hyperandrogenism is suspected, particularly in children ages 1 to 7 years who may have midchildhood acne (see Chap. 80). There are numerous clinical studies relating acne to elevated serum levels of androgens in both adolescents and adults. Among 623 prepubertal girls, girls with acne had increased levels of DHEAS as compared with age-matched control participants without acne.[105] DHEAS can serve as a precursor for testosterone and DHT. Elevated serum levels of androgens have been found in cases of severe nodular acne and in acne associated with a variety of endocrine conditions, including congenital adrenal hyperplasia (11β- and 21β-hydroxylase deficiencies), ovarian or adrenal tumors, and polycystic ovarian syndrome (PCOS). However, in the majority of patients with acne, serum androgens are within the normal range.[93,106]

Excess androgens may be produced by either the adrenal gland or ovary. The laboratory workup should include measurement of serum DHEAS, total testosterone, and free testosterone, with free testosterone considered the most sensitive test for PCOS.[107] Additional tests to consider include the luteinizing hormone (LH) to follicle-stimulating hormone (FSH) ratio or serum 17-hydroxyprogesterone to identify an adrenal source of androgens in cases in which testing does not clearly indicate an adrenal or ovarian source of androgens. Testing should be obtained just before or during the menstrual period, not midcycle at the time of ovulation. Patients taking contraceptives that prevent ovulation will need to discontinue their medication for at least 1 month before testing. Values of DHEAS in the range of 4000 to 8000 ng/mL (units may vary at different laboratories) may be associated with congenital adrenal hyperplasia. Patients with a serum level of DHEAS greater than 8000 ng/mL could have an adrenal tumor and should be referred to an endocrinologist for further evaluation. An ovarian source of excess androgens can be suspected in cases when the serum total testosterone is greater than 150 ng/dL. Serum total testosterone in the range of 150 to 200 ng/dL or an increased LH-to-FSH ratio (>2.0) can be found in cases of PCOS. Greater elevations in serum testosterone may indicate an ovarian tumor, and appropriate referral should be made. It is important to emphasize that there is a significant amount of variability in individual serum androgen levels. Therefore, in cases in which abnormal results are obtained, repeat testing should be considered before proceeding with additional workup or therapy.

PATHOLOGY

The histopathology of acne vulgaris varies with the clinical lesion. Early lesions, microcomedones, demonstrate a dilated follicle with a narrow follicular orifice filled with shed keratinocytes. Closed comedones show increased distension of the follicle, creating a cystic space that contains eosinophilic keratinous debris, hair, and bacteria. Open comedones show enlarged follicular ostia, with atrophic or absent sebaceous glands. Only mild perivascular inflammation is present at this stage.

As the cystic structure enlarges, its contents begin to infiltrate the dermis, inducing an inflammatory response with neutrophils. If the lesion does not resolve, it may develop a foreign body granulomatous reaction or scarring.

TABLE 78-1
Differential Diagnosis of Acne

Most Likely
- Closed comedonal acne
  - Milia
  - Sebaceous hyperplasia
- Open comedonal acne
  - Dilated pore of Winer
  - Favre–Racouchot syndrome
- Inflammatory acne
  - Rosacea
  - Perioral dermatitis
- Neonatal acne
  - Miliaria rubra
  - Neonatal cephalic pustulosis

Consider
- Closed comedonal acne
  - Osteoma cutis
  - Trichoepitheliomas
  - Trichodiscomas
  - Fibrofolliculomas
  - Eruptive vellus hair cysts, steatocystoma multiplex
  - Colloid milia
  - Flat warts
- Open comedonal acne
  - Trichostasis spinulosa
  - Nevus comedonicus
- Inflammatory acne
  - Pseudofolliculitis barbae, acne keloidalis nuchae
  - Keratosis pilaris
  - Neurotic excoriations/factitial
  - Lupus miliaris disseminatus faciei
- Neonatal acne
  - Sebaceous hyperplasia
  - Milia
  - Transient neonatal pustular melanosis

Always Rule Out
- Closed comedonal acne
  - Acne due to systemic agents (eg, corticosteroids)
  - Contact acne (eg, occupational acne)
  - Chloracne
- Open comedonal acne
  - Acne caused by systemic agents
  - Contact acne
  - Chloracne
- Inflammatory acne
  - Acne caused by systemic agents
  - Staphylococcal folliculitis
  - Gram-negative folliculitis
  - Eosinophilic folliculitis
  - Furuncle or carbuncle
  - Angiofibromas of tuberous sclerosis
- Neonatal acne
  - Candidal infections

DIFFERENTIAL DIAGNOSIS

Although one type of lesion may predominate, acne vulgaris is diagnosed by a variety of acne lesions (comedones, pustules, papules, and nodules) on the face, back, or chest (Table 78-1). The diagnosis is usually straightforward, but inflammatory acne may be confused with folliculitis, rosacea, or perioral dermatitis. Patients with tuberous sclerosis and facial angiofibromas have been misdiagnosed as having recalcitrant midfacial acne. Facial flat warts or milia are occasionally confused with closed comedones.

As discussed earlier, acne can be seen in association with endocrinologic abnormalities. Patients with hyperandrogenism may have acne plus other stigmata of increased androgen levels (ie, hirsutism, deepened voice, irregular menses). Endocrinologic disorders such as PCOS (including hyperandrogenism, insulin resistance, acanthosis nigricans [HAIR-AN] syndrome), congenital adrenal hyperplasia, and adrenal and ovarian neoplasms often have accompanying acne.

Variants of acne, as reviewed in Chap. 80, must also be differentiated from typical acne vulgaris to guide treatment. These types of acne include neonatal acne, infantile acne, midchildhood acne, acne fulminans, acne conglobata, acne with solid facial edema, and acne excoriée des jeunes filles.

Several less common acneiform eruptions can be confused with acne vulgaris. These mimickers include medication-induced acne, halogen acne, chloracne, acne mechanica, tropical acne, radiation acne, and other miscellaneous acneiform disorders that are discussed in Chap. 80.

CLINICAL COURSE AND PROGNOSIS

The typical age of onset of acne vulgaris varies considerably. It may start as early as 8 years of age or it may not appear until the age of 20 years or even later. The course generally lasts several years and is followed by spontaneous remission in most cases. Although the condition clears in the majority of patients by their early 20s, some have acne extending well into the third or fourth decades of life. The extent of involvement varies, and spontaneous fluctuations in the degree of involvement are the rule rather than the exception. In women, there is often variation in relation to the menstrual cycle, with a flare just before the onset of menstruation, especially in those older than 30 years of age.[108] Family history, body mass index, and diet may predict risk for development of moderate to severe acne.[109] Furthermore, prepubescent females with comedonal acne and females with high DHEAS levels are

TABLE 78-2
Treatment Algorithm for Acne Vulgaris

	MILD	MODERATE	SEVERE		
	COMEDONAL	PAPULAR OR PUSTULAR	PAPULAR OR PUSTULAR	NODULAR	CONGLOBATA OR FULMINANS
First	Topical retinoid or combination[a]	Topical retinoid + topical antimicrobial or combination[a]	Oral antibiotic + topical retinoid ± BPO or combination[a]	Oral antibiotic + topical retinoid ± BPO	Oral isotretinoin ± oral corticosteroids
Second	Topical dapsone or azelaic acid or salicylic acid	Topical dapsone or azelaic acid or salicylic acid	Oral antibiotic + topical retinoid ± BPO or combination[a]	Oral isotretinoin or oral antibiotic + topical retinoid ± BPO–azelaic acid or combination[a]	High-dose oral antibiotic + topical retinoid + BPO or combination[a]
Female	—	—	+ Oral contraceptive–antiandrogen	+ Oral contraceptive–antiandrogen	+ Oral contraceptive–antiandrogen
Additional options	Comedone extraction	Comedone extraction, Laser or light therapy, photodynamic therapy	Comedone extraction, laser or light therapy, photodynamic therapy	Comedone extraction; intralesional corticosteroid, laser or light therapy, photodynamic therapy	Intralesional corticosteroid, laser or light therapy, photodynamic therapy
Refractory to treatment	Check compliance	Check compliance Exclude gram-negative folliculitis Females: exclude PCOS, adrenal or ovarian tumors, CAH Males: exclude ECAH			
Maintenance	Topical retinoid ± BPO, or combination[a]	Topical retinoid ± BPO, or combination[a]	Topical retinoid ± BPO, or combination[a]	Topical retinoid ± BPO, or combination[a]	

[a]Manufactured combination products include benzoyl peroxide (BPO)–erythromycin, BPO–clindamycin, adapalene–BPO, and tretinoin–clindamycin.
CAH, congenital adrenal hyperplasia; PCOS, polycystic ovarian syndrome.
Adapted from Gollnick H, Cunliffe W, Berson D, et al. Management of acne: a report from a Global Alliance to improve outcomes in acne. *J Am Acad Dermatol.* 2003;49(1Suppl):S1.

more likely to develop severe or long-standing nodular acne.[110]

MANAGEMENT

Tailoring a patient's acne regimen with the knowledge of the pathogenesis of acne and the mechanism of action of the available acne treatments will ensure maximum therapeutic response. Treatment regimens should be initiated early and be sufficiently aggressive to prevent permanent sequelae. Often multiple treatments are used in combination so as to combat the various factors in the pathogenesis of acne (Table 78-2). The mechanism of action of the most common treatments for acne can be divided in the following categories as they relate to the pathophysiology:

1. Correct the altered pattern of follicular keratinization.
2. Decrease sebaceous gland activity.
3. Decrease the follicular bacterial population, particularly *P. acnes*.
4. Exert an antiinflammatory effect.

LOCAL THERAPY

CLEANSING

The importance of cleansing in the treatment of acne is generally intuitive. Twice-daily washing with a gentle cleanser followed by the application of acne treatments may encourage a routine and therefore better compliance. Overcleansing or use of harsh alkaline soaps are likely to increase the skin's pH, disrupt the cutaneous lipid barrier, and compound the irritancy potential of many topical acne treatments. Use of a syndet (synthetic detergent) will allow cleansing without disruption of the skin's normal pH. Medicated cleansers, containing benzoyl peroxide, salicylic acid, or sulfur, offer convenience as a wash and are excellent for hard-to-reach areas such as the back.

TOPICAL MEDICATIONS (SEE TABLE 78-3)

Retinoids: Retinoids are defined by their ability to bind to and activate retinoic acid receptors (RARs) and in turn activate specific gene transcription resulting in a biologic response. Some have chemical structures similar to tretinoin (all-*trans*-retinoic acid), but they may be entirely dissimilar, such as adapalene or tazarotene, and still potentiate a retinoid effect. In general, the binding of these agents to nuclear RAR affects the expression of genes involved in cell proliferation, differentiation, melanogenesis, and inflammation.[111,112] The result is modification of corneocyte accumulation and cohesion and inflammation. Thus, retinoids have both comedolytic and antiinflammatory properties.[112]

Tretinoin is commercially available in several strengths and formulations. Having both potent comedolytic and antiinflammatory properties, it is widely

TABLE 78-3
Commonly Available Prescription Acne Preparations—Topical

GENERIC	TRADE	VEHICLE	CONCENTRATION	SIZE
Retinoids—Topical				
Tretinoin	Retin-A	Cream	0.025%, 0.05%, 0.1%	20 g, 45 g
		Gel	0.01%, 0.025%	15 g, 45 g (0.025% only)
		Liquid	0.05%	28 mL
	Retin-A micro	Gel with microsponge	0.04%, 0.1%	20 g, 45 g
				50-g pump
	Avita	Cream	0.025%	20 g, 45 g
		Gel	0.025%	20 g, 45 g
	Refissa	Cream	0.05%	40 g
	Tretin-X	Cream	0.025%, 0.05%, 0.1%	35 g (kit with cleanser)
		Gel	0.025%, 0.1%	35 g (kit with cleanser)
	Generic	Cream	0.025%, 0.05%, 0.1%	20 g, 45 g
		Gel	0.01%, 0.025%, 0.05%	15 g, 45 g
Adapalene	Differin	Cream	0.1%	15 g, 45 g
		Gel	0.1%, 0.3%	15 g, 45 g
		Lotion	0.1%	2 oz
	Generic	Gel	0.1%	45 g
Tazarotene	Tazorac	Cream	0.1%	30 g, 60 g
		Gel	0.1%	30 g, 60 g
	Fabior	Foam	0.1%	50 g, 100 g
Retinoid Combinations—Topical				
Tretinoin–clindamycin	Ziana	Gel	0.025%/1.2%	30 g, 60 g
	Veltin	Gel	0.025%/1.2%	30 g, 60 g
Adapalene–benzoyl peroxide	Epiduo	Gel	2.5%/0.1%, 2.5%/0.3%	45 g

(Continued)

TABLE 78-3
Commonly Available Prescription Acne Preparations—Topical (*Continued*)

GENERIC	TRADE	VEHICLE	CONCENTRATION	SIZE
Antimicrobials—Topical				
Benzoyl peroxide	Benzac AC	Gel	2.5%, 5%, 10%	60 g
		Wash	2.5%, 5%, 10%	240 mL (2.5%), 226 mL
	Benzac W	Gel	2.5%, 5%, 10%	60 g
		Wash	5%, 10%	226 mL
	Benzashave	Cream	5%, 10%	113.4 g
	Benziq LS	Gel	5.25%	50 g
		Wash	5.25%	175 g
	Brevoxyl	Gel	4%, 8%	42.5 g
		Creamy wash	4%, 8%	170 g (kit with cleanser)
	BenzEFoam	Foam	5.3%, 9.8%	60 g, 100 g
	Clinac	Gel	7%	45 g
	Desquam-E	Gel	2.5%, 5%, 10%	42.5 g
	PanOxyl	Creamy wash	4%	6 oz
		Foamy wash	10%	5.5 oz
	Triaz	Gel	3%, 6%, 9%	42.5 g
		Cleanser	3%, 6%, 9%	6 oz, 12 oz
		Pads	3%, 6%, 9%	1 g (30 or 60/box)
		Foaming cloths	3%, 6%, 9%	3.2 g (30 or 60/box)
	ZoDerm	Cleanser	4.5%. 6.5%, 8.5%	400 mL
		Pads	4.5%. 6.5%, 8.5%	6 mL (30/box)
		Hydrating wash	5.75%	400 mL
	Generic	Gel	5%, 10%	45 g, 60 g, 90 g
		Wash	2.5%, 5%, 10%	142 g, 227 g
Erythromycin	Generic	Gel	2%	30 g, 60 g
		Ointment	2%	25 g
		Solution	2%	60 mL
		Pledget	2%	(60/box)
Clindamycin	Cleocin T	Gel	1%	30 g, 60 g
		Lotion	1%	60 mL
		Solution	1%	30 mL, 60 mL
		Pledget	1%	(60/box)
	Evoclin	Foam	1%	50 g, 100 g
	Clindagel	Gel	1%	40 mL, 75 mL
	ClindaMax	Gel	1%	30 g, 60 g
		Lotion	1%	60 mL
	Clindets	Pledget	1%	60 s
	Generic	Gel	1%	30 g, 60 g
		Lotion	1%	30 g, 60 g
		Solution	1%	30 g
Dapsone	Aczone	Gel	5%, 7.5%	30 g, 60 g, 90 g
Benzoyl peroxide–erythromycin	Benzamycin	Gel	5%/3%	46.6 g, 60/box
	Benzamycin Gel Pak			
	Generic	Gel	5%/3%	23.2 g, 46.6 g
Benzoyl peroxide/clindamycin	BenzaClin	Gel	5%/1%	25 g, 50 g
				50-g pump
	Duac	Gel	5%/1%	45 g
	Acanya	Gel	2.5%/1.2%	50 g
	Generic	Gel	5%/1%	50 g
Benzoyl peroxide/hydrocortisone	Vanoxide HC	Lotion	5%–0.5%	25 mL
Miscellaneous				
Sodium sulfacetamide	Klaron	Lotion	10%	4 oz
	Ovace	Foam	10%	70 g
		Wash	10%	6 oz, 12 oz, 16 oz
Sodium sulfacetamide/sulfur	Avar	Emollient cream	10%–5%	45 g, 2 oz
	Generic	Suspension (cleanser)	8%–4%, 9%–4%, 10%–5%	6 oz, 12 oz
		Foam	10%–5%	60 g60/box
		Topical pad	10%–5%	
Azelaic acid	Finacea	Gel	15%	50 g
	Azelex	Cream	20%	30 g, 50 g

used. In general, all retinoids can be contact irritants, with alcohol-based gels and solutions having the greatest irritancy potential. Some newer formulations use a microsphere delayed-delivery technology (Retin A Micro 0.04%, 0.08% or 0.1% gel) or are incorporated within a polyolprepolymer (PP-2; Avita cream) to decrease the irritancy potential of tretinoin while allowing greater concentration of medication. Advising patients to apply tretinoin on alternate nights during the first few weeks of treatment can help ensure greater tolerability. Patients must also be cautioned about sun exposure because of thinning of the stratum corneum, especially those with any irritant reaction. Regular use of a sunscreen should be advised. The comedolytic and antiinflammatory properties of topical retinoids make them ideal for maintenance therapy of acne. Generic tretinoin is inactivated by concomitant use of benzoyl peroxide and is photolabile. Therefore, patients should be counseled to apply tretinoin at bedtime and not at the same time as benzoyl peroxide.

Adapalene is a synthetic retinoid widely marketed for its greater tolerability. It specifically targets the RARγ receptor. It is both photostable and can be used in conjunction with benzoyl peroxide without degradation. Adapalene 0.1% gel has been shown in clinical trials to have greater or equal efficacy to tretinoin 0.025% gel with greater tolerability.[113,114] It is available at a 0.1% concentration in both a nonalcohol gel and cream and as a 0.3% gel. The 0.3% adapalene gel has been shown to have similar efficacy to tazarotene 0.1% gel with increased tolerability.[115] A combination topical agent containing adapalene (0.1% or 0.3%) and 2.5% benzoyl peroxide is also available.[116,117] Adapalene 0.1% gel is the only retinoid recently made available by the U.S. Food and Drug Administration (FDA) for over-the-counter (OTC) treatment of acne in those 12 years and older.[118]

Tazarotene, also a synthetic retinoid, exerts its action through its metabolite, tazarotenic acid, which in turn inhibits the RARγ receptor. It is a potent comedolytic agent and has been shown to be more effective than tretinoin 0.025% gel and tretinoin 0.1% microsphere gel.[119,120] Both the 0.1% cream and gel formulations are approved for the treatment of acne, as well as a 0.1% foam for the chest and back. The irritant properties of tazarotene can be minimized by the use of short-term contact therapy. In this regimen, the medication is applied for 5 minutes and then washed off with a gentle cleanser. The use of tazarotene is not recommended for use during pregnancy (formerly Pregnancy Category X classification), and female patients of childbearing age should be adequately counseled, with consideration of obtaining a negative pregnancy test result before initiation of therapy.

Benzoyl Peroxide: Benzoyl peroxide preparations are among the most common topical medications prescribed by dermatologists and are also readily available OTC. Benzoyl peroxide is a powerful antimicrobial agent, markedly reducing the bacterial population via release of free oxygen radicals.[121] It also has mild comedolytic properties. Benzoyl peroxide preparations are available in creams, lotions, gels, washes, foams, and pledgets in a variety of concentrations ranging from 2.5% to 10%. Products that are left on the skin, such as gels, are generally considered more effective, but data are lacking. Benzoyl peroxide can produce significant dryness and irritation and can bleach clothing and hair. Higher concentrations are not necessarily more efficacious and can cause increased irritation. Allergic contact dermatitis has been uncommonly reported. Of significance, bacteria are unable to develop resistance to benzoyl peroxide, making it the ideal agent for combination with topical or oral antibiotics.[122]

Topical Antibiotics: Erythromycin and clindamycin have historically been the most commonly used topical antibiotics for the treatment of acne. However, over the past few decades, the estimated global incidence rate of *P. acnes* resistance to antibiotics has increased from 20% (in 1978) to 62% (in 1996). In particular, high resistance to erythromycin has resulted in significant reduction in its use in recent years with preferential use of clindamycin. These two agents have also been used in combination preparations with benzoyl peroxide. The development of resistance is less likely in patients who are treated concurrently with benzoyl peroxide[123]; therefore, the combination of these two products is preferable over monotherapy with topical antibiotics. Topical dapsone 5% and 7.5% gel is the most recently approved topical antibiotic for acne. With twice-daily application, topical dapsone has shown better efficacy in controlling inflammatory lesions (58%) versus noninflammatory lesions (19%).[124,125] Unlike oral dapsone, topical dapsone is safe for use even in patients with a glucose-6-phosphate dehydrogenase (G6PD) deficiency.[126] It is generally well tolerated but should not be applied concomitantly with benzoyl peroxide, or it may impart an orange color on the skin.[127] As of submission of this chapter, a phase II clinical trial with topical minocycline 1% and 4% foam for the treatment of moderate to severe acne has been published and shows promising results.[128]

Salicylic Acid: Salicylic acid is a ubiquitous ingredient found in OTC acne preparations (gels and washes) in concentrations ranging from 0.5% to 2%. This lipid-soluble β-hydroxy acid has comedolytic properties but somewhat weaker than those of a retinoid. Salicylic acid also causes exfoliation of the stratum corneum through decreased cohesion of the keratinocytes. Mild irritant reactions may result. It is generally considered less effective than benzoyl peroxide.

Azelaic Acid: Azelaic acid is available by prescription in a 20% cream or 15% gel. This dicarboxylic acid has both antimicrobial and comedolytic properties[129] It is also a competitive inhibitor of tyrosinase and thus may decrease postinflammatory hyperpigmentation.[130] It is generally well tolerated, although transient burning can occur, and is considered safe in pregnancy.

Sulfur, Sodium Sulfacetamide, and Resorcinol: Products containing sulfur, sodium sulfacetamide, and resorcinol, once favored treatments for acne, are still found in several OTC and prescription niche formulations. Sulfonamides are thought to have antibacterial properties through their inhibition of *para*-aminobenzoic acid (PABA), an essential substance for *P. acnes* growth.[131] Sulfur also inhibits the formation of free fatty acids and has presumptive keratolytic properties. It is often combined with sodium sulfacetamide to enhance its cosmetic tolerability due to sulfur's distinctive odor. Resorcinol is also indicated for use in acne for its antimicrobial properties. It is generally found in a 2% concentration in combination with 5% sulfur.

An overview of topical agents for acne treatment is outlined in Table 78-3.

SYSTEMIC THERAPY

ANTIBIOTICS AND ANTIBACTERIAL AGENTS

Tetracyclines: Broad-spectrum antibiotics are widely used in the treatment of inflammatory acne. The tetracyclines are the most commonly used antibiotics in the treatment of acne. Although the oral administration of tetracyclines does not alter sebum production, it does decrease the concentration of free fatty acids while the esterified fatty acid content increases. Free fatty acids are inflammatory, and their level is an indication of the metabolic activity of *P. acnes* and its secretion of proinflammatory products. This reduction in free fatty acids may be through suppression of *P. acnes* and may take several weeks to become evident. Therefore, several weeks of therapy are often required to observe maximal clinical benefit. The effect, then, is one of prevention; the individual lesions require their usual time to undergo resolution. Decreases in free fatty acid formation also have been reported with erythromycin, demethylchlortetracycline, clindamycin, and minocycline.

Doxycycline and minocycline are the most commonly used tetracycline derivatives for the treatment of acne. They have the distinct advantage that they can be taken with food with minimal impaired absorption. Doxycycline is administered in dosages of 50 to 100 mg twice daily. Its major disadvantage is the potential risk of photosensitivity reactions, including photo-onycholysis, and patients may need to be switched to another antibiotic during summer months. Gastrointestinal (GI) upset is another common side effect; it can be minimized if medication is taken with food.

Minocycline is given in divided doses at a level of 100 to 200 mg/day. Patients taking minocycline should be monitored carefully because the drug can cause blue-black pigmentation, especially in acne scars, as well as the hard palate, alveolar ridge, and anterior shins. Vertigo has occasionally been described. Minocycline-induced autoimmune hepatitis and a systemic lupus erythematosus–like syndrome have been reported during minocycline therapy, but these side effects are very rare.[132,133] Of note, patients who develop lupus-like reactions can be safely switched to an alternative tetracycline. Serum sickness–like reactions and drug reaction with eosinophilia and systemic symptoms (DRESS) syndrome have also been reported with minocycline use.

Tetracycline is usually given initially in dosages of 500 to 1000 mg/day. Higher doses of up to 3500 mg/day have been used in severe cases, but prudent monitoring of liver function is warranted. Tetracycline should be taken on an empty stomach, 1 hour before or 2 hours after meals, to promote absorption; thus, compliance by adolescents with its administration can be challenging. GI upset is the most common side effect, with esophagitis and pancreatitis possible. Uncommon side effects include hepatotoxicity, hypersensitivity reactions, leukocytosis, thrombocytopenic purpura, and pseudotumor cerebri.

Tetracyclines should be used with caution in patients with renal disease because they may increase uremia. Tetracyclines have an affinity for rapidly mineralizing tissues and are deposited in developing teeth, where they may cause irreversible yellow-brown staining; also, tetracyclines have been reported to inhibit skeletal growth in fetuses. Therefore, they should not be administered to pregnant women, especially after the fourth month of gestation, and are not recommended for use in children younger than 9 years of age in the treatment of acne.

Macrolides: Because of the prevalence of erythromycin-resistant strains of *P. acnes*, the use of oral erythromycin is generally limited to pregnant women or children. Azithromycin has been used more often for acne, typically at dosages of 250 to 500 mg orally three times weekly.[134] Azithromycin undergoes hepatic metabolism with GI upset and diarrhea as the most common side effects.

Trimethoprim–Sulfamethoxazole: Trimethoprim–sulfamethoxazole combinations are also effective in acne. In general, because the potential for side effects is greater with their use, they should be used only in patients with severe acne who do not respond to other antibiotics. GI upset and cutaneous hypersensitivity reactions are common. Serious adverse reactions, including the Stevens-Johnson syndrome–toxic epidermal necrolysis spectrum and aplastic anemia, have been described. If trimethoprim–sulfamethoxazole is used, the patient should be monitored for potential hematologic suppression monthly.

Cephalexin: Cephalexin, a first-generation cephalosporin, has been shown in vitro to kill *P. acnes*. However, because it is hydrophilic and not lipophilic, it penetrates poorly into the pilosebaceous unit. Success with oral cephalexin[135] is most likely caused by its antiinflammatory rather than antimicrobial properties. Because of the risk of promoting the development of bacterial resistance, particularly to *Staphylococcus* spp., the authors discourage the use of cephalexin for acne.

Clindamycin and Dapsone: Less commonly used antibiotics include clindamycin and dapsone. Oral clindamycin had been used more readily in the past, but because of the risk of pseudomembranous colitis, it is now rarely used systemically for acne. It is still commonly used topically, however, often in combination with benzoyl peroxide. Dapsone (see Chap. 187), a sulfone often used for cutaneous neutrophilic disorders, may be beneficial in severe markedly inflammatory acne and select cases of resistant acne. It is used at doses of 50 to 100 mg daily for 3 months. G6PD levels should be examined before initiation of therapy, and regular monitoring for hemolysis and liver function abnormalities is warranted. Although not as reliably effective as isotretinoin, it is relatively low cost and should be considered in severe cases when isotretinoin is not an option.

Antibiotics and Bacterial Resistance: Antibiotic resistance is a growing concern worldwide and should be suspected in patients unresponsive to appropriate antibiotic therapy after 6 weeks of treatment. Increasing propionibacterium resistance has been documented to all macrolides and tetracyclines commonly used in the treatment of acne. A prevalence rate of 65% was documented in one study performed in the United Kingdom.[136] Overall, resistance is highest with erythromycin and lowest with the lipophilic tetracyclines, doxycycline, and minocycline.[63] The least resistance is noted with minocycline. To prevent resistance, prescribers should avoid antibiotic monotherapy, limit long-term use of antibiotics, and combine usage with benzoyl peroxide whenever possible.[137] Recent guidelines recommend limiting the duration of oral antibiotic therapy in acne to 3 to 6 months to reduce risk of resistance.[138]

HORMONAL THERAPY

The goal of hormonal therapy is to counteract the effects of androgens on the sebaceous gland. This can be accomplished with antiandrogens, or agents designed to decrease the endogenous production of androgens by the ovary or adrenal gland, including oral contraceptives, glucocorticoids, or gonadotropin-releasing hormone (GnRH) agonists.

TABLE 78-4
U.S. Food and Drug Administration–Approved Oral Contraceptives for Acne in Women

Ortho Tri-Cyclen (norgestimate + ethinyl estradiol)
Estrostep (norethindrone acetate + ethinyl estradiol)
Yaz (drospirenone + ethinyl estradiol)

Oral Contraceptives: Oral contraceptives can improve acne by four main mechanisms. First, they decrease the amount of gonadal androgen production by suppressing LH production. Second, they decrease the amount of free testosterone by increasing the production of sex hormone binding globulin. Third, they inhibit the activity of 5-α reductase activity, preventing the conversion of testosterone to the more potent DHT. Last, progestins that have an antiandrogenic effect can block the androgen receptors on keratinocytes and sebocytes. The third-generation progestins—gestodene (not available in the United States), desogestrel, and norgestimate—have the lowest intrinsic androgenic activity.[139] Two progestins have demonstrated antiandrogenic properties: (1) cyproterone acetate (not available in the United States) and (2) drospirenone. There are three oral contraceptives currently FDA approved for the treatment of acne: (1) Ortho Tri-Cyclen, (2) Estrostep, and (3) Yaz (Table 78-4). Ortho Tri-Cyclen is a triphasic oral contraceptive comprised of a norgestimate (180, 215, 250 mg)–ethinyl estradiol (35 μg) combination.[140] In an effort to reduce the estrogenic side effects of oral contraceptives, preparations with lower doses of estrogen (20 μg) have been developed for the treatment of acne. Estrostep contains a graduated dose of ethinyl estradiol (20–35 μg) in combination with norethindrone acetate (1 mg).[141] Yaz contains ethinyl estradiol (20 ug) and the antiandrogen drospirenone (3 mg). Drospirenone is a 17 α-spironolactone derivative that has both antimineralocorticoid and antiandrogenic properties, which may improve estrogen-related weight gain and bloating.[141] An oral contraceptive containing a low dose of estrogen (20 μg) in combination with levonorgestrel (Alesse) has also demonstrated efficacy in acne.[142] Side effects from oral contraceptives include nausea, vomiting, abnormal menses, weight gain, and breast tenderness. Rare but more serious complications include thrombophlebitis, pulmonary embolism, and hypertension. With the use of oral contraceptives containing estrogen and progestin rather than estrogen alone, side effects such as delayed menses, menorrhagia, and premenstrual cramps are uncommon. However, other side effects such as nausea, weight gain, spotting, breast tenderness, amenorrhea, and melasma can occur.

Glucocorticoids: Because of their antiinflammatory activity, high-dose systemic glucocorticoids may be of benefit in the treatment of acne. In practice, their use is usually restricted to severely involved patients, often overlapping with isotretinoin to limit any potential flaring from at the start of treatment. Furthermore, because of the potential side effects, these drugs are ordinarily used for limited periods of time, and recurrences after treatment are common. Prolonged use may result in the appearance of steroid acne. Glucocorticoids in low dosages are also indicated in female patients who have an elevation in serum DHEAS associated with an 11- or 21-hydroxylase deficiency or in other individuals with demonstrated androgen excess. Low-dose prednisone (2.5 mg or 5 mg) or dexamethasone can be given orally at bedtime to suppress adrenal androgen production.[106] The combined use of glucocorticoids and estrogens has been used in recalcitrant acne in women based on the inhibition of sebum production by this combination.[143] The mechanism of action is probably related to a greater reduction of plasma androgen levels by combined therapy than is produced by either drug alone.

Gonadotropin-Releasing Hormone Agonists: GnRH agonists, such as leuprolide (Lupron), act on the pituitary gland to disrupt its cyclic release of gonadotropins. The net effect is suppression of ovarian steroidogenesis in women. These agents are used in the treatment of ovarian hyperandrogenism. GnRH agonists have demonstrated efficacy in the treatment of acne and hirsutism in female patients both with and without endocrine disturbance.[144] However, their use is limited by their side effect profile, which includes menopausal symptoms and bone loss.

Antiandrogens: Spironolactone is an aldosterone antagonist and functions in acne as both an androgen-receptor blocker and inhibitor of 5-α reductase. In dosages of 50–100 mg twice a day, it has been shown to reduce sebum production and to improve acne.[145] Side effects include diuresis, potential hyperkalemia, irregular menstrual periods, breast tenderness, headache, and fatigue. Combining spironolactone treatment with an oral contraceptive can alleviate the symptoms of irregular menstrual bleeding. Although hyperkalemia is a risk of spironolactone, this risk has shown to be minimal, even when spironolactone is administered with other aldosterone antagonists (eg, drospirenone-containing oral contraceptives).[146] A recent study evaluating the usefulness of routine potassium monitoring in healthy young female patients taking spironolactone for acne showed that the rate of hyperkalemia was equivalent to that of the general population and therefore routine monitoring is of low utility.[147] As an antiandrogen, there is a risk of feminization of a male fetus if a pregnant woman takes this medication. Long-term studies in rats receiving high doses of spironolactone demonstrated an increased incidence of adenomas on endocrine organs and the liver, resulting in a black box warning by the FDA (http://www.drugs.com/pro/aldactone). The potential for spironolactone to induce estrogen-dependent malignancies still remains controversial. However, the available data suggest that there is no definitive documented association between breast carcinoma and spironolactone ingestion after more than 30 years of data on spironolactone.[148,149]

Cyproterone acetate is a progestational antiandrogen that blocks the androgen receptor. It is combined with ethinyl estradiol in an oral contraceptive formulation that is widely used in Europe for the treatment of acne. Cyproterone acetate is not available in the United States.

Flutamide, an androgen receptor blocker, has been used at doses of 250 mg twice a day in combination with oral contraceptives for treatment of acne or hirsutism in females.[150] Liver function tests should be monitored because cases of fatal hepatitis have been reported.[151] Pregnancy should be avoided. Use of flutamide in the treatment of acne may be limited by its side effect profile.

ISOTRETINOIN (SEE CHAP. 185)

The use of the oral retinoid isotretinoin has revolutionized the management of treatment-resistant acne.[152] It is approved for use in patients with severe recalcitrant nodular acne. However, it is commonly used in many other acne scenarios, including any significant acne that is unresponsive to treatment with oral antibiotics and acne that results in significant physical or emotional scarring. Isotretinoin is also effective in the treatment of gram-negative folliculitis, pyoderma faciale, and acne fulminans.[153] The remarkable aspects of isotretinoin therapy are the complete remission in almost all cases and the longevity of the remission, which lasts for months to years in the great majority of patients. However, because of its teratogenicity, its use has become highly regulated in the United States with the initiation of the iPledge program in 2006 to ensure that pregnancy-prevention procedures are followed.

The mechanism of action of isotretinoin is not completely known. The drug produces profound inhibition of sebaceous gland activity, and this undoubtedly is of great importance in the initial clearing.[154,155] In some patients, sebaceous gland inhibition continues for at least 1 year, but in the majority of patients, sebum production returns to normal after 2 to 4 months.[154] Thus, this action of the drug cannot be used to explain the long-term remissions. The *P. acnes* population is also decreased during isotretinoin therapy, but this decrease is generally transient.[155,156] Isotretinoin has no inhibitory effect on *P. acnes* in vitro. Therefore, the effect on the bacterial population is probably indirect, resulting from the decrease in intrafollicular lipids necessary for organism growth. Isotretinoin also has antiinflammatory activity and probably has an effect on the pattern of follicular keratinization. These effects also are temporary, and the explanation for long-term remissions remains obscure.

Given the ubiquitous distribution of RAR, isotretinoin almost always causes side effects, mimicking those seen in the chronic hypervitaminosis A syndrome.[157] In general, the severity of side effects tends to be dose dependent. The most common side effects are related to the skin and mucous membranes. Cheilitis of varying degrees is found in virtually all cases. Other side effects that are likely to be seen in more than 50% of patients are dryness of the mucous membranes and skin. An eczematous eruption is occasionally seen, particularly in cold, dry weather. Thinning of hair and granulomatous paronychial lesions are less common.

Ophthalmologic findings include xerophthalmia, night blindness, conjunctivitis, keratitis, and optic neuritis. Corneal opacities and hearing loss (both transient and persistent) have also been reported with isotretinoin use. Pseudotumor cerebri, also known as benign intracranial hypertension, is evidenced by severe headache, nausea, and visual changes. The risk of pseudotumor cerebri may be increased with concomitant use of tetracyclines and isotretinoin; therefore, these two medications should not be used together without careful prior consideration. If symptoms suggest benign intracranial hypertension, prompt neurologic evaluation for evidence of papilledema is required. Vague complaints of headache, fatigue, and lethargy are also frequent.

The relationship between isotretinoin use and psychiatric effects is currently being examined. Risks of depression, suicide, psychosis, and aggressive or violent behavior are all listed as possible side effects. Although no clear mechanism of action has been established, some evidence for biologic plausibility does exist. Psychiatric adverse events are described with high-dose vitamin A and etretinate. Also, retinoids have the demonstrated ability to enter the central nervous system (CNS) of rats and mice. And finally, there are documented case reports and studies linking isotretinoin use to depression in certain individuals.[158] A meta-analysis of nine studies looking at the possible link between isotretinoin and depression found that the incidence of depression in patients on isotretinoin ranged from 1% to 11%.[159] The authors importantly pointed out that this range is similar to control group patients taking oral antibiotics. Another author examining case-control studies on isotretinoin and depression found the relative risk to range from 0.9 to 2.7 with wide confidence intervals.[160] Some studies demonstrate that patients taking isotretinoin have an overall improvement in mood.[161] Retinoids have not been shown to activate genes to induce behavioral or psychiatric changes. Nor is there evidence demonstrating functionality of retinoid signaling pathways in the mature CNS. Large population-based studies have not supported causality. As dermatologists are often on the front line seeing adolescents at risk for depression, careful screening of adolescents is particularly needed because the risk of depression in this population is 10% to 20%.[162]

GI symptoms are generally uncommon, but nausea, esophagitis, gastritis, and colitis can occur. Acute hepatitis is rare, but liver function studies should be regularly monitored because elevations in liver enzymes can occur in 15% of patients, sometimes necessitating dose adjustments. Elevated levels of serum triglycerides occur in approximately 25% of patients taking isotretinoin. This elevation, which is dose related, typically occurs within the first 4 weeks of treatment and is often accompanied by an overall increase in cholesterol with a decrease in the high-density lipoprotein levels. The effect of this transient alteration on overall coronary artery health is unclear. Acute pancreatitis is a rare complication that may or may not be related to triglyceride levels. There are case reports documenting a potential link between isotretinoin and new-onset or flared inflammatory bowel disease (IBD). However, a study that critically examined these case reports found no grounds for a causal relationship between isotretinoin use and IBD.[163] A recent population-based case-control study found that patients with IBD were no more likely to have used isotretinoin than those without IBD.[164] Patients with a family history of IBD and those with a preexisting IBD should be counseled regarding the possibility of isotretinoin-induced IBD.

Isotretinoin has effects on bone mineralization as well. A single course of isotretinoin was not shown to have a significant effect on bone density.[165] However, chronic or repeated courses may result in significant osteopenia. Osteoporosis, bone fractures, and delayed healing of bone fractures have also been reported. The significance of reported hyperostosis is unclear, but the development of bony hyperostoses after isotretinoin therapy is more likely in patients who receive the drug for longer periods of time and in higher dosages, such as for disorders of keratinization.[166] Serial bone densitometry should be done in any patient on long-term isotretinoin. Myalgias are the most common musculoskeletal complaint, seen in 15% of patients. In severe cases, creatine phosphokinase levels should be evaluated for possible rhabdomyolysis.

Other laboratory abnormalities that have been reported with isotretinoin use are an elevated erythrocyte sedimentation rate and platelet count. Alterations in the red blood cell parameters with decreased white cell counts can occur. White blood cells in the urine have rarely been linked to isotretinoin use. Most laboratory changes are mild and spontaneously resolve upon discontinuation of medication use.

Laboratory monitoring while patients are taking isotretinoin includes obtaining a baseline complete blood count, liver function tests and lipid panel, with the greatest attention paid to following serum triglyceride levels. Baseline values for serum triglycerides should be obtained and repeated at 4 and 8 weeks of therapy. If the values are normal at 8 weeks, there is no need to repeat the test during the remaining course of therapy unless there are risk factors. If serum triglycerides increase above 500 mg/dL, the levels should be monitored frequently. Levels above 700 to 800 mg/dL are a reason for interrupting therapy or treating the patient with a lipid-lowering drug. Eruptive xanthomas or pancreatitis can occur at higher serum triglyceride levels.

A recent study evaluating the characteristics of lab abnormalities in 515 patients who underwent isotretinoin therapy for acne reported clinically insignificant leukopenia (1.4%) or thrombocytopenia (0.9%), infrequent transaminitis (1.9%) with the most significant elevations occurring with triglyceride (19.3%) and cholesterol (22.8%) levels. Recommendations for otherwise healthy patients with normal baseline labs are to repeat laboratory studies after 2 months taking isotretinoin therapy, and if results are normal, no further testing may be required. Routine complete blood count monitoring was also found to be unnecessary.[167]

The greatest concern during isotretinoin therapy is the risk of the drug being administered during pregnancy and thereby inducing teratogenic effects in the fetus.[168,169] The drug is not mutagenic; its effect is on organogenesis. Therefore, the production of retinoic embryopathy occurs very early in pregnancy, with a peak near the third week of gestation.[168,169] A significant number of fetal abnormalities have been reported after the use of isotretinoin. For this reason, it should be emphasized that isotretinoin should be given only to patients who have not responded to other therapy. Furthermore, women who are of childbearing age must be fully informed of the risk of pregnancy. The patient must use two highly effective contraception techniques such as the use of an oral contraceptive and condoms with a spermicidal jelly. Contraception must be started at least 1 month before isotretinoin therapy. Female patients must be thoroughly counseled and demonstrate an understanding of contraception techniques before starting isotretinoin. Two forms of contraception should be used throughout the course of isotretinoin and for 1 month after stopping treatment. No more than 1 month's supply of isotretinoin should be given to a female patient so that she can be counseled on a monthly basis on the hazards of pregnancy during isotretinoin therapy. A pregnancy test must be repeated monthly. Abstinence as the sole form of birth control should only be allowed in special instances. Because the drug is not mutagenic, there is no risk to a fetus conceived by a man who is taking isotretinoin. Although it may seem obvious, it is important to remind men who are taking isotretinoin not to give any of their medication to female companions under any circumstances or to donate blood while taking the medication.

The recommended daily dosage of isotretinoin is in the range of 0.5 to 1 mg/kg/day. A cumulative weight-based dosing formula may also be used with a total dose of 120 to 150 mg/kg of isotretinoin during a course of therapy.[170] This dosing regimen is of particular use in patients who have variable dosages or interrupted periods of treatment because achieving the total dose will ensure the greatest chance of long-term remission. Because back and chest lesions show less of a response than facial lesions, dosages as high as 2 mg/kg/day may be necessary in patients who have very severe truncal involvement. Patients with severe acne, particularly those with granulomatous lesions, often develop marked flares of their disease when isotretinoin is started. Therefore, the initial dosing should be low, even below 0.5 mg/kg/day. These patients often need pretreatment for 1 to 2 weeks with prednisone (40–60 mg/day), which may have to be continued for the first 2 weeks of therapy. A typical course of isotretinoin is 20 weeks, but the length of the course of treatment is not absolute; in patients who have not shown an adequate response, therapy can be extended. Additional improvement may be seen for 1 to 2 months after discontinuation, so that complete clearance may not be a necessary endpoint for determining when to discontinue therapy. Low-dose regimens, 0.1 to 0.4 mg/kg/day, have shown efficacy. However, with such dosages, the incidence of relapses after therapy is greater. Approximately 10% of patients treated with isotretinoin require a second course of the drug. The likelihood for repeat therapy is increased in patients younger than 16 to 17 years of age. It is standard practice to allow at least 2 to 3 months between courses of isotretinoin.

DIET

Several articles suggesting a role for diet in acne exist.[171,172] A recent review of these studies concluded that there may be some link between milk and acne as well as between high-glycemic index foods and acne.[173] Yet overall, the implications of these studies are not clear, and the role of chocolate, sweets, milk, high-glycemic index foods, and fatty foods in patients with acne requires further study. There is no evidence to support the value of elimination of these foods. However, restricting a food firmly thought by the patient to be a trigger is not harmful as long as the patient's nutritional well-being is not compromised.

PROCEDURES

ACNE SURGERY

Acne surgery, a mainstay of therapy in the past used for the removal of comedones and superficial pustules, aids in bringing about involution of individual acne lesions. However, with the advent of comedolytic agents, such as topical retinoids, its use is primarily restricted to patients who do not respond to comedolytic agents. Even in these patients, the comedones are removed with greater ease and less trauma if the patient is pretreated with a topical retinoid for 3 to 4 weeks. Acne surgery should not be performed at home because inaccurate placement of the comedo extractor may rupture the follicle and incite an inflammatory reaction. The Unna type of comedo extractor, which has a broad flat plate and no narrow sharp edges, is preferable. The removal of open comedones is desirable for cosmetic purposes but does not significantly influence the course of the disease. In contrast, closed comedones should be removed to prevent their rupture. Unfortunately, the orifice of closed comedones is often very small, and usually the material contained within the comedo can be removed only after the orifice is gently enlarged with a 25- or 30-gauge needle, lancet, or other suitable sharply pointed instrument. Cotton-tipped applicators are also useful to gently extract follicular content after the orifice is opened.

SUBCISION

Subcision is a minor surgical procedure used for treatment of depressed scars and is most effective for rolling acne scars (distensible, depressed scars with gentle sloping edges). This method involves the use of a small hypodermic needle that is inserted into the periphery of a scar with the sharp edges maneuvered under the defect to loosen the fibrotic adhesions, which results in release of the tethered scar to the underlying subcutaneous tissue and collagen formation during wound healing. Subcision has a reported success rate of 50% in the treatment of rolling scars.[174]

INTRALESIONAL INJECTION OF CORTICOSTEROIDS

Intralesional injection of corticosteroids can dramatically decrease the size of deep nodular lesions. The injection of 0.05 to 0.25 mL per lesion of a triamcinolone acetonide suspension (2.5–10 mg/mL) is recommended as the antiinflammatory agent. This is a very useful form of therapy in patients with nodular acne or for particularly persistent nodular lesions. A major advantage is that it can be done without incising or draining the lesions, thus avoiding the possibility of scar formation. Hypopigmentation, particularly in darker-skinned patients, and atrophy are risks.

CHEMICAL PEELS

Superficial chemical peels can be performed as an adjuvant to the pharmacologic treatment of facial acne or in patients with contraindications for other treatment modalities (eg, pregnancy). Superficial peels aim to remove the stratum corneum, enhancing physiologic cell turnover.[175] The most common peeling agents for use in acne are the α-hydroxy acids such as glycolic acid and trichloroacetic acid (TCA), β-hydroxy acid such as salicylic acid, and combination peels including Jessner solution. Glycolic acid reduces hyperkeratinization by decreasing cohesion of corneocytes at low concentrations and promoting desquamation and epidermolysis at higher concentrations,[176] with one study of 80 patients reporting glycolic acid peels effective at improving comedonal, papulopustular, and nodulocystic acne variants.[177] Salicylic acid is a lipophilic agent that also decreases corneocyte cohesion and promotes desquamation of the stratum corneum. Whereas low concentrations of salicylic acid are found in daily acne cleansers, concentrations of 20% to 30% are typically used for superficial peels, and similar to glycolic acid, have been reported to reduce the number of inflammatory and noninflammatory acne lesions.[178] The most common side effects of chemical peels include erythema, xerosis, exfoliation, burning, and increase in photosensitivity.

PHOTOTHERAPY AND LASERS

Various forms of phototherapy are under investigation for their use in treating acne vulgaris.[179] Ultraviolet (UV) light has long been thought to be beneficial in the treatment of acne. Up to 70% of patients report that sun exposure improves their acne.[180] This reported benefit may be attributable to camouflage by UV radiation–induced erythema and pigmentation, although it is likely that the sunlight has a biologic effect on the pilosebaceous unit and *P. acnes*. Although UVB can also kill *P. acnes* in vitro, UVB penetrates poorly to the dermal follicle, and only high doses causing sunburn have be shown to improve acne.[181,182] UV radiation may have antiinflammatory effects by inhibiting cytokine action.[183] Twice-weekly phototherapy sessions are needed for any clinical improvement. The therapeutic utility of UV radiation in acne is superseded by its carcinogenic potential.[179,184-187]

Other types of phototherapy for acne treatment use porphyrins. Treatment of acne with phototherapy works either by activating the endogenous porphyrins of *P. acnes* or by applying exogenous porphyrins. Coproporphyrin III is the major endogenous porphyrin of *P. acnes*. Coproporphyrin III can absorb light at the near-UV and blue light spectrum of 415 nm.[188] Irradiation of *P. acnes* with blue light leads to photoexcitation of endogenous bacterial porphyrins, singlet oxygen production, and subsequent bacterial destruction.[189] A visible light source—blue, red, or both—may be used to excite the endogenous porphyrins. The high-intensity, enhanced, narrowband (407–420 nm) blue light known as ClearLight (Lumenis) is currently FDA approved for the treatment of moderate inflammatory acne.[187] Red light may also be beneficial because it penetrates deeper into the dermis and has greater antiinflammatory properties but causes less photoactivation of the porphyrins. Therefore, the combination of blue and red light may prove the most beneficial. Treatments should be given twice weekly for 15-minute sessions for the face alone and 45 minutes for the face, chest, and back. A multicenter study has shown that 80% of patients treated with the ClearLight for 4 weeks had a 60% reduction in acne lesions. There was a gradual return of lesions over 3 to 6 months.[190]

The most consistent improvement in acne after light treatment has been demonstrated with photodynamic therapy.[191] Photodynamic therapy involves the topical application of aminolevulinic acid (ALA) 1 hour before exposure to a low-power light source. These sources include the pulsed-dye laser, intense pulsed light, or a broadband red light source. The topical ALA is taken up by the pilosebaceous unit and metabolized to protoporphyrin IX.[192] The protoporphyrin IX is targeted by the light and produces singlet oxygen species, which then damage the sebaceous glands.[193] Several studies using ALA-PDT maintained clinical improvement for up to 20 weeks.[194,195]

Although lasers are beginning to find a role in the treatment of acne, the authors consider them inferior to the traditional medical treatments. They work by emitting minimally divergent, coherent light that can be focused over a small area of tissue. The pulsed KTP laser (532 nm) has demonstrated a 35.9% decrease in acne lesions when used twice weekly for 2 weeks. Although there was no significant decrease in *P. acnes*, there was significantly lower sebum production even at 1 month.[196] The pulsed-dye laser (585 nm) can also be used at lower fluences to treat acne. Instead of ablating blood vessels and causing purpura, a lower fluence can stimulate procollagen production by heating dermal perivascular tissue.[193] The beneficial effects of a single treatment can last 12 weeks.[197] Some of the nonablative infrared lasers, such as the 1450- and 1320-nm laser, have shown to be helpful in improving acne.[198,199] These lasers work by causing thermal damage to the sebaceous glands. The concurrent use of a cryogen spray device protects the epidermis while the laser causes necrosis of the sebaceous gland.[200] In a pilot study, 14 of 15 patients treated with the 1450-nm laser had a significant reduction in inflammatory lesions that persisted for 6 months. The 1320-nm Nd:YAG (neodymium-doped yttrium aluminum garnet) and the 1540 erbium glass lasers have also been demonstrated to improve acne.[201] Multiple treatments are needed with either of these lasers to lessen acne lesions. These treatments tend to be painful and show a gradual modest improvement, limiting their utility.

One of the newer uses of light for treating acne is with a photopneumatic device (Isolaz, Solta Medical). This photopneumatic device has a handpiece that applies negative pressure (ie, suction) to the skin and then delivers a broadband-pulsed light (400–1200 nm). The suction is used to unplug the infundibulum of the pilosebaceous unit, and the light is delivered to activate the *P. acnes* porphyrins, thus releasing singlet oxygen species. Patients treated with this device may experience some posttreatment erythema or purpura. Results are modest and temporary, and the device is best for inflammatory lesions.[202,203] Although the light-based treatments are beneficial in that they avoid some of the side effects of the oral medications, the cost of these light and laser treatments tends to be prohibitive.

Lasers, however, can be useful for the treatment of acne scars.[204] Pulsed-dye lasers help improve persistent erythema from acne lesions and atrophic scars. Fractional photothermolysis lasers are approved for the treatment of acne scars by the FDA, and studies support improvement of various acne scars. The use of 1550-nm fractional photothermolysis two to six times in a 1-month interval showed the majority of patients achieving a 50% to 75% improvement in facial and back acne scarring, and some patients had greater than 75% in acne scarring. No adverse effects were found including in patients with Fitzpatrick Skin types III to V.[205] Another study showed a clinical improvement averaged 51% to 75% in nearly 90% of patients after three monthly laser treatments,[206] and a long-term improvement can be seen.[207] Ablative CO_2 and fractional CO_2 lasers have also been shown to improve acne scars,[208] but adverse effects can be more common and should be used with caution, particularly in darker skin types.

DERMABRASION

Dermabrasions are used less now since the development of new lasers, lights, and other devices. Dermabrasion is useful in treating larger atrophic scars,[209,210] but because physical removal of uninvolved skin must occur to reach the deeper scarred areas, this treatment is less favored given the prolonged recovery and increase in risk of complications. In particular, there is a greater chance of discoloration of skin in darker-skinned patients (Fitzpatrick types IV–VI). Microdermabrasion, however, has fewer adverse effects and can be used safely in most patients.[211]

MICRONEEDLING

Nonablative radiofrequency microneedling is a relatively novel technique for the treatment of both inflammatory acne lesions and acne scars. Microneedling is a minimally invasive procedure that uses fine needles to puncture the epidermis. The mechanism of action is primarily by reduction of sebaceous gland activity and remodeling of dermis through thermal stimulation.[212,213] The microwounds created also stimulate the release of growth factors and induce collagen production.[214,215] The epidermis remains relatively intact, therefore healing quickly and helping to limit adverse events. It has been shown to have a better safety profile in treating acne scars, particularly in darker skin types population (Fitzpatrick skin types IV–VI), compared with more conventional resurfacing modalities.[216] It has been shown that microneedling can be combined with various adjuvant treatments, including platelet-rich plasma, vitamin C, and glycolic acid, to enhance the clinical improvement of atrophic acne scars.[217,218]

FILLERS

The injection of dermal fillers to improve acne scars is based on soft tissue augmentation. Hyaluronic acid fillers are nonpermanent fillers that stimulate collagen production and are a safe and effective treatment for acne scars including atrophic scars. A stronger stimulation of collagen production is seen with semipermanent or biostimulatory fillers, such as poly-L-lactic acid (PLL) and calcium hydroxylapatite, and permanent fillers.[219,220]

Acne scars can be permanent and have a long-lasting impact on patients who have acne, even after active lesions resolve. In general, multiple and combination treatments using various available modalities can improve acne scars and address patients' physical and psychological concerns.

TABLE 78-5
Safety Ratings of Acne Medications in Pregnancy

MEDICATION	PREGNANCY CATEGORY[a]
Topical Therapies	
Azelaic acid	B
Clindamycin	B
Erythromycin	B
Metronidazole	B
Adapalene	C
Benzoyl peroxide	C
Dapsone	C
Salicylic acid	C
Sodium sulfacetamide	C
Tretinoin	C
Tazarotene	X
Oral Therapies	
Amoxicillin	B
Azithromycin	B
Cephalexin	B
Erythromycin	B
Cotrimoxazole	C
Levofloxacin	C
Spironolactone	C
Tetracyclines	D
Isotretinoin	X
Oral contraceptive pills	X
Physical Modalities	
ALA: photodynamic therapy	C
Glycolic acid peels	N
Blue-red light phototherapy	N

[a]Pregnancy categories:
A: Controlled studies show no risk. Adequate well-controlled studies in pregnant women have failed to demonstrate a risk to the fetus.
B: No evidence of risk. Animal reproduction studies have failed to demonstrate a risk to the fetus, and there are no adequate and well-controlled studies in pregnant women.
C: Risk cannot be ruled out. Animal reproduction studies have shown an adverse effect on the fetus, and there are no adequate and well-controlled studies in pregnant women, but use in pregnancy may be justified if potential benefits outweigh risks.
D: Positive evidence of human fetal risk. Investigational or marketing experience show risks to the fetus, but use in pregnancy may be justified if potential benefits outweigh risks.
X: Contraindicated in pregnancy. Studies in animals or humans and/or investigational or marketing experience have shown positive evidence for human fetal risk, which clearly outweighs potential benefits in the patient.
N: No pregnancy category has been assigned.

ACNE THERAPY IN PREGNANCY

Acne vulgaris is a common problem encountered by pregnant and lactating women. During pregnancy, acne may worsen as a result of a rise in serum maternal androgen levels. Inflammatory lesions tend to be more common than noninflammatory lesions, often with involvement of the trunk. Patients with a history of acne are more prone to developing acne during pregnancy.[221] Because pregnant or lactating women are often excluded from clinical trials, current evidence is limited to animal studies, retrospective studies, and case reports. As a general rule, topical agents are safer than oral medications for use during pregnancy and lactation because systemic absorption is lower.[222] Listed in Table 78-5 is a summary of common acne medications used and their safety in pregnancy. Of note, although benzoyl peroxide and salicylic acid are considered Pregnancy Category C, recent changes in pregnancy labeling of drugs suggest that more topical medications may be used during pregnancy, and although inadequate human data may be available, the risk of fetal harm is not expected based on expected limited systemic absorption. No reports of teratogenicity have been associated with either medication. For the retinoids, adapalene is categorized as "may use during pregnancy," but tretinoin is "consider avoiding use during pregnancy," and tazarotene is "use alternative during pregnancy" (Epocrates [2016], Dx version 16.11 [mobile application software]). Safety in lactation may be different from that in pregnancy. For example, the World Health Organization considers benzoyl peroxide compatible with breastfeeding (Micromedex Healthcare Series, version 5.1; Thompson Microdex, Greenwood Village, CO).

REFERENCES

1. White GM. Recent findings in the epidemiologic evidence, classification, and subtypes of acne vulgaris. *J Am Acad Dermatol*. 1998;39:S34-37.
2. Lynn DD, Umari T, Dunnick CA, Dellavalle RP. The epidemiology of acne vulgaris in late adolescence. *Adolesc Health Med Ther*. 2016;7:13-25.
3. Hay RJ, Johns NE, Williams HC, et al. The global burden of skin disease in 2010: an analysis of the prevalence and impact of skin conditions. *J Invest Dermatol*. 2014;134:1527-1534.
4. Davis SA, Narahari S, Feldman SR, et al. Top dermatologic conditions in patients of color: an analysis of nationally representative data. *J Drugs Dermatol*. 2012;11:466-473.
5. Yin NC, McMichael AJ. Acne in patients with skin of color: practical management. *Am J Clin Dermatol*. 2014;15:7-16.
6. Tan JK, Bhate K. A global perspective on the epidemiology of acne. *Br J Dermatol*. 2015;172(suppl 1): 3-12.
7. Schafer T, Nienhaus A, Vieluf D, et al. Epidemiology of

acne in the general population: the risk of smoking. *Br J Dermatol*. 2001;145:100-104.
8. Collier CN, Harper JC, Cafardi JA, et al. The prevalence of acne in adults 20 years and older. *J Am Acad Dermatol*. 2008;58:56-59.
9. Bhate K, Williams HC. Epidemiology of acne vulgaris. *Br J Dermatol*. 2013;168:474-485.
10. Wei B, Pang Y, Zhu H, et al. The epidemiology of adolescent acne in North East China. *J Eur Acad Dermatol Venereol*. 2010;24:953-957.
11. Dreno B, Jean-Decoster C, Georgescu V. Profile of patients with mild-to-moderate acne in Europe: a survey. *Eur J Dermatol*. 2016;26:177-184.
12. Wilkins JW Jr, Voorhees JJ. Prevalence of nodulocystic acne in white and Negro males. *Arch Dermatol*. 1970; 102:631-634.
13. Voorhees JJ, Wilkins J Jr, Hayes E, Harrell ER. The XYY syndrome in prisoners and outpatients with cystic acne. *Birth Defects Orig Artic Ser*. 1971;7:186-192.
14. Tian LM, Xie HF, Yang T, et al. Association study of tumor necrosis factor receptor type 2 M196R and toll-like receptor 2 Arg753Gln polymorphisms with acne vulgaris in a Chinese Han ethnic group. *Dermatology*. 2010;221:276-284.
15. Szabo K, Tax G, Teodorescu-Brinzeu D, et al. TNFalpha gene polymorphisms in the pathogenesis of acne vulgaris. *Arch Dermatol Res*. 2011;303:19-27.
16. Szabo K, Tax G, Kis K, Szegedi K, et al. Interleukin-1A +4845(G> T) polymorphism is a factor predisposing to acne vulgaris. *Tissue Antigens*. 2010;76:411-415.
17. He L, Yang Z, Yu H, et al. The relationship between CYP17 -34T/C polymorphism and acne in Chinese subjects revealed by sequencing. *Dermatology*. 2006; 212:338-342.
18. Grech I, Giatrakou S, Damoraki G, et al. Single nucleotide polymorphisms of toll-like receptor-4 protect against acne conglobata. *J Eur Acad Dermatol Venereol*. 2012;26:1538-1543.
19. Zhang M, Qureshi AA, Hunter DJ, et al. A genome-wide association study of severe teenage acne in European Americans. *Hum Genet*. 2014;133:259-264.
20. Khunger N, Kumar C. A clinico-epidemiological study of adult acne: is it different from adolescent acne? *Indian J Dermatol Venereol Leprol*. 2012;78:335-341.
21. Del Rosso JQ, Harper JC, Graber EM, et al. Status report from the American Acne & Rosacea Society on medical management of acne in adult women, part 1: overview, clinical characteristics, and laboratory evaluation. *Cutis*. 2015;96:236-241.
22. Scheffers CS, Armstrong S, Cantineau AE, et al. Dehydroepiandrosterone for women in the peri- or postmenopausal phase. *Cochrane Database Syst Rev*. 2015;1:CD011066.
23. Silverberg NB. Whey protein precipitating moderate to severe acne flares in 5 teenaged athletes. *Cutis*. 2012;90:70-72.
24. Do TT, Zarkhin S, Orringer JS, et al. Computer-assisted alignment and tracking of acne lesions indicate that most inflammatory lesions arise from comedones and de novo. *J Am Acad Dermatol*. 2008;58:603-608.
25. Kang S, Lozada VT, Bettoli V, et al. New atrophic acne scar classification: reliability of assessments based on size, shape, and number. *J Drugs Dermatol*. 2016;15:693-702.
26. Jacob CI, Dover JS, Kaminer MS. Acne scarring: a classification system and review of treatment options. *J Am Acad Dermatol*. 2001;45:109-117.
27. Wilson BB, Dent CH, Cooper PH. Papular acne scars. A common cutaneous finding. *Arch Dermatol*. 1990; 126:797-800.
28. Revol O, Milliez N, Gerard D. Psychological impact of acne on 21st-century adolescents: decoding for better care. *Br J Dermatol*. 2015;172(suppl 1):52-58.
29. Tan JK. Psychosocial impact of acne vulgaris: evaluating the evidence. *Skin Therapy Lett*. 2004;9:1-3.
30. Zaraa I, Belghith I, Ben Alaya N, et al. Severity of acne and its impact on quality of life. *Skinmed*. 2013;11:148-153.
31. Mooney T. Preventing psychological distress in patients with acne. *Nurs Stand*. 2014;28:42-48.
32. Niemeier V, Kupfer J, Demmelbauer-Ebner M, et al. Coping with acne vulgaris. Evaluation of the chronic skin disorder questionnaire in patients with acne. *Dermatology*. 1998;196:108-115.
33. Purvis D, Robinson E, Merry S, et al. Acne, anxiety, depression and suicide in teenagers: a cross-sectional survey of New Zealand secondary school students. *J Paediatr Child Health*. 2006;42:793-796.
34. Picardi A, Mazzotti E, Pasquini P. Prevalence and correlates of suicidal ideation among patients with skin disease. *J Am Acad Dermatol*. 2006;54:420-426.
35. Nagy I, Pivarcsi A, Kis K, et al. Propionibacterium acnes and lipopolysaccharide induce the expression of antimicrobial peptides and proinflammatory cytokines/chemokines in human sebocytes. *Microbes Infect*. 2006;8:2195-2205.
36. Thiboutot DM, Knaggs H, Gilliland K, et al. Activity of type 1 5 alpha-reductase is greater in the follicular infrainfundibulum compared with the epidermis. *Br J Dermatol*. 1997;136:166-17.
37. Thiboutot D, Knaggs H, Gilliland K, et al. Activity of 5-alpha-reductase and 17-beta-hydroxysteroid dehydrogenase in the infrainfundibulum of subjects with and without acne vulgaris. *Dermatology*. 1998;196:38-42.
38. Imperato-McGinley J, Gautier T, Cai LQ, et al. The androgen control of sebum production. Studies of subjects with dihydrotestosterone deficiency and complete androgen insensitivity. *J Clin Endocrinol Metab*. 1993;76:524-528.
39. Downing DT, Stewart ME, Wertz PW, et al. Essential fatty acids and acne. *J Am Acad Dermatol*. 1986;14:221-225.
40. Guy R, Green MR, Kealey T. Modeling acne in vitro. *J Invest Dermatol*. 1996;106:176-182.
41. Dinarello CA, Simon A, van der Meer JW. Treating inflammation by blocking interleukin-1 in a broad spectrum of diseases. *Nat Rev Drug Discov*. 2012;11: 633-652.
42. Munro CS, Wilkie AO. Epidermal mosaicism producing localised acne: somatic mutation in FGFR2. *Lancet*. 1998;352:704-705.
43. Melnik B, Schmitz G. FGFR2 signaling and the pathogenesis of acne. *J Dtsch Dermatol Ges*. 2008;6:721-728.
44. Thiboutot D, Harris G, Iles V, et al. Activity of the type 1 5 alpha-reductase exhibits regional differences in isolated sebaceous glands and whole skin. *J Invest Dermatol*. 1995;105:209-214.
45. Picardo M, Ottaviani M, Camera E, Mastrofrancesco A. Sebaceous gland lipids. *Dermatoendocrinol*. 2009; 1:68-71.
46. Harris HH, Downing DT, Stewart ME, et al. Sustainable rates of sebum secretion in acne patients and matched normal control subjects. *J Am Acad Dermatol*. 1983;8:200-203.

47. Kligman AM, Wheatley VR, Mills OH. Comedogenicity of human sebum. *Arch Dermatol*. 1970;102:267-275.
48. Ottaviani M, Alestas T, Flori E, et al. Peroxidated squalene induces the production of inflammatory mediators in HaCaT keratinocytes: a possible role in acne vulgaris. *J Invest Dermatol*. 2006;126:2430-2437.
49. Trivedi NR, Cong Z, Nelson AM, et al. Peroxisome proliferator-activated receptors increase human sebum production. *J Invest Dermatol*. 2006;126:2002-2009.
50. Pochi PE, Strauss JS. Sebaceous gland response in man to the administration of testosterone, delta-4-androstenedione, and dehydroisoandrosterone. *J Invest Dermatol*. 1969;52:32-36.
51. Thiboutot D, Gilliland K, Light J, et al. Androgen metabolism in sebaceous glands from subjects with and without acne. *Arch Dermatol*. 1999;135:1041-1045.
52. Lucky AW, Biro FM, Simbartl LA, et al. Predictors of severity of acne vulgaris in young adolescent girls: results of a five-year longitudinal study. *J Pediatr*. 1997;130:30-39.
53. Strauss JS, Pochi PE. Effect of cyclic progestin-estrogen therapy on sebum and acne in women. *JAMA*. 1964;190:815-819.
54. Thiboutot D. Regulation of human sebaceous glands. *J Invest Dermatol*. 2004;123:1-12.
55. Ganceviciene R, Graziene V, Fimmel S, et al. Involvement of the corticotropin-releasing hormone system in the pathogenesis of acne vulgaris. *Br J Dermatol*. 2009;160:345-352.
56. Norris JF, Cunliffe WJ. A histological and immunocytochemical study of early acne lesions. *Br J Dermatol*. 1988;118:651-659.
57. Jeremy AH, Holland DB, Roberts SG, et al. Inflammatory events are involved in acne lesion initiation. *J Invest Dermatol*. 2003;121:20-27.
58. Bek-Thomsen M, Lomholt HB, Kilian M. Acne is not associated with yet-uncultured bacteria. *J Clin Microbiol*. 2008;46:3355-3360.
59. Fitz-Gibbon S, Tomida S, Chiu BH, et al. Propionibacterium acnes strain populations in the human skin microbiome associated with acne. *J Invest Dermatol*. 2013;133:2152-2160.
60. Kim J, Ochoa MT, Krutzik SR, et al. Activation of toll-like receptor 2 in acne triggers inflammatory cytokine responses. *J Immunol*. 2002;169:1535-1541.
61. Leyden JJ, McGinley KJ, Mills OH, et al. Propionibacterium levels in patients with and without acne vulgaris. *J Invest Dermatol*. 1975;65:382-384.
62. Eady EA, Cove JH, Holland KT, et al. Erythromycin resistant propionibacteria in antibiotic treated acne patients: association with therapeutic failure. *Br J Dermatol*. 1989;121:51-57.
63. Ross J, Snelling A, Carnegie E, et al. Antibiotic-resistant acne: lessons from Europe. *Br J Dermatol*. 2003;148:467-478.
64. McDowell A, Nagy I, Magyari M, et al. The opportunistic pathogen Propionibacterium acnes: insights into typing, human disease, clonal diversification and CAMP factor evolution. *PLoS One*. 2013;8:e70897.
65. Lomholt HB, Kilian M. Population genetic analysis of Propionibacterium acnes identifies a subpopulation and epidemic clones associated with acne. *PLoS One*. 2010;5:e12277.
66. McDowell A, Gao A, Barnard E, et al. A novel multi-locus sequence typing scheme for the opportunistic pathogen Propionibacterium acnes and characterization of type I cell surface-associated antigens. *Microbiology*. 2011;157:1990-2003.
67. McDowell A, Barnard E, Nagy I, et al. An expanded multilocus sequence typing scheme for propionibacterium acnes: investigation of "pathogenic," "commensal" and antibiotic resistant strains. *PLoS One*. 7:e41480, 2012.
68. Tomida S, Nguyen L, Chiu BH, et al. Pan-genome and comparative genome analyses of propionibacterium acnes reveal its genomic diversity in the healthy and diseased human skin microbiome. *MBio*. 2013;4:e00003-00013.
69. Johnson T, Kang D, Barnard E, et al. Strain-level differences in porphyrin production and regulation in propionibacterium acnes elucidate disease associations. *mSphere*. 2016;1(1).e00023-15.
70. Kang D, Shi B, Erfe MC, et al. Vitamin B12 modulates the transcriptome of the skin microbiota in acne pathogenesis. *Sci Transl Med*. 2015;7:293ra103.
71. Yu Y, Champer J, Agak GW, et al. Different Propionibacterium acnes phylotypes induce distinct immune responses and express unique surface and secreted proteomes. *J Invest Dermatol*. 2016;136(11):2221-2228.
72. Webster GF, Indrisano JP, Leyden JJ. Antibody titers to Propionibacterium acnes cell wall carbohydrate in nodulocystic acne patients. *J Invest Dermatol*. 1985;84:496-500.
73. Webster GF, Leyden JJ, Nilsson UR. Complement activation in acne vulgaris: consumption of complement by comedones. *Infect Immun*. 1979;26:183-186.
74. Puhvel SM, Hoffman IK, Reisner RM, et al. Dermal hypersensitivity of patients with acne vulgaris to Corynebacterium acnes. *J Invest Dermatol*. 1967;49:154-158.
75. Abdel Fattah NS, Shaheen MA, Ebrahim AA, et al. Tissue and blood superoxide dismutase activities and malondialdehyde levels in different clinical severities of acne vulgaris. *Br J Dermatol*. 2008;159:1086-1091.
76. Vowels BR, Yang S, Leyden JJ. Induction of proinflammatory cytokines by a soluble factor of Propionibacterium acnes: implications for chronic inflammatory acne. *Infect Immun*. 1995;63:3158-3165.
77. Graham GM, Farrar MD, Cruse-Sawyer JE, et al. Proinflammatory cytokine production by human keratinocytes stimulated with Propionibacterium acnes and P. acnes GroEL. *Br J Dermatol*. 2004;150:421-428.
78. Nagy I, Pivarcsi A, Koreck A, et al. Distinct strains of Propionibacterium acnes induce selective human beta-defensin-2 and interleukin-8 expression in human keratinocytes through toll-like receptors. *J Invest Dermatol*. 2005;124:931-938.
79. Jugeau S, Tenaud I, Knol AC, et al. Induction of toll-like receptors by Propionibacterium acnes. *Br J Dermatol*. 2005;153:1105-1113.
80. Qin M, Pirouz A, Kim MH, et al. Propionibacterium acnes Induces IL-1beta secretion via the NLRP3 inflammasome in human monocytes. *J Invest Dermatol*. 2014;134:381-388.
81. Kistowska M, Gehrke S, Jankovic D, et al. IL-1beta drives inflammatory responses to propionibacterium acnes in vitro and in vivo. *J Invest Dermatol*. 2014;134:677-685.
82. Li ZJ, Choi DK, Sohn KC, et al. Propionibacterium acnes activates the NLRP3 inflammasome in human sebocytes. *J Invest Dermatol*. 2014;134:2747-2756.
83. Kamisango K, Saiki I, Tanio Y, et al. Structures and biological activities of peptidoglycans of Listeria monocytogenes and Propionibacterium acnes. *J Biochem*. 1982;92:23-33.

84. Inohara N, Ogura Y, Fontalba A, et al. Host recognition of bacterial muramyl dipeptide mediated through NOD2. Implications for Crohn's disease. *J Biol Chem*. 2003;278:5509-5512.
85. Girardin SE, Boneca IG, Viala J, et al. Nod2 is a general sensor of peptidoglycan through muramyl dipeptide (MDP) detection. *J Biol Chem*. 2003;278:8869-8872.
86. Martinon F, Agostini L, Meylan E, et al. Identification of bacterial muramyl dipeptide as activator of the NALP3/cryopyrin inflammasome. *Curr Biol*. 2004;14:1929-1934.
87. Lee DY, Huang CM, Nakatsuji T, et al. Histone H4 is a major component of the antimicrobial action of human sebocytes. *J Invest Dermatol*. 2009;129:2489-2496.
88. Lee DY, Yamasaki K, Rudsil J, et al. Sebocytes express functional cathelicidin antimicrobial peptides and can act to kill propionibacterium acnes. *J Invest Dermatol*. 2008;128:1863-1866.
89. Liu PT, Phan J, Tang D, et al. CD209(+) macrophages mediate host defense against Propionibacterium acnes. *J Immunol*. 2008;180:4919-4923.
90. Mouser PE, Baker BS, Seaton ED, et al. Propionibacterium acnes-reactive T helper-1 cells in the skin of patients with acne vulgaris. *J Invest Dermatol*. 2003;121:1226-1228.
91. Agak GW, Qin M, Nobe J, et al. Propionibacterium acnes Induces an IL-17 response in acne vulgaris that is regulated by vitamin a and vitamin D. *J Invest Dermatol*. 2014;134:366-373.
92. Kistowska M, Meier B, Proust T, et al. Propionibacterium acnes promotes Th17 and Th17/Th1 responses in acne patients. *J Invest Dermatol*. 2015;135:110-118.
93. Levell MJ, Cawood ML, Burke B, et al. Acne is not associated with abnormal plasma androgens. *Br J Dermatol*. 1989;120:649-654.
94. Chiu A, Chon SY, Kimball AB. The response of skin disease to stress: changes in the severity of acne vulgaris as affected by examination stress. *Arch Dermatol*. 2003;139:897-900.
95. Holland DB, Jeremy AH. The role of inflammation in the pathogenesis of acne and acne scarring. *Semin Cutan Med Surg*. 2005;24:79-83.
96. Holland DB, Jeremy AH, Roberts SG, et al. Inflammation in acne scarring: a comparison of the responses in lesions from patients prone and not prone to scar. *Br J Dermatol*. 2004;150:72-81.
97. Smith RN, Mann NJ, Braue A, et al. The effect of a high-protein, low glycemic-load diet versus a conventional, high glycemic-load diet on biochemical parameters associated with acne vulgaris: a randomized, investigator-masked, controlled trial. *J Am Acad Dermatol*. 2007;57:247-256.
98. Bowe WP, Joshi SS, Shalita AR. Diet and acne. *J Am Acad Dermatol*. 2010;63:124-141.
99. Berra B, Rizzo AM. Glycemic index, glycemic load: new evidence for a link with acne. *J Am Coll Nutr*. 2009;28(suppl):450S-454S.
100. Kaymak Y, Adisen E, Ilter N, et al. Dietary glycemic index and glucose, insulin, insulin-like growth factor-I, insulin-like growth factor binding protein 3, and leptin levels in patients with acne. *J Am Acad Dermatol*. 2007;57:819-823.
101. Reynolds RC, Lee S, Choi JY, et al. Effect of the glycemic index of carbohydrates on Acne vulgaris. *Nutrients*. 2010;2:1060-1070.
102. Hoyt G, Hickey MS, Cordain L. Dissociation of the glycaemic and insulinaemic responses to whole and skimmed milk. *Br J Nutr*. 2005;93:175-177.
103. Agamia NF, Abdallah DM, Sorour O, et al. Skin expression of mammalian target of rapamycin and forkhead box transcription factor O1, and serum insulin-like growth factor-1 in patients with acne vulgaris and their relationship with diet. *Br J Dermatol*. 2016;174:1299-1307.
104. Melnik BC, Zouboulis CC. Potential role of FoxO1 and mTORC1 in the pathogenesis of Western diet-induced acne. *Exp Dermatol*. 2013;22:311-315.
105. Lucky AW, Biro FM, Huster GA, et al. Acne vulgaris in premenarchal girls. An early sign of puberty associated with rising levels of dehydroepiandrosterone. *Arch Dermatol*. 1994;130:308-314.
106. Marynick SP, Chakmakjian ZH, McCaffree DL, et al. Androgen excess in cystic acne. *N Engl J Med*. 1983;308:981-986.
107. Goodman NF, Cobin RH, Futterweit W, et al. American Association of Clinical Endocrinologists, American College of Endocrinology, and Androgen Excess and PCOS Society disease state clinical review: guide to the best practices in the evaluation and treatment of polycystic ovary syndrome–part 1. *Endocr Pract*. 2015;21:1291-1300.
108. Stoll S, Shalita AR, Webster GF, et al. The effect of the menstrual cycle on acne. *J Am Acad Dermatol*. 2001;45:957-960.
109. Di Landro A, Cazzaniga S, Parazzini F, et al. Family history, body mass index, selected dietary factors, menstrual history, and risk of moderate to severe acne in adolescents and young adults. *J Am Acad Dermatol*. 2012;67:1129-1135.
110. Herane MI, Ando I. Acne in infancy and acne genetics. *Dermatology*. 2003;206:24-28.
111. Brecher AR, Orlow SJ. Oral retinoid therapy for dermatologic conditions in children and adolescents. *J Am Acad Dermatol*. 2003;49:171-182; quiz 183-176.
112. Fisher GJ, Voorhees JJ. Molecular mechanisms of retinoid actions in skin. *FASEB J*. 1996;10:1002-1013.
113. Shalita A, Weiss JS, Chalker DK, et al. A comparison of the efficacy and safety of adapalene gel 0.1% and tretinoin gel 0.025% in the treatment of acne vulgaris: a multicenter trial. *J Am Acad Dermatol*. 1996;34:482-485.
114. Cunliffe WJ, Caputo R, Dreno B, et al. Clinical efficacy and safety comparison of adapalene gel and tretinoin gel in the treatment of acne vulgaris: Europe and U.S. multicenter trials. *J Am Acad Dermatol*. 1997;36:S126-134.
115. Thiboutot D, Arsonnaud S, Soto P. Efficacy and tolerability of adapalene 0.3% gel compared to tazarotene 0.1% gel in the treatment of acne vulgaris. *J Drugs Dermatol*. 2008;7(6 suppl):S3-S10.
116. Tan JK. Adapalene 0.1% and benzoyl peroxide 2.5%: a novel combination for treatment of acne vulgaris. *Skin Therapy Lett*. 2009;14:4-5.
117. Thiboutot DM, Weiss J, Bucko A, et al. Adapalene-benzoyl peroxide, a fixed-dose combination for the treatment of acne vulgaris: results of a multicenter, randomized double-blind, controlled study. *J Am Acad Dermatol*. 2007;57:791-799.
118. Williams C, Layton AM. Persistent acne in women: implications for the patient and for therapy. *Am J Clin Dermatol*. 2006;7:281-290.
119. Webster GF, Berson D, Stein LF, et al. Efficacy and tolerability of once-daily tazarotene 0.1% gel versus once-daily tretinoin 0.025% gel in the treatment of facial acne vulgaris: a randomized trial. *Cutis*. 2001;67:4-9.
120. Leyden JJ, Tanghetti EA, Miller B, et al. Once-daily tazarotene 0.1 % gel versus once-daily tretinoin 0.1 % micro-

sponge gel for the treatment of facial acne vulgaris: a double-blind randomized trial. *Cutis*. 2002;69:12-19.
121. Hegemann L, Toso SM, Kitay K, et al. Anti-inflammatory actions of benzoyl peroxide: effects on the generation of reactive oxygen species by leucocytes and the activity of protein kinase C and calmodulin. *Br J Dermatol*. 1994;130:569-575.
122. Zaenglein AL, Pathy AL, Schlosser BJ, et al. Guidelines of care for the management of acne vulgaris. *J Am Acad Dermatol*. 2016;74:945-973 e933.
123. Eady EA, Bojar RA, Jones CE, et al. The effects of acne treatment with a combination of benzoyl peroxide and erythromycin on skin carriage of erythromycin-resistant propionibacteria. *Br J Dermatol*. 1996;134:107-113.
124. Raimer S, Maloney JM, Bourcier M, et al. Efficacy and safety of dapsone gel 5% for the treatment of acne vulgaris in adolescents. *Cutis*. 2008;81:171-178.
125. Lucky AW, Maloney JM, Roberts J, et al. Dapsone gel 5% for the treatment of acne vulgaris: safety and efficacy of long-term (1 year) treatment. *J Drugs Dermatol*. 2007;6:981-987.
126. Piette WW, Taylor S, Pariser D, et al. Hematologic safety of dapsone gel, 5%, for topical treatment of acne vulgaris. *Arch Dermatol*. 2008;144:1564-1570.
127. Dubina MI, Fleischer AB, Jr. Interaction of topical sulfacetamide and topical dapsone with benzoyl peroxide. *Arch Dermatol*. 2009;145:1027-1029.
128. Shemer A, Shiri J, Mashiah J, et al. Topical minocycline foam for moderate to severe acne vulgaris: phase 2 randomized double-blind, vehicle-controlled study results. *J Am Acad Dermatol*. 2016;74:1251-1252.
129. Gollnick H, Schramm M. Topical therapy in acne. *J Eur Acad Dermatol Venereol*. 1998;(11 suppl 1):S8-S12; discussion S28-S19.
130. Hjorth N, Graupe K. Azelaic acid for the treatment of acne. A clinical comparison with oral tetracycline. *Acta Derm Venereol Suppl (Stockh)*. 1989;143:45-48.
131. Kaminsky A. Less common methods to treat acne. *Dermatology*. 2003;206:68-73.
132. Gough A, Chapman S, Wagstaff K, et al. Minocycline induced autoimmune hepatitis and systemic lupus erythematosus-like syndrome. *BMJ*. 1996;312:169-172.
133. Goulden V, Glass D, Cunliffe WJ. Safety of long-term high-dose minocycline in the treatment of acne. *Br J Dermatol*. 1996;134:693-695.
134. Fernandez-Obregon AC. Azithromycin for the treatment of acne. *Int J Dermatol*. 2000;39:45-50.
135. Fenner JA, Wiss K, Levin NA. Oral cephalexin for acne vulgaris: clinical experience with 93 patients. *Pediatr Dermatol*. 2008;25:179-183.
136. Eady EA. Bacterial resistance in acne. *Dermatology*. 1998;196:59-66.
137. Gollnick H, Cunliffe W, Berson D, et al. Management of acne: a report from a Global Alliance to Improve Outcomes in Acne. *J Am Acad Dermatol*. 2003;49:S1-3.
138. Barbieri JS, Hoffstad O, Margolis DJ. Duration of oral tetracycline-class antibiotic therapy and use of topical retinoids for the treatment of acne among general practitioners (GP): a retrospective cohort study. *J Am Acad Dermatol*. 2016;75:1142-1150 e1141.
139. Speroff L, DeCherney A. Evaluation of a new generation of oral contraceptives. The Advisory Board for the New Progestins. *Obstet Gynecol*. 1993;81:1034-1047.
140. Lucky AW, Henderson TA, Olson WH, et al. Effectiveness of norgestimate and ethinyl estradiol in treating moderate acne vulgaris. *J Am Acad Dermatol*. 1997;37:746-754.
141. Maloney JM, Dietze P Jr, Watson D, et al. Treatment of acne using a 3-milligram drospirenone/20-microgram ethinyl estradiol oral contraceptive administered in a 24/4 regimen: a randomized controlled trial. *Obstet Gynecol*. 2008;112:773-781.
142. Thiboutot D, Archer DF, Lemay A, et al. A randomized, controlled trial of a low-dose contraceptive containing 20 microg of ethinyl estradiol and 100 microg of levonorgestrel for acne treatment. *Fertil Steril*. 2001;76:461-468.
143. Pochi PE, Strauss JS. Sebaceous gland inhibition from combined glucocorticoid-estrogen treatment. *Arch Dermatol*. 1976;112:1108-1109.
144. Faloia E, Filipponi S, Mancini V, et al. Treatment with a gonadotropin-releasing hormone agonist in acne or idiopathic hirsutism. *J Endocrinol Invest*. 1993;16:675-677.
145. Goodfellow A, Alaghband-Zadeh J, Carter G, et al. Oral spironolactone improves acne vulgaris and reduces sebum excretion. *Br J Dermatol*. 1984;111:209-214.
146. Krunic A, Ciurea A, Scheman A. Efficacy and tolerance of acne treatment using both spironolactone and a combined contraceptive containing drospirenone. *J Am Acad Dermatol*. 2008;58:60-62.
147. Plovanich M, Weng QY, Mostaghimi A. Low usefulness of potassium monitoring among healthy young women taking spironolactone for acne. *JAMA Dermatol*. 2015;151:941-944.
148. Kim GK, Del Rosso JQ. Oral spironolactone in post-teenage female patients with acne vulgaris: practical considerations for the clinician based on current data and clinical experience. *J Clin Aesthet Dermatol*. 2012;5:37-50.
149. Mackenzie IS, Morant SV, Wei L, et al. Spironolactone use and risk of incident cancers: a retrospective, matched cohort study. *Br J Clin Pharmacol*. 2017;83(3):653-663.
150. Cusan L, Dupont A, Belanger A, et al. Treatment of hirsutism with the pure antiandrogen flutamide. *J Am Acad Dermatol*. 1990;23:462-469.
151. Wysowski DK, Freiman JP, Tourtelot JB, Horton ML 3rd. Fatal and nonfatal hepatotoxicity associated with flutamide. *Ann Intern Med*. 1993;118:860-864.
152. Peck GL, Olsen TG, Yoder FW, et al. Prolonged remissions of cystic and conglobate acne with 13-cis-retinoic acid. *N Engl J Med*. 1979;300:329-333.
153. Pochi PE. The pathogenesis and treatment of acne. *Annu Rev Med*. 1990;41:187-198.
154. Strauss JS, Stranieri AM. Changes in long-term sebum production from isotretinoin therapy. *J Am Acad Dermatol*. 1982;6:751-756.
155. Leyden JJ, McGinley KJ. Effect of 13-cis-retinoic acid on sebum production and Propionibacterium acnes in severe nodulocystic acne. *Arch Dermatol Res*. 1982;272:331-337.
156. Weissmann A, Wagner A, Plewig G. Reduction of bacterial skin flora during oral treatment of severe acne with 13-cis retinoic acid. *Arch Dermatol Res*. 1981;270:179-183.
157. Windhorst DB, Nigra T. General clinical toxicology of oral retinoids. *J Am Acad Dermatol*. 1982;6:675-682.
158. Wysowski DK, Pitts M, Beitz J. An analysis of reports of depression and suicide in patients treated with isotretinoin. *J Am Acad Dermatol*. 2001;45:515-519.
159. Marqueling AL, Zane LT. Depression and suicidal behavior in acne patients treated with isotretinoin: a systematic review. *Semin Cutan Med Surg*. 2007;26:210-220.

160. Bigby M. Does isotretinoin increase the risk of depression? *Arch Dermatol*. 2008;144:1197-1199; discussion 1234-1195.
161. Kaymak Y, Taner E, Taner Y. Comparison of depression, anxiety and life quality in acne vulgaris patients who were treated with either isotretinoin or topical agents. *Int J Dermatol*. 2009;48:41-46.
162. Birmaher B, Ryan ND, Williamson DE, et al. Childhood and adolescent depression: a review of the past 10 years. Part II. *J Am Acad Child Adolesc Psychiatry*. 1996;35:1575-1583.
163. Crockett SD, Gulati A, Sandler RS, et al. A causal association between isotretinoin and inflammatory bowel disease has yet to be established. *Am J Gastroenterol*. 2009;104:2387-2393.
164. Bernstein CN, Nugent Z, Longobardi T, et al. Isotretinoin is not associated with inflammatory bowel disease: a population-based case-control study. *Am J Gastroenterol*. 2009;104:2774-2778.
165. DiGiovanna JJ, Langman CB, Tschen EH, et al. Effect of a single course of isotretinoin therapy on bone mineral density in adolescent patients with severe, recalcitrant, nodular acne. *J Am Acad Dermatol*. 2004;51:709-717.
166. Pittsley RA, Yoder FW. Retinoid hyperostosis. Skeletal toxicity associated with long-term administration of 13-cis-retinoic acid for refractory ichthyosis. *N Engl J Med*. 1983;308:1012-1014.
167. Hansen TJ, Lucking S, Miller JJ, et al. Standardized laboratory monitoring with use of isotretinoin in acne. *J Am Acad Dermatol*. 2016;75:323-328.
168. Stern RS, Rosa F, Baum C. Isotretinoin and pregnancy. *J Am Acad Dermatol*. 1984;10:851-854.
169. Fernhoff PM, Lammer EJ. Craniofacial features of isotretinoin embryopathy. *J Pediatr*. 1984;105:595-597.
170. Lehucher-Ceyrac D, Weber-Buisset MJ. Isotretinoin and acne in practice: a prospective analysis of 188 cases over 9 years. *Dermatology*. 1993;186:123-128.
171. Adebamowo CA, Spiegelman D, Danby FW, et al. High school dietary dairy intake and teenage acne. *J Am Acad Dermatol*. 2005;52:207-214.
172. Cordain L, Lindeberg S, Hurtado M, et al. Acne vulgaris: a disease of Western civilization. *Arch Dermatol*. 2002;138:1584-1590.
173. Spencer EH, Ferdowsian HR, Barnard ND. Diet and acne: a review of the evidence. *Int J Dermatol*. 2009;48:339-347.
174. Alam M, Omura N, Kaminer MS. Subcision for acne scarring: technique and outcomes in 40 patients. *Dermatol Surg*. 2005;31:310-317; discussion 317.
175. Kaminaka C, Uede M, Matsunaka H, et al. Clinical evaluation of glycolic acid chemical peeling in patients with acne vulgaris: a randomized, double-blind, placebo-controlled, split-face comparative study. *Dermatol Surg*. 2014;40:314-322.
176. Kim RH, Armstrong AW. Current state of acne treatment: highlighting lasers, photodynamic therapy, and chemical peels. *Dermatol Online J*. 2011;17:2.
177. Atzori L, Brundu MA, Orru A, et al. Glycolic acid peeling in the treatment of acne. *J Eur Acad Dermatol Venereol*. 1999;12:119-122.
178. Lee HS, Kim IH. Salicylic acid peels for the treatment of acne vulgaris in Asian patients. *Dermatol Surg*. 2003;29:1196-1199; discussion 1199.
179. Mills OH, Kligman AM. Ultraviolet phototherapy and photochemotherapy of acne vulgaris. *Arch Dermatol*. 1978;114:221-223.
180. Momen S, Al-Niaimi F. Acne vulgaris and light-based therapies. *J Cosmet Laser Ther*. 2015;17:122-128.
181. Sigurdsson V, Knulst AC, van Weelden H. Phototherapy of acne vulgaris with visible light. *Dermatology*. 1997;194:256-260.
182. Kjeldstad B, Johnsson A. An action spectrum for blue and near ultraviolet inactivation of Propionibacterium acnes; with emphasis on a possible porphyrin photosensitization. *Photochem Photobiol*. 1986;43:67-70.
183. Suh DH, Kwon TE, Youn JI. Changes of comedonal cytokines and sebum secretion after UV irradiation in acne patients. *Eur J Dermatol*. 2002;12:139-144.
184. Lassus A, Salo O, Forstrom L, et al. [Treatment of acne with selective UV-phototherapy (SUP). An open trial]. *Dermatol Monatsschr*. 1983;169:376-379.
185. Meffert H, Kolzsch J, Laubstein B, et al. [Phototherapy of acne vulgaris with the "TuR" UV 10 body section irradiation unit]. *Dermatol Monatsschr*. 1986;172:9-13.
186. Meffert H, Laubstein B, Kolzsch J, Sonnichsen N. [Phototherapy of acne vulgaris with the UVA irradiation instrument TBG 400]. *Dermatol Monatsschr*. 1986;172:105-106.
187. van Weelden H, de Gruijl FR, van der Putte SC, et al. carcinogenic risks of modern tanning equipment: is UV-A safer than UV-B? *Arch Dermatol Res*. 1988;280:300-307.
188. Lee WL, Shalita AR, Poh-Fitzpatrick MB. Comparative studies of porphyrin production in Propionibacterium acnes and Propionibacterium granulosum. *J Bacteriol*. 1978;133:811-815.
189. Arakane K, Ryu A, Hayashi C, et al. Singlet oxygen (1 delta g) generation from coproporphyrin in Propionibacterium acnes on irradiation. *Biochem Biophys Res Commun*. 1996;223:578-582.
190. Oberemok SS, Shalita AR. Acne vulgaris, II: treatment. *Cutis*. 2002;70:111-114.
191. Haedersdal M, Togsverd-Bo K, Wulf HC. Evidence-based review of lasers, light sources and photodynamic therapy in the treatment of acne vulgaris. *J Eur Acad Dermatol Venereol*. 2008;22:267-278.
192. Melo TB. Uptake of protoporphyrin and violet light photodestruction of Propionibacterium acnes. *Z Naturforsch C*. 1987;42:123-128.
193. Charakida A, Seaton ED, Charakida M, et al. Phototherapy in the treatment of acne vulgaris: what is its role? *Am J Clin Dermatol*. 2004;5:211-216.
194. Ibbotson SH. Topical 5-aminolaevulinic acid photodynamic therapy for the treatment of skin conditions other than non-melanoma skin cancer. *Br J Dermatol*. 2002;146:178-188.
195. Hongcharu W, Taylor CR, Chang Y, et al. Topical ALA-photodynamic therapy for the treatment of acne vulgaris. *J Invest Dermatol*. 2000;115:183-192.
196. Sadick N. An open-label, split-face study comparing the safety and efficacy of levulan kerastick (aminolevulonic acid) plus a 532 nm KTP laser to a 532 nm KTP laser alone for the treatment of moderate facial acne. *J Drugs Dermatol*. 2010;9:229-233.
197. Seaton ED, Charakida A, Mouser PE, et al. Pulsed-dye laser treatment for inflammatory acne vulgaris: randomised controlled trial. *Lancet*. 2003;362:1347-1352.
198. Paithankar DY, Ross EV, Saleh BA, et al. Acne treatment with a 1,450 nm wavelength laser and cryogen spray cooling. *Lasers Surg Med*. 2002;31:106-114.

199. Friedman PM, Jih MH, Kimyai-Asadi A, et al. Treatment of inflammatory facial acne vulgaris with the 1450-nm diode laser: a pilot study. *Dermatol Surg*. 2004;30:147-151.
200. Lloyd JR, Mirkov M. Selective photothermolysis of the sebaceous glands for acne treatment. *Lasers Surg Med*. 2002;31:115-120.
201. Angel S, Boineau D, Dahan S, et al. Treatment of active acne with an Er:Glass (1.54 microm) laser: a 2-year follow-up study. *J Cosmet Laser Ther*. 2006;8:171-177.
202. Wanitphakdeedecha R, Tanzi EL, Alster TS. Photopneumatic therapy for the treatment of acne. *J Drugs Dermatol*. 2009;8:239-241.
203. Gold MH, Biron J. Efficacy of a novel combination of pneumatic energy and broadband light for the treatment of acne. *J Drugs Dermatol*. 2008;7:639-642.
204. Cohen BE, Brauer JA, Geronemus RG. Acne scarring: a review of available therapeutic lasers. *Lasers Surg Med*. 2016;48:95-115.
205. Chrastil B, Glaich AS, Goldberg LH, et al. Second-generation 1,550-nm fractional photothermolysis for the treatment of acne scars. *Dermatol Surg*. 2008;34:1327-1332.
206. Alster TS, Tanzi EL, Lazarus M. The use of fractional laser photothermolysis for the treatment of atrophic scars. *Dermatol Surg*. 2007;33:295-299.
207. Tanzi EL, Wanitphakdeedecha R, Alster TS. Fraxel laser indications and long-term follow-up. *Aesthet Surg J*. 2008;28:675-678; discussion 679-680.
208. Omi T, Numano K. The role of the CO2 laser and fractional CO2 laser in dermatology. *Laser Ther*. 2014;23:49-60.
209. Levy LL, Zeichner JA. Management of acne scarring, part II: a comparative review of non-laser-based, minimally invasive approaches. *Am J Clin Dermatol*. 2012;13:331-340.
210. Tsao SS, Dover JS, Arndt KA, et al. Scar management: keloid, hypertrophic, atrophic, and acne scars. *Semin Cutan Med Surg*. 2002;21:46-75.
211. Spencer JM. Microdermabrasion. *Am J Clin Dermatol*. 2005;6:89-92.
212. Kim ST, Lee KH, Sim HJ, et al. Treatment of acne vulgaris with fractional radiofrequency microneedling. *J Dermatol*. 2014;41:586-591.
213. Lee SJ, Goo JW, Shin J, et al. Use of fractionated microneedle radiofrequency for the treatment of inflammatory acne vulgaris in 18 Korean patients. *Dermatol Surg*. 2012;38:400-405.
214. Hou A, Cohen B, Haimovic A, et al. Microneedling: a comprehensive review. *Dermatol Surg*. 2017;43(3):321-339.
215. Liebl H, Kloth LC. Skin cell proliferation stimulated by microneedles. *J Am Coll Clin Wound Spec*. 2012;4(1):2-6.
216. Cohen BE, Elbuluk N. Microneedling in skin of color: a review of uses and efficacy. *J Am Acad Dermatol*. 2016;74:348-355.
217. Asif M, Kanodia S, Singh K. Combined autologous platelet-rich plasma with microneedling verses microneedling with distilled water in the treatment of atrophic acne scars: a concurrent split-face study. *J Cosmet Dermatol*. 2016;15(4):434-443.
218. Sharad J. Combination of microneedling and glycolic acid peels for the treatment of acne scars in dark skin. *J Cosmet Dermatol*. 2011;10:317-323.
219. Hirsch RJ, Lewis AB. Treatment of acne scarring. *Semin Cutan Med Surg*. 2001;20:190-198.
220. Hirsch RJ, Cohen JL. Soft tissue augmentation. *Cutis*. 2006;78:165-172.
221. Murase JE, Heller MM, Butler DC. Safety of dermatologic medications in pregnancy and lactation: part I. Pregnancy. *J Am Acad Dermatol*. 2014;70:401 e401-414; quiz 415.
222. Kong YL, Tey HL. Treatment of acne vulgaris during pregnancy and lactation. *Drugs*. 2013;73:779-787.

Chapter 79 :: Rosacea
:: Martin Steinhoff & Jörg Buddenkotte

第七十九章
玫瑰痤疮

中文导读

玫瑰痤疮是一种好发于面中部皮肤的慢性炎症性皮肤病，本章从流行病学及疾病负担、临床表现、病因学和病理生理学、诊断、鉴别诊断和治疗六个方面全面讲述了玫瑰痤疮。

流行病学及疾病负担方面介绍了玫瑰痤疮在不同国家的患病率、患病人群的性别比例及典型玫瑰痤疮的发病年龄；由于该病好发于面部，严重损害了患者的心理健康和社交行为，但玫瑰痤疮的疾病负担并不仅仅是心理的，因为伴随着潮红和红斑，患者可能有严重的刺痛和灼热感。

临床表现方面讲述了玫瑰痤疮皮损在面部的分布特征，指出虽然不同患者其临床表现不同，但潮红（flushing）、暂时性红斑、持续性红斑、毛细血管扩张、丘疹、脓疱、赘生物、水肿、疼痛、刺痛和灼热感以及瘙痒是所有可能的症状和体征，同时分别就玫瑰痤疮持续性红斑、赘生物、潮红和暂时性红斑、毛细血管扩张、丘疹和脓疱及眼玫瑰痤疮的表现和特征进行了详细的描述，特别提出"blushing"与"flushing"的区别；并讨论了玫瑰痤疮的一些少见的亚型，包括类狼疮/肉芽肿型玫瑰痤疮、聚合性玫瑰痤疮、爆发性玫瑰痤疮、卤素性玫瑰痤疮、类固醇性玫瑰痤疮、革兰氏阴性菌性玫瑰痤疮、玫瑰痤疮持续性水肿等。

病因学和病理生理学方面指出玫瑰痤疮的发病机制不明，基因和环境因素均参与了发病；总结了与玫瑰痤疮发病相关的基因、合并症、环境触发因子（表79-1）等研究进展；从皮肤屏障的功能异常、Toll样受体、蛋白酶、抗菌肽、炎症小体和不平衡的适应性免疫讲述了玫瑰痤疮发病中的免疫反应，总结于图79-9；阐述了神经血管失调和神经炎症在玫瑰痤疮中的研究（图79-10），认为自主神经功能失调在潮红的发生中起了重要作用，并做了玫瑰痤疮潮红产生的可能机制的示意图（图79-11）；最后总结了赘生物改变、纤维化和皮脂腺增生（图79-12）以及毛细血管扩张的可能机制，并提出了幽门螺杆菌及SIBO综合征与玫瑰痤疮发病的关系。

玫瑰痤疮的诊断方面介绍了玫瑰痤疮不同表型皮损以及不同亚型玫瑰痤疮的组织病理改变并介绍了2002版和2017版的玫瑰痤疮分类系统（表79-2，79-3），同时描述了一些针对玫瑰痤疮主要特征的诊断工具（表79-4）和严重程度的分级，部分特征的分级标准列于表79-5和表79-6。

鉴别诊断方面介绍了玫瑰痤疮需要与脂溢性皮炎、寻常痤疮、慢性盘状红斑狼疮、多形性日光疹等疾病进行鉴别，鉴别要点列于表79-7；同时将各种表型，如鼻赘、持续性红斑、潮红、毛细血管扩张、丘疹脓疱的鉴别要点列于表79-8 — 表79-13；将各种少见玫瑰痤疮亚型的鉴别诊断要点列于表79-14 — 表79-16。

玫瑰痤疮的治疗方面，从一般的皮肤护理（表79-17）、一线、二线和超说明治疗等方面介绍了玫瑰痤疮治疗的基本原则，指出由于每种疾病特征的病理生理机制和严重程度不同，所用的一线治疗可能会不一样（图79-13，79-14），接着详细介绍了不同疾病特征的治疗方案，最后提出了维持治疗的重要性和物理/手术治疗在玫瑰痤疮中的运用（表79-18）。

〔李 吉〕

AT-A-GLANCE

- Rosacea is a common facial skin disease in many countries.
- Signs and symptoms for rosacea include flushing, transient erythema, persistent erythema, telangiectasia, papules, pustules, phymata, edema, pain, stinging or burning, and (very rarely) pruritus.
- The pathophysiology of rosacea is poorly understood; however, a genetic predisposition along with trigger factors activate a dysregulated neurovascular, innate immune, and adaptive immune system.
- Taking a thorough family and patient history and performing a clinical examination are crucial to diagnose rosacea.
- All clinical features have to be considered with severity scores for a proper treatment, combined with assessing patient's quality of life.
- Approved topical or systemic drugs exist for various, but not all, features of rosacea and should be used on the basis of pathophysiology and while considering efficacy and side effect profiles.
- Knowledge about the beneficial use of physical therapies and their limitations is important for best medical practice in patients with rosacea.
- Education about disease progress, general skin care, cosmetic usage and medication effects and potential adverse events is mandatory; teaching of proper topical use guarantees better treatment results.
- Education to prevent exacerbating "trigger factors" is critical for successful management of patients with rosacea.

INTRODUCTION

Rosacea is a common chronic inflammatory skin disease that almost exclusively affects the central facial skin and rarely affects the extrafacial (neck, forehead) skin. *Rosacea* derives from the Greek word meaning "rose-like," which describes the main symptomatology of repeated flushing alone or in combination with transient or persistent erythema. Clinically, the condition is characterized by prolonged flushing (transient erythema), persistent erythema, telangiectasia, papules, pustules, and phymatous changes, often accompanied by burning, stinging, or even migraine-like pain (cutaneous rosacea). Eyes can be also involved (ocular rosacea). Because of their different pathophysiologies, the terms *acne rosacea* and *adult acne* are no longer used to describe this disorder.[1,2]

Worldwide, more than 20 million patients are estimated to have rosacea, although reliable statistics are lacking.[3] Because of its obvious facial location, rosacea is associated with a significant disease burden and impaired quality of life.[4] The etiology and pathophysiology of rosacea are poorly understood, so the therapy of rosacea is still unsatisfactory; currently used treatment modalities mainly aim to control the clinical signs and symptoms rather than target causes or prevent disease.[5-9]

EPIDEMIOLOGY AND DISEASE BURDEN

In many countries, rosacea is more prevalent than asthma or diabetes. Depending on the country, rosacea affects at least 2% to 18% of individuals, with the highest level reported in Celtic populations. A Swedish study described a prevalence of 10% for rosacea,[10] and a German study found 12.3% of the population to be affected.[11] In 2010, an epidemiologic study from Ireland reported a prevalence of 13.9% for rosacea.[12] The prevalence of rosacea probably depends on the genetic make-up of the population being studied. The condition affects women more often than men (3:1) and typically starts a decade earlier in women than in men; the normal age of onset is generally considered to be 35 to 45 years in women and 45 to 55 years in men, although recent studies suggest an earlier clinical onset with flushing, which is often not recognized as an early sign of rosacea.[1,13,14] Research indicates that the first, often unrecognized, signs can occur in the second decade of a patient's life, more often in women than in men.

Rosacea is often misinterpreted as a disease of alcohol overconsumption or "lying," which can stigmatize patients. The facial distribution of the disease is generally recognized to have a significant negative psychological impact on patients, although the statistical evidence for this effect is poor. Patients report significantly impaired self-esteem and may become unemployed, stop socializing, get divorced, or develop depression.[15] However, not all of the disease burden is psychological because patients may also have potentially severe stinging or burning associated with the flushing or erythema.[3,16]

CLINICAL FINDINGS

Rosacea is, in most cases, a symmetric skin disease affecting the central face, nose, chin, central cheeks, and glabella; the forehead (more common in bald men), neck, and chest are only rarely affected. The perioral or periorbital regions, or areas behind the ears, are rarely affected. The clinical findings can vary substantially among rosacea-affected patients. In general, all possible signs or symptoms are flushing, transient erythema, persistent erythema, telangiectasia, papules, pustules, phymata, edema, pain, stinging or burning, and (very rarely) pruritus.[16-18] Although flushing is the hallmark of rosacea, some patients develop rosacea without much flushing. Classically, most patients describe the disease development as a "crescendo" manifestation with increased numbers of "flushes" after exposure to trigger factors. Sooner or later, most patients develop persistent erythema with or without telangiectasia. Notably, comedones are absent, which differentiates papulopustular rosacea from acne or Favre-Racouchot disease.

The clinical findings are gender and age dependent: in younger female and male patients, flushing and erythema are often the first symptoms; in older adult patients, telangiectasia can be a first sign. Rhinophyma is a characteristic of male patients. The clinical picture is also dependent on the special susceptibility of the patient toward trigger factors; for example, a patient who has high susceptibility to ultraviolet (UV) radiation as a trigger factor may have an asymmetric facial erythema caused by window exposure (eg, driver vs. co-driver). The progression of rosacea is relatively slow, evident only after thorough history taking.

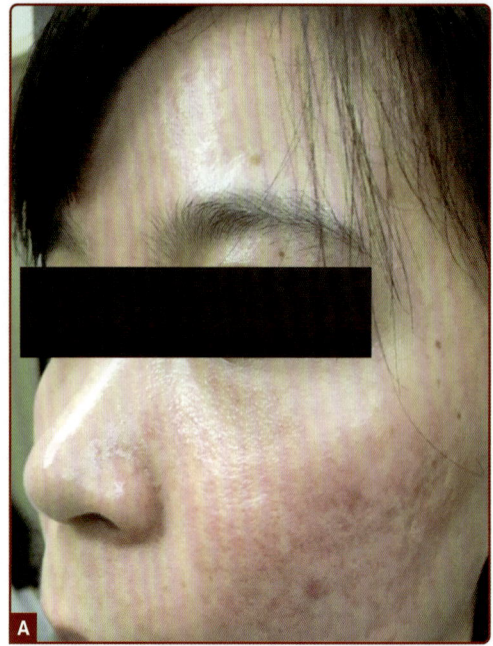

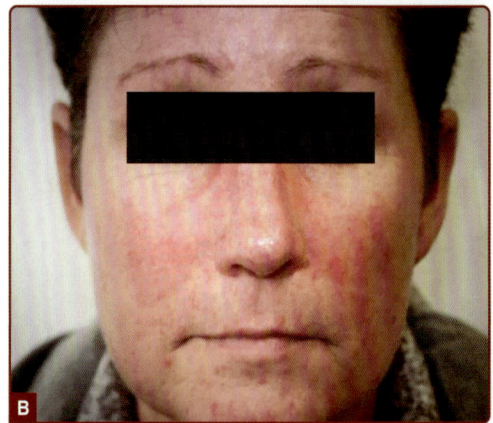

Figure 79-1 **A,** Persistent erythema in patients with rosacea. **B,** Although mostly symmetrical, persistent erythema can present with asymmetrical distribution and intensity based on underlying trigger factor. (Image A, used with permission from Professors H. Xie and J. Li, University Hospital Changsha, China.)

PERSISTENT ERYTHEMA

Persistent erythema (from Greek *erythros*, red) is defined as erythema that lasts for at least 3 months. It constitutes an abnormal redness of the skin or mucous membranes caused by vasodilation of arterioles or capillaries, resulting in increased perfusion and thus redness. Persistent (perilesional) erythema can be found around papules and pustules. Clinically, patients with persistent erythema present with a striking clinical appearance: there is profound central facial erythema predominant on the projecting facial anatomical features (Fig. 79-1). The erythema depth ranges from pink-red to deep burgundy red.

PHYMATA

Phymata (*phyma*, Greek meaning swelling, mass) represents a macroscopic lesion that is uniquely associated with rosacea. Phymatous rosacea is a persistent, firm, nonpainful, nonpitting swelling of the tissue of the nose (rhinophyma), chin (gnathophyma), forehead (metophyma), or eyelids (blepharophyma) that seldom begins before the age of 40 years. Phymatous changes, fortunately, are a rare malady in patients with rosacea, but affected patients are often involuntarily subjected to speculations about insalubrious alcohol consumption. Correspondingly, "brandy nose" has been used as a misleading label to describe rhinophyma. Typically, phymata do not resolve spontaneously.

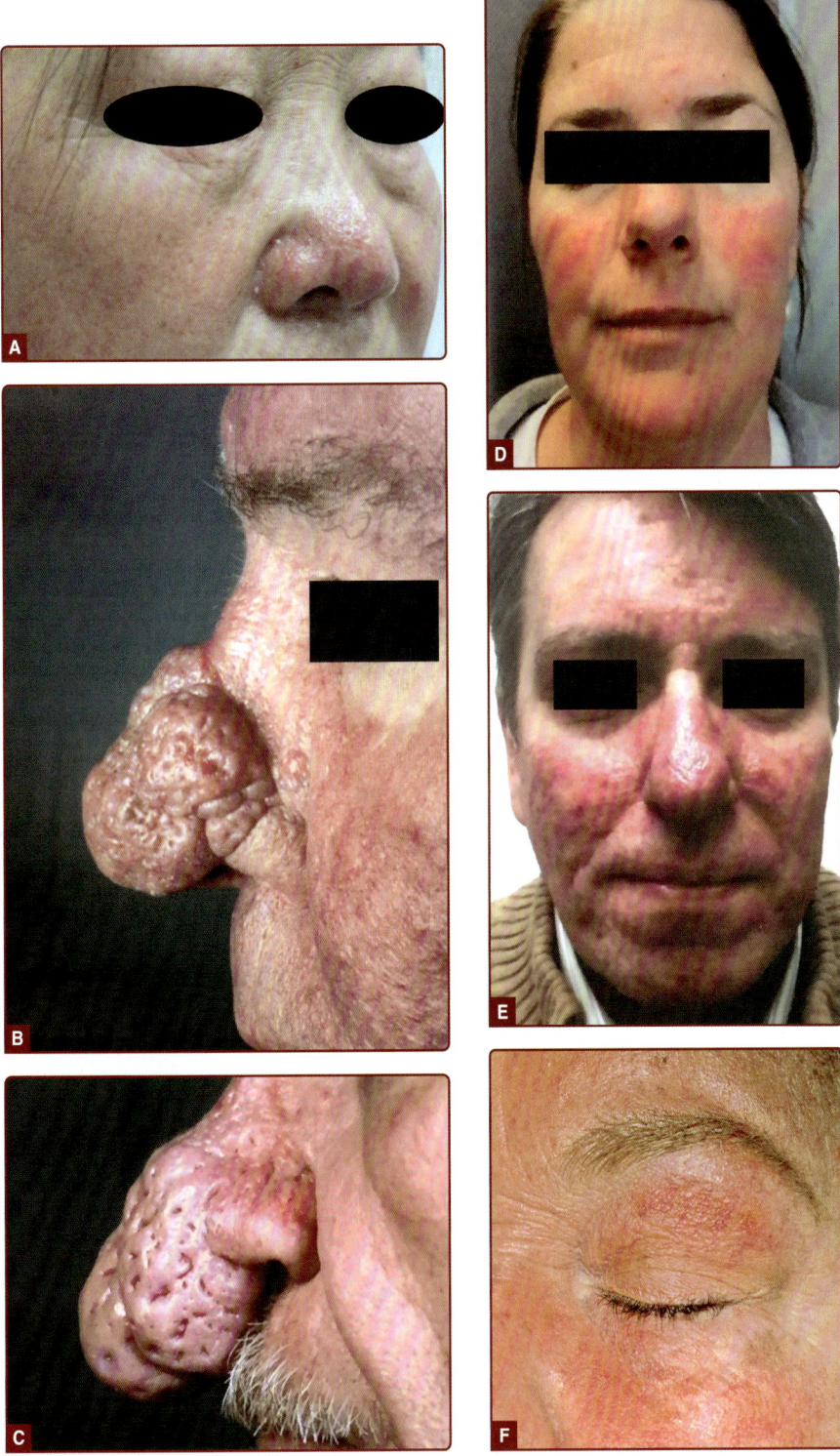

Figure 79-2 Phymata in patients with rosacea. **A,** In the initial stages, rhinophyma is often apparent only at the distal end of the nose as dilated patulous follicles or plaque. **B,** Marked rhinophyma. **C,** Asymmetric fibrous form of rhinophyma with asymmetrical clinical appearance. **D,** Mild gnathophyma. **E,** Metrophyma in combination with granulomatous plaques on the cheeks. **F,** Blepharophyma. (Image **A,** used with permission from Professors H. Xie and J. Li, University Hospital Changsha, China. Image **F,** used with permission from James E. Fitzpatrick.)

Rhinophyma, which occurs almost 20 times more often in male patients than in female patients, is often apparent initially in the skin of the alae nasi and at the distal end of the nose as dilated patulous follicles (Fig. 79-2A). Humps and grooves are prominent, resembling a "peau d'orange" appearance of the nose. Compression produces a white pasty matter that is composed of sebum, corneocytes, bacteria, and sometimes Demodex folliculorum mites. When rhinophyma becomes marked (Fig. 79-2B), it leads to the greatest deformity in this region and sometimes affects more proximal areas of the nose, as far as adjacent portions of the cheeks. Rhinophyma of the fibrous form (Fig. 79-2C) manifests with asymmetry of the nasal swelling caused by diffuse hyperplasia of connective tissue and sebaceous hyperplasia. Large actinic comedones can be prominent (sometimes called "potato nose"). In the fibroangiomatous form, the nose then appears copper to dark red, is grossly enlarged, and presents a network of ectatic veins and sometimes pustules. Although gross nasal distortion rarely occurs, the cosmetic impact is very significant in disease management. The incidence of both basal and squamous cell carcinomas has been reported to be higher in rhinophyma-affected skin than in nonlesional skin. However, this observation has not been unambiguously confirmed. There is no consistent relationship between the duration, severity, or any other feature of rosacea and the occurrence of rhinophyma; therefore, rhinophyma should be designated a condition of the skin that is closely associated with rosacea rather than a disorder that occurs as a consequence of the disease.

Gnathophyma (Fig. 79-2D) is a rare occurrence, with the central chin typically being involved, while the lower half of the helices of the ears and the lobes are mainly affected in otophyma. Edema in this region may be present in severe inflammatory papulopustular rosacea. Other locations of phymata can involve the forehead (metrophyma; Fig. 79-2E) and eyelids (blepharophyma; Fig. 79-2F).

The clinical picture of persistent edema and phymatous changes may overlap in some patients. Swelling is often associated with erythema and sometimes with other manifestations of rosacea (papules, pustules, telangiectasias) and occasionally ocular inflammation. Rhinophymata are particularly frequent when associated with seborrhea. Contrarily, seborrhea is not particularly associated with rhinophymata and often occurs in rosacea devoid of phyma.

FLUSHING AND TRANSIENT ERYTHEMA

Flushing involves reactive vascular changes in the face that can be observed in normal individuals for a few seconds or few minutes. Physiologically, it can occur in response to various stimuli, especially heat, certain foods, alcohol, exercising, or stressful emotional stimuli. By contrast, moderate cooling alleviates the redness and has a transient therapeutic effect. Prolonged or more frequent than normal nonphysiological flushing manifests itself over hours to days and can develop into persistent erythema.

Flushing in rosacea is a pathophysiological neurovascular process in the central face experienced for more than 5 to 10 minutes because of neuropeptide release. Because of its sudden noncontrollable appearance, it is embarrassing and very unpleasant for patients and is often associated with sensory symptoms such as stinging, burning pain. Flushing can be associated with persistent erythema, papules, pustules, or phymata or can occur as a single symptom. Both genders are equally susceptible to flushing without age preference, although in women, it is more frequent during menopause. Prolonged and frequent flushing is, with erythema, the most common complaint in patients with rosacea.

Rosacea flushing can often be linked to typical trigger factors, mostly heat, hot steam (kitchen, beverages), red wine and certain other alcoholic beverages, medications such as niacin or topical glucocorticosteroids, noxious cold, and hormonal changes (menopause), rarely systematic disease. It may be accompanied with systemic symptoms such as wheezing, diarrhea, or headache and may be associated with sweating, indicating a role of nerves and mast cells in flushing pathophysiology. In particular, the release of gastrin hormonal mediators from the gastrointestinal (GI) tract have a systematic effect leading to frequent facial flushing and then persistent vasodilatation and telangiectasias on the face.

Transient erythema is a prolonged unphysiological flushing that persists for more than 5 minutes and possibly as long as weeks or a few months but for no more than 3 months.

BLUSHING

Blushing is not a characteristic feature of rosacea. We are briefly mentioning it in this chapter because although different in many aspects, the terms "flushing," "transient erythema," "persistent erythema," and "blushing" are often inappropriately used to describe redness of the facial skin, which leads to confusion. Blushing, in contrast to flushing, is almost exclusively induced by emotionally stressful situations and not by spicy food or other rosacea trigger factors. Blushing has a more pinkish appearance than persistent erythema or flushing and is located on rosacea-atypical sites. It is characterized by sudden transient (mostly <5 minutes), pinkish involuntary redness of the peripheral cheeks, ears, retroauricular areas, neck, and chest, which can occur over years and often starts in early adulthood. "Pale islands" in between the salmon-like redness are also characteristic of blushing and cannot be found in flushing or transient or persistent erythema, indicating that a more autonomic neural process, often associated with enhanced sweating, also a sign of autonomic neural

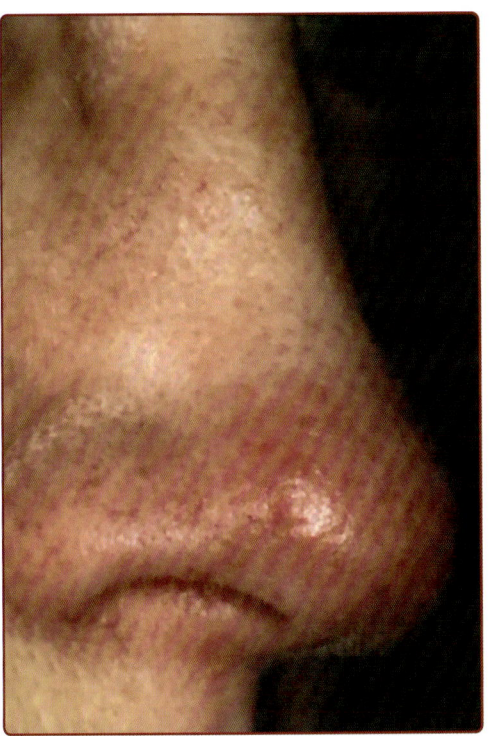

Figure 79-3 Telangiectasia in a patient with rosacea.

involvement. As with flushing, blushing can be also associated with skin sensations such as stinging or burning, as well as increased sweating but often milder than in flushing.

TELANGIECTASIA

Telangiectasia can be defined as a permanent visible dilated blood vessel on the skin or mucosal surface. Multiple telangiectatic blood vessels build the clinical picture of telangiectasia (Fig. 79-3), which can develop in the absence of any disease (genetically acquired, so-called primary or "essential" telangiectasia) or coexist or even precede skin (eg, rosacea) or systemic (eg, scleroderma) diseases, defined as secondary telangiectasia. In the new classification,[16,19] telangiectasia are classified as a primary feature of rosacea, which can coexist with or without any other rosacea features. They can occur very sparsely or densely and be widely distributed in patients with rosacea.

PAPULES AND PUSTULES

Papules (Fig. 79-4A and B) can occur with or without pustules and can develop into cysts and nodules (rosacea conglobate), depending on the cytokines and chemokines released.[20] Papules and pustules caused by rosacea can be easily recognized in most cases because

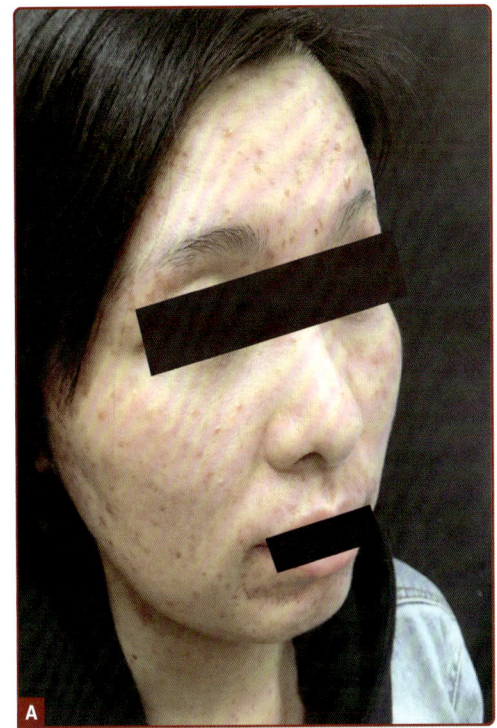

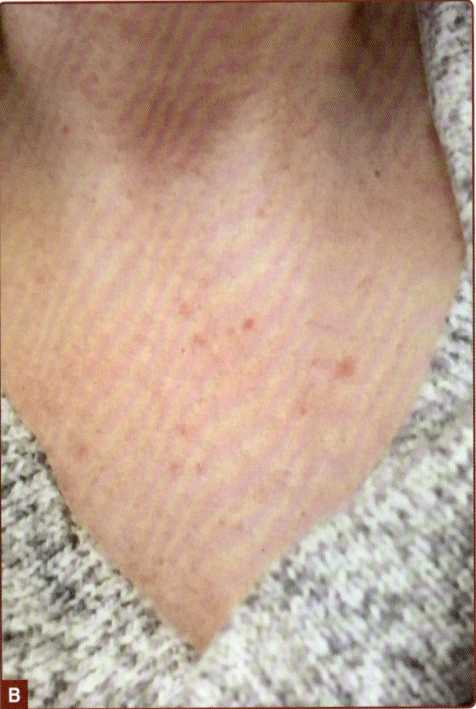

Figure 79-4 Individual with rosacea with mild chronic facial erythema and disseminated facial papules and pustules (**A**). Papules and pustules can develop extrafacially, mostly on the neck, trunk, or bald scalp, indicating ultraviolet light as a trigger factor on bald scalp rosacea (**B**). (Image **A**, used with permission from Professors H. Xie and J. Li, University Hospital Changsha, China.)

of their mostly centrofacial distribution and the lack of comedones and scales, although multiple differential diagnoses of course need to be considered (see Differential Diagnosis). The papules in rosacea are mostly small, low pain, dome shaped, and red in color and usually present as multiples. They can also develop into edematous plaques, resembling lupus erythematosus. The lesions tend to occur symmetrically on the centrofacial skin but can extend to the neck, chest (Fig. 79-4B), and forehead, even in children. Forehead rosacea almost exclusively develops in patients with male pattern baldness, supporting the concept that UV radiation is a trigger factor for rosacea.

Papules and pustules can, rarely, resolve spontaneously after 4 to 8 weeks, notably without scarring. The condition waxes and wanes because of trigger factors, emphasizing the value of maintenance therapy and tapering strategy.

Papules and pustules are often associated with erythema or flushing, which mostly remains after antibiotic therapy (see combination therapy). Telangiectasias, phymatous changes, and ocular rosacea can also accompany papules and pustules.

OCULAR ROSACEA

Ocular rosacea is a frequent, bothersome, and often underestimated feature of rosacea. It involves the eyelids, eyelashes, or eyes of patients with rosacea and, if left untreated, bears risk of blindness. Ocular rosacea occurs in 25% of all patients with rosacea and in as many as 50% of patients with papules and pustules.[21] Rosacea may affect many compartments of the eyes (Fig. 79-5), such as margins of the eyelids, glands of Zeiss, meibomian glands, lacrimal glands, conjunctiva, cornea, sclera, and iris.[9,16,22,23] Typically, patients report a "foreign body" sensation of itching, burning, and stinging in the eyes and grittiness around the eyes. Inspection of the eyes is important; they often have red, swollen, crusty, or scaly margins. Telangiectasia of the conjunctiva may also occur.

RARE SUBFORMS OF ROSACEA

LUPOID OR GRANULOMATOUS ROSACEA

Lupoid rosacea is a distinct subform of rosacea defined by chronic, therapy-resistant, 0.2- to 0.3-cm-sized, often follicular brown-red or red papules that can develop to epithelioid (lupoid), granulomatous plaques and nodules on the cheek, forehead, or chin. The skin appears thickened and erythematous. Typically, the centrofacial and perioral regions of the face are affected. The upper and lower eyelids are involved in some cases. Diascopy reveals a follicle-associated lupoid infiltrate. Rare cases of lupoid rosacea have been observed after treatment with infliximab or etanercept. Whether lupoid rosacea and lupus miliaris disseminates faciei depict distinct disease entities is not yet clarified.

ROSACEA CONGLOBATE

Rosacea conglobate (Fig. 79-6) is a rare, chronic, and severe form of rosacea that resembles acne conglobate with hemorrhagic nodular abscesses and indurated plaques on erythematous background.

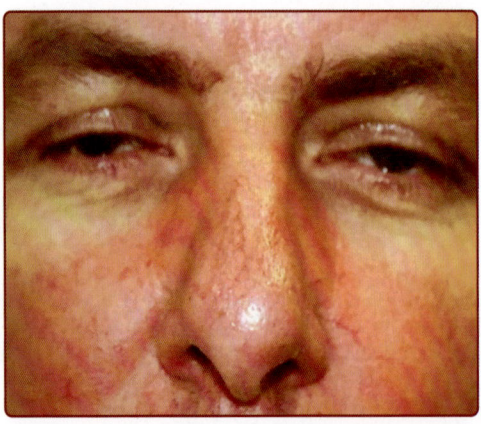

Figure 79-5 Ocular rosacea may affect many compartments of the eyes. Ophthalmology referral is advised, and systemic therapy is recommended in most cases.

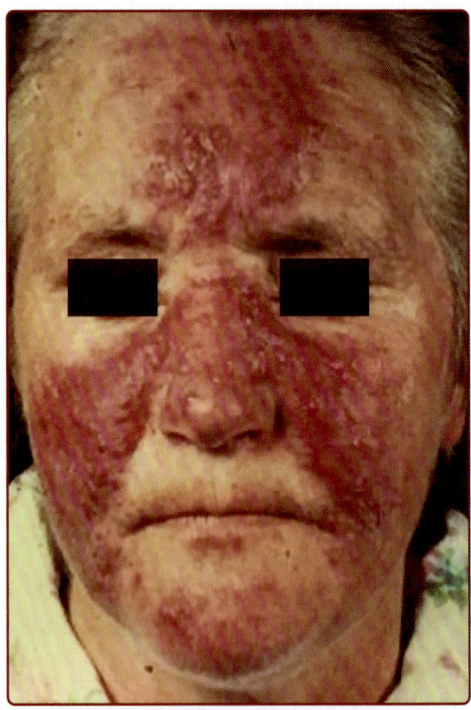

Figure 79-6 Conglobate form of rosacea, which can clinically resemble conglobate form of acne but occurs predominantly in older age groups more often than acne.

ROSACEA FULMINANS (PYODERMA FACIALE-O'LEARY)

Rosacea fulminans is a rare, acute or subacute, developing, maximal variant of rosacea with acne conglobate–like progression and predilection for postadolescent (20–30 years) women, particularly pregnant women; men are affected only rarely. Associations with seborrhoic dermatitis, a common inflammatory skin condition, and Crohn disease, a chronic inflammatory bowel disease, have been described without disclosing a mechanistic connection to rosacea fulminans. The clinical findings develop within days to weeks and can affect the complete face—particularly the chin, cheeks, forehead, and nose—or remain localized, especially when present on the neck or trunk. The lesions present papulopustules and coalescent purplish nodules as well as associated abscesses, which often form confluent fistulae that drain a serous, seropurulent, or mucoid discharge. Reddish to violaceous firm swelling of the face is commonly noted. Patients often report an oiliness of the skin before the outbreak of rosacea fulminans. Despite the horrendous clinical picture, systemic symptoms such as fatigue, fever, arthralgia, and anaemia are usually absent. When the disease is controlled, it does not recur.

HALOGEN ROSACEA

Ingestion of iodides or bromides might cause a rosacea-like reaction or deteriorate a persisting rosacea. The clinical findings resemble acne-like rashes or those described for rosacea conglobate. Patients can develop erythematous pustules, vegetative nodules, in extreme cases fungating nodules, small to large blisters, exudative plaques, ulcer (sometimes necrotic), a circumscribed panniculitis, or combinations of these presentations. Potential sources of halogen exposure are citrus-flavored soft drinks (cola drinks), (sea)food, diagnostic radiocontrast media, pool disinfectants, certain topical antiseptics, permanent hair wave formulations, and various products often not considered as potential sources, such as vitamin preparations and medications (eg, thyroid medication, chemotherapeutics). The amount of halogen required to cause a halogen rosacea is variable. The condition typically improves in 4 to 6 weeks after elimination of the exposure. Scarring and postinflammatory pigmentation might occur as residuals.

STEROID ROSACEA

When a patient with rosacea is treated with topical corticosteroids for a prolonged time, the atrophic side effects of the medication sometimes lead to an aggravation of the condition. The complexion changes to a deep flaming red or copper-red covered by a network of telangiectases (Fig. 79-7). The atrophic skin develops patches of scales, follicular papulopustules, nodules, and secondary comedones. The presentation is typically restricted to the area of corticosteroid application. Patients report a severe discomfort and nagging pain sensation.

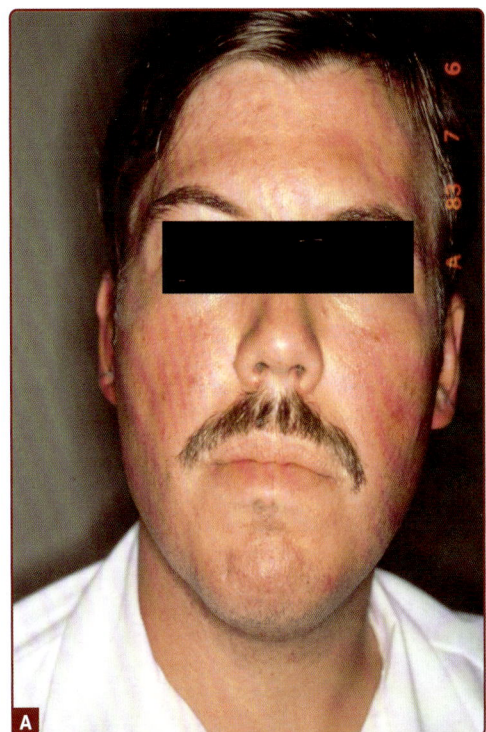

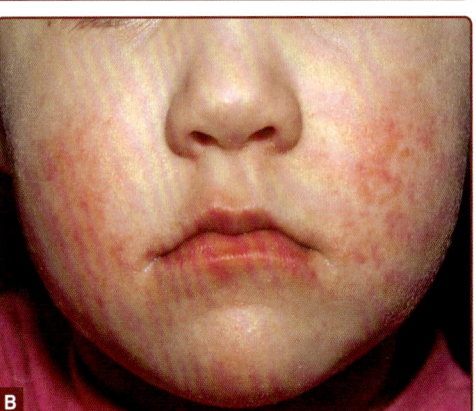

Figure 79-7 Steroid rosacea. **A,** An adult patient with primarily telangiectatic rosacea with rare acneiform papules that was the result of prolonged use of topical glucocorticosteroid (Valisone), which may increase colonization of *Demodex* mites because of immunosuppression. (From the Fitzsimons Army Medical Center Teaching Files.) **B,** A pediatric patient with steroid rosacea. (Used with permission from the William Weston Collection.)

GRAM-NEGATIVE ROSACEA

Prolonged treatment of a rosacea patient with a topical or systemic antibiotic that covers gram-positive bacteria will select gram-negative pathogens and thereby complicate the rosacea complexion. The characteristic clinical finding is the development of miniscule yellow pustules on a preexisting or newly formed erythema background. The clinical picture is not distinguishable from papulopustular rosacea. However, because of the difference in therapy, the discriminating it from (gram-positive) papulopustular rosacea is essential.

PERSISTENT EDEMA OF ROSACEA

Edema in rosacea should be distinguished from the diffuse idiopathic solid upper-facial edema (sometimes called Morbihan disease or edematous rosacea). Morbihan disease (Fig. 79-8; named after a region of northern France where patients with this problem were first identified) typically is not preceded by significant cutaneous inflammation. The cause of this type of facial swelling is unknown, and any relationship of chronic Morbihan disease to the typical pathophysiology of rosacea described later is doubtful. However, in rosacea, edema is present as hard, nonpitting swellings of mainly the caudal half of the face (ie, forehead, eyelids, cheeks, and nose) but also the glabella. Although the initial edema might not be constantly experienced, the later swelling is persistent and accompanied by erythema. In particular, swelling of the upper and lower eyelids causing visual difficulties is perceived as aggravating by the patient. Patients also report skin tightness and, infrequently, pruritus. Systemic reactions are profoundly absent. Edema in rosacea tends to become chronic, with flare-ups and periods of partial regression.

ETIOLOGY AND PATHOPHYSIOLOGY

Epidemiologic, clinical, and genetic studies indicate a genetic as well as environmental origin of rosacea; however, the pathophysiological mechanisms that initiate and perpetuate this chronic relapsing inflammatory skin disease are still poorly understood.

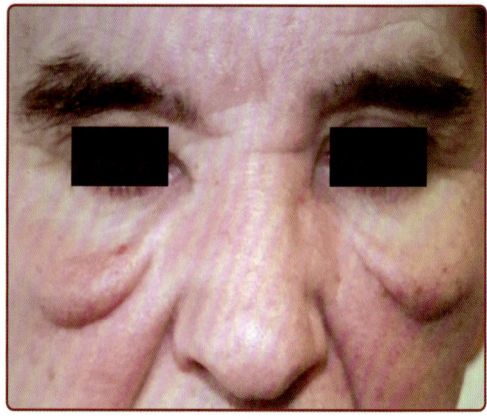

Figure 79-8 Morbihan disease. An adult patient with non to mild erythematous cushionlike edema of the lower eyelids. It may include the forehead, nose, glabella, and central cheeks. It can occur in men and women.

GENETICS AND ASSOCIATED CLUES REGARDING MECHANISMS OF DISEASE

A positive family history markedly increases the chances of developing rosacea. Moreover, monozygous twins with rosacea have a higher correlation of National Rosacea Society clinical score criteria than heterozygous twins.[24]

Null mutation polymorphisms in the glutathione S-transferase (GST) gene have been found in patients with rosacea, which indicates that increased oxidative stress may be associated with rosacea pathogenesis.[25,26] Two single-nucleotide polymorphisms (SNPs) found in patients with rosacea of European descent encode for butyrophilin-like 2 (BTNL2) and human leukocyte antigen (HLA)-DRA loci.[26,27] Whereas HLA-DRA showed strong staining at sites of perifollicular inflammatory infiltrates, epidermal Langerhans cells, and endothelial cells, staining using an anti-BTNL2 antibody revealed diffuse expression in keratinocytes, perifollicular inflammatory infiltrates, and endothelial cells of papulopustular patients with rosacea. A polymorphism in NOD2/CARD15 was observed in a patient with granulomatous rosacea;[28] the gene encodes a caspase recruitment protein involved in Toll-like receptor (TLR) function, including the function of TLR-2. Finally, a polymorphic variant of TACR3 was also observed in patients with rosacea;[29] this gene encodes a tachykinin receptor subtype that responds to substance P family members, a neuropeptide critically involved in neurogenic inflammation, flare, and edema.

COMORBIDITIES AND ASSOCIATED CLUES REGARDING MECHANISMS OF DISEASE

Recent studies indicate that an increased risk of rosacea may be associated with inflammatory diseases of the GI tract, such as Crohn's disease, ulcerative colitis, celiac disease or small intestinal bacterial overgrowth (SIBO) syndrome,[26,30-33] probably caused by shared disease susceptibility to the HLA-DRA locus. Other associations to metabolic diseases such as diabetes,[34] hypertension, dyslipidemia, and coronary artery disease[35-37] have been found, possibly owing to low levels of high-density lipoprotein–associated proteins or enzymes (eg, paraoxonase-1),[38,39] increased cathelicidin levels,[40] or endoplasmic reticulum stress.[40-42]

Patients with rosacea notably have various associations to neurologic disorders and neurodegenerative diseases, such as Alzheimer disease,[43] Parkinson disease,[44] migraine,[45] depression,[46] anxiety disorders,[47] complex regional pain syndrome, and glioma.[48]

TABLE 79-1
Common Rosacea Triggers and Their Activation Pathways

TRIGGER[a]	REPORTED INCIDENCE (%)	PUTATIVE RECEPTOR OR PATHWAY
Sun exposure	81	NALP3, TLR-2, TRPV4
Emotional stress	79	NALP3, TLR-2, TRPV1
Hot weather	75	TRPV1,2
Wind	57	NALP3, TLR2-, TRPV(?)
Heavy exercise	56	NALP3, TLR-2, TRPV1
Alcohol consumption	52	NALP3, TLR-2, TRPV1
Hot baths	51	TRPV1
Cold weather	46	TRPA1
Spicy foods	45	TRPV1
Humidity or osmotic changes	44	TRPV4
Indoor heat	41	TRPV1
Certain skin-care products	41	NALP3, TLR-2, TRPA1
Heated beverages (steam)	36	TRPV1
Certain cosmetics (eg, formaldehyde)	27	NALP3, TLR-2, TRPA1
Medications	15	NALP3, TLR-2, TRPV(?)
Microorganisms[b]	NR	NALP3, TLR-2
Garlic, mustard oil	NR	TRPA1
Noxious heat (52°C)	NR	TRPA1

[a]Most common patient-reported triggers adapted from the National Rosacea Society (NRS); http://www.rosacea.org/patients/materials/triggersgraph.php) and modified from Holmes and Steinhoff.[6]

[b]Microorganisms not reported as a known trigger in NRS survey.

NALP3, NACHT-, LRR-, and PYD, domains-containing protein 3; NR, not reported; TLR-2, Toll-like receptor 2; TRPA1, transient receptor potential ankyrin 1; TRPV, transient receptor potential vanilloid.

Modified from Holmes AD, Steinhoff M. Integrative concepts of rosacea pathophysiology, clinical presentation and new therapeutics. *Exp Dermatol.* 2017;26(8):659-67; with permission. Copyright © 2017, John Wiley & Sons.

ENVIRONMENTAL TRIGGER FACTORS AND ASSOCIATED CLUES REGARDING MECHANISMS OF DISEASE

Characteristic trigger factors for the initiation or aggravation of rosacea include heat (and, rarely, noxious cold), UV radiation, spicy food, certain alcoholic beverages (red wine more than white wine), stress, and microbial infestation on the face or in the gut (eg, demodex, bacterial overgrowth) (Table 79-1).[16,49] Demodex mites are particularly found in association with papulopustular lesions.[50]

Which and how trigger factors induce papules and pustules is still unclarified and may include demodex mites, cutaneous or GI bacteria, a dysbalanced microbiota system in the gut (eg, SIBO syndrome), or stomach infection (eg, *Helicobacter pylori*). Whether the classical rosacea triggers, such as heat, UV radiation, some alcoholic beverages, hormonal dysregulation, or stress, are capable of triggering these eruptions is unknown.

HEAT, NOXIOUS COLD

Recent transcriptome and quantitative immunohistochemistry data indicate a role of transient receptor potential (TRP) ion channels (eg, TRP vanilloid type 1 [TRPV1] and TRP ankyrin type 1 [TRPA1]), which can be activated by temperature changes (Fig. 79-9).[1,51] Whether any noxious cold receptor(s) may trigger rosacea is unknown.

ULTRAVIOLET RADIATION

Sun exposure is a well-accepted trigger factor for rosacea. Indeed, sun exposure may be the trigger factor for rosacea on the bald scalp. However, to what extent UVA, UVB, or temperature increases account for rosacea symptom induction is not clear. The fact that patients behind glass shields develop asymmetric rosacea erythema and flushing indicates a role for at least UVA in rosacea. UV radiation induces neuroinflammation, endoplasmic reticulum stress, and innate immune responses and promotes skin fibrosis or solar elastosis, characteristics of rosacea. UVB triggers TRP vanilloid type 4 (TRPV4) activation on keratinocytes and is increased in tissue of patients with chronic photodermatitis and rosacea, suggesting a molecular pathway of UVB-induced rosacea through TRPV channels (see Fig. 79-9).[52]

MICROORGANISMS

Whether a dysbalance of the skin or GI microbiota contributes to the pathophysiology of rosacea, and if so which microorganisms are involved, is still poorly understood. Demodex folliculorum is a commensal of human and animal skin, predominantly in oily skin close to the pilosebaceous glands,[53,54] and is increased in some patients with rosacea, predominantly in those with phymata as well as papules and pustules.[55] Whether demodex mites are significantly enhanced in erythematous skin is unknown,[56-58] but treatment that reduces demodex mite density positively correlates with clinical improvement.[59,60] Which molecules or substrates produced by, or associated with, demodex mites account for rosacea is unknown. Candidates include *Bacillus oleronius*, proteases or chitins, which can activate protease-activated receptors (eg, PAR-2)[61] or TLRs (eg, TLR-2),[62] thereby releasing cytokines, chemokines, and matrix metalloproteinases (MMPs)

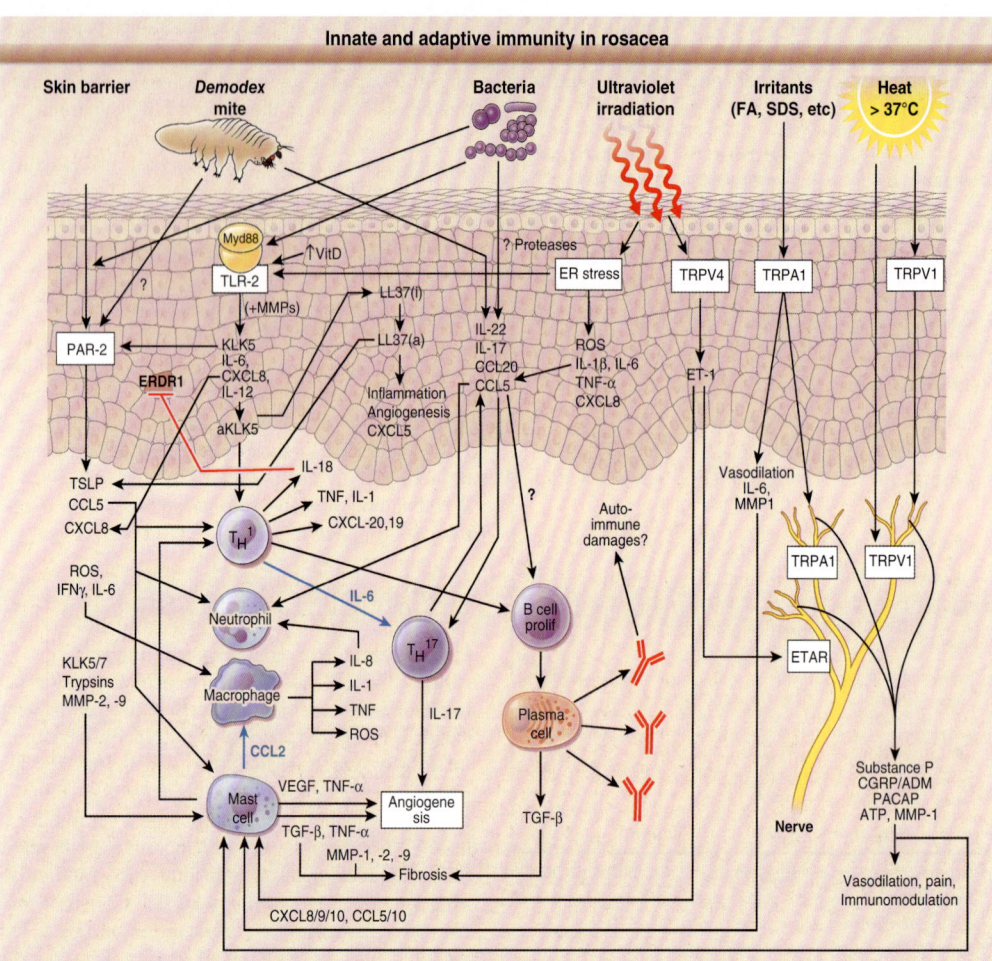

Figure 79-9 Dysregulation of innate and adaptive immune system in rosacea. Environmental triggers are shown at the top of the figure, with their known or assumed downstream signaling effects shown below. Protease-activated receptor-2 (PAR-2) not only induces neuroinflammation or pain but also stimulates release of cytokines such as interleukin (IL)-1, tumor necrosis factor (TNF), IL-6, IL-8, thymic stromal lymphopoietin (TSLP), chemokines, matrix metalloproteinases (MMPs), and prostaglandins; recruits neutrophils and T cells or macrophages to the site of inflammation; and induces mast cell release. Because PAR-2 is expressed by keratinocytes, endothelial cells, mast cells, macrophages, and neutrophils; is regulated by microbial products; and interacts with TLRs, a role of serine proteases and PARs in rosacea innate immune responses can be assumed.[119-124] Cytokine expression profiles of all skin rosacea phenotypes demonstrate elevation of the cytokine interferon (IFN)-γ,[20] which can be produced by type 1 helper T cells and natural killer cells, and because IFN-γ is a potent activator of macrophages, this is likely a close communication of the adaptive and innate immune networks in rosacea. TLR-2 is known to increase the expression of the serine protease KLK-5.[125] Notably, the lesional skin of patients with rosacea was shown to express more KLK-5 than the skin of healthy control participants.[40] In addition, Yamasaki and coworkers[41] revealed that the increased capacity for releasing KLK-5 is calcium dependent; the ligand for TLR-2 triggers an influx of calcium, which in turn induces the increased release of KLK-5. In this process, calcium functions as the stimulus for transcription of KLK-5, with TLR-2 regulating the functional release of KLK-5.[41] Via KLK-5, TLR-2 induces upregulation and activation of the innate immune peptide human cathelicidin (the active form of which is LL-37),[41] leading to erythema, immune response, and angiogenesis through release of serine proteases, MMPs, cytokines, chemokines, and proliferation of endothelial cells.[40,41,73,74,126] KLK-5 protein activity can also be regulated by serine protease inhibitors of Kazal-type (SPINKs).[72] Among these, SPINK6 was identified in human skin as a specific inhibitor of KLKs.[72] However, its putative role in rosacea should be further explored. KLK-5 is also mediated by MMPs. Specifically, the activation of KLK-5 occurs after the cleavage of its proenzyme form by MMP-9.[72] Notably, enhanced expression of MMP-2 and MMP-9 was observed in the skin of patients with rosacea.[127] Such increased expression of MMPs has potential implications for the solar-mediated degeneration that is observed in rosacea.[128] In addition, MMP-mediated initiation of KLK-5 activation leads to further activation of LL-37, the processed form of cathelicidin. Increased expression of transient receptor potential (TRP) channels of the vanilloid subfamily (TRPV1–4) was found in lesional skin of rosacea patients.[51] TRP channels are widely acknowledged as polymodal sensors of environmental and endogenous irritative signals and can be activated by typical rosacea triggers (eg, heat, ultraviolet B, temperature changes, pungent compounds from vegetable and spices, alcohol, mechanical stimuli, irritants). Activation of TRPs increases intracellular calcium concentrations

and prostanoids, and attracting immune cells (see Fig. 79-9).

MECHANISMS OF DISEASE

The already mentioned trigger factors probably initiate release of proinflammatory mediators from keratinocytes (eg, cathelicidin, vascular endothelial growth factor [VEGF], endothelin-1), endothelial cells (nitric oxide [NO], pituitary adenylate cyclase activating peptide [PACAP]), mast cells (cathelicidin, MMPs, tumor necrosis factor [TNF]-α), macrophages (interferon [IFN]-γ, TNF, MMPs, interleukin [IL]-26), helper-1 T (T_H1) cells (IFN-γ), and helper-17 T (T_H17) cells. Triggers such as heat, noxious cold, exercising, spicy food, ethanol (or other ingredients or certain alcoholic beverages), and pH changes can directly activate sensory nerves to release vasoactive and proinflammatory neuromediators. Likewise, exercising and ethanol can activate release of neurotransmitters such as acetylcholine or neuropeptides such as PACAP from autonomic nerves.

Some receptors that are responsive to rosacea trigger factors have indeed been discovered.[41,51,63] Most of the trigger factors activate TRP ion channels on sensory nerves to induce neurogenic inflammation through release of neuropeptides such as substance P or PACAP. Neuropeptides are potent inducers of edema and vasodilation, the basis of flushing and erythema.[56,64,65] The individual reactivity to otherwise innocuous triggers, however, is still not understood, but a genetic predisposition appears to influence this phenomenon. The genes involved have yet to be confirmed, but two SNPs have recently been identified and involve a major histocompatibility complex predisposition.[26] It may well transpire that several of these factors are relevant and that each of the rosacea subtypes has different factors that are important to their initiation and progression.

IMMUNE RESPONSES

Similar to psoriasis and atopic dermatitis, innate immunity is known to have an essential role in the initiation and maintenance of rosacea. However, recent results point also to an important role of cytotoxic T-cell response in the pathophysiology of rosacea.[6,66] How the adaptive and innate immune systems are connected in rosacea is still unclear (see Fig. 79-9).

Skin Barrier Dysfunction: Patients with rosacea suffer from increased transepidermal water loss (TEWL), as well as pH increase of the facial skin, both markers for skin barrier dysfunction.[67,68] Increased TEWL leads to enhanced epidermal "leakage" and thus access for microbes, and an alkali pH enhances enzyme activity, for example, of kallikreins (KLK), such as KLK-5,-6,-7 or -12, which are enhanced in rosacea skin.[1,5] KLK-5 activates LL-37 activity, which stimulates erythema, cytokine release, and angiogenesis.[40,69] In addition, KLKs-5,-7 (and probably others) activate PAR-2, which is involved in several inflammatory responses (see Fig. 79-9). Notably, both LL-37 and PAR-2 are upregulated in rosacea skin tissue, and PAR-2 upregulates LL-37 expression levels.[70] The precise role and therapeutic impact of skin barrier dysfunction and restoration awaits further clarification.

Toll-Like Receptors, Proteases, and Cathelicidin: TLR-2 is upregulated in patients with rosacea[41,71] and induces release of proinflammatory cytokines, chemokines, proangiogenic factors, and proteases.[56,63,72] TLR-2 induces upregulation and activation of the innate immune peptide cathelicidin via KLK-5 (see Fig. 79-9),[41] leading to erythema, immune response, and angiogenesis through release of serine proteases, MMPs, cytokines, chemokines, and proliferation of endothelial cells.[41,73,74] A role of cathelicidins in rosacea inflammation is now widely accepted,[40] although direct functional in vivo data in humans is still missing.

TLR-2 is also able to facilitate the activation of the NLRP3 inflammasome, which mediates IL-1β release and further inflammatory reactions.[75] IL-1β expression is elevated in rosacea and mediates inflammatory responses therein.

The upstream stimulator of TLR-2 in rosacea is still unknown. Microbes can activate TLRs on keratinocytes, although a direct link between demodex mites or certain bacteria, such as *Bacillus oleronius*, and TLRs in rosacea skin has not yet been demonstrated. Likewise, the connection between the intestinal microbiota flora

---

and release of neuropeptides such as substance P, calcitonin gene-related peptide (CGRP), adrenomedullin (ADM), and pituitary adenylate cyclase-activating polypeptide (PACAP), as well as adenosine triphosphate (ATP) from cutaneous sensory nerves, or endothelin-1 (ET-1) and IL-6 from keratinocytes. These products mediate an increase in vasodilation (flushing), vascular permeability (edema), or blood flow and enhance inflammatory circuits of adaptive and innate immune system, such as by leukocyte recruitment, T-cell or macrophage activation, and degranulation of mast cells. The released products of mast cell granules are especially involved in angiogenesis (vascular endothelial growth factor [VEGF], transforming growth factor [TGF]-β) and fibrosis (TGF-β, MMPs-1, -2, and -9). Substance P can induce release of chemokines from mast cells which can modulate function of TH1 cells (through CCL5, CXCL10), macrophages, or dendritic cells (via CCL2), thereby regulating adaptive immunity. It is furthermore known that activation of neuronal TRPA1, TRPV1, and TRPV4 lead to painful burning sensations, which may be similar to that observed in patients with rosacea. Of note, patients with rosacea rarely have pruritus as neural sensation. Through neural mediators, the sensory and autonomic nervous systems contribute to pain, vasodilation (flushing, erythema), plasma extravasation (edema), and immunomodulation (innate and adaptive immune cells). ETAR, endothelin receptor type A; FA, fatty acid; SDS, sodium dodecyl sulfate.

dysbalance and the inflammatory responses in the skin are also unknown. Notably, vitamin D is enhanced in patients with rosacea and has been demonstrated to increase TLR-2 and KLK-5 mRNA expression levels, thereby regulating TLR-2, KLK-5, and LL-37 levels in rosacea.[76]

Inflammasome: The inflammasome consists of the rosacea trigger–responsive NALP3, caspase-1, and the adaptor protein apoptosis-associated speck-like protein (ASC), and orchestrates cleavage and activation of an rosacea-upregulated IL-1.[56,75,77] Nucleotide-binding oligomerization domain (NOD)-like receptor (NALP3) is an integral member of the IL-1β inflammasome complex in keratinocytes that is required for inflammasome activation in rosacea.[56] Inflammasome activation results in neutrophil chemotaxis, IL-1- and TNF-mediated inflammation amplification, and prostaglandin E2 synthesis, which supports pustule formation, heat pain sensation, and vascular responses, respectively. The inflammasome-activated cellular network of keratinocytes, macrophages, mast cells, and neutrophils (in papulopustular rosacea) creates a highly inflammatory milieu in rosacea. The concomitant production of reactive oxygen species (ROS) and MMPs further contribute to tissue damage, vasorelaxation, vasopermeability, and late-onset fibrosis in rosacea.

Imbalanced Adaptive Immunity: Both, T and B lymphocytes play a role in rosacea. Histological analysis and transcriptome studies reveal the presence of predominantly CD4+ and to a lower extent CD8+ T cells and cytokines in rosacea skin,[20,78,79] with the dominance of CD4+ T_H1 and T_H17 cells and their corresponding cytokines. Cytokine expression profiles of all skin rosacea phenotypes demonstrate elevated T_H1 cytokines IFN-γ, TNF, and T_H17 cytokines IL-17A and IL-22.[20] T_H17 cells induce VEGF, which contributes to angiogenesis in rosacea (see Fig. 79-9). Because IFN-γ is a potent activator of macrophages, a close communication of adaptive and innate immune networks is likely to be present in rosacea.

Rosacea eruptions, however, are also associated with T-cell immunosuppression after infection[80] or therapeutic intervention (eg, corticosteroids, calcineurin inhibitors, phototherapy).[81-83] Patients with eruptions of rosacea commonly present with *Demodex* mite infestation, supporting a parallel between *Demodex* proliferation and T-cell activity, and antibodies against *Demodex* have been found in patients with rosacea.[80,81]

In rosacea, immunologic tolerance is well preserved through relative high numbers of tolerogenic (regulatory) T cells compared with other skin.[79] Other important molecules involved in rosacea pathophysiology through regulating adaptive immune responses are Erdr1[84] and IL-18,[85] supporting the concept that T_H1 immune responses, induction of ROS molecules,[86] and angiogenesis are all important contributors of rosacea.[87]

NEUROVASCULAR DYSREGULATION AND NEUROINFLAMMATION

Skin hypersensitivity and flushing are direct consequences of neural stimulation in any condition or disease, including rosacea.[88] The human face is to a certain extent physiologically unique because it is one of the few regions in the human skin where the blood vessels are under control of the sympathetic, parasympathetic, and sensory nerves. This fact implies that (nor)epinephrine, acetylcholine, and neuropeptides can modulate the state of the blood vessel diameter. Because autonomic nerves also release neuropeptides under certain circumstances and all mediators are involved in inflammatory processes and immune defense control, neuroinflammatory processes are involved in the perpetuation and maintenance of unphysiological ("diseased") flushing and transient erythema. To which extent early immune responses may also induce neurovascular dysregulation is currently unknown. Flushing in patients with rosacea is pathophysiologically neurogenic inflammation, as described by Jancso and Szolcsanyi 50 years ago.[89] Histopathologically, upper dermal edema and leukocytes can be found, which corresponds with neurogenic inflammation in animal ex vivo and in vivo studies. Thus, also not clearly shown in dermatopathological studies, transient erythema can be seen as an inflammatory process and cannot be explained by merely prolonged vasodilation.

The molecular basis of the "neurovascular" genes, mediators, and receptors activated in rosacea are partially clarified (Fig. 79-10). However, it is still unknown whether the neurovascular system is mechanistically up- or downstream of the inflammatory cascade. It is certain that flushing and erythema are part of the inflammatory process and not merely a dilated vessel and cosmetic problem. Prolonged flushing lasting longer than 5 minutes is always part of the neurogenic inflammation cascade[56,90] characterized by erythema (vasodilation), edema (postcapillary plasma extravasation), and recruitment of leukocytes to site of inflammation. Sensory neuron density is moderately increased in the erythematotelangiectatic rosacea.[51,90]

The various TRPs appear to render the thermal, chemical, and mechanical rosacea stimuli into clinical manifestations of rosacea.[91] Because TRP channels can cross-talk with neuropeptide receptors, the interaction between these two types of receptors may be involved in sustaining neurovascular responses and inflammation in rosacea, particularly TRPA1 and TRPV1.[1,51] TRPV1, TRPV2, TRPV3, TRPV4, and TRPA1 ion channels are broadly expressed on neuronal and non-neuronal cells in rosacea skin.[51] Thus, TRPs might thereby establish the neuroimmune and neurovascular communication observed in rosacea.

The variety of neuronal and vascular pathways that seem to be involved in rosacea neuroinflammation and pain, as well as skin hypersensitivity, explains the unique trigger profiles of individual

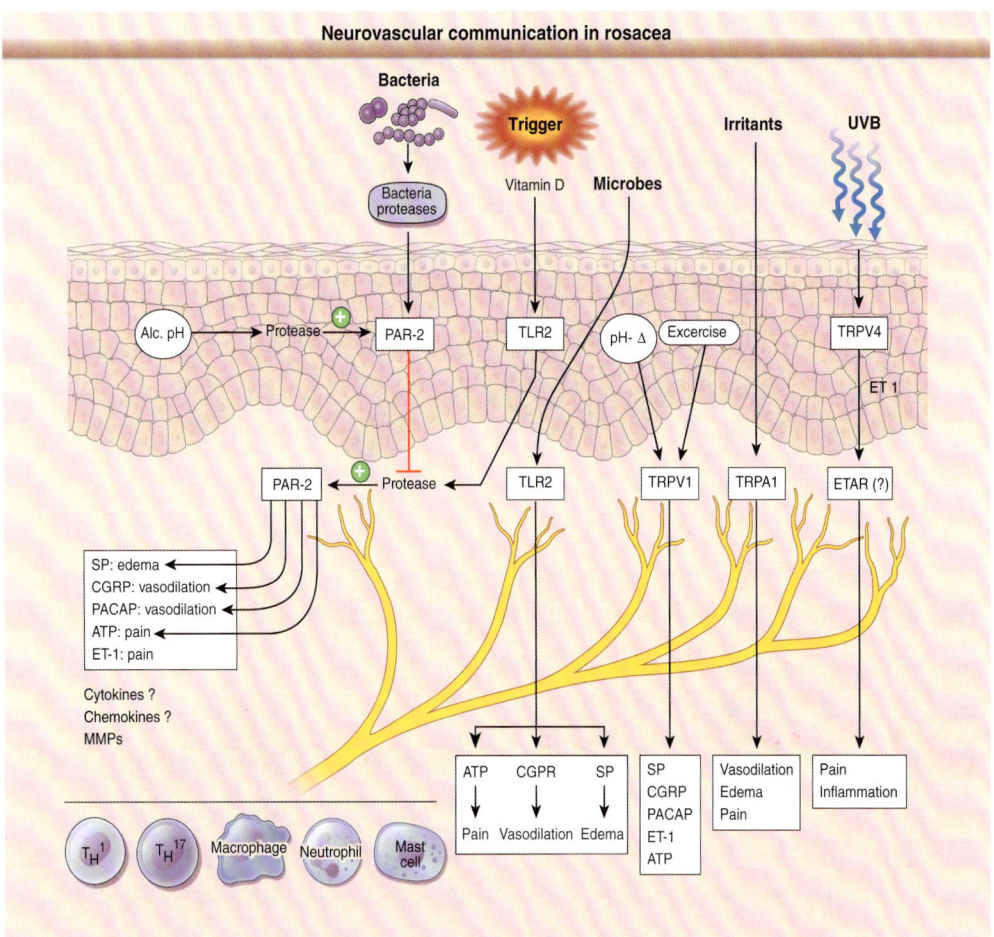

Figure 79-10 Neurovascular communication in rosacea. Notably, a polymorphism in the *TAC3* gene has been identified in rosacea, which encodes for neurokinin receptor-3 and induces neuroinflammation, pain, and immune responses in various tissues. Thus, overstimulation of neurokinin receptor-3 may contribute to neurovascular and neuroimmune changes in rosacea through substance P and other tachykinins.[129] Activation of neuronal transient receptor potential (TRP) ion channels through rosacea trigger factors can lead to release of vasoactive neuropeptides (eg, pituitary adenylate cyclase activating peptide [PACAP], substance P [SP], and calcitonin gene-related peptide [CGRP]),[91] which are involved in rosacea-associated vasodilation,[90] plasma extravasation, and leukocyte recruitment, also via induction of mast cell degranulation.[5] SP-positive nerve fibers are enhanced in patients with rosacea. Also, PACAP-positive nerves are anatomically closely associated with mast cells that release a number of vasoactive mediators.[65] Finally, agonist and one of the receptors for CGRP are increased at mRNA levels in patients with rosacea.[98] Because TRP channels can cross-talk with neuropeptide receptors, the interaction of both receptors may be involved in sustaining neurovascular responses and inflammation in rosacea, particularly TRP ankyrin type 1 (TRPA1) and TRP vanilloid type 1 (TRPV1).[1,51]

Proteases such as kallikreins (KLKs)-5, -6, and -7 activate protease-activated receptor-2 (PAR-2) on keratinocytes, endothelial cells, macrophages, mast cells, and sensory nerves, thereby contributing to innate and adaptive immune activation, vasoregulation and pain. PAR-2 induces release of various neuropeptides (SP, CGRP, PACAP) from nerves, as well as cytokines, chemokines, reactive oxygen species (ROS), and matrix metalloproteinases (MMPs) from cutaneous and immune cells. Although SP primarily promotes plasma extravasation (edema) and CGRP and PACAP vascular dilation, all can initiate pain sensations. PAR-2 is also regulated by various exogenous rosacea trigger factors as well as microbial agents and interacts with Toll-like receptors (TLRs).[119-124] TLRs are pattern recognition receptors (PRR) that sense pathogen-associated molecular patterns (PAMPs). Notably, TLR-2 is also upregulated in patients with rosacea[41,71] and induces release of neuropeptides, proinflammatory cytokines, chemokines, proangiogenic factors, and proteases such as KLK-5.[56,63,72] However, the stimulator of TLR-2 in rosacea is still unknown. Via KLK-5-release, TLR-2 can activate PAR-2 and activate the innate immune peptide cathelicidin,[41] leading to neuropeptide release and subsequent angiogenesis, erythema, plasma extravasation, and immune modulation. Thus, TLR and PAR-2 can be seen as a "forefront" of innate immunity in rosacea. ETAR, endothelin receptor type A; UV, ultraviolet.

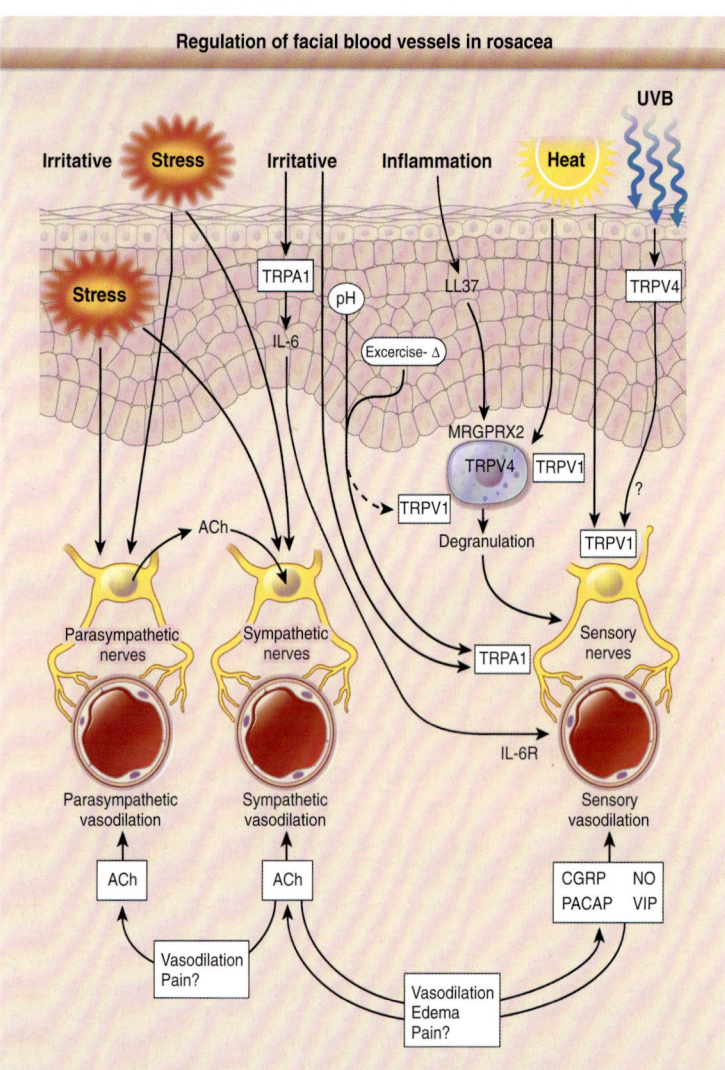

Figure 79-11 Potential pathomechanism of facial flushing in rosacea. Flushing involves an immediate (in contrast to persistent erythema) reactive vascular response to various "irritative" stimuli (within seconds to minutes), induced by trigger factors (eg, spicy food, certain alcohols [Alc], ultraviolet [UV] B, heat, noxious cold, exercising, or stressful emotional stimuli; top of the figure). Most of the trigger factors capably activate transient receptor potential (TRP) ion channels (eg, TRP vanilloid type 1 [TRPV1], TRP ankyrin type 1 [TRPA1], TRP vanilloid type 4 [TRPV4]) on keratinocytes, immune cells, or sensory nerves to induce neurogenic inflammation through release of neuropeptides such as substance P, calcitonin gene-related peptide (CGRP), adrenomedullin (ADM), pituitary adenylate cyclase activating peptide (PACAP), or vasointestinal peptide (VIP) from sensory nerves. Neuropeptide release from sensory nerves is either directly facilitated by the irritant stimulus or established via intermediate signals derived from keratinocytes (eg, interleukin [IL]-6), endothelial cells (eg, tumor necrosis factor [TNF]-α, IL-1), or immune cells (eg, mast cells). Neuropeptides are potent inducers of vasodilation, the basis of flushing and erythema, plasma extravasation (leading to edema), and pain. In addition, stressful stimuli also hyperstimulate the autonomic nervous system, especially sympathetic and parasympathetic vasodilator fibers, thereby regulating release of acetylcholine (ACh), for example, a potent vasoregulator and immunomodulator. NO, nitric oxide.

patients with rosacea (see Table 79-1 and Fig. 79-10). Furthermore, pathophysiological outcomes may differ depending on individual receptor activation profiles and downstream cellular activation targets, providing a hypothesis for the phenotypic variability seen in rosacea.

The autonomic nervous system, via stress-induced increase of the skin sympathetic nerve activity (SSNA), may also contribute to the pathophysiology of rosacea through increased blood flow (erythema), neuroinflammatory responses (cytokine release), and pain induction,[92,93] for example, through release of cortisol-releasing hormone (CRH),[94] PACAP,[65] or NO.[95] Clearly, autonomic dysregulation is involved in facial flushing (Fig. 79-11).[66,92,96] This may be due to release of neuropeptides such as PACAP. In contrast, the skin shows

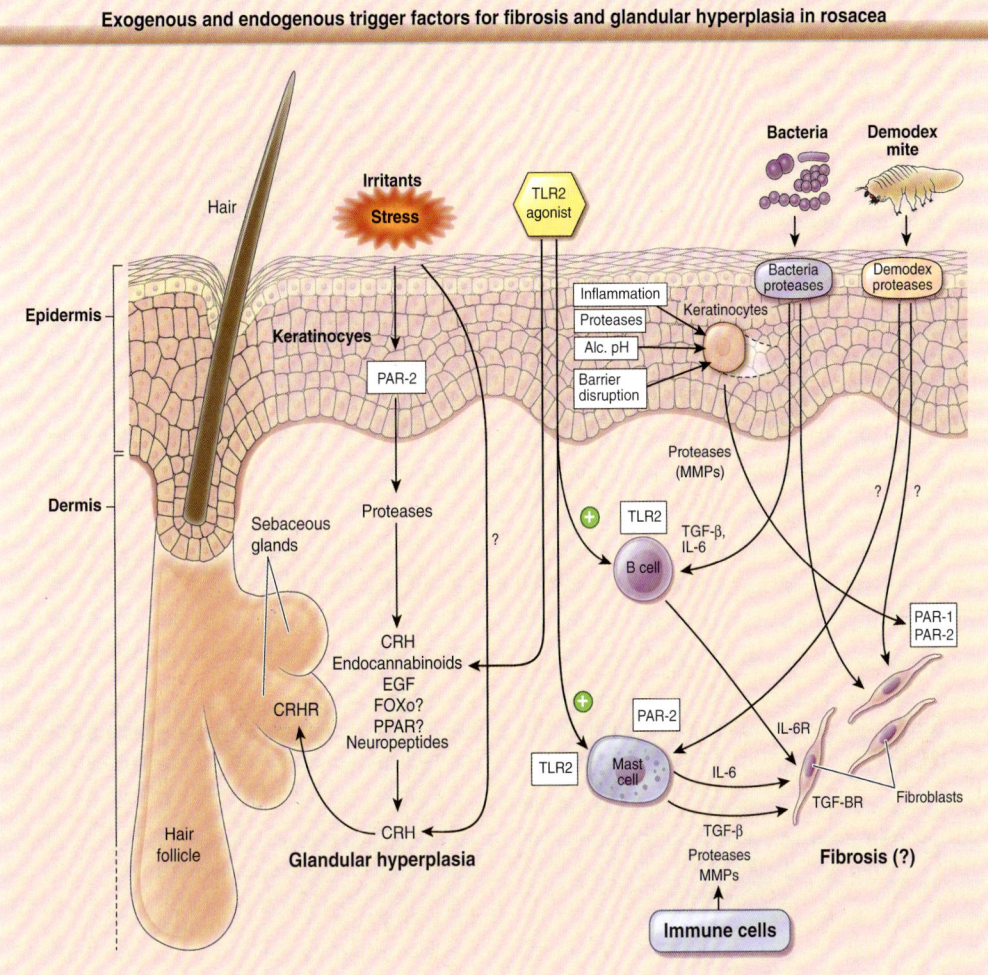

Figure 79-12 Pathomechanism and current therapy strategies for fibrosis and glandular hyperplasia in rosacea. Phymata are verrucous nodules and plaques based on glandular hyperplasia of sebaceous glands and fibroblast activation. They develop through either clinically visible chronic inflammation (chronic erythema, papules or pustules) or sometimes clinically unremarkable skin (subclinical phyma). In any case, they develop because of persistent inflammatory processes accompanied by edema. Histopathologically, phymata are characterized by a perivascular lymphocytic infiltrate, enlarged sebaceous glands and follicles, dilated vessels, remodeled myofibroblasts, and fibrosis. The dysregulated inflammatory process can be triggered by multiple exogenous and endogenous factors. Cell wall components are recognized by Toll-like receptor 2 (TLR2, CD282) leading to the activation of the innate immune system in form of macrophages and mast cell activation or adaptive immune cells (eg, B cells), which readily release a cocktail of profibrotic mediators (eg, interleukin [IL]-6, IL-4, transforming growth factor [TGF]-β, platelet-derived growth factor [PDGF]) that remodel and activate dermal fibroblasts to deposit excessive amounts of extracellular matrix, a hallmark of fibrosis. Demodex or bacterial-derived proteases or endogenous proteases (eg, kallikreins, matrix metalloproteinases) can engage in this fibrotic process by activating resident skin cell- (eg, keratinocytes, fibroblasts) and immune cells (eg, mast cells, macrophages) through cytokine receptors (IL-4, IL-6) growth factor receptors (eg, TGF-β, PDGF), protease-activated receptor-2 (PAR-2) or TLRs. Low pH and barrier disruption additionally activate keratinocytes to release profibrotic proteases that can target fibroblast-derived PAR-2. The precise pathomechanism of sebaceous glandular hyperplasia is far from being understood. An important signaling network appears to be triggered by stress that probably activates keratinocytic PAR-2, causing protease release, and might interfere with the corticotropin-releasing hormone and cannabinoid system, the modulation of epidermal growth factor (EGF) and neuropeptide abundance and peroxisome proliferator-activated receptor gamma (PPARγ) activation. Each target is involved in the regulation of lipid and glucose metabolism, cell proliferation and differentiation, or inflammation that fundamentally regulate sebogenesis, sebaceous gland proliferation, and consequently glandular hyperplasia. Alc, alcohol; CRH, cortisol-releasing hormone; MMP, matrix metalloproteinase.

normal vascular responses to application of epinephrine, norepinephrine, and acetylcholine in patients with rosacea.

PHYMATOUS CHANGES, FIBROSIS, AND GLANDULAR HYPERPLASIA

Although a significant percentage of male patients with rosacea develop phymata, mostly on the nose, a pathophysiological link of chronic inflammation and skin fibrosis or sebaceous hyperplasia is unknown. A role of seborrhea has not been demonstrated convincingly for patients with rosacea, and some even have "dry skin."

Mast cells and B cells are critical contributor to skin fibrosis through release of MMPs, which is one plausible pathway for the development of phymata through chronic inflammation.[20,97] The pathophysiological link between chronic inflammation and glandular hyperplasia is still enigmatic (Fig. 79-12).

TELANGIECTASIA

The pathophysiology of telangiectasia is unknown but differs from sun damage (chronic photodermatitis, heliodermatitis).[98] One possible explanation is that proteases, MMPs, and growth factors from the transforming growth factor or fibroblast growth factor family destroy the architecture of the extracellular matrix, thereby reducing the tissue resistance for blood vessels, which subsequently leads to irreversible vasodilation.[99] This, however, awaits further clarification through research.

GASTROINTESTINAL TRACT

The role of *H. pylori* in rosacea is controversial.[100,101] More convincing evidence derives from studies in which patients with SIBO syndrome (eg, after surgeries, metabolic diseases) develop a microbiota flora in favor of proinflammatory, instead of protective, bacteria in the GI tract.[102] Rifaximin, a drug that through T-cell modulation reinstalls the physiological flora in the GI tract, alleviates rosacea symptoms in the majority of cases (but not of patients with *H. pylori* through H⁺ pump blockers), which supports this hypothesis.[32,103,104]

DIAGNOSIS OF ROSACEA

The diagnosis of rosacea is led by the clinical features (see Clinical Findings) along with taking a thorough patient history (age, gender, trigger factors, hormonal changes, profession, hobbies, gut surgeries, *Demodex* infestation, exercising, heat exposure, noxious cold exposure, drinking and eating habits) and family history (positive family history). No diagnostic markers or laboratory workup exists to diagnose rosacea. To differentiate from other skin or systemic diseases, however, laboratory workup and diagnostic tools may be used. Histopathology, especially in the early erythematous stage, is often nonspecific; however, a biopsy may be helpful to exclude other differential diagnoses (see Differential Diagnosis).

HISTOPATHOLOGY OF ROSACEA

Histologically, rosacea is characterized by numerous features, depending on the presenting symptoms or subtype. In erythematous skin and telangiectasia, a perivascular inflammatory infiltrate consisting mainly of T_H1 and T_H17 cells, as well as macrophages and mast cells, can be observed;[5,20] depending on severity, these cells can be sparse to numerous. In addition, blood and lymphatic vessels are markedly dilated, and a microscopically visible dermal edema can be found in all stages but is rarely found clinically.

Papules consist of CD4⁺ T_H1 and T_H17 cells, macrophages, mast cells, and plasma cells. In pustules, additional neutrophils can be found.

In phymatous rosacea lesions, the infiltrate still consists of T_H1 and T_H17 cells, macrophages, mast cells, and more plasma cells than in nonphymatous rosacea. Glandular hyperplasia and follicular plugging without comedones can be found as well as fibrosis and increase in fibroblasts.[5] In phymatous rosacea and often follicular or perifollicular inflammation, *Demodex folliculorum* is present up to 50% of tissue specimen; these mites are most abundant in phymatous skin, which may account for the folliculitis and perifolliculitis.

Whether Langerhans cells or dendritic cells are enumerated in all lesions is still unclear. Some authors found increased Langerhans cell density but others not.[5]

In ocular rosacea, dilation of blood and lymphatic vessels as well as obstruction of the meibomian gland can be observed.

Granulomatous rosacea is characterized by dermal edema and vasodilation as well as dermal granulomas of the tuberculoid type with T cells and macrophages as well as multinucleated giant cells and plasma cells. The marked upper dermal vasodilation of blood and lymphatic vessels differentiates it from other granulomatous disorders such as lupus vulgaris.

In rosacea fulminans, besides the infiltrate mentioned earlier, numerous epithelioid cells as well as occasionally granulomas with multinucleated giant cells can be observed.

The histopathologic findings in patients with combined erythema and telangiectasia are relatively mild and not diagnostic. Upper dermal blood vessels usually appear prominent, and there may be a mild perivascular infiltrate composed mainly of lymphocytes with an admixture of histiocytes. The most consistent abnormality is a change in the collagen of the upper dermis, so-called "solar elastosis." This represents the result of chronic actinic damage.

The histopathological changes in some patients are characterized by marked fibrosis in the superficial and reticular dermis, accentuated around follicles and

TABLE 79-2
Classification from 2002 and 2004: Subtypes of Rosacea[17,106]

SUBTYPE (NUMBER AND NAME)[a]	CLINICAL CHARACTERISTICS
Subtype 1: erythematotelangiectatic	Persistent central facial erythema, frequent flushing; may be telangiectatic vessels
Subtype 2: papulopustular	Erythematous dome-shaped papules, some with surmounting postulation in a centrofacial distribution on a background of persistent erythema
Subtype 3: phymatous	Persistent facial swelling with hypertrophy of tissue (rhinophyma); different variants described
Subtype 4: OR	Ocular inflammation (eg, blepharitis, conjunctivitis, or meibomian gland dysfunction; chalazion)

[a]Each subtype can be graded as mild, moderate, and severe.

TABLE 79-3
Classification of Rosacea from 2016 and 2017: Diagnostic, Major, and Secondary Features of Rosacea

DIAGNOSTIC FEATURES[a]	MAJOR FEATURES	SECONDARY FEATURES
Persistent centrofacial erythema associated with periodic intensification by potential trigger factors	Flushing or transient erythema	Burning sensation of the skin
Phymatous changes	Inflammatory papules and pustules	Stinging sensation of the skin
	Telangiectasia	Edema
	Ocular manifestations ■ Eyelid margin telangiectasis ■ Blepharitis ■ Keratitis, conjunctivitis, or sclerokeratitis	Dry sensation of the skin

[a]All features can present as mild, moderate, or severe.
Modified from Tan J, Almeida LMC, Bewley A, et al. Updating the diagnosis, classification and assessment of rosacea: recommendations from the global ROSacea COnsensus (ROSCO) panel. *Br J Dermatol*. 2017;176(2):431-438 and Gallo RL, Granstein RD, Kang S, et al. Standard classification and pathophysiology of rosacea: The 2017 update by the National Rosacea Society Expert Committee. *J Am Acad Dermatol*. 2018;78(1):148-155.

increased number of fibroblasts, but others (especially the obstructive form) show deposition of mucin in the dermis. The collagen in the upper dermis often shows changes of solar elastosis, which is marked in patients with rhinophyma secondary to actinic damage.

CLASSIFICATION

Currently, two classification systems exist: The first, described in 2002, regards rosacea as a syndrome or typology with four distinct clinical subtypes: (1) erythematotelangiectatic, (2) papulopustular, (3) phymatous, and (4) ocular rosacea Table 79-2).[17,105] The severity can be graded as mild, moderate, or severe.[106] These subtypes may be discrete variants or may progress from one subtype to another, with overlaps observed. The improvement brought by this classification was to determine a more structured phenomenology into this enigmatic skin disease and helped physicians on a daily basis to monitor the therapeutic success of each subtype. The disadvantage is that the clinically accumulated symptoms (eg, erythema and telangiectasia) may be based on different pathophysiologies and are thus preventing a more pathophysiology-based understanding of the disease. Moreover, many patients present with an overlap of all subtypes (eg, papulopustular and ocular or phymatous with or without erythema), which complicates a clear-cut classification. Finally, a frequent, if not dominant symptom—flushing—is neglected or subclassified as erythema, which is pathophysiologically incorrect.

Consequently, a modified classification or grading system was introduced in 2016 to 2017,[16,19] emphasizing each possible symptom in rosacea and subclassifying them as diagnostic, major, or secondary features based on how important or selective the symptom is to make the diagnosis (eg, there are almost no differential diagnoses for a phymata or persistent central facial erythema) Table 79-3). Although also not perfect, the new classification considers more thoroughly the many overlap patients existing in the "real-world situation," outlying the subtype classification and leaving more room for a pathophysiology-based classification and therapy.[13,18,107] Thus, the new classification likely reflects more precisely the clinical reality of the disease presentation, although validating data are missing.[16,13]

A recent expert group assessed phymatous changes as an individually diagnostic sign of rosacea and persistent centrofacial erythema associated with periodic intensification by potential trigger factors as a minimum diagnostic sign of rosacea. Flushing, telangiectasia, and inflammatory papules or pustules are considered major features but are not diagnostic of rosacea. The centrofacial location of diagnostic and major features is essential for rosacea diagnosis. The bilateral facial location of a presentation is considered typical but not essential. Stinging sensation, edema, dry sensation, and burning sensation are considered secondary features (symptoms) of rosacea.

DIAGNOSTIC TOOLS

Diagnostic tools are available for some of the major features of rosacea Table 79-4).

TABLE 79-4
Diagnostic Tools for Different Clinical Features of Rosacea

CLINICAL MANIFESTATION	DIAGNOSTIC TOOL
Flushing	Flushing Assessment Tool (FAST)
	Global Flushing Severity Score (GFSS)
Persistent erythema	Investigator's Global Assessment (IGA)
	Clinician's Erythema Assessment (CEA)/
	Patient's Self-Assessment (PSA)
Telangiectasia	None
Papules or pustules	Lesion counts
	Investigator's Global Assessment
Phymatous changes	None
Ocular manifestations	Pending

Modified from Tan J, Almeida LMC, Bewley A, et al. Updating the diagnosis, classification and assessment of rosacea: recommendations from the global ROSacea COnsensus (ROSCO) panel. *Br J Dermatol*. 2017; 176(2):431-38.

TABLE 79-5
Classification of Rhinophymata

GROUP	PRESENTATION
1	Distal end, apex of nose
2	Distal half nose, apex, alae,
3	Distal half of nose, apex, alar nodules
4	Complete nose, including bridge and nasofacial sulci

Modified from Clark DP, Hanke CW. Electrosurgical treatment of rhinophyma. *J Am Acad Dermatol*. 1990;22(5 Pt 1):831-37.

THE GRADING OF SEVERITY OF ROSACEA

The grading of rosacea is divided into mild, moderate, and severe. The grading provides the physician with a practical tool to evaluate the patient's need for a certain therapy and helps to monitor the response to therapeutic intervention.[16]

A clinical scale based on the morphological involvement has been introduced for assessment of the severity of rhinophymata Table 79-5). No widely accepted classification exists for telangiectasia.[17,106] The severity of papules and pustules in rosacea may be graded according to the numbers of papules and pustules (few, several, or many) and whether plaques (confluent inflammatory lesions on a raised area of erythema) are present. Ocular rosacea should be graded Table 79-6), and ophthalmologic consultation should be initiated promptly in moderate to severe cases.

DIFFERENTIAL DIAGNOSIS

Clinically, the classical (vulgaris) rosacea has to be differentiated from various diseases and rarer rosacea forms Table 79-7), such as granulomatous, lupoid, fulminans, conglobata. Most prominent disorders that may be confused with rosacea are seborrheic dermatitis, acne vulgaris, chronic discoid lupus erythematosus, sarcoidosis, polymorphous light eruption, and erysipelas (see Table 79-7). Thorough examination may be necessary to exclude multisystem involvement if other diagnoses are suspected. The list of diseases mimicking the rosacea phenotype is vast and includes disorders of various etiopathologies. Consideration of the differential diagnoses on the basis of the main feature of skin presentation is therefore useful (Tables 79-8 to 79-16). Helpful observations to differentiate various forms of flushing are shown in Table 79-11.

MANAGEMENT OF ROSACEA

Before therapy, the features and severity of the disease should be rated to define the right therapy, although it should be remembered that some of the features may not be visible or present at consultation. Evaluation of the medical history (including steroids, topical calcineurin inhibitors, brome) should be undertaken, and drug triggers should be ceased. Trigger avoidance is important to improve the condition and protect from relapses and is thus as important as therapy (Fig. 79-13 and Table 79-17).

GENERAL SKIN CARE

Thorough education and instructions for proper general skin care is a critical component of adequate rosacea management because consequent application of adequate nonirritating skin care can significantly prevent or attenuate relapses or tone down dry skin or pain sensations (see Table 79-17). Moreover, educating patients about behavioral strategies and approaches to reduce the facial skin symptoms will reduce the psychological disease burden and significantly improve patient's quality of life and patient outcome.

Essential skin care advice elements are (1) avoidance of trigger factors, (2) usage of foundations and facial coverage without aggravating symptoms of rosacea, (3) use of sunscreen SPF (sun protection factor) of at least 30+, (4) frequent use of moisturizers if dry skin is

TABLE 79-6
Classification of Ocular Rosacea

Mild: mild itch, dryness or grittiness of the eyes; fine scaling of eyelid margins; telangiectasia and erythema of eyelid margins; mild conjunctival injection.
Moderate: burning of eyes; crusting or irregularity of eyelid margins with erythema and edema; formation of chalazion or hordeolum)
Severe: pain, photosensitivity, blurred vision, loss of eyelashes, severe conjunctival inflammation, corneal changes, scleritis or episcleritis, uveitis, iritis

TABLE 79-7
Most Prominent Differential Diagnosis to Rosacea and Investigations

DIFFERENTIAL DIAGNOSIS	INVESTIGATION	DIFFERENTIAL DIAGNOSIS	INVESTIGATION
Acne vulgaris	- Comedones, no flushing, different age peak, no phymatous changes	Facial atopic dermatitis	- Blood work (IL-16, ECP, IgE) - Skin biopsy and histopathologic examination - Anamnesis, patient history, eczema morphology, pruritus
Systemic lupus erythematosus (SLE)	- Patients with SLE often have other areas of cutaneous involvement such as the sides and V of the neck - Systemic reactions - ANA and anti-DNA (anti-Ro, anti-La) - Skin biopsy, histopathologic examination; direct and indirect immunofluorescence	Erysipelas	- Serology (leucocytosis, CRP) - ASO, ADB titer - Fever
		Steroid-induced acneiform folliculitis, steroid rosacea	- Medication - History
		Jessner lymphocytic infiltrate	- No pustules, distribution, history, histology
Chronic discoid lupus erythematosus (CDLE)	- Skin biopsy, histopathologic examination - Direct immunofluorescence (IgG, IgM, IgA, C_1, C_3) - Photosensitivity - UV-induced pruritus	Sarcoidosis	- Serology (ACE, sIL-2R, Neopterin, Ca^{2+}) - Serum electrophoresis (IgG) - Cell count - Histology
Photodamage (heliodermatitis)	- History, photosensitive eruptions, distribution more peripheral	Perioral dermatitis	- Unaffected perioral zone - History of "intensive" local therapy - No flushing; rarely, erythematous plaques
Allergic photoreaction	- Heliotropic macropattern - Diffusely bordered eczema - Eczematous "satellite" lesions - History, photopatch test	Obstruction of superior vena cava	- Facial swelling in the morning - Breathing difficulty - Upper limb edema - Neck edema - Pemberton's sign - Radiography, CT scan, bronchoscopy
Toxic photoreaction	- Heliotropic macropattern - Sharply bordered eczema - History		
Polymorphic light eruption	- More monomorphic - Photo provocation, early and late assessment - Skin biopsy, histopathologic examination	Syphilis	- Serology, - TPHA, VDRL, FTA(Abs) test - Liquor serology
Dermatomyositis	- Muscle weakness - Anti-Jo antibody	Tuberculosis	- Skin biopsy, Ziehl-Neelsen stain - QuantiFERON-TB GIT test - Radiography
Seborrheic dermatitis	- Slight yellow to orange tinge or scales on erythematous ground - More itch, less stinging or burning - Distribution and more eczematous	Haber syndrome	- Family history - Hereditary transmission (autosomal dominant - Burning sensation - Brownish pigmentation, induration
Contact dermatitis	- Morphology of eczema - Patient history - Exposition		

ADB, anti-DNase B; ACE, angiotensin converting enzyme; ANA, antinuclear antibody; ASO, anti-streptolysin O; CRP, C-reactive protein; CT, computed tomography; C1, complement component 1; C3, complement component 3; FTA(Abs), fluorescent treponemal antibody absorption; Ig, immunoglobulin; IL, interleukin; sIL-2R, soluble interleukin-2 receptor; TPHA, treponema pallidum hemagglutination assay; UV, ultraviolet; VDRL, Venereal Disease Research Laboratory.

TABLE 79-8
Differential Diagnosis of Rhinophyma

CONDITION	FEATURES
Lupus pernio (sarcoid of the nose)	Shiny brown, red, or violaceous, firm swelling of nose; can be monomorph and singular; may be asymmetrical; may extend to medial cheeks; diascopy reveals "apple jelly nodules" in lupus pernio; dermoscopy and biopsy help establish diagnosis; workup for systemic involvement required
Basal or squamous cell carcinoma	Age; histology; both mimic or occur in association with rhinophyma; rapid growth and surface erosion or ulceration requires biopsy
Lymphoma or angiosarcoma	Rare; intranasal biopsy may be necessary to diagnose lymphoma; nasal lymphomas may be mistaken for rhinophyma but do not show glandular hyperplasia but a shiny surface
Lupus vulgaris (TB)	Geographical differences of prevalence; can mimic rhinophyma, but scarring often present; also extrafacial; histology
Acrocyanosis	Bluish discoloration of nose, especially in cold weather; usually no deformity; no glandular hyperplasia
Lupus erythematosus	Erythema but no flushing history; scales (CDLE); tendency to scarring is a features of CDLE; more rarely, papules and pustules

CDLE, chronic discoid lupus erythematosus; TB, tuberculosis.

TABLE 79-9
Causes and Differential Diagnoses of Persistent Erythema

Rosacea
Demodicosis
Drug induced (eg, cortisone)
Contact dermatitis
Seborrheic dermatitis
Tinea
Dermatomyositis
Lupus erythematosus
Polymorphous light eruption
Disorders of flushing
Facial erysipelas, Jessner lymphocytic infiltrate, polymorphic light eruption
Granuloma faciale, lymphocytoma cutis, facial sarcoid
Heliodermatitis, atopic dermatitis, contact and photo contact dermatitis
Photodermatitis

---

an issue, (5) usage of drying cleansing for an oily nose, (6) regular use of gentle cleansers for the whole face, (7) use of matte green–toned foundations to mask skin redness, and (9) avoidance of rubbing the face.

FIRST-LINE, SECOND LINE, AND OFF-LABEL TREATMENTS

Based on new knowledge, a phenotype-driven treatment algorithm has recently been developed (see Fig. 79-13) relating to the major cutaneous features of flushing, transient erythema, persistent erythema, papules or pustules, telangiectasia, phymata, and pain sensations. For each feature, first-line therapies vary on the basis of their pathophysiology (Fig. 79-14) and

TABLE 79-10
Causes and Differential Diagnoses of Flushing

Rosacea
Benign causes: emotion (blushing), anxiety, stress, climacteric flushing, hyperthermia, temperature (both hot and cold), sun exposure, fever, exercise, fluorescent lights, foods, beverages, drugs, alcohol, sodium nitrate
Drug-induced (eg, bromindione), peptic ulcer episodes of diarrhea
Systemic diseases: carcinoid syndrome, mastocytosis, polycythemia vera, anaphylaxis, allergy, Zollinger-Ellison syndrome, Rovsing syndrome, Frey syndrome
Neurologic: see later
Tumors: medullary carcinoma of thyroid, renal carcinoma, pancreatic cell tumor (VIP, PACAP, and so on), pheochromocytoma, bronchogenic carcinoma
Postsurgical (gastric, prostate, orchiectomy)
Idiopathic

PACAP, pituitary adenylate cyclase activating peptide; VIP, vasoactive intestinal peptide.

TABLE 79-11
Helpful Observations to Differentiate Various Forms of Flushing

- Menopausal flushing is usually diffuse on the face and the skin often appears shiny because this type of flushing is typically associated with sweating (so-called "hot flushes"). The average hot flush lasts about 4 minutes. Women with hot flushes have an increased body core temperature and a reduced thermo-neutral zone (the body core temperature range above which sweating occurs and below which shivering occurs).[130]
- Hormonal therapy (eg, estrogen) is the standard treatment and can decrease the frequency and severity of hot flushes by up to 90%.
- The flushing that occurs with the carcinoid syndrome, mastocytosis, and pheochromocytoma is not usually accompanied by sweating and so fall into the category of "dry flushing."
- Flush associated with the carcinoid syndrome has been classified into four different patterns. One pattern involves the face and chest and is relatively brief, lasting less than 5 minutes. In other patients, the flush can be prolonged for more than 5 minutes. Persistent edema and "leonine facies" have been reported in a patient with longstanding carcinoid syndrome.[131]
- Flushing may occur in patients with mastocytosis after exercise, ingestion of alcohol or codeine, or injection of polymyxin B. Palpitations, diarrhea, and pruritus may accompany it. Dermatographia is often present.
- Hyperhidrosis, piloerection, and episodic hypertension in association with flushing can occur in patients with phaeochromocytoma. It affects the face, neck, chest, and trunk for 15 minutes to several hours.
- Flushing and severe pruritus or a burning sensation after a hot bath has been reported to patients who have polycythemia. This group appears plethoric and can associate with facial telangiectasias, which affect the face but also distal extremities. The veins of the sclera, retina, and oral mucosa may also be distended.

---

clinical severity. Given that the different symptoms derive from different pathophysiologies, the combination of various topical with systemic treatments or even topical with systemic treatments and physical therapy has to be considered (see Fig. 79-13).[7,108]

If one of the first-line therapies fails, alternative first-line options should be considered or second-line therapies chosen. These therapies should always be combined with an adequate general skin care and prevention therapy.

TABLE 79-12
Differential Diagnosis of Telangiectasias

Chronic discoid lupus erythematosus
Drug induced (eg, cortisone)
Senile atrophy
Basal cell carcinoma
Dermatomyositis
Haber syndrome
Carcinoid syndrome
Systemic lupus erythematosus
Heliodermatosis, polymorphous light eruption
Naevus flammeus
Poikiloderma
Sarcoidosis

TABLE 79-13
Differential Diagnosis of Papules and Pustules

Rosaceiform dermatitis (check drug history, eg, steroid, calcineurin inhibitor intake)
Acne vulgaris (comedones, cysts, and scarring on the chest and back in males)
Perioral dermatitis (check topical steroid usage)
Seborrheic dermatitis (pityriasis capitis is often marked)
Pityriasis folliculorum or demodicosis (skin scraping is helpful)
Tinea faciei, Candida spp. (scraping or swabs for culture), contact dermatitis (patch testing is helpful)
Ulerythema ophryogenes, Jessner lymphocytic infiltrate, lymphocytoma cutis, sarcoid (skin biopsy is helpful)
Morbihan disease, polycythemia, polymorphic light eruption, photosensitive eruption (blood tests and phototesting are helpful)
T. faciei

PERSISTENT ERYTHEMA

For persistent erythema, approved therapeutic regimens are topical brimonidine gel (1%) and oxymetazoline crème (1%). Beta-blockers such as carvedilol can be used off label and should be tapered down.[109] Intense pulse light as well as lasers can be used but should be avoided in patients with rosacea with somatosensations such as pain without pretreatment to avoid aggravation of pain symptoms through neuroinflammation Table 79-18).[8]

If erythema is associated with mild, moderate, or severe pain, topical or systemic analgesic therapy such as lidocaine gel (up to 4%), polidocanol cream (in mild cases), or even systemics such as nonsteroidal antiinflammatory drugs (eg, ibuprofen) should be applied; antidepressants or neuroleptics (eg, amitriptyline, gabapentin, pregabalin) may also need to be prescribed.[110] If suspicious of the cause of pain, consultation of a neurologists is advised to rule out other pain syndromes, such as trigeminal neuralgia, small-fiber neuropathy, or early multiple sclerosis.

FLUSHING AND TRANSIENT ERYTHEMA

Early rosacea is often associated with flushing or transient erythema. Laser therapy (see discussion of physical therapies) is the common treatment used (see Table 79-18). Off-label use of topical adrenergic receptor modulators (eg, brimonidine, oxymetazoline) may alleviate flushing intensity and frequency. Avoidance of triggers (see Table 79-1) is likely to prevent or alleviate flushing, and thus patients should be advised to keep a diary of events. If unsure with any topical agents, patients should test the medication or cosmetic on one spot on one side of the face first. If pain symptoms are associated, the same applies as for persistent erythema. In addition, topical lidocaine (4%) may be helpful.

TABLE 79-14
Differential Diagnosis of Lupoid Rosacea

Perioral dermatitis
Steroid rosacea
Small nodular sarcoidosis

TABLE 79-15
Differential Diagnosis of Rosacea Fulminans

Acne conglobate
Acne fulminans
Halogen rosacea
Gram-negative folliculitis

TELANGIECTASIA

Telangiectasia can only be treated with either laser therapy (see discussion of physical therapies) or 0.5% to 1.0% aethoxysclerol injections, similar to leg sclerotherapy. However, contraindications have to be considered, and the potential induction of vasoocclusion advocates for a cautious application by specialists. Steroid use and sun exposure should be avoided, and sunscreens are helpful to prevent sun damage followed by destruction of the extracellular matrix.

PAPULES AND PUSTULES

Papules and pustules are primary clinical signs and features of rosacea. The basic therapy (avoiding triggers or irritating substances on the affected skin, application of photoprotective agents, appropriate cosmetic coverage, stress management, and optimized skin cleansing and moisturizing routines) as outlined for patients with erythema also applies to patients who develop rosacea with papules and pustules.

In general, mild to moderate papules and pustules respond well to topical therapy such as ivermectin (1%), metronidazole (0.75%–1%), azelaic acid (15%), sodium sulfacetamide, and sulphur. Successful nonapproved (off-label) therapy has been described with topical erythromycin (2%), tretinoin or isotretinoin, clindamycin, and permethrin. However, good evidence indicates that papules and pustules resolve faster and longer using a combination therapy, for example. using the slow-release doxycycline and topical ivermectin. Off-label use with oxytetracycline 500 mg twice a day, doxycycline 100 mg twice a day,

TABLE 79-16
Differential Diagnosis of Halogen Rosacea

Acne vulgaris
Acneiform exanthema
Acneiform syphilid
Rosacea conglobate or fulminans
Follicular pyoderma
Tinea barbae

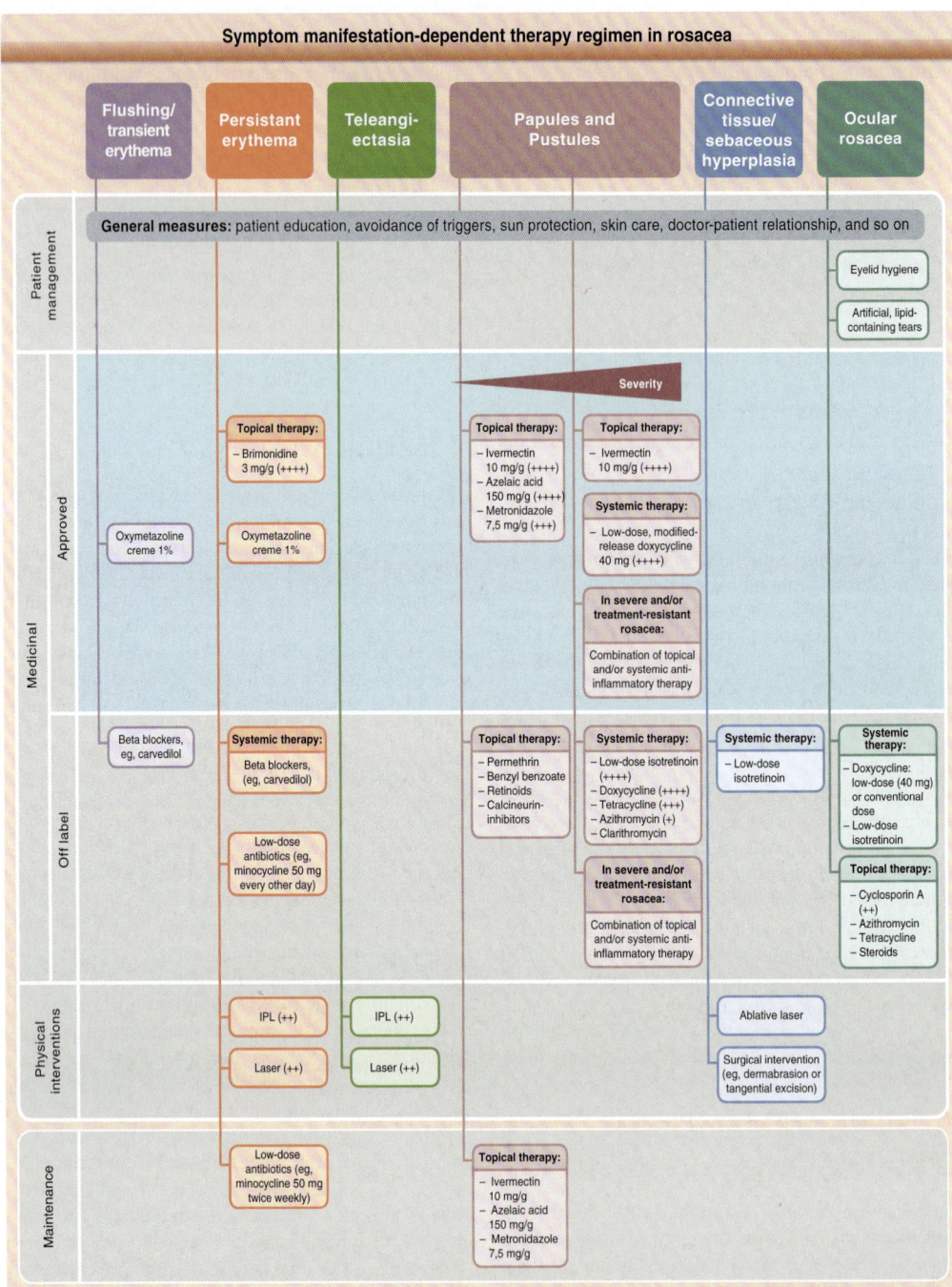

Figure 79-13 Symptom manifestation-dependent therapy regimen in rosacea. IPL, intense pulsed light. (Modified from Schaller M, Schöfer H, Homey B, et al. Rosacea management: update on general measures and topical treatment options. *J Dtsch Dermatol Ges.* 2016;14(Suppl 6):17-27; with permission. Copyright © 2016, John Wiley & Sons.)

minocycline 50 mg/day, erythromycin 500 mg twice a day has been reported with good success and tolerability. In severe or resistant cases, systemic metronidazole, clarithromycin, and azithromycin have relatively rapid onsets of efficacy and fewer tendencies for GI adverse effects than erythromycin and less hyperpigmentation tendency than minocycline. If *Demodex* mite numbers are increased, a short course of permethrin cream should be applied in addition to approved ivermectin cream therapy.

After 3 or 4 months, depending on improvement, systemic therapy can be tapered down while topical therapy is continued. If erythema remains an issue, topical adrenergic receptor blockers (brimonidine, oxy-

TABLE 79-17
Dos and Don'ts for General Rosacea Care

ALLOWED	NOT ALLOWED
Use powder cosmetics with a matte finish; the best is green (complementary color of red).	Use cream or liquid cosmetics.
Try cosmetics before buying them if possible.	Use old cosmetics.
Wear light earth tones (tan, peach, matte green) for eye shadow.	Wear deep eye shadows (blue, purple, red, or pink).
Apply a separate sunblock after topical medication and before cosmetics. Use moisturizer on dry skin with at least SPF20+.	Use cosmetics containing perfume.
Avoid cosmetics using formaldehyde, propylene glycol, alcohol, toners, and palmitic, oleic acid, and other irritants.	Purchase cosmetics with more than 10 ingredients.
Use a flat or soft brush applicator without rubbing.	Apply with a sponge or fingers. Massage creams into the skin. Use peeling "rejuvenating" agents.
Use facial foundation of power or cream variety with matte finish.	Use light-reflective powders containing mica.
Wear only black mascara.	Use nail polish.
Use pencil forms of eyeliner. Start applying new medications or cosmetics on weekends or vacations on one site and take photos to compare sites to reveal potential irritations.	Waterproof eye cosmetics are best avoided.

SPF, sun protection factor.

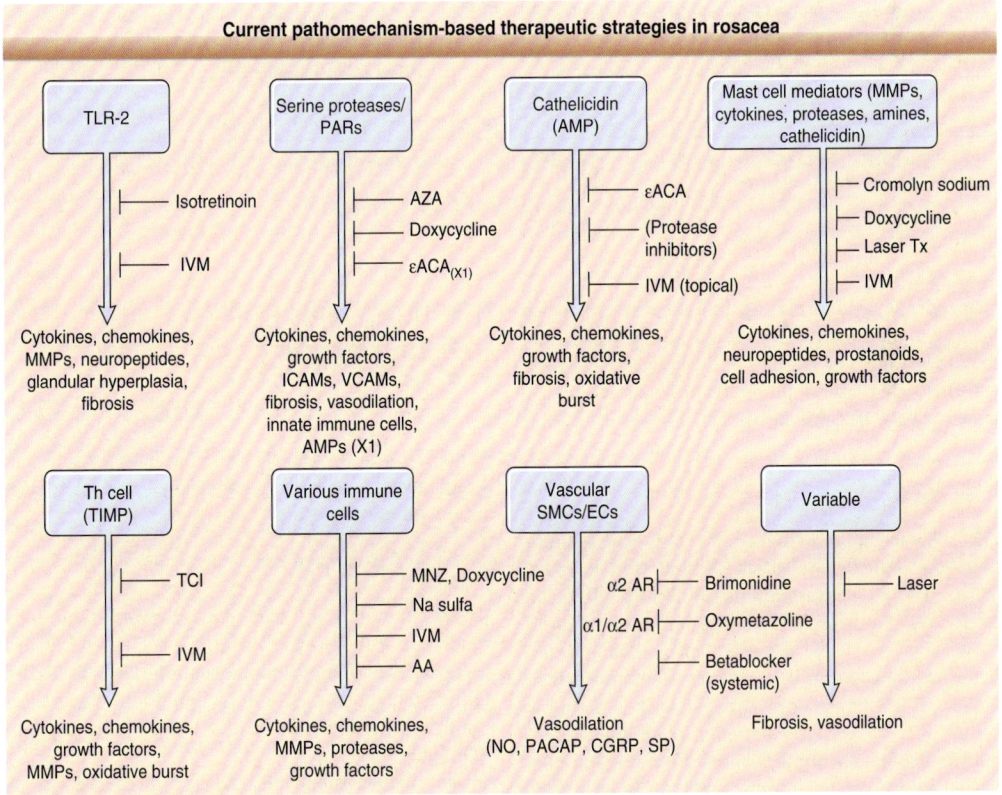

Figure 79-14 Current pathomechanism-based therapeutic strategies in rosacea. AA, azelaic acid; AMP, antimicrobial peptide; AZA, azathioprine; εACA, ε-aminocaproic acid; AR, adrenergic receptor; CGRP, calcitonin gene-related peptide; ECs, endothelial cells; ICAM, intercellular adhesion molecule; IVM, ivermectin; MMP, matrix metalloproteinase; MNZ, minocycline; NO, nitric oxide; PACAP, pituitary adenylate cyclase-activating peptide; PAR, protease-activated receptor; SMC, smooth muscle cell; SP, substance P; TCI, T cell inhibitor; TIMP, tissue inhibitor of metalloproteinases; Th, T helper; TLR, Toll-like receptor; Tx, treatment; VCAM, vascular cell adhesion protein.

TABLE 79-18
Physical Interventions in Rosacea Therapy

	METHOD	SYMPTOM TO TREAT	EVALUATION OR SIDE EFFECTS
Laser therapy	PDL laser	Erythema, telangiectatsia	Advantage over IPL: more selective treatment of blood vessels More effective than Nd:YAG Purpura induction with short pulse duration Prevention of purpura with longer pulse duration of 40–50 ms Side effects: hyper- or hypopigmentation
	PTP laser	Telangiectasia (erythema)	Short healing process, well tolerated Low risk of scaring Better for treatment of telangiectasia than erythema Good safety and tolerability profile
	Nd:YAG laser	Erythema, telangiectasia	Minor pain sensation Less painful than PDL Combination with PDL possible in therapy-resistant cases Risk for atrophic scars
Light therapy	IPL	Erythema, teleangiectatsia, papules or pustules	Good safety and tolerability profile Time-saving procedure
Surgical intervention	Dermabrasion	Phymata	Risk of bleeding
	Electrocautery	Phymata	Rapid procedure Potential side effect: cartilage damage Protracted wound healing disorder Atrophic scaring
	Laser (CO_2- or Er:YAG laser)	Phymata	CO_2: low risk for bleeding Er:YAG: low scaring risk CO_2–Er:YAG combination
	Scalpel excision	Phymata	Risk of intraoperative bleeding Deep tissue excisions or resections Risk: resection of excessive tissue

Er:YAG, erbium-doped yttrium aluminium garnet; IPL, intense pulsed light; Nd:YAG, neodymium-doped yttrium aluminum garnet; PDL laser, pulsed-dye laser; PTP, potassium–titanyl–phosphate.

Modified from Hofmann MA, Lehmann P. Physical modalities for the treatment of rosacea. J Dtsch Dermatol Ges. 2016;14(Suppl 6):38-43; with permission. Copyright © 2016, John Wiley & Sons.

metazoline) may be continued. Topical maintenance therapy may be beneficial to avoid reoccurrence. Successful treatment of papules and pustules have been reported using laser, light, or photodynamic therapy but remains to be clarified.[8]

PHYMATA

There is substantial evidence that low-dose isotretinoin has a beneficial effect in early as well as established rosacea because of its inhibitory effect on sebaceous glands as well as some antiinflammatory capacity.[111] This can be also used before laser and dermatosurgery procedures to reduce size and inflammation. It is often recommended to stop isotretinoin before surgery because isotretinoin inhibits keratinocyte-mediated wound healing. However, no controlled studies exist to inform whether this is also true for low-dose isotretinoin. Rarely, dapsone is used in these cases.

For laser treatment options or surgical therapy, including surgery, cryosurgery, radiofrequency ablation, electrosurgery, and thermosurgery, see the later discussion of physical and surgical procedures.

FACIAL LYMPH EDEMA (MORBIHAN DISEASE)

For facial edema based on lymphatic vessel dilation, no approved or standard therapy exists. Oral isotretinoin, Dapsone, hydroxychloroquine, minocycline, and combined doxycycline–prednisolone have each been tried with mixed results.[112-114]

OCULAR ROSACEA

Every patient with cutaneous rosacea should be questioned about eye symptoms, such as itchy, dry eyes with a foreign body sensation, and avoidance of light. Bloodshot eyes in combination with a thorough family and skin history is often indicative of the disorder.

The management of ocular rosacea has to be defined as a multidisciplinary effort with ophthalmologists and dermatologists involved with or without general practitioners. The severity can range from mild to severe and may lead to chronic defects, even blindness.[9,16,22,23]

General basic includes is eyelid hygiene (warm compresses, meibomian gland expression, dilute baby

TABLE 79-19
Treatment of Ocular Rosacea

THERAPY	COMMENT
Artificial tears	Frequently needed for "dry eyes" of ocular rosacea; use several times daily
Eyelid and eyelash hygiene	Using warm soaks or compresses; can use saline or dilute baby shampoo lavage; overnight creams soften scale and remove plugs from meibomian gland orifices
Expression of meibomian glands	Following hygiene gentle manual massage extrudes thickened, wormlike secretions from glands
Topical antibiotics	Effective treatment for infected blepharitis applied twice daily after eyelid hygiene
Topical steroids	Fucidic acid; metronidazole, erythromycin, and azelaic acid are main options; topical steroids should be used with caution; 1% hydrocortisone cream for blepharitis; may be used in antibiotic–steroid combination
Tacrolimus–cyclosporine	Insufficient evidence to know indications or role in therapy as yet
Systematic antibiotics	As used for PPR; minocycline, doxycycline, oxytetracycline, erythromycin commonly used; 6–12 wk of therapy; response begins after 2 wk; metronidazole used rarely; relapse common after course of therapy completed
Surgery	Incision and curettage for chalazion after eyelid everted; required for keratitis if impending perforation
Other therapies	Topical sulfur, zinc, and ichthammol preparations; hexachlorocyclohexane; vitamin B_2 orally or parentally; omega-3 fatty acid dietary supplementation; topically applied cold tea or tea tree oil

shampoo scrubs, and lubricating drops) and artificial tear substitutes for mild ocular burning or stinging followed by topical and systemic therapy in more severe cases Table 79-19). UV-blocking sunglasses can also be helpful. A proper education about general eye care improves success of treatment (see Table 79-19). In patients with ocular rosacea, screening for cutaneous features is obligatory.

PAIN

See the section on "Erythema and Flushing."

MAINTENANCE THERAPY

Compared with other inflammatory skin diseases, such as atopic dermatitis or psoriasis, the rosacea maintenance therapy regimen is poorly validated and depends on available modalities and the patient's expectance. In the authors' experience, maintenance therapy is superior to sudden discontinuation. General skin care should always be continued, as recommended earlier.

PHYSICAL AND SURGICAL THERAPIES IN ROSACEA

PHYSICAL METHODS

Physical methods such as light and laser therapies, as well as surgical interventions, are important and adequate additions to the often symptom-oriented topical or oral therapies used for rosacea. In an efficient and mostly long-lasting fashion, they supplement the conservative treatment and general skin care. Because several features coexist in many patients, multimodal therapy is often demanded. In patients with erythema and telangiectasia, for example, a combination of topical vasoconstrictors with light or laser therapy is incremental because telangiectasias do not respond to topical or systemic treatment. An initial medical therapy of erythema can also unmask telangiectasias, which are then easier to approach with physical methods.[7,115]

In general, long-term efficacy and safety data from controlled, blinded trials for many procedures are very sparse. However, repetitions of laser procedures are regarded as safe. In ablative procedures of phymata, the risk for scarring is enhanced compared with nonablative techniques; however, no scientific data exist that would validate this generally accepted observation.

For the treatment of erythema and telangiectasia, various light and laser systems exist (see Table 79-18). Laser systems are, for example, the frequency-doubled potassium-titanyl-phosphate laser (PTP; 532 nm), neodymium-doped yttrium aluminum garnet laser (Nd:YAG; 1.064 nm), and pulsed-dye laser (585–595 nm). They act in wavelengths, which are absorbed by hemoglobin and subsequently lead to blood vessel destruction.

Light lamps such as intense pulsed lights (spectrum range of 500-1.200 nm) operate using specific filters in the wavelength of hemoglobin absorption. Older laser generations, such as the argon laser, are out of date because the newer generation lasers exert lower adverse event profiles related to dyspigmentation, scaring, pain, and economic downtime.[8,116,117]

A recent Cochrane review performed a meta-analysis on various laser therapies and concluded for all studies a low to moderate evidence level.[118] However, pulsed-dye laser was superior to Nd:YAG laser and comparable to intense pulsed-light laser. Other studies were not comparable.

SURGICAL INTERVENTIONS

Surgical intervention therapies to treat phymata are scalpel excisions, dermabrasion, electrosurgery and CO_2- or erbium:YAG laser (see Table 79-18). The classical surgical excision and resection is a rapid option for large phymata, with a relatively high bleeding rate. This risk is lower with electrosurgery, which in contrast has a higher risk of deeper tissue destruction. Dermabrasion can be used in mild as well as severe phymata. A good option is also the CO_2 laser, which has a relatively lower risk of bleeding.[8]

REFERENCES

1. Steinhoff M, Buddenkotte J, Aubert J, et al. Clinical, cellular, and molecular aspects in the pathophysiology of rosacea. *J Investig Dermatology Symp Proc*. 2011;15(1):2-11.
2. Del Rosso JQ, Gallo RL, Tanghetti E, et al. An evaluation of potential correlations between pathophysiologic mechanisms, clinical manifestations, and management of rosacea. *Cutis*. 2013;91(3 suppl):1-8.
3. Tan J, Berg M. Rosacea: current state of epidemiology. *J Am Acad Dermatol*. 2013;69(6 suppl 1):S27-S35.
4. Huynh TT. Burden of Disease: the psychosocial impact of rosacea on a patient's quality of life. *Am Heal Drug Benefits*. 2013;6(6):348-354.
5. Schwab VD, Sulk M, Seeliger S, et al. Neurovascular and neuroimmune aspects in the pathophysiology of rosacea. *J Investig Dermatology Symp Proc*. 2011;15(1):53-62.
6. Holmes AD, Steinhoff M. Integrative concepts of rosacea pathophysiology, clinical presentation and new therapeutics. *Exp Dermatol*. 2017;26(8):659-667.
7. Schaller M, Schöfer H, Homey B, et al. State of the art: systemic rosacea management. *J Dtsch Dermatol Ges*. 2016;14
8. Hofmann MA, Lehmann P. Physical modalities for the treatment of rosacea. *J Dtsch Dermatol Ges*. 2016;14(suppl 6):38-43.
9. Schaller M, Almeida LMC, Bewley A, et al. Rosacea treatment update: recommendations from the global ROSacea COnsensus (ROSCO) panel. *Br J Dermatol*. 2017;176(2):465-471.
10. Berg M, Lidén S. An epidemiological study of rosacea. *Acta Derm Venereol*. 1989;69(5):419-423.
11. Tan J, Schöfer H, Araviiskaia E, et al. Prevalence of rosacea in the general population of Germany and Russia—the RISE study. *J Eur Acad Dermatol Venereol*. 2016;30(3):428-434.
12. McAleer MA, Fitzpatrick P, Powell FC. Papulopustular rosacea: prevalence and relationship to photodamage. *J Am Acad Dermatol*. 2010;63(1):33-39.
13. Tan J, Blume-Peytavi U, Ortonne JP, et al. An observational cross-sectional survey of rosacea: clinical associations and progression between subtypes. *Br J Dermatol*. 2013;169(3):555-562.
14. Docherty JR, Steinhoff M, Lorton D, et al. Multidisciplinary consideration of potential pathophysiologic mechanisms of paradoxical erythema with topical brimonidine therapy. *Adv Ther*. 2016;33(11):1885-1895.
15. Abram K, Silm H, Maaroos H-I, et al. Subjective disease perception and symptoms of depression in relation to healthcare-seeking behaviour in patients with rosacea. *Acta Derm Venereol*. 2009;89(5):488-491.
16. Tan J, Almeida LMC, Bewley A, et al. Updating the diagnosis, classification and assessment of rosacea: recommendations from the global ROSacea COnsensus (ROSCO) panel. *Br J Dermatol*. 2017;176(2):431-438.
17. Wilkin J, Dahl M, Detmar M, et al. Standard classification of rosacea: report of the National Rosacea Society Expert Committee on the Classification and Staging of Rosacea. *J Am Acad Dermatol*. 2002;46(4):584-587.
18. Powell FC. Clinical practice. Rosacea. *N Engl J Med*. 2005;352(8):793-803.
19. Gallo RL, Granstein RD, Kang S, et al. Standard classification and pathophysiology of rosacea: the 2017 update by the National Rosacea Society Expert Committee. *J Am Acad Dermatol*. 2018;78(1):148-155.
20. Buhl T, Sulk M, Nowak P, et al. Molecular and morphological characterization of inflammatory infiltrate in rosacea reveals activation of Th1/Th17 pathways. *J Invest Dermatol*. 2015;135(9):2198-2208.
21. Kligman AM. Ocular rosacea. Current concepts and therapy. *Arch Dermatol*. 1997;133(1):89-90.
22. Vieira AC, Mannis MJ. Ocular rosacea: common and commonly missed. *J Am Acad Dermatol*. 2013;69(6 suppl 1):S36-S41.
23. Geerling G, Baudouin C, Aragona P, et al. Emerging strategies for the diagnosis and treatment of meibomian gland dysfunction: proceedings of the OCEAN group meeting. *Ocul Surf*. 2017;15(2):179-192.
24. Aldrich N, Gerstenblith M, Fu P, et al. Genetic vs environmental factors that correlate with rosacea: a cohort-based survey of twins. *JAMA Dermatol*. 2015;151(11):1213-1219.
25. Yazici AC, Tamer L, Ikizoglu G, et al. GSTM1 and GSTT1 null genotypes as possible heritable factors of rosacea. *Photodermatol Photoimmunol Photomed*. 2006;22(4):208-210.
26. Chang ALS, Raber I, Xu J, et al. Assessment of the genetic basis of rosacea by genome-wide association study. *J Invest Dermatol*. 2015;135(6):1548-1555.
27. Woo YR, Lim JH, Cho DH, et al. Rosacea: molecular mechanisms and management of a chronic cutaneous inflammatory condition. *Int J Mol Sci*. 2016;17(9).
28. van Steensel MAM, Badeloe S, Winnepenninckx V, et al. Granulomatous rosacea and Crohn's disease in a patient homozygous for the Crohn-associated NOD2/CARD15 polymorphism R702W. *Exp Dermatol*. 2008;17(12):1057-1058.
29. Karpouzis A, Avgeridis P, Tripsianis G, et al. Assessment of tachykinin receptor 3' gene polymorphism rs3733631 in rosacea. *Int Sch Res Not*. 2015;2015:469402.
30. Silverberg MS, Cho JH, Rioux JD, et al. Ulcerative colitis-risk loci on chromosomes 1p36 and 12q15 found by genome-wide association study. *Nat Genet*. 2009;41(2):216-220.
31. Weinstock LB, Steinhoff M. Rosacea and small intestinal bacterial overgrowth: prevalence and response to rifaximin. *J Am Acad Dermatol*. 2013;68(5):875-876.
32. Drago F, De Col E, Agnoletti AF, et al. The role of small intestinal bacterial overgrowth in rosacea: a 3-year follow-up. *J Am Acad Dermatol*. 2016;75(3):e113-e115.
33. Spoendlin J, Karatas G, Furlano RI, et al. Rosacea in patients with ulcerative colitis and Crohn's disease: a population-based case-control Study. *Inflamm Bowel Dis*. 2016;22(3):680-687.
34. Akin Belli A, Ozbas Gok S, Akbaba G, et al. The relationship between rosacea and insulin resistance and metabolic syndrome. *Eur J Dermatol*. 2016;26(3):260-264.
35. Hua T-C, Chung P-I, Chen Y-J, et al. Cardiovascular comorbidities in patients with rosacea: a nationwide

36. Duman N, Ersoy Evans S, Atakan N. Rosacea and cardiovascular risk factors: a case control study. *J Eur Acad Dermatol Venereol*. 2014;28(9):1165-1169.
37. Rainer BM, Fischer AH, Luz Felipe da Silva D, et al. Rosacea is associated with chronic systemic diseases in a skin severity-dependent manner: results of a case-control study. *J Am Acad Dermatol*. 2015;73(4):604-608.
38. Takci Z, Bilgili SG, Karadag AS, et al. Decreased serum paraoxonase and arylesterase activities in patients with rosacea. *J Eur Acad Dermatol Venereol*. 2015;29(2):367-370.
39. Kota SK, Meher LK, Kota SK, et al. Implications of serum paraoxonase activity in obesity, diabetes mellitus, and dyslipidemia. *Indian J Endocrinol Metab*. 2013;17(3):402-412.
40. Yamasaki K, Di Nardo A, Bardan A, et al. Increased serine protease activity and cathelicidin promotes skin inflammation in rosacea. *Nat Med*. 2007;13(8):975-980.
41. Yamasaki K, Kanada K, Macleod DT, et al. TLR2 expression is increased in rosacea and stimulates enhanced serine protease production by keratinocytes. *J Invest Dermatol*. 2011;131(3):688-697.
42. Melnik BC. Endoplasmic reticulum stress: key promoter of rosacea pathogenesis. *Exp Dermatol*. 2014;23(12):868-873.
43. Egeberg A, Hansen PR, Gislason GH, et al. Patients with rosacea have increased risk of dementia. *Ann Neurol*. 2016;79(6):921-928.
44. Egeberg A, Hansen PR, Gislason GH, et al. Exploring the association between rosacea and Parkinson Disease: a Danish nationwide cohort study. *JAMA Neurol*. 2016;73(5):529-534.
45. Spoendlin J, Voegel JJ, Jick SS, et al. Migraine, triptans, and the risk of developing rosacea: a population-based study within the United Kingdom. *J Am Acad Dermatol*. 2013;69(3):399-406.
46. Gupta MA, Gupta AK, Chen SJ, et al. Comorbidity of rosacea and depression: an analysis of the National Ambulatory Medical Care Survey and National Hospital Ambulatory Care Survey—Outpatient Department data collected by the U.S. National Center for Health Statistics from 1995 to 2002. *Br J Dermatol*. 2005;153(6):1176-1181.
47. Egeberg A, Hansen PR, Gislason GH, et al. Patients with rosacea have increased risk of depression and anxiety disorders: a Danish nationwide cohort study. *Dermatology*. 2016;232(2):208-213.
48. Egeberg A, Hansen PR, Gislason GH, et al. Association of rosacea with risk for glioma in a Danish nationwide cohort study. *JAMA Dermatol*. 2016;152(5):541-545.
49. Jarmuda S, O'Reilly N, Zaba R, et al. Potential role of Demodex mites and bacteria in the induction of rosacea. *J Med Microbiol*. 2012;61(Pt 11):1504-1510.
50. Lazaridou E, Giannopoulou C, Fotiadou C, et al. The potential role of microorganisms in the development of rosacea. *J Dtsch Dermatol Ges*. 2011;9(1):21-25.
51. Sulk M, Seeliger S, Aubert J, et al. Distribution and expression of non-neuronal transient receptor potential (TRPV) ion channels in rosacea. *J Invest Dermatol*. 2012;132(4):1253-1262.
52. Moore C, Cevikbas F, Pasolli HA, et al. UVB radiation generates sunburn pain and affects skin by activating epidermal TRPV4 ion channels and triggering endothelin-1 signaling. *Proc Natl Acad Sci U S A*. 2013;110(34):E3225-E3234.
53. Bonnar E, Eustace P, Powell FC. The Demodex mite population in rosacea. *J Am Acad Dermatol*. 1993;28(3):443-448.
54. Forton F, Seys B. Density of Demodex folliculorum in rosacea: a case-control study using standardized skin-surface biopsy. *Br J Dermatol*. 1993;128(6):650-659.
55. Georgala S, Katoulis AC, Kylafis GD, et al. Increased density of Demodex folliculorum and evidence of delayed hypersensitivity reaction in subjects with papulopustular rosacea. *J Eur Acad Dermatol Venereol*. 2001;15(5):441-444.
56. Steinhoff M, Ständer S, Seeliger S, et al. Modern aspects of cutaneous neurogenic inflammation. *Arch Dermatol*. 2003;139(11):1479-1488.
57. Casas C, Paul C, Lahfa M, et al. Quantification of Demodex folliculorum by PCR in rosacea and its relationship to skin innate immune activation. *Exp Dermatol*. 2012;21(12):906-910.
58. Turgut Erdemir A, Gurel MS, Koku Aksu AE, et al. Demodex mites in acne rosacea: reflectance confocal microscopic study. *Australas J Dermatol*. 2017;58(2):e26-e30.
59. Forton FMN. Papulopustular rosacea, skin immunity and Demodex: pityriasis folliculorum as a missing link. *J Eur Acad Dermatol Venereol*. 2012;26(1):19-28.
60. Sattler EC, Hoffmann VS, Ruzicka T, et al. Reflectance confocal microscopy for monitoring the density of Demodex mites in patients with rosacea before and after treatment. *Br J Dermatol*. 2015;173(1):69-75.
61. Steinhoff M, Buddenkotte J, Shpacovitch V, et al. Proteinase-activated receptors: transducers of proteinase-mediated signaling in inflammation and immune response. *Endocr Rev*. 2005;26(1):1-43.
62. Koller B, Müller-Wiefel AS, Rupec R, et al. Chitin modulates innate immune responses of keratinocytes. *PLoS One*. 2011;6(2):e16594.
63. Gerber PA, Buhren BA, Steinhoff M, et al. Rosacea: the cytokine and chemokine network. *J Investig Dermatol Symp Proc*. 2011;15(1):40-47.
64. Steinhoff M, Vergnolle N, Young SH, et al. Agonists of proteinase-activated receptor 2 induce inflammation by a neurogenic mechanism. *Nat Med*. 2000;6(2):151-158.
65. Seeliger S, Buddenkotte J, Schmidt-Choudhury A, et al. Pituitary adenylate cyclase activating polypeptide: an important vascular regulator in human skin in vivo. *Am J Pathol*. 2010;177(5):2563-2575.
66. Steinhoff M, Schmelz M, Schauber J. Facial erythema of rosacea—aetiology, different pathophysiologies and treatment options. *Acta Derm Venereol*. 2016;96(5):579-586.
67. Dirschka T, Tronnier H, Fölster-Holst R. Epithelial barrier function and atopic diathesis in rosacea and perioral dermatitis. *Br J Dermatol*. 2004;150(6):1136-1141.
68. Ní Raghallaigh S, Powell FC. Epidermal hydration levels in patients with rosacea improve after minocycline therapy. *Br J Dermatol*. 2014;171(2):259-266.
69. Yamasaki K, Gallo RL. Rosacea as a disease of cathelicidins and skin innate immunity. *J Investig dermatology Symp Proc*. 2011;15(1):12-15.
70. Kim JY, Kim YJ, Lim BJ, et al. Increased expression of cathelicidin by direct activation of protease-activated receptor 2: possible implications on the pathogenesis of rosacea. *Yonsei Med J*. 2014;55(6):1648-1655.

71. Ozlu E, Karadag AS, Ozkanli S, et al. Comparison of TLR-2, TLR-4, and antimicrobial peptide levels in different lesions of acne vulgaris. *Cutan Ocul Toxicol*. 2016;35(4):300-309.
72. Meyer-Hoffert U, Schröder J-M. Epidermal proteases in the pathogenesis of rosacea. *J Investig Dermatology Symp Proc*. 2011;15(1):16-23.
73. Lee Y, Kim H, Kim S, et al. Activation of toll-like receptors 2, 3 or 5 induces matrix metalloproteinase-1 and -9 expression with the involvement of MAPKs and NF-kappaB in human epidermal keratinocytes. *Exp Dermatol*. 2010;19(8):e44-e49.
74. Kanada KN, Nakatsuji T, Gallo RL. Doxycycline indirectly inhibits proteolytic activation of tryptic kallikrein-related peptidases and activation of cathelicidin. *J Invest Dermatol*. 2012;132(5):1435-1442.
75. Segovia J, Sabbah A, Mgbemena V, et al. TLR2/MyD88/NF-κB pathway, reactive oxygen species, potassium efflux activates NLRP3/ASC inflammasome during respiratory syncytial virus infection. *PLoS One*. 2012;7(1):e29695.
76. Morizane S, Yamasaki K, Kabigting FD, et al. Kallikrein expression and cathelicidin processing are independently controlled in keratinocytes by calcium, vitamin D(3), and retinoic acid. *J Invest Dermatol*. 2010;130(5):1297-1306.
77. Tschopp J, Schroder K. NLRP3 inflammasome activation: the convergence of multiple signalling pathways on ROS production? *Nat Rev Immunol*. 2010; 10(3):210-215.
78. Rufli T, Büchner SA. T-cell subsets in acne rosacea lesions and the possible role of Demodex folliculorum. *Dermatologica*. 1984;169(1):1-5.
79. Brown TT, Choi E-YK, Thomas DG, et al. Comparative analysis of rosacea and cutaneous lupus erythematosus: histopathologic features, T-cell subsets, and plasmacytoid dendritic cells. *J Am Acad Dermatol*. 2014;71(1):100-107.
80. Jansen T, Kastner U, Kreuter A, et al. Rosacea-like demodicidosis associated with acquired immunodeficiency syndrome. *Br J Dermatol*. 2001;144(1):139-142.
81. Basta-Juzbašić A, Subić JS, Ljubojević S. Demodex folliculorum in development of dermatitis rosaceiformis steroidica and rosacea-related diseases. *Clin Dermatol*. 20(2):135-140.
82. Teraki Y, Hitomi K, Sato Y, et al. Tacrolimus-induced rosacea-like dermatitis: a clinical analysis of 16 cases associated with tacrolimus ointment application. *Dermatology*. 2012;224(4):309-314.
83. McFadden JP, Powles AV, Walker M. Rosacea induced by PUVA therapy. *Br J Dermatol*. 1989;121(3):413.
84. Kim M, Kim K-E, Jung HY, et al. Recombinant erythroid differentiation regulator 1 inhibits both inflammation and angiogenesis in a mouse model of rosacea. *Exp Dermatol*. 2015;24(9):680-685.
85. Salzer S, Ruzicka T, Schauber J. Face-to-face with anti-inflammatory therapy for rosacea. *Exp Dermatol*. 2014;23(6):379-381.
86. Jones D. Reactive oxygen species and rosacea. *Cutis*. 2004;74(3 suppl):17-20, 32-34.
87. Aroni K, Tsagroni E, Kavantzas N, et al. A study of the pathogenesis of rosacea: how angiogenesis and mast cells may participate in a complex multifactorial process. *Arch Dermatol Res*. 2008;300(3):125-131.
88. Drummond PD, Su D. Endothelial and axon reflex vasodilatation to acetylcholine in rosacea-affected skin. *Arch Dermatol Res*. 2012;304(2):133-137.
89. Jancsó N, Jancsó-Gábor A, Szolcsányi J. Direct evidence for neurogenic inflammation and its prevention by denervation and by pretreatment with capsaicin. *Br J Pharmacol ChemoTher*. 1967;31(1):138-151.
90. Aubdool AA, Brain SD. Neurovascular aspects of skin neurogenic inflammation. *J Investig dermatology Symp Proc*. 2011;15(1):33-39.
91. Baylie RL, Brayden JE. TRPV channels and vascular function. *Acta Physiol (Oxf)*. 2011;203(1):99-116.
92. Metzler-Wilson K, Toma K, Sammons DL, et al. Augmented supraorbital skin sympathetic nerve activity responses to symptom trigger events in rosacea patients. *J Neurophysiol*. 2015;114(3):1530-1537.
93. Black PH. Stress and the inflammatory response: a review of neurogenic inflammation. *Brain Behav Immun*. 2002;16(6):622-653.
94. Kim JE, Cho BK, Cho DH, et al. Expression of hypothalamic-pituitary-adrenal axis in common skin diseases: evidence of its association with stress-related disease activity. *Acta Derm Venereol*. 2013;93(4):387-393.
95. Johnson JM, Minson CT, Kellogg DL. Cutaneous vasodilator and vasoconstrictor mechanisms in temperature regulation. *Compr Physiol*. 2014;4(1):33-89.
96. Del Rosso JQ. Management of facial erythema of rosacea: what is the role of topical α-adrenergic receptor agonist therapy? *J Am Acad Dermatol*. 2013;69 (6 suppl 1):S44-S56.
97. Muto Y, Wang Z, Vanderberghe M, et al. Mast cells are key mediators of cathelicidin-initiated skin inflammation in rosacea. *J Invest Dermatol*. 2014;134(11):2728-2736.
98. Helfrich YR, Maier LE, Cui Y, et al. Clinical, histologic, and molecular analysis of differences between erythematotelangiectatic rosacea and telangiectatic photoaging. *JAMA dermatology*. 2015;151(8):825-836.
99. Mould TL, Roberts-Thomson PJ. Pathogenesis of telangiectasia in scleroderma. *Asian Pacific J Allergy Immunol*. 2000;18(4):195-200.
100. Holmes AD. Potential role of microorganisms in the pathogenesis of rosacea. *J Am Acad Dermatol*. 2013;69(6):1025-1032.
101. Haber R, El Gemayel M. Comorbidities in rosacea: a systematic review and update. *J Am Acad Dermatol*. 2018;78(4):786-792.e8.
102. Ciccarese G, Parodi A, Rebora A, et al. The usefulness of investigating the possible underlying conditions in rosacea. *J Eur Acad Dermatol Venereol*. 2018;32(3):e88-e89.
103. Parodi A, Paolino S, Greco A, et al. Small intestinal bacterial overgrowth in rosacea: clinical effectiveness of its eradication. *Clin Gastroenterol Hepatol*. 2008;6(7):759-764.
104. Drago F, Ciccarese G, Parodi A. Effects of the treatment for small intestine bacterial overgrowth on rosacea. *J Dermatol*. 2017;44(12):e321.
105. Crawford GH, Pelle MT, James WD. Rosacea: I. Etiology, pathogenesis, and subtype classification. *J Am Acad Dermatol*. 2004;51(3):327-414.
106. Wilkin J, Dahl M, Detmar M, et al. Standard grading system for rosacea: report of the National Rosacea Society Expert Committee on the classification and staging of rosacea. *J Am Acad Dermatol*. 2004;50(6):907-912.
107. Weinkle AP, Doktor V, Emer J. Update on the management of rosacea. *Clin Cosmet Investig Dermatol*. 2015;8:159-177.
108. Steinhoff M, Vocanson M, Voegel JJ, et al. Topical ivermectin 10 mg/g and oral doxycycline 40 mg modified-release: current evidence on the complementary use

of anti-inflammatory rosacea treatments. *Adv Ther*. 2016;33(9):1481-1501.
109. Pietschke K, Schaller M. Long-term management of distinct facial flushing and persistent erythema of rosacea by treatment with carvedilol. *J Dermatolog Treat*. 2017:1-4.
110. Scharschmidt TC, Yost JM, Truong SV, et al. Neurogenic rosacea: a distinct clinical subtype requiring a modified approach to treatment. *Arch Dermatol*. 2011;147(1):123-126.
111. Schmidt JB, Gebhart W, Raff M, et al. 13-cis-Retinoic acid in rosacea. Clinical and laboratory findings. *Acta Derm Venereol*. 1984;64(1):15-21.
112. Veraldi S, Persico MC, Francia C. Morbihan syndrome. *Indian Dermatol Online J*. 2013;4(2):122-124.
113. Fujimoto N, Mitsuru M, Tanaka T. Successful treatment of Morbihan disease with long-term minocycline and its association with mast cell infiltration. *Acta Derm Venereol*. 2015;95(3):368-369.
114. Ranu H, Lee J, Hee TH. Therapeutic hotline: successful treatment of Morbihan's disease with oral prednisolone and doxycycline. *Dermatol Ther*. 23(6):682-685.
115. Schaller M, Schöfer H, Homey B, et al. Rosacea management: update on general measures and topical treatment options. *J Dtsch Dermatol Ges*. 2016;14(suppl 6):17-27.
116. Arndt KA. Argon laser therapy of small cutaneous vascular lesions. *Arch Dermatol*. 1982;118(4):220-224.
117. Laube S, Lanigan SW. Laser treatment of rosacea. *J Cosmet Dermatol*. 2002;1(4):188-195.
118. van Zuuren EJ, Fedorowicz Z, Carter B, et al. Interventions for rosacea. *Cochrane database Syst Rev*. 2015;(4):CD003262.
119. Shpacovitch VM, Brzoska T, Buddenkotte J, et al. Agonists of proteinase-activated receptor 2 induce cytokine release and activation of nuclear transcription factor kappaB in human dermal microvascular endothelial cells. *J Invest Dermatol*. 2002;118(2):380-385.
120. Buddenkotte J, Stroh C, Engels IH, et al. Agonists of proteinase-activated receptor-2 stimulate upregulation of intercellular cell adhesion molecule-1 in primary human keratinocytes via activation of NF-kappa B. *J Invest Dermatol*. 2005;124(1):38-45.
121. Moormann C, Artuc M, Pohl E, et al. Functional characterization and expression analysis of the proteinase-activated receptor-2 in human cutaneous mast cells. *J Invest Dermatol*. 2006;126(4):746-755.
122. Rallabhandi P, Nhu QM, Toshchakov VY, et al. Analysis of proteinase-activated receptor 2 and TLR4 signal transduction: a novel paradigm for receptor cooperativity. *J Biol Chem*. 2008;283(36):24314-24325.
123. Shpacovitch VM, Varga G, Strey A, et al. Agonists of proteinase-activated receptor-2 modulate human neutrophil cytokine secretion, expression of cell adhesion molecules, and migration within 3-D collagen lattices. *J Leukoc Biol*. 2004;76(2):388-398.
124. Nakayama M, Niki Y, Kawasaki T, et al. IL-32-PAR2 axis is an innate immunity sensor providing alternative signaling for LPS-TRIF axis. *Sci Rep*. 2013;3:2960.
125. Yamasaki K, Schauber J, Coda A, et al. Kallikrein-mediated proteolysis regulates the antimicrobial effects of cathelicidins in skin. *FASEB J*. 2006;20(12):2068-2080.
126. Ramanathan B, Davis EG, Ross CR, et al. Cathelicidins: microbicidal activity, mechanisms of action, and roles in innate immunity. *Microbes Infect*. 2002;4(3):361-372.
127. Jang YH, Sim JH, Kang HY, et al. Immunohistochemical expression of matrix metalloproteinases in the granulomatous rosacea compared with the non-granulomatous rosacea. *J Eur Acad Dermatol Venereol*. 2011;25(5):544-548.
128. Tewari A, Grys K, Kollet J, et al. Upregulation of MMP12 and its activity by UVA1 in human skin: potential implications for photoaging. *J Invest Dermatol*. 2014;134(10):2598-2609.
129. Steinhoff MS, von Mentzer B, Geppetti P, et al. Tachykinins and their receptors: contributions to physiological control and the mechanisms of disease. *Physiol Rev*. 2014;94(1):265-301.
130. Freedman RR. Physiology of hot flashes. *Am J Hum Biol*. 2001;13(4):453-464.
131. Abreu Velez AM, Howard MS. Diagnosis and treatment of cutaneous paraneoplastic disorders. *Dermatol Ther*. 2010;23(6):662-675.

Chapter 80 :: Acne Variants and Acneiform Eruptions
:: Andrea L. Zaenglein, Emmy M. Graber, & Diane M. Thiboutot

第八十章
痤疮异型和痤疮样疹

中文导读

本章作者将临床各种痤疮异型、痤疮样疹及与之相关的综合症进行了详细的归纳和总结。

痤疮异型方面介绍了新生儿痤疮、婴儿痤疮、童年中期痤疮及其可能的发病机制，提醒医生接诊过程中应仔细体查，必要时应做相应的实验室检测；针对两种最严重的痤疮异型，聚合性痤疮和暴发性痤疮予以了详细介绍，推荐使用异维A酸和或糖皮质激素治疗；还提及了一些罕见痤疮异型，如实质性面部肿胀、SAPHO综合征、PAPA、PASH、PAPSH综合征、APERT综合征等，并引用相关文献阐述了综合征相关的可能发病机制及可能有效的治疗药物；另外提及因机械摩擦和心理行为所致的相关痤疮异型，分别是机械性痤疮和少女人为痤疮，其发病机制不明确，改变行为可使病情得到改善。虽然大部分寻常痤疮患者不伴有内分泌问题，但有少部分患者的皮损是可由内分泌异常促发或加重的，因此需仔细问问病史并做细致的体查，必要时应行实验室检查。

痤疮样疹方面详细列举了常见的痤疮样疹，如药物所致的类固醇毛囊炎、革兰阴性毛囊炎、EGFR抑制剂所致痤疮样疹（表80-1）以及各种因素所致的热带痤疮、放射性痤疮、夏季痤疮、鼻皱褶假痤疮、Apert综合征及口周皮炎，并详细介绍了与之相关的可能致病因素和预防治疗措施。特别是对于口周皮炎进行了详尽的介绍，认为目前关于此病的发病机制尚不明确，强调治疗应该避免局部使用糖皮质激素，可以外用抗生素和抗炎药物。

〔李 吉〕

AT-A-GLANCE

- Mid-childhood acne warrants evaluation for various causes of hyperandrogenism.
- Acne fulminans and isotretinoin-induced acne fulminans represent severe presentations of acne. Management should include both modified dosing of isotretinoin and systemic corticosteroids.
- Acne conglobata is a severe, nodular form of acne that heals with extensive scarring.
- Acne excoriee, or skin-picking disorder, is a psychological disorder, and patients should be comanaged with psychiatric providers.
- Periorificial dermatitis is a common acneiform eruption often caused by topical or inhaled corticosteroids.

ACNE VARIANTS

NEONATAL ACNE

Neonatal acne can occur in up to 20% of healthy newborns. Lesions usually appear around 2 weeks of age and resolve spontaneously within 3 months. Typically, small, inflamed papules congregate over the nasal bridge and cheeks (Fig. 80-1). Because comedo formation is absent, the pathogenesis of neonatal acne may be different than acne vulgaris. It has been shown that sebum excretion rates in newborns are transiently elevated in the perinatal period.[1] Additionally, *Malassezia sympodialis*, a normal commensal on human skin, may also play a role. Some reports have demonstrated positive cultures of the pustules with *Malassezia* spp. and improvement with ketoconazole cream.[2] Although there appears to be a strong association between *Malassezia* spp. and neonatal acne, definite causality has not yet been proven.[3] *Neonatal cephalic pustulosis* presents with similar but widespread papulopustular lesions over face, scalp, upper chest and back, and shoulders.

INFANTILE ACNE

Infantile acne presents at 3 to 6 months of age classically with open and closed comedones over the cheeks and chin. (Fig. 80-2). Papules, pustules, and nodules can also present on the face. Pitted scarring may occur even with relatively mild disease. Infantile acne is caused in part by the transient elevation of dehydroepiandrosterone (DHEA) produced by the immature adrenal gland.[4] Additionally, during the first 6 to 12 months of life, boys may also have an increased level of luteinizing hormone (LH) that stimulates testosterone production. Around 1 year of age, these hormone levels begin to stabilize until they surge again during adrenarche. As a result, infantile acne usually resolves around 1 to 2 years of age. Treatment gener-

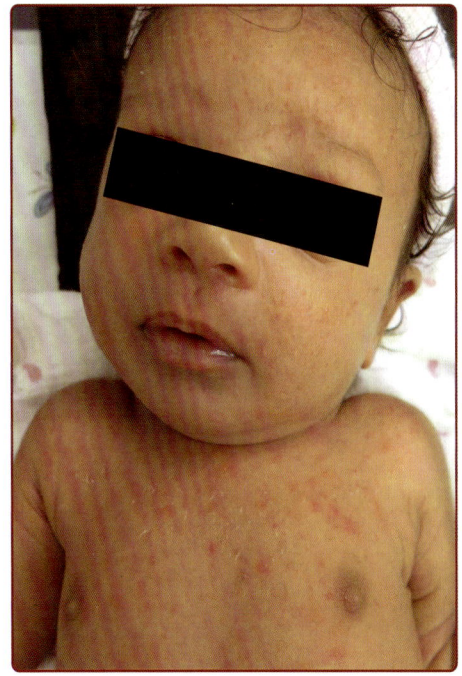

Figure 80-1 Neonatal acne. Small, erythematous papules and pustules over the face and chest in a newborn.

ally consists of topical retinoids and benzoyl peroxide. Oral therapy with erythromycin, azithromycin, trimethoprim, or isotretinoin can be used in severe or refractory cases.

MID-CHILDHOOD ACNE

Mid-childhood acne is defined as appearing between 1 and 7 years of age.[5] Typically, acne is very rare in this age group because the adrenal and gonadal production of androgens should be quiescent. Therefore, any child with acne in mid-childhood should be evaluated

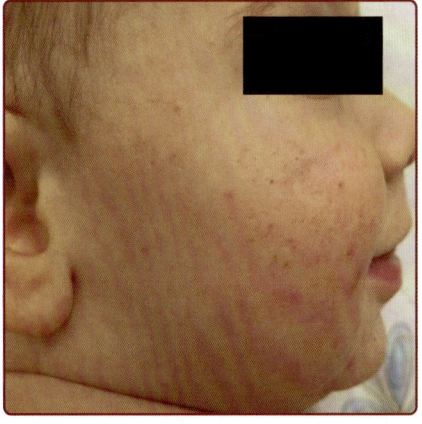

Figure 80-2 Infantile acne. Primarily open and closed comedones over the cheeks of a 5-month-old infant.

for other signs of hyperandrogenism (pubic or axillary hair, testicular enlargement or breast development). In addition, the child's growth chart should be compared with the bone age to determine if child's growth is accelerated as well. If any additional abnormalities are noted, further laboratory workup for hyperandrogenism is warranted with the input of a pediatric endocrinologist.

ACNE CONGLOBATA

This severe form of nodular acne is most common in teenage males but can occur in either sex and into adulthood. Acne conglobata (*conglobate* means shaped in a rounded mass or ball) is a mixture of comedones, papules, pustules, nodules, abscesses, and scars arising in a more generalized pattern over the back, buttocks, chest, and, to a lesser extent, on the abdomen, shoulders, neck, face, upper arms, and thighs (see Fig. 78-4). The comedones often have multiple openings. The inflammatory lesions are large, tender, and dusky colored. Draining lesions discharge a foul-smelling serous, purulent, or mucoid material. Subcutaneous dissection with the formation of multichanneled sinus tracts is common. Healing results in an admixture of depressed and keloidal scars. The management of these patients is challenging. The use of isotretinoin is highly effective in these patients. However, because severe flares may occur when isotretinoin is started, the initial dose should be 0.5 mg/kg/day or less, and systemic glucocorticoids are often required either before initiating isotretinoin therapy or as concomitant therapy. Systemic tetracyclines, intralesional glucocorticoids, systemic glucocorticoids, surgical debridement, surgical incision, and surgical excision may also be required to effectively control acne conglobata.

ACNE FULMINANS

Acne fulminans (also known as acute febrile ulcerative acne) is the most severe form of acne and may

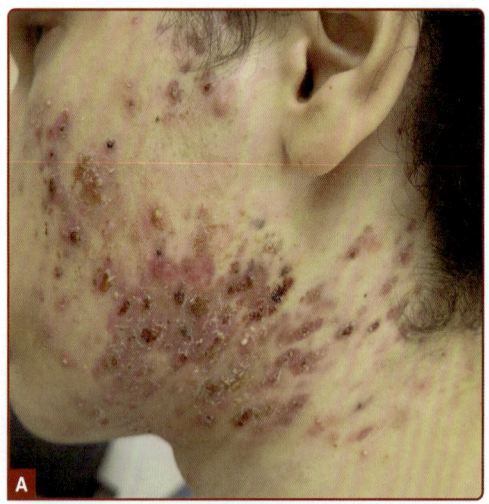
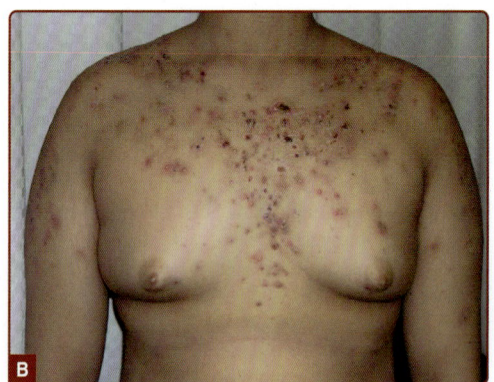
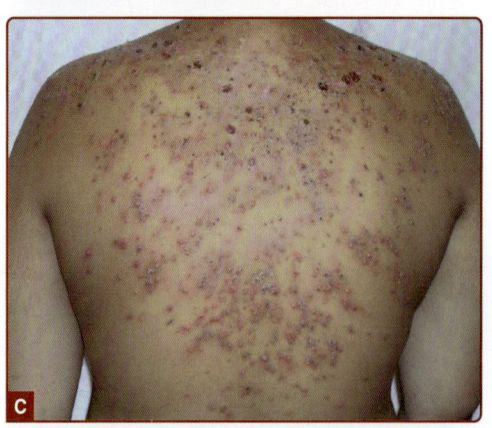
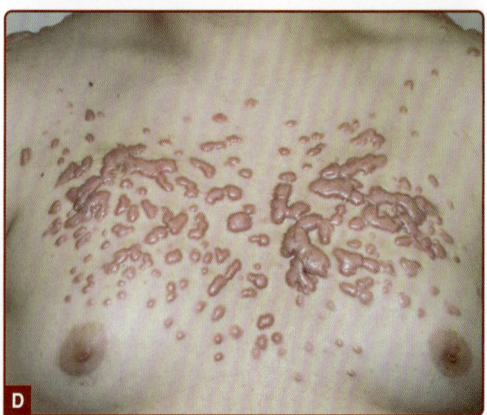

Figure 80-3 **A,** Acne fulminans. An eruptive form of acne with extensive inflammatory papules and nodules on the face, coalescing with ecchymoses and crusting. **B** and, Eruptive, uniform friable papules over the chest and back with crusting. **D,** Resultant keloid scars in the same patient.

occur with or without systemic symptoms. The sudden appearance of inflammatory, tender, oozing, friable plaques with hemorrhagic crusts characterizes this extreme presentation. The lesions predominate on the chest and back (Fig. 80-3) and rapidly become ulcerative and heal with scarring. The disease is reported to occur primarily in teenage boys. Systemic symptoms are often present. The patients are febrile; have a leukocytosis of 10,000 to 30,000/mm³ white blood cells; and usually have polyarthralgia, myalgia, hepatosplenomegaly, and anemia. Bone pain is common, especially at the clavicle and sternum. Radiologic examination may demonstrate lytic bone lesions. Occasionally, there is accompanying erythema nodosum. Although this disease is often classified with acne conglobata, there are basic differences. The onset of acne fulminans is more explosive; nodules and polymorphous comedones are less common; the face is not involved as frequently, and the neck is usually spared; ulcerative and crusted lesions are unique; and systemic symptoms are more common.

Systemic glucocorticoid therapy, along with intralesional glucocorticoids, is first-line treatment for acne fulminans. Systemic glucocorticoids (prednisone 0.5–1.0 mg/kg/day) are started before isotretinoin for 2 to 4 weeks, depending on the severity of systemic symptoms, and continued during the first few weeks to months of isotretinoin therapy. The initial dosing of isotretinoin should be quite low (0.1 mg/kg/day) during the initial weeks of therapy until the inflammation is controlled.[6] The daily dose of glucocorticoids should be slowly decreased as tolerated over weeks to months. Alternately, 0.5 mg/kg/day of isotretinoin started immediately with 10 mg of prednisolone three times daily has been recommended.[7] Dapsone in conjunction with isotretinoin has been reportedly beneficial in the treatment of acne fulminans associated with erythema nodosum.[8] Cyclosporine, anakinra, and tumor necrosis factor (TNF) inhibitors have also been used in difficult cases of acne fulminans.[9-11]

ISOTRETINOIN-INDUCED ACNE FULMINANS

In contrast to the de novo version, isotretinoin-induced acne fulminans arises after starting isotretinoin therapy for acne. An explosive flare of tender, oozing, friable plaques with hemorrhagic crusts occurs with or without associated systemic symptoms. The flaring typically arises within the first month of treatment but may occur later. The pharmacomechanism of this unfortunate adverse reaction is not fully understood. Patients with severe inflammatory acne in particular are at risk. Lower starting doses of isotretinoin (0.3 to 0.5 mg/kg/day) and the concomitant addition of systemic corticosteroids may prevent flaring. If isotretinoin-induced acne fulminans does occur, the isotretinoin dose should be lowered or discontinued and prednisone therapy immediately started, following the guidelines for the management of acne fulminans above.

SAPHO SYNDROME

SAPHO syndrome is manifested by synovitis, acne, pustulosis, hyperostosis, and osteitis. It is predominantly associated with hyperostosis of the anterior chest, palmoplantar pustulosis, hidradenitis suppurativa, and acne fulminans. Its cause is unknown. Reported successful treatments for SAPHO syndrome include nonsteroidal antiinflammatory drugs, sulfasalazine, infliximab, adalimumab, methotrexate.[12] Paradoxically, worsening of SAPHO skin manifestations can be seen with anti-TNF agents.[13,14] The bisphosphonates are beneficial for treating the associated bone pain.[15]

PAPA, PASH, AND PAPSH SYNDROME

PAPA (pyogenic arthritis, pyoderma gangrenosum and acne), PASH (pyoderma gangrenosum, acne and hidradenitis suppurativa) and PAPASH (pyogenic arthritis, acne, pyoderma gangrenosum and hidradenitis suppurativa) are a group of systemic autoinflammatory disorders resulting from dysregulation of the innate immune system and over production of interleukin (IL)-1.[16] Patients with these disorders have a variable combination of sterile neutrophilic skin lesions, including acne, pyogenic granuloma, and hidradenitis suppurativa, and pyogenic arthritis. They may also give a history of inflammatory bowel disease and pancytopenia after administration of sulfa-containing medications. Mutations in the protein serine–threonine phosphatase interacting protein (PSTPIP1) results in an increase in IL-1β production.[17] There have been reports of successful treatment with cyclosporine, dapsone, infliximab, and anakinra.[18,19]

ACNE EXCORIÉE

Acne excoriée (or acne excoriée des jeunes filles) is a variant of skin-picking disorder. Often quite mild acne is systematically and neurotically excoriated, leaving crusted erosions that may scar. It is more common in females. Acne excoriée and skin-picking disorder are now recognized as excoriation disorders by the American Psychiatric Association in the *Diagnostic and Statistical Manual of Mental Disorders*, 5th edition (DSM-5).[20] They are categorized under obsessive-compulsive disorders and as such should be comanaged with psychiatry to address both the acne and the underlying psychogenic excoriation. That said, many patients are lost to follow-up, and there is a low rate of referral to mental health providers.[21]

ACNE MECHANICA

Acneiform eruptions have been observed after repetitive physical trauma to the skin such as pressure, friction, or rubbing. Two types of reactions result, either a flare in acne with comedones and inflammatory papules ("acne mechanica") or follicular inflammatory lesions ("folliculitis mechanica").[22] This can occur from clothing (belts and straps), sports equipment (football helmets and shoulder pads), and with crutches and prosthetics.[23,24] A classic example of acne mechanica is "fiddler's neck," produced where the violin pad repetitively rubs against the player's lateral neck.[25] The pathogenesis of these reactions are not fully understood. Alterations in the barrier function, microbiome, and activation of innate immune system, as well as keratinocyte disruption and increase in IL-1a are purposed to play a role.[22,26]

ACNE WITH SOLID FACIAL EDEMA

A rare and disfiguring variant of acne vulgaris is acne with solid facial edema, also known as Morbihan disease. There is a woody edema of the mid third face with accompanying erythema and acne. Similar changes have been reported with rosacea and Melkerson-Rosenthal syndrome. There may be fluctuations in the severity of the edema, but spontaneous resolution does not occur. Diagnosis can be made clinically. The histology of solid facial edema is nonspecific with dermal edema, fibrosis, dilated blood vessels, and a mixed inflammatory infiltrate.[27] Oral antibiotic treatment in acne with solid facial edema is typically ineffective. Treatment with low-dose isotretinoin (0.2–0.5 mg/kg/day) alone or in combination with oral glucocorticoids, ketotifen (1–2 mg/day), or clofazimine for 4 to 5 months has been reported to be beneficial.[28-30]

ACNE WITH ASSOCIATED ENDOCRINOLOGY ABNORMALITIES

Although the majority of cases of acne vulgaris occur in patients without endocrinologic disturbances, there are specific populations whose acne is driven or worsened by endocrine abnormalities. As mentioned previously, it is important to screen patients for such abnormalities by taking a thorough history. In females, in addition to the presence of acne, hyperandrogenism may be marked by irregular menstrual cycles, a deepened voice, increased libido, and hirsutism. Laboratory work can help define an endocrinologic problem causing acne.

POLYCYSTIC OVARIAN SYNDROME

Polycystic ovarian syndrome (PCOS) occurs in roughly 5% to 10% of women. Hyperandrogenism, acne, insulin resistance, and acanthosis nigricans are clinical markers of this syndrome. PCOS should be suspected in women with any combination of oligomenorrhea, clinical or biochemical hyperandrogenism, or polycystic ovaries on ultrasound scan.[31] Premenarchal women with acne and hirsutism should be screened for PCOS with a serum free testosterone level.[32,33] Additional testing may be indicated if the result is abnormal. In typical cases, testing should be deferred until 2 years after menarche because of the lack of established laboratory norms and inherent irregularity of menstrual cycles in this age group.[34] Women with PCOS are at increased risk of infertility, impaired glucose tolerance, type 2 diabetes, dyslipidemia, endometrial cancer, and cardiovascular disease. Combined oral contraceptives with spironolactone can be helpful in controlling acne and hirsutism.[35,36] The addition of metformin can also beneficial.[37] Additional treatment consists of weight management, lipid control, regulation of insulin resistance, and fertility assistance.[32]

CONGENITAL ADRENAL HYPERPLASIA

Congenital adrenal hyperplasia (CAH) is an autosomal recessive disorder caused by varying enzyme defects in the cortisol production pathway. 21β-hydroxylase, deficiency can result in both a classic severe type and as a nonclassic mild type. Neonates are screened at birth for the classic type and typically present with ambiguous genitalia and salt wasting. The nonclassic type is not identified at birth and can present throughout childhood and adolescence. The prevalence of the nonclassic type in the white population is 0.1%. Patients with this type of CAH have normal cortisol levels but increased androgens. Female patients present with findings similar to PCOS, including precocious puberty, irregular menses, polycystic ovaries, hirsutism, and acne.[38] Values of dehydroepiandrosterone sulfate (DHEAS) in the range of 4000 to 8000 ng/mL are suggestive of CAH. Findings of CAH in males are often subtle and acne may be the only sign. CAH should be considered in patients who do not respond to treatment.[39] Treatment of patients with CAH consists of low-dose replacement of glucocorticoids, as well as oral contraceptives, spironolactone, or flutamide in females.

ACNEIFORM ERUPTIONS

STEROID FOLLICULITIS

As early as 2 weeks after initiation of systemic glucocorticoids or corticotropin, folliculitis may appear. Similar lesions may follow the prolonged application of topical glucocorticoids to the face or with inhaled steroids for asthma. The pathology of steroid acne is that of a focal folliculitis with a neutrophilic infiltrate in and around the follicle. This type of acne clearly differs from acne vulgaris in its distribution and in the type of lesions observed. The lesions, which are usually all in the same stage of development, consist of small pustules and red papules. In contrast to acne vulgaris, they appear mainly on the trunk, shoulders, and upper arms, with lesser involvement of the face. Postinflammatory hyperpigmentation may occur, but comedones, cysts, and scarring are unusual. Steroid folliculitis is uncommon in younger children. Treatment consists primarily of stopping any corticosteroid use. Typical acne treatments such as topical retinoids and antibiotics may also be helpful.

DRUG-INDUCED ACNE

In addition to glucocorticoids, other medicines can also cause a monomorphic, diffuse papular eruption that mimics steroid folliculitis. Such drugs include phenytoin, lithium, isoniazid, high doses of vitamin B complexes, halogenated compounds, and certain chemotherapy medications (Table 80-1). Halogenated compounds containing either bromides or iodides are often found in cold and asthma remedies, sedatives, radiopaque contrast material, kelp, and other vitamin and mineral combinations. With iodides, in particular, inflammation may be marked.[40,41] The iodine content of iodized salt is low and; therefore, it is extremely unlikely that enough iodized salt could be ingested to cause this type of acne.

EPIDERMAL GROWTH FACTOR RECEPTOR INHIBITOR ASSOCIATED ERUPTION

Epidermal growth factor receptor (EGFR) inhibitors may also cause a follicular-based eruption. EGFR inhibitors are primarily used to treat non–small-cell lung cancer, colorectal cancer, and breast cancer. Some of the EGFR inhibitors include the monoclonal antibodies cetuximab, panitumumab, necitumumab, pertuzumab, and small-molecule tyrosine kinase inhibitors gefitinib, erlotinib, afatinib, osimertinib, and lapatinib. A frequent side effect of the EGFR inhibitors is a perifollicular, papulopustular eruption distributed on the face and upper torso. The eruption occurs in up to 86% of patients treated with EGFR inhibitors.[42] An associated lateral paronychia may also occur. Histopathological sections of lesional skin show a noninfectious perifolliculitis. The cause of the acneiform eruption is not clear, but it may occur because EGFR is highly expressed in the basal cell layer of the epidermis, follicular keratinocytes, and the sebaceous epithelium. The presence and severity of the eruption correlates with a positive treatment response.[42,43] If the eruption is absent, dosing may be inadequate, or the patient's tumor may be unresponsive to EGFR inhibitor therapy. Treatment consists of managing pruritus with systemic antihistamines, γ-aminobutyric acid agonists, or aprepitant.[44] Management of the rash is based on the severity. The National Cancer Institute's Common Terminology Criteria for Adverse Events (CTCAE) grades the rash using a 1 to 5 scale based on body surface area involved, associated symptoms, and concomitant infection. For mild disease, topical hydrocortisone 2.5% cream or clindamycin 1% lotion is suggested. For more severe disease, higher strength topical steroids, doxycycline or minocycline, or low-dose isotretinoin is recommended.[45]

OCCUPATIONAL ACNE AND CHLORACNE

Several different groups of industrial compounds encountered in the workplace may cause acne. These include coal tar derivatives, insoluble cutting oils, and chlorinated hydrocarbons (chloronaphthalene, chlorobiphenyls, and chlorodiphenyloxide). Chloracne is the term that is used to describe occupational acne caused from chlorinated hydrocarbons. Occupational acne tends to be quite inflammatory and, in addition to large comedones, is characterized by papules, pustules, large nodules, and true cysts. Tar acne is often accompanied by hyperpigmentation.[46] The lesions of occupational acne are not restricted to the face and, in fact, are more common on covered areas with intimate contact to clothing saturated with the offending compound. Because cutting oils are so widely used, they are the most common cause of industrial acne. However, the chlorinated hydrocarbons, which cause chloracne, have posed a more difficult problem because of the severity of the disease induced with these compounds. Exposure can cause comedones, cysts, and pigmentary changes of the skin but can also affect the ophthalmic, nervous, and hepatic systems. Exposure to the dioxin Agent Orange predisposes to invasive nonmelanoma skin cancer as well.[47] Many cases have occurred as the result of massive exposure in industrial accidents.[48]

TABLE 80-1
Drug-Induced Acneiform Eruptions

- Glucocorticoids
- Phenytoin
- Lithium
- Isoniazid
- High-dose vitamin B complex
- Halogenated compounds
- Epidermal growth factor receptor inhibitors
- BRAF inhibitors

Chlorinated hydrocarbons are found in fungicides, insecticides, and wood preservatives. Chloracne classically affects the malar, retroauricular, and mandibular regions of the head and neck, as well as the axillae and scrotum. Pathology demonstrates multiple tiny infundibular cysts. Most chloracne lesions clear up within 2 years, providing exposure to the chemical has stopped. Treatment with topical or systemic retinoids or oral antibiotics may be beneficial.

GRAM-NEGATIVE FOLLICULITIS

Gram-negative folliculitis may occur in patients with preexisting acne vulgaris treated with long-term oral antibiotics, especially the tetracyclines. Patients usually give a history of initial success with oral tetracyclines followed by a worsening of their acne. Gram-negative folliculitis may appear as either papulopustules concentrated around the nose or as deep-seated nodules. Culture of these lesions may reveal *Enterobacter*, *Klebsiella*, or *Escherichia* spp. in the papulopustules or *Proteus* spp. in the nodules. An appropriate antimicrobial agent with adequate gram-negative coverage should be used. In recalcitrant cases, gram-negative folliculitis improves with oral isotretinoin for 4 to 5 months. Gram-negative bacteria require a moist environment for survival, and the drying action of isotretinoin will kill the bacteria.

RADIATION ACNE

Different types of radiation such as ionizing and ultraviolet (UV) may induce acneiform eruptions. Infrared radiation has been implicated recently as well.[49] Previous sites of therapeutic ionizing radiation (eg, external beam) can develop comedo-like papules.[50] These lesions begin to appear as the acute phase of radiation dermatitis is resolving. The ionizing rays induce epithelial metaplasia within the follicle, creating adherent hyperkeratotic plugs in the pilosebaceous unit. These keratotic plugs are resistant to extraction. Excessive exposure to UV radiation may produce a yellow, atrophic plaque studded with large open comedones. This condition is known as *Favre-Racouchot syndrome* but has also been called solar comedones, senile comedones, nodular cutaneous elastosis with cysts and comedones, and nodular elastoidosis with cysts and comedones. It has been estimated to occur in 6% of persons older than 50 years of age. The lesions are usually symmetrically distributed on the temporal and periorbital areas. Unilateral presentations have been reported depending on exposure. The exact pathogenesis of Favre-Racouchot syndrome is unknown, but it is suggested that extensive UV exposure as well as exposure to harsh climates and smoking may be risk factors. It can be treated with oral or topical retinoids as well as comedone extraction or CO_2 laser.[51,52]

TROPICAL ACNE

In extreme heat, a severe acneiform folliculitis may develop. This can be seen in tropical climates or in scorching occupational environments, as in furnace workers. This acneiform eruption is a major cause of dermatologic disability in military troops serving in tropical climates. Tropical acne occurs mainly on the trunk and buttocks. It has many deep, large, inflammatory nodules with multiple draining areas, resembling acne conglobata. The pathogenesis of this type of acne is unknown, although secondary infection with coagulase-positive staphylococci almost always ensues. Systemic antibiotics may be given but often removing the patient to a cooler environment is more important.

ACNE AESTIVALIS

This monomorphous eruption consists of multiple, uniform, red, papular lesions seen after sun exposure. It was initially called *Mallorca acne* because it occurred in many Scandinavians after they had been on a sunny vacation in Mallorca in southern Europe after a long, dark winter.[53] Almost all cases have occurred in women, mainly 20 to 30 years old. The lesions are common on the shoulders, arms, neck, and chest. Histologically, the lesions resemble steroid acne in that they show a focal follicular destruction with neutrophilic infiltrate. Comedones are not part of the clinical or histologic picture. The eruption is caused by the effects of UV radiation, primarily UVA. Rarely, a similar clinical picture can be observed after starting psoralen and UVA (PUVA) treatment. The eruption will subside if the patient is protected from UV light for several months. Oral antibiotics are ineffective in speeding up the resolution, but topical retinoids and benzoyl peroxide may be helpful. Like polymorphous light eruption, patients with acne aestivalis will flare on reexposure to UV light.[41]

PSEUDOACNE OF THE NASAL CREASE

The transverse nasal crease is an anatomic variant that appears as a transverse linear groove across the middle of the nose. Preadolescent patients develop comedones, milia, and acneiform red papules within the nasal crease (Fig. 80-4). It can be familial or associated with the "allergic salute." Histologic examination of the papules reveals keratin granulomas that may be derived from ruptured, inflamed milia. Because of its similarity in clinical appearance to acne but deviation

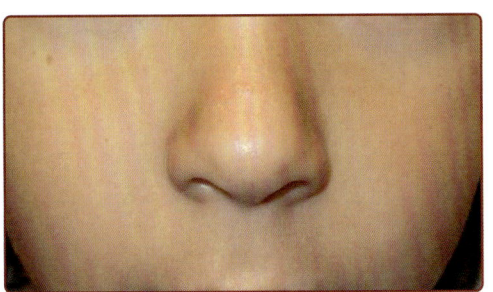

Figure 80-4 Pseudoacne of the nasal crease. Open and closed comedones and small papules line up along the transverse nasal crease.

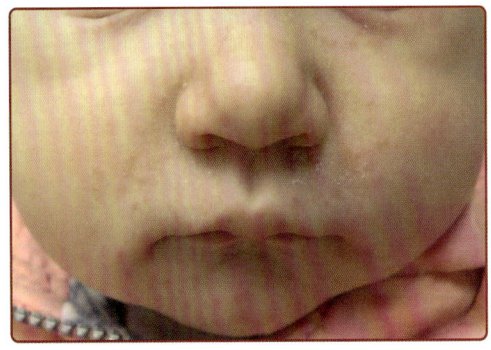

Figure 80-5 Periorificial dermatitis. An 8-month-old girl with perioral and perinasal 2-mm pink papules. Note a few lesions on the lower eyelid as well.

from acne histologically, it has been termed "pseudoacne of the nasal crease."[54]

APERT SYNDROME

Apert syndrome, also known as acrocephalosyndactyly, is an autosomal dominant disorder marked by synostoses of the cranium, vertebral bodies and hands and feet. It is caused by a mutation in the gene encoding FGFR-2. These patients have a diffuse acneiform eruption that often involves the arms, buttocks, and thighs. It is typically very resistant to treatment, but excellent responses to isotretinoin have been reported.[55] Patients with Apert syndrome may also present with severe seborrhea, nail dystrophy, and cutaneous and ocular hypopigmentation.

PERIORAL DERMATITIS (PERIORIFICIAL DERMATITIS)

Perioral dermatitis is an acneiform eruption that occurs in a bimodal distribution young children and young adults.[56] There is female predominance, mostly in adolescents and adults.[57] Small inflammatory papules and pustules group around the mouth in a typically well demarcated pattern, with sparing of the lip margin (Fig. 80-5). There is variable scaling and dryness. If the nose, eyes, or groin region is involved, it is called periforificial dermatitis. The neck, trunk, and extremities are rarely involved but have been reported in children with the disorder.[58,59] Usually perioral dermatitis is asymptomatic with occasional itchy or burning noted.

A severe variant is called periorificial granulomatous dermatitis. In this version, larger, granulomatous inflammatory papules coalesce into a well delineated plaque around the mouth with more likely involvement of the periocular, perinasal, and groin areas. Rarely, scarring can occur. Blepharitis and chalazion may accompany eye involvement.

The facial Afro-Caribbean eruption (FACE) is another variant of periorificial dermatitis characterized by uniform, granulomatous sarcoidal papules distributed over the typical periorificial areas.[60] (Fig. 80-6) Distinguishing features include involvement of the upper eyelids and helices of the ears.[61] Histology is similar to granulomatous perioral dermatitis.

The diagnosis of periorificial dermatitis is typically made by clinical evaluation, although a biopsy may be indicated in atypical cases. Histologically, periorificial dermatitis resembles rosacea with perifollicular and perivascular lymphohistiocytic infiltrate with variable perifollicular granulomas. In granulomatous periorificial dermatitis, histology is characterized by upper dermal and perifollicular granulomas admixed with lymphocytes, similar to sarcoidosis.

The pathogenesis of perioral dermatitis is not fully understood. The secondary eye changes along with the rosacea-like histology have prompted some to consider the disorder a form of rosacea.[62]

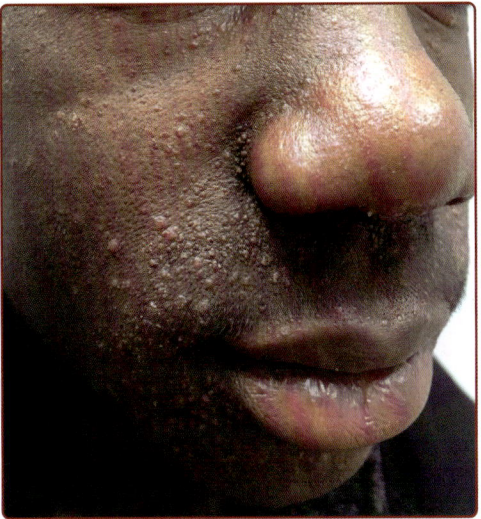

Figure 80-6 Facial Afro-Caribbean eruption, a variant of granulomatous periorificial dermatitis. Numerous inflammatory papules and pustules with overlying scale scattered around the mouth and nose extending to the lower eyelids.

Additionally, demodex may play a role in some cases of periorificial dermatitis, evidenced by response to antiparasitic agents. There are several known triggers for the disorders, including topical or inhaled corticosteroid use, particularly fluorinated steroids and fluoride in dentifrices.

The differential diagnosis of periorificial eruptions includes acne vulgaris, allergic contact or irritant dermatitis, demodicosis, lupus miliaris disseminatus faciei, molluscum, seborrheic dermatitis, systemic lupus erythematosus, and steroid-induced rosacea. For the granulomatous variant, the differential diagnosis would include other granulomatous disorders such as granulomatous rosacea, fungal or mycobacterial infection, familial juvenile systemic granulomatosis (Blau syndrome), and sarcoidosis.

The management of periorificial dermatitis in children and adults is similar. Topical corticosteroid use should be avoided because it tends to perpetuate the eruption. In mild cases resulting from corticosteroid use, discontinuation of steroid application can alone be effective. Alternate therapies include topical antimicrobial and antiinflammatory agents, including metronidazole cream or gel, clindamycin gel or lotion, erythromycin gel, azelaic acid cream, and sodium sulfacetamide lotion. Topical pimecrolimus cream or tacrolimus ointment has also been used in to treat periorificial dermatitis and to diminish flares from topical steroid withdrawal.[63,64] In children, oral erythromycin or azithromycin may be added for refractory or severe cases, but tetracyclines are commonly used in adolescents and adults.[65] Recently, the antiparasitic agents praziquantel and ivermectin (both topical and oral) have been successfully used.[66,67] Although spontaneous resolution upon discontinuation of a known trigger can occur, prolonged and refractory cases are not that uncommon.

REFERENCES

1. Henderson CA, Taylor J, Cunliffe WJ. Sebum excretion rates in mothers and neonates. *Br J Dermatol*. 2000;142(1):110-111.
2. Bernier V, Weill FX, Hirigoyen V, et al. Skin colonization by Malassezia species in neonates: a prospective study and relationship with neonatal cephalic pustulosis. *Arch Dermatol*. 2002;138(2):215-218.
3. Bergman JN, Eichenfield LF. Neonatal acne and cephalic pustulosis: is Malassezia the whole story? *Arch Dermatol*. 2002;138(2):255-257.
4. Lucky AW. A review of infantile and pediatric acne. *Dermatology*. 1998;196(1):95-97.
5. Eichenfield LF, Krakowski AC, Piggott C, et al. Evidence-based recommendations for the diagnosis and treatment of pediatric acne. *Pediatrics*. 2013; 131(suppl 3):S163-S186.
6. Greywal T, Zaenglein AL, Baldwin HE, et al. Evidence-based recommendations for the management of acne fulminans and its variants. *J Am Acad Dermatol*. 2017;77(1):109-117.
7. Massa AF, Burmeister L, Bass D, et al. Acne fulminans: treatment experience from 26 patients. *Dermatology*. 2017; 233(2-3):136-140.
8. Tan BB, Lear JT, Smith AG. Acne fulminans and erythema nodosum during isotretinoin therapy responding to dapsone. *Clin Exp Dermatol*. 1997;22(1):26-27.
9. Giavedoni P, Mascaró-Galy JM, Aguilera P, et al. Acne fulminans successfully treated with cyclosporine and isotretinoin. *J Am Acad Dermatol*. 2014;70(2):e38-39.
10. Oranges T, Insalaco A, Diociaiuti A, et al. Severe osteoarticular involvement in isotretinoin-triggered acne fulminans: two cases successfully treated with anakinra. *J Eur Acad Dermatol Venereol*. 2017;31(6): e277-e279.
11. Lages RB, Bona SH, Silva FV, et al. Acne fulminans successfully treated with prednisone and dapsone. *An Bras Dermatol*. 2012;87(4):612-614.
12. Iqbal M, Kolodney MS. Acne fulminans with synovitis-acne-pustulosis-hyperostosis-osteitis (SAPHO) syndrome treated with infliximab. *J Am Acad Dermatol*. 2005;52(5 suppl 1):S118-120.
13. Li C, Wu X, Cao Y, et al. Paradoxical skin lesions induced by anti-TNF-alpha agents in SAPHO syndrome. *Clin Rheumatol*. https://doi.org/10.1007/s10067-018-4083-5
14. Amano H, Matsuda R, Shibata T, et al. Paradoxical SAPHO syndrome observed during anti-TNFα therapy for Crohn's disease. *Biologics*. 2017;11:65-69.
15. Kerrison C, Davidson JE, Cleary AG, et al. Pamidronate in the treatment of childhood SAPHO syndrome. *Rheumatology (Oxford)*. 2004;43(10):1246-1251.
16. Cugno M, Borghi A, Marzano AV. PAPA, PASH and PAPASH syndromes: pathophysiology, presentation and treatment. *Am J Clin Dermatol*. 2017;18(4): 555-562.
17. Geusau A, Mothes-Luksch N, Nahavandi H, et al. Identification of a homozygous PSTPIP1 mutation in a patient with a PAPA-like syndrome responding to canakinumab treatment. *JAMA Dermatol*. 2013;149(2):209-215.
18. Staub J, Pfannschmidt N, Strohal R, et al. Successful treatment of PASH syndrome with infliximab, cyclosporine and dapsone. *J Eur Acad Dermatol Venereol*. 2015;29(11):2243-2247.
19. Jennings L, Molloy O, Quinlan C, et al. Treatment of pyoderma gangrenosum, acne, suppurative hidradenitis (PASH) with weight-based anakinra dosing in a Hepatitis B carrier. *Int J Dermatol*. 2017;56(6): e128-e129.
20. Force APAAPAD-T. *Diagnostic and Statistical Manual of Mental Disorders*, 5th ed. ed. Washington, DC: American Psychiatric Association; 2013.
21. Anzengruber F, Ruhwinkel K, Ghosh A, et al. Wide range of age of onset and low referral rates to psychiatry in a large cohort of acne excoriee at a Swiss tertiary hospital. *J Dermatolog Treat*. 2017:1-4.
22. Dreno B, Bettoli V, Perez M, et al. Cutaneous lesions caused by mechanical injury. *Eur J Dermatol*. 2015;25(2): 114-121.
23. Kang YC, Choi EH, Hwang SM, et al. Acne mechanica due to an orthopedic crutch. *Cutis*. 1999;64(2):97-98.
24. Strauss RM, Harrington CI. Stump acne: a new variant of acne mechanica and a cause of immobility. *Br J Dermatol*. 2001;144(3):647-648.
25. Knierim C, Goertz W, Reifenberger J, et al. [Fiddler's neck]. *Hautarzt*. 2013;64(10):724-726.
26. Bettoli V, Toni G, Zauli S, et al. Acne mechanica: probable role of IL-1alpha. *G Ital Dermatol Venereol*. 2016;151(6):720-721.
27. Kuhn-Régnier S, Mangana J, Kerl K, et al. A report of two cases of solid facial edema in acne. *Dermatol Ther (Heidelb)*. 2017;7(1):167-174.

28. Friedman SJ, Fox BJ, Albert HL. Solid facial edema as a complication of acne vulgaris: treatment with isotretinoin. *J Am Acad Dermatol*. 1986;15(2 Pt 1):286-289.
29. Jungfer B, Jansen T, Przybilla B, et al. Solid persistent facial edema of acne: successful treatment with isotretinoin and ketotifen. *Dermatology*. 1993;187(1):34-37.
30. Helander I, Aho HJ. Solid facial edema as a complication of acne vulgaris: treatment with isotretinoin and clofazimine. *Acta Derm Venereol*. 1987;67(6):535-537.
31. Rotterdam ESHRE/ASRM-Sponsored PCOS Consensus Workshop Group. Revised 2003 consensus on diagnostic criteria and long-term health risks related to polycystic ovary syndrome. *Fertil Steril*. 2004;81(1):19-25.
32. Goodman NF, Cobin RH, Futterweit W, et al. American Association of Clinical Endocrinologists, American College of Endocrinology, and Androgen Excess and PCOS Society disease state clinical review: guide to the best practices in the evaluation and treatment of polycystic ovary syndrome—part 2. *Endocr Pract*. 2015;21(12):1415-1426.
33. Goodman NF, Cobin RH, Futterweit W, et al. American Association of Clinical Endocrinologists, American College of Endocrinology, and Androgen Excess and PCOS Society disease state clinical review: guide to the best practices in the evaluation and treatment of polycystic ovary syndrome—part 1. *Endocr Pract*. 2015;21(11):1291-1300.
34. Ibanez L, Oberfield SE, Witchel S, et al. An international consortium update: pathophysiology, diagnosis, and treatment of polycystic ovarian syndrome in adolescence. *Horm Res Paediatr*. 2017;88(6):371-395.
35. Leelaphiwat S, Jongwutiwes T, Lertvikool S, et al. Comparison of desogestrel/ethinyl estradiol plus spironolactone versus cyproterone acetate/ethinyl estradiol in the treatment of polycystic ovary syndrome: a randomized controlled trial. *J Obstet Gynaecol Res*. 2015;41(3):402-410.
36. Hagag P, Steinschneider M, Weiss M. Role of the combination spironolactone-norgestimate-estrogen in Hirsute women with polycystic ovary syndrome. *J Reprod Med*. 2014;59(9-10):455-463.
37. Harborne L, Fleming R, Lyall H, et al. Metformin or antiandrogen in the treatment of hirsutism in polycystic ovary syndrome. *J Clin Endocrinol Metab*. 2003;88(9):4116-4123.
38. Falhammar H, Nordenström A. Nonclassic congenital adrenal hyperplasia due to 21-hydroxylase deficiency: clinical presentation, diagnosis, treatment, and outcome. *Endocrine*. 2015;50(1):32-50.
39. Degitz K, Placzek M, Arnold B, et al. Congenital adrenal hyperplasia and acne in male patients. *Br J Dermatol*. 2003;148(6):1263-1266.
40. Harrell B, Rudolph A. Kelp diet: a cause of acneiform eruption. *Arch Dermatol* 1976;112:560.
41. Plewig G, Jansen T. Acneiform dermatoses. *Dermatology*. 1998;196(1):102-107.
42. Perez-Soler R, Delord JP, Halpern A, et al. HER1/EGFR inhibitor-associated rash: future directions for management and investigation outcomes from the HER1/EGFR inhibitor rash management forum. *Oncologist*. 2005;10(5):345-356.
43. Nasu S, Suzuki H, Shiroyama T, et al. Skin rash can be a useful marker for afatinib efficacy. *Anticancer Res*. 2018;38(3):1783-1788.
44. Santini D, Vincenzi B, Guida FM, et al. Aprepitant for management of severe pruritus related to biological cancer treatments: a pilot study. *Lancet Oncol*. 2012;13(10):1020-1024.
45. Lacouture ME, Anadkat M, Jatoi A, et al. Dermatologic toxicity occurring during anti-EGFR monoclonal inhibitor therapy in patients with metastatic colorectal cancer: a systematic review. *Clin Colorectal Cancer*. 2018;17(2):85-96.
46. Leijs MM, Esser A, Amann PM, et al. Hyperpigmentation and higher incidence of cutaneous malignancies in moderate-high PCB- and dioxin exposed individuals. *Environ Res*. 2018;164:221-228.
47. Clemens MW, Kochuba AL, Carter ME, et al. Association between Agent Orange exposure and nonmelanotic invasive skin cancer: a pilot study. *Plast Reconstr Surg*. 2014;133(2):432-437.
48. Bertazzi PA, Bernucci I, Brambilla G, et al. The Seveso studies on early and long-term effects of dioxin exposure: a review. *Environ Health Perspect*. 1998;106(suppl 2):625-633.
49. Pizzati A, Passoni E, Nazzaro G. Monolateral Favre-Racouchot syndrome following long-term exposure to infrared waves. *JAMA Dermatol*. 2018;154(5):623-625.
50. Hubiche T, Sibaud V. Localized acne induced by radiation therapy. *Dermatol Online J*. 2014;20(2).
51. Rallis E, Karanikola E, Verros C. Successful treatment of Favre-Racouchot disease with 0.05% tazarotene gel. *Arch Dermatol*. 2007;143(6):810-812.
52. Mavilia L, Campolmi P, Santoro G, et al. Combined treatment of Favre-Racouchot syndrome with a superpulsed carbon dioxide laser: report of 50 cases. *Dermatol Ther*. 2010;23(suppl 1):S4-S6.
53. Hjorth N, Sjolin KE, Sylvest B, et al. Acne aestivalis—Mallorca acne. *Acta Derm Venereol*. 1972;52(1):61-63.
54. Risma KA, Lucky AW. Pseudoacne of the nasal crease: a new entity? *Pediatr Dermatol*. 2004;21(4):427-431.
55. Paradisi A, Ghitti F, Capizzi R, et al. Acne treatment with isotretinoin in a patient with Apert syndrome. *Eur J Dermatol*. 2011;21(4):611-612.
56. Hafeez ZH. Perioral dermatitis: an update. *Int J Dermatol*. 2003;42(7):514-517.
57. Lipozenčić J, Hadžavdić SL. Perioral dermatitis. *Clin Dermatol*. 2014;32(1):125-130.
58. Urbatsch AJ, Frieden I, Williams ML, et al. Extrafacial and generalized granulomatous periorificial dermatitis. *Arch Dermatol*. 2002;138(10):1354-1358.
59. Hansen KK, McTigue MK, Esterly NB. Multiple facial, neck, and upper trunk papules in a black child. Childhood granulomatous perioral dermatitis with involvement of the neck and upper trunk. *Arch Dermatol*. 1992;128(10):1396-1397,1399.
60. Cribier B, Lieber-Mbomeyo A, Lipsker D. [Clinical and histological study of a case of facial Afro-Caribbean childhood eruption (FACE)]. *Ann Dermatol Venereol*. 2008;135(10):663-667.
61. Williams HC, Ashworth J, Pembroke AC, et al. FACE—facial Afro-Caribbean childhood eruption. *Clin Exp Dermatol*. 1990;15(3):163-166.
62. Lucas CR, Korman NJ, Gilliam AC. Granulomatous periorificial dermatitis: a variant of granulomatous rosacea in children? *J Cutan Med Surg*. 2009;13(2):115-118.
63. Rodriguez-Martin M, Saez-Rodriguez M, Carnerero-Rodriguez A, et al. Treatment of perioral dermatitis with topical pimecrolimus. *J Am Acad Dermatol*. 2007;56(3):529-530.
64. Oppel T, Pavicic T, Kamann S, et al. Pimecrolimus cream (1%) efficacy in perioral dermatitis—results of a randomized, double-blind, vehicle-controlled

study in 40 patients. *J Eur Acad Dermatol Venereol.* 2007;21(9):1175-1180.
65. Goel NS, Burkhart CN, Morrell DS. Pediatric periorificial dermatitis: clinical course and treatment outcomes in 222 patients. *Pediatr Dermatol.* 2015;32(3):333-336.
66. Bribeche MR, Fedotov VP, Jillella A, et al. Topical praziquantel as a new treatment for perioral dermatitis: results of a randomized vehicle-controlled pilot study. *Clin Exp DermatolClin Exp Dermatol.* 2014;39(4):448-453.
67. Noguera-Morel L, Gerlero P, Torrelo A, et al. Ivermectin therapy for papulopustular rosacea and periorificial dermatitis in children: a series of 15 cases. *J Am Acad Dermatol.* 2017;76(3):567-570.

Disorders of Eccrine and Apocrine Sweat Glands

PART 15

第十五篇　汗腺疾病

Chapter 81 :: Hyperhidrosis and Anhidrosis :: Anastasia O. Kurta & Dee Anna Glaser

第八十一章
多汗症和无汗症

中文导读

汗液由神经内分泌网络调节；任何调节通路的紊乱，都能改变出汗。汗腺疾病主要分为两大类：过度出汗(多汗症)和出汗减少(少汗或无汗症)。本章着重于回顾几种可能导致局灶性、区域性或全身性出汗异常的疾病。表81-1列出了出汗异常的疾病分类。

1. 多汗症　多汗是指出汗过多，超过了维持正常体温的生理需要。作者将多汗症细分为原发性多汗症和继发性多汗症，分别讲述其临床特征、病因和发病机制、诊断、临床病程、预后及处理等。

（1）原发性多汗症又可细分为局灶性多汗症和泛发性多汗症。

原发性局灶多汗症是一种神经紊乱，表现为多种解剖部位出汗过多。其病因尚不清除，可能是交感神经过度兴奋的结果，其小汗腺结构并没有缺陷；也与遗传因素相关。

诊断上，应了解患者详细的临床病史，作者提到的病史包括发病年龄、出汗部位和对称性、加重和缓解因素、手术史、家族史以及目前可能加重病情的药物治疗等。诊断要点是多汗症状至少应持续6个月，且没有潜在的系统性疾病。出汗应至少包括以下特点中的两个：双侧对称性出汗，出汗影响了日常活动，每周至少有一次出汗经历，发病年龄小于25岁，阳性家族史，睡眠中出汗停止(表81-2)。关键要明确出汗是生理性的，出汗可以是持续性的(轻微的或严重的)或阶段性的，并会因特殊的诱因而加剧，如体温升高、焦虑、压力和体育活动等。

本章还提到两种常用的评价工具：皮肤病学生活质量指数(DLQI)和多汗症严重程度量表(HDSS)，用于评估多汗症对生活质量的影响，有助于指导治疗反应。治疗上，本章提出：应根据多汗部位和疾病的严重程度选择合适的治疗方式，并于表81-4讲述了原发性局灶多汗症的治疗选择。包括局部外用六水合氯化铝、局部注射A型肉毒杆菌毒素、水离子导入疗法、内窥镜胸交感神经切断术，以及口服抗胆碱药等，并分别详细讲述了这些治疗方法的适应症、副作用及操作注意事项等。

（2）继发性多汗症可由潜在疾病(先天性或后天)或药物/毒素的副作用而发生。患者可经历局灶性、区域性或全身性出汗，经常在睡眠期间持续发生。

首先，作者分别讲述了发生继发性局灶多汗症和继发性泛发多汗症的常见疾病。继发性局灶多汗症可由生理性或病理性的味觉性出汗、中枢或周围神经功能障碍、冷诱导出汗综合征、阵发性局部多汗症等而发生。继发性泛发多汗症可由代谢和其他系统性疾病、感染、发热、恶性肿瘤或中枢或周围自主神经功能紊乱以及药物或毒素的副作用引起。

接着讲述了继发性多汗症的临床特征、病因和发病机制、诊断、临床病程、预后及处理等。

在讲述继发性局灶多汗症的病因及发病机制时，讲到了味觉性出汗、小汗腺痣。前者是吃辛辣食物时，嘴唇、前额、头皮和鼻子局部出汗是很常见的，这是三叉神经血管反射的一种生理反应。后者是一种罕见的皮肤错构瘤，组织学上定义为小汗腺的局灶性增生或肥大。还提到了阵发性局部多汗症，以及已报道的与某些皮肤疾病有关的继发性局灶多汗症，并简要讲述了治疗方法。

而继发性泛发多汗症多由代谢、传染性或其他系统性疾病引起。既往报道多汗症与糖尿病、低血糖、甲状腺毒症、类癌综合征、垂体机能亢进(肢端肥大症)、充血性心力衰竭、倾泄综合征、更年期、恶性肿瘤和停药有关。本章还提到了Riley-Day综合征，认为它是遗传性感觉自主神经病变研究最为深入的疾病。

诊断上，同样需要彻底的临床病史和体格检查，尤其要关注的症状包括发烧、原因不明的体重减轻、发冷、盗汗、疲劳，以及内分泌和神经系统症状。本章提出，询问每日或必要时服用的处方、非处方药和补充剂有助于识别次要原因。与原发性多汗症相比，继发性多汗症必须进行基本的生命体征和实验室检查，必要时进行会诊。

治疗上，侧重于纠正或控制潜在疾病或停用可疑药物。

2. 无汗症　无汗症可由汗腺的先天性缺失而发生，如无汗性外胚层发育不良、遗传性代谢性疾病(法布里病)或后天原因(继发性或特发性无汗)。继发性无汗症或少汗症可发生于结缔组织疾病(干燥综合征)、外分泌腺的导管阻塞、潜在的神经障碍和自主神经功能障碍、周围神经病变、药物或毒素。作者简要介绍了其临床特征、病因和发病机制、诊断、临床病程、预后及处理等。

本章还简要讲述了ED-1基因突变导致X连锁少汗性外胚层发育不良、先天性无汗症(CIPA)、FABRY疾病、获得性特发性全身无汗症(AIGA)等多种无汗症疾病的病因及一些典型的病理表现。

诊断上，提出要仔细询问病史，尤其是药物治疗史、潜在疾病和家族史。皮肤检查虽然不能显示无汗体征，但代偿性多汗症可以有所提示。必要时，可对受影响区域进行活检以明确可能的汗腺异常。

无汗症的治疗方法是有限的。首先应该确定主要病因，并且停用可疑药物；让病人保持低温，避免过热危及生命；运动时穿湿衣服也有帮助。痱子的预防和治疗包括避免暴露在湿热环境下、治疗任何潜在的发热性疾病，以及去除覆盖衣物等。

〔刘芳芬〕

AT-A-GLANCE

Primary focal (essential) hyperhidrosis:
- Idiopathic and symmetric and can affect the palms, soles, axillae, craniofacial region, groin, other areas, or combination of body sites.
- Treatment is based on severity of symptoms and location and follows a stepwise approach.

Secondary hyperhidrosis:
- Can occur from underlying systemic illnesses, medications, or both (obtaining a detailed medical history is crucial).
- The pattern of sweating is classically generalized, but sometimes can be focal or regional if caused by neurologic disease or trauma, or a primary dermatologic cause (eg, eccrine nevus).
- Treatment should target the underlying disease process or eliminate or change medications that the patient takes, but this is often not feasible.

Anhidrosis:
- Anhidrosis may occur because of congenital or acquired causes (secondary or idiopathic anhidrosis).
- Can become a medical emergency leading to hyperthermia, heat stroke, or death.

INTRODUCTION

Eccrine sweating is regulated by neurohormonal mechanisms; a derangement in any part of the regulatory pathways, such as the thermal center, central or peripheral nerve transmission, or eccrine gland sweat secretion can alter sweating. Eccrine sweat glands are innervated by sympathetic nerve fibers; the main neurotransmitter, acetylcholine, binds to the muscarinic receptors on the eccrine sweat glands to produce sweating. Disorders of eccrine sweating can be subdivided into two main categories: excessive sweating (hyperhidrosis) and reduced sweating (hypohidrosis or anhidrosis). Hyperhidrosis is a condition of excessive sweating beyond what is physiologically necessary to maintain normal body temperature. The prevalence at 4.8%, represents around 15.3 million people in the United States.[1] Hyperhidrosis can be further subdivided into primary and secondary hyperhidrosis. Pathogenesis of primary or essential hyperhidrosis is poorly understood. Secondary hyperhidrosis can result from underlying systemic illnesses, including, but not limited to, central and peripheral neurologic dysfunctions, endocrine disorders, psychiatric disorders, hormonal imbalance, infections, malignancy, certain primary dermatologic disorders, and from medications or toxins.[2] Hyperhidrosis can adversely impact patients' daily activities, be occupationally restrictive, and interfere with interpersonal relationships.

Anhidrosis is characterized by the inability to normally generate sweat when physiologically necessary to dissipate heat. As a result, this can become a medical emergency, leading to hyperthermia, heat stroke, or death. This chapter focuses on reviewing several disorders that can cause focal, regional, and generalized abnormalities in sweating. Please refer to Table 81-1 for an inclusive list of disorders of the eccrine glands and sweating. A review of the normal anatomy and physiology of eccrine sweat glands and sweating may be found in Chap. 6.

PRIMARY FOCAL (ESSENTIAL) HYPERHIDROSIS

Primary focal hyperhidrosis is a neurologic disorder that manifests as excessive sweating at baseline in various anatomic locations, including, but not limited to, the palms and soles, axillae, craniofacial region, groin, or a combination of body sites. It affects males and females equally, typically begins in childhood (palmar-plantar) or during puberty (axillary), and continues to persist into adulthood, with rare reports of spontaneous improvement.

CLINICAL FEATURES

Patients may experience mild (moist or damp skin) to severe (dripping wet) excessive sweating in affected areas. Hyperhidrosis rarely presents with medical complications such as maceration or secondary infections, but it has been reported to predispose the patient to increased risk of cutaneous infection, such as pitted keratolysis, dermatophytosis, and verruca vulgaris or plantaris.[3]

ETIOLOGY AND PATHOGENESIS

The cause of primary focal hyperhidrosis is poorly understood, but is believed to be a result of sympathetic overactivity without structural defects of the eccrine glands. Evidence also suggests that hyperhidrosis has a familial component, proposing a possible genetic cause for the condition.[4-6]

DIAGNOSIS

A thorough clinical history should be obtained from the patient, including age of onset, location and symmetry of sweating, aggravating and alleviating factors, previous treatments, full past medical and surgical history, family history, and current medications that may exacerbate the condition. To establish a diagnosis of primary focal hyperhidrosis, symptoms should be present for at least 6 months without an underlying

TABLE 81-1
Classification of Disorders of Eccrine Sweating

Primary Focal (Essential) Hyperhidrosis
Palmoplantar, axillary, craniofacial, generalized hyperhidrosis

Secondary Causes of Focal Hyperhidrosis
Caused by cerebral infarction
- Frontal opercular infarct
- Brainstem stroke

Associated with spinal cord injury
- Autonomic dysreflexia
- Posttraumatic syringomyelia
- Orthostatic hypotension triggered

Associated with other central nervous system disorders
- Chiari type I and II malformation
- Myelopathies caused by infarction, syringomyelia, tumor
- Cold-induced sweating syndrome
- Olfactory hyperhidrosis

Associated with peripheral nervous system disorders
- Peripheral motor neuropathy with autonomic dysfunction
- Dermatomal or focal hyperhidrosis caused by nerve trunk irritation
- Compensatory segmental hyperhidrosis (postsympathectomy, Ross syndrome, pure autonomic failure)
- Gustatory sweating
- Physiologic
- Idiopathic
- Postherpetic
- Post nerve injury (postsurgical, diabetic autonomic neuropathy, postinfectious, tumor invasion)
- Lacrimal sweating
- Harlequin syndrome
- Idiopathic, localized hyperhidrosis
- Idiopathic unilateral circumscribed hyperhidrosis
- Postmenopausal localized hyperhidrosis

Associated with local skin disorders
- Blue rubber bleb nevi
- Eccrine angiomatous hamartoma
- Tufted angioma
- Glomus tumor
- Burning feet syndrome
- Pachydermoperiostosis
- Granulosis rubra nasi
- Pretibial myxedema
- POEMS (polyneuropathy, organomegaly, endocrinopathy, M protein, and skin changes) syndrome

Secondary Causes of Generalized Hyperhidrosis
Associated with central nervous system disorders
- Episodic hypothermia with hyperhidrosis (Hines-Bannick or Shapiro syndrome)
- Posttraumatic or posthemorrhagic "diencephalic epilepsy"
- Fatal familial insomnia and Parkinson disease

Associated with fever and chronic infection
- Tuberculosis, malaria, brucellosis, endocarditis

Associated with metabolic and systemic medical diseases
- Hyperthyroidism, diabetes mellitus, hypoglycemia, hypercortisolism, acromegaly

Associated with malignancy
- Leukemia, lymphoma, pheochromocytoma, Castleman disease, carcinoids, renal cell cancer

Medication induced
- See Table 81-4
- Neuroleptic malignant syndrome
- Serotonin syndrome, other medications

Toxic syndromes
- Alcohol, opioid withdrawal, delirium tremens

Associated with central and peripheral nervous system disorders
- Familial dysautonomia (Riley-Day), Morvan fibrillary chorea

Primary Autonomic Disorders with Acquired Anhidrosis
Isolated sudomotor disorders
- Progressive isolated segmental anhidrosis
- Idiopathic pure sudomotor failure
- Chronic idiopathic anhidrosis

Sudomotor plus other autonomic disorders
- Ross syndrome
- Pure autonomic failure
- Autoimmune autonomic neuropathy

Secondary Autonomic Disorders Associated with Anhidrosis
Central nervous system lesions (eg, stroke, tumor, infection, infiltration, trauma)
- Hypothalamic lesions
- Brainstem lesions
- Spinal cord lesions

Degenerative disorders
- Multiple system atrophy, dementia with Lewy body disease, Parkinson disease—autonomic failure

Peripheral Nerve Lesions Causing Anhidrosis
- Hereditary sensory and autonomic neuropathy types I, II, IV (congenital insensitivity to pain with anhidrosis)
- Guillain-Barré syndrome (acute inflammatory demyelinating polyneuropathy)
- Diabetic autonomic neuropathy
- Amyloidosis
- Lepromatous neuropathy
- Lambert-Eaton myasthenic syndrome
- Alcoholic neuropathy
- Fabry disease
- Idiopathic small-fiber neuropathy
- Erythromelalgia
- Sympathectomy and other surgical lesions
- Harlequin syndrome

Anhidrosis caused by toxins, pharmacologic agents, and heat exposure
- Botulism
- Ganglionic blockers, anticholinergics, carbonic anhydrase inhibitors
- Opioids
- Heat hyperpyrexia and heat stroke

Anhidrosis Associated with Diseases of Skin and Sweat Glands
Anhidrosis caused by physical agents damaging skin
- Trauma, burns, pressure, scar formation, radiation therapy

Anhidrosis caused by congenital and acquired skin diseases
- Fabry and other congenital metabolic diseases
- Congenital ectodermal dysplasia
- Ichthyosis
- Neutrophilic eccrine hidradenitis
- Sjögren syndrome
- Systemic sclerosis (scleroderma)
- Incontinentia pigmenti
- Segmental vitiligo
- Bazex-Dupre-Christol syndrome

Disorders affecting the sweat duct
- Miliaria
- Palmoplantar pustulosis
- Psoriasis
- Lichen planus
- Atopic dermatitis

Disorders with abnormal sweat composition
- Atopic dermatitis (reduced dermcidin levels)
- Cystic fibrosis (increased chloride concentration)

systemic cause and include at least two of the following characteristics: bilateral and symmetric sweating, impairment of daily activities because of sweating, at least one episode of sweating per week, age of onset younger than 25 years, positive family history, and cessation of sweating during sleep[7] (Table 81-2). In the authors' experience, it is key to understand if the reported sweating is physiologic or not. Sweating can be continuous (mild or severe) or phasic and can be intensified by typical triggers, such as increased temperature, anxiety, stress, and physical activity. A thorough physical examination is necessary and includes inspection for excessive moisture and any other secondary skin conditions, such as bacterial or fungal infections or skin maceration, as well as evidence of systemic findings that might indicate a secondary form of hyperhidrosis. A Minor starch-iodine test is helpful to identify the involved area of hyperhidrosis at baseline, but it does not provide any information on severity of the disease (Fig. 81-1). Gravimetric (weight-based) assessment is an objective measurement of the amount of sweat production, commonly performed in clinical research studies, but it is not practical for routine clinical use. The effect of hyperhidrosis on quality of life can be assessed in multiple ways and can help guide response to therapy. Two commonly used tools are the Dermatology Life Quality Index (DLQI) and The Hyperhidrosis Disease Severity Scale (HDSS), a 4-point scale that measures the severity of patients' hyperhidrosis based on how it affects daily activities[8] (Table 81-3). Both of these tools can also be used to follow the response to therapy. The diagnosis of primary focal hyperhidrosis is generally straight forward; however, based on medical history, review of systems, and physical examination, the differential diagnosis could include the possibility of underlying secondary cause(s), which are reviewed later in this chapter.

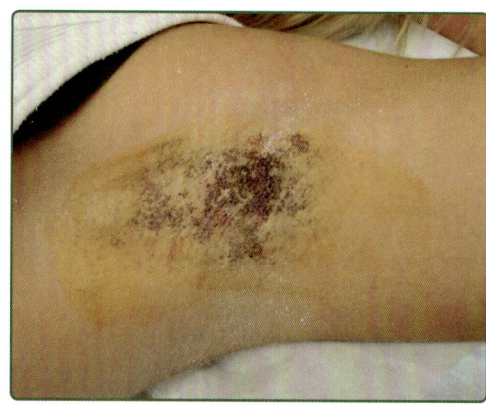

Figure 81-1 Positive starch iodine test result in a patient with primary axillary hyperhidrosis.

mental health.[1] There have been advancements in treatment options. Choosing the right treatment (Table 81-4) involves consideration of body location and severity of the disorder. Properly addressing patients' expectations is crucial in selecting the appropriate treatment and obtaining treatment compliance. First-line therapy includes over-the-counter (OTC) antiperspirants or aluminum chloride hexahydrate (10% to 35%). Aluminum chloride hexahydrate works best when applied to dry skin at bedtime and washed off after 6 to 8 hours. Patients should be counseled carefully on the proper application to reduce the risk of irritation. If moisture is present on the skin when aluminum chloride hexahydrate is applied, this can result in formation of a weak hydrochloric acid, which can cause symptoms of burning, irritation, or desquamation. If irritation occurs, it can usually be minimized by decreasing application to every other night or few times per week. However, this may also reduce efficacy. Thus, the authors recommend use of OTC clinical-strength antiperspirant on the nights when aluminum chloride hexahydrate is not being applied.

There have been several studies showing beneficial results with topical glycopyrrolate ranging in concentrations from 0.5% to 2%, particularly when used for craniofacial hyperhidrosis.[9,10] It is not yet commercially available in the United States at the time of writing this chapter, but it can be compounded at specialty pharmacies.

If the patient fails to respond to topical therapy, intradermal injection of botulinum toxin may be administered to areas of excessive sweating. Botulinum toxin

CLINICAL COURSE, PROGNOSIS, AND MANAGEMENT

Primary focal hyperhidrosis is a chronic disorder, and it does not affect life expectancy. It does, however, have a very negative impact on the quality of life, affecting all domains of social life, sense of well-being, and

TABLE 81-2
Primary Focal (Essential) Hyperhidrosis

Focal visible excessive sweating ≥6 months' duration without apparent cause and at least two of the following:
- Bilateral and relatively symmetric
- Age of onset typically before age of 25 years
- Cessation of sweating from the focal areas during sleep
- Frequency of at least once per week
- Positive family history
- Sweating impairs daily activities

TABLE 81-3
Hyperhidrosis Disease Severity Scale

	IMPACT OF SWEATING ON DAILY ACTIVITIES
4	Intolerable; always interferes
3	Barely tolerable; frequently interferes
2	Tolerable; sometimes interferes
1	Never noticeable; never interferes

TABLE 81-4
Treatment Options for Primary Focal Hyperhidrosis

First-Line Topical Options
- Over-the-counter antiperspirants and aluminum chloride hexahydrate (10%–35%)
- Topical glycopyrrolate (0.5%–2%)

Second-Line Agents
- Intradermal botulinum toxin injections
- Electromagnetic energy thermolysis
- Tap water iontophoresis

Severe or Refractory Cases
- Endoscopic thoracic sympathectomy

Systemic Medications
- Glycopyrrolate or oxybutynin
- Clonidine
- Propranolol
- Benzodiazepines

acts on the cholinergic synapses, inhibiting the release of acetylcholine. Numerous studies have demonstrated the efficacy and safety of several botulinum toxin A drugs as well as botulinum toxin B to treat hyperhidrosis. However, only onabotulinum toxin A (onabotA), (BOTOX; Allergan, Irvine, CA) was approved by the U.S. Food and Drug Administration (FDA) in 2004 for the treatment of severe primary axillary hyperhidrosis in adults 18 years and older. Although its approval is for adults, the efficacy and safety of onabotA can also be extended to adolescents. A large multicenter, nonrandomized, open-label study evaluated the efficacy and safety of onabotA in adolescents ages 12 to 17 years with severe primary axillary hyperhidrosis and demonstrated that 72% of patients experienced at least a two-grade improvement in the HDSS score at 4 and 8 weeks after each of the first two treatments.[11] The median duration of effect ranged from 4 to 5 months, and fewer than 6% of patients experienced treatment-related adverse effects.[11]

Botulinum toxin injections are also used off-label for treatment of other focal areas, such as the face or scalp, palms, soles, and inframammary and inguinal folds, with average efficacy duration of approximately 4 to 12 months.[12-14] Injections are placed at the dermal subcutaneous junction where the eccrine glands reside.

Electromagnetic energy thermolysis is a non-invasive procedure that can provide long-lasting reduction in axillary sweating; miraDry (Miramar Labs, Sunnyvale, CA) was cleared by the FDA in 2011 for adults with primary axillary hyperhidrosis. Microwave energy is readily absorbed by water molecules and as a result can easily target tissues with high water content, such as the eccrine glands. Eccrine glands do not regenerate, and their destruction theoretically reduces sweating in the treated area permanently. Side effects are generally minor and include edema, erythema, bruising from device vacuum suction, axillary tenderness or pain, paresthesia in the axilla or upper arm, and less commonly, blisters or burns at the treatment site, scar tissue formation, and patchy axillary alopecia (permanent).[15]

This technology cannot be applied to nonaxillary body sites at the time of writing this chapter.

Control of palmar-plantar hyperhidrosis can be obtained via tap water iontophoresis therapy, which uses the passage of a direct electrical current onto the skin. Although the underlying mechanism of iontophoresis remains unclear, a controlled trial of 112 patients with palmar hyperhidrosis showed that after eight treatments, sweating was reduced by 81.2% from baseline with use of iontophoresis therapy.[16] Treatments need to be maintained typically once to twice weekly for maximal improvement. An anticholinergic, such as glycopyrrolate, can be crushed and mixed with the water to enhance sweat reduction. Side effects are typically minor (erythema, mild pain or discomfort, and paresthesia in the treatment zone) and related to higher amperage. Severe cases of palmar hyperhidrosis that failed conservative management may be considered for endoscopic thoracic sympathectomy (ETS). This surgical procedure carries an increased risk of creating minor to severe compensatory sweating in body segments below the treated area, as well as less common complications such as Horner syndrome, bradycardia, pneumothorax requiring chest tube drainage, pleural effusion, acute bleeding or delayed hemothorax, chylothorax, and persistent intercostal neuralgia.[17]

Systemic medications can be used as monotherapy or to supplement the above therapies, especially when symptoms are multifocal. The oral agents that are commonly used are anticholinergics (glycopyrrolate and oxybutynin) or clonidine, a centrally acting α_2-adrenergic agonist.[18] Anticholinergic agents are contraindicated in those with myasthenia gravis, paralytic ileus, and pyloric stenosis and should be used with caution in patients with closed-angle glaucoma, bladder outflow obstruction, gastroesophageal reflux disease, and cardiac insufficiency.[19] They are also associated with many side effects, such as xerostomia, xerophthalmia, constipation, mydriasis, blurred vision, bradycardia (lower doses), tachycardia (higher doses), mental confusion (usually in children or older adults), and urinary hesitancy or retention. Glycopyrrolate is a quaternary amine and has limited passage across lipid membranes, such as the blood–brain barrier. Anticholinergic agents such as oxybutynin, atropine, and scopolamine are tertiary amines and can easily penetrate lipid barriers. This might explain why glycopyrrolate has fewer central nervous system side effects and may have less effect on the heart rate at lower doses.[19] β-Blockers, such as propranolol and benzodiazepines, are oral agents that can be useful in stress-induced hyperhidrosis. However, long-term use of benzodiazepines is not recommended.

SECONDARY HYPERHIDROSIS

Secondary hyperhidrosis can occur because of underlying medical conditions (congenital or acquired) or as a side effect from medications or toxins. Based on a retrospective chart review study conducted over a 13-year period (1993 to 2005) of all patients (children and adults) seen at a university-based outpatient dermatology department with a diagnosis of hyperhidrosis; in patients with secondary hyperhidrosis, endocrine disease accounted for 57% of cases (including diabetes mellitus, hyperthyroidism, and hyperpituitarism); neurologic disease accounted for 32% of cases and more commonly presented as asymmetric hyperhidrosis, and the remaining causes included malignancy (pheochromocytoma), respiratory disease, and psychiatric disease.[20] In this study, secondary hyperhidrosis was more often unilateral or asymmetric, generalized, and present nocturnally.

Localized secondary hyperhidrosis can occur because of physiologic or pathologic gustatory sweating, central or peripheral neurologic dysfunctions, cold-induced sweating syndrome, paroxysmal localized hyperhidrosis, intrathoracic neoplasms, or compensatory segmental hyperhidrosis (as in cases after ETS or as seen in Ross syndrome, which is a degenerative autonomic nervous system disorder). It can also be seen in association with certain cutaneous disorders.

Generalized secondary hyperhidrosis can result from metabolic and other systemic disorders, infections and fever, malignancy (eg, lymphoma or pheochromocytoma), or derangement in the central or peripheral autonomic nervous system (eg, Riley-Day syndrome, or familial dysautonomia) and as a side effect from medications or toxins. Pathogenesis varies depending on the underlying condition.

Several entities associated with secondary hyperhidrosis are highlighted below.

CLINICAL FEATURES

Patients with secondary hyperhidrosis can experience focal, regional, or generalized sweating that often persists during sleep. Although the onset of primary hyperhidrosis is often before age 25 years, secondary hyperhidrosis tends to present in adulthood, especially if it is caused by an underlying acquired disease; new symptoms of excessive sweating in adults should be carefully evaluated to ensure an underlying cause is not overlooked.[20]

ETIOLOGY AND PATHOGENESIS OF LOCALIZED (FOCAL OR REGIONAL) SECONDARY HYPERHIDROSIS

GUSTATORY SWEATING

It is common to experience localized sweating on the lips, forehead, scalp, and nose while eating hot and spicy foods as a physiologic response via trigeminovascular reflex. In contrast, pathologic gustatory sweating is usually asymmetric and intense and can occur in the distribution of the auriculotemporal nerve after injury or surgery in the region of the parotid gland; this is known as Frey syndrome (Fig. 81-2). The pathophysiology is not completely understood, but is thought to be caused by aberrant regeneration of autonomic fibers after local trauma to the auriculotemporal nerve.[21]

Frey syndrome can also be seen in infants and children, often after birth trauma with forceps delivery, but cases of familial, bilateral Frey syndrome without birth trauma have been reported.[22]

Gustatory sweating may also occur after upper thoracic and cervical sympathectomy,[23,24] facial herpes zoster, or chorda tympani injury[25] and has been described in association with cluster headache[26] and diabetes mellitus.[27]

Treatment with topical glycopyrrolate,[10] aluminum chloride, or botulinum toxin injection[27] can be effective; rarely, intracranial section of the glossopharyngeal nerve or tympanic neurectomy is needed.

PAROXYSMAL LOCALIZED HYPERHIDROSIS

Daytime paroxysmal hyperhidrosis affecting the head, neck and upper trunk can occasionally affect older postmenopausal women and less commonly, men. Hot flashes are typically not associated with paroxysmal

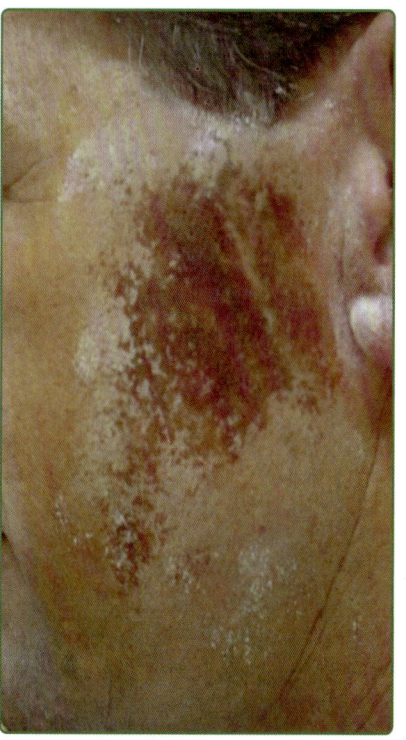

Figure 81-2 A patient with pathologic gustatory sweating and a positive starch iodine test result.

localized hyperhidrosis, and hormonal replacement therapy is usually ineffective. Reported history of sweating before menopause is normal, distinguishing the syndrome from craniofacial essential hyperhidrosis. Alterations in hypothalamic set point temperature range for sweating could be the contributing factor; however, the pathophysiology is not clearly understood. Symptomatic treatment with clonidine or topical or oral glycopyrrolate may be effective.[28]

LOCALIZED SECONDARY HYPERHIDROSIS ASSOCIATED WITH CUTANEOUS DISORDERS

Excessive sweating has also been reported in association with certain cutaneous disorders such as blue rubber bleb nevus syndrome, perilesional skin of a glomus tumor, tufted angioma, eccrine angiomatous hamartoma or eccrine nevus, Grierson-Gopalan disease, pachydermoperiostosis, and pretibial myxedema.

ECCRINE NEVUS

Eccrine nevus is a rare skin hamartoma histologically defined as focal hyperplasia or hypertrophy of eccrine glands.[29] Clinically, it presents as hyperhidrotic isolated patch of skin with no epidermal changes and is frequently located on the forearm. Treatment decisions depend on the severity of the hyperhidrotic area. Isolated case reports have shown successful response to botulinum toxin injections and topical glycopyrrolate.[29,30]

ETIOLOGY AND PATHOGENESIS OF GENERALIZED SECONDARY HYPERHIDROSIS

METABOLIC, INFECTIOUS, AND OTHER SYSTEMIC DISORDERS

Hyperhidrosis has been previously reported in association with diabetes mellitus, hypoglycemia, thyrotoxicosis, carcinoid syndrome, hyperpituitarism (acromegaly), congestive heart failure, dumping syndrome, menopause, malignancy, and drug withdrawal.

Exogenous bacterial pyrogens that stimulate production of interleukin (IL)-1, IL-6, tumor necrosis factor, and interferons can cause fever and subsequently hyperhidrosis. These inflammatory cytokines act in the brain to induce and increase the synthesis of prostaglandins, resulting in elevation of the thermal set point.[31] The simultaneous activation of antipyretic mechanisms eventually produces excessive sweating. Tuberculosis, malaria, brucellosis, and subacute bacterial endocarditis are some of the infectious etiologies that could present with generalized hyperhidrosis.

With regard to malignancy, excessive production of IL-6 by Hodgkin lymphoma cells has been shown to result in fever and subsequent night sweating.[32]

Riley-Day Syndrome: Familial dysautonomia (FD), also known as Riley-Day syndrome, is the most intensively studied of the hereditary sensory-autonomic neuropathies (designated as hereditary sensory and autonomic neuropathy [HSAN] type III). This is an autosomal recessive disorder that affects 1 in 3600 live births in the Ashkenazi Jewish population and is caused by mutations in the *IKAP* gene, located on chromosome 9.[33] FD is characterized by pronounced autonomic dysregulation with profuse sweating and salivation, diminished production of tears, red blotching of the skin, absence of fungiform papillae of the tongue, episodic orthostatic hypotension, arterial hypertension, reduced deep tendon reflexes, and behavioral abnormalities.[33]

MEDICATIONS AND TOXINS

Alteration in sweating can occur as a side effect from diverse classes of medications. Hyperhidrosis can be associated with serotonin (5-hydroxytryptamine) reuptake inhibitors, opioids, and prostaglandin inhibitors (naproxen). The mechanisms may relate to 5-hydroxytryptamine (2A) and dopamine receptor antagonism. Hyperhidrosis that commonly occurs during acute and chronic administration of opioids is mainly caused by stimulation of mast cell degranulation, resulting in the release of histamine.[34] In contrast, tricyclic antidepressants occasionally cause hyperhidrosis because of their sympathomimetic effect. The presumed mechanism is inhibited reuptake of norepinephrine, leading to stimulation of peripheral adrenergic receptors and a generalized diaphoretic response. Cholinergic agonists such as pilocarpine and bethanechol and reversible cholinesterase inhibitors such as pyridostigmine can increase sweating directly or indirectly via activation of M3 cholinergic receptors on sweat glands.

DIAGNOSIS

Just as with primary hyperhidrosis, a thorough clinical history and physical examination are crucial, particularly focusing on constitutional symptoms (fever, unexplained weight loss, chills, night sweats, fatigue) and endocrine and neurologic systems. Inquiring about prescription and OTC medications and supplements taken daily or as needed will also aid in recognizing secondary causes. Primary hyperhidrosis may be present in patients with underlying medical conditions, but generally with an onset of symptoms at a younger age and occurs in more classic focal locations as discussed previously. A Minor starch-iodine test may be used to assess the distribution of excessive sweating. If secondary hyperhidrosis is suspected, baseline vital signs and laboratory studies are warranted, and the patient should be referred to his primary care physician for an evaluation. Neurologic consultation may also be considered if suggested by the medical history or physical exam.

CLINICAL COURSE, PROGNOSIS, AND MANAGEMENT

Clinical course and prognosis will depend on the underlying disease that is manifesting symptoms of hyperhidrosis or discontinuing a culprit medication. Treatment should be focused on correcting or controlling the underlying disease, but symptoms may be reduced with any of the mentioned modalities listed previously.

ANHIDROSIS

Anhidrosis may occur because of congenital absence of sweat glands as in cases of hypohidrotic ectodermal dysplasia, hereditary metabolic disorders (Fabry disease), or acquired causes (secondary or idiopathic anhidrosis).

Secondary anhidrosis or hypohidrosis can result from connective tissue diseases (Sjögren syndrome), eccrine duct obstruction (from chronic dermatoses such as psoriasis or atopic dermatitis, or acute causes such as miliaria), underlying neurologic disorders with autonomic dysfunction (congenital insensitivity to pain with anhidrosis, multiple sclerosis, Shy-Drager syndrome), peripheral neuropathies, and medications or toxins.

CLINICAL FEATURES

Patients with focal or segmental anhidrosis may become aware of their disease because of compensatory hyperhidrosis in other regions (Fig. 81-3). Generalized anhidrosis or anhidrosis with large areas of involvement usually manifests as heat exhaustion, inability to tolerate increased physical activity in a hot environment, or dizziness upon exposure to heat.

HYPOHIDROTIC ECTODERMAL DYSPLASIA

Mutations in the *ED-1* gene encoding for ectodysplasin result in X-linked hypohidrotic ectodermal dysplasia, which is the most common form of the ectodermal dysplasias. These disorders are characterized by an abnormal development of eccrine sweat glands, hair, and teeth.[35] Autosomal-recessive and autosomal-dominant modes of inheritance have also been described.[36] Affected children are at risk of experiencing life-threatening hyperpyrexia because of their inability to sweat.

CONGENITAL INSENSITIVITY TO PAIN WITH ANHIDROSIS

Congenital insensitivity to pain with anhidrosis (CIPA), also known as HSAN type IV, is a rare autosomal recessive disorder characterized by the congenital insensitivity to noxious stimuli, anhidrosis, recurrent hyperpyrexia, mental retardation, and self-mutilating behavior.[37] CIPA is reported to occur because of loss-of-function variants in neurotrophic tyrosine receptor kinase 1 (NTRK1) gene. Nearly all of the associated symptoms can be attributed to the inability of NTRK1 signaling pathways to regulate the development of nociceptive, sympathetic, and central cholinergic neurons.[37]

FABRY DISEASE

Fabry disease is an inherited X-linked lysosomal storage disorder caused by deficient activity of α-galactosidase A. It presents during childhood in both male and female patients. Early manifestations include hypohidrosis, telangiectasia, angiokeratoma, acroparesthesia, and gastrointestinal symptoms.[38] Later in adolescence or adulthood, manifestations can include renal, cardiac, and central nervous system dysfunction. Hypohidrosis is the second most common symptom of Fabry disease; the pathogenesis is unclear

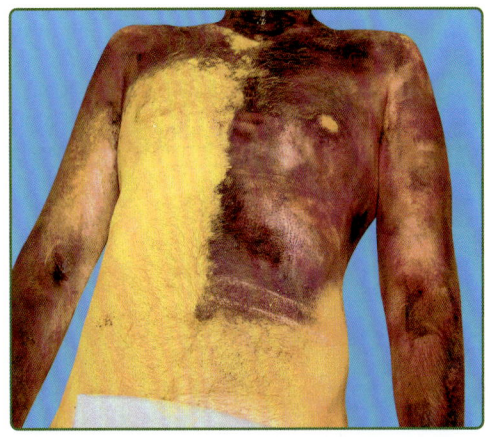

Figure 81-3 A patient with segmental anhidrosis (*yellow*) with compensatory left-sided hemihyperhidrosis (*purple*) caused by a right greater than left-sided upper thoracic spinal cord injury (sodium alizarin sulfate indicator powder).

ACQUIRED IDIOPATHIC GENERALIZED ANHIDROSIS

Acquired idiopathic generalized anhidrosis (AIGA) is a rare cause of anhidrosis that can result from idiopathic pure sudomotor failure, sudomotor neuropathy, or eccrine sweat gland failure.[40] The majority of AIGA cases, however, lack these pathologic abnormalities. Cases reported in literature affect primarily patients of Asian ethnicity, but it is not entirely clear if this is because of a genetic component or if AIGA is underreported in other populations. AIGA has a heterogenous clinical presentation and can include the following clinical features: acute onset, cholinergic urticaria, elevated serum immunoglobulin E levels, absence of other autonomic dysfunction, and marked response to glucocorticoids.[41] Spontaneous remission has been reported in some cases of AIGA, but anhidrosis tends to persist if it has been present for a long time. Patients with generalized or partial anhidrosis involving at least 30% to 40% of their body surface area should be advised against participation in activities requiring increased endurance or working in high ambient temperatures.[40]

MILIARIA

Miliaria results from obstruction of eccrine sweat ducts and occurs in conditions of increased heat and humidity. There are three types of clinically distinctive miliaria classified based on the level of the obstruction: miliaria crystallina, miliaria rubra, and miliaria profunda. In miliaria crystallina, ductal obstruction occurs at the stratum corneum. It presents as small, 1-mm, clear, fragile, vesicles that rupture easily (Fig. 81-4). They are commonly seen on the face and upper trunk in infants and on the trunk in adults. In miliaria rubra, obstruction occurs deeper within the epidermis and results in pruritic, 1- to 3-mm, nonfollicular, erythematous macules and papules on the upper trunk and neck. Sterile pustules may also develop and are termed *miliaria pustulosa*. When miliaria rubra becomes chronic or recurrent, occlusion of eccrine sweat ducts extends to a deeper level. In miliaria profunda, ductal obstruction occurs at the dermal–epidermal junction and produces asymptomatic, 1- to 3-mm white papules.

DIAGNOSIS

As with hyperhidrosis, a careful medical history is necessary, with special attention to medications, underlying medical conditions, and family history. Examination of the skin may not reveal the presence of anhidrosis, but could indicate compensatory hyperhidrosis. To identify possible sweat gland abnormalities, a biopsy specimen from the affected area should be obtained in patients with anhidrosis (Fig. 81-5).

CLINICAL COURSE, PROGNOSIS, AND MANAGEMENT

Unlike treatment of hyperhidrosis, options for anhidrosis are limited. The primary cause should be identified first, and any possible contributing medications

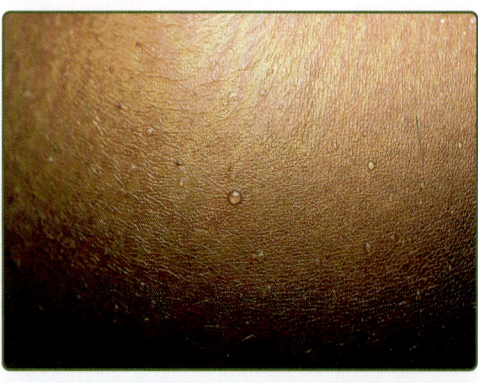

Figure 81-4 Miliaria crystallina with delicate, droplike vesicles and no underlying erythema.

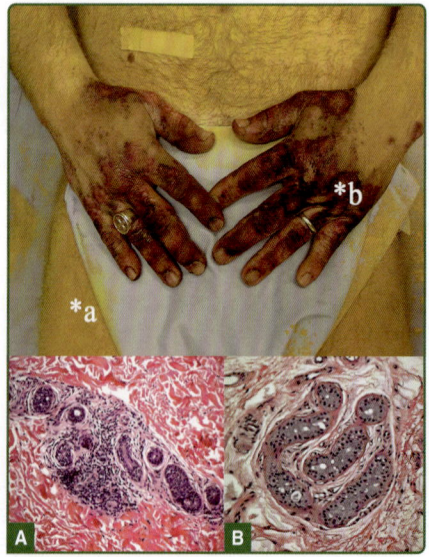

Figure 81-5 Punch skin biopsy from an anhidrotic skin site (**A**) shows marked perieccrine lymphocytic infiltration of sweat gland secretory coils, and sweating skin (**B**) shows normal sweat gland morphology.

should be discontinued. Keeping the patient in cool temperatures is crucial to avoid life-threatening overheating. It can also be helpful to wear wet clothing during physical activity; however, the effectiveness of external cooling may be compromised in patients with ectodermal dysplasia, presumably because of poor capillary dilation.[41,42] In cases of miliaria, treatment is usually not indicated for miliaria crystallina because of its self-limited nature. The topical application of anhydrous lanolin has resulted in dramatic improvement in patients with miliaria profunda.[43] Prevention and treatment of miliaria consists of controlling exposure to heat and humidity, treating any underlying febrile illnesses, and removing occlusive clothing.

ACKNOWLEDGMENTS

The authors acknowledge the contribution of Robert D. Fealey and Adelaide A. Hebert, the former authors of this chapter.

REFERENCES

1. Doolittle J, Walker P, Mills T, et al. Hyperhidrosis: an update on prevalence and severity in the United States. *Arch Dermatol Res*. 2016;308(10):743-749.
2. Sato K, Kang WH, Saga K, et al. Biology of sweat glands and their disorders. II. Disorders of sweat gland function. *J Am Acad Dermatol*. 1989;20(5):713-726.
3. Walling HW. Primary hyperhidrosis increases the risk of cutaneous infection: a case-control study of 387 patients. *J Am Acad Dermatol*. 2009;61(2):242-246.
4. Ro KN, Cantor RM, Lange KL, et al. Palmar hyperhidrosis: evidence of genetic transmission. *J Vasc Surg*. 2002;382-386.
5. Chen J, Lin M, Chen X, et al. A novel locus for primary focal hyperhidrosis mapped on chromosome 2q31.1. *Br J Dermatol*. 2015;172:1150-1164.
6. Kaufmann H, Saadia D, Polin C, et al. Primary hyperhidrosis: evidence for autosomal dominant inheritance. *Clin Auton Res*. 2003;13:96-98.
7. Hornberger J, Grimes K, Naumann M, et al. Recognition, diagnosis, and treatment of primary focal hyperhidrosis. *J Am Acad Dermatol*. 2004;51(2):274-286.
8. Solish N, Bertucci V, Dansereau A. A comprehensive approach to the recognition, diagnosis, and severity-based treatment of focal hyperhidrosis: recommendations of the Canadian Hyperhidrosis Advisory Committee. *Dermatol Surg*. 2007;908-923.
9. Kim WO, Kil HK, Yoon KB, et al. Topical glycopyrrolate for patients with facial hyperhidrosis. *Br J Dermatol*. 2008;158:1094-1097.
10. Hays LL. The Frey syndrome: a review and double blind evaluation of the topical use of a new anticholinergic agent. *Laryngoscope*. 1978;88:1796-1824.
11. Glaser DA, Pariser DM, Hebert AA, et al. A prospective, nonrandomized, open-label study of the efficacy and safety of onabotulinumtoxinA in adolescents with primary axillary hyperhidrosis. *Pediatr Dermatol*. 2015;32(5):609-617.
12. Kinklelin I, Hund M, Naumann M, et al. Effective treatment of frontal hyperhidrosis with botulinum toxin A. *Br J Dermatol*. 2000;143:824-827.
13. Shelley WB, Talanin NY, Shelley ED. Botulinum toxin therapy for palmar hyperhidrosis. *J Am Acad Dermatol*. 1998;38:227-229.
14. Hexsel DM, Dal'Forno T, Hexsel CL. Inguinal, or Hexsel's hyperhidrosis. *Clin Dermatol*. 2004;22(1):53-59.
15. Jacob C. Treatment of hyperhidrosis with microwave technology. *Semin Cutan Med Surg*. 2013;32(1):2-8.
16. Karakoc Y, Aydemir EH, Kalkan MT, et al. Safe control of palmoplantar hyperhidrosis with direct current. *Int J Dermatol*. 2002;41:602-605.
17. Cerfolio RJ, De Campos JRM, Bryant AS, et al. The Society of Thoracic Surgeons expert consensus for the surgical treatment of hyperhidrosis. *Ann Thorac Surg*. 2011;91:1642-1648.
18. Walling HW. Systemic therapy for primary hyperhidrosis: a retrospective study of 59 patients treated with glycopyrrolate or clonidine. *J Am Acad Dermatol*. 2012;66(3):387-392.
19. Bajaj V, Langtry JA. Use of oral glycopyrronium bromide in hyperhidrosis. *Br J Dermatol*. 2007;157:118-121.
20. Walling, HW. Clinical differentiation of primary from secondary hyperhidrosis. *J Am Acad Dermatol*. 2011;64(4):690-695.
21. Dunbar EM, Singer TW, Singer K, et al. Understanding gustatory sweating. What have we learned from Lucja Frey and her predecessors? *Clin Auton Res*. 2002;12:179-184.
22. Sethuraman G, Mancini AJ. Familial auriculotemporal nerve (Frey) syndrome. *Pediatr Dermatol*. 2009;26(3):302-305.
23. Kurchin A, Adar R, Zweig A, et al. Gustatory phenomena after upper dorsal sympathectomy. *Arch Neurol*. 1977;34:619-623.
24. Bloor K. Gustatory sweating and other responses after cervicothoracic sympathectomy. *Brain*. 1969;92:137-146.
25. Young AG. Unilateral sweating of the submental region after eating (chorda tympani syndrome). *Br Med J*. 1956;12:976-979.
26. Drummond PD. Autonomic disturbances in cluster headache. *Brain*. 1988;111:1199-1209.
27. Restivo DA, Lanza S, Patti F, et al. Improvement of diabetic autonomic gustatory sweating by botulinum toxin type A. *Neurology*. 2002;59:1971-1973.
28. Kuritzky A, Hering R, Goldhammer G, et al. Clonidine treatment in paroxysmal localized hyperhidrosis. *Arch Neurol*. 1984;41:1210-1211.
29. Lera M, Espana A, Idoate MA. Focal hyperhidrosis secondary to eccrine naevus successfully treated with botulinum toxin type A. *Clin Exp Dermatol*. 2015;40(6):640-643.
30. Dua J, Grabczynska S. Eccrine nevus affecting the forearm of an 11-year-old girl successfully controlled with topical glycopyrrolate. *Pediatr Dermatol*. 2004;31(5):611-612.
31. Netea MG, Kullberg BJ, Van der Meer JWM. Circulating cytokines as mediators of fever. *Clin Infect Dis*. 2000;31(5):S178-S184.
32. Nagel S, et al. HLXB9 activates IL6 in Hodgkin lymphoma cell lines and is regulated by PI3K signalling involving E2F3. *Leukemia*. 2005;19(5):841-846.
33. Dietrich P, Dragatsis I. Familial dysautonomia: mechanisms and models. *Genet Mol Biol*. 2016;39(4):497-514.
34. Ikeda T, Kurz A, Sessler DI, et al. The effect of opioids on thermoregulatory responses in humans and the special antishivering action of meperidine. *Ann N Y Acad Sci*. 1997;813:792-798.
35. Vincent MC, Biancalana V, Ginisty D, et al. Mutational spectrum of the ED1 gene in X-linked hypohidrotic

ectodermal dysplasia. *Eur J Hum Genet*. 2001;9:355-363.
36. Priolo M, Lagana C. Ectodermal dysplasias: a new clinical-genetic classification. *J Med Genet*. 2001;38:579-585.
37. Wang QL, Guo S, Duan G, et al. Phenotypes and genotypes in five children with congenital insensitivity to pain with anhidrosis. *Pediatr Neurol*. 2016;61:63-69.
38. Zampetti A, Orteu CH, Antuzzi D, et al. Angiokeratoma: decision-making aid for the diagnosis of Fabry disease. *Br J Dermatol*. 2012;166:712-720.
39. Orteu CH, Jansen T, Lidove O, et al. Fabry disease and the skin: data from FOS, the Fabry outcome survey. *Br J Dermatol*. 2007;157:331-317.
40. Tay LK, Chong WS. Acquired idiopathic anhidrosis: a diagnosis often missed. *J Am Acad Dermatol*. 2014;71(3):499-506.
41. Nakazato Y, Tamura N, Ohkuma A, et al. Idiopathic pure sudomotor failure anhidrosis due to deficits in cholinergic transmission. *Neurology*. 2004;63:1476-1480.
42. Brengelmann GL, Freund PR, Rowell LB, et al. Absence of active cutaneous vasodilation associated with congenital absence of sweat glands in human. *Am J Physiol*. 1981;240:H571-H575.
43. Kirk JF, Wilson BB, Chun W, et al. Miliaria profunda. *J Am Acad Dermatol*. 1996;35(5 Pt 2):854-856.

Chapter 82 :: Bromhidrosis and Chromhidrosis
:: Christos C. Zouboulis

第八十二章
腋臭和色汗

中文导读

本章分别讲述了腋臭和色汗的流行病学特征、病因和发病机制、临床研究成果、病理、鉴别诊断、治疗、预后与临床病程等。

一、腋臭

腋臭指的是身体散发出过多或令人不舒服的气味，主要来自大汗腺和汗腺，最常见于腋窝。本章从六个方面全面讲述了腋臭。

1. 流行病学　腋臭通常发生在青春期之后，男性的大汗腺功能比女性更活跃。虽然在夏季或温暖的气候时腋臭症状会加重，但该病并没有季节性或地域性；腋臭通常是一种个体疾病，而腋臭顶泌症有亚洲家族发病的报道。

2. 病因和发病机制　针对腋臭的发病机制，文章提出，大汗腺通过其分泌物的成分发挥主导作用。其中，有气味的激素，即信息素（pheromones），被认为是导致汗臭的原因。作者重点讲解了信息素5α-Reductase type-I在汗臭人群的大汗腺中表达增高，催化睾酮转化为5α-二氢睾酮，5α-二氢睾酮继而促进皮肤中的睾酮增高。

腋窝有多种细菌，以革兰氏阳性杆菌为主，腋臭与需氧棒状杆菌尤其有关。文中进一步讲解了细菌是如何将汗液中的无味前体转化为氨和恶臭的短链挥发性脂肪酸，从而产生独特气味的过程。

有研究还提出了大汗腺的常染色体显性遗传模式。较新的研究发现，腋臭和湿耳垢之间的密切关系与ABCC11基因的单核苷酸多态性rs17822931有关。

此外，多汗症对大汗腺分泌以及腋臭的影响尚不清楚。一些人认为，小汗腺广泛分布，其分泌物通常无臭，可以通过冲洗过量的汗液来改善腋臭大汗液。另一些人则认为汗液通过促进大汗腺分泌物成分的局部传播和加强细菌滋生的潮湿环境，从而增加了腋臭。也就是说，腋臭可能是由于细菌作用于被小汗腺分泌物软化的角蛋白而形成。本章还提到，足底汗臭是典型的小汗腺汗臭。某些食物、药物、毒素或代谢等原因也可导致小汗腺汗臭。

3. 临床研究成果　什么是"正常"量的体味在个人和种族群体中差异很大。在亚洲人群中，通常只有轻微的气味即被做出诊断。

腋臭的诊断主要靠临床症状。因为腋臭没有相关的实验室异常；在病理改变方面，尽管有些报告没有显示腋臭患者的大分泌腺有任何异常，但已有报道称大分泌腺的数量和大小是有所增加的。

4. 鉴别诊断　大汗腺臭汗症远比小汗腺臭汗症常见。文中，表82-1列出了腋臭的鉴别诊断，与外分泌腺的臭汗、肝衰竭、肾功能衰竭、卫生差、嗅幻觉、身体畸形恐惧等进行鉴别诊断。

5. 治疗　作者较为详细地总结了临床上

治疗腋臭的一般措施（如经常清洗、使用除臭剂或止汗剂、香水、换脏衣服、去除腋毛等）；还有局部注射A型肉毒杆菌毒素，掺钕钇铝石榴石激光等非手术治疗；还有负压抽吸刮除术、上胸交感神经切断术等手术治疗。

6．预后与临床病程　腋臭顶泌症是一种慢性且不能缓解的疾病。作者特别提出，患腋臭顶泌症的患者常常对自己的状况感到难为情和尴尬，并可能发展为社会心理功能障碍，而患有躯体畸形障碍的患者可能会声称患有腋臭。

二、色汗症

色汗症是一种罕见的疾病，其特征是分泌有颜色的汗液。本章从七个方面讲述了色汗症。

1．流行病学　世界范围内的流行情况尚不清楚，在非洲裔美国人中最常见，但地域性从未被描述过。汗腺的发病通常发生在青春期，但也有报道在婴儿期发病的罕见病例。文章指出，色汗症伴随人的一生，在老年人中有所改善。虽然文献报道的大多数病例涉及妇女，但目前缺乏足够的证据支持该病在女性人群中高发。

2．病因和发病机制　造成大汗腺色汗症的色素是脂褐素，它由大汗腺分泌细胞产生并分泌到皮肤表面。在色汗症中，脂褐素颗粒处于较高的氧化状态，从而产生各种颜色的色素，如黄色、绿色、蓝色或黑色。氧化状态越高，颜色越深。但为什么这种情况只发生在某些人身上的原因还不清楚。这里，作者提到了P物质（一种强大的血管扩张剂）可能在出汗和色汗症中发挥作用。

真正的小汗腺色汗症是非常罕见的。当水溶性色素从汗腺排泄后，摄入某些染料或药物，色汗形成。此外，小汗腺色汗症也被报道与尿黑酸症、高胆红素和血汗有关。

3．临床研究成果　既往研究包括，患有色汗症的人通常描述在大汗腺分泌前有温暖、刺痛的感觉。色汗的诱因通常与情绪或身体刺激有关。

作者还介绍了通过实验室检查排除出血素质、黑酸尿、假汗腺嗜铬等疾病；介绍了一些特殊的检测手段。

4．病理　作者描述了色汗症的特异性的病理学改变。

5．鉴别诊断　假性色汗症是指汗液表面的化合物或分子与汗液混合后产生的色素，色汗症必须与假性色汗症区别开来。作者列出了鉴别诊断表（表82-2），并举例说明。

6．治疗　色汗症缺乏有效的治疗方法。手动挤压使汗液分泌可在接下来的48到72小时内暂时改善症状。有报道，A型肉毒杆菌毒素、辣椒素等治疗面部色汗症有效。对于假性色汗症，合并到细菌感染的病例中，局部和口服红霉素似乎是有效的治疗方法。

7．预后与临床病程　大汗腺色汗症是一种慢性疾病，随着大汗腺活动的减少，它在老年期得到改善。发病率受患者的社会心理功能障碍的影响。

〔刘芳芬〕

BROMHIDROSIS

AT-A-GLANCE

- *Bromhidrosis* refers to an offensive or unpleasant body odor arising from apocrine or eccrine gland secretions.
- Chronic disorder that most often develops in the axillae, but may also involve the genitals or plantar aspect of the feet.
- The best-characterized short-chain fatty acid causing odor is ε-3-methyl-2-hexenoic acid.
- Surgical removal of affected glands may be effective.

Body odor, *osmidrosis*, is a common phenomenon in a postpubertal population. *Bromhidrosis* refers to offensive body odor that is excessive or particularly unpleasant, which prominently arises from apocrine and eccrine glands. Bromhidrosis is most often reported in the axillae (apocrine bromhidrosis). This condition may contribute to impairment of an individual's psychosocial functioning. The terminology in the literature is sometimes confusing, using *osmidrosis* to imply offensive odor, and *bromhidrosis* to imply osmidrosis in the setting of concomitant hyperhidrosis (excessive eccrine sweat gland secretion).[1]

EPIDEMIOLOGY

Apocrine bromhidrosis usually occurs after puberty. It exhibits a male predominance, which may be a reflection of greater apocrine gland activity in men than in women. There is no seasonal or geographic predilection, although summer months or warm climates may aggravate the disease. Poor personal hygiene also may be a contributing factor. Bromhidrosis is usually an individual condition, whereas apocrine bromhidrosis has been reported in asian families.[2]

ETIOLOGY AND PATHOGENESIS

Apocrine secretion is predominantly responsible for odor production, primarily through bacterial action on its components.[3] It is accepted that the odorous steroids, the so-called pheromones, among them 16-androstenes, 5α-androstenol, and 5α-androstenone, contribute to osmidrosis.[4,5] 5α-Reductase type I is expressed in apocrine glands. Individuals with osmidrosis have increased levels of 5α-reductase in their apocrine glands. Because this enzyme catalyzes the conversion of testosterone to 5α-dihydrotestosterone, levels of 5α-dihydrotestosterone may be greater than testosterone in the skin of affected individuals.[6] The biotransformation of these steroids is complex and further research is required to delineate these pathways.

Moreover, the axilla hosts many different bacteria, most of which are Gram-positive. Bromhidrosis has been particularly associated with the action of aerobic *Corynebacterium* species.[3] Axillary bacterial florae produce the distinctive axillary odor by transforming nonodoriferous precursors in sweat to ammonia and short-chain, malodorous, volatile fatty acids. The most common of these are ε-3-methyl-2-hexenoic acid and (RS)-3-hydroxy-3-methlyhexanoic acid, which are released through the action of a specific zinc-dependent N-alpha-acyl-glutamine aminoacylase from *Corynebacterium* species.[6,7] ε-3-Methyl-2-hexenoic acid is delivered to the surface of the skin on 2 binding proteins, apocrine-secretion binding proteins 1 (ASOB1) and 2 (ASOB2). ASOB2 has been identified as apolipoprotein D.[8]

One study proposed an autosomal dominant inheritance pattern for apocrine bromhidrosis. Newer studies have found a strong relationship between bromhidrosis and wet ear wax associated with the single nucleotide polymorphism rs 17822931 of the *ABCC11* gene.[9,10]

Eccrine secretions are distributed in a generalized fashion, are usually odorless, and serve a thermoregulatory function. The effect of hyperhidrosis on eccrine osmidrosis and bromhidrosis is unclear. Some advocate that excessive eccrine sweat improves apocrine bromhidrosis by flushing away excessive apocrine secretions. Others postulate that eccrine sweat augments apocrine bromhidrosis by encouraging local spread of apocrine sweat components and enhancing the moist environment in which bacteria flourish; that is, eccrine bromhidrosis may develop from the action of bacteria on keratin that has been softened by eccrine secretions. A plantar location is characteristic for eccrine bromhidrosis. Certain foods (garlic, curry, alcohol), drugs (bromides), toxins, or metabolic causes (disorders of amino acid metabolism) may result in eccrine bromhidrosis; the latter being fish odor syndrome (trimethylaminuria), phenylketonuria, cat syndrome, isovaleric acidemia, hypermethioninemia, and food, drug, toxin ingestion.[2]

CLINICAL FINDINGS

HISTORY

Patients complain of an unpleasant body odor. The axillae are the most commonly affected site, although the genitals or plantar feet also may be affected.[3] The diagnosis is usually clinical. What constitutes a "normal" amount of body odor varies considerably among individuals and ethnic groups. In Asian populations, only slight odor is often considered diagnostic.[11,12]

CUTANEOUS LESIONS

Physical examination of the affected individual is usually unremarkable.

LABORATORY TESTS

There are no associated laboratory abnormalities.

PATHOLOGY

Although some reports do not reveal any abnormalities in the apocrine glands of affected individuals, an increase in the numbers and size of apocrine glands has been reported.[11]

TABLE 82-1
Differential Diagnosis of Bromhidrosis[13]

- Apocrine bromhidrosis
- Eccrine bromhidrosis
  - Fish odor syndrome (trimethylaminuria)
  - Phenylketonuria
  - Sweaty feet syndrome
  - Odor of cat syndrome
  - Isovaleric acidemia
  - Hypermethioninemia
  - Food, drug, toxin ingestion
- Liver failure (fetor hepaticus)
- Renal failure
- Nasal foreign body in children
- Poor hygiene
- Olfactory hallucinations/Schisophenia
- Body dysmorphic disorder
- Erythrasma
- Trichomycosis axillaris

DIFFERENTIAL DIAGNOSIS

Apocrine bromhidrosis can be distinguished from eccrine bromhidrosis, which is far less common. Moreover, further conditions should be distinguished from bromhidrosis; Table 82-1 outlines the differential diagnosis of bromhidrosis.

TREATMENT

GENERAL MEASURES

Frequent washing of the axillae, use of a deodorant or antiperspirant (aluminum chloride hexahydrate), perfumes, and changing of soiled clothing can help. Removal of axillary hair may minimize odor by preventing bacteria and sweat accumulation on the hair shafts. Antibacterial soaps or topical antibacterial agents also may be beneficial.

NONSURGICAL THERAPY

The injection of botulinum toxin A has been reported to successfully treat genital[13] and axillary bromhidrosis.[14] The frequency-doubled, quality-switched neodymium:yttrium-aluminum-garnet laser also has been reported to be an effective noninvasive therapy for axillary bromhidrosis.[15]

SURGERY

Several surgical measures have been investigated in the treatment of apocrine bromhidrosis. Patient selection is important because surgery is potentially associated with postoperative scar formation, prolonged healing times, infection, and other complications. Upper thoracic sympathectomy has been successful in treating apocrine bromhidrosis either in isolation or in association with palmar hyperhidrosis.[1] Surgical removal of the culprit apocrine glands can be achieved either by the removal of subcutaneous tissue in isolation or in combination with axillary skin.[16-20] Surgical subcutaneous tissue removal also has been used in association with CO_2 laser ablation.[21,22] Although surgical excision may be highly efficacious, depending on the depth of tissue removed and surgical technique used, regeneration and return of apocrine function/osmidrosis and bromhidrosis may develop. Superficial liposuction,[21] tumescent superficial liposuction with curettage,[23] and ultrasound-assisted liposuction,[24] as well as their combinations,[25] have efficacy in the management of apocrine bromhidrosis. Liposuction curettage can be considered the primary choice among surgical procedures used to treat patients with bromhidrosis because of its fewer complications.[24] In a series of 375 patients, more than 90% reported a satisfactory reduction in odor after ultrasound-assisted liposuction.[26] This technique uses ultrasound to liquefy fat and sweat glands. In contrast, laser hair removal may be associated with intensification of bromhidrosis.[27] The newly reported treatment using a microwave-based device may be an effective alternative treatment for axillary hyperhidrosis/bromhidrosis.[28]

PROGNOSIS AND CLINICAL COURSE

Apocrine bromhidrosis is a chronic and nonremitting condition.[29] Patients with apocrine bromhidrosis often feel self-conscious and embarrassed by their condition and may develop a psychosocial functioning impairment. Patients with body dysmorphic disorders may present claiming bromhidrosis.

CHROMHIDROSIS

AT-A-GLANCE

- Rare, chronic condition characterized by the secretion of colored sweat.
- Axillary and facial involvement is most common. Areola involvement has been reported.
- Caused by an increased number of lipofuscin granules in the luminal secretory cells of the apocrine glands.
- Secretions may be yellow, blue, green, brown, or black.
- Wood light examination may demonstrate fluorescence of secretions and stained clothes.
- Adequate therapy is lacking. Reports of treatment efficacy with manual expression, capsaicin, and botulinum toxin.

Chromhidrosis is a rare condition characterized by the secretion of colored apocrine sweat. Two variants of apocrine chromhidrosis are recognized: axillary and facial.[29] Involvement of the mammary areola also has been described.[30,31] Yonge first recognized facial chromhidrosis in 1709. Shelley and Hurley described this entity in 1954 and associated it with an increased number of lipofuscin granules in apocrine glands.[32]

EPIDEMIOLOGY

Chromhidrosis is a rare disease. The worldwide prevalence is unknown. Onset of chromhidrosis is usually at puberty, at the time of increased apocrine gland activity. However, rare cases of onset in infancy have been reported.[33] The disease persists throughout life, improving in the aged. It is reported most commonly in African Americans.[29] Geographic predilections have never been described. Most of the cases reported in the literature involve women; however, there is a lack of sound scientific evidence supporting a female preponderance.

ETIOLOGY AND PATHOGENESIS

The pigment responsible for causing apocrine chromhidrosis is lipofuscins that are produced in the apocrine secretory cells and excreted to the skin surface. Lipofuscin is a golden-colored pigment that is not specific to apocrine glands. In chromhidrosis, the lipofuscin granules are in a higher state of oxidation, thereby imparting various colors of pigment, such as yellow, green, blue, or black. Higher states of oxidation produce darker colors.[29,34] It is uncertain why this only develops in some individuals. One case of facial chromhidrosis was successfully treated with capsaicin.[35] Nerve endings with receptors for substance P have been found around eccrine sweat glands, suggesting that substance P, a potent vasodilator, may play a role in sweat production and chromhidrosis.[29]

True eccrine chromhidrosis is very rare and occurs when water-soluble pigments are excreted from eccrine glands after the ingestion of certain dyes or drugs, such as quinine or cranberry juice.[34,36] Eccrine chromhidrosis also has been reported in association with alkaptonuria (ochronosis), hyperbilirubinemia[37,38] and hematohidrosis (bleeding diathesis).

CLINICAL FINDINGS

HISTORY

Individuals with chromhidrosis often describe a sensation of warmth, a prickling sensation, or tingling feeling before apocrine gland secretion. Triggers for colored sweating are usually emotional or physical stimuli.[29] The morbidity associated with chromhidrosis stems from the emotional distress experienced by affected individuals.[39] Staining of undershirts and handkerchiefs are common complaints.

CUTANEOUS LESIONS

Individuals with chromhidrosis develop colored sweat in the axillae, face, or mammary areolae area (Fig. 82-1).[29-31] The pigment produced ranges in color from yellow to blue, green, brown, or black. The quantity of pigmented sweat produced is usually quite small (approximately 0.001 mL at each follicular orifice).[41] The droplets are odorless and dry quickly. Dried secretions appear as dark flecks within affected areas. Axillary involvement causes staining of shirts and undergarments. Facial chromhidrosis commonly develops close to the lower eyelid, including the malar cheeks, and occasionally the forehead.[39,40] Colored sweat also can be manually expressed by squeezing in the affected area. Such a maneuver also may be therapeutic.[29]

SPECIAL TESTS

An examination of yellow, blue, or green secretions using a Wood light (360 nm) produces a characteristic yellow fluorescence. Black or brown pigment rarely autofluoresces.[29] Secretions can be manually

fungal cultures of affected areas to exclude pseudoeccrine chromhidrosis.[34]

PATHOLOGY

The luminal cells of the apocrine sweat glands have an eosinophilic cytoplasm, a large nucleus, and may contain lipofuscin, iron, lipid, or periodic acid–Schiff–positive and diastase-resistant granules.[42] Under light microscopy using hematoxylin-and-eosin staining, an increased number of (yellow to brown) lipofuscin granules may be present in the apical portion of luminal secretory cells of the apocrine glands. The number of granules varies. Additionally, autofluorescence of paraffin-embedded nonstained sections can be demonstrated using a 360-nm wavelength.[41] The granules are positive on periodic acid–Schiff stains. Schmorl stain also may be weakly positive.[43]

DIFFERENTIAL DIAGNOSIS

Chromhidrosis must be distinguished from pseudochromhidrosis (Table 82-2).[34,44] *Pseudoeccrine chromhidrosis* refers to the development of colored sweat when surface compounds or molecules mix with sweat to produce pigment. A classic example of this type is the formation of blue sweat in copper workers.[39] Extrinsic dyes, paints, fungi, and chromogenic bacteria (eg, *Corynebacterium* species) are other causes of pseudochromhidrosis.[29,34]

TREATMENT

Adequate therapy for chromhidrosis is lacking. Manual expression of colored secretions may result in a temporary improvement in symptoms for the following 48 to 72 hours.[35] Botulinum toxin type A has been reported as being successful in one patient with facial chromhidrosis. This patient experienced a substantial reduction in pigmented sweat and the results were sustained for 4 months.[45] Capsaicin is a topical cream that depletes and prevents reaccumulation of substance P levels in unmyelinated, slow-conducting type C sensory fibers. Case reports demonstrate the efficacy of capsaicin in the treatment of facial chromhidrosis.[35] For pseudochromhidrosis, topical and oral erythromycin seems to be the most effective treatment, both in unidentified and identified chromogenic bacteria cases.[44]

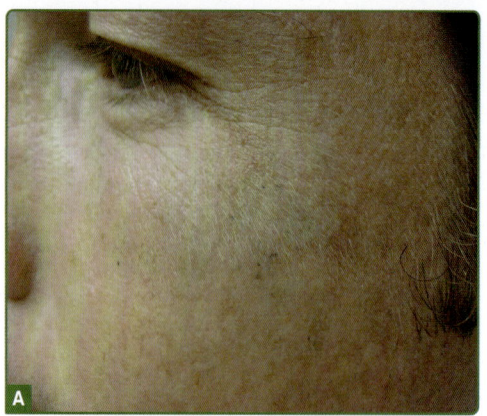
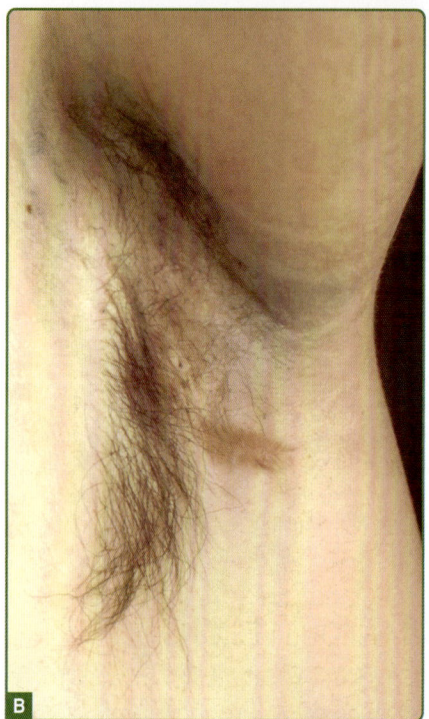

Figure 82-1 **A,** Blue-black sweat produced in a patient with facial apocrine chromhidrosis after gentle squeezing of the cheeks. (Reproduced with permission from Chang YC, Anderson N, Soeprono F. Bilateral facial pigmentation. *Dermatol Online J.* 2007;13[3]:16.) **B,** Blue-black apocrine pigmentation of the axilla and the inflammatory boils of a male patient with hidradenitis suppurativa.

expressed if not present at the time of examination. Stained clothing may also fluoresce with Wood lamp examination.[41] Apocrine glands can be stimulated to produce colored secretions by the injection of epinephrine or oxytocin.

LABORATORY TESTS

It is reasonable to check a complete blood cell count to exclude a bleeding diathesis, homogentisic levels in urine to exclude alkaptonuria, and bacterial and

TABLE 82-2
Differential Diagnosis of Chromhidrosis[34]
▪ Pseudoeccrine chromhidrosis[42]
▪ Blue sweat with copper exposure
▪ Extrinsic dyes, paints
▪ Chromogenic bacteria (eg, *Corynebacterium* species), *Pseudomonas*

PROGNOSIS AND CLINICAL COURSE

Apocrine chromhidrosis is a chronic disease that improves in old age as apocrine gland activity diminishes. Disease-associated morbidity is a result of psychosocial dysfunction experienced by affected individuals.

REFERENCES

1. Kao TH, Pan HC, Sun MH, et al. Upper thoracic sympathectomy for axillary osmidrosis or bromidrosis. *J Clin Neurosci*. 2004;11:719.
2. Teegee N, Rehmus W. Bromhidrosis. *Medscape*. Updated May 24, 2018. https://emedicine.medscape.com/article/1072342-overview.
3. Pinto M, Hundi GK, Bhat RM, et al. Clinical and epidemiological features of coryneform skin infections at a tertiary hospital. *Indian Dermatol Online J*. 2016;7:168.
4. Decréau RA, Marson CM, Smith KE, et al. Production of malodorous steroids from androsta-5, 16-dienes and androsta-4,16-dienes by Corynebacteria and other human axillary bacteria. *J Steroid Biochem Mol Biol*. 2003;87:327.
5. Austin C, Ellis J. Microbial pathways leading to steroidal malodour in the axilla. *J Steroid Biochem Mol Biol*. 2003;87:105.
6. Sato T, Sonoda T, Itami S, et al. Predominance of type I 5-reductase in apocrine sweat glands of patients with excessive or abnormal odour derived from apocrine sweat (osmidrosis). *Br J Dermatol*. 1998;139:806.
7. Spielman AI, Sunavala G, Harmony JA, et al. Identification and immunohistochemical localization of protein precursors to human axillary odors in apocrine glands and secretions. *Arch Dermatol*. 1998;134:813.
8. Zeng C, Spielman AI, Vowels BR, et al. A human axillary odorant is carried by apolipoprotein D. *Proc Natl Acad Sci U S A*. 1996;93:6626.
9. Nakano M, Miwa N, Hirano A, et al. A strong association of axillary osmidrosis with the wet earwax type determined by genotyping of the ABCC11 gene. *BMC Genet*. 2009;10:42.
10. Shang D, Zhang X, Sun M, et al. Strong association of the SNP rs17822931 with wet earwax and bromhidrosis in a Chinese family. *J Genet*. 2013;92:289.
11. Bang YH, Kim JH, Paik SW, et al. Histopathology of apocrine bromhidrosis. *Plast Reconstr Surg*. 1996;98:288.
12. Hurley HJ. Diseases of the apocrine sweat glands. In: Moschella SL, Hurley HJ, eds. *Dermatology*. 3rd ed. Philadelphia, PA: Saunders; 1992:1495.
13. He J, Wang T, Dong J. Effectiveness of botulinum toxin A injection for the treatment of secondary axillary bromhidrosis. *J Plast Reconstr Aesthet Surg*. 2017;70:1641.
14. Wang T, Dong J, He J. Long-term safety and efficacy of botulinum toxin A treatment in adolescent patients with axillary bromhidrosis. *Aesthetic Plast Surg*. 2018; 42:560.
15. Kunachak S, Wongwaisayawan S, Leelaudomlipi P. Non-invasive treatment of bromhidrosis by frequency doubled Q-switched Nd:YAG laser. *Aesthetic Plast Surg*. 2000;24:198.
16. Yoshikata R, Yanai A, Takei T, et al. Surgical treatment of axillary osmidrosis. *Br J Plast Surg*. 1990;43:483.
17. Breach NM. Axillary hyperhidrosis: surgical cure with aesthetic scars. *Ann R Coll Surg Engl*. 1979;61:295.
18. Endo T, Nakayama Y. Surgical treatment of axillary osmidrosis. *Ann Plast Surg*. 1993;30:136.
19. Zhao H, Li S, Nabi O, et al. Treatment of axillary bromhidrosis through a mini-incision with subdermal vascular preservation: a retrospective study in 396 patients. *Int J Dermatol*. 2016;55:919.
20. Dai Y, Xu AE, He J. A refined surgical treatment modality for bromhidrosis: subcutaneous scissor with micropore. *Dermatol Ther*. 2017;30:e12484.
21. Kim IH, Seo SL, Oh CH. Minimally invasive surgery for axillary osmidrosis: combined operation with CO_2 laser and subcutaneous tissue remover. *Dermatol Surg*. 1999;25:875.
22. Park JH, Cha SH, Park SD. Carbon dioxide laser treatment vs. subcutaneous resection of axillary osmidrosis. *Dermatol Surg*. 1997;23:247.
23. Seo SH, Jang BS, Oh CK, et al. Tumescent superficial liposuction with curettage for treatment of axillary bromhidrosis. *J Eur Acad Dermatol Venereol*. 2008; 22:30.
24. Zhang L, Chen F, Kong J, et al. The curative effect of liposuction curettage in the treatment of bromhidrosis: a meta-analysis. *Medicine (Baltimore)*. 2017;96: e7844.
25. He J, Wang T, Zhang Y, et al. Surgical treatment of axillary bromhidrosis by combining suction-curettage with subdermal undermining through a miniature incision. *J Plast Reconstr Aesthet Surg*. 2018;71:913.
26. Hong JP, Shin HW, Yoo SC. Ultrasound-assisted lipoplasty treatment for axillary bromhidrosis: clinical experience of 375 cases. *Plast Reconstr Surg*. 2004; 113:1264.
27. Hélou J, Soutou B, Jamous R, et al. Novel adverse effects of laser-assisted axillary hair removal [in French]. *Ann Dermatol Venereol*. 2009;136:495.
28. Hsu TH, Chen YT, Tu YK, et al. A systematic review of microwave-based therapy for axillary hyperhidrosis. *J Cosmet Laser Ther*. 2017;19:275.
29. Hurley SJ. Apocrine chromhidrosis. In: Freedberg MI, Eisen AZ, Wolff K, et al, eds. *Fitzpatrick's Dermatology in General Medicine*. 5th ed. MI New York, NY: McGraw-Hill; 1999:811.
30. Saff DM, Owens R, Kahn TA. Apocrine chromhidrosis involving the areolae in a 15-year-old amateur figure skater. *Pediatr Dermatol*. 1995;12:48.
31. Griffith JR. Isolated areolar apocrine chromhidrosis. *Pediatrics*. 2005;115:e239.
32. Shelley WD, Hurley HJ Jr. Localized chromhidrosis: a survey. *Arch Derm Syphilol*. 1954;69:449.
33. Yöntem A, Kör D, Hızlı-Karabacak B, et al. Blue-colored sweating: four infants with apocrine chromhidrosis. *Turk J Pediatr*. 2015;57:290.
34. Kim J, Rhemus W. Chromhidrosis. *Medscape*. Updated May 14, 2018. https://emedicine.medscape.com/article/1072254-overview.
35. Marks JG Jr. Treatment of apocrine chromhidrosis with topical capsaicin. *J Am Acad Dermatol*. 1989; 21:418.

36. Jaiswal AK, Ravikiran SP, Roy PK. Red eccrine chromhidrosis with review of literature. *Indian J Dermatol*. 2017;62:675.
37. Uzoma M, Singh G, Kohen L. Green palmoplantar vesicular eruption in a patient with hyperbilirubinemia. *JAAD Case Rep*. 2017;3:273.
38. Park JG, Prose NS, Garza R. Eccrine chromhidrosis in an adolescent with sickle cell disease. *Pediatr Dermatol*. 2017;34:e273.
39. Barankin B, Alanen K, Ting PT, et al. Bilateral facial apocrine chromhidrosis. *J Drugs Dermatol*. 2004;3:184.
40. Daoud MS, Dicken CH. Disorders of the apocrine sweat glands. In: Freedberg MI, Eisen AZ, Wolff K, et al, eds. *Fitzpatrick's Dermatology in General Medicine*. 6th ed. New York, NY: McGraw-Hill; 2003:708.
41. Cox NH, Popple AW, Large DM. Autofluorescence of clothing as an adjunct in the diagnosis of apocrine chromhidrosis. *Arch Dermatol*. 1992;128:275.
42. Urmacher CD. Normal skin. In: Sternberg SS, ed. *Histology for Pathologists*. 2nd ed. Philadelphia, PA: Lippincott-Raven; 1997:25.
43. Cilliers J, de Beer C. The case of the red lingerie—chromhidrosis revisited. *Dermatology*. 1999;199:149.
44. Tempark T, Wittayakornrerk S, Jirasukprasert L, et al. Pseudochromhidrosis: report and review of literature. *Int J Dermatol*. 2017;56:496.
45. Matarasso SL. Treatment of facial chromhidrosis with botulinum toxin type A. *J Am Acad Dermatol*. 2005;52:89.

Chapter 83 :: Fox-Fordyce Disease
:: Powell Perng & Inbal Sander

第八十三章
Fox-Fordyce病

中文导读

Fox-Fordyce病是一种慢性瘙痒性丘疹损害，累及身体富含顶泌汗腺区域。皮损特征是大量坚实的、肉色的丘疹群集性分布。本章从以下8节进行讲述：

1．流行病学　Fox-Fordyce病的发病率尚不清楚，流行病学研究表明，Fox-Fordyce病对女性的影响很大，很少报道在青春期前或绝经后发病。

2．临床表现　详细描述了Fox-Fordyce病的临床表现，并提出典型病变在青春期开始后，最常见的发病部位是腋窝。诊断通常要推迟数年，因为皮疹最初可能只是瘙痒，或者不伴有瘙痒。皮疹的数量会随着时间慢慢增多。瘙痒是间歇性和剧烈的。发痒会因交感神经的刺激而加重，这些刺激包括出汗、情绪紧张或兴奋以及温暖的天气。反复抓挠可引起局部感染等并发症。

3．病因和发病机制　Fox-Fordyce病的病因尚不清楚。Fox-Fordyce病倾向于青春期发病，绝经后缓解，提示激素在该病中发挥作用。但事实上，文献报道对2例Fox-Fordyce疾病患者的激素分析没有发现异常。遗传可能在Fox-Fordyce病中起作用，但没有明确的遗传缺陷或多态性的报道。有病例描述了激光脱毛后Fox-Fordyce病加重。

4．病理生理学　在大汗腺导管插入部位因毛囊漏斗部角化过度引起的阻塞被认为是主要的病理生理学改变。接着，作者还较为详细地对发病过程进行推断。然而，在实验环境中通过阻断大汗腺导管来重现疾病过程的尝试并没有出现类似的临床症状。

作者还提出了，有病例显示：Fox-Fordyce病组织学证明其表皮内汗管阻塞，提示大汗腺和/或小汗管阻塞可能是该疾病的另一诱因。

5．诊断　Fox-Fordyce病是一种基于仔细的病史和皮肤表现的临床诊断，影像学和实验室检测均没有诊断价值。组织病理学分析有助于诊断，但结果是可变的和非特异性的，并对组织病理学改变作了描述。横切面比常规的垂直切面能产生更多的毛囊单位，更容易显示Fox-Fordyce病的组织病理学特征。

6．鉴别诊断　Fox-Fordyce病可被误认为是刺激性接触性皮炎、淀粉样苔藓、颗粒状角化过度、糜烂性苔藓、发疹性汗管瘤或感染性毛囊炎（表83-1）。Fox-Fordyce病也应与早期化脓性汗腺炎区别开来。

7．临床病程与预后　Fox-Fordyce病是一种慢性疾病，难以治疗，而且没有绝对的治愈方法。有时，绝经后症状缓解。

8．管理　本章提到的保守和改善症状的治疗措施包括：减少压力和避免热量有助于减少瘙痒；口服第一代抗组胺药和低剂量的多塞平可以缓解瘙痒；避免使用会加重毛囊阻塞的厚重乳膏和洗液。

治疗上，外用类固醇药膏是一线疗法，还提及钙调磷酸酶抑制药以及维甲酸类等外用药的注意事项。其他药物治疗包括己烯雌酚、口服避孕药、睾酮、促肾上腺皮质激素、紫外线疗法、X光疗法、局部注射A型肉毒杆菌毒素等。

电灼、刮除吸脂术、微波热消融和激光切除均可治愈，但由于担心感染、增生性瘢痕和/或毁损，一般都是晚期的选择。表83-2总结了Fox-Fordyce病的治疗策略。

〔刘芳芬〕

AT-A-GLANCE

- A rare, itchy, chronic papular eruption localized to apocrine gland–bearing areas of the body with unclear etiology.
- Females are disproportionately affected compared to males (9:1), with age of onset most commonly between 13-35 years of age.
- Hyperkeratotic plugging of the follicular infundibulum at the apocrine gland duct insertion site is thought to be the primary pathophysiologic event, leading to duct dilation, rupture, inflammation, and pruritus.
- No definitive cure; oral antihistamines and topical clindamycin may help alleviate symptoms and induce remission.

Fox-Fordyce disease is a chronic, itchy, papular eruption involving apocrine gland–rich areas of the body. Lesions are characterized by numerous firm, flesh-colored, follicular-based papules arranged in a grouped configuration.[1] Fox-Fordyce disease was first described in 1902 by George Henry Fox and John Addison Fordyce in 2 patients with axillary disease.[2] The pubic, perineal, areolar, umbilicus, and sternal areas also can be involved.[3,4] Fox-Fordyce disease is otherwise known as *apocrine miliaria*; however, the centrality of apocrine gland dysfunction to the disease pathophysiology remains controversial.[1,5]

EPIDEMIOLOGY

The incidence of Fox-Fordyce disease is unknown; however, it is considered a rare disease. Epidemiologic studies suggest Fox-Fordyce disease disproportionately affects females.[3,6] Females between the ages of 13 and 35 years comprise more than 90% of cases. Fox-Fordyce disease is rarely reported before puberty or after menopause.[7] There is no known racial predilection for the disease.

CLINICAL FEATURES

HISTORY

Fox-Fordyce disease typically manifests after the onset of puberty, most commonly in the axillae. Patients may notice lesions for the first time with shaving.[8] Diagnosis is often delayed for years,[9-11] as the eruptions may only itch initially with onset[12] or not at all.[11] The number of lesions accumulate slowly over time.[13] Pruritus is intermittent and intense. Itchiness is made worse by sympathetic stimulation, including sweating, emotional stress or excitement, and warm weather.[13] Family history is usually unremarkable.

CUTANEOUS FINDINGS

Fox-Fordyce lesions manifest as grouped, symmetrically distributed, monomorphic, dome-shaped papules (1 to 3 mm) that are typically follicular based, flesh-colored to mildly erythematous, and intermittently pruritic (Figs. 83-1 and 83-2). Excoriations and lichenification are often present secondary to scratching. The axillae are most commonly affected. The pubic, perineal, areolar, umbilicus, and sternal areas also can be involved. Diminished sweat production is frequently observed in affected areas.[11]

COMPLICATIONS

Localized superinfections secondary to repeated scratching can be managed with antihistamines and standard antibiotic therapy. Although hidradenitis suppurativa has been observed in conjunction with Fox-

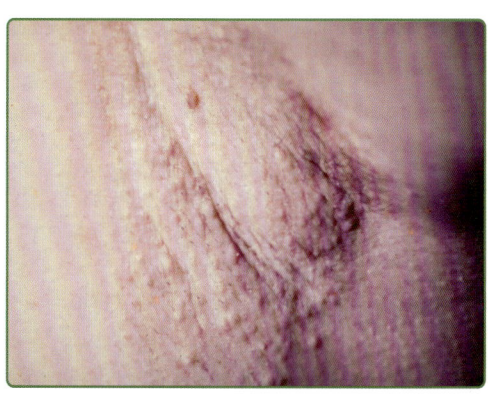

Figure 83-1 Fox-Fordyce disease with skin-colored papules involving the axilla. (Image used with permission from the Graham Library of Wake Forest Department of Dermatology.)

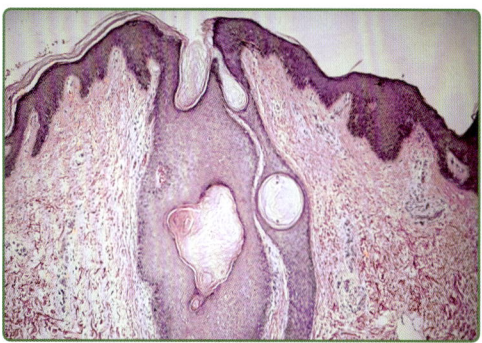

Figure 83-3 Follicular infundibular and excretory duct of apocrine gland with dilation, hyperkeratosis, and plugging. (Image used with permission from the Graham Library of Wake Forest Department of Dermatology.)

Fordyce disease, there is no evidence that Fox-Fordyce disease progresses to hidradenitis suppurativa.[6,14]

ETIOLOGY AND PATHOGENESIS

The etiology of Fox-Fordyce disease is unclear. The tendency of Fox-Fordyce disease to present at puberty and remit after menopause suggests a hormonal component to the disease.[15,16] Improvements also have been reported during pregnancy[16,17] and with use of oral contraceptives.[18,19] Alterations in follicle-stimulating hormone,[20] estrogen,[21] and premenstrual urinary gonadotropins[21] have been noted in case reports. Rarely, Fox-Fordyce disease has been observed in men,[13,20] preadolescent girls,[7,9,22] and postmenopausal women,[21] suggesting hormonal factors may not be responsible in all cases. In fact, hormonal analyses in 2 patients with Fox-Fordyce disease found no aberrations.[11,23]

Genetics likely play a role in Fox-Fordyce disease; however, no clear genetic defect or polymorphism has been reported. The disease has been observed among siblings[17] and monozygotic twins,[8,24] as well as sisters[17] and father and daughter.[25] Two patients with Turner syndrome[26] and 1 patient with a small deletion on chromosome 21 were also reported to have had Fox-Fordyce disease.[20]

Several case reports have described Fox-Fordyce–like eruptions developing after laser hair removal.[12,27,28] It is thought that laser-induced thermal damage to the follicular infundibulum causes altered keratinocyte maturation and subsequent plugging of the apocrine gland duct insertion site.[12] Eruptions tend to occur several months after initiating laser hair removal[27] and do not appear to be associated with particular laser wavelengths.[27]

PATHOPHYSIOLOGY

Hyperkeratotic obstruction of the follicular infundibulum at the apocrine gland duct insertion site is believed to be the primary pathophysiologic event.[4] The intraluminal obstruction leads to glandular distension and eventual ductal rupture. The subsequent expulsion of glandular contents into the surrounding dermis then causes an inflammatory response that manifests clinically as the intensely pruritic, dome-shaped, perifollicular papules. However, attempts to recreate the disease process by blocking the apocrine ducts in the experimental setting have failed to elicit the clinical manifestations.[29] Notably, Fox-Fordyce

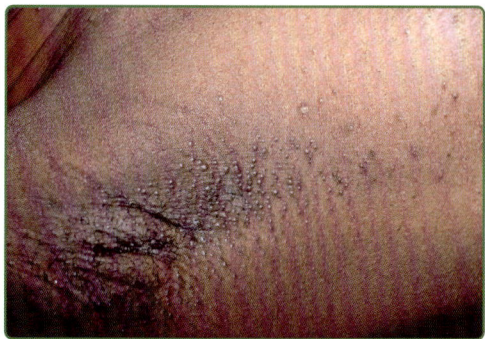

Figure 83-2 Fox-Fordyce in a dark-skin patient with well-demarcated papules on the axilla. (Image used with permission from the Graham Library of Wake Forest Department of Dermatology.)

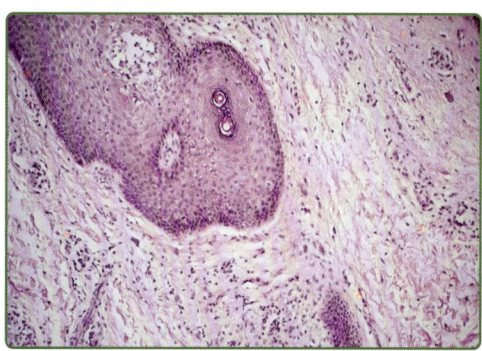

Figure 83-4 Fox-Fordyce disease in the nipple region. (Image used with permission from the Graham Library of Wake Forest Department of Dermatology.)

disease has been described in cases with histologic evidence of intraepidermal sweat duct obstruction, suggesting that apocrine and/or eccrine duct obstruction may be another trigger for the disease.[4,9]

DIAGNOSIS

Fox-Fordyce disease is a clinical diagnosis based on careful history and cutaneous findings. Histopathologic analysis can facilitate with diagnosis, but findings are variable and nonspecific. Imaging and laboratory testing are not useful.

HISTOPATHOLOGY

Histopathologic features of Fox-Fordyce lesions (Figs. 83-3 and 83-4) are variable and should not be relied upon for making or excluding the diagnosis.[1] The most consistent finding is hyperkeratosis of the infundibular epithelium and dilation of the follicular infundibulum (Fig. 83-3).[1] Perifollicular and periductal xanthomatosis cells are frequently seen.[30] Focal spongiosis of the upper infundibulum along with perifollicular adventitial fibrosis and lymphohistiocytic infiltrate also were consistently observed.[3,30] Other findings include vacuolar alterations at the dermato–epithelial junction of the infundibula; smatterings of dyskeratotic cells throughout the infundibula; and tiny columns of cornoid lamella-like parakeratosis in close proximity to the acrosyringium of the apocrine duct, with eosinophilic keratinocytes found underneath.[1] The existence of pathognomonic "sweat retention" vesicles described by Shelly and Levy[6] is controversial, as these vesicles are rarely demonstrated in histologic specimens. There is evidence that transverse sectioning, rather than conventional vertical sectioning, produces a higher yield of hair follicle units and more readily demonstrates the histopathologic features of Fox-Fordyce disease.[31]

DIFFERENTIAL DIAGNOSIS

Fox-Fordyce eruptions can be mistaken for irritant contact dermatitis, lichen amyloidosis, granular hyperkeratosis, lichen nitidus, eruptive syringoma, or infectious folliculitis (Table 83-1). Fox-Fordyce disease should also be distinguished from early stages of hidradenitis suppurativa,[6,14] a chronic pustular dermatosis that also localizes to apocrine gland–rich regions of the body; however, the purulence, discharge, and sinus tracking of hidradenitis suppurativa are not observed in Fox-Fordyce disease.

CLINICAL COURSE AND PROGNOSIS

Fox-Fordyce disease is chronic, difficult to treat, and has no definitive cure. On occasion, remission has occurred after menopause.[15,16]

MANAGEMENT

Therapeutic knowledge is derived primarily from case reports. Table 83-2 summarizes select therapeutic strategies for Fox-Fordyce disease.

CONSERVATIVE AND SYMPTOMATIC MEASURES

Stress reduction and heat avoidance may help minimize pruritus. First-generation oral antihistamines can be useful for alleviating itch, especially during the night. Low doses of doxepin (<10 mg), up to 3 times a day, can be used as an alternative to oral antihistamines.[32] There is no evidence to suggest that shaving or deodorant use worsen symptoms; however, thick creams and lotions, which can exacerbate follicular obstruction, should be avoided.

TABLE 83-1
Differential Diagnosis for Fox-Fordyce Disease

- Irritant contact dermatitis
- Chronic dermatitis
- Lichen amyloidosis
- Granular hyperkeratosis
- Lichen nitidus
- Syringoma
- Axillary papillary mucinosis
- Infectious folliculitis
- Early-stage hidradenitis suppurativa
- Scabies

TABLE 83-2
Select Therapeutic Strategies for Fox-Fordyce

Symptomatic therapies
- Oral antihistamines
- Low-dose doxepin

Topical therapies
- Short-term steroids
- Calcineurin inhibitors
- Tretinoin
- Adapalene
- Clindamycin in propylene glycol solution

Oral therapies
- Isotretinoin
- Oral contraceptives

Procedural therapies
- Intralesional steroid injection
- Intralesional botulinum toxin injection
- Surgical excision
- Microwave thermal ablation

TOPICAL AND MEDICAL THERAPIES

Topical steroid creams are first-line therapies and can temporarily relieve itching; however, continuous application for more than 10 to 14 days is discouraged because of the risk of skin thinning and formation of striae.[33] Intradermal triamcinolone[34] may help alleviate itching during acute flares, but can also cause cutaneous atrophy with repeated administrations. Topical calcineurin inhibitors (1% pimecrolimus cream, 0.1% tacrolimus) can be used as alternatives to steroids and will not thin the skin. Pimecrolimus 1% cream applied twice daily over 8 weeks induced complete remission in 1 patient and partial remissions in 2 patients.[35] Topical tretinoin can be effective[36] but is often abandoned because of excessive irritation of the skin. Topical 0.1% adapalene gel, which is better tolerated than tretinoin, produced mild-to-moderate improvements in itch and number of papules in 1 case when applied every other day for 2 months.[37] Side effects of adapalene included erythema and burning sensation.[37] In 2 cases, topical clindamycin in propylene glycol solution led to rapid resolution of papules after 1 month of treatment without recurrence at 6 to 9 months.[17,38]

Other medical therapies include diethylstilbestrol,[6] oral contraceptives,[19] testosterone,[39] corticotropin,[6] ultraviolet light therapy,[40] and X-ray therapy.[23] Oral isotretinoin dosed at 15 to 30 mg daily for 16 weeks induced near-complete remission of lesions and pruritus in 1 case[20]; however, lesions recurred 3 months after discontinuing therapy, accompanied by a more intense pruritus than before.[20] A one-time injection of botulinum toxin type A (2 units diluted into 2.5 mL of 0.9% saline at multiple points 2-cm apart in axillae) produced complete remission 15 days after injections without recurrence at 8 months of followup.[41]

PROCEDURAL THERAPIES

Case reports suggest different procedural therapies, including electrocautery, excision-liposuction with curettage, microwave thermal ablation,[42] and laser-based excisions,[43,44] can be curative, but are generally late-line options because of concern about infection, hypertrophic scarring, and/or disfiguration.[44]

REFERENCES

1. Boer A. Patterns histopathologic of Fox-Fordyce disease. *Am J Dermatopathol*. 2004;26(6):482-492.
2. Fox GH, Fordyce JA. Two cases of a rare, papular disease affecting the axilla region, with a report on the histopathology. *J Cutan Dis*. 1902;20:1-5.
3. Kao PH, Hsu CK, Lee JY. Clinicopathological study of Fox-Fordyce disease. *J Dermatol*. 2009;36(9):485-490.
4. Kamada A, Saga K, Jimbow K. Apoeccrine sweat duct obstruction as a cause for Fox-Fordyce disease. *J Am Acad Dermatol*. 2003;48(3):453-455.
5. Ackerman AB. *Resolving Quandaries in Dermatology, Pathology, and Dermatopathology*. Philadelphia, PA: Promethean Medical Press; 1995.
6. Shelley WB, Levy EJ. Apocrine sweat retention in man. II. Fox-Fordyce disease (apocrine miliaria). *AMA Arch Derm*. 1956;73(1):38-49.
7. Sandhu K, Gupta S, Kanwar AJ. Fox Fordyce disease in a prepubertal girl. *Pediatr Dermatol*. 2005;22(1):89-90.
8. Guiotoku MM, Lopes PT, Marques ME, et al. Fox-Fordyce disease in monozygotic female twins. *J Am Acad Dermatol*. 2011;65(1):229-230.
9. Ranalletta M, Rositto A, Drut R. Fox-Fordyce disease in two prepubertal girls: histopathologic demonstration of eccrine sweat gland involvement. *Pediatr Dermatol*. 1996;13(4):294-297.
10. Shackelton J, English JC 3rd. Fox-Fordyce disease (apocrine miliaria). *J Pediatr Adolesc Gynecol*. 2011;24(3):108-109.
11. Ballester I, Lopez-Avila A, Ortiz S. Fox-Fordyce disease with an atypical clinical presentation. *Actas Dermosifiliogr*. 2013;104(9):832-834.
12. Tetzlaff MT, Evans K, DeHoratius DM, et al. Fox-Fordyce disease following axillary laser hair removal. *Arch Dermatol*. 2011;147(5):573-576.
13. Alikhan A, Gorouhi F, Zargari O. Fox-Fordyce disease exacerbated by hyperhidrosis. *Pediatr Dermatol*. 2010;27(2):162-165.
14. Spiller RF, Knox JM. Fox-Fordyce disease with hidradenitis suppurativa. *J Invest Dermatol*. 1958;31(2):127-135.
15. Bolognia JL, Jorizzo JL, Rapini RP. *Dermatology*. London, UK: Mosby Elsevier; 2008.
16. Cornbleet T. Pregnancy and apocrine gland diseases: hidradenitis, Fox-Fordyce disease. *AMA Arch Derm Syphilol*. 1952;65(1):12-19.
17. Miller ML, Harford RR, Yeager JK. Fox-Fordyce disease treated with topical clindamycin solution. *Arch Dermatol*. 1995;131(10):1112-1113.
18. Yang CS, Teeple M, Muglia J, et al. Inflammatory and glandular skin disease in pregnancy. *Clin Dermatol*. 2016;34(3):335-343.
19. Kronthal HL, Pomeranz JR, Sitomer G. Fox-Fordyce disease: treatment with an oral contraceptive. *Arch Dermatol*. 1965;91:243-245.
20. Effendy I, Ossowski B, Happle R. Fox-Fordyce disease in a male patient—response to oral retinoid treatment. *Clin Exp Dermatol*. 1994;19(1):67-69.
21. Montes LF, Caplan RM, Riley GM, et al. Fox-Fordyce disease. An endocrinological study. *Arch Dermatol*. 1961;84:452-458.
22. Senear FE, Cornbleet T, Brunner M. Fox-Fordyce disease before puberty. *Arch Derm Syphilol*. 1948;57(3, pt 2):438.
23. Turner TW. Hormonal levels in Fox-Fordyce disease. *Br J Dermatol*. 1976;94(3):317-318.
24. Graham JH, Shafer JC, Helwig EB. Fox-Fordyce disease in male identical twins. *Arch Dermatol*. 1960;82:212-221.
25. Scroggins L, Kelly E, Kelly B. Fox-Fordyce disease in daughter and father. *Dermatology*. 2009;218(2):176-177.
26. Patrizi A, Orlandi C, Neri I, et al. Fox-Fordyce disease: two cases in patients with Turner syndrome. *Acta Derm Venereol*. 1999;79(1):83-84.
27. Sammour R, Nasser S, Debahy N, et al. Fox-Fordyce disease: an under-diagnosed adverse event of laser

hair removal? *J Eur Acad Dermatol Venereol*. 2016; 30(9):1578-1582.
28. Yazganoglu KD, Yazici S, Buyukbabani N, et al. Axillary Fox-Fordyce-like disease induced by laser hair removal therapy. *J Am Acad Dermatol*. 2012;67(4):e139-e140.
29. Hurley HJ Jr, Shelley WB. Apocrine sweat retention in man. I. Experimental production of asymptomatic form. *J Invest Dermatol*. 1954;22(5):397-404.
30. Bormate AB Jr, Leboit PE, McCalmont TH. Perifollicular xanthomatosis as the hallmark of axillary Fox-Fordyce disease: an evaluation of histopathologic features of 7 cases. *Arch Dermatol*. 2008;144(8):1020-1024.
31. Stashower ME, Krivda SJ, Turiansky GW. Fox-Fordyce disease: diagnosis with transverse histologic sections. *J Am Acad Dermatol*. 2000;42(1, pt 1):89-91.
32. Smith PF, Corelli RL. Doxepin in the management of pruritus associated with allergic cutaneous reactions. *Ann Pharmacother*. 1997;31(5):633-635.
33. Coondoo A, Phiske M, Verma S, et al. Side-effects of topical steroids: a long overdue revisit. *Indian Dermatol Online J*. 2014;5(4):416-425.
34. Helfman RJ. A new treatment of Fox-Fordyce disease. *South Med J*. 1962;55:681-684.
35. Pock L, Svrckova M, Machackova R, et al. Pimecrolimus is effective in Fox-Fordyce disease. *Int J Dermatol*. 2006;45(9):1134-1135.
36. Giacobetti R, Caro WA, Roenigk HH Jr. Fox-Fordyce disease. Control with tretinoin cream. *Arch Dermatol*. 1979;115(11):1365-1366.
37. Kassuga LE, Medrado MM, Chevrand NS, et al. Fox-Fordyce disease: response to adapalene 0.1%. *An Bras Dermatol*. 2012;87(2):329-331.
38. Feldmann R, Masouye I, Chavaz P, et al. Fox-Fordyce disease: successful treatment with topical clindamycin in alcoholic propylene glycol solution. *Dermatology*. 1992;184(4):310-313.
39. Cornbleet T. Testosterone for apocrine diseases: hidrosadenitis, Fox-Fordyce disease. *AMA Arch Derm Syphilol*. 1952;65(5):549-552.
40. Pinkus H. Treatment of Fox-Fordyce disease. *JAMA*. 1973;223(8):924.
41. Gonzalez-Ramos J, Alonso-Pacheco ML, Goiburu-Chenu B, et al. Successful treatment of refractory pruritic Fox-Fordyce disease with botulinum toxin type A. *Br J Dermatol*. 2016;174(2):458-459.
42. Taylor D, Au J, Boen M, et al. A novel modality using microwave technology for the treatment of Fox-Fordyce disease (FFD). *JAAD Case Rep*. 2016;2(1):1-3.
43. Ahmed Al-Qarqaz F, Al-Shannag R. Fox-Fordyce disease treatment with fractional CO_2 laser. *Int J Dermatol*. 2013;52(12):1571-1572.
44. Han HH, Lee JY, Rhie JW. Successful treatment of areolar Fox-Fordyce disease with surgical excision and 1550-nm fractionated erbium glass laser. *Int Wound J*. 2016;13(5):1016-1019.

Chapter 84 :: Hidradenitis Suppurativa
:: Ginette A. Okoye

第八十四章
化脓性汗腺炎

中文导读

化脓性汗腺炎（Hidradenitis Suppurativa，简称HS）是一种多因素的，发生于间擦区和肛门生殖器区域的慢性毛囊炎症。本章从以下8节进行讲述：

1. 流行病学　HS缺乏可靠的流行病学数据。截至撰写本文时，仅发表了一项以人群为基础的发病率研究。研究表明，女性发病率高于男性，腋窝和肛门生殖器部位高发，男性更容易发展为会阴和肛周疾病。作者还提到：在女性，月经、绝经和妊娠对HS的影响不一致，值得进一步研究。

2. 详细讲述了HS复发和缓解的临床症状及慢性的发病过程。还提到了长期疾病后遗症，包括皮肤挛缩和毁容，会对日常生活、社会功能和心理健康产生有害影响。

3. 首先提供了部分数据说明HS并发症对患者生活质量的影响。接着分别讲述了有报道的系统并发症和局部并发症。最后，作者还提到，与健康个体相比，HS患者患任何类型恶性肿瘤的风险都要高出50%。鳞状细胞癌(SCC)是一种罕见的长期慢性炎性病变的并发症。

4. 病因和发病机制　HS的病因是多因素的，作者从以下多个方面详细阐述了HS的病因和发病机制：首先，毛囊远端的角化闭塞是最主要的病理生理基础。进一步讲述了毛囊角化物形成，毛囊的闭塞、扩张、破裂，以及后续引起的淋巴组织细胞异物性炎症反应，吞噬了毛囊皮脂腺单位及其附属结构，最终引起临床表现的发病过程。其次，顶泌汗腺也参与了HS的发病过程。在附属器参与HS发病机制的研究进展时，还提到了皮脂腺萎缩似乎是HS发病的早期事件，先于淋巴细胞性毛囊炎症和漏斗部角化过度，但皮脂腺萎缩是原发性病变还是上游病变的继发改变仍有待确定。此外，家族遗传、雄激素、吸烟、肥胖、免疫失调、细菌感染等均是HS发病机制的组成部分，对此分别进行了阐述。

5. 共病和相关疾病　HS常与其他毛囊闭塞性疾病相关，包括HS四分体（The tetrad of HS）、聚合性痤疮、头皮蜂窝织炎和藏毛窦等。HS也是几种自身炎症综合征的一部分，包括PASH（坏疽性脓皮病、痤疮和HS），PAPASH(化脓性关节炎、坏疽性脓皮病、痤疮和HS)，和PsAPASH(银屑病性关节炎和PASH)。HS还与炎症性肠病有关，特别是肛周受累的患者。此外，血清反应阴性的脊椎关节炎、淀粉样变、遗传性角蛋白病、皮肤鳞状细胞癌患者也普遍患有HS。一些激素失衡和/或代谢失衡也与HS发作相关。

6. 诊断　首先总结了HS的3个临床症状的诊断标准(表84-1)，并且提出：所有这些标准都必须具备才能确诊。进一步详细讲述了以上三个标准，并指出在6个月内有2次复发被认为是慢性的，还提供了HS的诊断流程图（图84-10）。接着，从严重程度、临床分型、实验室检查、影像学、组织病理学等5个方面分别进行讲述：在讲述临床评估严重程度时，提出Hurley分期系统(表84-3)是评估疾病严重程度最广泛使用的方法。并进一步讲解了这一分期系统的使用及优缺点。HS的3种临床表型已被提出，详细讲述了三个临床亚型的形态、发病部位、发病率等，并相互之间进行了一定比较。实验室检查异常包括，急性病灶患者可表现为白细胞增多、血沉升高、血清铁含量低和血清电泳蛋白异常。对于发热或出现中毒症状的患者，应发送生化检测、全血细胞计数和血液培养。脓性引流物应送细菌培养和药敏检测。如果担心感染，应进行深部组织培养。超声和MRI等影像学典型的改变是皮下组织的皮肤增厚和硬化，可用于观察病变的分期以及制定手术计划。关于组织病理学改变，作者也进行了深入的阐述。

7. 临床过程和预后　HS通常发生在青春期之后，且与其他脓疱性皮肤病相似，诊断延迟7～12年并不少见。疾病活动一般在50岁后下降。在非吸烟者、已戒烟者和非肥胖者中，缓解症状的可能性更大。

8. 疾病管理　HS治疗的总体目标是减少疾病后遗症(如纤维化、挛缩、窦道)对生活质量的影响。文章提出，治疗手段取决于疾病的严重程度，并分期进行了简述。列表84-4、84-5和图84-11提出了基于HS疾病严重程度，选择治疗方案。接着，作者从生活方式、内科治疗、外科治疗、疼痛管理、心理健康管理等5个方面进行阐述：首先着重讲了对患者的生活方式进行管理，包括戒烟、控制体重是减轻疾病各阶段症状的重要组成部分；保守的措施，如减轻压力、温水浴、热敷和水疗，有助于缓解症状；避免穿紧身衣以及长时间暴露在湿热环境中。内科治疗方面，讲述了抗生素、生物制剂、免疫抑制剂、激素、二甲双胍、维甲酸等药物治疗的适应症，以及已报道的有效的用药方案等。手术治疗方面，认为手术切除是治疗慢性HS的基础，但术后复发非常常见，往往需要重复多次手术切除。激光作为治疗HS的辅助手段越来越多，通过消融组织减少肿胀，同时减少毛囊、皮脂腺和感染区域的细菌数量。其他外科治疗手段还包括冷冻治疗、放射治疗、A型肉毒毒素注射等。

治疗HS疼痛的方法来源于专家的意见和一般的疼痛管理指南。外用镇痛药、口服扑热息痛和非甾体类抗炎药被认为是治疗HS疼痛的一线用药。持续性和爆发性疼痛可口服阿片类镇痛药。针对神经性疼痛的药物治疗是有益的，因为它们可能同时改善抑郁和瘙痒。

最后提及HS患者的心理健康管理。虽然关于HS心理健康发病率的文献很少，但定性研究表明，大多数患者有抑郁症状。因此，对有抑郁症状的患者进行常规筛查和转诊很重要。

〔刘芳芬〕

AT-A-GLANCE

- Hidradenitis suppurativa is a chronic and debilitating inflammatory disorder of the hair follicles that localizes to intertriginous and anogenital regions of the body.
- Lesions are characterized by inflammatory nodules, subcutaneous abscesses, and sinus tracts.
- Reproductive-age women are disproportionately affected.
- Hyperkeratotic plugging of the terminal hair follicle is a consistent histologic finding of early disease and is thought to be the primary pathophysiologic event.

Hidradenitis suppurativa (HS), otherwise known as *acne inversa*, is a multifactorial, chronic inflammatory disorder of the hair follicles in intertriginous and anogenital regions of the body. HS is characterized by recurrent, deep-seated, painful, subcutaneous nodules, sinus tracts, and hypertrophic scarring. The long-term sequelae, including chronic pain, skin contractures, and disfigurement, can detrimentally impact activities of daily living, social functioning, and psychosocial well-being.[1,2]

EPIDEMIOLOGY

Robust epidemiologic data on HS is lacking. The reported point prevalence of HS worldwide is between 0.00033% and 4.1%.[3] As of this writing, only 1 population-based incidence study has been published.[4] Among residents of Olmsted County, Minnesota (population 144,000 in 2010), the overall annual age- and sex-adjusted incidence rate of HS was 6 per 100,000 person-years over a 40-year period.[4] Between 1970 and 2008, the age- and sex-adjusted incidence rate rose steadily from 4.3 per 100,000 person-years to 9.6 per 100,000 person-years.[4] The etiology of this trend is unclear but may be related to concomitant rises in risk factors among the general population, including obesity and metabolic syndrome, as well as improved physician recognition of HS.[5]

For unknown reasons, women are disproportionately affected (female-to-male ratio is 3.3:1) and more likely to develop axillary and genitofemoral lesions.[4] Men, on the other hand, tend to develop perineal and perianal disease.[4] Among women, the impact of menstruation, menopause, and pregnancy on the natural history of HS is inconsistent and warrants further study. Although unconfirmed by population-based studies, data suggests that black patients may be disproportionately affected by HS.[6-9]

CLINICAL FEATURES

HS is a chronic relapsing and remitting disease with an unpredictable clinical course, leading to detrimental impacts on quality of life. Lesions may begin as tenderness or pruritus that progresses to a tender papule or deep-rooted nodule (Fig. 84-1). Nodules can become quite large and painful. They may resolve slowly without drainage or progress to an abscess-like lesion that eventually ruptures and drains purulent material before involuting (Fig. 84-2). Involution may take 7 to 10 days,[10] but in some patients, healing may be delayed, resulting in persistent open wounds with variable amounts of granulation tissue (Fig. 84-3). The process then reoccurs in adjacent and/or other intertriginous sites. With repeated episodes, epithelial strands may develop from ruptured follicular epithelium,[11] leading to sinus tract formation and intermittent drainage of foul-smelling serosanguinous and/or purulent material (Fig. 84-4). Over time, the healing process leads to exuberant scar formation, depositing densely fibrotic dermal plaques and rope-like bands (Fig. 84-5). The long-term disease sequelae, including dermal contractures and disfigurement, can detrimentally impact activities of daily living, social functioning, and psychosocial well-being (Figs. 84-6 to 84-8).[1,2]

COMPLICATIONS

QUALITY OF LIFE

HS is a burdensome and distressing disease that has a detrimental impact on quality of life. The degree of quality-of-life impairment, as measured by the Dermatology Life Quality Index, is more severe for HS than for other dermatologic conditions, including alopecia, psoriatic arthritis, and chronic urticaria.[1,12] The highest single Dermatology Life Quality Index score is for disease-associated pain and discomfort.[12] Anogenital involvement is associated with a significantly worse Dermatology Life Quality Index score compared to other sites.[13] HS-associated debility may cause professional setbacks. In one report, HS resulted in work absences in 58.1% of patients.[13] Work absences occurred 1 to 10 times per year, totaling 33.6 days lost on average per patient per year (SD: 26.1 days).[13] Twenty-three percent of patients reported hindrance of professional advancement secondary to disease-related morbidity.[13]

SYSTEMIC COMPLICATIONS

A small number of patients (4% to 6%) may develop a normocytic and/or microcytic anemia of little clinical

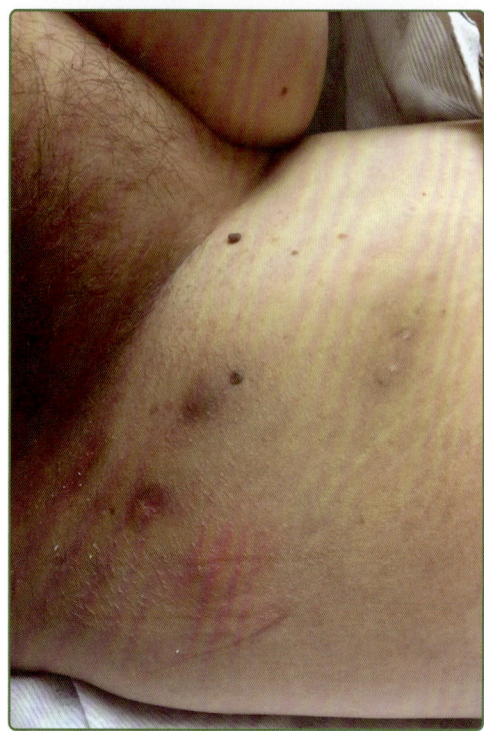

Figure 84-1 Inflammatory subcutaneous nodule of hidradenitis suppurativa with adjacent scars from previous lesions.

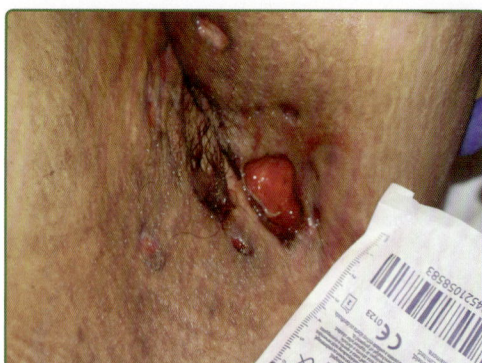

Figure 84-3 Inflammatory nodules of hidradenitis suppurativa rupture and drain, leaving behind persistent ulcerations in the axilla. (Copyright © Katherine Püttgen, MD. Used with permission.)

develop from chronic anogenital and perineal inflammation, leading to incontinence.[17] Urethral fistulization secondary to genital involvement has been reported.[8] Inflammation, scarring, and destruction of lymphatic drainage routes can lead to disfiguring elephantiasis (see Fig. 84-7)[18] and verrucous lymphangiomas,[19] requiring surgical reconstruction.

significance secondary to chronic inflammation.[14] Rare cases of renal amyloidosis associated with severe HS have been reported.[15] Sepsis arising from infected lesions is a rare but fatal complication.[16]

LOCAL COMPLICATIONS

Fibrosis and dermal contractures can limit joint mobility. Vaginal, urethral, and/or anal strictures can

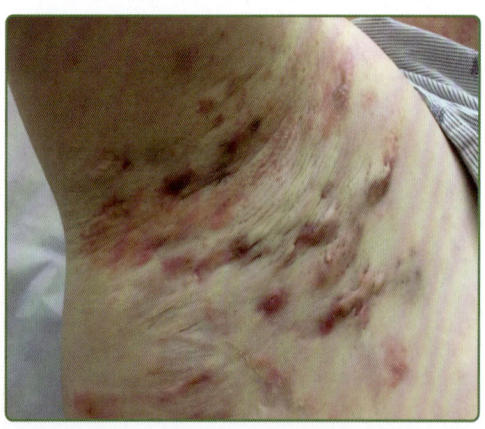

Figure 84-2 Multiple inflammatory nodules of hidradenitis suppurativa in the axilla.

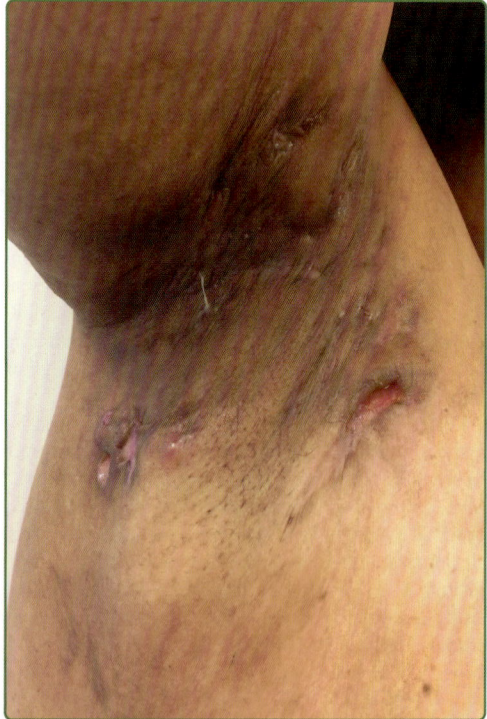

Figure 84-4 Sinus tracts and purulent drainage associated with chronic hidradenitis suppurativa in the axilla.

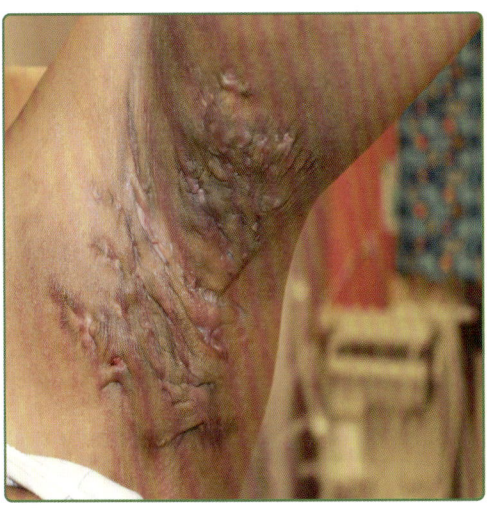

Figure 84-5 Dense fibrotic plaques and rope-like scars associated with chronic hidradenitis suppurativa in the axilla. (Copyright © Katherine Püttgen, MD. Used with permission.)

SQUAMOUS CELL CARCINOMA

Squamous cell carcinoma (SCC) is an infrequent complication of longstanding chronically inflamed lesions, occurring in 4.6% of HS cases (see Fig. 84-8).[20] As of this writing, a total of 86 cases of SCC arising from HS

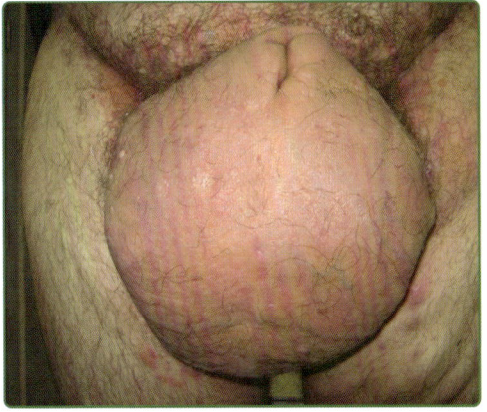

Figure 84-7 Scrotal lymphedema associated with long-term hidradenitis suppurativa in the inguinal folds.

lesions had been recorded in the literature.[21] Males with anogenital disease are preferentially affected.[20,21] HS-associated anogenital SCC is often associated with high-risk human papillomavirus strains, most commonly human papillomavirus-16.[22] HS-associated SCC also tends to be more locally aggressive and metastasizes to lymph nodes with greater frequency (50% of cases) than SCC from any cause (5% to 10% of cases).[20] Thus, practitioners should have a low threshold to biopsy any nonhealing wound in an area of chronic HS. Patients with HS are deemed to be at 50% greater risk of developing malignancies of any kind compared to the healthy individuals,[23] although smoking status is not accounted for in the calculation of this statistic.

ETIOLOGY AND PATHOGENESIS

The etiology of HS is multifactorial and remains to be fully elucidated. It is likely that a combination of factors, including genetic predisposition, aberrant immunity, hormonal dysregulation, and environmental modifiers, are involved in the pathophysiology of this complex disease.

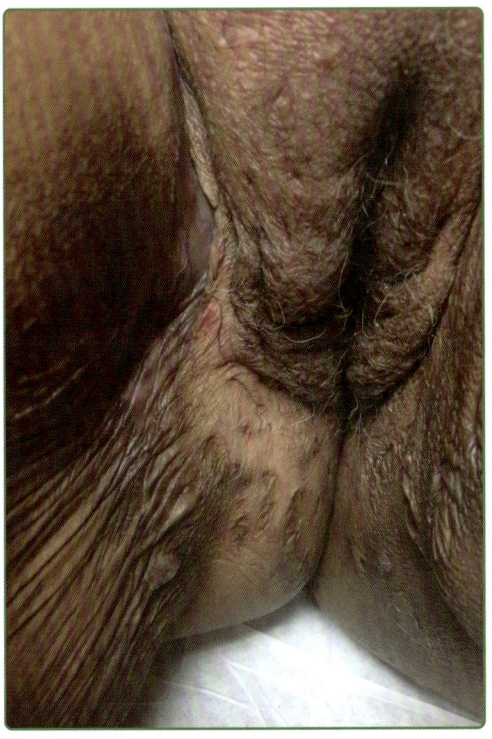

Figure 84-6 Disfiguring atrophic scars in the groin from recurrent lesions of hidradenitis suppurativa.

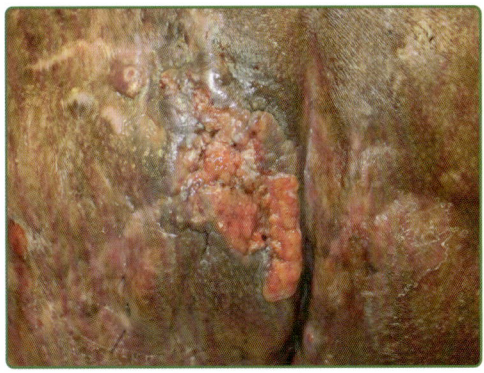

Figure 84-8 Squamous cell carcinoma arising in long-standing hidradenitis suppurativa on the buttocks.

FOLLICULAR OCCLUSION

Keratinous occlusion of the terminal hair follicle is a consistent histologic finding of early HS[24] and is thought to be the primary pathophysiologic event.[25] An aberrant immune response to commensal flora[25] and/or shear forces causing microtrauma to the deep part of the hair follicles in intertriginous skin[26] are believed to contribute to the initial lymphocytic perifolliculitis, hyperkeratosis, and hyperplasia of the infundibular epithelium.[24] This accumulation of keratinous debris leads to plugging and dilation of hair follicles. With subsequent rupture, follicles expel their contents (keratin, hair, sebum, bacteria) into the surrounding dermis. This incites a florid lymphohistiocytic foreign-body–type inflammatory response that engulfs the pilosebaceous units and adnexal structures, giving rise to the clinical findings.

ADNEXAL STRUCTURES

HS was once thought to originate in the apocrine glands. It is now clear, however, that the apocrine glands are only secondarily involved.[27] On the other hand, sebaceous gland atrophy appears to be an early event in disease pathogenesis, preceding the onset of lymphocytic follicular inflammation and hyperkeratosis of the infundibulum.[28] Whether sebaceous gland atrophy represents a primary event or is a reflection of upstream processes remains to be determined.

GENETICS

HS can develop sporadically or be inherited in familial forms. One-third of patients with HS report a positive family history of the disease.[29] Familial forms are thought to arise from autosomal dominant inheritance of highly penetrant single gene mutations, whereas sporadic cases are thought to result from defects in several genes.[29,30] Loss-of-function mutations in the genes encoding subunit proteins of the γ-secretase complex—presenilin (PSEN1/PSEN2), presenilin enhancer-2 (PSENEN), nicastrin (NCSTN)—also have been identified in families with HS.[31,32] In animal models, γ-secretase deficiency leads to sebaceous gland atrophy, a histologic finding in HS, as well as epidermal cyst formation.[33] Defective γ-secretase also impairs the Notch signaling pathway, which mediates normal hair follicle development, promotes antiinflammatory regulatory T-cell activity, and suppresses toll-like-receptor–induced proinflammatory responses.[34,35] Together, these data suggest that defective γ-secretase and/or Notch signaling may serve a pathophysiologic role in HS. No associations between human leukocyte antigen antigens and HS have been reported.[36,37]

SMOKING

According to a multivariate analysis, the odds of having HS are substantially higher among current smokers than nonsmokers (odds ratio [OR] 12.55; 95% confidence interval [CI] 8.58 to 18.38).[38] Smoking also is associated with the development of more-severe disease.[39] Whether smoking is merely a risk factor or plays a direct role in disease pathogenesis is still controversial. Nicotine is thought to promote follicular occlusion by increasing sweat gland secretion and inducing hyperplasia of the follicular infundibulum.[39] Nicotine is also thought to induce neutrophil chemotaxis and stimulate release of proinflammatory cytokines.[40] Smoking cessation may improve symptoms[41] as well as reduce the rates of de novo lesion formation following excisional surgery.[42]

ANDROGENS

The propensity for HS to develop after puberty suggests an androgenic basis for the disease. However, the role of androgen remains unclear. Androgen modulation therapy has demonstrated therapeutic benefit equivalent to that of oral antibiotic therapy.[43] Yet, after adjusting for body mass index, there was no significant difference in the level of circulating androgens between women with HS and healthy controls.[44,45] Additionally, the expression of androgen receptors[46] and the 5-α-reductase enzyme[47] on the apocrine glands is similar in HS lesions and healthy skin.

OBESITY

A higher body mass index is associated with greater odds of having HS (OR 1.12; 95% CI 1.08 to 1.15).[38] Obesity is likely not causative but rather exacerbates HS via augmenting tissue mechanics, that is, promoting sweat retention and occlusion, and increasing friction and maceration in skinfolds.[39] Greater adiposity may also alter the androgenic milieu by reducing global levels of sex hormone-binding globulin[44] and/or augmenting peripheral conversion of sex hormones.[47,48] Weight loss is recommended in overweight patients with HS. A study found that weight loss of more than 15% after bariatric surgery was associated with a 20% reduction in active disease.[41]

IMMUNE DYSREGULATION

A growing body of literature implicates immune dysregulation as an integral part of disease pathogenesis.[49] The proinflammatory cytokine, tumor necrosis factor (TNF)-α, is markedly elevated in HS lesions and in the serum of patients with HS compared to healthy controls.[50] Interleukin (IL)-1β, another potent proinflammatory cytokine, is also strikingly elevated in lesional and perilesional skin (34- to 115-fold higher in lesional compared to healthy skin).[49] IL-1β can promote inflammation by driving differentiation of IL-17–secreting CD4+ helper T cells (Th17) cells. The IL-23/Th17 pathway is implicated in numerous autoimmune diseases, including rheumatoid arthritis, lupus, multiple sclerosis, and psoriasis.[51] Levels of IL-12 and IL-23 are significantly elevated (2.6- to 5.2-fold) in lesional HS skin compared to that of healthy controls,[52] with an increased number of Th17 cells infiltrating the dermis in the lesional HS skin compared to healthy skin.[52]

BACTERIA

Whether bacterial involvement of HS lesions is a primary or secondary pathophysiologic event remains controversial. Traditional bacterial cultures taken from involved sites are often negative or grow commensal skin flora.[53] Coagulase-negative staphylococcus and anaerobic bacteria are the most frequently isolated organisms.[53] Deep-tissue samples from the dermis grow a preponderance of coagulase-negative staphylococcus.[53] It has been postulated that an overzealous immune response to commensal flora within hair follicles triggers the initial follicular inflammation.[25,54] Topical and oral antibiotics tend to improve symptoms in most patients; however, long courses of therapy are often needed, and relapse is common. Bacterial biofilm formation may help explain the intractability of skin lesions despite long-term antibiotic therapies.[55]

COMORBIDITIES AND ASSOCIATED DISEASES

HS is frequently associated with other diseases of follicular occlusion. The tetrad of HS, acne conglobata, dissecting cellulitis of the scalp, and pilonidal cysts is well documented.[56] HS also has been described as a component of several autoinflammatory syndromes, including PASH (pyoderma gangrenosum, acne, and HS),[57] PAPASH (pyogenic arthritis, pyoderma gangrenosum, acne, and HS),[58] and PsAPASH (psoriatic arthritis and PASH).[59] Mutations in the NCSTN[60] and PSTPIP1 (proline-serine-threonine phosphatase interacting protein 1)[61] genes have been observed in PASH. Improvement of PASH and PAPASH with IL-1 receptor antagonist therapy suggests IL-1β may also play a pathogenic role.[57,58] HS is also associated with inflammatory bowel disease.[62,63] Twenty-six percent of patients with Crohn disease and 18% of patients with ulcerative colitis reported having HS.[62] Coexistence of Crohn disease and HS is associated with a more fulminant disease course, especially in patients with perianal involvement.[64] However, patients with HS do not appear to harbor CARD15/NOD2 polymorphisms associated with the inflammatory pathways of Crohn disease.[65,66] Clinical improvement of concurrent Crohn disease and HS with anti–TNF-α therapy has been reported.[67] Seronegative spondyloarthropathies, amyloidosis, genetic keratin disorders, and SCCs are also commonly cited in patients with HS.[56] Several large studies have demonstrated that disease of hormonal and/or metabolic disequilibrium are frequently comorbid with HS.[68-70] Patients with HS had significantly higher odds of also having metabolic syndrome (OR 1.61; 95% CI 1.36 to 1.89), diabetes mellitus (OR 1.41; 95% CI 1.19 to 1.66), obesity (OR 1.71; 95% CI 1.53 to 1.91), and hypertension (OR 1.14; 95% CI 1.02 to 1.28).[70]

DIAGNOSIS

HS is a clinical diagnosis based on 3 criteria (Table 84-1), all of which must be present for the definitive diagnosis. First, typical lesions must be present. These include deep-seated painful nodules, abscesses, draining sinuses, double-open comedones (Fig. 84-9), and bridged scars. It is important to distinguish HS lesions from common mimickers, including simple folliculitis and bacterial furunculosis (Table 84-2 outlines the differential diagnosis for HS). Second, lesions must exhibit a typical distribution, with 1 or more typical lesions in the axillae, groin, buttocks, perineal, or inframammary region. Nonclassical or ectopic sites may be present (eg, thighs, abdominal skinfolds) but must be accompanied by lesions in typical areas. Sites of involvement, in decreasing frequency, are: axillary, inguinal, perineal and perianal, mammary and inframammary, buttock, pubic region, chest, scalp, retroauricular, and eyelid.[71] Third, there must be a clear history of symptom chronicity and recurrence.[38,72] No formal guidelines for the clear history criteria exist. Delays in diagnosis are not uncommon, with 7 years being the average time from symptom onset to diagnosis.[10] Having 2 recurrences over a 6-month period has been suggested as one measure of chronicity.[3] Figure 84-10 provides an example of a proposed diagnostic algorithm.[73]

SEVERITY

The Hurley staging system (Table 84-3) is the most widely used approach to assessing disease severity.

TABLE 84-1
Diagnostic Criteria

1. **Typical lesion (1 or more):** painful nodules, abscesses, draining sinuses, double-open comedones, bridged scars
2. **Typical distribution[a]:** axillae, groin, buttocks, perineal, and inframammary regions
3. **Chronicity and recurrence** of symptoms

[a]Atypical or ectopic sites may be affected but at least 1 typical area must be involved.

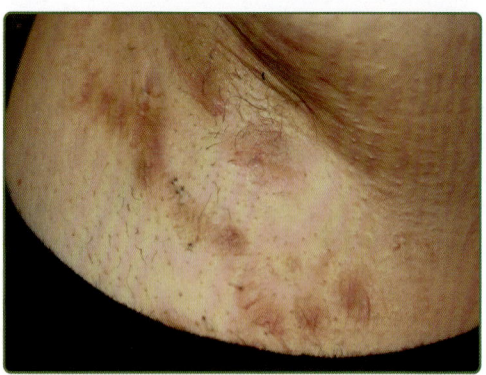

Figure 84-9 Atrophic scars and double-open comedones associated with hidradenitis suppurativa in the axilla.

Stage I is defined by recurrent abscesses without scarring or sinus tracts; stage II is defined by recurrent abscesses with scarring and sinus tract(s), separated by normal skin; and stage III is defined by recurrent abscesses with diffuse scarring and interconnected sinus tracts with minimal to no normal skin between lesions.[74] The vast majority of HS patients (68%) have stage I disease; stage II and stage III disease develop in 28% and 4% of HS patients, respectively.[74,75]

Although useful for rapid classification of disease severity, the Hurley system does not account for the dynamic changes of lesion progression and regression, which are important for assessing therapeutic response. Other scoring systems have been developed to more accurately capture disease nuance. These systems include the Sartorius score,[76] an HS-specific Physician Global Assessment,[77] the HS Severity Index,[78] and the HS Clinical Response Score.[79] These systems, however, are generally considered too cumbersome for clinical practice but remain useful in research settings.

CLINICAL PHENOTYPES

Several clinical phenotypes of HS have been proposed.[72,80] Using latent class analysis (a multivariate regression model) without any a priori hypotheses, Canoui-Poitrine and colleagues identified 3 distinct phenotypes from a large, prospective cross-sectional study of 618 patients.[80] The classic "axillary–mammary" subtype, characterized by breast and axillary involvement with hypertrophic scarring, accounted for 48% of the patients. The "follicular" subtype, characterized by a predilection for follicular lesions (eg, epidermal cysts, pilonidal sinus, comedones, severe acne) and atypical topography involving the ears, chest, back, or legs, comprised 26% of the patients. Compared to those of the classic axillary–mammary subtype, patients of the follicular subtype were also more likely to be male smokers with a family history of HS and greater disease severity.[80] The "gluteal" subtype, characterized by follicular papules, folliculitis, and gluteal involvement, comprised 26% of patients. Patients with the gluteal subtype tended to be smokers with lower body mass indexes and more indolent disease compared to the axillary–mammary subtype.[80]

LABORATORY TESTING

Patients with acute lesions may exhibit leukocytosis, elevated erythrocyte sedimentation rate, low serum iron levels, and serum protein abnormalities on serum electrophoresis.[81] Chemistries, complete blood counts, and blood cultures should be sent for patients who are febrile or appear toxic.[81] Purulent drainage should be sent for bacterial cultures and sensitivities.[81] If there is a concern for infection, a deep-tissue culture should be sent for bacterial and fungal organisms.

IMAGING

Ultrasonography and MRI may be used to visualize lesions for staging and surgical planning, although these strategies are rarely used.[82] Ultrasonography features may reveal subclinical fluid collections in 76.4% of the patients, fistulous tracts in 29.4%, dermal pseudocysts in 70.6%, and widening of the hair follicles in 100%.[83] MRI findings are nonspecific. Skin thickening and induration of subcutaneous tissue that are low signal on T1-weighted images and high-signal on T2-weighted and short tau inversion recovery (STIR) images are typical.[84] With IV contrast, abscesses appear as subcutaneous rim-enhancing collections that are low signal on T1-weighted images and high-signal on T2-weighted and STIR images.[84]

TABLE 84-2
Differential Diagnosis for Hidradenitis Suppurativa

EARLY LESIONS	LATE LESIONS
Acne vulgaris	Actinomycosis
Carbuncle	Anal fistula
Cellulitis	Cat scratch disease
Cutaneous blastomycosis	Crohn disease
Dermoid cyst	Granuloma inguinale
Erysipelas	Ischiorectal abscess
Folliculitis	Lymphogranuloma venereum
Furuncle	*Nocardia* infection
Inflamed epidermoid cysts	Noduloulcerative syphilis
Lymphadenopathy	Pilonidal disease
Perirectal abscess	Tuberculosis abscess
Pilonidal cyst	Tularemia

Adapted from Alikhan A, Lynch PJ, Eisen DB. Hidradenitis suppurativa: a comprehensive review. *J Am Acad Dermatol*. 2009;60(4):539-61.

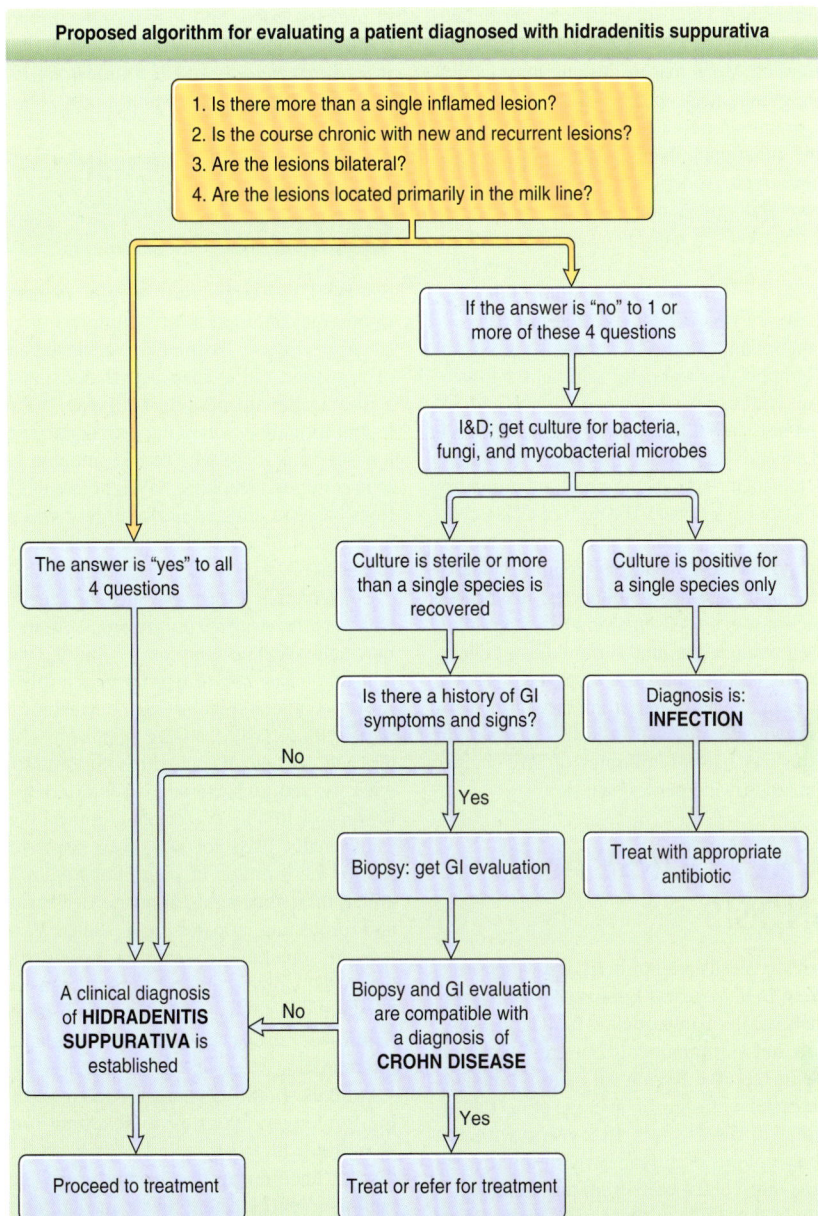

Figure 84-10 Proposed algorithm for evaluating a patient in whom a diagnosis of hidradenitis suppurativa is being considered. I&D, incision and drainage. (From Alikhan A, Lynch PJ, Eisen DB. Hidradenitis suppurativa: a comprehensive review. *J Am Acad Dermatol*. 2009;60[4]:539-561, with permission. Copyright © American Academy of Dermatology.)

TABLE 84-3
Hurley Staging

HURLEY STAGE	CHARACTERISTICS
I	Recurrent abscesses without scarring or sinus tract formation
II	Recurrent abscesses with scarring and sinus tract formation separated by normal skin
III	Recurrent abscesses, diffuse scarring, and interconnecting sinus tracts with minimal to no normal skin between lesions

HISTOPATHOLOGY

Follicular occlusion is a nonspecific but universal histopathologic finding in HS irrespective of disease duration.[85] Early lesions are characterized by follicular hyperkeratosis of the terminal hair follicles, hyperplasia of the follicular infundibulum, and perifolliculitis.[24,86] These processes lead to keratinous plugging of the terminal hair follicles, a consistent histologic finding that precedes follicular dilation and rupture.[24] Epidermal psoriasiform hyperplasia (lacking parakeratosis) and subepidermal perifollicular collections of lymphocytes also have been observed in early disease.[24] More mature lesions may exhibit noncaseating granulomas, abscesses, epidermal cysts, sinus tracts, granulation tissue, and dermal fibrosis.[27,87] Subcutaneous inflammation, fibrosis, and fat necrosis also can be observed. Apocrinitis may occur by extension; however, apocrine gland involvement is seen in 12% to 30% of cases.[27,85,87] However, secondary inflammation of the eccrine glands is more often present (19% to 32% of cases).[27,85,87] Primary inflammation of the apocrine glands is rare, occurring in 5% of lesions.[27,85,87]

Acutely, the inflammatory infiltrate is largely comprised of T-lymphocytes and neutrophils at the follicular epithelium with variable extension into the adnexal structures.[24] A histopathologic analysis of surgical specimens found a marked CD8+ T-lymphocyte epitheliotropism in the follicular and subepidermal inflammatory infiltrates of early HS lesions.[24] The ratio of CD8+ cytotoxic T-lymphocytes to CD4+ helper T-lymphocytes also appears to increase over the lifetime of active lesions.[86] In chronic lesions, lymphocytes, histiocytes, and multinucleated giant cells predominate, generating foreign-body granulomas around ruptured hair follicles and skin adnexa.[88] Eosinophils and plasma cells are also seen on occasion.[87] Notably, recent immunohistochemistry studies report elevated IL-17 and IL-23 expression along with distinct dermal infiltrates of Th17 helper T cells within lesional and perilesional skin.[49,52]

CLINICAL COURSE AND PROGNOSIS

Disease onset is typically after puberty, with a reported age range from 16 to 81 years.[4] Because HS can resemble other pustular dermatoses, delays in diagnosis of 7 to 12 years are not uncommon.[89] In one cross-sectional survey, patients reported having 4.6 painful boils per month, with each boil lasting an average of 6.9 days.[90] Mean duration of disease was 18.8 years, with the most-severe symptoms occurring early in the disease course (after a mean of 6.4 years from disease onset).[90] Disease activity generally declines after 50 years of age.[38] Remissions are significantly more likely in nonsmokers, those who have quit smoking, and in nonobese individuals.[41]

MANAGEMENT

HS is a complex, heterogeneous disease with unpredictable responses to therapy. Therefore, formal treatment guidelines for HS do not exist, and therapeutic decisions are generally guided by disease severity. Hurley stage I disease (mild) is typically amenable to medical therapy alone; Hurley stage II disease (moderate) may require both medical therapy and localized surgical excisions; Hurley stage III disease (severe) often requires extensive, wide excisional surgical procedures with advanced grafting and flap procedures. There is no cure for HS. The overall goals of therapy are to prevent formation of primary lesions and to reduce the impact of disease sequelae (eg, fibrosis, contractures, sinus tracts) on quality of life. Tables 84-4 and 84-5 and Fig. 84-11 offer a proposed management algorithm.

LIFESTYLE MODIFICATIONS AND HOME REMEDIES

Smoking cessation and weight management are important components of symptom mitigation at all stages of disease. Nonsmokers achieved a higher rate of remission (40%) than active smokers (29%) over a mean followup period of 22 years.[41] Rates of new lesion formation following excisional surgery were lower among those who ceased smoking versus those who continued smoking.[42] Weight loss of 15% or more from baseline after bariatric surgery was also associated with a 20% reduction in number of active, eruptive sites.[41]

Conservative measures, such as stress reduction, warm baths, warm compresses, and hydrotherapy, may help alleviate symptoms.[91] Taking "bleach baths" (ie, one-quarter cup of regular bleach diluted in a full tub or 40 gallons of water) and/or washing the affected areas with topical cleansing agents (eg, chlorhexidine gluconate or benzoyl peroxide solution) 2 to 3 times per week can reduce bacterial load and decrease malodor.[9] Resorcinol 10% to 15% cream, a topical peeling agent traditionally used for acne, can improve pain and reduce the duration of painful abscesses.[92] Dressings are useful for managing drainage, decreasing malodor, and protecting apparel from stains. Wound dressings are sometimes covered by insurance; abdominal (eg, ABD) gauze pads and sanitary pads can be used as alternatives. Short courses of nonsteroidal antiinflammatory drugs can help alleviate pain and reduce inflammation.

Patients should be counseled to avoid tight clothing, prolonged exposure to heat and humidity, and shaving, if these are noted as triggers.[90] Consumption of insulinotropic milk and dairy products, as well as hyperglycemic foods, upregulate the PI3K/Akt-signaling pathway, leading to nuclear deficiency of FoxO1 transcription factor.[93,94] Deficiency in FoxO1 is thought to play a role in acne vulgaris and acne-like eruptions.[94] Further research is needed in this area, but decreasing exposure to dairy and high-glycemic-index foods may be an adjunct to medical therapy, either directly or indirectly, by promoting weight loss.

Applying minced turmeric root as a poultice to active sites or ingesting diluted turmeric (1 teaspoon of turmeric powder diluted in one-quarter cup liquid) 3 times daily has had anecdotal success in ameliorating symptoms. Curcumin, the active ingredient in turmeric, may help reduce inflammation via suppression of TNF-α.[95]

A 6-month course of high-dose zinc gluconate supplementation (90 mg daily, tapered by 15 mg every 2 months) improved clinical status in a cohort

TABLE 84-4
Ratings of Select Therapies for Hidradenitis Suppurativa Based on Category of Evidence and Strength of Recommendation

THERAPY	CATEGORY OF EVIDENCE	STRENGTH OF RECOMMENDATION
First-line		
• Clindamycin (topical)[a]	IIb	Possible B
• Clindamycin/rifampicin (oral)[b]	III	C
• Adalimumab (subcutaneous)[c]	I	A
• Tetracycline (oral)	IIb	B
Second-line		
• Zinc gluconate	III	C
• Resorcinol (cream)	III	C
• Intralesional corticosteroid	IV	D
• Systemic corticosteroid	IV	D
• Infliximab	Ib/IIa	B
• Acitretin/etretinate	III	C
Third-line		
• Colchicine	IV	D
• Botulinum toxin (subcutaneous)	IV	D
• Isotretinoin	IV	D
• Dapsone	IV	D
• Cyclosporine	IV	D
• Hormones	IV	D
Surgery		
• Excision or curettage of individual lesions	III	C
• Total excision of lesions and surrounding hair-bearing skin	IIb	B
• Secondary intension healing	IIb	B
• Primary closure	III	C
• Reconstruction with skin grafting and negative pressure wound therapy	III	C
• Reconstruction with flap plasty	Ia/IIa	A/B
• Deroofing	IV	D
• CO_2 laser therapy	Ib	A
• Neodymium:yttrium-aluminum-garnet (Nd:YAG) laser	Ib	A
• Intense pulsed light	IV	D
Pain Control		
• Nonsteroidal antiinflammatory drugs	IV	D
• Opiates	IV	D
Dressings		
• No studies have been published as of this writing on the use of specific dressings or wound care methodology in hidradenitis suppurativa; choice of dressing is based on clinical experience	IV	D

[a]Single double-blind, placebo-controlled, randomized trial. Hurley stages I to II.
[b]Evaluated in case series.
[c]Multiple prospective, randomized, double-blind, placebo-controlled trials (Pioneer 1 and 2).
Adapted from Gulliver W, Zouboulis CC, Prens E, et al. Evidence-based approach to the treatment of hidradenitis suppurativa/acne inversa, based on the European guidelines for hidradenitis suppurativa. *Rev Endocr Metab Disord*. 2016;17(3):343-351, with permission.

TABLE 84-5
Category of Evidence/Strength of Recommendation Grading Scale

CATEGORY OF EVIDENCE	STRENGTH OF RECOMMENDATION
Ia: Metaanalysis of randomized controlled trials Ib: Randomized controlled trial	A: Category I evidence
IIa: Controlled study without randomization IIb: Quasiexperimental study	B: Category II evidence or extrapolated from category I evidence
III: Nonexperimental descriptive studies such as comparative, correlation, and case-control studies	C: Category III evidence or extrapolated from category I or II evidence
IV: Expert committee reports or opinion or clinical experience of respected authorities, or both	D: Category IV evidence or extrapolated from category II or III evidence

Data from Guyatt G, Oxman AD, Vist GE, et al. GRADE: An emerging consensus on rating quality of evidence and strength of recommendations. *BMJ*. 2008;336:924; and from Gulliver W, Zouboulis CC, Prens E, et al. Evidence-based approach to the treatment of hidradenitis suppurativa/acne inversa, based on the European guidelines for hidradenitis suppurativa. *Rev Endocr Metab Disord*. 2016;17(3):343-351, with permission.

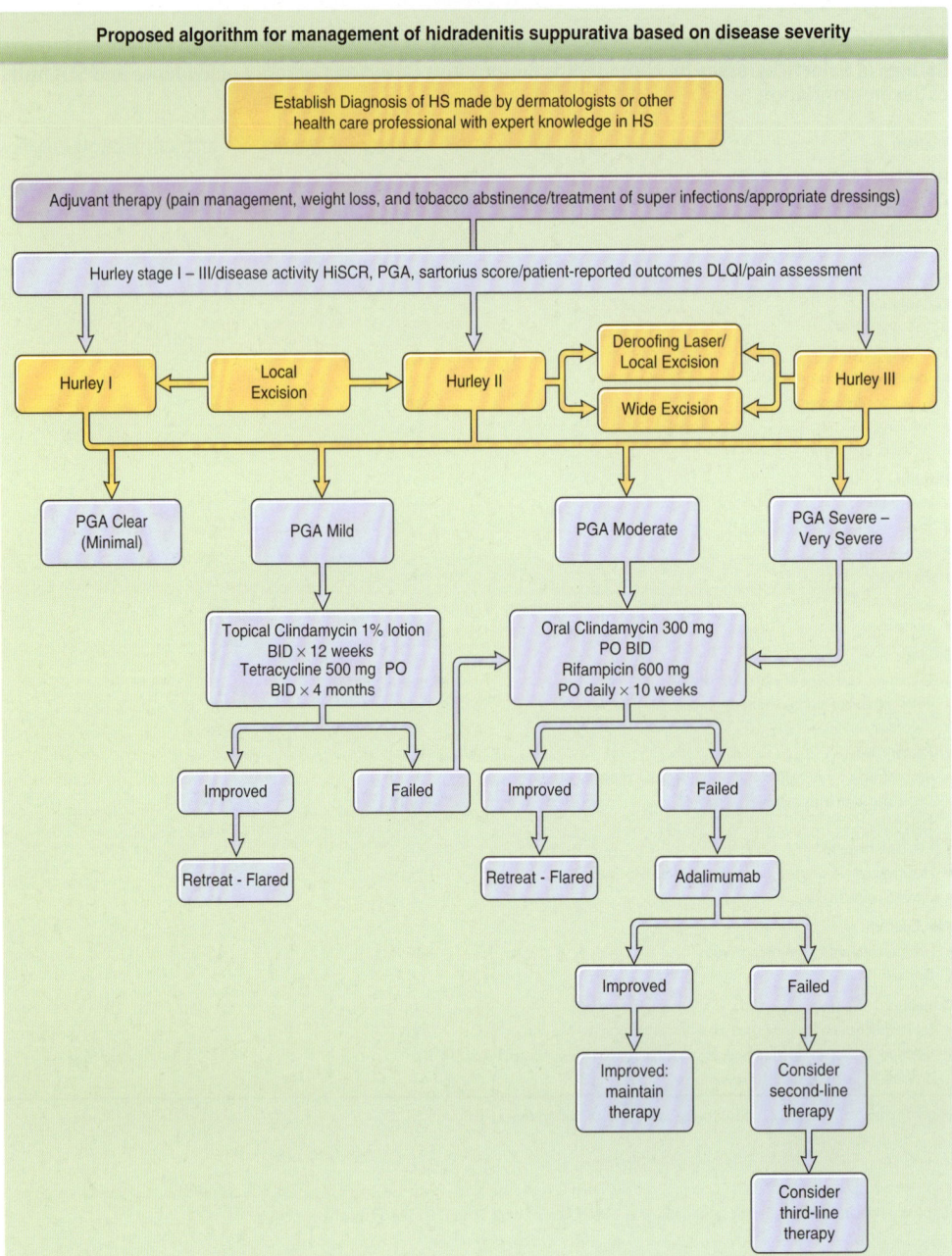

Figure 84-11 Proposed algorithm for management of hidradenitis suppurativa (HS) based on disease severity. BID, twice daily; DLQI, Dermatology Life Quality Index; HiSCR, Hidradenitis Suppurativa Clinical Response; OD, once daily; PGA, Physician Global Assessment; PO, by mouth. (From Gulliver W, Zouboulis CC, Prens E, et al. Evidence-based approach to the treatment of hidradenitis suppurativa/acne inversa, based on the European guidelines for hidradenitis suppurativa. *Rev Endocr Metab Disord.* 2016;17[3]:343-351, with permission.)

of 22 patients with therapy-resistant mild-to-moderate HS.[96] Eight patients achieved complete remission while 14 patients achieved partial remission.[96] Mild side effects (nausea, vomiting, abdominal distension, esophagitis) were reported in 14% of patients.[96] Therapeutic benefit is thought to derive from the antioxidant and antiinflammatory properties of zinc gluconate.

MEDICAL THERAPY

ANTIBIOTIC THERAPY

Topical and oral antibiotic therapy are the mainstays of management of mild-to-moderate HS. A randomized, double-blind, placebo-controlled trial demonstrated that clindamycin 1% lotion applied twice daily to affected areas reduced the number of pustules, inflammatory nodules, and abscesses in patients with Hurley stage I and mild stage II disease.[97,98] Topical metronidazole 0.75% or erythromycin 2% can be trialed as alternatives to clindamycin. A 4-month trial of oral tetracyclines can be used for their antiinflammatory effect in any disease stage.

For more-severe disease (Hurley stage II) that is refractory to topical clindamycin and/or oral tetracyclines, a regimen of 300 mg of clindamycin and 300 mg of rifampin taken 2 to 3 times daily may be effective.[99] Triple therapy with rifampin (10 mg/kg/day), moxifloxacin (400 mg/day), and metronidazole (500 mg 3 times daily) can be used as an alternative antibiotic regimen for resistant or severe disease.[100] There is weak-to-moderate evidence supporting a course of dapsone (50 to 200 mg daily for 4 to 12 weeks) in refractory HS.[101]

BIOLOGIC THERAPY

Patients with moderate-to-severe HS who are unresponsive to, or intolerant of, antibiotic therapy may benefit from 40 mg weekly subcutaneous adalimumab, a monoclonal antibody specific to TNF-α.[77] Nonresponders to adalimumab therapy may benefit from infliximab, a chimeric monoclonal antibody inhibitor of TNF-α, dosed at 5 mg/kg at weeks 0, 2, and 6, followed by every 8 weeks thereafter.[78] Ustekinumab (an IL-12 and IL-23 inhibitor) and anakinra (an IL-1α and IL-1β inhibitor) have been used in small numbers of patients for HS with anecdotal success.[102,103]

IMMUNOSUPPRESSANT THERAPY

Overall, there is weak evidence supporting use of oral glucocorticoids, colchicine, cyclosporine, azathioprine,[104] and methotrexate in HS.[105] Intralesional steroid injections of triamcinolone acetonide suspension, 5 to 10 mg/mL, can decrease inflammation in acutely flaring lesions, but is not an effective long-term strategy.[105,106]

HORMONAL THERAPY

Androgen modulation therapy can be trialed as second-line therapy for patients with mild-to-moderate HS. Small case series have shown improvement with spironolactone 100 to 150 mg daily,[107] as well as finasteride 5 mg daily.[108]

METFORMIN

Metformin, an insulin-sensitizing biguanide agent used in Type 2 diabetes mellitus, is an appealing second-line option for women with HS and comorbid polycystic ovarian syndrome and/or metabolic syndrome. By improving insulin sensitivity, metformin is thought to counter insulin resistance–induced ovarian androgen production. In a small prospective study of 25 patients with HS who had failed standard-line therapies, metformin dosed at 500 mg to 1500 mg daily reduced clinical severity and improved quality of life in 72% of patients over a course for 24 weeks.[109]

RETINOIDS

Topical tretinoin and oral isotretinoin are largely ineffective for HS[110] but are still commonly prescribed.[111] In a retrospective study of 88 patients with HS who had been treated with oral isotretinoin (dosing range 20 to 140 mg/kg/day) over a mean duration of 7.8 months, only 14 (16%) demonstrated clinical response.[112] Case reports suggest that acitretin, a second-generation retinoid, may have better efficacy in HS compared to isotretinoin.[110] In 1 retrospective study, 12 of 12 patients treated with 0.25 to 0.88 mg/kg acitretin for 9 to 12 months showed clinical improvement.[113] More recently, alitretinoin, a first-generation retinoid with similar properties to acitretin, produced 50% reduction in Sartorius score in 6 of 14 patients when dosed at 10 mg daily for 24 weeks.[114]

SURGICAL THERAPY

EXCISIONAL SURGERY

Excisional surgical interventions are a cornerstone for managing chronic HS. The vast majority of patients (>90%) are satisfied with results after surgery.[115] For milder disease, simple incision and drainage procedures, local excisions, and/or deroofing of sinus tracts typically suffice.[116] More-severe disease will likely require wide local excisions with primary closure, split-thickness grafting, flap advancements, and/or healing by secondary intention.[117] Optimal surgical closure is controversial and depends on characteristics of the surgical site, a topic that has been well reviewed elsewhere.[117]

Unfortunately, disease recurrence is common after surgery and many patients will require reexcisions throughout the lifetime of the disease.[118] A recent systematic review of surgical interventions for HS reported a 13% recurrence rate for wide local excisions; 22% recurrence rate for local incision; and 27% recurrence rate after deroofing.[119] Interestingly, the recurrence rate after wide local excision was lower for graft (6%) and flap (8%) closure than for primary closure (15%).[119] Some authors maintain, however, that disease recurrence after surgery is likely related to the adequacy of original excision and/or severity of disease rather than type of surgical closure.[120]

LASER THERAPY

Lasers are growing in use as adjunctive therapies for HS. Laser therapies mitigate flares by debulking tissue as well as reducing the number of hair follicles, sebaceous glands, and bacteria in affected areas.[121] Long-pulse 1065-nm neodymium-doped yttrium aluminum garnet (Nd:YAG) laser surgery, and both ablative and fractional CO_2 laser surgery have been used successfully in the management of HS[122] and are amenable to outpatient settings.

OTHER THERAPY OPTIONS

Cryotherapy improved symptoms in 8 of 10 patients with limited, painful nodules[123]; however, most patients reported significant pain with the procedure, postprocedure ulceration and/or infection, and long healing times (average of 25 days).[123]

Radiotherapy for HS was popular in the past but fell out of favor in the 1970s following the advent of cheaper, more easily administered topical and oral therapies.[124] Recent case series have reported moderate success among patients with chronic HS who have failed medical and traditional surgical therapies.[124,125] Prospective studies are needed to better evaluate its efficacy in chronic HS.

Intralesional botulinum toxin A injections may have efficacy for HS.[126] Botulinum toxin A is thought to alleviate HS by diminishing or even abolishing eccrine, apocrine, and pilosebaceous gland function,[126] which prevents excretions and follicular rupture. Substantive trials are lacking.

PAIN MANAGEMENT

Current approaches to managing pain in HS derive from expert opinions as well as general pain management guidelines.[127] Topical analgesics, oral acetaminophen, and oral nonsteroidal antiinflammatory drugs are considered first-line therapy for pain in HS.[127] Persistent and breakthrough pain may require stepup therapy with oral opioid analgesics. Pharmacotherapy targeting neuropathic pain pathways may be beneficial, especially given that they may concomitantly ameliorate comorbid depression and itch.[127] More studies are needed to determine optimal pain regimens for patients with HS as well as to educate dermatologists, pain management specialists, and general practitioners about the pain associated with HS.

MENTAL HEALTH

Literature concerning the management of mental health morbidity in HS is scant. Qualitative studies indicate that a majority of patients feel symptoms of depression.[128] Whether incidence of clinical depression is higher among patients with HS compared to patients without HS is unclear.[129] A cross-sectional study in Israel reported that the incidence of depression (5.9% vs 3.5%) and anxiety (3.9% vs 2.4%) were significantly higher among patients with HS when compared to age- and gender-matched controls without HS.[130] No formal management guidelines exist for the psychosocial comorbidities of HS. Nevertheless, routine screening and referral of patients with signs of depression to mental health specialists are important. Patient support groups and forums also may be beneficial.

ACKNOWLEDGMENTS

The author would like to acknowledge Powell Perng, BS, for his invaluable contribution to this chapter.

REFERENCES

1. Matusiak L, Bieniek A, Szepietowski JC. Psychophysical aspects of hidradenitis suppurativa. *Acta Derm Venereol*. 2010;90(3):264-268.
2. Wolkenstein P, Loundou A, Barrau K, et al; Quality of Life Group of the French Society of Dermatology. Quality of life impairment in hidradenitis suppurativa: a study of 61 cases. *J Am Acad Dermatol*. 2007;56(4):621-623.
3. Vinding GR, Miller IM, Zarchi K, et al. The prevalence of inverse recurrent suppuration: a population-based study of possible hidradenitis suppurativa. *Br J Dermatol*. 2014;170(4):884-889.
4. Vazquez BG, Alikhan A, Weaver AL, et al. Incidence of hidradenitis suppurativa and associated factors: a population-based study of Olmsted County, Minnesota. *J Invest Dermatol*. 2013;133(1):97-103.
5. Sung S, Kimball AB. Counterpoint: analysis of patient claims data to determine the prevalence of hidradenitis suppurativa in the United States. *J Am Acad Dermatol*. 2013;69(5):818-819.
6. Vlassova N, Kuhn D, Okoye GA. Hidradenitis suppurativa disproportionately affects African Americans: a single-center retrospective analysis. *Acta Derm Venereol*. 2015;95(8):990-991.
7. Anderson BB, Cadogan CA, Gangadharam D. Hidradenitis suppurativa of the perineum, scrotum, and gluteal area: presentation, complications, and treatment. *J Natl Med Assoc*. 1982;74(10):999-1003.
8. Chaikin DC, Volz LR, Broderick G. An unusual presentation of hidradenitis suppurativa: case report and review of the literature. *Urology*. 1994;44(4):606-608.
9. Paletta C, Jurkiewicz MJ. Hidradenitis suppurativa. *Clin Plast Surg*. 1987;14(2):383-390.
10. Jemec GB. Clinical practice. Hidradenitis suppurativa. *N Engl J Med*. 2012;366(2):158-164.
11. Mortimer PS, Lunniss PJ. Hidradenitis suppurativa. *J R Soc Med*. 2000;93(8):420-422.
12. von der Werth JM, Jemec GB. Morbidity in patients with hidradenitis suppurativa. *Br J Dermatol*. 2001;144(4):809-813.
13. Matusiak L, Bieniek A, Szepietowski JC. Hidradenitis suppurativa markedly decreases quality of life and professional activity. *J Am Acad Dermatol*. 2010;62(4):706-708, 708.e1.
14. Miller IM, Johansen ME, Mogensen UB, et al. Is hidradenitis suppurativa associated with anaemia?: a population-based and hospital-based cross-sectional study from Denmark. *J Eur Acad Dermatol Venereol*. 2016;30(8):1366-1372.

15. Utrera-Busquets M, Romero-Mate A, Castano A, et al. Severe hidradenitis suppurativa complicated by renal AA amyloidosis. *Clin Exp Dermatol*. 2016; 41(3):287-289.
16. Verdelli A, Antiga E, Bonciani D, et al. A fatal case of hidradenitis suppurativa associated with sepsis and squamous cell carcinoma. *Int J Dermatol*. 2016; 55(1):e52-e53.
17. Williams ST, Busby RC, DeMuth RJ, et al. Perineal hidradenitis suppurativa: presentation of two unusual complications and a review. *Ann Plast Surg*. 1991; 26(5):456-462.
18. Good LM, Francis SO, High WA. Scrotal elephantiasis secondary to hidradenitis suppurativa. *J Am Acad Dermatol*. 2011;64(5):993-994.
19. Chu EY, Kovarik CL, Lee RA. Lymphedematous verrucous changes simulating squamous cell carcinoma in long-standing hidradenitis suppurativa. *Int J Dermatol*. 2013;52(7):808-812.
20. Lavogiez C, Delaporte E, Darras-Vercambre S, et al. Clinicopathological study of 13 cases of squamous cell carcinoma complicating hidradenitis suppurativa. *Dermatology*. 2010;220(2):147-153.
21. Pena ZG, Sivamani RK, Konia TH, et al. Squamous cell carcinoma in the setting of chronic hidradenitis suppurativa; report of a patient and update of the literature. *Dermatol Online J*. 2015;21(4).
22. De Vuyst H, Clifford GM, Nascimento MC, et al. Prevalence and type distribution of human papillomavirus in carcinoma and intraepithelial neoplasia of the vulva, vagina and anus: a meta-analysis. *Int J Cancer*. 2009;124(7):1626-1636.
23. Lapins J, Ye W, Nyren O, et al. Incidence of cancer among patients with hidradenitis suppurativa. *Arch Dermatol*. 2001;137(6):730-734.
24. von Laffert M, Helmbold P, Wohlrab J, et al. Hidradenitis suppurativa (acne inversa): early inflammatory events at terminal follicles and at interfollicular epidermis. *Exp Dermatol*. 2010;19(6):533-537.
25. Prens E, Deckers I. Pathophysiology of hidradenitis suppurativa: an update. *J Am Acad Dermatol*. 2015;73(5)(suppl 1):S8-S11.
26. Danby FW, Jemec GB, Marsch W, et al. Preliminary findings suggest hidradenitis suppurativa may be due to defective follicular support. *Br J Dermatol*. 2013; 168(5):1034-1039.
27. Jemec GB, Hansen U. Histology of hidradenitis suppurativa. *J Am Acad Dermatol*. 1996;34(6):994-999.
28. Kamp S, Fiehn AM, Stenderup K, et al. Hidradenitis suppurativa: a disease of the absent sebaceous gland? Sebaceous gland number and volume are significantly reduced in uninvolved hair follicles from patients with hidradenitis suppurativa. *Br J Dermatol*. 2011;164(5):1017-1022.
29. Fitzsimmons JS, Guilbert PR, Fitzsimmons EM. Evidence of genetic factors in hidradenitis suppurativa. *Br J Dermatol*. 1985;113(1):1-8.
30. Fitzsimmons JS, Guilbert PR. A family study of hidradenitis suppurativa. *J Med Genet*. 1985;22(5):367-373.
31. Ingram JR. The genetics of hidradenitis suppurativa. *Dermatol Clin*. 2016;34(1):23-28.
32. Chen S, Mattei P, You J, et al. γ-Secretase mutation in an African American family with hidradenitis suppurativa. *JAMA Dermatol*. 2015;151(6):668-670.
33. Pan Y, Lin MH, Tian X, et al. Gamma-secretase functions through Notch signaling to maintain skin appendages but is not required for their patterning or initial morphogenesis. *Dev Cell*. 2004;7(5):731-743.
34. Radtke F, Fasnacht N, Macdonald HR. Notch signaling in the immune system. *Immunity*. 2010;32(1):14-27.
35. Zhang Q, Wang C, Liu Z, et al. Notch signal suppresses toll-like receptor-triggered inflammatory responses in macrophages by inhibiting extracellular signal-regulated kinase 1/2-mediated nuclear factor kappaB activation. *J Biol Chem*. 2012;287(9):6208-6217.
36. Lapins J, Olerup O, Emtestam L. No human leukocyte antigen-A, -B or -DR association in Swedish patients with hidradenitis suppurativa. *Acta Derm Venereol*. 2001;81(1):28-30.
37. O'Loughlin S, Woods R, Kirke PN, et al. Hidradenitis suppurativa. Glucose tolerance, clinical, microbiologic, and immunologic features and HLA frequencies in 27 patients. *Arch Dermatol*. 1988;124(7):1043-1046.
38. Revuz JE, Canoui-Poitrine F, Wolkenstein P, et al. Prevalence and factors associated with hidradenitis suppurativa: results from two case-control studies. *J Am Acad Dermatol*. 2008;59(4):596-601.
39. Woodruff CM, Charlie AM, Leslie KS. Hidradenitis suppurativa: a guide for the practicing physician. *Mayo Clin Proc*. 2015;90(12):1679-1693.
40. Totti N 3rd, McCusker KT, Campbell EJ, et al. Nicotine is chemotactic for neutrophils and enhances neutrophil responsiveness to chemotactic peptides. *Science*. 1984;223(4632):169-171.
41. Kromann CB, Deckers IE, Esmann S, et al. Risk factors, clinical course and long-term prognosis in hidradenitis suppurativa: a cross-sectional study. *Br J Dermatol*. 2014;171(4):819-824.
42. Kurzen H, Schönfelder-Funcke, S, Hartschuh W. Surgical treatment of acne inversa at the University of Heidelberg. *Coloproctology*. 2000;22:76-80.
43. Kraft JN, Searles GE. Hidradenitis suppurativa in 64 female patients: retrospective study comparing oral antibiotics and antiandrogen therapy. *J Cutan Med Surg*. 2007;11(4):125-131.
44. Barth JH, Layton AM, Cunliffe WJ. Endocrine factors in pre- and postmenopausal women with hidradenitis suppurativa. *Br J Dermatol*. 1996;134(6):1057-1059.
45. Jemec GB. The symptomatology of hidradenitis suppurativa in women. *Br J Dermatol*. 1988;119(3): 345-350.
46. Buimer MG, Wobbes T, Klinkenbijl JH, et al. Immunohistochemical analysis of steroid hormone receptors in hidradenitis suppurativa. *Am J Dermatopathol*. 2015;37(2):129-132.
47. Barth JH, Kealey T. Androgen metabolism by isolated human axillary apocrine glands in hidradenitis suppurativa. *Br J Dermatol*. 1991;125(4):304-308.
48. Kurzen H, Kurokawa I, Jemec GB, et al. What causes hidradenitis suppurativa? *Exp Dermatol*. 2008;17(5): 455-456; discussion 457-472.
49. Kelly G, Prens EP. Inflammatory mechanisms in hidradenitis suppurativa. *Dermatol Clin*. 2016;34(1): 51-58.
50. Kelly G, Sweeney CM, Tobin AM, et al. Hidradenitis suppurativa: the role of immune dysregulation. *Int J Dermatol*. 2014;53(10):1186-1196.
51. Waite JC, Skokos D. Th17 response and inflammatory autoimmune diseases. *Int J Inflam*. 2012;2012: 819467.
52. Schlapbach C, Hanni T, Yawalkar N, et al. Expression of the IL-23/Th17 pathway in lesions of hidradenitis suppurativa. *J Am Acad Dermatol*. 2011;65(4): 790-798.
53. Ring HC, Emtestam L. The microbiology of hidradenitis suppurativa. *Dermatol Clin*. 2016;34(1):29-35.

54. van der Zee HH, Laman JD, Boer J, et al. Hidradenitis suppurativa: viewpoint on clinical phenotyping, pathogenesis and novel treatments. *Exp Dermatol*. 2012;21(10):735-739.
55. Kathju S, Lasko LA, Stoodley P. Considering hidradenitis suppurativa as a bacterial biofilm disease. *FEMS Immunol Med Microbiol*. 2012;65(2):385-389.
56. Scheinfeld N. Diseases associated with hidradenitis suppurativa: part 2 of a series on hidradenitis. *Dermatol Online J*. 2013;19(6):18558.
57. Braun-Falco M, Kovnerystyy O, Lohse P, et al. Pyoderma gangrenosum, acne, and suppurative hidradenitis (PASH)—a new autoinflammatory syndrome distinct from PAPA syndrome. *J Am Acad Dermatol*. 2012;66(3):409-415.
58. Marzano AV, Trevisan V, Gattorno M, et al. Pyogenic arthritis, pyoderma gangrenosum, acne, and hidradenitis suppurativa (PAPASH): a new autoinflammatory syndrome associated with a novel mutation of the PSTPIP1 gene. *JAMA Dermatol*. 2013;149(6):762-764.
59. Saraceno R, Babino G, Chiricozzi A, et al. PsAPASH: a new syndrome associated with hidradenitis suppurativa with response to tumor necrosis factor inhibition. *J Am Acad Dermatol*. 2015;72(1):e42-e44.
60. Duchatelet S, Miskinyte S, Join-Lambert O, et al. First nicastrin mutation in PASH (pyoderma gangrenosum, acne and suppurative hidradenitis) syndrome. *Br J Dermatol*. 2015;173(2):610-612.
61. Calderon-Castrat X, Bancalari-Diaz D, Roman-Curto C, et al. PSTPIP1 gene mutation in a pyoderma gangrenosum, acne and suppurative hidradenitis (PASH) syndrome. *Br J Dermatol*. 2016;175(1):194-198.
62. van der Zee HH, de Winter K, van der Woude CJ, et al. The prevalence of hidradenitis suppurativa in 1093 patients with inflammatory bowel disease. *Br J Dermatol*. 2014;171(3):673-675.
63. van der Zee HH, van der Woude CJ, Florencia EF, et al. Hidradenitis suppurativa and inflammatory bowel disease: are they associated? Results of a pilot study. *Br J Dermatol*. 2010;162(1):195-197.
64. Burrows NP, Jones RR. Crohn's disease in association with hidradenitis suppurativa. *Br J Dermatol*. 1992;126(5):523.
65. Nassar D, Hugot JP, Wolkenstein P, et al. Lack of association between CARD15 gene polymorphisms and hidradenitis suppurativa: a pilot study. *Dermatology*. 2007;215(4):359.
66. van Rappard DC, Mekkes JR. Hidradenitis suppurativa not associated with CARD15/NOD2 mutation: a case series. *Int J Dermatol*. 2014;53(1):e77-e79.
67. Martinez F, Nos P, Benlloch S, et al. Hidradenitis suppurativa and Crohn's disease: response to treatment with infliximab. *Inflamm Bowel Dis*. 2001;7(4):323-326.
68. Shlyankevich J, Chen AJ, Kim GE, et al. Hidradenitis suppurativa is a systemic disease with substantial comorbidity burden: a chart-verified case-control analysis. *J Am Acad Dermatol*. 2014;71(6):1144-1150.
69. Miller IM, Ellervik C, Vinding GR, et al. Association of metabolic syndrome and hidradenitis suppurativa. *JAMA Dermatol*. 2014;150(12):1273-1280.
70. Shalom G, Freud T, Harman-Boehm I, et al. Hidradenitis suppurativa and metabolic syndrome: a comparative cross-sectional study of 3207 patients. *Br J Dermatol*. 2015;173(2):464-470.
71. Slade DE, Powell BW, Mortimer PS. Hidradenitis suppurativa: pathogenesis and management. *Br J Plast Surg*. 2003;56(5):451-461.
72. van der Zee HH, Jemec GB. New insights into the diagnosis of hidradenitis suppurativa: Clinical presentations and phenotypes. *J Am Acad Dermatol*. 2015;73(5)(suppl 1):S23-S26.
73. Alikhan A, Lynch PJ, Eisen DB. Hidradenitis suppurativa: a comprehensive review. *J Am Acad Dermatol*. 2009;60(4):539-561; quiz 562-563.
74. Canoui-Poitrine F, Revuz JE, Wolkenstein P, et al. Clinical characteristics of a series of 302 French patients with hidradenitis suppurativa, with an analysis of factors associated with disease severity. *J Am Acad Dermatol*. 2009;61(1):51-57.
75. Hurley HJ. Axillary hyperhidrosis, apocrine bromhidrosis, hidradenitis suppurativa, and familial benign pemphigus: surgical approach. In: Roenigk RK, Roenigk HH, eds. *Dermatologic Surgery*. New York, NY: Marcel Dekker; 1989:729-739.
76. Sartorius K, Lapins J, Emtestam L, et al. Suggestions for uniform outcome variables when reporting treatment effects in hidradenitis suppurativa. *Br J Dermatol*. 2003;149(1):211-213.
77. Kimball AB, Kerdel F, Adams D, et al. Adalimumab for the treatment of moderate to severe Hidradenitis suppurativa: a parallel randomized trial. *Ann Intern Med*. 2012;157(12):846-855.
78. Grant A, Gonzalez T, Montgomery MO, et al. Infliximab therapy for patients with moderate to severe hidradenitis suppurativa: a randomized, double-blind, placebo-controlled crossover trial. *J Am Acad Dermatol*. 2010;62(2):205-217.
79. Kimball AB, Jemec GB, Yang M, et al. Assessing the validity, responsiveness and meaningfulness of the Hidradenitis Suppurativa Clinical Response (HiSCR) as the clinical endpoint for hidradenitis suppurativa treatment. *Br J Dermatol*. 2014;171(6):1434-1442.
80. Canoui-Poitrine F, Le Thuaut A, Revuz JE, et al. Identification of three hidradenitis suppurativa phenotypes: latent class analysis of a cross-sectional study. *J Invest Dermatol*. 2013;133(6):1506-1511.
81. Ferri FF. Hidradenitis suppurativa. In: *Ferri's Clinical Advisor 2017*. St. Louis, MO: Elsevier; 2017:588-589.
82. Wortsman X. Imaging of hidradenitis suppurativa. *Dermatol Clin*. 2016;34(1):59-68.
83. Wortsman X, Jemec G. A 3D ultrasound study of sinus tract formation in hidradenitis suppurativa. *Dermatol Online J*. 2013;19(6):18564.
84. Kelly AM, Cronin P. MRI features of hidradenitis suppurativa and review of the literature. *AJR Am J Roentgenol*. 2005;185(5):1201-1204.
85. Attanoos RL, Appleton MA, Douglas-Jones AG. The pathogenesis of hidradenitis suppurativa: a closer look at apocrine and apoeccrine glands. *Br J Dermatol*. 1995;133(2):254-258.
86. Boer J, Weltevreden EF. Hidradenitis suppurativa or acne inversa. A clinicopathological study of early lesions. *Br J Dermatol*. 1996;135(5):721-725.
87. Jemec GB, Thomsen BM, Hansen U. The homogeneity of hidradenitis suppurativa lesions. A histological study of intra-individual variation. *APMIS*. 1997;105(5):378-383.
88. Fismen S, Ingvarsson G, Moseng D, et al. A clinical-pathological review of hidradenitis suppurativa: using immunohistochemistry one disease becomes two. *APMIS*. 2012;120(6):433-440.
89. Poli F, Jemec GB, Revuz J. Clinical presentation. In: *Hidradenitis Suppurativa*. Heidelberg, Germany: Springer; 2006:11-24.

90. von der Werth JM, Williams HC. The natural history of hidradenitis suppurativa. *J Eur Acad Dermatol Venereol.* 2000;14(5):389-392.
91. Shah N. Hidradenitis suppurativa: a treatment challenge. *Am Fam Physician.* 2005;72(8):1547-1552.
92. Boer J, Jemec GB. Resorcinol peels as a possible self-treatment of painful nodules in hidradenitis suppurativa. *Clin Exp Dermatol.* 2010;35(1):36-40.
93. Kumari R, Thappa DM. Role of insulin resistance and diet in acne. *Indian J Dermatol Venereol Leprol.* 2013;79(3):291-299.
94. Melnik BC. Acneigenic stimuli converge in phosphoinositol-3 kinase/Akt/Foxo1 signal transduction. *J Clin Exp Dermatol Res.* 2010;1(1):1-8.
95. Sahebkar A, Cicero AF, Simental-Mendia LE, et al. Curcumin downregulates human tumor necrosis factor-alpha levels: a systematic review and meta-analysis of randomized controlled trials. *Pharmacol Res.* 2016;107:234-242.
96. Brocard A, Knol AC, Khammari A, et al. Hidradenitis suppurativa and zinc: a new therapeutic approach. A pilot study. *Dermatology.* 2007;214(4):325-327.
97. Clemmensen OJ. Topical treatment of hidradenitis suppurativa with clindamycin. *Int J Dermatol.* 1983;22(5):325-328.
98. Jemec GB, Wendelboe P. Topical clindamycin versus systemic tetracycline in the treatment of hidradenitis suppurativa. *J Am Acad Dermatol.* 1998;39(6):971-974.
99. Bettoli V, Zauli S, Borghi A, et al. Oral clindamycin and rifampicin in the treatment of hidradenitis suppurativa-acne inversa: a prospective study on 23 patients. *J Eur Acad Dermatol Venereol.* 2014;28(1):125-126.
100. Join-Lambert O, Coignard H, Jais JP, et al. Efficacy of rifampin-moxifloxacin-metronidazole combination therapy in hidradenitis suppurativa. *Dermatology.* 2011;222(1):49-58.
101. Yazdanyar S, Boer J, Ingvarsson G, et al. Dapsone therapy for hidradenitis suppurativa: a series of 24 patients. *Dermatology.* 2011;222(4):342-346.
102. Tzanetakou V, Kanni T, Giatrakou S, et al. Safety and efficacy of anakinra in severe hidradenitis suppurativa: a randomized clinical trial. *JAMA Dermatol.* 2016;152(1):52-59.
103. Gulliver WP, Jemec GB, Baker KA. Experience with ustekinumab for the treatment of moderate to severe hidradenitis suppurativa. *J Eur Acad Dermatol Venereol.* 2012;26(7):911-914.
104. Nazary M, Prens EP, Boer J. Azathioprine lacks efficacy in hidradenitis suppurativa: a retrospective study of nine patients. *Br J Dermatol.* 2016;174(3):639-641.
105. Lam J, Krakowski AC, Friedlander SF. Hidradenitis suppurativa (acne inversa): management of a recalcitrant disease. *Pediatr Dermatol.* 2007;24(5):465-473.
106. Revuz J. Hidradenitis suppurativa. *J Eur Acad Dermatol Venereol.* 2009;23(9):985-998.
107. Lee A, Fischer G. A case series of 20 women with hidradenitis suppurativa treated with spironolactone. *Australas J Dermatol.* 2015;56(3):192-196.
108. Joseph MA, Jayaseelan E, Ganapathi B, et al. Hidradenitis suppurativa treated with finasteride. *J Dermatolog Treat.* 2005;16(2):75-78.
109. Verdolini R, Clayton N, Smith A, et al. Metformin for the treatment of hidradenitis suppurativa: a little help along the way. *J Eur Acad Dermatol Venereol.* 2013;27(9):1101-1108.
110. Boer J, van Gemert MJ. Long-term results of isotretinoin in the treatment of 68 patients with hidradenitis suppurativa. *J Am Acad Dermatol.* 1999;40(1):73-76.
111. Ingram JR, McPhee M. Management of hidradenitis suppurativa: a U.K. survey of current practice. *Br J Dermatol.* 2015;173(4):1070-1072.
112. Soria A, Canoui-Poitrine F, Wolkenstein P, et al. Absence of efficacy of oral isotretinoin in hidradenitis suppurativa: a retrospective study based on patients' outcome assessment. *Dermatology.* 2009;218(2):134-135.
113. Boer J, Nazary M. Long-term results of acitretin therapy for hidradenitis suppurativa. Is acne inversa also a misnomer? *Br J Dermatol.* 2011;164(1):170-175.
114. Verdolini R, Simonacci F, Menon S, et al. Alitretinoin: a useful agent in the treatment of hidradenitis suppurativa, especially in women of child-bearing age. *G Ital Dermatol Venereol.* 2015;150(2):155-162.
115. Harrison BJ, Mudge M, Hughes LE. Recurrence after surgical treatment of hidradenitis suppurativa. *Br Med J (Clin Res Ed).* 1987;294(6570):487-489.
116. van der Zee HH, Prens EP, Boer J. Deroofing: a tissue-saving surgical technique for the treatment of mild to moderate hidradenitis suppurativa lesions. *J Am Acad Dermatol.* 2010;63(3):475-480.
117. Mitchell KM, Beck DE. Hidradenitis suppurativa. *Surg Clin North Am.* 2002;82(6):1187-1197.
118. Mandal A, Watson J. Experience with different treatment modules in hidradenitis suppuritiva: a study of 106 cases. *Surgeon.* 2005;3(1):23-26.
119. Mehdizadeh A, Hazen PG, Bechara FG, et al. Recurrence of hidradenitis suppurativa after surgical management: a systematic review and meta-analysis. *J Am Acad Dermatol.* 2015;73(5 Suppl 1):S70-S77.
120. Rompel R, Petres J. Long-term results of wide surgical excision in 106 patients with hidradenitis suppurativa. *Dermatol Surg.* 2000;26(7):638-643.
121. Hamzavi IH, Griffith JL, Riyaz F, et al. Laser and light-based treatment options for hidradenitis suppurativa. *J Am Acad Dermatol.* 2015;73(5)(suppl 1):S78-S81.
122. Gulliver W, Zouboulis CC, Prens E, et al. Evidence-based approach to the treatment of hidradenitis suppurativa/acne inversa, based on the European guidelines for hidradenitis suppurativa. *Rev Endocr Metab Disord.* 2016;17(3):343-351.
123. Bong JL, Shalders K, Saihan E. Treatment of persistent painful nodules of hidradenitis suppurativa with cryotherapy. *Clin Exp Dermatol.* 2003;28(3):241-244.
124. Patel SH, Robbins JR, Hamzavi I. Radiation therapy for chronic hidradenitis suppurativa. *J Nucl Med Radiat Ther.* 2013;4(146).
125. Trombetta M, Werts ED, Parda D. The role of radiotherapy in the treatment of hidradenitis suppurativa: case report and review of the literature. *Dermatol Online J.* 2010;16(2):16.
126. Khoo AB, Burova EP. Hidradenitis suppurativa treated with *Clostridium botulinum* toxin A. *Clin Exp Dermatol.* 2014;39(6):749-750.
127. Horvath B, Janse IC, Sibbald GR. Pain management in patients with hidradenitis suppurativa. *J Am Acad Dermatol.* 2015;73(5)(suppl 1):S47-S51.
128. Esmann S, Jemec GB. Psychosocial impact of hidradenitis suppurativa: a qualitative study. *Acta Derm Venereol.* 2011;91(3):328-332.
129. Onderdijk AJ, van der Zee HH, Esmann S, et al. Depression in patients with hidradenitis suppurativa. *J Eur Acad Dermatol Venereol.* 2013;27(4):473-478.
130. Shavit E, Dreiher J, Freud T, et al. Psychiatric comorbidities in 3207 patients with hidradenitis suppurativa. *J Eur Acad Dermatol Venereol.* 2015;29(2):371-376.

Disorders of the Hair and Nails

PART 16

第十六篇　毛发和甲疾病

Chapter 85 :: Androgenetic Alopecia
:: Ulrike Blume-Peytavi & Varvara Kanti

第八十五章

雄激素性脱发

中文导读

雄激素性脱发（AGA）是一种非进行性的毛囊小型化，是最常见的脱发类型。

第一节介绍了AGA在不同国家的患病率、患病人群的性别比例及发病年龄阶段，提到了在青春期后随着年龄的增长，此病的发病率也在增加，且AGA女性发病率低于男性。

第二节介绍了不同类型的脱发。男性脱发，又叫汉密尔顿-诺伍德型（HAMILTON-NORWOOD型）(Figs. 85-1 and 85-2)；女性脱发，包括路德维希型（LUDWIG型）(Fig. 85-3 、Fig. 85-4、 Fig. 85-5)、圣诞树型(Fig. 85-6)。

男性脱发：额叶发际线衰退，主要呈三角形，随后顶点逐渐变薄，直至头皮顶部完全秃顶，但枕骨区和头皮两侧不受影响；女性脱发，路德维希型（LUDWIG型）是在保持额叶发线的情况下，中央-顶区弥漫性变薄，它是女性中最常见的AGA类型；圣诞树型是显示出弥漫性的中央-顶间皮变薄，类似于路德维希型，额叶发线有额外的断裂。

第三节介绍了AGA的病因，其是多因素和多基因的，激素水平也是很重要的一个病因，作者分别介绍男性、女性的病因。男性脱发是多基因导致的，在本文中，有12个基因区域被认为与男性AGA有关，与父系的秃顶有很大的遗传关系，且具有雄激素依赖性特征。雌性AGA中雄激素的作用不如男性那么确定，女性脱发可能与雌激素作用、高雄激素血症及其相关激素失调有关。

第四节介绍了AGA的诊断，它基于病史和临床检查。其中临床检查包括头皮皮肤、头发密度（见图85-1至图85-6）及毛发拉拔试验（Sabouraud动作）、面部和体毛、指甲检查，其中的指甲检查主要用于鉴别诊断。继续讲述了诊断工具，包括皮肤镜、全方位摄影、毛发密度和生长/休止期毛发的自动数字化系统等。AGA很少活检，活检仅在怀疑有瘢痕性脱发或弥漫性脱发的鉴别诊断时才使用。此外，除了病史和临床检查，可能需要额外的诊断来排除鉴别诊断：例如，铁蛋白水平或甲状腺刺激激素扩散性流出物或有高雄激素血症症状的妇女内分泌检查。最后，综合以上诊断介绍了由欧洲共识小组提出的一份AGA的临床诊断评估程序（图85-8）。

第五节介绍了雄激素性脱发需要与休止期脱发、弥漫性斑秃、中央离心性瘢痕性脱发、额叶纤维化性脱发、牵引性脱发、遗传性单发性低毛症进行鉴别，鉴别要点列于表85-1；

第六节介绍了药物治疗、毛发移植、假发、低强度激光治疗等措施，药物治疗中局部外用米诺地尔是相对有效的治疗手段，但需至少使用6个月后再评估治疗疗效，还有针对女性脱发和男性脱发的不同药物治疗方法。在手术治疗中，毛发移植可获得满意的美容效果。

〔简　丹〕

AT-A-GLANCE

- Androgenetic alopecia (AGA) is a nonscarring progressive miniaturization of the hair follicle in genetically predisposed men and women, usually in a specific pattern distribution.
- AGA onset may be at any age following puberty, showing an increasing frequency with age.
- The etiology of AGA is multifactorial and polygenic with, as of this writing, 12 genetic regions recognized to associate with AGA in men. In men, AGA is an androgen-dependent trait. Even though the role of androgens in female AGA is less certain than in men, there is a subset of women with AGA and associated hormonal dysregulation.
- Generally, diagnosis of AGA is based on history and clinical examination. Depending on patient history and clinical evaluation, however, additional diagnostics may become necessary to exclude differential diagnoses; for example, ferritin level or thyroid-stimulating hormone in diffuse effluvium or endocrinologic workup in women with signs of hyperandrogenism.
- Biopsy is very rarely indicated in AGA. Biopsy is indicated only if, for example, the differential diagnoses cicatricial alopecia or diffuse alopecia areata are suspected.
- AGA has a naturally progressive course, meaning that the main therapeutic aim is the prevention of disease progression or enhancement of hair growth during the early, mild to moderate stages of the disease.
- The best clinical evidence according to current study data exists for topical application of minoxidil in both genders and for the oral intake of finasteride in men. Alternatively, cosmetically satisfactory results can be achieved using hair transplantation in nonprogressive stable AGA with sufficient available donor area.

DEFINITION

Androgenetic alopecia (AGA) is the most common type of hair loss, a nonscarring progressive miniaturization of the hair follicle with shortening of the anagen phase in genetically predisposed men and women, usually in a specific pattern distribution.[1] Life quality may be significantly impaired in affected individuals, independent of severity, age, or gender.

EPIDEMIOLOGY

Although AGA onset may be at any age following puberty, there is an increasing frequency with age. Reportedly, approximately 50% to 60% of men are affected by the age of 50 years increasing to approximately 80% by the age of 70 years and beyond.[2,3] The prevalence of AGA is reportedly lower and its severity less among Asians, Native Americans, and African Americans compared to the European population.[4,5] Approximately 10% to 20% of Chinese men are affected by the age of 40 to 49 years, rising to 40% to 60% by the age of 70 years and beyond.[6,7]

The frequency and severity of AGA is lower in women than in men, but it still affects a sizeable proportion of the population. Reported prevalence rates in white women in the United Kingdom and United States range between 3% and 6% in women younger than 30 years of age, increasing to 29% to 42% in women 70 years of age and older.[8,9] AGA is less common and appears to start later in life in Asian women with a reported prevalence of 25% in Korean[10] and of 12% to 15% in Chinese women 70 years of age and older.[6,7]

CLINICAL FEATURES

MALE PATTERN HAIR LOSS

MALE PATTERN, HAMILTON-NORWOOD TYPE

This is the most frequent clinical pattern in men with AGA, and only occasionally observed in women. Recession of the frontal hairline, mainly in a triangular pattern is the characteristic finding, later followed by a vertex thinning with progression until the top of the scalp is completely bald (Figs. 85-1 and 85-2). Occipital area and sides of the scalp are spared even in long-standing male pattern hair loss.

FEMALE PATTERN HAIR LOSS

FEMALE PATTERN, LUDWIG TYPE

The so-called female pattern hair loss is characterized by a diffuse thinning of the centroparietal region with maintenance of the frontal hair line (Fig. 85-3). It is the most common type of AGA in women; it is occasionally observed in men. There are 2 scales describing this pattern, the 3-point Ludwig scale (Fig. 85-4) and the 5-point Sinclair scale (Fig. 85-5).

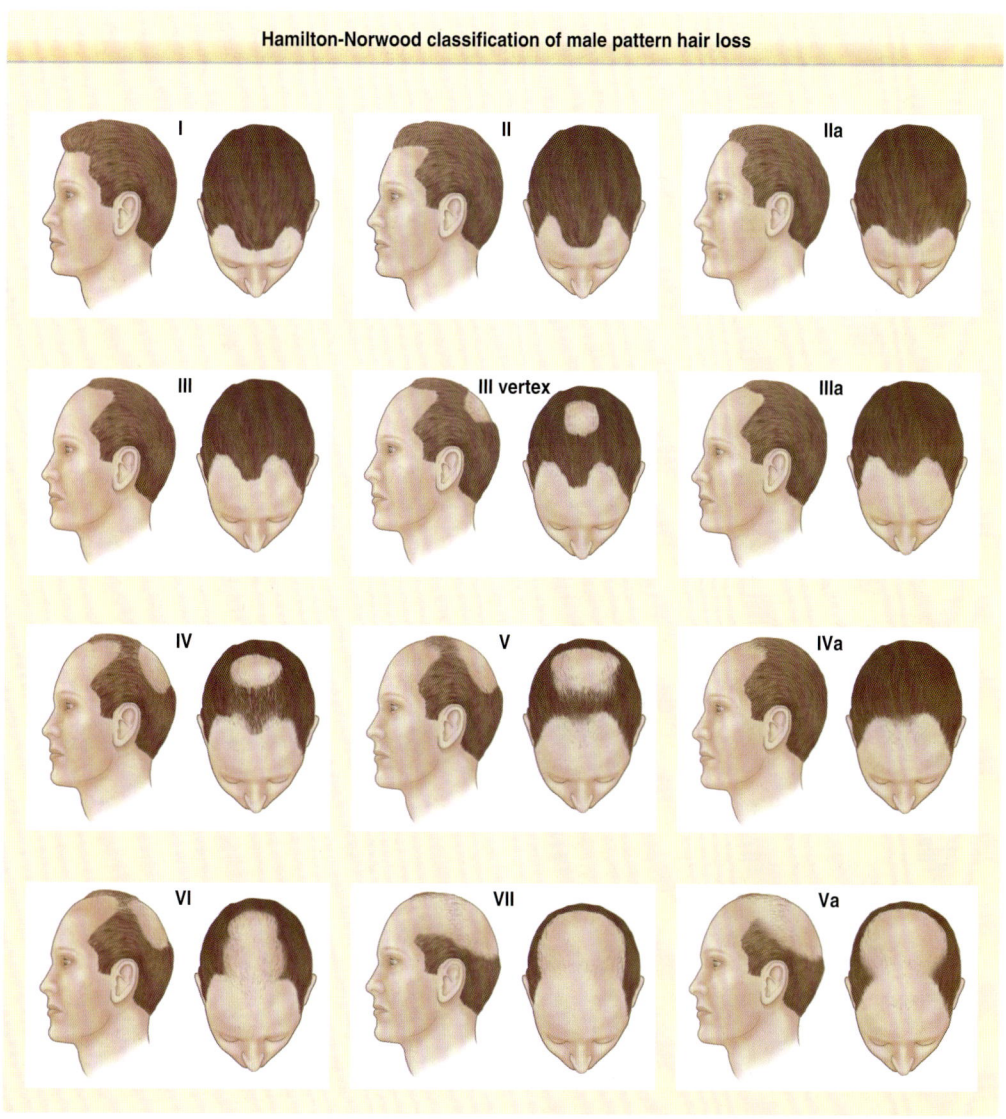

Figure 85-1 Hamilton-Norwood classification. (Redrawn from Blume-Peytavi U, Blumeyer A, Tosti A, et al. S1 guideline for diagnostic evaluation in androgenetic alopecia in men, women and adolescents. *Br J Dermatol*. 2011;164[1]:5-15.)

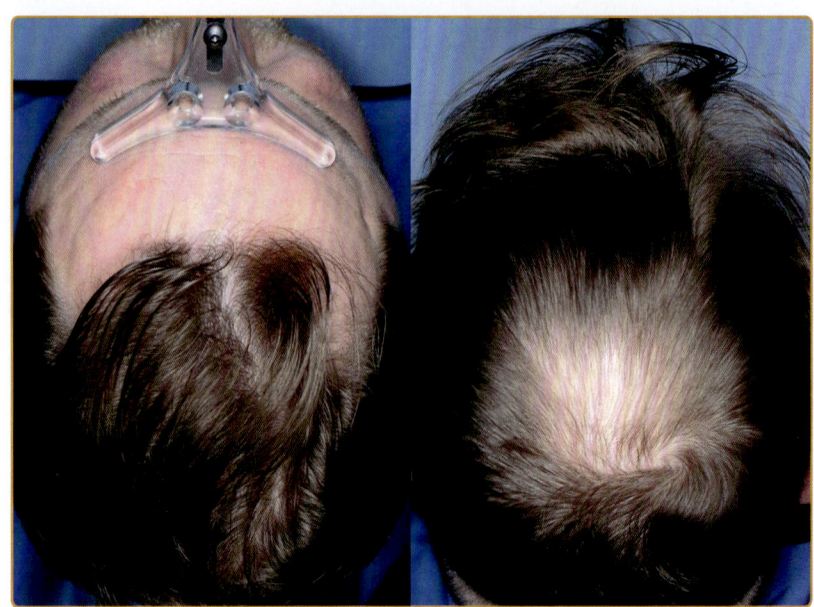

Figure 85-2 Male-pattern androgenetic alopecia, grade III vertex according to the Hamilton-Norwood classification. Standardized global photography overview (Canfield system).

CHRISTMAS TREE PATTERN

Frequently observed in women, the Christmas tree pattern shows diffuse centroparietal thinning similar to the Ludwig pattern with an additional breaching of the frontal hair line (Fig. 85-6).

ETIOLOGY AND PATHOGENESIS

RISK FACTORS

The etiology of AGA is multifactorial and polygenic.[1]

MEN

Male AGA is largely determined by genetic factors.[11,12] There is a strong paternal influence on the risk of balding.[3] Although once thought to be an autosomal dominant trait, it is now clear that AGA has a complex polygenic basis. As of this writing, molecular studies

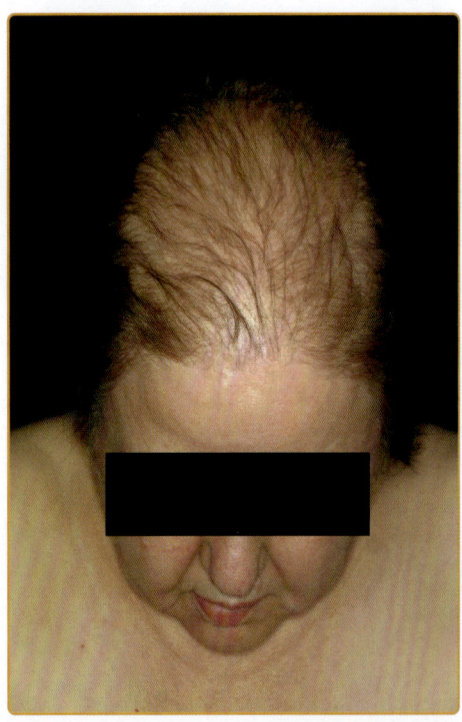

Figure 85-3 Female pattern androgenetic alopecia, grade III according to the Ludwig classification.

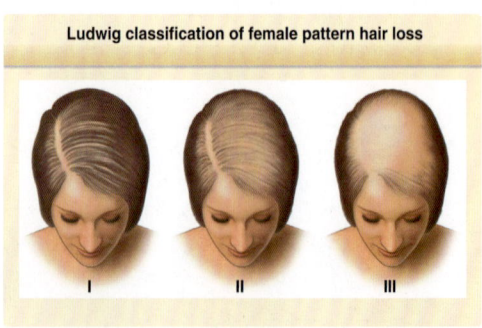

Figure 85-4 Ludwig pattern of hair loss (3-point scale). (Redrawn from Blume-Peytavi U, Blumeyer A, Tosti A, et al. S1 guideline for diagnostic evaluation in androgenetic alopecia in men, women and adolescents. *Br J Dermatol.* 2011;164[1]:5-15.)

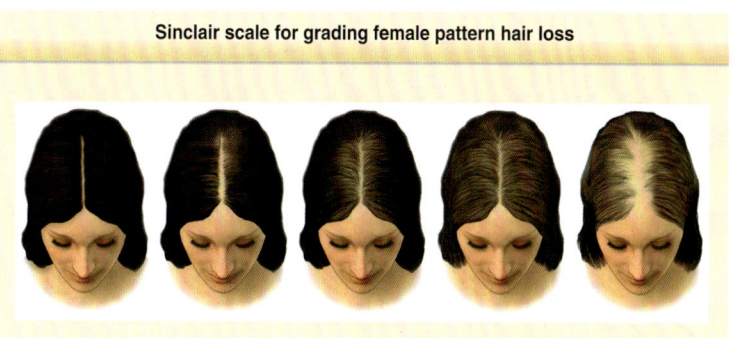

Figure 85-5 Sinclair scale for grading female pattern hair loss (5-point scale). (Redrawn from Blume-Peytavi U, Blumeyer A, Tosti A, et al. S1 guideline for diagnostic evaluation in androgenetic alopecia in men, women and adolescents. *Br J Dermatol.* 2011;164[1]:5-15.)

have recognized 12 genetic regions associated with AGA. Candidate genes include genes for the androgen receptor (*AR*), histone-deacetylases (*HDAC*) 4 and 9, and the WNT molecule *WNT10A*.[13]

In men, AGA is an androgen-dependent trait.[14] Dihydrotestosterone is the androgen chiefly responsible for the follicular pathology. Dihydrotestosterone probably acts primarily on dermal papilla, the predominant site of androgen receptor and type II 5α-reductase expression within the hair follicle. A number of signaling molecules have been implicated in the inhibition of hair growth in AGA including transforming growth factor (TGF)-$β_1$ and transforming growth factor-$β_2$,[14] dickkopf 1 (a member of the WNT signaling family),[15] and interleukin-6.[16] There is also evidence for involvement of prostaglandins in AGA. The enzyme prostaglandin D_2 synthase and its product prostaglandin D_2 are elevated in balding scalp skin; prostaglandin D_2 has an inhibitory effect on hair growth in animal and in in vitro experiments.[17]

WOMEN

Less is known about the etiology of AGA in women. There is an increased frequency of balding in first-degree male relatives of women with AGA, which suggests there is at least some genetic commonality between female and male AGA.[18] Case-control gene-association studies have found a weak association between the *AR/EDA2* locus and early-onset female AGA, but no association with the 11 autosomal loci that associate with male AGA.[19-21] There is a weak association with the gene for estrogen receptor 2 (*ESR2*), which suggests the involvement of estrogenic pathways in female AGA.[22,23] As of this writing there have been no genome-wide studies in women.

The role of androgens in female AGA is also less certain than in men. Nevertheless, there is a subset of women with AGA and associated hormonal dysregulation.

DIAGNOSIS

Generally, AGA is a clinical diagnosis. Depending on patient history and clinical evaluation, further diagnostics may be necessary.

PATIENT HISTORY

Patient and family history of the first manifestation of hair loss and of the course of hair loss (chronic or intermittent) should be documented. Patients with AGA usually complain about a longstanding, slowly progressing reduction of hair density, sometimes even without noticing significant hair loss. Patients typically describe hair thinning with an accentuation of the frontal, parietal, or vertex region, but diffuse thinning is possible as well. Pruritus and trichodynia may present as initial signs of AGA. The family history for AGA is often positive. A positive family history for other hair disorders may facilitate differential diagnostic conclusions and lead to further diagnostic procedures.

In women, especially in those with peripheral signs of hyperandrogenism (Fig. 85-7), a gynecologic history is recommended, including among other possibilities, menstrual cycle disturbances and intake of hormonal contraception.

Furthermore, a detailed patient history should be performed to rule out other causes for the hair loss or

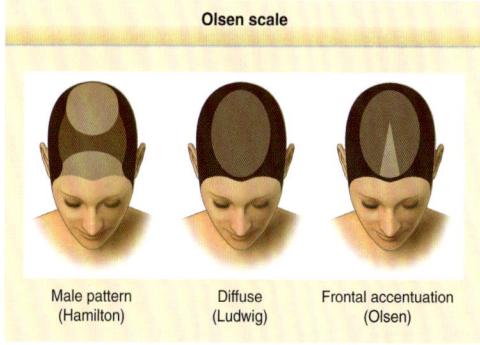

Figure 85-6 Olsen scale: Christmas tree pattern in female pattern hair loss. (Redrawn from Blume-Peytavi U, Blumeyer A, Tosti A, et al. S1 guideline for diagnostic evaluation in androgenetic alopecia in men, women and adolescents. *Br J Dermatol.* 2011;164[1]:5-15.)

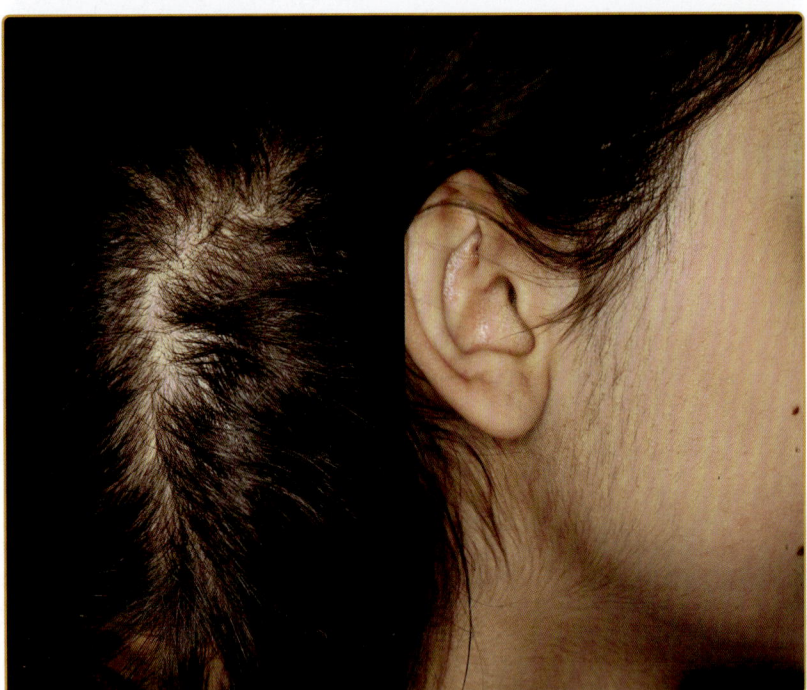

Figure 85-7 Female pattern androgenetic alopecia, facial hypertrichosis, and seborrhea oleosa in an adolescent 15-year old girl.

aggravating factors. Patient interview should include systemic and newly diagnosed diseases (eg, infections, thyroid function disorders, and surgical procedures) that occurred 6 months to 1 year prior to the first signs of hair loss, and nutritional behavior (especially chronic deficient diet or rapid significant weight loss) possibly leading to diffuse effluvium (see section "Differential Diagnosis"). Lifestyle procedures, such as special hairstyles causing traction, and environmental factors like smoking and ultraviolet radiation exposure should be considered.[1] A drug history should be taken to identify a possibly drug-related hair loss, such as after treatment with chemotherapeutic agents, hormones with proandrogenic or antithyroid action, intake of anabolic steroids, or supplemental androgens. Allergies and intolerances should be recorded as they might be important for the choice of the appropriate therapy (eg, contact dermatitis caused by propylene glycol in topical solutions)[1] as well as cosmetic habits (eg, hair care and color, hair style).

CLINICAL EXAMINATION

Clinical examination should involve the scalp skin and hair, facial and body hair, and skin, as well as the nails.

SCALP EXAMINATION

The scalp skin usually appears normal in AGA, but frequently associated findings include seborrhea and/or seborrheic dermatitis.[1] Inflammatory or infectious diseases, as well as alopecia areata and scarring alopecia like lichen planopilaris or frontal fibrosing alopecia, which can mimic AGA, should be considered (see section "Differential Diagnosis"). Balding scalp examination should include checking for photodamage and field cancerization. Thus, clinical examination of the scalp should focus on possible signs of inflammation, like erythema, scaling, or hyperkeratosis, and signs of scarring, such as skin atrophy and loss of hair follicle ostia. However, atrophy of scalp skin also may be present in longstanding AGA.[1]

HAIR EXAMINATION

Scalp Hair: Hair should be parted to assess scalp hair density. Part width should be compared between the frontal, occipital, and temporal regions to examine the distribution of alopecia (see Figs. 85-1 through 85-6, Hamilton-Norwood, Ludwig, and Olsen scales). Dermoscopy/trichoscopy can be helpful in assessing hair follicle openings to exclude scarring alopecia and in identifying short and fine miniaturized hairs. Hair caliber variations might also be present.

The hair pull test (Sabouraud maneuver) can be implemented to provide information on hair shedding. For this test, approximately 50 to 60 hairs are grasped between the thumb, index, and middle fingers from the base of the hairs near the scalp and firmly, but not forcefully, tugged away from the scalp. If more than 10% of the grasped hairs are pulled away from the scalp, this constitutes a positive pull test and confirms active hair shedding.[1] In AGA, the hair pull test may be positive in the frontal region, while it is typically negative in the occipital region.

Facial and Body Hair Examination: Facial and body hair density and/or distribution changes can be found as a result of ethnic hypertrichosis, hypertrichosis caused by medications, or hirsutism. Signs of acne, seborrhea, oily skin, and obesity might present peripheral signs of hyperandrogenism. Even though some women with AGA complain of reduction of eyebrows or eyelashes, this finding points to other types of alopecia, like alopecia areata or frontal fibrosing alopecia (see section "Differential Diagnosis")[24] rather than to AGA.

NAIL EXAMINATION

Nail abnormalities are not characteristic for AGA, but may contribute to differential work up of alopecia areata, certain deficiencies, and lichen planus.[1]

DIAGNOSTIC TOOLS

DERMOSCOPY

Dermoscopy, a noninvasive technique, improves examination of scalp skin and hair shafts by magnification (eg, assessment of hair follicle openings, hair shaft caliber variations). The findings can be saved for future comparison using videodermoscopy. In AGA, hair diameter variations, loss of trio groups with single terminal hairs, and an increased number of vellus hairs can be seen.

GLOBAL PHOTOGRAPHY

Global photographs are helpful tools for the objective evaluation of the course of hair growth, hair volume, and hair density in clinical studies, and for long-term followup in daily practice. For followup assessment, a standardized technique should be implemented, for example, by using a stereotactic device assuring a constant view, magnification, and lighting.

AUTOMATIC DIGITALIZED SYSTEM FOR HAIR DENSITY AND ANAGEN/TELOGEN HAIRS (PHOTOTRICHOGRAM)

These systems allow measurement of hair density and the anagen-to-telogen ratio for diagnostic and followup purposes, but they are mainly used for standardized and reproducible tools in clinical studies. Typical findings in AGA are reduced hair density in a pattern distribution compared to the occipital area. The anagen-to-telogen ratio is normal or decreased when comparing frontal or vertex to the occiput. These techniques are helpful for long-term followup and quantification of hair density.

TRICHOGRAM

The trichogram is not indicated as a routine diagnostic tool in AGA. It should only be considered in individual cases to rule out other differential diagnoses or comorbidities.[1] The trichogram should only be performed by dermatologists who are familiar with this technique and perform it routinely.

BIOPSY

A biopsy, mostly performed as a deep, 4-mm, cylindrical punch, is indicated in AGA only in cases where the diagnosis is uncertain, such as where scalp changes are suggestive of cicatricial alopecia or diffuse alopecia areata. Scalp biopsies should be evaluated by dermatopathologists who are experienced in hair pathology using both vertical and horizontal sectioning. The preferred area for biopsy is the central scalp in an area representative of the hair loss process. Biopsies should not be taken from the bitemporal area as miniaturized hairs may be present in this region independent of AGA.[1] Histologically AGA presents an increased number and proportion of miniaturized (vellus-like) hair follicles with a typically less than 3:1 ratio of terminal to vellus-like hair follicles, compared with a greater than 7:1 ratio in the normal scalp. Other features include an increased telogen-to-anagen ratio and an increase in the number of follicular stelae (tracts beneath miniaturized follicles). A mild perifollicular lymphohistiocytic infiltration, primarily around the upper hair follicle, also may be present, as well as perifollicular fibrosis, in longstanding AGA.

LABORATORY TESTING

In men, laboratory testing for the diagnosis of AGA is not necessary, except if the history or clinical examination indicate another underlying disorder or associated disease. Literature data indicate a possible positive association between AGA and insulin resistance, metabolic syndrome, hypertension, and benign prostate hyperplasia in men.[25] Furthermore, laboratory testing might be indicated before introducing specific therapies (eg, measurement of the prostate-specific antigen value before introducing finasteride therapy; see section "Medications").

In women, an extensive endocrinologic workup is not necessary, except if the history and clinical examination indicate androgen excess. In this case, an interdisciplinary approach involving gynecologists, endocrinologists, and dermatologists is recommended to rule out/distinguish between the different causes associated with hyperandrogenism, such as polycystic ovary syndrome, congenital adrenal hyperplasia, androgen-secreting tumors, or Cushing syndrome. For this purpose the free androgen index, sex hormone-binding globulin, and prolactin should be determined and further laboratory testing (eg, 17-OH-progesterone, follicle-stimulating hormone, estradiol, or cortisol) should be considered. The measurements should be optimally taken between 8:00 and 9:00 AM, ideally between the second and fifth day of the menstrual cycle, in order to standardize and facilitate interpretation. Furthermore, it is advisable to perform blood hormone testing at least 2 months after stopping any hormonal intake, including oral contraception, as estrogens lead to elevated sex hormone-binding globulin levels and consequently falsify the outcome of the free androgen index.[1]

Measurement of ferritin level or thyroid-stimulating hormone may be considered depending on patient history, especially when diffuse effluvium is suspected. Literature data indicate a possible supportive role of adequate serum ferritin levels during treatment of diffuse androgen-dependent alopecia in women, even though contradictory data also have been published.[1]

Interdisciplinary evaluation must be decided individually, based on age, clinical findings, and associated findings. Especially in children and adolescents with premature onset of AGA, an interdisciplinary approach involving the dermatologist and pediatric endocrinologist should be taken. If significant psychological distress is observed, especially in women and young patients with early onset of AGA, psychological referral should be considered for the development of coping strategies.

DIAGNOSTIC ALGORITHM

A diagnostic evaluation form for AGA has been proposed by the European Consensus Group that includes history, clinical examination, laboratory and hair examination tests, diagnostic techniques and clinical documentation (Fig. 85-8).[1]

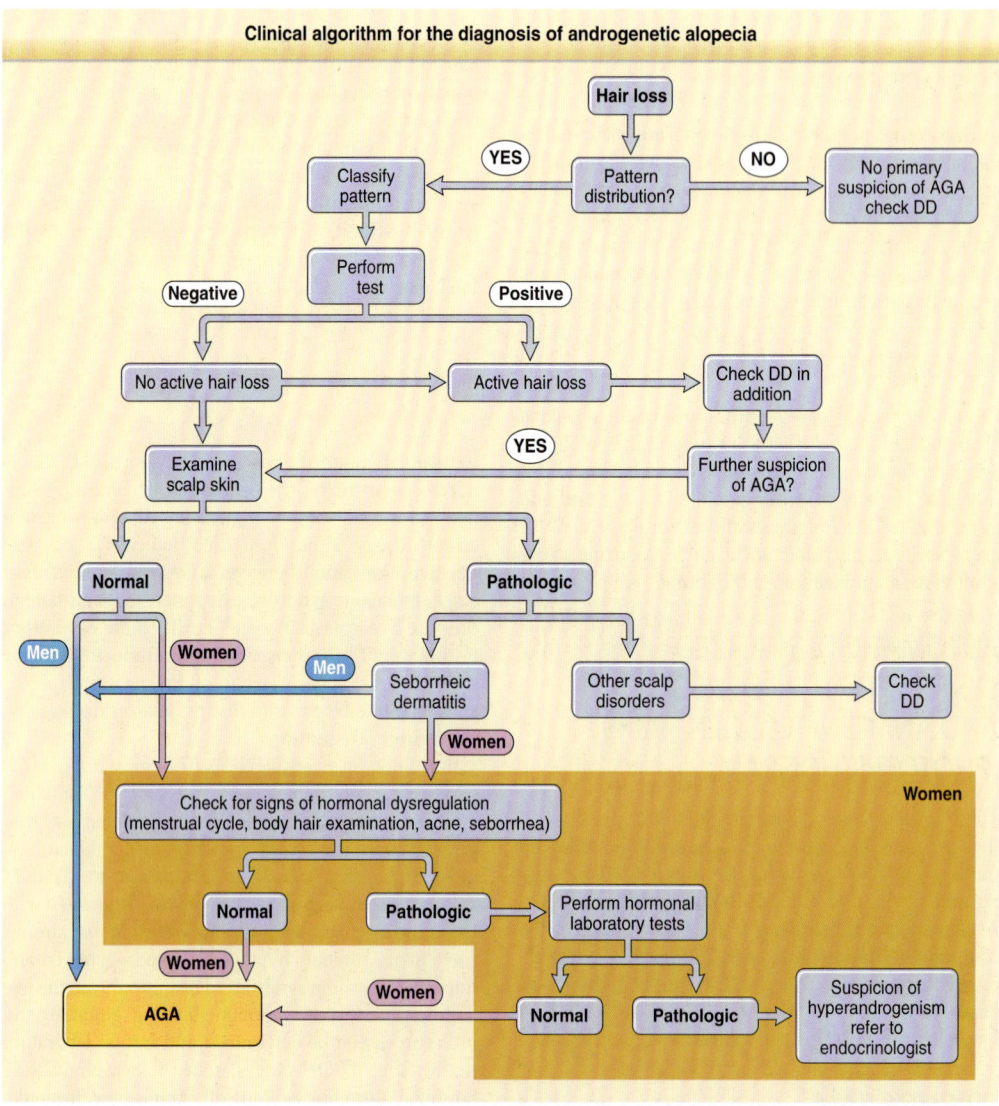

Figure 85-8 Clinical algorithm for the diagnosis of androgenetic alopecia (AGA). DD, differential diagnosis. (Adapted from Blume-Peytavi U, Blumeyer A, Tosti A, et al. S1 guideline for diagnostic evaluation in androgenetic alopecia in men, women and adolescents. *Br J Dermatol*. 2011;164[1]:5-15, with permission. Copyright © 2011 John Wiley & Sons.)

DIFFERENTIAL DIAGNOSIS

Table 85-1 outlines the differential diagnosis of AGA. Multiple hair and scalp disorders may present with clinical features that resemble or coexist with AGA.

TELOGEN EFFLUVIUM

Telogen effluvium is an acute or chronic diffuse hair loss caused by an increased number of hair follicles in telogen, possibly leading in the time course to a reduced hair density over the entire scalp. Telogen effluvium is usually associated with a precipitating event, like a severe illness or psychological trauma, crash diet or certain medications, and the results of the hair pull test are diffusely positive (Fig. 85-9B).

DIFFUSE ALOPECIA AREATA

Diffuse alopecia areata typically does not follow a patterned distribution. Although not always present, a personal or family history of alopecia areata, the detection of patchy or total hair loss, hair loss in other body sites, and nail abnormalities offer support to this diagnosis. A biopsy is useful for confirming the diagnosis if clinically not distinct (see Fig. 85-9A).

CENTRAL CENTRIFUGAL CICATRICIAL ALOPECIA

Central centrifugal cicatricial alopecia is a scarring alopecia of the vertex region that most commonly occurs in women of African descent (Fig. 85-10A). The dermoscopic detection of loss of follicular ostia confirms the scarring type. Biopsies can be useful to confirm the diagnosis.

FRONTAL FIBROSING ALOPECIA

Frontal fibrosing alopecia is a frontotemporal band-like scarring alopecia, characterized by frontotemporal band like recession, loss of eyebrows, perifollicular erythema and hyperkeratosis (see Fig. 85-10C, D). The detection of clinical and histologic signs consistent with a lymphocytic scarring alopecia aid in diagnosis.

TRACTION ALOPECIA

Traction alopecia occurs as a result of chronic tension on the hair shaft (see Fig. 85-10B). Although the hair loss is reversible initially, hair loss may become permanent if tension on the hair follicles continues. History of tight braiding of the hair is useful for diagnosis.

HYPOTRICHOSIS SIMPLEX OR ECTODERMAL DYSPLASIA

It is important to differentiate between congenital or acquired hair loss in adolescents. Hereditary hypotrichosis simplex is characterized by diffuse and progressive hair loss of the scalp and the body, beginning during early childhood. There are no anomalies of the skin, nails, or teeth. The group of ectodermal dysplasias comprise a large, heterogenous group of inherited disorders involving the skin, its appendages, nails, and teeth. Delayed physical/psychological development and sweating disorders may be present.

CLINICAL COURSE AND PROGNOSIS

The course of AGA is naturally progressive, meaning that the main therapeutic aim is the improvement or even merely prevention of disease progression. This can mainly be achieved during the early, mild to

---

TABLE 85-1
Differential Diagnoses for Androgenetic Alopecia

Telogen Effluvium
- Associated with precipitating event
- Hair pull test diffusely positive

Diffuse Alopecia Areata
- No pattern of distribution
- Personal or family history of alopecia areata
- Hair loss in other body sites
- Nail changes

Central Centrifugal Cicatricial Alopecia
- Scarring alopecia of the vertex region
- Most commonly in women of African descent
- Dermoscopy and histologic evaluation shows scarring alopecia

Frontal Fibrosing Alopecia
- Frontotemporal, band-like scarring
- Associated with loss of eyebrows
- Perifollicular erythema and hyperkeratosis
- Histology shows lymphocytic scarring alopecia

Early Traction Alopecia
- History of chronic tension in the hair shaft (tight braiding)

Hypotrichosis Simplex
- Diffuse, progressive loss of scalp and body hair from early childhood
- No anomalies of skin, nails, or teeth

Ectodermal Dysplasia
- Skin, appendages, nails, and teeth associated
- Delayed physical/psychological development and sweating disorders

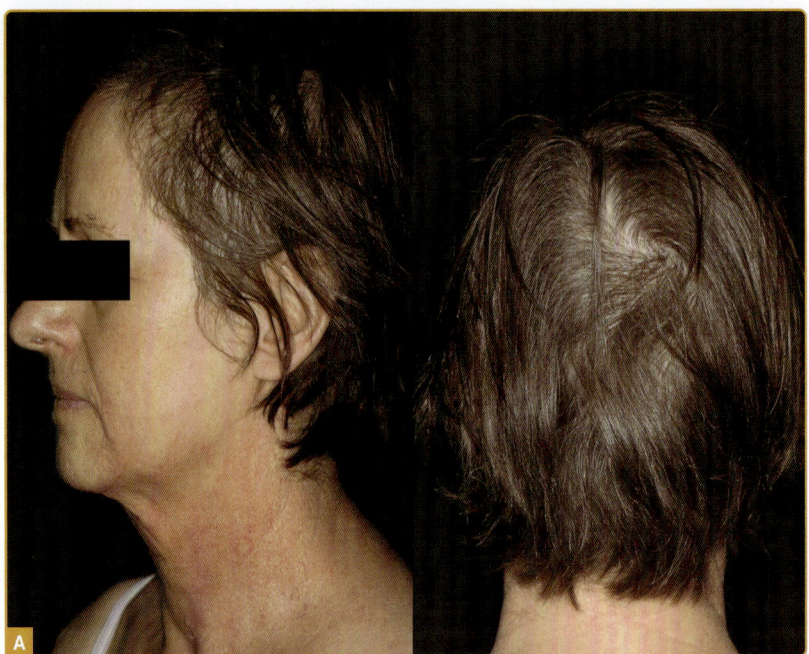

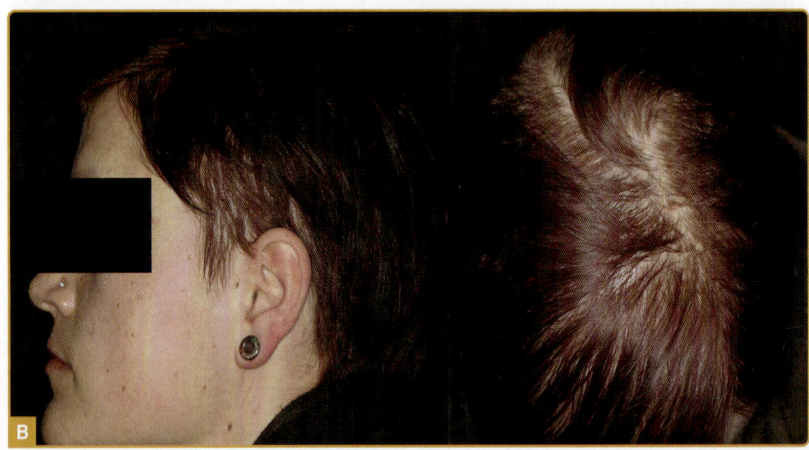

Figure 85-9 Differential diagnosis between female pattern androgenetic alopecia and (**A**) diffuse alopecia areata or (**B**) diffuse effluvium may present a challenge; a detailed patient and family history, laboratory testing and/or biopsy might be necessary.

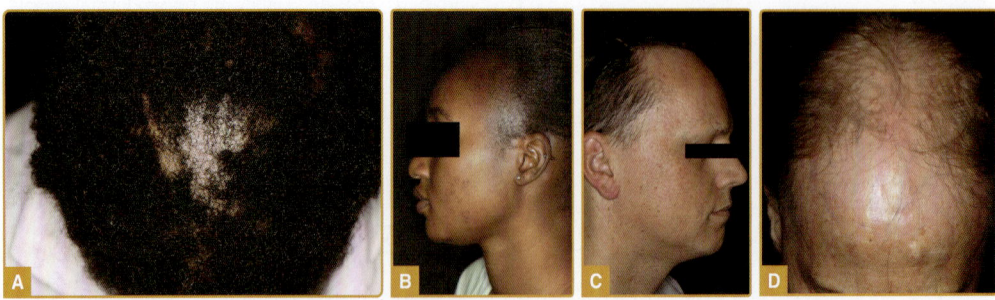

Figure 85-10 Hair disorders mimicking androgenetic alopecia. **A**, Central centrifugal cicatricial alopecia; **B**, traction alopecia; **C**, frontal fibrosing alopecia; and **D**, coexisting frontal fibrosing alopecia and androgenetic alopecia Ludwig grade III in a postmenopausal woman.

moderate stages of the disease. Irrespective of its clinical progression, AGA provokes significant distress and has an often underestimated psychosocial impact on the affected patients.[26]

MANAGEMENT

MEDICATIONS

The best clinical evidence according to current study data concerns the topical application of minoxidil. Minoxidil prevents further progression of the disease and leads to an increase in hair density and hair thickness both in male patients older than 18 years of age with mild to moderate AGA (2% to 5% solution; 1 mL or half a cap of 5% foam twice daily) and female patients older than 18 years of age (2% solution; 1 mL twice daily or half a cap of 5% foam once daily). The response to treatment should be assessed at 6 months. If successful, treatment needs to be continued to maintain efficacy.[27]

The patients should be informed about transitory increased telogen hair shedding, usually appearing within the first 8 weeks of therapy initiation. Furthermore, after end of therapy with topical minoxidil, increased hair loss follows.

The main side effect of topical minoxidil is hypertrichosis, mostly from local spreading or excessive continuous topical application. To avoid contamination of the pillow with subsequent facial contact patients should be advised to apply the drug at least 2 hours before going to bed. Irritant and allergic contact dermatitis may also occur. Irritation is more common with the 5% solution because of its higher content in propylene glycol. Contact dermatitis resulting from propylene glycol or from minoxidil itself should be confirmed by patch testing. It is recommended to pause topical minoxidil use during pregnancy and lactation, owing to the lack of data during this period.[27]

In male patients older than 18 years of age with mild to moderate AGA, a systemic therapy with the 5α-reductase type 2 inhibitor finasteride (1 mg/day) improves or to prevents progression of AGA. For greater efficacy, the combination of oral finasteride (1 mg once daily) and topical minoxidil can be considered. Patients under treatment with finasteride should be aware of reduction of prostate-specific antigen, which is important in prostate cancer screening in men. Further reported side effects of finasteride are impaired sexual function, including erectile dysfunction, ejaculation dysfunction, reduced ejaculate volume, and loss of libido. A possible negative impact of finasteride on those who have a constitutive predisposition to psychological disorders, leading to alteration of mood/depression has been reported; gynecomastia; testicular pain; hypersensitivity reactions; and possible negative impact on spermatogenesis in those men with preexisting conditions relating to infertility should be mentioned. Post-finasteride syndrome, defined as various symptoms persisting for months or years after discontinuation of finasteride treatment, including sexual dysfunction, loss of libido, depression, suicidal ideation, impaired cognition, fatigue, and decreased penile sensitivity, probably occurring in men with a history of sexual dysfunction or a personal or family history of psychiatric illness, are also discussed in the literature. Consequently, finasteride is contraindicated in patients with active depression or current sexual dysfunction.

The response to treatment should be assessed at 6 months, although in some men it may not become evident before 12 months. If successful, treatment needs to be continued to maintain efficacy. In case of ineffective treatment with 1 mg finasteride over 12 months, the off-label use of the 5α-reductase inhibitor dutasteride, which inhibits the isoenzymes type 1 and type 2, at a dose of 0.5 mg a day can be considered.

Finasteride is not indicated in women and is contraindicated in pregnant women and women of childbearing potential, because of the risk of feminization of a male fetus. Finasteride-treated men must avoid donating their blood.[27]

In female postmenopausal patients, finasteride 1 mg failed to show efficacy; however, finasteride 5 mg may be effective in female normoandrogenic premenopausal and postmenopausal patients. However, no placebo-controlled trials are available in this population. In women of childbearing age, the use of a safe contraceptive method is indispensable.[27]

Clinical studies on the efficacy of topical finasteride preparations are currently underway.

Antiandrogens and estrogenic drugs are being used in the treatment of AGA, although evidence of efficacy for any of these treatments is insufficient. In male patients, the use of systemic estrogens or androgen-receptor antagonists is not recommended. In women with AGA and clinical or biochemical evidence of hyperandrogenism, the use of oral antiandrogens (chlormadinone acetate, cyproterone acetate, drospirenone, spironolactone, flutamide) in combination with an estrogen as an oral contraceptive pill can be considered. Side effects of cyproterone acetate include depressive mood changes and liver toxicity. There is an increased risk of venous thromboembolism in patients taking estrogen-containing oral contraceptives, which may be greater in those taking cyproterone acetate than other oral contraceptives. Spironolactone 100 to 200 mg per day taken continuously is an alternative option because of its antiandrogenic effect, but should also be combined with a safe contraceptive in women of childbearing age. Side effects include menstrual disturbances and hyperkalaemia.[27]

As of this writing, there is insufficient literature evidence on the effect of topical alfatradiol, topical natural estrogens or progesterones, or topical fluridil.[27]

PROCEDURES

SURGERY

In AGA, hairless or thinning areas can be cosmetically covered, albeit with a decreased density, using hair restoration surgery. Hair restoration surgery involves hair transplantation, scalp reduction surgery, or a combination of both. Hair transplantation is less invasive than scalp reduction surgery. Over the last decades, hair transplantation has evolved into a microsurgical procedure. Follicular units of 1 to 4 hairs are transplanted in large numbers and high densities. Hair surgery, especially follicular unit transplantation, can be considered to improve AGA in suitable patients with sufficient donor hair supply and medically controlled or spontaneously stabilized AGA, especially in the frontoparietal area. The result greatly depends on the skills of the surgical team and the adjustment of the surgical plan to individual patient characteristics. As hair surgery does not influence progression of AGA, long-term results in early stages depend on spontaneous or medical stabilization of AGA. In men, a combination of finasteride 1 mg and/or topical minoxidil with follicular unit transplantation may reduce postoperative progression of AGA.[27]

NONPERMANENT HAIR REPLACEMENT MEASURES

Nonsurgical hair replacement methods include, in addition to full and partial hair replacement measures (wigs), various hair-binding techniques and hair extension and supplementation techniques, either performed by the patients themselves (eg, sprinkle hair) or by specialized personnel (eg, camouflage techniques, bonding).[28]

INTERVENTIONS

Low-Level Laser Therapy: Low-level laser therapy, including the exposure of tissues to low levels of visible or near infrared light, can be used as an ancillary treatment for AGA. Low-level laser therapy can be performed at home, using a LaserComb or wearing for a certain amount of time a helmet whose power cord is plugged into a standard outlet. Duration of therapy and frequency varies for the different devices. Current studies evaluating laser devices show inconsistent results thus providing low quality evidence.[27] However, an improvement in total hair count has been partly reported after using such devices.[29,30]

MISCELLANEOUS

Besides the above-mentioned evidence-based therapeutic approaches, there is a wide range of molecules, products, and interventions claiming to promote hair growth in AGA. These include platelet-rich plasma, mesotherapy, botulinum toxin injections, pulsed electromagnetic/static field devices, topically applied caffeine, melatonin, retinoids, biochanin A, adenosine, prostaglandin analogs, herbal preparations, and nutritional supplements (eg, biotin, zinc, copper, amino acids, micronutrients and combination preparations). For most of these products controlled clinical studies are scarce and largely of low evidence level. Detailed information on these products and the available literature can be found in the current S3 guidelines for the treatment of AGA in women and in men.[27] Based on currently available literature data no evidence-based recommendation can be given for these miscellaneous products. Their use as a supportive strategy within an individually tailored management approach is at the discretion of the treating dermatologist and the decision of the patient. Further controlled studies to prove the relevance of these and other new approaches in the treatment of AGA are needed.

COUNSELING

AGA is the most common hair loss disorder, affecting both men and women. Taking into account the high prevalence and the psychosocial burden and the often significant impairment of life of affected patients, the need for competent counseling and development of a trusting patient–physician relationship becomes apparent. To enhance therapy compliance, the patient must be informed in detail about the therapeutic goal, the possible treatment options, and their potential side effects. The naturally progressive nature of the disease should be pointed out, as well as the often limited response to therapy, particularly in advanced AGA. Practical counseling with tips on handling the disease in daily life should be offered. In individual cases with high emotional overlay, particularly in women, professional psychological help might be helpful. Overall, counseling dermatologists should develop a therapeutic personalized plan for each patient based on clinical status, demands, needs, and complaints. The individualized concept should comprise pharmacologic evidence-based recommendations, hair care and cosmetic tips, and psychological counseling. The physician and patient must decide together on the best suited individualized therapy, considering the expected results, practicality, and compliance.

SCREENING

Early diagnosis and treatment to prevent progression of AGA is important in genetically predisposed families. In patients with longstanding advanced AGA, especially in male pattern baldness, scalp examination should include screening for benign and malignant skin lesions, such as actinic keratoses, squamous cell carcinoma or basal cell carcinoma as a result of increased ultraviolet exposure of the balding scalp and the lack of protecting full hair.

REFERENCES

1. Blume-Peytavi U, Blumeyer A, Tosti A, et al. S1 guideline for diagnostic evaluation in androgenetic alopecia in men, women and adolescents. *Br J Dermatol.* 2011;164(1):5-15.
2. Norwood OT. Male pattern baldness: classification and incidence. *South Med J.* 1975;68(11):1359-1365.
3. Birch MP, Messenger AG. Genetic factors predispose to balding and non-balding in men. *Eur J Dermatol.* 2001;11:309-314.
4. Tsuboi R, Arano O, Nishikawa T, et al. Randomized clinical trial comparing 5% and 1% topical minoxidil for the treatment of androgenetic alopecia in Japanese men. *J Dermatol.* 2009;36(8):437-446.
5. Hoffmann R, Happle R. Current understanding of androgenetic alopecia. Part II: clinical aspects and treatment. *Eur J Dermatol.* 2000;10(5):410-417.
6. Xu F, Sheng YY, Mu ZL, et al. Prevalence and types of androgenetic alopecia in Shanghai, China: a community-based study. *Br J Dermatol.* 2009;160(3):629-632.
7. Wang TL, Zhou C, Shen YW, et al. Prevalence of androgenetic alopecia in China: a community-based study in six cities. *Br J Dermatol.* 2010;162(4):843-847.
8. Birch MP, Messenger JF, Messenger AG. Hair density, hair diameter and the prevalence of female pattern hair loss. *Br J Dermatol.* 2001;144:297-304.
9. Norwood OT. Incidence of female androgenetic alopecia (female pattern alopecia). *Dermatol Surg.* 2001;27(1):53-54.
10. Paik JH, Yoon JB, Sim WY, et al. The prevalence and types of androgenetic alopecia in Korean men and women. *Br J Dermatol.* 2001;145(1):95-99.
11. Nyholt DR, Gillespie NA, Heath AC, et al. Genetic basis of male pattern baldness. *J Invest Dermatol.* 2003;121(6):1561-1564.
12. Rexbye H, Petersen I, Iachina M, et al. Hair loss among elderly men: etiology and impact on perceived age. *J Gerontol A Biol Sci Med Sci.* 2005;60(8):1077-1082.
13. Heilmann-Heimbach S, Hochfeld LM, Paus R, et al. Hunting the genes in male-pattern alopecia: how important are they, how close are we and what will they tell us? *Exp Dermatol.* 2016;25(4):251-257.
14. Inui S, Itami S. Androgen actions on the human hair follicle: perspectives. *Exp Dermatol.* 2013;22(3):168-171.
15. Kwack MH, Kim MK, Kim JC, et al. Dickkopf 1 promotes regression of hair follicles. *J Invest Dermatol.* 2012;132(6):1554-1560.
16. Kwack MH, Ahn JS, Kim MK, et al. Dihydrotestosterone-inducible IL-6 inhibits elongation of human hair shafts by suppressing matrix cell proliferation and promotes regression of hair follicles in mice. *J Invest Dermatol.* 2012;132(1):43-49.
17. Garza LA, Liu Y, Yang Z, et al. Prostaglandin D2 inhibits hair growth and is elevated in bald scalp of men with androgenetic alopecia. *Sci Transl Med.* 2012;4(126):126ra34.
18. Smith MA, Wells RS. Male-type alopecia, alopecia areata, and normal hair in women. *Arch Dermatol.* 1964;89:155-158.
19. Redler S, Brockschmidt FF, Tazi-Ahnini R, et al. Investigation of the male pattern baldness major genetic susceptibility loci AR/EDA2R and 20p11 in female pattern hair loss. *Br J Dermatol.* 2012;166(6):1314-1318.
20. Heilmann S, Kiefer AK, Fricker N, et al. Androgenetic alopecia: identification of four genetic risk loci and evidence for the contribution of WNT signaling to its etiology. *J Invest Dermatol.* 2013;133(6):1489-1496.
21. Redler S, Dobson K, Drichel D, et al. Investigation of six novel susceptibility loci for male androgenetic alopecia in women with female pattern hair loss. *J Dermatol Sci.* 2013;72(2):186-188.
22. Yip L, Zaloumis S, Irwin D, et al. Association analysis of oestrogen receptor beta gene (*ESR2*) polymorphisms with female pattern hair loss. *Br J Dermatol.* 2012;166(5):1131-1134.
23. Redler S, Birch P, Drichel D, et al. The oestrogen receptor 2 (*ESR2*) gene in female-pattern hair loss: replication of association with rs10137185 in German patients. *Br J Dermatol.* 2014;170(4):982-985.
24. Badawy A, Elnashar A. Treatment options for polycystic ovary syndrome. *Int J Womens Health.* 2011;3(1):25-35.
25. Agamia NF, Abou Youssif T, El-Hadidy A, et al. Benign prostatic hyperplasia, metabolic syndrome and androgenic alopecia: is there a possible relationship? *Arab J Urol.* 2016;14(2):157-162.
26. Harth W, Blume-Peytavi U. Psychotrichology: psychosomatic aspects of hair diseases. *J Dtsch Dermatol Ges.* 2013;11(2):125-135.
27. Kanti V, Messenger A, Dobos G, et al. Evidence-based (S3) guideline for the treatment of androgenetic alopecia in women and in men–short version. *J Eur Acad Dermatol Venereol.* 2018;32(1):11-22.
28. Blume-Peytavi U, Vogt A. Current standards in the diagnostics and therapy of hair diseases-hair consultation. *J Dtsch Dermatol Ges.* 2011;9(5):394-410; quiz 411-412.
29. Leavitt M, Charles G, Heyman E, et al. HairMax LaserComb laser phototherapy device in the treatment of male androgenetic alopecia: a randomized, double-blind, sham device-controlled, multicentre trial. *Clin Drug Investig.* 2009;29(5):283-292.
30. Avci P, Gupta GK, Clark J, et al. Low-level laser (light) therapy (LLLT) for treatment of hair loss. *Lasers Surg Med.* 2014;46(2):144-151.

Chapter 86 :: Telogen Effluvium
:: Manabu Ohyama

第八十六章
休止期脱发

中文导读

休止期脱发（TE）是毛囊生长期提前终止，导致休止期毛发增多的疾病，是弥漫性脱发最常见的原因。

第一节介绍了休止期脱发的流行病学，强调很难估计其实际发病率或患病率，因为很多病例可能是亚临床的。

第二节介绍了TE的三大分类：典型急性休止期脱发、慢性弥漫性休止期脱发、慢性休止期脱发，并分别列其潜在病因于表86-1。

第三节介绍了其病因及发病机制。在病因方面，作者分别整理三类休止期脱发的潜在病因于表86-1，且列出了新生儿脱发、热病、外科手术、怀孕、甲状腺疾病、老化、减肥、营养不良、缺铁、缺锌、系统性疾病、性传播疾病、药物、全身性疾病、心理压力等因素，其中可引起脱发的药物见表86-2。根据Headington提出的5种不同的致病机制来解释TE：毛发生长期过早终止、生长期延长并突然进入终止期、生长期变短、休止期过早结束、休止期延长和被调控的外显子。

第四节介绍了休止期脱发的诊断主要依据病史和检查，其中检查包括：头发外观、脱发计数、头发拉力试验、毛发图、光毛图和毛扫描、皮肤镜、组织病理学检查。头发拉力试验较为经济快捷，拉扯下来的毛发根部可见棒状结构有助于诊断，皮肤镜有助于鉴别其他脱发，而组织病理学检查结果最为可靠。休止期脱发的病因可通过病史和实验室检查来确定。

第五节介绍了休止期脱发须与其他引起弥漫性脱发的疾病相鉴别，如女性脱发、斑秃、精神性假性脱发。

第六节介绍了其特点是：一旦病因被发现并消除，可自限并可预测正常毛发再生时间。

〔简　丹〕

AT-A-GLANCE

- Telogen effluvium is characterized by increased telogen club hair shedding.
- Telogen effluvium is the most common cause of diffuse hair loss.
- Telogen effluvium is subdivided into acute telogen effluvium, chronic diffuse telogen hair loss, and chronic telogen effluvium.
- Differential diagnoses include alopecia areata incognita and psychogenic pseudoeffluvium.
- Spontaneous recovery can be expected once a cause is identified and eliminated.

INTRODUCTION

Telogen effluvium (TE) was originally described by Kligman in 1961.[1] TE is best characterized by a premature termination of the anagen (growing) phase of hair follicles, with a resultant increase in telogen (resting) phase hairs leading to excessive and diffuse loss of club hairs.[1] Classically, TE refers to an acute hair loss subsequent to a variety of stresses including those caused by febrile diseases, childbirth, emotional disturbance, chronic systemic diseases, or the administration of heparin.[1] TE can be a physiologic event in the newborn.[1] Later studies revealed that the trigger and manifestation of TE were variable.[2,3] TE represents the most common cause of diffuse hair loss.[3] In clinics, truly diffuse hair loss is not often encountered.[4] The most common reason bringing TE patients to the clinic is the increase in hair shedding after shampooing or brushing alone.[4] Typically, TE is self-limiting, and full recovery can be expected once the specific causes are identified and corrected.[3,4] However, especially in nonclassical chronic TE in women, distinction between female pattern hair loss is often challenging.[5] In this chapter, the clinical features, pathophysiology, and differential diagnoses of TE are discussed.

EPIDEMIOLOGY

Approximately, the loss of more than 25% of scalp hairs has been reported to be necessary to clinically detect diffuse hair loss.[1] Therefore, most TE cases are likely to be subclinical, making estimation of its real incidence or prevalence quite difficult.[2,4] Female predominance has been noted in TE, probably because of stronger awareness of daily hair conditions and more dynamic hormonal changes including menstruation and gestation.[4,6] In theory, incidence of classic acute TE following known triggering events would not be distinct between the sexes.[4] TE can occur in children but the incidence has been reported to be low.[7] Elderly women are more likely to suffer from classic acute TE.[4] Chronic TE (CTE) represents a unique form of unknown etiology that affects the whole scalp and is mostly seen in middle-aged women.[8,9]

CLINICAL FEATURES

Depending on the clinical course and symptoms, TE can be subdivided into 3 subgroups: classic acute TE,[1] chronic diffuse telogen hair loss,[2,4,10] and chronic telogen effluvium[8,9] (Table 86-1). Irrespective of clinical subtypes, the most representative manifestation of TE is diffuse excessive shedding of club hairs.[1,2,4,8,9] It should be noted that in severe TE cases, apparent diffuse or bitemporal hair thinning can be observed; however, hair loss is often subclinical and increased hair shedding can be the only objective sign in TE.[1,4] In some cases, hair shedding has already peaked out and shed hairs carried by a patient alone is indicative of TE history.[4] The clinical features of each subset are listed below.

ACUTE TE

This is the most classic type of TE originally described by Kligman in 1961.[1] Typically, acute and diffuse hair shedding is noted 2 to 4 months from causative events.[1-3] The presence of this latency period, probably reflecting the duration of catagen and telogen periods, has been considered to be characteristic for this type of TE.[1] No sign of inflammation or scarring is observed on the scalp.[3] Usually, shed hairs demonstrate the morphology of club hairs in the late stage of telogen without an enclosing sac (root sheath cells) and pigmentation.[1] The amount of shedding hairs is significantly influenced by age, gender, race, or sampling methods, yet, in the original study by Kligman, the average number of hairs shed daily during classic TE ranged from 109 (postpartum case) to 646 (heparin-induced case).[1] Usually gradual decrease and termination of hair shedding and the regrowth of new anagen hairs can be expected by 3 to 6 months.[1,2]

CHRONIC DIFFUSE TELOGEN HAIR LOSS

A temporal insult usually triggers sudden-onset diffuse hair shedding as seen in acute TE, which recovers after the elimination of triggering stress.[2] However, telogen hair shedding may last longer than 6 months.[2,4] Chronic diffuse telogen hair loss (CDTHL) is one such condition that is secondary to various causes, including thyroid disorders, acrodermatitis enteropathica, malnutrition, and drugs (Fig. 86-1).[2,4,10] The relation between CDTHL and the causative factors needs to be reversible and reproducible.

TABLE 86-1
Clinical Subtypes and Potential Etiologies of Telogen Effluvium

CLINICAL SUBTYPE	ETIOLOGY[a]
Acute telogen effluvium (acute TE)	Effluvium of the newborn
	Febrile illness
	Surgery
	Pregnancy
	Weight loss (crash diet)
	Drugs (may cause CDTHL)
Chronic diffuse telogen hair loss (CDTHL)	Thyroid disease
	Aging
	Malnutrition
	Iron deficiency (controversial)
	Zinc deficiency (severe cases)
	Systemic illness
	Psychological stress (controversial)
	STD (HIV infection and syphilis)
	Miscellaneous
Chronic telogen effluvium (CTE)	Idiopathic (shortening of anagen)

[a]Each etiology may explain both acute TE and CDTHL.

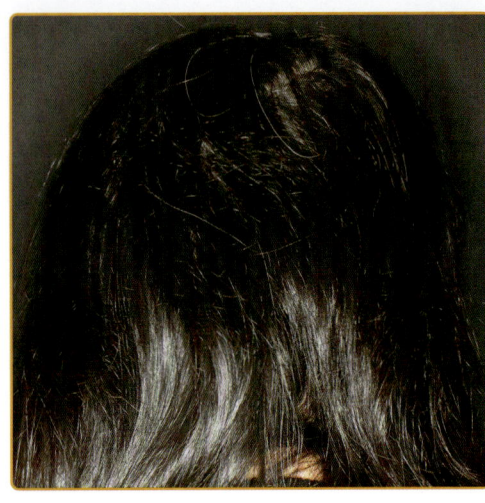

Figure 86-2 Chronic telogen effluvium in a middle-aged woman.

CHRONIC TELOGEN EFFLUVIUM

CTE is an idiopathic form of diffuse club hair loss seen in middle-aged women in their fourth to sixth decade (Fig. 86-2).[8,9] Telogen hair shedding extends more than 6 months to several years with fluctuation. The patient tends to have denser hair than average before the onset and could have been able to grow very long hair, especially in their childhood,[8,11,12] implying that anagen duration is intrinsically prolonged.[2] Typically, the onset of CTE is abrupt, and the amount of shed hairs is quite large. The patient may claim that the shed hairs block the drain after shower or bring a sack of shed hair to convince excessive hair loss.[8] Telogen club hairs can be pulled out easily from the vertex and occipital areas.[2] Marked bitemporal recession of hair is frequently observed.[8,9] Female pattern hair loss needs to be excluded. A rare male case of CTE also has been reported.[13]

ETIOLOGY AND PATHOGENESIS

ETIOLOGY

In the normal human scalp, the number of total hair follicles and the ratio between anagen and telogen hair are maintained as constant.[14] On average, telogen hair accounts for around 10% of scalp hairs.[15] Any factors that affect the duration of each phase of hair cycles with resultant abnormal increase of club hair loss can be potential TE triggers. As described above, TE consists of heterogeneous subsets with distinct pathophysiology, and therefore it is technically difficult to fully delineate the etiology. However, past observations listed definitive/probable causative factors (Table 86-1).

EFFLUVIUM OF THE NEWBORN

Physiologic type of TE can be seen in infants.[1] The shedding starts within 4 months after birth. This type of effluvium may be regarded as "total replacement of the first pelage completed before the first 6 month of life."[1] Telogen counts in this form of effluvium are around 60% to 80% and higher than other pathogenic TEs. The hair loss pattern may resemble that of androgenetic alopecia in some cases.[1]

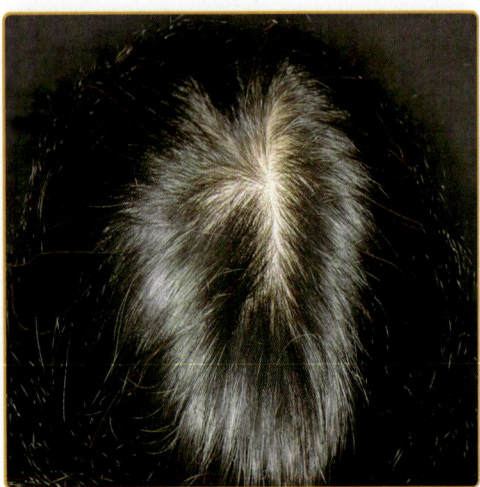

Figure 86-1 Chronic diffuse telogen hair loss due to Hashimoto disease.

FEBRILE ILLNESS

Hair loss in the influenza epidemic of 1971 has been described.[16] Kligman reported 4 pediatric cases of acute TE that developed after pertussis, pneumonia, and influenza.[1] Hair shedding appeared 3 to 4 months after the illness and continued for 3 to 4 weeks. Complete hair regrowth was achieved in these cases. Febrile illness was probably a common cause of TE in the preantibiotic era, and it still needs to be counted as a trigger in critically ill patients, including those with acute sepsis.[16] High fever can cause physiologic stress to hair-producing matrix cells and lead to early anagen release,[14] or alternatively, high levels of interferons may contribute to the development of acute TE.[17,18]

SURGERY

Major surgery can trigger postoperative TE.[15,19] It is a matter of debate whether surgery alone or other factors accompanying surgery, for example, fever; general anesthesia; and changes in hormone, cytokine, or nutrition levels triggered acute TE. Rhytidectomy has been reported to cause "local" TE.[20]

PREGNANCY

Postpartum alopecia or telogen gravidarum is probably the most widely recognized form of classic TE observed 2 to 3 months after childbirth.[14,21] Using a trichogram (forced plucking of hairs), progressive increase in anagen hairs during pregnancy has been reported.[21,22] Lynfiend reported a high anagen hair rate (94.4% on average) during the second and third trimesters, whereas telogen hairs accounted for 25.5% at 6 weeks postpartum.[21] A recent analysis of 116 pregnant women with digital image analysis software (Trichoscan) has confirmed the increase in anagen rate during pregnancy.[23] However, the increase in telogen rate after delivery was only 3% and the authors suggested that postpartum TE may not be as frequent as generally thought.[23] This observation is supported by other investigators.[24,25] Accumulated clinical observations suggest that postpartum TE exists[1]; however, as most descriptions are based on studies conducted in the 1960s, further revisit and dissection of the pathophysiology using modern technology is needed to draw definitive conclusions.

THYROID DISEASE

Association between hypothyroidism and TE has been well established.[26] The manifestation is more likely to be CDTHL rather than acute TE (Fig. 86-1).[4] Hair regrowth can be observed around 8 weeks after the initiation of thyroid hormone replacement in patients with hypothyroidism, with telogen hair loss clearly indicating their link.[27] No correlation between the severity of thyroid dysfunction and the degree of effluvium has been demonstrated.[26]

Compared with hypothyroidism, the role of hyperthyroidism in TE, especially in CDTHL, is less clear and requires further investigation.[26,28]

AGING

Diffuse hair loss in the scalp and body can be seen in elderly subjects with histopathologic increase in telogen ratio.[29] Incidence of TE tends to be higher in elder individuals.[30] Senility may be a risk factor for TE or CDTHL.

WEIGHT LOSS (CRASH DIET)

A vigorous weight loss (11.7 to 24.75 kg within 3 weeks to 3 months) can result in remarkable increase in telogen counts (25% to 50%) and lead to acute TE (Fig. 86-3).[31] Calorie restriction of 0 to 1200 kcal per day has been reported to be associated with hair loss.[26]

MALNUTRITION

An increase in telogen hair ratio has been noted in protein-deficient elderly subjects and children with protein-calorie malnutrition, though only in severely affected cases.[32,33] The effect of malnutrition on the hair cycle may be variable, and CDTHL may be observed in those seriously malnourished.[26]

IRON DEFICIENCY

Iron deficiency has been implicated in the pathogenesis of TE.[26] Previous studies demonstrated that iron supplementation to CTE patients resulted in a reduction of hair shed or a decrease in telogen rate.[34] Recent studies revealed that serum ferritin levels were reduced in

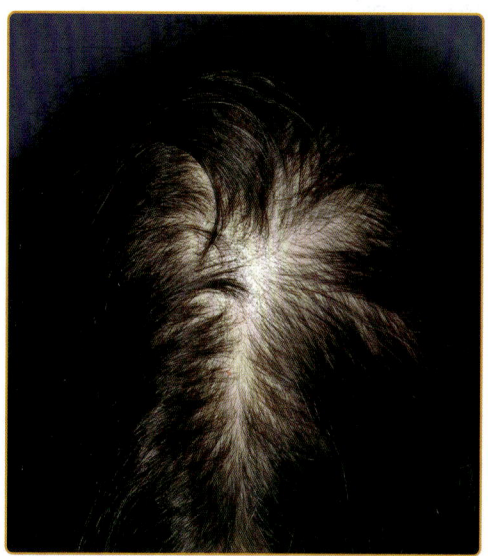

Figure 86-3 Acute telogen effluvium started 3 months after crash diet (weight loss of more than 10 kg within 2 to 3 months).

women but not significantly in CTE patients compared with control subjects.[35,36] Thus, the role of iron deficiency in TE is still controversial, and the efficacy of iron supplementation in CDTHL or CTE needs to be assessed in further clinical trials. A serum ferritin level less than 40 ng/ml may be considered as iron deficient in the general population.[35]

ZINC DEFICIENCY

Acrodermatitis enteropathica is an autosomal recessive disorder characterized by zinc malabsorption with resultant hair loss, acral and periorificial dermatitis, diarrhea, immunodeficiency, mental and neurologic disturbances, and growth retardation.[26] CDTHL is a typical pathophysiology for hair loss.[4] Supplemental zinc should improve all symptoms, including hair loss.[26]

Acquired zinc deficiency resembling acrodermatitis enteropathica may develop in parenteral alimentation, GI tract surgery, pancreatitis, inflammatory bowel disease, or AIDS nephropathy as well as in premature infants[26] and cause acute TE or CDTHL.

In contrast, the contribution of moderately low serum zinc levels to the development of CTE remains elusive.[36]

SYSTEMIC DISEASE

In addition to one-time-only febrile illness or endocrine/metabolic disorders, a variety of systemic diseases have been reported to be associated with diffuse hair loss.[26] CDTHL in connection with lymphoproliferative disease, advanced malignancy, collagen disease (systemic lupus erythematosus and dermatomyositis), hepatic disease, chronic renal failure, systemic amyloidosis, eosinophilia-myalgia syndrome, and inflammatory bowel disease have been reported.[4,26] Extensive acute TE has been reported to be characteristic for Cronkhite-Canada syndrome but full recovery can be expected once the underlying condition is healed.[37]

PSYCHOLOGICAL STRESS

The general perception is that psychological stress can play a role in the increase in hair shedding. In fact, Kligman in his original report of TE mentioned about psychological events as a potential cause of effluvium.[1] The contribution of psychological stress to the development of TE has been suggested; however, it is not fully supported by a high level of scientific evidence.[26]

SEXUALLY TRANSMITTED DISEASES

HIV infection and secondary syphilis have been reported to be associated with CDTHL.[4] The mechanism is not fully elucidated but the observations suggest that HIV and syphilis tests need to be included when screening for TE causes.

DRUGS

Many drugs have been reported to cause TE (Table 86-2).[4,26,38-42] However, exact incidence rates have not been documented in most agents.[26] To conclude an etiologic role of some drug in TE, other potential causes of TE need to be excluded and the hair loss should resolve after the discontinuation of the medication.[26,41] The cause-effect relationship can further be supported with the reappearance of TE when a drug is readministered. Early entry of anagen hair follicles into telogen (immediate anagen release) represents a main mechanism of drug-induced TE.[41] In many cases, the shedding starts 2 to 3 months after the initiation of the medication.[1,41] Usually, the recovery from TE can be expected around 3 months after the termination of a causative drug.[41]

TABLE 86-2
Representative Drugs Cause Telogen Effluvium

Androgen hormone (testosterone, anabolic steroids, proandrogenic supplements [DHEA], contraceptives containing progesterone)
Anticoagulants (heparins, warfarin, [possible; dabigatran, rivaroxaban])
Antihistamines (cimetidine, ranitidine)
Anti-infective agents
    Antifungals (clotrimazole, fluconazole, itraconazole, terbinafine)
    Antivirals (acyclovir, imiquimod, indinavir)
    Antituberculosis (ethambutol, isoniazid)
    Antiparasitic drug (albendazole, mebendazole)
Antimitotic agents (colchicine, methotrexate)
Antithyroid agents (propylthiouracil, methimazole)
Cardiovascular drugs
    ACE inhibitors (captopril, enalapril, moexipril, ramipril)
    Beta-adrenoceptor antagonists (metoprolol, propranolol)
Disease-modifying antirheumatic drug (leflunomide)
HPV vaccine
Dopamine precursor and agonists (levodopa, bromocriptine, pergolide pramipexole,)
Interferons (interferon a-2b, γ)
Intravenous immunoglobulin
Metabolic disease therapeutics (allopurinol, cholestyramine, clofibrate, fenofibrate, triparanol, nicotinic acid)
Minoxidil (at initiation or withdrawal)
Nonsteroidal antiinflammatories (ibuprofen, naproxen, salicylates)
Oral contraceptives (cyproterone, drospirenone)
Psychotropics
    Amphetamines
    Anticonvulsants (lamotrigine, phenytoin, valproic acid)
    Antidepressants (fluoxetine, sertraline, tricyclic antidepressants)
    Mood stabilizers (lithium, sodium valproate)
Pyridostigmine bromide
Retinoid, vitamin A and its derivatives (acitretin, etretinate, isotretinoin)
Spironolactone
Sulfasalazine

ACE; angiotensin-converting enzyme.

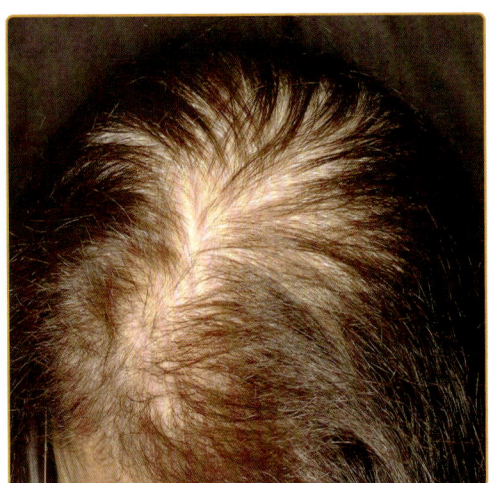

Figure 86-4 Acute telogen effluvium triggered by the administration of warfarin.

Anticoagulants, such as heparin and warfarin, have been recognized as a trigger of TE (Fig. 86-4).[1,42] Other important TE inducers include antiinfective agents, cardiovascular drugs, psychotropics, oral contraceptives, and retinoids (Table 86-2).[4,26,41,42]

MISCELLANEOUS

Biotin or fatty acid deficiency; exposure to heavy metals including arsenic, thallium, and selenium; sunlight and UV ray exposure; and contact dermatitis are reported to be possible triggers for TE.[4]

PATHOGENESIS

Exact mechanisms modulating hair cycle to increase telogen hairs have not been fully delineated. Headington proposed 5 distinct pathogeneses accounting for TE.[14] Recently, the concept that exogen, a hair-shedding process, is an actively controlled biochemical event independent from each phase of hair cycle has been widely accepted,[43,44] which sheds new light on the pathophysiology of TE.

IMMEDIATE ANAGEN RELEASE

Premature termination of anagen and entry into telogen can be a common mechanism for acute TE.[14] Many drug- or stress-induced TE respectively represented by those induced by heparin and drugs in the heparin family or febrile illness[1] can be explained by this phenomenon.[14] Recovery can be expected once external insults are withdrawn and the normal hair cycle restarts.[14]

DELAYED ANAGEN RELEASE

The anagen period is prolonged in most hair follicles but eventually terminated, resulting in an abrupt increase in telogen hairs. This may cause synchronous telogen hair shedding.[14] Delayed anagen release has been observed in the postpartum period[21,23]; however, whether or not this prolongation truly leads to TE remains an open question.[23-25]

SHORT ANAGEN

Headington suggested that idiopathic anagen shortening could be observed in some individuals (a short anagen syndrome).[14] Theoretically, shorter anagen results in a higher telogen rate, with resultant effluvium. An example of this phenomenon is a decrease in anagen period in etretinate-treated patients.[45]

IMMEDIATE TELOGEN RELEASE

The hair follicle is programmed to release club hair to approximately 100 days after the end of previous anagen and enters into new anagen.[46] TE may result from earlier entry into anagen as the frequency of hair shedding should increase.[14] The shedding phase observed at the initiation of topical minoxidil can be explained by this mechanism.[46]

DELAYED TELOGEN RELEASE

The telogen phase is sustained in this case but immediately after, the anagen is initiated, resulting in an increase in shedding club hairs.[14] This situation is observed in seasonal molting in mammals and, probably, in humans traveling from low-daylight to high-daylight conditions.[14]

MODULATED EXOGEN (PROVISIONAL)

Exogen refers to a term during which club hairs are shed from the telogen root sheath sac.[44] Recent studies have suggested that exogen is not a passive process cued by the new anagen hair shaft but a step characterized by proteolytic activity.[47] In rodents, the club hair is retained in the hair follicle even after the initiation of new anagen and contributes to protection from external insults.[44] In the human scalp, exogen is believed to take place sometime around the transition between telogen and anagen.[44] The presence of "kenogen" follicles, the telogen hair follicle without the hair shaft, suggests that shedding of club hair and the anagen-telogen transition do not always keep their orders.[44]

To what extent does exogen play a role in the pathogenesis of TE remains elusive. Technically, immediate or delayed telogen release also can be explained by accelerated or delayed exogen. Consideration of the role of exogen may enable further dissection of TE pathophysiology

DIAGNOSIS

TE should be suspected when a patient claims diffuse hair shedding exclusively consisting of club hairs. In typical acute TE cases with large amounts of telogen hair loss, detailed history attempting to identify possible triggers as described above in the preceding 3 to 4 months is helpful for the diagnosis of TE.[3] It should be noted that triggering events are not identifiable in up to 33% of acute TE cases.[14,48] The diagnosis of TE needs to be made based on the medical history and the findings implying increased telogen hair shedding obtained by the examinations listed below.

HAIR EXAMINATION

HAIR APPEARANCE

The assessment of global hair thickness and part width may be useful; however, as described above, TE can be subclinical in many cases and needs to be evaluated by quantitative approaches.

HAIR LOSS COUNT

Patients often bring shed hairs collected after shampooing or brushing during a certain period. Counting shed hair in such way can be quantitative with patient cooperation and skilled hands[49] but usually not. At the same time, hair loss count alone can allow making the diagnosis in severe TE cases. In addition, it gives an idea for the patient condition and further evaluation. Thus, hair loss count still provides valuable information for clinicians.

Despite hard efforts by investigators, the definitive "normal hair loss count" has not been fixed.[4] In his landmark study, Kligman reported that daily telogen hair loss by regular combing and brushing was 11 to 113, varying considerably among individuals, with an average number of 47.[1] A later study reports the daily shed count to be 40 to 180.[50] A daily telogen hair loss more than 100 has been widely used as the "gold standard" for distinguishing abnormal hair loss.[1,50] This number can be a useful yardstick. Yet, it should be noted that the score is not fully supported by scientific evidence.[50]

HAIR PULL TEST

To be strict, the hair pull test is performed in a patient who has not shampooed for more than 24 hours prior to examination.[51] About 40 to 60 hairs are grasped between the thumb and fingers and pulled firmly alongside with hair shafts.[51] The process needs to be repeated in at least 3 scalp areas, including the frontal, occipital, and temporal regions.[52] Active hair shedding is indicated when more than 10% of tested hairs were collected.[51] Careful attention needs to be paid to the morphology of hair roots as positive findings can

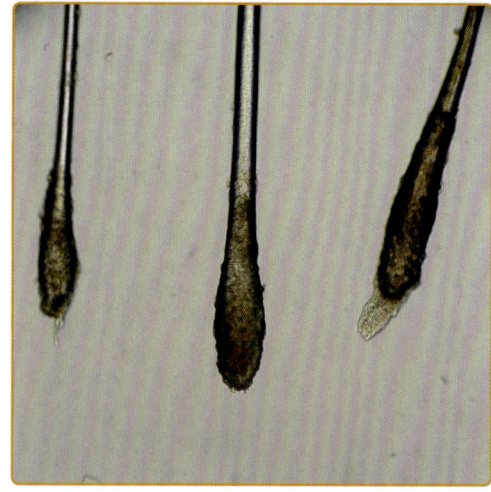

Figure 86-5 Telogen club hairs with intact hair roots collected by hair pull test.

be observed in other hair loss disorders (Fig. 86-5).[4] Of note, the presence of tapered "pencil point" hairs suggests alopecia areata.[4]

In clinics, the hair pull test can be more casually adopted to patients at any time to check if effluvium is present. Perhaps, the increase in hair loss is suggested when more than 5 to 6 hairs were consistently pulled from 2 or more areas. The examiner should be aware that negative hair pull does not exclude TE.[4]

TRICHOGRAM

Trichogram is a semiinvasive technique and represents the most commonly used technique to evaluate hair cycles in the past.[4,52] The patient undergoing this procedure should not wash her or his hair 3 to 5 days before examination.[4,52] Fifty to 100 hairs were clumped by rubber-armed forceps or needle holder and forcibly plucked and investigated for the root morphology under a light microscope.[1,4,52] Usually, sites 2 cm from the front line and midline are sampled.[52] The procedure may yield artifacts if an examiner is unskilled and if it is uncomfortable for the patient, but it provides the telogen-anagen ratio, which is crucial for TE diagnosis.[4,52] Normal values vary among the reports: telogen 13% ranging from 4 to 20% may set a standard.[1] Acute TE can be suggested if the telogen rate exceeds 25%.[1]

PHOTOTRICHOGRAM AND TRICHOSCAN

The phototrichogram is basically a comparison of sequential photographs of a shaved scalp area to detect growing hairs.[52] The procedure is noninvasive but, as it requires shaving, can be refused by a patient. The method provides little quantitative information with regard to the hair cycle phase and may be useful when a remarkable increase in telogen (nongrowing) hairs is observed.[52] Trichoscan is an automated version of phototrichogram using digital software for analyzing dermoscopy images.[52] These techniques are more frequently adopted for the evaluation of hair growth (in clinical trials) rather than effluvium.

TRICHOSCOPY (DERMOSCOPY)

Recently, trichoscopy (dermoscopy without immersion gel; dry-dermoscopy) attracts great interest as a method for the diagnosis of hair disorders.[53] The technique enables the distinction of clinically resembling disorders including TE, androgenetic alopecia (AGA) and diffuse alopecia areata (AA).[53] The decrease in hair density and empty hair openings (active phase) or short-vellus hairs (recovery phase) may be seen in TE (Fig. 86-6). Other signs suggestive of AGA or AA, such as hair diameter diversity, broken hairs, black dots, and tapering hairs, should be absent. In this sense, the diagnosis of TE by this technique is rather based on the exclusion.[54] Trichoscopy is useful for early detection of regrowth of short vellus hairs in the recovery phase of TE.

HISTOLOGY

Histopathologic examination is an invasive but most reliable and informative method for the evaluation of hair loss disorders.[15] For the diagnosis of TE, a quantitative assessment by means of hair counts (eg, total hair numbers, terminal vs vellus hair ratio [indicating miniaturization], telogen-anagen ratio) is indispensable, which can be achieved by horizontal sectioning of a 4-mm punch biopsy specimen at the level between reticular dermis and subcutaneous tissue.[9,55]

The histopathologic findings of TE are a normal total hair count, an increase in telogen hair ratio, normal hair size, and absence of significant inflammation or fibrotic changes.[55] The telogen count greater than 20% support the diagnosis of TE; however, the number can vary depending on the baseline of each patient.[55] In CTE, histologically-detectable increase in telogen hairs can be moderate, around 11% on average.[9] Again, the number can be variable, and multiple biopsies can enhance the accuracy of the diagnosis.[56]

GENERAL EXAMINATION

MEDICAL HISTORY AND PHYSICAL EXAMINATION

Interview of medical history and daily medication potentially associated with telogen hair loss can be beneficial, especially in CDTHL cases. Varying degrees of trichodynia has been reported to be seen in TE and may help the diagnosis.[57] Physical examination for thyroid swelling, skin, and nail condition can be performed to detect subclinical thyroid or collagen disease.

LABORATORY EXAMINATION

A battery of laboratory tests should be performed when the cause is not identified or needs to be evaluated for its status. Recommended items include urine analysis, complete blood count, erythrocyte sedimentation rate, total protein and albumin, aspartate transaminase and alanine transaminase, blood urea nitrogen/creatinine, lactate dehydrogenase, serum ferritin and zinc, T3, T4, thyroid-stimulating hormone, antinuclear antibody, sex hormones (testosterone, luteinizing hormone, and follicle-stimulating hormone in females), prolactin, C-reactive protein, syphilis, and HIV tests.[3,4]

DIFFERENTIAL DIAGNOSIS

A condition that possibly manifests diffuse hair loss needs to be included in the differential diagnoses. Of note, female pattern hair loss, alopecia areata incognita, and psychogenic pseudoeffluvium can present quite similar clinical features and thus should be excluded.[4,46] Their distinction can be very challenging, especially in women.[46,56]

FEMALE PATTERN HAIR LOSS

Female pattern hair loss (FPHL) preferentially affects the top of the scalp, and the frontal hairline is usually preserved.[46] Some patients can demonstrate a triangular reduction in hair density in the frontal scalp behind a preserved fringe resembling a Christmas tree.[46] FPHL can be distinguished from TE in cases at an advanced stage with typical "patterned" hair loss. However, an early-stage FPHL without apparent hair loss may

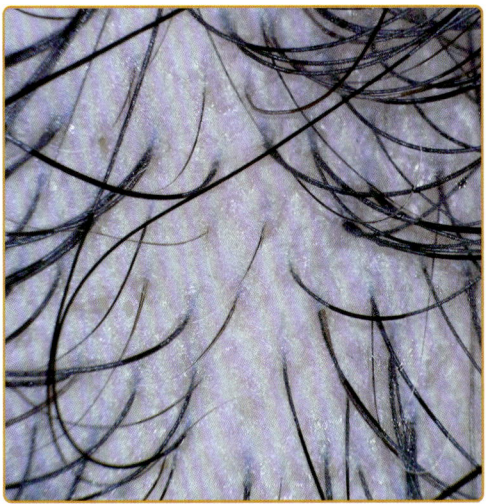

Figure 86-6 The most characteristic dermoscopic finding of telogen effluvium is an increase in short-vellus hairs.

report an increase in hair shedding with diffuse distribution similar to that in CTE.[46,56] The history and common approaches, such as hair pull test, trichogram, as well as laboratory investigation are usually not valuable in distinction.[2,4,46,52] Dermoscopic investigation of an affected area may enable the differentiation when characteristic FPHL signs, including hair diameter diversity, peripilar signs (a brown halo around the follicular ostium), and empty follicles, are present.[46] A quantitative histopathologic examination using horizontal sections adopting the terminal to vellus-like hair ratio (FPHL<CTE) can help confirm the diagnosis; however, multiple biopsies are necessary for diagnostic accuracy.[56]

ALOPECIA AREATA INCOGNITA

Alopecia areata incognita is a rare variant of alopecia areata characterized by acute and diffuse loss of hairs without apparent alopecic patches.[58] Hair pull test is strongly positive and collects telogen hairs.[59] Exclamation mark hairs with dystrophic roots are hardly found.[4] The diagnosis can be challenging.[4,46] Detection of numerous yellow dots of various size and uniform in color by dermoscopy or peribulbar lymphocytic infiltration by histopathologic examination can help establish the diagnosis.[4,46,59]

PSYCHOGENIC PSEUDOEFFLUVIUM

Psychogenic pseudoeffluvium is typically seen in women aged between 35 and 50 years or in men under 35 years.[4] The affected individuals claim hair shedding; however, clinicopathologic examinations fail to detect any evidence of active hair loss.[4,46] The condition is included in body dysmorphic disorder and, in some cases, underlying depressive or anxiety disorders may be present which require appropriate psychiatric management.[4,46]

CLINICAL COURSE, PROGNOSIS, AND MANAGEMENT

Clinical course and prognosis of TE can be variable. However, normal hair regrowth can be expected within several months once a triggering cause is successfully identified and eliminated.[1,4,46] In some cases, the hair texture may be altered.[46] CTE represents an idiopathic form of TE, and its chronology remains elusive.[4] A long-term follow-up of CTE cases reported no visible reduction in hair density even after continuous and fluctuating hair loss for more than 7 to 8 years, suggesting a favorable prognosis.[60]

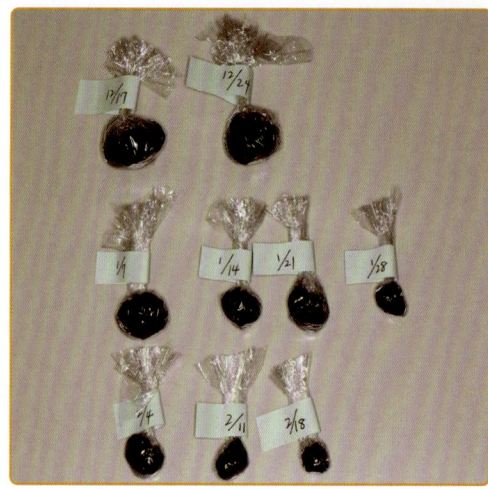

Figure 86-7 Packs of shed hairs collected by periodical sampling confirm spontaneous resolution.

In principle, the management of TE consists of observation until spontaneous resolution, reassurance that hair loss should terminate and not lead to total baldness and psychological support represented by counseling.[1,2,4,46] The explanation of hair cycle and the pathophysiology of TE may help reducing frustration and anxiety of the patients. For those not convinced, periodical sampling of shed hairs under a constant condition (eg, after shampooing everyday [Fig. 86-7]) or demonstration of an image of regrowing hairs can enable a patient to realize the recovery.

Distinction between CDTHL and CTE requires exclusion of etiologic factors.[2] Well-organized clinical and laboratory examinations assessing possible causes listed above should be performed. Medications tend to be less regarded as a cause and needs to be fully evaluated.[2]

Currently, treatment options for CTE are limited.[4,46] Topical minoxidil may be beneficial; however, increase in telogen hair loss may be experienced 2 to 6 weeks after treatment initiation.[26]

Further dissection of the pathophysiology of TE, especially that of CTE, and the elucidation of the mechanism of exogen are indispensable to better manage this common hair loss.

ACKNOWLEDGMENTS

The author would like to thank the Department of Dermatology, Keio University School of Medicine, for permitting the use of images.

REFERENCES

1. Kligman AM. Pathologic dynamics of human hair loss. I. Telogen effuvium. *Arch Dermatol.* 1961;83:175-198.
2. Harrison S, Sinclair R. Telogen effluvium. *Clin Exp Dermatol.* 2002;27(5):389-385.

3. Malkud S. Telogen effluvium: a review. *J Clin Diagn Res.* 2015;9(9):WE01-WE03.
4. Grover C, Khurana A. Telogen effluvium. *Indian J Dermatol Venereol Leprol.* 2013;79(5):591-603.
5. Rebora A. Telogen effluvium. *Dermatology.* 1997;195(3):209-212.
6. Mirmirani P. Managing hair loss in midlife women. *Maturitas.* 2013;74(2):119-122.
7. Nnoruka EN, Obiagboso I, Maduechesi C. Hair loss in children in South-East Nigeria: common and uncommon cases. *Int J Dermatol.* 2007;46(suppl 1):18-22.
8. Whiting DA. Chronic telogen effluvium. *Dermatol Clin.* 1996;14(4):723-731.
9. Whiting DA. Chronic telogen effluvium: increased scalp hair shedding in middle-aged women. *J Am Acad Dermatol.* 1996;35(6):899-906.
10. Dawber RPR, Simpson NB, Barth JH. Diffuse alopeica: endocrine, metabolic and chemical influences on the follicular cycle. In: Dawber RP, ed. *Disease of the Hair and Scalp.* Oxford, UK: Blackwell Science; 1997.
11. Sinclair R. Diffuse hair loss. *Int J Dermatol.* 1999;38(suppl 1):8-18.
12. Rushton DH, Ramsay ID, James KC, et al. Biochemical and trichological characterization of diffuse alopecia in women. *Br J Dermatol.* 1990;123(2):187-197.
13. Thai KE, Sinclair RD. Chronic telogen effluvium in a man. *J Am Acad Dermatol.* 2002;47(4):605-607.
14. Headington JT. Telogen effluvium. New concepts and review. *Arch Dermatol.* 1993;129(3):356-363.
15. Sperling LC. Hair and systemic disease. *Dermatol Clin.* 2001;19(4):711-726, ix.
16. Bernstein GM, Crollick JS, Hassett JM Jr. Postfebrile telogen effluvium in critically ill patients. *Crit Care Med.* 1988;16(1):98-99.
17. Brown TD, Koeller J, Beougher K, et al. A phase I clinical trial of recombinant DNA gamma interferon. *J Clin Oncol.* 1987;5(5):790-798.
18. Olsen EA, Rosen ST, Vollmer RT, et al. Interferon alfa-2a in the treatment of cutaneous T cell lymphoma. *J Am Acad Dermatol.* 1989;20(3):395-407.
19. Desai SP, Roaf ER. Telogen effluvium after anesthesia and surgery. *Anesth Analg.* 1984;63(1):83-84.
20. Kim JH, Lew BL, Sim WY. Localized telogen effluvium after face lift surgery. *Ann Dermatol.* 2015;27(1):119-120.
21. Lynfield YL. Effect of pregnancy on the human hair cycle. *J Invest Dermatol.* 1960;35:323-327.
22. Pecoraro V, Barman JM, Astore I. The normal trichogram of pregnant women. *Adv Biol Skin.* 1967;9:203-210.
23. Gizlenti S, Ekmekci TR. The changes in the hair cycle during gestation and the post-partum period. *J Eur Acad Dermatol Venereol.* 2014;28(7):878-881.
24. Mirallas O, Grimalt R. The postpartum telogen effluvium fallacy. *Skin Appendage Disord.* 2016;1(4):198-201.
25. Rebora A, Guarrera M, Drago F. Postpartum telogen effluvium. *J Eur Acad Dermatol Venereol.* 2016;30(3):518.
26. Fiedler VC, Gray AC. Diffuse alopecia: telogen hair loss. In: Olsen EA, ed. *Disorders of Hair Growth: Diagnosis and Treatment.* 2nd ed. New York, NY: McGraw-Hill; 2003:303-320.
27. Freinkel RK, Freinkel N. Hair growth and alopecia in hypothyroidism. *Arch Dermatol.* 1972;106(3):349-352.
28. Baldari M, Guarrera M, Rebora A. Thyroid peroxidase antibodies in patients with telogen effluvium. *J Eur Acad Dermatol Venereol.* 2010;24(8):980-982.
29. Kligman AM. The comparative histopathology of male-pattern baldness and senescent baldness. *Clin Dermatol.* 1988;6(4):108-118.
30. Reszke R, Pelka D, Walasek A, et al. Skin disorders in elderly subjects. *Int J Dermatol.* 2015;54(9):e332-e338.
31. Goette DK, Odom RB. Alopecia in crash dieters. *JAMA.* 1976;235(24):2622-2623.
32. Jordan VE. Protein status of the elderly as measured by dietary intake, hair tissue, and serum albumin. *Am J Clin Nutr.* 1976;29(5):522-528.
33. Johnson AA, Latham MC, Roe DA. An evaluation of the use of changes in hair root morphology in the assessment of protein-calorie malnutrition. *Am J Clin Nutr.* 1976;29(5):502-511.
34. Trost LB, Bergfeld WF, Calogeras E. The diagnosis and treatment of iron deficiency and its potential relationship to hair loss. *J Am Acad Dermatol.* 2006;54(5):824-844.
35. Olsen EA, Reed KB, Cacchio PB, et al. Iron deficiency in female pattern hair loss, chronic telogen effluvium, and control groups. *J Am Acad Dermatol.* 2010;63(6):991-999.
36. Abdel Aziz AM, Sh Hamed S, Gaballah MA. Possible relationship between chronic telogen effluvium and changes in lead, cadmium, zinc, and iron total blood levels in females: a case-control study. *Int J Trichol.* 2015;7(3):100-106.
37. Watanabe-Okada E, Inazumi T, Matsukawa H, et al. Histopathological insights into hair loss in Cronkhite-Canada syndrome: diffuse anagen-telogen conversion precedes clinical hair loss progression. *Australas J Dermatol.* 2014;55(2):145-148.
38. Tosti A, Pazzaglia M. Drug reactions affecting hair: diagnosis. *Dermatol Clin.* 2007;25(2):223-231, vii.
39. Conde J, Davis K, Ntuen E, et al. A case of imiquimod-induced alopecia. *J Dermatolog Treat.* 2010;21(2):122-124.
40. Sperling LC. Telogen effluvium. In: Sperling LC, Cowper SE, Knopp EA, eds. *An Atlas of Hair Pathology With Clinical Correlation.* 2nd ed. New York: CRC Press; 2012:53-59.
41. Patel M, Harrison S, Sinclair R. Drugs and hair loss. *Dermatol Clin.* 2013;31(1):67-73.
42. Watras MM, Patel JP, Arya R. Traditional anticoagulants and hair loss: a role for direct oral anticoagulants? A Review of the Literature. *Drugs Real World Outcomes.* 2016;3(1):1-6.
43. Milner Y, Sudnik J, Filippi M, et al. Exogen, shedding phase of the hair growth cycle: characterization of a mouse model. *J Invest Dermatol.* 2002;119(3):639-644.
44. Higgins CA, Westgate GE, Jahoda CA. From telogen to exogen: mechanisms underlying formation and subsequent loss of the hair club fiber. *J Invest Dermatol.* 2009;129(9):2100-2108.
45. Berth-Jones J, Hutchinson PE. Novel cycle changes in scalp hair are caused by etretinate therapy. *Br J Dermatol.* 1995;132(3):367-375.
46. Trueb RM. Systematic approach to hair loss in women. *J Dtsch Dermatol Ges.* 2010;8(4):284-297, 284-298.
47. Higgins CA, Westgate GE, Jahoda CA. Modulation in proteolytic activity is identified as a hallmark of exogen by transcriptional profiling of hair follicles. *J Invest Dermatol.* 2011;131(12):2349-2357.
48. Harrison S, Sinclair R. Optimal management of hair loss (alopecia) in children. *Am J Clin Dermatol.* 2003;4(11):757-770.
49. Guarrera M, Fiorucci MC, Rebora A. Methods of hair loss evaluation: a comparison of TrichoScan((R)) with the modified wash test. *Exp Dermatol.* 2013;22(7):482-484.

50. Van Neste MD. Assessment of hair loss: clinical relevance of hair growth evaluation methods. *Clin Exp Dermatol.* 2002;27(5):358-365.
51. Pierard GE, Pierard-Franchimont C, Marks R, et al. EEMCO guidance for the assessment of hair shedding and alopecia. *Skin Pharmacol Physiol.* 2004;17(2):98-110.
52. Olszewska M, Warszawik O, Rakowska A, et al. Methods of hair loss evaluation in patients with endocrine disorders. *Endokrynol Pol.* 2010;61(4):406-411.
53. Inui S. Trichoscopy for common hair loss diseases: algorithmic method for diagnosis. *J Dermatol.* 2011;38(1):71-75.
54. Jain N, Doshi B, Khopkar U. Trichoscopy in alopecias: diagnosis simplified. *Int J Trichology.* 2013;5(4):170-178.
55. Sperling LC, Lupton GP. Histopathology of non-scarring alopecia. *J Cutan Pathol.* 1995;22(2):97-114.
56. Sinclair R, Jolley D, Mallari R, et al. The reliability of horizontally sectioned scalp biopsies in the diagnosis of chronic diffuse telogen hair loss in women. *J Am Acad Dermatol.* 2004;51(2):189-199.
57. Rebora A. Trichodynia: a review of the literature. *Int J Dermatol.* 2016;55(4):382-384.
58. Rebora A. Alopecia areata incognita: a hypothesis. *Dermatologica.* 1987;174(5):214-218.
59. Tosti A, Whiting D, Iorizzo M, et al. The role of scalp dermoscopy in the diagnosis of alopecia areata incognita. *J Am Acad Dermatol.* 2008;59(1):64-67.
60. Sinclair R. Chronic telogen effluvium: a study of 5 patients over 7 years. *J Am Acad Dermatol.* 2005;52(2)(suppl 1):12-16.

Chapter 87 :: Alopecia Areata
:: Nina Otberg & Jerry Shapiro

第八十七章

斑秃

中文导读

斑秃是一种常见的自身免疫性、无瘢痕的毛发疾病。此疾病在男女中均有发生，可影响每个年龄组，但在较年轻年龄组中发病率较高；是儿童脱发中最常见的一种。在斑秃患者中，5%出现全头皮脱发(全秃)，1%出现全身脱发(全身脱发)。

第一节讲述了斑秃的大体外观，发生部位，之后讲述了其临床特点是黑点、感叹号发，甚至指甲受累，还可伴有其他自身免疫疾病。

第二节从自身免疫反应、遗传、情绪压力、氧化应激方面讲述其病因及发病机制。自体细胞毒CD8 T细胞和干扰素-g驱动的针对毛囊或指甲的免疫反应；斑秃的遗传倾向；脱发前的情绪压力；氧化应激的影响都在本章的陈述内容中。

第三节从斑秃的临床特点、体格检查、皮肤镜下毛发毛囊的特点、家族史，甚至头皮活检来诊断此病，强调需要使用实验室检查排除其他疾病。

第四节指出其组织病理学具有阶段性，其典型的炎性浸润在亚急性或慢性时可能缺失或明显减少，但在急性期斑秃的特征是以毛球为中心的球周免疫细胞浸润。

第五节提到斑秃需要与暂时性三角型脱发、头癣、早期瘢痕性脱发、拔毛癣、二期梅毒(斑秃)、雄激素性脱发、休止期脱发、生长期脱发相鉴别（表87-1）。

第六节指出此疾病的并发症：复发、进展到全秃或全身性脱发、毛发的缺失致晒伤和皮肤癌，对于心理情绪的影响也是很显著的。

第七节提到该病病程多变，并以不规则的复发过程为特征，介绍了不同时间段的头发再生和此病复发率，以及进展到全头皮脱发和全身脱发的可能性。

第八节指出目前还没有一种疗法可以改变疾病的自然过程。所有治疗斑秃的有效方法都是姑息性的，只控制正在发生的脱发，而不治疗脱发本身。之后把治疗分为保守治疗、局部外用糖皮质激素、皮损内注射糖皮质激素、血小板血浆治疗、系统用糖皮质激素、前列腺类似物治疗、局部米诺地尔、蒽林药物、局部免疫疗法、光动力治疗、环孢素治疗、JANUS激酶抑制药以及假发或化妆。其中强调皮质类固醇（曲安奈德或己曲安奈德）注射是治疗50%以下头皮受累的成人患者的一线疗法。并提出了局部免疫治疗虽然没有通过FAD批准，但却有一定疗效。并且提出系统用糖皮质激素、联合使用米诺地尔有效；光动力治疗手段相对较少使用。最后通过图 87-6，从患者年龄、头皮毛发受累面积以及治疗后的反应疗效来实施斑秃的治疗程序，并使用对应的治疗手段。

〔简　丹〕

AT-A-GLANCE

- Alopecia areata is a nonscarring hair disorder.
- It occurs in both genders equally and can affect every age group, although incidence at in younger age groups is higher.
- It is the most common form of hair loss in children. Clinically, it presents with well-demarcated round or oval bald spots on the scalp or other parts of the body.
- Of patients with alopecia areata, 5% develop hair loss of their entire scalp hair (alopecia areata totalis) and 1% develop alopecia areata universalis (loss of total body hair).
- Nail changes include pitting or sandpaper nails.
- Alopecia areata is thought to be an autoimmune disease with a possible hereditary component.
- In general, alopecia areata is a medically friendly condition, but it can coexist with other autoimmune disorders such as Hashimoto thyroiditis and vitiligo.

Alopecia areata is a common autoimmune hair disorder. This nonscarring, usually patchy hair loss condition can affect any hair-bearing area. At any given time, approximately 0.2% of the world population is suffering from alopecia areata. It has an estimated lifetime risk of 1.7%[1,2]; it is a common cause of abrupt-onset hair loss, but occurs less often than androgenetic alopecia or telogen effluvium. Both sexes are equally affected. Although it may occur at any age, incidence at younger ages is higher. Alopecia areata is the most common form of alopecia seen in children. The familial occurrence is approximately 15%, but expression of the disorder is variable between different family members. Of patients suffering from alopecia areata, 5% develop hair loss of their entire scalp hair (alopecia areata totalis) and 1% develop alopecia areata universalis (loss of total body hair).

CLINICAL FEATURES

Alopecia areata is characterized by an acute onset. It typically presents with oval- or round-shaped, well-circumscribed, bald, patches with a smooth surface in a diffuse distribution (Figs. 87-1 and 87-2). Alopecia totalis results in the loss of the entire scalp hair and may occur suddenly or follow partial alopecia (Fig. 87-3). Partial alopecia may be observed in other areas of the body as well. Loss of total body hair is called *alopecia areata universalis* and may occur suddenly or follow longstanding partial alopecia.

Characteristic hallmarks of alopecia areata are so-called black dots (cadaver hairs, point noir), resulting from hair that breaks off by the time it reaches the skin surface. Exclamation point hairs, which have a blunt distal end and taper proximally, appear when the broken hairs (black dots) are pushed out of the follicle. Localization of the initial patch occurs most often on the scalp, but may occur on any hair-bearing part of the body. Patches are usually without further symptoms, but may cause mild itching and erythema. In addition to this well-demarcated localized form, alopecia areata can also present in a diffuse generalized pattern that resembles androgenic alopecia or telogen effluvium. Involvement of nails can occur with nail pitting and a sandpaper-like appearance.

Alopecia areata has been described in association with a variety of other disorders, including cataracts, thyroid disease, vitiligo, atopic dermatitis, psoriasis, Cronkhite-Canada, and Down syndrome.[3,4]

ETIOLOGY AND PATHOGENESIS

Alopecia areata is a chronic, organ-specific autoimmune disease. Autoactive cytotoxic CD8 T cells, which affect hair follicles and sometimes nails,[5-11] and an interferon-γ–driven immune response, which includes interferon-γ and interferon-γ–induced chemokines, have been identified as the main drivers of disease pathogenesis.[12] The importance of a cytotoxic subset of CD8+ NKG2D+ (natural-killer group 2 member D-positive) T cells within the inflammatory infiltrate in alopecia areata and an upregulation in the hair follicle itself of 2 NKG2D ligands have been discovered in several studies.[10,11] Furthermore, other cell types, including natural killer cells, may play a regulatory role in alopecia areata.[5,8,13,14]

Patients with alopecia areata seem to have a genetic predisposition to the disease. There is a high frequency of a positive family history of alopecia areata in affected individuals, ranging from 10% to 42% of cases,[15] and a much higher incidence of a positive family history in early-onset alopecia areata.[16] A genome-wide association study[10] and a large genome-wide association study metaanalysis[17] have identified numerous loci that imply a strong role for variants in genes that direct and influence immune responses.[13]

Many patients report the experience of major emotional stress prior to the onset of alopecia. Stress perception seems to be a risk factor that may influence the onset and exacerbation of alopecia areata.[18] Moreover, an antioxidant–oxidant imbalance can be found in many autoimmune disorders as well as in patients suffering from emotional and environmental stress. Several studies support an association between oxidative stress and alopecia areata.[19-24]

DIAGNOSIS

Clinical features, such as shape and look of the patches, presence of exclamation point hairs, and nail changes (pitting or sandpaper nails), lead to the diagnosis of alopecia areata (Fig. 87-4). In most patients the physical findings are so characteristic that the diagnosis is

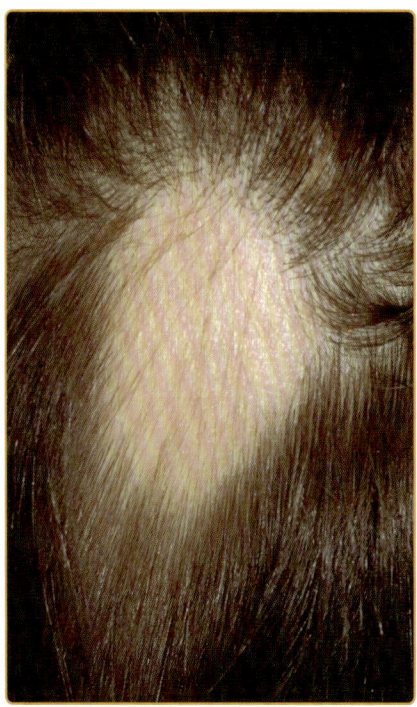

Figure 87-1 Patch of alopecia areata with mild peachy erythema and some fine residual hairs.

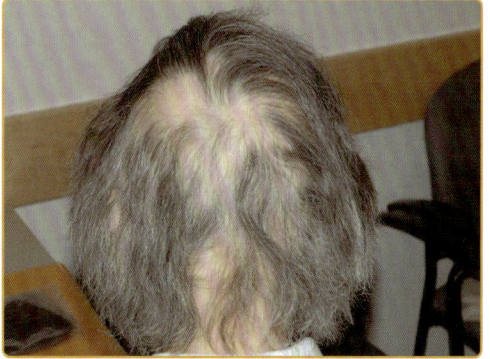

Figure 87-2 Patient with patchy alopecia areata.

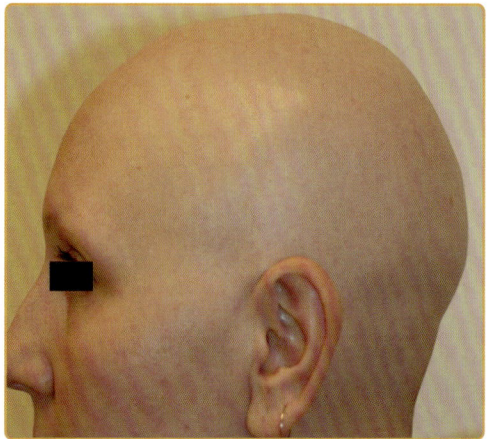

Figure 87-3 Patient with alopecia areata totalis.

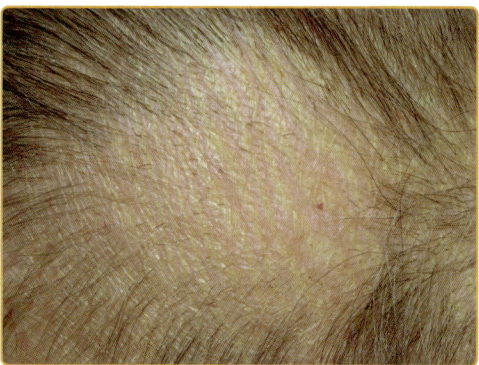

Figure 87-4 Patch of alopecia area with exclamation point hair.

obvious. Patchy or complete loss of eyebrows and eyelashes can also lead to the diagnosis of alopecia areata (Fig. 87-5). Sudden and rapid loss of the entire scalp hair (alopecia areata totalis) or the entire body hair (alopecia areata universalis) are diagnostic for alopecia areata. A dermatoscopic evaluation will help to support the diagnosis by showing the presence of follicular ostia. The presence of either follicular ostia, exclamation point hair, cadaver hair (residual hair shafts visible as black dots in the follicular ostia), or yellow dots that will confirm the diagnosis. These features are even more visible with a trichoscopic evaluation at higher magnification.[25,26] In the acute stages gentle pulling from the periphery of bald areas will yield more than 10 hairs. White hairs are sometimes spared by the disease. This can lead to canities subita, a sudden whiting of the hair. In this case, all pigmented hairs fall out and the patient is left with only white hair. Moreover, positive family history and/or the presence of associated diseases may give further evidence. Diffuse alopecia areata can be very difficult to diagnose. In cases of doubt, a scalp biopsy (a 4-mm punch processed for horizontal sections) should be taken to confirm the diagnosis of alopecia areata.

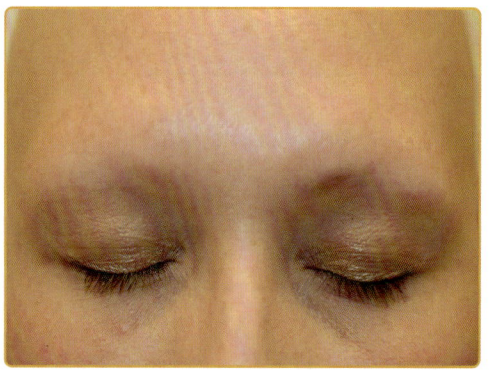

Figure 87-5 Patient with alopecia areata of the eyebrows.

Additionally, laboratory tests should be performed to rule out thyroid dysfunction[27] and iron or vitamin deficiencies.

PATHOLOGY

Scalp biopsy reveals a generalized miniaturization and a marked increase in catagen and telogen hair follicles. In the acute phase, alopecia areata is characterized by a peribulbar immune infiltrate centered around the hair bulb which has been described as a "swarm of bees." This infiltrate is made up of predominantly CD4 and CD8 T cells and natural killer cells.[28] Sometimes mast cell, plasma cells and eosinophils also can be seen.[13,14,29] The histopathologic features of alopecia areata, however, are stage-dependent. The classic inflammatory infiltrate may be missing or markedly less in subacute or chronic forms.[30] Sometimes an immune infiltrate is visible around the bulb of miniaturized hairs in the upper dermis.[30] Alopecia areata should be in the differential diagnosis whenever high percentages of telogen hairs or miniaturized hairs are present, even in the absence of peribulbar inflammation.

DIFFERENTIAL DIAGNOSIS

Table 87-1 outlines the differential diagnosis of alopecia areata.

COMPLICATIONS

Relapsing course and progress of hair loss to severe forms of alopecia totalis or universalis are dreaded complications. Missing hair on the scalp and face, including nasal hair and eyelashes and eyebrows can increase incidence of sunburns and skin cancers, as well as of nasopharyngeal and ophthalmologic inflammation. Although the condition is not life threatening, changes in appearance frequently cause a diminished sense of personal well-being and self-esteem, leading to severe depressive mood and withdrawal from social situations.

TABLE 87-1
Differential Diagnosis

- Temporal triangular alopecia
- Tinea capitis
- Early scarring alopecia
- Trichotillomania
- Secondary syphilis (alopecia areolaris)
- Androgenetic alopecia
- Telogen effluvium
- Anagen effluvium

PROGNOSIS AND CLINICAL COURSE

The course of the disease is very variable and characterized by an irregular relapsing course, with approximately 25% of affected individuals having a solitary episode. Spontaneous regrowth of hair is common. Different body areas appear to regrow independently. Approximately 60% of patients have at least a partial regrowth by 1 year, but this is often followed by repeated episodes of hair loss. Approximately 40% of the relapses occur within the first year, but a large percentage of patients may relapse after 5 years. Hair can regrow white but may change to the patient's natural color over time. Poor prognosis is linked to involvement of the occiput and/or hairline, chronic relapsing course, presence of nail changes, and when onset is in childhood.[31-33]

Patients with alopecia areata have a 5% risk of losing their entire scalp hair (alopecia areata totalis) and an estimated 1% risk for progressing to alopecia areata universalis, characterized by total body and scalp hair loss. The number of patients progressing to alopecia areata totalis is higher in the younger age groups, and in patients with hair loss from the trunk and extremities.

TREATMENT

Very little evidence-based data is available for the treatment of alopecia areata; recommendations are mainly based on case series and clinical experience (Fig. 87-6). At this time there is no single therapy that can alter the natural course of the disease. All available treatments for alopecia areata are palliative, only controlling the ongoing episode of hair loss and not curing the condition itself. However, helpful treatment guidelines have been published.[31-33]

CONSERVATIVE MANAGEMENT

Alopecia areata shows a high rate of spontaneous remission, especially in those patients with a short history and limited scalp involvement. On the other hand, in alopecia areata totalis and universalis, treatments have a high failure rate. After the discussion of possible risks and benefits of all options, no treatment may be a legitimate option for some patients.

TOPICAL CORTICOSTEROIDS

Superpotent (class I) and potent (class II) topical corticosteroids are widely used to treat alopecia areata. Evidence of efficacy has been proven for class I corticosteroids when applied under occlusion[34] and for class II corticosteroids when used in combination with minoxidil.[35]

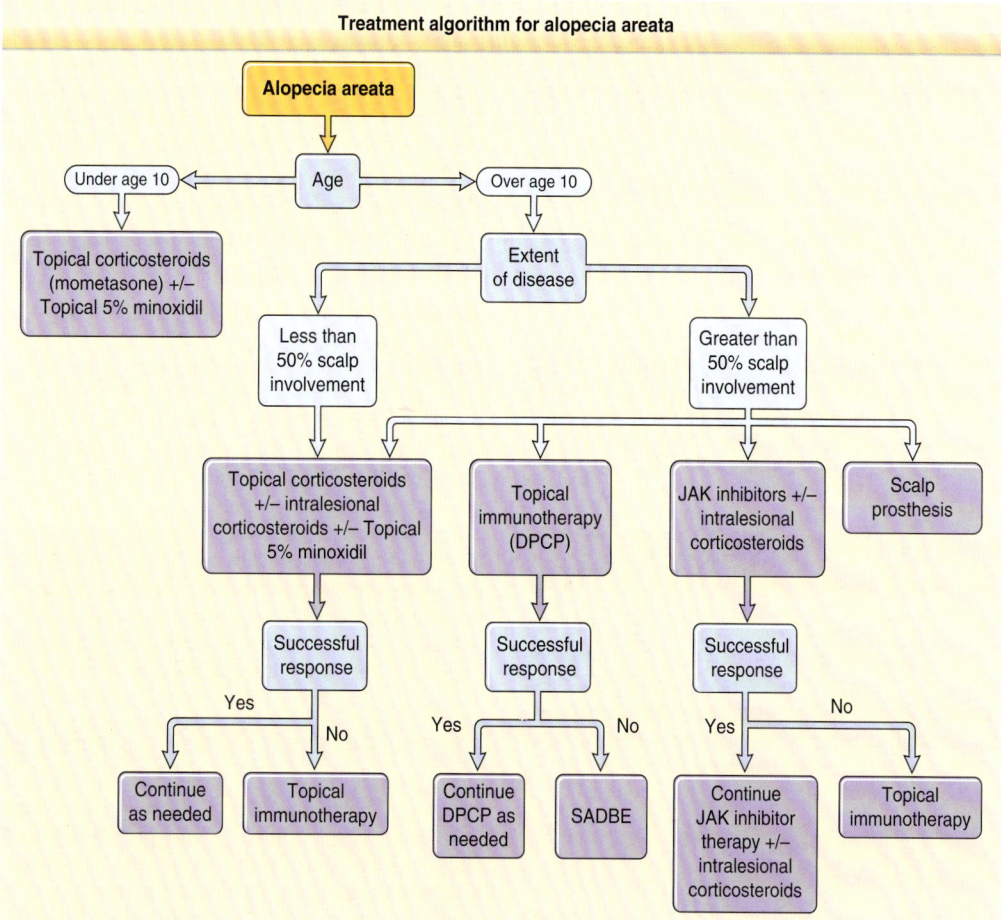

Figure 87-6 Treatment algorithm for alopecia areata. DNCB, dinitrochlorobenzene; DPCP, diphenylcyclopropenone; PUVA, psoralen and ultraviolet A; SADBE, squaric acid dibutylester. (From Strazzulla LC, Wang EHC, Avila L et al. Alopecia areata: An appraisal of new treatment approaches and overview of current therapies. J Am Acad Dermatol. 2018;78:15-24. Copyright © Lauren Strazzulla, Lorena Avila, and Jerry Shapiro, with permission.)

INTRALESIONAL CORTICOSTEROIDS

Intralesional corticosteroid (triamcinolone acetonide or triamcinolone hexacetonide) injection is first-line therapy for adult patients with less than 50% scalp involvement. Triamcinolone acetonide is used at concentrations from 2.5 to 10 mg/mL. Treatment is repeated every 4 to 6 weeks; the total amount injected per session varies from 15 to 40 mg.[31-33,36-38] An initial response is often seen after 4 to 8 weeks. Some patients experience indentation of the scalp skin in the injection sites as the result of a nonpermanent atrophy of the subcutaneous fat. Permanent skin atrophy can occur if the same skin area is injected repeatedly over months and years. If no regrowth can be seen after 4 months of treatment, other treatment options should be considered. Intralesional corticosteroids injections are usually used on the scalp, eyebrows and beard area and can be combined with topical treatment.

PLATELET-RICH PLASMA

Reports state that the use of platelet-rich plasma injections as monotherapy or in combination with other therapies are beneficial in the treatment of alopecia areata.[39-41] In a double-blind trial, platelet-rich plasma was superior to low-dose triamcinolone acetonide and placebo injection.[42,43] Further studies are necessary to determine the effectiveness of platelet-rich plasma in the therapy of alopecia areata.[41]

SYSTEMIC CORTICOSTEROIDS

Systemic corticosteroids are effective in the treatment of alopecia areata. However, the regrown hair frequently falls out again when the treatment is discontinued. The use of systemic corticosteroids is controversial. They should not be used as routine treatments because they do not alter the long-term prognosis and can cause side effects, such as striae, acne, obesity, cataracts, and hypertension. Dosages vary from an initial 20 to 40 mg dose of prednisone daily, with tapering down to 5 mg daily in a few weeks or different pulse therapies regimens with short-term high doses of oral prednisolone (100 to 300 mg) or IV methylprednisolone (250 mg).[31,32,34,36]

TOPICAL MINOXIDIL

There is some evidence of clinically acceptable hair regrowth using topical minoxidil 5% solution.[44,45] Better results can be achieved when minoxidil is used in combination with class I or class II topical corticosteroids or anthralin.[35] Minoxidil shows little efficacy in alopecia areata totalis and universalis.

PROSTAGLANDIN ANALOGS

Prostaglandin analogs like latanoprost and bimatoprost have been studied for their use in the treatment of alopecia areata of eyelashes and eyebrows. Some studies showed hair regrowth of eyelashes and eyebrows after the treatment with prostaglandin analogs.[46] However, several reports showed a negative outcome after the use of latanoprost and bimatoprost.[47-49] Prostaglandin analogs may have some use as an adjuvant therapy.

ANTHRALIN

Anthralin is an irritant that may have a nonspecific immunomodulating effect (anti–Langerhans cell) and is usually used in the treatment of psoriasis.[50] Several studies have shown efficacy in the treatment of alopecia areata with cosmetically acceptable varying from 20% to 25% for patchy alopecia areata.[51,52] Anthralin is used as a 0.2% to 1% cream or ointment. It is usually applied daily to the affected scalp areas and left on for 20 to 30 minutes for the first 2 weeks, and then for 45 minutes daily for 2 weeks, up to a maximum of 1 hour daily. Some patient may tolerate overnight therapy.[36,51] When therapy is effective, new hair growth can usually be seen after 2 to 3 months of treatment. Because of its good safety profile, anthralin is a good treatment choice for children. Side effects of anthralin are irritation, scaling, folliculitis, and regional lymphadenopathy. Anthralin is not suitable for the treatment of eyebrows and the beard area. Patients should be cautious not to get anthralin in the eyes and to protect the treated skin areas from ultraviolet radiation. Brown discoloration of the treated skin and brown staining of clothes and linen may occur. The patient should be advised to rinse off the anthralin with cool or lukewarm water, as hot water increases the likelihood of brown stains of tiles and bathtub.

TOPICAL IMMUNOTHERAPY

Although not approved by the U.S. Food and Drug Administration (FDA), topical immunotherapy seems to be a very effective therapeutic option with a good safety profile in the treatment of chronic severe alopecia areata. The exact mechanism of action is not fully understood. A decrease in the peribulbar CD4+/CD8+ lymphocyte ratio and a shift in the position of T-lymphocytes away from the perifollicular area to the interfollicular area and dermis are thought to be responsible for the immunomodulating effect.[53-55] The desired effect of the treatment is the creation of a contact dermatitis. Diphenylcyclopropenone is the most commonly used contact sensitizer. Diphenylcyclopropenone is compounded in an acetone base and stored in opaque bottles to protect the solution from photodegradation. Applying a small amount of a 2% solution to a small scalp area 1 week prior to treatment start, sensitizes the patient. The diphenylcyclopropenone solution is then applied weekly to the scalp, starting at a concentration of 0.0001%. The scalp should not be washed for 48 hours after treatment and should be protected from ultraviolet radiation. Carefully increase the concentration every week until the patient develops a mild erythema and mild itching. The treatment is continued with this concentration; the usual highest concentration used is 2%. Success rates vary from 17% to 75%, with the lowest success rates being in patients with alopecia areata totalis and universalis.[56] Side effects include lymphadenopathy in 100% of patients, severe contact eczema, discoloration of the skin including vitiliginous patches and hyperpigmentation on the scalp and other parts of the body. Extreme caution is indicated in patients with atopic dermatitis and dark skin types.

PHOTO(CHEMO)THERAPY

Ultraviolet B light has been reported to be useful in some patients with alopecia areata.[57] Further therapeutic options include both oral and topical administration of psoralen followed by ultraviolet A irradiation. Psoralen and ultraviolet A therapy may affect T-cell function and antigen presentation, and possibly inhibit the local immunologic attack against the hair follicle by depleting Langerhans cells.[58] Photo(chemo)therapy shows a very high relapse rate, especially after tapering the treatment. Today's major concern about long-term ultraviolet irradiation of any kind is its promotion of all types of skin cancer, including melanoma. Consequently, phototherapy should only be considered in exceptional cases.[56]

CYCLOSPORINE

Systemic cyclosporine at doses of 4 to 6 mg/kg/day has been shown to have a beneficial effect in some patients with alopecia areata.[56,59] Side effects of oral cyclosporine include elevated serum transaminases and cholesterol levels, as well as headaches, dysesthesia, fatigue, diarrhea, gingival hyperplasia, flushing, and myalgia. Cyclosporine can be combined with low-dose oral prednisone and may be considered in patients with severe atopic dermatitis and alopecia areata. However, because of its side-effect profile and the high recurrence rate observed after discontinuation, cyclosporine seems to be a relatively impractical treatment for alopecia areata.

JANUS KINASE INHIBITORS

Recent mechanistic data support a role for Janus kinase (JAK)-mediated pathways in alopecia areata[11,60] Interferon-γ, interleukin-2, and interleukin-15 play a significant role in maintaining the autoreactive CD8+ T-cell infiltrate in alopecia areata. Their receptors signal through JAK1, JAK2, and JAK3. The inhibition of these cytokine receptors with JAK inhibitors can lead to a reversal of alopecia areata.

Several case reports show that JAK inhibitors are a promising class of drugs for alopecia areata even in cases of severe or widespread disease. Oral baricitinib and tofacitinib citrate (approved by the FDA for mild rheumatoid arthritis) and oral ruxolitinib (approved by the FDA for myelofibrosis) have shown a good treatment outcome with full regrowth of scalp hair in widespread alopecia areata.[61-65]

CAMOUFLAGE, WIGS, AND HAIRPIECES

When despite treatment alopecia is progressive and there is no hope for hair regrowth, permanent adaptation to the disease is necessary. Extensive alopecia areata of the scalp can be camouflaged with wigs and hair pieces. In women with alopecia areata of the eyebrows, permanent makeup may be considered.

The treating physician should provide psychological support. Local alopecia areata support groups and annual meetings of the National Alopecia Areata Foundation (www.naaf.org) can be very helpful for patients and their relatives.

REFERENCES

1. Price VH. Alopecia areata: clinical aspects. *J Invest Dermatol.* 1991;96(5):S68.
2. Safavi K. Prevalence of alopecia areata in the First National Health and Nutrition Examination Survey. *Arch Dermatol.* 1992;128:702.
3. Allbritton J, Simmons-O'Brien E, Hutcheons D, et al. Cronkhite-Canada syndrome: report of two cases, biopsy findings in the associated alopecia, and a new treatment option. *Cutis.* 1998;61(4):229-232.
4. Sethuraman G, Malhotra AK, Sharma VK. Alopecia universalis in Down syndrome: response to therapy. *Indian J Dermatol Venereol Leprol.* 2006;72(6):454-455.
5. Gilhar A, Kalish RS. Alopecia areata: a tissue specific autoimmune disease of the hair follicle. *Autoimmun Rev.* 2006;5:64.
6. Gilhar A, Paus R, Kalish R. Lymphocytes, neuropeptides, and genes involved in alopecia areata. *J Clin Invest.* 2007;111:2019.
7. McDonagh AJ, Messenger AG. The pathogenesis of alopecia areata. *Dermatol Clin.* 1996;14:661.
8. Paus R, Nickoloff BJ, Ito T. A "hairy" privilege. *Trends Immunol.* 2005;26:32.
9. McElwee KJ, Freyschmidt-Paul P, Hoffmann R, et al. Transfer of CD8(+) cells induces localized hair loss whereas CD4(+)/CD25(−) cells promote systemic alopecia areata and CD4(+)/CD25(+) cells blockade disease onset in the C3H/HeJ mouse model. *J Invest Dermatol.* 2005;124:947-957.
10. Petukhova L, Duvic M, Hordinsky M, et al. Genome-wide association study in alopecia areata implicates both innate and adaptive immunity. *Nature.* 2010;466:113-117.
11. Xing L, Dai Z, Jabbari A, et al. Alopecia areata is driven by cytotoxic T lymphocytes and is reversed by JAK inhibition. *Nat Med.* 2014;20(9):1043-1049.
12. Rork JF, Rashighi M, Harris JE. Understanding autoimmunity of vitiligo and alopecia areata. *Curr Opin Pediatr.* 2016;28(4):463-469.
13. Jabbari A, Cerise JE, Chen JC, et al. Molecular signatures define alopecia areata subtypes and transcriptional biomarkers. *EBioMedicine.* 2016;7:240-247.
14. Kaufman G, d'Ovidio R, Kaldawy A, et al. An unexpected twist in alopecia areata pathogenesis: are NK cells protective and CD49b+ T cells pathogenic? *Exp Dermatol.* 2010;19(8):e347-e349.
15. Shellow WV, Edwards JE, Koo JY. Profile of alopecia areata: a questionnaire analysis of patient and family. *Int J Dermatol.* 1992;31(3):186-189.
16. Price VH, Colombe BW. Heritable factors distinguish two types of alopecia areata. *Dermatol Clin.* 1996;14(4):679-689.
17. Betz RC, Petukhova L, Ripke S, et al. Genome-wide meta-analysis in alopecia areata resolves HLA associations and reveals two new susceptibility loci. *Nat Commun.* 2015;22(6):5966.
18. Brajac I, Tkalcic M, Dragojević DM, et al. Roles of stress, stress perception and trait-anxiety in the onset and course of alopecia areata. *J Dermatol.* 2003; 30(12):871-878.
19. Prie BE, Voiculescu VM, Ionescu-Bozdog OB, et al. Oxidative stress and alopecia areata. *J Med Life.* 2015; 8(spec issue):43-46.
20. Abdel Fattah NS, Ebrahim AA, El Okda ES. Lipid peroxidation/antioxidant activity in patients with alopecia areata. *J Eur Acad Dermatol Venereol.* 2011;25:403-408.
21. Akar A, Arca E, Erbil H, et al. Antioxidant enzymes and lipid peroxidation in the scalp of patients with alopecia areata. *J Dermatol Sci.* 2002;29:85-90.

22. Bakry OA, Elshazly RM, Shoeib MA, et al. Oxidative stress in alopecia areata: a case-control study. *Am J Clin Dermatol.* 2014;15:57-64.
23. Naziroglu M, Kokcam I. Antioxidants and lipid peroxidation status in the blood of patients with alopecia. *Cell Biochem Funct.* 2000;18:169-173.
24. Motor S, Ozturk S, Ozcan O, et al. Evaluation of total antioxidant status, total oxidant status and oxidative stress index in patients with alopecia areata. *Int J Clin Exp Med.* 2014;7:1089-1093.
25. Rudnicka L, Olszewska M, Rakowska A, et al. Trichoscopy update 2011. *J Dermatol Case Rep.* 2011;5(4):82-88.
26. Gordon KA, Tosti A. Alopecia: evaluation and treatment. *Clin Cosmet Investig Dermatol.* 2011;4:101-106.
27. Saylam Kurtipek G, Cihan FG, Erayman Demirbaş Ş, et al. The frequency of autoimmune thyroid disease in alopecia areata and vitiligo patients. *Biomed Res Int.* 2015;2015:435947.
28. Todes-Taylor N, Turner R, Wood GS. T cell subpopulations in alopecia areata. *J Am Acad Dermatol.* 1984;11(2):216-223.
29. Sperling LC, Lupton GP. Histopathology of nonscarring alopecia. *J Cutan Pathol.* 1995;22(2):97-114.
30. Whiting DA. Histopathologic features of alopecia areata: a new look. *Arch Dermatol.* 2003;139(12):1555-1559.
31. Alkhalifah A, Alsantali A, Wang E, et al. Alopecia areata update: part I. Clinical picture, histopathology, and pathogenesis. *J Am Acad Dermatol.* 2010;62(2):177-188.
32. Alkhalifah A, Alsantali A, Wang E, et al. Alopecia areata update: part II. Treatment. *J Am Acad Dermatol.* 2010;62(2):191-202.
33. Shapiro J. Alopecia areata. Update on therapy. *Dermatol Clin.* 1993;11(1):35-46.
34. Friedli A, Labarthe MP, Engelhardt E, et al. Pulse methylprednisolone therapy for severe alopecia areata: an open prospective study of 45 patients. *J Am Acad Dermatol.* 1998;39(4, pt 1):597-602.
35. Fiedler VC. Alopecia areata: current therapy. *J Invest Dermatol.* 1991;96(5):S69-S70.
36. Price VH. Treatment of hair loss. *N Engl J Med.* 1999;341(13):964-973.
37. Whiting DA. The treatment of alopecia areata. *Cutis.* 1987;40(3):247-250.
38. Chu TW, AlJasser M, Alharbi A, et al. Benefit of different concentrations of intralesional triamcinolone acetonide in alopecia areata: an intrasubject pilot study. *J Am Acad Dermatol.* 2015;73(2):338-340.
39. Singh S. Role of platelet-rich plasma in chronic alopecia areata: our centre experience. *Indian J Plast Surg.* 2015;48(1):57-59.
40. Donovan J. Successful treatment of corticosteroid-resistant ophiasis-type alopecia areata (AA) with platelet-rich plasma (PRP). *JAAD Case Rep.* 2015;1(5):305-307.
41. Bagherani N. Is platelet-rich plasma effective in the treatment of alopecia areata? *Dermatol Ther.* 2016;29(4):284.
42. Spano F, Donovan JC. Alopecia areata: part 2: treatment. *Can Fam Physician.* 2015;61(9):757-761.
43. Trink A, Sorbellini E, Bezzola P, et al. A randomized, double-blind, placebo- and active-controlled, half-head study to evaluate the effects of platelet-rich plasma on alopecia areata. *Br J Dermatol.* 2013;169(3):690-694.
44. Price VH. Topical minoxidil in extensive alopecia areata, including 3-year follow-up. *Dermatologica.* 1987;175(suppl 2):36-41.
45. Price VH. Double-blind, placebo-controlled evaluation of topical minoxidil in extensive alopecia areata. *J Am Acad Dermatol.* 1987;16(3, pt 2):730-736.
46. Vila TO, Camacho Martinez FM. Bimatoprost in the treatment of eyelash universalis alopecia areata. *Int J Trichology.* 2010;2(2):86-88.
47. Ross EK, Bolduc C, Lui H, et al. Lack of efficacy of topical latanoprost in the treatment of eyebrow alopecia areata. *J Am Acad Dermatol.* 2005;53(6):1095-1096.
48. Roseborough I, Lee H, Chwalek J, et al. Lack of efficacy of topical latanoprost and bimatoprost ophthalmic solutions in promoting eyelash growth in patients with alopecia areata. *J Am Acad Dermatol.* 2009;60(4):705-706.
49. Faghihi G, Andalib F, Asilian A. The efficacy of latanoprost in the treatment of alopecia areata of eyelashes and eyebrows. *Eur J Dermatol.* 2009;19(6):586-587.
50. Morhenn VB, Orenberg EK, Kaplan J, et al. Inhibition of a Langerhans cell-mediated immune response by treatment modalities useful in psoriasis. *J Invest Dermatol.* 1983;81(1):23-27.
51. Fiedler-Weiss VC, Buys CM. Evaluation of anthralin in the treatment of alopecia areata. *Arch Dermatol.* 1987;123(11):1491-1493.
52. Schmoeckel C, Weissmann I, Plewig G, et al. Treatment of alopecia areata by anthralin-induced dermatitis. *Arch Dermatol.* 1979;115(10):1254-1255.
53. Happle R, Klein HM, Macher E. Topical immunotherapy changes the composition of the peribulbar infiltrate in alopecia areata. *Arch Dermatol Res.* 1986;278(3):214-218.
54. MacDonald N, Wiseman MC, Shapiro J. Alopecia areata: topical immunotherapy—application and practical problems. *J Cutan Med Surg.* 1999;3(suppl 3):S36-S40.
55. Shapiro J, Sundberg JP, Bissonnette R, et al. Alopecia areata-like hair loss in C3H/HeJ mice and DEBR rats can be reversed using topical diphencyprone. *J Investig Dermatol Symp Proc.* 1999;4(3):239.
56. Shapiro J. Assessment of the patient with alopecia. In: *Hair Loss: Principles of Diagnosis and Management of Alopecia.* London, UK: Martin Dunitz; 2002.
57. Krook G. Treatment of alopecia areata with Kromayer's ultra-violet lamp. *Acta Derm Venereol.* 1961;41:178-181.
58. Mitchell AJ, Douglass MC. Topical photochemotherapy for alopecia areata. *J Am Acad Dermatol.* 1985;12(4):644-649.
59. Gupta AK, Ellis CN, Cooper KD, et al. Oral cyclosporine for the treatment of alopecia areata. A clinical and immunohistochemical analysis. *J Am Acad Dermatol.* 1990;22(2, pt 1):242-250.
60. Jabbari A, Dai Z, Xing L, et al. Reversal of alopecia areata following treatment with the JAK1/2 inhibitor baricitinib. *EBioMedicine.* 2015;2(4):351-355.
61. Harris JE, Rashighi M, Nguyen N, et al. Rapid skin repigmentation on oral ruxolitinib in a patient with coexistent vitiligo and alopecia areata (AA). *J Am Acad Dermatol.* 2016;74(2):370-371.
62. Anzengruber F, Maul JT, Kamarachev J, et al. Transient efficacy of tofacitinib in alopecia areata universalis. *Case Rep Dermatol.* 2016;8(1):102-106.
63. Higgins E, Al Shehri T, McAleer MA, et al. Use of ruxolitinib to successfully treat chronic mucocutaneous candidiasis caused by gain-of-function signal transducer and activator of transcription 1 (STAT1) mutation. *J Allergy Clin Immunol.* 2015;135:551-553.
64. Pieri L, Guglielmelli P, Vannucchi AM. Ruxolitinib-induced reversal of alopecia universalis in a patient with essential thrombocythemia. *Am J Hematol.* 2015;90:82-83.
65. Craiglow BG, King BA. Killing two birds with one stone: oral tofacitinib reverses alopecia universalis in a patient with plaque psoriasis. *J Invest Dermatol.* 2014;134:2988-2990.

Chapter 88 :: Cicatricial Alopecias :: Nina Otberg & Jerry Shapiro

第八十八章

瘢痕性脱发

中文导读

瘢痕性脱发是指一组特发性炎症性疾病，炎症过程导致毛囊干细胞结构的永久性破坏，再被纤维组织替代。瘢痕性脱发是一组导致永久性脱发的头皮疾病。图88-1展示了脱发的亚型及瘢痕性脱发的分型。把瘢痕性脱发分为原发性瘢痕性脱发和继发性瘢痕性脱发两部分来讲述。

第一部分：原发性瘢痕性脱发，从流行病学、分型、病因及发病机制、临床特点、诊断、预后/临床病程、治疗及其对应的常见皮肤疾病等方面来进行介绍。

疾病分为三型：淋巴细胞为主型、中性粒细胞为主型及混合型，具体见表88-1；流行病学方面是未知的；病因及发病机制也尚不明确，本章讲述了毛囊各部分炎症浸润可能导致的脱发情况，有推测认为是毛囊峡部炎症浸润损伤引起的；临床特点方面，介绍了从体格检查中此病常发生的头皮部位、脱发斑块肉眼可见情况到其镜下改变；原发性瘢痕性脱发诊断要依据病史、头皮检查，尤其头皮活检是必要的；强调了一旦毛囊被纤维组织破坏和取代，毛发就没有再生的希望，更严重的甚至会产生永久性脱发所致的美容方面问题。治疗方面，先讲述了治疗原则，强调主要目的是阻止炎症和疾病的进一步发展，如果脱发已经很严重和/或药物治疗失败，应建议患者使用伪装技术，而头发修复术是主要治疗方式，但治疗后存在复发的可能。

接下来，详细介绍了各型对应的常见皮肤疾病的临床表现、组织病理及其治疗管理。首先是淋巴细胞为主的原发性瘢痕性脱发：慢性皮肤红斑狼疮（盘状红斑狼疮）、扁平苔藓和额叶纤维化性脱发、经典的布罗克假性脱发、中央离心性瘢痕性脱发、粘蛋白性脱发、棘突毛囊角化病；其次是中性粒细胞为主的原发性瘢痕性脱发：脱发性毛囊炎、解剖性毛囊炎；最后介绍了混合型原发性瘢痕性脱发：颈项部瘢痕性痤疮、坏死型痤疮、糜烂性脓疱性皮肤病。最后通过表88-2提出了需要与原发性瘢痕性脱发相鉴别的其他疾病。

第二部分：继发性瘢痕性脱发，从病因及发病机制、临床特点、诊断、预后/临床病程、治疗及其对应的常见皮肤疾病等方面来进行介绍。

病因和发病机制方面，提出其是由头皮的各种其他改变引起的，而与毛囊无关，病因发生在毛囊单位之外，只引起毛囊的偶然破坏。详细病因分类作者列于表88-3。临床特点中至关重要的是病史；而有广泛的疤痕伴纤维化，弹性纤维和附件结构消失的组织学特点也是一个重要诊断条件。预后及临床病程主要取决于基础疾病的进程，作者强调一旦毛囊被纤维组织破坏和取代，毛发就没有再生的希望。治疗分为疾病早期和后期，在疾病早期主要是针对病因的治疗，疾病后期则主要采用头发修复术。与原发性瘢痕性脱发类似，列出了导致继发性瘢痕性脱发的常见疾病。

首先介绍头癣病因、临床表现、诊断及其治疗。接下来是创伤性脱发，包括外伤、牵引性脱发、拔毛癖、压力性脱发。通过表88-4提出了需要与继发性瘢痕性脱发相鉴别的其他疾病。

〔简 丹〕

AT-A-GLANCE

- Scarring alopecia occurs in a heterogeneous etiologic group of various disorders.
- The inflammatory process leads to permanent destruction of hair follicular stem cell structure and subsequent replacement with fibrous tissue.
- The destructive process can occur as a primary or secondary cicatricial alopecia.
- Loss of hair-producing attribute finalizes this process and results clinically in permanent alopecia.
- No evidence-based treatment is available.

Cicatricial or scarring alopecias comprise a diverse group of scalp disorders that result in permanent hair loss (Fig. 88-1). The destructive process can occur as a primary or secondary cicatricial alopecia. *Primary cicatricial alopecia* refers to a group of idiopathic inflammatory diseases, characterized by a folliculocentric inflammatory process that ultimately destroys the hair follicle. *Secondary cicatricial alopecias* can be caused by almost any cutaneous inflammatory process of the scalp skin or by physical trauma, which injures the skin and skin appendages. Regardless of whether a cicatricial alopecia is primary or secondary in nature, all scarring alopecias are characterized clinically by a loss of follicular ostia and pathologically by a replacement of hair follicles with fibrous tissue.

Cicatricial alopecias are psychosocially distressing for the affected patient and medico-surgically challenging for the treating physician.

PRIMARY CICATRICIAL ALOPECIAS

EPIDEMIOLOGY

Inflammatory cicatricial alopecias are rare skin diseases. The epidemiology is basically unknown.

CLASSIFICATION[1]

Table 88-1 outlines the classification of primary cicatricial alopecias.

ETIOLOGY AND PATHOGENESIS

Little is known about most of the etiologies. Hence the exact mechanisms that cause follicle stem cell destruction are not completely understood, and there is no cure as of this writing. Primary cicatricial alopecias are characterized by an inflammatory infiltrate affecting the upper, permanent portion of the follicle referred to as the infundibulum, and below it, the isthmus of the follicle. The isthmus is the home of pluripotent hair stem cells, which are found in the bulge region where the arrector pili muscle attaches to the outer root sheath. Pluripotent hair follicle stem cells are responsible for the renewal of the upper part of the hair follicle and sebaceous glands, and for the restoration of the lower cyclical component of the follicles at the onset of a new anagen period.[1,2] Damage to the bulge area and the sebaceous gland with the isthmus may result in an incomplete hair cycle and can be associated with chronic follicular inflammation and foreign-body reaction.[3] It has been assumed that scarring hair loss is a consequence of damage to the isthmus, affecting either stem cells or sebaceous glands.[4-7]

CLINICAL FEATURES

Primary cicatricial alopecia usually affects the central and parietal scalp before progressing to other sites of the scalp. Isolated alopecic patches showing atrophy and a lack of follicular ostia with inflammatory changes, such as diffuse or perifollicular erythema, follicular hyperkeratosis, pigment changes, tufting, and pustules, provide hints to the diagnosis.[8,9] However, clinically visible inflammatory change might be absent in the affected lesions and may present histologically

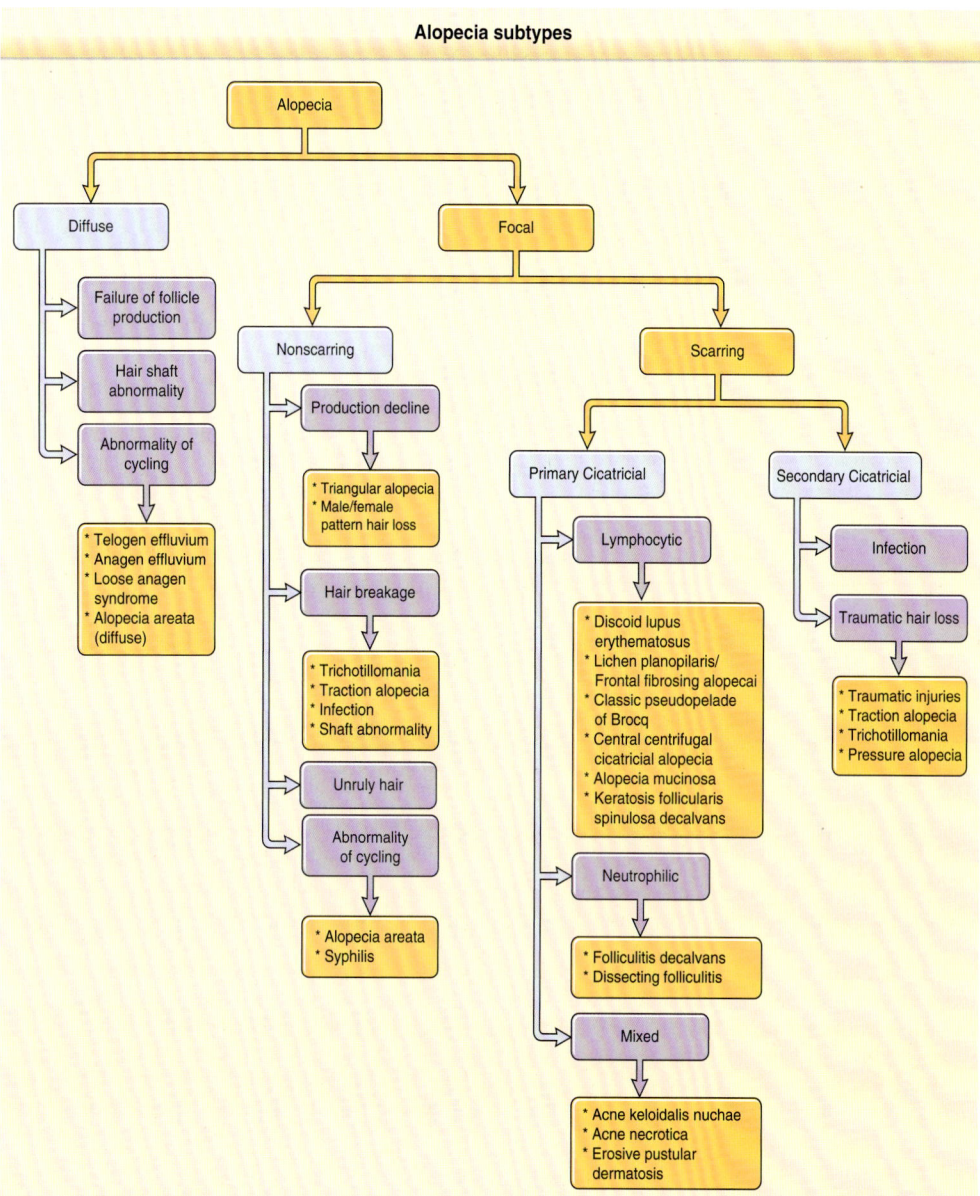

Figure 88-1 Alopecia subtypes.

as inflammatory infiltrates in the deep dermis and subcutaneous tissue.

DIAGNOSIS

Diagnostic tools such as a 10-fold magnifying dermatoscope with and without polarized light can help to identify the presence or absence of follicular ostia, perifollicular erythema, and follicular hyperkeratosis in the affected areas.

A thorough examination of the entire scalp, a detailed clinical history, as well as skin biopsies of an active lesion are crucial in the correct diagnosis of most cicatricial alopecias. Patient-reported symptoms, such as itching or pain, might be used as approximate indicators of disease activity but also can be completely absent. Presence of other indirectly related symptoms, such as sun sensitivity, can also help support a particular diagnosis (eg, discoid lupus erythematosus [DLE]).

A scalp biopsy is necessary to confirm a scarring alopecia diagnosis. The following recommendations were developed at the consensus meeting on cicatricial alopecia[1] in February 2001: One 4-mm punch biopsy including subcutaneous tissue should be taken from a clinically active area, processed for horizontal sections and stained with hematoxylin and eosin. Elastin (acid alcoholic orcein), mucin, and periodic acid–Schiff stains may provide additional diagnosis-defining information.

TABLE 88-1
Classification of Primary Cicatricial Alopecias

Lymphocytic Primary Cicatricial Alopecia
- Chronic cutaneous lupus erythematosus (discoid lupus erythematosus)
- Lichen planopilaris
- Classic lichen planopilaris
- Frontal fibrosing alopecia
- Graham-Little syndrome
- Classic pseudopelade of Brocq
- Central centrifugal cicatricial alopecia
- Alopecia mucinosa
- Keratosis follicularis spinulosa decalvans

Neutrophilic Primary Cicatricial Alopecia
- Folliculitis decalvans
- Dissecting cellulites/folliculitis (perifolliculitis abscedens et suffodiens)

Mixed Cicatricial Alopecia
- Folliculitis (acne) keloidalis
- Folliculitis (acne) necrotica
- Erosive pustular dermatosis

A second 4-mm punch biopsy from a clinically active disease-affected area should be cut vertically into 2 equal pieces. One half provides tissue for transverse cut routine histologic sections, and the other half can be used for direct immunofluorescence studies.[10-12]

PROGNOSIS/CLINICAL COURSE

Once the hair follicle is destroyed and replaced by fibrous tissue, there is no hope for hair regrowth. Various medical treatment options may fail and the inflammatory process may continue and leave the patient with a disfiguring permanent alopecia.

TREATMENT

The main goal in treating primary cicatricial alopecia is to stop the inflammation and further progression of the disease. If hair loss is already extensive and/or medical treatment fails, patients should be advised about camouflage techniques, such as hairpieces and wigs. Women with extensive scarring lesion on the crown and vertex benefit highly from a well-designed hairpiece, which can look very natural, particularly if the frontal hair line is preserved and is usually more comfortable to wear than a full wig.

Hair restoration surgery, including hair transplantation and scalp reduction, can be an option for burned out cicatricial alopecia. No disease activity should occur on the scalp for at least 1 year after therapy after which hair restoration surgery can begin. The patient has to be warned about a possible limited graft survival and disease recurrence, which seems to be higher in neutrophilic primary scarring alopecia.

LYMPHOCYTIC PRIMARY CICATRICIAL ALOPECIAS

CHRONIC CUTANEOUS LUPUS ERYTHEMATOSUS (DISCOID LUPUS ERYTHEMATOSUS)

DLE, together with lichen planopilaris (LPP), is the most common cause of inflammatory cicatricial alopecia.[8] Females are more often affected than males and the disease is more common in adults (with first onset typically at 20 to 40 years of age) than in children.[13-15] Of patients with DLE, approximately 26% to 31% of children and 5% to 10% of adults will develop systemic lupus erythematosus.[15,16] Patients with DLE also have a higher incidence of concurrent alopecia areata. Moreover, DLE also is associated with verruciform xanthoma and papulonodular dermal mucinosis.[17]

Clinical Presentation: DLE usually presents with 1 or more erythematous, atrophic, and alopecic patches on the scalp. Follicular hyperkeratosis, hyperpigmentation, hypopigmentation, and telangiectasia can be present.[3,18] Hyperpigmentation is frequently found in the center of the lesion. Active lesions can be sensitive or pruritic, and the patient might report a worsening after ultraviolet light exposure (Fig. 88-2).

Pathology: Characteristic features of early, active DLE lesions are lymphocyte-mediated interface dermatitis with vacuolar degeneration of the basal cell layer and necrotic keratinocytes, a thickening of the basement membrane and destruction of sebaceous glands. Elastic fibers are frequently destroyed throughout the reticular dermis.[5,10] The lymphocytic infiltrate is predominantly found in the upper part of the follicle but also can be found in deeper parts of the follicle, in the interfollicular epidermis, and around the periadnexal vessels.[19-22] Direct immunofluorescence typically shows a linear granular deposition of immunoglobulin (Ig) G and C3 at the dermoepidermal junction. IgM, C1q, and, rarely, IgA also can be found.

Management and Treatment: Hydroxychloroquine at a dose of 200 to 400 mg daily in adults or 4

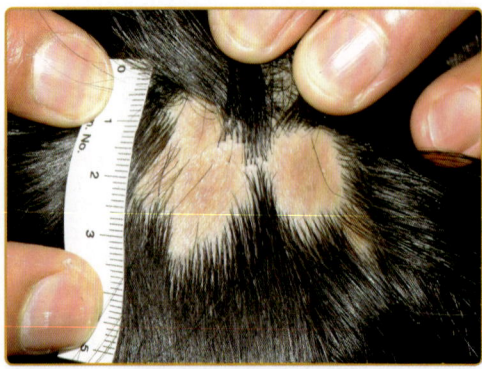

Figure 88-2 Discoid lupus erythematosus.

to 6 mg/kg in children is highly effective at managing. A baseline ophthalmologic examination and complete blood count is required before the therapy is started.[13,15] Bridge therapy with oral prednisone (1 mg/kg) tapered over the first 8 weeks of treatment might be helpful in adult patients with rapidly progressive disease.[8,9] In limited or slowly progressive DLE, intralesional triamcinolone acetonide should be used at a concentration of 10 mg/mL every 4 to 6 weeks, alone or in addition to oral therapy.[8] Intralesional triamcinolone acetonide can be used with or without topical class I or class II corticosteroids. Topical corticosteroids alone also are effective at managing in milder forms of DLE.[9,10,15,20] Oral acitretin and isotretinoin have also shown some effectiveness at managing.[23,24] Immunosuppressive therapies, such as mycophenolate mofetil, methotrexate, and azathioprine, should only be considered if the above therapies fail. Multimodal aggressive therapy in rapidly progressive DLE might reverse early alopecic patches and save hair follicles from the destructive process.[25]

LICHEN PLANOPILARIS AND FRONTAL FIBROSING ALOPECIA

LPP is a follicular variant of lichen planus. Together with DLE, this is the most common cause of primary cicatricial alopecia. LPP can be divided into classic LPP, Graham-Little syndrome, and frontal fibrosing alopecia (FFA). The typical age of onset of classic LPP is around the fifth decade, and women are more often affected than men. Extracranial lichen planus may occur in up to 28% of patients.[6,26,27] Graham-Little syndrome is a very rare condition that predominantly affects female adults. It is characterized by LPP of the scalp, noncicatricial of the eyebrows, axilla, and groin, and keratosis pilaris.

FFA was first described by Kossard in 1992.[28] FFA predominantly affects postmenopausal women. However, some cases of affected men or premenopausal women are reported.[29-31] Although as of this writing there are no epidemiologic data on the incidence or prevalence of FFA, FFA seems to be fast on the rise. In many hair clinics, FFA has become the most frequently seen form of cicatricial alopecia.[32] Causes and trigger factors and whether FFA is a variant of LPP or its own entity is as of this writing unknown.

Lichenoid drug eruptions can be triggered by many drugs. Some of the most common drugs that cause lichenoid drug eruption are gold, antimalarials, and captopril. Actinic lichenoid drug eruption is confined to sun-exposed sites. The most likely drugs to cause lichenoid drug eruption are quinine and thiazide diuretics.[33-35] Whether drugs play a role as trigger factors in LPP and FFA is not clear.

Clinical Presentations of Lichen Planopilaris and Frontal Fibrosing Alopecia:
Classic LPP typically starts at the crown and vertex area. In classic LPP, the affected areas usually show perifollicular erythema and follicular hyperkeratosis. The alopecic areas of LPP are often smaller, irregularly shaped and interconnected, which can lead to a reticulated clinical pattern as compared to DLE. However, overlapping clinical features with those of DLE are frequently seen. Patients complain about itching, burning sensations and sensitivity of the scalp (Fig. 88-3).

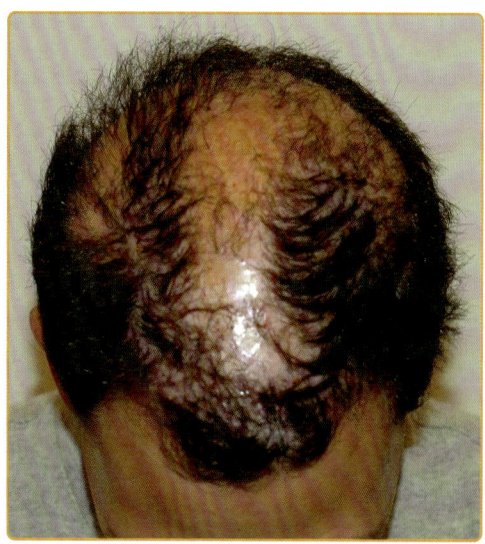

Figure 88-3 Extensive lichen planopilaris.

FFA is characterized by a frontal, band-like or circumferential scarring alopecia.[5] In some cases, a few hairs are spared in the original frontal hairline. Follicular hyperkeratosis and perifollicular erythema may be found in a band-like pattern in the frontal hairline. Alopecia of the eyebrows is also frequently seen in FFA (Fig. 88-4).

Graham-Little syndrome presents with lesions of classic LPP on the scalp, nonscarring alopecia of axillae, pubic area, and eyebrows, as well as keratosis pilaris of the trunk and extremities.

Pathology: LPP and FFA show similar histopathologic features. A lymphocytic infiltrate and interface dermatitis are predominantly found in and around the upper permanent part of the hair follicle. Unlike DLE, the vascular plexus is not affected by inflammation

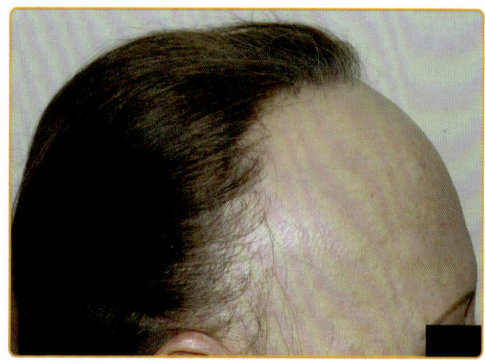

Figure 88-4 Frontal fibrosing alopecia.

and mucin deposits are absent.[5] Direct immunofluorescence typically shows globular cytoid depositions of IgM, and, rarely, IgA, IgG, or C3, in the dermis around the infundibulum.[36]

Management and Treatment: First-line treatment for moderately active classic LPP lesions is intralesional triamcinolone acetonide at a concentration of 10 mg/mL every 4 to 6 weeks or in combination with topical class I or class II corticosteroids.[8,24] For FFA near the face, triamcinolone acetonide at 2.5 mg/mL injected 1 cm behind the hair line should be used. Topical minoxidil may be given in patients with concomitant androgenetic alopecia to improve thickness of the remaining hair. Newer studies suggest preliminarily that injections of platelet-rich plasma might be useful as additional treatment.[37] More studies are required. Studies on the efficacy of oral medication are limited. Oral cyclosporine, retinoids, antimalarials, and griseofulvin[3,18,38-41] have a positive effect in patients with rapidly progressive LPP. Oral corticosteroids as bridge therapy in the first weeks of treatment might be considered in very active cases. The treatment of Graham-Little syndrome is typically similar to the management of classic LPP. In FFA a lower dose of intralesional triamcinolone acetonide (2.5 to 5 mg/mL) and topical application of minoxidil or topical tacrolimus can be considered, although no effective treatment has yet been reported.

CLASSIC PSEUDOPELADE OF BROCQ

Pseudopelade of Brocq (PPB) is classified as an idiopathic lymphocytic primary cicatricial alopecia that predominantly affects the scalp. Women between 30 and 50 years of age are most frequently affected.[6]

Clinical Presentation: PPB usually affects the vertex and occipital area of the scalp. It presents with small flesh-toned alopecic patches with irregular margins. This pattern has been described as "foot prints in the snow."[42] PPB can also present as a noninflammatory, centrifugally spreading, patch of alopecia, which might be seen as a variant of central centrifugal cicatricial alopecia (CCCA) in whites. Follicular hyperkeratosis and perifollicular or diffuse erythema are mostly absent.[18] Clinically, the features may overlap with LPP.

Pathology: Early PPB lesions typically show a sparse to moderate lymphocytic infiltrate around the follicular infundibulum with a complete destruction of the sebaceous glands.[43] In later disease stages, hair follicles are completely replaced by fibrous tracts. Unlike DLE and LPP, interface dermatitis is usually absent and the elastic fibers are preserved and thickened in PPB.[44]

Management and Treatment: Intralesional triamcinolone acetonide at a concentration of 10 mg/mL every 4 to 6 weeks in combination with topical corticosteroids is the treatment of first choice. Hydroxychloroquine, oral prednisone, and isotretinoin have shown some effectiveness in treating PPB.[6,18,45,46]

CENTRAL CENTRIFUGAL CICATRICIAL ALOPECIA

CCCA is the most common form of primary cicatricial alopecia in women of African descent. The etiology of CCCA is not fully understood. An autosomal mode of inheritance, chemical hair grooming practices, and traction-inducing hair styles seem to be the major pathogenic factors.[20,47-50] CCCA is rarely seen in whites (sometimes called "central elliptical pseudopelade") and African American men. Because of clinical and histopathologic similarities, there is a debate as to whether or not CCCA is a variant of PPB.

Clinical Presentation: CCCA presents with a skin-colored patch of scarring alopecia on the crown, gradually progressing centrifugally to the parietal areas. In 2008, Olsen and associates developed a photographic scale to identify the pattern and severity of CCCA in the general community.[51] Perifollicular hyperpigmentation and polytrichia might be present.[8] Patients may complain about pain, itching, tenderness, and "pins-and-needle" sensations (Fig. 88-5).[52]

Pathology: Pathologic features of CCCA include dermal hyalinization, hair fiber granulomas, loss of follicular epithelium, follicular lymphocytic inflammation of the lower infundibulum and up to the isthmus, premature desquamation of the inner root sheath, and fibrous connective tissue. Similarities to PPB have been discussed.[3,20]

Management and Treatment: Early diagnosis is crucial in the management of CCCA. Early screening is suggested because CCCA has been described in children.[53] More natural, less traumatizing hair care practices are recommended.[10,18,54,55] Screening of family members also may be useful

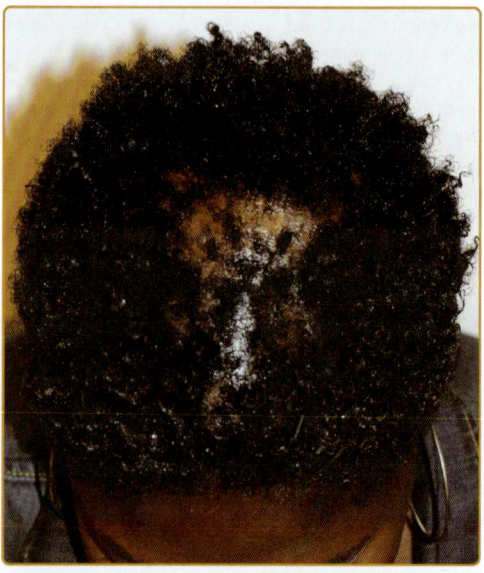

Figure 88-5 Central centrifugal cicatricial alopecia.

because of the genetic pathogenicity.[48] Topical and intralesional corticosteroids, and tetracycline are effective in active progressive cases.[20] Systemic treatment with tetracyclines, hydroxychloroquine, immunosuppressive medication (eg, mycophenolate mofetil and cyclosporine), and antiandrogens also have been described to be successful.[55] Wigs and hairpieces can help camouflage the alopecia and are frequently used by women with CCCA.

ALOPECIA MUCINOSA

Alopecia mucinosa can present as indurated, well-demarcated erythematosus or skin-colored patches of scarring or nonscarring alopecia that can be accompanied by diffuse hair loss[56] and alopecia of the eyebrows.[57] Grouped follicular papules, follicular cysts, and follicular hyperkeratosis may be present in some cases. Early lesions of alopecia mucinosa show mucin deposition in the outer root sheath and replacement of the entire pilosebaceous unit by pools of mucin in more advanced lesions.[5,57] Strictly speaking, alopecia mucinosa is not a primary cicatricial alopecia because the hair follicle is not replaced by a true scar.[5]

Alopecia mucinosa can occur idiopathically or in the setting of cutaneous T-cell lymphoma or mycosis fungoides.[58] Cell atypia and monoclonal populations of T-lymphocytes can be present in the idiopathic form of alopecia mucinosa as well as in mycosis fungoides.[58]

Management and Treatment: A complete workup is necessary to rule out an underlying malignancy such as mycosis fungoides and Sézary syndrome, its advanced end point. Oral corticosteroids, minocycline, and isotretinoin are effective. Topical and intralesional corticosteroids, dapsone, indomethacin, and light therapy also have been used with variable outcomes.[59]

KERATOSIS FOLLICULARIS SPINULOSA DECALVANS

Keratosis follicularis spinulosa decalvans together with keratosis atrophicans faciei (also called *ulerythema ophryogenes* or *keratosis pilaris rubra atrophicans faciei*) and atrophoderma vermiculata belongs to a heterogeneous group of congenital follicular keratinizing disorders. Keratosis follicularis spinulosa decalvans is X-linked, usually develops during adolescence, and mostly presents with scarring alopecic patches, follicular hyperkeratosis, and, rarely, pustules.[5] Eyebrow and eyelash involvement also can be present.

Keratosis follicularis spinulosa decalvans shows an inflammatory infiltrate consisting of lymphocytes and neutrophils in the infundibular area in early lesions. Later, the infiltrate is predominantly lymphocytic and the follicle is eventually replaced by fibrous tissue.

The condition may improve with age. Careful calculation of risks and benefits in the treatment of children, teenagers, and young adults is important. Topical and intralesional corticosteroids as well as oral retinoids have shown some effectiveness.[60]

NEUTROPHILIC PRIMARY CICATRICIAL ALOPECIA

FOLLICULITIS DECALVANS

Approximately, 11% of all primary cicatricial alopecia cases are diagnosed with folliculitis decalvans (FD).[3,6] FD predominantly occurs in young and middle-aged adults with a slight preference for the male gender.

A bacterial infection involving *Staphylococcus aureus*, in combination with hypersensitivity reaction to "superantigens" and defect in host cell–mediated immunity have all been suspected as possible pathogenetic factors.[3,61,62]

Clinical Presentation: FD frequently starts at the vertex area of the scalp with erythematous alopecic patches, follicular pustules and follicular hyperkeratosis. Tufted folliculitis is typically found in FD but can also occur in other cicatricial inflammatory alopecias. Tufted folliculitis is characterized by multiple hairs (5 to 15) emerging from a single, dilated, follicular orifice. In older lesions, pustules might be absent but progressive scarring may still continue (Fig. 88-6). An overlap with acne keloidalis is possible as some patients with acne keloidalis not only develop cicatricial lesion on the nape of the neck but also develop progressive cicatricial alopecia that resembles FD in other areas of the scalp. Patients frequently complain about pain, itching, and/or burning sensations.

Pathology: Early lesions are characterized by keratin aggregation in the infundibulum with numerous intraluminal neutrophils, as well as an intrafollicular and perifollicular neutrophilic infiltrate.[3,5,18] Sebaceous glands are destroyed early. In advanced lesions, the infiltrate may consist of neutrophils, lymphocytes, and plasma cells, and extend into the dermis.[8,18] Hair-shaft granulomas with foreign-body giant cells are frequently found.[3,18] In end-stage lesions, follicular and interstitial dermal fibrosis, as well as hypertrophic scarring, can be observed.[18]

Management and Treatment: Treatment of FD in general is difficult and disease activity can be

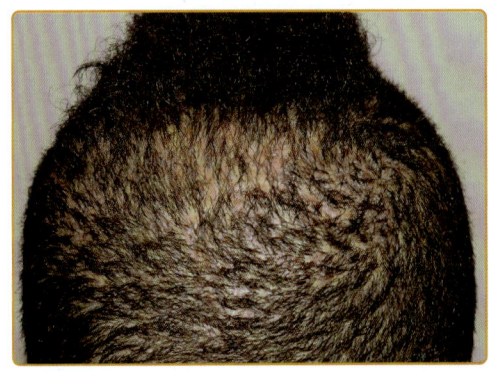

Figure 88-6 Folliculitis decalvans.

noted over many years. Bacterial cultures with the testing of antibiotic sensitivities are recommended. Eradication of *S. aureus* with minocycline, erythromycin, cephalosporins, and sulfamethoxazole-trimethoprim has shown some effectiveness. Relapse can often be observed after the antibiotics are discontinued.[9,61,63] If so, the patient might have to stay on low-dose antibiotics for many years. Although rifampin in combination with clindamycin has shown good response, this combination also has shown a higher incidence of side effects.[61,64] Oral fucidic acid alone or in combination with other agents has also shown to be effective in some patients.[65] Oral therapy should be combined with topical antibiotics such as mupirocin, 1.5% fusidic acid, and 2% erythromycin,[64,65] and antibacterial cleansers. Intralesional triamcinolone acetonide at a concentration of 10 mg/mL every 4 to 6 weeks might help to reduce the inflammation and symptoms such as itching, burning, and pain.[6,9] Intranasal eradication of *S. aureus* with topical antibacterial agents are described as useful.[18]

DISSECTING FOLLICULITIS

Dissecting folliculitis (or *dissecting cellulites* or *perifolliculitis capitis abscedens et suffodiens of Hoffman*) is related to acne conglobata and hidradenitis suppurativa. These 3 diseases have been described as the follicular occlusion triad. Dissecting folliculitis predominantly occurs in young men between 18 and 40 years of age.[8] African American men seem to be more commonly affected than white men. The pathogenesis of dissecting folliculitis may include follicular occlusion, seborrhea, androgens, and secondary bacterial overpopulation, as well as an abnormal host response to bacterial antigens.[66-73]

Clinical Presentation: Dissecting folliculitis typically presents with fluctuating nodules, abscesses, and sinuses, which frequently show spontaneous discharge of pus, as well as with erythematous, follicular papules and pustules. Initial lesions are mostly found on the vertex and occipital scalp. Multifocal lesions can form an intercommunicating ridge and seropurulent exudates can be discharged when pressure is applied to 1 region of the scalp (Fig. 88-7). The lesions can be pruritic and tender. Chronic and relapsing courses results in cicatricial alopecia that can occur as hypertrophic or keloidal scars.[73]

Pathology: The main histologic feature is an intrafollicular and perifollicular neutrophilic infiltrate with follicular occlusion in early lesions.[5] In more advanced stages, interconnecting sinus tracts lined by squamous epithelium, follicular perforation, and perifollicular and deep dermal abscesses are typical findings.[5,18,22]

Management and Treatment: Multimodal treatment has been reported with successful results, such as systemic antibiotics (minocycline, tetracycline, cloxacillin, erythromycin, cephalosporin, or clindamycin with or without rifampin), intralesional corticosteroids, and oral prednisolone.[74,75] The benefits of systemic antibiotics are most likely a result of their antiinflammatory effects rather than their antibacterial action. Isotretinoin at a dose of 0.5 to 1 mg/kg/day prolongs remission.[76,77] Incision and drainage of therapy-resistant, painful nodules, marsupialization with curettage of the cyst wall, and complete scalp extirpation with skin grafting have been reported, but should be an exception for extreme and therapy refractory cases.[77-80]

MIXED PRIMARY CICATRICIAL ALOPECIAS

ACNE KELOIDALIS NUCHAE

Acne keloidalis nuchae predominantly occurs in African American men 14 to 25 years of age. This idiopathic primary cicatricial alopecia might be triggered by trauma (shirt collars) or infection (*Demodex* or bacteria). Clinically, acne keloidalis nuchae presents with skin-colored follicular papules, pustules, and plaques, as well as keloid-like scarred lesions in the occipital scalp (Fig. 88-8). Histologically, acne keloidalis is characterized by an acute inflammation with neutrophilic

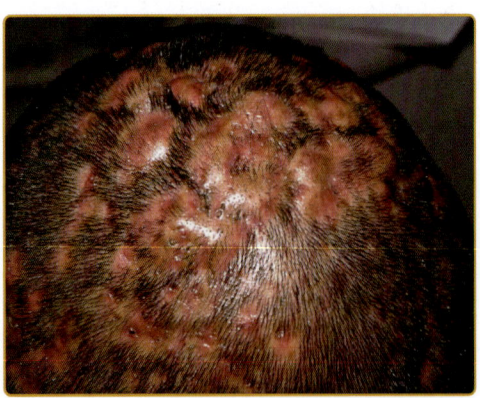

Figure 88-7 Dissecting cellulitis.

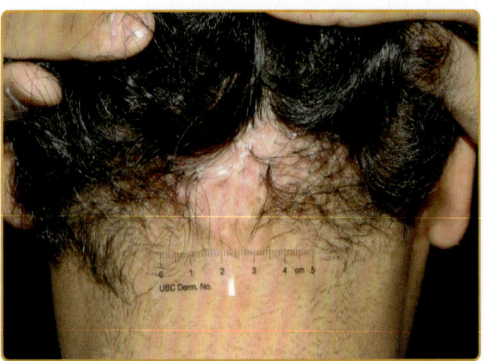

Figure 88-8 Acne keloidalis nuchae.

or lymphocytic infiltration and chronic granulomatous inflammation around the isthmus and the lower infundibulum. Monthly intralesional triamcinolone acetonide (10 to 40 mg/mL) alone or combined with topical 2% clindamycin or oral (tetracyclines) antibiotics is the treatment of first choice.[3,10,20,81,82] Class I or class II topical steroids alone or in combination with topical antibiotics for mild cases of acne keloidalis nuchae, as well as topical retinoids, cryotherapy, and laser therapy, have shown some success. Surgical excision of extensive keloidal lesions may be considered but should be reserved for therapy refractory, extensive, and symptomatic cases.

ACNE NECROTICA (VARIOLIFORMIS)

Acne necrotica varioliformis is a very rare, chronic condition, which predominantly occurs in adults. Frontal and parietal scalp, as well as seborrheic areas of the face are most commonly affected. Acne necrotica presents with umbilicated, pruritic, or painful papules that undergo central necrosis. The condition leaves varioliform, or smallpox-like scars.[83,84] Histology shows a suppurative, necrotic, infundibular folliculitis with lymphocytic or mixed inflammatory infiltrate.[84]

Oral antibiotics, isotretinoin, and intralesional or topical corticosteroids have shown success.[85] Excision of larger scarred areas can be considered.

EROSIVE PUSTULAR DERMATOSIS

Erosive pustular dermatosis is an uncommon disorder predominantly occurring in elderly women.[86,87] The characteristic lesion is a suppurative, necrotic, erosive papule or plaque.[86,88] Histology of early lesions is nonspecific, but older lesions show an extensive, chronic, mixed inflammatory infiltrate in the dermis, and later dermal fibrosis. Treatment includes class I or class II topical steroids with or without topical antibiotics, systemic antibiotics, and oral isotretinoin.[86,88]

DIFFERENTIAL DIAGNOSIS

Table 88-2 outlines the differential diagnosis of primary cicatricial alopecias.

TABLE 88-2
Differential Diagnosis for Primary Cicatricial Alopecias

- Alopecia areata
- Secondary cicatricial alopecia
- Temporal triangular alopecia
- Trichotillomania
- Secondary syphilis (alopecia areolaris)

SECONDARY CICATRICIAL ALOPECIA

ETIOLOGY AND PATHOGENESIS

In secondary cicatricial alopecias, permanent hair loss is caused by various other scalp conditions not related to the hair follicle. In these conditions, the primary event develops outside the follicular unit, and leads to incidental destruction of the follicle. Possible causes are congenital defects, trauma, inflammatory conditions, infections, neoplasms, and, rarely, drugs (Table 88-3). Permanent, chronic traction alopecia and scars from surgery can be considered secondary scarring alopecias as well.[89]

CLINICAL FEATURES

A thorough clinical history is crucial in the diagnosis of secondary cicatricial alopecia. Diagnosis in early stages can sometimes be made based on specific clinical and histologic features of the underlying disorder. Follicular orifices are lost clinically, and histology shows extensive scarring with fibrosis, loss of elastic fibers and adnexal structures.[89]

PROGNOSIS AND CLINICAL COURSE

Prognosis and clinical course of secondary cicatricial alopecia depend on the underlying disease. Once scar tissue has formed and the adnexal structures are destroyed no hair regrowth can be expected.

TREATMENT

Treatment is specific in active conditions, whereas in localized end-stage lesions, specific medical treatment is no longer efficient and hair restoration surgery techniques become the mainstay of therapy.

TINEA CAPITIS

Tinea capitis is a common cause of hair loss in children secondary to an infection with dermatophytes species. The etiologic agent varies in different parts of the world. Presently, *Trichophyton tonsurans* accounts for approximately 90% of cases of tinea capitis in the United States and United Kingdom.[90]

TABLE 88-3
Secondary Cicatricial (Permanent) Alopecias: A Classification Based on Etiology

Genodermatoses and developmental defects with permanent alopecia (excluding congenital hypotrichoses and atrichias)	• Ectodermal dysplasias • Aplasia cutis congenita • Incontinentia pigmenti • Porokeratosis of Mibelli • Ichthyosis • Hereditary epidermolysis bullosa • Meningocele • Hamartoma • Organoid nevi (sebaceous, epidermal) vascular malformations • Darier disease • Fibrodysplasia	Inflammatory dermatoses	• Psoriasis (rarely) • Pityriasis amiantacea • Arteritis temporalis • Pyoderma gangrenosum • Graft-versus-host disease ***Sclerosing*** • Morphea • Scleroderma en coup de sabre and Parry-Romberg syndrome • Lichen sclerosus et atrophicus ***Bullous*** • Cicatricial pemphigoid • Porphyria cutanea tarda • Acquired epidermolysis bullosa ***Granulomatous*** • Sarcoidosis • Granuloma anulare • Necrobiosis lipoidica (including Miescher granulomatosis)
Physical and chemical injury	• Mechanical trauma and pressure • Scratching • Burns • Freezing • Chemical injury • Insect bites • Radiation		
Infections	***Bacterial*** • Carbuncle • Leprosy • Tertiary syphilis • Tuberculosis–lupus vulgaris ***Viral*** • Zoster • Varicella ***Tinea capitis*** • Kerion • Favus ***Protozoal*** • *Leishmania*	Neoplastic	***Infiltration*** • Lymphoproliferative disorders • Mastocytosis ***Benign solid neoplasms*** • Cysts • Vascular tumors • Adnexal tumors • Plasmacytoma ***Malignant solid tumors*** • Angiosarcoma • Dermatofibrosarcoma protuberans • Malignant fibrous histiocytoma • Melanoma • Squamous cell carcinoma • Basal cell carcinoma • Metastasis (alopecia neoplastica) • Lymphoma

Adapted by permission from Springer: Finner AM, Shapiro J. Secondary cicatricial and other permanent alopecias. In: Blume-Peytavi U, Tosti A, Whiting DA, et al, eds. *Hair Growth and Disorders*. Berlin, Germany: Springer-Verlag; 2008:229, Table 12.1. Copyright © 2008.

Ectothrix infection, most commonly caused by *Microsporum* spp. (especially *Microsporum canis*) and *Epidermophyton* spp. destroy the hair cuticle and masses of spores are located outside of the hair shaft. The alopecic patches usually show signs of inflammation and scaling with brittle grayish hair stumps. The areas may show a yellow-green fluorescence under Wood light examination. Endothrix infections are most commonly caused by *Trichophyton* spp. (especially *T. tonsurans* subspecies *sulfureum*).[91,92] The fungus is capable of invading the hair and masses of spores can be found within the hair shaft on microscopic examination. The hair breaks off directly at the skin surface, which clinically presents as "black dots." Hair loss, inflammation, and scaling may be minimal; consequently, this type of tinea capitis is often dismissed as seborrheic or atopic dermatitis. Favus is a specific type of tinea capitis characterized by patelliform scales (scutula), which are sulfuric-yellow concretions of hyphae and skin debris in the follicular orifices and exhibit a distinct malodorous smell. A kerion is a deep, highly inflammatory fungal infection of the scalp. It presents as a highly suppurative, boggy, nodular, deep folliculitis with fistulas and pus secretion. To establish a diagnosis, hair shafts should be plugged out and cultured, as well as examined after potassium hydroxide preparation. Favus and kerion may lead to scarring hair loss and should be treated aggressively.[93-96]

Systemic antifungal treatment such as terbinafine, itraconazole, ketoconazole, griseofulvin, and fluconazole is indispensable to treat tinea capitis. The choice of the systemic antifungal agent depends on the type of fungus.[95,97,98] Especially in children, social contacts must be sought and treated to prevent reinfection. Topical sporicidal agents, such as selenium or ketoconazole help to limit the spread of the infectious spores.[99]

TRAUMATIC HAIR LOSS

An acute or chronic mechanical insult to the scalp hair may lead to reversible or irreversible alopecia of the scalp. Traumatic alopecias are usually of 3 types: acute trauma, prolonged traction, and pressure.

TRAUMATIC INJURIES

Minimal or severe injuries to the scalp can result in alopecia. It usually presents with fine streaks of hair loss in the injured scalp area, but if the wound borders undergo contusion or destruction, this may result in irregular and large patches of hair loss. Traumatic hair loss can occur after scalp surgery, especially after extensive scalp reduction or large donor strip harvesting in hair restoration surgery, if too much tension is applied with wound closure. This type of hair loss is usually reversible but also can be permanent. Traumatic birth induced alopecia is infrequent; causes include mechanical extractor marks, tears or contusions or resulting infections. Aplasia cutis congenita should be considered in the differential diagnosis of cicatricial alopecia at birth.[100]

TRACTION ALOPECIA

Prolonged traction of the hair may lead to transient or if continued over a period of time, may lead to follicular atrophy, resulting in cicatricial alopecia. Chronic traction can be caused by tight pony tails, braids, heavy dead locks or extensive use of rollers. As a consequence of ethnic differences in hair fragility and cultural differences in hair-styling practices, marginal traction alopecia is more commonly seen in African American women from hair braiding and weaving procedures (Fig. 88-9).[101] Patchy traction alopecia in the frontal hairline or temples is commonly seen in Sikh boys, whose hair is usually tight up in a "topknot."[102] Cicatricial alopecia caused by prolonged traction can be treated with hair transplantation, if the patient discontinues the injuring hairstyles and sufficient donor hair supply is available.

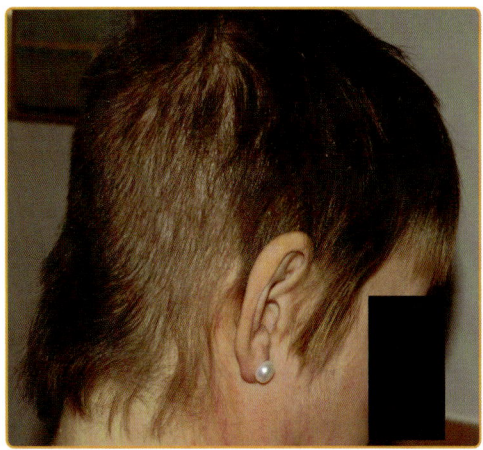

Figure 88-10 Trichotillomania.

TRICHOTILLOMANIA (HAIR PULLING DISORDER)

Trichotillomania (greek: *tricho* = hair, *tillo* = pull, *mania* = excessive excitement) is a form of traumatic alopecia caused by an irresistible compulsion to pull out or twist or break of one's own hair. Two forms of trichotillomania can be distinguished: infantile or early-onset trichotillomania, which starts in early childhood, is typically of short duration and may resolve spontaneously or with simple interventions.[103,104] The clinical presentation is usually quite distinctive with a single or multiple asymmetrical, occasionally geometrically shaped, areas of hair loss on the scalp or other areas of the body (Fig. 88-10). The areas are not smoothly devoid of hairs, as seen in alopecia areata, but display short or bristly anagen hair. Most important in the therapy of trichotillomania is the education of patient and/or parents, and in late-onset trichotillomania, the treatment of the underlying psychopathology. Especially if patients deny the self-inflicting nature of their hair loss, a referral to a psychiatrist or psychologist is usually refused and treatment becomes difficult.

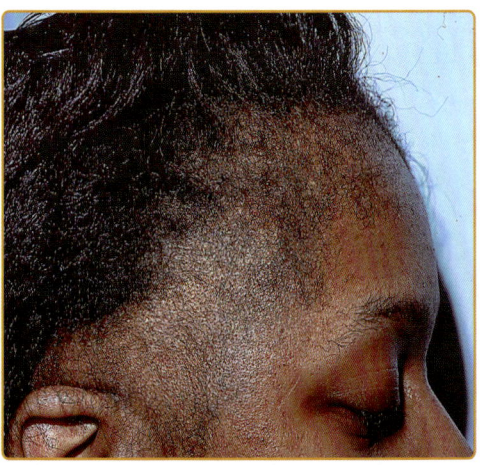

Figure 88-9 Traction alopecia.

TABLE 88-4

Differential Diagnosis for Secondary Cicatricial Alopecias

- Primary cicatricial alopecia
- Alopecia areata
- Temporal triangular alopecia
- Trichotillomania
- Secondary syphilis (alopecia areolaris)

PRESSURE ALOPECIA

Pressure alopecia can occur after a patient was unconscious and completely immobile for a certain length of time. Hair loss is presumably a result of ischemia caused by the pressure of the body weight to a certain scalp area. The ischemic injury may lead to permanent hair loss.

DIFFERENTIAL DIAGNOSIS

Table 88-4 outlines the differential diagnosis of secondary cicatricial alopecias.

REFERENCES

1. Olsen EA, Bergfeld WF, Cotsarelis G, et al. Summary of North American Hair Research Society (NAHRS)-sponsored Workshop on Cicatricial Alopecia, Duke University Medical Center, February 10 and 11, 2001. *J Am Acad Dermatol.* 2003;48(1):103-110.
2. Olsen E, Stenn K, Bergfeld W, et al. Update on cicatricial alopecia. *J Investig Dermatol Symp Proc.* 2003; 8(1):18-19.
3. Whiting DA. Cicatricial alopecia: clinico-pathological findings and treatment. *Clin Dermatol.* 2001;19(2): 211-215.
4. Cotsarelis G, Sun TT, Lavker RM. Label-retaining cells reside in the bulge area of pilosebaceous unit: implications for follicular stem cells, hair cycle, and skin carcinogenesis. *Cell.* 1990;61(7):1329-1337.
5. Sellheyer K, Bergfeld WF. Histopathologic evaluation of alopecias. *Am J Dermatopathol.* 2006;28(3):236-259.
6. Tan E, Martinka M, Ball N, et al. Primary cicatricial alopecias: clinicopathology of 112 cases. *J Am Acad Dermatol.* 2004;50(1):25-32.
7. Taylor G, Lehrer MS, Jensen PJ, et al. Involvement of follicular stem cells in forming not only the follicle but also the epidermis. *Cell.* 2000;102(4):451-461.
8. Ross EK, Tan E, Shapiro J. Update on primary cicatricial alopecias. *J Am Acad Dermatol.* 2005;53(3):1-37.
9. Shapiro J. Assessment of the patient with alopecia. In: *Hair Loss: Principles of Diagnosis and Management of Alopecia.* London, UK: Martin Dunitz, 2002.
10. Bergfeld WF, Elston DM. Cicatricial alopecia. In: Olsen EA, ed. *Disorders of Hair Growth: Diagnosis and Treatment.* 2nd ed. New York, NY: McGraw-Hill; 2003:363-398.
11. Otberg N, Wu WY, McElwee KJ, et al. Diagnosis and management of primary cicatricial alopecia: part I. *Skinmed.* 2008;7(1):19-26.
12. Wu WY, Otberg N, McElwee KJ, et al. Diagnosis and management of primary cicatricial alopecia: part II. *Skinmed.* 2008;7(2):78-83.
13. Callen JP. Chronic cutaneous lupus erythematosus. Clinical, laboratory, therapeutic, and prognostic examination of 62 patients. *Arch Dermatol.* 1982;118(6): 412-416.
14. Wilson CL, Burge SM, Dean D, et al. Scarring alopecia in discoid lupus erythematosus. *Br J Dermatol.* 1992; 126(4):307-314.
15. George PM, Tunnessen WW Jr. Childhood discoid lupus erythematosus. *Arch Dermatol.* 1993;129(5):613-617.
16. Moises-Alfaro C, Berrón-Pérez R, Carrasco-Daza D, et al. Discoid lupus erythematosus in children: clinical, histopathologic, and follow-up features in 27 cases. *Pediatr Dermatol.* 2003;20(2):103-107.
17. Meyers DC, Woosley JT, Reddick RL. Verruciform xanthoma in association with discoid lupus erythematosus. *J Cutan Pathol.* 1992;19(2):156-158.
18. Headington JT. Cicatricial alopecia. *Dermatol Clin.* 1996;14(4):773-782.
19. Kossard S. Lymphocytic mediated alopecia: histological classification by pattern analysis. *Clin Dermatol.* 2001;19(2):201-210.
20. Sperling LC. Hair density in African Americans. *Arch Dermatol.* 1999;135:656-658.
21. Solomon AR. The transversely sectioned scalp biopsy specimen: the technique and an algorithm for its use in the diagnosis of alopecia. *Adv Dermatol.* 1994;9: 127-157.
22. Templeton SF, Solomon AR. Scarring alopecia: a classification based on microscopic criteria. *J Cutan Pathol.* 1994;21(2):97-109.
23. Ruzicka T, Sommerburg C, Goerz G, et al. Treatment of cutaneous lupus erythematosus with acitretin and hydroxychloroquine. *Br J Dermatol.* 1992;127(5): 513-518.
24. Newton RC, Jorizzo JL, Solomon AR Jr, et al. Mechanism-oriented assessment of isotretinoin in chronic or subacute cutaneous lupus erythematosus. *Arch Dermatol.* 1986;122(2):170-176.
25. Hamilton T, Otberg N, Wu WY, et al. Successful hair regrowth with multimodal treatment of early cicatricial alopecia in discoid lupus erythematosus. *Acta Derm Venereol.* 2009;89(4):417-418.
26. Eisen D. The evaluation of cutaneous, genital, scalp, nail, esophageal, and ocular involvement in patients with lichen planus. *Oral Surg Oral Med Oral Pathol Oral Radiol Endod.* 1999;88(4):431-436.
27. Chieregato C, Zini A, Barba A, et al. Lichen planopilaris: report of 30 cases and review of the literature. *Int J Dermatol.* 2003;74(6):784-786.
28. Kossard S. Postmenopausal frontal fibrosing alopecia. Scarring alopecia in a pattern distribution. *Arch Dermatol.* 1994;130(6):770-774.
29. Atarguine H, Hocar O, Hamdaoui A, et al. Frontal fibrosing alopecia: report on three pediatric cases [in French]. *Arch Pediatr.* 2016;23(8):832-835.
30. Ormaechea-Pérez N, López-Pestaña A, Zubizarreta-Salvador J, et al. Frontal fibrosing alopecia in men: presentations in 12 cases and a review of the literature. *Actas Dermosifiliogr.* 2016;7310(16):30260-30265.
31. Vañó-Galván S, Molina-Ruiz AM, Serrano-Falcón C, et al. Frontal fibrosing alopecia: a multicenter review of 355 patients. *J Am Acad Dermatol.* 2014; 70(4):670-678.
32. Holmes S. Frontal fibrosing alopecia. *Skin Therapy Lett.* 2016;21(4):5-7.
33. Phillips WG, Vaughan-Jones S, Jenkins R, et al. Captopril-induced lichenoid eruption. *Clin Exp Dermatol.* 1994;19(4):317-320.
34. Katta R. Lichen planus. *Am Fam Physician.* 2000; 61(11):3319-3324.
35. Kang H, Alzolibani AA, Otberg N, et al. Lichen planopilaris. *Dermatol Ther.* 2008;21(4):249-256.
36. Mehregan DA, Van Hale HM, Muller SA. Lichen planopilaris: clinical and pathologic study of forty-five patients. *J Am Acad Dermatol.* 1992;27(6):935-942.
37. Bolanča Ž, Goren A, Getaldić-Švarc B, et al. Platelet-rich plasma as a novel treatment for lichen planopilaris. *Dermatol Ther.* 2016;29(4):233-235.

38. Ott F, Bollag W, Geiger JM. Efficacy of oral low-dose tretinoin (all-trans-retinoic acid) in lichen planus. *Dermatology.* 1997;192(4):334-336.
39. Mirmirani P, Willey A, Price VH. Short course of oral cyclosporine in lichen planopilaris. *J Am Acad Dermatol.* 2003;49(4):667-671.
40. Cribier B, Frances C, Chosidow O. Treatment of lichen planus. An evidence-based medicine analysis of efficacy. *Arch Dermatol.* 1998;134(12):1521-1530.
41. Massa MC, Rogers RS 3rd. Griseofulvin therapy of lichen planus. *Acta Derm Venereol.* 1981;61(6):547-550.
42. Ronchese F. Pseudopelade. *Arch Dermatol.* 1960;82:336-343.
43. Schmoeckel C, Weissmann I, Plewig G, et al. Treatment of alopecia areata by anthralin-induced dermatitis. *Arch Dermatol.* 1979; 115(10):1254-1255.
44. Elston DM, McCollough ML, Warschaw KE, et al. Elastic tissue in scars and alopecia. *J Cutan Pathol.* 2000;27(3):147-152.
45. Bulengo-Ransby SM, Headington JT. Pseudopelade of Brocq in a child. *J Am Acad Dermatol.* 1990; 23(5):944-945.
46. Alzolibani AA, Kang H, Otberg N, et al. Pseudopelade of Brocq. *Dermatol Ther.* 2008;21(4):257-263.
47. Olsen EA. Disorders of hair growth. In: Cotsarelis G, Millar SE, Chan EF, eds. *Embryology and Anatomy of the Hair Follicle.* 2nd ed. Vol. 1. New York, NY: McGraw-Hill; 2003:544.
48. Dlova NC, Jordaan FH, Sarig O, et al. Autosomal dominant inheritance of central centrifugal cicatricial alopecia in black South Africans. *J Am Acad Dermatol.* 2014;70(4):679-682.
49. Dlova NC, Salkey KS, Callender VD, et al. Central centrifugal cicatricial alopecia: new insights and a call for action. *J Investig Dermatol Symp Proc.* 2017; 18(2):S54-S56.
50. Suchonwanit P, Hector CE, Bin Saif GA, et al. Factors affecting the severity of central centrifugal cicatricial alopecia. *Int J Dermatol.* 2016;55(6):e338-e343.
51. Olsen EA, Callender V, Sperling L, et al. Central scalp alopecia photographic scale in African American women. *Dermatol Ther.* 2008;21(4):264-267.
52. Sperling LC, Sau P. The follicular degeneration syndrome in black patients. "Hot comb alopecia" revisited and revised. *Arch Dermatol.* 1992;128(1):68-74.
53. Eginli AN, Dlova NC, McMichael A. Central centrifugal cicatricial alopecia in children: a case series and review of the literature. *Pediatr Dermatol.* 2017;34(2):133-137.
54. Callender VD, McMichael AJ, Cohen GF. Medical and surgical therapies for alopecias in black women. *Dermatol Ther.* 2004;17(2):164-176.
55. Ogunleye TA, McMichael A, Olsen EA. Central centrifugal cicatricial alopecia: what has been achieved, current clues for future research. *Dermatol Clin.* 2014;32(2):173-181.
56. Gibson LE, Muller SA, Peters MS. Follicular mucinosis of childhood and adolescence. *Pediatr Dermatol.* 1988;5(4):231-235.
57. van Doorn R, Scheffer E, Willemze R. Follicular mycosis fungoides, a distinct disease entity with or without associated follicular mucinosis: a clinicopathologic and follow-up study of 51 patients. *Arch Dermatol.* 2002; 138(2):191-198.
58. Boer A, Guo Y, Ackerman AB. Alopecia mucinosa is mycosis fungoides. *Am J Dermatopathol.* 2004;26(1):33-52.
59. Emmerson RW. Follicular mucinosis. A study of 47 patients. *Br J Dermatol.* 1969;81(6):395.
60. Baden HP, Byers HR. Clinical findings, cutaneous pathology, and response to therapy in 21 patients with keratosis pilaris atrophicans. *Arch Dermatol.* 1994;130(4):469-475.
61. Powell JJ, Dawber RP, Gatter K. Folliculitis decalvans including tufted folliculitis: clinical, histological and therapeutic findings. *Br J Dermatol.* 1999;140(2):328-333.
62. Powell J, Dawber RP. Successful treatment regime for folliculitis decalvans despite uncertainty of all aetiological factors. *Br J Dermatol.* 2001;144:428-429.
63. Brooke RC, Griffiths CE. Folliculitis decalvans. *Clin Exp Dermatol.* 2001;26(1):120-122.
64. Brozena SJ, Cohen LE, Fenske NA. Folliculitis decalvans: response to rifampin. *Cutis.* 1988;42:512-515.
65. Abeck D, Korting HC, Braun-Falco O. Folliculitis decalvans. Long-lasting response to combined therapy with fusidic acid and zinc. *Acta Derm Venereol.* 1992;72(2):143-145.
66. Sivakumaran S, Meyer P, Burrows NP. Dissecting folliculitis of the scalp with marginal keratitis. *Clin Exp Dermatol.* 2001;26:490-492.
67. Ramasastry SS, Granick MS, Boyd JB, et al. Severe perifolliculitis capitis with osteomyelitis. *Ann Plast Surg.* 1987;18:241-244.
68. Ongchi DR, Fleming MG, Harris CA. Sternocostoclavicular hyperostosis: two cases with differing dermatologic syndromes. *J Rheumatol.* 1990;17:1415-1418.
69. Libow L, Friar DA. Arthropathy associated with cystic acne, hidradenitis suppurativa, and perifolliculitis capitis abscedens et suffodiens: treatment with isotretinoin. *Cutis.* 1999;64:87-90.
70. Curry SS, Gaither DH, King LE Jr. Squamous cell carcinoma arising in dissecting perifolliculitis of the scalp. A case report and review of secondary squamous cell carcinomas. *J Am Acad Dermatol.* 1981;4:673-678.
71. Boyd AS, Zemtsov A. A case of pyoderma vegetans and the follicular occlusion triad. *J Dermatol.* 1992;19(1):61-63.
72. Bergeron JR, Stone OJ. Follicular occlusion triad in a follicular blocking disease (pityriasis rubra pilaris). *Dermatologica.* 1968;136(5):362-367.
73. Scheinfeld NS. A case of dissecting cellulitis and a review of the literature. *Dermatol Online J.* 2003;9(1):8.
74. Goldsmith PC, Dowd PM. Successful therapy of the follicular occlusion triad in a young woman with high dose oral antiandrogens and minocycline. *J R Soc Med.* 1993;86:729-730.
75. Adrian RM, Arndt KA. Perifolliculitis capitis: successful control with alternate-day corticosteroids. *Ann Plast Surg.* 1980;4:166-169.
76. Scerri L, Williams HC, Allen BR. Dissecting cellulitis of the scalp: response to isotretinoin. *Br J Dermatol.* 1996;134:1105-1108.
77. Koca R, Altinyazar HC, Ozen OI, et al. Dissecting cellulitis in a white male: response to isotretinoin. *Int J Dermatol.* 2002;41:509-513.
78. Stites PC, Boyd AS. Dissecting cellulitis in a white male: a case report and review of the literature. *Cutis.* 2001;67:37-40.
79. Otberg N, Kang H, Alzolibani AA, et al. Folliculitis decalvans. *Dermatol Ther.* 2008;21(4):238-244.
80. Scheinfeld N. Dissecting cellulitis (perifolliculitis capitis abscedens et suffodiens): a comprehensive review focusing on new treatments and findings of the last decade with commentary comparing the therapies

and causes of dissecting cellulitis to hidradenitis suppurativa. *Dermatol Online J.* 2014;20(5):22692.
81. Halder RM. Pseudofolliculitis barbae and related disorders. *Dermatol Clin.* 1988;6:407-412.
82. Dinehart SM, Herzberg AJ, Kerns BJ, et al. Acne keloidalis: a review. *J Dermatol Surg Oncol.* 1989;15:642-647.
83. Stritzler C, Friedman R, Loveman AB. Acne necrotica; relation to acne necrotica miliaris and response to penicillin and other antibiotics. *Arch Derm Syphilol.* 1951;64:464-469.
84. Kossard S, Collins A, McCrossin I. Necrotizing lymphocytic folliculitis: the early lesion of acne necrotica (varioliformis). *J Am Acad Dermatol.* 1987;16(1):1007-1014.
85. Maibach HI. Acne necroticans (varioliformis) versus *Propionibacterium acnes* folliculitis. *J Am Acad Dermatol.* 1989;21:323.
86. Grattan CE, Peachey RD, Boon A, Evidence for a role of local trauma in the pathogenesis of erosive pustular dermatosis of the scalp. *Clin Exp Dermatol.* 1988;13:7-10.
87. Ena P, Lissia M, Doneddu GM, et al. Erosive pustular dermatosis of the scalp in skin grafts: report of three cases. *Dermatology.* 1997;194:80-84.
88. Pye RJ, Peachey RD, Burton JL. Erosive pustular dermatosis of the scalp. *Br J Dermatol.* 1979;100:559-566.
89. Finner AM, Otberg N, Shapiro J. Secondary cicatricial and other permanent alopecias. *Dermatol Ther.* 2008;21(4):279-294.
90. Elewski BE. Tinea capitis: a current perspective. *J Am Acad Dermatol.* 2000;42:1.
91. Hebert AA. Tinea capitis. Current concepts. *Arch Dermatol.* 1988;124(10):1554-1557.
92. Tanz RR, Hebert AA, Esterly NB. Treating tinea capitis: should ketoconazole replace griseofulvin? *J Pediatr.* 1988;112(6):987-991.
93. Fiedler L, Rückauer K, Faber M, et al. Surgical and ketoconazole treatment of a kerion Celsi caused by *Trichophyton mentagrophytes* and *Candida tropicalis*. *Mycoses.* 1988;(suppl 1):81-87.
94. Kron C, Oger P, Traxer O, et al. Bulky superinfected tinea capitis of the scalp. Treatment by surgical resection and reconstruction by cutaneous expansion [in French]. *Arch Pediatr.* 1998;5:992-995.
95. Otberg N, Tietz HJ, Henz BM, et al. Kerion due to *Trichophyton mentagrophytes*: responsiveness to fluconazole versus terbinafine in a child. *Acta Derm Venereol.* 2001;81(6):444-445.
96. Thoma-Greber E, Zenker S, Röcken M, et al. Surgical treatment of tinea capitis in childhood. *Mycoses.* 2003;46(8):351-354.
97. Chen X, Jiang X, Yang M, et al. Systemic antifungal therapy for tinea capitis in children: an abridged Cochrane Review. *J Am Acad Dermatol.* 2017;76(2):368-374.
98. Kaul S, Yadav S, Dogra S. Treatment of dermatophytosis in elderly, children, and pregnant women. *Indian Dermatol Online J.* 2017;8(5):310-318.
99. Trovato MJ, Schwartz RA, Janniger CK. Tinea capitis: current concepts in clinical practice. *Cutis.* 2006;77:93.
100. Roberts JL, De Villez R. Infectious, and physical, and inflammatory causes of hair and scalp abnormalities. In: Olsen EA, ed. *Disorders of Hair Growth.* 2nd ed. Vol. 1. New York, NY: McGraw-Hill; 2003.
101. Wilborn WS. Disorders of hair growth in African-Americans. In: Olsen EA, ed. *Disorders of Hair Growth.* 2nd ed. Vol. 1. New York, NY: McGraw-Hill; 2003.
102. Singh G, Traction alopecia in Sikh boys. *Br J Dermatol.* 1975;92:232.
103. Swedo SE, Leonard HL. Trichotillomania. An obsessive compulsive spectrum disorder? *Psychiatr Clin North Am.* 1992;15(4):777-790.
104. Winchel RM, Jones JS, Stanley B, et al. Clinical characteristics of trichotillomania and its response to fluoxetine. *J Clin Psychiatry.* 1992;53(9):304-308.

Chapter 89 :: Hair Shaft Disorders
:: Leslie Castelo-Soccio & Deepa Patel

第八十九章

毛干疾病

中文导读

传统上，毛干疾病分为毛干断裂和毛干紊乱两类疾病，还有未归入上两类的其他毛干疾病。各个疾病都从流行病学、临床特征、病因及危险因素、诊断、鉴别诊断、临床病程与预后、治疗管理这7个方面来陈述。

第一部分介绍与毛发断裂相关的毛发疾病，分别介绍结节性脆发症、毛发分裂症和毛发硫营养不良、毛卷曲、套叠性脆发症、念珠状发。

第一节介绍结节性脆发症（TN），流行病学提示此病是最常见的与毛发断裂相关的毛干疾病，再介绍其临床特点。此病病因或危险因素包括先天遗传或后天获得，并通过表89-1回顾了与TN相关的其他代谢和先天性综合征。诊断方面则强调通过光镜或电镜观察呈八字油漆刷状的发干；作者再通过表89-2列出需要与此病相鉴别的疾病。临床病程、预后和治疗管理强调防止外部创伤，减少断发出现的频率和次数。

第二节介绍毛发分裂症和毛发硫营养不良，流行病学提示此病罕见且与基因和外部创伤都有一定的关系。表89-3列出与此病相关的6种遗传性疾病及其对应的临床特点；讲述了遗传基因、外部创伤这些病因及危险因素。诊断方面则强调显微镜下因毛发含硫量导致的"虎尾"现象。最后讲述了鉴别诊断、临床病程、预后及治疗管理。

第三节介绍毛卷曲（"扭曲的头发"），头发轴为扁平的是其特点，并沿其长轴扭曲180度。并从流行病学、临床特征、病因及危险因素、诊断、鉴别诊断、临床病程与预后、治疗管理这7个方面来陈述。表89-4列出了与毛卷曲相关的综合征，表89-5列出需要与毛卷曲相鉴别的其他疾病。

第四、第五节介绍套叠性脆发症、念珠状发，它们都是较为罕见的疾病。套叠性脆发症（竹毛）通常与Netherton综合征有关，其特征是远端发干内陷到近端。念珠状发伴随着脆弱性的增加和病理学上的串珠状毛发的出现，文中也陈述了此疾病的7个方面。其中表89-6列出需要与念珠状发相鉴别的其他疾病。

第二部分介绍毛干紊乱，提出其与不受约束的头发有关，但没有或很少有毛发断裂，包括不规则毛发综合征、Marie-Unna遗传性少毛症（MUHH）、羊毛状发、遗传性单纯性少毛症（HHS）。表89-7、表89-8、表89-9分别概述了不规则毛发综合征、MUHH、羊毛状发的鉴别诊断。对于遗传性单纯性少毛症（HHS），作者通过表89-10列出其10种亚型，及其相对应的遗传模式、缺陷基因（和）或基因位置。

第三部分介绍其他毛干疾病，包括疏松发综合征（LAS）、环状发。其中表89-11列出需要与疏松发综合征（LAS）相鉴别的其他疾病。

在第四部分总结结节性脆发症(TN)、毛发分裂症和毛发硫营养不良(TTD)、毛卷曲、套叠性脆发症、念珠状发、不规则毛发综合征、Marie-Unna遗传性少毛症、羊毛状发、遗传性单纯性少毛症（HHS）、疏松发综合征（LAS）、环状发等毛干疾病的病因/危险因素/遗传模式、临床表现、诊断、临床病程管理、相关症状，并通过表89-12列出。

〔简　丹〕

AT-A-GLANCE

- Hair shaft disorders associated with hair breakage include trichorrhexis nodosa, trichoschisis, pili torti, trichorrhexis invaginata, and monilethrix.
- Hair shaft disorders associated with unruly hair, but none or little hair breakage, include uncombable hair syndrome, wooly hair, Marie Unna hereditary hypotrichosis, and hypotrichosis.
- Other hair shaft disorders that don't distinctly fall into either of the above categories are loose anagen syndrome and pili annulati.

Hair shaft disorders can be classified as primary and secondary. A primary disorder is caused by a gene defect that changes the shape or composition of the hair shaft, and a secondary disorder is caused by external factors applied to the hair leading to weakness and often breakage of the hair shaft. Classically, hair shaft disorders are also divided into those that cause hair breakage and those that cause unruly hair, although there can be overlap between the 2 categories.

HAIR SHAFT DISORDERS ASSOCIATED WITH HAIR BREAKAGE

TRICHORRHEXIS NODOSA

EPIDEMIOLOGY

Trichorrhexis nodosa (TN) is the most common hair shaft disorder associated with breakage.

CLINICAL FEATURES

TN presents as brittle, easily broken, and lusterless hair with white nodular swellings at irregular intervals along the hair shaft.[1] Patients with TN often complain of inability to grow hair past a certain length.

ETIOLOGY/RISK FACTORS

TN can either be acquired or inherited. Acquired TN is the more common subtype and is caused by external trauma, which includes mechanical, chemical, and thermal injury. Acquired TN has been divided into 3 groups based on localized, proximal, or distal location.[2] Localized TN usually presents as isolated patches that occurs from mechanical trauma secondary to a pruritic dermatosis.[1] Proximal TN has primarily been observed in the African American population where the use of strong chemical and heat-straightening treatments is more common. Distal TN is described in white and Asian populations and is associated with frequent shampoo use, brushing, and chemical treatments such as bleaching. Other causes of acquired disease include malnutrition, iron deficiency, and hypothyroidism.

There are also instances where TN is either inherited or congenital. When TN is inherited, it occurs at birth or within a few months of birth and is an isolated autosomal dominant condition. Congenital TN can be associated with ectodermal dysplasias or with metabolic disorders such as arginosuccinic aciduria. Arginosuccinic aciduria leads to a buildup of toxic levels of ammonia and presents within a few days of birth with infants displaying lethargy, temperature instability and ataxia.[3] Occasionally, an individual may inherit a milder form of the disorder where ammonia builds up in the bloodstream only during periods of illness. The gene defect is in the *ASL* gene, which provides instructions for making the protein arginosuccinase lyase. Testing for this disorder is included in many state newborn screens. Workup includes genetic testing for *ASL* gene as well as a complete metabolic panel looking for acidosis, hyperammonemia, and low serum arginine. Treatment results in resolution to normal hair and involves supplementation with arginine and dietary restriction of protein.

Table 89-1 reviews additional metabolic and congenital syndromes that are associated with TN.

TABLE 89-1
Syndromes Associated with Trichorrhexis Nodosa

CONDITION	INHERITANCE PATTERN AND GENE DEFECT	CLINICAL FEATURES	TREATMENT AND PROGNOSIS
Multiple carboxylase deficiency	Autosomal recessive Early onset: holocarboxylase synthetase gene (*HLCS*) Late onset: biotinidase gene (*BTD*)	Hypotonia, failure to thrive, seizures, TN, and generalized rash	Most features, including hair symptoms, will resolve with biotin supplementation
Trichohepatoenteric syndrome (THE)	Autosomal recessive *TTC37* gene	Intractable diarrhea, facial dysmorphism, intrauterine growth restriction, immune system dysfunction, and hair that is wooly or easily removable	Supportive care; total parenteral nutrition (TPN) for nutrition; prognosis poor with main complications that include infection and severe liver disease
Menkes syndrome	X-linked recessive ATP7A copper-transporter gene defect	Hypotonia, failure to thrive, seizures, developmental delay, pale skin, and sparse, coarse, lighter-colored hair	Early copper supplementation may be of some benefit, but most patients will not live past age 3 years
Goltz syndrome	X-linked dominant ectodermal dysplasia *PORCN* (porcupine O-acyltransferase) mutation	Craniofacial, skeletal, ocular, renal, and GI involvement can occur, as well as hair shaft abnormalities	Corrective treatment and medical management of various associated anomalies
Netherton syndrome	Autosomal recessive *SPINK5* (serine peptidase inhibitor, Kazal type 5) gene	Atopic diathesis, severe dehydration, growth retardation, ichthyosis linearis circumflexa, and hair shaft abnormalities, including trichorrhexis nodosa, trichorrhexis invaginata, and pili torti	No known cure, but intravenous immunoglobulin has become treatment of choice along with supportive care
Wooly hair	Autosomal dominant *KRT74* (keratin 74) gene	Hair shaft disorder with fine, tightly curled hair; can display associated structural anomalies such as trichorrhexis nodosa	No effective treatments have been found; avoidance of harsh chemicals and application of oils can make hair more manageable
Trichothiodystrophy (TTD)	Autosomal recessive There are 4 known gene mutations: MPLKIP (M-phase specific PLK1 interacting protein), ERCC2 (ERCC excision repair 2), ERCC3 (ERCC excision repair 3), GTF2H5 (general transcription factor IIH subunit 5)	Severe forms may be associated with developmental delay, short stature, dry skin, abnormal toenails and fingernails, congenital cataracts, and increased risk for respiratory tract infections; milder forms can be limited to hair changes and are associated with both trichorrhexis nodosa and trichoschisis	No effective treatments have been found for TTD; avoidance of trauma may prevent further hair breakage or loss

DIAGNOSIS

Diagnosis of TN can be made with light and electron microscopy. The characteristic finding is a splayed paint brush bristle appearance (Fig. 89-1), which is caused by a breach in the cuticle leading to exposure of the fibers and increasing their susceptibility to fracture. Additional analysis of hair shaft, as well as blood tests such as complete blood count, thyroid function, and copper levels, may reveal other acquired or congenital causes of TN.

DIFFERENTIAL DIAGNOSIS

Differential diagnosis for TN (Table 89-2) includes conditions associated with hair loss and increased hair fra-

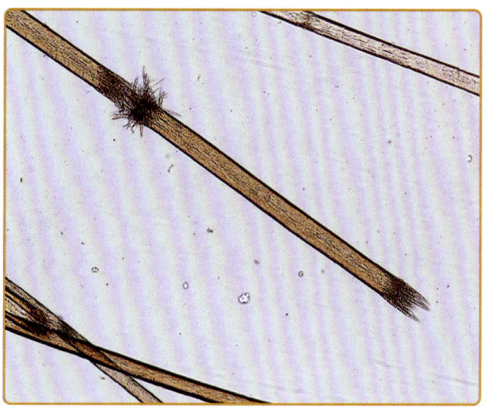

Figure 89-1 Microscopic findings of trichorrhexis nodosa.

TABLE 89-2
Differential Diagnosis of Trichorrhexis Nodosa

- Alopecia areata
- Androgenic alopecia
- Monilethrix
- Piedra
- Seborrheic dermatitis
- Telogen effluvium
- Trichotillomania

gility, as well as the associated syndromes discussed above.

CLINICAL COURSE AND PROGNOSIS

Patients with inherited causes of TN have a varying course. Those with external causes can improve with removal of the external trauma to the hair shaft.

MANAGEMENT

Acquired TN is often a self-limited and reversible disease. Management involves avoiding harsh chemical treatments, excessive hair brushing, heat exposure, and mechanical trauma such as rubbing or scratching. Resolution to normal hair will occur within 2 to 4 years. Additional use of a protein-enriched shampoo, as well as cutting the hair in cases of distal damage, may prevent future reoccurrence of TN.[1]

TRICHOSCHISIS AND TRICHOTHIODYSTROPHY

Trichoschisis refers to a localized absence of cuticle that leads to exposure and a clean transverse fracture of the hair shaft. Trichoschisis is associated with low-sulfur-containing hair seen in trichothiodystrophy (TTD), but can also occur secondary to external trauma.

EPIDEMIOLOGY

TTD is an extremely rare condition occurring in 1 in 1 million live births.[4] TTD is associated with defects in genes involved in DNA repair and transcription and occurs as part of multiple inherited syndromes.

In addition to being a characteristic finding in TTD, trichoschisis can more frequently be caused by external trauma from heat, chemicals, relaxants, and excessive brushing.

CLINICAL FEATURES

Trichoschisis is characterized by brittle, easily broken hair as well as short, brittle eyebrows and eyelashes. When trichoschisis occurs as part of TTD, possible clinical features include cutaneous findings such as lamellar ichthyosis, brittle nails, short stature, mental retardation, facial dysmorphisms, and gonadal dysgenesis.[4,5] A recent review of the literature noted an increased risk for severe infections in patients with TTD, especially of the respiratory tract.[6] Photosensitivity is seen in some forms of TTD although no accompanying increased risk for skin cancer has been found.[6] Associated abnormalities seen in TTD are specific to each group of inherited disorders and are outlined in Table 89-3.

ETIOLOGY/RISK FACTORS

The localized absence of cuticle seen in trichoschisis can be a consequence of mechanical trauma from excessive styling, brushing, or combing. Chemical treatments, such as dye or bleach, may strip away the cuticle and cause local breakage. When it occurs congenitally, trichoschisis is seen in TTD and is associated with sulfur-deficient and cysteine-deficient hair. TTD is an autosomal recessive disorder that is linked to 4 major genes: *ERCC2 (XPD)*, *ERCC3 (XPB)*, *p8 (TTDA)*, and *C7Orf11 (TTDN1* or *MPLKIP)*.[7] The photosensitive forms of TTD are clinically grouped into 1 class and include alterations in the *XPD*, *XPB*, and *TTDA* genes. These genes encode a subunit of the transcription factor II H (TFIIH) complex, which initiates

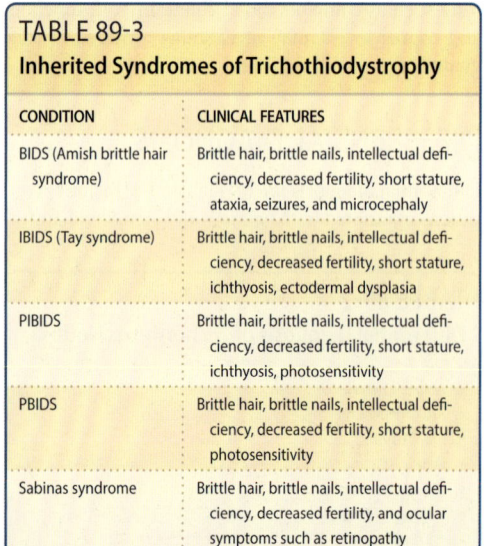

TABLE 89-3
Inherited Syndromes of Trichothiodystrophy

CONDITION	CLINICAL FEATURES
BIDS (Amish brittle hair syndrome)	Brittle hair, brittle nails, intellectual deficiency, decreased fertility, short stature, ataxia, seizures, and microcephaly
IBIDS (Tay syndrome)	Brittle hair, brittle nails, intellectual deficiency, decreased fertility, short stature, ichthyosis, ectodermal dysplasia
PIBIDS	Brittle hair, brittle nails, intellectual deficiency, decreased fertility, short stature, ichthyosis, photosensitivity
PBIDS	Brittle hair, brittle nails, intellectual deficiency, decreased fertility, short stature, photosensitivity
Sabinas syndrome	Brittle hair, brittle nails, intellectual deficiency, decreased fertility, and ocular symptoms such as retinopathy

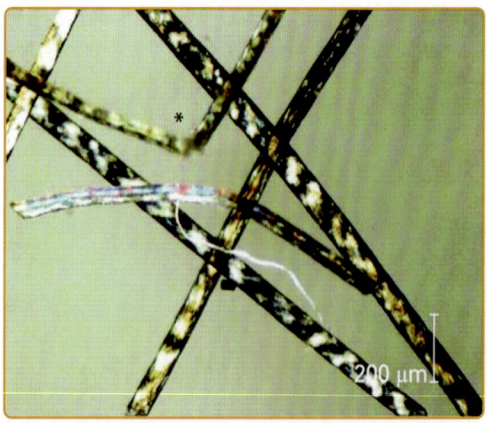

Figure 89-2 Tiger tail pattern seen with trichoschisis in trichothiodystrophy. (From Faghri S, Tamura D, Kraemer KH, et al. Trichothiodystrophy: a systematic review of 112 published cases characterises a wide spectrum of clinical manifestations. *J Med Genet*. 2008;45(10):609-21, with permission from BMJ Publishing Group Ltd.)

nucleotide excision repair when damage in the DNA is detected. The photosensitivity in this group is thus caused by a defect in nucleotide excision repair that prevents removal of modified or damaged DNA secondary to ultraviolet light. Nonphotosensitive forms of TTD are linked to patients with TTDN1 mutations. Although the exact function of TTDN1 is unknown, it is thought to regulate the cell cycle, namely mitosis and cytokinesis.[8]

DIAGNOSIS

In TTD, "tiger tail" hair with light and dark alternating bands is seen on polarized light microscopy (Fig. 89-2). This alternating pattern is related to irregular sulfur content of the hair, with lighter areas representing lower sulfur concentrations. Diagnosis can be confirmed by genetic testing of the genes described above or by sulfur and amino acid analysis of the hair shaft. The hair cysteine and sulfur content in TTD is less than 50% of normal in the cuticle and the cortex of the hair.[5]

DIFFERENTIAL DIAGNOSIS

Because of variation in presentation and potential effects on multiple organ systems, TTD has an extensive differential diagnosis. Most commonly, xeroderma pigmentosum and Cockayne syndrome are considered because of the increased photosensitivity of TTD, as well as the mechanism of defect in the DNA repair pathway. However, clinical presentation, low sulfur content, and hair pathology all help to distinguish TTD from other disorders.

CLINICAL COURSE AND PROGNOSIS

Patients with acquired trichoschisis often have good clinical prognosis with return to normal hair after reduction in mechanical or chemical trauma. Those with TTD have varying phenotypes that result in a spectrum from mild disease with only hair involvement to severe disease with profound developmental delay and high mortality. A systemic review of the literature found a 20-fold higher rate of mortality in children younger than the age of 10 years with TTD when compared to the general U.S. population.[6] The majority of these cases were the result of complications from severe infections. This same literature review by Faghri et al noted that patients can develop complications such as intellectual impairment (86%), short stature (73%), ocular abnormalities (51%), and ichthyosis (65%) at any point during their lifetime.[6]

MANAGEMENT

If trichoschisis is acquired, reducing hair manipulation can result in resolution of symptoms. In cases of TTD, no effective treatment modality has been identified. However, potential complications of TTD can be man-

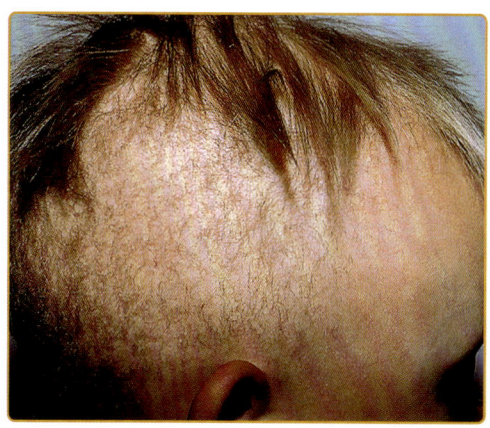

Figure 89-3 Brittle and broke hair typical of pili torti.

aged by regular monitoring of patients. Because of the extensive systemic effects of TTD, a multidisciplinary approach including, but not limited to, dermatologic, ophthalmologic, audiologic, skeletal, and developmental evaluations is required.

PILI TORTI

Pili torti ("twisted hair") is characterized by hair shafts that are flattened and twisted 180 degrees along their long axis.

EPIDEMIOLOGY

Pili torti often presents within the first 3 years of life. A less common, postpubertal form has been described.[9]

CLINICAL FEATURES

Hair is brittle, dry, and appears spangled as a result of uneven light reflections (Fig. 89-3). Fractures within the weak points of the twists result in shorter hair with increased fragility. Coarse hair or areas of alopecia are especially prevalent in the parietal and occipital areas. Hair is fair in appearance, except in postpubertal cases where darker hair, areas of alopecia, and late-onset intellectual disability is observed.[9] The scalp is the primary area affected, but eyebrows, eyelashes, and other body hairs may be involved. Neurologic disorders, hearing loss, and ectodermal dysplasia may be found in cases of pili torti.[10] Pili torti occurring as a feature of a clinical syndrome is associated with many cutaneous and extracutaneous features (Table 89-4).

ETIOLOGY/RISK FACTORS

Pili torti is either inherited or acquired. Isolated inherited cases occur in an autosomal dominant pattern, but can also be autosomal recessive or sporadic.[10] When occurring as part of a clinical syndrome, inheri-

TABLE 89-4
Syndromes Associated with Pili Torti

CONDITION	INHERITANCE PATTERN AND GENE DEFECT	CLINICAL FEATURES
Menkes syndrome	X-linked recessive ATP7A gene encoding copper transporter	Hypotonia, failure to thrive, seizures, developmental delay, pale skin, and sparse, coarse, lighter-colored hair
Bazex syndrome	X-linked dominant Xq24-27	Follicular atrophoderma, facial milia, sweating disorders, and congenital hypotrichosis with pili torti
Beare syndrome	Autosomal dominant Chromosome 10q26.13 FGFR2 gene	Alopecia after puberty, decreased beard and body hair, and pili torti
Björnstad syndrome	Autosomal recessive Chromosome 2q35 BCS1L gene	Sensorineural deafness and pili torti
Crandall syndrome	Autosomal recessive	Sensorineural deafness, hypopituitarism, and congenital hypotrichosis with pili torti
Goltz syndrome (focal dermal hypoplasia)	X-linked dominant PORCN gene	Facial abnormalities (asymmetry of the face, narrow nasal bridge), short stature, skeletal features (adactyly, claw hands, clinodactyly), cognitive impairment, CNS (seizures, microcephaly), ocular abnormalities (heterochromia, aniridia, colobomas), malformation of ears, atopic dermatitis, hypohidrosis, alteration in pigment, photosensitivity, nail changes (V-nicking, micronychia), GI features (omphalocele, gastric polyps), genitourinary findings (horseshoe kidney, hypoplasia, or absent kidney) hair shaft disorders (pili torti, pili trianguli et canaliculi, trichorrhexis nodosa)
Netherton syndrome	Autosomal recessive Chromosome 5q32 SPINK5 gene, serine protease inhibitor	Ichthyosis linearis circumflexa, atopic diathesis, and hair shaft abnormalities (pili torti, trichorrhexis nodosa, trichorrhexis invaginata)
Rapp-Hodgkin syndrome	Autosomal dominant Chromosome 3q28 TP63 gene	Anhidrotic ectodermal dysplasia, cleft lip and palate, hypodontia, nail abnormalities, hypospadia, and pili torti
Ronchese syndrome	X-linked recessive EDA gene	Ichthyosis, keratosis pilaris, nail dystrophy, dental abnormalities, leukonychia, and pili torti
Trichothiodystrophy (TTD1), photosensitive type	Autosomal recessive Chromosome 19q13 ERCC2/XPD gene	Ichthyosiform erythroderma, mental delay, short stature, brittle nails, brittle hair (torti pili or trichorrhexis nodosa)

tance patterns of pili torti vary. Acquired cases of pili torti have been seen in cases of anorexia nervosa, malnutrition, after oral retinoid treatment, and with inflammatory conditions affecting the scalp such as alopecia areata.[10] Pathogenesis is most likely caused by abnormalities of the inner root sheath and perifollicular fibrosis in cases of acquired pili torti.[11,12] Pili torti is seen in Menkes syndrome in combination with other hair shaft disorders including TN, trichoclasis, and trichoptilosis. Menkes is an X-linked recessive disorder occurring secondary to a defect in the ATP7A gene encoding for a copper transporter. Clinical signs become apparent in infancy with hypopigmentation of the skin, mental disability, depigmented hair, and neurologic impairment. Diagnosis is made by low copper and ceruloplasmin levels. Prognosis for Menkes is poor with most patients dying by age 3 years. Immediate supplementation with copper-histidine may have some benefit in preventing severe neurologic features.

DIAGNOSIS

Diagnosis of pili torti is made with light microscopy. Microscopic examination reveals flattened, twisted hair occurring at irregular intervals along the hair shaft (Fig. 89-4). Twists occur in groups of 3 to 10 and are 0.4 to 0.9 mm wide.[12,13] With scanning electron microscopy, a spiral pattern of the hair follicle is evident.[11]

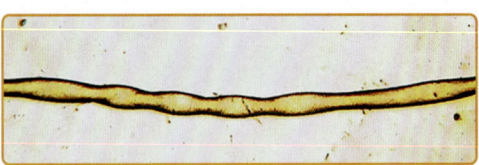

Figure 89-4 Pili torti under light microscopy: irregularly spaced 180-degree twists.

TABLE 89-5
Differential Diagnosis of Pili Torti

- Hypotrichosis
- Monilethrix
- Pseudomonilethrix
- Trichorrhexis nodosa

DIFFERENTIAL DIAGNOSIS

In addition to the associated syndromes discussed above, other hair shaft disorders are considered in the differential diagnosis for pili torti (Table 89-5).

CLINICAL COURSE AND PROGNOSIS

In most cases, hair spontaneously improves after puberty.

MANAGEMENT

No effective treatment for pili torti has been identified. Chemical and/or mechanical trauma should be reduced to avoid further breakage.

TRICHORRHEXIS INVAGINATA

Trichorrhexis invaginata (bamboo hair) is commonly associated with Netherton syndrome and is characterized by invagination of the distal hair shaft into the proximal portion. It may also occur as an isolated condition or sporadically with other hair shaft abnormalities.

EPIDEMIOLOGY

Isolated trichorrhexis invaginata is a rare condition. Incidence of Netherton syndrome is estimated to be 1 in 200,000 live births.

CLINICAL FEATURES

Hair has a dry, lusterless, brittle appearance with increased fragility. Areas of diffuse thinning with some instances of complete alopecia are present. Eyebrows and eyelashes are also affected. The Netherton syndrome clinical triad includes atopic diathesis, ichthyosiform erythroderma, and trichorrhexis invaginata. Few cases of Netherton syndrome with only ichthyosis linearis circumflexa and no other clinical features have been described.[14] Atopic diathesis occurs in approximately 75% of Netherton syndrome cases,[15] and includes atopic dermatitis, asthma, allergic rhinitis, angioedema, urticarial, hypereosinophilia, and elevated immunoglobulin E levels.[16] Hair shaft abnormalities become clinically apparent after infancy in Netherton syndrome with trichorrhexis invaginata being the most common, but abnormalities may also include pili torti and trichorrhexis invaginata. Ichthyosis appears at birth as a collodion baby or during the first few months of life with ichthyosis linearis circumflexa, which is classically described as migratory hyperkeratosis with polycyclic and serpiginous erythematous plaques that have double-edged margins at the scale. Additional extracutaneous include recurrent infections, hypogammaglobulinemia, neurologic deficits, hypernatremia, hypothermia, mental disability, delayed growth, and short stature.[17,18]

ETIOLOGY/RISK FACTORS

Netherton syndrome is an autosomal recessive disorder involving the gene serine protease inhibitor, Kazal type-5 (*SPINK5*). The *SPINK5* gene is located on chromosome 5q32 and encodes an inhibitor of lymphoepithelial Kazal-type–related inhibitor (LEKTI). As a serine protease enzyme, LEKTI is responsible for the breakdown of intracellular adhesions resulting in desquamation of epidermal cells.[16] LEKTI is also present in the inner root sheaths of hair follicles. Hair shaft abnormalities seen in Netherton syndrome may be the result of intermittent incomplete formation of disulfide bonds in the keratogenous zone.[16,19]

DIAGNOSIS

Under light microscopy, intussusception of the distal hair shaft into the proximal portion, which is soft and incompletely keratinized, leads to a "golf-tee" deformity (Fig. 89-5).[20] Because of increased fragility in these areas, nodular fractures can also be seen along the shafts at irregular intervals.[17] Electron microscopy reveals defects in keratinization of the inner root sheath.[21] Trichoscopic examination of the hair shaft also has been proposed as an accurate and quick diagnostic tool.[22] Additional laboratory findings that may aid in diagnosis include immunohistochemistry of skin biopsies to detect LEKTI deficiency, elevated levels of immunoglobulin E, and moderate eosinophilia.[18]

DIFFERENTIAL DIAGNOSIS

Differential diagnosis for trichorrhexis invaginata includes black piedra, monilethrix, and TN.[21] When diagnosing Netherton syndrome, additional disorders to consider include Leiner disease, acrodermatitis enteropathica, erythrokeratoderma variabilis, generalized seborrheic dermatitis, erythrodermic psoriasis, staphylococcal scalded skin syndrome, and nonbullous ichthyosiform erythroderma.[17,18,21]

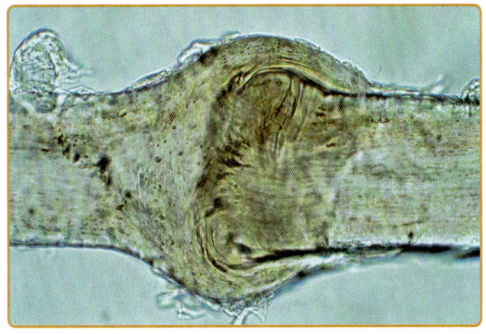

Figure 89-5 Golf-tee appearance of hair shaft under light microscopy.

CLINICAL COURSE AND PROGNOSIS

Those with milder phenotypes in Netherton syndrome often see improvement of their condition with age in addition to resolution of hair anomalies. Patients with more-severe phenotypes with erythroderma have a more persistent and severe disease course. Recurrent infections, as well as early mortality, are commonly observed in these cases.

MANAGEMENT

Cutaneous features of Netherton syndrome are managed with the use of emollients, topical steroids, and topical immunomodulators such as tacrolimus and pimecrolimus. Caution is taken when using these treatments as patients with Netherton syndrome have an increased susceptibility to absorption of topical medications.[16] Systemic therapies include low-dose corticosteroids, retinoids, and phototherapy.[16]

MONILETHRIX

Monilethrix is a rare genetic disorder associated with increased fragility and a pathognomonic beaded hair appearance (Fig. 89-6).

EPIDEMIOLOGY

Monilethrix appears early in infancy and generally occurs in an autosomal dominant pattern, although reports of autosomal recessive inheritance have been documented.[23,24] Clinical presentation varies widely with mild involvement involving only a few follicles to severe disease with complete alopecia.

CLINICAL FEATURES

Monilethrix becomes clinically apparent within the first few months of life after lanugo hair is shed and replaced with short, dry, and lusterless hair. Hair is sparse with increased fragility. Beaded hairs emerge from keratotic follicular papules that are primarily seen in the occiput.[25] Mild disease may involve only the scalp, but more severe forms can affect eyebrows, eyelashes, and generalized body hair.[26] Cases resulting in scarring alopecia also have been reported.[26] Monilethrix may occur as an isolated condition or in association with keratosis pilaris, nail defects (koilonychias), cataracts, teeth abnormalities, syndactyly, oligophrenia, and mental disability.[25,26]

ETIOLOGY/RISK FACTORS

Autosomal dominant forms of monilethrix are associated with mutations in genes for type II hair keratins including hHb1 (KRT81), hHb3 (KRT83), and hHb6 (KRT86).[24,27] These genes have been mapped to chromosome 12q11-q13.[24,26] Rare cases of autosomal recessive inheritance are linked to mutations in desmoglein 4.[26,28]

DIAGNOSIS

Light microscopy reveals a pearl necklace appearance with areas of knots and narrowing along the hair shaft. Nonmedullated elliptical nodes can be seen at regular intervals, 0.7 to 1 mm apart.[29] Trichoscopy of the hair shaft will show both dilated nodes and constricted internodes.

DIFFERENTIAL DIAGNOSIS

Table 89-6 outlines the differential diagnosis of monilethrix. Pseudomonilethrix presents with the same beaded morphology as monilethrix. However, unlike monilethrix, elliptical nodes are not seen at regular intervals along the hair shaft and keratotic follicular papules are not seen on physical examination.

CLINICAL COURSE AND PROGNOSIS

Clinical course is variable although hair often improves with age.[27]

MANAGEMENT

No definitive treatment has been identified.[30] Oral retinoids and topical minoxidil may be of some benefit.[31,32] N-acetyl cysteine provides initial improvement but its effects do not persist long-term.[24]

UNRULY HAIR

UNCOMBABLE HAIR SYNDROME

Uncombable hair syndrome (pili trianguli et canaliculi or spun glass hair) is a rare disorder of the scalp hair that is characterized by a structural anomaly of the inner and outer hair sheath.[33,34]

TABLE 89-6
Differential Diagnosis of Monilethrix

- Alopecia areata
- Alopecia secondary to chemotherapy
- Monilethrix-like autosomal recessive hypotrichosis
- Pseudomonilethrix
- Trichorrhexis nodosa

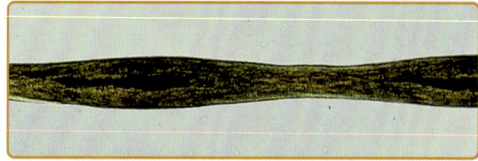

Figure 89-6 Typical beaded appearance of hair as seen under light microscopy in monilethrix.

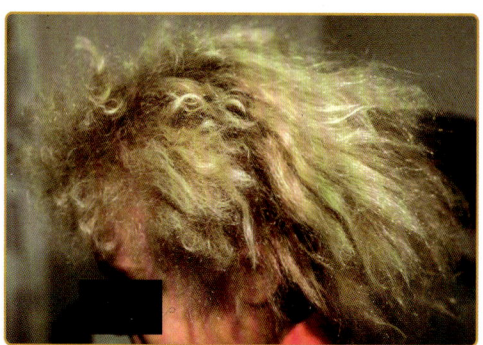

Figure 89-7 Clinical appearance of uncombable hair syndrome.

TABLE 89-7
Differential Diagnosis of Uncombable Hair
▪ Acquired progressive hair kinking
▪ Drug-induced kinking
▪ Loose anagen syndrome
▪ Marie Unna hypotrichosis
▪ Monilethrix
▪ Pili torti
▪ Rapp-Hodgkin syndrome
▪ Wooly hair

EPIDEMIOLOGY

Uncombable hair most commonly presents within the first few months, but can occur up to 12 years of age.[35] It affects males and females equally. The majority of cases are autosomal dominant with complete or incomplete penetrance though sporadic forms of uncombable hair have been observed. Acquired forms are more common in dark, curly hair individuals and tend to occur later in life. A partial variant with patchy, well-demarcated involvement, typically in frontal and occipital areas also has been described.

CLINICAL FEATURES

Patients with familial uncombable hair have unruly, frizzy, and dry hair that sticks out from scalp and is difficult to comb flat (Fig. 89-7). Hair is normally red-blond to light blond in color and has a spangled appearance. There is no increased fragility and hair is generally normal in both quantity and length. Eyebrows, eyelashes, and body hair are not affected. Several systemic disorders have been known to present concurrently with uncombable hair, including various forms of ectodermal dysplasia such as Bork syndrome, multiple epiphyseal dysplasia, and type I neurofibromatosis.[33,34,36-38] Other conditions, such as digital abnormalities, juvenile cataracts, retinal dysplasia, pigmentary dystrophy, tooth enamel anomalies, oligodontia, and phalangoepiphyseal dysplasia, have been reported.[37]

ETIOLOGY/RISK FACTORS

In 2016, 3 genes were implicated in the autosomal recessive variants: PADI3 (peptidylarginine deiminase 3), TGM3 (transglutaminase 3), and TCHH (trichohyalin).[38A] Premature keratinization or a structural anomaly of the dermal papillae of the inner and outer hair shaft of the follicle may result in the rigid configuration that is characteristic of uncombable hair.[39,40]

DIAGNOSIS

Under closer analysis of hair cross-sections with electron microscopy, the affected hairs exhibit a triangular or kidney shape with shallow longitudinal grooving. It is thought that this longitudinal grooving is responsible for the physical manifestation of the hair's appearance. In normal hair, the largest amount of light refraction occurs at the center of the hair because of the dark longitudinal band. However, in uncombable hair, the presence of longitudinal hair grooving of the hair shaft causes hair to have more of a characteristically glistening appearance at the edges of the hair strand.[41]

DIFFERENTIAL DIAGNOSIS

Table 89-7 outlines the differential diagnosis of uncombable hair syndrome. Other closely associated hair disorders may mimic the clinical features of uncombable hair syndrome.

CLINICAL COURSE AND PROGNOSIS

Hair typically improves with age and most cases resolve after puberty.

MANAGEMENT

No treatment has been identified and is generally not necessary. Biotin supplementation has been reported to have a positive effect on uncombable hair.[39,41,42]

MARIE-UNNA HEREDITARY HYPOTRICHOSIS

Marie-Unna hereditary hypotrichosis (MUHH) is an autosomal dominant condition that presents at birth with sparse or absent hair.

EPIDEMIOLOGY

MUHH is most commonly seen in those of European descent but occurrences in China have been reported.[43] Males and females are equally affected. Clinical features are normally seen at birth. A single case series, notes a few individuals with normal hair at birth with later progression to hair loss.[43]

TABLE 89-8

Differential Diagnosis of Marie Unna Hereditary Hypotrichosis

- Androgenetic alopecia
- Alopecia areata
- Congenital atrichia with popular lesions
- Hereditary hypotrichosis simplex
- Loose anagen syndrome
- Uncombable hair syndrome

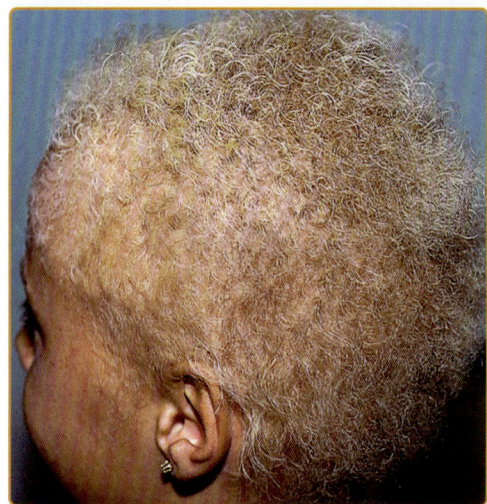

Figure 89-8 Wooly hair syndrome clinical presentation.

CLINICAL FEATURES

Clinical features vary over time. Hair is typically sparse or completely absent at birth with regrowth of coarse, wiry, and unruly hair during childhood. Around puberty, nonscarring hair loss is again seen. Pattern of hair loss may be similar to androgenic alopecia with thick hair scattered in thinning areas that are especially noted on vertex, parietal, and occipital regions.[44] Total alopecia may be observed. Scalp, eyebrows, eyelashes, secondary sexual hairs, and generalized body hair are affected. Other cutaneous features associated with MUHH include milia-like lesions on the face as well as follicular hyperkeratosis.[43]

ETIOLOGY/RISK FACTORS

MUHH is inherited in an autosomal dominant pattern. MUHH is caused by a heterozygous mutation in *U2HR*, which is an upstream open reading frame that normally acts to inhibit the *HR* gene on chromosome 8p21. Up to 17 different mutations in the *U2HR* gene are described in the literature.[45]

DIAGNOSIS

Clinical examination reveals multiple anagen hairs on pull test. Scalp biopsy may show a reduced number of follicles with inflammation, but no fibrosis or scarring.[43] Both light and electron microscopy reveal irregular twisting of the hair along with longitudinal ridges and peeling of the cuticle.[51]

DIFFERENTIAL DIAGNOSIS

Table 89-8 outlines the differential diagnosis of MUHH. Hereditary hypotrichosis has a large clinical overlap with MUHH, but is distinguished by normal hair at birth as well as no associated hair shaft abnormalities. The characteristic clinical course of MUHH, as well as the twisted hair morphology, differentiates MUHH from other disorders.[43]

CLINICAL COURSE/PROGNOSIS

Hair features of MUHH are persistent.

MANAGEMENT

There is no known treatment.

WOOLY HAIR

Wooly hair is a congenital disorder that is characterized by unruly and tightly coiled hair (Fig. 89-8).[46]

EPIDEMIOLOGY

Wooly hair is a rare condition although exact incidence has not been reported. It is primarily seen in white and Asian individuals and appears during childhood or adolescence.[47] Males and females are affected equally.[48] Autosomal dominant and recessive forms of wooly hair have been described, although it can occur sporadically.[46]

CLINICAL FEATURES

Hair is characterized by tight curls that have an average diameter of 0.5 cm. Hair may occasionally be shorter because of a briefer anagen phase, although rate of growth and telogen-to-anagen ratio is often normal.[49] Brittle hair with no increased fragility is observed. Wooly hair can also show signs of TN.[49]

Four variants have been identified including hereditary wooly hair, familial wooly hair, symmetrical circumscribed allotrichia, and wooly hair nevus.[50] Hereditary wooly hair (autosomal dominant) is often associated with ocular anomalies such as persistent pupillary membranes, retinal defects, and cataracts.[51] Familial wooly hair (autosomal recessive) may occur concomitantly with palmoplantar hyperkeratosis and cardiac anomalies.[52] Naxos disease and Carvajal syn-

TABLE 89-9
Differential Diagnosis of Wooly Hair

- Acquired progressive kinky hair
- Allotrichia circumscripta symmetrica
- Drug-induced kinky hair

TABLE 89-10
Subtypes of Hypotrichosis

SUBTYPE	INHERITANCE PATTERN	GENE DEFECT AND/OR LOCATION
HYPT1	Autosomal dominant	Heterozygous mutation APCDD1 Chromosome 18p1
HYPT2	Autosomal dominant	Heterozygous mutation CDSN Chromosome 6p21.3
HYPT3	Autosomal dominant	Heterozygous mutation KRT74 Chromosome 12q13
HYPT4	Autosomal dominant	Heterozygous mutation 5′ UTR (untranslated region) region of *HR* gene Chromosome 8p21.3
HYPT5	Autosomal recessive	Chromosome 1p21.1-q21.3
HYPT6	Autosomal recessive	Homozygous or compound heterozygous mutation DSG4 Chromosome 18q12
HYPT7 Wooly hair autosomal recessive II	Autosomal recessive	Homozygous or compound heterozygous mutation LIPH Chromosome 3q27
HYPT8 Wooly hair autosomal recessive I	Autosomal recessive	Homozygous or compound heterozygous mutation P2RY5 Chromosome 13q14
HYPT9	Autosomal recessive	Chromosome 10q11.23-q22.3
HYPT10	Autosomal recessive	Chromosome 7p22.3-p21.3

drome are 2 variants of this association. Naxos disease is caused by a plakoglobin gene mutation and is characterized by wooly hair, right ventricular cardiomyopathy, and nonepidermolytic diffuse palmoplantar keratoderma (Vörner-Unna-Thost type).[53] Carvajal syndrome is caused by a defect in desmoplakin and also presents with wooly hair, but presents with left ventricular dilated cardiomyopathy and striate palmoplantar keratoderma.[52] Wooly hair nevus can be accompanied by melanocytic or epidermal nevi in addition to delayed bone growth, periodontal changes, and developmental delay.[54] Noonan syndrome, cardiofaciocutaneous syndrome, and keratosis pilaris also have been reported with wooly hair.[49]

ETIOLOGY/RISK FACTORS

Autosomal dominant forms occur as a result of a mutation in the keratin gene, *KRT71*, on chromosome 12q13.[54] There are 2 forms of autosomal recessive disease, both of which occur with or without hypotrichosis. Autosomal recessive wooly hair type I is caused by a mutation of the P2RY5 or LPAR6 gene on chromosome 13q14 that encodes for a G-protein–coupled receptor that is known to play a role in hair growth.[55] Autosomal recessive wooly hair type II is caused by a mutation in the *LIPH* gene, which is found on chromosome 3q27.[56]

DIAGNOSIS

Diagnosis is made by clinical presentation. Light microscopy and scalp biopsy are normal.

DIFFERENTIAL DIAGNOSIS

Table 89-9 outlines the differential diagnosis of wooly hair.

CLINICAL COURSE AND PROGNOSIS

Wooly hair appearance is most pronounced in childhood and becomes significantly less evident in adulthood.

MANAGEMENT

No treatment has been established for wooly hair. Harsh chemical and physical injury should be avoided.

HYPOTRICHOSIS

Hereditary hypotrichosis simplex (HHS) is a nonsyndromic hereditary condition that presents with normal hair at birth and progressively thins with age.

EPIDEMIOLOGY

Prevalence is unknown. Both genders are affected equally.

CLINICAL FEATURES

HHS is characterized by diffusely sparse, fine, short hairs. Follicular miniaturization and noninflammatory alopecia are characteristic of the disease. It can either affect the scalp only or can be more generalized with complete body hair involvement. HHS occurs as an isolated condition with no reports of associated cutaneous or extracutaneous anomalies.

ETIOLOGY/RISK FACTOR

Ten subtypes of HHS have been identified based on gene mutations, including 4 autosomal dominant (HYPT1 to HYPT4) and 6 autosomal recessive forms (HYPT5 to HYPT10) (Table 89-10).[57]

DIAGNOSIS

Light and electron microscopy of HHS show normal findings in early stages and later may reveal focal areas of defect in the cuticle.[58] Scalp biopsy in HHS demonstrates a decreased number of follicles in the telogen phase.[58]

DIFFERENTIAL DIAGNOSIS

Hypotrichosis has been identified as a feature of many other conditions including wooly hair and MUHH. HHS must be distinguished from other hair shaft abnormalities that may have similar clinical presentations.

CLINICAL COURSE AND PROGNOSIS

Hair becomes progressively thinner with age. Most patients have complete baldness by 30 years of age.[59]

MANAGEMENT

No treatment is available.

OTHER

LOOSE ANAGEN SYNDROME

Loose anagen syndrome (LAS) is a sporadic or inherited hair condition characterized by hair that is loosely attached to the scalp. Hair loss in this condition is nonscarring and noninflammatory.

EPIDEMIOLOGY

LAS is most often diagnosed in children between the ages of 2 and 6 years[60] and may present for the first time in adulthood. LAS has been reported to occur in a 6:1 female-to-male ratio,[61] although cases in males are underreported because of differences in hairstyles.[62] Classically described in lighter skin and hair individuals, those with darker skin and hair can also be affected.[63-65] The diagnosis should be considered in all presentations with scant, thinning hair.

CLINICAL FEATURES

Hair in LAS is diffusely sparse and is easily pulled from the scalp without pain. Inability to grow long hair and rare need for a haircut is common. LAS is especially evident in the posterior scalp where hair becomes matted. Hair has no increased fragility, although it can be unruly and difficult to comb. Three groups of LAS have been established based on phenotype.[63,66] LAS type A is characterized by sparse, dull, and unruly hair that does not grow long. Patients with LAS type B have diffuse or patchy unruly hair and patients with type C LAS typically present as adults with excessive shedding.[63,66]

Most cases of LAS are isolated although associated systemic diseases have been identified. Atopic diseases such as eczema and asthma are most commonly seen with LAS. Other concomitant disorders reported in the literature include coloboma, ectodermal dysplasia, ectrodactyly-ectodermal dysplasia-clefting syndrome, trichorhinophalangeal syndrome, nail-patella syndrome, neurofibromatosis, trichotillomania, wooly hair, AIDS, and alopecia areata.[67] Noonan syndrome and Noonan-like syndrome also have been linked to LAS.[68]

ETIOLOGY/RISK FACTORS

When it occurs in a familial pattern, LAS has an autosomal dominant inheritance.[69] LAS presents secondary to defects in keratinization of the inner root sheath, which impairs adhesion to the cuticle of the hair shaft. Studies suggest an E337K mutation in the K6HF keratin gene, although other genes may be involved.[66] LAS with Noonan-like syndrome is linked to a heterozygous mutation of SHOC2 gene on chromosome 10q25.[68]

DIAGNOSIS

Diagnosis of LAS is made by pull-test, examination of hair under microscope, and trichogram analysis. Pull-test typically results in 3 to 10 hairs that are easily and painlessly plucked from hair. Light microscopy reveals predominantly anagen hairs with distorted hair bulbs and abnormal keratinization of root sheaths. Flattening of hair and longitudinal grooving can be found on electron microscope.[70] Cuticles are also characteristically ruffled, baggy, twisted, and have a floppy sock appearance. Trichogram shows at least 70% anagen hairs.[71] Trichoscopy also may be helpful in diagnosing LAS with typical features including solitary rectangular black granular structures, solitary yellow dots, and follicles with single hairs.[72]

DIFFERENTIAL DIAGNOSIS

Table 89-11 outlines the differential diagnosis of LAS. Any type of diffuse, nonscarring alopecia is considered in the differential diagnosis for LAS. Clinical findings, as well as evaluation with trichography, will help differentiate LAS from the other conditions.

CLINICAL COURSE AND PROGNOSIS

LAS typically resolves with age. If it presents at an older age, hair loss is more likely to be persistent.

TABLE 89-11
Differential Diagnosis of Loose Anagen Syndrome

- Alopecia areata
- Hypothyroidism or hyperthyroidism
- Iron-deficiency anemia
- Medication related hair loss
- Telogen effluvium
- Traction alopecia
- Trichotillomania
- Uncombable hair syndrome

MANAGEMENT

No treatment specific for LAS is available. Gentle hair care is advised to prevent further shedding of hair. Biotin use has been suggested, although there is no evidence of benefit in the literature. Use of topical 5% minoxidil has been used successfully in some severe cases of LAS.[73]

PILI ANNULATI

Pili annulati presents with ringed hair that is not usually associated with increased fragility. Hair in pili annulati is characterized by alternating light and dark bands.[74]

EPIDEMIOLOGY

Pili annulati typically presents at birth or during infancy, but can appear later in life. Familial patterns show an autosomal dominant inheritance pattern with both reduced and variable penetrance. Pili annulati can be sporadic and isolated, but also has been observed in patients with woolly hair and alopecia areata.[75] Patients with light blond or brown hair present more often with pili annulati in comparison to darker hair individuals where the banding pattern characteristic of this condition is difficult to detect.

CLINICAL FEATURES

Alternating shiny and dull segments gives the hair an overall shiny, speckled appearance. The scalp is the primary site affected with involvement of 20% to 80% of hair and a decrease in number of bands distally. Localized involvement of axillary, pubic, and beard hair also has been reported.[76-78] Hair strength and growth are typically normal, although 6 cases of increased fragility with pili annulati have been found in the literature.[79-82] Conditions previously associated with pili annulati include alopecia areata, blue nevi, syndactyly, polydactylism, and leukonychia.[83] More commonly, however, pili annulati is limited to the hair shaft with no associated cutaneous or extracutaneous features.

ETIOLOGY/RISK FACTORS

In inherited cases, pili annulati is caused by a single defect on chromosome 12q24.33.[74,84] A recent study mapped the gene locus to a 2.9-Mb region between D12S343 and the telomeric end of chromosome 12. This region contains 24 genes for hair expression.[84] Exact pathology has yet to be established although proposed mechanisms include defects in cytokeratin, abnormal matrix formation, and a malfunction of the protein that regulates the structure of the extracellular matrix.[76,84-87]

Pili annulati is not frequently associated with increased fragility, but some cases have been reported in the literature.[79-82] In these cases, analysis of amino acid content revealed an elevated lysine and decreased cysteine content in affected hair when compared to normal.[79,88] These findings suggest a role for biochemical makeup in the pathogenesis of pili annulati. Exogenous trauma such as from rigorous brushing also contribute to the changes that are seen in instances of fragility in pili annulati.[79-81]

DIAGNOSIS

Trichoscopy of pili annulati demonstrates alternating white and dark bands along the hair shaft with lighter segments representing air-filled cavities. Under light microscope, the visual effects are switched with clinically light bands appearing dark under microscopy, a result of air cavities scattering the light.[79] With the addition of potassium hydroxide for mounting, banding in hair disappears as the liquid fills the cavities.[79] Transmission electron microscopy and scanning electron microscopy will further reveal air cavities of varying sizes and shapes as well as a cobblestone appearance of the cuticle.[86] In some cases, scanning electron microscopy and transmission electron microscopy may also demonstrate areas of cuticle weathering.[79-82]

DIFFERENTIAL DIAGNOSIS

Because of the similar clinical appearance of color banding, pseudopili annulati is important to consider for the differential diagnosis. Pseudopili annulati, however, is not caused by an underlying physical defect, but instead occurs from periodic twisting of the hair. Unlike in pili annulati, in pseudopili annulati, light microscopy, scanning electron microscopy, and transmission electron microscopy of hair all demonstrate normal findings. Other conditions to consider for differential diagnosis include fragmented medulla, bubble hair, and pseudopili torti.

TABLE 89-12
Summary of Hair Shaft Disorders

	ETIOLOGY/RISK FACTORS/MODE OF INHERITANCE	CLINICAL MANIFESTATION	DIAGNOSIS	CLINICAL COURSE	MANAGEMENT	RELATED SYNDROMES & CONDITIONS
Associated with Hair Breakage						
Trichorrhexis nodosa (TN)	Acquired—external trauma	Brittle, lusterless hair with white nodular swellings along hair shaft	Light and electron microscopy: splayed paint brush bristle appearance (see Fig. 89-1)	Acquired TN may improve with removal of external trauma. Inherited TN may have varying courses	For acquired TN, avoidance of harsh chemical treatments	None
	Inherited—autosomal dominant Congenital—ectodermal dysplasias, or metabolic disorders					None Ectodermal dysplasias, arginosuccinic aciduria and other metabolic disorders
Trichoschisis & trichothiodystrophy (TTD)	Trichoschisis—may occur from external trauma or secondary to TTD	Brittle, easily broken hair with short, brittle eyebrows and eyelashes; clinical and cutaneous features of TTD may accompany hair findings	Polarized light microscopy: "tiger tail" hair. Genetic testing and amino acid analysis of the hair shaft: low cysteine and sulfur content (<50% of normal)	Acquired trichoschisis improves with removal of external trauma; course of TTD depends on the clinical phenotype	For acquired trichoschisis, reducing hair manipulation is helpful. TTD with systemic effects requires multidisciplinary care	See Table 89-3
	TTD—congenital (autosomal recessive; ERCC2, ERCC3, p8, C7Orf11); photosensitive types (XPD, XPB, TTDA genes); nonphotosensitive types (TTDN1)					
Pili torti	Acquired—anorexia nervosa, severe malnutrition, oral retinoid treatment, inflammatory scalp conditions	Brittle, dry, and spangled from uneven light reflections	Light microscopy: flattened, twisted hair occurring at irregular intervals along the hair shaft	Most cases show spontaneous improvement after puberty	Although no effective treatment, mechanical trauma should be reduced	Menke syndrome
	Isolated cases may be autosomal dominant, autosomal recessive, or sporadic. Menke syndrome is X-linked recessive					

(Continued)

TABLE 89-12
Summary of Hair Shaft Disorders (Continued)

	ETIOLOGY/RISK FACTORS/MODE OF INHERITANCE	CLINICAL MANIFESTATION	DIAGNOSIS	CLINICAL COURSE	MANAGEMENT	RELATED SYNDROMES & CONDITIONS
Trichorrhexis invaginata	Isolated cases; inherited (as in Netherton syndrome–autosomal recessive disorder; SPINK5)	Dry, lusterless, brittle appearance with increased fragility. Eyebrows and eyelashes are also affected	Light microscopy: intussusception of the distal hair shaft into the proximal portion; "golf tee" deformity Trichoscopy may be helpful	Milder phenotypes of Netherton syndrome may improve with age; severe phenotypes have a persistent and severe course	Treatment for cutaneous features of Netherton syndrome are available	Netherton syndrome
Monilethrix	Autosomal dominant inheritance (KRT81, KRT83, KRT86) Rarely, autosomal recessive (DSG4)	Short, dry, lusterless hair. Beaded hairs emerge from keratotic follicular papules. Eyebrows, eyelashes, and body hair may be affected	Light microscopy: "pearl necklace" appearance with areas of knots and narrowing along the hair shaft Trichoscopy: dilated nodes and constricted internodes	Variable; hair often improves with age	Oral retinoids and topical minoxidil. No definitive treatment	May have associated cutaneous, renal, and dental abnormalities
Unruly Hair						
Uncombable hair syndrome (pili trianguli et canaliculi; spun glass hair)	Autosomal dominant Acquired forms are common in dark, curly haired individuals	Unruly, frizzy, dry hair. No increased fragility. Eyebrows, eyelashes, and body hair are not affected	Electron microscopy: triangular/kidney-shaped cross-sectional appearance with longitudinal grooving	Usually resolves after puberty	Biotin supplementation may be of help. Treatment is generally not necessary	Ectodermal dysplasia syndrome, Bork syndrome, multiple epiphyseal dysplasia, type I neurofibromatosis
Marie-Unna hereditary hypotrichosis	Autosomal dominant condition (U2HR)	Sparse, absent hair; regrowth may be coarse, wiry and unruly in childhood, but hair loss may recur at puberty Total alopecia may be present Associated milia-like lesions and follicular hyperkeratosis	Pull test: multiple anagen hairs Scalp biopsy: reduced number of follicles and no evidence of fibrosis. Light and electron microscopy: irregular twisting of the hair, with longitudinal ridging and peeling of the cuticle	Persistent	No known treatment	None
Wooly hair	Autosomal dominant (KRT71) and autosomal recessive (type I: P2RY5 or LPAR6, type II: LIPH), as well as sporadic forms	Tight curls with an average diameter of 0.5 cm; brittle hair with no increased fragility. Trichorrhexis nodosa may be seen	Clinical presentation Light microscopy and scalp biopsy are normal	Less pronounced in adulthood	No treatment, but harsh chemical and mechanical injury should be avoided	Hereditary wooly hair Naxos disease Carvajal syndrome Noonan syndrome
Hereditary hypotrichosis simplex (HHS)	4 Autosomal dominant subtypes (HYPT1-4) and 6 autosomal recessive subtypes (HYPT 5-10)	Diffusely sparse, fine, short hairs. Follicular miniaturization and inflammatory alopecia; body hair may be involved	Light and electron microscopy: focal areas of defect in cuticle Scalp biopsy: decreased number of follicles	Complete baldness by age 30 years	No treatment available	None

Other					
Loose anagen syndrome (LAS)	Sporadic and inherited condition (autosomal dominant; K6HF gene)	Hair is diffusely sparse, and easily pulled from the scalp without pain. Individuals rarely need a haircut. No increased hair fragility, but hair may be difficult to comb. LAS has 3 phenotypes	Pull test: increased anagen hairs. Light microscopy: anagen hairs with distorted bulbs, cuticles have a "floppy sock" appearance. Trichogram: 70% anagen hairs	Resolves with age; when LAS presents late, hair loss more likely to be persistent	Gentle hair care, 5% minoxidil	Atopic diseases Ectodermal dysplasia Nail-patella syndrome Neurofibromatosis Noonan syndrome Noonan-like syndrome
Pili annulati	Sporadic, or inherited (autosomal dominant, single defect on chromosome 12q24.33)	Characterized by alternating light and dark bands; hair has a "speckled" appearance	Trichoscopy: alternating white and dark bands; light microscopy: reversal of white and dark bands; electron microscopy: shows a cobblestone appearance of the cuticle	Clinical features become more prominent with age; course is benign	Gentle hair care practices; no specific treatment available	None

CLINICAL COURSE AND PROGNOSIS

Pili annulati frequently goes undiagnosed because of its subtle clinical features. Although it is a lifelong condition, lack of abnormalities in skin and other organs make its course relatively benign. Clinical features do become more prominent with age,[83] but the shiny appearance of hair is often appealing to patients.

MANAGEMENT

Specific treatment of pili annulati is not available. Gentle hair care practices should be employed to prevent further weathering.

SUMMARY

Table 89-12 summarizes hair shaft disorders.

REFERENCES

1. Sisto T, Bussoletti C, D'amore A. Inability to grow long hair: a presentation of trichorrhexis nodosa. *Cutis*. 2015;95(4):E15-E16.
2. Whiting DA. Structural abnormalities of hair shaft. *J Am Acad Dermatol*. 1987;16(1, pt 1):1-25.
3. Allan, JD, Cusworth, DC, Dent, CE, et al. A disease, probably hereditary, characterized by severe mental deficiency and a constant gross abnormality of amino acid metabolism. *Lancet*. 1958;271:182-187.
4. Moslehi R, Signore C, Tamura D, et al. Adverse effects of trichothiodystrophy DNA repair and transcription gene disorder on human fetal development. *Clin Genet*. 2010;77(4):365-373.
5. Hansen LK, Wulff K, Brandrup F. Trichothiodystrophy. Hair examination as a diagnostic tool. *Ugeskr Laeger*. 1993;155(25):1949-1952.
6. Faghri S, Tamura D, Kraemer KH, et al. Trichothiodystrophy: a systematic review of 112 published cases characterises a wide spectrum of clinical manifestations. *J Med Genet*. 2008;45:609-621.
7. Stefanini M, Botta E, Lanzafame M, et al. Trichothiodystrophy: from basic mechanisms to clinical implications. *DNA Repair (Amst)*. 2010 2;9(1):2-10.
8. Heller ER, Khan SG, Kuschal C, et al. Mutations in the TTDN1 gene are associated with a distinct trichothiodystrophy phenotype. *J Invest Dermatol*. 2015;135(3):734-741.
9. Beare JM. Congenital pilar defect showing features of pili torti. *Br J Dermatol*. 1952;64:366-372.
10. Yang JJ, Cade KV, Rezende FC, et al. Clinical presentation of pili torti—case report. *An Bras Dermatol*. 2015;90(3)(suppl 1):29-31.
11. Maruyama T, Toyoda M, Kanei A, et al. Pathogenesis in pili torti: morphological study. *J Dermatol Sci*. 1994;7:S5-S12.
12. Whiting DA. Hair shaft defects. In: Olsen EA, ed. *Disorders of Hair Growth: Diagnosis and Treatment*. 2nd ed. New York, NY: McGraw-Hill; 2003:123-175.
13. Price V. Structural anomalies of the hair shaft: pili torti. In: Orfanos CE, Happle R, eds. *Hair and Hair Diseases*. Heidelberg, Germany: Springer-Verlag; 1990:384-390.
14. Guerra L, Fortugno P, Pedicelli C, et al. Ichthyosis linearis circumflexa as the only clinical manifestation of Netherton syndrome. *Acta Derm Venereol*. 2015;95(6):720-724.
15. Salodkar AD, Choudhary SV, Jadwani G, et al. Bamboo hair in Netherton's syndrome. *Int J Trichology*. 2009;1:143-144.
16. Kumar R, Abhinandan HB, Mehta P, et al. Netherton's syndrome. *Indian J Paediatr Dermatol*. 2014;15:120-122.
17. Blume-Peytavi U. Hair loss in children. In: *Hair Growth and Disorders*. Berlin, Germany: Springer; 2008:273-309.
18. Tadini G, Brena M, Gelmetti C, et al. Icthyoses. In: *Atlas of Genodermatoses*, 2nd ed. Milan, Italy: CRC Press; June 2015:65-69.
19. Jain SP, Jain PA, Pandey N. The arid melancholy-Netherton syndrome with protein energy malnutrition. *J Clin Diagn Res*. 2016;10(4):WD01-WD02.
20. Elewski BE. Tinea capitis: a current perspective. *J Am Acad Dermatol*. 2000;42:1.
21. Bittencourt Mde J, Moure ER, Pies OT, et al. Trichoscopy as a diagnostic tool in trichorrhexis invaginata and Netherton syndrome. *An Bras Dermatol*. 2015;90(1):114-116.
22. Burk C, Hu S, Lee C, et al. Netherton syndrome and trichorrhexis invaginata—a novel diagnostic approach. *Pediatr Dermatol*. 2008;25:287-288.
23. Kljuic A, Bazzi H, Sundberg JP, et al. Desmoglein 4 in hair follicle differentiation and epidermal adhesion: evidence from inherited hypotrichosis and acquired pemphigus vulgaris. *Cell*. 2003;113:249-260.
24. Vikramkumar AG, Kuruvila S, Ganguly S. Monilethrix: a rare hereditary condition. *Indian J Dermatol*. 2013;58(3):243.
25. Olsen EA. Hair disorders. In: Irvine AD, Hoeger PH, Yan AC, eds. *Harper's Textbook of Pediatric Dermatology*. Oxford, UK: Wiley-Blackwell; 2011:148-149.
26. Ferrando J, Galve J, Torres-Puente M, et al. Monilethrix: a new family with the novel mutation in KRT81 gene. *Int J Trichology*. 2012;4:53-55.
27. De Oliveira EF, Araripe AL. Monilethrix: a typical case report with microscopic and dermatoscopic findings. *An Bras Dermatol*. 2015;90(1):126-127.
28. Jain N, Khopkar U. Monilethrix in pattern of distribution in siblings: diagnosis by trichoscopy. *Int J Trichology*. 2010;2:56-59.
29. Rogers M, Tay YK, Wong LC. Hair disorders. In: Schachner LA, Hansen RC, eds. *Pediatric Dermatology*. Philadelphia, PA: Mosby Elsevier; 2011:752-753.
30. Narmatha GR, Chithra S, Balasubramanian N. Monilethrix. *Indian J Dermatol Venereol Leprol*. 2002;68:220-221.
31. Rossi A, Iorio A, Scali E, et al. Monilethrix treated with minoxidil. *Int J Immunopathol Pharmacol*. 2011;24:239-242.
32. Karincaoglu Y, Coskun BK, Seyhan ME, et al. Monilethrix: improvement with acitretin. *Am J Clin Dermatol*. 2005;6:407-410.
33. Rieubland C, de Viragh PA, Addor MC. Uncombable hair syndrome: a clinical report. *Eur J Med Genet*. 2007;50:309-314.
34. Kiliç A, Oğuz D, Can A, et al. A case of uncombable hair syndrome: light microscopy, trichoscopy, and scanning electron microscopy. *Acta Dermatovenerol Croat*. 2013;21(3):209-211.

35. Wagner AM, Cunningham BB, Weinstein JM, et al. Uncombable hair syndrome: light microscopy diagnosis. *Pediatr Dermatol*. 2005;22:369-370.
36. Jarell AD, Hall MA, Sperling LC. Uncombable hair syndrome. *Pediatr Dermatol*. 2007;24(4):436-438.
37. Fritz TM, Trueb RM. Uncombable hair syndrome with angel-shaped phalango-epiphyseal dysplasia. *Pediatr Dermatol*. 2000;17(1):21-24.
38. Schena D, Germi L, Zamperetti MR, et al. Uncombable hair syndrome, mental retardation, single palmar crease and arched palate in a patient with neurofibromatosis type 1. *Pediatr Dermatol*. 2007;24(5):E73-E75.
38A. Ü Basmanav FB, Cau L, Tafazzoli A, Méchin MC, Wolf S, Romano MT, et al. Mutations in three genes encoding proteins involved in hair shaft formation cause uncombable hair syndrome. *Am J Hum Genet*. 2016;99 (6):1292-1304.
39. Boccaletti, Zendri E, Giordano G, et al. Familial uncombable hair syndrome: ultra-structural hair study and response to biotin. *Pediatr Dermatol*. 2007;24(3):e14-e16.
40. Ahmed I, Subtil A, Thomas D. Pili trianguli et canaliculi is a defect of inner root sheath keratinization: ultrastructural observations of anomalous tonofilament organization in a case. *Am J Dermatopathol*. 2005;27(3):232-236.
41. Hicks J, Metry DW, Barrish J, et al. Uncombable hair (cheveux incoiffables, pili trianguli et canaliculi) syndrome: brief review and role of scanning electron microscopy in diagnosis. *Ultrastruct Pathol*. 2001;25: 99-103.
42. Shelley WB, Shelley ED. Uncombable hair syndrome: observations on response to biotin and occurrence in siblings with ectodermal dysplasia. *J Am Acad Dermatol*. 1985;13:97-102.
43. Srinivas SM, Hiremagalore R. Marie-Unna hereditary hypotrichosis. *Int J Trichology*. 2014;6(4):182-184.
44. Roberts JL, Whiting DA, Henry D, et al. Marie Unna congenital hypotrichosis: clinical description, histopathology, scanning electron microscopy of a previously unreported large pedigree. *J Investig Dermatol Symp Proc*. 1999;4:261-267.
45. Yun SK, Cho YG, Song KH, et al. Identification of a novel U2HR mutation in a Korean woman with Marie Unna hereditary hypotrichosis. *Int J Dermatol*. 2014;53(11):1358-1361.
46. Venugopal V, Karthikeyan S, Gnanaraj P, et al. Woolly hair nevus: a rare entity. *Int J Trichology*. 2012;4(1):42-43.
47. Prasad GK. Familial woolly hair. *Indian J Dermatol Venereol Leprol*. 2002;68:157.
48. Stieler W, Otte HG, Stadler R. Multiple woolly hair nevi with linear epidermal nevus and persistent pupillary membrane [in German]. *Hautarzt*. 1992;43:441-445.
49. Singh SK, Manchanda K, Kumar A, et al. Familial woolly hair: a rare entity. *Int J Trichology*. 2012;4(4):288-289.
50. Hutchinson PE, Cairns RJ, Wells RS. Woolly hair. Clinical and general aspects. *Trans St Johns Hosp Dermatol Soc*. 1974;60:160-177.
51. Taylor AE. Hereditary woolly hair with ocular involvement. *Br J Dermatol*. 1990;123:523-525.
52. Chien AJ, Valentine MC, Sybert VP. Hereditary woolly hair and keratosis pilaris. *J Am Acad Dermatol*. 2006;54:S35-S39.
53. McKoy G, Protonotarios N, Crosby A, et al. Identification of a deletion in plakoglobin in arrhythmogenic right ventricular cardiomyopathy with palmoplantar keratoderma and woolly hair (Naxos disease) *Lancet*. 2000;355:2119-2124.
54. Fujimoto A, Farooq M, Fujikawa H, et al. A missense mutation within the helix initiation motif of the keratin K71 gene underlies autosomal dominant woolly hair/hypotrichosis. *J Invest Dermatol*. 2012;132:2342-2349.
55. Azeem Z, Jelani M, Naz G, et al. Novel mutations in G protein-coupled receptor gene (P2RY5) in families with autosomal recessive hypotrichosis (LAH3). *Hum Genet*. 2008;123:515-519.
56. Ali G, Chishti MS, Raza SI, et al. A mutation in the lipase H (LIPH) gene underlie autosomal recessive hypotrichosis. *Hum Genet*. 2007;121:319-325.
57. Al Aboud D, Al Aboud K, Al Hawsawi K, et al. Hereditary hypotrichosis simplex of the scalp: a report of 2 additional families. *Sudan J Dermatol*. 2005;3:128-131.
58. Betz RC, Lee, YA, Bygum, A, et al. A gene for hypotrichosis simplex of the scalp maps to chromosome 6p21.3. *Am J Hum Genet*. 2000;66:1979-1983.
59. Toribio J, Quinones PA. Hereditary hypotrichosis simplex of the scalp: evidence for autosomal dominant inheritance. *Br J Dermatol*. 1974;91:687-696.
60. Srinivas SM. Loose anagen hair syndrome. *Int J Trichology*. 2015;7(3):138-139.
61. Sinclair R, Cargnello J, Chow CW. Loose anagen syndrome. *Exp Dermatol*. 1999;8 297-298.
62. Pham CM, Krejci-Manwaring J. Loose anagen hair syndrome: an underdiagnosed condition in males. *Pediatr Dermatol*. 2010;27:408-409.
63. Dey V, Thawani M. Loose anagen hair syndrome in black-haired Indian children. *Pediatr Dermatol*. 2013;30:579-583.
64. Agi C, Cohen B. A case of loose anagen syndrome in an African American girl. *Pediatr Dermatol*. 2015;32:128-129.
65. Swink SM, Castelo-Soccio L. Loose anagen syndrome: a retrospective chart review of 37 cases. *Pediatr Dermatol*. 2016;33:507-510.
66. Chapalain V, Winter H, Langbein L, et al. Is the loose anagen hair syndrome a keratin disorder? A clinical and molecular study. *Arch Dermatol*. 2002;138:501-506.
67. Dey VK, Thawani M. Loose anagen hair syndrome: is there any association with atopic dermatitis? *Indian Dermatol Online J*. 2016;7(1):56-57.
68. Mazzanti L, Cacciari E, Cicognani A, et al. Noonan-like syndrome with loose anagen hair: a new syndrome? *Am J Med Genet*. 2003;118A:279-286.
69. Baden HP, Kvedar JC, Magro CM. Loose anagen hair as a cause of hereditary hair loss in children. *Arch Dermatol*. 1992;128:1349-1353.
70. Hamm H, Traupe H. Loose anagen hair of childhood: the phenomenon of easily pluckable hair. *J Am Acad Dermatol*. 1989;20:242-248.
71. Tosti A, Piraccini BM. Loose anagen hair syndrome and loose anagen hair. *Arch Dermatol*. 2002;138:521-522.
72. Rakowska A, Zadurska M, Czuwara J, et al. Trichoscopy findings in loose anagen hair syndrome: rectangular granular structures and solitary yellow dots. *J Dermatol Case Rep*. 2015;9(1):1-5.
73. Chandran NS, Oranje AP. Minoxidil 5% solution for topical treatment of loose anagen hair syndrome. *Pediatr Dermatol*. 2014;31:389-390.
74. Green J, Fitzpatrick E, de Berker D, et al. A gene for pili annulati maps to the telomeric region of

chromosome 12q. *J Invest Dermatol*. 2004;123: 1070-1072.
75. Castelli E, Fiorella S, Caputo V. Pili annulati coincident with alopecia areata, autoimmune thyroid disease, and primary IgA deficiency: case report and considerations on the literature. *Case Rep Dermatol*. 2012;4(3):250-255.
76. Musso LA. Pili annulati. *Australas J Dermatol*. 1970;11:67-75.
77. Amichai B, Grunwald MH, Halevy S. Hair abnormality present since childhood. Pili annulati. *Arch Dermatol*. 1996;132:575, 578.
78. Montgomery RM, Binder AI. Ringed hair. *Arch Derm Syphilol*. 1970;58:177-179.
79. Giehl KA, Ferguson DJ, Dawber RP, et al. Update on detection, morphology and fragility in pili annulati in three kindreds. *J Eur Acad Dermatol Venereol*. 2004;18:654-658.
80. Werner K, St-Surin-Lord S, Sperling LC. Pili annulati associated with hair fragility: cause or coincidence? *Cutis*. 2013;91:36-38.
81. Akoglu G, Emre S, Metin A, et al. Pili annulati with fragility: electron microscopic findings of a case. *Int J Trichology*. 2012;4(2):89-92.
82. Feldmann KA, Dawber RP, Pittelkow MR, et al. Newly described weathering pattern in pili annulati hair shafts: a scanning electron microscopic study. *J Am Acad Dermatol*. 2001;45:625-627.
83. Green J, Sinclair RD, de Bereker D. Disappearance of pili annulati following an episode of alopecia areata. *Clin Exp Dermatol*. 2002;27:458-460.
84. Giehl KA, Rogers MA, Radivojkov M, et al. Pili annulati: refinement of the locos on chromosome 12q24.33 to a 2.9-MB interval and candidate gene analysis. *Br J Dermatol*. 2009;160:527-533.
85. Giehl KA, Ferguson DJ, Dean D, et al. Alterations in the basement membrane zone in pili annulati hair follicles as demonstrated by electron microscopy and immunohistochemistry. *Br J Dermatol*. 2004;150:722-727.
86. Gummer CL, Dawber RP. Pili annulati: electron histochemical studies on affected hairs. *Br J Dermatol*. 1981;105:303-309.
87. Ito M, Hashimoto K, Sakamoto F, et al. Pathogenesis of pili annulati. *Arch Dermatol Res*. 1988;280:308-318.
88. Dawber R. Investigations of a family with pili annulati associated with blue naevi. *Trans St Johns Hosp Dermatol Soc*. 1972;58:51-58.

Chapter 90 :: Hirsutism and Hypertrichosis
:: Thusanth Thuraisingam & Amy J. McMichael

第九十章
多毛和多毛症

中文导读

第一部分介绍多毛。多毛是指女性过多的毛发以男性分布的方式生长，主要的驱动因素是高于正常水平的雄激素水平。而多毛症患者的毛发分布更广泛，与雄激素无关。多囊卵巢综合征（PCOS）、非经典先天性肾上腺增生症（CAH）和肾上腺或卵巢肿瘤是主要原因，或者是特发性的。本章指出多毛影响个人精神情绪和社交状况。分为6个部分：①流行病学；②发病机制；③临床特点和诊断；④多毛相关病因；⑤评估；⑥治疗。

第一节指出种族、家族遗传影响、不同国家人群、不同年龄对多毛的发病率都有影响。

第二节提出两种情况，一种是高于正常的雄激素水平，另一种却没有雄激素过高的证据。于是先介绍第一种情况，即先简述毛发生长的基本原理，指出毛发的成熟是毛囊中雄激素，尤其是二氢睾酮与其受体激活的结果，引出高雄激素这种发病机制；而另一种机制则可能是局部因素和终末器官敏感性的差异导致的。

第三节中先通过表90-1列出导致多毛的疾病、相对应的临床特点及诊断的要点，如特发性多毛、多囊卵巢综合症、非典型的先天性肾上腺增生等，并在下文有分开介绍。并给出评估女性九个部位多毛程度的方法——改良Ferriman-and-Gallwey（mFG）评分量表，见图90-1，并把评分为8分或以上的女性视为多毛。

第四节提到多毛相关病因：特发性多毛、多囊卵巢综合症及其一个亚型HAIR-AN、SAHA综合症、肾上腺和卵巢引起的多毛、甚至可能与内分泌疾病有关。其中多囊卵巢综合征是最常见的引起高雄激素血症的疾病，是引起多毛的常见次要原因。

第五节指出评估此疾病的方法，主要是寻找病因、诊断，及相对应的治疗方法。先通过mFG评分量表诊断是否为多毛，再通过问诊月经情况、性激素检查、肾上腺、卵巢及妊娠相关妇科检查、甲状腺及胰岛素相关检查来寻找病因。其具体诊断治疗流程见图90-5。

第六节提出主要的治疗方案可分两种，一种为病人接受的物理治疗，如剃须和脱毛，另一种是由医生或美容师指导的治疗，如口服药物、电解和激光治疗。当然，心理辅助治疗是必要的，因为多毛可导致美容方面的困扰。接下来介绍多毛的一线药物治疗为口服避孕药（OCPs），通常与抗雄激素联合使用，如螺内酯和氟他胺。本章列出总共7种药物治疗：口服避孕药、安体舒通、醋酸环丙孕酮、促性腺激素释放激素（GnRH）激动剂、酮康唑、非那雄胺、二甲双胍，及对应作用机制、剂量、副作用及治疗注意事项，见表90-2。

第二部分介绍多毛症。多毛症是指在非男性第二性征的身体部位，因年龄、性别或种族差异而导致的胎毛、绒毛或末梢毛的过度生长。并分成三种情况分别讲述：先天性多毛症（弥漫型）、先天性局限型多毛症、其他获得性多毛症。总结了多毛症的先天性、代谢性、药物及其他获得性疾病的病因，见于表90-3。

首先指出多毛症是许多遗传综合征的常见症状，在先天性多毛症（弥漫型）中讲述了四种较为常见的遗传综合征：先天性多毛症(CHL)和先天性全身性多毛症，骨软骨发育不良伴多毛症（也称为Cantu综合征），以及伴多毛症的牙龈纤维瘤病。

其次提到先天性局限型多毛症是指过度生长的毛发局限于单个身体部位，再者指出其他获得性多毛症主要是药物及代谢紊乱导致的，最后指出其主要治疗手段是脱毛，包括仅脱去毛干和毛干毛球皆脱去的两种脱毛方法。

〔简　丹〕

HIRSUTISM

AT-A-GLANCE

- Hirsutism is defined as terminal body hair growth in women in a male distribution.
- Women with a Ferriman-Gallwey score of 8 or higher are considered hirsute.
- Women with mild to moderate hirsutism and regular menstrual cycles are most likely diagnosed with idiopathic hirsutism; hormone testing is not necessary.
- Hormone testing is necessary in women with moderate to severe hirsutism and all women with hirsutism and irregular menstrual cycles or signs of virilisation.

INTRODUCTION

Hirsutism is a condition in which excessive hair in women grows in a male pattern distribution. It has a significant psychosocial impact on the affected individual as well as a number of medical consequences for the skin. The main driving factors are the higher-than-normal androgen levels, either in circulation or locally, and an increased sensitivity of the hair follicle to androgens. This condition differs from hypertrichosis in which the excess hair has a more generalized distribution and independent of androgens. Hirsutism may result from various causes, with polycystic ovarian syndrome (PCOS), nonclassical congenital adrenal hyperplasia (CAH), and adrenal or ovarian tumors being among the major causes, or hirsutism may be idiopathic.

Hirsutism can cause the affected individual embarrassment, leading to social withdrawal and even depression.[1,2] A recent study has identified that patients view their condition as more severe than do their clinicians, which is associated with a negative effect on their quality of life.[3] The authors suggest that treatment be guided by the level of patient's distress with the hair growth.

EPIDEMIOLOGY

The prevalence of hirsutism is unknown. Approximately 5% to 15% of the female population of reproductive age is thought to be affected by hirsutism, and it is one of the most common complaints of patients presenting to dermatology offices.[4,5] The variability in concentration of hair follicles is influenced by ethnicity and strong family inheritance. Asians, with lower hair concentration, are much less likely to present with hirsutism resulting from an androgen excess state compared with their Mediterranean counterparts.[6] As a result, the cut-off value for diagnosis of hirsutism varies among different ethnic populations. The prevalences of hirsutism were estimated to be 38% in Greece, 21.2% in Australia, 10.8% in Iran, 10.5% in India, 8.3% in Turkey, 7.1% in Spain, and 2% in Thailanand.[7,8] A study of North American women with hirsutism identified that 25% to 33% of white women have terminal hairs on the upper lip and periareolar area, as well as the linear alba, with normal androgen levels. The degree of facial and body terminal hair was similar in black and white women in North America with a prevalence of 4.3% and 5.4%, respectively.[9] Hirsutism may also be influenced by age. Most of the patients are women of reproductive age, and the growth pattern is heaviest at a younger age compared with older age.[10]

PATHOGENESIS

The hair growth cycle is made up of three phases: anagen (growth phase), catagen (involution), and telogen (rest phase). The cycle is under hormonal influence in a site-specific pattern. The maturation of vellus (small, straight, and nonpigmented) hair to terminal (long, curlier, and pigmented) hair is the result of the activation of androgen receptors in the hair follicle.[11] During puberty, an increase in androgen levels drives vellus hair to differentiate into terminal hair, as well as sebaceous gland development (see Chap. 6 for more detail).

In women, the androgens are produced in the ovaries and adrenal glands and are subject to peripheral conversion. Enzymatic conversion of cholesterol to pregnenolone is the rate-limiting step of all steroid hormone production. This step is under the influence of luteinizing hormone (LH) in the ovary and adrenocorticotropic hormone (ACTH) in the adrenal cortex.[11] Although both testosterone and dihydrotestosterone (DHT) are capable of converting vellus hair to terminal hair, DHT is the most potent androgen. DHT is produced from the peripheral enzymatic conversion of testosterone by 5α-reductase within the hair follicle.[11] Binding of DHT to its nuclear receptor activates genes responsible for conversion of vellus hair to terminal hair in androgen sensitive areas of the body. However, excess circulating androgens alone do not explain the pathogenesis of hirsutism because some women have hirsutism without evidence of androgen excess (idiopathic hirsutism; see below).[12] In these individuals, local factors and variability in end-organ sensitivity are thought to be the underlying cause.

CLINICAL FINDINGS AND DIAGNOSIS

Hirsutism can be categorized as primary or idiopathic in 5% to 15% of affected patients with regular menstrual cycles and normal levels of circulating androgens[12] versus secondary hirsutism associated with underlying causes (Table 90-1). In evaluating patients, it is important to obtain a thorough history of their symptoms and signs. Apart from hirsutism, other cutaneous signs of hyperandrogenism include acne, acanthosis nigricans, androgenetic alopecia,

TABLE 90-1
Causes of Hirsutism

ETIOLOGY	FINDINGS	COMMENT
Idiopathic hirsutism (IH)	Regular ovulation and normal to slightly elevated androgen levels Often presents with mild to moderate hirsutism	Mean age, BMI, and hip and waist circumference higher in IH vs patients with metabolic disturbance[13]
Polycystic ovarian syndrome (PCOS)	Hyperandrogenism; menstrual irregularities, including oligomenorrhea, amenorrhea, and infertility; and impaired glucose tolerance, hyperlipidemia, and obesity	Cutaneous findings of acanthosis nigricans may also be observed in 5% of obese women with insulin resistance Warrants endocrinology evaluation for impaired glucose tolerance as increased risk for type 2 diabetes mellitus[16,18]
Nonclassic congenital adrenal hyperplasia	Autosomal recessive inheritance of 21-hydroxylase deficiency Rarely secondary to 11β-hydroxylase deficiency Hirsutism, acne, alopecia, anovulation, and menstrual dysfunction	Patients often present accelerated bone age maturation and increased basal or stimulated 17-OHP
HAIR-AN	Hyperandrogenism (HA), insulin resistance (IR), and acanthosis nigricans (AN) Considered a subtype of PCOS	Insulin elevated; elevated or high-normal levels of testosterone and androstenedione but normal levels of LH and prolactin[30]
SAHA	Seborrhea (S), acne (A), hirsutism (H), and alopecia (A)	
Hyperprolactinemia	Presents with amenorrhoea, galactorrhea, and infertility	Associated with stress, pituitary adenoma, pregnancy, drug intake, and primary hypothyroidism with elevated TSH
Cushing syndrome	Centripetal fat distribution, thinning of the skin with striae, glucose intolerance, osteoporosis, and proximal muscle weakness; signs and symptoms of hyperandrogenism and menstrual irregularities	▪ Multiple causes: ▪ Adrenal neoplasm ▪ Ectopic ACTH-secreting tumor ▪ Pituitary tumor (Cushing disease)
Pregnancy	Most common areas involved are the upper abdomen, lower abdomen, lower back, upper lip, and thighs[52]	Serum total testosterone levels and mFG score increase with the progression of pregnancy Associated with physiological changes of pregnancy
Acromegaly	Elevated random serum GH and IGF-1	Patients can present with abnormal growth of the hands and feet, arthritis, sleep apnea, headache, and impaired vision

ACTH, adrenocorticotropic hormone; BMI, body mass index; GH, growth hormone; HCG, human chorionic gonadotropin; IGF, insulin-like growth factor; LH, luteinizing hormone; mFG, modified Ferriman and Gallwey; 17-OHP, 17-hydroxyprogesterone; TSH, thyroid-stimulating hormone.

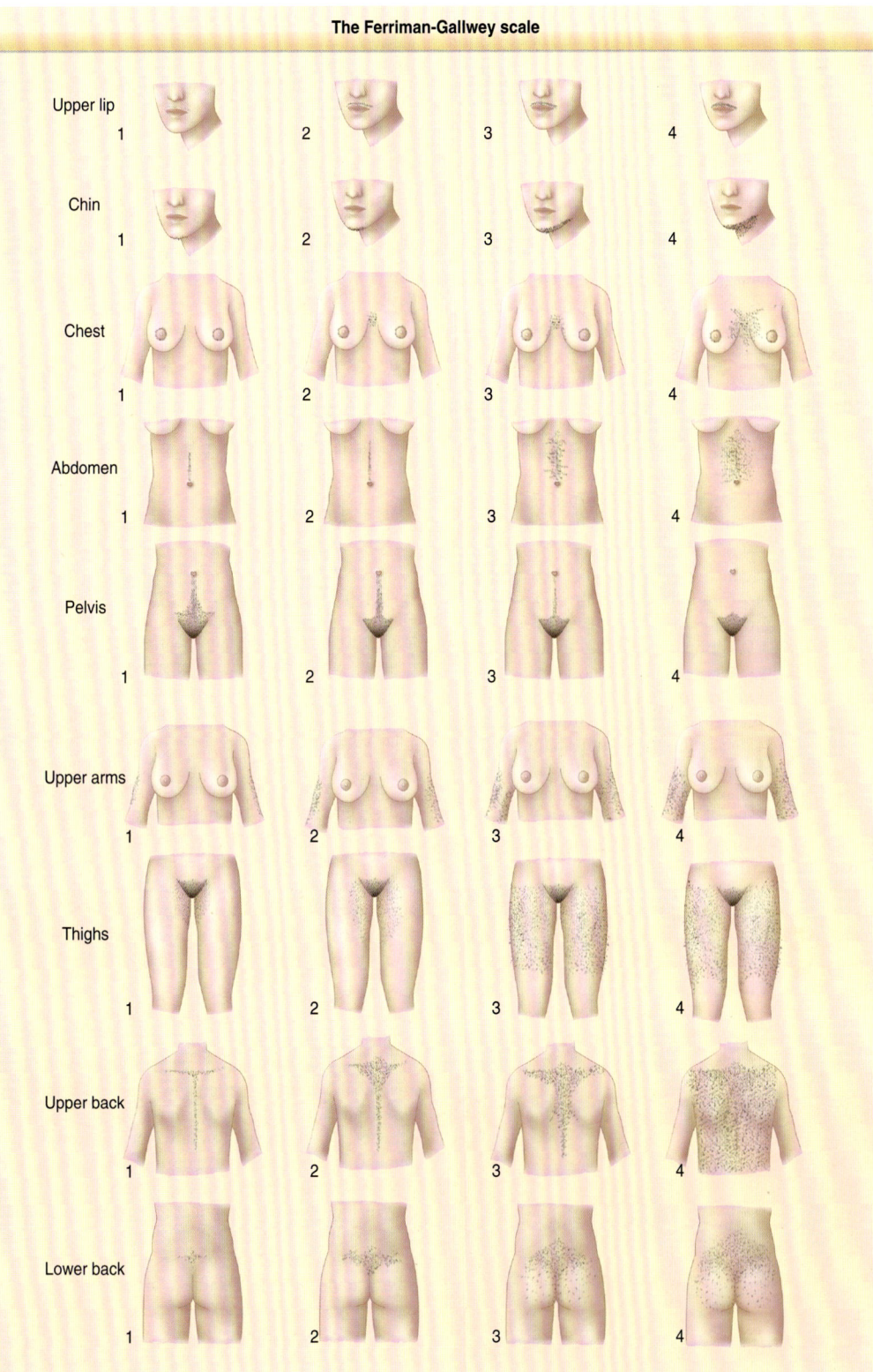

Figure 90-1 The Ferriman-Gallwey scale.

seborrheic dermatitis, and signs of virilization. Signs of virilization include clitoromegaly, male pattern balding, deepening voice, or decreased breast size.[13] It is also important to review the patient's list of medications and supplements to be assured that these are not contributing to androgen excess. The abrupt and rapid onset of hirsutism should raise suspicion of malignancy. The most commonly involved areas are the upper lip > thighs > lower abdomen > upper back.[14]

The modified Ferriman and Gallwey (mFG) scoring scale is a systematic assessment tool for the degree of hirsutism of nine body locations, which when combined, allow for an overall diagnosis of hirsutism. It was developed by Ferriman in 1961 and later modified by Hatch in 1981.[15,16] It assigns a score of 1 to 4 in nine body areas, with an increasing numeric score corresponding to greater hair density (Fig. 90-1). Excess hair distribution in the nine anatomical areas evaluated by the mFG scale (upper lip, chin and cheeks, chest, abdomen, pubic area and lower abdomen, arms, legs, upper back and lower back, and buttocks) characterize patients with hirsutism.[15,17] The score varies from 0 (no hair) to 4 (extensive hair growth) in each area. Normal hair growth is defined by a score of 8 or less, mild hirsutism is defined by a score of 8 to 14, and a score of greater than 15 indicates moderate to severe hirsutism.[18] The anatomical distribution and the extent of body involvement may vary among individual patients. An alternative simplified scoring system with three body parts (upper abdomen, lower abdomen, and chin) with a cut-off score of 3 was able to distinguish hirsute from nonhirsute women with an accuracy of 87.5%.[19]

The diagnosis of hirsutism can be challenging because many physicians are not familiar with the Ferriman and Gallwey scoring scale and, among those who are, discrepancies exist in their interpretation of the scoring value. Furthermore, the diagnostic score varies among different ethnic populations: for example, 2 or 3 or greater for Asians and 9 to 10 or greater for Mediterraneans.[7,20] Also, there is no consensus on how many body regions are to be included in the scoring system. Another challenge is that most patients presenting for evaluation will have used

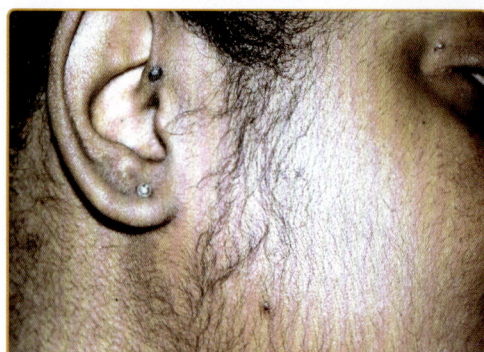

Figure 90-3 Hirsutism of the lateral face and jawline in the young woman.

various cosmetic measures to remove excess hair, thus leading to an inaccurate assessment.

ASSOCIATED CAUSES

IDIOPATHIC HIRSUTISM

Idiopathic hirsutism occurs in a subgroup of hirsute patients who present with hirsutism, regular ovulation, and normal to slightly elevated androgen levels in the absence of features that suggest other causes of hirsutism. Its prevalence is 4% to 7%, and it is a diagnosis of exclusion[21] (Figs. 90-2 and 90-3). The pathogenesis remains unclear. The intrinsic hyperresponsiveness of androgen receptors to normal circulating levels of androgens and increased activity of the 5α-reductase enzyme at the hair follicle are postulated thoeries.[12] The increased local circulation of androgens is caused by increased gene expression of the steroid-converting enzymes 17β-hydroxysteroid dehydrogenase and steroid sulfatase, resulting in decreased levels of estradiol/testosterone.[22]

POLYCYSTIC OVARIAN SYNDROME

Polycystic ovarian syndrome, also known as Stein-Leventhal syndrome after the clinicians who first described the condition, is the most common associated cause of hyperandrogenism in women of reproductive age and is a common secondary cause of hirsutism[23] (Fig. 90-4). The other clinical characteristics of PCOS can include chronic anovulation, insulin resistance, and infertility.[24] Apart from hirsutism, the hyperandrogenic state causes PCOS patients to also present with other cutaneous manifestations, including acne, acanthosis nigricans, alopecia, and seborrheic dermatitis.[25] More than 50% of women with PCOS present with hirsutism that tends to have a more truncal distribution.[26] Alternatively, individuals of certain ethnicities may lack the feature of hirsutism, as in the Asian patient with PCOS.[20,27] PCOS increases the risk of type 2 diabetes mellitus and cardiovascular dysfunction. Both the reproductive and the metabolic manifestations of PCOS are exacerbated by being overweight or obese.[28]

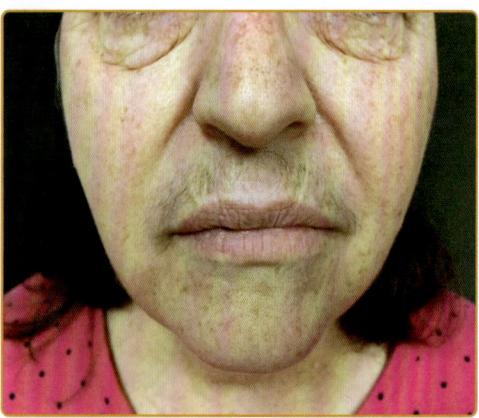

Figure 90-2 Dark terminal hair of the upper lip and chin in a middle-age woman.

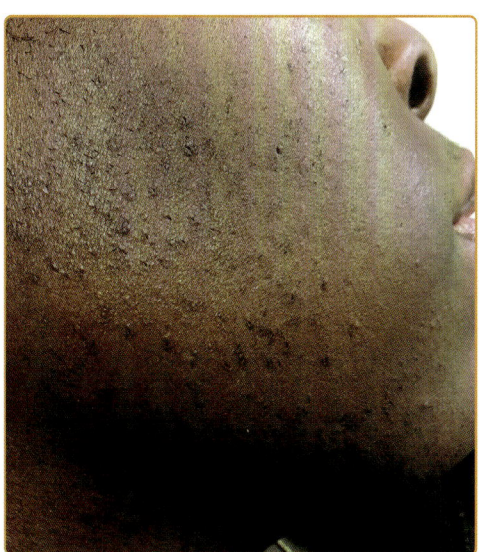

Figure 90-4 Hirsutism of the chin with associated pseudofolliculitis barbae.

HAIR-AN

A subset of PCOS patients are classified as HAIR-AN because of the presence of hyperandrogenism (HA), insulin resistance (IR), and acanthosis nigricans (AN). This syndrome is found in 1% to 5% in women presenting with hyperandrogenism. The underlying cause is associated with insulin resistance with compensatory hyperinsulinemia.[29] The clinical presentation can include various combinations of oily skin, hirsutism, acne, menstrual irregularities, androgenic alopecia, signs of virilization (deepening of voice, clitoromegaly and changes in muscle mass), insulin resistance with diabetic symptoms, as well as acanthosis nigricans.[30] If ovarian biopsy is performed, the most consistent histopathologic finding is islands of hyperplastic theca cells in ovarian stroma known as hyperthecosis, with normal adrenal function. There are reports of association with other autoimmune or endocrine diseases such as Hashimoto thyroiditis, Graves disease, vitiligo, Cushing syndrome, Cohen syndrome, acromegaly, CAH, and insulinoma.[30,31]

SAHA SYNDROME

The constellation of cutaneous manifestations such as seborrhea, acne, hirsutism, and androgenetic alopecia is identified as SAHA syndrome. Apart from seborrhea, which is present in 100% of the cases, the other conditions can be variable in presentation. The condition is further divided into idiopathic, ovarian, adrenal, and hyperprolactinemic types,[32] and it can be associated with PCOS, cystic mastitis, obesity, and infertility. SAHA syndrome is prevalent in 17.7 % of PCOS patients, and this variety of PCOS is associated with greater insulin resistance.[33]

ADRENAL AND OVARIAN HIRSUTISM

Adrenal hyperplasia is associated with a defect in the enzyme responsible for the synthesis of cortisol, which leads to the accumulation of precursors that are diverted into androgen synthesis. Late onset or nonclassic CAH is an autosomal recessive disorder caused by mutations in the *CYP21A2* gene, which causes deficiency in 21 hydroxylases. This results in the defective conversion of 17-hydroxyprogesterone (17-OHP) to 11-deoxycortisol. Rarely, it also can be caused by a deficiency in 11–hydroxylase. It is often diagnosed after the age of 10 years and can present with peripubertal hirsutism, oligomenorrhea, acne, infertility, alopecia, primary amenorrhea, and premature pubarche.[34] An elevated 17-OHP, substrate of 21-hydroxylase, level is the biochemical hallmark of the disease. Increased circulation of ACTH as in Cushing syndrome (pituitary origin) or ectopic origin can also be associated with overstimulation of adrenal androgens production.

Adrenal tumors are a rare cause of hirsutism. Whereas adrenal adenomas secrete testosterone, adrenal carcinomas secrete testosterone, dehydroepiandrosterone sulfate (DHEAS), and cortisol. Symptoms may be acute and quite severe.

Hirsutism with galactorrhea must raise suspicions of hyperprolactinemia. Hyperprolactinemia may be associated with various conditions, either physiological or nonphysiological. Whereas some drugs (phenothiazines, benzodiazepines, and others) as well as prolactinoma, hypothyroidism, or idiopathic hyperprolactinemia are nonphysiological, lactation and stress represent physiological causes.

Apart from PCOS, in women of reproductive age, pregnancy as a possible cause of hirsutism should also be ruled out. The excess androgens produced during pregnancy can be caused by luteoma of pregnancy, hyperreactio luteinalis, or aromatase deficiency in the fetus.

Sertoli-Leydig cell tumors, granulosa-theca cell tumors, and hilus cell tumors are the ovarian tumors known to secrete excess androgens. They have low metastatic potential, and the treatment is surgical.

Hirsutism can also be associated with other endocrinopathies, including acromegaly, hyperprolactinemia, and thyroid dysfunction.

EVALUATION

To determine the cause of hirsutism, a detailed clinical, medication, and family history with physical examination is needed. After diagnosing hirsutism by an increased mFG score, diagnostic studies should focus on identification of the most likely cause (see Table 90-1). Functional causes almost always have a peripubertal onset with slow progression. Signs of virilization such as clitoromegaly or balding or of defemi-

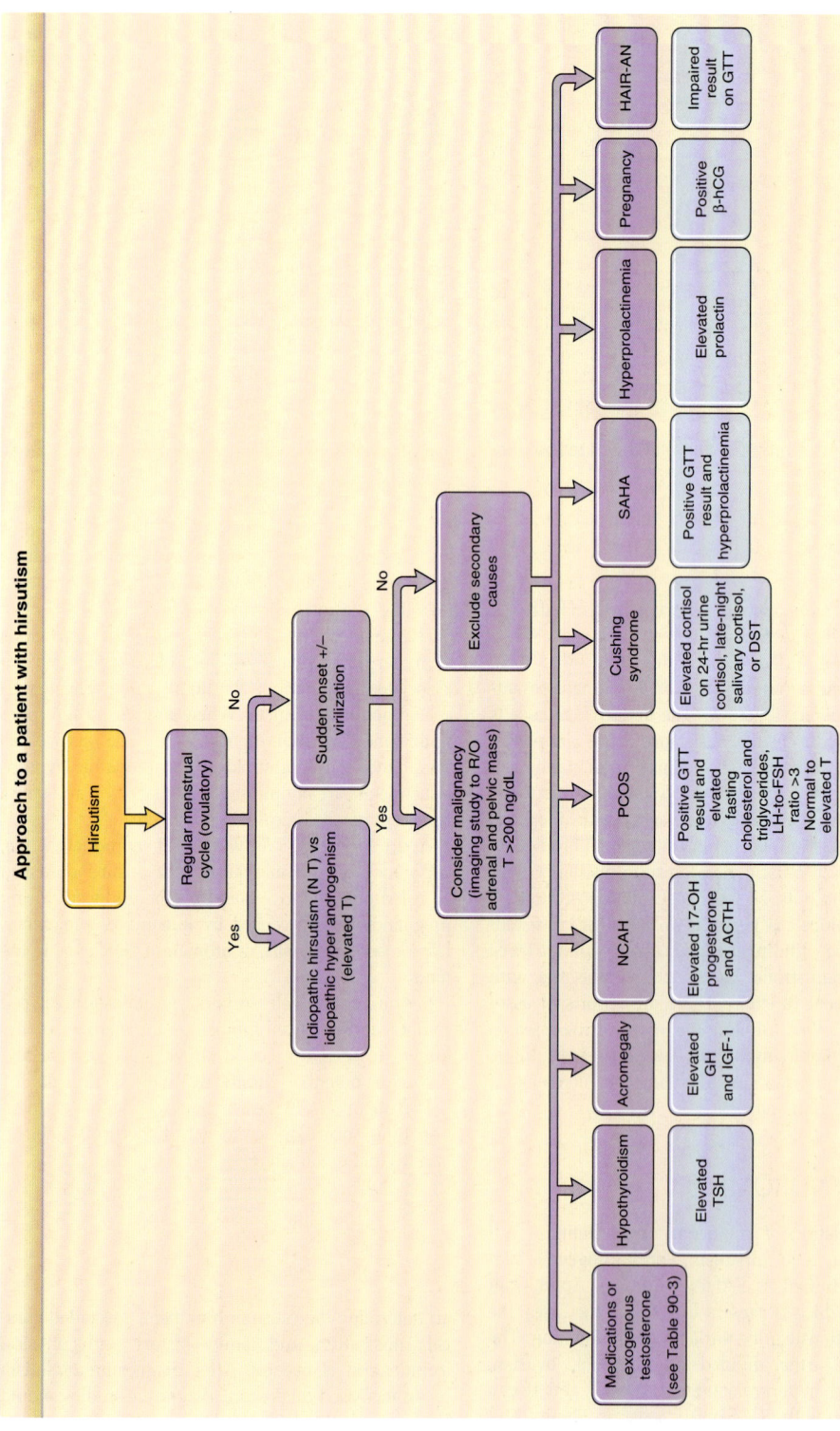

Figure 90-5 Approach to a patient with hirsutism. ACTH, adrenocorticotropic hormone; DST, dexamethasone suppression test; FSH, follicle-stimulating hormone; GH, growth hormone; GTT, glucose tolerance test; HCG, human chorionic gonadotropin; IGF, insulin-like growth factor; LH, luteinizing hormone; NCAH, non-classical adrenal hyperplasia; NT, normal testosterone; PCOS, polycystic ovarian syndrome; R/O, rule out; SAHA, seborrhea, acne, hirsutism, and androgenetic alopecia; 17-OH, 17-hydroxyprogesterone; T, testosterone; TSH, thyroid-stimulating hormone. (Source: References 36 to 38.)

nization such as breast tissue atrophy are extremely rare.³⁵ Often, the severity of the hirsutism does not correlate well with the magnitude of androgen excess. Signs of infertility with oligo- or amenorrhea, insulin resistance, abdominal obesity, or acanthosis nigricans favor PCOS.

The chronicity of the symptoms may direct the investigation. If the hirsutism is long standing and mild to moderate, testosterone or androstenedione measurements are recommended. Free testosterone is a more sensitive biochemical marker of hyperandrogenism than total testosterone, but as stated earlier, the levels can be normal in women with hirsutism. With sudden onset of hirsutism, with or without virilization or high testosterone levels, other measurement of adrenal marker levels (cortisol and DHEAS) and ovarian and adrenal imaging are highly recommended (Fig. 90-5).

After androgen excess is confirmed, further tests should be considered such as a pregnancy test (if the patient has amenorrhea), pelvic ultrasonography (if an ovarian neoplasm or PCOS is suspected), measurement of DHEAS and early morning 17-OHP (if CAH or adrenal neoplasm is suspected), and a prolactin level. Further testing may also include measurement of thyroid function, adrenocortical function, and insulin-like growth factor 1. Further workup typically begins with dexamethasone suppression testing to determine the source of androgen excess production. If androgen excess is not suppressible by dexamethasone, the presence of Cushing syndrome, neoplasm, and PCOS must be considered. If androgen excess is dexamethasone suppressible, an ACTH test for CAH is indicated. A serum testosterone level greater than 200 ng/dL is highly suggestive of adrenal or ovarian tumor, and further imaging studies may be warranted, such as abdominal computed tomography for adrenal or ovarian neoplasm.

TREATMENTS

The cultural norm of absence of hair as being more desirable in females has driven hirsute women to seek various methods of removing excess body and facial hair. Patients affected by hirsutism have lower quality of life and symptoms of both anxiety and depression.³⁹ Along with treatment options directed at excess unwanted hair, patients should be evaluated for their social support, and psychological treatment should be offered when necessary.³⁹,⁴⁰ Before the onset of therapy, it is important to advise patients that treatment will never be curative, and the effects of any drug or treatment will not likely become evident for several months; thus, chronic treatment will be necessary.⁷

The major treatment options can be categorized as physical modalities that are patient administered, such as shaving and depilation, versus physician- or aesthetician-directed therapy such as oral medications, electrolysis, and laser therapy (Table 90-2). The pharmacologic strategies aim to control the dermatologic symptoms by both lowering androgen levels and controlling the effect of androgens at the tissue level. Lifestyle modification with weight loss and diet changes in patients with PCOS may improve insulin resistance,⁴⁴ menstrual regularity, and hirsutism score.⁴⁵

Direct hair removal can be achieved with nonpermanent techniques such as shaving, depilatories (last 12 hours to a few days), waxing, threading and sugaring (last up to 4 weeks), and photoepilation (intense pulsed light), or permanent hair reduction techniques such as electrolysis and laser (photodestruction). Bleaching hair in the affected areas to a similar color as the skin is a form of camouflage used to make hair less obvious. In patients with moderate to severe hirsutism and women with androgen excess, additional medical therapy may be necessary.

There is only one prescription medication that is approved for the treatment of unwanted facial hair in women. This drug, topical eflornithine, has been shown to slow down the hair growth cycle and can be used in combination with other hair removal techniques. Eflornithine works through inhibiting ornithine decarboxylase, which results in a shortening of the anagen phase of the hair growth cycle. The major adverse effects of topical eflornithine are burning or tingling of the treated area.

First-line medical therapy of hirsutism is oral contraceptives (OCPs), usually in combination with antiandrogens, such as spironolactone and flutamide. Studies with oral ethinyl-estradiol plus cyproterone acetate showed this combination to be superior at control of hyperandrogenism and for the restoration of menstrual regularity in patients with PCOS compared with metformin alone in PCOS patients.⁴⁶ In studies in which various forms of oral antiandrogens were compared, the effectiveness of finasteride, cyproterone acetate, and flutamide were shown to be equally effective in decreasing hirsutism.⁴⁷ Glucocorticoids can be considered for women with hirsutism caused by nonclassic CAH who have a suboptimal response to or cannot tolerate oral contraceptives or antiandrogens or who are seeking ovulation induction. In women with severe forms of hyperandrogenemia, such as ovarian hyperthecosis, who have a suboptimal response to oral contraceptives and antiandrogens, gonadotropin-releasing hormone (GnRH) agonists can also be considered. Although the benefit of such therapy can be maintained long term, the initial response may not be evident until 6 to 12 months after the start of therapy. Therefore, to manage patient expectations and to emphasize the importance of maintaining chronic long-term treatment, patients must be made aware of slow clinical response of oral therapies and be followed closely by trained physicians.³⁵

ANDROGEN SUPPRESSION

The androgenic symptoms that may be attenuated by OCPs treatment include hirsutism and acne, primarily through the ability of OCPs to raise sex hormone–binding globulin and lower free testosterone levels.

TABLE 90-2
Pharmacologic Treatment of Hirsutism

	MECHANISM OF ACTION	DOSAGE	ADVERSE EFFECTS	COMMENTS
Oral contraceptive pills (OCPs)	Suppress ovarian androgen synthesis Increase SHBG	Single pill a day	Headaches Migraines Risk of VTE Melasma Alopecia (upon discontinuation)	First-line therapy (in women not seeking to conceive) Contradictions: • Uncontrolled HTN • Thromboembolic disorder • Breast cancer • Active smoker (absolutely if older than 35 yr) • Cardiovascular disease
Spironolactone	Competitive inhibitor of AR and 5α-reductase Increases SHBG Decreases androgen synthesis	Starting dosage is 50 mg twice daily and may be increased to a total daily dose of 200 mg	Polyuria Hypotension Headaches Fatigue Syncope Hyperkalemia Irregular menses Teratogen Decreased libido	Avoid combination with other potassium-sparing diuretics and thiazides Contraindicated in patients with renal failure Recommend combination with OCPs Pregnancy Category C
Cyproterone acetate	Competes with DHT for binding to the androgen receptor	Low dose (2 mg) in OCPs 12.5–100 mg as monotherapy or with estrogen	Fluid retention Depression Menstrual irregularities Teratogen Increased risk of liver dysfunction	Not available in the United States Contraindicated during pregnancy and breastfeeding and with liver diseases
Flutamide and bicalutamide	Nonsteroidal competitive inhibitor of androgen receptor binding	Flutamide: 62.5–250mg, twice daily Bicalutamide: 25 mg/day	Teratogen Hepatotoxicity Diarrhea Nausea Vomiting	Recommend combination with OCPs Pregnancy Category D
Glucocorticoids	Suppress adrenal function	Prednisone: 5-7.5 mg by mouth at bedtime Dexamethasone: 0.5 mg at bedtime	Hyperglycemia Hypertension Cushingoid changes Esophageal reflux and peptic ulcer disease Psychosis and agitation Increased risk of infections Adrenal suppression	Indicated for hirsutism secondary to CAH Not recommended in patients with uncontrolled diabetes and hypertension When used as monotherapy, does not significantly improve hirsutism Pregnancy Category C
GnRH agonist (Leuprolide acetate, depot suspension)	Suppresses gonadotropin and ovarian androgen secretion	7.5 mg monthly intramuscularly, with 25–50 ug of transdermal estradiol	Osteoporosis if not combined with estrogen–progestin	Pregnancy Category X
Ketoconazole	Cytochrome P450 enzyme inhibitor and decreases adrenal steroid production	400–600 mg by mouth daily	Headache Nausea Hair loss	Pregnancy Category C
Finasteride	Inhibits 5α-reductase	1–5 mg by mouth	Headaches Decreased libido	Pregnancy Category X
Metformin	Insulin-sensitizing agent	850 mg twice a day or 500 mg three times a day	Rare lactic acidosis GI distress	Must ensure normal renal function before starting Pregnancy Category B

AR, androgen receptor; CAH, congenital adrenal hyperplasia; GI, gastrointestinal; GnRH, gonadotropin-releasing hormone; HTN, hypertension; SHBG, sex hormone–binding globulin; VTE, venous thromboembolic event.
Data from Refs. 38 and 41 to 43.

When treating mild to moderate alopecia or hirsutism, combination with an androgen antagonist should be considered as OCPs as monotherapy are not very effective. OCPs containing the second-generation progestin levonorgestrel have been associated with lower venous thromboembolic risk than those containing other progestins.[48] When combined with estrogen, Leuprolide, a long-acting GnRH analog, has been shown to decrease hirsutism significantly over OCPs alone,[49] and this benefit was greater in PCOS than in idiopathic hirsutism.[36]

The biological activity of androgens can also be inhibited by androgen receptor blockers. Antiandrogens (cyproterone acetate, chlormadinone acetate, drospirenone, spironolactone, flutamide, and bicalutamide) prevent androgen cellular action by blocking intracellular androgen receptors.[50,51] Cyproterone acetate and chlormadinone acetate block androgen receptors in target organs (ovaries and adrenal gland) but also reduce 5α-reductase, which converts testosterone to 5α-dihydrotestosterone, a more potent androgen. Cyproterone acetate has steroidal side effects and can cause abnormalities in liver function and menstrual irregularity. Because of its progestin activity, it needs to be combined with estrogens in women who have a uterus.

Spironolactone, a potassium-sparing diuretic that acts as an aldosterone antagonist, is the most studied of the androgen receptor blockers for hirsutism. Because of its androgen-antagonizing activity, it is also used as a therapeutic modality in androgenetic alopecia in postmenopausal women. It is usually administered in conjunction with OCPs to help to minimize the dysfunctional uterine bleeding that is one of the major side effects of this medication. The beneficial effect may take up to 6 months to observe.

Flutamide is used in dosages of 62.5 to 500 mg/day. Because liver toxicity is a potential side effect, serum transaminases should be measured frequently. Other side effects that have been reported include dry skin, diarrhea, nausea, and vomiting.

Bicalutamide (a dosage of 25 mg/day) is a new and potent, well-tolerated nonsteroidal pure antiandrogen. It was developed for treating prostate cancer. It has been shown effective in the treatment of patients with PCOS-induced and idiopathic hirsutism.[52] However, hepatotoxic effects in the treatment of prostate cancer have been reported starting at doses of 50 mg/day.[53]

The oral medications finasteride and dutasteride, both 5α-reductase inhibitors, may improve hirsutism by antagonizing the production or biological activity of DHT.

ELECTROLYSIS AND LASERS

Electrolysis and laser hair reduction are the only hair removal methods that may provide permanent hair reduction or long-lasting results. Electrolysis uses a fine needle insertion into individual follicles to destroy the hair follicle via current (galvanic electrolysis), a high-frequency alternating current (thermolysis), or a blend of the two.[54] Major disadvantages of this technique include potential scarring, follicular hyperpigmentation, and pain. Because this technique is time consuming, especially with extensive hair growth, and requires a well-trained operator, it can become costly. The regrowth rate of hair with this technique is approximately 40%.[50]

There have recently been major advances in the field of laser hair removal. Laser treatments remove dark hair quickly through photothermolysis by selectively damaging the pigmented part of the hair follicle. It may take 3 to 6 months before regrowth is evident. Several treatment cycles are required with the spacing between treatments depending on the body area being treated. The most commonly used devices are 755-nm alexandrite laser, 800-nm diode laser, and 1064-nm Nd:YAG (neodymium-doped yttrium aluminum garnet) laser and intense pulsed light sources.[55] Laser treatments are less painful and much quicker than electrolysis. Electrolysis is the favored method of treatment for lightly pigmented hair because only anagen hair follicles with dark bulb areas can be destroyed by the light source of laser. The major adverse effects of laser and intense pulsed light include postinflammatory pigmentary change, folliculitis, reactivation of herpes simplex, and paradoxical hypertrichosis, although these are all rare complications when laser is performed by properly trained providers.

HYPERTRICHOSIS

AT-A-GLANCE

- Hypertrichosis is defined as hair growth that is excessive in a localized or diffuse pattern not considered to be in a male pattern distribution.
- The hair growth in hypertrichosis can be lanugo, vellus, or terminal.
- Many genetic syndromes have hypertrichosis as a common finding.
- Metabolic disorders and medications can contribute to the development of hypertrichosis.
- Therapy should always consist of direct hair removal with or without medical therapy.

INTRODUCTION

Hypertrichosis is defined as hair growth that is considered excessive for age, sex, or ethnicity in areas of the body not considered to be in a pattern of male secondary characteristic. However, it can be seen in both sexual and nonsexual areas.[56] Hypertrichosis can be congenital or acquired, and causes include familial factors, medications, and metabolic disorders.[57] The hair types seen in hypertrichosis can be lanugo, vellus, or terminal.

TABLE 90-3
Causes of Hypertrichosis

ETIOLOGY	SPECIFIC DISORDERS
Congenital Disorders	
Diffuse	Congenital hypertrichosis lanuginosa
	Congenital generalized hypertrichosis
	Cantú syndrome
	Gingival fibromatosis with hypertrichosis
	Congenital syndromes with secondary hypertrichosis
	• Cornelia de Lange syndrome
	• Mucopolysaccharidosis disorders
	▪ Hurler Syndrome
	▪ Hunter Syndrome
	▪ Sanfilippo Syndrome
	• Stiff skin syndrome
Localized	• Winchester syndrome
	• Rubinstein-Taybi syndrome
	• Schinzel-Giedion syndrome
	• Barber-Say syndrome
	• Coffin-Siris syndrome
	• Lawrence-Seip syndrome
	• Hemimaxillofacial dysplasia
	• Craniofacial dysostosis
	• Hypomelanosis of Ito
	Spinal dysraphism
	Faun tail deformity
	Congenital nevocellular nevus
	Congenital Becker nevus
	Smooth muscle hamartoma
	Nevoid hypertrichosis
	Underlying neurofibroma
	Hypertrichosis cubiti
	Hemihypertrophy
	Hairy congenital malformation of palms and soles
	Hairy pinnae
	Anterior cervical hypertrichosis
Metabolic Disorders	Thyroid disorders
	Anorexia nervosa
	Porphyria
	Malignancy
	Fetal alcohol syndrome
	Malnutrition
Medications	Dilantin
	Cyclosporine
	Glucocorticoids
	Minoxidil
	Diazoxide
	Phenytoin
	Anabolic steroids
	Danazol
	Penicillamine
	Psoralens
	Streptomycin
	Isotretinoin
	Cetuximab
	Testosterone
	Valproic acid.
	Topical prostaglandin inhibitors
Other Acquired	Post-laser hair removal
	Local pressure or inflammation: casts, lichen simplex, biting, insect bites
	Human immunodeficiency virus: trichomegaly
	Acrodynia
	Infection
	Dermatomyositis

CONGENITAL FORMS OF HYPERTRICHOSIS

Congenital forms of hypertrichosis can be localized or diffuse (Table 90-3). The generalized (diffuse) forms tend to occur as a secondary characteristic in a number of well-described syndromes except in the four cases in which the syndrome is defined by the condition of hypertrichosis. The hypertrichosis-defined conditions are congenital hypertrichosis lanuginosa (CHL) and congenital generalized hypertrichosis, osteochondrodysplasia with hypertrichosis (also known as Cantú syndrome), and gingival fibromatosis with hypertrichosis.

Congenital hypertrichosis lanuginosa, at times controversially referred to as Ambras syndrome, is a rare, inherited disorder in which an excess of lanugo hair remains over the entire body after birth or may develop in the first few months of life.[58] Only the palms, soles, mucous membranes, and glans penis are spared. Some of these patients lose the hair during childhood, but others retain the excess body hair. The disease is very rare with the first reports appearing in the German literature in the 1870s, approximately 50 cases reported in the current world literature, and an estimated incidence of 1 in 10,000,000.[59,60] CHL is associated with genetic abnormalities in chromosome 8q (insertion 8q23-24 and deletion 8q23), although other chromosomal abnormalities have been reported.[61]

Congenital generalized hypertrichosis is similar to CHL in presentation but with terminal hair growth on the body instead of lanugo hair. Only one family has been reported in the literature with this disorder, which is thought to be X-linked with gene mapping to X24-q27.1.[62,63]

Osteochondrodysplasia with hypertrichosis (Cantú syndrome) is an autosomal dominant disorder characterized by newborns with thick scalp hair and excessive hair growth on the forehead, face, back, and extremities. Some have thick or curly eyelashes. The hypertrichosis usually persists over time. Associated findings include skeletal abnormalities and a variety of cardiac abnormalities.[64] The diagnosis is established based on clinical findings and confirmed by detection of a heterozygous pathogenic variant in *ABCC9* or *KCNJ8*.[65,66]

Gingival fibromatosis with hypertrichosis is a rare genetic syndrome characterized by severe overgrowth of the hair and gums.[67,68] Seizures have been reported as part of the syndrome.[69] Overlap of the characteristics of this condition with other syndromes have been reported, making the diagnosis of this form of hypertrichosis complicated.[70]

Of the syndromes in which hypertrichosis is a secondary characteristic, the most commonly reported is Cornelia de Lange syndrome, also known as Brachmann-de Lange syndrome. It is characterized by severe mental retardation, cutis marmorata, frequent limb abnormalities, and characteristic facial features (micrognathia, high palate, low frontal hair line) with the hypertrichosis most prominent as thickened convergent (synophrys) eyebrows with hypertrichotic eyelashes.[71,72]

The most commonly reported genetic cause of Cornelia De Lange syndrome is a mutation in *NIPBL*, which accounts for up to 80% of cases, although other gene mutations have been reported to account for the rest of the cases. All the causative genes for this disorder are thought to encode proteins related to cohesion complex function.[73,74]

The mucopolysaccharidoses (MPS) are a constellation of disorders that result from a deficiency of lysosomal enzymes responsible for glycosaminoglycan metabolism. Several of the MPS are considered to have associated hypertrichosis: Hurler syndrome, Hunter syndrome, and Sanfilippo syndrome.[75]

Other less common syndromes with the secondary characteristic of diffuse hypertrichosis are listed in Table 90-3.

LOCALIZED CONGENITAL HYPERTRICHOSIS

Congenital hypertrichoses localized to a single body part include hypertrichosis cubiti (hairy elbows), hairy pinna, anterior cervical hypertrichosis, hairy polythelia (hair tufts along the mammary line), overlying plexiform neurofibromas with spinal dysraphism (when presenting over the sacral midline, it is called "faun tail deformity") in association with congenital nevi, and occasionally in association with Becker nevi.[76] They can be present at birth or soon thereafter, but many of these disorders present later in childhood.[77] When any of these disorders are found in the midline, it is imperative to look for underlying neurologic deficits and spinal deformities.[78]

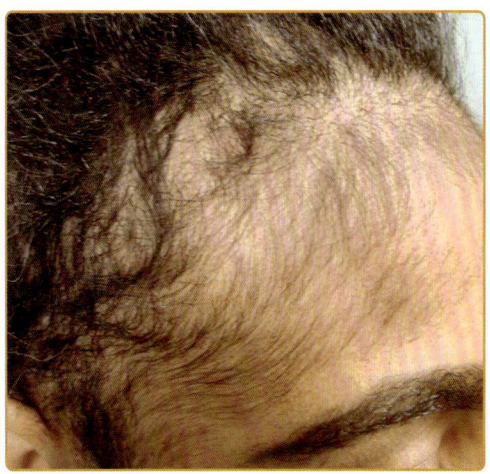

Figure 90-6 Hypertrichosis of the forehead in a patient applying topical minoxidil to the scalp.

OTHER ACQUIRED FORMS OF HYPERTRICHOSIS

There is a long list of medications that can cause hypertrichosis (see Table 90-3), so a full medical history can easily identify the culprit (Fig. 90-6). Porphyria and other metabolic disorders are important forms of acquired hypertrichosis. The most common porphyrias to cause hypertrichosis are porphyria cutanea tarda and erythropoietic porphyria (Gunther disease), but hereditary coproporphyria and variegate porphyria may produce excessive hair growth as well.[79]

TREATMENT

The treatment of hypertrichosis mirrors that of hirsutism. The general approach to treatment will differ based on the patient age, ethnicity, and extent of hair.[80] For situations when there is an underlying metabolic process or a medication is involved, the underlying cause should be addressed. For other conditions in which the hair is persistent, treatments can be divided into depilatory methods (removal of hair along the hair shaft) and epilatory methods (removal of the entire hair shaft including the hair bulb).[75] Depilatory methods include mechanical and chemical methods of removal, such as shaving, waxing, sugaring, threading, tweezing, and chemical depilation. These methods are all temporizing and can produce mild to moderate pain or irritation of the treated skin.

For more permanent hair removal, electrolysis and laser can be used. Although permanent hair reduction has improved in efficacy over the past 2 decades, the achievement of complete permanent hair removal remains elusive. Electrolysis for extensive cases can be time consuming, and appropriately trained operators can be difficult to find.[81]

Laser hair reduction has been used successfully in treating various forms of hypertrichosis but can also be time consuming and expensive.[82,83]

Laser hair epilation can rarely lead to paradoxical hypertrichosis, so this must be considered as well.[84]

When considering recommendations for hair removal, it is important to underscore the possibility of injury with both in-the-home and professionally performed treatments. Between the years 1994 and 2014, there were nearly 300,000 hair removal–related injuries seen in U.S. emergency departments. There were nearly equal numbers of men and women presenting for injuries, with 60% of the injuries occurring at home. Because this study only examined the injuries severe enough to present for treatment and tabulated only injuries caused by scissors, clippers, and razors, it is likely that hair-removal injury rates are actually much higher than reported.[85]

REFERENCES

1. Lipton MG, Sherr L, Elford J, et al. Women living with facial hair: the psychological and behavioral burden. *J Psychosom Res.* 2006;61(2):161-168.
2. Keegan A, Liao LM, Boyle M. "Hirsutism": a psychological analysis. *J Health Psychol.* 2003;8(3):327-345.
3. Pasch L, He SY, Huddleston H, et al. Clinician vs self-ratings of hirsutism in patients with polycystic ovarian syndrome: associations with quality of life and depression. *JAMA Dermatol.* 2016;152(7):783-738.
4. Knochenhauer ES, Key TJ, Kahsar-Miller M, et al. Prevalence of the polycystic ovary syndrome in unselected black and white women of the southeastern United States: a prospective study. *J Clin Endocrinol Metab.* 1998;83(9):3078-3082.
5. Azziz R. The evaluation and management of hirsutism. *Obstet Gynecol.* 2003;101(5 Pt 1):995-1007.
6. Cheewadhanaraks S, Peeyananjarassri K, Choksuchat C. Clinical diagnosis of hirsutism in Thai women. *J Med Assoc Thai.* 2004;87(5):459-463.
7. Escobar-Morreale HF, Carmina E, Dewailly D, et al. Epidemiology, diagnosis and management of hirsutism: a consensus statement by the Androgen Excess and Polycystic Ovary Syndrome Society. *Hum Reprod Update.* 2012;18(2):146-170.
8. Javorsky E, Perkins AC, Hillebrand G, et al. Race, rather than skin pigmentation, predicts facial hair growth in women. *J Clin Aesthet Dermatol.* 2014;7(5):24-26.
9. DeUgarte CM, Woods KS, Bartolucci AA, et al. Degree of facial and body terminal hair growth in unselected black and white women: toward a populational definition of hirsutism. *J Clin Endocrinol Metab.* 2006;91(4):1345-1350.
10. Li R, Qiao J, Yang D, et al. Epidemiology of hirsutism among women of reproductive age in the community: a simplified scoring system. *Eur J Obstet Gynecol Reprod Biol.* 2012;163(2):165-169.
11. Breitkopf T, Leung G, Yu M, et al. The basic science of hair biology: what are the causal mechanisms for the disordered hair follicle? *Dermatol Clin.* 2013;31(1):1-19.
12. Azziz R, Carmina E, Sawaya ME. Idiopathic hirsutism. *Endocr Rev.* 2000;21(4):347-362.
13. Azziz R, Sanchez LA, Knochenhauer ES, et al. Androgen excess in women: experience with over 1000 consecutive patients. *J Clin Endocrinol Metab.* 2004;89(2):453-462.
14. Wong M, Zhao X, Hong Y, et al. Semiquantitative assessment of hirsutism in 850 PCOS patients and 2,988 controls in China. *Endokrynol Pol.* 2014;65(5):365-370.
15. Ferriman D, Gallwey JD. Clinical assessment of body hair growth in women. *J Clin Endocrinol Metab.* 1961;21:1440-1447.
16. Hatch R, Rosenfield RL, Kim MH, et al. Hirsutism: implications, etiology, and management. *Am J Obstet Gynecol.* 1981;140(7):815-830.
17. Minooee S, Ramezani Tehrani F, Azizi F. Hirsutism region and the likelihood of metabolic syndrome: is there a link? *Endocrine.* 2016;53(2):607-609.
18. Bode D, Seehusen DA, Baird D. Hirsutism in women. *Am Fam Physician.* 2012;85(4):373-380.
19. Cook H, Brennan K, Azziz R. Reanalyzing the modified Ferriman-Gallwey score: is there a simpler method for assessing the extent of hirsutism? *Fertil Steril.* 2011;96(5):1266-1270.e1261.
20. Huang Z, Yong EL. Ethnic differences: is there an Asian phenotype for polycystic ovarian syndrome? *Best Pract Res Clin Obstet Gynaecol.* 2016;37:46-55.
21. Carmina E, Rosato F, Janni A, et al. Extensive clinical experience: relative prevalence of different androgen excess disorders in 950 women referred because of clinical hyperandrogenism. *J Clin Endocrinol Metab.* 2006;91(1):2-6.
22. Taheri S, Zararsiz G, Karaburgu S, et al. Is idiopathic hirsutism (IH) really idiopathic? mRNA expressions of skin steroidogenic enzymes in women with IH. *Eur J Endocrinol.* 2015;173(4):447-454.
23. Housman E, Reynolds RV. Polycystic ovary syndrome: a review for dermatologists: part I. Diagnosis and manifestations. *J Am Acad Dermatol.* 2014;71(5): 847, e841-847, e810; quiz 857-848.
24. Falsetti L, Gambera A, Andrico S, et al. Acne and hirsutism in polycystic ovary syndrome: clinical, endocrine-metabolic and ultrasonographic differences. *Gynecol Endocrinol.* 2002;16(4):275-284.
25. Lee AT, Zane LT. Dermatologic manifestations of polycystic ovary syndrome. *Am J Clin Dermatol.* 2007;8(4):201-219.
26. Schmidt TH, Khanijow K, Cedars MI, et al. Cutaneous findings and systemic associations in women with polycystic ovary syndrome. *JAMA Dermatol.* 2016;152(4):391-398.
27. Carmina E, Koyama T, Chang L, et al. Does ethnicity influence the prevalence of adrenal hyperandrogenism and insulin resistance in polycystic ovary syndrome? *Am J Obstet Gynecol.* 1992;167(6):1807-1812.
28. Jayasena CN, Franks S. The management of patients with polycystic ovary syndrome. *Nat Rev Endocrinol.* 2014;10(10):624-636.
29. Amesse LS, Ding X, Pfaff-Amesse T. From HAIR-AN to eternity. *J Pediatr Adolesc Gynecol.* 2002;15(4):235-240.
30. Elmer KB, George RM. HAIR-AN syndrome: a multisystem challenge. *Am Fam Physician.* 2001;63(12):2385-2390.
31. Chen W, Obermayer-Pietsch B, Hong JB, et al. Acne-associated syndromes: models for better understanding of acne pathogenesis. *J Eur Acad Dermatol Venereol.* 2011;25(6):637-646.
32. Orfanos CE, Adler YD, Zouboulis CC. The SAHA syndrome. *Horm Res.* 2000;54(5-6):251-258.
33. Dalamaga M, Papadavid E, Basios G, et al. Ovarian SAHA syndrome is associated with a more insulin-resistant profile and represents an independent risk factor for glucose abnormalities in women with polycystic ovary syndrome: a prospective controlled study. *J Am Acad Dermatol.* 2013;69(6):922-930.
34. Bidet M, Bellanne-Chantelot C, Galand-Portier MB, et al. Clinical and molecular characterization of a cohort of 161 unrelated women with nonclassical congenital adrenal hyperplasia due to 21-hydroxylase deficiency and 330 family members. *J Clin Endocrinol Metab.* 2009;94(5):1570-1578.
35. Escobar-Morreale HF. Diagnosis and management of hirsutism. *Ann N Y Acad Sci.* 2010;1205:166-174.
36. Falsetti L, Pasinetti E. Treatment of moderate and severe hirsutism by gonadotropin-releasing hormone agonists in women with polycystic ovary syndrome and idiopathic hirsutism. *Fertil Steril.* 1994;61(5):817-822.
37. Ramezani Tehrani F, Behboudi-Gandevani S, Simbar M, et al. A population-based study of the relationship between idiopathic hirsutism and metabolic disturbances. *J Endocrinol Invest.* 2015;38(2):155-162.
38. Rosenfield RL. Clinical practice. Hirsutism. *N Engl J Med.* 2005;353(24):2578-2588.

39. Ekback MP, Lindberg M, Benzein E, et al. Health-related quality of life, depression and anxiety correlate with the degree of hirsutism. *Dermatology*. 2013;227(3):278-284.
40. Ekback MP, Lindberg M, Benzein E, et al. Social support: an important factor for quality of life in women with hirsutism. *Health Qual Life Outcomes*. 2014;12:183.
41. Schmidt TH, Shinkai K. Evidence-based approach to cutaneous hyperandrogenism in women. *J Am Acad Dermatol*. 2015;73(4):672-690.
42. Akalin S. Effects of ketoconazole in hirsute women. *Acta Endocrinol*. 1991;124(1):19-22.
43. Isik AZ, Gokmen O, Zeyneloglu HB, et al. Low dose ketoconazole is an effective and a relatively safe alternative in the treatment of hirsutism. *Aust N Z J Obstet Gynaecol*. 1996;36(4):487-489.
44. Lizneva D, Gavrilova-Jordan L, Walker W, et al. Androgen excess: investigations and management. *Best Pract Res Clin Obstet Gynaecol*. 2016;37:98-118.
45. Marzouk TM, Sayed Ahmed WA. Effect of dietary weight loss on menstrual regularity in obese young adult women with polycystic ovary syndrome. *J Pediatr Adolesc Gynecol*. 2015;28(6):457-461.
46. Luque-Ramirez M, Alvarez-Blasco F, Botella-Carretero JI, et al. Comparison of ethinyl-estradiol plus cyproterone acetate versus metformin effects on classic metabolic cardiovascular risk factors in women with the polycystic ovary syndrome. *J Clin Endocrinol Metab*. 2007;92(7):2453-2461.
47. Fruzzetti F, Bersi C, Parrini D, et al. Treatment of hirsutism: comparisons between different antiandrogens with central and peripheral effects. *Fertil Steril*. 1999;71(3):445-451.
48. Evans G, Sutton EL. Oral contraception. *Med Clin North Am*. 2015;99(3):479-503.
49. Azziz R, Ochoa TM, Bradley EL Jr, et al. Leuprolide and estrogen versus oral contraceptive pills for the treatment of hirsutism: a prospective randomized study. *J Clin Endocrinol Metab*. 1995;80(12):3406-3411.
50. Blume-Peytavi U. How to diagnose and treat medically women with excessive hair. *Dermatol Clin*. 2013;31(1):57-65.
51. Blume-Peytavi U, Hahn S. Medical treatment of hirsutism. *Dermatol Ther*. 2008;21:329-339.
52. Muderris II, Bayram F, Ozcelik B, et al. New alternative treatment in hirsutism: bicalutamide 25 mg/day. *Gynecol Endocrinol*. 2002;16(1):63-66.
53. Hussain S, Haider A, Bloom RE, et al. Bicalutamide-induced hepatotoxicity: a rare adverse effect. *Am J Case Rep*. 2014;15:266-270.
54. Kercher KR, McMichael AJ. Hirsutism and hypertrichosis. In: McMichael A, Hordinsky MK, eds. Hair and Scalp Diseases: Medical, Surgical, and Cosmetic Treatments.: New York: Informa Healthcare; 2008:218.
55. Gan SD, Graber EM. Laser hair removal: a review. *Dermatol Surg*. 2013;39(6):823-838.
56. Deplewski D, Rosenfield RL. Role of hormones in pilosebaceous unit development. *Endocr Rev*. 2000;21(4):363.
57. Pavone P, Practico AD, Falsaperla R, et al. Congenital generalized hypertrichosis: the skin as a clue to complex malformation syndromes. *Ital J Pediatr*. 2015;41-55.
58. Chen W, Ring J, Happle R. Congenital generalized hypertrichosis terminalis:a proposed classification and a plea to avoid the ambiguous term "Ambras syndrome." *Eur J Dermatol*. 2015;25(3):223-227.
59. Silveira LM, Ramos AN, Amaral IR, et al. Do you know this syndrome? *An Bras Dermatol*. 2013;88(3):473-475.
60. Shah IH, Zeerak S, Sajad P, et al. Congenital hypertrichosis lanuginose. *Indian J Dermatol Venereol Leprol*. 2018;84:248.
61. Tadin M, Braverman E, Cianfarani S, et al. Complex cytogenetic rearrangement of chromosome 8q in a case of Ambras syndrome. *Am J Med Genet*. 2001;102:100-104.
62. Tadin-Strapps M, Salas-Alanis JC, Moreno L, et al. Congenital universal hypertrichosis with deafness and dental anomalies inherited as an X-linked trait. *Clin Genet*. 2003;63(5):418-22.
63. DeStefano GM, Fantauzzo KA, Petukhova L, et al. Position effect on FGF13 associated with X-linked congenital generalized hypertrichosis. *Proc Natl Acad Sci U S A*. 2013;110(19):7790-5.
64. Grange DK, Nichols CG, Singh GK. Cantú syndrome and related disorders. In: Adam MP, Ardinger HH, Pagon RA, et al, eds. *GeneReviews*. Seattle, University of Washington, Seattle; 2014.
65. van Bon BW, Gilissen C, Grange DK, et al. Cantú syndrome is caused by mutations in ABCC9. *Am J Hum Genet*. 2012;90(6):1094-1101.
66. Cooper PE, Reutter H, Woelfle J, et al. Cantú syndrome resulting from activating mutation in the KCNJ8 gene. *Human Mutat*. 2014;35(7):809-813.
67. Balaji P, Balaji SM. Gingival fibromatosis with hypertrichosis syndrome: case series of rare syndrome. *Indian J Dent Res*. 2017;28(4):457-460.
68. Ishita A, Sujatha GP, Pramod GV, et al. Ambras syndrome: a rare case report. *J Indian Soc Pedod Prev Dent*. 2016;34:189-189.
69. Snyder CH. Syndrome of gingival hyperplasia, hirsutism, and convulsions. *J Pediatr*. 1965;67:499-502.
70. Lacombe D, Bioulac-Sage P, Sibout M, et al. Congenital marked hypertrichosis and Laband syndrome in a child: overlap between the gingival fibromatosis-hypertrichosis and Laband syndromes. *Genet Couns*. 1994;5(3):251-256.
71. De Lange C. Sur un type nouveau de generation (Typus amstelodamensis). *Arch Med Enfant*. 1933;36:713.
72. Salazar FN. Dermatological manifestations of the Cornelia de Lange syndrome. *Arch Dermatol*. 1966;94(1):38-43.
74. Krantz ID, McCallum J, DeScipio C, et al. Cornelia de Lange syndrome is caused by mutations in NIBPL, the human homolog of *Drosophila melanogaster* Nipped-B. *Nat Genet*. 2004;36(6):631-635
74. Huisman SA, Redeker EJW, Maas SM, et al. High rate of mosaicism in individuals with Cornelia de Lange syndrome. *J Med Genet*. 2013;50(5):339-344.
75. Wendelin DS, Pope DN, Mallory S. Hypertrichosis. *J Am Acad Dermatol* 2003;48:161-179.
76. Guggisberg D, Hadj-Rabia S, Viney C, et al. Skin markers of occult spinal dysraphism in children: a review of 54 cases. *Arch Dermatol*. 2004;140(9):1109-1115.
77. Vashi RA, Mancini AJ, Paller AS. Primary generalized and localized hypertrichosis in children. *Arch Dermatol*. 2001;137(7):877-884.
78. Olsen E. Hypertrichosis. In: Olsen E, ed. Disorders of Hair Growth: Diagnosis and Treatment. New York: McGraw-Hill;1993:326-329.
79. Grossman ME, Bickers DR, Poh-Fitzpatrick MB, et al. Porphyria cutea tarda. Clinical features and laboratory findings in 40 patients. *Am J Med*. 1979;67(2):277-286.
80. Vachiramon V, McMichael AJ. Laser hair removal in ethnic skin: principles and practical aspects. *J Drugs*

81. Ellis FA. Electrolysis versus high frequency currents in the treatment of hypertrichosis: a comparative histologic and clinical study. *Arch Derm Syphilol*. 1947;56(3):291-305.
82. Salas-Alanis JC, Lopez-Cepeda LD, Elizondo-Rodriguez A, et al. Hypertrichosis lanuginose congenita treated with diode laser epilation during infancy. *Pediatr Dermatol*. 2014;31(4):529-530.
83. Benmously MR, Ben Hamida M, Hammami H, et al. Long-pulsed Nd:YAG laser in the treatment of facial hypertrichosis during topical minoxidil therapy. *J Cosmet Laser Ther*. 2013;15(4):217-218.
84. Alajlan A, Shapiro J, Rivers JK, et al. Paradoxical hypertrichosis after laser epilation. *J Am Acad Dermatol*. 2005;53(1):85-88.
85. Swain TA, Tully AS, Redford T, et al. Hair removal-related injuries in the United States, 1991-2014. *J Cosmet Dermatol*. 2016;15(4)444-451.

Chapter 91 :: Nail Disorders
:: Eckart Haneke

第九十一章
甲疾病

中文导读

本章将甲疾病分为两个方面：甲的病变和引起甲病变的疾病。

第一部分介绍甲的病变及其对应的临床表现、常伴发于哪些疾病和治疗。①无甲；②少甲和双甲；③甲颜色变化；④甲下血肿；⑤裂片样出血；⑥甲剥离；⑦甲下角化过度和甲癣；⑧翼状胬肉；⑨倒向翼状胬肉；⑩Beau线和甲脱落；⑪脆甲；⑫甲内嵌；⑬反甲；⑭甲过度弯曲；⑮甲美容治疗的影响。

第二部分介绍引起甲改变的甲疾病，分为炎症性疾病、感染性疾病、其他一般疾病中的甲改变、影响指甲的遗传性皮肤病及甲肿瘤5大板块进行讲述。主要是各个疾病的临床特征、发病机制、诊断、鉴别诊断、疾病关联、临床病程、预后和治疗。

第一节介绍炎症性甲疾病：分别介绍了银屑病、湿疹、斑秃、扁平苔藓、自身免疫性大疱性疾病、结缔组织病、血管炎和血管病变7种。

第二节介绍感染性甲疾病：分为病毒感染、细菌感染及真菌感染三个方面。

第三节介绍其他一般疾病中的甲改变：介绍了心血管疾病和肺部疾病（如杵状指）、肠道和肝疾病、泌尿生殖疾病（如对半甲）、淀粉样变、心理精神疾病、中毒引起的甲改变。

第四节介绍药物反应引起的甲改变，包括细胞抑制和靶向治疗、博来霉素、逆转录酶抑制药、阿昔洛韦、β受体阻滞药、维生素A和高剂量维生素A、补骨脂素和紫外线A的光化疗药物，并且总结于表91-9。

第五节介绍影响甲的遗传性皮肤病，讲述先天性厚甲症、外胚层发育不良、遗传性大疱性表皮松解症、甲-髌综合征、先天性角化不良、角化病（孟德尔角化病）、先天性踇趾甲排列不良及其对应的临床表现和涉及的基因。

第六节介绍甲肿瘤，分为良性肿瘤和恶性肿瘤，尤其提出黑甲——良性黑色素痣和甲黑色素瘤，为了便于色素性黑色素瘤的诊断，提出了一种考虑多种因素的ABCDEF诊断法（表91-11），但需注意它不适用于儿童的无黑色素的黑色素瘤和纵向黑甲(LM)。甲黑色素瘤主要采用手术治疗。

〔简　丹〕

The diagnosis and treatment of nail diseases require an in-depth knowledge of the anatomy, physiology, and pathology of the nail unit (see Chap. 8). It is an integral part of the tip of the digit, and its anatomy, growth characteristics, and functions vary between the different fingers and toes, which have to be considered when faced with a diseased nail. There are different ways to classify nail disorders and a compromise between a scientifically based etiologic classification and a more clinico-morphologically based one appears to be a practical approach to nail disorders. This chapter discusses specific nail changes either resulting from particular nail disorders or from dermatologic or systemic diseases, the peculiarities, including etiopathogenetic aspects, of which are not repeated here if they are not specific for the nail lesions.

NAIL SIGNS AND NAIL-SPECIFIC CONDITIONS

ANONYCHIA, HYPONYCHIA, AND DOUBLE NAIL

Complete or almost complete lack of the nail is called anonychia, severe hypoplasia, or hyponychia. The condition is usually inborn, may be a genetic trait or the result of drug or toxin-induced lack of nail formation during embryogenesis. Several different types are known, ranging from a round tip of the digit without any visible change of the skin to an area that may correspond to the nail field, or a hyperkeratosis. When there is no terminal phalanx and no nail growth this is called Cooks syndrome or atelephalangia with anonychia. Hyponychia may be on all or several digits and is more common. A particular form with half-side index fingernail hypoplasia and a Y-shaped radiologic alteration of the distal phalanx is characteristic for Iso-Kikuchi syndrome.

Micronychia may be a sign of phenytoin and alcohol fetopathy and is a constant feature of congenital onychodysplasia of Iso-Kikuchi (COIF [congenital onychodysplasia of index finger] syndrome).

Racket nail is a short wide nail, mostly of the thumb, which develops from the age of 12 years on and is the result of a premature ossification of the epiphysis of the distal phalanx. The bone cannot grow longitudinally but continues to get broader because of apposition on the sides. This condition is autosomal dominant with variable expression and penetrance.

Very short nails (brachyonychia) may develop in patients under chronic hemodialysis who develop a tertiary hyperparathyroidism with resorption of the bone of the terminal phalanx.

A rudimentary double nail of the fifth toe is a relatively frequent finding in subjects of all races. The nail may be slightly wider and have a slight longitudinal indentation or be discernable as a complete accessory nail (Fig. 91-1).[1]

TABLE 91-1
Nail Discolorations (Chromonychia)

White–Leukonychia
- **True leukonychia:** hereditary, acquired; punctate, striate, diffuse (total, subtotal), multiple narrow white longitudinal lines: Hailey-Hailey disease, Darier disease
- **Causes:** idiopathic, microtrauma, manicure induced, liver disease, renal insufficiency
- **Apparent leukonychia:** pale nail bed in anemia, Raynaud syndrome, scleroderma
- **Pseudoleukonychia:** superficial white onychomycosis

Brown to Black–Melanonychia
- **Melanin:** activation of matrix melanocytes (functional melanonychia), matrix lentigo, nevus, melanoma
- **Microbial pigments:** *Proteus* spp, *Klebsiella* spp, melanin-producing fungi
- **Exogenous:** silver nitrate, potassium permanganate, heavy smoking, dirt
- **Blood:** acute or chronic trauma, friction

Green–Chloronychia
- *Pseudomonas aeruginosa* (pyocyanin)

Red–Erythronychia
- **Red lunula:** spotted or diffuse: acute nail involvement in several dermatoses such as erythema multiforme, alopecia areata, psoriasis, lupus erythematosus
- **Longitudinal erythronychia:** onychopapilloma, Bowen disease; multiple narrow red lines: dyskeratosis follicularis of Darier (often with some white lines in between).

Yellow–Xanthonychia
- All very thick nails appear yellow, often also onycholytic nails are yellow
- Yellow nail syndrome (triad of chronic bronchopulmonary infection, edema of the distal extremities, and extremely slow-growing yellow nails)

Blue–Azure Nail (Glauconychia)
- Copper sulfate; gray-blue lunulae: ingestion of silver nitrate

CHROMONYCHIA

The nail may show a variety of color changes that may be caused by true coloration of the nail plate or alterations of the matrix and nail bed shining through the nail plate (Table 91-1).

Leukonychia is the most common color change. It is caused by alterations in the keratinization of the nail plate with the nail cells being parakeratotic and/or having an eosinophilic cytoplasm in histologic sections. Often, these changes slowly disappear so that the free margin of the nail plate appears normal. Morphologically, there may be small patches or transverse bands, mainly seen in children and youngsters, probably the result of an overzealous manicure (Fig. 91-2). Total diffuse leukonychia (Fig. 91-3) is inborn in most cases. Subtotal diffuse leukonychia is sometimes seen in chronic liver disease. Many longitudinal white bands are characteristic for Hailey-Hailey disease.

Apparent leukonychia is a result of nail bed pallor. It may disappear with temperature change or pressure.

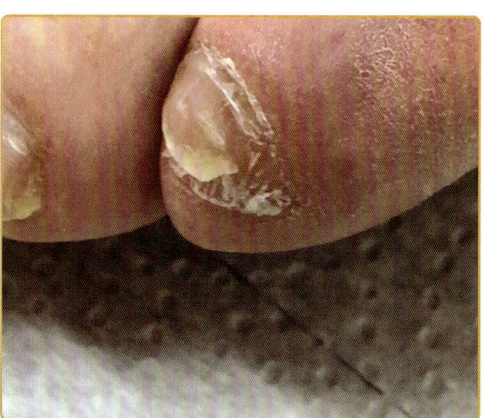

Figure 91-1 Rudimentary double nail of the little toe.

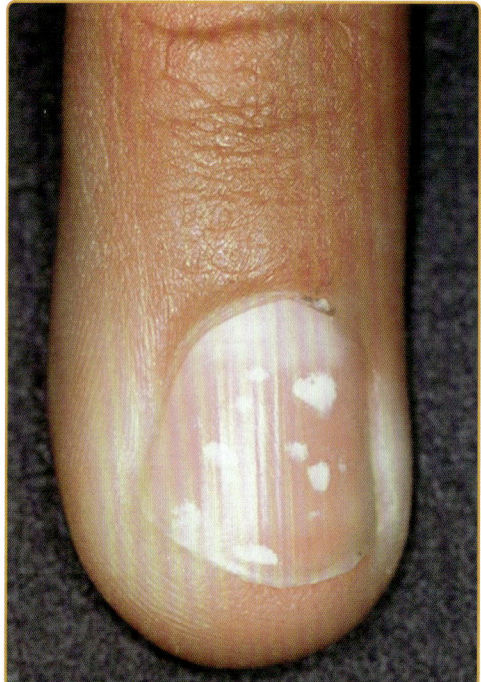

Figure 91-2 Leukonychia punctata.

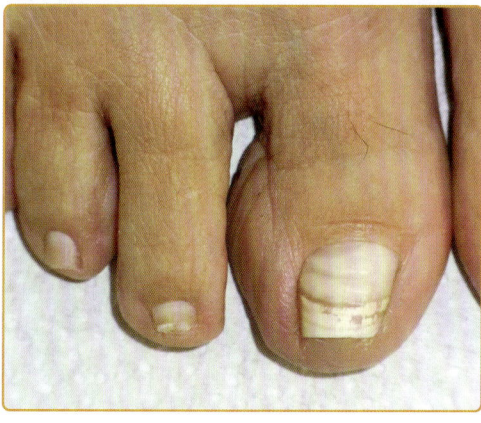

Muehrcke lines are a pair of 2 whitish transverse lines and are said to be a sign of hypalbuminemia (Fig. 91-4).

Pseudoleukonychia is the white surface of the nail, which is infected by fungi. It was also termed (pseudo) leukonychia trichophytica although nondermatophyte molds also may be causative (Fig. 91-5).

Erythronychia is the term for red nails. It may appear as red spots in the matrix (Fig. 91-6),[2] one or more longitudinal streaks in the distal matrix and nail bed (Figs. 91-7 and 91-8). Multiple red bands are commonly caused by inflammatory conditions such as lichen planus, whereas a single red band may represent specific tumors such as onychopapilloma (Fig. 91-7) or Bowen disease; hence a biopsy is indicated. Alternating narrow white and red bands are seen in Darier disease.

Chloronychia is the term for green nails. In almost all cases, it is caused by a colonization of the nail by *Pseudomonas aeruginosa*. Often, 1 margin of the nail is involved with circumscribed swelling and detachment of the proximal nailfold, lack of the cuticle, and lateral onycholysis (Fig. 91-9). However, it is also seen in distal onycholysis and onycholysis over subungual tumors. Although *Pseudomonas* colonization is harmless for the patient, it may pose a risk for immunosuppressed individuals and these patients should not work in kitchens, bakeries, other food industry jobs, or in surgery, premature, and newborn wards and intensive care units. The treatment of choice of *P. aeruginosa* colonization is soaking in diluted white vinegar, 2 or 3 times daily for 10 minutes, then brushing the fingers dry. Household bleach for fingertip baths can be used undiluted or 1:1 diluted in water. Other disinfective agents may be used in addition. Topical antibiotics such as gentamycin are sometimes used, but are no more efficacious. Systemic antibiotics do not reach the site of infection because *Pseudomonas* mainly colonizes an onycholytic nail. In rare cases, systemic treatment with ciprofloxacin may be indicated.

Blue nails were seen developing in persons swimming in water with copper sulfate as a disinfective agent.

Slate-gray to bluish nail matrix is a sign of *argyria*.[3]

Melanonychia denotes brown-to-black nail pigmentation. Although this term is generally used for melanin pigmentation of the nail, many other agents may stain the nail brown, such as potassium permanganate or tobacco smoke. Silver nitrate makes the nail jet-black (Fig. 91-10). Some bacteria cause dirty grayish discoloration (Fig. 91-11). Melanonychia may be diffuse and total, transverse or longitudinal. Usually, a brown-to-black band develops in the nail running from the proximal nailfold into the free margin of the nail plate. It is caused by melanocyte activation, a lentigo, nevus, or melanoma of the matrix. Multiple melanonychias in several or all digits are common in dark-skinned individuals and Asians and are a physiologic phenomenon seen in almost all African Americans (Fig. 91-12). Pregnancy, a variety of drugs, vitamin B_{12} deficiency, Addison disease, HIV infection, some dermatoses such as ungual lichen planus, and Bowen disease of the nail (particularly when associated with human papillomavirus [HPV] Type 56) may exhibit melanonychias. The association of lenticular labial, oral, and genital mucosal

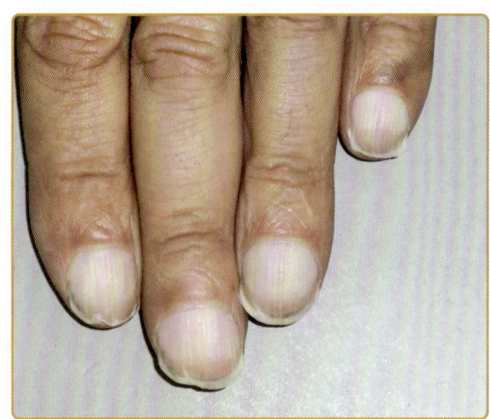

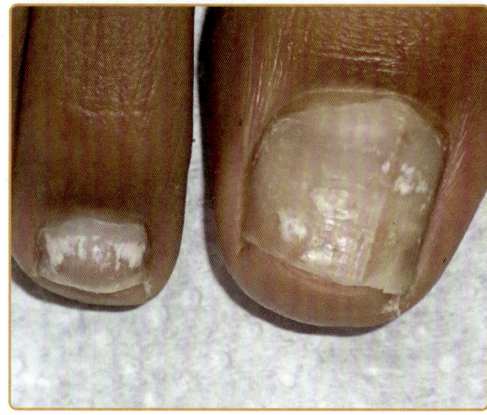

Figure 91-5 Pseudoleukonychia in superficial white onychomycosis; the white spots are on the surface of the nail plate.

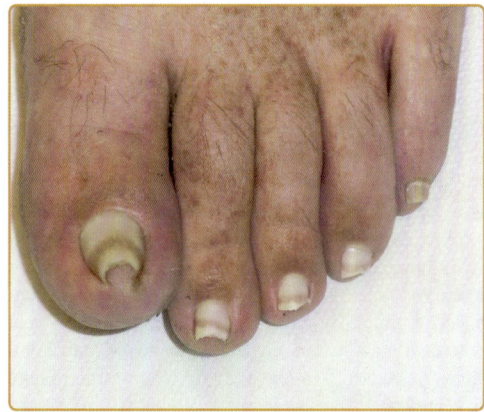

Figure 91-3 Diffuse leukonychia.

nail melanoma and requires a meticulous evaluation. Single-digit melanonychia in an adult requires a biopsy.

SUBUNGUAL HEMATOMA

A single, heavy trauma that is usually well-remembered because of its intense pain, or repeated microtraumas, most commonly from ill-fitting shoes or particular sports activities, lead to bleeding under the

brown spots with melanonychias is characteristic for Laugier-Hunziker-Baran syndrome. Friction from rubbing shoes may cause longitudinal melanonychia of the little or big toenail, and onychophagia may cause melanocyte activation with subsequent melanonychia. Longitudinal nail pigmentation is the most frequent sign of

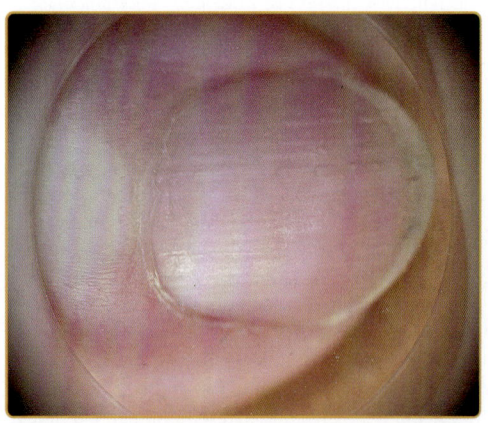

Figure 91-4 Muehrcke lines in hypoalbuminemia after more than 7 weeks of high fever.

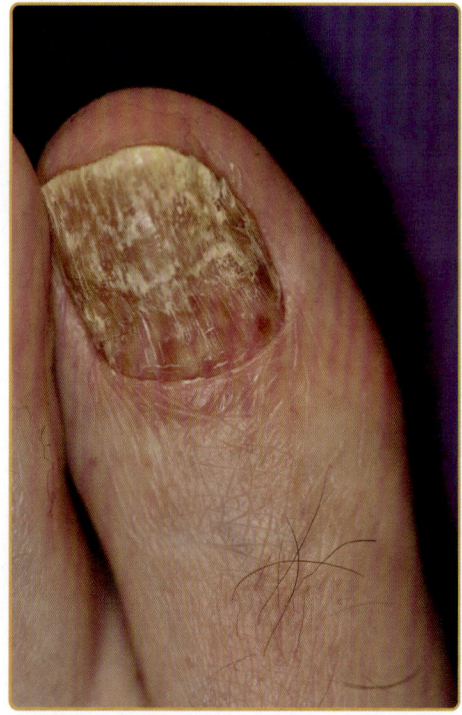

Figure 91-6 Red spot in the lunula of a patient with acute nail psoriasis.

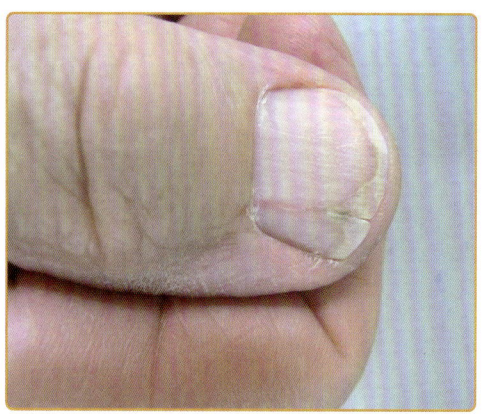

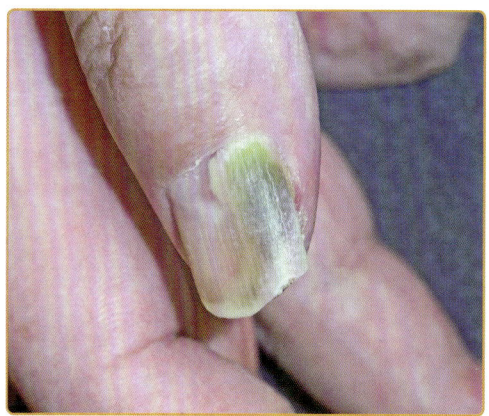

Figure 91-9 Green nail caused by *Pseudomonas* abscess under the nail.

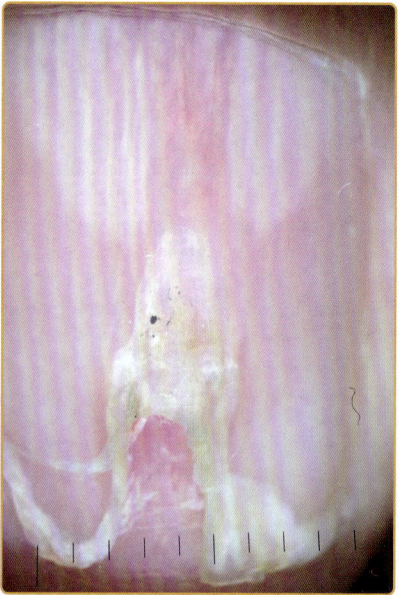

Figure 91-7 Longitudinal erythronychia caused by an onychopapilloma.

nail (Fig. 91-13). The blood is located between the overlying nail and the underlying matrix and nail bed epithelium and is therefore not degraded to hemosiderin by macrophages; consequently, it remains Prussian blue–negative or Perls stain–negative. With time it is included into the newly formed nail. It takes some months to slowly grow out but, in contrast to melanonychia, it never reaches into the free margin of the nail plate; this is one of the most reliable criteria for differential diagnosis. It also does not form a regular longitudinal band and when growing out a normal nail reappears. Dermatoscopy shows round red to dark-brown globules. Acute subungual hematoma can be drained by drilling a small hole into the nail plate to release the blood. Hematomas occupying more than 50% of the nail field are commonly associated with a fracture of the distal phalanx.

SPLINTER HEMORRHAGES

Splinter hemorrhages are narrow red to almost black longitudinal lines in the distal nail bed and are caused by blood that is enclosed in the subungual keratin (Fig. 91-14). They develop either from thrombosed or ruptured capillaries that run longitudinally in the nail

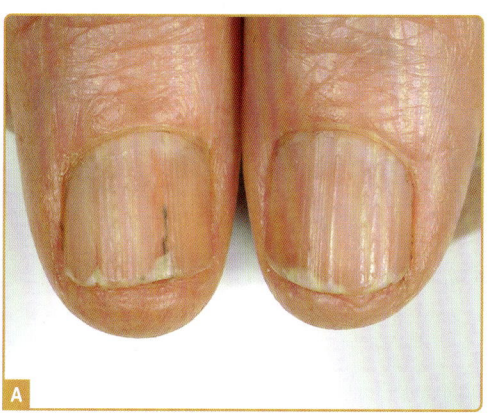

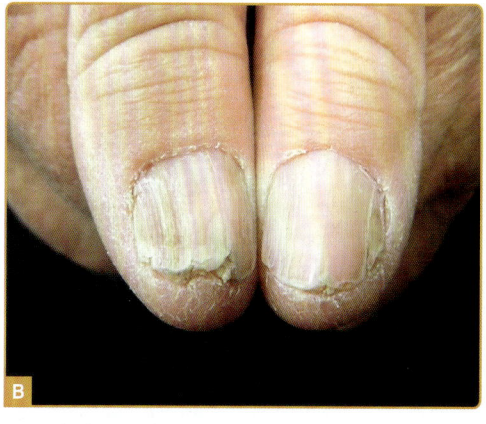

Figure 91-8 Multiple red lines in dyskeratosis follicularis Darier (**A**) and white lines in Hailey-Hailey disease (**B**).

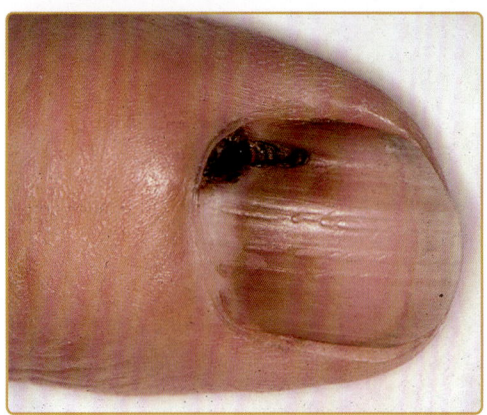

Figure 91-10 Jet-black nail surface stain from 5% silver nitrate solution used to etch what was thought to be granulation tissue protruding from under the proximal nailfold.

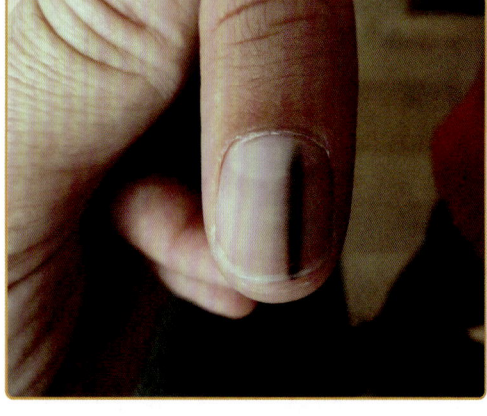

Figure 91-12 Melanonychia caused by melanin production in the matrix of a dark-skinned person.

bed. They are characteristic for trauma, psoriasis, and some other inflammatory nail and systemic diseases, such as scleroderma, systemic lupus erythematosus, rheumatoid arthritis, antiphospholipid syndrome, and hematologic malignancies. Splinter hemorrhages also are characteristic for bacterial endocarditis with subsepsis lenta (39%) where they may occur together with Osler nodes (6.7%), Janeway lesions (2.2%), and retinal hemorrhages called Roth spots (3%). Oblique splinter hemorrhages may be a sign of trichinosis.

ONYCHOLYSIS

Detachment of the nail from the distal nail bed is called onycholysis. All conditions with abnormal subungual hyperkeratosis will eventually cause onycholysis. These may be inflammatory nail diseases such as psoriasis (Fig. 91-15), lichen planus (Fig. 91-16), atopic dermatitis, and pityriasis rubra pilaris, or infections such as onychomycoses, or tumors of the nail bed. Direct trauma resulting from overzealous nail cleaning is the cause of onycholysis semilunaris (Fig. 91-17). This is characterized by sharply delimited proximal margins that may look like a half moon. Repeated frictional trauma is another cause, particularly in the asymmetric gait nail unit syndrome (see below). Onycholysis is usually colonized by a variety of microorganisms, both bacteria and fungi. Treatment is the avoiding of moisture, cutting the nail back to the adherent part, brushing the nail bed twice daily with a disinfective solution, and applying an antimicrobial cream. Approximately one-half of the regrowing nail will remain attached to the nail bed; however, once having been onycholytic, a nail remains susceptible to reoccurrence of onycholysis.

SUBUNGUAL HYPERKERATOSIS AND ONYCHOGRYPOSIS

Hyperkeratosis of the nail bed is a frequent event (Fig. 91-18). It is characteristic for onychomycoses

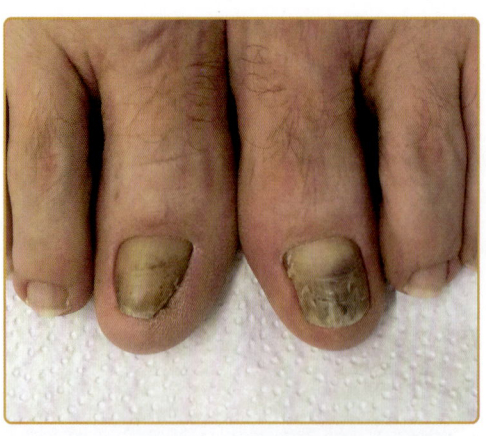

Figure 91-11 Dirty grayish nail discoloration caused by *Proteus* spp.

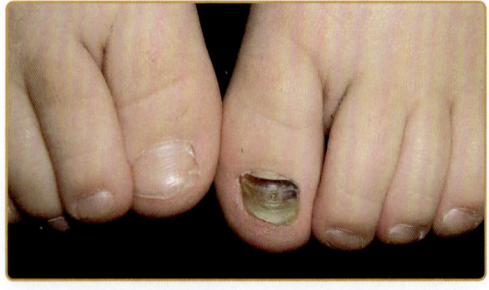

Figure 91-13 Subungual hematoma in a little boy with congenital malalignment of the big toenail. This condition is often associated with large subungual hematomas from minor trauma. The figure shows that the hematoma grows out with its proximal border being parallel to the presumed lunula border and free nail end.

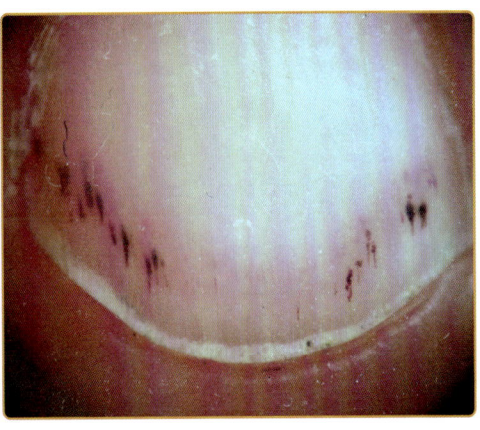

Figure 91-14 Splinter hemorrhages in a patient with chronic diarrhea.

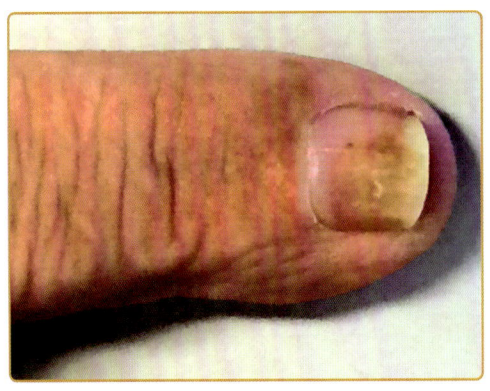

Figure 91-16 Lichen planus of the nail bed causing onycholysis.

where it contains most of the fungi, and for psoriasis. Other frequent causes are trauma, allergic and toxic contact, and atopic dermatitis. It is virtually always associated with onycholysis, except in pachyonychia congenita, where the nail covers an excessive nail bed hyperkeratosis in a horseshoe-like fashion.

Onychogryposis (the common spelling, *onychogryphosis*, is etymologically incorrect as *gryphos* means a mythical animal that is half bird–half lion, whereas *grypos* means horn, hence it should be written *onychogryposis*) is an exaggeration of nail bed and matrix hyperkeratosis. It consists of innumerable stacks of keratin layers piled up one over the other, grows upward, is opaque and often has the shape of a ram's horn. There is usually no contact with the nail bed anymore and the nail pocket is extremely short. It is mainly seen in elderly, neglected, and debilitated individuals (Fig. 91-19). Treatment is by nail avulsion, often completed by nail matrix cauterization to prevent regrowth of a gryptotic nail.

PTERYGIUM

Pterygium (from Greek for wing formation) is the bridging of the nail pocket by connective tissue, in most cases scars. It is very common in lichen planus (Fig. 91-20), but is occasionally seen in other conditions, such as bullous pemphigoid, but particularly also after trauma. It first divides the nail into 2 parts, but may lead to complete nail destruction when it occupies almost the entire nail pocket.

PTERYGIUM INVERSUM

When the nail plate does not separate correctly from the nail plate at the hyponychium and remains attached, a painful hyperkeratosis obliterates the distal groove. This is quite common in acral scleroderma and Raynaud syndrome, but also may be idiopathic (Fig. 91-21). Nail trimming can be very difficult and painful.

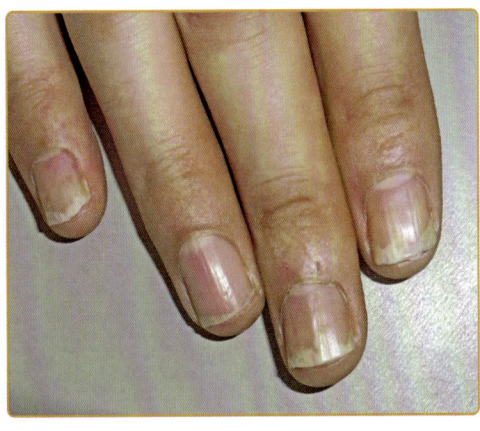

Figure 91-15 Psoriatic onycholysis.

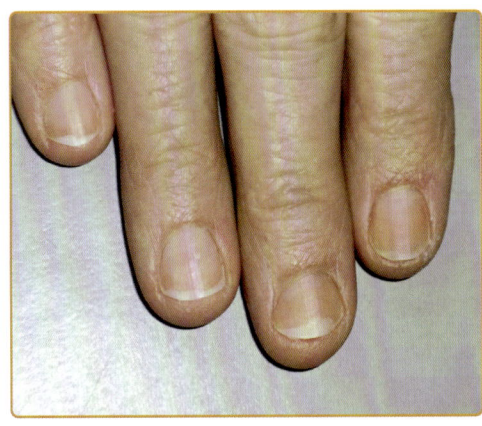

Figure 91-17 Onycholysis semilunaris induced by overzealous manicure.

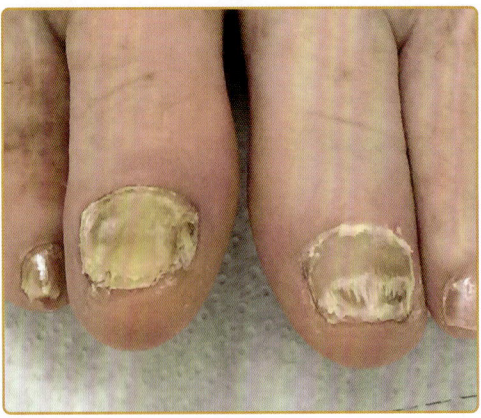

Figure 91-18 Hyperkeratosis of the nail bed.

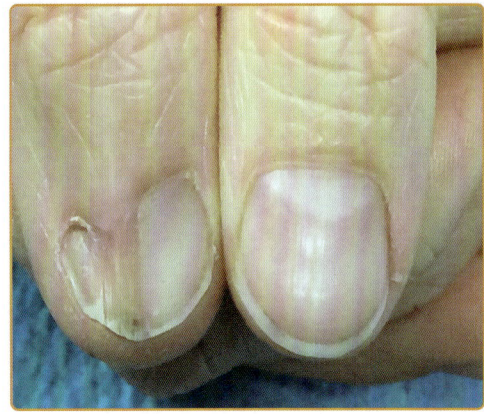

Figure 91-20 Pterygium in nail lichen planus.

BEAU LINES AND ONYCHOMADESIS

A temporary slowdown or even arrest of nail formation results in a transverse groove that runs parallel to the lunula border (Fig. 91-22). It may be shallow at the lateral portions and deeper centrally. Onychomadesis is the result of a longer-lasting arrest of nail matrix proliferation that eventually results in a proximal gap in the nail and proximal onycholysis (Fig. 91-23). It may end up in loss of the nail. The faster a nail grows the more pronounced the lesion; hence Beau lines and onychomadesis are much more common in fingernails than in toenails. Repeated Beau lines indicate repeated trauma, such as chemotherapy cycles. Equally distributed Beau lines hint at a general cause, whereas one-sided lines are seen after surgery of the extremity or a single-digit line at previous finger or toe surgery. A great many different causes are known, ranging from high fever to other serious diseases. Localized Beau lines and onychomadesis were also seen several weeks after hand-foot-and-mouth disease (coxcackievirus infection). Trauma, cosmetic manipulations, onychophagia, and onychotillomania are other causes and explain why the fingernails are predominantly affected (Table 91-2).

PITTING AND TRACHYONYCHIA

Pits are small depressions in the nail surface resulting from minute foci of abnormal keratinization in the apical matrix. This produces small mounds of parakeratosis that tend to break away from the nail when this emerges from under the proximal nailfold. Sometimes, the parakeratosis is not shed and small ivory-colored spots are seen. Pits are the most frequent sign of nail psoriasis (Fig. 91-24) where they are deep and of regular size, whereas those developing in alopecia areata and atopic dermatitis are more shallow and less-well delimited. Large surface defects are typical for pustular psoriasis and are called elkonyxis (Table 91-3).

Trachyonychia is the term for rough nails (Fig. 91-25). In addition to multiple pits, longitudinal striations and ridges such as seen in ungual lichen planus may cause

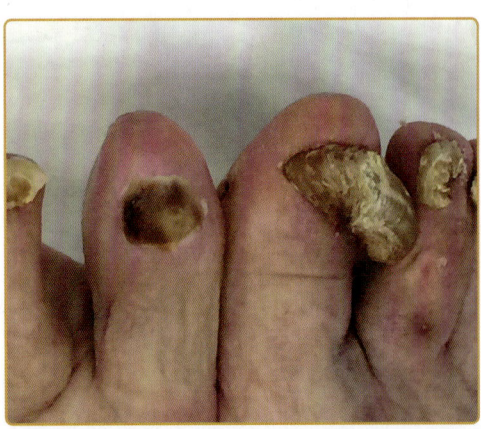

Figure 91-19 Onychogryphosis in a 63-year-old woman.

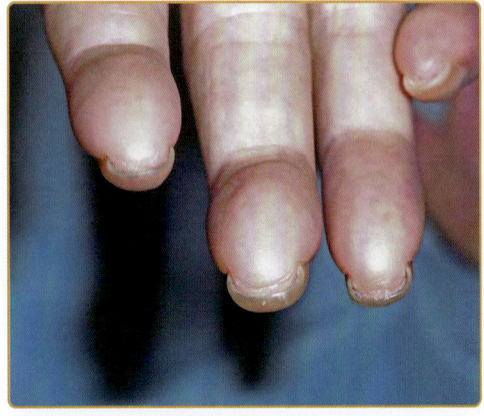

Figure 91-21 Pterygium inversum in a 54-year-old patient with Guillain-Barré syndrome.

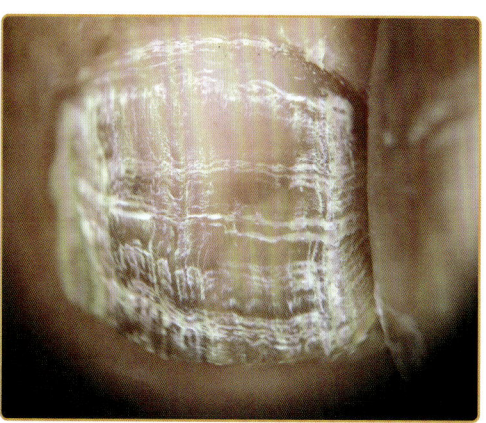

Figure 91-22 Multiple Beau lines in a patient under cyclic chemotherapy. (Used with permission from Dr. Patricia Chang, Guatemala.)

this condition. When many nails are affected the diagnosis of 20-nail syndrome can be made.

Longitudinal grooves are the result of pressure on the nail matrix, which is usually the result of a small tumor in the proximal nailfold (Fig. 91-26).

BRITTLE NAILS

Brittle nails are a very common complaint in daily practice, particularly by women. Multiple longitudinal fissures, often associated with nail thinning and ridges, are the hallmark of *onychorrhexis* (Fig. 91-27). Defective keratinization is thought to be one of the causes.

Onychoschizia is the lamellar splitting of the nail at its free end (Fig. 91-28). It is usually confined to fingernails and occurs much more often in women than in men, pointing to the importance of environmental factors, such as frequent water contact that results in hydration and dehydration of the nail, which leaks cementing lipoproteins out. In babies with koilonychia of the big toenail, onychoschizia is common. Other causes are some dermatoses, onychomycosis, peripheral

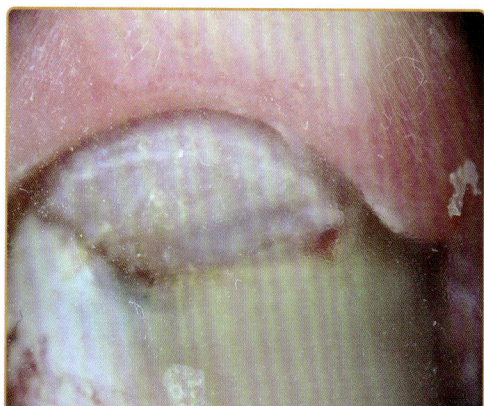

Figure 91-23 Onychomadesis after hand-foot-and-mouth disease.

TABLE 91-2
Causes of Beau lines and Onychomadesis

- **Generalized:** Acute severe diseases, high fever, some drugs (retinoids), zinc deficiency, autoimmune bullous diseases, menstruation (often repeated)
- **One extremity:** carpal tunnel syndrome (hand), surgery with extremity tourniquet, reflex sympathetic dystrophy (regional pain syndrome)
- **One or several digits:** nail surgery, hand-foot-and-mouth disease, trauma

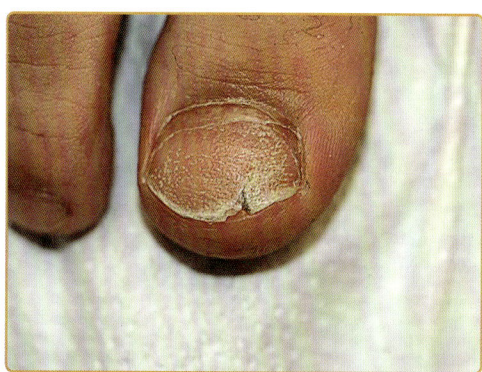

Figure 91-24 Psoriatic pitting.

TABLE 91-3
Causes of Pitting and Trachyonychia

- Psoriasis
- Eczema
- Alopecia areata
- Lichen planus
- Graft-versus-host disease
- Rheumatoid arthritis

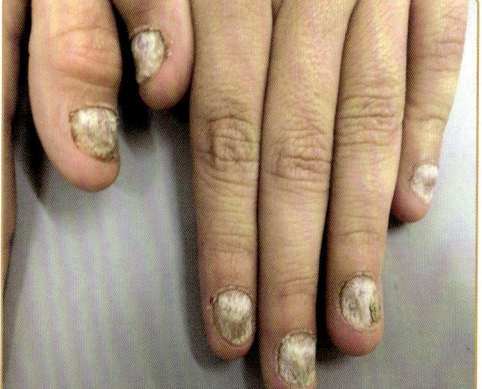

Figure 91-25 Trachyonychia in an 11-year-old boy with atopic dermatitis.

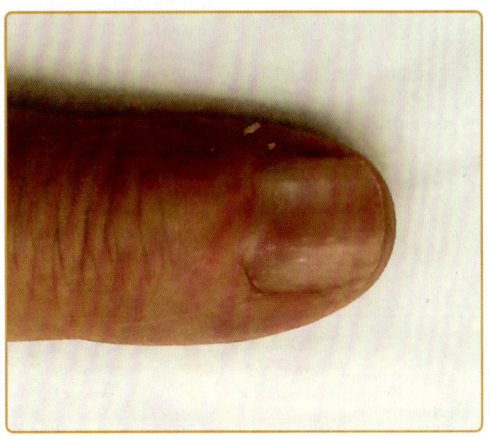

Figure 91-26 Longitudinal groove in a patient with a myxoid pseudocyst.

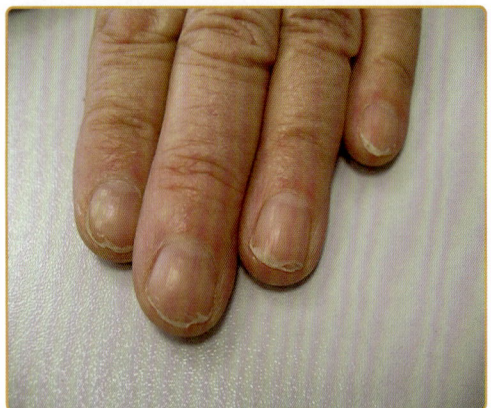

Figure 91-28 Onychoschizia.

neuropathies and vascular disease, occupational traumas, and a variety of drugs, particularly those interfering with nail growth (Table 91-4). The role of nutrition is frequently overestimated.[4]

INGROWN NAILS

Ingrown nails also affect adults and the elderly, but to a much lesser degree in terms of frequency. The most common type is distal–lateral ingrowing of the edge of the big toenail (Fig. 91-29), rarely of neighboring toes, and even less frequently of fingers (Fig. 91-30). There are many theories as to why and how ingrown nails develop and several are not exclusive of another one. Commonly, there is a discrepancy between too wide a nail plate and too narrow a nail bed. Usually, this is true for the distal portion where most pressure from shoes acts on the toes. The tip is compressed, it hurts, and the patient tries to cut the edge away, thereby leaving a kind of a spicule behind that pierces into the soft tissue of the distal portion of the nail sulcus causing pain, suppuration, granulation tissue, swelling, and,

with time, fibrosis of the nailfold.[5] Further etiologic factors are tight socks, hyperhidrosis, and overcurvature of the nails. Treatment is either conservative with insertion of a wisp of cotton between the offending nail and the nail sulcus, taping to pull the soft tissue away from the nail, or protection of the soft tissue from the nail margin by a gutter, which requires a local anesthesia. There are many more conservative approaches; however, all require consistent compliance from both the physician and the patient. Surgery is either to narrow the nail or to remove the swollen soft tissue (see Chap. 205).

RETRONYCHIA

Proximal ingrowing of the nail is called retronychia. It is caused by a single strong or repeated minor trauma to the nail that eventually results in a backward movement of the nail plate. Most patients are children, adolescents, and young adults with 1 or 2 swollen, bluish, proximal nailfolds of their big toes (Fig. 91-31). The lunula is no longer present. On pressure, granulation tissue may emerge from under the nailfold. Careful clinical examination reveals that there is a major onycholysis of the nail that allows the plate to be pushed backward. This leads to a horizontal split in the matrix. As the nail bed is mainly responsible for the forward growth

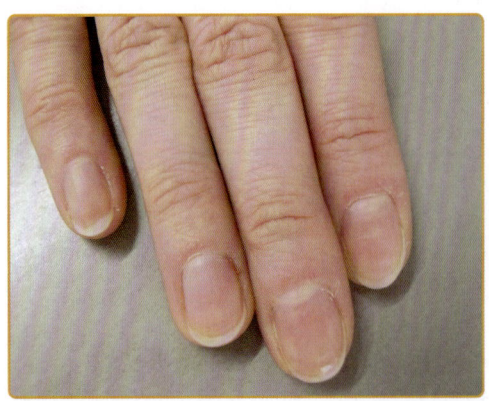

Figure 91-27 Onychorrhexis.

TABLE 91-4
Causes of Brittle Nails

Note: General disorders tend to affect all nails; fingernail-only involvement points at an etiology linked to wet work. Single-digit nail splitting is most likely a circumscribed disease or tumor.

- Chronic anemia; iron deficiency; zinc deficiency; vitamins A, B_6, and C deficiencies; hypervitaminosis A; genetic diseases with disturbance of keratin formation
- Local damage from trauma, alkalis, detergents, overzealous manicure

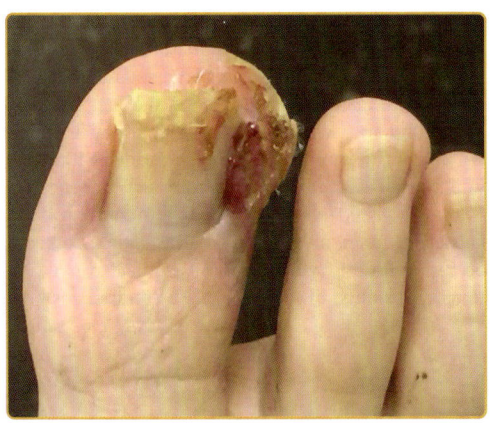

Figure 91-29 Ingrown nail of the big toe.

of the nail, this mechanism may no longer function and 1 or more new nails will be formed under the old proximal nail portion lifting this up. Its margin is very hard and sharp so that it cuts into the undersurface of the proximal nailfold with each step. The Y-shaped, W-shaped, or serrated proximal nail margin is well seen when the nail is avulsed, which is the treatment of choice.[6]

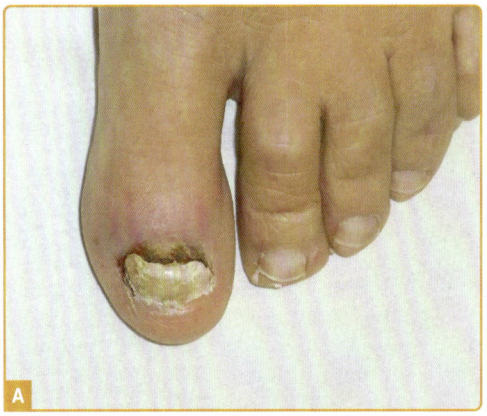

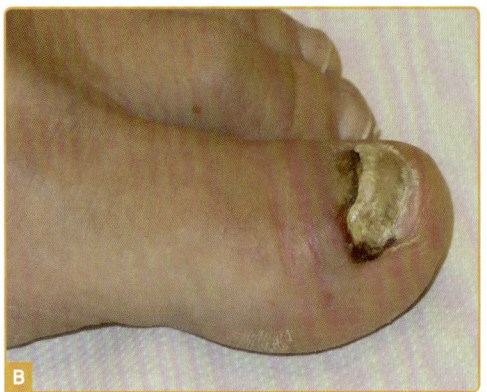

Figure 91-31 Retronychia of the big toe in a 17-year-old girl. **A,** Dorsal view. **B,** Oblique view.

PINCER NAILS (NAIL OVERCURVATURE)

Overcurvature of the nails is commonly called pincer nails, tubed nails, trumpet nails, and the like. The most common variant shows a distally increasing curvature (Fig. 91-32), but it may also remain at the same degree (tile nail) or exhibit sharp lateral bends. Half-side overcurvature is quite common. There are 2 types: *acquired* as a result of foot deformation, degenerative distal interphalangeal osteoarthritis (mainly in fingers), and some dermatoses, and *hereditary* with symmetrical involvement of the big toenails and often some, but very rarely all, lesser toenails. The big toenails show lateral deviation, the affected lesser nails are medially deviated. The base of the distal phalanx is widened, which can be felt by sliding palpation of the toe. Systematic radiographic examinations of the toes show that the distal phalanx is asymmetrical and often shows distally pointing exophytes that may correspond to the insertion of the interosseous ligament; they are much more pronounced medially than laterally, which explains in part the increasing lateral deviation of the nail plate. Furthermore, a distal dorsal traction osteophyte is commonly seen, which has to be removed when surgically flattening and spreading out the nail bed. In the distal portion,

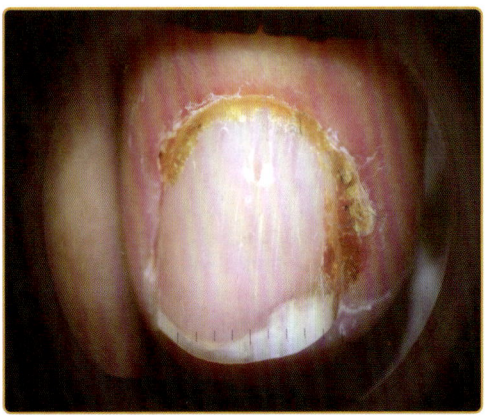

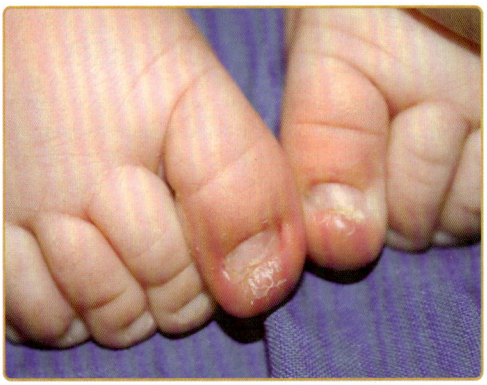

Figure 91-30 Ingrown nail of the finger in a patient under targeted anticancer treatment with cetuximab.

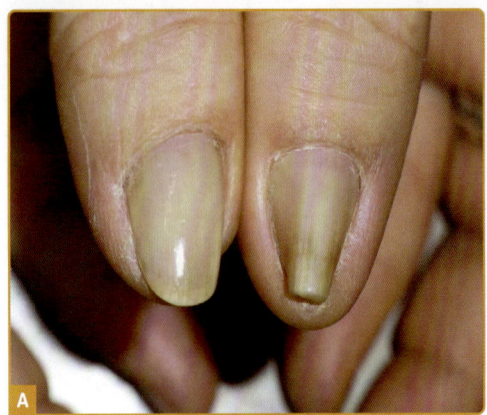

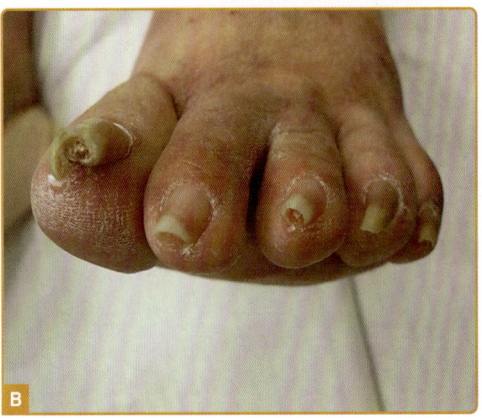

Figure 91-32 **A,** Pincer nails of the thumbs in a 53-year-old woman. **B,** Pincer nails of the toes in a 38-year-old woman.

the overcurved nail pinches the nail bed and heaps it up, resulting in a reactive subungual hyperkeratosis.[7] Treatment is by long-term application of nail braces to decrease the curvature, or a surgical procedure.

EFFECTS OF NAIL TREATMENT

The nails are not only subject to many environmental and traumatic influences, but also the target of cosmetic and medical treatments that often have a profound effect on the integrity of the nail. Nail hardeners are frequently prescribed for brittle nails. They contain formaldehyde that renders the nails harder and decreases their elasticity. Nail varnish is usually well tolerated but the tosyl formaldehyde resin may be the cause of allergic contact dermatitis. Artificial nails made from acrylics or cyanoacrylates may also cause contact dermatitis, often in the face and neck, less frequently of the nails; here, the reaction may persist for a long time, even after removal of the artificial nails, and be associated with long-lasting or even persisting pain. Gel nails are presently very popular. They are very hard and their removal requires harsh treatment with a coarse file that thins the nail plate and thus damages

it. Chemical peels of the nail with 70% glycolic acid to improve their surface have been described[8]; their rationale remains to be clarified. Overzealous manicure is the cause of many untoward effects such as onycholysis semilunaris, wavy nail surface, loss of the cuticle with penetration of foreign substances under the proximal nailfold and subsequent paronychia, and bacterial colonization and infection. Urea in high concentrations is used to soften mycotic nails; urea 40% paste under occlusion for 3 to 5 days makes the infected nail portions soft enough to allow them to be scraped off.

INFLAMMATORY NAIL DISORDERS

PSORIASIS

AT-A-GLANCE

- Psoriasis is the dermatosis with the most frequent nail involvement.
- Approximately 50% of all psoriatics have nail changes at a given time, but 90% will have nail alterations at least once in their life.
- Nail involvement is even more frequent in psoriatic arthritis.
- The most frequent nail changes are pits, subungual hyperkeratosis, onycholysis, salmon spots, red lunulae, splinter hemorrhages, leukoplakia, and psoriatic paronychia.
- Infection with pathogenic fungi is frequent and should be treated first.

Psoriasis is the skin disease with the most frequent nail involvement. At the time of consultation, approximately 50% of the patients present with nail changes. Over their lifetime, up to 90% of all psoriatics will develop nail alterations. The prevalence is even higher in psoriatic arthritis.

ETIOLOGY AND PATHOGENESIS

There appears to be neither a gender nor race predilection. In contrast to skin, there is no association of human leukocyte antigen (HLA)-C0602 with nail and joint involvement, and nail psoriasis is often associated with inflammation at the insertion points of tendons and ligaments, giving rise to enthesitis. The nail lesions were thought to represent an aberrant response to tissue stressing of the integrated nail–joint apparatus, rather than being the result of an autoimmunity. The nail-and-joint disease may be linked to tissue-specific factors, including tissue biomechanical stressing and microtrauma that lead to activation of aberrant innate immune responses.[9]

CLINICAL FEATURES

Psoriasis causes both very specific and ambiguous nail lesions (Figs. 91-33 to 91-35). The most characteristic and most frequent signs are pits representing small, sharply delimited depressions in the nail surface of remarkably even size and depth. They may be haphazardly arranged or sometimes show parallel transverse or short longitudinal lines (Fig. 91-33). They are thought to arise from tiny psoriatic lesions in the apical matrix leading to parakeratosis that breaks off leaving these hole-like lesions. When the parakeratosis remains it is seen as an ivory-colored spot in the proximal third of the nail plate (Fig. 91-34). Pits may be single, which is not yet psoriasis specific, or multiple. Ten pits per nail or more than 50 pits on all nails are seen as proof of nail psoriasis. Rarely, red spots are seen in the lunula usually representing a very active psoriasis lesion with dilation of the capillaries and thinning of the suprapapillary plate.[10] Complete nail destruction following crumbling of the plate is a sign of total matrix affection (Fig. 91-35). Leukonychia is seen when the psoriatic lesion is in the mid to distal matrix and parakeratotic cells are incorporated into the nail plate, making it optically appear white. It is commonly an ill-defined white transverse band, but other morphologies are possible. Splinter hemorrhages are some millimeters long, reddish–dark-brown to black

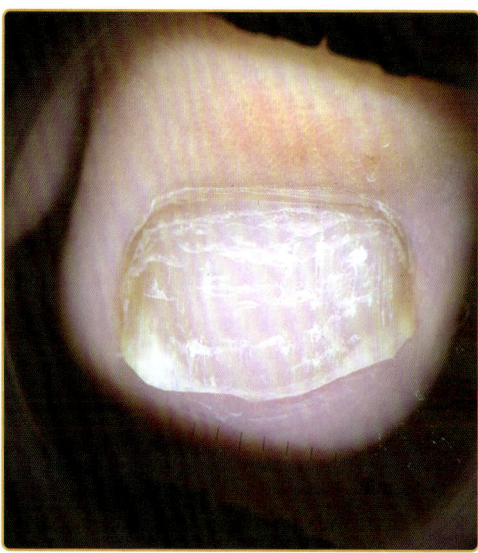

Figure 91-34 Nail psoriasis with pits and spots on the surface.

streaks of barely 1 mm in diameter. They are analogous to the Auspitz phenomenon on the skin and result from damage to the dilated capillaries in the nail bed causing the blood to clot in these longitudinally arranged small vessels. Salmon spots are frequent. They represent psoriatic plaques in the distal matrix

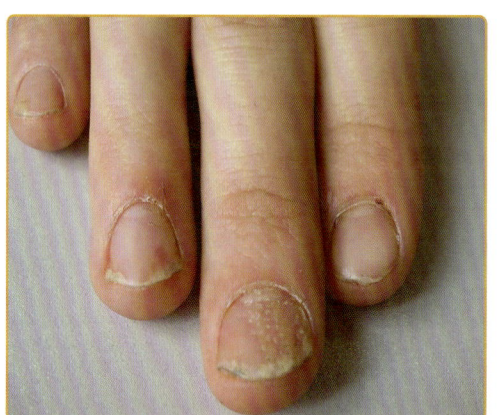

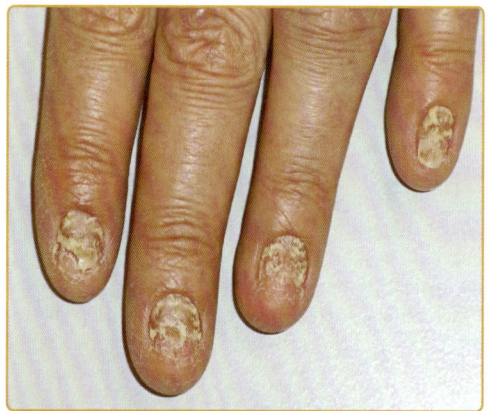

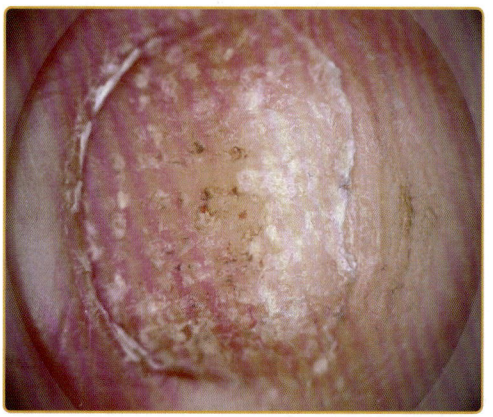

Figure 91-33 Nail psoriasis with pits arranged in a line.

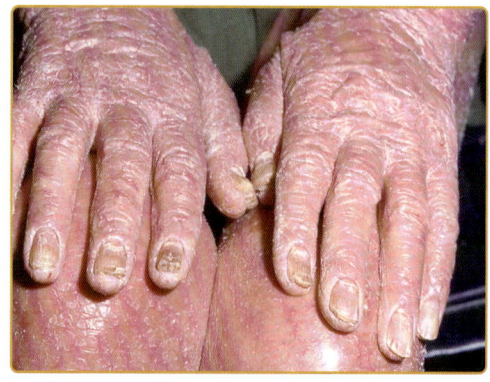

Figure 91-35 Nail psoriasis destroying the entire nail.

and the nail bed. The nail looks like paper on which a drop of oil has fallen: A yellowish-brownish spot with a red margin shines through the plate. The reason for this is that the squames of the psoriasis lesion are imbibed with serum and compressed under the nail. When such a salmon spot reaches the hyponychium, part of the parakeratosis breaks out and psoriatic onycholysis develops, which typically has a reddish proximal margin differentiating it from most other causes of onycholysis. In addition, there is often subungual hyperparakeratosis without oil-drop phenomenon causing onycholysis. Psoriatic hyperkeratosis may be marked and sometimes so extreme that it resembles pachyonychia congenita. Psoriasis involving both the dorsal and ventral surface of the proximal nailfold causes thickening and rounding of its free edge, which, in turn, are associated with loss of the cuticle, thus giving the pattern of chronic paronychia.

In *psoriatic arthritis*, nail involvement is often severe with psoriatic paronychia, complete nail destruction, and swelling of the distal interphalangeal joint.

Psoriatic pachydermoperiostosis is a condition closely related to psoriatic arthritis but usually without obvious nail changes. Mainly the big toe is considerably thickened and often painful.

Pustular psoriasis occurs in 3 different forms, all of which also involve the nail. In the *palmar plantar pustular psoriasis of Barber-Königsbeck*, all nail changes described above as well as larger surface defects called elkonyxis, plus subungual yellow spots representing large Munro abscesses may be seen (Fig. 91-36). Generalized pustular psoriasis of von Zumbusch occasionally causes red areas with a rim of small pustules that may affect the nail. Subungual abscesses are frequent. The most notorious form of pustular psoriasis is *acrodermatitis continua suppurativa of Hallopeau*. Often beginning with a single digit, the skin of the distal phalanx becomes red, develops some pustules that migrate under the nail and cause nail dystrophy, which, with time, may lead to complete disappearance of the nail unit so that only a red smooth digit tip is left until the disease slowly wanes off. However, acrodermatitis continua suppurativa may also initially involve several fingers and toes and run a very severe course

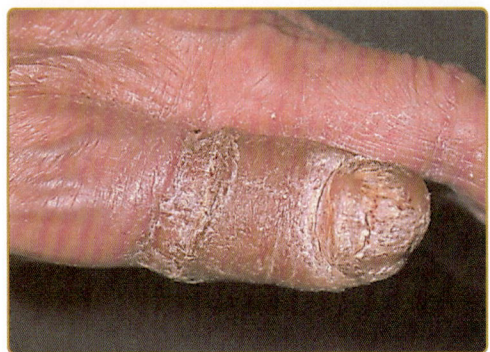

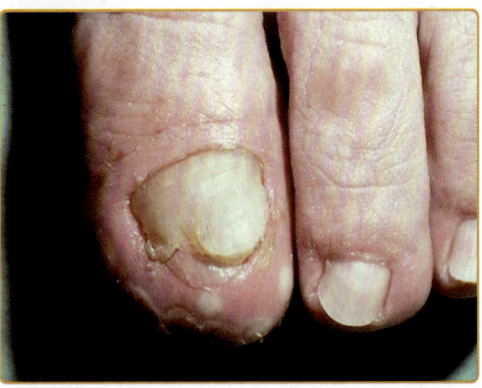

Figure 91-37 Acrodermatitis continua suppurativa of Hallopeau.

(Fig. 91-37). A mutation in the gene for the interleukin-36 receptor antagonist leading to a defect in interleukin-36 receptor antagonist was found in generalized pustular psoriasis and acrodermatitis continua suppurativa, supporting the assumption that these conditions belong to the group of autoinflammatory diseases.[11,12]

Reiter disease, also known as reactive arthritis, is a systemic condition with characteristic joint, mucosal, eye, genitourinary, skin, and nail changes. The latter are very similar to pustular psoriasis although they usually have a more brownish tint because of the content of erythrocytes in the pustules (Fig. 91-38). Histopathology also shows spongiform pustules.

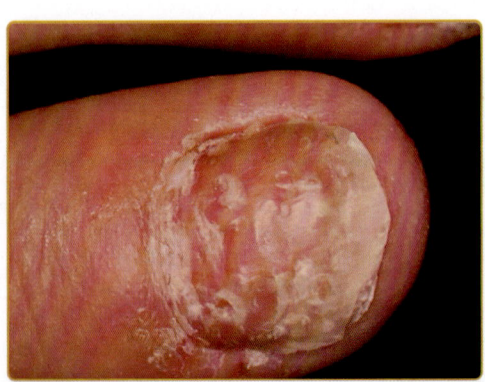

Figure 91-36 Nail involvement in pustular psoriasis of Barber-Königsbeck.

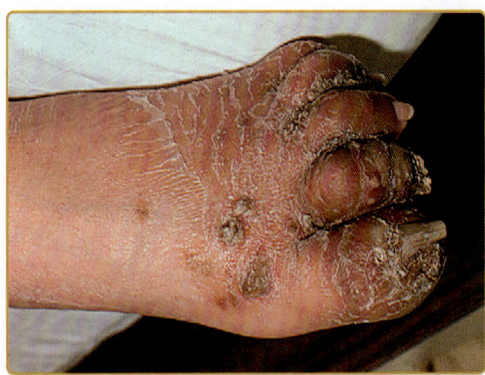

Figure 91-38 Nail changes in Reiter disease. (Used with permission from Dr. Robert Baran, France.)

TABLE 91-5
Differential Diagnosis of Nail Psoriasis and Onychomycosis

	PSORIASIS	ONYCHOMYCOSIS
Frequency	High, most common dermatosis with nail involvement	Very high: up to 30% to 40% of all nail diseases
Course	Chronic, often recurrent	Chronic, often progressive
Symptoms	Usually embarrassing cosmetically and functionally	Embarrassing, sometimes pain
Signs ▪ Pits ▪ Onycholysis ▪ Discoloration ▪ Spores and hyphae ▪ Transverse furrows ▪ Skin lesions elsewhere	Variable, depending on nail structure involved ▪ Very common, regular ▪ Common ▪ None to yellow ▪ Rarely spores ▪ Rare ▪ Very common	Variable, depending on severity and type of onychomycosis ▪ Rare, irregular ▪ Common ▪ Yellow to brown ▪ Very frequent ▪ Rare ▪ Often tinea
Trauma	May induce Köbner phenomenon	Important predisposing factor
Heredity	Strong hereditary component, particularly in juvenile onset psoriasis	Autosomal dominant susceptibility to develop onychomycosis

DIAGNOSIS

In most cases, nail psoriasis is diagnosed on clinical grounds. Skin lesions elsewhere plus 1 or several psoriatic nail features suggest the correct diagnosis. Histopathology is usually pathognomonic and helps to delineate nail psoriasis from other conditions, particularly onychomycosis. Reiter disease requires additional laboratory examinations.

DIFFERENTIAL DIAGNOSIS

Table 91-5 outlines the differential diagnosis of nail psoriasis and onychomycosis.

ASSOCIATIONS

Psoriasis is a frequent skin disease. Hence co-occurrence with other dermatoses that may also involve the nail is not exceptional. The most important association is that with onychomycosis as both conditions may look very similar, but a psoriatic nail may be colonized with pathogenic fungi and a true infection of the psoriatic nail is not infrequent (see Table 91-1).

COURSE

Why nail psoriasis often improves and worsens is unknown, although trauma may play an important role in the exacerbation of nail psoriasis. There may be periods without any nail alterations.

TREATMENT

Nail psoriasis is very resistant to almost all topical treatments whereas systemic therapies clearing the skin are usually also effective in nail psoriasis. The problem of all topical treatments is the penetration of the drug to the diseased tissue: through the nail plate in nail bed psoriasis, through all layers of the proximal nailfold plus the underlying nail in matrix lesions. Hence, pits, even though often being rather inconspicuous, are the most resistant to treatment. Nevertheless, a 3-month trial of a combination of a vitamin D_3 derivative with a potent corticosteroid is warranted. The less of the nail is present, the easier is penetration of the drug to the very psoriatic lesion. The list of other drugs tried is long and mostly comprises anecdotal reports and small case series. Injections of triamcinolone acetonide crystal suspension, 10 mg/mL every 6 weeks, into the proximal nailfold often improves nail psoriasis, but is painful and cumbersome for the patient. Methotrexate injections were also given with some success; however, this cytostatic drug may slow down nail growth and make an improvement visible only very late. The best treatment results are those with systemic antipsoriatic therapies, including biologics (see Chap. 28 for details).[13]

ECZEMA

AT-A-GLANCE

- *Eczema* is a traditional dermatologic term denoting a frequent reaction of the epidermis to a large variety of different stimuli; it is often used synonymously with "dermatitis."
- Virtually all nail components may show eczematous changes: matrix, nail bed, periungual skin.
- Allergic contact dermatitis may be the result of nail cosmetics, particularly acrylic nails; this type of contact dermatitis may last longer than the actual duration of exposition.

(Continued)

AT-A-GLANCE (Continued)

- Toxic contact dermatitis may be indistinguishable from allergic dermatitis and psoriasis.
- Atopic dermatitis may cause rough nails when the matrix is involved, or very shiny nails when they are used to rub the itchy skin.
- Nummular eczema is occasionally seen on the proximal nailfold.

In this context, the term *eczema* is used as a collective one comprising allergic contact dermatitis, toxic/irritant contact dermatitis, atopic dermatitis, and nummular eczema; seborrheic eczema does not occur in the nail unit. They have a common denominator, the so-called spongiotic dermatitis.

CLINICAL FEATURES

Although differing in typical cases the clinical features may be similar between the different forms of eczema (Fig. 91-39), particularly in chronic eczema. *Acute allergic contact dermatitis* exhibits redness of the periungual skin with tiny vesicles that tend to break and ooze. Serous crusts follow. Secondary infection with pyogenic micrococci leads to impetiginization. With time, oozing disappears, the redness decreases, and desquamation develops followed by cracking, particularly of the volar aspects and transition to the hyponychium and lateral nailfolds. The nails may become grossly deformed with deep asymmetric transverse furrows and ridges. Matrix and nail bed involvement is rather rare, but when present, for example, in patients with an allergy to artificial nails, may be painful. The nail itself loses its transparency as the spongiotic dermatitis of the matrix leads to inclusion of serum in the plate. The nail bed appears to be hyperkeratotic, even though this is a mixture of subungual keratin with serum inclusions. Chronic allergic contact dermatitis of the proximal nailfold leads to swelling, loss of the acute angle of its free margin with disappearance of the cuticle and separation of the underlying nail plate.

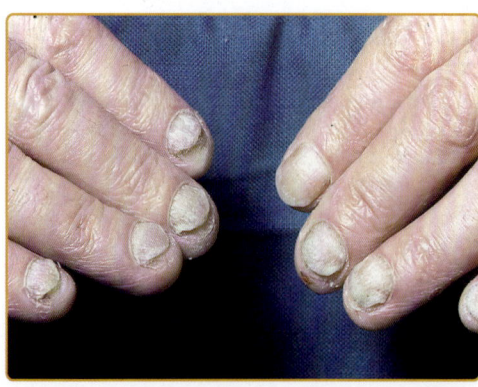

Figure 91-39 Nail eczema in a gardener handling tulips.

Toxic contact dermatitis rarely begins acute with erythema, vesicle formation, and oozing, such as from certain plants like garlic. Chronic irritant contact dermatitis is characterized by redness, scaling, fissures, and paronychia. It is often indistinguishable from chronic allergic dermatitis.

Nummular eczema of the nail region mainly involves the proximal nailfold with round red infiltrated plaques exhibiting tiny papules that are covered with a small serosanguinolent crust.

Atopic dermatitis may affect the nail in different ways. Shiny nails are characteristic in chronic itchy atopic dermatitis of children and young and middle-aged adults. These individuals "learned" not to harm their skin by scratching with the free margin of the nails and to relieve the itch by rubbing with the back of the distal phalanx. The use of emollients may enhance the polishing action of this habit. Atopic pulpitis sicca demonstrates desquamation and cracking of the finger and toe tips and is often also a feature of atopic winter feet. Painful cracks starting in the lateral nail groove of the thumbs and extending to pulp are often seen in elderly atopics. Frank "eczematous" changes are exceptional.

Trachyonychia is the term for rough nails and a hallmark of the so-called 20-nail dystrophy. In author's experience, most cases are caused by atopic dermatitis, although psoriasis, alopecia areata, and nail lichen planus were also found as the underlying disorder.[14] Many nails, rarely all 20 nails, are affected, but often 1 or more nails remain normal despite progression of the alterations. The nails become very rough, lose their shine and transparency, often turn partly koilocytotic, and the cuticles become thickened and ragged. Most cases are children between 6 and 10 years of age, sometimes younger. The condition usually runs a protracted course until, in many cases, the nails become normal from age of 14 to 16 years on.

ETIOLOGY AND PATHOGENESIS

The rare occurrence of allergic and irritant contact dermatitis on toenails as compared to fingernails points at the importance of nail cosmetics as well as a number of household allergens. The household allergens are complicated by the fact that (immediate-type) contact allergy to food may be chronic and superimposed by chronic irritation as well as colonization with yeasts.[15] Painful matrix and nail bed dermatitis is characteristic for acrylate allergy. The exact etiopathogenesis of nummular eczema is not yet fully elucidated.

DIAGNOSIS

Acute allergic contact dermatitis is usually diagnostic, although rare cases of acute irritant contact dermatitis may look identical. Skin tests are commonly applied both to make the diagnosis as well as find out the responsible allergen. In acrylate allergy, ectopic skin lesions may characteristically be found on the neck, décolleté, and around the eyes, a result of vapors of the acrylic monomer. Atopic dermatitis almost invariably demonstrates lesions on other body sites that may vary according to the age of the patient. In nummular eczema, lesions are commonly seen on the forearms and lower legs. Twenty-nail dystrophy is diagnosed in children when more than 10 nails are involved.

Histopathology shows a spongiotic dermatitis in acute cases, but a more psoriasiform epidermal hyperplasia in chronic eczema. Persistent allergic contact dermatitis caused by acrylates exhibits a dense, often band-like lymphocytic infiltrate, exocytosis, and spongiosis with massive acanthosis of the matrix and nail bed epithelium as well as lymphocytes and serum in the nail plate. Nummular lesions show spongiotic vesicles in the upper half of the epidermis with clotted serum on top. In trachyonychia, there is a very severe spongiotic inflammation with strong exocytosis of T lymphocytes that migrate upward and become part of the nail plate.

DIFFERENTIAL DIAGNOSIS

Chronic allergic and irritative contact dermatitis are difficult to distinguish from each other, as well as from psoriasis, ungual lichen planus, and alopecia areata. Careful examination of the entire skin is a must for each dermatologist. Chronic paronychia occurs in all contact dermatitides. Parakeratosis pustulosa is a rare condition that mainly occurs in young girls and exhibits vesiculopustular lesions of the hyponychium extending into the distal nail bed. After some weeks the condition resembles an eczema or psoriasis. Twenty-nail dystrophy usually represents an eczematous reaction.

CLINICAL COURSE, PROGNOSIS, AND MANAGEMENT

Except for acute allergic contact dermatitis, all other eczemas usually run a protracted course. However, even grossly distorted nails may become completely normal when the cause is found and eliminated and the condition adequately treated, which may be difficult in persons who have to handle food and/or expose their hands to a harsh environment. In addition, smoking and nail cosmetics, as well as particular habits, often complicate treatment. Twenty-nail dystrophy is a disease of children and said to disappear spontaneously at the age of approximately 16 years.

Periungual eczematous lesions respond to topical steroids, but chronic paronychia may require intralesional steroid injections. Very severe and painful lesions may have to be treated systemically as transungual penetration is insufficient for matrix and nail bed involvement. Very recalcitrant paronychia can be treated surgically by a beveled excision of the thickened part of the proximal nailfold.

ALOPECIA AREATA

AT-A-GLANCE

- Nail involvement in alopecia areata is frequent: the more severe the alopecia areata, the more frequent the nail involvement.
- The nails are rough, as if sandpapered, with innumerable small pits.
- The surface may keep its shine or have lost it.
- The nails often lose their transparence due to inclusion of serum globules, this makes them also brittle.

CLINICAL FEATURES

Alopecia areata (AA) affects between 6 and 7 million individuals in the United States. The prevalence of nail abnormalities varies between 10% and 65%. They may precede, occur concurrently with, or follow hair loss activity. There is no known age, race, or ethnic preponderance. In contrast to other autoimmune diseases, the hair follicle does not usually sustain permanent injury and maintains its potential to regrow hair.

AA often affects the nails; the more severe the AA, the more likely is nail involvement. Thus nail changes are rare in the most frequent mild type of AA with only a few bald patches and a high rate of spontaneous resolution, whereas nail changes are rather the rule in AA universalis. However, it is generally accepted that there may be nail AA without hair loss. Two types of nail alterations are seen: rough nails that have lost their shine and pitted nails with surface shine (Fig. 91-40). The nails may lose their transparence, get thicker, become brittle and split distally. The cuticles may become ragged. Koilonychia is a sign of very severe nail involvement.

ETIOLOGY AND PATHOGENESIS

AA is an autoimmune disease mediated by natural-killer group 2 member D expressing CD8+ lymphocytes and it can be assumed that the etiology of nail AA is not different from that of hairy skin. However, the pathogenesis appears to be variable as nails do not fall off in contrast to hair, and the histopathologic pattern of inflammation in hair follicles and nails are different; exact data are not yet known. AA preferentially affects pigmented hairs, and the hair of AA patients frequently shows a change in color when it regrows following an acute episode of AA. Although this might indicate a relationship between AA, pigmentation, and melanin-concentrating hormone signaling nails are usually not pigmented in light-skinned individuals. Whether or not duplications in *MCHR2*[16] are important for the involvement in nail AA pathogenesis remains to be elucidated.

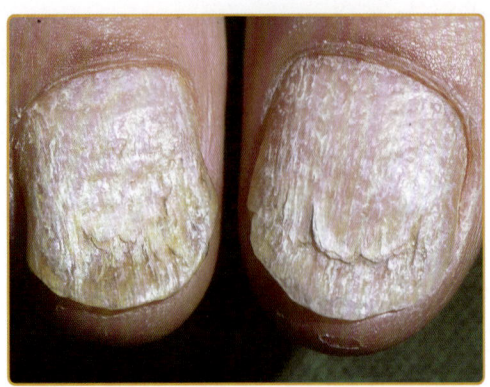

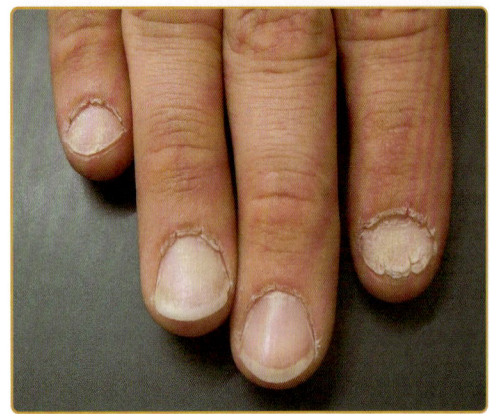

Figure 91-40 Alopecia areata of the nail.

CLINICAL COURSE, PROGNOSIS, AND MANAGEMENT

Occurring more commonly in severe AA, the nail changes usually run a protracted course over years. Successful systemic treatments will greatly improve the nails. Tofacitinib is a Janus kinase inhibitor with a good effect on hair loss and nail changes in nail AA. It is assumed that other Janus kinase inhibitors also might be beneficial for the treatment of nail changes in AA.[19] Apremilast did not induce hair regrowth in severe AA. Topical treatments with steroids or steroid–calcipotriol combinations are often tried, but mostly in vain. Injections of triamcinolone acetonide crystal suspension, 0.5 to 1 mg per proximal nailfold, have to be repeated every 4 to 6 weeks, but are cumbersome and painful.

The prognosis of nail AA is linked to that of AA in general. The nail lesions may persist longer than the hair loss. Permanent nail dystrophy after resolution of the AA is not observed.

The patient has to be counseled concerning the nature of the disorder and the chronicity of nail lesions in AA. This is particularly important in children where the parents require detailed information as to the natural course of AA and its nail alterations.

DIAGNOSIS

In the typical case, the diagnosis is self-evident. However, AA is a relatively frequent disorder and associations with other conditions potentially affecting the nail are possible. Thus, ruling out atopic dermatitis, psoriasis, lichen planus, or onychomycosis may be warranted. The real problem is to make the diagnosis of isolated nail AA. Nail biopsy shows a spongiotic dermatitis with lymphocyte exocytosis involving the matrix; thus the histopathologic pattern is different from that of the scalp. The nail surface is wavy and often serum inclusions are seen in the nail plate.[17] There are no laboratory examinations that help make the diagnosis of nail AA.

DIFFERENTIAL DIAGNOSIS

In the presence of round bald spots on the scalp, the diagnosis of a pitted nail is obvious. However, pits were also observed in different eczemas, lichen planus, ichthyosis vulgaris, and, above all, psoriasis. In psoriasis, the pits are deeper and a bit larger.[18]

DISEASE ASSOCIATIONS

Asthma, allergic rhinitis, atopic dermatitis, thyroid disease, and autoimmune diseases, such as thyroiditis and vitiligo are common associated diseases.

LICHEN PLANUS OF THE NAILS

AT-A-GLANCE

- Lichen planus rarely affects the periungual skin, most commonly the proximal matrix and less frequently the nail bed.
- Matrix involvement leads to longitudinal ridging and splitting until the distal nail plate breaks away and a pterygium develops.
- Nail bed affection causes subungual hyperkeratosis with onycholysis.
- Postlichen atrophy is the end stage of ungual lichen planus.
- Variants of ungual lichen planus include pigmented lichen planus, ulcerated lichen planus, and bullous lichen planus.

CLINICAL FEATURES

Nail lichen planus is a chronic disease that usually occurs in association with typical skin lesions (Figs. 91-41 and 91-42). Depending on the particular structure of the nail apparatus affected, variable clinical alterations develop. Most commonly, the apical matrix is involved leading to ridging, rough nails, loss of nail shine, longitudinal

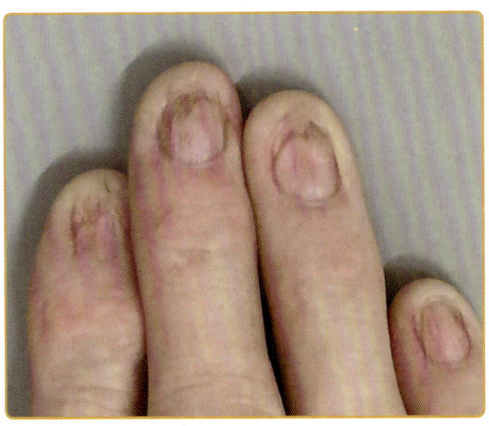
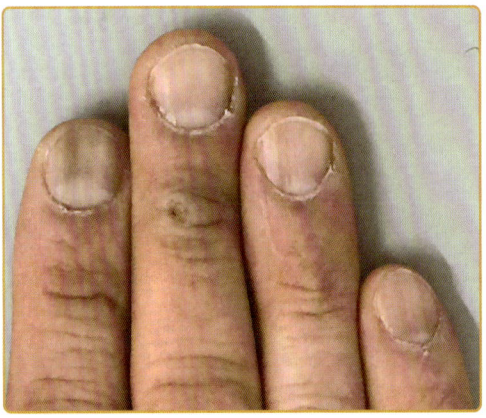
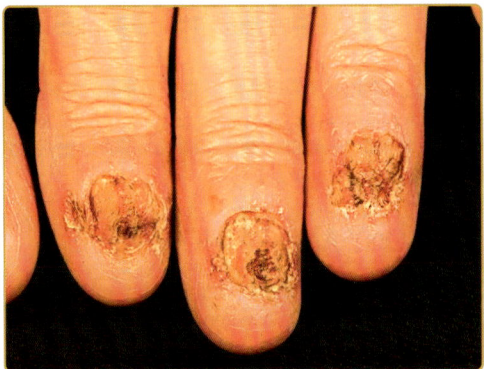
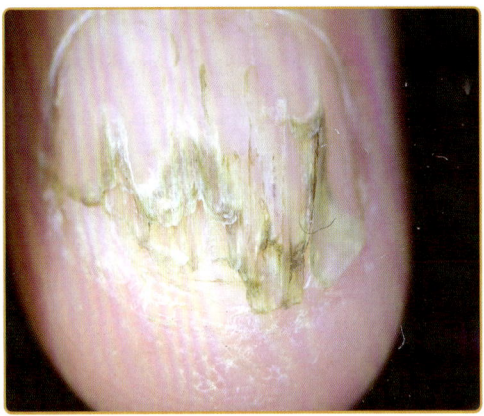

Figure 91-41 Lichen planus of the nails.

Figure 91-42 Lichen planus of the nails.

surface defects, and splits. Nail bed lichen planus is rare; it may cause subungual orthokeratosis with subsequent onycholysis. Even bullous lichen planus of the nails is possible.[20] Involvement of the proximal nailfold results in a bluish-red discoloration, sometimes associated with swelling. Longstanding nail lichen planus may lead to nail thinning and obliteration of the nail pocket with pterygium formation. The nail edge may look frayed. As the apical matrix is the site of the nail stem cells,[21] scarring with permanent nail dystrophy may occur. Ulcerating nail lichen planus is very rare. Finally, a progressive nail atrophy may develop characterized by nail thinning and extreme fragility thus very similar to nails in amyloidosis.

ETIOLOGY AND PATHOGENESIS

The similarity of clinical and histopathologic nail alterations in graft-versus-host disease with those of lichen planus has supported the view that it is an autoimmune disorder. Nonwhites appear to have nail lichen planus more frequently. There is a high frequency of HLA-A3, HLA-A5, HLA-B7, HLA-DR1, and HLA-DR10.

The histopathology of nail lichen planus is characteristic. There is a dense epitheliotropic lymphocytic infiltrate around the apical matrix leading to vacuolar basal cell degeneration with thinning of the epithelium and impaired nail substance formation. As this is not evenly distributed over the width of the matrix longitudinal furrows and splits develop. Severe infiltration causes epithelial consumption and, finally, deficient nail formation, obliteration of the nail cul-de-sac, and pterygium.

DIAGNOSIS

Nail lichen planus is usually diagnosed clinically. There are no blood tests. Lichen planus lesions on the skin, oral, and genital mucosa should be looked for. Ultimately, a nail biopsy can confirm the diagnosis. Bullous nail lichen planus may mimic yellow nail syndrome.

DIFFERENTIAL DIAGNOSIS

All nail conditions causing rough nails with longitudinal ridging and surface defects have to be considered. The diagnosis is more obvious with fingernail than toenail lesions. Amyloidosis involving the nails looks very similar.

DISEASE ASSOCIATIONS

These are the same as with cutaneous lichen planus: AA, vitiligo, localized scleroderma, Castleman tumor with pemphigus vulgaris, and chronic liver disease.

CLINICAL COURSE, PROGNOSIS, AND MANAGEMENT

Nail lichen planus is particularly chronic and stubbornly resistant to almost all topical treatments. Slight variations in the disease intensity may be observed. Some patients have mild disease with almost no progression whereas others may experience rapid exacerbation with cicatricial nail dystrophy. Once a pterygium has developed, nail lichen planus is no longer amenable to treatment. Furthermore, there may be a Koebner phenomenon when using harsh treatment methods. Despite the lack of controlled studies for topical treatment modalities, the combination of a steroid with calcipotriol is recommended, which may induce some improvement or stop disease progression. Perimatricial injections of triamcinolone acetonide every 4 to 8 weeks, either with or without a needle, are often successful and may be continued by IM injections, 0.5 to 1 mg/kg bodyweight. However, up to 50% of the responders may experience a recurrence.[22] Biologics are highly effective in recalcitrant cases.[23]

AUTOIMMUNE BULLOUS DISEASES

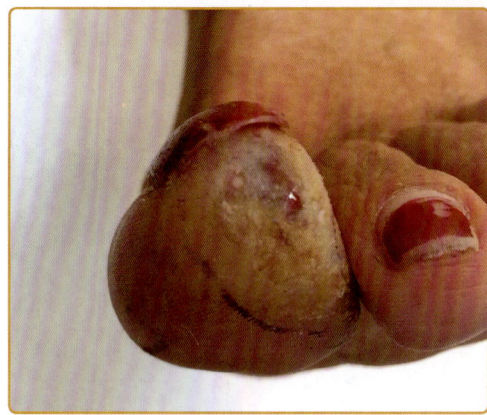

Figure 91-43 Bullous pemphigoid of the nail.

AT-A-GLANCE

- Even though all autoimmune bullous disease can affect the nail unit, the clinical changes are nonspecific and do not permit a conclusive diagnosis.
- Chronic paronychia, hyperkeratosis, and oozing with crusting are common to all autoimmune bullous diseases.

Among the autoimmune bullous diseases, pemphigus vulgaris, pemphigus vegetans, bullous pemphigoid, cicatricial pemphigoid, and epidermolysis bullosa acquisita may affect the nails. However, nail lesions are rarely specific enough as to allow the exact diagnosis to be made. Associated skin lesions may suggest a blistering disease.

CLINICAL FEATURES

Chronic paronychia with oozing and crust formation are the most common initial signs (Fig. 91-43), followed by onychomadesis (see Fig. 91-23) and sometimes by loss of the nail, of nail involvement. Pterygium formation and permanent nail loss were observed in bullous pemphigoid, cicatricial pemphigoid, and acquired epidermolysis bullosa. Large clear periungual blisters are occasionally seen in bullous pemphigoid. They may be followed by erosions with crusting and sometimes superficial impetiginization. Pemphigus vegetans of the distal phalanx may resemble a very severe form of acrodermatitis continua suppurativa of Hallopeau with extensive pustulation and often a markedly pronounced pustular margin.

ETIOLOGY AND PATHOGENESIS

They are dealt with in the chapters on autoimmune bullous disorders. It was once thought that nail involvement in pemphigus vulgaris might be a sign of a particularly aggressive course or even a special subtype; however, this has not been substantiated.

DIAGNOSIS

The diagnosis may be suspected in case of a longstanding oozing and crusting paronychia with development of onychomadesis and even nail loss. However, serologic investigations including enzyme-linked immunosorbent assay tests and indirect immunofluorescence, and in case of skin lesions, a biopsy, are usually necessary to make the diagnosis.

DIFFERENTIAL DIAGNOSIS

The various autoimmune bullous diseases require immunoserologic and histopathologic examinations for their differentiation.

DISEASE ASSOCIATIONS

Other autoimmune phenomena and diseases may be associated.

CLINICAL COURSE, PROGNOSIS, AND MANAGEMENT

The course of the nail lesions is linked to that of the cutaneous and mucous membrane lesions. Their efficacious therapy will also control the nail alterations albeit with some delay. Nail lesions take between 6 and 18 months to grow out. Pterygium is permanent.

SO-CALLED CONNECTIVE TISSUE DISEASES

Lupus erythematosus and its particular form of chilblain lupus, dermatomyositis, and scleroderma may affect the nail unit.

CLINICAL FEATURES

All these disorders may cause alterations of the nailfold capillaries. They may be reduced in number, dilated, tortuous, shorter, and show aneurysms and bleeding. This is easily seen when using a fluorescent dye that gives evidence of vessel leakage. However, even though often stressed in the rheumatologic literature, most of these changes do not allow a safe distinction to be made between them. Some changes are more typical for dermatomyositis, which is also characterized by Gottron papules of the dorsal aspect of phalanx, less frequently on the distal phalanx (Fig. 91-44). Periungual erythema and red lunula may be seen in acute lupus erythematosus whereas in chilblain lupus the changes reach from pernio-like nonspecific violaceous-blue hue with some telangiectasias to ulceration of the tip of the toe and the nail unit. Chronic discoid lupus erythematosus may cause red streaks in the nail bed, ridging of the nail, and dystrophy. White bands were seen in the diffusely brown nail of a black patient who had leukoderma of the head as a result of chronic discoid lupus erythematosus. Onycholysis, pterygium, and clubbing are nonspecific signs.[24]

Scleroderma with its acral variant often shows ulceration of the pulp and narrowing of the tip of the finger. The nail insidiously bends volarly giving the aspect of a parrot beak. The nail surface is dull and may show pronounced ridging. The plate is often nontransparent.

ETIOLOGY AND PATHOGENESIS

The etiology is that of the cutaneous involvement. Infarctions of the nailfold capillaries may lead to necrosis and scars. The degree of matrix affection determines that of the nail changes. Most sclerodermatous nail alterations are said to be secondary to the associated vascular damage.

DIAGNOSIS

As isolated nail changes in these connective tissue diseases are exceptional, the diagnosis is usually made by their skin lesions and immunoserologically (Fig. 91-45). Capillary alterations are easily seen by dermatoscopy and laser scanning confocal microscopy; the latter also permits the blood flow to be observed.

DIFFERENTIAL DIAGNOSIS

Capillary microscopy of the nailfold may give a hint at the diagnosis of an autoimmune disease; however, despite many claims, it is very difficult to differentiate them purely on capillary microscopy. Nail plate changes may have to be distinguished from lichen planus. Red lunulae are seen in acute AA of the nail and some other diseases, as well as in drug reactions. Periungual erythema may be caused by HIV infection or treatment with cytotoxic agents.

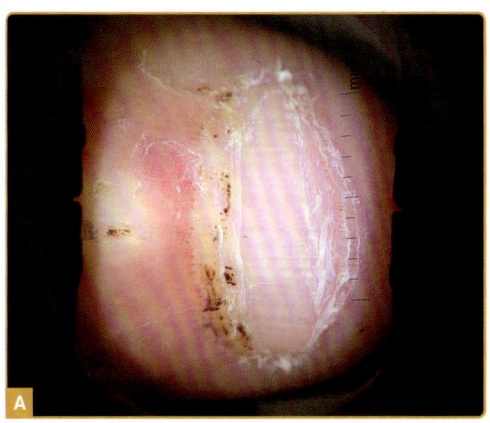
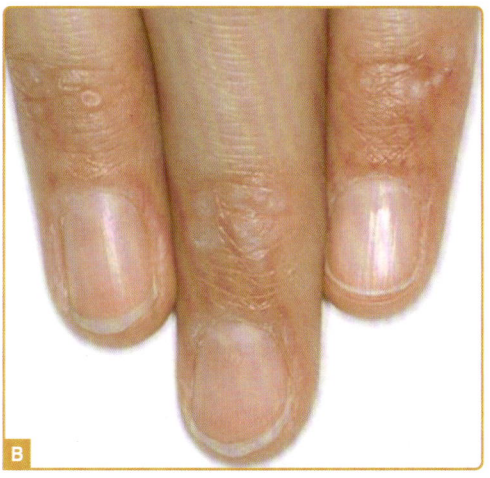

Figure 91-44 Dermatomyositis. **A,** Capillary microscopy shows avascular areas and aneurysms. **B,** Gottron papules on the distal phalanges.

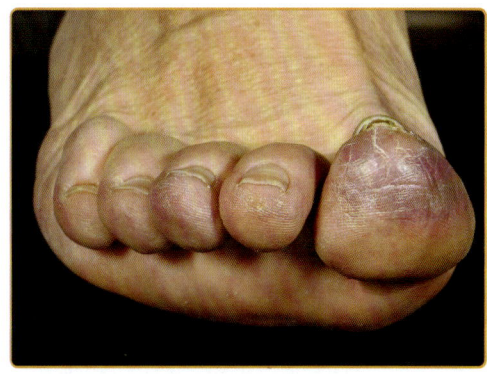

Figure 91-45 Chilblain lupus of the toes.

DISEASE ASSOCIATIONS

Mixed connective tissue disease exhibits features of lupus erythematosus plus dermatomyositis and sometimes even scleroderma. Other immune disorders may be associated. The association with erythema multiforme is called Rowell syndrome. Vasculitis accompanies systemic lupus erythematosus in 10% to 20% of patients.

CLINICAL COURSE, PROGNOSIS, AND MANAGEMENT

The clinical course, prognosis and management are those of the skin lesions, however, the nail alterations usually take longer to respond.

VASCULITIS AND VASCULOPATHIES

Nail changes of the "true" vasculitides, as well as of occlusive and infectious vasculopathies, are mentioned.

CLINICAL FEATURES

Leukocytoclastic vasculitis may affect the distal phalanx with the nail unit, particularly of the toes. Dark red small palpable spots develop both on the proximal nailfold and the pulp, which have a tendency to leave small necroses and tiny scars. Under the nail, they are seen as dark red spots and may be painful.

In "benign" gonococcal sepsis, small hemorrhagic papules may develop on the distal phalanx, involving also the proximal nailfold. Similar lesions were also observed in pneumococcal and meningococcal sepsis; however, these are very serious diseases that are not diagnosed by their nail involvement.

Livedoid vasculopathy, also called livedo reticularis, is a typical disorder of the legs that causes painful torpid ulcers. It is often called atrophie blanche when located in the ankle region.[25] It may affect the free margin of the proximal nailfold of toes, exhibiting lichenoid papules with reddening and white lines (Fig. 91-46).

ETIOLOGY AND PATHOGENESIS

The etiology and pathogenesis of the vasculitides and vasculopathies are not different from those of the skin lesions. Hypercoagulability in association with stasis are assumed to underlie livedoid vasculopathy. In infectious vasculitides, microbial thrombi are said to be responsible, but a general toxic response has also to be discussed.

DIAGNOSIS

The diagnosis of the nail lesions depends on that of the skin disease.

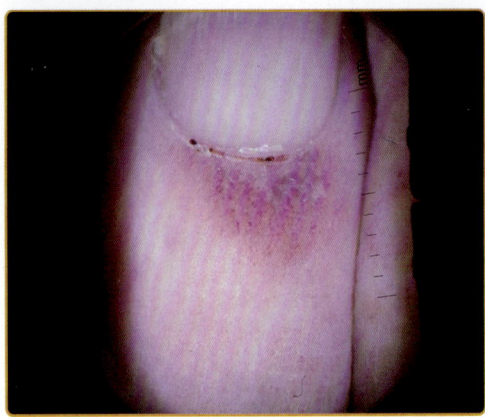

Figure 91-46 Livedoid vasculopathy involving the proximal nailfold.

DIFFERENTIAL DIAGNOSIS

Osler nodules are small painful nodules and bleedings in the fingertips in bacterial endocarditis.

DISEASE ASSOCIATIONS

Vasculitis is often seen in conjunction with systemic lupus erythematosus, but may also occur in a variety of infections and as a drug reaction.

CLINICAL COURSE, PROGNOSIS, AND MANAGEMENT

The clinical course depends on whether or not the cause of the vasculitis is found and removed. Large necrotic lesions heal with scars that may distort the nail.

INFECTIOUS NAIL DISEASES

AT-A-GLANCE

- Otherwise banal infections are often disproportionately painful, for instance digital herpes simplex.
- Subungual warts may be very painful because of pressure on the bone; those under the proximal nailfold mimic chronic paronychia.
- In hand-foot-and-mouth disease, small oval blisters may occur around the nail, and possibly also in the matrix region, causing late onychomadesis.
- Bullous impetigo presents as a blister with a stable roof that may extend around the nail.

(Continued)

AT-A-GLANCE (Continued)

- Deep bacterial infections may reach down to the bone; these whitlows (felons) cause pain and require surgical exploration.
- Syphilis may occur as a primary chancre, which also may be atypically painful, or as a subungual papular exanthem causing onycholysis.
- Both tuberculosis, leprosy and atypical mycobacterioses occur in the nail unit and cannot be diagnosed on clinical grounds alone.
- Fungal nail infections are extremely common. Independent of the pathogen, the clinical types look similar; hence cultural identification is warranted.
- Leishmaniasis can present as ulcerating paronychia.
- Nail infestation by *Sarcoptes scabiei* is very often overlooked as it may mimic psoriasis or acrokeratosis paraneoplastica of Bazex; it is refractory if not treated correctly and often the source of reinfection and small institutional epidemics.

VIRAL INFECTIONS

A variety of viruses may infect the nail and periungual skin and cause skin lesions that are sometimes different from what is seen on normal skin.

HERPES VIRUS INFECTIONS

The most important Herpesviridae affecting the nail are herpes simplex virus Type 1 (HHV1), Type 2 (HHV2), varicella-zoster virus (HHV3), and HHV8 found in Kaposi sarcoma.

Herpes Simplex of the Nail Apparatus—Clinical Features: The primary herpes simplex infection rarely causes nail lesions although virus inoculation may take place during the disease in finger-sucking babies. Recurrent digital herpes simplex is occasionally seen in children, adolescents, and in certain professions, such as dentists (before they started routinely wearing gloves). Small vesicles are seen to develop that first have a clear content, which, after some days, becomes yellowish while the blisters tend to merge (Fig. 91-47). From the beginning, a visible red streak is commonly seen extending from the finger to the arm; this lymphangitis is usually associated with pain. After 7 to 10 days, the tenderness decreases, and the blister content may turn hemorrhagic and finally dry. After 2 to 3 weeks, the blister roof sheds.

Herpes Simplex of the Nail Apparatus—Etiology and Pathogenesis: In children, recurrent digital herpes simplex is usually caused by HHV1 whereas in adults, HHV1 and HHV2 are the

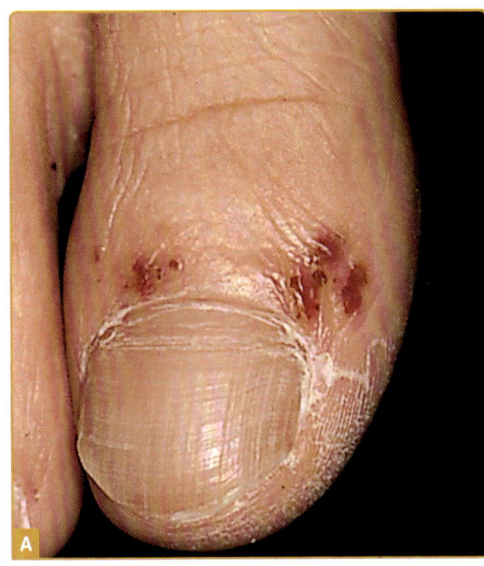
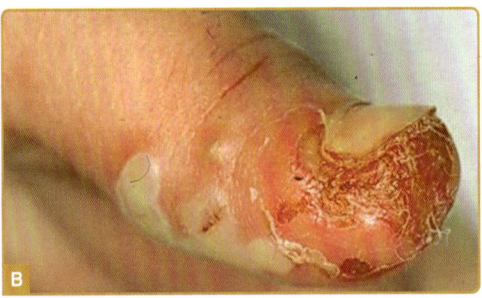
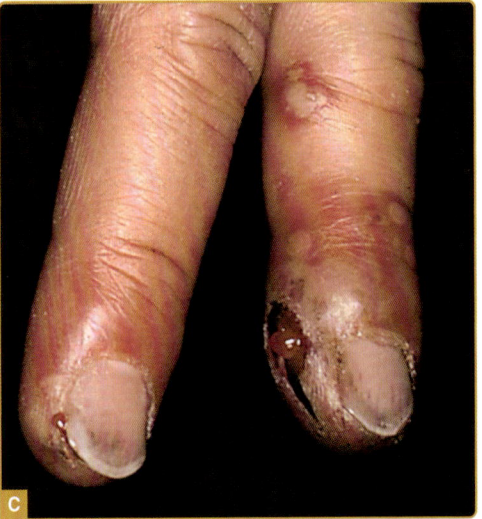

Figure 91-47 Recurrent herpes simplex of the toe (**A**), thumb (**B**), and fingers (**C**).

causative agents, with each being the cause in approximately 50% of patients.

Herpes Simplex of the Nail Apparatus—Diagnosis: The diagnosis is made clinically by an experienced dermatologist. A classical Tzanck smear is helpful in the early stage. Immunofluorescence with specific HHV antibodies not only confirms the diagnosis but may also distinguish infections caused by HHV1 from those caused by HHV2. Immunohistochemistry with HHV1 and HHV2 antibodies on histologic sections is also positive. Polymerase chain reaction is another option. However, when the lesion is too old, all tests may fail.

Herpes Simplex of the Nail Apparatus—Differential Diagnosis: Acute paronychia, bullous impetigo (runaround), whitlow (felon), and other bacterial infections have to be considered as part of the differential diagnosis. However, the repetitive nature of digital herpes simplex and its painful course are typical.

Herpes Simplex of the Nail Apparatus—Disease Associations: Severe and even ulcerative herpes simplex is seen in immunocompromised individuals.

Herpes Simplex of the Nail Apparatus—Clinical Course, Prognosis, and Management: Recurrent digital herpes simplex is frequently misdiagnosed as an acute paronychia. The patients consult their family physician or a surgeon who treat it as an acute whitlow by opening the blisters, disinfection, antiseptic baths, systemic antibiotics and splinting of the digit. Only after repeated recurrences may the patient be referred to a dermatologist who can make the diagnosis from the clinical course. Recurrences may come in waves: several waves in relatively short intervals that then become longer and finally turn into a herpes-free period for several months or even some years until the recurrences restart. There are no controlled studies proving the value of long-term antiviral prophylaxis.

Varicella and Herpes Zoster: Varicella may involve the nail region with a few characteristic vesicles, and herpes zoster may, although rarely, extend to the distal digits. The diagnosis is made from the skin lesions (Fig. 91-48). However, onychomadesis was observed in children several weeks after chickenpox; it may be assumed that unnoticed viral blisters of the matrix were the cause. Treatment follows the general rules of HHV3 therapy.

HUMAN PAPILLOMAVIRUS INFECTIONS

Clinical Features: Common warts belong to the most frequent infections of humans. On the proximal nailfold, they are round papules with a rough keratotic surface; on the lateral folds they are often oval (Fig. 91-49). Subungual warts have an unspecific appearance often lifting the nail up and they are commonly painful. Under the proximal nailfold they raise it from the underlying nail and cause a marked swelling. At the hyponychium there may just be a rim-like thickening of the keratin that swells after 5 minutes in water.

Etiology and Pathogenesis: Infection with HPV types 1, 2, 3, 4, and 7 is the most common cause for viral warts of the nail unit. It is believed that infectious virus particles get into the epidermis via microwounds; however, how this exactly happens is still not fully understood.

Diagnosis: The diagnosis of viral warts is clinical. Histopathology is characteristic in young warts, but may be very inconspicuous in old ones. Immunohistochemistry with an antibody against a common papillomavirus antigen can be helpful. Serologic studies do not help. Polymerase chain reaction and in situ hybridization help to identify the HPV type.

Differential Diagnosis: The differential diagnosis of ungual warts is extensive and depends also on the localization within the nail unit. Subungual warts, particularly when painful, may be mistaken for a subungual exostosis. Other subungual tumors and inflammatory processes may have to be considered.

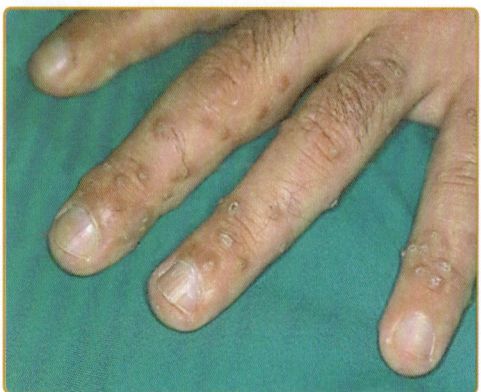

Figure 91-48 Generalized verrucous herpes zoster in a patient with advanced Hodgkin disease.

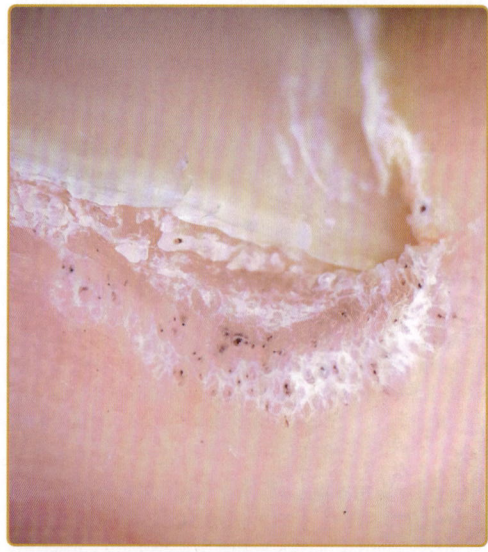

Figure 91-49 Viral warts of the hyponychium and nailfolds.

Disease Associations: Periungual warts are common in children and adolescents. However, severe immunodeficiency states and iatrogenic immunosuppression may be associated with innumerable warts in many locations.

Clinical Course, Prognosis, and Management: It is said that the average life span of a banal wart is approximately 2 years. However, clinical experience shows that periungual warts—like palmar and plantar ones—often exist much longer and may give rise to new ones during this period. They often grow very fast to a certain size and then remain stable for many months or years. The prognosis is good as the no-risk HPV types do not progress to carcinoma.

Management of periungual and subungual warts is difficult. There are surprisingly few randomized controlled studies, but they all show that aggressive keratolysis with salicylic acid is superior to wait-and-see. Salicylic acid plus cryotherapy is more efficacious than cryosurgery alone. Second-line treatments are laser, either ablative with CO_2 laser or with nonablative lasers. One regimen using the pulsed-dye laser to coagulate the vessels to the wart has been shown to be efficacious in more than two-thirds of cases. A variety of immune therapies, such as contact allergens and different vaccines, have been used with variable effect. Imiquimod may be tried off-label after aggressive keratolysis; however, the 3-times weekly regimen recommended for condylomata acuminata is not enough for ungual warts. Here, a daily treatment under occlusion is necessary, eliciting a marked inflammatory reaction. Third-line treatments comprise compounded cidofovir as a topical therapy; however, cidofovir is very expensive and therefore rarely used except in cases of an excessively large number of ungual warts.

ENTEROVIRUS INFECTIONS

A variety of different enteroviruses may cause periungual erythema; however, this is not specific enough to allow a particular diagnosis to be made. The most characteristic infection is hand-foot-and-mouth disease.

Clinical Features: Hand-foot-and-mouth disease is a vesicular disease characterized by intraoral aphthoid lesions that cause less discomfort than common aphthous ulcers, with small vesicles on the palms, soles, and around the nails (Fig. 91-50). They are usually oval in shape, the covering epidermis is gray from necrosis, and surrounded by a narrow erythematous rim. In ridged skin, the long axis of the vesicles is along the dermatoglyphics. Mild fever may be present in the beginning. Small outbreaks of this infection typically occur in spring and autumn. Many infections remain virtually asymptomatic and escape notice.

After approximately 6 weeks, some patients develop onychomadesis of single nails, probably as a sign of direct matrix involvement.[26]

Etiology and Pathogenesis: In most cases, the cause of hand-foot-and-mouth disease is an

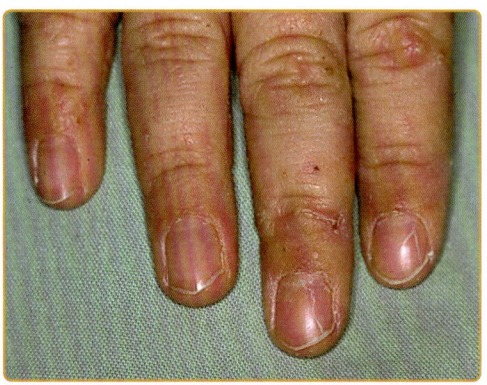

Figure 91-50 Hand-foot-and-mouth disease.

infection with enterovirus Type 71 and Coxsackieviruses, mainly Types A5 and A16, and rarely B or other enteroviruses. The infected cells swell, necrose, form a reticular, and, finally, a multilocular vesicle. After some days, this dries out and leaves a dry scab of necrotic epidermis and serum.

Diagnosis: The characteristic slightly oval vesicles with a gray blister roof and a narrow red margin, together with oral lesions reminiscent of aphthous ulcers, permit the diagnosis to be made. Serology may confirm the serotype.

Differential Diagnosis: As skin vesicles may be scarce the oral mucosal lesions may be mistaken for viral lesions of other enteroviruses, for example, herpangina.

Disease Associations: There are no characteristic disease associations.

Clinical Course, Prognosis, and Management: The clinical course is self-limited. The vesicles usually disappear within 7 to 10 days. The prognosis is good. There is no specific antiviral therapy.

BACTERIAL INFECTIONS

Most bacterial infections are caused by streptococci or staphylococci. Enterobacteria are mainly seen in toes. Clinical variants of impetigo are the most common bacterial infections. Paronychias and whitlows are also seen.

COCCAL INFECTIONS

Clinical Features: The most characteristic bacterial infection is a bullous impetigo (Fig. 91-51) that runs around the proximal part of the nail, hence the common term *runaround*. It starts with a clear blister of the proximal and lateral nailfold that soon becomes putrid and often also hemorrhagic. Pain is usually mild. Extension under the nail is exceptional in adults, but may occur in children and is seen as a yellowish lake of pus under the nail. It is commonly painful.

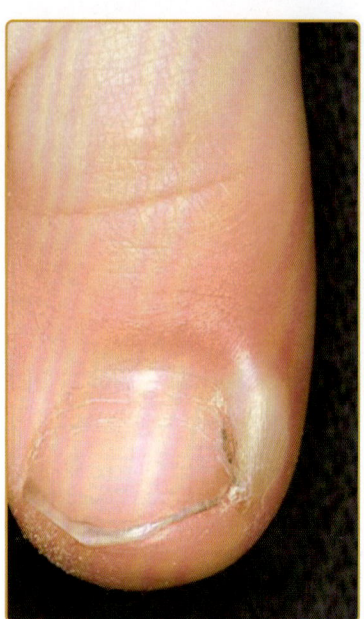

Figure 91-51 Bullous impetigo of the nailfold, so-called runaround.

When the infection occurs primarily under the nail it is called a subungual whitlow. It exhibits the features of an abscess. Deep soft-tissue infections cause considerable pain and are usually treated by surgeons with incisions and pus evacuation.

Etiology and Pathogenesis: Most of these infections are caused by staphylococci, rarely by streptococci. Subungual *P. aeruginosa* infections are rare. Small lacerations often from hangnails and other minor wounds are the portal of entry.

Diagnosis: The course of the infections is sufficiently characteristic to make the correct diagnosis. Bacterial swabs may confirm the infection.

Differential Diagnosis: The main differential diagnosis is recurrent digital herpes simplex, which is more painful, develops a lymphangitis, and starts with a group of small clear blisters that coalesce and later becomes putrid.

Disease Associations: There are no specific disease associations.

Clinical Course, Prognosis, and Management: When treated early the lesions disappear within 1 to 2 weeks. The prognosis of most cases is excellent. Uncomplicated bullous impetigo of the nail is treated with opening of the blister, disinfective baths twice a day, and antimicrobial creams. However, extension under the nail, particularly in children, should immediately prompt institution of systemic *Staphylococcus*-fast antibiotics that may be changed according to the sensitivity profile of the bacteria cultured from a swab. This is essential as the matrix in children may be permanently damaged within 24 to 48 hours in a subungual whitlow.

PSEUDOMONAS INFECTION

Clinical Features: *P. aeruginosa* is a ubiquitous pathogen quite frequently seen in the nail apparatus. Most cases are colonizations causing a green to brownish-black nail and often a localized marginal paronychia as evidenced by circumscribed swelling and loss of the cuticle (Fig. 91-52). Deep infections are rare in immunocompetent subjects.

Etiology and Pathogenesis: The dorsal and ventral surfaces of the nails may be severely colonized by *P. aeruginosa*, which can form a bacterial biofilm.

Diagnosis: The greenish color of the nail is very characteristic so that bacterial cultures are usually not needed to make the diagnosis. The color can be scraped off in most cases, but soon returns if the bacteria are not addressed.

Differential Diagnosis: Both exogenous and other enterobacteria causing a grayish discoloration, particularly *Klebsiella* spp. and *Proteus* spp., may have to be considered.

Disease Associations: It appears that coinfection with yeasts and/or dermatophytes makes the nails more susceptible to *Pseudomonas* colonization.

Clinical Course, Prognosis, and Management: The clinical course is chronic with insidious aggravation. The prognosis for the immunocompetent is very good. However, these individuals should not work as doctors or nurses in newborn, cancer, or gnotobiotic units, or as scrub nurses in the surgical theater as they can spread their infection. It is also advisable that they do not work in the food industry, in bakeries, butcheries, or other professions with direct contact with foods, such as chefs. The management is usually not complicated. Baths with diluted white vinegar 2 or 3 times a day for 5 to 10 minutes, then brushing the digits dry, are often sufficient. This may be completed with a topical antimicrobial drug or

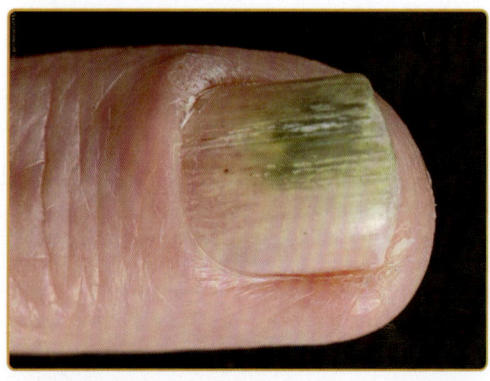

Figure 91-52 *Pseudomonas aeruginosa* colonization of the nail in a patient with an onychomatricoma.

disinfective. Topical antibiotics like gentamycin may be used in addition. Systemic antibiotics are not the first choice for 2 reasons: (a) the bacterial biofilm is approximately 1000 times less sensitive to antibiotics than isolated bacteria of the same species, and (b) the green nail is almost always onycholytic, thus not in contact with the nail bed so that the antibiotic cannot reach the biofilm. Ciprofloxacin, levofloxacin, and polymyxin B show the highest activity against *Pseudomonas*, followed by gentamicin and ofloxacin, whereas the bactericidal antibiotic cefuroxime and the bacteriostatic antibiotic chloramphenicol are less active.

FUNGAL INFECTIONS

The nail apparatus is an extremely frequent site of infection for a great variety of different fungi. They may cause various acute, subacute and chronic infections. Fungal infections may be classified according to their pathogens into dermatophyte, yeast, and nondermatophyte mold infections, according to their time course (acute, subacute, subchronic, chronic), and, above all, according to their mechanism of infection (Table 91-6).

Onychomycoses affect toenails 7 to 10 times more frequently than they affect fingernails, which is thought to be attributable to the 3 times faster growth of fingernails as compared to toenails.

CLINICAL FEATURES

Onychomycoses are often seen as the most frequent nail disorders making up approximately 40% to 50% of all nail diseases. The vast majority are distal or distal–lateral subungual onychomycoses (Fig. 91-53). In the beginning, there is a distal subungual keratosis with an irregular border toward the nail bed. This slowly and insidiously progresses proximally while the nail may become discolored, nontransparent, and break distally. After some months or years, there is often no more progression but the subungual hyperkeratosis may continue to thicken. Often, there is a mild and inconspicuous desquamation around the nail or even an obvious tinea pedis is observed. Sometimes, a yellow streak develops that is formed like a narrow wedge in proximal direction. The lateral edge of the nail is frequently onycholytic.

Superficial white onychomycosis is a condition mostly seen on the toenails as chalky-white patches with no shine of the nail surface (Fig. 91-54). When

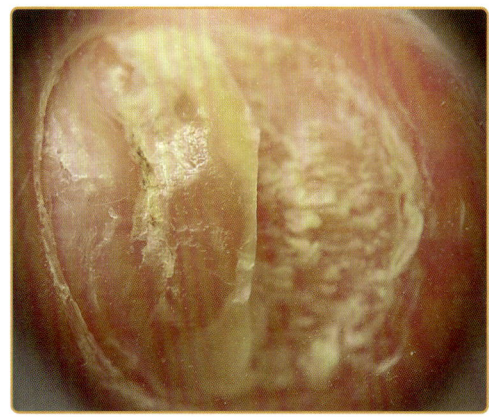

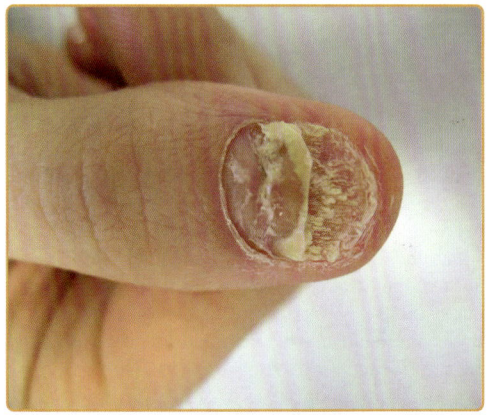

Figure 91-53 Distal–lateral subungual onychomycosis.

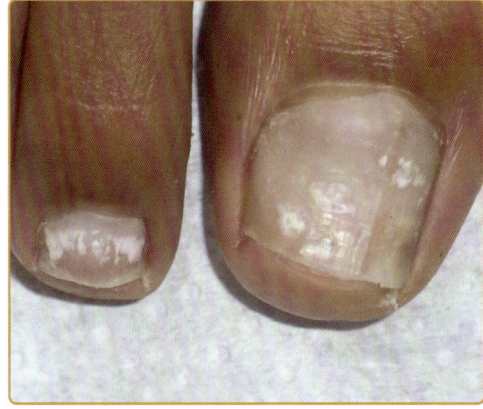

Figure 91-54 White superficial onychomycosis, caused by *Fusarium* spp, of the toe in an immunocompetent person.

TABLE 91-6
Onychomycosis Facts

Onychomycoses According to Pathogens
- Dermatophytes
- Yeasts
- Nondermatophyte molds

Onychomycosis According to the Entry of the Fungi
- Distal and distal–lateral subungual onychomycosis
- Proximal white subungual onychomycosis: with/without paronychia
- Superficial white/black onychomycosis: superficial form, deep form
- Endonyx onychomycosis
- Total dystrophic onychomycosis: secondary to any of the above forms, primary in chronic mucocutaneous candidiasis

Most Important Differential Diagnoses
- Nail psoriasis, asymmetric gait nail unit syndrome, chronic nail dystrophy in the elderly, in chronic venous insufficiency, in impaired arterial circulation, ungual lichen planus, eczema

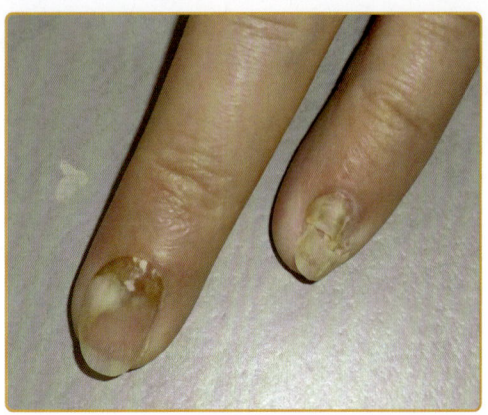

Figure 91-55 Superficial white onychomycosis caused by *Trichophyton rubrum* in an AIDS patient.

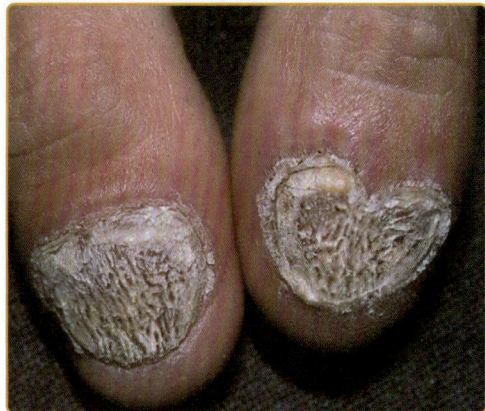

Figure 91-57 Total dystrophic onychomycosis in a 10-year-old boy with chronic mucocutaneous candidiasis.

occurring on fingernails, the white discoloration is inhomogeneous and more cloudy, but the nail surface remains shiny; this is the typical form of HIV infections (Fig. 91-55).

Proximal subungual onychomycosis is also rare. Clinically, it is seen as a white to yellowish discoloration of the nail that grows out from under the proximal nailfold (Fig. 91-56). The plate may be onycholytic under the whitish area. Repeated arched white lines are seen as recurrences from an internal focus.

Endonyx onychomycosis is a rare form in which the fungus only grows in the nail plate without affecting the subungual tissue. The nail is nontransparent, discolored, and dermatoscopy may show air-filled channels in the nail plate.

All these different onychomycoses may lead to total dystrophic onychomycosis where the nail is substituted by irregular keratotic debris full of fungi. Primary total dystrophic onychomycosis is characteristic for chronic mucocutaneous candidiasis (Fig. 91-57), which represents a group of immune defects with impaired defense against *Candida albicans*. Chronic oral lesions, involvement of the scalp and other regions, and granulomatous lesions coexist.

ETIOLOGY AND PATHOGENESIS

The most common causes of onychomycoses are dermatophytes, particularly *Trichophyton rubrum*, *Trichophyton mentagrophytes* var *interdigitale*, much more rarely *Epidermophyton floccosum*, *Trichophyton violaceum*, and *Trichophyton soudanense*. In warm climates, *C. albicans* can cause a clinically identical nail infection as it has enzymes that also degrade keratin. Other yeasts may be found, but their pathogenic role is often not clear. Nondermatophyte molds were mainly seen in tropical climates but are now emerging pathogens in Central Europe.

The pathogenesis is characteristic for each of the onychomycosis forms described. The pathogenic fungus grows from the tip of the digit through the hyponychium toward the nail bed in *distal–lateral subungual onychomycosis*. The nail bed reacts with a hyperkeratosis that harbors the vast majority of the fungi, whereas the overlying nail plate is a barrier for the fungi rather than their site of infection. When the fungus advances proximally, an inflammatory infiltrate develops in the nail bed and epithelium with accumulations of neutrophils very similar to Munro microabscesses; however, there is much less parakeratosis in onychomycosis. Often, a yellow streak or narrow wedge is seen under the nail extending from the distal nail bed proximally. Here, huge amounts of compressed, mostly very thick-walled fungi are seen; this phenomenon is called *dermatophytoma*. In *proximal subungual (white) onychomycosis*, the fungus infects first the undersurface of the proximal nailfold via the cuticle and grows toward the matrix. When this is reached, the fungi are included into the newly formed nail substance and can be found in all layers of the nail plate. *Superficial white onychomycosis* is a rare form of infection of the dorsal surface of the nail plate. In temperate climates, it is mainly caused by *T. mentagrophytes*. Histologically, chains of small spores and, rarely, short slender hyphae are seen on the nail. When this infection extends under the proximal nailfold it may invade deeper layers of the nail plate. In HIV patients, fungi are seen directly under

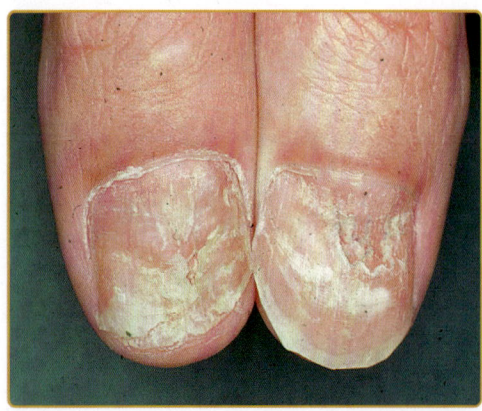

Figure 91-56 Proximal white subungual onychomycosis.

the surface, showing both spores and short hyphae; they are commonly *T. rubrum*. Endonyx onychomycosis is a rare infection, mainly caused by *T. soudanense* or *T. violaceum* that are exclusively found within the nail plate. All these forms may progress to *total dystrophic onychomycosis*, although in a variable frequency. The nail is completely destroyed and substituted by irregular keratotic debris. The nail bed and matrix often show papillomatosis and acanthosis. Rarely, this is found as an acute infection.

DIAGNOSIS

Although most onychomycoses can be diagnosed clinically they should be confirmed by direct microscopy, after clearing of the subungual keratotic debris with 10% to 20% potassium hydroxide, culture, and histopathology. The rate of false-negative results, particularly for cultures, is very high, commonly between 30% and 60%, but histopathology has proved to be doubly sensitive. Furthermore, it can distinguish between colonization and true infection; however, species identification is not possible. Modern methods to confirm a fungal infection comprise polymerase chain reaction and matrix-assisted laser desorption/ionization–time-of-flight spectroscopy. These methods are expensive and require reference DNA and proteins, respectively.

DIFFERENTIAL DIAGNOSIS

Onychomycosis make up approximately 40% to 60% of all nail diseases. Consequently, it is frequently diagnosed without laboratory proof, risking that roughly 50% of the diagnoses are not correct. The most important differential diagnosis is nail psoriasis. Both are frequent, may involve the nails only, cause discoloration, loss of nail transparency, brittle nails, and subungual hyperkeratosis; however, the most frequent sign of nail psoriasis, the pits, are rare in onychomycoses. Onycholysis in psoriasis often has a brownish-reddish proximal margin corresponding to the salmon spot, which is not seen in onychomycosis. Dermatoscopy of this margin exhibits a proximal border that is irregularly serrated and was called the "aurora borealis" sign. Histologically, subungual hyperkeratosis and neutrophil accumulations in the subungual hyperkeratosis are seen in both conditions and called Munro microabscesses; in psoriasis, there is more parakeratosis around them, which is mostly arranged as obliquely ascending columns.

The "asymmetric gait nail unit syndrome" is a condition of toenails,[27] in which onycholysis usually affects 1 corner of the big toenail. It is a result of orthopedic abnormalities leading to rubbing and pressure against shoes. It is very often confounded with onychomycosis, but regularly negative for fungi in all laboratory tests. Additional important differential diagnoses are nail lichen planus, nail eczema, trachyonychia, pityriasis rubra pilaris, nail changes in cutaneous lymphomas, and, above all, nonspecific nail dystrophy in the elderly, persons with chronic venous and lymphatic stasis, peripheral neuropathy, impaired arterial blood supply, and repeated trauma in sportsmen like soccer players, particularly when the big toenails are involved.

DISEASE ASSOCIATIONS

Onychomycoses are usually associated with tinea of the hand and/or feet. They are more frequent in patients with nail psoriasis. Particularly severe and fast progressing onychomycoses are observed in immunosuppression. Peripheral neuropathy, arterial and venous insufficiency, and traumatically damaged nails are risk factors for onychomycoses and hence often associated. Onychomycoses are more frequently seen in diabetic patients. In the two-feet-one-hand syndrome, the tinea of both soles and 1 palm is very often accompanied by onychomycosis, most frequently *T. rubrum*. It is thought that scratching habits are the cause of the unilateral hand involvement.[28]

CLINICAL COURSE, PROGNOSIS, AND MANAGEMENT

Most onychomycoses run a chronic protracted course. For unknown reasons, they may stop progressing after years and remain virtually unchanged for decades if not treated. The prognosis as to the nail destruction is good in more than 90% of patients, and complete recovery, even after severe total dystrophic onychomycosis, is possible. In contrast to this, the management of most onychomycoses is still challenging. Any associated fungal skin infection has to be treated. Hygienic measures, such as regular disinfection of shoes and socks, wearing open shoes whenever possible, changing the footwear daily, and washing socks at 60°C (140°F) are of paramount importance. Infected nail material and subungual keratosis should be removed as much as possible. This can be accomplished with a nail clipper and later with the application of 40% urea paste under occlusion for 3 to 5 days. This softens the infected keratin and allows it to be scraped off atraumatically. Usually, this procedure has to be repeated 2 or 3 times. Surgical nail avulsion should be abandoned as it represents a severe iatrogenic trauma to the nail apparatus, rendering it more susceptible to fungal infection. In cases of less than 50% involvement of the nail or when the matrix is not affected, topical treatment with 8% ciclopirox lacquer (Penlac), 10% efinaconazole (Jublia) and 5% tavaborole (Kerydin) solution or 5% amorolfine (Loceryl, not marketed in the United States) follows for many months, including some months beyond clinically visible clearing. However, even the new antifungal drugs have complete cure rates lower than 20%. When more than 50% of the nail is affected or the infection reaches the matrix at any point, systemic treatment is indicated. Dermatophytes respond best to terbinafine (Lamisil) 250 mg daily, whereas yeasts and some nondermatophyte molds are better treated with itraconazole 400 mg/day for 1 week

TABLE 91-7
Onychomycosis Treatments Approved by the U.S. Food and Drug Administration and Their Response Rates

TREATMENT MODALITY	INDICATION	MYCOLOGIC CURE	COMPLETE CURE
Ciclopirox 8% lacquer	*Trichophyton rubrum* onychomycosis	29%, 36%	6%, 9%
Efinaconazole 5% solution	Dermatophyte onychomycosis	55%, 53%	18%, 15%
Tavaborole 8% solution	Dermatophyte onychomycosis	31%, 36%	7%, 9%
Itraconazole	Dermatophyte onychomycosis	63%, 66%	22%, 22%
Terbinafine	Dermatophyte onychomycosis	60%	46%, 44%
Neodymium:yttrium-aluminum-garnet (Nd:YAG) laser	Temporary increase in clear nail	11%	–

Compiled from Gupta AK, Versteeg SG, Shear NH. Onychomycosis in the 21st century: an update on diagnosis, epidemiology, and treatment. *J Cutan Med Surg.* 2017;21:525-39.

every 4 weeks. This pulse therapy has been shown to be at least as efficacious as continuous itraconazole 200 mg/day. Fluconazole was given once at 150 mg per week, but this dose appears to be too low for individuals weighing more than 70 kg (154 lbs). Controlled trials have shown that the combination of topical plus systemic treatment can reduce the failure rate of systemic therapy alone by 50%.[29] Nevertheless, even combined treatments have cure rates not better than 70% to 75%. Results of combined treatment with systemic and the new antifungals are not yet available. Lasers were approved by the U.S. Food and Drug Administration for the temporary increase in clear nail. Their mycologic cure rate was 11% with no complete cure rates given. Photodynamic treatment of onychomycoses is still in an experimental phase (Table 91-7).

Recurrences are very frequent. The reasons may be the persisting risk factors including the hereditary susceptibility to fungal nail infection and the potential to reinfect in the own household and public sports facilities.

NAILS IN GENERAL DISEASE

Nail alterations in systemic diseases usually affect all digits but they may vary in intensity according to the growth characteristics of the individual nails.

CARDIOVASCULAR AND PULMONARY DISEASES

Clubbing is a characteristic sign of chronic hypoxemia and thus frequently indicates a cor pulmonale. The finger tips and often also the toe tips are enlarged, giving the look of a drumstick. The nail size is increased and both the longitudinal and transverse curvatures are more pronounced so that the nail is round like a watch glass (Fig. 91-58). Quite often, the lunula is very big. Nail bed and lunula are cyanotic. The angle between the proximal nailfold and the nail plate (angle of Lovibond) is greater than 180 degrees. When the 2 opposite fingers are held together, there is a narrow lozenge space between the proximal nail areas in normal persons whereas this diamond-shaped window is absent in clubbed nails, and the angle between the free nail margins is greater than 30 degrees (Schamroth sign). In addition, many other conditions are associated with clubbing (Table 91-8). Unilateral clubbing may hint at arterial insufficiency of this extremity. The cause of clubbing is still not known, but the prevailing hypothesis is that megakaryocytes are incompletely degraded to normal-size platelets in the lungs and may strand in the capillary network of the digits where they disintegrate and release their various growth factors.

Splinter hemorrhages were once seen as an indicator of bacterial endocarditis. However, there is a plethora of other associations.

Yellow nail syndrome (YNS) is a characteristic triad of signs: yellow, thick, extremely slow-growing nails with onycholysis, often also spontaneous nail loss and complete disappearance of the cuticle (Fig. 91-59), chronic sinus-bronchopulmonary infection and edema of the distal extremities. Chronic GI diseases and a variety of internal cancers also have been observed in association with the yellow nail syndrome.

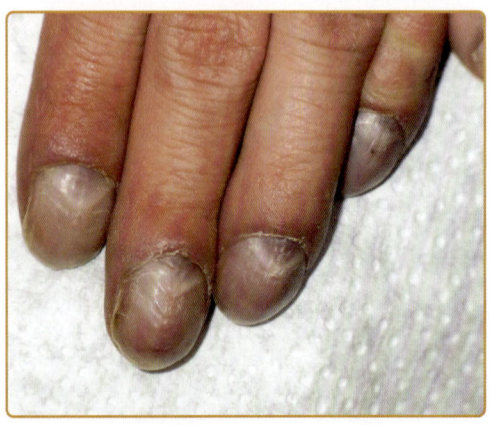

Figure 91-58 Clubbing in a patient with trisomy 21 and Eisenmenger complex.

TABLE 91-8
Causes of Digit Clubbing

Cardiovascular
- Cor pulmonale
- Cardiac insufficiency
- Open foramen ovale, Eisenmenger complex
- Aortic aneurysm

Bronchopulmonary
- Chronic obstructive and suppurative pulmonary diseases
- Intrathoracic tumors
- Hypertrophic pulmonary osteoarthropathy

Gastrointestinal
- Hepatic disorders
- Inflammatory bowel diseases
- Polyposis intestini
- GI neoplasms
- Bacillary and amebic dysentery

Blood Dyscrasias
- Chronic methemoglobinemia (eg, in heavy smokers)

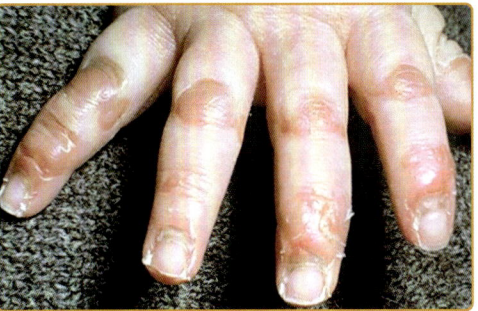

Figure 91-60 Acrodermatitis enteropathica with blisters and erosions on the periungual skin.

UROGENITAL DISEASES

So-called half-and-half nails are seen in chronic renal insufficiency and under long-term hemodialysis. The proximal half of the nail is whitish, the distal half tends to be brownish (Fig. 91-61).

INTESTINAL AND HEPATIC DISEASES

AMYLOIDOSIS

Most nail changes seen in malnutrition, anorexia nervosa, bulimia, or kwashiorkor are nonspecific: the nails may be thin, brittle, and have lost their shine. In acrodermatitis enteropathica and acquired zinc deficiency there are often periungual erosions with crusting, the nail edges may break through the epidermis of the nail grooves and cause granulation tissue (Fig. 91-60). Very similar lesions are seen in glucagonoma dermatitis.

In severe liver disease, the nails may turn white and opaque. In Terry nails, a distal normal-colored band remains. Muehrcke lines are 2 parallel white bands in the middle of the nail bed that do not move out and are seen in severe hypoalbuminemia.

The nails may turn bluish in Wilson disease.

Systemic amyloidosis may have profound effects on the cutaneous appendages including the nails. They insidiously become thinner, fragile, ridged, and lose their shine, resembling late ungual lichen planus (Fig. 91-62). Subungual hemorrhage may occur.

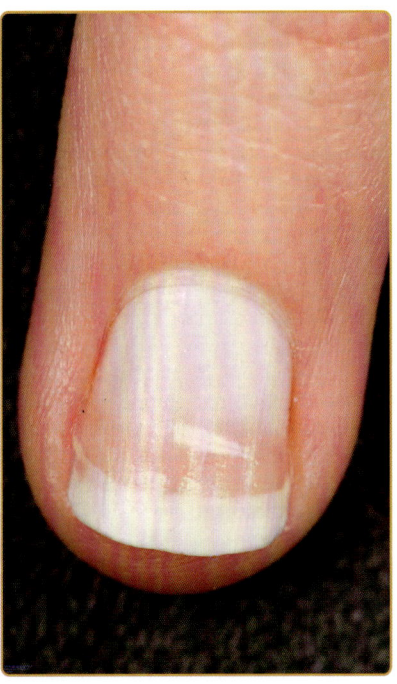

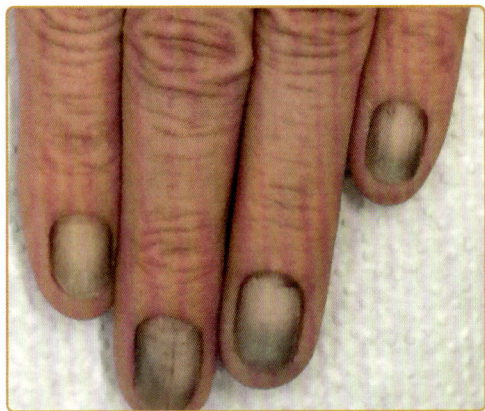

Figure 91-59 Yellow nail syndrome.

Figure 91-61 Half-and-half nail in a patient with renal insufficiency.

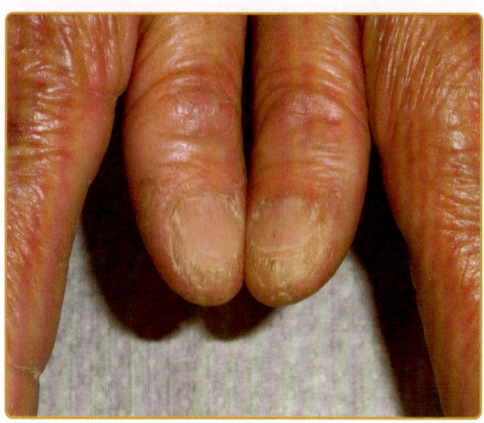

Figure 91-62 Severely dystrophic nails in systemic amyloidosis.

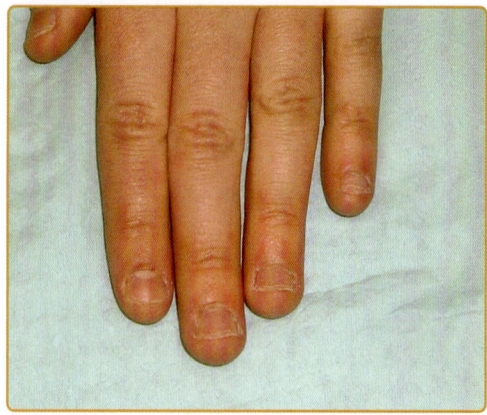

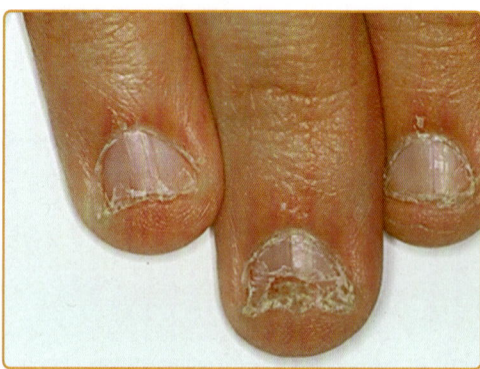

Figure 91-63 Onychophagia.

PSYCHOLOGICAL DISORDERS

A number of autoaggressive nail conditions are known that are commonly described as psychological disorders. Some are extremely frequent, such as chewing of the nails (onychophagia), picking of the periungual skin (perionychotillomania) and habitual pushing back of the cuticle and pressing on the lunula with another fingernail. *Onychophagia* is frequent in children, but it often lasts into adulthood (Fig. 91-63). *Perionychotillomania* is more a condition of adults who continuously pull off hangnails and other tiny skin tags. This habit tic results in a central depression of the nail with a washboard aspect, an unusually long lunula and loss of the cuticle (Fig. 91-64). This must not be confused with the *Heller's median canaliform dystrophy* of the thumb nails, which is characterized by a median split in the nail plate that starts in the proximal portion, extends distally, and typically shows oblique furrows running proximally on both sides, thus giving the aspect of a Christmas tree (Fig. 91-65). Trauma is also the main cause. More-severe autoaggressive behaviors are *onychoteiromania* where the nails are virtually rubbed away, *onychotillomania* where the nail is pulled out in pieces (Fig. 91-66), and *onychotemnomania* where a cutting device is used to remove all the nail. *Onychodaknomania* is a frankly psychotic behavior; the patients bite on their nails in the lunula or proximal nail bed region to produce pain. Many of these patients have a deprivation syndrome.[30] All these behavioral abnormalities are difficult to treat. Psychological support may be necessary. N-acetyl cysteine in a dose of 1800 to 2400 mg/day has been successfully used in a number of obsessive-compulsive disorders, including autoaggressive nail conditions. Nail chewing may spread periungual warts and lead to melanocyte activation with the development of brown streaks in the nails.

INTOXICATIONS

High doses of arsenic cause transverse white nail discoloration. The high arsenic content is important for medicolegal reasons. Cadmium and other heavy metals, as well as many drugs, can be recovered from nails many months after their intake. Toxic doses of vitamin A are destructive of the nail.

DRUG REACTIONS

Some drugs cause characteristic, although rarely specific, nail alterations (Table 91-9). They are most often observed under the treatment with cytostatic drugs. They may cause white lines, Beau lines, or onychomadesis, with the white lines being the least-severe and onychomadesis being the most-severe form of a similar reaction pattern, namely, growth retardation. Brown nail pigmentation may occur and represents an activation of matrix melanocytes. Taxanes cause painful subungual hemorrhagic abscesses that may require withdrawal of the drug. The use of frozen gloves and socks may partially prevent these adverse effects. Targeted anticancer therapies, particularly with epidermal growth factor receptor inhibitors and multiple kinase inhibitors, render the skin very fragile, leading the nail edge to break through and cause granulation tissue that looks similar to pyogenic granulomas.

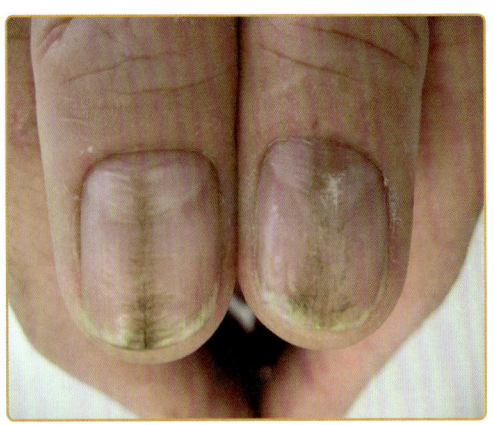

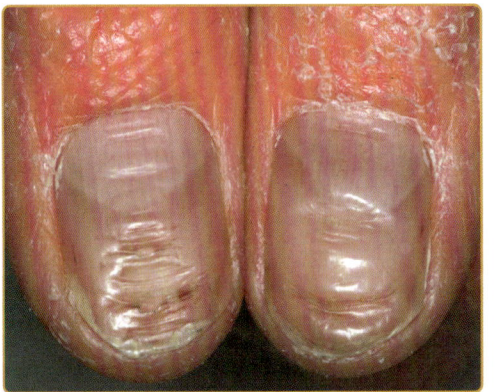

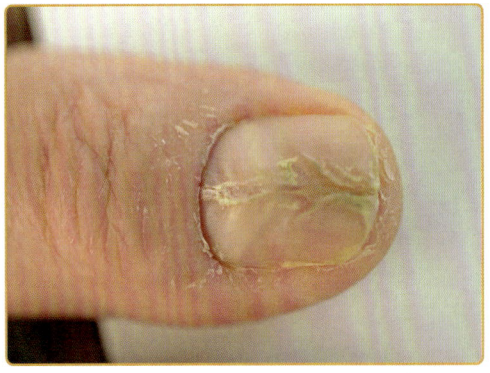

Figure 91-65 The Heller's median canaliform dystrophy of the thumbnail.

may be hemorrhagic, and occurs in the central nail bed of 1 or more nails. Its pathomechanism remains dubious as the nail plate absorbs almost all ultraviolet B and more than 95% of ultraviolet A light, and the skin is often not affected. Acyclovir does induce longitudinal melanonychias.

GENODERMATOSES AFFECTING THE NAIL

Nail involvement in hereditary and congenital disorders is very frequent. Some are highly specific and characterize the genodermatosis, others are frequently seen, many may accompany other severe diseases.

PACHYONYCHIA CONGENITA

Pachyonychia congenita is a group of 5 molecular biologically well-defined diseases of cytokeratins *KRT6a*, *KRT6b*, *KRT6c*, *KRT16*, and *KRT17*. Its traditional

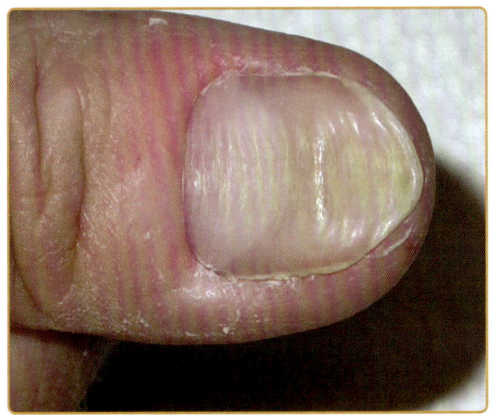

Figure 91-64 Perionychotillomania (habit tic): habitual pushing back of the proximal nailfold.

This phenomenon is also seen under therapy with indinavir, a reverse transcriptase inhibitor, and retinoids. Retinoids are also associated with fragile nails and paronychia. Beta-blockers induce acral ischemia. Bleomycin may also lead to digital ischemia, and permanent nail loss was repeatedly seen after bleomycin treatment of periungual warts. Photochemotherapy with psoralens and ultraviolet A can induce multiple longitudinal brown streaks in several nails. Photoonycholysis is rarely seen during administration of some tetracyclines and fluoroquinolones, as it is painful,

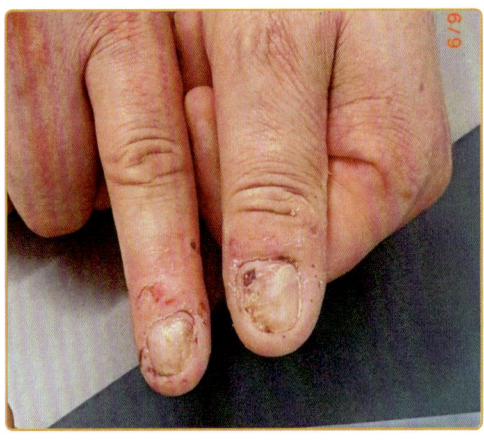

Figure 91-66 Onychotillomania.

TABLE 91-9
Drug-Induced Nail Alterations

Cytostatic and Targeted Therapies
- White lines
- Beau lines
- Onychomadesis
- Muehrcke lines
- Hemorrhagic onycholysis and subungual abscesses
- Melanonychia
- Granulation tissue

Bleomycin
- Permanent nail loss

Reverse Transcriptase Inhibitors
- Granulation tissue

Acyclovir
- Melanonychia

β-Blockers
- Digital ischemia
- Lichenoid-psoriasiform changes

Retinoids and High-Dose Vitamin A
- Brittle nails
- Paronychia
- Granulation tissue

Photochemotherapy with Psoralens and Ultraviolet A
- Melanonychia
- Photoonycholysis

ECTODERMAL DYSPLASIAS

By definition, any hereditary disorder involving at least 2 of the cutaneous adnexa—hair, nails, sweat glands, and teeth—are ectodermal dysplasias. Roughly 30 of the more than 200 ectodermal dysplasias are now molecular biologically defined. For clinical convenience, the ectodermal dysplasias are subdivided into hidrotic and hypohidrotic ectodermal dysplasias. The most frequent ectodermal dysplasias are characterized by hair and nail involvement with normal sweat gland function and normal teeth, particularly the Clouston type, with dysplastic nails that often exhibit distally increasing plications, and are short, thickened, or brittle (Fig. 91-68). Three types of hypohidrotic ectodermal dysplasias are known, autosomal recessive, X-linked recessive, and autosomal dominant. Clinically, they

classification into Type 1 Jadassohn-Lewandowsky syndrome and Type 2 Jackson-Lawler syndrome has now been abandoned as there were too many overlaps. Clinically, pachyonychia congenita shows painful callus-like palmar and plantar hyperkeratoses, monstrous thickening of the subungual hyperkeratosis that is covered by a horseshoe-like nail usually of normal thickness (Fig. 91-67), oral leukokeratosis with no potential for malignant degeneration, natal teeth, and vellus hair cysts. These cysts are mainly seen in *KRT17* and *KRT6a* mutations. Nail changes occur in more than 80% of the patients and develop during infancy. Whether a late-onset pachyonychia congenita exists is not yet clear. Virtually all nails are affected. They are dark, appear thick (although this is the subungual keratosis), and the nail itself is overcurved and difficult to trim.

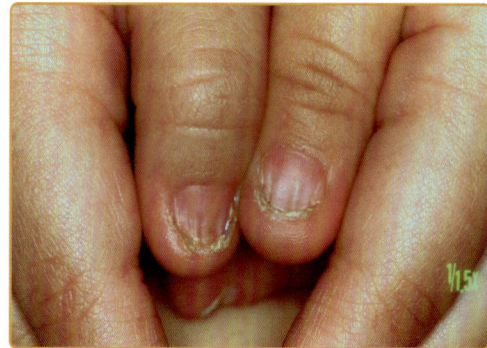
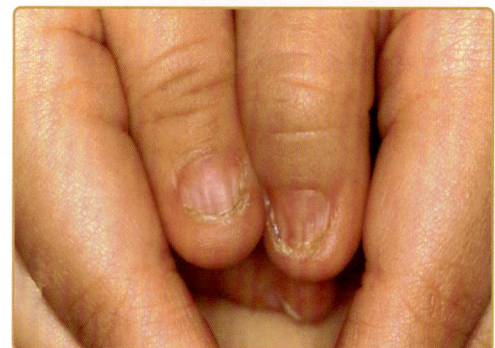
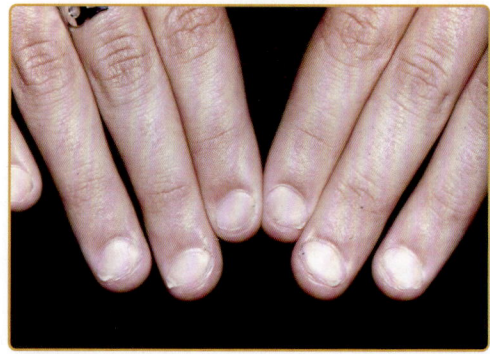

Figure 91-68 Hidrotic ectodermal dysplasia with folded nails.

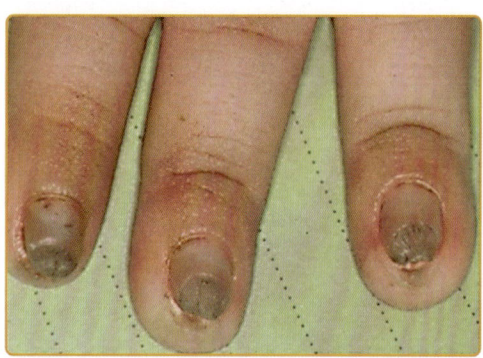

Figure 91-67 Pachyonychia congenita.

present with hypoplastic nails, hypodontia, hypotrichosis, and inability to sweat adequately, which renders the babies at risk for hyperthermia when they are kept too warm. Frontal bossing and the characteristic midface hypoplasia give the affected individuals a very similar appearance, even when they belong to different races.

BULLOUS EPIDERMOLYSIS GROUP

There are 3 distinct, large groups of hereditary bullous epidermolyses: simplex, junctional, and dystrophic. Nail lesions in the simplex types are rare, but are quite common in the course of the junctional and dystrophic bullous epidermolyses. Anonychia is the consequence of repeated blistering of the nail organ and leaves smooth digit tips covered with a shiny epidermis. One dystrophic epidermolysis bullosa is characterized by predominant nail lesions and hence called the nail type (Fig. 91-69). It may be identical with epidermolysis bullosa pruriginosa and pretibial epidermolysis bullosa. The big toenails are dystrophic and thickened; later the other toenails may follow. A pretibial reticular hyperkeratosis with tendency to develop blisters, and often itch, may be seen.

NAIL-PATELLA SYNDROME

Nail-patella syndrome is caused by a mutation in the homeobox gene *LMXB1*, which is necessary for the anterior–posterior orientation during organogenesis. In nail-patella syndrome, nail involvement is characterized by hypoplasia, which is more marked on the thumbs, decreasing toward the fifth digit, and on the medial side of the nail. The lunula exhibits a triangular shape. The patella is hypoplastic or may be absent. Radiographs often show iliac horns. There may be eye involvement and a severe membranous glomerulopathy with protein loss.

DYSKERATOSIS CONGENITA

Dyskeratosis congenita is characterized by pigmentary abnormalities of the skin, nail dystrophy, oral leukoplakias with a tendency to malignant degeneration and severe immune deficiency that is similar, but not identical, to Fanconi anemia.

DISEASES OF CORNIFICATION

The group of *ichthyoses* is now called mendelian disorders of cornification. Nail changes are rare and not specific, such as rough nails and loss of surface shine.

Severe subungual hyperkeratoses similar to those of pachyonychia congenita were observed in a case of *epidermolytic palmar plantar keratosis*; however, the affected nail also exhibited a fungal infection, which might have triggered the hyperkeratosis (Fig. 91-70).

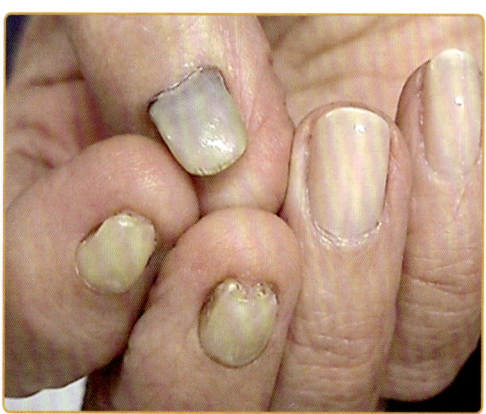

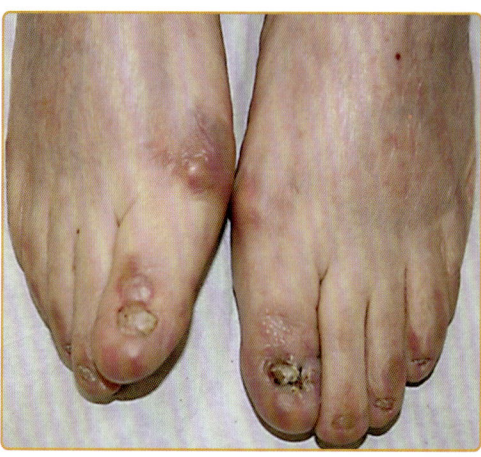

Figure 91-69 Epidermolysis bullosa hereditaria dystrophica ("epidermolysis pruriginosa").

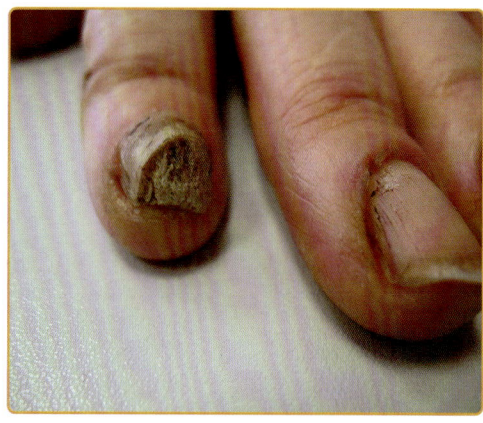

Figure 91-70 Epidermolytic keratosis palmaris et plantaris with nail involvement.

CONGENITAL MALALIGNMENT OF THE BIG TOENAIL

Congenital malalignment of the hallux nail, first described as congenital nail dystrophy, is a fairly common condition. The child may be born with normal nails and develop the condition later, or the nails may be abnormal at birth. Apparently, the disorder can also appear later in life, precipitated by a trauma in an individual with lateral deviation of the distal phalanx of the hallux. Sometimes only one side is affected. Identical twins may have identical unilateral involvement. In classical cases, the affected nail is triangular, thickened, oyster shell–like, discolored, and onycholytic. There is a false distal nailfold and a considerably shortened nail bed (Fig. 91-71). The degree of onycholysis and nail bed shrinkage determine the chances of spontaneous resolution and also of any type of treatment. If resolution has not started by the age of 2 years, it will likely not occur. Symptoms are rare and the children are often only presented to the dermatologist around puberty when the ugly nails are seen as an esthetic problem. Systematic radiographic examinations in more than 40 of our patients have shown that there is virtually always a lateral deviation of the distal phalanx called *hallux valgus interphalangeus*, a lateral deviation of the proximal great toe phalanx leading to classical hallux valgus, and a medial deviation of the first metatarsal bone because of an oblique distal surface of the first cuneiform bone. This forms an arch of the first ray, which self-perpetuates as a result of the action of the flexor and extensor hallux tendons. Early treatment by taping of this orthopedic abnormality is beneficial in those cases where the nail bed shrinkage, onycholysis, and distal nailfold are not too pronounced.

NAIL TUMORS

Tumors of the nail apparatus may originate from all tissue components present in the distal phalanx. Hence, more than 130 different tumors and tumor-like lesions under and around the nail unit have been described. Most of them are rare and their clinical appearance is often not pathognomonic. Analogous to the hair follicle, a few tumors are nail-specific, but these neoplasms have only been described since 30 years.

Tumors of the nail unit exhibit certain growth patterns that allow some of their components to be diagnosed. Tumors in the proximal nailfold exert pressure on the matrix, resulting in a furrow in the nail plate. Lesions under the matrix may cause bulging with increased curvature of one half of the nail. Nail bed neoplasms may cause onycholysis and elevation of the nail plate from the bed. Slow-growing benign tumors usually alter the nail shape, whereas fast-growing tumors may destroy the nail.

BENIGN NAIL TUMORS

Only the most important nail tumors are dealt with here.

EPITHELIAL AND FIBROEPITHELIAL TUMORS

Onychocytic Matricoma: First described under the name *subungual seborrheic keratosis*, this name has now been abandoned in favor of *onychocytic matricoma*.[31] Clinically, there is a longitudinal brownish to dirty-yellow lesion under the nail that shines through the plate. Looking under the free margin of the nail reveals a thickening of keratotic material (Fig. 91-72). Surgical removal demonstrates an acanthoma histologically made up of mainly basaloid cells. Round keratin inclusions are similar to squamous eddies but their keratinization mode is via a keratogenous zone like normal nail formation.

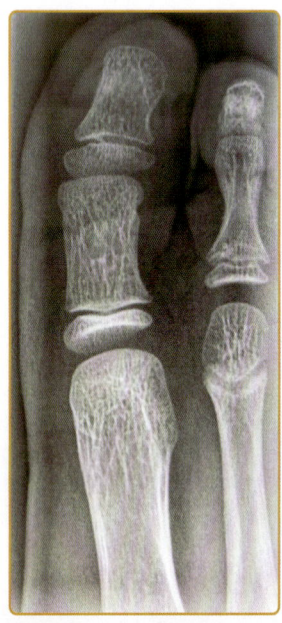

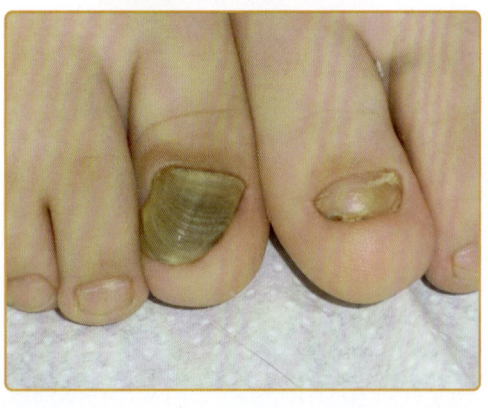

Figure 91-71 Congenital malalignment of the big toenail.

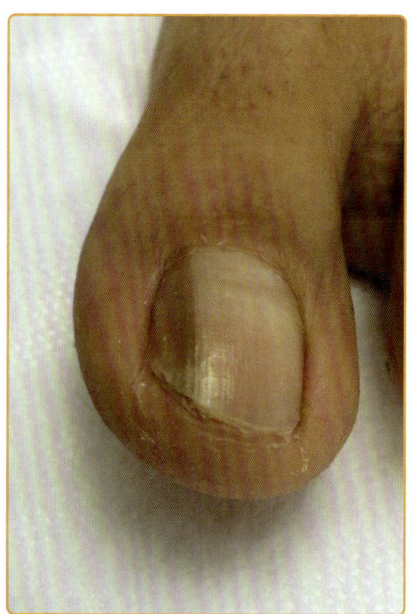

Figure 91-72 Onychocytic matricoma.

Onychomatricoma: More than 200 cases of onychomatricoma have been reported since its first description in 1992.[32] It is a fibroepithelial neoplasm originating from the matrix. The nail is thickened, funnel-shaped, yellow, striated, and may show splinter hemorrhages (Fig. 91-73). At the free end of the plate, small holes can be recognized. Dermatoscopy shows that the tunnels contain capillaries that may run a long distance distally in the nail; in rare cases they remain patent, and may cause bleeding upon nail trimming. This clinical appearance is caused by a densely cellular fibrous stroma with long filiform projections that are all covered with normal matrix epithelium extending into the nail. Thus the surface of nail-producing matrix is massively enlarged causing the nail thickening. Variants of this tumor are myxoid onychomatricoma and pigmented onychomatricoma, with pigmented onychomatricoma being an important differential diagnosis of subungual melanoma.

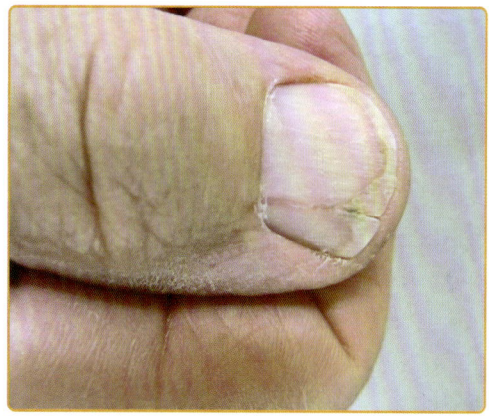

Figure 91-74 Onychopapilloma.

Onychopapilloma: This is another recently described nail-specific tumor that arises from the distal matrix and produces a thread of abnormal keratin. Clinically, it is seen as a whitish, ivory-colored, yellowish, reddish, or light-brown band of 4 to 8 mm in width in the nail, similar to onychocytic matricoma (Fig. 91-74). End-on dermatoscopy of the nail shows, however, a circumscribed thinning of the nail plate over the keratotic distal end of the onychopapilloma. Often, the nail tends to break here and a V-shaped onycholysis develops in the distal nail bed. Treatment is by tangential excision of the entire lesion from the hyponychium to the mid-matrix.[33]

Subungual Filamentous Tumor: Subungual filamentous tumor is clinically seen as a whitish to yellowish line of 1 to 2 mm that does not widen with time. The nail may show a short longitudinal fissure at its free margin. A tiny round keratotic tip is seen under the nail. Its relation to onychopapilloma is not clear.

Ungual Fibrokeratoma: Fibrokeratomas of the nail unit are quite common. They are sausage-like lesions with a keratotic tip. Most arise from under the proximal nailfold and remain lying on it causing a longitudinal groove (Fig. 91-75). When a fibrokeratoma originates from the mid-matrix, it grows within the nail

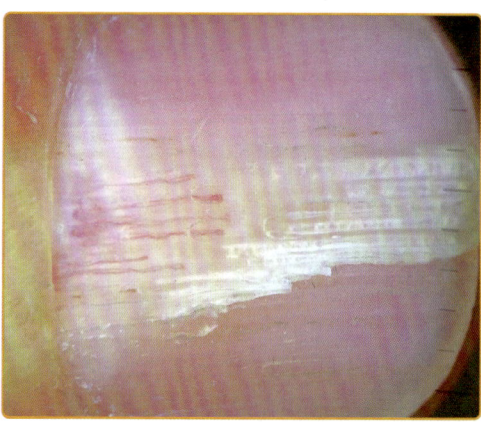

Figure 91-73 Onychomatricoma.

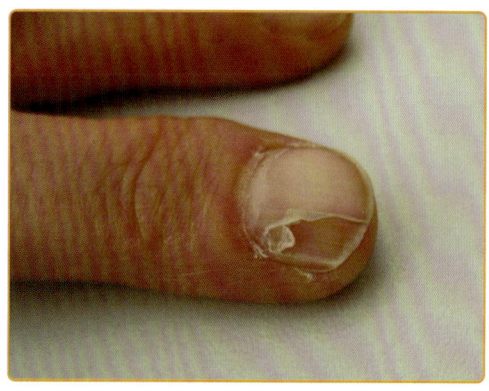

Figure 91-75 Fibrokeratoma of the nail.

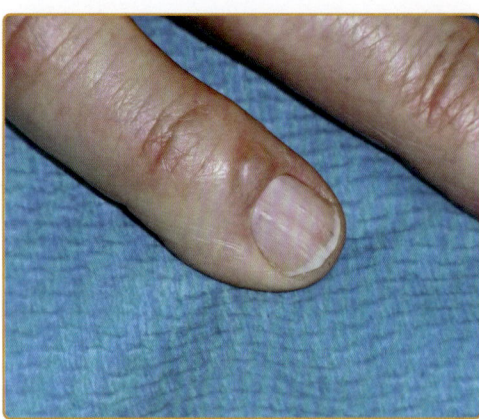

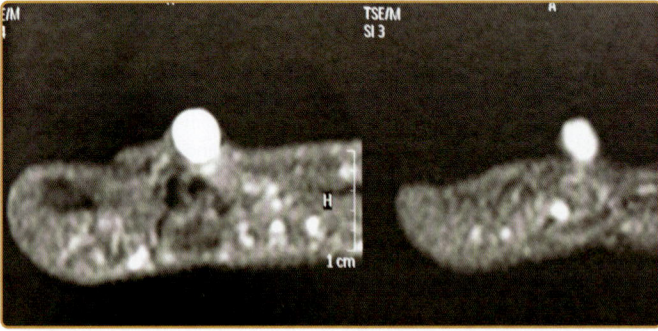

Figure 91-76 Myxoid pseudocyst in the proximal nailfold causing a longitudinal groove in the nail. In the magnetic resonance tomography, the content of the myxoid pseudocyst stands out due to its high water content. A connecting stalk is seen as a sinuous narrow band extending from the lesion to the joint.

plate until the overlying nail lamella breaks away and a sharply delimited groove remains. Subungual fibrokeratomas arise from the most distal matrix or nail bed and cause a ridge. Multiple ungual fibrokeratomas, so-called Koenen tumors, are a sign of the tuberous sclerosis complex and occur in approximately 50% of these patients after the age of 12 years. Treatment is by incision around the tumor down to the bone and extirpation.

Myxoid Pseudocysts: These lesions are very common pseudotumors of middle-aged and elderly individuals and were known as "dorsal finger cysts." Most occur in the proximal nailfold of the fingers, rarely on toes, where they exert pressure on the underlying matrix, resulting in a regular longitudinal groove (Fig. 91-76). When the lesion drains into the nail pocket the groove is very irregular, mirroring the periods of increased and released pressure. Subungual localization is rare and often seen as a violaceous lesion on one side of the matrix associated with hemi-overcurvature. Women are more frequently affected. Degenerative distal interphalangeal osteoarthritis with Heberden nodes is usually seen. Treatments vary from repeated punctures and expression of the viscous gelatinous mucin, to injection of steroids or sclerosants, infrared or laser coagulation, cryotherapy, and surgery. The recurrence rate is high except for the technique with intraarticular injection of methylene blue to visualize a potential connecting stalk to the joint, ligation of it, and meticulous extirpation of the myxoid material.

Glomus Tumor: Although rare, this is the best-known nail tumor because of its highly characteristic symptoms. Patients usually present with the complaint of an extremely painful digit tip. Clinical examination reveals a violaceous red spot under the nail of a finger, from which a reddish line may sometimes extend distally (Fig. 91-77). The slightest shock and cold precipitate the pain that radiates into the arm. Probing allows to exactly locate the tumor, but variable high-frequency ultrasound and magnetic resonance tomography may sometimes be needed. Treatment is by meticulous enucleation of the tumor and repair of the matrix and nail bed.

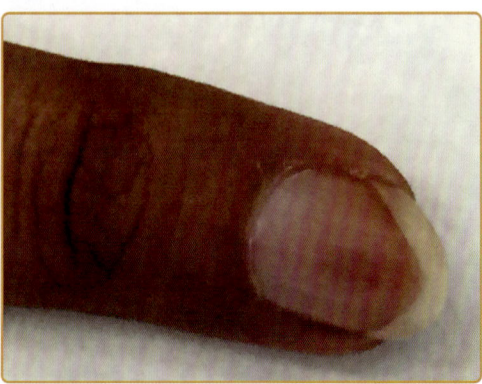

Figure 91-77 Glomus tumor.

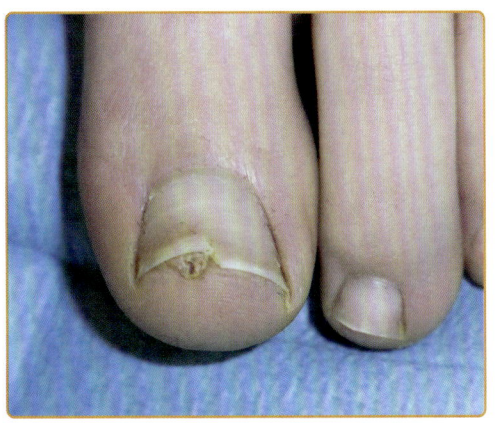

Figure 91-78 Subungual exostosis of the big toe.

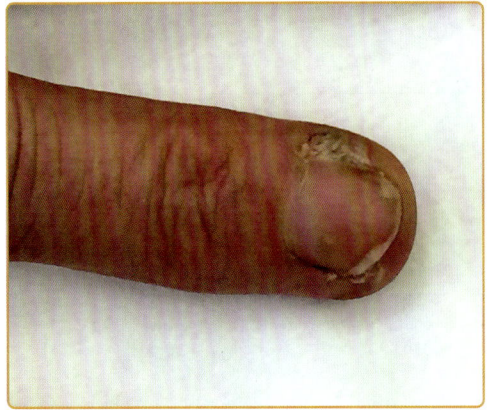

Figure 91-79 Bowen disease' of the nail.

Subungual Exostosis and Subungual Osteochondroma: Both lesions are often seen as being the same condition and are confounded, although there are important differences. Osteochondromas arise from the epiphysis region of the distal phalanx and have a hyaline cartilage cap, whereas subungual exostoses originate from the corona unguicularis, are thus more distal, and have a fibrous cap. The nail plate is lifted up by a stone-hard nodule that, in case of exostosis, has a characteristic collarette-like margin representing the former border of the hyponychium (Fig. 91-78). Most subungual exostoses occur in children and young adults, commonly the big toe. Trauma was thought to be the cause. The recent finding of a chromosome translocation suggests a true tumor nature; however, it is not clear whether the examined lesions were exostoses or osteochondromas. A radiograph confirms the diagnosis and helps to preoperatively estimate the extent of surgery.

MALIGNANT NAIL TUMORS

SQUAMOUS CELL CARCINOMA

Squamous cell carcinoma is the most frequent malignant neoplasm of the nail. Its in situ form is Bowen disease. Most commonly seen around fingernails, Bowen disease may clinically resemble a flat agglomeration of warts (Fig. 91-79). Paronychia may be associated. Melanonychia is a feature in dark-skinned persons and association with HPV56. Other high-risk HPV are HPV16, HPV18, and HPV35, but many more were found, hinting at a possible genitodigital transmission. Bowen disease is slowly and insidiously growing and may result in large irregular periungual areas of velvety, red and scaling skin. Extension under the nail to the nail bed and matrix are common, and leukonychia is characteristic for matrix involvement. Ulceration and crust formation indicate invasive growth (Fig. 91-80), which is, however, a late event. Bone invasion and metastases are rare in the Bowen type of squamous cell carcinoma, but occur in the common squamous cell carcinoma type.

Treatment of choice is Mohs surgery, but amputation is required in case of bone invasion.

OTHER MALIGNANT NAIL TUMORS

Basal cell carcinoma is exceedingly rare in the nail unit.

Onycholemmal carcinoma is a very slow-growing subungual tumor that clinically presents as a longstanding oozing mass. The diagnosis is made by histopathology.

THE MELANONYCHIA PROBLEM

The challenging problem of brown nail pigmentation is dealt with here. This is important as nail melanoma is the most serious nail condition and the rate of misdiagnoses and diagnostic delays is very high.

BENIGN MELANONYCHIAS

A brown streaky pigmentation of the nail is called *longitudinal melanonychia* (LM). LM does not primarily

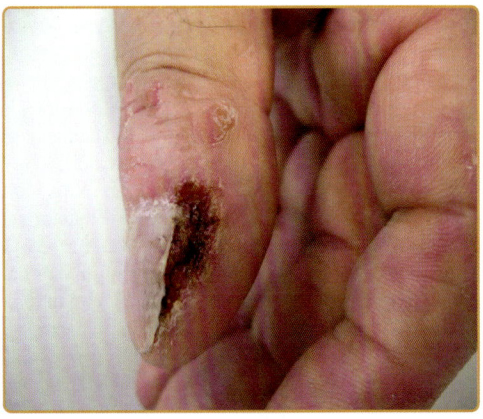

Figure 91-80 Bowen disease' of the nail with an invasive component.

TABLE 91-10
Differential Diagnosis of Longitudinal Melanonychia

Age at Onset
- Babies—benign
- Children—mostly benign
- Adolescents—probably benign
- Adults until age 30 to 35 years—suspicious
- Adults older than age 40 years—highly suspicious
- Adults older than age 50 years—probably melanoma

Color and Internal Structure of the Brown Band
- Regular light-brown band on a gray background—functional LM
- Regular brown band on a brown background—lentigo
- Regular brown band with dark brown spots on brown background—nevus
- Irregular brown band with asymmetric, unevenly spaced lines of variable length, proximal widening of the band—melanoma

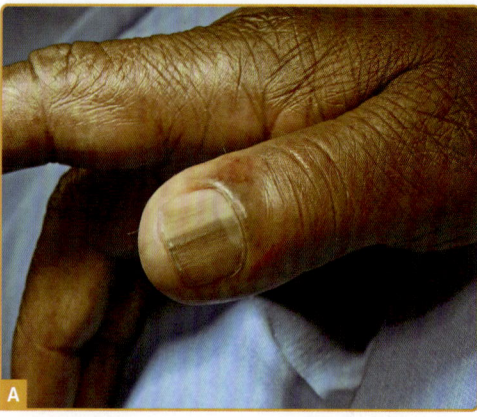
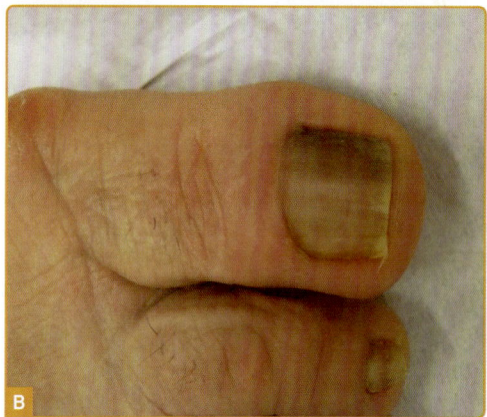
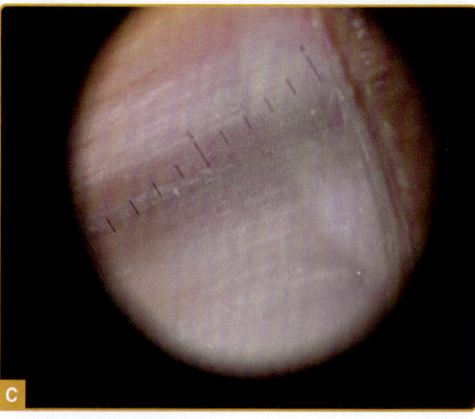

Figure 91-81 **A,** Functional melanonychia in a dark skinned person. **B,** due to friction. **C,** drug-induced functional melanonychia.

include the type of pigment responsible for it. Bacterial, fungal, blood, and various exogenous pigments can cause band-like or diffuse brown to black nail pigmentations. It is the color itself, not its intensity, that is important; the internal architecture of a pigmented streak, its extension in the nail, whether it is associated with nail dystrophy or onycholysis, its time course and development, the patient's age, gender, skin type, and profession are all important for the evaluation of LM (Table 91-10).

Four lesion types can induce a true LM: *melanocyte activation* in the matrix results in functional melanonychia. This is the rule for LM in pigmented persons, including many children (Fig. 91-81), because of repeated trauma, such as friction or onychophagia, during pregnancy, under chemotherapy, and a variety of other drugs. A *matrix lentigo* is a numerical increase in melanin-producing cells (Fig. 91-82). A *matrix nevus* is characterized by the nest-like agglomeration of melanocytes in the matrix; most are seen in children and are junctional (Fig. 91-83). Pigmented *melanoma* of the matrix also causes LM (Fig. 91-84). None of the underlying pathologic processes can be safely distinguished on clinical grounds alone although dermatoscopy may help in certain respects. An LM with regular color and banding, symmetrical diameter, and no nail dystrophy is most likely benign. Periungual pigmentation in children may be a sign of a congenital nevus. LM in children and adolescents is commonly regarded as being benign. Particularly in children, an LM may fade with age, but rarely may become darker, particularly in children with skin types IV to VI. Although childhood nail melanoma is extremely rare, a single rapidly increasing LM in a light-skinned child is best excised. The tangential excision technique can prevent postsurgical nail dystrophy. It is recommended to tangentially excise all acquired matrix melanocyte proliferations in adults, and if parents insist, also in children. This approach and the growing awareness of nail melanomas among dermatologists have now led to fewer advanced nail melanomas among the author's patients.

UNGUAL MELANOMA

Nail melanoma is a subtype of acral melanoma. It makes up 1.5% to 2.5% of all melanomas in light-skinned individuals, 10% to 20% in Asians, and up to 25% in Africans, although the absolute numbers are very similar. With nails representing less than 1% of the body surface area the nail is overrepresented as a site for melanomas.[34] In fact, as subungual melanomas with melanonychia derive from the matrix, which represents only one-quarter to one-third of the nail field,

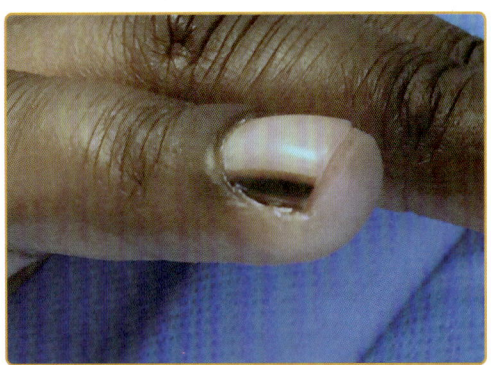

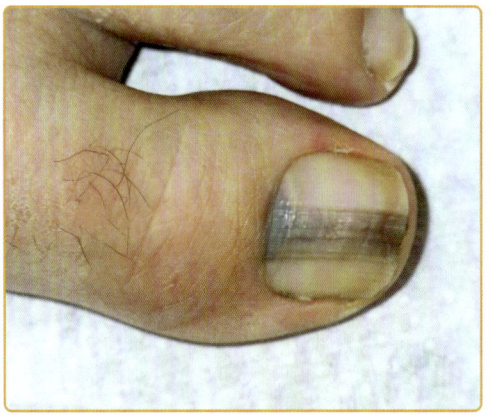

Figure 91-84 Matrix melanoma causing longitudinal melanonychia with irregular outline.

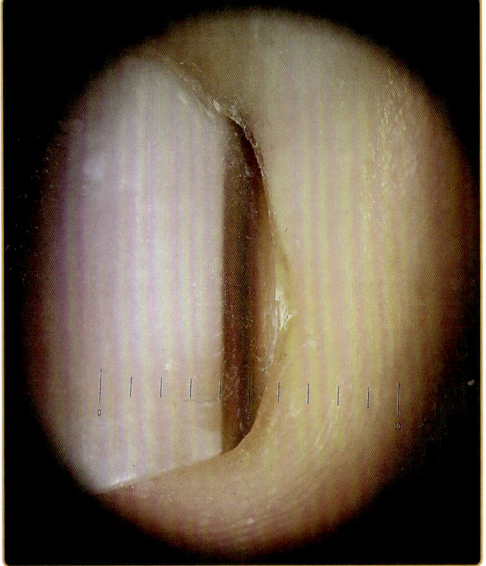

Figure 91-82 Melanonychia caused by a matrix lentigo.

this is a particular area of concentration of melanoma development.

The peak incidence of nail melanoma is from the fifth to seventh decades of life, but nail melanomas may occur in children and in the very old. There is no clear-cut gender predominance. Thumbs, big toes, index fingers, and middle fingers are the most common sites.

Periungual pigmentation is called the Hutchinson sign and represents periungual spread of the in situ component (Fig. 91-85). Most subungual melanomas are pigmented and start with an LM, which is irregular in contrast to benign LMs (see Table 91-10). Proximal widening indicates rapid growth of the lesion. Nail dystrophy is a sign of an advanced melanoma. Dermatoscopy helps to determine the internal structure of the LM and allows a micro-Hutchinson sign to be seen. Approximately 25% to 33% of nail melanomas are amelanotic and pose great diagnostic challenges (Fig. 91-86). They usually arise from the nail bed, cause onycholysis that may ooze, and are frequently misdiagnosed as a pyogenic granuloma, ingrown nail, or wart, or even onychomycosis. Unfortunately, even pigmented nail melanomas are usually diagnosed very late with a diagnostic delay of years to decades. This is why the prognosis of nail melanomas is so poor, with 5-year survival rates of 15% to 20% for invasive nail melanomas.

Diagnosis: A diagnostic algorithm considering several factors was proposed to facilitate the diagnosis of pigmented melanoma (Table 91-11); it is not useful for amelanotic melanomas and LM in children.[35]

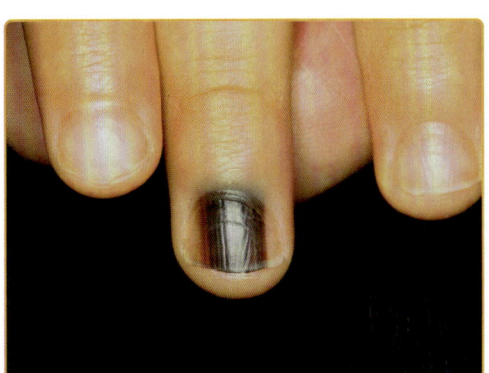

Figure 91-83 Melanonychia caused by a matrix nevus.

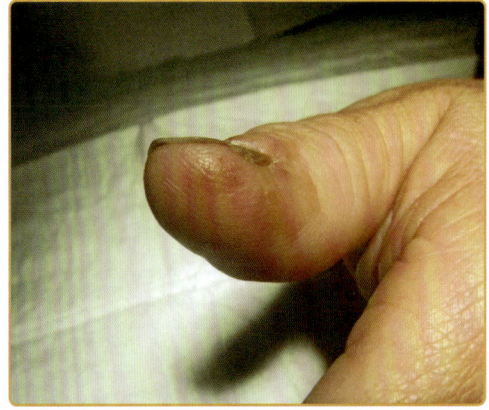

Figure 91-85 Subungual melanoma with Hutchinson sign.

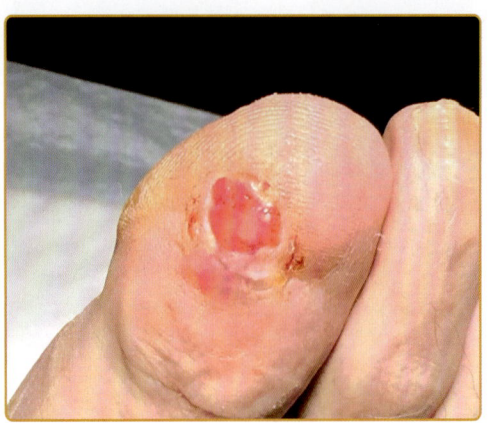

Figure 91-86 Amelanotic melanoma of the nail bed.

Treatment: Treatment of nail melanoma is by surgery. In situ and early invasive melanomas can be removed by wide local excision with preservation of the digit,[36,37] whereas distal amputation is recommended for advanced melanomas. Hutchinson sign responds to topical immunotherapy with imiquimod.[38]

Disease Associations: Ungual melanomas occur more frequently in those subjects with a personal or family history of melanoma. Ultraviolet exposure is not associated with nail melanoma. Histopathologically, there is a frequent association with multiple subungual onycholemmal cysts, which must not be mistaken for subungual squamous cell carcinoma.[39,40]

Clinical Course, Prognosis, and Management: As the diagnostic delay is often years or even decades many melanoma patients come late with advanced tumors, although this is exceptional in the author's practice. The list of misdiagnoses is long and often incomprehensible for an experienced dermatologist.

In situ and early invasive melanomas have a very good prognosis; however, advanced and metastatic melanomas have a 5-year survival rate of 15% to 24%.

There are no controlled studies concerning the efficacy of new targeted and immune checkpoint inhibitor therapies on nail melanoma, although there is no reason not to assume that they will have a similar activity.

Postoperatively, patients are seen for followup examinations at regular intervals, depending on tumor thickness and stage. It has to be stressed that ungual melanomas are not particularly aggressive and that it is the delay in diagnosis and treatment that makes their prognosis so poor.

REFERENCES

1. Haneke E. The double nail of the little toe. *Skin Appendage Disord*. 2015;1:163-167.
2. Peña-Romero AG, Domínguez-Cherit J, Guzmán-Abrego AC. Under-reported finding in acral erythema multiforme. *Indian J Dermatol*. 2015;60:636.
3. Molina-Hernandez AI, Diaz-Gonzalez JM, Saeb-Lima M, et al. Argyria after silver nitrate intake: case report and brief review of literature. *Indian J Dermatol*. 2015;60:520.
4. van de Kerkhof PC, Pasch MC, Scher RK, et al. Brittle nail syndrome: a pathogenesis-based approach with a proposed grading system. *J Am Acad Dermatol*. 2005;53:644-651.
5. Haneke E. Controversies in the treatment of ingrown nails. *Dermatol Res Pract*. 2012;2012:1-12.
6. Baumgartner M, Haneke E. Retronychia: diagnosis and treatment. *Dermatol Surg*. 2010;36:1610-1613.
7. Haneke E. Etiopathogénie et traitement de l'hypercourbure transversale de l'ongle du gros orteil. *J Méd Esth Chir Dermatol*. 1992;19:123-127.
8. Banga G, Patel K. Glycolic acid peels for nail rejuvenation. *J Cutan Aesthet Surg*. 2014;7:198-201.
9. McGonagle D, Tan AL, Benjamin M. The nail as a musculoskeletal appendage-implications for an improved understanding of the link between psoriasis and arthritis. *Dermatology*. 2009;218:97-102.
10. Morrissey KA, Rubin AI. Histopathology of the red lunula: new histologic features and clinical correlations of a rare type of erythronychia. *J Cutan Pathol*. 2013;40:972-975.
11. Marrakchi S, Guigue P, Renshaw BR, et al. Interleukin-36-receptor antagonist deficiency and generalized pustular psoriasis. *N Engl J Med*. 2011;365:620-628.
12. Abbas O, Itani S, Ghosn S, et al. Acrodermatitis continua of Hallopeau: a clinical phenotype of DITRA: evidence that it is a variant of pustular psoriasis. *Dermatology*. 2013;226:28-31.
13. Baran R, Rigopoulos D. *Nail Therapies*. London, UK: Informa Healthcare; 2012.
14. Scheinfeld NS. Trachyonychia: a case report and review of manifestations, associations, and treatments. *Cutis*. 2003;71:299-302.
15. Tosti Piraccini BM, Ghetti E, Colombo MD. Topical steroids versus systemic antifungals in the treatment of chronic paronychia: an open, randomized double-blind and double dummy study. *J Am Acad Dermatol*. 2002;47:73-76.
16. Fischer J, Degenhardt F, Hofmann A, et al. Genome-wide analysis of copy number variants in alopecia areata in a Central European cohort reveals association with MCHR2. *Exp Dermatol*. 2017;26(6):536-541.

TABLE 91-11

Diagnostic Algorithm for Nail Melanomas—The ABCDEF Rule

- **A**—**A**ge: most ungual melanomas occur between 40 and 70 years of age; **A**frican **A**mericans, native **A**mericans, **A**sians: a higher percentage of nail melanomas
- **B**—**B**rown to **b**lack **b**and in the nail, **b**readth over 3 mm, irregular or blurred **b**order
- **C**—**C**hange: Rapid increase in width and growth rate, nail dystrophy does not improve despite adequate therapy; **c**olor
- **D**—**D**igit: thumb > big toe > index finger; single-digit involvement; very rarely more affected
- **E**—**E**xtension of pigmentation: Hutchinson sign
- **F**—**F**amily or personal history of melanoma or so-called dysplastic nevi

17. Haneke E. Non-infectious inflammatory disorders of the nail apparatus. *J Dtsch Dermatol Ges.* 2009;7:787-797.
18. Baran R, Haneke E. *The Nail in Differential Diagnosis.* Abingdon, UK: Informa Healthcare, 2007.
19. Dhayalan A, King BA. Tofacitinib citrate for the treatment of nail dystrophy associated with alopecia universalis. *JAMA Dermatol.* 2016;152:492-493.
20. Haneke E. Isolated bullous lichen planus of the nails mimicking yellow nail syndrome. *Clin Exp Dermatol.* 1983;8:425-428.
21. Sellheyer K, Nelson P. The ventral proximal nail fold: stem cell niche of the nail and equivalent to the follicular bulge–a study on developing human skin. *J Cutan Pathol.* 2012;39:835-843.
22. Piraccini BM, Saccani E, Starace M, et al. Nail lichen planus: response to treatment and long term follow-up. *Eur J Dermatol.* 2010;20:489-496.
23. Irla N, Schneiter T, Haneke E, et al. Nail lichen planus: successful treatment with etanercept. *Case Rep Dermatol.* 2010;2:173-176.
24. Bouaziz JD, Barete S, Le Pelletier F, et al. Cutaneous lesions of the digits in systemic lupus erythematosus: 50 cases. *Lupus.* 2007;16:163-167.
25. Obermoser G, Sontheimer RD, Zelger B. Overview of common, rare and atypical manifestations of cutaneous lupus erythematosus and histopathological correlates. *Lupus.* 2010;19:1050-1070.
26. Haneke E. Onychomadesis and hand, foot and mouth disease—is there a connection? *Euro Surveill.* 2010;15(37).
27. Zaias N, Rebell G, Escovar S. Asymmetric gait nail unit syndrome: the most common worldwide toenail abnormality and onychomycosis. *Skinmed.* 2014;12:217-223.
28. Zhan P, Ge YP, Lu XL, et al. A case-control analysis and laboratory study of the two feet-one hand syndrome in two dermatology hospitals in China. *Clin Exp Dermatol.* 2010;35:468-472.
29. Baran R, Feuilhade M, Combemale P, et al. A randomized trial of amorolfine 5% solution nail lacquer combined with oral terbinafine compared with terbinafine alone in the treatment of dermatophytic toenail onychomycoses affecting the matrix region. *Br J Dermatol.* 2000;142:1177-1183.
30. Haneke E. Autoaggressive nail disorders. *Dermatol Rev Mex.* 2013;57:225-234.
31. Perrin C, Cannata GE, Bossard C, et al. Onychocytic matricoma presenting as pachymelanonychia longitudinal. A new entity (report of five cases). *Am J Dermatopathol.* 2012;34:54-59.
32. Baran R, Kint A. Onychomatrixoma. Filamentous tufted tumour in the matrix of a funnel-shaped nail: a new entity. *Br J Dermatol.* 1992;126:510-515.
33. Jellinek NJ. Longitudinal erythronychia: suggestions for evaluation and management. *J Am Acad Dermatol.* 2011;64:167.e1-.e11.
34. Haneke E. Ungual melanoma—controversies in diagnosis and treatment. *Dermatol Ther.* 2012;25:510-524.
35. Levit EK, Kagen MH, Scher RK, et al. The ABC rule for clinical detection of subungual melanoma. *J Am Acad Dermatol.* 2000;42:269-274.
36. Haneke E, Binder D. Subunguales Melanom mit streifiger Nagelpigmentierung [in German]. *Hautarzt.* 1978;29:389-391.
37. Moehrle M, Metzger S, Schippert W, et al. "Functional" surgery in subungual melanoma. *Dermatol Surg.* 2003;29:366-374.
38. Ocampo-Garza J, Gioia Di Chiacchio N, Haneke E, et al. Subungual melanoma in situ treated with imiquimod 5% cream after conservative surgery recurrence. *J Drugs Dermatol.* 2017;16:268-270.
39. Boespflug A, Debarbieux S, Depaepe L, et al. Association of subungual melanoma and subungual squamous cell carcinoma: a case series. *J Am Acad Dermatol.* 2018;78(4):760-768.
40. Haneke E. *Histopathology of the nail - Onychopathology.* CRC Press Boca Raton 2018.

PART 17 Disorders Due to the Environment

第十七篇 环境引起的皮肤病

Chapter 92 :: Polymorphic Light Eruption :: Alexandra Gruber-Wackernagel & Peter Wolf

第九十二章 多形性日光疹

中文导读

多形性日光疹（PMLE）是最常见的光敏性疾病，女性多见，通常出现在春季或夏初。本章主要从该病的流行病学、临床特征、病因和发病机制、诊断、鉴别诊断、临床病程和预后、处理等方面来进行介绍。在临床特征方面，分别从皮肤表现、引起病变的波长、非皮肤表现以及可能出现的并发症四方面进行了介绍。提出本病的确切病因和发病机制尚不清楚，可能与免疫学、皮肤抗原、遗传、激素因素、抗菌肽等有关。可以根据病史、实验室检查、组织病理学、光测试和光激发试验等进行诊断，并总结了主要的鉴别诊断以及PMLE的诊断思路。此外，还提出预防是PMLE的重要措施方法，并介绍了轻症和重症患者的治疗。

〔易 梅〕

AT-A-GLANCE

- Polymorphic light eruption is the most common photodermatosis with a female preponderance typically presenting in the spring.
- *Clinical presentation:* A pruritic, erythematous, symmetrically distributed, eruption of variable interindividual morphology (in most cases papular) on sun-exposed skin areas, within hours to days of exposure, with full resolution in several days.
- *Histopathology:* Epidermal spongiosis with a superficial and deep dermal, perivascular, mixed-cell infiltrate and papillary dermal edema.
- *Etiology and Pathogenesis:* A resistance to ultraviolet (UV)-induced immune suppression with subsequent delayed-type hypersensitivity reaction against UV-induced antigen(s).
- *Prevention and Therapy:* Responds to broad-spectrum sunscreen use, oral or topical steroids, and prophylactic low-dose immunosuppressive phototherapy.

DEFINITIONS

Polymorphic light eruption (PMLE) is the most common photodermatosis, with a high prevalence, particularly among young women, in temperate climates. As the name of the condition implies, itchy lesions of variable morphology appear on sun-exposed skin after the first exposure to an intense dose of sunlight in spring or early summer. The exact etiology and pathogenesis of PMLE is unknown, but a resistance to ultraviolet (UV)-induced immune suppression (a physiologic phenomenon in healthy individuals) and a subsequent immune reaction to UV-modified elements in the skin are suggested.

HISTORICAL PERSPECTIVE

Clinical symptoms of PMLE were first described under the term of *Prurigo aestivalis* in 1888 by Hutchinson.[1,2] In 1942, Epstein suggested a photoallergic pathophysiology for photodermatoses.[2] In 1984, Moncada and colleagues found a predominance of T-helper (Th) cells and cells expressing high levels of Ia antigens in the dermal cell infiltrate of PMLE, suggesting that an abnormal immune response is responsible for the pathophysiology of the disease.[3] Consistently, histologic features with an early influx of CD4+ T lymphocytes, followed by CD8+ T cells in established lesions, were described in PMLE by Norris and colleagues, pointing to a cellular-mediated immune response.[4]

EPIDEMIOLOGY

PMLE has a wide geographic distribution, but is described as being seen more frequently in temperate latitudes and rarely in equatorial latitudes. The incidence rate of PMLE in the United Kingdom has been described as being approximately 15%, compared with less than 5% in Australia.[5] However, a recent large-scale cross-sectional study with individuals residing from the Mediterranean to Scandinavia found no correlation between PMLE incidence and increasing latitude, with an average prevalence of PMLE in 18% of Europeans.[6] PMLE occurs in all skin types and racial groups.[7,8] Similar to many autoimmune disorders PMLE usually has its onset within the first 3 decades of life and affects females approximately 4 times more often than males.[8-10] Symptoms also may begin in early childhood or late adulthood, but onset during childhood is less commonly seen in PMLE than for instance in other photodermatoses like actinic prurigo.[7] Fitzpatrick skin type is described to influence the risk of developing PMLE. In a pan-European study of PMLE patients with skin types I to IV, PMLE had the highest prevalence in individuals with skin type I and the lowest prevalence in people with skin type IV.[6] However, a specific variant of PMLE (pinpoint papular variant) has been linked to the African American population of the northern states of the United States (Michigan)[11,12] and dark-skinned individuals in Asia (eg, Singapore, Taiwan, and India).[13,14]

CLINICAL FEATURES

CUTANEOUS FINDINGS

Within several hours to days, but usually not less than 30 minutes, after the first exposure to an intense dose of sunlight, usually in spring or early summer, itchy skin lesions of variable morphology appear on sun-exposed skin. Many patients also suffer from flares during summer holidays.[6] Once UV exposure ceases, all lesions gradually resolve fully without scarring over several days, occasionally taking 7 to 10 days. As summer progresses, following repetitive exposures to sunlight, many individuals show a hardening effect. Skin lesions are then less likely to occur or are less severe, permitting the individual to tolerate prolonged sun exposure. PMLE can also occur after recreational sunbed use. It is rare in winter except after extended outdoor recreational activities. Sufficient exposure may also occur through window glass. Sunburn is not mandatory for the development of a PMLE skin rash. Itching may be noted as the first sign of an impending PMLE eruption.

In any given patient, PMLE outbreaks tend to affect the same exposed sites. The distribution is generally symmetric. Only some areas of the exposed skin are usually affected and large areas may be spared. Particularly sun-exposed areas that are normally covered during winter such as the upper chest and the extensor aspects of the arms are most affected (Figs. 92-1 through 92-6). In contrast, the face and the hands of patients with PMLE are typically spared, presumably because of continuous natural hardening resulting from daily sun exposure.

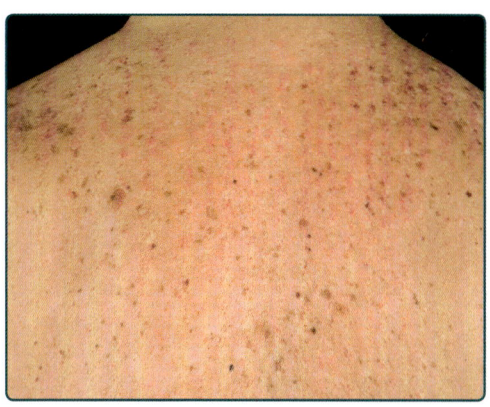

Figure 92-1 Macular polymorphic light eruption on the back of a middle-aged woman.

As the name of the condition implies, PMLE has many morphologic forms of skin lesions, all probably with similar pathogenesis and prognosis. The term *polymorphous* describes the variability in lesion morphology observed among different patients with the eruption. In general, in an individual patient the lesions are usually quite monomorphous. Macular, papular, papulovesicular, vesiculobullous, urticarial, plaque, insect bite, and erythema multiforme–like forms have been described (see Figs. 92-1 to 92-6). The papular form, characterized by large or small separate or confluent erythematous and edematous papules that may form clusters, is most common. Papulovesicular and plaque variants occur less frequently, and the other forms are rare. A pinpoint papular variant (Fig. 92-7) of PMLE has been described in people with skin phototypes IV to VI, which is characterized by the development of very small papules on sun-exposed areas, including the face.[15] The existence of a localized variant of PMLE, with erythematous–edematous papules and plaques, located on both elbows, has been suggested.[16] Another potential localized subtype of PMLE may be juvenile spring eruption,[17] which tends to affect boys in the spring and is characterized by pruritic papules and vesicles on their ear helices (Fig. 92-8), although typical features of PMLE sometimes coexist. Another potential rare variant of PMLE with manifestation predominantly on the lower legs is solar purpura (Fig. 92-9).[8] Benign summer light eruption and PMLE sine eruption, with extensive pruritus on sun-exposed skin but without visible skin changes are other potential variants of PMLE.[18,19]

CAUSING WAVEBANDS

UVA radiation (320 to 400 nm) usually seems more causative than UVB (290 to 320 nm) at initiating PMLE, but lesions also can be induced with UVB alone and sometimes with both waveband ranges.[8] Even visible light may be responsible on rare occasions.[20] The role of UVA in triggering the eruption is substantiated by phototest findings and the observation that most patients with PMLE exhibit sensitivity to sunlight through window glass,[8] and by the lack of protection from pure UVB-absorbing sunscreens.[21] As a result, paradoxically, some patients may note that the use of sunscreens, which tend preferentially to remove UVB while transmitting some UVA and all visible light, may have a PMLE-enhancing effect if exposure times are lengthened.

NONCUTANEOUS FINDINGS

Systemic symptoms in PMLE are rare, but headache, fever, chills, malaise, and nausea may occur.[7,22] These systemic symptoms may result from UV-induced release of cytokines with pyrogenic activity related to an accompanying sunburn reaction.[23,24]

COMPLICATIONS

Patients with PMLE may experience significant disease-related psychosocial morbidity. The rate of both anxiety and depression in patients with PMLE are twice that of the general population, and these rates are similar to those observed in patients with psoriasis and atopic dermatitis.[25] A shared pathogenesis for lupus erythematosus and PMLE has been suggested.[26-28] PMLE lesions may precede the development of lupus,[27] and progression of PMLE to lupus has been proposed in some cases, but long-term followup studies have not shown a general increased rate of lupus in PMLE patients.[29,30] A resistance to UV-induced immune suppression in PMLE may be responsible for the photoaggravation of other diseases, such as coexisting psoriasis, commonly responding beneficial to UV radiation from sunlight or artificial sources.[31] In an epidemiologic study, 43% of all patients suffering from photosensitive psoriasis were concluded to have a history of PMLE with secondary exacerbation of psoriatic lesions.[32] PMLE patients with coexisting psoriasis may not experience the beneficial antipsoriatic effects of UV, but rather induction and/or worsening of psoriatic disease after UV exposure. UV radiation may induce innate immunity in these patients, resulting in psoriatic lesions when there is simultaneous resistance against UV-induced suppression of the adaptive immune response (like in PMLE) that would otherwise counteract.[31]

ETIOLOGY AND PATHOGENESIS

IMMUNOLOGIC ASPECTS

The exact etiology and pathogenesis of PMLE are unknown, but a resistance to UV-induced immune suppression and a subsequent delayed-type hyper-

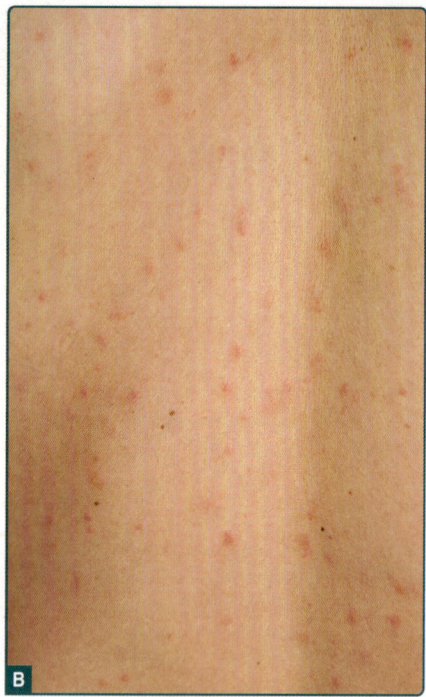
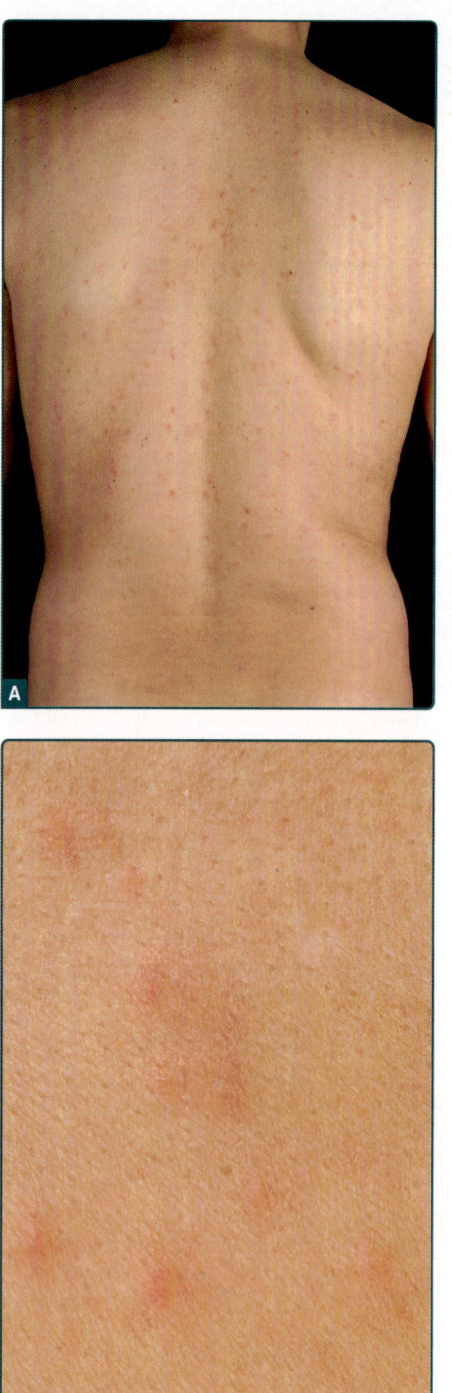

Figure 92-2 Maculopapular polymorphic light eruption on the back of a young man undergoing ultraviolet B broadband hardening after several exposures. **A,** Overview image. **B** and **C,** Details of lesions.

sensitivity response to UV-modified elements of the skin have been suggested.[8] A photoallergic response to a sunlight-induced antigen in the skin was first suggested in 1942.[2] Histologic features with an initial influx of CD4+ T lymphocytes for up to 72 hours in early PMLE lesions, followed by CD8+ T cells in established lesions, are consistent with a cellular-mediated immune response.[4] Increased numbers of Langerhans cells and dermal macrophages are also present in lesions of PMLE. An immunologic basis of the pathophysiology of the disease is also supported by immunohistologic findings, showing similarities to delayed-type hypersensitivity in the expression of adhesion molecules, comparing UVB-induced ery-

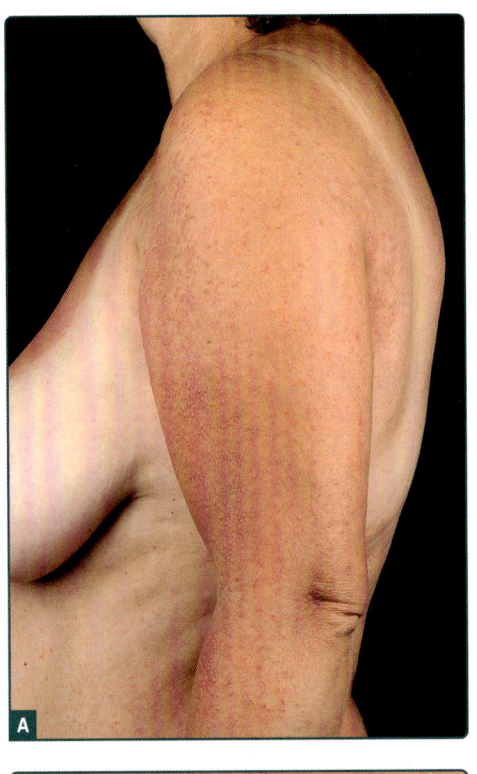
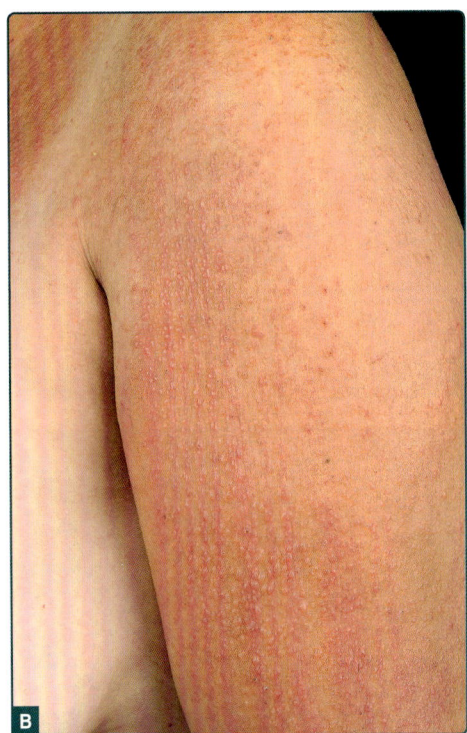
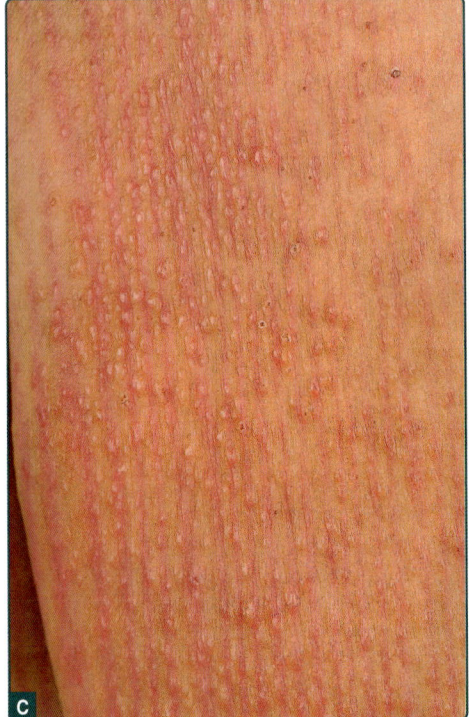

Figure 92-3 Papular polymorphic light eruption in a young woman on the trunk and arms. **A,** Overview image. **B** and **C,** Details of lesions.

thema, delayed-type hypersensitivity response, and PMLE lesions.[33,34]

UVB irradiation of the skin modifies cellular organic molecules such as proteins and DNA, creating antigens that the immune system may recognize as foreign and that may provoke (auto)immunoreactivity.[35,36] Such adverse immune reactions are prevented in UV-exposed healthy skin by the immunosuppressive properties of UV radiation, inducing an immunosuppressive Th2 micromilieu in UV-exposed healthy skin,

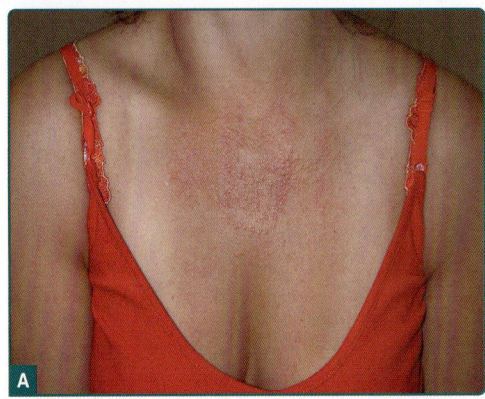
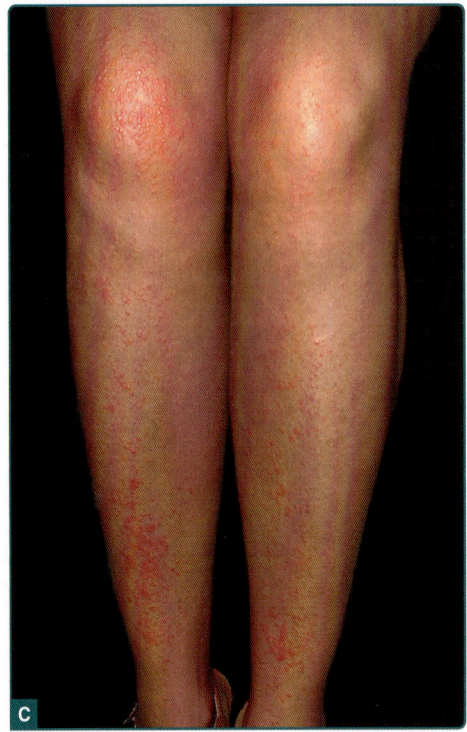
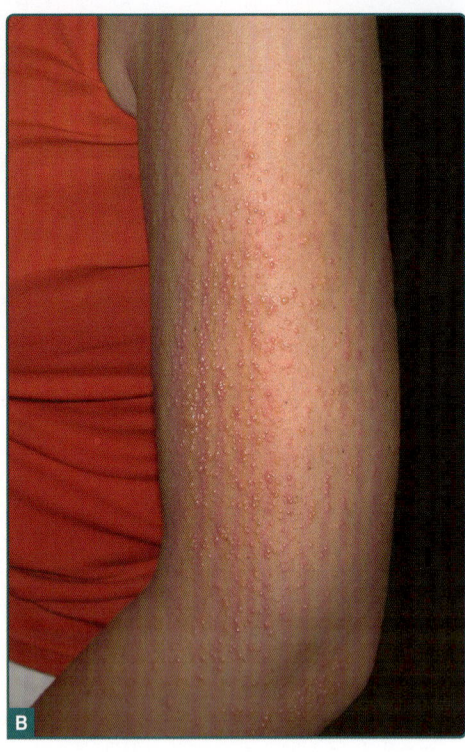

Figure 92-4 Papulovesicular polymorphic light eruption in a young woman on the trunk and extremities. Typical lesions (**A**) in the V-neck, (**B**) on the left arm, and (**C**) on the extensor sites of the legs.

accompanied by depletion of epidermal Langerhans cells,[37] neutrophilic infiltration, and the release of immunosuppressive cytokines, including interleukin (IL)-4 and IL-10.[38,39] Immune suppression after UV exposure is clinically demonstrated in studies, showing suppression of the induction of contact hypersensitivity in UV-exposed healthy skin and the induction of hapten-specific tolerance.[40-42]

However, in models of contact hypersensitivity, patients with PMLE show a resistance to UV-induced immune suppression, favoring immune response to potential UV-induced antigens under certain circumstances.[43,44] Additionally, the UV-induced tolerance to a contact allergen is impaired in PMLE.[45] On the other hand, the elicitation phase of allergic contact responses to dinitrochlorobenzene in previously sensitized PMLE patients and normal persons were equally suppressed by UV irradiation.[46]

Whereas an immunosuppressive Th2 cytokine (IL4+, IL10+) milieu is induced in normal skin following irradiation, in patients with PMLE a Th1 cytokine profile is favored.[47] In UV-exposed PMLE skin cell migration is deficient, with persistence of CD1a+ Langerhans cells[48] and impaired neutrophilic infiltration,[47,49] leading to reduced IL-4 and IL-10 release. It is thought that this creates an environment in which hypersensitivity responses to 1 or more photoinduced antigens are permissible. Photohardening therapy or desensitization, a frequently performed therapeutic approach in PMLE, is said to work by restoring the impaired UV-induced Langerhans cells depletion and neutrophil influx in PMLE.[50]

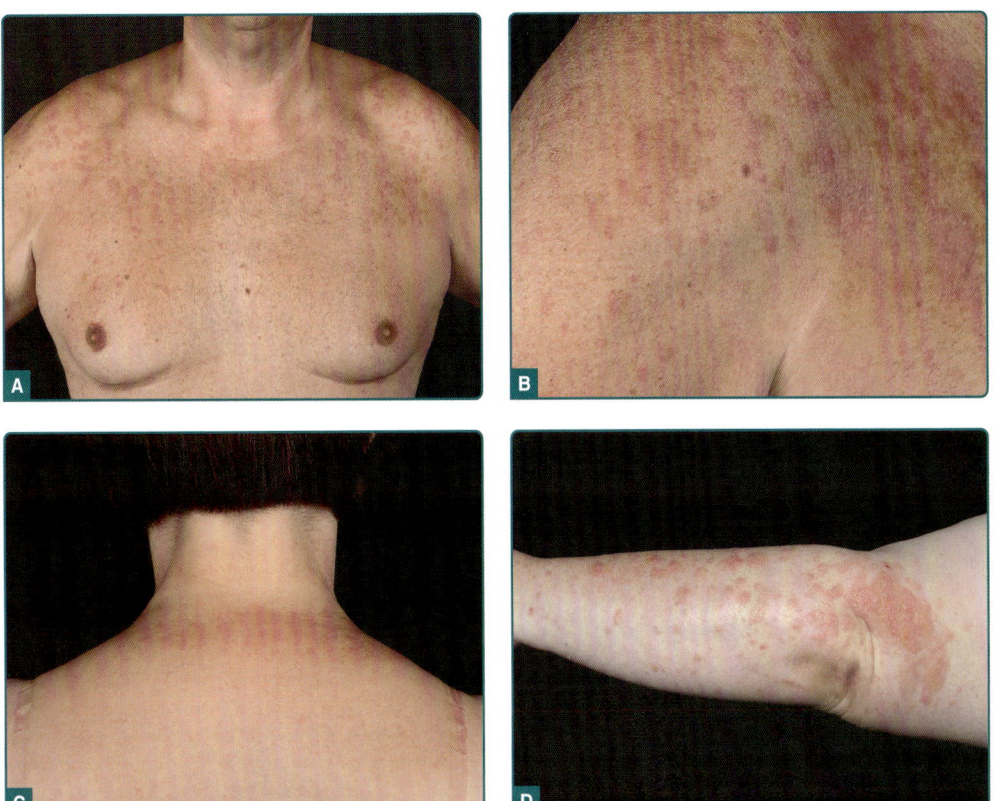

Figure 92-5 Plaque type of polymorphic light eruption (PMLE). **A,** Typical urticarial plaques and papules on the chest and shoulders occurring during a summer holiday in a young man. **B,** Detail of these lesions. **C,** Band-like PMLE lesions on the sun-exposed neck of a young woman. **D,** Elevated thick plaques on the sun-exposed extensor site of the arm in another woman. Note the involvement of the elbow.

Additionally, the impaired neutrophil responsiveness to chemoattractants in PMLE was found to be restored after photohardening.[51] Overall, abnormal baseline levels of proinflammatory cytokines, such as IL-1 family members, have been reported in PMLE.[52,53]

POSSIBLE PHOTOANTIGENS

The suggested photo-induced skin antigens that initiate PMLE have not been identified, but evidence for the existence of these antigens comes from experiments, in which UV-irradiated epidermal cells derived from the skin of PMLE patients stimulated strongly autologous peripheral blood mononuclear cells, suggesting that an immune-sensitizing agent is induced by UV exposure in PMLE skin.[54] As a possible photoantigen, expression of heat shock protein (HSP65), related to autoimmune processes such as lupus erythematosus, is described in experimentally induced PMLE lesions.[55] A recent study described a genetic deficiency in clearing apoptotic keratinocytes, resulting in a possible autoantigen source as well as altered immune function, both promoting PMLE.[56] Moreover, the hypothesis has been proposed, that microbial elements are the initial triggers of PMLE.[57] Direct UV-induced DNA damage to the microbiome[58] and a specific pattern of expression of antimicrobial peptides may be involved.[59]

RELATION TO SKIN CARCINOGENESIS

Skin cancer patients show a higher susceptibility to the immunosuppressive effects of UV radiation as a potential risk factor for skin cancer.[42] Consistent with the reported resistance to UV-induced immune suppression in PMLE, its prevalence has been found to be lower in patients with skin cancer.[60] In addition, a trend for decreased skin cancer prevalence was observed in PMLE patients compared to matched controls.[60] Together, this makes PMLE a potential skin cancer protective condition.

GENETICS

Genetic factors seem to play a role in PMLE, as a polygenic model indicated PMLE inheritance.[61,62] Familial

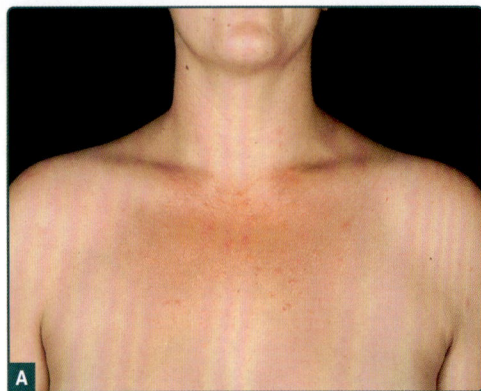

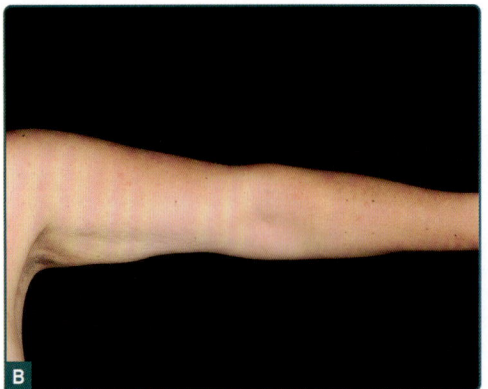

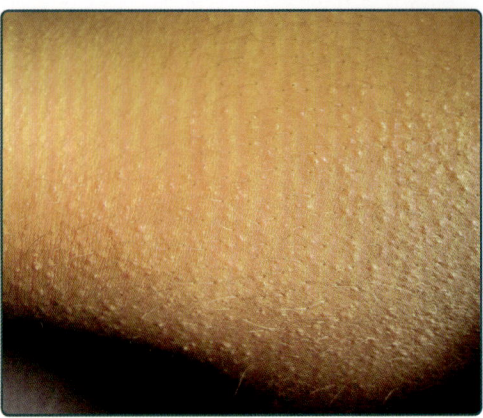

Figure 92-7 Pinpoint variant of PMLE in dark skin. (Used with permission from Henry W. Lim, MD. Department of Dermatology, Henry Ford Hospital, Detroit, Michigan, USA.)

HORMONAL FACTORS

Regarding the disproportionate incidence observed in females, the role of hormonal factors was investigated. Compared to males, females are described to be relatively resistant to the immunosuppressive effects of UV radiation, requiring more than 3 times the amount to achieve the same level of immune

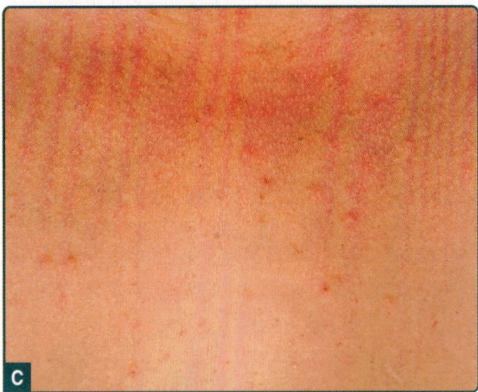

Figure 92-6 Insect bite polymorphic light eruption lesion in a young woman undergoing ultraviolet B 311-nm hardening therapy after a few exposures. **A,** Typical lesions in the V-neck and **(B)** on the arm. **C,** Detail of lesions. (Part A was taken from Gruber-Wackernagel A, Byrne S N, Wolf P. Polymorphous light eruption: clinic aspects and pathogenesis. *Dermatol Clin*. 2014;32:315-334, viii, Fig. 6. Copyright © Elsevier.)

clustering is evident as family history of PMLE in first-degree relatives is present in 12% of affected twins, compared with 4% in unaffected twins.[62] A positive family history is present in approximately 20% of patients.[61] Across the pedigrees of 23 PMLE patients a 21% prevalence of photosensitivity was observed among first-degree relatives.[61]

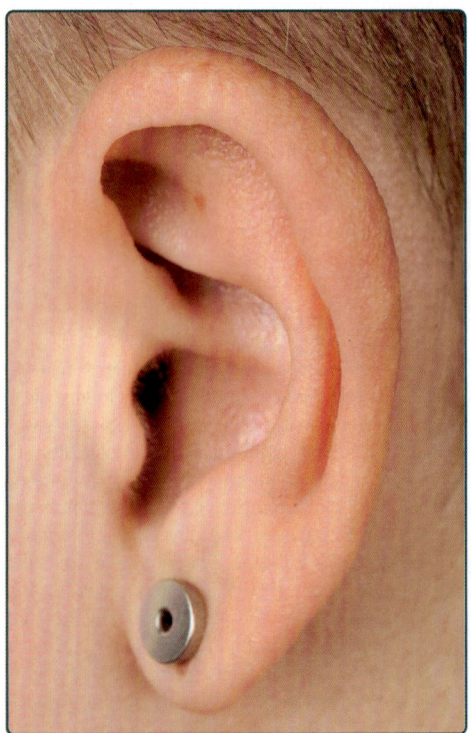

Figure 92-8 Juvenile spring eruption on the ear of a young boy.

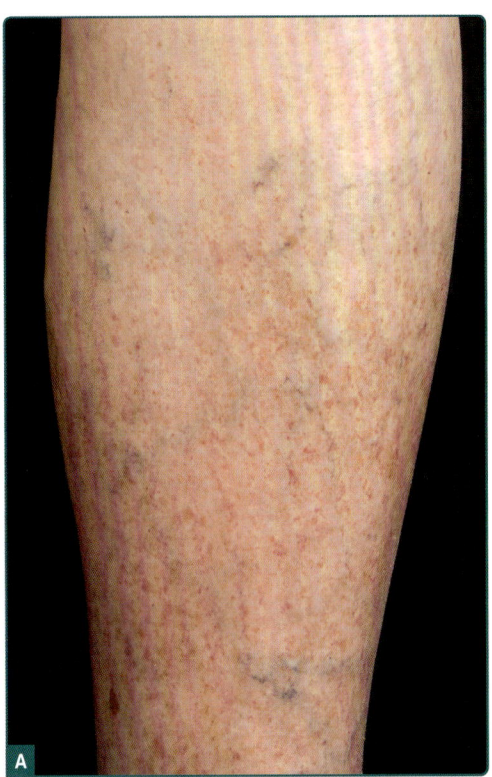
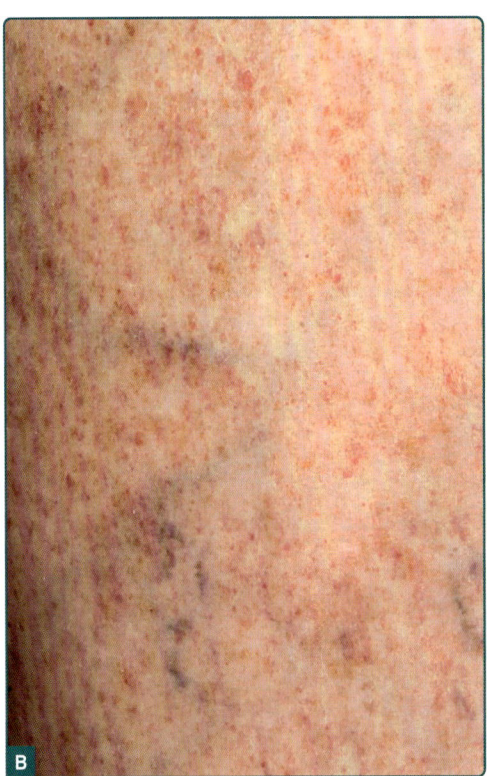

Figure 92-9 Purpura solaris on the extensor sites of a middle-aged woman. **A,** Overview image. **B,** Detail of lesions.

suppression as men.[63] This may explain the higher incidence of PMLE in women. The female hormone 17β-estradiol, which can prevent UV radiation-induced immune suppression by limiting the release of IL-10 from keratinocytes, is likely to be involved.[64,65] However, the role of oral hormonal contraceptives is controversial,[66,67] and there is no clear relationship between their use and PMLE.

ANTIMICROBIAL PEPTIDES

In addition to their potent antimicrobial activity, antimicrobial peptides, guarding the body environment interface as part of the innate immune system, can also modulate inflammatory and immune responses by modulating the production and release of cytokines and chemokines and the induction of regulatory T cells.[8] In PMLE, skin UV induction of antimicrobial peptides occurred in an atypical manner, with greater upregulation and altered expression of antimicrobial peptides, particularly in the early stages of the development of PMLE lesions.[68] Dysregulated expression of antimicrobial peptides such as cathelicidin peptide LL-37 following UV radiation may play a particular role in the described failure of immune suppression in PMLE.[31]

DIAGNOSIS

PATIENT HISTORY

An exact anamnesis, especially concerning the time of occurrence of skin rash after UV exposure, the persistence and the described morphology of skin lesions, and the affected body sites is a relevant diagnostic tool. Diagnostic criteria are the delayed occurrence of skin lesions after UV exposure (within hours to days, but not less than 30 minutes), the persistence of the skin lesions for several days (up to 10 days) and the monomorphous clinical presentation on predilection sites (Table 92-1).

TABLE 92-1
Diagnostic Criteria for Polymorphic Light Eruption

1. Delayed occurrence of skin lesions after ultraviolet (UV) exposure (within hours to days; but not <30 minutes).
2. Lesions persist for several days after exposure (up to 10 days after cessation of UV exposure).
3. *Monomorphous* clinical presentation on sites of predilection (upper chest, extensor arms, with sparing of the face and hands).

LABORATORY TESTING

Assessment for circulating antinuclear antibodies and antibodies against extractable nuclear antigens, including anti double-stranded DNA and anti-SSA/Ro or anti-SSB/La antibodies is advisable to exclude subacute cutaneous or other forms of lupus erythematosus. In one study, 11% of patients with PMLE were antinuclear antibody–positive, with the vast majority having insignificant titers of less than 1:160.[69] An even smaller fraction (less than 1%) of patients with PMLE had anti-Ro antibodies.[69] In certain cases, assessment of red blood cell protoporphyrins can help to exclude erythropoietic protoporphyria.

PATHOLOGY

The histologic features of PMLE are characteristic but not pathognomonic and they vary with clinical presentation.[70] There is generally a moderate to dense mixed perivascular infiltrate in the upper and mid dermis in all forms (Fig. 92-10). The infiltrate consists predominantly of T cells, with neutrophils and infrequent eosinophils. Other common features are papillary, dermal, and perivascular edema with endothelial cell swelling. Epidermal change, which is not always present, may include variable spongiosis and occasional dyskeratosis, exocytosis, and basal cell vacuolization.

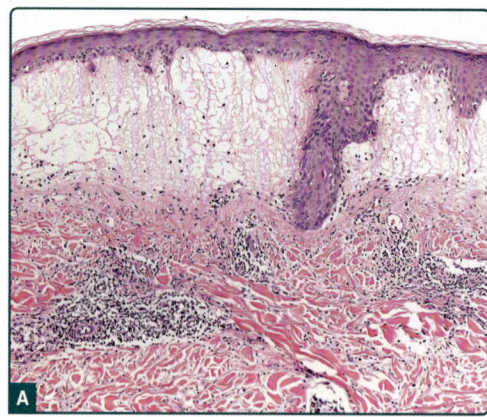
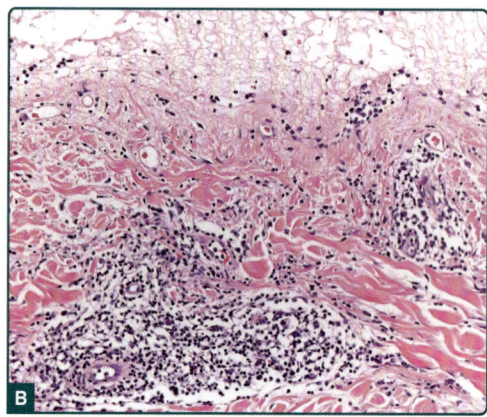

Figure 92-10 Histology of polymorphic light eruption. **A,** Hematoxylin and eosin staining shows a pronounced edema in the papillary dermis, leading to just beginning subepidermal vesiculation. **B,** Higher magnification illustrates rather dense, predominantly perivascular superficial mixed-cell infiltrates.

PHOTOTESTING AND PHOTOPROVOCATION

Patients with PMLE do not exhibit an abnormal sensitivity to develop (physiologic) erythema upon UV exposure. When tested for their UVB-induced or UVA-induced minimal erythema dose, they show normal values (Fig. 92-11). To confirm the diagnosis when the history and clinical features are not diagnostic, photoprovocation is performed in clinical practice to reproduce PMLE lesions, allowing also a subsequent skin biopsy. Repeated daily suberythemal exposures of the same skin area (at a predilection site) to UVA or UVB are necessary to provoke PMLE lesions in situ (Fig. 92-12).[71] In addition to the site of photoprovocation, the time of season of photoprovocation is critical. Photoprovocation is best performed before the beginning of the sunny summer season, preferentially in early spring, to avoid the false-negative results that may occur when the test is done too late in the season (ie, late spring or summer) because of tolerance induction through natural photohardening.[7] In general, the principles of photoprovocation are as follows: 2 symmetrically located test areas at predilection sites, preferably on previously involved skin, are exposed daily for 4 to 5 days to increasing suberythemal or near-erythemal doses of UVA or UVB radiation (or solar-simulated UV radiation). Depending on the method, PMLE lesions can be reproduced in 60% to 90% of affected subjects, most of them exhibiting sensitivity to UVA, and some to UVB or both wavebands.[7-9] Negative test areas of photoprovocation should be evaluated and monitored up to several weeks for a delayed eruption of possible lupus lesions, most often evolving 10 to 14 days after start of provocation. Additionally, phototesting can be performed with visible light (single irradiation of a single test area), in particular to exclude solar urticaria. Photopatch test can be used to exclude chronic actinic dermatitis or photoaggravated eczema.

DIAGNOSTIC ALGORITHM

Sometimes patients present with a manifested rash of skin lesions. Then primary diagnostic tools are patient history, clinical evaluation and in selected cases a skin biopsy. If the patient presents without (typical)

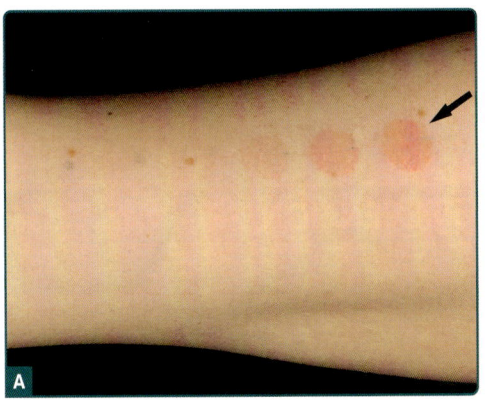
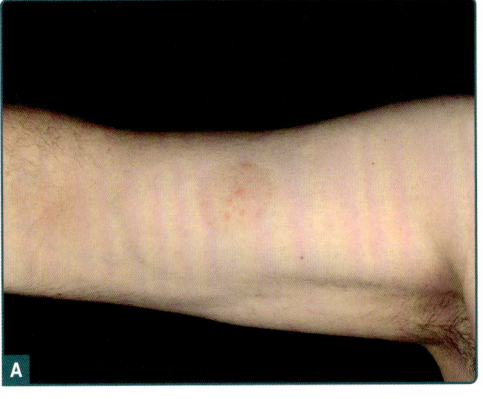
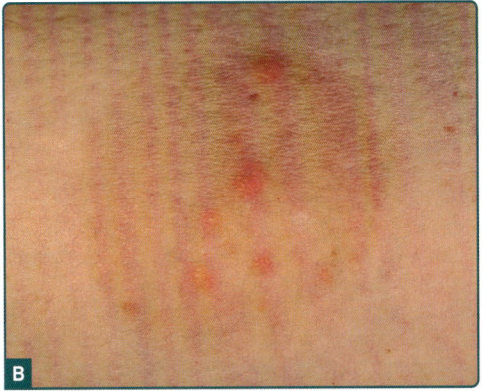
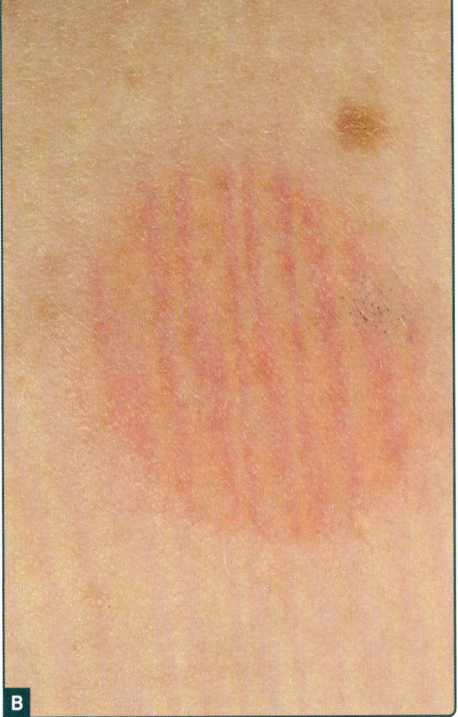

Figure 92-12 Positive photoprovocation result in a man with a history of recurrent sun-exposure–related skin rash. **A,** Typical papular lesions occurring after 4 days of suberythemal ultraviolet B exposure within the test field, clinically consistent with polymorphic light eruption. **B,** Detail of lesions.

Figure 92-11 A, Normal physiologic minimal erythema dose response in a polymorphic light eruption (PMLE) patient tested with an ultraviolet (UV) solar-simulated radiation ladder of 6 fields at 24 hours after exposure. Note the irregular dark erythematous small macules representing early PMLE lesions inside the erythematous test field exposed to the highest UV dose of the ladder (*arrow*). **B,** Detail of this test field. (Part A was taken from Gruber-Wackernagel A, Bambach I, Legat FJ, et al. Randomized double-blinded placebo-controlled intra-individual trial on topical treatment with a 1,25-dihydroxyvitamin D analogue in polymorphic light eruption. *Br J Dermatol.* 2011;165:152-163, Fig. 3. Used with permission. Copyright © 2011 John Wiley & Sons.)

skin rash, an exact patient history (concerning time of occurrence and persistence of skin lesions after UV exposure, morphology of skin lesions, and affected body sites) is most relevant and in many cases sufficient for diagnosis. In certain cases photoprovocation is needed, also allowing a skin biopsy if there is any doubt in the clinical diagnosis of eventually provoked lesions. In all cases of not unambiguous clinical diagnosis laboratory tests (antinuclear antibodies, extractable nuclear antigens) should be done.

DIFFERENTIAL DIAGNOSIS

Table 92-2 and Fig. 92-13 outline the most important differential diagnoses of PMLE and their characteristics.

Other photosensitive conditions can be usually differentiated from PMLE by clinical features and morphology of skin lesions. Mallorca acne (acne aestivalis), characterized by long-persisting acneiform, follicular papules on sun-exposed neck and shoulder belt area[72] may represent a separate entity (Fig. 92-14). This condition occurs within or follows a summer holiday with long and intensive sun exposure and sunscreen use. A link to the use of too oily vehicles of sunscreen has been suggested. Prurigo actinica shows prurigo lesions in chronic UV-exposed skin areas, mainly in the face, associated with cheilitis, most often starting in childhood. Whereas in childhood the disease shows a seasonal character, later in adulthood the lesions may persist perennially with occurrence also on nonexposed skin.[73] Hydroa vaccineforme usually is easily differentiated from PMLE by its early onset in childhood and intermittent occurrence of papulovesicular or bullous hemorrhagic skin lesions, which are most commonly located on the face, ears, and dorsum of the hands.[74,75] Residual vacciniform scarring is typical and association with Epstein-Barr virus has been reported in some cases.[74]

Persistent erythematous plaques, mostly on the face, may be lesions of lymphocytic infiltration (Jessner-Kanof).[76] Lymphocytic infiltration typically occurs on the cheeks and earlobes, but also on the neck and upper trunk or proximal extremities of men. Lesions persist for months or years, and can resolve spontaneously without treatment, but often recur. Whether this condition is a separate entity or identical with lupus tumidus is still a matter of debate. Other forms of lupus, such as chronic discoid lupus erythematosus, can usually be easy differentiated from PMLE by its clinical morphology.

Eczematous morphology of skin lesions is atypical for PMLE and rather refers to chronic actinic dermatitis or photoaggravated atopic dermatitis.[77] Chronic actinic dermatitis[78] or photoaggravated eczema can be usually excluded in the differential diagnosis of PMLE by typical lesion morphology, patient history, and results of (photo)patch testing. An exact patient history concerning drugs can be necessary in certain cases to exclude phototoxic or photoallergic drug eruption.

CLINICAL COURSE AND PROGNOSIS

PMLE is chronic in nature and in most affected patients the disease has a persistent course with a slow tendency to amelioration.[29,30] In a study with a followup time span of 7 years, 64 of 114 PMLE patients reported steadily diminishing sun sensitivity and 12 patients no further sun-precipitated rashes.[29] In another study, Hasan and colleagues found that after an average of 32 years after the onset of PMLE symptoms, 23 (24%) of 94 patients were considered cured, 48 (51%) reported alleviation of symptoms, and the remaining 23 (24%) had noticed equal or stronger symptoms than before.[30]

MANAGEMENT

PREVENTION/PROPHYLAXIS

Prophylaxis is an important therapeutic approach in PMLE, and mild cases respond well to basic photoprotective measures such as avoiding sun exposure, the use of broad-spectrum sunscreens with effective UVA protection capacity, and wearing protective clothing.[79] Whereas sunscreens with high UVA and UVB protection may prevent PMLE eruptions in photoprovocable patients,[80] sunscreens with moderate UVA protection are often ineffective. For instance, a sun protection factor 45 sunscreen with high UVA protection was able to protect most patients from the development of UV-provoked PMLE even at a low sunscreen concentration of 1 mg/cm^2.[81]

MEDICATIONS

After the eruption of PMLE lesions, topical steroids and, occasionally, oral antihistamines can be used to reduce inflammation, alleviate itch, and shorten the duration of the eruption.[7,8,82,83] Further PMLE treatment depends on the severity of the disease. Patients who have outbreaks only infrequently, such as on vacations, usually respond well to short courses of oral steroids that are prescribed to use in the event of an eruption.[84] If PMLE does develop, approximately 20 to 30 mg prednisone taken initially at the first sign of pruritus and then each morning at tapered doses until the eruption clears usually provides relief within several days, and recurrences are then uncommon during the same vacation. This treatment, if well tolerated, may be repeated safely. Alternatively, oral prednisolone also can be given prophylactically, starting 1 to 2 days before expected sun exposure to prevent flares, when patients go to sunny locations for vacation.

PHOTOHARDENING

More-severely affected individuals, who experience repeated attacks of PMLE throughout the summer, may require prophylactic medical photohardening courses each spring before the first intense sun exposure to prevent attacks. Broadband UVB (290 to 320 nm), narrowband UVB (311 nm), or psoralen plus UVA photochemotherapy are effective in photohardening of PMLE.[8] Phototherapy, usually given 2 to 3 times per week for 4 to 6 weeks with suberythemal doses, simulates the naturally occurring phenomenon of hardening and aims to induce photoadaption. Photochemotherapy appears to be more

TABLE 92-2
Most Important Clinical Differential Diagnoses of Polymorphic Light Eruption (Characteristics)

- Solar urticaria (occurrence of wheals at any sun-exposed body site within minutes after ultraviolet (UV) exposure and fading within hours)
- Lupus erythematosus, especially subacute cutaneous lupus erythematosus (delayed occurrence of skin lesions on exposed sites within 10-14 days or later after UV exposure and persisting for several weeks)
- Erythropoietic protoporphyria (painful skin redness and swelling within minutes of sun exposure starting in early childhood)
- Photoaggravated erythema multiforme (photodistributed erythema multiforme-like skin lesions, often associated with herpes simplex virus infection)

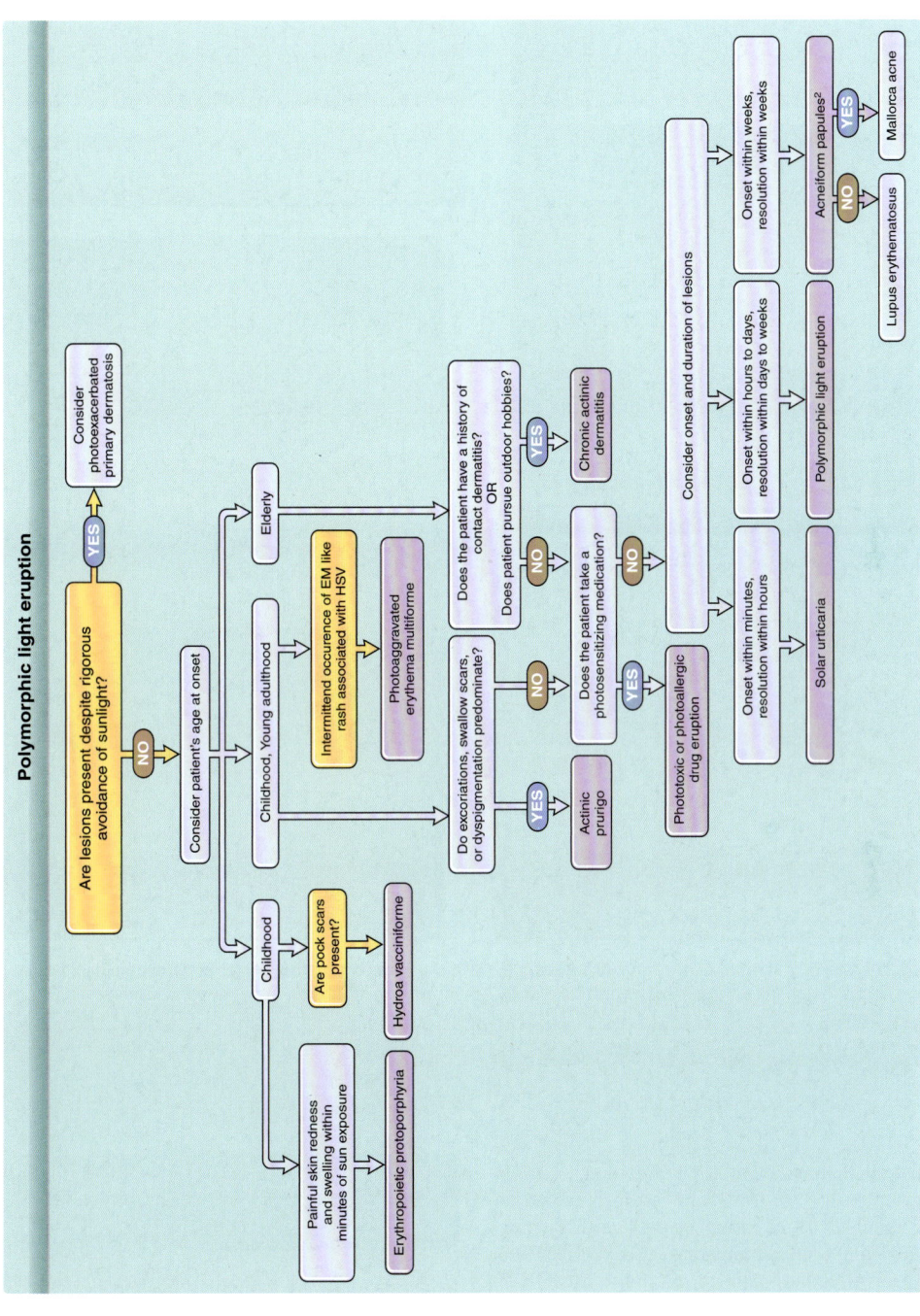

Figure 92-13 Algorithm of polymorphic light eruption diagnosis. HSV, herpes simplex virus.

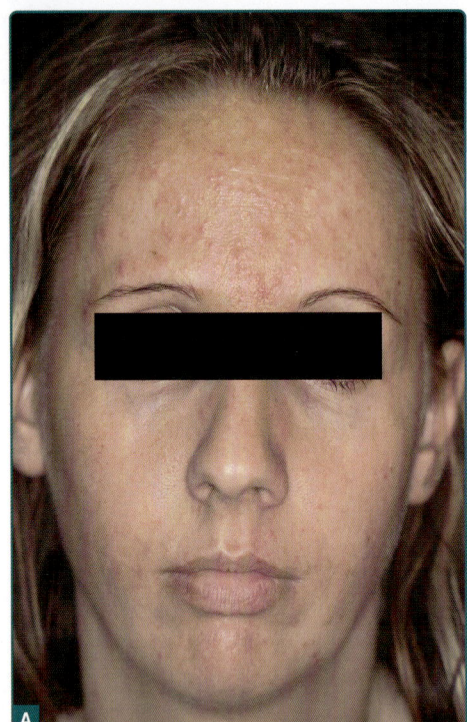
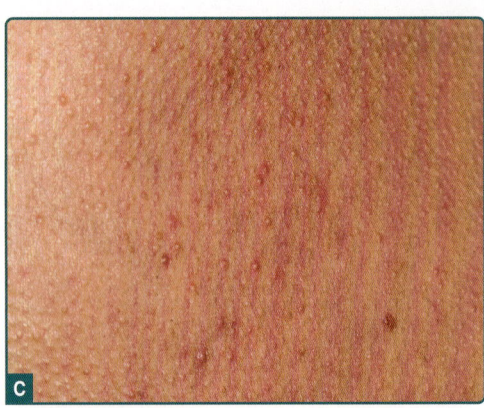
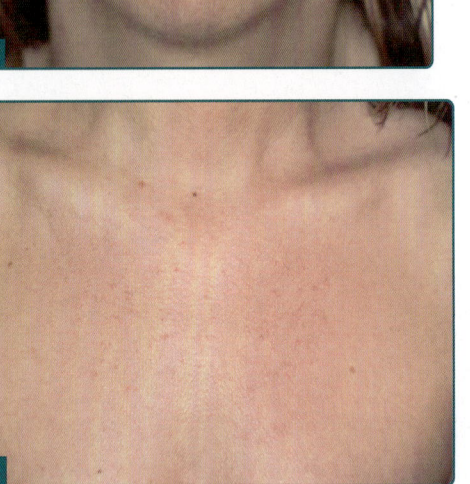
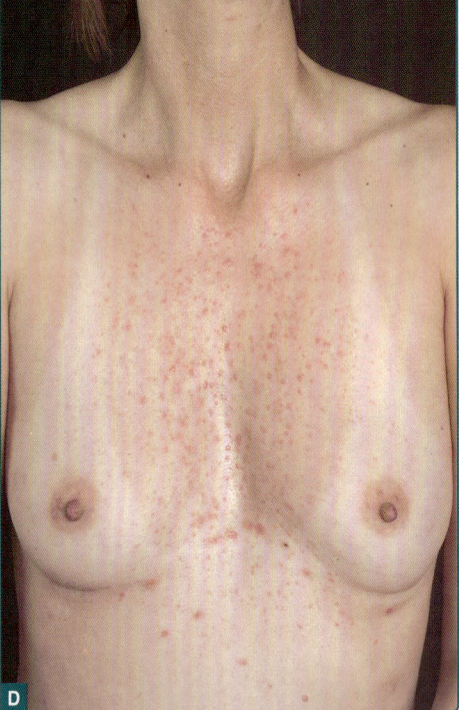

Figure 92-14 Mallorca acne. **A,** Acneiform skin lesions in the face of a young woman. **B,** Follicular papulopustular lesions in the V-neck of this patient. **C,** Higher magnification of **B**. **D,** Acneiform skin lesions on sun-exposed upper chest of another young woman.

effective than broadband UVB radiation, controlling symptoms in up to 90% of cases, compared to approximately 60% of cases,[85] respectively. Narrow-band (311-nm) UVB phototherapy, effective in 70% to 80% of cases, is the treatment of choice because of ease of administration.[86] The mechanisms underlying the photohardening effect include melanization in the skin, thickening of the stratum corneum, and restoration of immunologic susceptibility,[87-89] especially the impaired UV-induced Langerhans cells depletion, neutrophil infiltration,[50] and neutrophil responsiveness to chemoattractants.[51]

TREATMENTS FOR SEVERE CASES

In cases with severe symptoms, treatment can involve administration of azathioprin,[90] thalidomide,[91] or antimalarials, such as choloroquine or hydroxychloroquine, with immunomodulatory and antiinflammatory properties.[92-94] Efficacy of immune suppressive therapy in PMLE is consistent with the observation of reduced prevalence of PMLE in iatrogenically immunosuppressed individuals.[95]

EXPERIMENTAL APPROACHES

Oral administration of supplements (containing lycopene, beta-carotene, and *Lactobacillus johnsonii*) or extracts (*Polypodium leucotomos*, a natural extract from tropical fern leaves) with antioxidant and anti-inflammatory effects have been described to prevent eruption of PMLE and diminish PMLE symptoms.[96-98] Topical application of DNA repair enzymes incorporated in an after-sun lotion diminished PMLE symptoms in an experimental study,[99] possibly by enhancing removal of UV-induced DNA photoproducts as an antigenic immune trigger in UV-exposed PMLE skin.

ACKNOWLEDGMENTS

The current authors (Alexandra Gruber-Wackernagel and Peter Wolf) are grateful to Travis W. Vandergriff and Paul R. Bergstresser as authors of this chapter in the previous edition for leaving behind an outstanding framework that they employed as their starting point for this updated edition. The authors thank Helmut Kerl for advice and help in histology, Angelika Hofer and Franz J. Legat for support in identifying clinical images, and Werner Stieber for professional support in preparing the illustrations of this chapter.

REFERENCES

1. Sellei J, Liebner E. Über Prurigo aestivalis. *Arch Dermatol Syph*. 1926;152:19-33.
2. Epstein S. Studies in abnormal human sensitivity to light. IV. Photoallergic concept of prurigo aestivalis. *J Invest Dermatol*. 1942;5:289-298.
3. Moncada B, Gonzalez-Amaro R, Baranda ML, et al. Immunopathology of polymorphous light eruption. T lymphocytes in blood and skin. *J Am Acad Dermatol*. 1984;10(6):970-973.
4. Norris PG, Morris J, McGibbon DM, et al. Polymorphic light eruption: an immunopathological study of evolving lesions. *Br J Dermatol*. 1989;120(2):173-183.
5. Pao C, Norris PG, Corbett M, et al. Polymorphic light eruption: prevalence in Australia and England. *Br J Dermatol*. 1994;130(1):62-64.
6. Rhodes LE, Bock M, Janssens AS, et al. Polymorphic light eruption occurs in 18% of Europeans and does not show higher prevalence with increasing latitude: multicenter survey of 6,895 individuals residing from the Mediterranean to Scandinavia. *J Invest Dermatol*. 2010;130(2):626-628.
7. Stratigos AJ, Antoniou C, Katsambas AD. Polymorphous light eruption. *J Eur Acad Dermatol Venereol*. 2002;16(3):193-206.
8. Gruber-Wackernagel A, Byrne SN, Wolf P. Polymorphous light eruption: clinic aspects and pathogenesis. *Dermatol Clin*. 2014;32(3):315-334, viii.
9. Gruber-Wackernagel A, Byrne SN, Wolf P. Pathogenic mechanisms of polymorphic light eruption. *Front Biosci (Elite Ed)*. 2009;1:341-354.
10. Wolf P, Byrne SN, Gruber-Wackernagel A. New insights into the mechanisms of polymorphic light eruption: resistance to ultraviolet radiation-induced immune suppression as an aetiological factor. *Exp Dermatol*. 2009;18(4):350-356.
11. Kerr HA, Lim HW. Photodermatoses in African Americans: a retrospective analysis of 135 patients over a 7-year period. *J Am Acad Dermatol*. 2007;57(4):638-643.
12. Nakamura M, Henderson M, Jacobsen G, et al. Comparison of photodermatoses in African-Americans and Caucasians: a follow-up study. *Photodermatol Photoimmunol Photomed*. 2014;30(5):231-236.
13. Wadhwani AR, Sharma VK, Ramam M, et al. A clinical study of the spectrum of photodermatoses in dark-skinned populations. *Clin Exp Dermatol*. 2013;38(8):823-829.
14. Chiam LY, Chong WS. Pinpoint papular polymorphous light eruption in Asian skin: a variant in darker-skinned individuals. *Photodermatol Photoimmunol Photomed*. 2009;25(2):71-74.
15. Isedeh P, Lim HW. Polymorphic light eruption presenting as pinhead papular eruption on the face. *J Drugs Dermatol*. 2013;12(11):1285-1286.
16. Molina-Ruiz AM, Sanmartin O, Santonja C, et al. Spring and summer eruption of the elbows: a peculiar localized variant of polymorphous light eruption. *J Am Acad Dermatol*. 2013;68(2):306-312.
17. Hawk J. Juvenile spring eruption is a variant of polymorphic light eruption. *N Z Med J*. 1996;109(1031):389.
18. Guarrera M, Cardo P, Rebora AE, et al. Polymorphic light eruption and benign summer light eruption in Italy. *Photodermatol Photoimmunol Photomed*. 2011;27(1):35-39.
19. Dover JS, Hawk JL. Polymorphic light eruption sine eruption. *Br J Dermatol*. 1988;118(1):73-76.
20. Piletta PA, Salomon D, Beani JC, et al. A pilot with an itchy rash. *Lancet*. 1996;348(9035):1142.
21. Diffey BL, Farr PM. An evaluation of sunscreens in patients with broad action-spectrum photosensitivity. *Br J Dermatol*. 1985;112(1):83-86.
22. Jansen CT. Heredity of chronic polymorphous light eruptions. *Arch Dermatol*. 1978;114(2):188-190.
23. Granstein RD, Sauder DN. Whole-body exposure to ultraviolet radiation results in increased serum interleukin-1 activity in humans. *Lymphokine Res*. 1987;6(3):187-193.
24. Urbanski A, Schwarz T, Neuner P, et al. Ultraviolet light induces increased circulating interleukin-6 in humans. *J Invest Dermatol*. 1990;94(6):808-811.
25. Richards HL, Ling TC, Evangelou G, et al. Evidence of high levels of anxiety and depression in polymorphic light eruption and their association with clinical and demographic variables. *Br J Dermatol*. 2008;159(2):439-444.
26. Petzelbauer P, Binder M, Nikolakis P, et al. Severe sun sensitivity and the presence of antinuclear antibodies in patients with polymorphous light eruption-like lesions. A form fruste of photosensitive lupus erythematosus? *J Am Acad Dermatol*. 1992;26(1):68-74.
27. Nyberg F, Hasan T, Puska P, et al. Occurrence of polymorphous light eruption in lupus erythematosus. *Br J Dermatol*. 1997;136(2):217-221.
28. Millard TP, Lewis CM, Khamashta MA, et al. Familial clustering of polymorphic light eruption in relatives of patients with lupus erythematosus:

evidence of a shared pathogenesis. *Br J Dermatol*. 2001; 144(2):334-338.
29. Jansen CT, Karvonen J. Polymorphous light eruption. A seven-year follow-up evaluation of 114 patients. *Arch Dermatol*. 1984;120(7):862-865.
30. Hasan T, Ranki A, Jansen CT, et al. Disease associations in polymorphous light eruption. A long-term follow-up study of 94 patients. *Arch Dermatol*. 1998; 134(9):1081-1085.
31. Wolf P, Weger W, Patra V, et al. Desired response to phototherapy versus photo-aggravation in psoriasis: what makes the difference? *Exp Dermatol*. 2016; 25(12):937-944.
32. Ros AM, Eklund G. Photosensitive psoriasis. An epidemiologic study. *J Am Acad Dermatol*. 1987;17(5, pt 1): 752-758.
33. Norris PG, Barker JN, Allen MH, et al. Adhesion molecule expression in polymorphic light eruption. *J Invest Dermatol*. 1992;99(4):504-508.
34. Norris P, Poston RN, Thomas DS, et al. The expression of endothelial leukocyte adhesion molecule-1 (ELAM-1), intercellular adhesion molecule-1 (ICAM-1), and vascular cell adhesion molecule-1 (VCAM-1) in experimental cutaneous inflammation: a comparison of ultraviolet B erythema and delayed hypersensitivity. *J Invest Dermatol*. 1991;96(5):763-770.
35. de Gruijl FR. Health effects from solar UV radiation. *Radiat Prot Dosimetry*. 1997;72:177-196.
36. Jung EG, Bohnert E, Krutmann J, et al. *Photobiology of Ultraviolet Induced DNA Damage*. Vol 3. Cambridge, UK: Cambridge University Press; 1995.
37. Kolgen W, Both H, van Weelden H, et al. Epidermal Langerhans cell depletion after artificial ultraviolet B irradiation of human skin in vivo: apoptosis versus migration. *J Invest Dermatol*. 2002;118(5): 812-817.
38. Teunissen MB, Piskin G, di Nuzzo S, et al. Ultraviolet B radiation induces a transient appearance of IL-4+ neutrophils, which support the development of Th2 responses. *J Immunol*. 2002;168(8):3732-3739.
39. Piskin G, Bos JD, Teunissen MB. Neutrophils infiltrating ultraviolet B-irradiated normal human skin display high IL-10 expression. *Arch Dermatol Res*. 2005;296(7):339-342.
40. Cooper KD, Oberhelman L, Hamilton TA, et al. UV exposure reduces immunization rates and promotes tolerance to epicutaneous antigens in humans: relationship to dose, CD1a-DR+ epidermal macrophage induction, and Langerhans cell depletion. *Proc Natl Acad Sci U S A*. 1992;89(18):8497-8501.
41. Cooper KD. Cell-mediated immunosuppressive mechanisms induced by UV radiation. *Photochem Photobiol*. 1996;63(4):400-406.
42. Yoshikawa T, Rae V, Bruins-Slot W, et al. Susceptibility to effects of UVB radiation on induction of contact hypersensitivity as a risk factor for skin cancer in humans. *J Invest Dermatol*. 1990;95(5):530-536.
43. Palmer RA, Friedmann PS. Ultraviolet radiation causes less immunosuppression in patients with polymorphic light eruption than in controls. *J Invest Dermatol*. 2004;122(2):291-294.
44. van de Pas CB, Kelly DA, Seed PT, et al. Ultraviolet-radiation-induced erythema and suppression of contact hypersensitivity responses in patients with polymorphic light eruption. *J Invest Dermatol*. 2004; 122(2):295-299.
45. Koulu LM, Laihia JK, Peltoniemi HH, et al. UV-induced tolerance to a contact allergen is impaired in polymorphic light eruption. *J Invest Dermatol*. 2010; 130(11):2578-2582.
46. Palmer RA, Hawk JL, Young AR, et al. The effect of solar-simulated radiation on the elicitation phase of contact hypersensitivity does not differ between controls and patients with polymorphic light eruption. *J Invest Dermatol*. 2005;124(6):1308-1312.
47. Kolgen W, van Meurs M, Jongsma M, et al. Differential expression of cytokines in UV-B-exposed skin of patients with polymorphous light eruption: correlation with Langerhans cell migration and immunosuppression. *Arch Dermatol*. 2004;140(3): 295-302.
48. Kolgen W, Van Weelden H, Den Hengst S, et al. CD11b+ cells and ultraviolet-B-resistant CD1a+ cells in skin of patients with polymorphous light eruption. *J Invest Dermatol*. 1999;113(1):4-10.
49. Schornagel IJ, Sigurdsson V, Nijhuis EH, et al. Decreased neutrophil skin infiltration after UVB exposure in patients with polymorphous light eruption. *J Invest Dermatol*. 2004;123(1):202-206.
50. Janssens AS, Pavel S, Out-Luiting JJ, et al. Normalized ultraviolet (UV) induction of Langerhans cell depletion and neutrophil infiltrates after artificial UVB hardening of patients with polymorphic light eruption. *Br J Dermatol*. 2005;152(6):1268-1274.
51. Gruber-Wackernagel A, Heinemann A, Konya V, et al. Photohardening restores the impaired neutrophil responsiveness to chemoattractants leukotriene B4 and formyl-methionyl-leucyl-phenylalanin in patients with polymorphic light eruption. *Exp Dermatol*. 2011; 20(6):473-476.
52. Wolf P, Gruber-Wackernagel A, Rinner B, et al. Phototherapeutic hardening modulates systemic cytokine levels in patients with polymorphic light eruption. *Photochem Photobiol Sci*. 2013;12(1):166-173.
53. Lembo S, Caiazzo G, Balato N, et al. Polymorphic light eruption and IL-1 family members: any difference with allergic contact dermatitis? *Photochem Photobiol Sci*. 2017;16(9):1471-1479.
54. Gonzalez-Amaro R, Baranda L, Salazar-Gonzalez JF, et al. Immune sensitization against epidermal antigens in polymorphous light eruption. *J Am Acad Dermatol*. 1991;24(1):70-73.
55. McFadden JP, Norris PG, Cerio R, et al. Heat shock protein 65 immunoreactivity in experimentally induced polymorphic light eruption. *Acta Derm Venereol*. 1994;74(4):283-285.
56. Lembo S, Hawk JL, Murphy GM, et al. Aberrant gene expression with deficient apoptotic keratinocyte clearance may predispose to polymorphic light eruption. *Br J Dermatol*. 2017;177(5):1450-1453.
57. Patra V, Wolf P. Microbial elements as the initial triggers in the pathogenesis of polymorphic light eruption? *Exp Dermatol*. 2016;25(12):999-1001.
58. Patra V, Byrne SN, Wolf P. The skin microbiome: is it affected by UV-induced immune suppression? *Front Microbiol*. 2016;7:1235.
59. Patra V, Mayer G, Gruber-Wackernagel A, et al. Unique profile of antimicrobial peptide expression in polymorphic light eruption lesions compared to healthy skin, atopic dermatitis, and psoriasis. *Photodermatol Photoimmunol Photomed*. 2018;34(2):137-144.
60. Lembo S, Fallon J, O'Kelly P, et al. Polymorphic light eruption and skin cancer prevalence: is one protective against the other? *Br J Dermatol*. 2008; 159(6):1342-1347.

61. McGregor JM, Grabczynska S, Vaughan R, et al. Genetic modeling of abnormal photosensitivity in families with polymorphic light eruption and actinic prurigo. *J Invest Dermatol.* 2000;115(3):471-476.
62. Millard TP, Bataille V, Snieder H, et al. The heritability of polymorphic light eruption. *J Invest Dermatol.* 2000;115(3):467-470.
63. Damian DL, Patterson CR, Stapelberg M, et al. UV radiation-induced immunosuppression is greater in men and prevented by topical nicotinamide. *J Invest Dermatol.* 2008;128(2):447-454.
64. Aubin F. Why is polymorphous light eruption so common in young women? *Arch Dermatol Res.* 2004; 296(5):240-241.
65. Hiramoto K, Tanaka H, Yanagihara N, et al. Effect of 17beta-estradiol on immunosuppression induced by ultraviolet B irradiation. *Arch Dermatol Res.* 2004; 295(8-9):307-311.
66. Mentens G, Lambert J, Nijsten T. Polymorphic light eruption may be associated with cigarette smoking and alcohol consumption. *Photodermatol Photoimmunol Photomed.* 2006;22(2):87-92.
67. Neumann R. Polymorphous light eruption and oral contraceptives. *Photodermatol.* 1988;5(1):40-42.
68. Felton S, Navid F, Schwarz A, et al. Ultraviolet radiation-induced upregulation of antimicrobial proteins in health and disease. *Photochem Photobiol Sci.* 2013;12(1):29-36.
69. Tzaneva S, Volc-Platzer B, Kittler H, et al. Antinuclear antibodies in patients with polymorphic light eruption: a long-term follow-up study. *Br J Dermatol.* 2008;158(5):1050-1054.
70. Hawk JL. The photosensitive disorders. In: Elder DE, Johnson B Jr, Elenitsas R, et al, eds. *Lever's Histopathology of the Skin*. 9th ed. Baltimore, MD: Lippincott Williams & Wilkins; 2005.
71. Epstein JH. Polymorphic light eruptions; phototest technique studies. *Arch Dermatol.* 1962;85:502-504.
72. Hjorth N, Sjolin KE, Sylvest B, et al. Acne aestivalis—Mallorca acne. *Acta Derm Venereol.* 1972;52(1):61-63.
73. Grabczynska SA, McGregor JM, Kondeatis E, et al. Actinic prurigo and polymorphic light eruption: common pathogenesis and the importance of HLA-DR4/DRB1*0407. *Br J Dermatol.* 1999;140(2): 232-236.
74. Cho KH, Kim CW, Heo DS, et al. Epstein-Barr virus-associated peripheral T-cell lymphoma in adults with hydroa vacciniforme-like lesions. *Clin Exp Dermatol.* 2001;26(3):242-247.
75. Sonnex TS, Hawk JL. Hydroa vacciniforme: a review of ten cases. *Br J Dermatol.* 1988;118(1):101-108.
76. Kaatz M, Zelger B, Norgauer J, et al. Lymphocytic infiltration (Jessner-Kanof): lupus erythematosus tumidus or a manifestation of borreliosis? *Br J Dermatol.* 2007;157(2):403-405.
77. O'Gorman SM, Murphy GM. Photoaggravated disorders. *Dermatol Clin.* 2014;32(3):385-398, ix.
78. Lim HW, Paek SY. Photodermatology. *Dermatol Clin.* 2014;32(3):xiii.
79. Fesq H, Ring J, Abeck D. Management of polymorphous light eruption: clinical course, pathogenesis, diagnosis and intervention. *Am J Clin Dermatol.* 2003;4(6):399-406.
80. Schleyer V, Weber O, Yazdi A, et al. Prevention of polymorphic light eruption with a sunscreen of very high protection level against UVB and UVA radiation under standardized photodiagnostic conditions. *Acta Derm Venereol.* 2008;88(6):555-560.
81. Bissonnette R, Nigen S, Bolduc C. Influence of the quantity of sunscreen applied on the ability to protect against ultraviolet-induced polymorphous light eruption. *Photodermatol Photoimmunol Photomed.* 2012; 28(5):240-243.
82. Naleway AL. Polymorphous light eruption. *Int J Dermatol.* 2002;41(7):377-383.
83. Millard TP. Treatment of polymorphic light eruption. *J Dermatolog Treat.* 2000;11:195-199.
84. Patel DC, Bellaney GJ, Seed PT, et al. Efficacy of short-course oral prednisolone in polymorphic light eruption: a randomized controlled trial. *Br J Dermatol.* 2000;143(4):828-831.
85. Murphy GM, Logan RA, Lovell CR, et al. Prophylactic PUVA and UVB therapy in polymorphic light eruption—a controlled trial. *Br J Dermatol.* 1987;116(4):531-538.
86. Bilsland D, George SA, Gibbs NK, et al. A comparison of narrow band phototherapy (TL-01) and photochemotherapy (PUVA) in the management of polymorphic light eruption. *Br J Dermatol.* 1993;129(6):708-712.
87. Norris PG, Hawk JL. Polymorphic light eruption. *Photodermatol Photoimmunol Photomed.* 1990;7(5):186-191.
88. Wolf R, Oumeish OY. Photodermatoses. *Clin Dermatol.* 1998;16(1):41-57.
89. Ferguson J, Ibbotson S. The idiopathic photodermatoses. *Semin Cutan Med Surg.* 1999;18(4):257-273.
90. Norris PG, Hawk JL. Successful treatment of severe polymorphous light eruption with azathioprine. *Arch Dermatol.* 1989;125(10):1377-1379.
91. Saul A, Flores O, Novales J. Polymorphous light eruption: Treatment with thalidomide. *Australas J Dermatol.* 1976;17(1):17-21.
92. Holzle E, Plewig G, von Kries R, et al. Polymorphous light eruption. *J Invest Dermatol.* 1987;88(3)(suppl): 32s-38s.
93. Corbett MF, Hawk JL, Herxheimer A, et al. Controlled therapeutic trials in polymorphic light eruption. *Br J Dermatol.* 1982;107(5):571-581.
94. Murphy GM, Hawk JL, Magnus IA. Hydroxychloroquine in polymorphic light eruption: a controlled trial with drug and visual sensitivity monitoring. *Br J Dermatol.* 1987;116(3):379-386.
95. Benanni B, Bruckner T, Bock M, et al. Low incidence of polymorphous light eruption in renal transplant recipients. *Acta Derm Venereol.* 2007;87(4):372-374.
96. Marini A, Jaenicke T, Grether-Beck S, et al. Prevention of polymorphic light eruption by oral administration of a nutritional supplement containing lycopene, β-carotene and *Lactobacillus johnsonii*: results from a randomized, placebo-controlled, double-blinded study. *Photodermatol Photoimmunol Photomed.* 2014; 30(4):189-194.
97. Tanew A, Radakovic S, Gonzalez S, et al. Oral administration of a hydrophilic extract of *Polypodium leucotomos* for the prevention of polymorphic light eruption. *J Am Acad Dermatol.* 2012;66(1):58-62.
98. Caccialanza M, Percivalle S, Piccinno R, et al. Photoprotective activity of oral *Polypodium leucotomos* extract in 25 patients with idiopathic photodermatoses. *Photodermatol Photoimmunol Photomed.* 2007;23(1): 46-47.
99. Hofer A, Legat FJ, Gruber-Wackernagel A, et al. Topical liposomal DNA-repair enzymes in polymorphic light eruption. *Photochem Photobiol Sci.* 2011;10(7): 1118-1128.

Chapter 93 :: Actinic Prurigo
:: Travis Vandergriff

第九十三章
光化性痒疹

中文导读

光化性痒疹（AP）是一种由日光照射引起的慢性瘙痒性皮肤病，皮损以丘疹或结节为主，主要分布在暴露部位，通常儿童期起病，春季发病，夏季加重，在冬季可消退。本章主要从该病的流行病学、临床特征、病因和发病机制、诊断、鉴别诊断、临床病程和预后、处理等方面来进行介绍。在临床特征方面，分别从病史、皮肤表现、非皮肤表现来进行描述。该病主要依据病史、实验室检查、光试验、组织病理学来进行诊断，并总结了诊断思路，提出了与多形性日光疹的皮疹的鉴别诊断。此外，防晒和避光预防是处理AP的基石，并提供了治疗思路。

〔易　梅〕

AT-A-GLANCE

- A rare chronic pruritic and excoriated papular or nodular eruption of sun-exposed and, to a lesser extent, nonexposed skin.
- Beginning in childhood, it may remit at puberty, exacerbate most often in summer, and fade in winter.
- Indigenous peoples of North and South America are disproportionately affected.
- Association with HLA-DR4, specifically the HLA-DRB1*0407 and DRB1*0401 variants
- Prevention through avoidance of sunlight is the first-line therapy; thalidomide or other immunosuppressive agents may be required.

INTRODUCTION

DEFINITION

Actinic prurigo (AP) is a chronic sunlight-induced pruritic eruption characterized by papules or nodules, many of which are excoriated. Lesions are distributed mostly on sun-exposed skin but may also occur in sun-protected sites. A family history of the disease may be reported by patients. Indigenous peoples of the Americas are most often affected, and strong associations with specific human leukocyte antigen (HLA) types have been identified.

HISTORICAL PERSPECTIVE

AP was first described by Hutchinson in 1878 and was designated by him as "summer prurigo." Other historical terms for the disease include solar eczema, prurigo solar, hereditary polymorphic light eruption, and hydroa aestivale.[1]

EPIDEMIOLOGY

AP occurs throughout much of the world. The indigenous populations of North and South America are particularly affected. The disease is estimated to occur in 2% of the Canadian Inuit population.[2] In Mexico, AP is seen most commonly in the indigenous and Mestizo (mixed native and European descent) populations living at altitudes greater than 1000 m.[3] Less commonly, inhabitants of Europe, United States, Australia, and Asia are reported to develop AP. In Scotland, less than 1% of all patients evaluated in a specialized photodiagnostic unit were diagnosed with AP.[4]

In most populations, females are affected more frequently than males, in a ratio ranging from 2:1 to 4:1.[5] In Asians, there is a male predominance.[6] The eruption has its onset in childhood, usually present by age 10 years.[7] The onset of disease appears to occur earliest in Native American populations, at 4 to 5 years of age.[5] A positive family history of either AP or polymorphous light eruption is present in about a fifth of patients.[8]

CLINICAL FEATURES

HISTORY

The eruption is often present all year round, but it is commonly worse in summer. About one third of patients experience symptoms in wintertime.[9] Very rarely it is worse in winter, with immunologic tolerance presumably developing during the summer. Exacerbations tend to begin gradually during sunny weather in general rather than after specific sun exposure, although PMLE-like outbreaks may also occur. Patients may not be aware that lesions are provoked by sun exposure.

Pruritus is universally present and is typically severe.[5,10] Pain or tingling sensations also may be reported, especially in patients with cheilitis.[10,11] When conjunctivitis is present, patients report pruritus, photophobia, and lacrimation.[5,12]

CUTANEOUS FINDINGS

The primary lesion of AP is a pruritic papule or nodule that occurs singly or in clusters (Fig. 93-1). Papules and nodules are often excoriated and crusted, and plaques may assume a lichenified or eczematous appearance (Fig. 93-2). Vesicles are not seen unless superinfection is present.[5] Sun-exposed areas are most often affected, particularly the forehead, chin, cheeks, ears, and forearms. There is a gradual fading toward habitually covered skin, and the sacral area and buttocks may be mildly affected. Although primary lesions of AP do not lead to scarring, healed facial lesions may leave dyspigmentation, and scarring can occur secondary to excoriations (Fig. 93-3).

NONCUTANEOUS FINDINGS

Mucosal involvement is not typically seen in Asian patients.[6] Cheilitis may be the sole manifestation in more than half of Native American patients and is evident by edema, scale, crust, and fissures of lip mucosa. Conjunctivitis leads to hyperemia, pterygium, pinguecula, and Trantas dots along the limbus.[12]

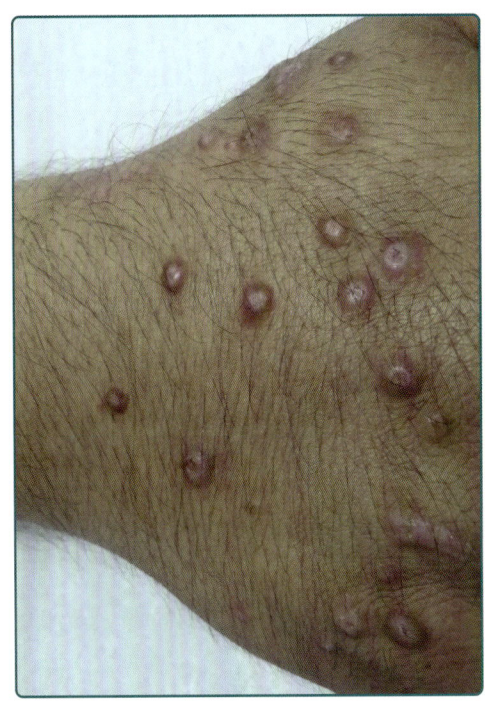

Figure 93-1 Primary lesions are excoriated or lichenified papules or nodules, predominantly on sun-exposed skin.

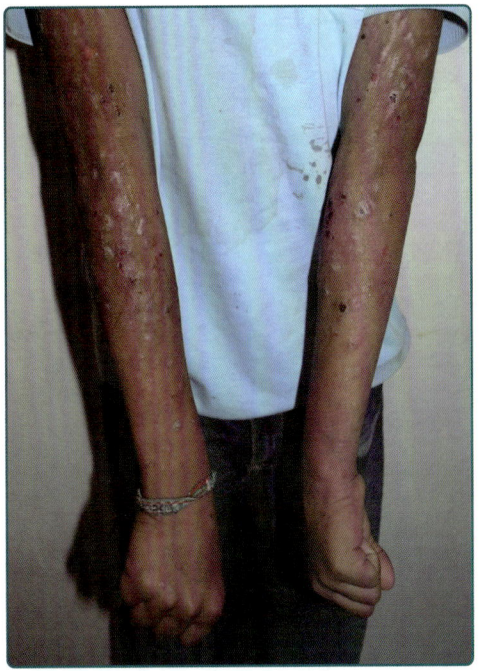

Figure 93-2 Excoriated and lichenified papules and nodules on the forearms of a child with Amerindian ancestry. (Photograph used with permission from Arturo R. Dominguez, MD.)

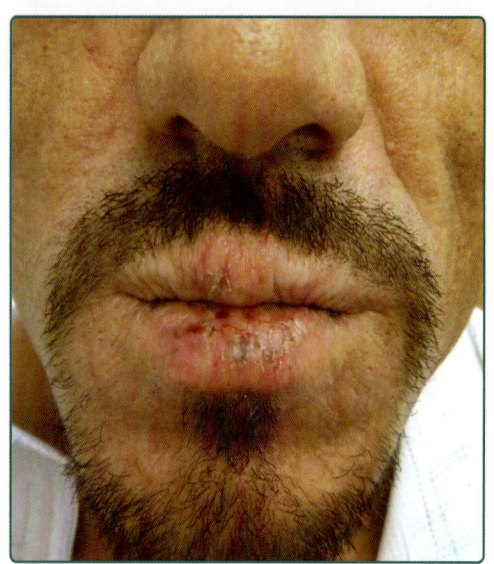

Figure 93-3 Cheilitis of actinic prurigo seen in a Mexican landscape gardener.

COMPLICATIONS

Mild scarring, especially on the face, and hypopigmentation may result from excoriations associated with AP. Additionally, 2 cases of primary cutaneous B-cell lymphoma arising on the face in patients with AP have been reported.[14]

ETIOLOGY AND PATHOGENESIS

AP appears to be induced by ultraviolet radiation in that it is more severe in spring and summer and predominates on sun-exposed skin. Additionally, patients with AP often demonstrate abnormal skin phototest responses to UVB and/or UVA radiation.[7] UVA is implicated more often than UVB, with most patients demonstrating reduced minimal erythema doses in the UVA or combined UVA/UVB ranges.[5,15] The cytokine TNF-α is overexpressed by keratinocytes in lesions of AP, creating a proinflammatory environment.[3] There is a concomitant increase in the number of dermal dendrocytes, and lymphocytes with a TH1 phenotype are recruited to lesional skin.[3]

Sunlight exposure and solar simulating irradiation may sometimes induce an eruption resembling polymorphous light eruption (PMLE) in patients with AP, and many patients have close relatives with PMLE.[8] Therefore, AP may be a slowly evolving, chronic, and excoriated variant of PMLE, and thus also a delayed hypersensitivity reaction.

A distinct genetic predisposition to AP has been identified for patients with specific human leukocyte antigen (HLA) subtypes. HLA-DR4 is found most commonly.[16] The frequency of the HLA-DR4 allele exceeds 90% in patients from Mexico.[17] Specific variants of HLA-DR4 are closely linked to AP, namely, DRB1*0407 and DRB1*0401. DRB1*0407 (DR4) is found in 60% to 70% of patients with AP but in only 4% to 8% of normal DR4-positive controls.[5] Additionally, HLA DRB1*0401 is found in approximately 20% of affected individuals.[5] Less frequently identified risk alleles include HLA-A24,[18] HLA-A28,[17] HLA-B39,[17] HLA-B40,[19] HLA-Cw3,[19] HLA-Cw4,[18,20] and HLA-DRB1*14.[2] These immunogenetic features may well be responsible for modulating conventional PMLE into AP. In addition, in some patients, AP appears to transform into PMLE and, in others, PMLE appears to transform into AP,[21] all of which suggests a relationship between the 2 disorders. The cutaneous UVR chromophores responsible for the eruption are not known, but they are likely to be diverse.

RISK FACTORS

Genetic risk factors for the development of AP include the aforementioned specific HLA haplotypes. Patients with these genotypes may report a family history of AP or other photosensitive disorder. Environmental risk factors have been explored, and in the Mexican population those risk factors include burning firewood, living with farm animals, and living with animals in the house.[10]

DIAGNOSIS

SUPPORTIVE STUDIES

LABORATORY TESTING

Assessment of ANA and ENA should be undertaken to exclude subacute cutaneous or other forms of cutaneous LE. The finding of HLA DR4, type DRB1*0401 or DRB1*0407 (especially the latter), supports the diagnosis of AP. Patients with moderate or severe presentations of AP may also have elevated serum immunoglobulin E (IgE) levels.[22]

PHOTOTESTING

Cutaneous phototesting with a monochromator confirms light sensitivity in up to half of cases,[7] but, as in PMLE, does not differentiate other photodermatoses. Most patients with positive monochromator testing have reduced minimal erythema doses (MEDs) in the UVA spectrum or in the combined UVA/UVB spectra.[4,5,15] Provocation testing with a solar simulator or other broadband sources induces typical lesions of AP in about two-thirds of patients.[4,5]

PATHOLOGY

Early papular lesions show changes similar to those of PMLE, namely, mild acanthosis, exocytosis of lymphocytes, spongiosis, and mild basilar vacuolar degeneration.[23] In the dermis, there is a moderate lymphohistiocytic superficial and middermal perivascular infiltrate, along with papillary dermal edema.[23] Chronic lesions of AP show more acanthosis and hyperkeratosis. Infiltrates of eosinophils may be seen (Fig. 93-4). Histopathologic findings in AP cheilitis tend to be more distinct and specific. Namely, there is a dense nodular lymphoid infiltrate in the lamina propria with formation of lymphoid follicles and expanded germinal centers[11] (Fig. 93-5). Eosinophilic spongiosis is also common.[11] In persistent lesions, however, excoriations, more acanthosis, variable lichenification, and a dense mononuclear cell infiltrate produce a nonspecific appearance.

DIAGNOSTIC ALGORITHM

See Fig. 93-6.

DIFFERENTIAL DIAGNOSIS

The most challenging diagnosis to distinguish from AP is PMLE, and some consider the 2 diagnoses to be chronicity variants. Some of the clinical features that suggest a diagnosis of AP rather than PMLE include disease onset in childhood, presence of lesions on both exposed and sun-protected skin, involvement of lip mucosa and conjunctiva, persistence of lesions beyond 4 weeks, occurrence in wintertime, excoriations, and scarring.[21] Previously mentioned HLA restrictions are seen in AP but not in PMLE. In a subgroup of patients, overlapping features are seen and a distinction is not possible. Diagnoses to distinguish from AP appear in Table 93-1.

CLINICAL COURSE AND PROGNOSIS

AP commonly arises in childhood and often improves or resolves in adolescence, although persistence into adult life is possible. When the disease begins in childhood (less than age 20 years), eruptions tend to be more severe and acute but remission in adulthood is more likely. When disease begins in adulthood, a milder but more persistent course is seen.[9] Persistent cases may assume features of PMLE in adulthood.

MANAGEMENT

INTERVENTIONS

MEDICATIONS

Controlled clinical trials evaluating medical management of AP are lacking. Higher-potency topical corticosteroids or topical calcineurin inhibitors may be used to relieve the inflammation and pruritus associated with the disease. Oral antihistamines also may be used for treatment of pruritus. Unlike some of the other photoexacerbated dermatoses, antimalarials seem to be ineffective for AP.[5]

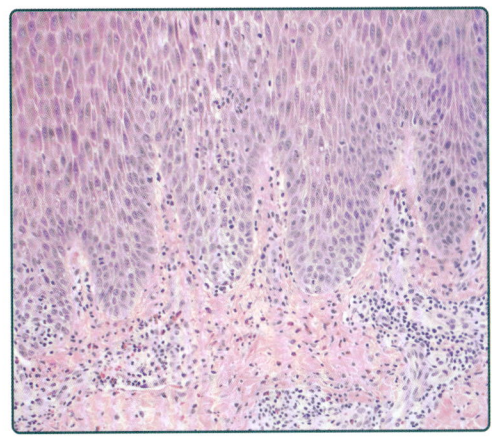

Figure 93-4 Histopathologic features are relatively nonspecific but may show acanthosis, spongiosis, exocytosis of lymphocytes, and an infiltrate of eosinophils.

The treatment of choice in more severe or recalcitrant cases is thalidomide, with initial doses of 50 to 100 mg daily for children and 100 to 200 mg daily for adults, preferably given intermittently.[5,24] Responses to thalidomide are evident in most patients within several weeks. The most serious complication associated with thalidomide is teratogenicity, so pregnancy must be rigorously avoided. Other potential adverse effects are typically mild, including drowsiness, headache, constipation, and weight gain. An increased risk of thromboembolism and dose-related peripheral (mostly sensory) neuropathy are other potential adverse effects of thalidomide. In cases where thalidomide is unavailable or otherwise not appropriate, oral immunosuppressive therapy with azathioprine or cyclosporine also may be considered.

PROCEDURES

Phototherapy with narrowband UVB or PUVA may occasionally help, but the treatment response is

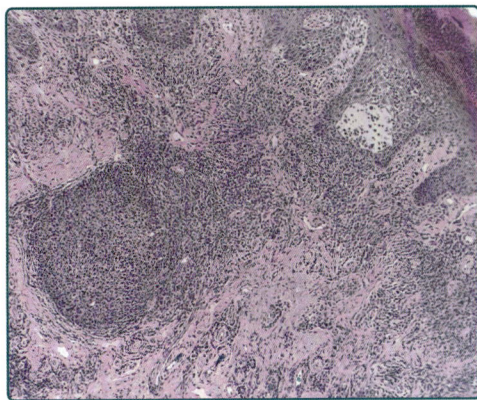

Figure 93-5 Lip biopsy from a patient with actinic prurigo shows a dense lymphohistiocytic infiltrate as well as a lymphoid follicle in the lamina propria.

limited to exposed areas, indicating that phototherapy does not alter the underlying photosensitive process.25

COUNSELING

Sun protection and avoidance strategies represent the cornerstone of management for AP. In less severe cases of AP, sufficient relief may be achieved by restricting sun exposure and by using broad-spectrum, high-protection-factor sunscreens alone.15

TABLE 93-1
Differential Diagnosis of Actinic Prurigo

Most Likely
- Polymorphic light eruption
- Atopic eczema
- Photoexacerbated atopic or seborrheic eczema
- Insect bites
- Prurigo nodularis

Always Rule Out
- Scabies

TREATMENT ALGORITHM

See Fig. 93-7.

PREVENTION

Prevention of AP flares begins by restricting midday sunlight exposure, wearing sun-protective clothing,

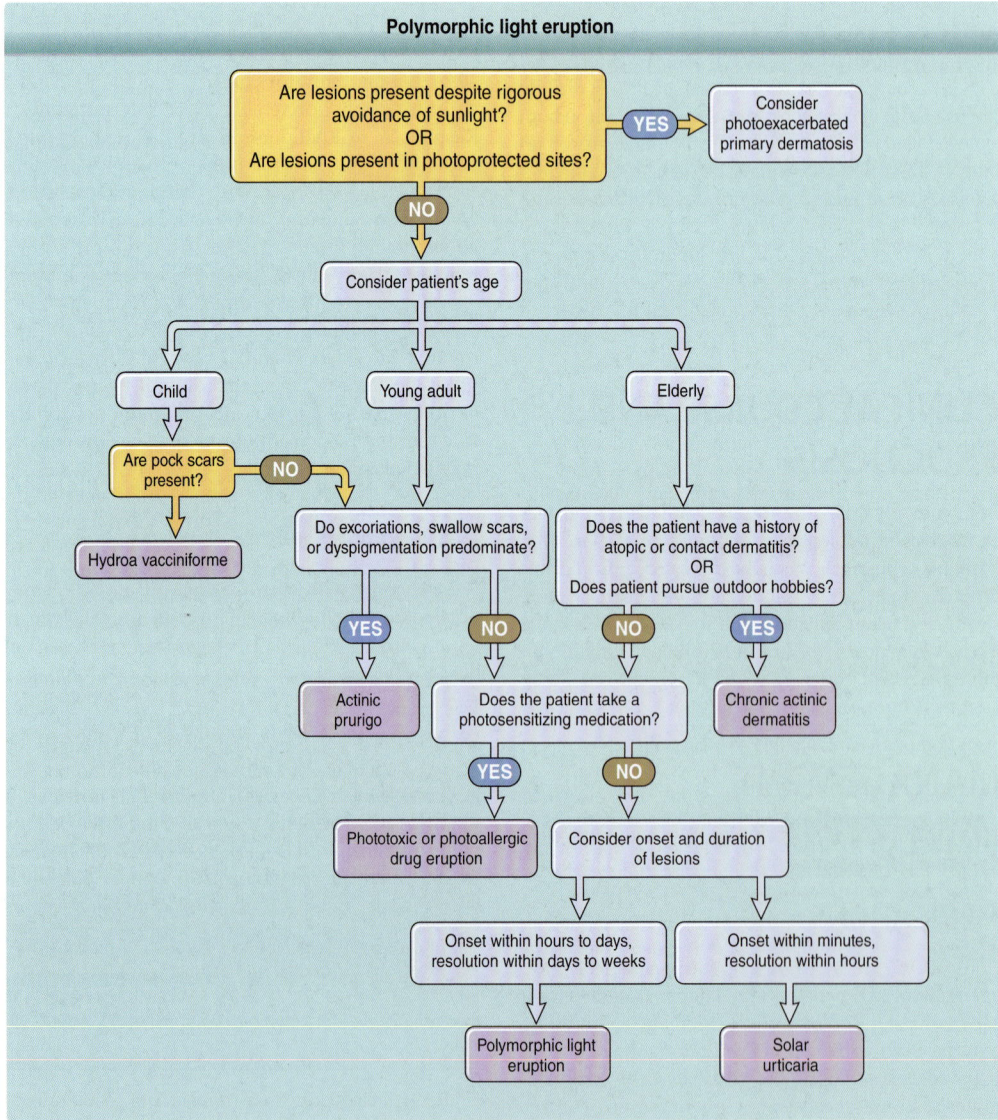

Figure 93-6 Diagnostic algorithm for abnormal responses to ultraviolet radiation.

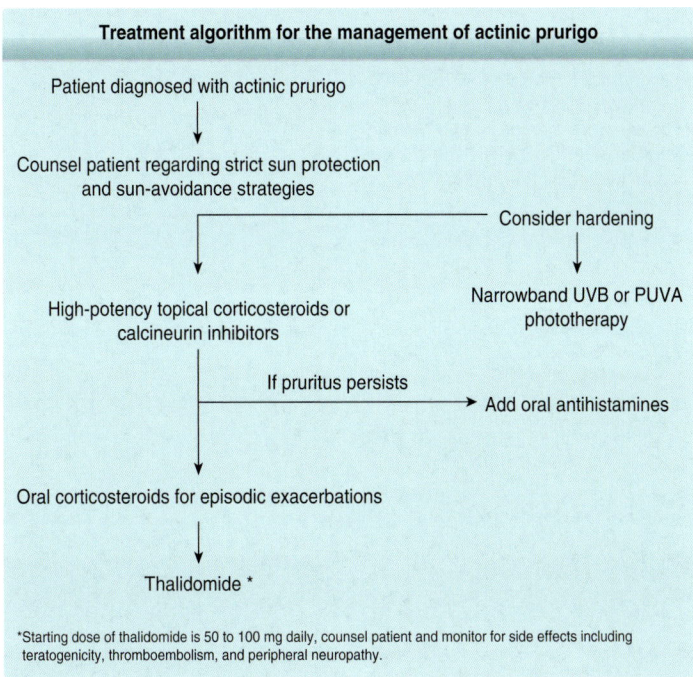

Figure 93-7 Treatment algorithm for the management of actinic prurigo.

and using of broad-spectrum sunscreens. There is no known way to prevent its initial onset.

REFERENCES

1. Scheen SR 3rd, Connolly SM, Dicken CH. Actinic prurigo. *J Am Acad Dermatol.* 1981;5(2):183-190.
2. Wiseman MC, Orr PH, Macdonald SM, et al. Actinic prurigo: clinical features and HLA associations in a Canadian Inuit population. *J Am Acad Dermatol.* 2001;44(6):952-956.
3. Arrese JE, Dominguez-Soto L, Hojyo-Tomoka MT, et al. Effectors of inflammation in actinic prurigo. *J Am Acad Dermatol.* 2001;44(6):957-961.
4. Macfarlane L, Hawkey S, Naasan H, et al. Characteristics of actinic prurigo in Scotland: 24 cases seen between 2001 and 2015. *Br J Dermatol.* 2016;174(6):1411-1414.
5. Ross G, Foley P, Baker C. Actinic prurigo. *Photodermatol Photoimmunol Photomed.* 2008;24(5):272-275.
6. Ker KJ, Chong WS, Theng CT. Clinical characteristics of adult-onset actinic prurigo in Asians: a case series. *Indian J Dermatol Venereol Leprol.* 2013;79(6):783-788.
7. Lim HW, Hönigsmann H, Hawk JLM. *Photodermatology. Basic and Clinical Dermatology.* New York: Informa Healthcare USA; 2007.
8. McGregor JM, Grabczynska S, Vaughan R, et al. Genetic modeling of abnormal photosensitivity in families with polymorphic light eruption and actinic prurigo. *J Invest Dermatol.* 2000;115(3):471-476.
9. Lane PR, Hogan DJ, Martel MJ, et al. Actinic prurigo: clinical features and prognosis. *J Am Acad Dermatol.* 1992;26(5, pt 1):683-692.
10. Vera Izaguirre DS, Zuloaga Salcedo S, González Sánchez PC, et al. Actinic prurigo: a case-control study of risk factors. *Int J Dermatol.* 2014;53(9):1080-1085.
11. Plaza JA, Toussaint S, Prieto VG, et al. Actinic prurigo cheilitis: a clinicopathologic review of 75 cases. *Am J Dermatopathol.* 2016;38(6):418-422.
12. Magana M, Mendez Y, Rodriguez A, et al. The conjunctivitis of solar (actinic) prurigo. *Pediatr Dermatol.* 2000;17(6):432-435.
13. Birt AR, Davis RA. Photodermatitis in North American Indians: familial actinic prurigo. *Int J Dermatol.* 1971;10(2):107-114.
14. Perrett CM, Harwood CA, Khorshid M, et al. Primary cutaneous B-cell lymphoma associated with actinic prurigo. *Br J Dermatol.* 2005;153(1):186-189.
15. Crouch R, Foley P, Baker C. Actinic prurigo: a retrospective analysis of 21 cases referred to an Australian photobiology clinic. *Australas J Dermatol.* 2002;43(2):128-132.
16. Dawe RS, Collins P, Ferguson J, et al. Actinic prurigo and HLA-DR4. *J Invest Dermatol.* 1997;108(2):233-234.
17. Hojyo-Tomoka T, Granados J, Vargas-Alarcón G, et al. Further evidence of the role of HLA-DR4 in the genetic susceptibility to actinic prurigo. *J Am Acad Dermatol.* 1997;36(6, pt 1):935-937.
18. Sheridan DP, Lane PR, Irvine J, et al. HLA typing in actinic prurigo. *J Am Acad Dermatol.* 1990;22(6, pt 1):1019-1023.
19. Bernal JE, Duran de Rueda MM, de Brigard D. Human lymphocyte antigen in actinic prurigo. *J Am Acad Dermatol.* 1988;18(2, pt 1):310-312.
20. Bernal JE, Duran de Rueda MM, Ordonez CP, et al. Actinic prurigo among the Chimila Indians in Colombia: HLA studies. *J Am Acad Dermatol.* 1990;22(6, pt 1):1049-1051.

21. Grabczynska SA, McGregor JM, Kondeatis E, et al. Actinic prurigo and polymorphic light eruption: common pathogenesis and the importance of HLA-DR4/DRB1*0407. *Br J Dermatol*. 1999;140(2):232-236.
22. Cuevas-Gonzalez JC, Lievanos-Estrada Z, Vega-Memije ME, et al. Correlation of serum IgE levels and clinical manifestations in patients with actinic prurigo. *An Bras Dermatol*. 2016;91(1):23-26.
23. Lane PR, Murphy F, Hogan DJ, et al. Histopathology of actinic prurigo. *Am J Dermatopathol*. 1993;15(4):326-331.
24. Lovell CR, Hawk JL, Calnan CD, et al. Thalidomide in actinic prurigo. *Br J Dermatol*. 1983;108(4):467-471.
25. Farr PM, Diffey BL. Treatment of actinic prurigo with PUVA: mechanism of action. *Br J Dermatol*. 1989;120(3):411-418.

Chapter 94 :: Hydroa Vacciniforme
:: Travis Vandergriff

第九十四章
种痘样水疱病

中文导读

种痘样水疱病（HV）是罕见的儿童光感性皮肤病，特点是日光暴露的皮肤出现水疱性病变，最终愈合会遗留凹陷性瘢痕。本章主要从该病的流行病学、临床特征、病因和发病机制、诊断、鉴别诊断、临床病程和预后、处理等方面来进行介绍。在临床特征方面，分别从病史、皮肤表现、非皮肤表现、并发症来进行描述。指出HV确切的发病机制尚不明确，可能与EB病毒感染有关。依据病史、实验室检查、光试验、组织病理学来进行诊断，并总结了诊断思路。提出必须与水痘样淋巴瘤（HVLL）进行鉴别。此外，HV是一种难治性疾病，本章提出了可能有效的治疗方法。

〔易　梅〕

AT-A-GLANCE

- A rare, chronic, scarring photodermatosis sometimes associated with Epstein-Barr virus infection.
- Characterized by recurrent sunlight-induced crops of papulovesicles and vesicles, most commonly on the face and dorsa of the hands.
- Onset commonly in childhood, remitting most often at puberty.
- May be a scarring variant of polymorphic light eruption.
- Focal intraepidermal vesiculation, reticular degeneration of the epidermis, epidermal and upper dermal necrosis, and sometimes ulceration are typical histologic changes.
- Avoidance of ultraviolet radiation including the use of broad-spectrum sunscreens is the only established therapy, but there may be a role for antivirals.
- A severe, often fatal lymphoma resembling hydroa vacciniforme is distinguished by fever, facial edema, and systemic symptoms.

DEFINITION

Hydroa vacciniforme (HV) is a rare, chronic photodermatosis with onset typically occurring in childhood and a tendency to remission in adolescence. HV is characterized by photoinduced papules and vesicles that invariably scar after healing.

HISTORICAL PERSPECTIVE

HV was first described in 1862 by Bazin.

EPIDEMIOLOGY

HV is reported most often in North America, Europe, and Japan but is known to occur globally. The disease has its onset in childhood, most often presenting before age 8 years; presentation in adulthood is unusual. Patients with light pigmentation are affected preferentially. The disease is rare, with one estimate of the prevalence of HV being 0.34 cases per 100,000 individuals with an approximately equal sex ratio.[1] There is male predominance for severe forms, whereas milder disease is more common in females.[1,2] Cases of HV are normally sporadic, and familial incidence is exceptional.

CLINICAL FEATURES

HISTORY

HV commonly develops in early childhood and resolves spontaneously by puberty, although, in some patients, it is lifelong. HV eruptions typically occur in summer,[3] often with an intense burning or stinging sensation followed by the appearance of individual or confluent papules and then vesicles, all within hours of sunlight exposure (Fig. 94-1). This is followed by umbilication, crusting, and progression to permanent pock scarring within weeks.

CUTANEOUS FINDINGS

HV is characterized initially by erythema, sometimes with swelling, followed by the eruption of tender papules and vesicles within 24 hours of sun exposure. The eruption affects the cheeks and to a lesser extent other areas of the face, as well as the backs of the hands and dorsal aspects of the arms. The distribution tends to be symmetrical. Vesicles may occasionally become confluent and hemorrhagic. Later, papules and vesicles umbilicate and develop ulceration. Within weeks to months, lesions heal leaving permanent, depressed, hypopigmented scars. These scars are invariably present and resemble those seen in vaccinia ("pock marks"), hence the "vacciniforme" nomenclature.

NONCUTANEOUS FINDINGS

Oral ulcers and eye involvement also occur in HV.[4-6] Ophthalmologic complications include conjunctival hyperemia, corneal erosions or ulcerations, iritis, keratitis, and uveitis.[6-8] Oral involvement presents as ulceration resembling aphthae or as gingivitis.[6,9]

COMPLICATIONS

Scars invariably ensue eruptions of HV. A quality-of-life study indicates that HV causes embarrassment and self-consciousness among children with the disease.[10] The negative impact of HV on quality of life exceeds previously reported indices for atopic dermatitis and psoriasis.[10]

Patients with severe presentations of HV-like eruptions along with systemic symptoms may develop a lymphoproliferative disorder with sometimes fatal systemic lymphoma. This entity (HV-like lymphoma) is later addressed in the section "Differential Diagnosis".

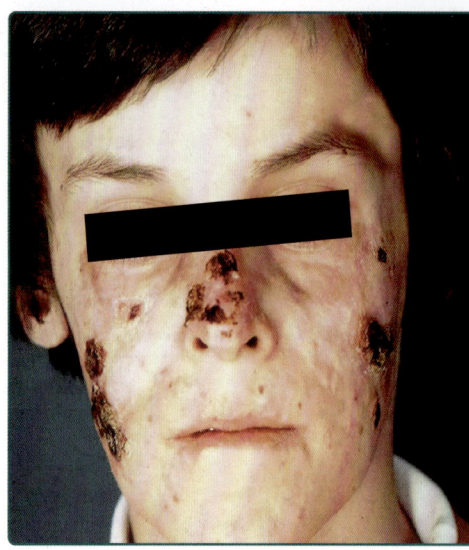

Figure 94-1 Hydroa vacciniforme. Vesicular, bullous, and crusted facial lesions, which heal with vacciniform scars.

ETIOLOGY AND PATHOGENESIS

The exact pathogenesis of HV is not known. No chromophores have been identified, and although ultraviolet B minimal erythema dose responses are normal in most patients, some have increased ultraviolet A sensitivity.[2] Nevertheless, its clear relationship to sunlight exposure, its distribution, and its early clinical appearances are all similar to that of polymorphous light eruption (PMLE), which suggests a relationship with that disease. On the other hand, fully developed HV eruptions are more severe than those found in PMLE, are associated with permanent scarring, and are unresponsive to treatments ordinarily effective in PMLE, apart perhaps from sunscreens and, occasionally, prophylactic phototherapy.

It is now widely recognized that chronic infection by Epstein-Barr virus (EBV) plays a role in the pathogenesis of HV in many cases,[11-13] although a relationship between EBV and HV in all populations has not been established. EBV nucleic acids are found in the cutaneous lesions of HV in 85% to 95% of patients, but not in lesional skin of control patients.[12,14] By electron microscopy, virions can be detected within lymphocytes as well as keratinocytes.[13] EBV DNA is found consistently in the peripheral blood of patients with HV, and higher levels correlate with disease activity and severity.[13,15] Patients with HV are also found to have higher percentages of circulating γδ T-cells, with demonstrable EBV infection of those cells.[15]

DIAGNOSIS

SUPPORTIVE STUDIES

LABORATORY TESTING

Blood, urine, and stool porphyrin concentrations should be assessed to exclude cutaneous porphyria, and an antinuclear antibody and extractable nuclear antibody to exclude the small possibility of cutaneous lupus erythematosus. Evidence of EBV viremia may support the diagnosis or indicate disease activity.

PHOTOTESTING

Phototesting may show increased sensitivity to short-wavelength ultraviolet A in some patients.[2,16,17] However, phototesting usually does not discriminate HV from other photodermatoses. Simulated solar irradiation may also induce erythema at reduced doses or occasionally provoke the typical vesiculation of HV (Fig. 94-2).

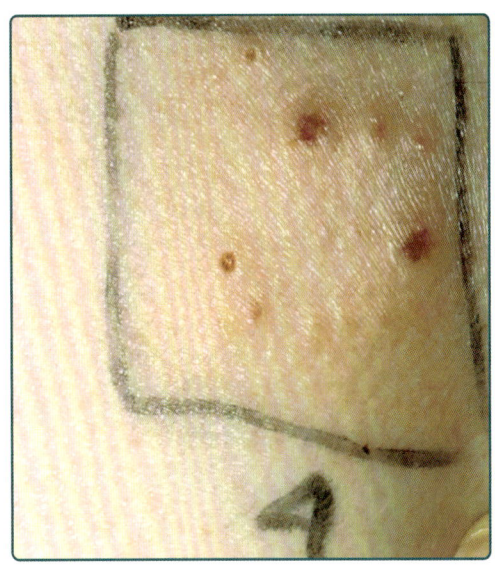

Figure 94-2 Hydroa vacciniforme. Induction of papulovesicles by ultraviolet A exposure.

PATHOLOGY

Early histologic changes include intraepidermal vesicle formation with spongiosis and subsequent focal epidermal keratinocyte necrosis. There is a dermal perivascular neutrophil and lymphocyte infiltrate. The lymphocytes are predominantly T cells, and approximately 5% to 20% of infiltrating lymphocytes may show evidence of EBV integration on in situ hybridization.[15] Older lesions show necrosis, ulceration, and scarring. Vasculitic features have been reported.[2] In some cases, there also may be a septal or lobular panniculitis. Healed pock-like lesions show dermal fibrosis in the pattern of a scar.

OTHER TESTS

Viral studies for herpes infection or other viral disorders should be undertaken if photoexacerbation or photoinduction of these other disorders seems at all possible.

DIAGNOSTIC ALGORITHM

Figure 94-3 shows an algorithm for abnormal responses to ultraviolet radiation.

DIFFERENTIAL DIAGNOSIS

Table 94-1 outlines the differential diagnosis of HV. Importantly, HV must be distinguished from a similar entity designated by the World Health Organization as hydroa vacciniforme–like lymphoma (HVLL).[18] The nomenclature of this entity is somewhat controversial, as some reports in the literature describe a "severe HV-like eruption" occurring in patients with chronic EBV infection and other associated disorders, such as hypersensitivity to mosquito bites and the hemophagocytic syndrome. HVLL has been identified mostly in children and young adults from Latin America and Asia.[19] HVLL eruptions are distinguished from true HV by the development of lesions in both exposed and sun-protected skin and by the presence of systemic symptoms such as fever, hepatosplenomegaly, and lymphadenopathy.[12,18,20] Facial edema with swelling of the lips and nose is common in HVLL, as is an eruption of papulovesicles on the legs.[19,21] Histologically, HVLL is distinguished by an angiocentric/angiodestructive infiltrate of atypical cytotoxic lymphocytes.[18,19,21] Clonal rearrangement of the T-cell receptor gene typifies HVLL but not HV.[18] The distinction between an HVLL and true HV is important because patients with a HVLL have a grave prognosis, with the possibility of fulminant and rapidly fatal disease.[19,21,22]

CLINICAL COURSE AND PROGNOSIS

HV often resolves in adolescence but may occasionally persist into adult life. Males have a later onset and longer duration of the disorder than females.[1] Age of onset appears to have prognostic value. Isolated cutaneous HV tends to present in early childhood, with a median age of onset around age 5 years.[23] Conversely, "severe" variants of HV and HVLL have their onset later in the first or second decade of life,[19,21,23] with one study identifying onset at age 9 years or later as significantly associated with mortality.[23]

MANAGEMENT

INTERVENTIONS

MEDICATIONS

HV often proves to be a refractory disease. Controlled clinical trials evaluating medical management of HV have not been performed. Occasionally, antimalarials appear to have helped, but their true value has not been established. Topical steroids, topical calcineurin inhibitors, and oral immunosuppressive medication tend to prove ineffective. In patients with chronic EBV infection, antiviral therapy with acyclovir and valacyclovir was reported in a small series of patients to reduce the frequency and severity of eruptions.[24] Improvement also has been reported in isolated cases with administration of dietary fish oil.[25,26]

TABLE 94-1
Differential Diagnosis of Hydroa Vacciniforme

- Photoexacerbated viral dermatoses such as herpes simplex
- Erythropoietic protoporphyria
- Polymorphic light eruption
- Actinic prurigo
- Subacute cutaneous lupus
- Xeroderma pigmentosum
- Hydroa vacciniforme-like lymphoma

PROCEDURES

As with PMLE, prophylactic phototherapy with narrowband ultraviolet B or psoralen and ultraviolet A, particularly psoralen and ultraviolet A, may be helpful but must be administered with care to avoid disease exacerbation.[2,13,27]

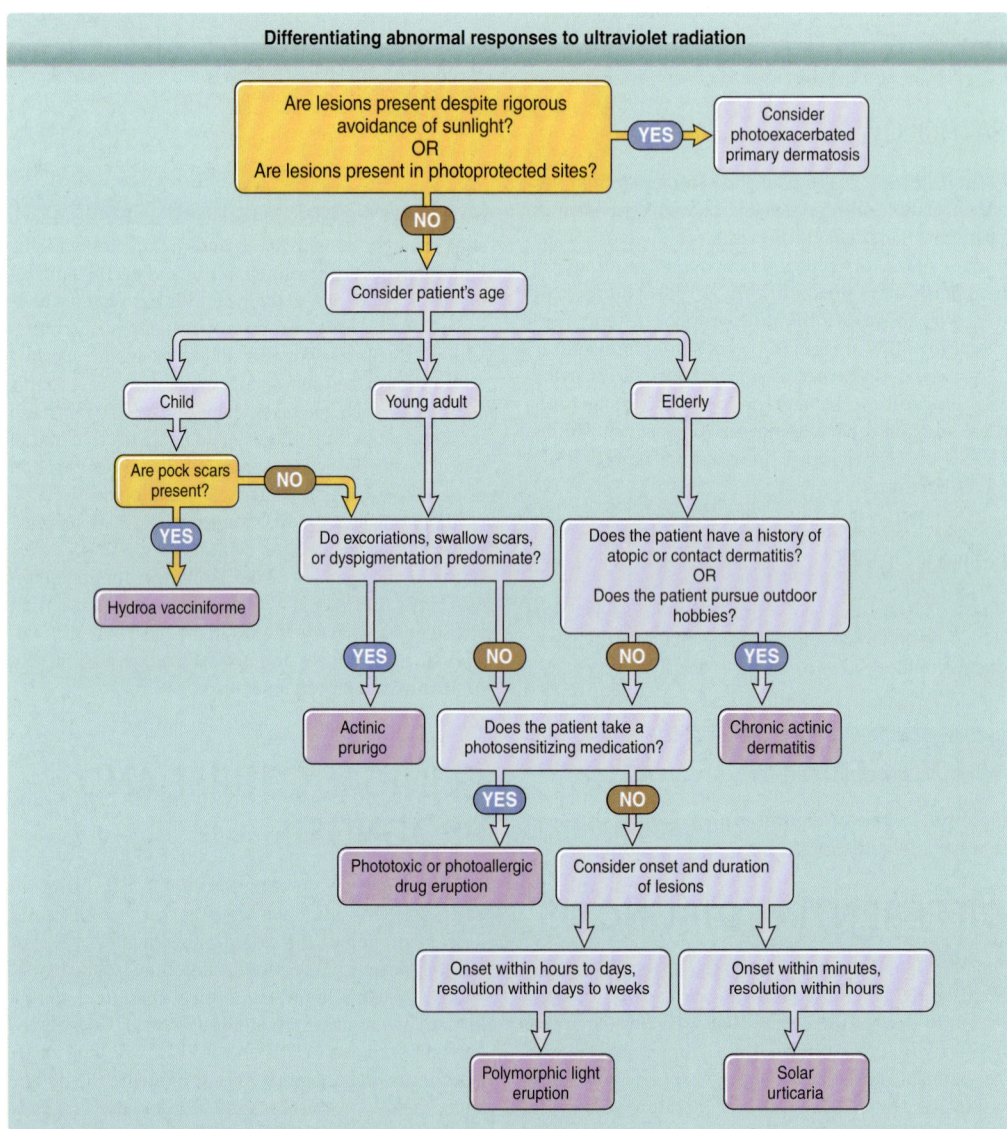

Figure 94-3 Diagnostic algorithm for abnormal responses to ultraviolet radiation.

COUNSELING

The mainstay of treatment of patients with HV relates to counseling regarding strict sun protection and avoidance strategies, including the use of broad-spectrum sunscreens.

PREVENTION

In mild cases of HV, sun avoidance and sunscreen use prevent HV eruptions.

REFERENCES

1. Gupta G, Man I, Kemmett D. Hydroa vacciniforme: a clinical and follow-up study of 17 cases. *J Am Acad Dermatol*. 2000;42(2, pt 1):208-213.
2. Sonnex TS, Hawk, JL. Hydroa vacciniforme: a review of ten cases. *Br J Dermatol*. 1988;118(1):101-108.
3. Lim HW, Hönigsmann H, Hawk JLM. *Photodermatology. Basic and Clinical Dermatology*. New York, NY: Informa Healthcare USA; 2007.
4. Yesudian PD, Sharpe GR. Hydroa vacciniforme with oral mucosal involvement. *Pediatr Dermatol*. 2004; 21(5):555-557.
5. Jeng BH, Margolis TP, Chandra NS, et al. Ocular findings as a presenting sign of hydroa vacciniforme. *Br J Ophthalmol*. 2004;88(11):1478-1479.
6. Yamamoto T, Hirai Y, Miyake T, et al. Oculomucosal and gastrointestinal involvement in Epstein-Barr virus-associated hydroa vacciniforme. *Eur J Dermatol*. 2012; 22(3):380-383.
7. Bennion SD, Johnson C, Weston WL. Hydroa vacciniforme with inflammatory keratitis and secondary anterior uveitis. *Pediatr Dermatol*. 1987;4(4):320-324.
8. Mortazavi H, Hejazi P, Aghazadeh N, et al., Hydroa vacciniforme with eye involvement: report of two cases. *Pediatr Dermatol*. 2015;32(1):e39-e41.
9. Wierzbicka E, Malthieu F, Villers A, et al. Oral involvement in hydroa vacciniforme. *Arch Dermatol*. 2006; 142(5):651.
10. Huggins RH, Leithauser LA, Eide MJ, et al. Quality of life assessment and disease experience of patient members of a web-based hydroa vacciniforme support group. *Photodermatol Photoimmunol Photomed*. 2009;25(4):209-215.
11. Iwatsuki K, Xu Z, Takata M, et al. The association of latent Epstein-Barr virus infection with hydroa vacciniforme. *Br J Dermatol*. 1999;140(4):715-721.
12. Iwatsuki K, Satoh M, Yamamoto T, et al. Pathogenic link between hydroa vacciniforme and Epstein-Barr virus-associated hematologic disorders. *Arch Dermatol*. 2006;142(5):587-595.
13. Verneuil L, Gouarin S, Comoz F, et al. Epstein-Barr virus involvement in the pathogenesis of hydroa vacciniforme: an assessment of seven adult patients with long-term follow-up. *Br J Dermatol*. 2010;163(1): 174-182.
14. Yamamoto T, Tsuji K, Suzuki D, et al. A novel, noninvasive diagnostic probe for hydroa vacciniforme and related disorders: detection of latency-associated Epstein-Barr virus transcripts in the crusts. *J Microbiol Methods*. 2007;68(2):403-407.
15. Hirai Y, Yamamoto T, Kimura H, et al. Hydroa vacciniforme is associated with increased numbers of Epstein-Barr virus-infected gammadeltaT cells. *J Invest Dermatol*. 2012;132(5):1401-1408.
16. Halasz CL, Leach EE, Walther RR, et al. Hydroa vacciniforme: induction of lesions with ultraviolet A. *J Am Acad Dermatol*. 1983;8(2):171-176.
17. Sunohara A, Mizuno N, Sakai M, et al. Action spectrum for UV erythema and reproduction of the skin lesions in hydroa vacciniforme. *Photodermatol*. 1988;5(3): 139-145.
18. Quintanilla-Martinez L, Ridaura C, Nagl F, et al. Hydroa vacciniforme-like lymphoma: a chronic EBV+ lymphoproliferative disorder with risk to develop a systemic lymphoma. *Blood*. 2013;122(18):3101-3110.
19. Sangueza M, Plaza JA. Hydroa vacciniforme-like cutaneous T-cell lymphoma: clinicopathologic and immunohistochemical study of 12 cases. *J Am Acad Dermatol*. 2013;69(1):112-119.
20. Cho KH, Lee SH, Kim CW, et al. Epstein-Barr virus-associated lymphoproliferative lesions presenting as a hydroa vacciniforme-like eruption: an analysis of six cases. *Br J Dermatol*. 2004;151(2):372-380.
21. Magaña M, Massone C, Magaña P, et al. Clinicopathologic features of hydroa vacciniforme-like lymphoma: a series of 9 patients. *Am J Dermatopathol*. 2016;38(1):20-25.
22. Cho KH, Kim CW, Heo DS, et al. Epstein-Barr virus-associated peripheral T-cell lymphoma in adults with hydroa vacciniforme-like lesions. *Clin Exp Dermatol*. 2001;26(3):242-247.
23. Miyake T, Yamamoto T, Hirai Y, et al. Survival rates and prognostic factors of Epstein-Barr virus-associated hydroa vacciniforme and hypersensitivity to mosquito bites. *Br J Dermatol*. 2015;172(1):56-63.
24. Lysell J, Wiegleb Edström D, Annika L, et al. Antiviral therapy in children with hydroa vacciniforme. *Acta Derm Venereol*. 2009;89(4):393-397.
25. Durbec F, Reguiaï Z, Léonard F, et al. Efficacy of omega-3 polyunsaturated fatty acids for the treatment of refractory hydroa vacciniforme. *Pediatr Dermatol*. 2012;29(1):118-119.
26. Rhodes LE, White SI. Dietary fish oil as a photoprotective agent in hydroa vacciniforme. *Br J Dermatol*. 1998;138(1):173-178.
27. Jaschke E, Honigsmann H. Hydroa vacciniforme-action spectrum. UV-tolerance following photochemotherapy [in German]. *Hautarzt*. 1981;32(7):350-353.

Chapter 95 :: Actinic Dermatitis
:: Robert S. Dawe

第九十五章
光化性皮炎

中文导读

本章主要介绍慢性光化性皮炎（CAD），它是一种罕见、持续影响暴露皮肤的光诱导性湿疹，常累及有严重日光暴露史的年长男性。本章节主要从该病的流行病学、病因和发病机制、临床特征、诊断、鉴别诊断、临床病程和预后、处理等方面来进行介绍。指出了CAD是类似于过敏性接触性皮炎的迟发型超敏反应。在临床特征方面，分别从病史、皮肤表现来进行描述。本章指出可以通过实验室检查、组织病理学、光测试、斑贴和光斑贴试验对CAD进行诊断，并概述了CAD的鉴别诊断以及可能出现的并发症。也指出CAD的治疗困难，预防是关键，并列出了有效的治疗方法。此外，本章还对光暴露部位皮肤病患者进行了探讨。

〔易　梅〕

Many diseases are caused by abnormal responses to ultraviolet radiation (UVR) and visible light exposure. This textbook includes separate chapters on other idiopathic (usually presumed immune-mediated) photodermatoses, including polymorphic light eruption/polymorphous light eruption (PLE/PMLE), actinic prurigo, hydroa vacciniforme (HV), and solar urticaria, and photodermatoses as a manifestation of metabolic diseases such as the cutaneous porphyrias. This chapter discusses conditions with a dermatitis on exposed sites, whether or not covered sites are also affected. These conditions include chronic actinic dermatitis, photoallergic contact dermatitis, drug-induced photosensitivity, and manifest as a dermatitis (eg, caused by thiazides) and photoaggravation of other dermatitides (atopic eczema, seborrheic dermatitis, and, often when caused by an airborne allergen, allergic contact dermatitis). Frequently, clinical assessment alone is insufficient to distinguish between true abnormal cutaneous photosensitivity (as in chronic actinic dermatitis) and photoaggravation, not true photosensitivity, of another dermatitis, and investigation with some form of photo-testing can be necessary for definitive diagnosis, with important implications for management.

CHRONIC ACTINIC DERMATITIS

AT-A-GLANCE

- Chronic actinic dermatitis is a rare, acquired, persistent eczematous eruption of exposed skin, sometimes having pseudolymphomatous (reticuloid) features.
- It commonly affects older men, but is increasingly recognized in women and in younger people, including children.
- Histologic features are eczematous, but pseudolymphomatous forms may be virtually indistinguishable from cutaneous T-cell lymphoma.

- It usually involves severe ultraviolet B sensitivity but often also involves ultraviolet A sensitivity and sometimes sensitivity to visible light.
- Persistent light reaction, actinic reticuloid, photosensitive eczema, and photosensitivity dermatitis are all considered either clinical variants or old diagnostic terms.
- It is likely the result of a delayed-type hypersensitivity reaction against an endogenous photoinduced epidermal antigen(s).
- Therapy consists of strict avoidance of the relevant ultraviolet and visible rays, along with topical and intermittent oral steroids, and topical calcineurin inhibitors. Occasionally, phototherapy (ultraviolet B, broadband ultraviolet A, ultraviolet A1, or psoralen-ultraviolet A photochemotherapy) can be used, guided by the findings of investigation, particularly phototesting. If these measures are insufficient, or cause too much disruption to quality of life, then systemic immunosuppression (such as azathioprine or methotrexate) is required.

EPIDEMIOLOGY

Chronic actinic dermatitis (CAD),[1] formerly called the photosensitivity dermatitis/actinic reticuloid syndrome,[2] occurs across the world.[3-5] As it is frequently impossible to definitively diagnose CAD without some form of phototesting, it is likely that some persons with this condition are being labeled as having photoaggravated atopic eczema. CAD is possibly more common in people of darker-skin phototypes, but can be found in all peoples.[4,6] Perhaps, melanin plays a part in causing this condition. CAD has not been reported in people with albinism.

ETIOLOGY AND PATHOGENESIS

Studies of the clinical, histologic, and immunohistochemical features of CAD all show it to resemble the delayed-type hypersensitivity reaction of allergic contact dermatitis,[7,8] even in its severe pseudolymphomatous form (formerly called *actinic reticuloid*), in which the clinical and histologic features duplicate those seen in longstanding allergic contact dermatitis. It is highly probable that CAD is an allergic reaction. In addition to hypersensitivity to cutaneous photoantigens, patients with CAD often have concomitant allergic contact dermatitis to airborne and other ubiquitous allergens, including plant compounds, fragrances, and medicaments.[8-18] Commonly implicated allergens include sesquiterpene lactones from plants of the Compositae family and sunscreens.[16] The percentages with contact allergy as part of CAD vary according to the report; it seems likely that the relevant allergens will differ in different parts of the world and that the more locally relevant patch test agents are tested the higher will be the percentages with identified contact allergy. Although photopatch testing is impossible in some persons with CAD (because the ultraviolet A photosensitivity can be too severe to allow irradiation of a photopatch test series), it can sometimes be done using an ultraviolet A minimal erythema dose assessment to determine a safe dose of ultraviolet A for this testing. This can be performed in those in whom it is helpful to determine whether or not there is photoallergy.[4]

When CAD occurs in the absence of an obvious contact allergen, the relevant novel antigen must be either directly radiation-induced or formed indirectly as a result of secondary oxidative metabolism. Important support for the latter possibility comes from the fact that albumin can become antigenic in vitro through photooxidation of its histidine moieties. There is no evidence for a genetic susceptibility to CAD; however, one stimulus for the acquisition of skin reactivity may be concurrent allergic contact dermatitis to recognized exogenous sensitizers or photosensitizers. These sensitizers are often airborne and may predispose by altering cutaneous immunity, and thus permit immunologic recognition of an endogenous photoantigen. Longstanding endogenous eczema, drug-induced photosensitivity, HIV infection,[19] and *possibly* PLE/PMLE also may play similar roles. On the other hand, in addition or instead, chronic photodamage in frequently sun-exposed elderly outdoor enthusiasts may impair normal UVR-induced skin immunosuppression sufficiently for endogenous UVR-induced photoantigens to be recognized, as apparently also occurs for genetic reasons in PLE/PMLE.[20] There is much work left to be done to identify the immunologic mechanisms that account for CAD.

Determining the action spectrum for CAD should theoretically help identify the postulated antigens, and the action spectra for CAD have been shown to resemble that of sunburn in many patients.[21] However, the eruption in CAD is eczematous, and much lower doses of UVR are required to evoke CAD than to produce erythema. In any event, the ultraviolet chromophore for some patients may be the same as that of sunburn, namely DNA,[21] with UVR-damaged DNA serving directly as an antigen in CAD. In other patients with CAD, however, the photoallergen must be different, because a few patients react only to ultraviolet A (UVA) radiation,[22] and some patients react only to visible light.[23]

In summary, CAD appears to be an allergic contact dermatitis-like reaction against UVR-altered DNA or similar or associated molecules, perhaps as a result of enhanced immune reactivity resulting from concomitant airborne contact dermatitis, or other longstanding preexisting dermatitis, or a reduced immunosuppressive capacity in ultraviolet-exposed skin.

CLINICAL FEATURES

HISTORY

CAD may arise de novo in apparently normal skin or in the skin of patients with previous endogenous eczema (often atopic or seborrheic eczema), photoallergic or allergic contact dermatitis, or, rarely, PLE/PMLE. Concurrent allergic contact sensitivity to plant allergens, fragrances, or sunscreens is common. The condition classically affects middle-aged and elderly men; however, CAD is increasingly recognized in younger people, particularly in those with atopic eczema,[24-27] although it is rarely present in children. The disorder is usually worse in summer in countries with marked seasonal variations, developing within minutes to hours after sunlight exposure and producing an itchy confluent erythematous eruption that occasionally remits over several days with scaling as long as exposure ceases and the reaction is mild. However, severely affected patients sometimes do not recognize that exacerbations are related to sunlight exposure, especially when affected all year round and when the wavelengths of sensitivity extend to longer UVA or visible wavelengths not associated with normal sunburn.

CUTANEOUS LESIONS

The lesions of CAD are eczematous, patchy or confluent, and acute, subacute, or chronic (Figs. 95-1 and 95-2). In severe cases, lichenification is common. Less commonly, scattered or widespread erythematous, shiny, infiltrated pseudolymphomatous papules or plaques are present on a background of erythematous, eczematous, or normal skin. Habitually exposed areas are most often affected, commonly with sharp cutoff at clothing lines. There is sparing of deep skin creases, upper eyelids, finger webs, and skin behind the earlobes. In severe disease, eczema of the palms and soles also may be found. Eyebrows, eyelashes, and scalp hair may be stubbly or altogether lost from constant rubbing and scratching. Erythroderma, usually accentuated on exposed sites, rarely supervenes. Variable, sometimes geographic, sparing of exposed areas of the face or elsewhere, as well as irregular hyperpigmentation and hypopigmentation, sometimes vitiligo-like, may also occasionally be found.

LABORATORY TESTS

HISTOLOGY

Histologic features include epidermal spongiosis and acanthosis, sometimes with hyperplasia. There is usually a predominantly perivascular lymphocytic cellular infiltrate confined to the upper dermis that in milder cases may resemble chronic eczema.[28] CAD cannot be diagnosed on histopathology but a biopsy of the eruption, whether naturally occurring or provoked on phototesting, can be helpful in confirming an eczema and not another pattern of inflammation. Severe CAD, however, may mimic cutaneous T-cell lymphoma (CTCL), on occasion being virtually indistinguishable. Features mimicking CTCL include epidermal Pautrier-like microabscesses and deep, dense epidermotropic mononuclear cell infiltration, sometimes with atypia. Typically, there is no marked increase in mitoses. T-cell receptor gene rearrangement studies are normally done if there is suspicion of CTCL. However, T-cell receptor clonality also may be observed in benign dermatoses, so even identification of a clone does not completely rule out CAD, rather than lymphoma, as the diagnosis.

BLOOD TESTS

Assessment of lupus autoantibodies is usually done to exclude the unlikely possibility of cutaneous lupus erythematosus. In severe or erythrodermic CAD, there may be large numbers of circulating CD8+ Sézary cells without other suggestions of malignancy.[29] HIV status should be assessed if there is suspicion that this may be a predisposing or associated factor. Serum immunoglobulin E may be elevated (even among those whose CAD has not supervened upon atopic eczema), with higher levels of immunoglobulin E correlating with more-severe disease.

PHOTOTESTING

Phototesting is essential to make the diagnosis of CAD. Almost invariably one finds low erythemal thresholds and eczematous or pseudolymphomatous responses

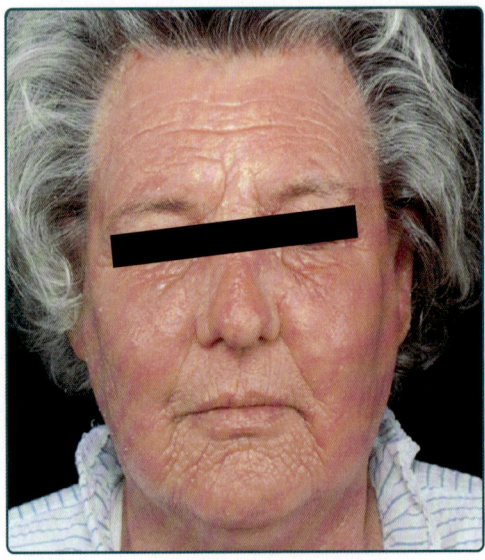

Figure 95-1 Chronic actinic dermatitis: infiltrated eczematous eruption on the face.

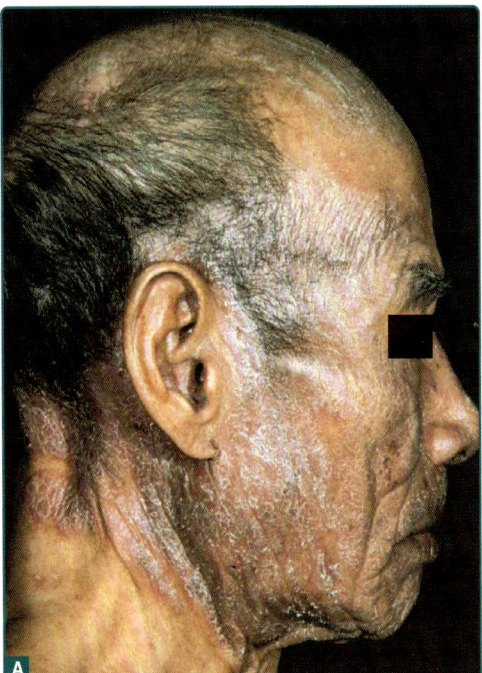
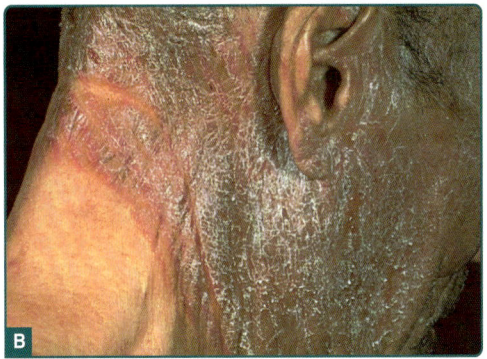
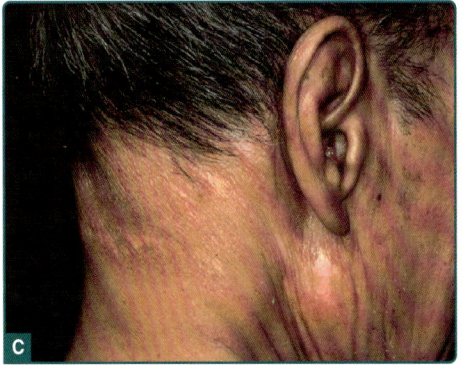
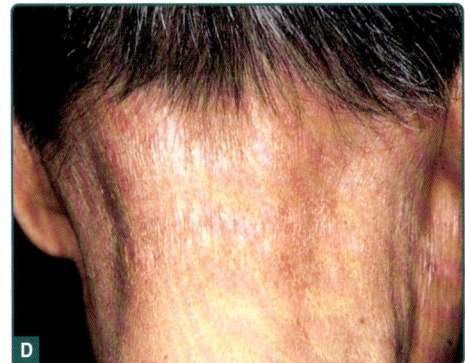

Figure 95-2 Chronic actinic dermatitis: **A** and **B,** Severe ultraviolet and light-induced eczema of the face and neck. **C** and **D,** Patient in full remission after low-dose psoralen plus ultraviolet A irradiation over weeks, with initial high-dose oral steroid cover to prevent initial exacerbation.

after irradiation with ultraviolet B (UVB), usually with UVA, and frequently also with visible wavelengths (accounting for presentations such as described after a tungsten light was used when ear cleaning).[30] A small number of patients genuinely seem to react only to UVA (although the possibility of another diagnosis such as drug reaction must be revisited if only UVA sensitivity is found), and fewer still only to visible light, in which case, drug photosensitivity must also be considered. Testing should be done on uninvolved skin of the back with no topical or systemic steroid therapy for at least the preceding few days to avoid false-negative results.[31,32] Various sources can be used for phototesting, including the irradiation monochromator, which allows the delivery of different doses of different ultraviolet and visible wavebands (which can be fairly narrow but which are not truly monochromatic).[33-36] If an irradiation monochromator is not available, then a series of different sources with filters can be used to sample through at least UVB and UVA (for which phototherapy treatment sources can be used) and visible light (such as using a slide projector). When such fairly elaborate equipment is not available, sunlight can be used (at least in warmer parts of the world) with a template devised to allow small areas of skin to have different durations of exposure and using a piece of window glass to filter out UVB, which enables testing with whole-spectrum sunlight and sunlight minus UVB. The output from the sun can be very variable, but the severity of abnormal photosensitivity in CAD is usually severe, so as long as a control population has been tested to establish what is normal, then such relatively crude testing is useful.

Monochromatic and broad-spectrum sources both induce abnormal responses, with monochromatic sources determining the action spectrum for disease induction and broad-spectrum sources tending to demonstrate acute eczema.

PATCH AND PHOTOPATCH TESTING

Patch testing and photopatch testing (when possible; sometimes the sensitivity to UVA on its own precludes irradiating with even a tiny dose of UVA for photopatch testing) are also important in suspected CAD, because contact sensitivity, including to airborne allergens such as Compositae oleoresins (including, where it occurs, parthenium),[16,37-39] colophony,[40,41] and methylisothiazolinone (the airborne dermatitis of which can be photoaggravated),[42,43] alone may resemble CAD or even coexist with CAD. In addition, occasional secondary contact or photocontact sensitivity to sunscreens or other topical therapies may complicate the clinical picture.[44]

DIFFERENTIAL DIAGNOSIS

Table 95-1 outlines the differential diagnosis of CAD.

COMPLICATIONS

A relationship to CTCL was considered a possibility.[45] However, when this was studied at a population level (and misclassifications in diagnostic databases were corrected) it was found that CTCL and CAD did not coexist more than would be expected by chance.[46] Results of T-cell receptor, immunoglobulin gene rearrangement, and other studies are usually negative in CAD.[47] In addition, CAD gradually resolves in many patients, there is no higher incidence of malignancies, and life expectancies are thought to be normal.[48] However, CTCL itself may present very rarely with severe CAD-like photosensitivity, and careful investigation to exclude CTCL is necessary when the disease suspected.[49-51]

PROGNOSIS AND CLINICAL COURSE

Once established, CAD usually persists for years before resolving gradually (Dawe et al).[48] Particularly severe phototest sensitivity and a number of completely separate contact allergens seem to be predictors of a poorer prognosis for resolution. In that study, young age and female sex were also associated with a poorer prognosis for resolution but when that study was done, CAD was considered to be a disease of old men so was likely more often not diagnosed in younger people and in women (and only diagnosed in the more severely affected young people and women).[48]

TREATMENT

Treatment of CAD is often difficult and not fully effective. Rigorous avoidance of UVR and exacerbating contact allergens is essential, along with regular application of high-protection-factor broad-spectrum topical sunscreens of low irritancy and allergenic potential. Ideally, sunscreen photoprotection should be guided by knowledge of the wavelengths (UVB, UVB and UVA, or UVB, UVA, and visible) implicated in each individual. Strong topical corticosteroids, such as clobetasol propionate 0.05%, are also often needed and frequently produce marked symptomatic relief without adverse effects, even after long-term use, if confined to affected skin. Occasional oral steroid use is often helpful for disease flares. In more-resistant disease, the topical calcineurin inhibitors—tacrolimus and pimecrolimus—sometimes produce good results if tolerated.[52-58] For refractory CAD, however, oral immunosuppressive therapy is often necessary and generally helpful if tolerated. Azathioprine 1.5 to 2.5 mg/kg/day can produce remission in months,[59-65] after which it may be reduced in dosage, or perhaps discontinued in the winter. While less studied for this indication, methotrexate is also used, especially when CAD has arisen on a background of atopic eczema. Cyclosporine 3.5 to 5 mg/kg/day can be rapidly effective,[66,67] but is more likely to produce adverse effects, and so is generally not a good long-term treatment. Mycophenolate mofetil is less often used.[68,69] More localized skin immunosuppression by psoralen activated by UVA treatment also can be effective,[70,71] and is often initially accompanied by oral and topical corticosteroid therapy to reduce disease flares.[71]

PREVENTION

The risk of CAD can *possibly* be reduced by moderating outdoor pursuits, especially those associated with plant allergen exposure, such as gardening, even more so for individuals who already have a tendency to develop eczematous eruptions in exposed areas. In those persons who are already developing CAD, avoidance of UVR is critical, and patients should be aware that indoor lighting with fluorescent lamps, including compact fluorescent energy-saving lamps, is also a source of UVA and UVB.[72,73]

TABLE 95-1
Differential Diagnosis of Chronic Actinic Dermatitis

- Photoexacerbated atopic or seborrheic eczema
- Drug or chemical photosensitivity
- Cutaneous T-cell lymphoma
- Eczematized actinic prurigo
- Photoallergic contact dermatitis
- Photoaggravated airborne contact allergic dermatitis

Note: The other conditions described in the text as capable of causing an exposed-site dermatosis do not cause a dermatitis unless the dermatitis is superimposed, such as someone who has PLE/PMLE but develops superimposed dermatitis changes perhaps because of having atopic eczema.

PHOTOEXACERBATED DERMATITIS

Several dermatoses that are not caused by UVR may be worsened by it (Table 95-2). Mechanisms of this phenomenon, termed *photoexacerbation*, have rarely been studied. The initial condition may be severely worsened even if it was originally only mild or subclinical. These disorders are relatively common. Such conditions, especially the eczemas, psoriasis, and acne, improve with sunlight exposure in most patients, perhaps because cutaneous reactivity is reduced, but in a small proportion of individuals, it is instead aggravated. If photoexacerbation does occur, the new eruption generally develops or worsens initially at sites typical of the basic disorder (Fig. 95-3), followed at times by extension to other areas. In photoexacerbated seborrheic eczema, however, an unpleasant sensation at the exposed sites may be the first or only feature. Treatment consists of minimizing sunlight exposure, protection with suitable clothing, application of high-protection-factor broad-spectrum sunscreens, and careful treatment of the underlying disorder. Taking these steps alone often improves the problem. If these actions are inadequate, phototherapy often helps, for example, in seborrheic or atopic eczema and psoriasis. Often a particular value in distinguishing between photoaggravation and true photosensitivity in these conditions is to decide whether or not phototherapy can be used. Phototherapy is contraindicated in cutaneous lupus erythematosus or dermatomyositis becauseaggravation of the systemic disease is a risk. Photoexacerbated acne commonly requires treatment with oral isotretinoin.

TABLE 95-2
Selection of Diseases Sometimes Exacerbated by Ultraviolet Irradiation

- Acne
- Atopic eczema
- Carcinoid syndrome
- Cutaneous T-cell lymphoma
- Dermatomyositis
- Disseminated superficial actinic porokeratosis
- Erythema multiforme
- Familial benign chronic pemphigus (Hailey-Hailey disease)
- Keratosis follicularis (Darier disease)
- Lichen planus
- Lupus erythematosus
- Pellagra
- Pemphigus foliaceus (erythematosus)
- Pityriasis rubra pilaris
- Psoriasis
- Reticulate erythematous mucinosis syndrome
- Rosacea
- Seborrheic eczema
- Transient acantholytic dermatosis (Grover disease)
- Viral infections

and the appearance of lesions; duration of the eruption after exposure ceases; effects of sunlight received through window glass (implicating UVA and visible light); presence of systemic symptoms; and patient-assessed morphologies (progression of the disease before the clinic visit).

In terms of age and sex, young women are more likely to develop PLE/PMLE; women or girls more commonly develop actinic prurigo; children of either

APPROACH TO THE PATIENT WITH A DERMATOSIS ON PHOTOEXPOSED SITES

CLINICAL FEATURES

Patients with abnormal photosensitivity present in 3 ways: (a) sporadic or (b) persistent eruptions in sunlight-exposed areas (Fig. 95-4), or, infrequently, (c) erythroderma. When sporadic, the patient usually considers sunlight exposure to be responsible; when persistent, the physician often must identify the association. Careful history taking is essential, first to confirm that sunlight exposure is responsible and then to make a diagnosis. Information of considerable importance are age at disease onset, gender, family history, previous sunlight sensitivity, occupation, leisure pursuits, and systemic and topical drug (or chemical) use. Additional relevant details include distribution of lesions; effects of season; exposure times required for induction; time between exposure

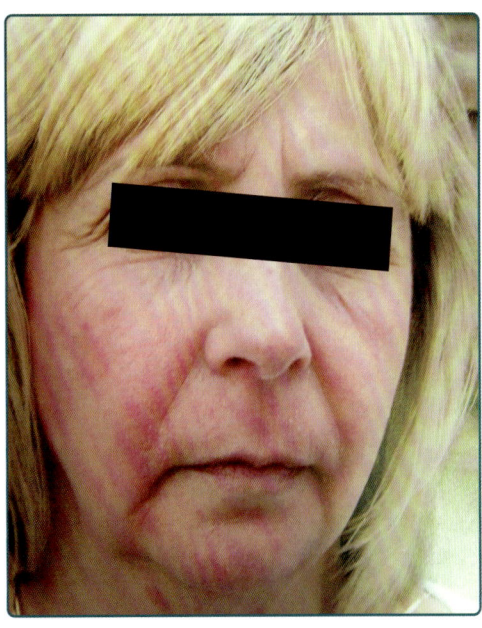

Figure 95-3 Photoexacerbated seborrheic dermatitis, affecting the face only at sites of predilection for the seborrheic eruption.

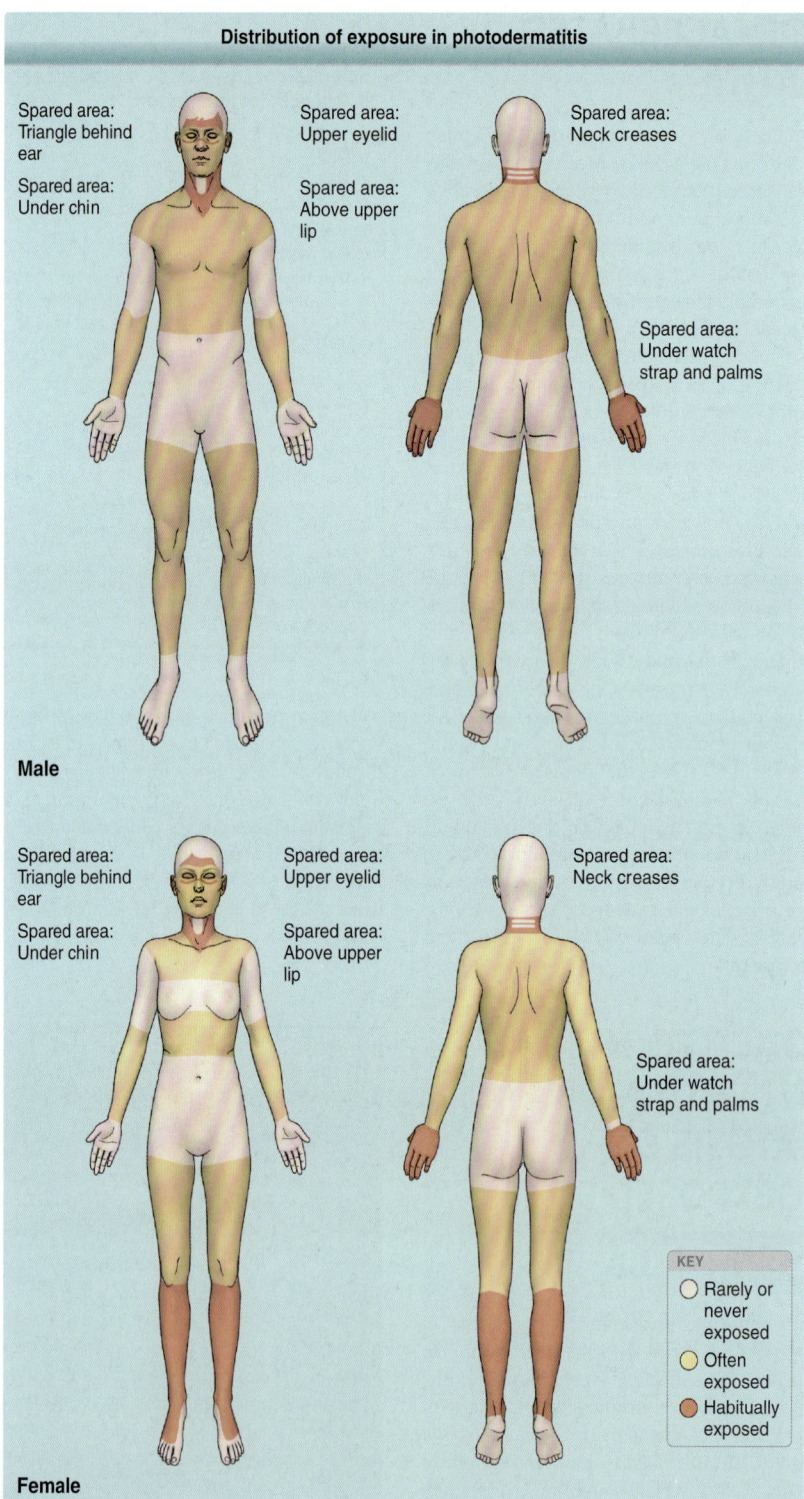

Figure 95-4 Distribution of exposure in photodermatitis. (From Wolff K, Johnson RA, Saavedra AP, et al. *Fitzpatrick's Color Atlas and Synopsis of Clinical Dermatology*, 8th ed. New York, NY: McGraw-Hill; 2017, with permission.)

gender may have HV, xeroderma pigmentosum, or erythropoietic protoporphyria; elderly men or younger individuals with a history of eczema most often develop CAD.

A family history of sunlight sensitivity may be present in patients with PMLE/PLE, actinic prurigo, xeroderma pigmentosum, and the porphyrias. CAD is common in outdoor enthusiasts exposed to both sunlight and airborne allergens (it is important to also consider it in patients from other demographics), although exacerbations of disease, despite sunscreen use, invoke the possibility of sunscreen allergy. An eruption appearing in minutes and remitting within 2 hours suggests solar urticaria or, occasionally, photosensitivity to drugs, such as amiodarone. Onset within 20 minutes to several hours, with resolution over days suggests PLE/PMLE, HV, erythropoietic protoporphyria, cutaneous lupus erythematosus, or other photoexacerbated dermatoses, or other drug photosensitivities, such as to thiazides. Systemic malaise is uncommon, but well recognized, in PMLE/PLE, HV, and solar urticaria. Development of lesions after exposure through window glass suggests an inducing spectrum that includes UVA and/or visible light.

The eruption described by patients with PMLE/PLE is generally that of small or large, elevated, pruritic, red or skin-colored, and often clumped spots of papules, sometimes confluent, that usually involve several, but not all exposed sites. In HV, blistering with scar formation occurs, and in solar urticaria, elevated pruritic wheals are often confluent. In erythropoietic protoporphyria and amiodarone drug photosensitivity, a marked burning sensation, without visible change, has been reported. In erythropoietic protoporphyria, relatively lengthy exposure may lead to firm, colorless or pink, diffuse swelling. In most drug photosensitivity reactions and in xeroderma pigmentosum, an exaggerated sunburn-like reaction is possible, which in many forms of xeroderma pigmentosum is maximal at 2 to 3 days. Finally, in photoexacerbated dermatoses, the eruption resembles that of the primary disorder.

Photosensitivity eruptions are usually present on some, and occasionally all, of the forehead; nose; upper cheeks; tip of the chin; rims of the pinnae; back and sides of the neck; upper chest; backs of the hands and feet; and extensor aspects of the limbs. Covered areas also may be involved, but to a lesser extent. On the other hand, portions of the face protected by hair or customarily in shadow, such as upper eyelids, finger webs, skin creases, and skin under the nose, lower lip, chin, and backs of earlobes, are frequently unaffected, except when there is associated airborne contact dermatitis. Excoriated papules suggest actinic prurigo, whereas eczematous lesions or, very rarely, light-associated erythrodermas suggest CAD, photoexacerbated atopic, or seborrheic eczema. Finally, skin fragility, bulla formation, and atrophic superficial scarring suggest hepatic porphyria or pseudoporphyria, especially if there has been drug or excessive alcohol intake.

Clinical appraisal along with the history usually results in a diagnosis, although for complete certainty, several of the studies listed below may be appropriate.

LABORATORY STUDIES

If the diagnosis is not certain, appropriate additional studies include an assessment of the antinuclear antibody and extractable nuclear antibody panel. If present at significant titers, cutaneous lupus erythematosus should be considered. In addition, examination of blood, urine, and stools for porphyrins should be considered.

Biopsies may be helpful. Lesional histologic features are characteristic in several photodermatoses, especially PMLE, HV, and CAD. However, with the exception of HV, histopathologic changes in photodermatoses are rarely entirely diagnostic. These are reviewed in the preceding disease descriptions.

Phototesting of normal back skin with a monochromator in CAD and solar urticaria often produces the papules or wheals of the condition itself, frequently at low irradiation doses, and this also may identify the action spectrum. Phototesting also helps to confirm xeroderma pigmentosum through the delayed development of erythema over 2 to 3 days, with an abnormally low-dose threshold, often eventuating in blister formation (Table 95-3). In eczematous photosensitivity, patch and photopatch testing are also essential to identify relevant allergens. Finally, special techniques, such as the assessment of DNA excision repair or of RNA synthesis recovery rate in cultured fibroblasts after UVR exposure, are essential for the diagnoses of certain genophotodermatoses.

PHOTOTESTING

Techniques of phototesting vary greatly from country to country and from center to center. Although it is the investigational technique of choice for photodermatoses when the diagnosis is uncertain or when details of the inducting action spectrum are required, phototesting remains unavailable in many clinical centers. The cost of the equipment and its infrequent use in most clinical practices means that patients should be referred for consultation to such centers whenever indicated.

Phototesting falls into 2 categories: (a) monochromator phototesting (testing to wavebands, it is not strictly monochromatic, produced by an irradiation monochromator),[35] usually of the upper back with selected wavebands and selected doses to identify the action spectrum for the disorder and to provoke the eruption (frequently responses at 24 hours and later after irradiating small circles of back skin with a monochromator look eczematous in CAD), and (b) photoprovocation with a broad-spectrum source to induce the eruption for its clinical appearance and subsequent biopsy if indicated. Table 95-3 lists the disorders for which monochromatic testing may be helpful.

For precise characterization of the wavelength dependency of a disorder, monochromator testing, preferably with a xenon arc irradiation monochromator, should be

TABLE 95-3
Usual Monochromatic Phototest Responses in Idiopathic, Probably Immunologic, Photodermatoses

DISEASE	ACTION SPECTRUM	FREQUENCY OF ABNORMAL FINDINGS
Polymorphic light eruption	UVA more often than UVB	Only sometimes
Actinic prurigo	UVA more often than UVB	Only sometimes
Hydroa vacciniforme	More often UVA	Only sometimes
Chronic actinic dermatitis	UVB ± UVA ± visible light	Virtually always
Solar urticaria	UVB, UVA, or visible, or combination	Usual
Xeroderma pigmentosum	UVB	Usual
Photoexacerbated dermatoses	UVB, UVA, or combination	Rare

UVA, ultraviolet A radiation; UVB, ultraviolet B radiation.

employed. For photoprovocation, the favored device is often a solar simulator, usually a xenon arc-filtered source that produces a spectrum that resembles the terrestrial sunlight spectrum at noon at sea level on a cloudless midsummer's day in temperate regions of the world. Keep in mind that the terrestrial spectrum at noon in June varies considerably between Iceland and Kenya, as it also does between high elevations and sea level. So, a solar simulator is only ever a simulator of a certain "type" of sunlight. Several suitable protocols also have been described for using simple broad-spectrum metal halide or fluorescent light sources with filters if necessary. In some parts of the world, sunlight with filters also has been used, although this method is generally too unpredictable for clinical use.

The mainstay of phototesting is a monochromator. It is composed of a high-pressure xenon arc source that emits radiation along a pathway incorporating a diffraction grating angled to produce the required waveband at the exit slit. Such equipment needs regular calibration of output and wavelength. Because even large centers cannot always afford such equipment, lesser alternatives have been created, such as metal halide or fluorescent light sources of sufficient output intensity. With such sources, the UVB, UVA, and visible light components of patient photosensitivity can be studied, based on deviation from normal erythemal reactions throughout the UVR spectrum.

Monochromator phototesting is preferably performed on unaffected skin of the upper back, lateral to the paravertebral groove whereas lesion induction, except when done relatively easily with the monochromator, as in solar urticaria and CAD, is best undertaken using broadband sources with output directed over larger areas of skin known to be susceptible to the eruption. PLE/PMLE, actinic prurigo, and HV are conditions in which repeated irradiation with UVA-emitting or UVB-emitting or combined sources is often required to reproduce the disease.

It is important that the use of potent topical and systemic steroids be avoided when possible for at least several days before phototesting to prevent false-negative results.[31,32] It is not certain how much the other oral immunosuppressive agents affect testing (and in CAD severe abnormal sensitivity can still be seen in those on azathioprine, methotrexate, or ciclosporin), but they should be stopped whenever possible as well. False-positive results may also occur in patients with widespread disease (with the possibility of photoaggravation of an underlying process being mistaken for true photosensitivity), and the eruption should first be well-controlled whenever possible, if necessary by keeping the patient in a reduced-light environment. However, it is often difficult to fulfill these requirements if the eruption is active, and in such circumstances, testing may need to be undertaken with knowledge of its limitations.

All phototesting should be undertaken at carefully standardized sequential doses (often a geometric series) and wavelengths, and the results read at consistent times after exposure in carefully controlled conditions of light and temperature. Furthermore, because testing involves UVR exposure, potentially harmful to both skin and eyes, the patient and the investigator should be protected with appropriate clothing, shielding and goggles.

PHOTOPATCH TESTING

Chapter 97 discusses photopatch testing in greater detail. Photopatch testing is an established investigational tool designed to identify photoallergic contact dermatitis, although it also can be employed to help identify phototoxic agents. It is essentially a more complex version of patch testing, and it is used in patients with exposed-site eczema, whether or not they also have another photodermatosis, to determine whether photoallergy is also present.

The methodology of photopatch testing has received less attention than allergen testing or phototesting, as it resides between the 2 specialty areas of photodermatology and contact dermatology. However, consensus methodology is now available.[74-78]

Using this approach, test materials (usually sunscreens, topical nonsteroidal, and antiinflammatory agents in Europe and North America—it is important to consider what might be locally relevant, eg, some antiseptics still used in soap in parts of the world—and other possible causative agents) are applied in duplicate for 24 to 48 hours to normal skin. One set of test sites is then uncovered and irradiated with a broad-spectrum UVA source, usually at 5 J/cm^2 from fluorescent UVA lamps (as used for psoralen activated by UVA), and the results read 24 and 48 hours later. Ideally, at the time of application of the patch tests (if 24 hours before planned irradiation), irradiations to determine the minimal erythemal dose with the planned UVA source should be conducted, especially if severe photosensitivity such as in CAD is possible. Sometimes if the minimal erythemal dose is extremely low the results preclude irradiation with any UVA, but sometimes they allow photopatch testing to proceed using a dose lower than the standard 5 J/cm^2. Strongly positive reactions at sites exposed to both chemical agent and UVA, with no reactions at the covered control sites, confirms a diagnosis of photoallergy. Occasionally, however, contact irritation or contact allergy occurs in both sites, making a diagnosis of photoallergy uncertain. One should also be alert to the possibility that all irradiated sites may become positive (especially if the patient is photosensitive and a UVA minimal erythemal dose was not done), suggesting that underlying widespread UVA photosensitivity is responsible. Furthermore, the identification of potential photoallergens is still primitive, often with separation of phototoxicity from photoallergy uncertain. Once again, testing for photoallergy is best conducted in regional centers or by physicians with appropriate experience.

ACKNOWLEDGMENTS

The author is grateful to the previous authors for the earlier versions of this chapter, Travis W. Vandergriff, Paul R. Bergstresser, John L. M. Hawk, and James Ferguson. I have not made changes for "changes sake," but I have added to or changed the text where new knowledge is available, where extra information might be useful, and to make this chapter as useful as possible in all parts of the world.

REFERENCES

1. Hawk JL, Magnus IA. Chronic actinic dermatitis—an idiopathic photosensitivity syndrome including actinic reticuloid and photosensitive eczema [proceedings]. *Br J Dermatol.* 1979;101(suppl 17):24.
2. Frain-Bell W, Lakshmipathi T, Rogers J, et al. The syndrome of chronic photosensitivity dermatitis and actinic reticuloid. *Br J Dermatol.* 1974;91:617-634.
3. Khoo SW, Tay YK, Tham SN. Photodermatoses in a Singapore skin referral centre. *Clin Exp Dermatol.* 1996;21:263-268.
4. Tan KW, Haylett AK, Ling TC, et al. Comparison of demographic and photobiological features of chronic actinic dermatitis in patients with lighter vs darker skin types. *JAMA Dermatol.* 2017;153:427-435.
5. Que SK, Brauer JA, Soter NA, et al. Chronic actinic dermatitis: an analysis at a single institution over 25 years. *Dermatitis.* 2011;22:147-154.
6. Kerr HA, Lim HW. Photodermatoses in African Americans: a retrospective analysis of 135 patients over a 7-year period. *J Am Acad Dermatol.* 2007;57:638-643.
7. Fujita M, Miyachi Y, Horio T, et al. Immunohistochemical comparison of actinic reticuloid with allergic contact dermatitis. *J Dermatol Sci.* 1990;1:289-296.
8. Hannuksela M, Suhonen R, Forstrom L. Delayed contact allergies in patients with photosensitivity dermatitis. *Acta Derm Venereol.* 1981;61:303-306.
9. Schauder S, Schroder W, Geier J. Olaquindox-induced airborne photoallergic contact dermatitis followed by transient or persistent light reactions in 15 pig breeders. *Contact Dermatitis.* 1996;35:344-354.
10. Thune P. Contact and photocontact allergy to sunscreens. *Photodermatol.* 1984;1:5-9.
11. Thune P. Photosensitivity and allergy to cosmetics. *Contact Dermatitis.* 1981;7:54-55.
12. Wahlberg JE, Wennersten G. Light sensitivity and chromium dermatitis. *Br J Dermatol.* 1977;97:411-416.
13. Thune P. Contact allergy due to lichens in patients with a history of photosensitivity. *Contact Dermatitis.* 1977;3:267-272.
14. du P Menagé H, Hawk JL, White IR. Sesquiterpene lactone mix contact sensitivity and its relationship to chronic actinic dermatitis: a follow-up study. *Contact Dermatitis.* 1998;39:119-122.
15. Frain-Bell W. Photosensitivity and compositae dermatitis. *Clin Dermatol.* 1986;4:122-126.
16. Addo HA, Sharma SC, Ferguson J, et al. A study of compositae plant extract reactions in photosensitivity dermatitis. *Photodermatol.* 1985;2:68-79.
17. Addo HA, Ferguson J, Johnson BE, et al. The relationship between exposure to fragrance materials and persistent light reaction in the photosensitivity dermatitis with actinic reticuloid syndrome. *Br J Dermatol.* 1982;107:261-274.
18. Frain-Bell W, Johnson BE. Contact allergic sensitivity to plants and the photosensitivity dermatitis and actinic reticuloid syndrome. *Br J Dermatol.* 1979;101:503-512.
19. Vin-Christian K, Epstein JH, Maurer TA, et al. Photosensitivity in HIV-infected individuals. *J Dermatol.* 2000;27:361-369.
20. Palmer RA, Friedmann PS. Ultraviolet radiation causes less immunosuppression in patients with polymorphic light eruption than in controls. *J Invest Dermatol.* 2004;122:291-294.
21. Menage HD, Harrison GI, Potten CS, et al. The action spectrum for induction of chronic actinic dermatitis is similar to that for sunburn inflammation. *Photochem Photobiol.* 1995;62:976-979.
22. ten Berge O, van Weelden H, Bruijnzeel-Koomen CA, et al. Throwing a light on photosensitivity in atopic dermatitis: a retrospective study. *Am J Clin Dermatol.* 2009;10:119-123.
23. Healy E, Rogers S. Photosensitivity dermatitis/actinic reticuloid syndrome in an Irish population: a review and some unusual features. *Acta Derm Venereol.* 1995;75:72-74.
24. Russell SC, Dawe RS, Collins P, et al. The photosensitivity dermatitis and actinic reticuloid syndrome (chronic actinic dermatitis) occurring in seven young atopic dermatitis patients. *Br J Dermatol.* 1998;138:496-501.
25. Ogboli MI, Rhodes LE. Chronic actinic dermatitis in young atopic dermatitis sufferers. *Br J Dermatol.* 2000;142:845.
26. Creamer D, McGregor JM, Hawk JL. Chronic actinic dermatitis occurring in young patients with atopic dermatitis. *Br J Dermatol.* 1998;139:1112-1113.
27. Kurumaji Y, Kondo S, Fukuro S, et al. Chronic actinic dermatitis in a young patient with atopic dermatitis. *J Am Acad Dermatol.* 1994;31:667-669.
28. Sidiropoulos M, Deonizio J, Martinez-Escala ME, et al. Chronic actinic dermatitis/actinic reticuloid: a clinicopathologic and immunohistochemical analysis of 37 cases. *Am J Dermatopathol.* 2014;36:875-881.
29. Zugerman C, Beeaff D, Roenigk HH Jr. Photosensitivity and Sezary syndrome. *Cutis.* 1980;25:495-499.
30. Hu SC, Lan CE. Tungsten lamp and chronic actinic dermatitis. *Australas J Dermatol.* 2017;58:e14-e16.

31. Ferguson J, Ibbotson SH. A case of false-negative monochromator phototesting in a patient with chronic actinic dermatitis taking prednisolone. *Br J Dermatol.* 2012;167:214-215.
32. Kerr AC, Dawe RS, Lowe G, et al. False-negative monochromator phototesting in chronic actinic dermatitis. *Br J Dermatol.* 2010;162:1406-1408.
33. Cripps DJ. Instrumentation and action spectra in light-associated diseases. *J Invest Dermatol.* 1981;77:20-31.
34. DeLeo V, Gonzalez E, Kim J, et al. Phototesting and photopatch testing: when to do it and when not to do it. *Am J Contact Dermat.* 2000;11:57-61.
35. Bilsland D, Diffey BL, Farr PM, et al. Diagnostic phototesting in the United Kingdom. British Photodermatology Group. *Br J Dermatol.* 1992;127:297-299.
36. MacKenzie LA, Frain-Bell W. The construction and development of a grating monochromator and its application to the study of the reaction of the skin to light. *Br J Dermatol.* 1973;89:251-264.
37. Agarwal KK, D'Souza M. Airborne contact dermatitis induced by parthenium: a study of 50 cases in South India. *Clin Exp Dermatol.* 2009;34:e4-e6.
38. Ross JS, du Peloux Menage H, Hawk JL, et al. Sesquiterpene lactone contact sensitivity: clinical patterns of Compositae dermatitis and relationship to chronic actinic dermatitis. *Contact Dermatitis.* 1993;29:84-87.
39. Dawe RS, Green CM, MacLeod TM, et al. Daisy, dandelion and thistle contact allergy in the photosensitivity dermatitis and actinic reticuloid syndrome. *Contact Dermatitis.* 1996;35:109-110.
40. Kuno Y, Kato M. Photosensitivity from colophony in a case of chronic actinic dermatitis associated with contact allergy from colophony. *Acta Derm Venereol.* 2001;81:442-443.
41. Krutmann J, Rzany B, Schopf E, et al. Airborne contact dermatitis from colophony: phototoxic reaction? *Contact Dermatitis.* 1989;21:275-276.
42. Pirmez R, Fernandes AL, Melo MG. Photoaggravated contact dermatitis to Kathon CG (methylchloroisothiazolinone/methylisothiazolinone): a novel pattern of involvement in a growing epidemic? *Br J Dermatol.* 2015;173:1343-1344.
43. Trokoudes D, Banerjee P, Fityan A, et al. Photoaggravated contact dermatitis caused by methylisothiazolinone. *Contact Dermatitis.* 2017;76:303-304.
44. Bilsland D, Ferguson J. Contact allergy to sunscreen chemicals in photosensitivity dermatitis/actinic reticuloid syndrome (PD/AR) and polymorphic light eruption (PLE). *Contact Dermatitis.* 1993;29:70-73.
45. Jensen NE, Sneddon IB. Actinic reticuloid with lymphoma. *Br J Dermatol.* 1970;82:287-291.
46. Bilsland D, Crombie IK, Ferguson J. The photosensitivity dermatitis and actinic reticuloid syndrome: no association with lymphoreticular malignancy. *Br J Dermatol.* 1994;131:209-214.
47. Bakels V, van Oostveen JW, Preesman AH, et al. Differentiation between actinic reticuloid and cutaneous T cell lymphoma by T cell receptor gamma gene rearrangement analysis and immunophenotyping. *J Clin Pathol.* 1998;51:154-158.
48. Dawe RS, Crombie IK, Ferguson J. The natural history of chronic actinic dermatitis. *Arch Dermatol.* 2000;136:1215-1220.
49. Neill SM, Du Vivier A. A case of mycosis fungoides mimicking actinic reticuloid. *Br J Dermatol.* 1985;113:497-500.
50. Volden G. A study of the photosensitive factor in relation to skin lesions of mycosis fungoides patients. *Dermatologica.* 1980;161:89-92.
51. Agar N, Morris S, Russell-Jones R, et al. Case report of four patients with erythrodermic cutaneous T-cell lymphoma and severe photosensitivity mimicking chronic actinic dermatitis. *Br J Dermatol.* 2009;160:698-703.
52. Bhari N, Gupta S. Tacrolimus 0.1% ointment applied under occlusion using cling film clears chronic actinic dermatitis resistant to systemic treatment. *Int J Dermatol.* 2017;56:e139-e141.
53. Ma Y, Lu Z. Treatment with topical tacrolimus favors chronic actinic dermatitis: a clinical and immunopathological study. *J Dermatolog Treat.* 2010;21:171-177.
54. Larangeira de Almeida H Jr. Successful treatment of chronic actinic dermatitis with topical pimecrolimus. *Int J Dermatol.* 2005;44:343-344.
55. Baldo A, Prizio E, Mansueto G, et al. A case of chronic actinic dermatitis treated with topical tacrolimus. *J Dermatolog Treat.* 2005;16:245-248.
56. McCall CO. Treatment of chronic actinic dermatitis with tacrolimus ointment. *J Am Acad Dermatol.* 2003;49:775; author reply 775-776.
57. Suga Y, Hashimoto Y, Matsuba S, et al. Topical tacrolimus for chronic actinic dermatitis. *J Am Acad Dermatol.* 2002;46:321-323.
58. Abe R, Shimizu T, Tsuji A, et al. Severe refractory chronic actinic dermatitis successfully treated with tacrolimus ointment. *Br J Dermatol.* 2002;147:1273-1275.
59. Dawe RS. Chronic actinic dermatitis in the elderly: recognition and treatment. *Drugs Aging.* 2005;22:201-207.
60. Yap LM, Foley P, Crouch R, et al. Chronic actinic dermatitis: a retrospective analysis of 44 cases referred to an Australian photobiology clinic. *Australas J Dermatol.* 2003;44:256-262.
61. Lim HW, Morison WL, Kamide R, et al. Chronic actinic dermatitis. An analysis of 51 patients evaluated in the United States and Japan. *Arch Dermatol.* 1994;130:1284-1289.
62. Murphy GM, Maurice PD, Norris PG, et al. Azathioprine treatment in chronic actinic dermatitis: a double-blind controlled trial with monitoring of exposure to ultraviolet radiation. *Br J Dermatol.* 1989;121:639-646.
63. Kingston TP, Lowe NJ, Sofen HL, et al. Actinic reticuloid in a black man: successful therapy with azathioprine. *J Am Acad Dermatol.* 1987;16:1079-1083.
64. Leigh IM, Hawk JL. Treatment of chronic actinic dermatitis with azathioprine. *Br J Dermatol.* 1984;110:691-695.
65. Haynes HA, Bernhard JD, Gange RW. Actinic reticuloid. Response to combination treatment with azathioprine, hydroxychloroquine, and prednisone. *J Am Acad Dermatol.* 1984;10:947-952.
66. Norris PG, Camp RD, Hawk JL. Actinic reticuloid: response to cyclosporine. *J Am Acad Dermatol.* 1989;21:307-309.
67. Duschet P, Schwarz T, Oppolzer G, et al. Persistent light reaction. Successful treatment with cyclosporin A. *Acta Derm Venereol.* 1988;68:176-178.
68. Thomson MA, Stewart DG, Lewis HM. Chronic actinic dermatitis treated with mycophenolate mofetil. *Br J Dermatol.* 2005;152:784-786.
69. Nousari HC, Anhalt GJ, Morison WL. Mycophenolate in psoralen-UV-A desensitization therapy for chronic actinic dermatitis. *Arch Dermatol.* 1999;135:1128-1129.
70. Hindson C, Spiro J, Downey A. PUVA therapy of chronic actinic dermatitis. *Br J Dermatol.* 1985;113:157-160.
71. Chee SN, Novakovic L, Fassihi H, et al. Chronic actinic dermatitis: successful treatment with PUVA photochemotherapy. *Br J Dermatol.* 2018;178(3):e189-e190.
72. Fenton L, Ferguson J, Ibbotson S, et al. Energy-saving lamps and their impact on photosensitive and normal individuals. *Br J Dermatol.* 2013;169:910-915.

73. Eadie E, Ferguson J, Moseley H. A preliminary investigation into the effect of exposure of photosensitive individuals to light from compact fluorescent lamps. *Br J Dermatol.* 2009;160:659-664.
74. European Multicentre Photopatch Test Study (EMCPPTS) Taskforce. A European multicentre photopatch test study. *Br J Dermatol.* 2012;166:1002-1009.
75. Bryden AM, Moseley H, Ibbotson SH, et al. Photopatch testing of 1155 patients: results of the U.K. multicentre photopatch study group. *Br J Dermatol.* 2006;155:737-747.
76. Chuah SY, Leow YH, Goon AT, et al. Photopatch testing in Asians: a 5-year experience in Singapore. *Photodermatol Photoimmunol Photomed.* 2013;29:116-120.
77. Jindal N, Sharma NL, Mahajan VK, et al. Evaluation of photopatch test allergens for Indian patients of photodermatitis: preliminary results. *Indian J Dermatol Venereol Leprol.* 2011;77:148-155.
78. Sharma VK, Sethuraman G, Bansal A. Evaluation of photopatch test series in India. *Contact Dermatitis.* 2007;56:168-169.

Chapter 96 :: Solar Urticaria
:: Marcus Maurer, Joachim W. Fluhr, & Karsten Weller

第九十六章
日光性荨麻疹

中文导读

　　日光性荨麻疹（SolU）是一种罕见的慢性诱导性荨麻疹，是一种特殊类型的物理性荨麻疹，主要特征是阳光照射后几分钟内出现红斑和瘙痒，几小时内可自行消退。本章节主要从该病的流行病学、病因和发病机制、临床特征、诊断、鉴别诊断、临床病程和预后、处理等方面来进行介绍。在临床特征方面，本章分别从皮肤表现、非皮肤表现对SolU进行描述。还提出可能出现的病因和发病机制，依据病史、实验室检查、光试验进行诊断，并总结了诊断思路，概述了鉴别诊断。此外，本章对治疗方法进行了总结。

〔易　梅〕

AT-A-GLANCE

- An uncommon form of chronic inducible urticaria
- Erythema and itchy wheals occur within minutes of sunlight exposure and resolve within hours.
- May be disabling and, rarely, life threatening.
- Phototesting confirms the diagnosis, determines the trigger threshold, and identifies the eliciting wave lengths.
- Sensitivity may be to ultraviolet B, ultraviolet A, visible light, and/or any combination, but most commonly to ultraviolet A and visible light.
- Sunlight avoidance, high-protection factor broad-spectrum sunscreens, and antihistamines may help.
- Omalizumab may be a helpful second-line treatment
- Phototherapy may also help but is usually not feasible as long-term treatment

INTRODUCTION

DEFINITIONS

Solar urticaria (SolU) is defined by the appearance of a whealing response within minutes of exposure to sunlight.[1] SolU is a rare type of physical urticaria. Physical urticarias, together with cholinergic urticaria, contact urticaria, and aquagenic urticaria, are subforms of chronic inducible urticaria, one of the 2 forms of chronic urticaria, the other one being chronic spontaneous urticaria. SolU usually is primary, where the cause is unknown. Very rarely, SolU is linked to cutaneous porphyria or systemic lupus erythematosus (SLE) and is then termed secondary SolU.

HISTORICAL PERSPECTIVE

Chronic inducible urticaria and their characteristic features, that is, wheal responses at skin sites exposed to urticariogenic triggers, were first described by Hippocrates.[2] The first reports of SolU are from the 18th century, and in 1887, SolU was identified as being sunlight-dependent.[3,4]

EPIDEMIOLOGY

The prevalence of SolU is low, but conclusive prevalence data are missing. It has been estimated that 3 in 100,000 are affected.[5] SolU reportedly accounts for 7% of all photodermatoses[6] and for less than 0.5% of all chronic urticaria cases.[7] SolU predominantly affects women in the third decade of life. Most patients show symptoms perennially, some only during spring to autumn.[5]

CLINICAL FEATURES

CUTANEOUS FINDINGS

SolU is characterized by erythema and itchy wheals that develop rapidly at skin sites exposed to sun or artificial light (Fig. 96-1). Light-exposed skin first shows diffuse erythema, followed by whealing associated with itch and/or, less frequently, burning and stinging. Wheals in SolU generally develop within a few minutes up to 1 hour of exposure and disappear usually within 1 hour and after a maximum of 24 hours of cessation of exposure, without leaving visible changes of the skin. SolU typically affects skin areas that are normally shielded by clothing and it spares skin sites that are frequently exposed to light such as the hands and the face, presumably because chronically sun-exposed areas show "hardening" or tolerance. SolU patients typically experience their first signs and symptoms after prolonged sun exposure on the first sunny days in spring. Rare variants include fixed SolU, which is characterized by the reoccurrence of light-induced whealing in the same location[8] and delayed SolU, where the onset of signs and symptoms after UV exposure is delayed by up to several hours. In some SolU patients, bruised skin is more sensitive to light.[9] Light-induced angioedema may occur.

NONCUTANEOUS FINDINGS AND COMPLICATIONS

Systemic involvement is rare and only occurs when large areas of skin are affected. Generalized signs and symptoms include malaise, nausea, dizziness, headaches, wheezing, dyspnea, loss of consciousness, and even anaphylactic shock, which is rarely fatal.

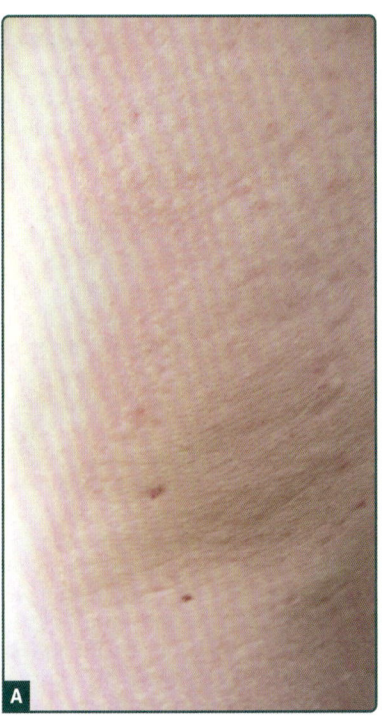
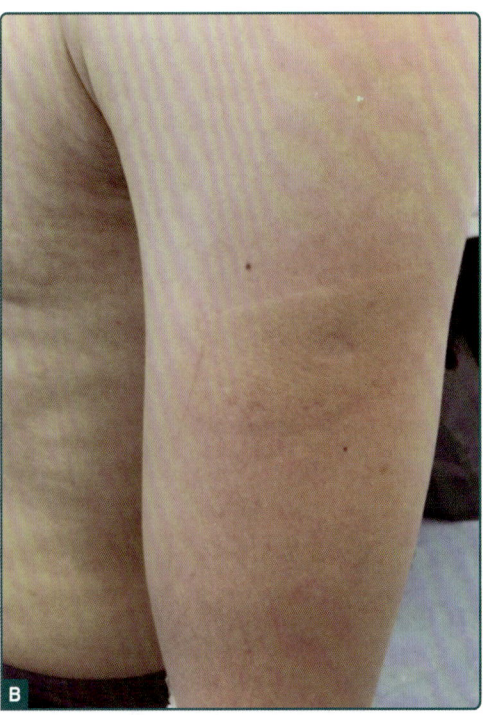

Figure 96-1 Solar urticaria. Pruritic wheals with a surrounding flare occurring 20 minutes after outdoor sun exposure at the arm. **A,** Close-up of the wheal. **B,** Lateral arm overview.

ETIOLOGY AND PATHOGENESIS

The signs and symptoms of SolU are due to the degranulation of skin mast cells and their subsequent release of histamine and other proinflammatory mediators. These mediators cause vasodilation (erythema) and increased extravasation (wheals, angioedema) and activate sensory nerves of the skin (itch). Widespread light-induced whealing in SolU patients can result in transiently increased blood levels of histamine.[10]

Skin mast cell degranulation in SolU is due to exposure of the skin to UVA (320 to 400 nm), visible (400 to 600 nm), less commonly UVB (280 to 320 nm), and, rarely, infrared (>600 nm) radiation. The underlying mechanism of mast cell degranulation has not been characterized in detail but is held to involve IgE that is specific for photo-induced neoantigens that act as autoallergens. This IgE is bound to the high-affinity IgE-receptor, FceRI, on cutaneous mast cells, which get activated by neoantigen-mediated crosslinking of IgE and FceRI. The wide range of relevant wavelengths is explained by the contribution of several different neoantigens/photoautoallergens with unique action spectra.[11,12] The range of eliciting wavelengths can narrow or broaden during the course of the disease, suggesting that the relevant neoantigens may vary over time. In some patients, skin exposure to distinct wavelength radiation, the so-called inhibition spectrum, can inhibit whealing in response to the eliciting wavelength spectrum.

RISK FACTORS

Specific risk factors for SolU or predictors for the severity or course of the disease have not yet been identified. SolU affects both genders and shows a female preponderance. The peak age of onset of symptoms is 20 to 40 years. There appears to be no influence of the skin type on the occurrence or severity of SolU.[13,14]

DIAGNOSIS

SUPPORTIVE STUDIES

The diagnosis of SolU is based on a thorough history. All patients who present with a history of rapid development of itching and whealing after exposure to light, should be investigated for SolU. Patients who report the occurrence of recurring itchy wheals should be asked if whealing can be induced, for example, by sun exposure. Patients who report the development of sunlight-induced skin lesions should be asked if these lesions resemble wheals, for example, if they are itchy, accompanied by erythema, short-lived, and transient. Photodocumentation including self-documentation with smartphone cameras of skin lesions at the time of occurrence is helpful.

LABORATORY TESTING

In SolU, routine laboratory tests are all within normal limits and not helpful for diagnosing the disease. Porphyria and SLE should be excluded by tests for antinuclear antibody (ANA) / extractable antinuclear antibody (ENA) and blood, urine and stool testing for porphyrins, respectively.

PATHOLOGY

SolU skin lesions, within the first hours after elicitation by irradiation, show vasodilation, edema, and perivascular neutrophils and eosinophils in the upper dermis. After 24 hours, mononuclear cells are the dominating infiltrating cells.[15] The histopathologic features of SolU do not allow for its distinction from other forms of urticaria.

PHOTOTESTING

Phototesting is essential for confirming the diagnosis of SolU. It also assesses disease activity by determining trigger thresholds and defines individual eliciting and inhibition spectra. Phototesting is performed by exposing patients to ultraviolet radiation and visible light at skin sites that have been protected from light for several days, most commonly the buttocks. No sunscreens, photoactive medications, or urticaria treatments should be used before phototesting, and the washout phase for antihistaminic and immunosuppressive medication prior to test needs to be adequate.

Phototesting is done with the help of solar simulators with filters (UVA and UVB) or monochromators (UVA and UVB, visible light) separately for UVA at 6 J/cm,^{2} UVB at 60 mJ/cm,^{2} and visible light. The test is considered positive if the test site exhibits a palpable and clearly visible itchy wheal and flare reaction at 10 minutes after phototesting. In patients with a positive phototest reaction, threshold testing is done with a range of doses of the eliciting wavelengths, for example, with UVA at 2.4, 3.3, 4.2, 5.1, and 6.0 J/cm^2 and with UVB at 24, 33, 42, 51, and 60 mJ/cm^2 (Fig. 96-2). Threshold testing determines the minimal urticarial dose, a marker of disease activity and response to therapy. In patients with a negative phototest and convincing history of light-induced whealing, SolU should not be excluded, and sunlight phototesting is recommended. Reasons for a negative phototest in patients with SolU include mild disease activity, with variable occurrence of signs and symptoms limited to erythema in some patients, prior intake of antihistamines or other medications that inhibit the development of wheals,

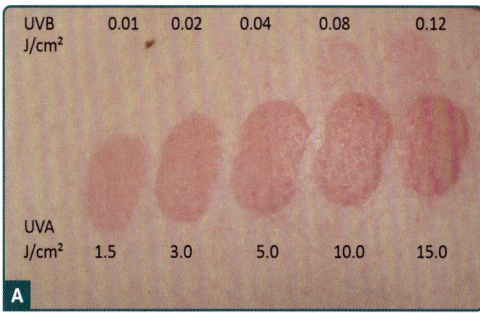
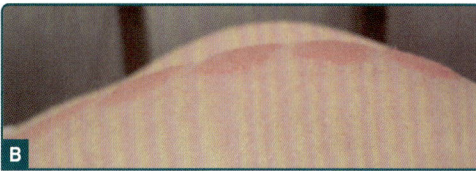

Figure 96-2 UVA and UVB testing with a solar simulator. **A,** Overview. **B,** lateral photography to demonstrate the elevation of the wheals.

and/or refractoriness of the skin due to previous light exposure of the test site.

DIAGNOSTIC ALGORITHM

See Fig. 96-3.

DIFFERENTIAL DIAGNOSIS

See Table 96-1.

CLINICAL COURSE AND PROGNOSIS

The mean duration of SolU is 5 to 7 years, but cases with disease duration of up to 50 years have been reported.[16] In a recent study, the median duration from disease onset to disease resolution was 63 months, and 50% of patients experienced complete spontaneous remission within 5 years of disease onset.[17] In contrast, older studies found rates of resolution of 12%, 26%, and 46% after 5, 10, and 15 years, respectively.[5,18]

MANAGEMENT

AVOIDANCE OF THE TRIGGER

All SolU patients should avoid the sun, wear protective clothing, and use high-protection broad-spectrum sunscreens, especially when the threshold is in the ultraviolet spectrum.

MEDICATIONS

Treatment with nonsedating H1 antihistamines at standard dose is the recommended first-line treatment. Evidence for the efficacy and safety of antihistamine treatment in SolU comes from controlled and uncontrolled studies,[19,20] case series and reports, as well as clinical experience. In case of insufficient response to treatment with a standard-dosed nonsedating second-generation antihistamine, doses should be increased up to 4-fold. This recommendation is largely based on the results of studies of other forms of inducible urticaria. Antihistamines work, but not in all patients. Updosing is needed in many.

Treatment with omalizumab, a monoclonal antibody directed against IgE, is recommended in patients who do not achieve sufficient control with the combined use of sunscreens and antihistamine treatment. For omalizumab, a complete or partial response in doses of up to 450 mg every 4 to 8 weeks has been reported in several case studies.[21-30] The best evidence comes from a recent open-label French multicentric Phase II study with 10 patients[31] that shows that omalizumab, at 300 mg every 4 weeks, is of benefit in half of the treated patients. Two reports showed no improvement.[32,33]

Other therapies that have been reported to be effective in some but not all patients include ciclosporin[34] and intravenous high-dose immunoglobins.[35,36] Afamelanotide, an alpha-MSH analog and melanocortin receptor agonist recently licensed for the treatment of erythropoietic protoporphyria, was shown to protect SolU patients from the development of signs and symptoms in a small open-label study.[37]

PROCEDURES

Tolerance to UV light can be achieved by desensitization achieved by phototherapy. This treatment is cumbersome and requires high patient compliance.[38] Phototherapy needs to be continued to maintain its effect. Discontinuation of phototherapy, in virtually all patients, results in the loss of protection from light-induced whealing.[39]

Phototherapy carries the usual risks of long-term phototherapy and should be done with caution because of the risk of anaphylaxis, particularly in severely affected individuals. So-called rush hardening protocols have been described (multiple UVA exposures with increasing doses during the same day) and may help some patients.[40,41]

COUNSELING

Avoidance of sun exposure and the use of high-protection factor broad-spectrum sunscreens and

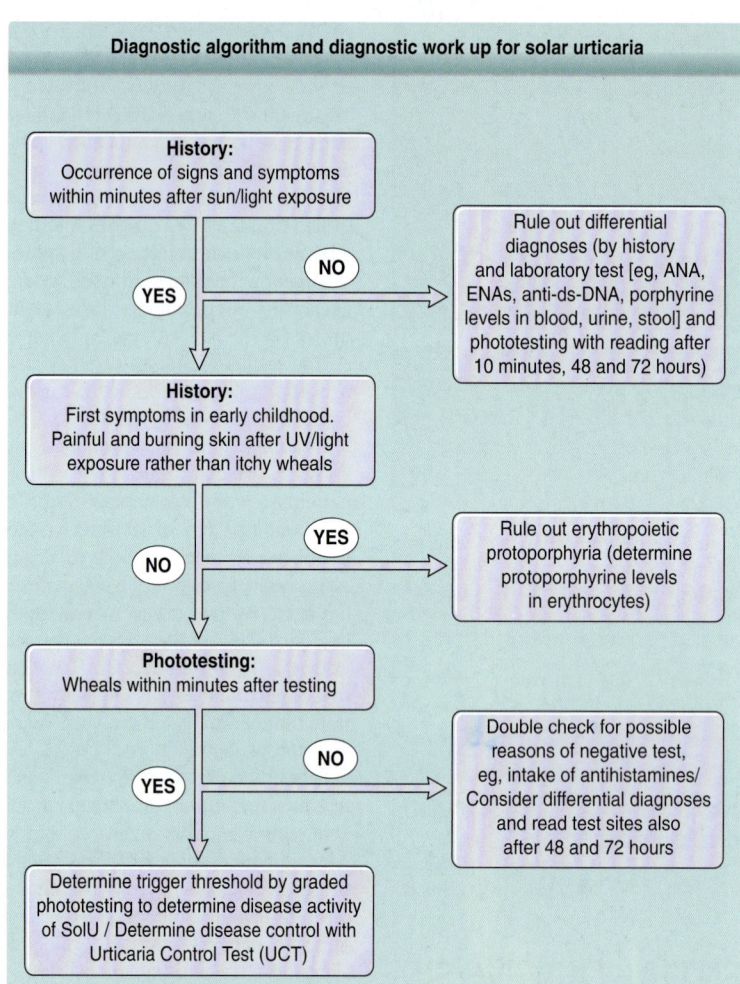

Figure 96-3 Diagnostic algorithm and diagnostic workup for solar urticaria.

appropriate clothing can help to prevent the development of SolU signs and symptoms.

MONITORING OF TREATMENT RESPONSES AND DISEASE ACTIVITY

Disease activity and control as well as response to treatment should be assessed at every patient visits. Suitable ways to do so include the urticaria control test (UCT) and trigger threshold phototesting.[42,43]

TREATMENT ALGORITHM

See Fig. 96-4.

ACKNOWLEDGMENTS

The authors acknowledge that this contribution is based, in part, on some of the content of the chapter by Travis W. Vandergriff and Paul R. Bergstresser on "Abnormal Responses to Ultraviolet Radiation: Idiopathic, Presumed Immunologic, and Photoexacerbated" in the 8th edition of *Fitzpatrick's Dermatology in General Medicine*.

REFERENCES

1. Magerl M, Altrichter S, Borzova E, et al. The definition, diagnostic testing, and management of chronic inducible urticarias—The EAACI/GA(2) LEN/EDF/UNEV consensus recommendations 2016 update and revision. *Allergy*. 2016;71(6):780-802.
2. Maurer M. Urticaria and angioedema. *Chem Immunol Allergy*. 2014;100:101-104.

TABLE 96-1
Differential Diagnosis of Solar Urticaria

DISORDER	DISTINGUISHING FEATURES	COMMON FEATURES
Polymorphic light eruption	Skin lesions: Papules, papulovesicles, eczematous appearance; occur within hours to days after UV exposure (not within minutes); resolve within several days (not minutes to hours).	May spare face and hands (hardening).
Lupus erythematosus	Skin lesions: Occur within days to weeks after UV exposure (not within minutes); resolve within weeks (not minutes to hours). ANAs are positive.	Skin lesions with wheallike appearance.
Photoexacerbated eczema (atopic, seborrheic)	Skin lesions: No wheals; occur within hours to days after UV exposure (not within minutes); resolve within several days (not minutes to hours).	
Photoallergic/phototoxic contact dermatitis	Skin lesions: No wheals; occur within hours to days after UV exposure (not within minutes); resolve within several days (not minutes to hours). Photoallergic contact dermatitis: Photopatchtest is positive.	
Erythropoietic protoporphyria	First symptoms in early childhood and lifelong persistence. Skin (lesions) is/are painful/burning but not itchy. The pain/burning often persists for hours to days. Elevated levels of protoporphyrin in erythrocytes.	Onset within minutes after UV exposure. Skin lesions may be wheallike.
Porphyria cutanea tarda	Increased skin vulnerability in UV-exposed areas. Skin lesions comprise blisters, erosions, scars, milia, hyper- and hypopigmentation, hypertrichosis, elastosis (but not wheals). Elevated porphyrin levels in urine. Liver enzymes frequently elevated.	
Drug or chemical photosensitivity	Patient uses medication. Skin lesions: Occur within hours to days after UV exposure (not within minutes); resolve within several days (not minutes to hours).	
Heat urticaria	Phototesting is negative; heat testing is positive.	Signs/symptoms identical to SolU.

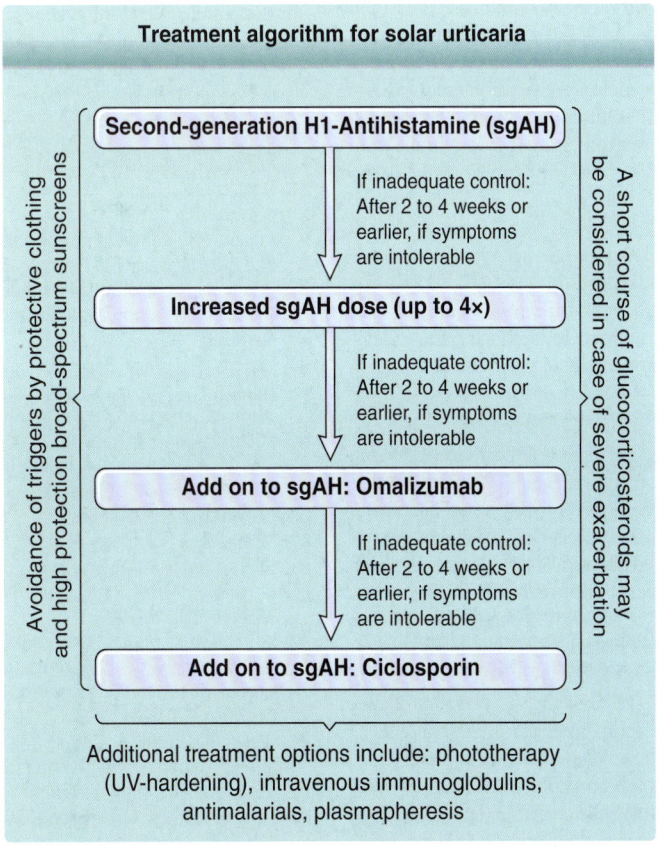

Figure 96-4 Treatment algorithm for solar urticarial.

3. Borsch JF. De purpura urticata, quam vocant "die Nesselsucht"; med diss, Halle. 1719.
4. Veiel T. Über einen Fall von Eczema solare. *Arch Derm Syph (Berlin)*. 1887;19(1113).
5. Beattie PE, Dawe RS, Ibbotson SH, et al. Characteristics and prognosis of idiopathic solar urticaria: a cohort of 87 cases. *Arch Dermatol*. 2003;139(9):1149-1154.
6. Chong WS, Khoo SW. Solar urticaria in Singapore: an uncommon photodermatosis seen in a tertiary dermatology center over a 10-year period. *Photodermatol Photoimmunol Photomed*. 2004;20(2):101-104.
7. Champion RH. Urticaria: then and now. *Br J Dermatol*. 1988;119(4):427-436.
8. Reinauer S, Leenutaphong V, Holzle E. Fixed solar urticaria. *J Am Acad Dermatol*. 1993;29(2, pt 1):161-165.
9. Norris PG, Hawk JL. Bruising and susceptibility to solar urticaria. *Br J Dermatol*. 1991;124(4):393.
10. Hawk JL, Eady RA, Challoner AV, et al. Elevated blood histamine levels and mast cell degranulation in solar urticaria. *Br J Clin Pharmacol*. 1980;9(2):183-186.
11. Kojima M, Horiko T, Nakamura Y, et al. Solar urticaria. The relationship of photoallergen and action spectrum. *Arch Dermatol*. 1986;122(5):550-555.
12. Miyauchi H, Horio T. Detection of action, inhibition and augmentation spectra in solar urticaria. *Dermatology*. 1995;191(4):286-291.
13. Du-Thanh A, Debu A, Lalheve P, et al. Solar urticaria: a time-extended retrospective series of 61 patients and review of literature. *Eur J Dermatol*. 2013;23(2):202-207.
14. Pérez-Ferriols A, Barnadas M, Gardeazábal J, et al. Solar urticaria: epidemiology and clinical phenotypes in a Spanish series of 224 patients [in Spanish]. *Actas Dermosifiliogr*. 2017;108(2):132-139.
15. Norris PG, Murphy GM, Hawk JL, et al. A histological study of the evolution of solar urticaria. *Arch Dermatol*. 1988;124(1):80-83.
16. Ive H, Lloyd J, Magnus IA. Action spectra in idiopathic solar urticaria. A study of 17 cases with a monochromator. *Br J Dermatol*. 1965;77:229-243.
17. Silpa-Archa N, Wongpraparut C, Leenutaphong V. Analysis of solar urticaria in Thai patients. *Asian Pac J Allergy Immunol*. 2016;34(2):146-152.
18. Botto NC, Warshaw EM. Solar urticaria. *J Am Acad Dermatol*. 2008;59(6):909-920; quiz 921-922.
19. Bilsland D, Ferguson J. A comparison of cetirizine and terfenadine in the management of solar urticaria. *Photodermatol Photoimmunol Photomed*. 1991;8(2):62-64.
20. Monfrecola G, Masturzo E, Riccardo AM, et al. Cetirizine for solar urticaria in the visible spectrum. *Dermatology*. 2000;200(4):334-335.
21. Guzelbey O, Ardelean E, Magerl M, et al. Successful treatment of solar urticaria with anti-immunoglobulin E therapy. *Allergy*. 2008;63(11):1563-1565.
22. Levi A, Tal Y, Dranitzki Z, et al. Successful omalizumab treatment of severe solar urticaria in a 6-year-old child. *Pediatr Allergy Immunol*. 2015;26(6):588-590.
23. Metz M, Ohanyan T, Church MK, et al. Omalizumab is an effective and rapidly acting therapy in difficult-to-treat chronic urticaria: a retrospective clinical analysis. *J Dermatol Sci*. 2014;73(1):57-62.
24. Waibel KH, Reese DA, Hamilton RG, et al. Partial improvement of solar urticaria after omalizumab. *J Allergy Clin Immunol*. 2010;125(2):490-491.
25. Baliu-Pique C, Aguilera Peiro P. Three cases of solar urticaria successfully treated with omalizumab. *J Eur Acad Dermatol Venereol*. 2016;30(4):704-706.
26. Arasi S, Crisafulli G, Caminiti L, et al. Treatment with omalizumab in a 16-year-old Caucasian girl with refractory solar urticaria. *Pediatr Allergy Immunol*. 2015;26(6):583-585.
27. Kowalzick L, Thiel W, Bielfeld C, et al. Partial response of solar urticaria to omalizumab therapy [in German]. *Hautarzt*. 2017;68(6):492-496.
28. Brüning JH, Ziemer M, Pemler S, et al. Successful treatment of solar urticaria with omalizumab. *J Dtsch Dermatol Ges*. 2016;14(9):936-937.
29. de Dios-Velázquez Á, González-de Arriba M, Beteta-Gorriti V, et al. Effectiveness of omalizumab in severe solar urticaria. *Ann Allergy Asthma Immunol*. 2016;116(3):260-262.
30. Terrani I, Bircher AJ, Scherer Hofmeier K. Solar urticaria induced by visible light: successful treatment with omalizumab. *Clin Exp Dermatol*. 2016;41(8):890-892.
31. Aubin F, Avenel-Audran M, Jeanmougin M, et al. Omalizumab in patients with severe and refractory solar urticaria: a phase II multicentric study. *J Am Acad Dermatol*. 2016;74(3):574-575.
32. Muller S, Schempp CM, Jakob T. Failure of omalizumab in the treatment of solar urticaria. *J Eur Acad Dermatol Venereol*. 2016;30(3):524-525.
33. Duchini G, Bäumler W, Bircher AJ, et al. Failure of omalizumab (Xolair(R)) in the treatment of a case of solar urticaria caused by ultraviolet A and visible light. *Photodermatol Photoimmunol Photomed*. 2011; 27(6):336-337.
34. Hurabielle C, Bedane C, Avenel-Audran M, et al. No major effect of cyclosporin A in patients with severe solar urticaria: a French retrospective case series. *Acta Derm Venereol*. 2015;95(8):1030-1031.
35. Correia I, Silva J, Filipe P, et al. Solar urticaria treated successfully with intravenous high-dose immunoglobulin: a case report. *Photodermatol Photoimmunol Photomed*. 2008;24(6):330-331.
36. Aubin F, Porcher R, Jeanmougin M, et al. Severe and refractory solar urticaria treated with intravenous immunoglobulins: a phase II multicenter study. *J Am Acad Dermatol*. 2014;71(5):948-953.e1.
37. Haylett AK, Nie Z, Brownrigg M, et al. Systemic photoprotection in solar urticaria with alpha-melanocyte-stimulating hormone analogue [Nle4-D-Phe7]-alpha-MSH. *Br J Dermatol*. 2011;164(2):407-414.
38. Dawe RS, Ferguson J. Prolonged benefit following ultraviolet A phototherapy for solar urticaria. *Br J Dermatol*. 1997;137(1):144-148.
39. Wolf R, Herzinger T, Grahovac M, et al. Solar urticaria: long-term rush hardening by inhibition spectrum narrow-band UVB 311 nm. *Clin Exp Dermatol*. 2013;38(4):446-447.
40. Beissert S, Stander H, Schwarz T. UVA rush hardening for the treatment of solar urticaria. *J Am Acad Dermatol*. 2000;42(6):1030-1032.
41. Masuoka E, Fukunaga A, Kishigami K, et al. Successful and long-lasting treatment of solar urticaria with ultraviolet A rush hardening therapy. *Br J Dermatol*. 2012;167(1):198-201.
42. Kulthanan K, Chularojanamontri L, Tuchinda P, et al. Validity, reliability and interpretability of the Thai version of the urticaria control test (UCT). *Health Qual Life Outcomes*. 2016;14:61.
43. Weller K, Groffik A, Church MK, et al. Development and validation of the Urticaria Control Test: a patient-reported outcome instrument for assessing urticaria control. *J Allergy Clin Immunol*. 2014;133(5):1365-1372, 1372.e1-1372.e6.

Chapter 97 :: Phototoxicity and Photoallergy :: Henry W. Lim

第九十七章
光毒性与光过敏

中文导读

本章节主要介绍外源性引起的光敏反应，包括光毒性与光过敏。光毒性是由光毒性物质和辐射引起的直接组织损伤，光过敏主要是一种Ⅳ型变态反应，只在致敏个体中发生。本章节主要从流行病学、病因和发病机制、临床特征、诊断、鉴别诊断、临床病程和预后、处理等方面分别对光毒性、光过敏进行了阐述。

〔易 梅〕

AT-A-GLANCE

- Photosensitivity to exogenous agents is broadly divided into phototoxicity and photoallergy; it is caused by topical or systemic agents that absorb ultraviolet A (UVA) radiation.
- Phototoxicity occurs in anyone exposed to sufficient doses of phototoxic agent and UV radiation; it usually manifests as an exaggerated sunburn reaction.
- Photoallergy is an immune reaction to a UVA-modified chemical, commonly topical sunscreen agents and antimicrobials in the United States and the United Kingdom, and topical nonsteroidal antiinflammatory agents in Europe. It presents as eczematous eruption on sun-exposed areas.
- Phototoxicity and photoallergy do occur in patients with skin of color, frequently resulting in postinflammatory hyperpigmentation.
- History taking is an important part of the evaluation; phototesting and photopatch testing are sometimes helpful.
- Differential diagnosis includes contact allergic or contact irritant dermatitis, airborne contact dermatitis, and other photodermatoses.
- Management consists of identification and avoidance of the precipitating agent, photoprotection, and symptomatic therapy.

Photosensitivity may be caused by exogenous or endogenous agents. It occurs when a compound, classically one with unsaturated double bonds in a 6-carbon ring, absorbs radiation energy in its action spectrum, usually ultraviolet A (UVA) wavelengths. Exogenous photosensitizers can be agents administered systemically or applied topically. Well-characterized examples of photosensitivity induced by endogenous photosensitizers are the cutaneous porphyrias, which are associated with enzymatic defects in heme biosynthetic pathways that result in elevated levels of porphyrins, known phototoxic agents. This is covered in Chap. 124.

This chapter focuses on photosensitivity induced by exogenous agents, which can be divided into phototoxicity and photoallergy. Phototoxicity is the result of direct tissue injury caused by the phototoxic agent and radiation. It can occur in all individuals exposed to adequate doses of the agent and the activating wavelengths of radiation (Table 97-1). In contrast,

TABLE 97-1
Characteristics of Phototoxicity and Photoallergy

	PHOTOTOXICITY	PHOTOALLERGY
Clinical presentation	Exaggerated sunburn reaction: erythema, edema, vesicles, and bullae; burning, stinging; frequently resolves with hyperpigmentation	Eczematous lesions; usually pruritic
Histologic features	Eosinophilic keratinocytes, epidermal necrosis, dermal edema, sparse dermal infiltrate of lymphocytes, macrophages, and neutrophils	Spongiotic dermatitis, dermal lymphohistiocytic infiltrate
Pathophysiology	Direct tissue injury	Type IV delayed hypersensitivity response
Occurrence after first exposure	Yes	No
Onset after exposure	Minutes to hours	24-48 hours
Dose of agent needed for reaction	Large	Small
Cross-reactivity with other agents	None	Common
Diagnosis		
Topical agent	Clinical	Photopatch tests
Systemic agent	Clinical + phototests	Clinical + phototests; possibly photopatch tests

photoallergy is a type IV delayed hypersensitivity response to a molecule that has been modified by absorption of photons. It has a sensitization phase, occurs only in sensitized individuals, and requires only a minimal concentration of the photoallergen (Table 97-1).

PREVALENCE

Even though hundreds of medications in the United States are reported to cause photosensitivity, only a small number of them induce reactions frequently or have been well studied (Tables 97-2 to 97-5).[1] In evaluations performed at photodermatology centers in New York City, Melbourne, Singapore, and Detroit, photosensitivity induced by systemic drugs was documented in 5% to 16% of the referred patients.[2-5] These data from different parts of the world indicate that photoallergy and phototoxicity do occur in patients with skin of color, frequently resulting in postinflammatory hyperpigmentation. Studies on photopatch testing published between 2011 and 2016 from different parts of the world showed from 1.5% to 74% of patients who had photopatch testing performed had positive response.[6-12]

Most of the photosensitivity induced by systemic medications are phototoxicity, whereas those induced by topical agents are photoallergy. However, it should be noted that clinically, it is not always possible to clearly differentiate between phototoxicity and photoallergy. Because many drug-induced photosensitivity has not been well-studied, it is possible that it is underestimated.[1,13]

PHOTOTOXICITY

CLINICAL FEATURES

ACUTE PHOTOTOXICITY

This occurs within hours of exposure to the phototoxic agent and UV radiation. Symptoms are drug-dose and UV-dose dependent; at sufficient doses, the patient complains of a burning and stinging sensation on exposed areas, such as forehead, nose, V area of the neck, and dorsa of the hands (Fig. 97-1). Erythema and edema may appear within hours of exposure; in severe cases, vesicles and bullae may develop accompanied by pruritus. Protected areas, such as nasolabial folds, postauricular and submental areas, and areas covered by clothing, are spared. A notable exception to these kinetics is psoralen-induced pho-

TABLE 97-2
Topical Phototoxic and Photosensitizing Agents

AGENT	EXPOSURE
Phototoxic Agents	
Fluorescein	Used topically to visualize the anterior surface of the eye
Furocoumarins	Occur naturally in plants (especially *Compositae* species), including fruits and vegetables (lime, lemon, celery, fig, parsley, and parsnip); used in topical photochemotherapy
Rose bengal	Used in ophthalmologic examinations
Tar	Used as topical therapeutic agent; found in roofing materials
Photosensitizing Agents[a]	
Fluorouracil[a]	Topical treatment of actinic keratoses
Retinoids[a]	For treatment of acne and photoaging

[a]Induces exaggerated ultraviolet response because of skin irritancy.

TABLE 97-3
Systemic Phototoxic Agents

CLASS	GENERIC NAME (COMMON U.S. TRADE NAMES)[a]	CLASS	GENERIC NAME (COMMON U.S. TRADE NAMES)[a]
Antiandrogen	Bicalutamide (Casodex)	Immunosuppressant	Acetic acid derivative
	Flutamide (Eulexin)	Nonsteroidal antiinflammatory drugs	Diclofenac (Cambia, Cataflam, Flector, Pennsaid, Solaraze, Voltaren, Zipsor)
Antifibrotic agent	Pirfenidone (Esbriet)		
Antifungal agents	Griseofulvin (Fulvicin, Grifulvin V, Gris-PEG)[b]		
	Voriconazole (Vfend)[c]		Alkanone derivative
Antimalarials	Chloroquine (Aralen)		Nabumetone (Relafen)[c,d]
	Quinine[b]		Anthranilic acid derivative
Antimicrobials	Sulfonamides		Mefenamic acid (Ponstel)
	Tetracyclines		Cyclooxygenase-2 inhibitor
	Demeclocycline (Declomycin)[c]		Celecoxib (Celebrex)
	Doxycycline (Adoxa, Doryx, Monodox, Periostat, Vibra-Tabs, Vibramycin)[c]		Enolic acid derivative
			Piroxicam (Feldene)[b,c]
	Minocycline (Arestin, Dynacin, Minocin)		Propionic acid derivatives
	Tetracycline (Helidac, Sumycin)		Ibuprofen (Advil, Medipren, Motrin, Nuprin)
	Trimethoprim (Bactrim, Polytrim, Primsol, Septra)[c]		
			Ketoprofen[b]
	Quinolones		Naproxen (Aleve, Anaprox, Naprelan, Midol, Naprosyn, Rugby, Select)[c]
	Ciprofloxacin (Cipro)		
	Enoxacin (Penetrex)[b]		Oxaprozin (Daypro)
	Gemifloxacin (Factive)		Tiaprofenic acid (Surgam, Surgamyl, Tiaprofen)
	Lomefloxacin (Maxaquin, Okacyn, Uniquin)[b,c]		
	Moxifloxacin (Avelox, Moxeza, Vigamox)		Salicylic acid derivative
	Nalidixic acid (NegGram)[b,c]		Diflunisal (Dolobid)
	Norfloxacin (Noroxin, Chibroxin–ophthalmic solution)		Capecitabine (Xeloda)
		Oncologic drugs	Crizotinib (Xalkori)
	Ofloxacin (Floxin, Ocuflox–ophthalmic solution)		Dacarbazine (DTIC, DTIC-Dome)
			Dabrafenib (Tafinlar)
	Sparfloxacin (Zagam)[c,d]		Docetaxel (Docefrez, Taxotere)
			Fluorouracil (Adrucil)
Cardiac drugs	Amiodarone (Cordarone, Nexterone, Pacerone)[c]		Methotrexate (Rheumatrex)[e]
	Quinidine (Quinaglute, Quinidex)[b]		Paclitaxel (Abraxane, Onxol, Taxol)
Diuretics	Furosemide (Lasix)[c]		Vemurafenib (Zelboraf)[c]
	Thiazides		Vinblastine (Velban)
	Bendroflumethiazide (Aprinox, Naturetin)	Photodynamic therapy agents	Porfimer (Photofrin)[c]
	Bendroflumethiazide/Nadolol (Corzide)		Verteporfin (Visudyne)[c]
	Chlorothiazide (Diuril)[c]	Psychotropic drugs	Alprazolam (Niravam, Xanax)
	Hydrochlorothiazide (Apo-Hydro, Aquazide, BPZide, Dichlotride, Esidrex, Hydrochlorot, HydroDIURIL, HydroSaluric, Hypothiazid, Microzide, Oretic, and others; frequently used as a fixed dose combination with other classes of hypertensive drugs)[c]		Chlordiazepoxide (Librium)
			Clozapine (Clozaril, FazaClo)
			Phenothiazines
			Chlorpromazine (Largactil, Thorazine)[c]
			Perphenazine (Trilafon)
			Prochlorperazine (Compazine, Compro)[c]
Dyes	Fluorescein (Ful-Glo, Fluorescite, AK-Fluor)		Thioridazine (Mellaril)
	Methylene blue		Trifluoperazine (Stelazine)
Furocoumarins	Psoralens		Tricyclics
	5-Methoxypsoralen[c]		Amitriptyline (Elavil)
	8-Methoxypsoralen (Oxsoralen-Ultra)[c]		Amitriptyline/Perphenazine (Duo-Vil, Etrafon, Triavil, Triptafen)
Hypoglycemics	Sulfonylureas		
	Chlorpropamide (Diabinese)		Desipramine (Norpramin)
	Glipizide (Glucotrol)		Imipramine (Tofranil)
	Glipizide/Metformin (Metaglip)		Dapsone
	Glyburide (DiaBeta, Glynase, Micronase)	Other	Hypericin (St John's wort)
	Glyburide/Metformin (Glucovance)		Pyridoxine (vitamin B_6)
	Tolazamide (Tolinase)		Ranitidine (Zantac)
	Tolbutamide (Orinase)[c]		
	Azathioprine (Azasan, Imuran)		

[a]Although it is the policy not to use trade names in this book, exceptions are made in cases in which we consider this information to be highly useful.
[b]Also reported as a systemic photoallergen.
[c]Commonly reported.
[d]Withdrawn from the United States market.
[e]Induces erythema on previously ultraviolet-exposed sites.

TABLE 97-4
Topical Photoallergens

GROUP	CHEMICAL NAME (TRADE NAME)[a]
Sunscreens (see Chap. 197)	Benzophenones
	Benzophenone-3 (oxybenzone)[b]
	Benzophenone-4 (sulisobenzone)
	Para-aminobenzoic acid (PABA) derivatives
	Ethylhexyl dimethyl PABA (padimate O)[b]
	PABA[b]
	Cinnamates
	Ethylhexyl methoxycinnamate (octinoxate)[b]
	Ethoxyethyl methoxycinnamate (cinoxate)
	Others
	Butyl methoxydibenzoylmethane (avobenzone, Parsol 1789)[b]
	Octocrylene (octocrylene)[b]
	Octyl triazone
	Phenylbenzimidazole sulfonic acid (ensulizole)
Fragrances	6-Methylcoumarin[b]
	Musk ambrette[b]
	Sandalwood oil
Antiinfective agents	Surface disinfectants: halogenated salicylanilides
	Dibromosalicylanilide (dibromsalan, DBS)[b]
	Tetrochlorosalicylanilide (Irgasan BS200)[b]
	Tribromosalicylanilide (tribromsalan, TBS)[b]
	Skin cleansers
	Chlorhexidine (Hibiclens)
	Hexachlorophene (pHisoHex)
	Pesticides
	Bithionol (thiobis-dichlorophenol)[b]
	Dichlorophene (G4, Korium, Teniatol)
	Dimethylol dimethyl hydantoin
	Fenticlor (*bis*-hydroxy-chlorophenyl sulfide)[b]
	Personal care products
	Triclosan (Irgasan DP300, Microban, Lexol 300)
	Topical antifungals
	Buclosamide (Jadit, butylchlorosalicylamide)
	Multifungin (bromochlorosalicylanilide, BCSA)
Others	Antibiotic for cattle
	Olaquindox[b]
	Nonsteroidal antiinflammatory agents (topical)
	Etofenamate
	Fepradinol
	Flufenamic acid
	Ketoprofen (Oruvail gel, Powergel, Tiloket gel)[b]
	Phenothiazines
	Chlorpromazine (Thorazine)[b]
	Promethazine (Phenergan)[b]
	Miscellaneous
	Acyclovir cream (Zovirax)
	Clioquinol (Vioform, iodochlorhydroxyquin)
	Cadmium sulfide
	Cinchocaine (Dibucaine)
	Thiourea (thiocarbamide, sulfourea)

[a]Although it is the policy not to use trade names in this book, exceptions are made in cases in which we consider this information to be highly useful.
[b]Commonly reported to be photoallergens.

TABLE 97-5
Systemic Photoallergens

PROPERTY	GENERIC NAME (U.S. TRADE NAME[a])
Antifungal	Griseofulvin (Fulvicin, Grifulvin V, Gris-PEG)
Antimalarial	Quinine
Antimicrobials	Quinolone
	Enoxacin (Penetrex)
Cardiac medication	Quinidine (Quinaglute, Quinidex)
Nonsteroidal antiinflammatory drugs	Ketoprofen
	Piroxicam (Feldene)
Vitamin	Pyridoxine hydrochloride (vitamin B_6)

[a]Although it is the policy not to use trade names in this book, exceptions are made in cases in which we consider this information to be highly useful.

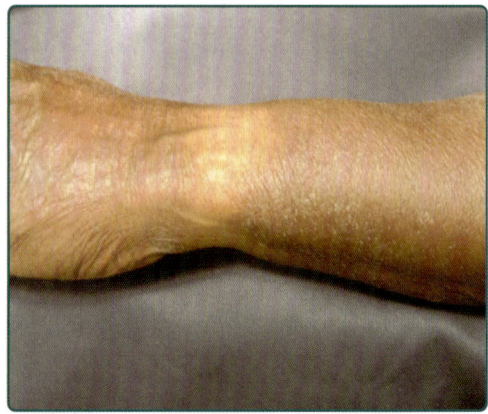

Figure 97-1 Sulfamethoxazole-trimethoprim–induced phototoxicity. Note the resolving erythema and fine scales on dorsum hand and forearm, and sparing of area covered by watch on the wrist.

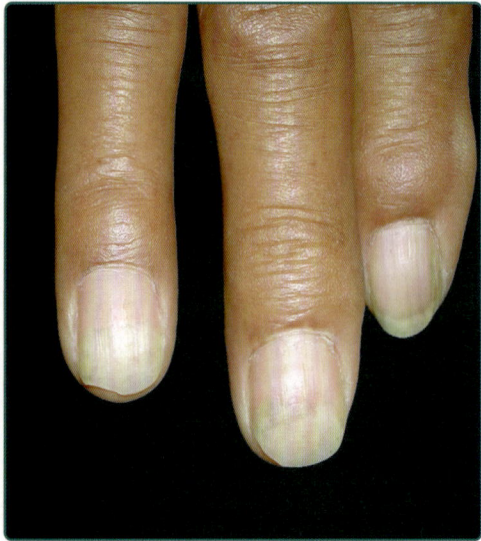

Figure 97-2 Distal onycholysis in a patient receiving psoralen plus ultraviolet A therapy.

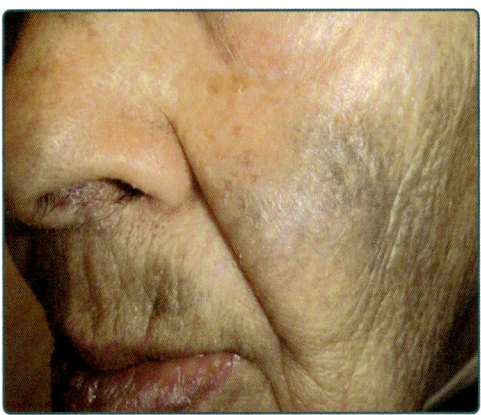

Figure 97-3 Minocycline-induced blue-gray pigmentation on cheeks and upper lip.

SLATE-GRAY PIGMENTATION

Asymptomatic blue-gray pigmentation on sun-exposed areas is associated with exposure to several agents.[14-16] These agents include amiodarone, chlorpromazine, clozapine, imipramine and, less commonly, desipramine. A drug metabolite–melanin complex is postulated to be the cause of this alteration. Minocycline can induce blue-gray pigmentation on sun-exposed areas such as face (Fig. 97-3), frequently on sites of acne scars, forearms, and shins; however, it also has been reported in non–sun-exposed sites such as mucosal surface, trachea, tympanic membrane, teeth, and cartilage. Chronic exposure to diltiazem, a benzothiazepine calcium channel blocker, has resulted in photodistributed, reticulated, slate-gray pigmentation. Slate-gray pigmentation seen in argyria involves the nail lunulae, mucous membranes, and sclerae. A photochemical reaction, in which silver granules are deposited in the dermis, results in these pigmentary alterations.

totoxicity, in which the acute response first appears after 24 hours, and peaks at 48 to 72 hours; this is the rationale for administering psoralen plus UVA (PUVA) photochemotherapy treatments 48 to 72 hours apart. The phototoxic response resolves with a varying degree of hyperpigmentation, which may last for months. At lower drug/UV doses, gradual tanning only, without preceding sunburn-like reaction, can be seen.

PHOTOONYCHOLYSIS

Separation of the distal nail from the nail bed, which could be asymptomatic, is a manifestation of acute phototoxicity, with the nail plate serving as a lens to focus UV energy on the nail bed. It has been reported with doxycycline and other tetracyclines,[13] fluoroquinolones, psoralens, benoxaprofen, clorazepate dipotassium, olanzapine, aripiprazole, indapamide, and quinine (Fig. 97-2).

PSEUDOPORPHYRIA

The development of porphyria cutanea tarda–like cutaneous changes of skin fragility, vesicles, and subepidermal blisters is associated with several phototoxic agents (Fig. 97-4). In contrast to porphyria cutanea tarda, the porphyrin profile is normal or in the upper range of normal in these patients. Naproxen is the most commonly reported causative agent. Other drugs and treatment modality incriminated include amiodarone, β-lactam antibiotics, celecoxib, ciprofloxacin, cyclosporine, diflunisal, etretinate,

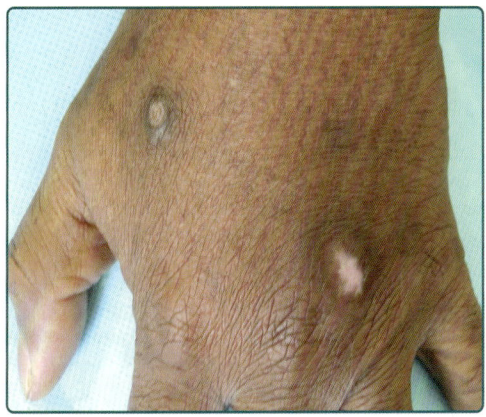

Figure 97-4 Pseudoporphyria. Crusted erosion and healed hypopigmented scar on dorsum of hand.

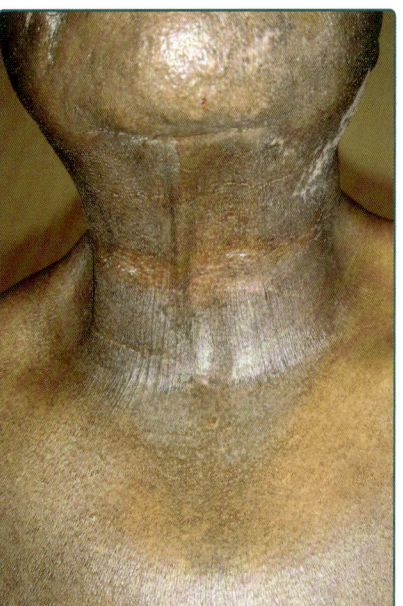

Figure 97-5 Chronic actinic dermatitis. Note the lichenification and hyperpigmentation on sun-exposed areas, and sparing of skin folds.

furosemide, imatinib, nabumetone, nalidixic acid, narrowband UVB, oral contraceptives, oxaprozin, ketoprofen, mefenamic acid, the tetracyclines, tiaprofenic acid, torsemide, and voriconazole.[17,18]

ACCELERATED PHOTO-INDUCED CHANGES

This has been uniquely described with voriconazole, a broad-spectrum antifungal agent.[18] Immunosuppressed patients receiving voriconazole for longer than 12 weeks can develop photosensitivity, pseudoporphyria, photoaging, lentigines, or premature dermatoheliosis; in addition, squamous cell carcinoma and melanoma have been described in patients who were on voriconazole for longer than 12 months.

PHOTODISTRIBUTED TELANGIECTASIA

This has been reported with calcium channel blockers, including nifedipine, amlodipine, felodipine, and diltiazem, with the antibiotic cefotaxime, and with the antidepressants venlafaxine and escitalopram.[19]

LICHENOID PHOTOSENSITIVE ERUPTION

This has been reported with doxycycline, capecitabine,[20] and other agents.

PERSISTENCE OF PHOTOSENSITIVITY AND EVOLUTION TO CHRONIC ACTINIC DERMATITIS

Phototoxicity usually resolves after discontinuation of the causative agent; however, persistence of photosensitivity for many years after the cessation of exposure, resulting in the development of chronic actinic dermatitis has been reported (Fig. 97-5). This has been reported with thiazides, quinidine, quinine, and amiodarone.

CHRONIC EFFECTS

These are best exemplified by the manifestations in patients who have received long-term PUVA photochemotherapy. These effects include premature aging of the skin, lentigines, squamous cell and basal cell carcinomas, and melanoma.

PHOTOTOXIC AGENTS

TOPICAL AGENTS

Table 97-2 lists the major topical phototoxic and photosensitizing agents. It should be noted that *fluorouracil* and *retinoids* induce exaggerated UV response as a result of their irritant effect on the skin, although systemically administered fluorouracil can induce phototoxicity. Topical exposures to *furocoumarins*, which are present in limes, celery, figs, and parsnips, may occur in individuals coming into regular contact with them (bartenders, salad chefs, gardeners) and in patients receiving topical photochemotherapy with psoralens. *Crude coal tar*, although no longer commonly used in dermatologic therapy, is well documented to produce a burning and stinging sensation on exposure to UVA (known as "tar smarts").

SYSTEMIC AGENTS

Table 97-3 lists the major systemic phototoxic agents.[1,21] The most commonly reported drugs are vemurafenib, voriconazole, doxycycline, hydrochlorothiazide, amiodarone, and chlorpromazine.[1] These agents produce an exaggerated sunburn reaction, but may also induce an eczematous response in a small percentage of users, especially after topical exposure. As a rule, the action spectra are in the UVA range; notable exceptions are the porphyrins, fluorescein, and other dyes, whose action spectra are in the visible light range.

PATHOPHYSIOLOGY

Several pathways eventuate in the development of phototoxic tissue damage, and for many phototoxic agents more than one pathway is responsible.[21]

PHOTODYNAMIC PROCESSES

This involves absorption of radiation energy by the photosensitizer and formation of an excited molecule. Subsequent generation of reactive oxygen species result in tissue injury. Phototoxicities induced by porphyrins, quinolones, nonsteroidal antiinflammatory agents, tetracyclines, amitriptyline, imipramine, sulfonylureas, hydrochlorothiazide, furosemide, and chlorpromazine are examples of photodynamic phototoxic reactions.

GENERATION OF PHOTOPRODUCTS

Stable photoproducts induced by exposure to radiation can be responsible for tissue injury. Phototoxic products have been demonstrated on irradiation of phenothiazines, chlorpromazine, tetracyclines, quinolones, and nonsteroidal antiinflammatory agents.

BINDING TO SUBSTRATE

An example of this mechanism is the covalent binding of 8-methoxypsoralen to pyrimidine bases of the DNA molecules upon exposure to UVA, which results in the formation of a crosslink between the DNA strands.

INFLAMMATORY MEDIATORS

Mediators of inflammation and inflammatory cells participate in phototoxic tissue injury. Biologically active products of complement activation, mast cell-derived mediators, eicosanoids, proteases, and polymorphonuclear leukocytes contribute to the development of phototoxicity induced by porphyrins, demeclocycline, and chlorpromazine.

APOPTOSIS

In addition to generating reactive oxygen species, photodynamic therapy also is a potent inducer of apoptosis.[22] This is discussed in detail in Chap. 199.

HISTOPATHOLOGY

Acute phototoxicity is characterized by individual necrotic keratinocytes and, in severe cases, epidermal necrosis (see Table 97-1). There may be epidermal spongiosis, dermal edema, and a mild infiltrate consisting of neutrophils, lymphocytes, and macrophages. Slate-gray pigmentation is associated with increased dermal melanin and dermal deposits of the drug or its metabolite.[23] Histologic features of lichenoid eruptions are similar to those of idiopathic lichen planus; however, there may be a greater degree of spongiosis and dermal eosinophilic and plasma cell infiltrates, and a larger number of necrotic keratinocytes and cytoid bodies. In pseudoporphyria, as in porphyria cutanea tarda, there is dermal–epidermal separation at the lamina lucida and deposits of immunoglobulins at the dermal–epidermal junction and surrounding blood vessel walls.

MANAGEMENT

Identification and avoidance of the causative phototoxic agent, along with rigorous photoprotection, are the most important steps in management.

Photoprotection includes seeking shade when outdoors, wearing photoprotective clothing, a wide-brimmed hat, sunglasses, and applying sunscreen to exposed areas.[24] Because the action spectrum for most agents is in the UVA range, high sun protection factor, broad-spectrum sunscreens should be used (see Chap. 197). Acute phototoxicity can be managed with topical corticosteroids and compresses; systemic corticosteroids can be used for the most severely affected patients. Management of patients with slate-gray pigmentation, lichenoid eruption, pseudoporphyria, and photodistributed telangiectasia is symptomatic only, and patients should be advised that it will take months after the discontinuation of the offending agent for the condition to resolve. For patients with slate-gray pigmentation, hydroquinone or hydroquinone-containing combination products can be used; however, because the location of pigments is in the dermis, these products are not completely effective. Patients with nonsteroidal antiinflammatory drug-induced pseudoporphyria who require nonsteroidal antiinflammatory drugs should be switched to a different class of agents or to those that are less photosensitizing, such as indomethacin or sulindac.[17]

PHOTOALLERGY

CLINICAL MANIFESTATIONS

In sensitized individuals, exposure to the photoallergen and sunlight results in the development of a pruritic, eczematous eruption within 24 to 48 hours after exposure (see Table 97-1). Although the morphology is clinically indistinguishable from that of allergic contact dermatitis, the distribution of the eruption in photoallergy is predominantly confined to sun-exposed areas; however, in severe cases, it may spread to the covered areas, albeit at a lower intensity. Unlike the lesions in phototoxicity in fair-skinned individuals, those in photoallergy usually resolve without significant postinflammatory hyperpigmentation. Lichenoid eruption also has been reported.

As with phototoxicity, persistence of photosensitivity and evolution to chronic actinic dermatitis (see Chap. 95) have been reported after exposure to photoallergens, including chlorpromazine, dioxopromethazine, halogenated salicylanilides, ketoprofen, musk ambrette, olaquindox, and quinidine.[25] A proposed mechanism is that UV radiation alters the carrier protein that originally binds the photoallergen; this results in the formation of a neoantigen that stimulates the immune system over the long term. This hypothesis is supported by the observation that the histidine moiety in albumin can undergo oxidation in the presence of salicylanilide, which binds to albumin.

PHOTOALLERGENS

TOPICAL AGENTS

In the United States, Canada, Europe, and the United Kingdom, common photoallergens include UV filters (benzophenone-3, octocrylene, avobenzone, octinoxate), and topical nonsteroidal antiinflammatory drugs (ketoprofen, etofenamate).[7-11,26] In China, chlorpromazine and para-aminobenzoic acid were the most common photoallergens in a 10-year study.[12] Table 97-4 lists the common photoallergens.

SYSTEMIC AGENTS

These are listed in Table 97-5. Photoallergy caused by systemic agents is not as well documented nor studied. All but one of the photoallergens (pyridoxine) are also phototoxic and were discussed earlier in this chapter (see "Phototoxic Agents: Systemic Agents" and Table 97-3).

HISTOPATHOLOGY

The histologic features are similar to those of allergic contact dermatitis. There is epidermal spongiosis associated with infiltrate of mononuclear cells in the dermis (see Table 97-1).

PATHOPHYSIOLOGY

Photoallergy is a type IV delayed hypersensitivity response requiring the presence of both photoallergen and the activating wavelengths of radiation (UVA)[27]; this is the reason that photopatch testing is done using UVA as a light source. After the absorption of UV energy, a photoallergen may be converted to an excited state molecule, which subsequently reverts to ground state by releasing the energy. In this process, the molecule may conjugate with a carrier protein to form a complete antigen. This is thought to be the mechanism of photoallergy induced by halogenated salicylanilides, chlorpromazine, and para-aminobenzoic acid. Alternatively, a photoallergen may form a stable photoproduct on exposure to radiation, which in turn may conjugate with a carrier protein to form a complete antigen. Sulfanilamide and chlorpromazine have both been shown to participate in this reaction.

Once the complete antigen is formed, the mechanism of photoallergy is identical to that of contact allergy. The antigen is taken up and processed by epidermal Langerhans cells, which then migrate to regional lymph nodes to present the antigen to T lymphocytes. Cutaneous lesions develop when the activated T lymphocytes circulate to the exposed site to initiate an inflammatory response.

MANAGEMENT

Management is identical to that of phototoxicity: identification and avoidance of the photoallergen, sun-protective measures, and symptomatic therapy.

EVALUATION OF PATIENTS WITH PHOTOTOXICITY AND PHOTOALLERGY

The evaluation of patients with phototoxicity and photoallergy is similar to the evaluation of patients with other photosensitivity disorders. A history of exposure to known photosensitizers is most important. It is also helpful to ascertain whether window glass-filtered sunlight can induce the cutaneous eruption, because UVB is filtered out by window glass. Distribution of the cutaneous eruption is a helpful clue to the type of photosensitizer responsible. Widespread eruption suggests systemic photosensitizers, whereas topical photosensitizers produce lesions only in areas that have been exposed to both sensitizers and radiation. Vesicular and bullous eruptions are most commonly associated with phototoxicity, whereas eczematous eruptions strongly suggest photoallergy; usually, phototoxicity is associated with a burning sensation, and photoallergy with pruritus. Skin biopsy findings also may be helpful in differentiating these 2 conditions: necrotic keratinocytes are commonly seen in phototoxicity, whereas spongiotic dermatitis is associated with photoallergy (see Table 97-1).

Phototests and photopatch tests are an integral part of the evaluation of photosensitivity when history and physical examination alone are insufficient to determine the responsible agent. Approximately 10% to 20% of patients who undergo photopatch testing have clinically relevant positive results, which leads to the diagnosis of photoallergic contact dermatitis.[2,9]

The procedures for phototesting and photopatch testing are generally as follows, although there are variations in testing methods. On day 1, exposure to UVB and UVA to determine minimal erythema doses is carried out, and duplicate sets of photoallergens are applied symmetrically to different sites on the back and covered by an opaque tape. On day 2, the minimal erythema doses are determined. One of the duplicate set of photoallergens is exposed to 10 J/cm^2 of UVA or 50% of the minimal erythema dose to UVA, whichever is lower. After irradiation, the exposed site is covered again with an opaque tape. On day 3, both irradiated and nonirradiated test sites are uncovered, and the reactions are graded. On day 5 or day 8, the irradiated and nonirradiated sites are evaluated for delayed reactions. Reaction only at an irradiated site indicates photoallergy. Reaction of equal intensity at both irradiated and covered sites indicates allergic contact dermatitis. Reaction at both sites, but with higher intensity at the irradiated site, signifies both photoallergy and allergic contact dermatitis. Well-defined erythema that resolves promptly indicates an irritant dermatitis.

DIFFERENTIAL DIAGNOSIS OF PHOTOTOXICITY AND PHOTOALLERGY

Airborne allergic contact dermatitis is characterized by involvement of skinfolds on exposed areas, such as the nasolabial folds and the eyelids that receive minimal direct sunlight. It also involves exposed areas that are relatively sun protected, such as the postauricular areas and area under the chin. Allergic contact dermatitis and irritant contact dermatitis occur at sites of contact, in both sun-exposed and sun-protected areas.

Other photodermatoses can be differentiated from phototoxicity and photoallergy by their characteristic time course and morphology and lack of exposure to photosensitizers. Polymorphous light eruption manifests itself within a few hours of sun exposure as pruritic papules, plaques, and, uncommonly, vesicles on sun-exposed sites and resolves in a few days. Chronic actinic dermatitis presents as chronically lichenified plaques on sun-exposed areas. Lesions of solar urticaria appear within minutes of sun exposure as mildly pruritic urticaria and resolve within a few hours.

REFERENCES

1. Kim WB, Shelley AJ, Novice K, et al. Drug-Induced Phototoxicity: A Systematic Review. *J Am Acad Dermatol*. 2018 Jul 9. [Epub ahead of print]
2. Fotiades J, Soter NA, Lim HW. Results of evaluation of 203 patients for photosensitivity in a 7.3-year period. *J Am Acad Dermatol*. 1995;33:597-602.
3. Crouch RB, Foley PA, Baker CS. Analysis of patients with suspected photosensitivity referred for Investigation to an Australian photodermatology clinic. *J Am Acad Dermatol*. 2003;48(5):714-720.
4. Wong SN, Khoo LS. Analysis of photodermatoses seen in a predominantly Asian population at a photodermatology clinic in Singapore. *Photodermatol Photoimmunol Photomed*. 2005;21:40-44.
5. Nakamura M, Henderson M, Jacobsen G, et al. Comparison of photodermatoses in African-Americans and Caucasians: a follow-up study. *Photodermatol Photoimmunol Photomed*. 2014;30(5):231-236.
6. Sharma VK, Bhari N, Wadhwani AR, et al. Photo-patch and patch tests in patients with dermatitis over the photo-exposed areas: a study of 101 cases from a tertiary care centre in India. *Australas J Dermatol*. 2018;59(1):e1-e5.
7. Greenspoon J, Ahluwalia R, Juma N, et al. Allergic and photoallergic contact dermatitis: a 10-year experience. *Dermatitis*. 2013;24(1):29-32.
8. Chuah SY, Leow YH, Goon AT, et al. Photopatch testing in Asians: a 5-year experience in Singapore. *Photodermatol Photoimmunol Photomed*. 2013;29(3):116-120.
9. European Multicentre Photopatch Test Study (EMCPPTS) Taskforce. A European multicentre photopatch test study. *Br J Dermatol*. 2012;166(5):1002-1009.
10. Haylett AK, Chiang YZ, Nie Z, et al. Sunscreen photopatch testing: a series of 157 children. *Br J Dermatol*. 2014;171(2):370-375.
11. Valbuena Mesa MC, Hoyos Jiménez EV. Photopatch testing in Bogota (Colombia): 2011-2013. *Contact Dermatitis*. 2016;74(1):11-17.
12. Hu Y, Wang D, Shen Y, et al. Photopatch testing in Chinese patients over 10 years. *Dermatitis*. 2016;27(3):137-142.
13. Wlodek C, Narayan S. A reminder about photo-onycholysis induced by tetracycline, and the first report of a case induced by lymecycline. *Clin Exp Dermatol*. 2014;39(6):746-747.
14. D'Agostino ML, Risser J, Robinson-Bostom L. Imipramine-induced hyperpigmentation: a case report and review of the literature. *J Cutan Pathol*. 2009;36(7):799-803.
15. Campbell M, Ahluwalia J, Watson AC. Diltiazem-associated hyperpigmentation. *J Gen Intern Med*. 2013;28(12):1676.
16. Imafuku K, Natsuga K, Aoyagi S, et al. Mucosal hyperpigmentation from prophylactic minocycline for EGFR inhibitor. *J Eur Acad Dermatol Venereol*. 2016;30(4):690-692.
17. Markova A, Lester J, Wang J, et al. Diagnosis of common dermopathies in dialysis patients: a review and update. *Semin Dial*. 2012;25(4):408-418.
18. Alberdi Soto M, Aguado Gil L, Pretel Irazabal M, et al. Accelerated photoaging induced by voriconazole treated with Q-switched Nd:YAG laser: case report and review of the literature. *J Cosmet Laser Ther*. 2014;16(6):314-316.
19. Bakkour W, Haylett AK, Gibbs NK, et al. Photodistributed telangiectasia induced by calcium channel blockers: case report and review of the literature. *Photodermatol Photoimmunol Photomed*. 2013;29(5):272-275.
20. Walker G, Lane N, Parekh P. Photosensitive lichenoid drug eruption to capecitabine. *J Am Acad Dermatol*. 2014;71(2):e52-e53.
21. Dawe RS, Ibbotson SH. Drug-induced photosensitivity. *Dermatol Clin*. 2014;32(3):363-368.
22. Ozog DM, Rkein AM, Fabi SG, et al. Photodynamic therapy: a clinical consensus guide. *Dermatol Surg*. 2016;42(7):804-827.
23. Eichenfield DZ, Cohen P. Amitriptyline-induced cutaneous hyperpigmentation: case report and review of psychotropic drug-associated mucocutaneous hyperpigmentation. *Dermatol Online J*. 2016;22(2).
24. Jansen R, Osterwalder U, Wang SQ, et al. Photoprotection: part II. Sunscreen: development, efficacy, and controversies. *J Am Acad Dermatol*. 2013;69(6):867-882.
25. Emmert B, Schauder S, Palm H, et al. Disabling work-related persistent photosensitivity following photoallergic contact dermatitis from chlorpromazine and olaquindox in a pig breeder. *Ann Agric Environ Med*. 2007;14(2):329-333.
26. Heurung AR, Raju SI, Warshaw EM. Adverse reactions to sunscreen agents: epidemiology, responsible irritants and allergens, clinical characteristics, and management. *Dermatitis*. 2014;25(6):289-326.
27. Kerr A, Ferguson J. Photoallergic contact dermatitis. *Photodermatol Photoimmunol Photomed*. 2010;26(2):56-65.

Chapter 98 :: Cold Injuries
:: Ashley N. Millard, Clayton B. Green, & Erik J. Stratman

第九十八章
冻伤

中文导读

许多生理行为和环境因素容易导致冻伤，对流、传导或辐射热损失的显著增加是冷暴露的直接影响。寒冷的环境会对皮肤造成威胁，并可能导致随后的核心体温下降。本章分为9节：①体温调节与冷生理反应；②皮肤冻伤的分类；③冻伤；④医源性冷损伤；⑤冬季干燥；⑥手足发绀；⑦冻疮；⑧冷性荨麻疹与多形性冷疹；⑨寒冷性脂膜炎及其相关疾病。分别介绍了这类疾病的临床特征、病因和发病机制、诊断、临床病程及治疗。

〔易 梅〕

AT-A-GLANCE

- Skin is important for maintaining core body temperature within a narrow physiologic range.
- Cold weather, wind, humidity, dampness, and altitude combine to inflict skin damage.
- Freezing and nonfreezing conditions can both produce cold injuries.
- Frostbite occurs after exposure to intensely cold air, liquids, or metals. Several degrees of frostbite are recognized.
- Self-inflicted freeze injuries from inhalant abuse and peer challenges are emerging.
- Winter xerosis and acrocyanosis are common consequences of prolonged exposure to cold.
- Pernio is an acral eruption of edematous violaceous papules occurring in cool rather than freezing exposures, and seen more frequently in lean persons.
- Cold urticaria is rare and occurs at the sites of localized cooling.
- Cold panniculitis typically occurs on legs and cheeks.

Many physiologic, behavioral, and environmental factors predispose to cold injuries. Marked increases in convective, conductive, or radiant heat loss are responsible for the immediate effects of cold exposure. A cold environment can be a threat to the skin, and can lead to subsequent fall in core body temperature. Cold injuries are becoming more prevalent among the general population.[1] Outdoor work, winter sports, windy conditions, humidity, altitude, and skin contact with cold objects are environmental factors that may predispose an individual to cold damage.[2] Insulation from clothing is insufficient when garments are too light, wet, tight, permeable to wind, or inadequate to cover the cold sensitive body parts. Frostbite prevails among winter sport enthusiasts, such as cross-country skiers and backpackers, who get lost or trapped in a snowstorm.[3-8] Accidental exposure to liquefied gas is an emerging cause of severe cold injuries.[9]

The human capacity for physiologic adaptation to cold is minimal. This deficiency may cause problems because seasonal changes in the outdoor environment can be quite dramatic, even in the temperate zones of the world. Skin is important in thermoregulation. Cutaneous blood flow and the resulting skin temperature may vary widely to preserve the core body temperature.[10,11] In fact, the body can maintain a constant core temperature of approximately 37°C (98.6°F) over a range of external temperatures between 15°C and 54°C (59°F and 129.2°F). In addition to external temperature, physiologic, behavioral, and environmental factors modulate skin responses to cold exposure.

THERMOREGULATION AND PHYSIOLOGIC RESPONSE TO COLD

Cutaneous thermoregulation is complex. As external temperature decreases, central thermoregulation centers in the hypothalamus signal other hypothalamic control centers to generate or conserve heat. Core body temperature is prioritized and maintained largely by controlling cutaneous blood flow. Arteriovenous anastomoses are abundant in acral areas, and they regulate the volume of blood passing through the skin. When the skin is cooled, there is usually an immediate vasoconstrictive response to reduce the amount of blood flowing at the skin surface. Without this vasoconstriction there would be significant heat transfer from the blood flowing in the skin to the environment, leading eventually to core temperature drop. The parallel arrangement of large arteries and veins in the limbs allows countercurrent exchange of heat. Vasoconstriction caused by cold results in shunting of blood from the superficial to the deep venous system, and heat is transferred from arteries to veins. Thus, the venous blood returning to the heart has already received heat transferred from the arteries before the heat can be lost to the environment.

In prolonged cold exposures, the skin experiences a paradoxical cyclic vasodilation known as the *hunting reaction of Lewis*, to protect against skin necrosis from prolonged vasoconstriction.[12,13] If cold exposure continues, there is an eventual reflex constriction of the arteries and veins in the extremities resulting in increased venous pressure, decreased capillary perfusion, sludging, hypoxia, microvascular thrombus formation, and surrounding tissue damage.[14] Segmental vascular necrosis ensues in areas of erythrostasis.

The rate of tissue freezing impacts the nature of cold injury.[15] Slow freezing results in extracellular formation of ice whereas fast freezing tends to produce intracellular ice. Extracellular ice crystals alter the osmotic properties of tissues and disturb the flow of water and electrolytes across the cell membranes. Thawing may be as damaging as the freezing itself, and repeated freeze and thaw cycles, as may occur in accidental injury, compound the damage. The rewarming rate is also important. In slow rewarming, ice crystals become larger and more destructive.

Other biologic factors influence vasoconstriction and tissue damage besides temperature. Painful stimuli, mental stress, arousal stimuli, deep breaths, and other stimuli of the autonomic nervous system can produce cutaneous vasoconstriction in warm subjects.[16,17] Increased blood viscosity (vascular sludging) also influences the negative effects of cold on the skin. Blood viscosity is strongly influenced by blood flow rates, hematocrit, platelet adhesiveness, concentrations of proteins, and the presence of abnormal proteins, such as fibrinogen.

Individual factors predisposing to cold injuries include skin conditions with transepidermal water loss (eg, atopic dermatitis), physical injuries, leanness, low physical fitness level, fatigue, dehydration, previous cold injuries, sickness, trauma, poor peripheral circulation, poor clothing insulation, and old age.[2] Newborns, the elderly, and individuals with acute or chronic impaired mental faculties remain the most vulnerable (Fig. 98-1). Many cases are associated with alcohol consumption, homelessness in urban centers, and car breakdown. Smoking and psychotropic drug use can also increase injury.

Given the presence of many cold-adapted enzymes, the skin may function more effectively when slightly cooled. In the case of adipose tissue, mild long-term exposure to cooling may lead to progressively better insulation. Consequently, overweight persons are more likely to survive prolonged accidental cold exposure.[18] Habitually cold-exposed skin also develops a more efficient system for shunting blood away from the surface. These adaptive mechanisms are most flexible during the first years of life. Tissues in the aged are less able to develop new shunts. In contrast, individuals who have experienced previous severe cold injury may have a profoundly delayed or absent hunting reaction in the affected limbs, making them more susceptible to recurrent cold injury with pain, hyperesthesia, or paresthesia.[19,20] Some of these individuals also have chronically cool skin.

CLASSIFICATION OF SKIN COLD INJURIES

Skin cold injuries can be divided into freezing and nonfreezing cold injuries. Although freezing injuries

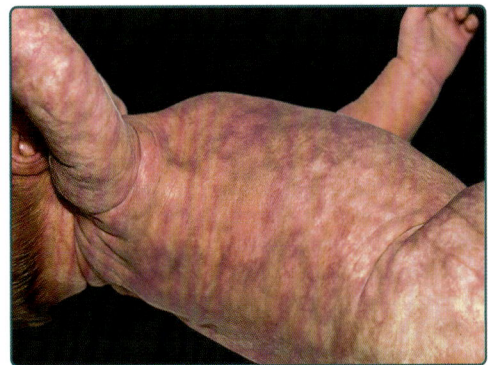

Figure 98-1 Reticulate appearance of cooled skin in a newborn resulting from the anatomic pattern of the blood supply and factors influencing flow, such as arteriolar vasoconstriction and the increased viscosity of cooled blood.

typically have clear associations with cold exposure by patient history, exposures that cause nonfreezing skin conditions are less likely to be associated or recounted by patients. Some of these conditions involve many variables other than temperature. Clinical recognition is generally easy, but awareness of potential uncommon associated disorders is important.

Table 98-1 outlines the classification of nonfreezing cold injuries. Treatment, both physical and pharmacologic, is aimed at keeping the body warm and maintaining vasodilation.

FROSTBITE

Frostbite occurs when tissue freezes after exposure to extremely cold air, liquids, or metals. The clinical effects of accidental injury that lead to the death of tissues are similar to those caused by cryosurgery.[21] Tissue injury results from initial vasoconstriction followed by intracellular and extracellular ice crystal formation.[10] This causes metabolic derangements in cells, electrolyte imbalances, membrane lysis, and cell death. Thawing can further exacerbate tissue damage through ischemia–reperfusion and increasing inflammation. Vascular stasis then occurs, followed lastly by a late ischemic phase that results in the eventual infarction of tissues, largely from damage to microcirculation.

Frostbite commonly affects fingers, toes, ears, nose, and cheeks.[22,23] Extreme and often conductive heat loss at a given body site freezes the tissues and results in localized blistering and necrosis (Fig. 98-2). The clinical presentation of frostbite falls into 3 categories that correspond to frostnip (mild frostbite), superficial frostbite, and deep frostbite with tissue loss.

Frostnip involves only the skin and damage is reversible (Fig. 98-3). There is a sensation of severe cold progressing to numbness followed by pain. Erythema is usually present on the cheeks, ears, nose, fingers, and toes. There is no edema or bleb formation. Frostnip is the only form of frostbite that can be treated safely in the field with first aid measures.

Superficial frostbite involves the skin and immediately subcutaneous tissues. It includes the previously described signs but with the pain subsiding to feelings of warmth. This is a sign of severe involvement. The skin has a waxy appearance, but deeper tissues remain soft and resilient. Clear blebs form, accompanied by edema and erythema within 24 to 36 hours after thawing. Lesions may become eroded (Fig. 98-4).

Deep frostbite extends to the deep subcutaneous tissue. The injured skin becomes white or bluish white with a variable degree of anesthesia. Most often the affected skin becomes deceptively pain free, and the discomfort of feeling cold vanishes. The tissue is totally numb, indurated with immobility of joints and extremities. Muscles may be paralyzed. Nerves, large blood vessels, and even bone may be damaged. Large blisters form 1 to 2 days after rewarming, and they can be classified according to depth, as in heat-induced burns (Fig. 98-5). Frostbite blister fluid contains high amounts of prostaglandins, including prostaglandin

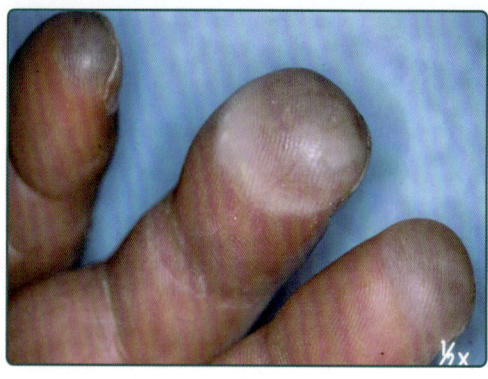

Figure 98-2 Bullous frostbite following contact with a cold steel sheet.

TABLE 98-1
Classification of Nonfreezing Cold Injuries to the Skin

- Vasoconstriction
- Hunting reaction
- Immersion foot
- Pulling-boat hands
- Acrocyanosis
- Chilblains
- Cold urticaria
- Cold panniculitis
- Erythromelalgia
- Raynaud phenomenon
- Sclerema neonatorum
- Subcutaneous fat necrosis of the newborn
- Livedo reticularis
- Cryoglobulinemia
- Cold agglutinins
- Cryofibrinogenemia

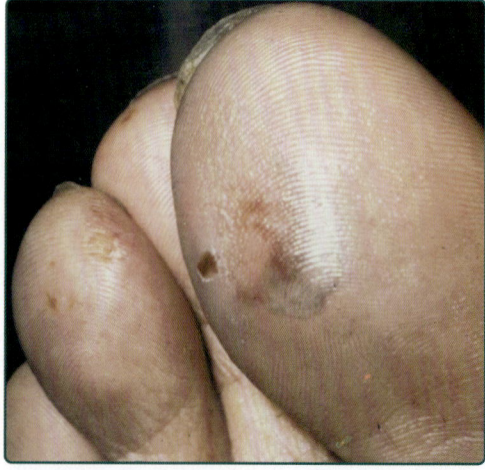

Figure 98-3 Frostnip.

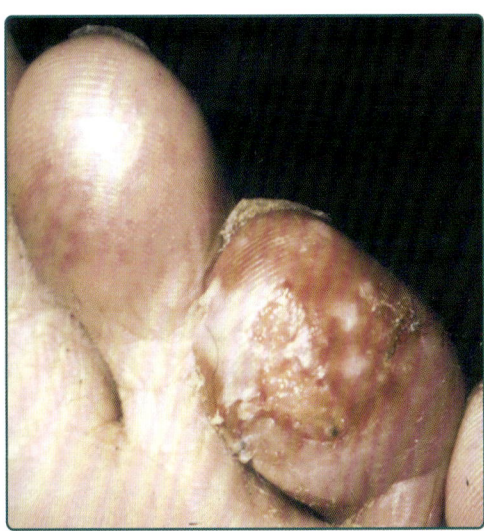

Figure 98-4 Superficial frostbite.

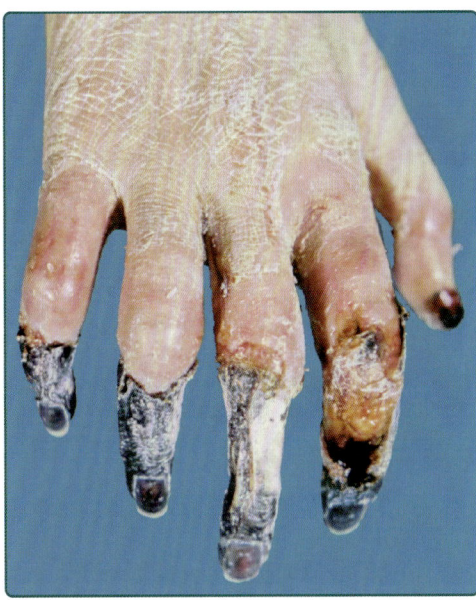

Figure 98-6 Dry gangrene of all fingers in a mountain climber 5 weeks after being caught in a snowstorm.

$F_{2\alpha}$ and thromboxane A_2. These mediators may contribute to increased vasoconstriction, platelet aggregation, leukocyte adhesiveness, and, ultimately, progressive tissue injury. The blister fluid begins to be resorbed within 5 to 10 days, which leads to the formation of hard, black gangrene. Weeks later, a line of demarcation occurs, and the tissues distal to the line undergo autoamputation (Fig. 98-6).

Prevention is key to protecting individuals from the effects of cold weather; frostbite, frostnip, and hypothermia always should be taken seriously. Table 98-2 lists prognostic factors.[7,8,24-26] Wearing protective clothing, a warm hat, earflaps, and scarf, together with preventive behavior, such as turning bare areas away from the wind, are the most important procedures for preventing frostbite. Nonmedicated waterless ointments are traditionally used for protection against facial frostbite, but their benefit is undocumented. The thermal insulation they provide is indeed minimal.[22,23] The use of protective emollients may lead to a false sense of safety and increased risk of frostbite, probably through neglect of other, more efficient protective measures.[27-29] In less-extreme conditions, however, some specific topical formulations bring beneficial effects.[30] The most effective products are those reducing transepidermal water loss and perspiration because these biologic functions cause emission of body thermal energy and further cool the skin.

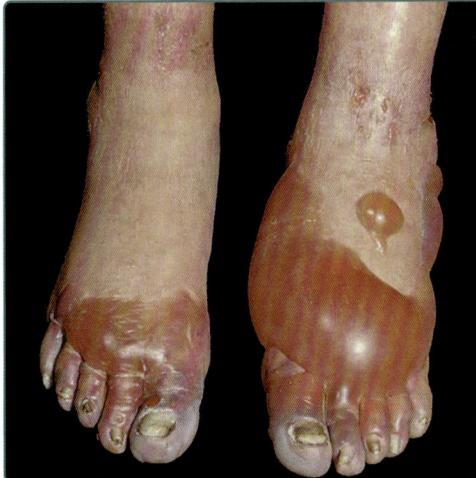

Figure 98-5 Deep frostbite after rewarming. Large blisters have formed. Note cyanosis of the toes as a sign of impending necrosis. This cold injury occurred in a homeless person who was found on the street after heavy alcohol consumption and overnight snowfall.

TABLE 98-2 Prognostic Signs of Frostbite	
Good prognostic signs	Large, clear blebs extending to the tips of the digits
	Rapid return of sensation
	Rapid return of normal (warm) temperature to the injured area
	Rapid capillary filling time after pressure blanching
	Pink skin after rewarming
Poor prognostic signs	Hard, white, cold, insensitive skin
	Cold and cyanotic skin without blebs after rewarming
	Dark hemorrhagic blebs
	Early evidence of mummification
	Constitutional signs of tissue necrosis, such as fever and tachycardia
	Cyanotic or dark red skin persisting after pressure
	Freeze–thaw–refreeze injury

The first consideration in frostbite treatment is to be aware that the victim may be suffering from hypothermia.[7,14,31,32] Prompt recognition and treatment are of paramount importance, because many hypothermia victims can recover from very low body temperatures. Treatment in an adequate medical facility can make the difference between full recovery and lifelong problems. Even if the victim appears to be dead from exposure to cold, resuscitative efforts should be started and continued until the proper core body temperature is reached.[14]

Because of the difficulty in assessing the depth of frostbite injury, conservative waiting after the frostbite episode is often encouraged in an attempt to delineate the extent of tissue loss. Care providers should avoid trauma, friction, pressure, massaging with snow, and refreezing. Slow rewarming increases tissue damage, making rapid rewarming the keystone of treatment.[33] Rewarming should be performed in a water bath between 37°C and 39°C (98.6°F and 102.2°F) until the most distal parts of the body are flushed.[29,34,35] Large amounts of analgesics may be required. The damaged part should be elevated, and blisters should be left intact. Surgical debridement is often best delayed until 1 to 3 months after demarcation. However, triple-phase bone scans, MRI, and magnetic resonance angiography can be used to predict ultimate tissue loss and to assess the possibility of earlier surgical intervention.[36-38]

There is no uniformly accepted protocol for other measures allegedly beneficial in the treatment of frostbite injury.[32] Intraarterial reserpine and sympathectomy have been used to reverse vasospasm, which may contribute to tissue loss. Their role is controversial, although some patients have benefited from this therapy. To counteract vasoconstriction caused by local release of inflammatory mediators, the use of topical aloe vera, which inhibits thromboxane synthetase, and oral ibuprofen, which inhibits cyclooxygenase, has been advocated. Oxpentifylline has been presented as an advanced therapy.[39] In addition, several adjunctive therapies, including vasodilators, thrombolysis, and hyperbaric oxygen, are sometimes useful.[40] Tetanus toxoid should be given in the case of open wounds. Surgery and amputation remain the ultimate strategies to help the victims.[41]

Sequelae of frostbite include permanent hypersensitivity to cold and, less often, hyperhidrosis.[42] Squamous cell carcinoma is a rare outcome, usually occurring on the heel 20 to 30 years later.[43] Epiphyseal plate damage or premature fusion may occur in children. Premature fusion can result in shortened digits, joint deviation, and dystrophic nails. In addition, frostbite arthritis, resembling osteoarthritis, may occur weeks to years later. Frostbite may also lead to ossification of one or both ears.[44]

IATROGENIC COLD INJURY

The most common in-office procedure performed in dermatology in the United States is cryodestruction using liquid nitrogen.[45] This destructive therapy causes localized cutaneous tissue freezing in a series of freeze–thaw cycles, leading to cell death in the targeted lesions, similar to a localized frostbite reaction. Vigorous tissue responses and overly aggressive treatments may lead to significant reactions, pain, and patient concern in the days following treatment. Vesicles and even large bullae, including hemorrhagic bullae, can occur acutely (Fig. 98-7). This can be followed by hemorrhagic crusting, hypopigmentation, and even scarring.

SELF-INFLICTED COLD INJURY

While accidental or incidental exposure to cool, cold, or freezing temperatures is the cause of many cold injuries and dermatoses, such injuries also may be self-inflicted by patients. Intentional and unintentional contact with cold substances, often through the misuse of household and industrial chemicals, can induce damage to the skin. Chemicals that are capable of cold-induced skin injury include the fluorinated hydrocarbons in propellants, refrigerants, and liquefied petroleum gases (eg, propane, butane), which are used as solvents and fuels.[46,47] Although these compounds can cause injury through accidental spray or drip exposures from pressurized canisters, such as occupational exposure to liquid nitrogen or pressurized ammonia,[48] they also may be intentionally abused for the purpose of achieving an altered mental state.

Inhalant abuse, which involves deliberately breathing volatile substances through the nose or mouth to achieve "a high" has been an emerging problem since the 1960s.[49] Slang terms for inhalant abuse include huffing, sniffing, snorting, dusting, glading, and bagging, depending on the substance involved and mode of inhalation.[50] The peak ages of inhalant abuse has been reported to be 14 to 15 years.[50] Individuals at increased risk include persons of low socioeconomic status and those with a history of criminal behavior, incarceration, depression, suicidal ideation, antisocial personality traits, unstable home life, or other drug use. The problem has been particularly widespread among Native American and Alaskan Native youth. Inhalation of amyl nitrite or butyl nitrite to augment sexual pleasure, referred to as "popping" or "snapping," also has been a practice among certain cultural groups, including men who have sex with men.[51]

Because of the low temperatures of inhalants, frostbite has been observed on the face, fingers, forearms, oral, laryngeal, and tracheal surfaces (Fig. 98-8A).[46-49] This may present as well-demarcated edema, erythema, cyanosis, and vesiculation concentrated around the nose, mouth, or even periorbital area (Fig. 98-8B).[49] Other skin findings may include a perioral or perinasal dermatitis with pyoderma ("huffer's rash"), contact dermatitis, yellow-stained facial dermatitis caused by nitrites,[52] and ichthyosis-like dermatitis from paradichlorobenzene in mothballs.[53] Extracutaneous manifestations of inhalant abuse can include conjunctival injection, headache, drowsiness, slurred speech, ataxia, disorientation, arrhythmia, vomiting, increased secretions, respiratory difficulty, and syncope.[50]

Pressurized gasses are not the only source of self-inflicted cold injury. Around 2012, a social media fad emerged in which teens applied table salt and ice cubes to the skin, challenging each other to see who could withstand the painful contact the longest.[54] Similar to salting an icy winter road, the salt rapidly decreases the freezing point of water to below 0°C (32°F), enhancing the ability to induce local frostbite.[55,56] A series of case reports have emerged in the literature in which teenage patients have presented to clinicians with factitial skin damage from the "salt-and-ice challenge." Lesions consist of painful, sharply demarcated, geometric or drip pattern, dusky erythematous patches, which may become bullous (Fig. 98-9).[54,56] Common locations include the palmar hands, forearms, and back.[54-56] Pathology on hematoxylin-and-eosin stain shows an interface dermatitis with extensive epidermal necrosis.[56] When confronted about possible self-infliction, patients frequently deny such behaviors, especially in the presence of parents or family members.

NONFREEZING COLD INJURY AND DAMPNESS

Nonfreezing cold injury occurs when tissues are cooled to temperatures between 0°C and 15°C (32°F and 59°F) for hours to days.[35] This type of injury, historically known as "trench foot," is exacerbated by dampness and has claimed numerous casualties in warfare. Cold, wet conditions at temperatures above freezing and limb dependency resulting from immobility and constrictive footwear are important pathogenic factors. Although classically thought to affect feet, nonfreezing cold injury can occur in other areas of the body.[35] Persistent erythema of the face and the hands is not a rare finding (Fig. 98-10).

WINTER XEROSIS

Minor but long-term cold exposure combined with environmental desiccation may have profound effects on the biology of the epidermis, leading, for example, to winter xerosis.[57,58] Many individuals present with dryness of the skin, particularly on the lower extremities, during wintertime (Fig. 98-11). The hands, forearms, cheeks, lips, and trunk also may be affected. Itching, a dry appearance, chapping, and cracking of the stratum corneum can be prominent. The condition is markedly influenced by cold environments, especially in combination with low humidity.[42,59] Predisposing factors include atopic dermatitis, ichthyosis, and increasing age. Excessive washing exacerbates winter xerosis. Indeed, irritant dermatitis of the hands worsens in a cold and dry environment.[60] Emollients and improvement in the environmental temperature and humidity are helpful in controlling this condition.

ACROCYANOSIS

Vasoconstriction can alter both skin temperature and skin color, resulting in a blue to violaceous acrocyanosis, a bilateral dusky mottled or confluent red to blue discoloration of the hands, feet, nailbeds, and sometimes the face (Fig. 98-12). It is persistent and accentuated by cold exposure. When the temperature is very low, the skin may be bright red. Trophic changes and pain do not occur, and pulses are present. This condition must be distinguished from obstructive arterial disease (see Chap. 148) and Raynaud phenomenon (see Chap. 145), which is clearly episodic, often segmental, and painful.

Acrocyanosis is genetically determined and usually starts in adolescence. Chronic vasospasm of small cutaneous arterioles or venules with a secondary dilation of the capillaries and subpapillary venous plexus

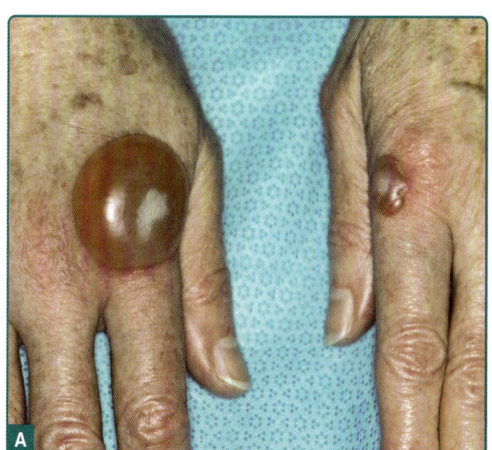
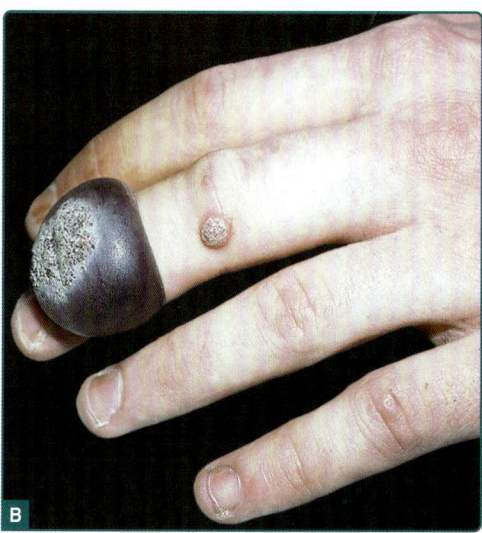

Figure 98-7 Iatrogenic bullae from liquid nitrogen treatment. Blister fluid may range from clear (**A**) to hemorrhagic (**B**) in appearance.

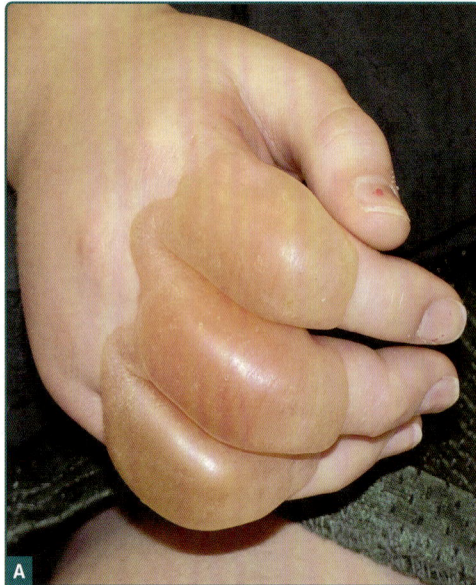

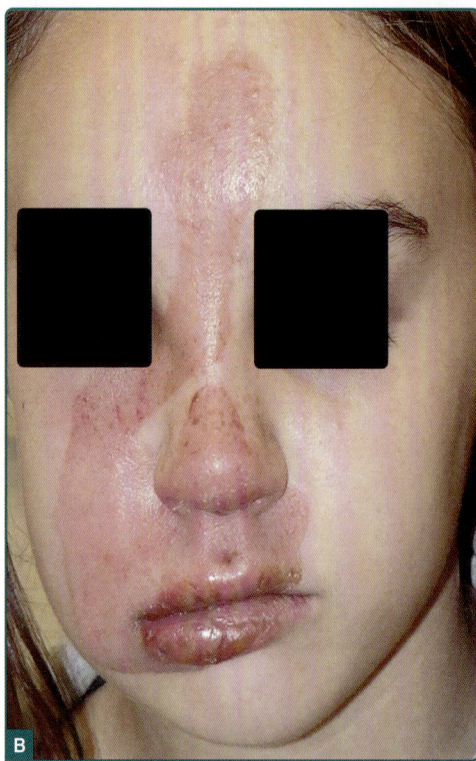

Figure 98-8 **A,** Dorsal hand frostbite and **(B)** "huffer rash" from inhalant abuse.

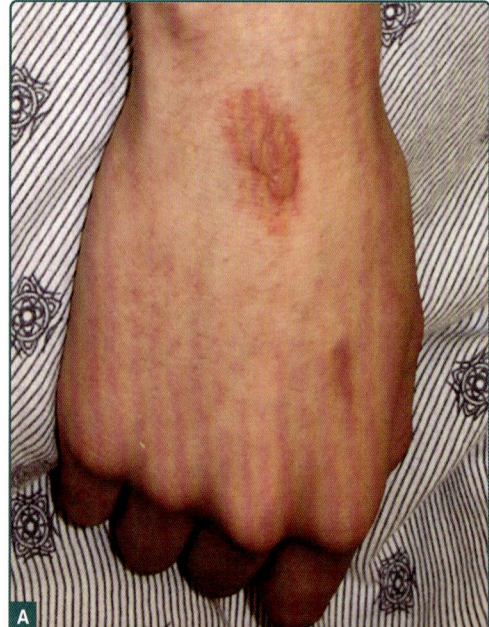

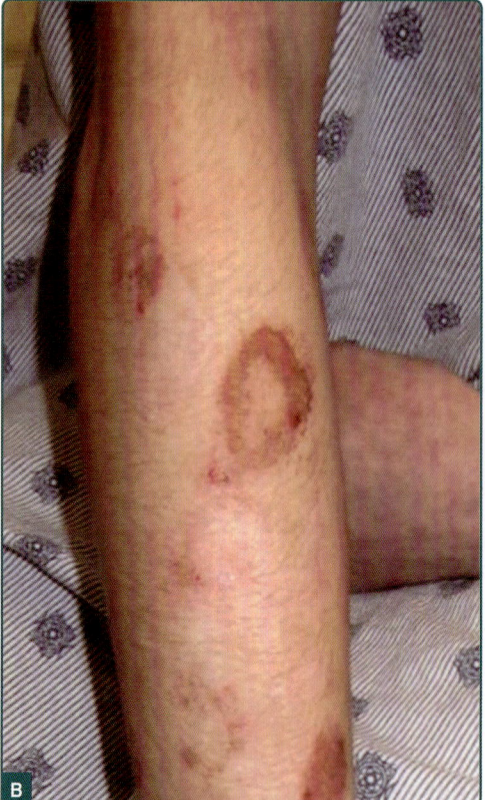

Figure 98-9 **A** and **B,** Acute, subacute, and chronic lesions inflicted by the "salt-and-ice challenge."

has been postulated. Stasis in the papillary loops with aneurysmal dilation at the tips redistributes blood flow to the subpapillary venous plexus. The blood flow may be compromised by altered erythrocyte flexibility, increased platelet adhesiveness, and other plasma viscosity factors. Cold agglutinins may exacerbate the acrocyanosis manifestations.[61,62] The "puffy hand syndrome" is defined by the presence of hand edema superposed on acrocyanosis.[63]

Tissues are less sclerotic in acrocyanosis than in Raynaud phenomenon. In cases developing for the

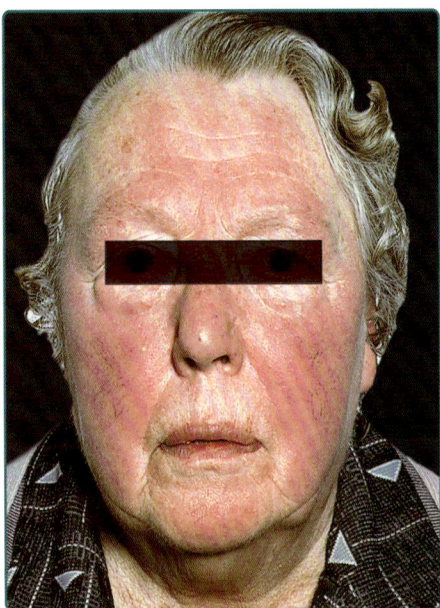

Figure 98-10 Facial redness in a person exposed to cold winters in a temperate climate.

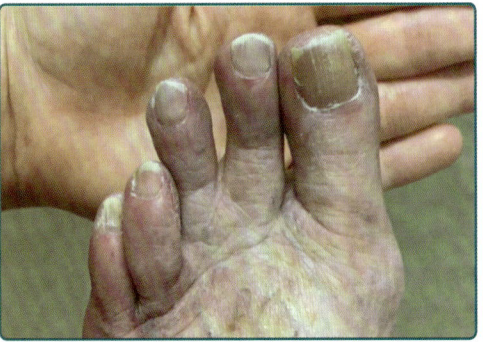

Figure 98-12 Acrocyanosis of the toes of an elderly woman with peripheral vascular disease. Note the contrast with the examiner's palmar skin in the background.

first time late in life, an underlying myeloproliferative disorder should be excluded. Remittent necrotizing acrocyanosis is associated with enhanced susceptibility to cooling and pain, as well as ulceration and gangrene of the fingers. Arteriolar occlusion by thrombi or intimal proliferation may occur. Cold pain should be distinguished from cold allodynia and cold hyperalgesia.

There is no effective treatment for acrocyanosis. Supportive measures to keep the skin warm are helpful.

PERNIO (CHILBLAINS)

Pernio, also called *perniosis* or *chilblains*, is a condition of localized inflammatory lesions caused by continued exposure to cool temperatures (above freezing).[64,65] Dampness and wind contribute to disease flares by increasing thermal conductivity and convection. Absolute temperature is less important than the cooling of nonadapted tissue. Abnormal vascular response to cold and minor trauma are believed to play a role.[66] The condition shows a genetic predisposition. It has been described most often in temperate regions, where winters are commonly cold and damp. Pernio is seen less often in very cold climates, where well-heated houses and warm clothing are available. When occurring in these colder regions, it is more common to occur during the cool early spring season rather than winter. Pernio is more common in children, women, and persons with low body mass index. Spontaneous remission is common when spring arrives, and relapse is frequent during the following winters.

Pernio develops acutely as single or multiple, burning, erythematous to violaceous macules, edematous papules, plaques, and nodules (Fig. 98-13). Patients may complain of itching, burning, or pain. In severe cases, blisters, pustules, and ulceration may occur. Characteristic locations include the dorsal and plantar surfaces of the toes, but the fingers, heels, nose, ears, and other sites, like the calves and thighs, can be affected.[67,68] Lesions usually resolve in 1 to 3 weeks but may become chronic in elderly people with venous stasis. A papular form of pernio resembling erythema multiforme can occur at all times of the year, usually in crops on the sides of the fingers,[69] often superimposed on a background of acrocyanosis.

Idiopathic perniosis is characterized histologically by edema of the papillary dermis and by the presence of superficial and deep perivascular lymphocytic infiltrates. Necrotic keratinocytes and lymphocytic vasculitis also have been reported. Thickening of blood vessel walls with intimal proliferation may lead to obliteration of the vascular lumen.[70-72]

A peculiar clinical presentation may occur in young women riding horses for several hours daily during winter.[73,74] Indurated red-to-violet tender plaques develop on the lateral calves and thighs (see Fig. 98-13D). The condition is quite similar to the nodular perniotic lesions described in adolescent girls with erythrocyanosis. For prophylaxis, experienced riders usually wear baggy riding pants that provide insulation and are not tight enough to compromise the circulation.

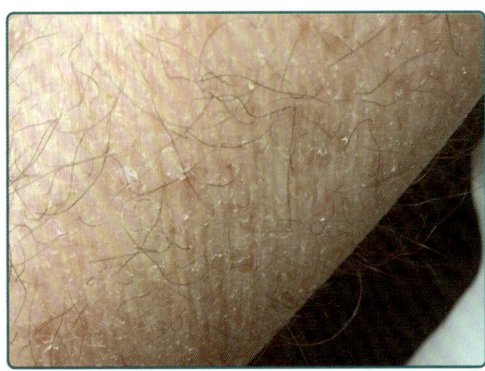

Figure 98-11 Xerosis of the legs of an elderly man in winter.

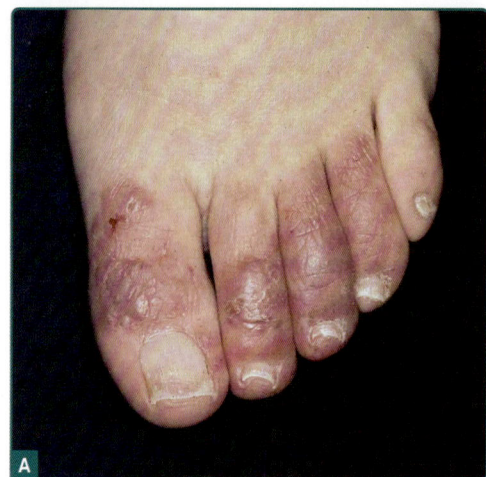
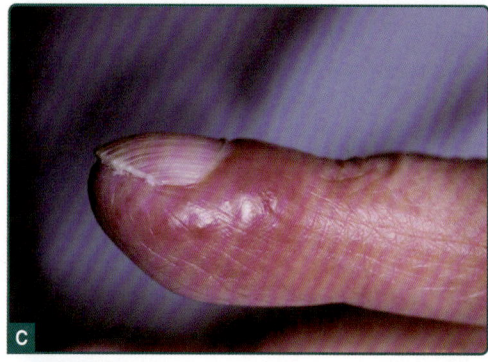
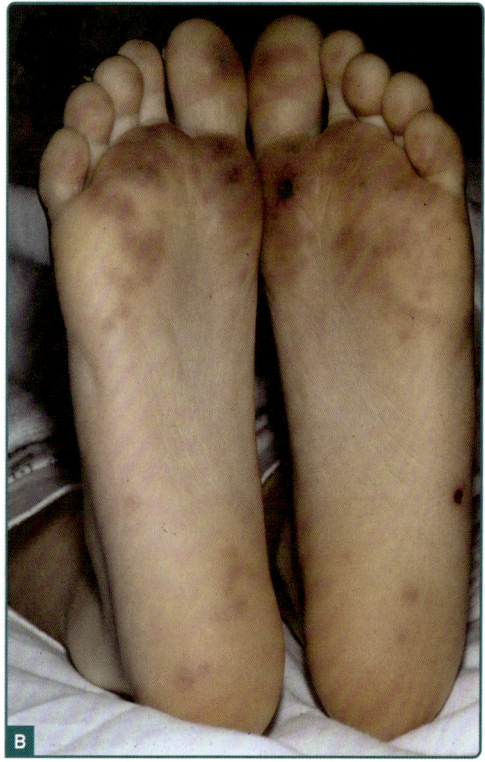
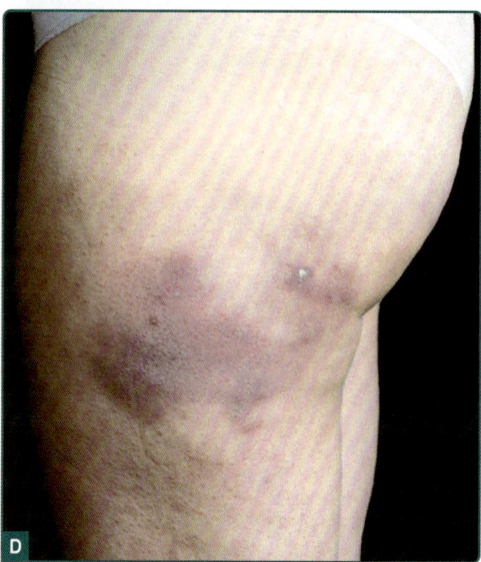

Figure 98-13 Pernio is common at sites such as the hands and feet when they are exposed to cooling, moisture, and tight garments. **A,** Pernio of the dorsal toes. **B,** Pernio of the plantar feet. **C,** Pernio of the fingertip. **D,** Equestrian chilblains from horse riding on a cold morning with inadequate clothing.

Perniotic lesions have been described in association with myeloproliferative disorders,[75] probably as a consequence of blood flow changes, presence of cold agglutinins, and altered inflammatory response on cooling. Chilblains lupus is a distinct disease in which lesions occur as a variant of chronic cutaneous lupus or in the setting of systemic lupus erythematosus.[72] Additional associations reported in cases of secondary pernio include connective tissue diseases other than lupus, monoclonal gammopathies, hyperviscosity syndromes, cryoglobulinemia, antiphospholipid positivity, and viral infections.[72,76] Of note, lupus pernio is a variant of sarcoidosis (see Chap. 35) and is unrelated to cold injuries.

The unfamiliarity of physicians with pernio sometimes gives rise to unnecessary hospital admissions with expensive laboratory and radiologic evaluations and, at times, hazardous therapy. All patients with pernio should undergo a detailed history, review of systems, and physical examination with or without a skin biopsy based on the degree of clinical certainty.[76] Laboratory workup (eg, complete blood count with peripheral smear, serum protein electrophoresis, antinuclear and extractable nuclear antigen antibodies, rheumatoid factor, cold agglutinins, and antiphospholipid antibodies) should be conducted only if the history and physical suggest a possible underlying systemic disease.

Pernio demonstrating a chronic course (continuous for at least 4 weeks and, in some cases, 8 weeks or longer, or episodic in nature), persistence into warm weather months, and onset in the elderly may be suggestive of an associated connective tissue disease, hematologic malignancy, or other systemic condition.[66,72,76,77]

The most important point in management of pernio is prevention through the use of adequate, loose, insulating clothing and appropriate warm housing and workplace. Tight garments, such as gloves, stockings, and shoes, are especially to be avoided in cases in which there is concomitant peripheral vascular disease. Instead, mittens can be useful for the hands. Minimizing moisture and maintaining blood circulation by avoiding immobility are also helpful.

Once pernio occurs, treatment is symptomatic with rest and warmth. Other conservative measures include smoking cessation and application of a midpotency topical steroid up to twice daily until lesions resolve. Associated systemic diseases, if present, should be treated. Second-line therapy for pernio consists of the addition of a calcium channel blocker, such as nifedipine 20 to 60 mg/day. Third-line and alternative management options include aspirin, pentoxifylline, nicotinamide, topical minoxidil, topical nitroglycerin, and tacrolimus ointment.

A related condition known as *pulling-boat hands* has been described, characterized by the presence of erythematous macules and plaques on the dorsum of the hands and fingers of sailors aboard rowboats.[78] Small vesicles developed later, accompanied by itching, burning, and tenderness. These individuals were exposed to long periods of high humidity, cool air, and wind, an ideal setting for the development of nonfreezing cold injury. In addition, hours of vigorous rowing daily produced repetitive hand trauma.

COLD URTICARIA AND POLYMORPHOUS COLD ERUPTION

Acquired cold urticaria is a form of physical urticaria. Lesions occur at sites of localized cooling, usually when the area is rewarmed. The disease is recognized by wheal and flare-type reactions and/or angioedema. Its morphology is indistinguishable from other forms of urticaria. The condition may be idiopathic or associated with some serologic abnormality.[79-83] It accounts for approximately 2% of cases of urticaria (see Chap. 41). Immunoglobulin E and, more rarely, immunoglobulin M have been implicated in the pathogenesis. Histamine from mast cell degranulation is one of the most important mediators, but leukotrienes, platelet-activating factor, and others also have been implicated.

Familial cold urticaria is a rare autosomal dominant condition with onset at an early age and persistence throughout life.[84-86] Urticaria develops when the patient is exposed to generalized cooling, particularly chilling wind, rather than local cold application. In addition to urticaria, headache, fever, arthralgia, leukocytosis, and swelling of the oral mucosa and esophagus can occur. The delayed type of familial cold urticaria is characterized by localized angioedema developing 24 to 72 hours after cold exposure. Coexistence with dermatographism or cholinergic urticaria is common. Alarming signs resembling histamine shock may lead to loss of consciousness. Death while swimming in cold water has been reported. A mutation in the CIAS1 gene, which is responsible for cold-induced autoinflammatory syndrome, has been identified.[85]

Cold urticaria may occur in 3% to 4% of patients with cryoglobulinemia, and it also may be associated with cold agglutinins, cryofibrinogens, and cold hemolysins. It has been reported in cases of infectious mononucleosis in association with either cryoglobulins or cold agglutinins, but such occurrences are rare. Cold urticaria also may be a sign of the Muckle-Wells syndrome that associates urticaria, deafness, and amyloidosis.[87] In this rare genetic disorder, recurrent bouts of urticaria, fever, chills, and malaise may occur from birth and persist throughout life. *Helicobacter pylori* has been suggested as a causative agent in some cases of acquired cold urticaria.[88]

Diagnosis of cold urticaria is confirmed by a cold challenge induced by an ice cube wrapped in a plastic bag placed on the skin of the forearm for periods varying from 30 seconds to 10 minutes (Fig. 98-14). Wheals form on rewarming. Sometimes water at 7°C (44.6°F) is more effective, presumably because it causes less-severe vasoconstriction. Peltier effect-based temperature challenge appears to be an improved method for diagnosis.[89] The Peltier effect relies on using 2 different sufficiently cold, microprocessor-controlled heat-transferring metals to generate a precise skin surface temperature to induce lesions.

Avoiding cold wind exposure and swimming in cold water are important preventive measures in cold

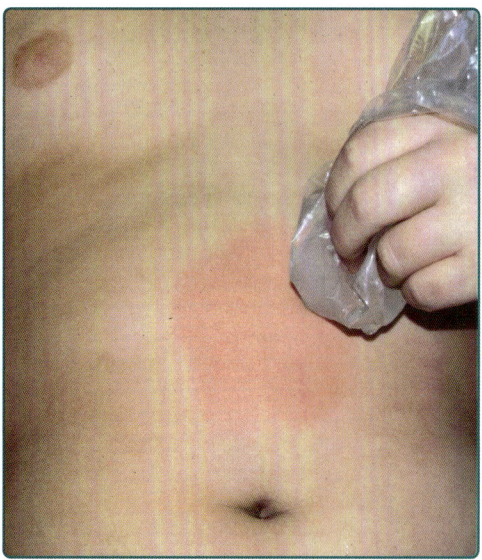

Figure 98-14 Cold urticaria induced by the application of ice to the skin.

urticaria. In the acquired form, 50% of cases improve or resolve within 5 to 6 years.[86] Second-generation H_1 antihistamines, up to 4 times the standard dose, are first-line for treatment.[86] Adjunctive agents and therapies for refractory cases include sedating antihistamines, H_2 blockers, montelukast, omalizumab, cyclosporine, and other immunosuppressives. Patients should also be considered for epinephrine pen prescription because of the anaphylaxis risk. Desensitization to cold is possible by immersing 1 arm into water at 15°C (59°F) for 5 minutes daily.

Cold erythema seems to be a related disorder with erythema and pain but without urticaria. Familial polymorphous cold eruption is a rare autosomal dominant disease characterized by childhood onset of nonpruritic, erythematous patches often accompanied by influenza-like symptoms and leukocytosis after generalized exposure to cold. Results of the ice cube test are negative. The pathogenesis remains unknown. The disease frequently has been referred to as *familial cold urticaria*, although the skin lesions are not urticarial.[90]

COLD PANNICULITIS AND RELATED ENTITIES

Nonfreezing injuries also can lead to inflammatory reactions in the subcutaneous fat layers, a condition called *cold panniculitis*. This condition is more common in children than in adults. It most commonly affects the cheeks and legs. Eating popsicles is a common trigger in children who develop the condition on the cheeks, so this entity is sometimes referred to as "popsicle panniculitis." Tender erythematous subcutaneous nodules appear 1 to 3 days after exposure. Delayed presentation in an adult has been reported 10 days after initiation of post–surgical procedure cold therapy.[91] Because of the adipocyte apoptosis that can result from the cold temperature, mild subcutaneous atrophy in the form of dimpling can occasionally follow cold panniculitis. Cosmetic device manufacturers have capitalized on this fat loss effect to manufacture and market fat-cooling devices to reduce fat layers for improved cosmetic contouring.[92] When suspecting cold panniculitis, an ice cube challenge to the patient's skin for 10 minutes should result in the development of an erythematous subcutaneous plaque 12 to 18 hours later.

A perivascular mixed infiltrate with neutrophils, lymphocytes, and histiocytes is present at the dermal–subcutaneous junction after 24 hours, followed by a well-developed, primarily lobular panniculitis at 48 to 72 hours. An overlying superficial and deep perivascular dermal lymphocytic infiltrate also may be seen. Some adipocytes are necrotic and rupture to form cystic spaces.

Infants have a higher content of saturated fatty acids in adipose tissue than do adults, and this may result in solidification at less-cold temperatures.[93,94] Cold panniculitis should be distinguished from other related disorders, including erythrocyanosis with nodules, sclerema neonatorum, and subcutaneous fat necrosis of the newborn. When the diagnosis is clear from history, biopsy to confirm cold panniculitis is not usually necessary, and care usually consists of reassurance and supportive analgesia as necessary. Lesions typically subside spontaneously within 2 to 3 weeks.

SCLEREMA NEONATORUM AND SUBCUTANEOUS FAT NECROSIS OF THE NEWBORN

See Chaps. 64 and 103.

RAYNAUD PHENOMENON

See Chap. 145.

CRYOGLOBULINEMIA

See Chap. 144.

LIVEDO RETICULARIS

See Chap. 148.

ERYTHROMELALGIA

See Chap. 148.

ACKNOWLEDGMENTS

We would like to thank Gérald E. Piérard, Pascale Quatresooz, and Claudine Piérard-Franchimont, the authors of the previous version of this chapter.

REFERENCES

1. Imray CH, Oakley EH. Cold still kills: cold-related illnesses in military practice freezing and nonfreezing cold injury. *J R Army Med Corps*. 2005;151:218.
2. Rintamaki H. Predisposing factors and prevention of frostbite. *Int J Circumpolar Health*. 2000;59:114.
3. Claes G, Henry F, Letawe C, et al. Skin, cold and winter sports [in French]. *Rev Med Liege*. 2001;56:257.
4. Long WB 3rd, Edlich RF, Winters KL, et al. Cold injuries. *J Long Term Eff Med Implants*. 2005;15:67.
5. Schindera ST, Triller J, Steinbach LS, et al. Spectrum of injuries from glacial sports. *Wilderness Environ Med*. 2005;16:33.
6. Miller BJ, Chasmar LR. Frostbite in Saskatoon: a review of 10 winters. *Can J Surg*. 1980;23:423.

7. Fritz RL, Perrin DH. Cold exposure injuries: prevention and treatment. *Clin Sports Med.* 1989;8:111.
8. Harirchi I, Arvin A, Vash JH, et al. Frostbite: Incidence and predisposing factors in mountaineers. *Br J Sports Med.* 2005;39:898.
9. Wright TC, Kim JB, Currie LJ, et al. Leakage of liquefied petroleum gas during motor vehicle refuelling—a new cause of cold injury. *Burns.* 2006;32:132.
10. Page EH, Shear NH. Temperature-dependent skin disorders. *J Am Acad Dermatol.* 1988;18:1003.
11. Quatresooz P, Piérard-Franchimont C, Paquet P, et al. It's a bit chilly, cold is stinging and skin is going to suffer [in French]. *Rev Med Liege.* 2008;63:18.
12. Dana AS Jr, Rex IH Jr, Samitz MH. The hunting reaction. *Arch Dermatol.* 1969;99:441.
13. O'Brien C. Reproducibility of the cold-induced vasodilation response in the human finger. *J Appl Physiol.* 2005;98:1334.
14. Arvesen A, Rosén L, Eltvik LP, et al. Skin microcirculation in patients with sequelae from local cold injuries. *Int J Microcirc Clin Exp.* 1994;14:335.
15. Gage AA. What temperature is lethal for cells? *J Dermatol Surg Oncol.* 1979;5:459.
16. Oberle J, Elam M, Karlsson T, et al. Temperature-dependent interaction between vasoconstrictor and vasodilator mechanisms in human skin. *Acta Physiol Scand.* 1988;132:149.
17. Hornstein OP, Heyer G. Responses of skin temperature to different thermic stimuli. *Acta Derm Venereol Suppl (Stockh).* 1989;144(suppl):149.
18. Keatinge WR, Coleshaw SR, Millard CE, et al. Exceptional case of survival in cold water. *Br Med J (Clin Res Ed).* 1986;292:171.
19. Foray J. Mountain frostbite: current trends in prognosis and treatment (from results concerning 1261 cases). *Int J Sports Med.* 1992;13(suppl 1):193.
20. Burge S, Shepherd JP, Dawber RP. Effect of freezing the helix and rim or edge of the human and pig ear. *J Dermatol Surg Oncol.* 1984;10:816.
21. Dawber R. Cold kills. *Clin Exp Dermatol.* 1988;13:137.
22. Lehmuskallio E, Anttonen H. Thermophysical effects of ointments in cold: an experimental study with a skin model. *Acta Derm Venereol.* 1999;79:33.
23. Lehmuskallio E. Cold protecting ointments and frostbite. A questionnaire study of 830 conscripts in Finland. *Acta Derm Venereol.* 1999;79:67.
24. Hamlet MP. Prevention and treatment of cold injury. *Int J Circumpolar Health.* 2000;59:108.
25. Ervasti O, Juopperi K, Kettunen P, et al. The occurrence of frostbite and its risk factors in young men. *Int J Circumpolar Health.* 2004;63:71.
26. Daanen HA, van der Struijs NR. Resistance index of frostbite as a predictor of cold injury in arctic operations. *Aviat Space Environ Med.* 2005;76:1119.
27. Lehmuskallio E. Emollients in the prevention of frostbite. *Int J Circumpolar Health.* 2000;59:122.
28. Lehmuskallio E, Rintamäki H, Anttonen H. Thermal effects of emollients on facial skin in the cold. *Acta Derm Venereol.* 2000;80:203.
29. De Buck E. BET 1: does the use of emollients prevent frostbite to the face? *Emerg Med J.* 2017;34:763.
30. Claes G, Piérard GE. Biometrological assessment of skin protectors against moderate cold threat. *Exog Dermatol.* 2002;1:92.
31. Hirvonen J. Some aspects on death in the cold and concomitant frostbites. *Int J Circumpolar Health.* 2000;59:131.
32. Koljonen V, Andersson K, Mikkonen K, et al. Frostbite injuries treated in the Helsinki area from 1995 to 2002. *J Trauma.* 2004;57:1315.
33. Murphy JV, Banwell PE, Roberts AH, et al. Frostbite: pathogenesis and treatment. *J Trauma.* 2000;48:171.
34. McIntosh SE, Opacic M, Freer L, et al. Wilderness Medical Society practice guidelines for the prevention and treatment of frostbite: 2014 Update. *Wilderness Environ Med.* 2014;25(4 suppl):S43.
35. Heil K, Thomas R, Robertson G, et al. Freezing and non-freezing cold weather injuries: a systematic review. *Br Med Bull.* 2016;117:79.
36. Kibbi AG, Tannous Z. Skin diseases caused by heat and cold. *Clin Dermatol.* 1998;16:91.
37. Mehta RC, Wilson MA. Frostbite injury: prediction of tissue viability with triple-phase bone scanning. *Radiology.* 1989;170:511.
38. Barker JR, Haws MJ, Brown RE, et al. Magnetic resonance imaging of severe frostbite injuries. *Ann Plast Surg.* 1997;38:275.
39. Probst F, Cox N, Anderson M. Oxpentifylline: an advance in the treatment of frostbite. *Emerg Nurse.* 2003;11:22.
40. Twomey JA, Peltier GL, Zera RT. An open-label study to evaluate the safety and efficacy of tissue plasminogen activator in treatment of severe frostbite. *J Trauma.* 2005;59:1350.
41. Petrone P, Kuncir EJ, Asensio JA. Surgical management and strategies in the treatment of hypothermia and cold injury. *Emerg Med Clin North Am.* 2003;21:1165.
42. Irwin MS, Sanders R, Green CJ, et al. Neuropathy in non-freezing cold injury (trench foot). *J R Soc Med.* 1997;90:433.
43. Uysal A, Koçer U, Sungur N, et al. Marjolin's ulcer on frostbite. *Burns.* 2005;31:792.
44. Manni JJ, Berénos-Riley LC. Ossification of the external ear: a case report and review of the literature. *Eur Arch Otorhinolaryngol.* 2005;262:961.
45. Tan SY, Tsoucas D, Mostaghimi A. Association of dermatologist density with the volume and costs of dermatology procedures among Medicare beneficiaries. *JAMA Dermatol.* 2018;154:73.
46. Bonamonte D, Profeta G, Conserva A, et al. Cold burn from contact with a propane and butane gas blend inside a spray canister used as a hooter. *Contact Dermatitis.* 2008;59:61.
47. Kuspis DA, Krenzelok EP. Oral frostbite injury from intentional abuse of a fluorinated hydrocarbon. *J Toxicol Clin Toxicol.* 1999;37:873.
48. Stefanutti G, Yee J, Sparnon AL. Cryogenic burns from intentional use of aerosol spray in children: an emerging phenomenon. *Burns.* 2010;36:e65.
49. Kurbat RS, Pollack CV. Facial injury and airway threat from inhalant abuse: a case report. *J Emerg Med.* 1998;16:167.
50. Williams JF, Storck M. Inhalant abuse. *Pediatrics.* 2007;119:1009.
51. Fischer AA. "Poppers" or "snappers" dermatitis in homosexual men. *Cutis.* 1984;34:118.
52. Fregert S, Poulsen J, Trulsson L. Yellow stained skin from sodium nitrite in etching agent. *Contact Dermatitis.* 1980;6:296.
53. Feuillet L, Mallet S, Spadari M. Twin girls with neurocutaneous symptoms caused by mothball intoxication. *N Engl J Med.* 2016;355:423.
54. Templeton D. Boy, 12, badly injured in 'salt-and-ice' challenge. *Pittsburg Post-Gazette.* June 29, 2012: http://www.post-gazette.com/local/city/2012/06/29/Boy-12-badly-injured-in-salt-and-ice-challenge/stories/201206290188. Accessed February 28, 2018.

55. Vosbikian MM, Ty JM. The ice and salt challenge: an atypical presentation of a cold injury: a case report. *JBJS Case Connect.* 2015;5:e11.
56. Zack JM, Fults M, Saxena H, et al. Factitial dermatitis due to the "salt and ice challenge". *Pediatr Dermatol.* 2014;31:252.
57. Middleton JB, Allen BM. The influence of temperature and humidity on stratum corneum and its relation to skin chapping. *J Soc Cosmet Chem.* 1974;24:239.
58. Piérard-Franchimont C, Piérard GE. Beyond a glimpse at seasonal dry skin: a review. *Exog Dermatol.* 2002;1:3.
59. Ervasti O, Hassi J, Rintamäki H, et al. Sequelae of moderate finger frostbite as assessed by subjective sensations, clinical signs, and thermophysiological responses. *Int J Circumpolar Health.* 2000;59:137.
60. Uter W, Gefeller O, Schwanitz HJ. An epidemiological study of the influence of season (cold and dry air) on the occurrence of irritant skin changes of the hands. *Br J Dermatol.* 1998;138:266.
61. Cholongitas E, Ioannidou D. Acrocyanosis due to cold agglutinins in a patient with rheumatoid arthritis. *J Clin Rheumatol.* 2009;15:375.
62. Shirafuji Y, Maeda Y, Iwatsuki K. Cold agglutinin-induced acrocyanosis in a patient with subclinical chronic lymphocytic leukemia; a beneficial response to rituximab. *Eur J Dermatol.* 2010;20:394.
63. Del Giudice P, Durant J, Dellamonica P. Hand edema and acrocyanosis: "puffy hand syndrome". *Arch Dermatol.* 2006;142:1084.
64. Goette DK. Chilbain (perniosis). *J Am Acad Dermatol.* 1990;23:257.
65. Simon TD, Soep JB, Hollister JR. Pernio in pediatrics. *Pediatrics.* 2005;116:472.
66. Guadagni M, Nazzari G. Acute perniosis in elderly people: a predictive sign of systemic disease? *Acta Derm Venereol.* 2010;90:544.
67. Price RD, Murdoch DR. Perniosis (chilblains) of the thigh: report of five cases, including four following river crossings. *High Alt Med Biol.* 2001;2:535.
68. Brown PJ, Zirwas MJ, English JC 3rd. The purple digit: an algorithmic approach to diagnosis. *Am J Clin Dermatol.* 2010;11:103.
69. Wessagowit P, Asawanonda P, Noppakun N. Papular perniosis mimicking erythema multiforme: the first case report in Thailand. *Int J Dermatol.* 2000;39:527.
70. Wall LM, Smith NP. Perniosis: a histopathological review. *Clin Exp Dermatol.* 1981;6:263.
71. Cribier B, Djeridi N, Peltre B, et al. A histologic and immunohistochemical study of chilblains. *J Am Acad Dermatol.* 2001;45:924.
72. Viguier M, Pinquier L, Cavelier-Balloy B, et al. Clinical and histopathologic features and immunologic variables in patients with severe chilblains. A study of the relationship to lupus erythematosus. *Medicine (Baltimore).* 2001;80:180.
73. Dowd PM, Rustin MH, Lanigan S, et al. Nifedipine in the treatment of chilblains. *Br Med J (Clin Res Ed).* 1986;293:923.
74. Beacham BE, Cooper PH, Buchanan CS, et al. Equestrian cold panniculitis in women. *Arch Dermatol.* 1980;116:1025.
75. Kelly JW, Dowling JP. Pernio: a possible association with chronic myelomonocytic leukemia. *Arch Dermatol.* 1985;121:1048.
76. Cappel JA, Wetter DA. Clinical characteristics, etiologic associations, laboratory findings, treatment, and proposal of diagnostic criteria of pernio (chilblains) in a series of 104 patients at Mayo Clinic, 2000 to 2011. *Mayo Clinic Proc.* 2014;89(2):207-215.
77. Takci Z, Vahaboglu G, Eksioglu H. Epidemiological patterns of perniosis, and its association with systemic disorder. *Clin Exp Dermatol.* 2012;37:844.
78. Toback AC, Korson R, Krusinski PA. Pulling boat hands: a unique dermatosis from coastal New England. *J Am Acad Dermatol.* 1985;12:649.
79. Wanderer AA. Cold urticaria syndromes: historical background, diagnostic classification, clinical and laboratory characteristics, pathogenesis, and management. *J Allergy Clin Immunol.* 1990;85:965.
80. Alangari AA, Twarog FJ, Shih MC, et al. Clinical features and anaphylaxis in children with cold urticaria. *Pediatrics.* 2004;113:e313.
81. Kozel MM, Sabroe RA. Chronic urticaria: aetiology, management and current and future treatment options. *Drugs.* 2004;64:2515.
82. La Shell MS, Tankersley MS, Kobayashi M. Cold urticaria: a case report and review of the literature. *Cutis.* 2005;76:257.
83. Buss YL, Sticherling M. Cold urticaria; disease course and outcome—an investigation of 85 patients before and after therapy. *Br J Dermatol.* 2005;153:440.
84. Hoffman HM, Rosengren S, Boyle DL, et al. Prevention of cold-associated acute inflammation in familial cold autoinflammatory syndrome by interleukin-1 receptor antagonist. *Lancet.* 2004;364:1779.
85. Shpall RL, Jeffes EW, Hoffman HM. A case of familial cold autoinflammatory syndrome confirmed by the presence of a CIAS1 mutation. *Br J Dermatol.* 2004;150:1029.
86. Singleton R, Halverstam C. Diagnosis and management of cold urticaria. *Cutis.* 2016;97:59.
87. Haas N, Küster W, Zuberbier T, et al. Muckle-Wells syndrome: clinical and histological skin findings compatible with cold air urticaria in a large kindred. *Br J Dermatol.* 2004;151:99.
88. Kränke B, Mayr-Kanhäuser S, Aberer W. *Helicobacter pylori* in acquired cold urticaria. *Contact Dermatitis.* 2001;44:57.
89. Siebenhaar F, Staubach P, Metz M, et al. Peltier effect-based temperature challenge: an improved method for diagnosing cold urticaria. *J Allergy Clin Immunol.* 2004;114:1224.
90. Urano Y, Shikiji T, Sasaki S, et al. An unusual reaction to cold: a sporadic case of familial polymorphous cold eruption? *Br J Dermatol.* 1998;139:504.
91. Lipke MM, Cutlan JE, Smith AC. Cold panniculitis: delayed onset in an adult. *Cutis.* 2015;95:21.
92. Garibyan L, Sipprell WH 3rd, Jalian HR, et al. Three-dimensional volumetric quantification of fat loss following cryolipolysis. *Lasers Surg Med.* 2014;46:75.
93. Requena L. Normal subcutaneous fat, necrosis of adipocytes and classification of the panniculitides. *Semin Cutan Med Surg.* 2007;26:66.
94. Quesada-Cortés A, Campos-Muñoz L, Díaz-Díaz RM, et al. Cold panniculitis. *Dermatol Clin.* 2008;26:485.

Chapter 99 :: Burns
:: Benjamin Levi & Stewart Wang

第九十九章
烧伤

中文导读

本章节从烧伤的流行病学、临床特征、并发症、病因和发病机制、诊断、处理等方面进行了详细的描述。指出烧伤的临床表现主要取决于组织破坏的深度和广度，对一度烧伤、二度烧伤、三度烧伤进行分类，提出烧伤可能出现的并发症。从病理生理学角度描述了烧伤的病因，对火焰烧伤、烫伤、电灼伤、化学性灼烧、Stevens-Johnson综合征、中毒性表皮坏死松解症等原因引起的烧伤进行阐述。提出对烧伤的诊断需要进行灼伤评估、气道评估、液体复苏、伤口护理评估等，总结了烧伤处理的要点。对于可能出现的症状及烧伤后瘢痕形成的处理进行了详细的描述。

〔易 梅〕

AT-A-GLANCE

- Burns are common in adults and kids; most are small and managed in the outpatient setting with dressing changes.
- Serious burns require inpatient care, ideally in a verified burn center.
- Large burns are managed in 4 general phases:
  - Initial evaluation and resuscitation.
  - Wound debridement and biologic closure.
  - Rehabilitation and reconstruction.
  - Long-term outcome quality tends to be very good in patients surviving large burns.

EPIDEMIOLOGY

In the year 2016, 486,000 patients in the United States received medical care for burns. In other words, 3 of every 3000 persons in the United States sustained a burn injury requiring medical attention.[1] Although the incidence of burn injury appears large, it has actually decreased by 60% since the early 1990s as the result of safety implementations, reduction in tobacco use and alcohol abuse, prevention education programs, change in home cooking practices, and decreased industrial employment.[2] Although some professions carry an increased risk of burn injury, the majority of burns occur at home. Males sustain the majority of burn injuries, and are twice as likely as females to require admission to a specialized burn center. Sadly, almost every 2.5 hours someone dies as a result of a fire, making the likelihood of fire-related death in the United States 1.5:1000.[1]

Of all United States patients receiving medical care for burns, only 5% to 10% are hospitalized for burn care, illustrating the tremendous role of outpatient care in the management of disease burden.[1,3] While not all of the other 90% to 95% patients receiving medical care for burns will require outpatient followup, of those who do, 30% will ultimately be admitted to the hospital for pain management or surgery (thus the importance of educating outpatient providers). Outpatient providers are most familiar with scald burns, as this is the most common mechanism of injury in the outpatient setting, whereas flame burns are the majority of inpatient burns.[4] Only 60% of hospitalized burn patients receive care at one of the 128 burn centers in the United States, which average about 200 patients per burn center each year. The organization of specialized, accredited burn centers has been arguably the most effective intervention in improving mortality of burn patients in the last half-century, with burn center survival rates now higher than 96%.[1,5]

Worldwide, burn injury poses a far more dramatic societal burden with much less optimistic outcomes. Yearly, 11 million people require treatment for burn injuries—more than the combined incidence of tuberculosis and HIV, and slightly less than the incidence of all combined malignant neoplasms—with 300,000 deaths annually. Socioeconomic disparities in treatment are vast, with 90% of all burn deaths sustained in low- to middle-income countries. Worldwide, injury is the cause of death in 1 in 10 persons, with burns as the fourth leading cause of injury-related death. For children who survive burn injury, 15% sustain long-term temporary disability, and 8% permanent disability—rates only superseded by near-drowning. In low- to middle-income countries, the prevalence of permanent disability attributable to burn injury is 12.5 times higher than in high-income countries. The aforementioned disparities likely arise from a mixture of inadequate safety measures, limited prevention outreach, lack of specialized burn centers, and deficiencies in training and resources necessary to provide impactful burn care.

CLINICAL FEATURES

Clinical manifestations of burn injury are determined by depth and breadth of tissue destruction (Table 99-1). Two independent systems of describing the depth of burn injury exist: that of "degrees" and of "thickness." Patients tend to be more familiar with the degrees system, whereas most medical and surgical providers will communicate using the thickness system. Both are interchangeable and should be used with awareness of one's audience.

SUPERFICIAL BURN (FIRST-DEGREE BURN)

Superficial burns involve only the epidermis. Like a sunburn, the skin is warm, erythematous, painful, blanching, and dry without blisters or eschar (Fig. 99-1). The epithelium remains intact, but will begin to slough within 7 to 14 days. They are self-limited and have no potential for scar.

PARTIAL-THICKNESS BURN (SECOND-DEGREE BURN)

Partial thickness burns involve the epidermis and penetrate to the dermis, but do not completely penetrate through the dermis or down to the subcutaneous tissue. These burns appear wet, weeping, and erythematous, and are exquisitely painful, with blisters or sloughing epidermal remnant (Fig. 99-2). They are further divided into 2 categories:

- *Superficial partial thickness burn:* blanching, more painful, hyperemic and erythematous, typically heal in approximately 2 weeks with appropriate wound care, low risk of scar and pigment change. Involves epidermis and papillary dermis. These can be managed conservatively with dressing changes or xenograft.
- *Deep partial-thickness burn:* nonblanching, less painful, pink or pale, require more than 3 weeks to heal, high risk of hypertrophic scar and pigment change, outcomes may be improved by excision and grafting. Involves epidermis, papillary dermis, and

TABLE 99-1
Clinical Manifestations of Burn Injury Are Determined by Depth and Breadth of Tissue Destruction

		FIRST-DEGREE BURN (SUPERFICIAL)	SECOND-DEGREE BURN (SUPERFICIAL PARTIAL THICKNESS)	SECOND-DEGREE BURN (DEEP PARTIAL THICKNESS)	THIRD-DEGREE BURN (FULL THICKNESS)
Clinical appearance		Painful, dry burn with no blisters or eschar formation, blanching	Exquisitely painful, wet, weeping burn, blanching	Less painful, pale, nonblanching	Insensate, dry, waxy, nonblanching with eschar formation
Epidermis		+	+	+	+
Dermis	Papillary	–	+	+	+
	Reticular	–	–	+	+
Subcutaneous tissue		–	–	–	+
Prognosis		Self-limited with sloughing within 7-14 days; no risk of scarring	Heals in 2 weeks with proper wound care; low risk of scarring	>3 weeks to heal; debridement and grafting may be necessary; high risk for scarring and pigmentary changes	Surgical excision with skin grafting necessary for healing; contractures, hypertrophic scars are common

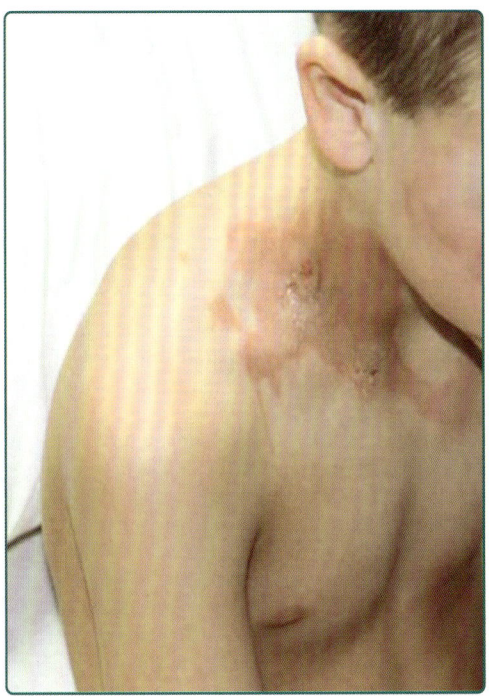

Figure 99-1 Superficial burn to the right aspect of the neck, in this case superficial area largely on the perimeter of the burn. Blistering represents partial-thickness burn of central area.

reticular dermis. These typically require debridement and grafting.

FULL-THICKNESS BURN (THIRD-DEGREE BURN)

Full-thickness burns penetrate to the subcutaneous tissue and beyond, affecting all dermal layers. These burns are dry, leathery, waxy, nonblanching, insensate, and eschar is frequently shades of brown, white, gray, or black. The transition from adjacent partial-thickness burn is clear by the lack of tissue edema. They will not heal without surgical excision with skin grafting or tissue transposition. Sequela, such as contractures and hypertrophic scars, are common.[6,7] Of note, "fourth-degree burn" has been used to refer to burn injuries that penetrate to and/or expose deep structures (eg, bone, muscle, tendon) (Fig. 99-3). Skin grafting alone is not adequate treatment for burns of this severity, and limb loss may occur.[8]

Breadth of injury is described as a percentage of total body surface area (TBSA) that is affected; its measurement is addressed in section "Fluid Resuscitation". Damaged tissues in burn wounds are almost always heterogeneous. Characterization of different regions of burns also can be described as the zone of coagulation (cell death), zone of stasis (cell injury that can either recover or transform into zone of coagulation), or

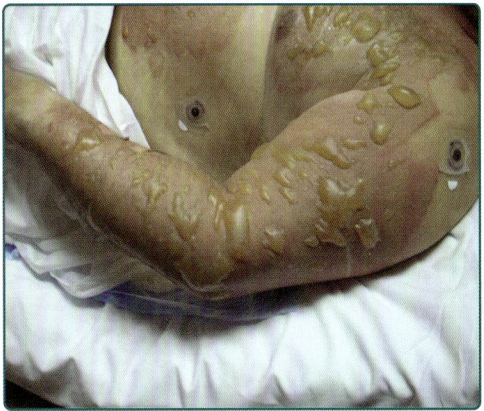

Figure 99-2 Partial-thickness burn of the left arm with blistering. Blisters are flaccid and contain serous fluid; burns of this degree are the most painful.

zone of hyperemia (cells that will recover from injury) (Fig. 99-4). Despite multiple classifications for burn depth, no objective measure of burn depth exists, leaving clinicians to rely on subjective assessments. Third-degree burns should be debrided within the first 3 to 5 days to avoid cellulitis and wound infections.

COMPLICATIONS

While it may appear that the sequelae of burn injury are limited to the integumentary system, there are many other systemic and local sequelae that must be considered when evaluating burn patients. Burns sustained in structural fires have a high incidence of smoke inhalation injury, wherein the pulmonary epithelium sustains direct thermal injury with ensuing edema and airway obstruction. Perioral burns and the presence of ashes and soot around or within the mouth

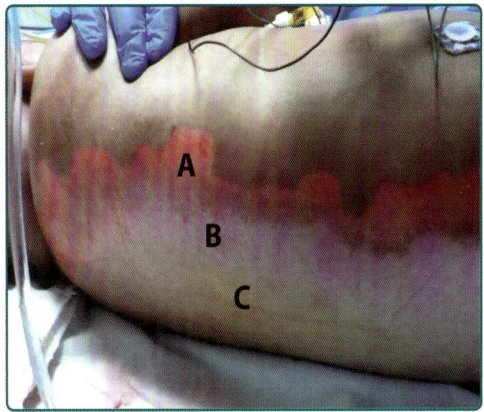

Figure 99-3 Full-thickness burn of the back demonstrating zones of injury according to Jackson's thermal wound theory. **A,** Zone of hyperemia (cells that will recover from injury); **B,** zone of stasis (cell injury that can either recover or transform into zone of coagulation); **C,** zone of coagulation (cell death).

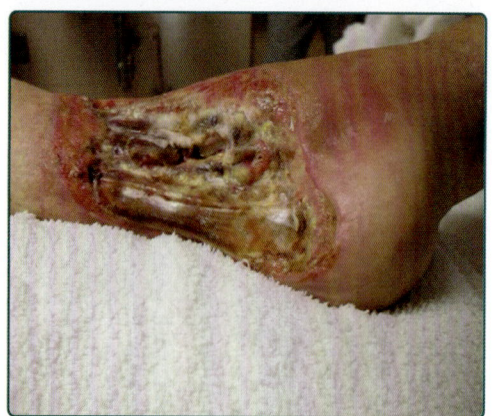

Figure 99-4 Fourth-degree burn of ankle with exposed tendon and muscle.

and oropharynx are highly suspicious for inhalation injury and require emergent intervention to protect the airway. Carbon monoxide and cyanide toxicity are also associated with smoke inhalation injury, and the presence of inhalation injury alone doubles the mortality rate of burn injury.[9] Circumferential burns of the extremities are at risk for the development of compartment syndrome as the underlying tissues becomes increasingly swollen and edematous and constricted by the eschar. If untreated, pressures can cause nerve impingement and vascular compromise. In electrical injuries, the muscle tissues swell and become restricted by the overlying fascia at which point the fascia muscle be surgically released. Similarly, full-thickness burns of the trunk restrict and compromise respiratory function, particularly in children, necessitating escharotomy of the chest to improve ventilation. Finally, excess resuscitation can cause abdominal compartment syndrome, which is defined as bladder pressure over 30 mm Hg. Patients often present with oliguria and abdominal distension. In these patients, first steps include escharotomy of the abdominal full-thickness burns, as well as paralysis and laying the patient flat. Fluids should be immediately decreased and diuresis or continuous renal replacement therapy should be considered to avoid a decompressive laparotomy. If these noninvasive measures fail to relieve the abdominal compartment syndrome, then a laparotomy might be required.

Acute stress gastritis (Curling ulcer) with accompanying bleeding may develop in the gastric or duodenal mucosa as a result of intravascular volume depletion. Acute renal failure may occur following inadequate resuscitation or thermal injury to muscle as a consequence of massive myoglobinuria, particularly in electrical burns. Ectopic bone formation known as heterotopic ossification may develop in patients with large TBSA burns causing severe pain, contractures, and restricting range of motion.[10] This most commonly occurs in the elbow and is more frequent if the burn injury includes the upper extremity.[11-13] Burns induce a hypermetabolic state which is proportional to the size of burn injury, leading to muscle catabolism, hyper-glycemia, and increased lipid liberalization with consequent steatosis. Finally, infection and sepsis are the most common cause of death in burn patients.[14]

ETIOLOGY AND PATHOGENESIS

BURN PATHOPHYSIOLOGY

The pathophysiology of burn injury can be appreciated by considering 2 paradigms: loss of skin organ function and production of an inflammatory response.

First, skin as an organ serves many functional purposes, not the least of which includes barrier protection against microbes, absorption and mitigation of mutagenic electromagnetic radiation, water and vapor impermeability, body thermoregulation, sensory perception, and motion-enabling elasticity balanced with sheer-resistant tensile strength. When skin is burned, these functions are lost. Microbe translocation into tissue or blood is unimpeded, leading to cellulitis, bacteremia, and sepsis. Unprotected from ultraviolet radiation, melanin-deficient burn scars are prone to squamous cell carcinoma development (eg, Marjolin ulcer). Loss of both the lamellar bodies of the stratum granulosum and the keratin-rich epidermal stratum lucidum and stratum corneum permits unregulated insensible vapor losses from transudates and interstitial fluid, causing intravascular volume depletion. Destruction of the dermal papillary plexus and eccrine sweat glands hinders autonomic hypothalamic regulation of body temperature and increased sensitivity to temperature fluctuations, especially in patients with high TBSA burns. Mechanoreceptor damage leads to long-term sensory loss, even in mild partial-thickness burns.[15] Destruction of native tissue elastin and migration and proliferation of fibroblasts in the wound site, with subsequent myofibroblast differentiation and deposition of irregular collagen bundles, produce function-limiting contractures and inelastic scar with only 80% tensile strength of native tissue.

Second, the inflammatory response to burn injury is profound and biphasic; an initial insult of inflammatory mediator release from necrotic tissue is followed by bacterial eschar invasion and establishment of a nidus. Local inflammatory response causes vasodilation and increased capillary permeability, promoting transudate production and insensible fluid losses. In burns greater than 20% TBSA, the initial insult from inflammatory mediator release triggers a systemic inflammatory response, manifesting as fever, hyperdynamic circulation, increased basal metabolic rate, and muscle catabolism.[7] Depending on the severity of insult, in some patients this state will persist for 1 or 2 years postburn.[16] Initially, burn wounds are sterile, but during the first week after injury, eschar becomes colonized and toxin exposure increases. In burns greater than 40% TBSA, bacterial load becomes so large that without intervention, sepsis and death are imminent. Beyond the colonization of the eschar, the excess dead tissue stimulates a massive inflammatory response which can lead to cardiovascular collapse.

FLAME BURN

Thermal injuries, caused by fire or flames, are the most common burn etiology reported over the past decade.[1] Thermal injuries are associated with the highest risk of death and complications compared to all other burn etiologies. Flame burns most commonly occur at home (64%), while work fires and recreational fire burns account for 12% and 6% of flame burns, respectively. When considering thermal injuries, it is important to consider smoke inhalation as it significantly impacts the morbidity and mortality of patients recovering from flame burns. The majority of inhalation injuries occur while the patient was indoors or in an enclosed space, and very few occur in patients who were burned while outside. Inhalation injury is present in 17% of patients with flame burns. The presence of smoke inhalation in burn patients is associated with an overall mortality rate of 24%, compared to the mortality rate of 4% in those patients without smoke inhalation damage.

SCALD BURN

Scalds are the second leading cause of burn injuries and are the most common mechanism of burns in the pediatric population. More than 50% of scalds are associated with food preparation or consumption, with a smaller proportion associated with bathing.[17,18] Common mechanisms, including pulling a tablecloth, reaching up and tipping a container near the edge of a counter, pulling electric cords attached to kitchen appliances, and carrying containers with hot liquids.[19,20] Contact burns from touching a hot object are extremely common in the pediatric population as well. Overall, contact burns make up 9% of burns reported, but they are the third leading cause of burns in children. Scald burns tend to cause a greater inflammatory response than flame burns.

ELECTRICAL BURN

Although only 4% of burns admitted to burn centers are caused by electricity, they pose the greatest diagnostic, therapeutic, and prognostic challenge among burn mechanisms. Notably, TBSA is an unreliable surrogate for burn severity, as it does not reflect the degree of internal tissue and organ damage caused after skin penetration by electrical current. To pass through dry human skin, a current must either surmount a huge amount of resistance, gain access to internal tissues through skin deficits such as cuts or burns, or induce skin breakdown (common above 500 volts [V]). Electrocution injuries are traditionally classified as low voltage (<1000 V) or high voltage (>1000 V), but ultimately it is the current (amperage) of the electricity and its direction of travel that ultimately determine ensuing tissue damage and lethality. For example, only 20 milliamperes (mA) are required to paralyze respiratory muscles, and only 100 mA to induce ventricular fibrillation. Typical North American alternating current outlets have an average amperage of 15 to 20 amperes.[21] Although TBSA does not represent burn severity, duration of contact with electrical source is proportional to tissue destruction. During electric shock by alternating current, both flexor and extensor muscles are stimulated, but the strength of flexors is greater than that of extensors, causing the "no let-go" phenomenon, and increasing contact time and tissue destruction.

Primary electrical tissue injury is greatest in areas with the least cross-sectional area, such as digits, wrist, and toes. Burn injuries will often be present at the entrance and exit sites of the current, indicating a general path through the internal structures. For example, electrical shocks that cross the thorax are more likely to induce ventricular fibrillation, and limbs with entrance and exit sites are those at risk for compartment syndrome. Current will pass through highly conducting soft tissues, contact bone, and then continue along bone until exit. Bone has the greatest resistance of all body tissues, and therefore generates the most heat as current flows through it. Bone heating leads to severe thermal injury of deep invested muscles and tendon insertions which can cause swelling and compartment syndrome. All compartments between the entrance and exit wound should be monitored closely by examination and direct measurement of compartment pressures if concern for compartment syndrome exists. If compartment pressures are greater than 30 mm Hg, then fasciotomies should be performed. Massive myoglobinuria may result, necessitating renal protective fluid resuscitation. Damaged endothelium in major vessels leads to thrombosis. Cataracts may also develop. Apart from current flow, electrical burns are also caused by electrical arcs (temperatures upwards of 4000°C [7232°F]) and flame injury from ignited clothing. Secondary electrical injury can result from explosive shock waves generated by electric arcs, causing blunt trauma and tympanic membrane rupture. Long-term complications of high-voltage electrical injury also includes cataracts, and these patients should followup with ophthalmology as an outpatient. Lightning strike is exceedingly rare but can be catastrophic. Typically, patients who survive a lightning strike are at high risk for arrhythmias and compartment syndrome between the entry and exit points.[22]

CHEMICAL BURN

Slightly more than 3% of burn center admissions are chemical burns, and with equal proportions occurring at work and at home. According to the Centers for Disease Control and Prevention, carbon monoxide, ammonia, chlorine, hydrochloric acid, and sulfuric acid are the chemicals with the highest frequency of associated injury, although carbon monoxide is likely not directly burn related.[23] Important clinical categories of chemical burns include alkali, acid, hydrofluoric acid, phenol, and white phosphorous. Acids induce burn damage through binding of hydrogen ions to proteins, inducing coagulation. Alkali burns are typically deeper and more serious than acid burns, as hydroxide ion saponification of fats induces liquefactive necrosis and permits further depth of chemical penetration. Mortality from chemical injury is low, and treatment cost is small relative to other injury mechanisms.

Chemical burns are unique in that they will continue to progress after the initial insult until the offending agent is eliminated. Initiating immediate treatment in the field is associated with reduced injury severity and shorter hospital stay. Great care must be taken to protect health care personnel from exposure upon intake of patients, wherein clothing and accessories should be removed. It is advisable for solids or powders to be removed by brushes or dusting, as wetting with irrigation may provoke injuries in some cases (eg, calcium oxide, alkali metals). Otherwise, irrigation of the wound with copious amounts of water or saline should be initiated immediately. Attempts at neutralizing pH with a complementary chemical should not be undertaken, as heat from the consequent exothermic reaction can worsen the severity of the burn.[24] Management of certain chemical exposures, such as hydrofluoric acid, white phosphorous, and phenol, require specialized therapy, and toxicology should be consulted. Although chemicals should not be neutralized, certain chemicals require specific treatments. Hydrofluoric acid is toxic because of the fluoride ion that binds calcium, but can be neutralized with topical calcium gel (1 ampule of calcium gluconate in 100 g of lubricating jelly). If symptoms persist, you can consider intraarterial calcium infusion (10 mL calcium gluconate diluted in 80 mL of saline, infused over 4 hours) and/or subeschar injection of dilute (10%) calcium gluconate solution. Phenol is commonly used in disinfectants and chemical solvents with poor water solubility. Phenol causes protein disruption and denaturation that result in coagulation necrosis. Treatment of phenol exposure includes copious water irrigation and cleansing with 30% polyethylene glycol or ethyl alcohol.[22]

STEVENS-JOHNSON SYNDROME AND TOXIC EPIDERMAL NECROLYSIS

Given the expertise of burn teams taking care of large body surface area burns, patients with desquamating skin processes, such as Stevens-Johnson syndrome (SJS) and toxic epidermal necrolysis (TEN), are often transferred to the burn unit. These are acquired blistering disorders of cutaneous and mucosal surfaces that are differentiated only by the affected TBSA: SJS less than 20% often with mucosal involvement, and TEN greater than 40%. Through an unknown mechanism of presumed immunologic origin, the epidermal–dermal junction begins to separate after starting new medications (particularly antiepileptic drugs or nonsteroidal antiinflammatory agents). The combined incidence of SJS and TEN in the United States is approximately 3800 per year, or 12 cases per million persons per year.[25] Diagnosis should be made by biopsy as analyzed by dermatology or a dermatopathologist. Steroids and IV immunoglobulin are controversial for SJS and TEN, and much of the burn literature does not support its use. Treatment is supportive and patients should have a robust airway assessment and should be flagged as "difficult airway" patients. Severe intraoral swelling may require intubation. If there is ocular involvement, ophthalmology should examine these patients and any vaginal mucosal involvement warrants evaluation by an obstetrician-gynecologist. For wound care, a nonadherent antimicrobial gauze such as Acticoat is preferred and mineral oil should be used on the skin to keep it from shearing off.

DIAGNOSIS

ASSESSING THE BURN

The initial care of a burn patient can be likened to that of any trauma patient. Over time, guidelines such as Advanced Trauma Life Support and Advanced Burn Life Support have standardized the care of trauma patients and have improved overall patient outcomes. Thus, given the extent of injuries that a burn patient may present with, it is important to follow a standard algorithm. A complete history and physical should be performed with specific focus placed on the cause and timing of the injury, concomitant injuries, and treatments received prior to arrival. The ultimate goal is to stabilize the patient and ensure a proper assessment of the burn so that further care can be transitioned to a burn center, if necessary.

AIRWAY ASSESSMENT

Assessment should begin with evaluation of the airway, breathing, and circulation. Inhalation injuries can occur in approximately 10% of all burn patients, but are notably present in 70% of those who eventually die of their burn.[26] Thus, it is important to specifically note such findings as soon as the patient presents with nasal passage or posterior pharynx blockage, facial burns, changes in voice quality, shortness of breath, and carbonaceous sputum in the nasal or oral passages. If there is any concern that the airway is compromised, a nasopharyngeal scope or bronchoscope can be used to directly visualize the airway. Some clinicians consider the use of these tools to be mandatory in any patient who presents with facial burns no matter the extent of the burn itself. Although patients may not present with obvious airway compromise by manifesting the symptoms as stated above, airway edema can progress very quickly making an intubation that would have been easily performed on initial presentation very difficult because of progressive swelling and obliteration of anatomic landmarks. Endotracheal intubation may be required for several days until edema subsides as the mucosal slough and secretions accumulate, obstructing the airway and atelectasis progresses. In these patients, frequent bronchoscopic suctioning should be performed until soot no longer exists. Although the data are inconclusive, most centers also recommend inhaled heparin-albuterol-Mucomyst to treat airway swelling and clots. Systemic steroids can be considered if there are no other burns outside of the inhalation injury. If inhalation injury progresses to acute respiratory distress syndrome, typical acute respiratory distress syndrome protocols should be followed, including lung-protective ventilation (keeping keep pressures less than 30 mm Hg) with permissive hypercapnia.

In some instances, identifying both the causative agent and the extent of the injury may aid in the recovery process. In particular, the possibility of carbon monoxide (CO) poisoning must also be assessed. Given the increased affinity of CO for hemoglobin molecules, oxygen (O_2) becomes displaced which creates a hypoxic environment in the body. Formal diagnosis of CO poisoning is based on CO levels in the blood. Symptoms of CO poisoning typically begin with headaches at levels of approximately 10%, whereas CO in the blood becomes toxic at levels of approximately 50% to 70%. While the half-life of CO is normally 4 hours at room air, its half-life is shortened with treatment. It is recommended to treat CO poisoning empirically, especially in those patients presenting with agitation, reddish appearance of mucous membranes, and altered consciousness, given that delivery of 100% O_2 (fraction of inspired O_2 [FiO_2] 100%) reduces the half-life of CO to 30 to 90 minutes. In patients with toxic levels of CO in the blood, more extreme measures are necessary, including the use of hyperbaric O_2 at 2.5 atmospheres with 100% O_2. Hyperbaric O_2 will reduce the half-life of CO to 15 to 23 minutes. Consequently, prompt and aggressive evaluation and maintenance of the airway is the most important initial step in management of a burn patient. Finally, cyanide poisoning can cause severe complications and Cyanokit can be given in the field by paramedics as prophylaxis.

FLUID RESUSCITATION

After initial stabilization of the patient has been performed, the next step is to determine the extent of the burn injury. For superficial burns, treatment of the burn wound oftentimes requires both topical antimicrobial agents and corticosteroids to minimize inflammation.[27] Microorganisms proliferate rapidly in burn wounds, particularly in patients with impaired immune function caused by the burn. Topical antimicrobial agents delay the interval between injury and colonization and maintain low levels of wound flora. The specific antibiotics and antiseptics for topical therapy in minor burns were discussed earlier in section "Wound Care". Antibiotics, however, should not be given unless signs of infection exist.

For full-thickness burns and some deep partial-thickness burns, identifying the extent of the burn injury is crucial. TBSA is used to design fluid administration regimens and defines overall prognosis of patients. Criteria for transfer to a burn center are also based on this concept.[28] Only partial-thickness and full-thickness burns are totaled to calculate TBSA. If small areas in various distributions are affected, it may be easier to use the patient as a ruler with one palm size representing 1% TBSA. Most emergency departments and burn units also have body surface charts available for use (the Lund & Browder Chart), but also follow the "rule of nines," wherein the body is partitioned into areas and each region constitutes 9% of the TBSA (Fig. 99-5). Regions on the adult that constitutes 9% of the TBSA include the head and arms, while the legs, anterior trunk, and posterior trunk account for 18% of TBSA each. In children, the arms each account for 9% of the TBSA, while the legs account for 14%. The head and neck region, the anterior trunk, and the posterior trunk each account for 18% in children. Careful estimation of TBSA is essential for proper early management of burn patients, as patients who have burns of more than 20% TBSA commonly require IV fluid resuscitation.

The Parkland Formula (Table 99-2; 4 mL × % TBSA × weight [kg]) is most commonly used to calculate fluid requirements within the first 24 hours.[29] It is extremely important to note that the original timing of the injury is what is used in the calculation, not the time of initial presentation. Half of this volume is administered in the first 8 hours after the injury and the second half is administered over the next 16 hours. For example, if a 70-kg (154-lb) patient with 10% TBSA burns sustained at 10 AM presents at 12 PM, the fluid to be administered in the first 8 hours is calculated using the following formula: [(4 mL × 10% × 70 kg)/2]/6 hours. Lactated Ringer solution is recommended to avoid complications associated with metabolic acidosis with normal saline or abnormal fluid shifts with colloid fluids.[29] Then, dextrose 5% in lactated Ringer solution is commonly used as maintenance fluids. Although such formulas exist, it is important to note that proper resuscitation is based on overall fluid status as represented by urine output, with the goal of 0.5 mL/kg/h in adults and 1 mL/kg/h in children, and fluids should be adjusted accordingly. Given the immobility associated with severe burn injuries and the abnormal fluid shifts that occur, aggressive hydration also accounts for potential rhabdomyolysis, leading to acute kidney injury that can occur in this setting. Pulmonary status is also an indicator of fluid status but in more of a delayed fashion. Complications such as pulmonary edema result from fluid overload and necessitate daily evaluation of O_2 requirements and ventilator settings.

Once the Parkland Formula (see Table 99-2) is begun, the patient's vital signs and urine output should be closely monitored and laboratory studies should be drawn frequently. Fluids should be increased or decreased based on the response of the patient. Although the urine output is considered a "gold standard," early urine output can be slow while the patient is in shock and if tailoring fluids only to urine output, overresuscitation may occur. In addition, close monitoring of the patient's laboratories are necessary to determine the trend in organ perfusion. Laboratory values that might help assess organ perfusion include lactate, base deficit, central venous O_2, and/or pH. Although any one of these values alone does not provide a sensitive marker of the patient status, trending these values during resuscitation can help direct if the current fluid rate is causing a positive trend. If the organs are perfused, decreases in lactate and base deficit as well as increases in central venous O_2 and normalization of pH should be observed. Finally, a monitor of cardiac output during large resuscitations can help guide fluid and assess for early cardiac failure. Such cardiac output monitors include esophageal Doppler monitors, pulse pressure variation monitors (FloTrac) and thermodilution monitors (PiCCO).

In large burns that involve the face, an ophthalmologic consultation should be obtained. As the patient becomes edematous from the resuscitation, it is imperative that the globe is kept moisturized with a lubricant. Ophthalmologic consultants can help assess globe pressure, injury to the cornea and glaucoma, which often occur in electrical injury.

Thus, even though burn injuries may initially appear to be a focal area of trauma, the assessment of all systematic manifestations is paramount and must be stabilized before the burn itself is addressed.

TABLE 99-2
Parkland Formula for Fluid Administration in the First 24 Hours

(4 mL × % TBSA × weight [kg])/2
= first half to be administered in the first 8 hours
= second half to be administered over the following 16 hours

TBSA, total body surface area.

WOUND CARE ASSESSMENT AND TREATMENT

As previously discussed, the depth, location, size, and duration of the burn injury are the most important

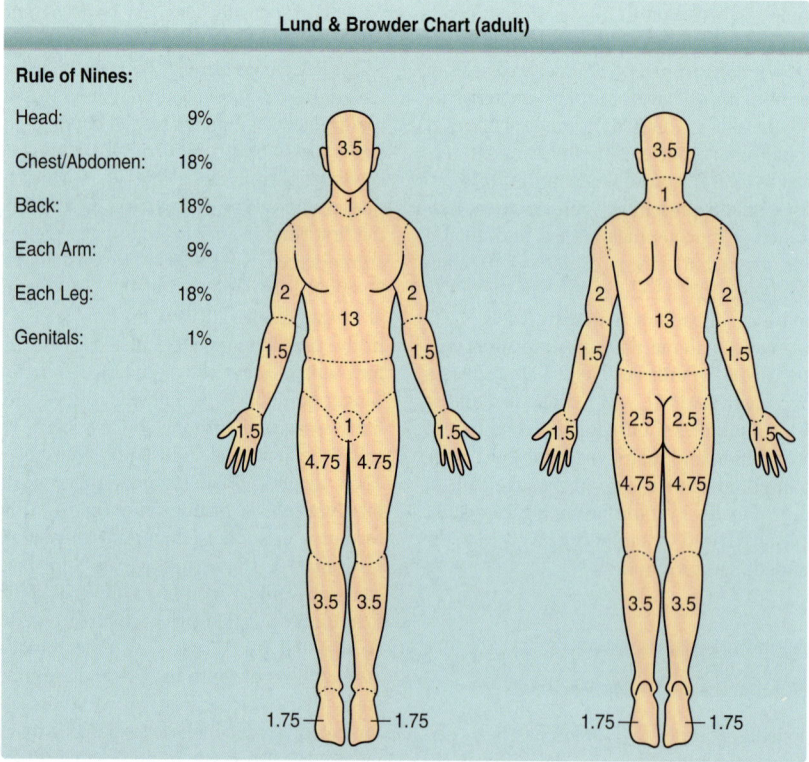

Figure 99-5 Rule of nines and the Lund & Browder Chart are methods commonly employed to estimate the total body surface area (TBSA) of a burn. Numbers in Lund & Browder Chart indicate percent TBSA of body region.

factors to consider in the assessment of a burn. Burns can present for reconstruction in the acute or chronic phase, and reconstructive options are very different depending upon when a patient presents.

Acute burn injuries require prompt intervention and serial examinations. On initial evaluation, it is important to rule out and prevent the development of circumferential burns that can lead to tissue ischemia and subsequent necrosis by limiting perfusion to the distal tissues.[26] The overarching concept, however, in acute burn reconstruction is early debridement and grafting. All blisters and nonviable tissue must be debrided upon presentation. After the initial debridement, dressing changes are initiated while the patient is stabilized from a systemic standpoint.

There are a variety of options for dressing materials (Table 99-3), and the appearance of the burn is mainly what dictates this choice. Although the indications for systemic antibiotic therapy have not been clearly defined within the literature, use of antimicrobial dressings is recommended. Silvadene is a silver-containing cream that has broad-spectrum coverage against both Gram-negative and Gram-positive bacteria that needs to be changed on a daily basis. Although its use is contraindicated in patients with sulfa allergies and over wounds near the eyes, Silvadene is commonly used over both partial-thickness and full-thickness injuries.[30] Laboratory values, including complete blood counts, must be followed while patients are using this medication in the acute phase because of possible leukopenia, which is a known side effect of this medication. If leukopenia develops, Silvadene should be stopped; however, patients rarely develop any serious complications. Additionally, Gram-negative infections can cause leukopenia and should be ruled out if this arises. Sulfamylon is an analogous agent that is used over cartilaginous areas such as the nose or ear because of increased penetration of this dressing over these areas as compared to other dressing types. As topical Sulfamylon cream can be used without dressings, it can be used for open burn wound therapy and regular examination of the burn wound surface. However, both the cream and a 5% solution of Sulfamylon are equally effective.[31] Sulfamylon has better penetration than Silvadene but may also cause increased pain. Patients should be monitored for complications such as hyperchloremic metabolic acidosis that can occur with use of this dressing as a result of its mechanism of action. Finally, chronic Sulfamylon can lead to fungal infection given that it does not cover any fungal species. This can be avoided by mixing with amphotericin.

Silver nitrate also can be used by soaking dressings in 0.5% to 1% concentration and applied 3 to 4 times a day. Unlike Sulfamylon, silver nitrate does cover fungal species and thus may be preferable postoperatively if concern for infection exists. Typically, silver nitrate is applied as a soak to a dressing 2 to 3 times per day. It can cause leaching of cations causing hyponatremia. Additionally, it stains the skin as well as the floor and any equipment it comes in contact with.

Bacitracin and Xeroform are additional examples of antimicrobial-type dressing regimens and should be changed every day or every other day. Even though both can be used anywhere on the body, bacitracin is commonly used for facial burns, whereas Xeroform is often used for partial-thickness skin graft donor sites. Regardless of the type of dressing used, wounds should be examined daily, given the predisposition of this wound niche to become infected.

For patients who are at lower risk of infection based on the appearance of wounds, dressings may be changed with less frequency to achieve a balance between pain control and the need for wound coverage. Acticoat is one such option that is mainly used in partial-thickness injuries. This dressing consists of silver-impregnated sheets that have antimicrobial properties and can be changed less frequently, reducing pain and cutting cost and only needs to be changed every 5 days.[32] The nanocrystalline particles in Acticoat are able to reduce wound infection and promote wound

TABLE 99-3
Wound Dressing Options

	INDICATIONS	MECHANISM OF ACTION	PRECAUTIONS
Silvadene	Partial- and full-thickness injuries	Broad-spectrum coverage vs Gram-positive and Gram-negative bacteria	Contraindicated in sulfa-allergic patients; avoid use near eyes Leukopenia known side effect
Sulfamylon	Burns over cartilaginous areas; for open burn wound therapy	Broad-spectrum coverage vs Gram-positive and Gram-negative bacteria	Associated with increased pain; risk for hyperchloremic metabolic acidosis; chronic use at risk for fungal infection
Silver nitrate	Soaking dressings, 2-4 times a day	Antifungal coverage	Hyponatremia Stains skin, adjacent surfaces
Bacitracin	Facial burns Dressings changed daily or every other day	Antibacterial	Daily dressing change required
Xeroform	Partial-thickness skin graft donor sites Dressings changed daily or every other day	Antibacterial	Daily dressing change required
Acticoat	Partial-thickness injuries with low risk of infection Dressings changed every 5 days	Antimicrobial silver impregnated dressings	

healing compared to older silver products, including silver nitrate.³³ When using Acticoat, it is important to remember to activate it with water and not normal saline as the sodium can leech out the silver.

While dressing changes are sometimes used to nourish and optimize a wound before and after operative interventions, dressings also have the potential to completely heal a wound without the need for surgical intervention depending on the overall appearance of the burn and patient as a whole. Thus, a proper wound care team must not only include a critical care physician and surgeon, but it must also include a specialized wound care nurse to appropriately address this central modality of care for any burn patient.

MANAGEMENT

Table 99-4 outlines the essentials of burn management.

TRIAGE

Upon presentation for care, a primary and secondary trauma survey should be performed, with special attention paid to signs of airway involvement and injury. Examination should be performed looking for intraoral swelling, hoarse voice, soot or singed nasal hairs. Nasopharyngeal scope examination can be performed in the emergency department for confirmation of airway involvement. Early intubation is recommended for patients with severe airway involvement or patients with large TBSA burns (>20% deep partial or full thickness) that will require Parkland large fluid resuscitation. Large-bore IV access should also be obtained in nonburned regions and arterial access, central line access and Foley catheter should be established to help guide resuscitation. Access to a burn center is crucial to optimize outcomes given the intricacies of airway management and complex resuscitative strategies.

TABLE 99-4
Essentials of Burn Management

- Burn location, size, extent, depth, and circumferential components influence decisions regarding outpatient care, hospitalization, or transfer.
- Burn percentage is best estimated using the Lund & Browder diagram that compensates for the changes in body proportions with age. An alternative is a "rule-of-nines" for adults and children.
- In the adult rule-of-nines, the head and neck is given 9%, each lower extremity is given 18%, each upper extremity is given 9%, and the anterior and posterior torso are each given 18%.
- In the pediatric rule-of-nines, the head and neck is given 18%, each lower extremity is given 15%, each upper extremity is given 10%, and the anterior and posterior torso are each given 16%.
- For scattered or irregular burns, the entire palmar surface of the patient's hand represents approximately 1% of the body surface over all ages.

OUTPATIENT CARE

In outpatient setting or prior to transfer, the clinician must ensure the burn process has stopped by removing all potentially hot or constricting items such as clothes, rings, or belts. Patient should also undergo decontamination and steps to ensure all chemicals are sufficiently diluted. Once at a burn center, the burns should be scrubbed with antimicrobial soap and subsequently wrapped in an antimicrobial dressing for transport. Practice patterns vary between centers but certain characteristics are universal. The wound should be kept clean and inspected for infection. Desiccated exudates and topical medications should be cleansed at least once daily. Burns selected for outpatient management are small and superficial with a corresponding low risk of infection, so clean rather than sterile technique is reasonable. If topical agents rather than membrane dressings are used, wounds may be cleansed with lukewarm tap water and a bland antimicrobial soap. Soaking adherent dressings prior to change will decrease the pain associated with daily wound care. It is important to instruct each patient to return promptly if erythema, swelling, increased tenderness, lymphangitis, odor, or drainage develops so that infectious complications can be addressed early. Pain and anxiety can be an issue for many. Some will benefit from pain medicine given 30 to 60 minutes prior to a planned dressing change. Increasing pain and anxiety associated with dressing changes; inability to keep scheduled followup appointments; delayed healing; signs of infection or a wound that appears deeper than appreciated at the time of the initial examination should prompt early return and specialty evaluation. Finally, wounds of the face, ears, hands, genitals, and feet have functional and cosmetic importance. Early specialty evaluation may be warranted, as initial care can have an impact on long-term outcome.

VACCINATION

A tetanus toxoid vaccine should be given to all burn patients with partial-thickness or full-thickness burns.³⁴ In very young children and persons with high-risk tetanus wounds (ie, burn older than 6 hours at presentation, immunodeficiency, or soil contamination in wound), tetanus immunoglobulin should also be administered (tetanus toxoid is not given in children younger than age 4 years).³⁵

PAIN

Burn pain is multifactorial and frequently severe, particularly in patients with partial-thickness burns. As burn wounds heal, they initially become increasingly painful. Scheduled narcotics are first-line medications for the management of outpatient burn pain, and acetaminophen and nonsteroidal antiinflammatory drugs should play a secondary role in management. Scheduled dosing of narcotics provides superior pain control in burn patients as compared to as needed dosing, and allows for tapering down as the healing process progresses.

Despite this, some patients may have inadequate control on short-acting narcotics. In this case, the patient should be interrogated about the nature of their pain. Frequently, pain intolerance is associated with wound dressing changes, which often occur daily. Anticipatory administration of narcotics before dressing changes can improve pain. Silver-coated dressings require less-frequent dressing changes, and if available, may aid in pain management. Furthermore, anxiety or acute stress disorders associated with dressing changes exacerbates pain, and scheduled administration of low-dose anxiolytics may manage pain without increased narcotic dosages. Pulsing or throbbing pain accompanied by warmth at the wound site may be associated with inflammatory progression, and in this case nonsteroidal antiinflammatory drugs may be appropriate. Otherwise, therapy may be escalated to long-acting scheduled narcotics. If pain cannot be controlled at home, the patient should be admitted for pain management.[36,37]

INFECTION

The infection rate of burns managed in the outpatient setting is 5%, which increases to 11% to 15% in diabetic patients. Usually these infections develop in the first 7 to 10 days, and normal flora organisms, such as *Staphylococcus*, are usually the culprits. Wound culture or quantitative culture is not necessary, as these infections present as cellulitis and may be reliably diagnosed clinically, with good response to first-generation cephalosporins. Infections occurring after the first 10 days, however, are more likely caused by Gram-negative rods, and patients benefit from wound culture and empiric coverage with ciprofloxacin. If symptoms progress to a combination of fever, chills, weakness, nausea, and/or vomiting, inpatient admission should be considered. Although burn wound infection looms as a feared complication, antibiotic prophylaxis is not appropriate and evidence does not support its use.[36]

Patients should be instructed to measure temperatures once or twice daily, with a measurement above 38°C (100.4°F) warranting urgent clinical evaluation. The wound should be well dressed with limited exposure to the environment. An antimicrobial barrier at the burn site should be maintained through application of silver-impregnated dressings or antimicrobial creams and ointments. Patients should avoid swimming in rivers, lakes, oceans, and even hot-tubs in order to avoid possible exposure to more virulent bacteria such as *Pseudomonas*. Tissue edema creates a nidus for infection, a risk factor easily managed by extremity elevation or a compression wrap (eg, ACE bandage). Patients should be educated about signs of infection, and if black or gray spots develop on the healing wound they should present immediately for evaluation. If undergoing treatment for infection, followup must be frequent (multiple visits weekly), and if hindered by provider availability, patient availability or travel, or suspected patient adherence, then admission for inpatient care may be appropriate.

PRURITUS

The majority of burn patients with both deep and superficial burns will experience clinically significant pruritus during their recovery. Regardless of severity, 90% of patients will experience pruritus during the first month after being burned. In 40% of patients, it will persist for at least 2 years, and roughly half of these chronic pruritus patients will experience consequent sleep disturbance. Risk factors for developing chronic pruritus include female gender, young age, skin grafting, raised or thick scars, and dry skin.[38]

The differentiation between transient and chronic postinjury pruritus can be understood by their distinguishable pathophysiologies. Mast cells produce and release histamine in response to the acute inflammatory burn reaction immediately following injury. As healing ensues, mast cell degranulation frequency decreases, and the majority of patients experience resolution. In full-thickness or grafted burns, however, afferent pathways have been destroyed, leading to general hypoesthesia. Despite this, such injuries predispose patients to the highest risk for chronic pruritus. Experts suggest that a neuropathic state of effective nociceptive hyperinnervation may develop in the setting of deafferentation because of release of selective neuropeptides from healing burn scar and degeneration of central inhibitory pathways regulating nociception.[39] Exact pathophysiologic mechanisms of chronic pruritus, however, remain unknown.

Evidence for treatment of burn pruritus is limited to 3 categories: topicals, antihistamines, and neuropathic agents. Selection of therapy generally follows aforementioned pathophysiologic reasoning. Nonetheless, the contribution of dry skin to pruritus should not be underestimated, and care should be taken for topical, bland, nonfragranced moisturizers to be applied to healed wound sites. Frequency of application is more important to achieve therapeutic effect than the product type, and patients should be advised to apply the moisturizer multiple times daily. When combined with antihistamines such as diphenhydramine, cetirizine, and hydroxyzine, early pruritus can be effectively managed. Cetirizine, a selective H_1-blocker, is more effective than general antihistamines such as diphenhydramine.[40] In patients with chronic pruritus, therapy with gabapentin and pregabalin is indicated—therapy that aligns with presumed neuropathic mechanisms. Similar to pain management, both antihistamines and neuropathic agents exhibit superior clinical benefits when doses are scheduled.[6]

SCAR

Thermal burn injuries can cause tremendous morbidity, leaving the patient with not only cosmetic but also functional impairments. Hypertrophic scarring is a major complication after burn injury with a prevalence of 32% to 72%. Several risk factors have been identified that contribute to its development, including the localization of the burn injury, burn depth, time to heal, and skin color.[41,42] Although the precise mechanism by which hypertrophic scarring occurs remains unclear, strong and persistent expression of transforming growth factor-β and its receptors is associated with postburn hypertrophic scarring. Furthermore, a critical step in the healing process that is altered is the transition from granulation tissue into normal scarring. During this remodeling process, wound epithelization and scar collagen is formed, but accompany a gradual decrease in cellularity as a result of apoptosis. However, early immature hypertrophic scars caused by burns are hypercellular and during the process of remodeling and maturing, fibroblast density does not resemble that of normal healing.[43] More specifically, apoptosis of myofibroblasts occurs 12 days after injury in normal wound healing, but in hypertrophic scar tissue, the maximum apoptosis occurs much later—at 19 to 30 months.[44] These events result in a significantly higher percentage of myofibroblasts and the hypertrophy of the scar tissue following severe burn injuries.

Although hypertrophic scarring often cannot be avoided, there are several steps that can optimize a burn scar:

1. Wound closure of a burn that is likely not to heal on its own in 3 weeks;
2. Avoidance of sun contact of the scar during the first 6 months;
3. Compression garments for those who can tolerate treatment for up to 1 year; and
4. Keeping the scar moist.

One of the key pathologic factors that needs to be addressed in any hypertrophic scar is tension. A new concept of "scar rejuvenation" has emerged with the key idea being to improve the environment of the scar without actual excision of the scar. The most important step in rejuvenating the scar is release of the tension. Rather than excising, the scar, this involves just releasing the area of greatest tension. Despite not removing any tissue, a large defect is often created once the tension is released. This defect can then be treated by adding new tissue such as a full-thickness skin graft or a thick split-thickness skin graft. Additional ways to relieve tension involve the use of tissue rearrangements such as a Z-plasty. A Z-plasty lengthens the scar at the expense of width, thereby alleviating tension along the central access of the hypertrophic scar. In general, Z-plasty rearrangements are made with 60-degree angles to maximize tissue gain without causing excess tension on the donor-site closure. The corner can be made at 90 degrees and then the rest of the limb at 60 degrees to improve blood flow to the tip of the flap and to avoid flap necrosis. Additionally, flaps should be kept thick to avoid flap ischemia. Alternative V-Y advancements are useful if there is healthy surrounding tissue and a combination of Z-plasty and V-Y advancement flaps, as in a 5-flap jumping man, are helpful for web spaces.[45]

Current treatment strategies for hypertrophic scars include surgical manipulation, intralesional corticosteroid injections, cryotherapy, and laser therapy. Surgical manipulation to remove the excess skin remains the traditional treatment for hypertrophic scar. Newer studies investigating the role of fat grafting into scars have shown promise to further improve function and appearance.[46] Patients who have undergone fat transfer report satisfactory results 6 months after the procedure, indicating considerable improvement in the features of the skin, skin texture, and thickness. Histologic examination demonstrated new collagen deposition, neovascularization, and dermal hyperplasia in regions treated with fat grafting, which mimicked surrounding undamaged skin. Additionally, intralesional corticosteroids suppress the inflammatory process in wounds, diminish collagen synthesis, and enhance collagen degradation.[47] Conversely, cryotherapy induces vascular damage that leads to anoxia and, ultimately, tissue necrosis, and has yielded marked improvement of hypertrophic scars.[48] However, its efficacy is limited to the management of small scars. Lastly, since the introduction of laser treatment in the mid-1980s, the therapeutic use of additional lasers with different wavelengths have been employed. The most encouraging results have been obtained with the 585-nm wavelength pulsed-dye laser, which has been recognized as an excellent therapeutic option for the treatment of younger hypertrophic scars.[49] Pulsed-dye laser induces the dissociation of disulfide bonds in collagen fibers and leads to collagen fiber realignment, decreased fibroblast proliferation, and neocollagenesis. However, it is necessary for repeated treatments, generally between 2 and 6 treatments, for optimal resolution.

Newer, exciting research has demonstrated the benefit of fractional photothermolysis in the treatment of hypertrophic scarring. Although the exact mechanism is unknown, this concept uses a CO_2 laser, which is an ablative laser that targets water in the underlying tissues (10,600 nm). The laser creates columns of tissue destruction, which stimulates collagen production in adjacent uninjured columns of tissue. The adjacent uninjured tissue allows for more rapid tissue regeneration from their follicles and sweat glands. Overall, this creates a smoother appearance and enables meshed grafts to appear less obvious.[10] Patients have described less tightness as well as decreased pruritus.[50] The key to this treatment modality is the fractionated nature of the laser, which allows for remodeling of the disorganized collagen without undue thermal injury to the surface. Different strategies are used for fractional CO_2 lasers with some clinicians preferring high density and low energy and others preferring low density and high energy.

ACKNOWLEDGMENTS

We would like to thank Dr. Joshua Peterson, MD for his assistance and guidance in figure and textual development of this chapter.

REFERENCES

1. American Burn Association. *Burn Incidence Fact Sheet: Burn Incidence and Treatment in the United States: 2016.* http://ameriburn.org/resources_factsheet.php. Accessed November 16, 2017.
2. Brigham P, McLoughlin E. Burn incidence and medical care use in the US: estimates, trends, and data souces. *J Burn Care Rehabil.* 1996;17(2):95-107.
3. Peck MD. Epidemiology of burns throughout the world. Part I: distribution and risk factors. *Burns.* 2011;37(7):1087-1100.
4. Kahn SA, Bell DE, Hutchins P, et al. Outpatient burn data: an untapped resource. *Burns.* 2013;39(7): 1351-1354.
5. Tompkins RG. Survival from burns in the new millennium: 70 years' experience from a single institution. *Ann Surg.* 2015;261(2):263-268.
6. Lloyd EC, Rodgers BC, Michener M, et al. Outpatient burns: prevention and care. *Am Fam Physician.* 2012; 85(1):25-32.
7. Grunwald TB, Garner WL. Acute burns. *Plast Reconstr Surg.* 2008;121(5):311e-319e.
8. U.S. Department of Health and Human Services, Radiation Emergency Medical Management. *Burn Triage and Treatment: Thermal Injuries—Diagnosis of Burns.* https://www.remm.nlm.gov/burns.htm#diagnosis. Accessed July 25, 2018.
9. Colohan SM. Predicting prognosis in thermal burns with associated inhalational injury: a systematic review of prognostic factors in adult burn victims. *J Burn Care Res.* 2010;31(4):529-539.
10. Agarwal S, Sorkin M, Levi B. Heterotopic ossification and hypertrophic scars. *Clin Plast Surg.* 2017;44(4):749-755.
11. Levi B, Jayakumar P, Giladi A, et al. Risk factors for the development of heterotopic ossification in seriously burned adults: a National Institute on Disability, Independent Living and Rehabilitation Research burn model system database analysis. *J Trauma Acute Care Surg.* 2015;79(5):870-876.
12. Ranganathan K, Loder S, Agarwal S, et al. Heterotopic ossification: basic-science principles and clinical correlates. *J Bone Joint Surg Am.* 2015;97(13):1101-1111.
13. Agarwal S, Loder S, Levi B. Heterotopic ossification following upper extremity injury. *Hand Clin.* 2017;33(2):363-373.
14. Williams FN, Herndon DN, Hawkins HK, et al. The leading causes of death after burn injury in a single pediatric burn center. *Crit Care.* 2009;13(6):R183.
15. Lim JY, Lum CH, Tan AJ, et al. Long term sensory function after minor partial thickness burn: a pilot study to determine if recovery is complete or incomplete. *Burns.* 2014;40(8):1538-1543.
16. Abu-Sittah GS, Sarhane KA, Dibo SA, et al. Cardiovascular dysfunction in burns: review of the literature. *Ann Burns Fire Disasters.* 2012;25(1):26-37.
17. Lowell G, Quinlan K, Gottlieb LJ. Preventing unintentional scald burns: moving beyond tap water. *Pediatrics.* 2008;122(4):799-804.
18. Rimmer RB, Weigand S, Foster KN, et al. Scald burns in young children—a review of Arizona Burn Center pediatric patients and a proposal for prevention in the Hispanic community. *J Burn Care Res.* 2008;29(4): 595-605.
19. Dissanaike S, Boshart K, Coleman A, et al. Cooking-related pediatric burns: risk factors and the role of differential cooling rates among commonly implicated substances. *J Burn Care Res.* 2009;30(4):593-598.
20. Drago DA. Kitchen scalds and thermal burns in children five years and younger. *Pediatrics.* 2005;115(1):10-16.
21. Fish RM, Geddes LA. Conduction of electrical current to and through the human body: a review. *Eplasty.* 2009;9:e44.
22. Friedstat J, Brown DA, Levi B. Chemical, electrical, and radiation injuries. *Clin Plast Surg.* 2017;44(3):657-669.
23. Orr MF, Wu J, Sloop SL; Centers for Disease Control and Prevention (CDC). Acute chemical incidents surveillance—Hazardous Substances Emergency Events Surveillance, nine states, 1999-2008. *MMWR Suppl.* 2015;64(2):1-9.
24. Palao R, Monge I, Ruiz M, et al. Chemical burns: pathophysiology and treatment. *Burns.* 2010;36(3): 295-304.
25. White ML, Chodosh J, Jang J, et al. Incidence of Stevens-Johnson syndrome and chemical burns to the eye. *Cornea.* 2015;34(12):1527-1533.
26. Bezuhly M, Fish JS. Acute burn care. *Plast Reconstr Surg.* 2012;130(2):349e-358e.
27. Posluszny JA, Conrad P, Halerz M, et al. Surgical burn wound infections and their clinical implications. *J Burn Care Res.* 2011;32(2):324-333.
28. Brown DL, Borschel GH, Levi B. *Michigan Manual of Plastic Surgery.* 2nd ed. Philadelphia, PA: Lippincott Williams & Wilkins; 2014.
29. Thorne CH, Chung KC, Gosain AK, et al, eds. *Grabb and Smith's Plastic Surgery.* 7th ed. Philadelphia, PA: Lippincott Williams & Wilkins; 2014.
30. Atiyeh BS, Costagliola M, Hayek SN, et al. Effect of silver on burn wound infection control and healing: review of the literature. *Burns.* 2007;33(2):139-148.
31. Falcone P, Harrison H, Sowemimo G, et al. Mafenide acetate concentrations and bacteriostasis in experimental burn wounds treated with a three-layered laminated famenide-saline dressing. *Ann Plast Surg.* 1980;5(4):226-229.
32. Fong J, Wood F. Nanocrystalline silver dressings in wound management: a review. *Int J Nanomedicine.* 2006;1(4):441-449.
33. Gravante G, Caruso R, Sorge R, et al. Nanocrystalline silver: a systematic review of randomized trials conducted on burned patients and an evidence-based assessment of potential advantages over older silver formulations. *Ann Plast Surg.* 2009;63(2):201-205.
34. Riddick-Grisham S, Deming L. *Pediatric Life Care Planning and Case Management.* 2nd ed. New York, NY: Routledge; 2011:993.
35. EMed. *Tetanus Prophylaxis.* http://www.emed.ie/Trauma/Wounds/Tetanus.php. Accessed July 25, 2018.

36. Warner PM, Coffee TL, Yowler CJ. Outpatient burn management. *Surg Clin North Am.* 2014;94(4):879-892.
37. Griggs C, Goverman J, Bittner EA, et al. Sedation and pain management in burn patients. *Clin Plast Surg.* 2017;44(3):535-540.
38. Carrougher GJ, Martinez EM, McMullen KS, et al. Pruritus in adult burn survivors. *J Burn Care Res.* 2013;34(1):94-101.
39. Goutos I. Neuropathic mechanisms in the pathophysiology of burns pruritus: redefining directions for therapy and research. *J Burn Care Res.* 2013;34(1):82-93.
40. Bell P, Gabriel V. Evidence based review for the treatment of post-burn pruritus. *J Burn Care Res.* 2009;30(1):55-61.
41. Lawrence JW, Mason ST, Schomer K, et al. Epidemiology and impact of scarring after burn injury. *J Burn Care Res.* 2012;33(1):136-146.
42. Gangemi EN, Gregori D, Berchialla P, et al. Epidemiology and risk factors for pathologic scarring after burn wounds. *Arch Facial Plast Surg.* 2008;10(2):93-102.
43. Nedelec B, Shankowsky H, Scott PG, et al. Myofibroblasts and apoptosis in human hypertrophic scars: the effect of interferon-α2b. *Surgery.* 2001; 130(5):798-808.
44. Armour A, Scott PG, Tredget EE. Cellular and molecular pathology of HTS: basis for treatment. *Wound Repair Regen.* 2007;15(s1):S6-S17.
45. Sorkin M, Cholok D, Levi B. Scar management of the burned hand. *Hand Clin.* 2017;33(2):305-315.
46. Parnell LK, Nedelec B, Rachelska G, et al. Assessment of pruritus characteristics and impact on burn survivors. *J Burn Care Res.* 2012;33(3):407-418.
47. Reish RG, Eriksson E. Scar treatments: preclinical and clinical studies. *J Am Coll Surg.* 2008;206(4):719-730.
48. Zouboulis CC, Blume U, Büttner P, et al. Outcomes of cryosurgery in keloids and hypertrophic scars. A prospective consecutive trial of case series. *Arch Dermatol.* 1993;129(9):1146-1151.
49. Alster TS, Handrick C. Laser treatment of hypertrophic scars, keloids, and striae. *Semin Cutan Med Surg.* 2000;19(4):287-292.
50. Manstein D, Herron GS, Sink RK, et al. Fractional photothermolysis: a new concept for cutaneous remodeling using microscopic patterns of thermal injury. *Lasers Surg Med.* 2004;34(5):426-438.

Psychosocial Skin Disease PART 18

第十八篇　心理社会性皮肤病

Chapter 100 :: Delusional, Obsessive-Compulsive, and Factitious Skin Diseases
:: Mio Nakamura, Josie Howard, & John Y. M. Koo

第一百章
妄想、强迫症和人为皮肤病

中文导读

　　本章开始介绍了原发性精神疾病和继发性精神疾病的定义，提出了皮肤感觉障碍是指病人在没有任何可诊断的皮肤病、神经病学、内科学或精神病学情况下的皮肤感觉异常。并对心身性皮肤疾病进行了分类，指出这类疾病有可能出现重叠或共存。本章着重对妄想性皮肤疾病中的寄生虫性妄想症、强迫症和相关皮肤疾病的体象障碍、抓痕、拔毛症、神经性表皮剥脱、人为疾病中的人工皮炎，从流行病学、临床表现、病因和发病机制、诊断、鉴别诊断、临床病程和预后、临床管理、治疗等方面进行介绍。

〔易　梅〕

MORGELLONS PSYCHODERMATOLOGY

It is estimated that approximately one-third of patients seeking treatment of skin complaints have associated psychological stress or psychiatric disease.[1] The field of psychodermatology studies the overlap of psychology/psychiatry and dermatology.[2] Psychophysiologic skin disorders are primary skin diseases that can be precipitated or exacerbated by psychosocial stress, such as psoriasis, atopic dermatitis, and acne. Such skin diseases are also known to lead to and/or exacerbate psychiatric disorders such as anxiety and depression,[3-5] which are referred to as secondary psychiatric disorders. On the other hand, in primary psychiatric skin disorders, there is an underlying psychiatric component that causes self-induced physical findings on the skin.[6] Underlying psychiatric issues, such as anxiety, depression, obsessive-compulsive disorder (OCD), and psychosis, result in destructive manipulation of the skin, hair, or nails, often as an expression of highly dysregulated emotions.[7] Lastly, cutaneous sensory disorders are conditions in which the patient has various abnormal sensations on the skin, such as itching, burning, stinging, biting, and crawling, in the absence of any diagnosable dermatologic, neurologic, medical, or psychiatric diagnosis.[8] Table 100-1 shows the categorization of psychodermatologic disorders. Although these categories are extremely useful in conceptualizing psychodermatologic disorders, it is important to note that there can be considerable overlap or coexistence of these conditions. This chapter focuses on primary psychiatric skin disease, which broadly includes delusional, obsessive-compulsive, and factitious skin disorders (Table 100-2).

DELUSIONAL SKIN DISORDERS

AT-A-GLANCE

- Monosymptomatic hypochondriacal diseases are characterized by the presence of usually 1 fixed, false belief, which includes delusions of parasitosis, Morgellons disease, and other rare types of hypochondriacal delusional ideations.
- Secondary skin findings of excoriation and manipulation of the skin, hair, or nails are seen in delusions of parasitosis and Morgellons disease.
- Treatment and management are challenging as patients often have low to absent levels of insight and, consequently, are not open to psychiatric treatment or referral. Establishing rapport is key.
- Treatment of choice for delusions of parasitosis is pimozide, followed by atypical antipsychotics.

Delusional skin disorders are characterized by the presence of usually one fixed, false belief. Delusional patients by definition lack insight; consequently, they primarily seek care from a dermatologist rather than a psychiatrist. Delusional patients are among the most difficult cases to manage successfully as they can be distrusting and unaccepting of treatments and psychiatric referral, which makes it critical to establish therapeutic rapport with these patients.

DELUSIONS OF PARASITOSIS (DELUSIONS OF INFESTATIONS, MORGELLONS DISEASE)

Delusions of parasitosis, also known as delusions of infestation, is a type of monosymptomatic hypochondriacal psychosis characterized by a false, fixed belief that one is infested with living organisms or inanimate materials in the absence of objective proof. Morgellons disease is a variant of delusions of parasitosis characterized by a fixed belief that there are fibers or solid material extruding from the skin.

CLINICAL FEATURES

Patients with delusions of parasitosis and Morgellons disease experience sensations of formication, including crawling, biting, and stinging, which they believe are symptoms caused by cutaneous infestation by parasites (parasitosis) or emergence of fibers from the skin (Morgellons disease). They may attempt to pick the "parasites" or "fibers" out of their skin. They frequently collect specimens they claim to have extracted from their skin, which may include scabs, skin flakes, hair, clothing fibers, and even real insects that actually have nothing to do with their symptoms. The specimens are brought in various containers, such as in an empty matchbox or Ziploc bags, which is referred to as the *matchbox sign*, *Ziploc sign*, or *specimen sign*.[9] In the age of the smartphone, it is also becoming increasingly common for patients to bring in what they believe to be photographic evidence of their infestation, often with an exhaustive photographic account of their skin and miscellaneous debris, which they interpret to be insects or fibers infiltrating their skin. Patients have often tried many courses of antiparasitic therapies such as permethrin and ivermectin. Many have had their homes exterminated, gotten rid of all of their belongings and pets, or moved out of their homes in an attempt to eradicate the parasites with only short-lasting relief or no improvement at all. A family member or friend may come in with the patient to confirm the patient's delusion. Physical examination often reveals evidence of self-mutilation, which can vary from minor excoriations to deep, gouged-out, irregular appearing ulcers. The skin lesions typically spare areas out of reach for the patients such as the interscapular region.

ETIOLOGY AND PATHOGENESIS

Delusions of parasitosis originates from a fixed, false belief that is encapsulated, meaning that the patient is otherwise seemingly "normal" aside from the delusion that they are infested by parasites. This is quite

TABLE 100-1
Psychodermatology: Categorization of Psychodermatologic Disorders[2]

PSYCHOPHYSIOLOGIC SKIN DISORDERS	PRIMARY PSYCHIATRIC SKIN DISORDERS	SECONDARY PSYCHIATRIC DISORDERS	CUTANEOUS SENSORY DISORDERS
- Psoriasis - Atopic dermatitis - Acne vulgaris - Seborrheic dermatitis - Hyperhidrosis - Lichen simplex chronicus	Delusional disorders - Delusions of parasitosis - Morgellons disease Obsessive-compulsive and related disorders - Body dysmorphic disorder - Trichotillomania - Excoriation disorder - Other body-focused repetitive behavior disorders Factitious disorders - Dermatitis artefacta	- Anxiety - Depression - Social phobia	- Cutaneous dysesthesia - "Central" pruritus - Formication

different from schizophrenia and other delusional disorders, which involve multiple functional defects, including auditory hallucinations, social isolation, flat or inappropriate affect, in addition to delusional ideation.

DIAGNOSIS

The diagnosis of delusions of parasitosis is a diagnosis of exclusion, meaning it cannot be diagnosed if the condition is better explained by a different disorder. It can only be made when the patient has an encapsulated delusion of infestation without presence of any organic cause. All other psychiatric disorders must also be ruled out prior to making the diagnosis of delusions of parasitosis. If the delusional ideation is part of a broader underlying psychosis such as schizophrenia or psychotic depression, then a separate diagnosis of delusions of parasitosis cannot be made. The diagnosis can be made by history, physical examination, and appropriate laboratory testing or imaging to rule out other causes of the patient's symptoms and skin findings (see section "Differential Diagnosis"). Even though a biopsy is likely to be non-diagnostic, there is merit in using a biopsy as a means of providing further objective evidence against an infestation and to optimize trust and therapeutic rapport with the patient.

DIFFERENTIAL DIAGNOSIS

First, a real infestation with parasites, such as scabies, must be excluded.[10] Second, any organic causes of symptoms of formication should be ruled out. Medical conditions associated with formication, pruritus, or paresthesia include endocrine disorders (diabetes mellitus, hyperthyroidism or hypothyroidism), renal disease (uremic pruritus), nutritional deficiencies (B_1, niacin, folic acid, B_{12}, iron), neurologic disorders (neuropathy, multiple sclerosis), and infections (syphilis). Laboratory tests, including comprehensive metabolic panel, thyroid function, serum vitamin levels, and ferritin level, can effectively rule out many of these medical etiologies. For cases in which there is suspicion of an underlying neurologic disease, a referral to a neurologist with appropriate workup, such as CT or MRI of the brain or spine, may be necessary. Infectious workup may be indicated in some cases. The patient's medication list should also be reviewed for pruritus-inducing medications such as opiates and stimulants. Third, recreational drug use must also be ruled out as substances such as cocaine, methamphetamine, and narcotics can cause formication. Therefore, a urine toxicology screen may be helpful.

Lastly, underlying, more global psychiatric diseases must be ruled out. The psychiatric differential diagnosis includes schizophrenia, psychotic depression, psychosis with florid mania, and drug-induced psychosis. In some patients, there is no ideation of infestation, in which case the patient has a diagnosis of simply "formication" rather than delusions of parasitosis.

CLINICAL COURSE, PROGNOSIS, AND MANAGEMENT

Early intervention is important in delusions of parasitosis, as patients with a shorter duration of active delusion have an increased probability of achieving remission following treatment.[11] On the other hand, when untreated, patients tend to further isolate themselves and subsequently progress into a more severe delusional state.[12,13]

Management of patients with delusions of parasitosis is challenging. Ultimately, the only therapy that consistently works is antipsychotic medications.

TABLE 100-2
Primary Psychiatric Skin Disorders

	CHARACTERISTICS	UNDERLYING PSYCHOPATHOLOGY	DIFFERENTIAL DIAGNOSES	TREATMENTS
Delusions of parasitosis, Morgellons disease	- Formication (crawling, biting, stinging) attributed to infestation by parasites or fibers emerging from the skin - Specimens collected and brought in - Impervious to rational explanation - Absent to low level of insight	- "Encapsulated" delusion of infestation (otherwise functional or "normal-appearing")	- Real infestations scabies, arthropod bites, etc. - Endocrine: diabetes, thyroid disease - Renal: uremia - Nutritional deficiencies: vitamin B_1/B_{12}, niacin, folate, iron - Neurologic: multiple sclerosis, neuropathy - Infections: syphilis - Drug use: cocaine, amphetamines, opiates - Medication-induced: opioids, psychostimulants - Psychiatric: schizophrenia, psychotic depression, psychosis with florid mania, and drug-induced psychosis	- Pimozide - Atypical antipsychotics (eg, risperidone, aripiprazole, olanzapine)
Body dysmorphic disorder	- Preoccupation with an imagined or minor physical flaw - Excessive time spent attempting to fix or conceal the "flaw" - Significant distress and dysfunction - None to low level of insight	- Obsession about a physical flaw - Comorbid depression, anxiety, or OCD	- Concern about a real physical defect - Anorexia nervosa - Bulimia nervosa - Primary psychiatric disease (depression anxiety, psychosis) - Somatic delusion	- SSRIs - CBT
Trichotillomania	- Repetitive action of hair-pulling - Irregular, nonscarring alopecia with excoriations - May acknowledge self-inflicted nature, relatively high level of insight	- OCD - Comorbid anxiety, depression, psychosis	- Alopecia areata, androgenic alopecia, alopecia mucinosa - Tinea capitis - Lichen planopilaris - Folliculitis decalvans - Discoid lupus erythematosus	- SSRIs - TCAs (eg, clomipramine) - HRT
Neurotic excoriations	- Self-induced scratching, picking, or rubbing of the skin - May acknowledge self-inflicted nature of skin lesions, relatively high level of insight and associated shame	- Psychosocial stressor - Comorbid depression, anxiety, OCD, BPD, or psychosis	- Medical causes of pruritus: cutaneous dysesthesia, urticaria, uremia, hepatitis, xerosis, thyroid disease, etc - Delusions of parasitosis - Dermatitis artefacta - Malingering	- Wound care - SSRIs - TCAs (eg, doxepin) - HRT - Psychotherapy
Dermatitis artefacta	- Self-induced injury using instruments (sharp objects, lighters, cigarettes, corrosive chemicals) - Deny self-inflicted nature of skin lesions	- Psychosocial stressor - History of physical, emotional, or sexual abuse - Outlet of anger - Comorbid depression, anxiety, OCD, or BPD	- Malingering - Delusions of parasitosis - Neurotic excoriation - Psychiatric: OCD, depression, suicide, Munchausen syndrome - Primary dermatologic diseases: pyoderma gangrenosum, collagen vascular diseases, vasculitis, arthropod bites	- Wound care - SSRIs - Antipsychotics - Psychotherapy (including DBT)

BPD, borderline personality disorder; CBT, cognitive behavioral therapy; DBT, dialectical behavioral therapy; HRT, habit reversal therapy; OCD, obsessive-compulsive disorder; SSRI, selective serotonin reuptake inhibitor; TCA, tricyclic antidepressant.

However, when the patient presents to the dermatologist's office, it is highly likely that the patient has already been seen by other physicians and is disillusioned with the care received. This negativity is often projected to the new provider. Patients are often hesitant to start antipsychotic therapy and may not be willing to see a psychiatrist for the presumed skin disease. Therefore, it is extremely important to first establish rapport with the patient. Until rapport is established, interactions should be focused on support, empathy, and validation before the patient comes to trust the dermatologist, thereby making it possible to begin discussing therapeutic options. Furthermore, the desperation to be relieved from symptoms may override the need for validation; therefore, the patient may eventually be receptive to pharmacologic treatment.

The antipsychotic agent pimozide (Orap) is the most studied pharmacologic agent for the treatment of delusions of parasitosis. In a review of 53 patients with delusions of parasitosis who received pimozide, 50 (94%) achieved partial or complete remission from delusional symptoms.[14] It is believed that at low doses, the dopamine-blocking effects of pimozide address psychotic symptoms, while its opioid antagonism effects alleviate cutaneous sensations.[15] Notable adverse effects of pimozide include extrapyramidal symptoms such as akathisia (restlessness) and pseudoparkinsonian symptoms. Patients should be educated on these symptoms, which can be treated with as-needed diphenhydramine (Benadryl) or benztropine (Cogentin). Another adverse effect of pimozide is QT prolongation. Obtaining a baseline EKG and medical clearance is recommended in patients who are older or have a cardiac history.

Risperidone (Risperdal) is both the most-studied atypical antipsychotic agent for delusions of parasitosis and efficacious. In a study of 35 patients receiving risperidone, 24 (69%) achieved partial or complete remission.[16] Risperidone is less likely to induce extrapyramidal symptoms than pimozide, but is associated with other side effects, such as galactorrhea, and periodic monitoring of prolactin levels may be indicated. Other reportedly efficacious antipsychotic medications include olanzapine (Zyprexa) and aripiprazole (Abilify).[16,17] Adverse effects to be aware of include significant weight gain with olanzapine and akathisia or agitation with aripiprazole. Table 100-3 shows the dosing and common adverse effects of various antipsychotic medications that can be used to treat delusions of parasitosis. When the patient begins to experience the clinical benefit of an antipsychotic, adherence to the medication generally increases. Most patients can be treated on an episodic basis and can be tapered off of the antipsychotic after several months while maintaining remission. However, there are some patients who require long-term, low-dose maintenance treatment.

OTHER DELUSIONAL DISORDERS

Other types of monosymptomatic hypochondriacal diseases are uncommon and include olfactory reference syndrome or delusion of bromosis, a preoccupation with body odor that is not perceived by others, leading to the substantial distress and disability.[18]

OBSESSIVE-COMPULSIVE AND RELATED DISORDERS

AT-A-GLANCE

- OCDs include intrusive, unwanted urges, often necessitating repetitive compulsive behaviors.
- Body dysmorphic disorder (BDD) is characterized by preoccupation with an imagined defect with excessive time spent attempting to conceal or fix the defect. Treatment of choice for BDD is high-dose selective serotonin reuptake inhibitors (SSRIs) and cognitive behavioral therapy (CBT).
- Hair pulling disorder is the repetitive action of pulling out hair, resulting in significant hair loss, which appears as nonscarring, patchy alopecia. The most effective treatment for this disorder is habit-reversal training (HRT). SSRIs can also be effective.
- Neurotic excoriations or psychogenic excoriations is a disorder characterized by self-induced cutaneous lesions resulting from the uncontrollable impulse to excessively pick, rub, or scratch normal skin or skin with minor surface irregularities. Treatment includes addressing the underlying psychiatric illness.

OCDs and related disorders are characterized by obsessive preoccupations and/or repetitive, compulsive behaviors. OCDs include intrusive thoughts or urges that are experienced as unwanted (obsession), often necessitating repetitive behaviors or rituals to help alleviate the otherwise intolerable anxiety (compulsion).[19] In the *Diagnostic and Statistical Manual of Mental Disorders*, 5th edition (DSM-5), the presence of either one or both obsessions and compulsions is necessary to make the diagnosis. OCDs and related skin disorders include body dysmorphic disorder (BDD), excoriations, and hair pulling disorder.

BODY DYSMORPHIC DISORDER

BDD is a somatoform disorder characterized by preoccupation with a nonexistent or minor physical flaw, estimated to affect 1.8% to 2.4% of the general population, which is likely an underestimate as patients with BDD often experience embarrassment and deliberately avoid confiding in the provider.[20,21] There is a slightly higher prevalence of this disease in women compared to men, and BDD can appear as early as childhood with a mean age of onset of 16 years old.[22]

TABLE 100-3
Summary of Psychopharmacologic Agents Used for the Management of Primary Psychodermatologic Conditions

		COMMON DERMATOLOGIC DOSAGE				
	CLASS	STARTING	TITRATION	MAXIMUM	ADVERSE REACTIONS	RECOMMENDED MONITORING
Pimozide (Orap)	Typical antipsychotic	0.5 mg/day	0.5-1 mg every 2-4 weeks	5 mg/day[a]	Sedation, arrhythmia (QT prolongation), orthostatic hypotension, seizure, EPS, NMS, leukopenia, neutropenia	EKG, potassium and magnesium levels
Risperidone (Risperdal)	Atypical antipsychotic	0.5 mg/day	0.5 mg every 2-4 weeks	4-6 mg/day	Sedation, QT prolongation, weight gain, hyperglycemia, galactorrhea, seizures, EPS, NMS, leukopenia	EKG, weight, fasting glucose, prolactin, CBC
Olanzapine (Zyprexa)	Atypical antipsychotic	2.5 mg/day	5 mg/day PRN	20 mg/day	Weight gain, diabetes, hyperglycemia, hyperlipidemia, galactorrhea, seizures, EPS, NMS, neutropenia, anemia	Weight, fasting glucose, lipids, prolactin, CBC
Aripiprazole (Abilify)	Atypical antipsychotic	2-5 mg/day	up to 5 mg/day qweek	30 mg/day	Akathisia, agitation, weight gain, headache, seizures, diabetes, hypertension, neutropenia	Weight, fasting glucose, CBC
Sertraline (Zoloft)	SSRI[c]	25 mg/day	25-50 mg/day qweek	200 mg/day	Nausea, diarrhea, dyspepsia, headache, sexual dysfunction, suicidality[b], hyponatremia	Clinical signs of suicidality
Paroxetine (Paxil)	SSRI[c]	20 mg/day	10 mg/day qweek	60 mg/day	Nausea, diarrhea, constipation, headache, dizziness, insomnia, sexual dysfunction, suicidality[b]	Clinical signs of suicidality
Fluoxetine (Prozac)	SSRI[c]	10 mg/day	Up to 80 mg/day	80 mg/day	Nausea, diarrhea, dyspepsia, headache, sexual dysfunction, suicidality[b], QT prolongation	Clinical signs of suicidality, EKG
Fluvoxamine (Luvox)	SSRI[c]	50 mg/day	50 mg/day q4-7 days	300 mg/day	Nausea, diarrhea, dyspepsia, headache, sexual dysfunction, suicidality[b], hyponatremia	Clinical signs of suicidality
Doxepin (Sinequan)	TCA	10 mg/day	q5-7 days up to lowest effective therapeutic dose	300 mg/day	Sedation, anticholinergic effects, QT prolongation, seizures, xerostomia, increased appetite, suicidality[b]	Clinical signs of suicidality, EKG
Clomipramine (Anafranil)	TCA	25 mg/day	25 mg/day q4-7 days	100 mg/day in first 2 weeks, 250 mg/day for maintenance tx	Headache, constipation, orthostatic hypotension, anticholinergic effects, QT prolongation, seizures, suicidality[b]	Clinical signs of suicidality, EKG, LFT

[a]This is the usual maximum, not the absolute maximum.
[b]The reported increased risk of suicidality appears situational and mostly in patients younger than 18 years of age.[53]
[c]Note that before starting an SSRI, underlying bipolar illness should be ruled out as SSRIs can unmask or precipitate a manic episode in bipolar patients. Signs of bipolar illness include periods of increased energy, risk-taking behaviors, and decreased need for sleep. Monitoring is recommended in high-risk or symptomatic patients.
CBC, complete blood count; EPS, extrapyramidal symptoms; LFT, liver function tests; NMS, neuroleptic malignant syndrome; SSRI, selective serotonin reuptake inhibitor; TCA, tricyclic antidepressant.

CLINICAL FEATURES

Patients with BDD fixate on a specific aspect of their appearance that they find to be unattractive or "deformed." The face is commonly involved; however, body parts such as the hips, breasts, abdomen and buttocks can also be the focus of concern. Patients will present to a dermatologist or plastic surgeon with a complaint regarding the skin (wrinkles, scarring, color), hair (excessive facial or body hair, loss of hair), or part of the body (breasts, hips, abdomen, buttocks). While the alleged defects cause overwhelming anxiety and distress to the patient, the site of complaint is unremarkable in appearance to others, and thus the defect appears to be a perceptual distortion or imagined by the patient. The distress manifests as excessive time spent thinking about the defect and attempting to conceal it. Patients with BDD often perform repetitive behaviors such as mirror checking, excessive grooming, and skin picking. Seeking repeated reassurance, but receiving little to no relief from that reassurance, is also common.

ETIOLOGY AND PATHOGENESIS

The etiology of BDD is poorly understood. Some psychoanalysts believe that there may be an underlying emotional conflict that is reflected to a particular body part, as patients can have comorbid anxiety, depression, and OCD.[22] Others believe that the disease originates from social and cultural pressures to look a certain way.[23] Studies also show that patients with BDD may have neurochemical alterations responsible for visual processing in the frontostriatal system of the brain.[24]

DIAGNOSIS

BDD is diagnosed clinically and is a diagnosis of exclusion, meaning it cannot be diagnosed if the condition is better explained by a different disorder.

DIFFERENTIAL DIAGNOSES

In BDD, the defect of concern must not be a genuinely significant defect in appearance. Psychiatric differential diagnoses also include anorexia nervosa or bulimia nervosa if body weight is the concern.[25] Primary psychiatric conditions such as anxiety, depression, and psychosis may be the cause and must be ruled out prior to diagnosing BDD.

CLINICAL COURSE, PROGNOSIS, AND MANAGEMENT

Many patients with BDD seek cosmetic correction for their perceived physical flaws. Unfortunately, cosmetic intervention generally does not result in patient satisfaction. In a cross-sectional survey study of BDD, 81% of patients reported dissatisfaction with the outcome of the consultation or surgery.[26] It is possible for a patient's delusional state to spontaneously lessen or even remit, as disordered thinking can fluctuate in severity. Therefore, it is best if unnecessary procedures are not performed in order to avoid a situation in which the patient is more dissatisfied following the intervention compared to before. High-dose selective serotonin reuptake inhibitors (SSRIs) (see Table 100-3) and cognitive behavioral therapy, alone and in combination, are 2 efficacious treatments in BDD.[27] The poor insight that is characteristic of BDD leads to poor adherence to the aforementioned interventions, making treatment and management, as well as psychiatric referral of these patients difficult.

HAIR PULLING DISORDER

Hair pulling disorder (formerly known as trichotillomania) is the repetitive action of pulling out hair, resulting in significant hair loss. Any region of the body with hair can be involved, with the scalp, eyebrows, and eyelashes comprising the most common sites. The reported prevalence of hair pulling disorder varies, with survey studies reporting prevalence rates ranging from 0.6% to 13.3%.[28,29] It is predominantly observed in females, with an early age of onset (averaging between 10.7 and 13 years).[30,31]

CLINICAL FEATURES

Patients with hair pulling disorder present with alopecia that is generally irregular and nonscarring. Broken, sparse hair on a background of excoriations is often observed. Hairs are broken at different lengths on the scalp (Fig. 100-1). Patients often endorse a

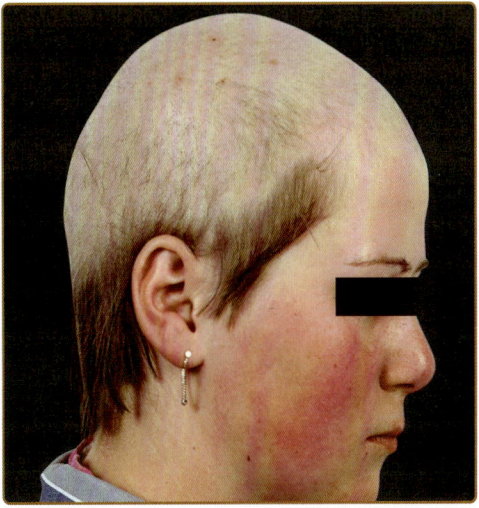

Figure 100-1 Trichotillomania. This extensive alopecia resulted from pulling and plucking hairs by the 17-year-old patient. Hairs are broken at different lengths throughout the scalp. (From Wolff K, Johnson R, Saavedra AP, et al. *Fitzpatrick's Color Atlas and Synopsis of Clinical Dermatology*, 8th ed. New York, NY: McGraw-Hill; 2017, with permission.)

history of hair pulling; however, some patients will not acknowledge the self-inflicted nature of their skin findings because of the profound shame that often accompanies the disorder. Furthermore, many sufferers engage in the behavior unconsciously at least part of the time, so they are not aware of their own contribution to the hair loss.

In rare cases, the patient may also eat the hair root (trichorhizophagia) as a secretive activity, and in even rarer cases the whole hair is eaten (trichophagia). It is possible to develop GI hairballs (trichobezoars), which have a high morbidity and can also be fatal. Children with hair pulling disorder who present with episodes of obscure abdominal pain, weight loss, nausea, vomiting, anorexia, and foul breath should be investigated for gastric trichobezoars, which may cause intestinal bleeding, pancreatitis, or obstructive symptoms.

ETIOLOGY AND PATHOGENESIS

In DSM-5, hair pulling disorder is placed under the category of "obsessive compulsive disorder," which is a change from the previous editions of DSM where the condition was previously called trichotillomania and categorized under "impulse disorders." In hair pulling disorder, the patient's obsession can be characterized by building up of tension prior to pulling hair, and the compulsion is characterized by feeling of pleasure, relief, or gratification following hair removal. Many patients with hair pulling disorder have psychiatric comorbidities. In a recent, large, population-based study, psychiatric disorder was seen in 75.5% of patients presenting to a medical facility with diagnosis of hair pulling disorder, with depressive disorder being the most common comorbidity observed in approximately 40% of these patients.[32]

DIAGNOSIS

The diagnosis of hair pulling disorder can be made on a clinical basis with careful examination of the scalp. The use of dermoscopy can be useful to detect irregularly broken hairs, V-sign (2 or more hairs emerging from 1 follicular unit are broken at the same length), flame hairs (semitransparent, wavy, cone-shaped hair residues), hair powder (sprinkled hair residue), and coiled hairs.[33] Dermoscopy findings such as exclamation point hairs, which are rare in hair pulling disorder, can overlap with other causes of alopecia such as alopecia areata; consequently, a skin biopsy may be indicated in some cases. Hair pulling disorder presents histologically as an increased number of catagen hairs, traumatized hair bulbs in the absence of perifollicular inflammation (trichomalacia), empty follicles, follicular keratin debris, and melanin pigment casts.[34]

DIFFERENTIAL DIAGNOSIS

Dermatologic differential diagnoses include alopecia areata, androgenic alopecia, alopecia mucinosa, tinea capitis, lichen planopilaris, folliculitis decalvans, syphilis-related alopecia, and discoid lupus erythematosus. Tinea capitis may be ruled out by the absence of scaling and negative fungal culture.

CLINICAL COURSE, PROGNOSIS, AND MANAGEMENT

Hair pulling disorder can cause significant social isolation and psychological disability, making treatment of this disorder important to restore the patient's quality of life. The most effective treatment is behavioral therapy, specifically habit reversal therapy. Habit reversal training is a form of behavioral therapy that focuses on 4 key aspects: awareness (increase awareness of hair-pulling behavior), competing response training (perform a specific action when there is an urge to pull hair), social support or contingency management (a person who reinforces the former), and stimulus control (minimize the influence of environmental factors on pulling behavior).[35] Children can benefit from behavioral therapy to prevent worsening of their disease into adulthood.[36] Habit reversal training does decrease repetitive, self-inflicted behaviors.[37]

Effective pharmacologic treatments involve treating the underlying psychiatric disease, and the first-line pharmaceutical approach depends on the nature of the involved underlying psychopathology. Frequently, these patients are treated with an antidepressant, such as tricyclic antidepressants (TCAs) or SSRIs (see Table 100-1). The TCA clomipramine (Anafranil), also indicated for OCD, is the most-studied medication for hair pulling disorder, and it reduces the frequency of hair-pulling urges.[38] SSRIs, such as sertraline (Zoloft), paroxetine (Paxil), and fluoxetine (Prozac), are also commonly used, although their effectiveness for the treatment of hair pulling disorder is unclear. The combination of pharmacotherapy and habit reversal training is effective in decreasing the frequency of hair pulling.[39,40]

NEUROTIC EXCORIATION

Neurotic excoriations, also called *psychogenic excoriations*,[2] is a disorder characterized by self-induced cutaneous lesions resulting from the uncontrollable impulse to excessively pick, rub, or scratch normal skin or skin with minor surface irregularities. Neurotic excoriations is estimated to occur in 2% of dermatology patients, although the disease is underreported.[41] The patient population is predominantly female, with the typical age of onset ranging from 15 to 45 years.[42]

CLINICAL FEATURES

Neurotic excoriations cause self-inflicted ulcers, abscesses, or scars that can ultimately become disfiguring (Figs. 100-2 and 100-3). There also may be atrophic, hyperpigmented or hypopigmented scars and lichenification, characteristics of older, healing lesions.

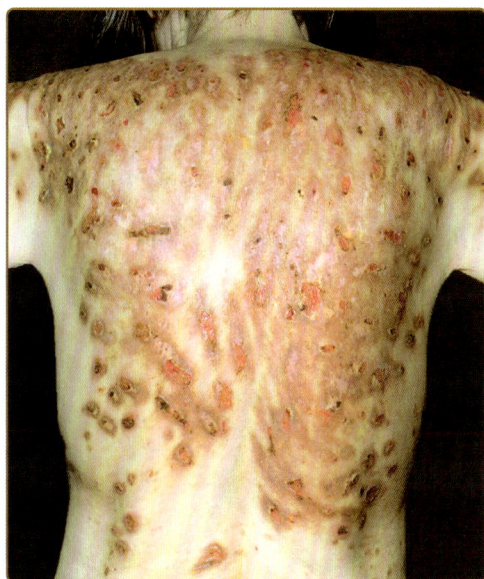

Figure 100-2 Neurotic excoriations: back. Excoriations of the upper and midback and linear areas of postinflammatory hyperpigmentation, crusting, and scarring in a 66-year-old female with diabetes. There is sparing in the interscapular region of the back. (From Wolff K, Johnson R, Saavedra AP, et al. *Fitzpatrick's Color Atlas and Synopsis of Clinical Dermatology*, 8th ed. New York, NY: McGraw-Hill; 2017, with permission.)

The skin lesions are distributed in accessible areas of the body such as the face, arms, legs, and upper back. The classic "butterfly sign," in which there are characteristic areas of sparing in the unreachable areas of the interscapular area, may be present. Patients with neurotic excoriations may openly acknowledge that the lesions are self-induced.

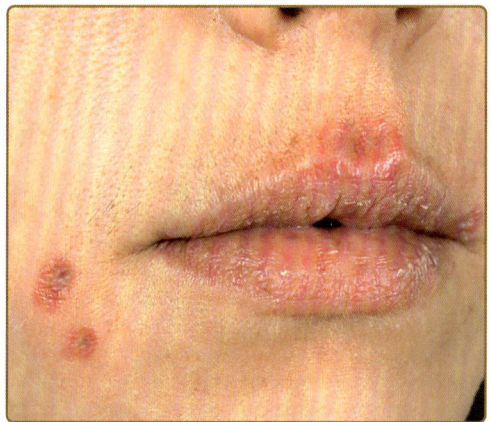

Figure 100-3 Neurotic excoriations/acne excoriee. Several erythematous and crusted macules and erosions on the lower cheek and upper lip of a 19-year-old female with mild facial acne. No primary lesions are seen. (From Wolff K, Johnson R, Saavedra AP, et al. *Fitzpatrick's Color Atlas and Synopsis of Clinical Dermatology*, 8th ed. New York, NY: McGraw-Hill; 2017, with permission.)

ETIOLOGY AND PATHOGENESIS

Although traditionally called "neurotic excoriation," the underlying psychopathology may not be neurosis but another underlying psychiatric illness such as depression, anxiety, OCD, or even psychosis. Psychiatric comorbidity, such as mood and anxiety disorders, is commonly observed in patients with neurotic excoriations, and the skin-picking behavior is a manifestation of the underlying psychopathology.[43] There may be triggers, such as stress or anxiety, or they may occur as a result of an unconscious tendency. Other important triggers are dermatologic in nature, such as mild to moderate acne, keratosis pilaris, pruritus, and even minor textural differences on the skin surface, which causes significant distress and subsequent manipulation of the skin. In these cases, there is a notable disconnect between the severity of the dermatologic manifestation and the level of distress, and it is important to address both the skin condition and the psychological impact.

DIAGNOSIS

A thorough history and physical examination, as well as appropriate laboratory tests should be performed as needed to rule out any potential medical or psychiatric causes.

DIFFERENTIAL DIAGNOSIS

Medical explanations for pruritus may be the underlying cause, trigger, or precipitant of excoriations. The differential diagnosis is broad and includes cutaneous dysesthesia, urticaria, uremia, hepatitis, xerosis, thyroid disease, and many other conditions that can cause pruritus without primary skin lesion. Cutaneous dysesthesia, abnormal sensations on the skin such as itching, burning, stinging, biting, and crawling, in the absence of any diagnosable dermatologic, neurologic, medical, or psychiatric diagnosis, can manifest as neurotic excoriations. The psychodermatologic differential diagnosis includes dermatitis artefacta, delusions of parasitosis, and malingering. It is important to note that there is often a concurrence of a dermatologic diagnosis as well as a psychiatric condition.

CLINICAL COURSE, PROGNOSIS, AND MANAGEMENT

Skin lesions in neurotic excoriations can be managed with topical treatment, such as topical corticosteroids or antipruritic agents, if there is underlying pruritus. The lesions should be evaluated for secondary infections and treated with topical or oral antibiotics if necessary.

When managing patients with neurotic excoriations, it is important to first assess psychosocial factors and the emotional well-being of the patient. If the patient has a comorbid psychiatric disorder such as anxiety, depression, OCD, or psychosis, it should be treated accordingly. Regardless of whether the psychiatric illness is considered to be the etiology for neurotic excoriations, it can exacerbate the tendency for skin picking. Patients with neurotic excoriations frequently acknowledge that they are self-inducing the lesions and have more insight compared to those with delusional disorders; consequently, patients may be more agreeable to pharmacologic intervention or a referral to a psychiatrist.

If referral to a psychiatrist is possible, patients may benefit from psychotherapy. If the patient is receptive to pharmacologic therapy, SSRIs such as paroxetine (Paxil), fluoxetine (Prozac), sertraline (Zoloft), and fluvoxamine (Luvox), are thought to decrease the compulsive tendencies frequently associated with this disorder (see Table 100-3). The TCA doxepin (Sinequan) is useful for neurotic excoriations because of its dual antipruritic and antianxiety effects. High-dose doxepin is particularly useful if the underlying psychopathology is major depression. With higher doses there is increasing risk of cardiac arrhythmia; therefore, a periodic EKG is recommended for elderly patients or any patient with a past history of cardiac dysrhythmia.

OTHER OBSESSIVE-COMPULSIVE AND RELATED DISORDERS

With the advent of DSM-5, a new diagnostic terminology of "body-focused repetitive behavior disorders" has been introduced. Body-focused repetitive behavior disorders are characterized by repetitive, damaging, and seemingly nonfunctional habits, such as hair pulling, skin picking, and nail biting, which cause significant distress and functional impairment.[44] Although neurotic excoriations and hair pulling disorder fall under this category of disorders, onychophagia (nail biting) and onychotillomania (nail picking) are also included. The treatment and management of these conditions are similar and focus on treating the underlying psychopathology.

Although rare, there are other forms of obsessive-compulsive skin disorders, such as hypochondriacal syndrome, whereby patients believe they are afflicted by a particular disease, infected, or contaminated. Fear of contamination and acquiring disease through physical contact may lead to compulsive handwashing rituals; as a result, these patients may present with physical findings typical of irritant hand dermatitis. Another hypochondriacal syndrome is AIDS phobia, which involves irrational fear of contracting the AIDS. Patients with AIDS phobia often seek dermatologic evaluation and multiple skin biopsies of every minor blemish to rule out Kaposi sarcoma.

FACTITIOUS DISORDERS

AT-A-GLANCE

- A psychodermatologic skin disorder characterized by self-inflicted injury to the skin, hair, or nails is called *dermatitis artefacta*.
- Secondary skin findings of abnormal-appearing lacerations, excoriations, ulcerations, scarring, and other injuries in reachable areas of the body are observed.
- Treatment is largely supportive including wound care, as well as treating the underlying psychiatric illness using both pharmacologic and nonpharmacologic interventions.

Factitious disorders are characterized by self-inflicted dermatologic lesions. The primary psychocutaneous disorder of dermatitis artefacta falls under this category of psychodermatologic disorders.

DERMATITIS ARTEFACTA

Dermatitis artefacta or factitial dermatitis is characterized by self-induced injury to the skin caused by instruments such as sharp objects, cigarettes, lighters, and corrosive materials. Although the incidence of this disease is difficult to assess, in a study evaluating 35 psychodermatology patients, nearly one-third were diagnosed with factitial dermatitis.[45] Female predominance is observed.

CLINICAL FEATURES

Patients with dermatitis artefacta generally deny that their skin injuries are self-inflicted. Furthermore, there is a "hollow history," meaning that the story of how the lesions came about is often vague and lacking in sufficient detail. Lesions, which have no recognizable characteristics of primary skin disease, are found on physically reachable areas of the body such as the face, upper trunk, and extremities. The appearance of the lesions depends upon the manner in which they are created, and can range from minor cuts to large areas of trauma, but is usually characterized by abnormally shaped superficial erosions with angulated borders surrounded by normal-looking skin.[46] Chemical or thermal burns, injection of foreign materials, circulatory occlusion, and tampering with old lesions, such as existing scars or prior surgical incision sites, are also some common methods of self-injury. More serious wounds can result in abscesses, gangrene, or even life-threatening infection.

ETIOLOGY AND PATHOGENESIS

Self-injurious behavior is often triggered by a psychosocial stressor and represents an outlet for expressing anger or satisfying internal emotional needs. The motive for creating the lesions can be a conscious or unconscious psychological need to seek attention or medical care as a result of childhood feelings of abandonment or neglect. Patients often report a history of physical, emotional, or sexual abuse. Recent studies suggest that a large proportion of patients with dermatitis artefacta may also have comorbid generalized anxiety, major depression, or borderline personality disorder.[47] In fact, self-injurious behavior such as cutting is part of the diagnostic criteria for borderline personality disorder.

DIAGNOSIS

Diagnosis is based on presenting clinical features. Skin biopsies are often nonspecific. If the self-inflicting injury is due to injection of foreign material into the skin, a foreign body reaction can be seen histologically.

DIFFERENTIAL DIAGNOSIS

First, it is imperative to rule out malingering as the etiology of the skin lesions. Malingering involves the conscious motivation of secondary gain, such as obtaining disability or insurance benefits. If malingering is suspected, the case is no longer considered psychiatric in nature; rather, it is considered a criminal act that may require legal actions. Once malingering is ruled out, dermatologic differential diagnoses include pyoderma gangrenosum, collagen vascular disorder, vasculitis, and arthropod bites.[48] Psychocutaneous differential diagnoses include delusions of parasitosis and neurotic excoriations. Primary psychiatric disease such as OCD, depression, and Munchausen syndrome should also be considered.

CLINICAL COURSE, PROGNOSIS, AND MANAGEMENT

The management of patients with dermatitis artefacta is generally supportive therapy, which includes both physical and emotional aspects. Treatment of the skin lesions should largely consist of wound care, such as irrigation, debridement, and topical or oral antibiotics, as needed. Covering the wounds with occlusive dressings may also help by discouraging the patient from further self-mutilation.

Emotional support should be provided, starting with avoiding confronting the patient's physical role in producing the lesions.[49] Rather, the focus should be placed on understanding the underlying psychiatric etiology of the self-harming behavior. Adjuvant psychiatric therapy should include both pharmacologic and nonpharmacologic interventions, depending on the nature of the underlying psychiatric illness (see Table 100-3). High-dose SSRIs may be beneficial for patients with primary or secondary depression. SSRIs can also help to decrease underlying compulsive tendencies. As dopaminergic dysfunction is believed to contribute to self-injurious behavior, antipsychotic drugs such as pimozide and risperidone may decrease the self-induced injuries.[47] Newer atypical antipsychotics, such as olanzapine and aripiprazole, have also shown benefit in a small number of cases.[50,51] Patients with more-severe presentations or comorbid borderline personality disorder could benefit from intensive psychotherapy.[52] If borderline personality disorder is diagnosed (or suspected), there is a significant body of evidence supporting the use of dialectical behavioral therapy for treatment of the disorder. Dialectical behavioral therapy involves a specially trained team of mental health practitioners using a manualized therapy specifically designed to treat borderline personality disorder.

Most patients with dermatitis artefacta will have a chronic, waxing-and-waning course of disease. Regular visits, whether or not lesions are present, will help the patient feel cared for and diminish the need for self-mutilation as a "call for help." Thus, even when the condition is under control, the physician should still follow the patient at regular intervals to ensure that the self-destructive behavior does not relapse.

REFERENCES

1. Gupta MA. Commentary: psychodermatology. *Clin Dermatol*. 2013;31(1):1-2.
2. Koo J. Psychodermatology: a practical manual for clinicians. *Curr Probl Dermatol*. 1995;7:199-234.
3. Kurd SK, Troxel AB, Crits-Christoph P, et al. The risk of depression, anxiety, and suicidality in patients with psoriasis: a population-based cohort study. *Arch Dermatol*. 2010;146:891-895.
4. Halvorsen JA, Lien L, Dalgard F, et al. Suicidal ideation, mental health problems, and social function in adolescents with eczema: a population-based study. *J Invest Dermatol*. 2014;134:1847-1854.
5. Purvis D, Robinson E, Merry S, et al. Acne, anxiety, depression and suicide in teenagers: a cross-sectional survey of New Zealand secondary school students. *J Paediatr Child Health*. 2006;42:793-796.
6. Brown GE, Malakouti M, Sorenson E, et al. Psychodermatology. *Adv Psychosom Med*. 2015;34:123-134.
7. Gupta MA. Emotional regulation, dissociation, and the self-induced dermatoses: clinical features and implications for treatment with mood stabilizers. *Clin Dermatol*. 2013;31(1):110-117.
8. Koo J, Gambla C. Cutaneous sensory disorder. *Dermatol Clin*. 1996;14(3):497-502.
9. Freudenmann RW, Lepping P. Delusional infestation. *Clin Microbiol Rev*. 2009;22:690-732.
10. Heller MM, Wong JW, Lee ES, et al. Delusional infestations: clinical presentation, diagnosis and treatment. *Int J Dermatol*. 2013;52:775-783.
11. Trabert W. 100 Years of delusional parasitosis. Metaanalysis of 1,223 case reports. *Psychopathology*. 1995;28:238-246.

12. Reichenberg JS, Magid M, Jesser CA, et al. Patients labeled with delusions of parasitosis compose a heterogeneous group: a retrospective study from a referral center. *J Am Acad Dermatol*. 2013;68:41-46, 46.e1-46.e2.
13. Brown GE, Sorenson E, Malakouti M, et al. The spectrum of ideation in patients with symptoms of infestation: from overvalued ideas to the terminal delusional state. *J Clin Exp Dermatol Res*. 2015;5(6):1-2.
14. Lepping P, Russell I, Freudenmann RW. Antipsychotic treatment of primary delusional parasitosis: systematic review. *Br J Psychiatry*. 2007;191:198-205.
15. Heller MM, Koo JYM. *Contemporary Diagnosis and Management in Psychodermatology*. Newton, PA: Handbooks in Health Care; 2011.
16. Freudenmann RW, Lepping P. Second-generation antipsychotics in primary and secondary delusional parasitosis: outcome and efficacy. *J Clin Psychopharmacol*. 2008;28:500-508.
17. Ladizinski B, Busse KL, Bhutani T, et al. Aripiprazole as a viable alternative for treating delusions of parasitosis. *J Drugs Dermatol*. 2010;9(12):1531-1532.
18. Feunser JD, Phillips KA, Stein DJ. Olfactory reference syndrome: issues for DMS-V. *Depress Anxiety*. 2010;27(6):592-599.
19. American Psychiatric Association: Obsessive-compulsive and related disorders. In: *Diagnostic and Statistical Manual of Mental Disorders: DSM-5*. 5th ed. Washington, DC: American Psychiatric Association; 2013:235-264.
20. Koran LM, Abujaoude E, Large MD, et al. The prevalence of body dysmorphic disorder in the United States adult population. *CNS Spectr*. 2008;13:316-322.
21. Conroy M, Menard W, Fleming-Ives K, et al. Prevalence and clinical characteristics of body dysmorphic disorder in an adult inpatient setting. *Gen Hosp Psychiatry*. 2008;30:67-72.
22. Phillips KA, Menard W, Fay C, et al. Demographic characteristics, phenomenology, comorbidity, and family history in 200 individuals with body dysmorphic disorder. *Psychosomatics*. 2005;46:317-325.
23. Varma A, Rastogi R. Recognizing body dysmorphic disorders (dysmorphophobia). *J Cutan Aesthet Surg*. 2015;8(3):165-168.
24. Fuesner JD, Moody T, Hembacher E, et al. Abnormalities of visual processing and frontostriatal systems in body dysmorphic disorder. *Arch Gen Psychiatry*. 2010;67:197-205.
25. Phillips KA, Kaye WH. The relationship of body dysmorphic disorder and eating disorders to obsessive-compulsive disorder. *CNS Spectr*. 2007;12:347-358.
26. Veale D, Boocock A, Gournay K, et al. Body dysmorphic disorder. A survey of fifty cases. *Br J Psychiatry*. 1996;169:196-201.
27. Wilhelm S, Otto MW, Lohr B, et al. Cognitive behavior group therapy for body dysmorphic disorder: a case series. *Behav Res Ther*. 1999;37:71-75.
28. Christenson GA, Pyle RL, Mitchell JE. Estimated lifetime prevalence of trichotillomania in college students. *J Clin Psychiatry*. 1991;52:415-417.
29. Rothbaum BO, Shaw L, Morris R, et al. Prevalence of trichotillomania in a college freshman population. *J Clin Psychiatry*. 1993;54:72-73.
30. Cohen LJ, Stein DJ, Simeon D, et al. Clinical profile, comorbidity, and treatment history in 123 hair pullers: a survey study. *J Clin Psychiatry*. 1995;56:319-326.
31. Christenson GA, MacKenzie TB, Mitchell JE. Adult men and women with trichotillomania. A comparison of male and female characteristics. *Psychosomatics*. 1994;35:142-149.
32. Gupta MA, Gupta AK, Knapp K. Trichotillomania: demographic and clinical features from a nationally representative US sample. *Skinmed*. 2015;13(6):455-460.
33. Rakowska A, Slowinska M, Olszewska M, et al. New trichoscopy findings in trichotillomania: flame hairs, V-sign, hook hairs, hair powder, tulip hairs. *Acta Derm Venereol*. 2014;94(3):303-306.
34. Muller SA. Trichotillomania: a histopathological study in 66 patients. *J Am Acad Dermatol*. 1990;23:56-62.
35. Snorrason I, Berlin GS, Lee HJ. Optimizing psychological interventions for trichotillomania (hair-pulling disorder): an update on current empirical status. *Psychol Res Behav Manag*. 2015;7(8):105-113.
36. Franklin ME, Edson AL, Ledley DA, et al. Behavior therapy for pediatric trichotillomania: a randomized controlled trial. *J Am Acad Child Adolesc Psychiatry*. 2011;50(8):763-771.
37. Morris SH, Zickgraf HF, Dingfelder HE, et al. Habit reversal training in trichotillomania: guide for the clinician. *Expert Rev Neurother*. 2013;13:1069-1077.
38. Swedo SE, Leonard HL, Rapoport JL, et al. A double-blind comparison of clomipramine and desipramine in the treatment of trichotillomania (hair pulling). *N Engl J Med*. 1989;321:497-501.
39. Dougherty D. Single modality versus dual modality treatment for trichotillomania. *J Clin Psychiatry*. 2006;67:1086-1092.
40. Walsh KH, McDougle CJ. Trichotillomania. Presentation, etiology, diagnosis and therapy. *Am J Clin Dermatol*. 2001;2:327-333.
41. Arnold LM, Auchenbach MB, McElroy SL. Psychogenic excoriation. Clinical features, proposed diagnostic criteria, epidemiology and approaches to treatment. *CNS Drugs*. 2001;15:351-359.
42. Wilhelm S, Keuthen NJ, Deckersbach T, et al. Self-injurious skin picking: clinical characteristics and comorbidity. *J Clin Psychiatry*. 1999;60:454-459.
43. Arnold LM, McElroy SL, Mutasim DF, et al. Characteristics of 34 adults with psychogenic excoriation. *J Clin Psychiatry*. 1998;59:509-514.
44. Roberts S, O'Connor K, Aardema F, et al. The impact of emotions on body-focused repetitive behaviors: evidence from a nontreatment-seeking sample. *J Behav Ther Exp Psychiatry*. 2015;46:189-197.
45. Sheppard NP, O'Loughlin S, Malone JP. Psychogenic skin disease: a review of 35 cases. *Br J Psychiatry*. 1986;149:636-643.
46. Gattu S, Rashid RM, Khachemoune A. Self-induced skin lesions: a review of dermatitis artefacta. *Cutis*. 2009;84:247-251.
47. Koblenzer CS. Dermatitis artefacta. Clinical features and approaches to treatment. *Am J Clin Dermatol*. 2000;1:47-55.
48. Koblenzer CS. Neurotic excoriations and dermatitis artefacta. *Dermatol Clin*. 1996;14:447-455.
49. Nielsen K, Jeppesen M, Simmelsgaard L, et al. Self-inflicted skin diseases. A retrospective analysis of 57 patients with dermatitis artefacta seen in a dermatology department. *Acta Derm Venereol*. 2005;85:512-515.
50. Garnis-Jones S, Collins S, Rosenthal D. Treatment of self-mutilation with olanzapine. *J Cutan Med Surg*. 2000;4:161-163.
51. Koblenzer CS. The current management of delusional parasitosis and dermatitis artefacta. *Skin Therapy Lett*. 2010;15:1-3.

52. Klobenzer CS. Psychosomatic concepts in dermatology. A dermatologist-psychoanalyst's viewpoint. *Arch Dermatol*. 1983;119:501-512.
53. Umetsu R, Abe J, Ueda N, et al. Association between selective serotonin reuptake inhibitor therapy and suicidality: analysis of U.S. Food and Drug Administration adverse event reporting system data. *Biol Pharm Bull*. 2015;38(11):1689-1699.

Chapter 101 :: Drug Abuse
:: Nicholas Frank, Cara Hennings, & Jami L. Miller

第一百零一章

药物滥用

中文导读

药物滥用是指经常使用非法药物或滥用非处方药或处方药导致了消极的后果。而药物成瘾的特征是生理依赖和无法持续戒除药物。本章介绍了药物滥用的流行病学、病因及发病机制、诊断、临床症状和治疗策略。诊断方面，药物检测是诊断药物滥用的金标准，包括血液、尿液、唾液等体液和头发都可以用于检测。本章节分别从静脉注射毒品、吸入剂的滥用、特殊的非法药物和添加剂、合法滥用药物方面介绍了可能出现的皮肤症状及非皮肤问题。此外，本章提出了对待药物滥用和成瘾的关键是尽早干预，对本病的治疗主要是采用药物治疗、精神治疗、针灸和冥想等替代疗法。

〔易 梅〕

AT-A-GLANCE

- Drug use is a growing problem in the United States and around the world. There are many cutaneous findings that suggest use, abuse, and addiction to drugs.
- Specific findings in affected patients include dental caries, madarosis, presence of scarring, tattooing, and staining in the skin.
- Levamisole causes a unique syndrome characterized by retiform purpura of the ears associated with neutropenia, perinuclear antineutrophil cytoplasmic antibody and anti-MPO3 antibodies.
- Less-specific findings of drug use include morbilliform eruptions, vasculitis, and formation of autoantibodies.
- Drug-use–related infections predominantly affect the skin and soft tissues. Staphylococcal species are the most common organisms, followed by streptococcal species, oral pathogens, and Candida.
- Other sequelae of drug use include increased risk of infections including HIV, hepatitides B and C, and syphilis.

DEFINITION

The term *drug* is defined as a medication or other substance, other than food, that has a physiologic effect when ingested or otherwise introduced into the body. Modern society is rife with medications that affect function or structure in the body, caffeine being the most widely used psychoactive substance in the world. *Drug abuse* is defined as the recurrent use of illegal drugs, or the misuse of nonprescription or prescription drugs, that results in negative consequences. *Drug addiction* is characterized by physiologic dependence and inability to consistently abstain from the drug. Tobacco and alcohol, although not illegal in the United States and most of the western world, are also considered substances of addiction and abuse.

HISTORICAL PERSPECTIVE

Drugs have been used and abused for thousands of years and all over the world. Use in religious ceremonies, for healing, or by the general population for recreation has occurred since ancient times. There is evidence that opium has been used since 5000 BC and alcohol since 3500 BC. References to those and other medications are found in the Bible and other religious and historical texts. Columbus and his crew introduced tobacco into Europe when they returned from the New World.

EPIDEMIOLOGY

Based on estimates released in the United Nations Office of Drugs and Crime's (UNODC) *2015 World Drug Report*, 246 million people worldwide—1 of 20 people between 15 and 64 years of age—used an illicit drug in the year 2015, which corresponds to a global prevalence of 5.2%.[1] With the exception of caffeine, cannabis is the most widely used drug in the world, and its' use is increasing. Amphetamines are the second most commonly used drugs worldwide, and their use is also increasing. The use of cocaine was in decline for several years but it too is now on the rise. Opiates, particularly prescription opioids cause the highest negative health impact.

Approximately 29.5 million people suffer from drug dependancy world wide, with the highest prevalence of illicit drug use is among those 18 to 25 years of age (1 in 5 persons in this age group). Marijuana was used by 8.2% of the population, making it the most commonly used illicit drug; it is commonly referred to as the "gateway drug" because marijuana use often leads to using other drugs. Prescription pain relievers were the second most commonly used drug, followed in decreasing prevalence by sedatives, stimulants, cocaine, hallucinogens, inhalants, heroin, and sedatives. Approximately 66.9 million people were current tobacco users, a decrease over previous years. An estimated 139.7 million people were current alcohol drinkers (52.7%), including 60.9 million binge alcohol users and 16.3 million heavy alcohol users.

ETIOLOGY AND PATHOGENESIS

The biologic and environmental mechanisms by which an individual comes to abuse certain licit and illicit substances is complex and studies suggest varying levels of genetic and environmental influence. Even though the biochemical changes in the brain that lead to drug abuse are intricate, dopaminergic neural pathways involved in motivation, reward, and habit formation play a central role in many neuropsychiatric conditions, including substance addiction.[2] Twin studies suggest that at least some component of drug abuse and dependence is driven by genetic preponderance. Environmental risk factors include easy access to the drug, poor school bonding, and peer use. Trauma, both physical and psychological, parental use and family conflict in the home are associated with use. Several protective factors also have been illustrated, including religiosity and strong family support, as well as social involvement in community organizations.[3]

DIAGNOSIS

Recognition of signs and symptoms associated with drug use is crucial and potentially lifesaving. Drug testing is the gold standard for diagnosis of most legal and illegal agents. Bodily fluids, including blood, urine, saliva, and hair can be used for drug detection. Suspected infections should be cultured by swab and, when necessary, tissue specimens. Serologic evaluation for transmissible infection, such as HIV, hepatitis, and sexually transmitted diseases, should be considered in appropriate patients.

CLINICAL FEATURES OF DRUG ABUSE (TABLE 101-1)

SIGNS OF INTRAVENOUS DRUG USE

TRACK MARKS

Track marks are the result of venous thrombosis with subsequent scarring (Fig. 101-1) and pigmentation of the veins (Fig. 101-2). Damage results from repeated injections, use of blunt needles, and irritation from chemicals that are added to the injected material. Early lesions show crusting and ecchymosis along the course of a vein; linear cords form with chronic use. The most common site is the medial vein in the antecubital fossa of the nondominant arm.[4] However, many people inject in less-visible places, such as the popliteal fossa, dorsal veins of the feet, and inguinal veins.[5] As these veins scar, intravenous drug users (IDUs) find other access points and will inject into hemorrhoids, the dorsal vein of the penis, the ventral surface of the tongue, or the internal jugular vein.[6] It is important to remember that a lack of track marks does not preclude IV drug use. Scarring is usually associated with a longer duration of drug use[7] and cocaine does not normally induce track marks because it does not typically contain the sclerosing chemicals that are added to other drugs such as heroin.[8]

SCARS RESULTING FROM SKIN POPPING

Sometimes drug users inject intradermally or subcutaneously. This is done accidentally or when veins can no longer be found and used. Some prefer this method of delivery instead of injecting intravenously. This is called *skin popping*. It leaves irregular, leukodermic, atrophic, punched out scars that result from irreversible tissue injury. Hypertrophic scars or keloids can develop over these areas.[9]

PANNICULITIS

Inflammation of the dermis and subcutaneous fat may occur with injection into the skin itself or with extravasation of intended IV administration. Sclerosants, particularly pentazocine, and additives, such as talc, may induce subcutaneous nodules. A lobular panniculitis is often seen on histopathology and the injected material may leave spaces in the tissue after fixation or cause birefringence on tissue polarization.[10]

HYPERPIGMENTATION

Sooting tattoos are also stigmata of drug abuse. Sooting tattoos are caused by cooking the drugs and flaming the needles with matches. Carbon and soot then deposit into the dermis. Users may cover these with commercial tattoos so they are hidden. Hyperpigmentation can also develop at tourniquet sites when placed too tightly and left on for too long, causing inflammation and subsequent hyperpigmentation.[11]

SKIN AND SOFT-TISSUE INFECTIONS

Skin and soft tissue infections (SSTIs) are very common among IDUs (Fig. 101-3). SSTIs are the most common disease for which users are usually admitted to the hospital.[12] Sepsis, rather than overdose, is the usual acute complication seen in this population.

The increased risk of SSTI in IDUs is multifactorial. Independent risk factors were found to be skin popping, the use of nonsterile needles, "speedball" (mixture of heroin and cocaine) injections, and "booting" (drawing back a small amount of blood usually into a dirty syringe prior to injection).[11] Skin popping has a fivefold greater risk of infection when compared to IV injection.[13] Infections associated with skin popping tend to be multilobulated, deeper, and have more extensive necrosis than those in non-IDUs.[8] Females

TABLE 101-1
Cutaneous Signs of Drug Use

SIGN	MOST COMMON DRUG	SPECIFIC FINDINGS
Track marks Skin popping Soot tattoos	Cocaine Heroin	Scarring along veins and skin
Madarosis	Cocaine Heroin Methamphetamine	Loss of lateral eyebrows
Hand dermatitis, puffiness, or discoloration	Cocaine Heroin Inhalants Cannabis Tobacco	Erythema, fissuring, edema, or staining
Acne	Anabolic steroids MDMA (methylenedioxymethamphetamine) Methamphetamine Cannabis	Pustules and nodules May be severe
Vasculitis	Cocaine Levamisole Cannabis Tobacco	Cocaine—urticarial vasculitis, midline nasal destruction Levamisole—retiform purpura of ears and elsewhere associated with p-ANCA (perinuclear antineutrophil cytoplasmic antibody) and MPO (myeloperoxidase) Cannabis—cannabis arteritis and thromboangiitis obliterans Tobacco—thromboangiitis obliterans and peripheral vascular disease
Formication and/or pruritus	Methamphetamine and amphetamines Cocaine Heroin/opiates Alcohol	Excoriations Prurigo nodules Ulcerations

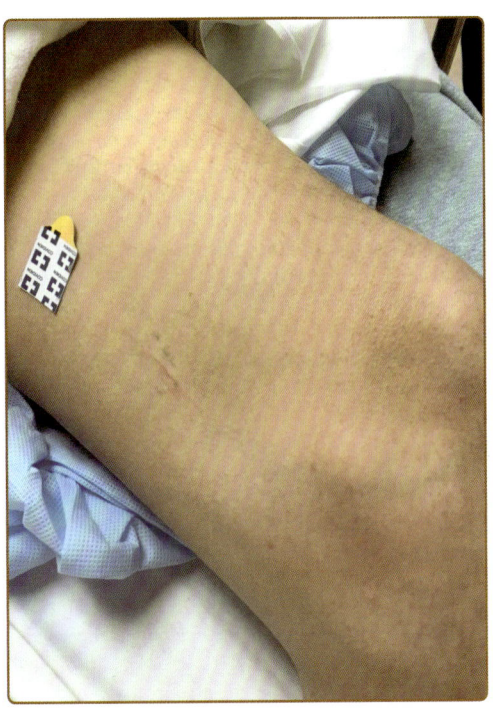

Figure 101-1 Track marks. Examples of track marks from intravenous drug use on the upper extremity.

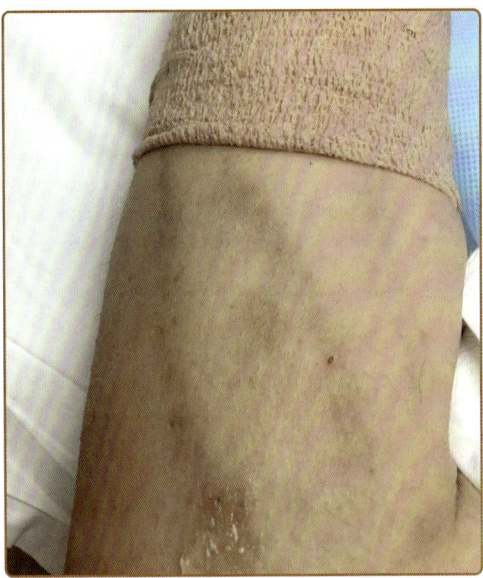

Figure 101-2 Hyperpigmentation. Intravenous drug use–induced hyperpigmentation on the dorsal forearm and hand.

also have an increased risk of SSTIs as compared to male IDUs, which is most likely a consequence of their less-prominent veins leading to more sticks to gain access.[14] Any type of immunocompromised state, such as AIDS, increases the risk of SSTIs. The local anesthetic properties of many illegal drugs can also make it difficult for users to feel the injury or realize they are developing an infection.

Many different pathogens are responsible for SSTIs in IDUs. Blood cultures are often negative in SSTIs, making it harder to identify the causative organism unless a culture can be performed of an abscess or ulceration. One pathogen is cultured in 50% of the cases, and more than 1 is found in 33% to 45% of cases.

The etiologic organism(s) in most SSTIs appear to be from the skin or oral cavity of the user rather than from the drug or paraphernalia used.[15] This correlates with other studies demonstrating *Staphylococcus* species (particularly *Staphylococcus aureus*) as the most frequently cultured organism, followed by group A β-hemolytic *Streptococcus* and other streptococcal species and then oral or skin pathogens.[16,17] Oral pathogens, including *Eikenella corrodens*, are also a cause of infection, as IDUs sometimes "clean" their needle or skin prior to injection with their saliva. Drug dealers have also hidden drug containers in their mouths, which was the source of an outbreak of a clonal strain of *Streptococcus pyogenes*.[18] Gram-negative bacteria and anaerobes also may be a cause of infection and the classic signs of anaerobic infections, such as free air bubbles on radiograph or foul smell, may not be present.

There have been numerous reports of SSTIs caused by uncommon pathogens. Quinine, which is usually added to heroin, increases the risk of tetanus.[19] *Clostridium botulinum* and *Clostridium tetani* are unusual organisms except in IDUs who skin pop. Wound botulism most commonly occurs from injection of

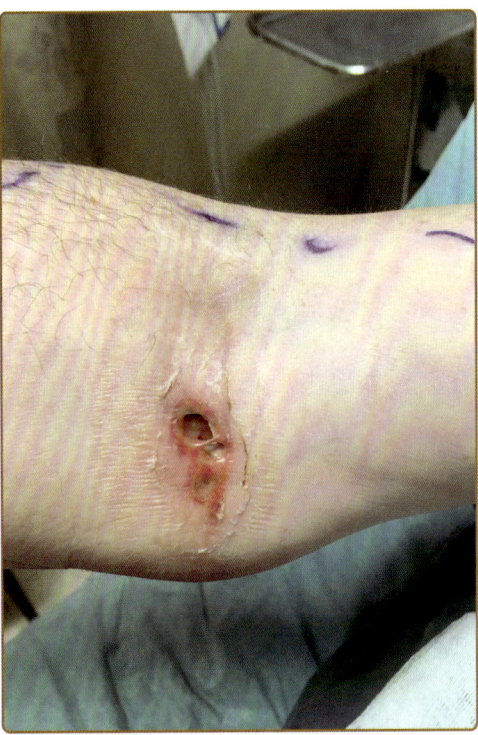

Figure 101-3 Infection. Sequelae following soft-tissue infection as a result of intravenous drug abuse.

black tar heroin, which is cut with dirt and is ideal for the growth of botulism because of its high water content. Heating the drug prior to injection actually stimulates the spores to germinate. Wound botulism in IDUs can present with symptoms of blurred vision, diplopia, and ptosis without any mental status changes. The patient may or may not have a visible cellulitis and may only present with pain, swelling, and tenderness. Approximately 85% of the cases of wound botulism at the time of presentation had wounds that were grossly infected and 65% had *C. botulinum* isolated from the wound. The diagnostic test of choice is detecting the toxin by standard mouse bioassay of the serum. Treatment includes the antitoxin and high-dose penicillin along with surgical debridement.[20] Other *Clostridium* species, including *Clostridium novyi*, *Clostridium perfringens*, *Clostridium sordellii*, and *Clostridium histolyticum*, have been reported to be the cause of serious illness or deaths among IDUs.

Necrotizing fasciitis (Fig. 101-4) is also common among IDUs. Chen et al reported 55% cases were in IDUs. IDUs with necrotizing fasciitis most commonly present with severe pain disproportionate to the examination (94%) or an abnormal temperature (88%).[21,22] They may show the classic findings of hemorrhagic bullae, systemic toxicity, or palpable crepitans. The pain complaints may be mistaken as a "drug-seeking" behavior, which could be deadly. Surgical exploration needs to be done in IDUs with cellulitis and unexplained severe pain.[23]

Fungal infections, including dermatophytes, are commonly seen in IDUs. Disseminated candidiasis has been reported among IV heroin users who used lemon juice to dissolve the heroin. The lemon juice was contaminated with *Candida albicans* and the patients developed high fevers, myalgias, and headaches with negative blood cultures. Painful nodules later developed on the scalp which resolved with alopecia. They also had ocular disease (*Candida endophthalmitis*), pleuritis, and costochondritis. It has been suggested that physicians should specifically ask IDUs who present with cutaneous, ophthalmologic and osteoarticular disease about a history of using lemon juice. Aspergillosis and zygomycosis also have been reported among IDUs.

In addition to SSTIs, IDUs may present with pseudoaneurysms, which may be mistaken for a cutaneous abscess, especially when they present as a nonpulsatile inflammatory mass. These usually manifest as a pulsatile mass located in the area of major arteries. They can develop if an IDU injects accidentally or purposefully into an artery. Gangrene can also develop after intraarterial injection and present as swelling cyanosis, and extreme pain.

CUTANEOUS SIGNS OF ENDOCARDITIS

A link between endocarditis and IDU has long been established. Cutaneous signs include Janeway lesions and Osler nodes. Chapter 155 provides a more detailed discussion of the link between endocarditis and IDU.

SIGNS OF INHALANT ABUSE

Euphoria and delirium can be achieved through the use of inhalants; adolescents are the most common population to abuse them. Inhalants represent a diverse group of readily vaporized chemical compounds with variable properties and have a wide range of potential clinical consequences. Common inhalants of abuse can be subdivided into 3 groups defined as: volatile solvents, fuels, and anesthetics; nitrous oxide; and volatile alkyl nitrites. These compounds can be found in readily available household products such as paint thinner, glues, lighter fluid, spray paint, and nail polish remover.[24] Inhaling these products from their original container through the nose ("sniffing"), a soaked rag ("huffing"), or a bag ("bagging") can lead to myriad clinical presentations resulting from mucous membrane irritation: rhinorrhea, epistaxis, sneezing, coughing, excess salivation, conjunctival injection, dyspnea, and wheezing, as well as dermatitic eruptions in the perioral and/or perinasal distribution. One specific condition that has been described includes "huffer's rash," which is perioral or perinasal dermatitis with pyoderma.

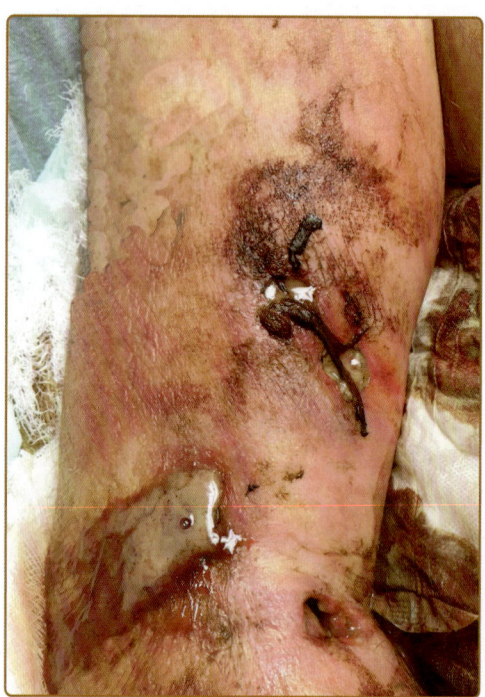

Figure 101-4 Necrotizing fasciitis. Photographic depiction of necrotizing fasciitis following intravenous drug use.

Frostbite on the face or oral/nasal cavity can be seen following inhalation of refrigerants or coolants (eg, chlorofluorohydrocarbon propellants in computer duster spray).[25] A helpful clinical clue to inhalant-induced hand and/or face dermatitis is the appearance of a yellow crust when it is caused by nitrites.

SPECIFIC ILLEGAL DRUGS AND ADDITIVES

COCAINE (ALSO KNOWN AS "COKE," "C," "SNOW," "FLAKE," OR "BLOW")

Cocaine is a sympathomimetic that creates feelings of euphoria and causes tachycardia, altered mental status, hypertension, and mydriasis. It is extracted and refined from the *Erythroxylum coca* plant leaves in the form of a coca paste. The paste is then treated with numerous chemicals to purify it into a water-soluble cocaine hydrochloride powder that is close to 100% pure. By the time the user buys it, the street dealer has generally diluted it with inert or active substances. Cocaine sold on the streets is a fine, bitter, white, crystalline powder that can be injected, inhaled as a powder, or ingested orally, but cannot be smoked. The free base form, also called *crack*, is processed with ammonia or sodium bicarbonate (baking soda) and water, and then heated to produce a smokable substance. The feelings of euphoria are more intense when inhaled and thus crack is more addictive. Smoking crack stimulates the user in seconds as opposed to snorting cocaine, which takes approximately 15 minutes.

There are many cutaneous signs of cocaine abuse, including halitosis, frequent lip smacking, cuts and burns on the lips from broken or chipped crack pipes, madarosis (lateral loss of the eyebrow) from the hot steam rising from the crack pipe,[26] palmar and digital hyperkeratosis from holding the hot crack pipe,[27] and midline destructive lesions of the nasal septum which result from snorting the cocaine.[8] "Snorter's warts" are nasal verrucae that can develop in cocaine abusers. They are caused by the human papillomavirus transmitted on items such as dollar bills that are used to snort the cocaine. The dollars bills are passed from person to person transmitting the human papillomavirus infection.[28]

Many types of vasculitis have been described in cocaine abusers, including urticarial vasculitis,[29] Churg-Strauss vasculitis,[30] necrotizing granulomatous vasculitis,[31] palpable purpura, and Buerger disease.[32-34] Cocaine-induced midline destructive lesions may cause aggressive nasal deformity that can sometimes be misdiagnosed as Wegener granulomatosis.[35] The cause is thought to be vascular ischemia and inflammation. Anti–human neutrophil elastase antibodies are also found in most patients with cocaine-induced midline-destructive lesions.[36]

Drug eruptions also have been documented, including acute generalized exanthematous pustulosis and Stevens-Johnson syndrome.[37,38] Cocaine also has been reported to unmask or cause scleroderma[39,40] and has been implicated in the development of Raynaud phenomenon.

Cocaine abuse can cause formication, a tactile hallucination of insects crawling underneath the skin, which leads to delusions of parasitosis and/or neurotic excoriations. Cocaine abuse should be suspected in a patient who develops these symptoms, especially if the patient has a vague medical history, labile affect, and delusional behavior.[9,41]

Levamisole: Levamisole has been discovered as a common adulterant added to cocaine. Unlike other cutting agents, levamisole is added at the onset of manufacturing in the countries of origin and is readily available and inexpensive. Levamisole adds bulk and weight to the cocaine and goes unnoticed by cocaine users because it has a similar appearance, taste, and melting point as pure cocaine. It also has its own stimulant effects and enhances the euphoric effects of cocaine.

Levamisole was used in humans as treatment of colon cancer, nephritic syndrome, and rheumatoid arthritis because of its immunomodulating effects, but it was withdrawn from the market in 2000 because of neutropenia, agranulocytosis, and vasculitis. Currently, it can only be used in veterinary medicine as an antihelminthic medication.

Side effects of levamisole-adulterated cocaine are widely reported. Most specific is *l*evamisole-*i*nduced *n*ecrosis *s*yndrome (**LINES**), which should be considered in patients who present with a distinctive retiform purpura on the ears (Fig. 101-5) with or without lesions elsewhere (particularly on the nose, cheeks, and extremities); the retiform purpura may also present with hemorrhagic bullae or ulceration. This is usually associated with leukopenia (especially neutropenia) and high titers of perinuclear antineutrophil antibodies and anti-myeloperoxidase antibodies, which are present in more than 70% of cases. Other testing that suggests LINES includes presence of cytoplasmic antineutrophil antibodies and anti–proteinase-3 antibodies, which are present in approximately 50% of cases. Other serologic studies may be positive for antinuclear antibodies, antiphospholipid antibodies, and the lupus anticoagulant. Biopsy specimens show leukocytoclastic vasculitis, thrombotic vasculopathy, vascular occlusion, or a combination of these. Vascular deposits of immunoglobulin M, immunoglobulin A, immunoglobulin G, and complement C3 on immunofluorescence studies point toward a vasculitis caused by levamisole-adulterated cocaine.

There also have been reports of pyoderma gangrenosum in patients using levamisole-adulterated cocaine. The lesions are consistent with classic pyoderma gangrenosum, but patients have serologic profiles that are similar to those seen in LINES.[42]

Unfortunately, levamisole is difficult to detect because of its short half-life (5 to 6 hours) and requires specific testing that is not readily available. Treatment consists of removing levamisole exposure, and mild organ involvement usually is managed with corticosteroids.[43]

HEROIN (ALSO KNOWN AS "SMACK," "H", "SKA", OR "JUNK")

Heroin is an opiate that causes euphoria, addiction, respiratory depression, and miosis. It is synthesized from morphine, a naturally occurring substance extracted from the seed pod of the Asian opium poppy plant. It is typically sold as a white or brownish powder or as a black sticky substance called *black tar heroin*. Heroin base (common in Europe) can only dissolve in water when mixed with an acid; the most commonly used are citric acid powder and lemon juice. Hydrochloride salt, mainly found in the United States, requires only water to dissolve. Most of the time, heroin is heated, drawn into a syringe or eyedropper through cotton, and then injected. A heroin abuser may inject up to 4 times a day. Because of decreasing prices and the increases in purity, heroin may now be snorted or smoked by inhaling its vapors, either with tobacco in a rolled cigarette or by heating the drug on aluminum foil.

There are many cutaneous signs of heroin abuse. Because it is often injected, the signs listed above for IDUs are the most common cutaneous evidence of use. Four percent of addicts develop urticaria, which can last for days. They can develop a "high pruritus," which is intense itching, especially on their genitals and on their face. "Puffy hand syndrome" (Fig. 101-6) is the condition where edema develops in the dorsal hands but not the fingers. This is mainly caused by lymphatic damage resulting from quinine, which is an adulterant that is added to heroin.[12] There have been a few cases of penile ulcers and necrotizing cellulitis of the scrotum when heroin was injected into the dorsal vein of the penis.[44] Pemphigus vegetans,[45] fixed drug eruptions, toxic epidermal necrolysis, necrolytic migratory erythema not associated with glucagonoma, and acanthosis nigracans[11] have all been described with heroin abuse.[8] Sometimes users resort to other drugs when heroin is not available. One of the commonly used alternatives to heroin is tripelennamine with pentazocine (called *Ts and blues*). Injection causes severe ulceration with hyperkeratosis that follows a linear pattern.

"CLUB DRUGS"

Methylenedioxymethamphetamine (MDMA, Ecstasy): The main active ingredient in the popular club drug ecstasy is 3,4-methylenedioxymethamphetamine (MDMA), which is used for its ability to induce a sense of euphoria and enhance sensory perception via effects on multiple neurochemical pathways.[46] MDMA is typically ingested as a tablet. When prepared in its pure powder form it is referred to as "molly" and can be snorted or orally ingested. MDMA is often combined with a wide variety of other drugs, such as amphetamine derivatives, caffeine, and aspirin, when manufactured in tablet form for ingestion. Few cutaneous manifestations following use/abuse have been reported as its deleterious adverse effects on the kidney, liver, and neuropsychiatric systems are more commonly encountered and studied. An acneiform eruption aptly labeled "ecstasy pimples" has been described,[47] as has a widespread guttate psoriasiform eruption.

γ-Hydroxybutyrate (also known as "Liquid Ecstasy," "Liquid X," or "Fantasy"): γ-Hydroxybutyrate (GHB) is a popular "party drug" based on its euphoric and aphrodisiac properties. It is also used as a "rape drug" in the nightclub scene based on its ability to induce a reversible coma as well as short term memory loss. Specific cutaneous features following its use are not well described. However, GHB use can cause an overdose syndrome in which pale skin is prominent and should prompt immediate medical attention if use is suspected.[48]

Methamphetmine (also known as "Speed," "Meth," "Chalk," "Ice," "Crystal," "Crank," or "Glass"): Methamphetamine is made by the reduction of ephedrine or pseudoephedrine in "meth labs." It can be made in a single 2-L bottle using

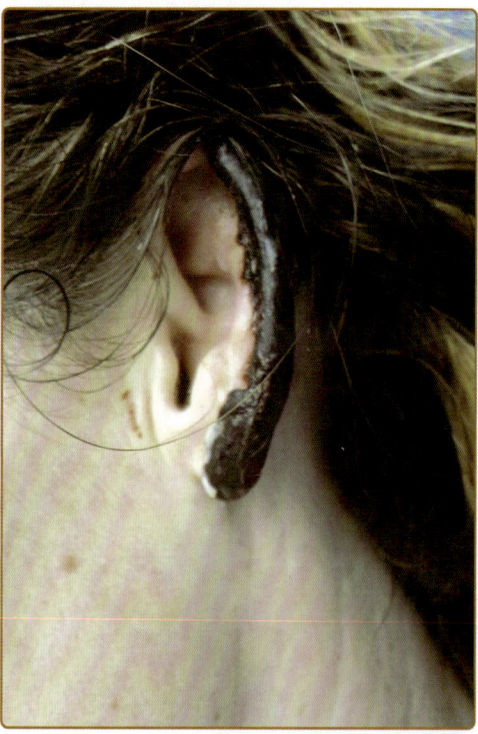

Figure 101-5 Levamisole. Characteristic purpuric eruption on the ear following levamisole toxicity. (Reproduced with permission from Hennings C, Miller J. Illicit drugs: what dermatologists need to know. *J Am Acad Dermatol*. 2013;69:135-142.)

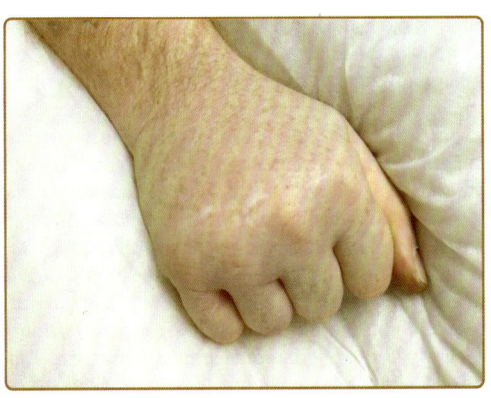

Figure 101-6 Puffy hand syndrome. Example of dorsal hand edema following intravenous drug use.

batteries and fertilizer, which makes meth labs more mobile and the drug more accessible. The process of making methamphetamine is very toxic and flammable. It causes euphoria, increased energy, anxiety, aggression, hallucinations, and severe withdrawal. It may be injected, smoked, or snorted.[8] Signs of methamphetamine abuse are intense pruritus, body odor, weight loss, premature aging, and hyperhidrosis. "Meth mouth", which consists of numerous dental caries and enamel erosions starting at the gum line, develops in users.[49] It is caused by a combination of xerostomia, bruxism (clenching and grinding of the teeth), and poor dental hygiene. Formication may also develop, especially on the face. Acne excoriee and lichenoid drug eruptions have been reported from methamphetamine use.[50]

Other Amphetamines and Methylphenidate—Uppers, Speed, Eye Openers, Pick Me Ups: The CNS stimulants amphetamine and methylphenidate are used for narcolepsy to improve alertness and appear to decrease abnormalities in brain structure and function found in attention deficit hyperactivity disorder.[51] Formication and obsessive skin-picking, as well as urticaria and acne, have been reported.

Hallucinogens—Lysergic Acid Diethylamide, Mushrooms: Lysergic acid diethylamide (LSD, acid) is found in ergot, a fungus cultivated from rye and other grains, which is often ingested in liquid form for its ability to alter one's sense of time and sensory perception. Psilocybin and its active metabolite psilocin (4-hydroxy-*N,N*- dimethyltryptamine) are the psychoactive compounds of various forms of hallucinogenic mushrooms ingested for their mind altering properties.[52] Dry mouth appears to be the main cutaneous effect.

Sedatives: Cutaneous reactions to sedatives are rare. The sedative class of drugs includes cannabis, benzodiazepines, and hydroxybutyrate. Drug reactions are rarely associated with benzodiazepines, including morbilliform hypersensitivity eruptions, erythema multiforme to clonazepam, and acute generalized exanthematous pustulosis.

CANNABIS (ALSO KNOWN AS "MARIJUANA," "POT," "WEED," OR "MARY JANE")

Cannabis is a mixture of dried shredded leaves and flowers of the *Cannabis sativa* plant. The psychoactive chemical compound is Δ9-tetrahydrocannabinol (THC). The potency of marijuana has increased over the years and is now 5 times stronger than the marijuana used in the 1970s. Since its legalization in some states of the United States, marijuana use has increased in those states by approximately 20% according to early data. Although recreational use tends to be for its ability to produce euphoria, medicinal use is gaining acceptance. Treatment of pain, glaucoma, muscle spasm, nausea, seizures, poor appetite, and inflammation are only a few of the disorders for which cannabinoids are being used and investigated. There are topical formulations that profess to improve the appearance of aging skin.

There are 4 ways to consume marijuana: inhalation, oral, sublingual or topical application. Inhalation causes an effect within minutes, peaks at approximately 1 hour, and wanes in approximately 2 hours. Inhalation occurs via smoking or vaporization (*vaping*). Marijuana can be smoked in joints (hand-rolled cigarettes), bongs (pipes), or blunts (marijuana cigars). Other drugs, such as cocaine, may be mixed with it. Vaping (see below) is also gaining popularity. Oral ingestion is becoming more common as cannabis is used for medical purposes and is legal in several states. Onset of action for oral consumption is slower than for inhalation, with initial effects taking 30 minutes or longer and peaking at approximately 2 hours; total duration of effects can be as long as 6 hours. The effects from oral consumption have been described as more "intense" than those from inhalation. Dosage of marijuana taken orally can be difficult to titrate; irregular effects and overdose are more common with this form. Cannabis edibles include the classic brownies and cookies, as well as other formulations, including lollipops, fudge, "cannabutter," oils and tinctures, and baked in breads and pizza. Sublingual use includes product in dissolvable strips, lozenges, and sublingual sprays. Onset of action may be earlier than in oral consumption. Finally, cannabis can be delivered topically via transdermal patches, oils, salves, lotions, and bath salts. Transdermal patches may deliver enough active ingredient to cause a "high" but usually only produce local effects.

There are few cutaneous signs of cannabis use. Acne, ranging from mild to severe, has been described. Allergic reactions, including contact dermatitis, also have been reported. Cannabis arteritis is a serious vascular complication that can occur with chronic use. Cannabis arteritis is rare, with approximately 50 cases reported in the literature despite more than 5 million daily users worldwide. It presents as peripheral ischemia and necrosis, most often of the lower limbs. Cannabis arteritis is one of the most frequent causes of peripheral arterial disease in adults younger than age 50 years and is a subtype of thromboangiitis obliterans.[53] It may present with Raynaud phenomenon and digital necrosis. Cannabis arteritis is thought to be caused by the combined vasoconstrictive effects of THC and arsenic, arsenic being a common contaminant in marijuana.[54] Claudication may present before the development of ulcers or gangrene.[55] Duplex ultrasound can be used to differentiate between cannabis arteritis and atherosclerosis. Cannabis arteritis shows occlusion of peripheral arteries below the knee, whereas atherosclerosis has calcified plaques in the iliofemoral arteries. Treatment is for the patient to stop cannabis use and to take low-dose (81 mg) aspirin. For severe cases, iloprost (0.5 to 2 ng/kg/min), which is a prostaglandin analog, can be given.[56]

CUTTING AGENTS

Drugs of abuse often contain additional ingredients besides the active compound the user desires to consume. These ingredients can be added intentionally to increase the volume of the product for additional profit, or, it may be unintentionally included in the final product as a result of the chemical manufacturing process. So-called cutting agents can be divided into diluents and adulterants. Diluents, such as dirt, baking soda, talc, and mannitol, are added to expand the volume of the drug for increased distribution.[57] Adulterants, such as caffeine, hydroxyzine, diltiazem, levamisole, and phenacetin, are added to enhance the effect of the main active ingredient or facilitate administration of the drug.

Several cutting agents deserve special mention because of their potential to induce cutaneous manifestations following exposure. Most notable among these is levamisole in cocaine and arsenic in cannabis. Diluents such as talc and starch are reported to cause foreign-body granulomas after parenteral use with various drugs (Fig. 101-7).[58] Another example of an emerging adulterant leading to adverse outcomes with heroin use is clenbuterol. Although unremarkable for its skin manifestations, several case series have described dangerous cardiac events.[59]

BETEL

Betel is a common drug of abuse in the Asian and Southeast Asian cultures. *Betel quid* is a combination of areca nut, betel leaf, slaked lime, and other ingredients. Psychoactive alkaloids appear to be the main stimulant. It is usually ingested by mucosal absorption similar to chewing tobacco. Chewing of the betel mixture causes maceration, erosions, and fissures of the oral commissures, which can be mistaken for other disorders such as angular cheilitis, candidiasis, or vitamin deficiencies. *Chewer's mucosa* is a brownish-red discoloration of the buccal mucosa associated with irregular desquamation. Lichenoid lesions may also appear. *Oral submucous fibrosis* is characterized by a prodrome of oral dysesthesia followed by palpable vertical fibrous bands that may require surgical interventions for opening of the mouth. Oral carcinoma can occur, usually on the buccal areas of the tongue and labial mucosa.[60]

KROKODIL

Desomorphine, a synthetic opioid derivative, manufactured using chemically altered codeine with several household ingredients, goes by the street name "Krokodil" and is reportedly ten times more potent than heroin. The drug acquired its name from the thick, scaly, green-black skin changes seen in its users.[61] The injectable drug is highly addictive and known for inducing widespread necrotizing skin lesions. It gained its popularity as a drug of abuse in Russia and cases of its adverse effects have been documented recently throughout Europe and only rarely in the United States. Besides skin color and texture change, cutaneous manifestations include swelling and pain at sites where the drug is subcutaneously injected followed by extremely aggressive necrotic ulcerations, which commonly involve muscle and cartilaginous tissue. Destructive infections often ensue and lead to extremely morbid sequelae. Alarmingly, these reactions are typically reported after short periods of use and the analgesic effects of the medicine can cause delay in the user seeking medical attention.

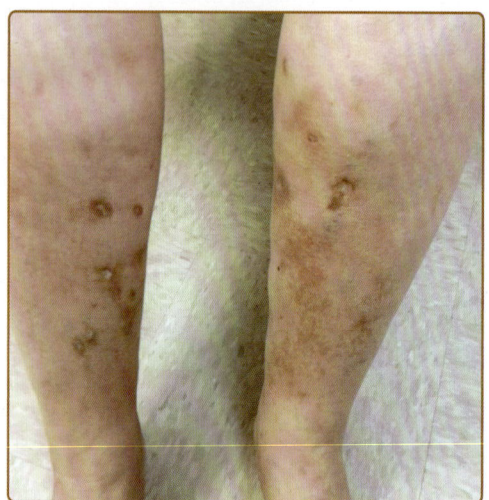

Figure 101-7 Talc granulomas. Multiple granulomas on the bilateral legs from intravenous use of drugs containing talc as a cutting agent.

LEGAL DRUGS OF ABUSE

ALCOHOL

Cutaneous manifestations of alcohol consumption comprise a wide spectrum of clinical presentations. Vascular lesions are some of the most easily recognizable skin findings seen in patients who abuse alcohol; they occur secondary to alcohol's effects on the vasodilatory properties of blood vessels as well as hormonal changes induced by alterations in liver metabolism.[62] Spider angiomata, palmar erythema, and telangiectasia are examples of common cutaneous signs in alcohol abuse. More subtle findings include corkscrew scleral vessels. Other signs of liver insufficiency include dilated periumbilical veins on the abdominal wall (caput medusae) and unilateral nevoid telangiectasia, a vascular proliferative syndrome. Nevoid telangiectasias have been proposed as latent congenital nevi that present in the setting of alcohol-induced hyperestrogenism. They appear on the upper body in the C3–C4 dermatomal distribution as thread-like collections of fine telangiectasias. Systemic jaundice is typically seen after serum bilirubin levels reach greater than 2.5 mg/dL.[63] Generalized pruritus is another end-stage sequelae of liver dysfunction and may present clinically as nonspecific excoriations or as prurigo nodules if areas are chronically scratched. Several nail abnormalities to both the nail plate and nail bed have been described in the setting of alcohol abuse and concomitant liver dysfunction. The classic nail change seen in these patients are "Terry's nails" in which the proximal nail is nontranslucent white while the distal nail remains pink. One study reported that 80% of patients with cirrhosis will manifest this finding. Furthermore, nail findings previously described in the literature include transverse white bands and red lunulae in the setting of cirrhosis with congestive heart failure.

There are many chronic skin conditions that can be induced or exacerbated by alcohol abuse. One hallmark cutaneous condition associated with alcohol abuse is porphyria cutanea tarda, which is discussed in Chap. 125. Other notable alcohol-associated conditions include Dupuytren contracture, as well as Madelung disease, psoriasis, rosacea, nummular eczema, and seborrheic dermatitis, although the exact connection with these conditions is unclear.

TOBACCO (CIGARETTES, CHEWING TOBACCO, ORAL TOBACCO, SPIT OR SPITTING TOBACCO, DIP, CHEW, SNUFF, OR SNOOZE)

Tobacco is made from the leaves of plants of the genus *Nicotiana*. Tobacco is usually smoked, but can be chewed (ie, absorbed via the oral mucosa when placed between the buccal and gingival mucosa) or sniffed. "Vaping" is a relatively new phenomenon where the tobacco is inhaled through a vaporizer that infuses water into the smoke. Nicotine in tobacco in particular is known to be addictive because of its mood-boosting effects; it is also known to suppress appetite.

There are many signs and symptoms of tobacco use. Yellow-brown staining of the teeth, fingers and fingernails from nicotine is clearly visible in many smokers. One of the most-well-established effects of tobacco smoking on the skin is premature aging. Although this association has been appreciated for decades, studies in the late 20th century confirmed the link between wrinkles on tobacco and further identified that the association is proportional to the tobacco load of the patient.[64] Some of the mechanisms by which this occurs have been described. One such mechanism is the increase in elastic fiber content of the reticular dermis along with upregulation of enzymes crucial to skin remodeling and repair essentially creating the effect of solar elastosis. Tobacco's effects on fibroblasts and the microvasculature impair wound healing.

There are more than 7000 chemicals found in cigarette smoke, more than 70 of which are known to be carcinogenic.[65] Although many studies have sought to identify a potential relationship between tobacco use and skin cancers, they have failed to identify a definitive causal relationship. One study did show an increased prevalence of keratoacanthomas in smokers compared to nonsmokers. Tobacco use also has been linked to hand dermatitis.[66]

Use of tobacco incites or worsens chronic skin conditions, including psoriasis (particularly the palmoplantar pustular variant), hidradenitis suppurativa, and subacute and chronic cutaneous lupus erythematosus. Smoking tobacco impairs the efficacy of antimalarial therapy in patients with lupus, making treatment of these patients more difficult.[67] Also, smokers should not use beta-carotene supplements because of the higher risk of lung cancer.

Chemical effects include peripheral vasoconstriction, platelet aggregation, and decrease in prostacyclin formation, which increase the risk of cardiovascular disease. Thromboangiitis obliterans (Buerger disease) is an inflammatory arteritis of the medium and small vessels of the upper and lower extremities. It typically presents with pain and necrosis of the digits in young male tobacco smokers. Carbon monoxide also increases risk of cardiovascular problems, as well as peripheral ischemia, in end organs such as the skin and digits.[68]

Both cigarette smoking and chewing are associated with several conditions of the oral mucosa. This includes *leukokeratosis nicotinica palati* (nicotine stomatitis, smoker's palate) which is characterized by uniform keratosis of the hard palate with multiple umbilicated erythematous papules that are the inflamed orifices of minor salivary glands. *Leukokeratosis nicotinica glossae* is a homogeneous white plaque that affects the anterior two-thirds of the dorsal tongue. Oral verrucous carcinoma, oral warty dyskeratoma, and oral melanosis (brown-black pigmentation of the oral mucosa) are also associated with tobacco use.[69]

PRESCRIPTION OPIATES

Hydrocodone, oxycodone, morphine, and codeine are legally prescribed analgesics that can produce euphoria. CNS depression is the most common side effect. Because they are taken orally, these medications do not produce the signs listed above for heroin. Urticaria and pruritus are the most common cutaneous effects.

ANABOLIC STEROIDS

Anabolic steroids are synthetic hormones similar to testosterone. They can be ingested or injected and have many legal indications. Illicit use is usually to build muscle and augment athletic performance. Cutaneous side effects are common and should be suspected in any patient who presents with acne vulgaris, hair growth on the body and loss on the scalp, and striae. Increased body hair, increased oil in the skin and hair, and premature androgenetic alopecia are also common.[70] Steroid acne is most commonly distributed on the face, chest, back, and shoulders. Women may demonstrate androgen-mediated effects, including androgenetic alopecia, deepening of the voice, clitoral enlargement, and menstrual irregularity. Men may experience gynecomastia, testicular atrophy, and infertility. Teenage use can induce precocious puberty and growth stunting. Side effects may not reverse upon discontinuation of the drug.[71] Striae may develop from muscle hypertrophy. Acne fulminans, psoriasis, familial angiolipomas and exacerbation of coproporphyria also have been reported. Systemic side effects also may be present, including hepatic enzyme elevations, jaundice, hypertension, and lipid abnormalities.

NONCUTANEOUS ISSUES

Noncutaneous complications and sequelae of drug use are extensive. In particular, bloodborne or sexually transmitted diseases, such as HIV and hepatitides B and C virus, are well-established comorbidities of IV drug use. There is data to suggest that illicit drug use is associated with premature mortality in young adults both from trauma and suicide.[72]

MANAGEMENT

The key to managing drug use, abuse and addiction is as early intervention as possible. The dermatologist may be able to help with recognition of the problem. Relatively recently, drug addiction has been recognized as a multifactorial disease and therapies ranging from medications, psychiatric treatment, and alternative treatments, including acupuncture and meditation, are being implemented.

REFERENCES

1. United Nations Office on Drugs and Crime. *World Drug Report 2017*. New York, NY: United Nations. http://www.unodc.org/wdr2015/.
2. Kim S, Kwok S, Mayes LC, et al. Early adverse experience and substance addiction: dopamine, oxytocin, and glucocorticoid pathways. *Ann N Y Acad Sci*. 2017;1394(1):74-91.
3. Beyers JM, Toumbourou JW, Catalano RF, et al. A cross-national comparison of risk and protective factors for adolescent substance use: the United States and Australia. *J Adolesc Health*. 2004;35:3-16.
4. Sim M, Hulse G, Khong E. Injecting drug use and skin lesions. *Aust Fam Physician*. 2004;33:519-522.
5. Hennings C, Miller J. Illicit drugs: what dermatologists need to know. *J Am Acad Dermatol*. 2013;69:135-142.
6. Bennet RG, Leyden JJ, Decherd JW. The heroin ulcer: new addition to the differential diagnosis of ulcers of the penis. *Arch Dermatol*. 1973;107:121-122.
7. Horowitz HW. Learning to recognize scarring among drug users: a tool for HIV risk reduction. *Am J Public Health*. 1997;87:1233-1234.
8. Bergstrom K. Cutaneous clues to drug addictions. *J Drugs Dermatol*. 2008;7:303-306.
9. Young AW Jr, Sweeney EW. Cutaneous clues to heroin addiction. *Am Fam Physician*. 1973;7:79-87.
10. Kathuria S, Ramesh V, Singh A. Pentazocine induced ulceration of the buttocks. *Indian J Dermatol Venereol Leprol*. 2012;78(4):521.
11. Murphy EL, DeVita D, Liu H, et al. Risk factors for skin and soft-tissue abscesses among injection drug users: a case-control study. *Clin Infect Dis*. 2001;33:35-40.
12. Orangio GR, Pitlick SD, Della Latta P, et al. Soft tissue infections in parental drug abusers. *Ann Surg*. 1984;199:97-100.
13. Binswanger IA, Kral AH, Bultenthal RN, et al. High prevalence of abscesses and cellulitis among community-recruited injection drug users in San Francisco. *Clin Infect Dis*. 2000;30:579-581.
14. Spijkerman IJ, Langendam MW, van Ameijden EJ, et al. Gender differences in clinical manifestations before AIDS diagnosis among injecting drug users. *Eur J Epidemiol*. 1998;14(3):213-218.
15. Tuazon CU, Cardella TA, Sheagren JN. Staphylococcal endocarditis in drug users. Clinical and microbiologic aspects. *Arch Intern Med*. 1975;135(12):1555-1561.
16. Cherubin CE, Sapira JD. The medical complications of drug addiction and the medical assessment of the intravenous drug user: 25 years later. *Ann Intern Med*. 1993;119:1017-1028.
17. Brown PD, Ebright JR. Skin and soft tissue infections in injection drug users. *Curr Infect Dis Rep*. 2002;4:415-419.
18. Bohlen L, Muhlemann K, Dubuis O. Outbreak among drug users caused by a clonal strain of group A streptococcus. *Emerg Infect Dis*. 2000;6:175-179.
19. Centers for Disease Control. Tetanus among injecting-drug users—California, 1997. *MMWR Morb Mortal Wkly Rep*. 1998;47:149-151.
20. Werner SB, Passaro D, McGee J, et al. Wound botulism in California, 1951-1998: recent epidemic in heroin injectors. *Clin Infect Dis*. 2000;31:1018-1024.
21. Chen JL, Fullerton KE, Flynn NM. Necrotizing fasciitis associated with injection drug use. *Clin Infect Dis*. 2001;33:6-15.

22. Sudarsky LA, Laschinger JC, Coppa GF, et al. Improved results from a standardized approach in treating patients with necrotizing fasciitis. *Ann Surg*. 1987;206:661-665.
23. Callahan TE, Schecter WP, Horn JK. Necrotizing soft tissue infection masquerading as cutaneous abscess following illicit drug injection. *Arch Surg*. 1998;133:812-818.
24. Anderson CE, Loomis GA. Recognition and prevention of inhalant drug abuse. *Am Fam Physician*. 2003;68(5):869-874.
25. Strock M, Black L, Liddell M. Inhalant abuse and dextromethorphan. *Child Adolesc Psychiatr Clin N Am*. 2016;25:497-508.
26. Tames SM, Goldenring JM. Madarosis from cocaine use. *N Engl J Med*. 1986;314:1324.
27. Feeney CM, Briggs S. Crack hands: a dermatologic effect of smoking crack cocaine. *Cutis*. 1989;44:223-225.
28. Schuster DS. Snorters' warts. *Arch Dermatol*. 1987;123:571.
29. Hofbauer GF, Hafner J, Trueb RM. Urticarial vasculitis following cocaine use. *Br J Dermatol*. 1999;141:600-601.
30. Orriols R, Munoz X, Ferrer J, et al. Cocaine-induced Churg-Strauss vasculitis. *Eur Respir J*. 1996;9:175-177.
31. Gertner E, Hamlar D. Necrotizing granulomatous vasculitis associated with cocaine use. *J Rheumatol*. 2002;29:1795-1797.
32. Brewer J, Meves A, Bostwick M, et al. Cocaine abuse: dermatologic manifestations and therapeutic approaches. *J Am Acad Dermatol*. 2008;59:483-487.
33. Marder VJ, Mellinghoff IK. Cocaine and Buerger disease: is there a pathogenetic association? *Arch Intern Med*. 2000;13:2057-2060.
34. Bozkurt AK. The role of cocaine in the etiology of Buerger disease is questionable. *Arch Intern Med*. 2001;161:486.
35. Friedman D, Wolfsthal S. Cocaine-induced pseudovasculitis. *Mayo Clin Proc*. 2005;80:671-673.
36. Specks U. The growing complexity of the pathology associated with cocaine use. *J Clin Rheumatol*. 2011;7(4):167-168.
37. Lu LK, High WA. Acute generalized exanthematous pustulosis caused by illicit street drugs? *Arch Dermatol*. 2007;143:430-431.
38. Hofbauer GF, Burg G, Nestle FO. Cocaine-related Stevens-Johnson syndrome. *J Am Acad Dermatol*. 1994;53:97-98.
39. Kerr HD. Cocaine and scleroderma. *South Med J*. 1989;10:1275-1276.
40. Attoussi S, Faulkner ML, Oso A, et al. Cocaine-induced scleroderma and scleroderma renal crisis. *South Med J*. 1998; 91:961-963.
41. Elpern DJ. Cocaine abuse and delusions of parasitosis. *Cutis*. 1988;42:273-274.
42. Jeong HS, Layher H, Cao L, et al. Pyoderma gangrenosum (PG) associated with levamisole-adulterated cocaine: clinical, serologic, and histopathologic findings in a cohort of patients. *J Am Acad Dermatol*. 2016;74(5):892-898.
43. Strazzula L, Brown KK, Brieva JC, et al. Levamisole toxicity mimicking autoimmune disease. *J Am Acad Dermatol*. 2013;69(6):954-959.
44. Alguire PC. Necrotizing cellulitis of the scrotum: a new complication of heroin addiction. *Cutis*. 1984;43:93-95.
45. Downie J, Dicostanzo D, Cohen S. Pemphigus vegetans-Neumann variant associated with intranasal heroin abuse. *J Am Acad Dermatol*. 1998;39:872-875.
46. Gowing LR, Henry-Edwards SM, Irvine RJ, et al. The health effects of ecstasy: a literature review. *Drug Alcohol Rev*. 2002; 21:53-63.
47. Wollina U, Kammler HJ, Hesselbarth N, et al. Ecstasy pimples a new facial dermatosis. *Dermatology*. 1998; 197:171-173.
48. Stromberg MW, Knudsen K, Stomberg H, et al. Symptoms and signs in interpreting gamma-hydroxybutyrate (GHB) intoxication—an explorative study. *Scand J Trauma Resusc Emerg Med*. 2014;22:27.
49. Hamamoto DT, Rhodus NL. Methamphetamine abuse and dentistry. *Oral Dis*. 2009;15:27-37.
50. Deloach-Banta LJ. Lichenoid drug eruption: crystal methamphetamine or adulterants? *Cutis*. 1992;50: 193-194.
51. Spencer TJ, Brown A, Seidman LJ, et al. Effect of psychostimulants on brain structure and function in ADHD: a qualitative literature review of MRI-based neuroimaging studies. *J Clin Psychiatry*. 2013;74(9):902-917.
52. Dos Santos RG, Osorio FL, Crippa JA, et al. Antidepressive, anxiolytic, and antiaddictive effects of ayahuasca, psilocybin and lysergic acid diethylamide (LSD): a systematic review of clinical trials published in the last 25 years. *Ther Adv Psychopharmacol*. 2016;6(3):193-213.
52. Sauvanier M, Constans J, Skopinski S, et al. Lower limb occlusive arteriopathy: retrospective analysis of 73 patients with onset before the age of 50 years [in French]. *J Mal Vasc*. 2002;27:69-76.
54. Peyrot I, Garsaud A-M, Saint-Cyr I et al: Cannabis arteritis: a new case report and a review of literature. *J Eur Acad Dermatol Venereol*. 2007;21:388-391.
55. Cazalets C, Laurat E, Cador B, et al. Cannabis arteritis: four new cases [in French]. *Rev Med Interne*. 2003;24:127-130.
56. Noel B, Ruf I, Panizzon G. Cannabis arteritis. *J Am Acad Dermatol*. 2008;58(suppl):S65.
57. Broseus J, Gentile N, Esseiva P. The cutting of cocaine and heroin: a critical review. *Forensic Sci Int*. 2016;262:73-83.
58. Del Giudice P: Cutaneous complications of intravenous drug abuse. *Br J Dermatol*. 2004;150:1-10.
59. Hieger MA, Emswiler MP, Maskell KF, et al. A case series of clenbuterol toxicity caused by adulterated heroin. *J Emerg Med*. 2016;51(3):259-261.
60. Lee CH, Ko A, Warnakulasuriya S, et al. Population burden of betel quid abuse and its relation to oral premalignant disorders in South, Southeast, and East Asia: an Asian Betel-Quid Consortium Study. *Am J Public Health*. 2012;102(3)e17-e24.
61. Haskin A, Kim N, Aguh C. A new drug with a nasty bite: a case of krokodil-induced skin necrosis. *JAAD Case Rep*. 2016;2:174-176.
62. Smith KE, Fenske NA. Cutaneous manifestations of alcohol abuse. *J Am Acad Dermatol*. 2000;43:1-16.
63. Liu SW, Lien MH, Fenske NA. The effects of alcohol and drug abuse on the skin. *Clin Dermatol*. 2010; 28:391-399.
64. Metelitsa AI, Lauzon GJ. Tobacco and the skin. *Clin Dermatol*. 2010;28:384-390.
65. Didkowska J, Wojciechowska U, Mańczuk M, et al. Lung cancer epidemiology: contemporary and future challenges worldwide. *Ann Transl Med*. 2016;4(8):150.
66. Lai YC, Yew YW. Smoking and hand dermatitis in the United States adult population. *Ann Dermatol*. 2016;28(2):164-171.
67. Boeckler P, Cosnes A, Frances C, et al. Association of cigarette smoking but not alcohol consumption with cutaneous lupus erythematosus. *Arch Dermatol*. 2009;145(9):1012-1016.

68. Hoffman D, Hoffman I. The changing cigarette, 1950-1995. *J Toxicol Environ Health*. 1997;50(4):307-364.
69. Alkan A, Bulut E, Gunhan O, et al. Oral verrucous carcinoma: a study of 12 cases. *Eur J Dent*. 2010;4(2):202-207.
70. Yesalis CE 3rd, Herrick RT, Buckley WE, et al. Self-reported use of anabolic-androgenic steroids by elite powerlifters. *Phys Sportsmed*. 1988;16:91-99.
71. Nieschlag E, Vorona E. Doping with anabolic androgenic steroids (AAS): adverse effects on non-reproductive organs and functions. *Rev Endocr Metab Disord*. 2015;16(3):199-211.
72. Meader N, King K, Moe-Byrne T, et al. A systematic review on the clustering and co-occurrence of multiple high-risk behaviors. *BMC Public Health*. 2016;16:657.

Chapter 102 :: Physical Abuse
:: Kelly M. MacArthur & Annie Grossberg

第一百零二章
身体虐待

中文导读

　　虐待是一个世界性的医学问题，特别是对于那些既不能提供可靠的病史(尤其是儿童、老年或认知障碍患者)，又害怕报告虐待的后果(与任何虐待受害者有关)的人来说，是很难诊断的。本章节主要从流行病学、病因及发病机制/危险因素、临床特征、诊断、鉴别诊断、临床进程和预后等方面分别对受虐待老人、受虐待儿童、家庭暴力进行阐述。从皮肤的形态学、部位、分布特点分别对受虐待老人、受虐待儿童、家庭暴力进行了描述。详尽的病史、体格检查、实验室检测以及影像学检查都可用于对疾病的诊断。本章提出早期识别和及时的诊断能够允许适当的医疗进行迅速的干预。采取措施提供保护，使其免受犯罪者的侵害，有助于预防再发生和优化预后。

〔易　梅〕

AT-A-GLANCE

- Child abuse, elder abuse, and domestic violence are common and affect patients of all socioeconomic classes and races.
- Identifying specific cutaneous findings concerning for physical abuse allows for early intervention to impact outcomes.
- Bruising on soft padded areas of the body and patterned bruising that are multiple and in different stages of healing are suspicious of abuse.
- Burns that are bilateral and uniform are suspicious of abuse.
- Law mandates the reporting of all suspected cases of child abuse and, in some states, elder abuse.

INTRODUCTION

Abuse is a world-wide medical issue that is notoriously difficult to diagnose in those who are either not able to provide reliable histories (especially seen in pediatric, geriatric, or cognitively impaired patients) or those who fear the ramifications of reporting abuse (pertinent to any victim of abuse).

The main diagnostic challenge lies in the various manifestations of physical abuse due to great diversity of patients and range of means used to inflict trauma. Injuries can result from primary trauma (abrasions, hematomas, choke marks) or secondary effects of an initial trauma (such as in thermal injuries). Superficial cutaneous signs can also indicate the presence and extent of internal injury. Both severe penetrating and blunt trauma can cause bone fractures, torn ligaments, and joint instability. Internal organ hemorrhage can produce fatal consequences and are especially of concern in (though not exclusive to) head and abdominal injuries. Identifying specific cutaneous findings concerning for physical abuse may allow for early intervention to impact outcomes.

EPIDEMIOLOGY

Types of abuse and their respective incidence rates are listed in Table 102-1. More than 1 type of abuse can occur simultaneously.[9,10]

TABLE 102-1
Types of Elder Abuse

- Neglect: 55%
- Physical abuse: 15%
- Financial and material abuse: 12%
- Emotional or psychological abuse: 8%
- Sexual abuse: 1%
- Unspecified forms of abuse: 9%

CHILD ABUSE

Despite potentially severe morbid and even fatal consequences, child abuse remains under-identified and thus under-reported.[1,2] In the United States, child abuse/neglect annual incidence is 700,000 to 1.25 million children, with approximately 18% of cases involving physical abuse.[3-5] Among the United States and developed countries of Europe, the prevalence of physical abuse anytime throughout childhood ranges from 5% to 16%, with only 5% of all episodes estimated to be reported to child protective services.[6,7] It is estimated that more than 300,000 children suffer from sexual abuse each year in the United States. The lifetime risk of sexual abuse is approximately 25% to 40% for girls and approximately 10% for males.

ELDER ABUSE

Elder abuse is one of the fastest-growing forms of abuse. Although statistics vary, the National Center on Elder Abuse in Washington, DC, estimates that 1 to 2 million Americans 65 years of age or older are victims of various forms of abuse each year. Abuse may affect a range of 2% to 10% of the elderly population. Those older than age 80 years are 2 to 3 times more likely to suffer abuse, and the American population in this age range continues to increase each year. True prevalence is difficult to determine as diagnoses can be often missed, with one study claiming that for every case of reported elder abuse, at least another 5 cases go undetected.[8] All segments of society are affected.

DOMESTIC ABUSE

Conservative estimates say that in the United States approximately 1 million people suffer domestic violence each year, but the actual number likely approaches 4 million. Women comprise approximately 90% to 95% of all victims, and men account for 95% of all perpetrators. Forty percent to 60% of men who abuse their partner or spouse are also abusing their children. In the United States, approximately 1 in 3 women suffers at least 1 physical assault during her life, and 1500 women are murdered by their husbands or boyfriends each year.[11,12]

CLINICAL FEATURES—CUTANEOUS FINDINGS

Because many forms of physical abuse have external manifestations, the skin examination may serve as important evidence that abuse is taking place. Implausible history can provide the first warning sign, particularly when the clinical examination and extent of injury does not match up with the proposed mechanism of trauma. Explanations for injury should be both comprehensible and coherent; providers should seek to identify congruence between history provided and physical examination findings.[13] Because of the significant heterogeneity of cutaneous clinical findings, morphology as well as traditional diagnostic criteria (localization, patterned injuries, repeated injuries, clustered injuries) helps to identify concerning lesions suspicious for abuse. In particular, morphology and localization are key features in forensic classification of abuse.[13]

MORPHOLOGY

Just as in all other facets of dermatology, morphology is key to accurate diagnosis. Examination of secondary lesions to determine concern for abuse requires inspection of size, shape (discussed in the section "Patterned Injuries"), color, and location (discussed in the section "Localization"), but also palpation to determine texture and degree of pain. These clinical features can vary based on the anatomic site, the degree of force used, the firmness of the object delivering the force, and the underlying health of the injured individual.

Although penetrating wounds develop from trauma due to sharp objects, bruises result from blunt injury. Multiple bruises of differing colors may indicate repeated trauma rather than one isolated incident. Determining time of injury based on bruise characteristics is challenging as bruise color depends on the intensity, depth, and location of the injury. However, evidence suggests that a bruise with a yellow hue is likely older than 18 hours, but a bruise may be red, blue, or purple/black throughout its life span, from onset to resolution. Bruises of identical age and cause on the same person may not appear as the same color and may not change at the same rate.[14] Faint bruising can be better appreciated with use of a Wood lamp.

CHILD ABUSE

Confounding early identification and diagnosis of abuse in this population, active children (especially toddlers) are prone to multiple accidental bruises. Although there are no absolute features to differentiate accidental bruising from intentionally inflicted bruising, location can be the most helpful for identifying abuse (see below).

ELDERLY ABUSE

Cutaneous morphologies that are more unique and specific to elderly abuse include bed sores and strangely patterned alopecia.

LOCATION

Injury distribution can vary. Although the head is a common target of physical abuse in children, centrally located injuries are more common in domestic abuse. Perpetrators in any cases of abuse may choose to injure hidden areas, such as the breast or genitals, to deter detection. Black eyes are often seen in accidental injuries but are more suspicious if they are bilateral or are unaccompanied by evidence of trauma to the nose or superior orbital ridge. Accidental bruising or other injuries to the oral mucous membranes are unusual and should be considered as suspect.

CHILD ABUSE

Because young children tend to explore in a forward direction, accidental bruises more frequently occur on the distal arms and legs, knees, elbows, and forehead. Soft, padded, posterior, and protected areas of the body are far less likely to be accidentally injured. Bruises on the trunk, buttocks (Fig. 102-1), neck folds, palms/soles, thighs, genitalia, ear lobes, neck, and cheeks are uncommon, so marks in these areas should raise concern. Trauma to the oral cavity including mucosal surfaces, posterior pharynx, teeth, and lingual/labial frenula are concerning findings that warrant abuse consideration.

Face: Subconjunctival hemorrhages can be seen in 0.5% to 13.0% of typical newborns, but a large subconjunctival hemorrhage beyond 1 and 2 weeks of life is suspicious of abuse. Petechiae in the periorbital region have been seen in children with abuse-related retinal hemorrhages.

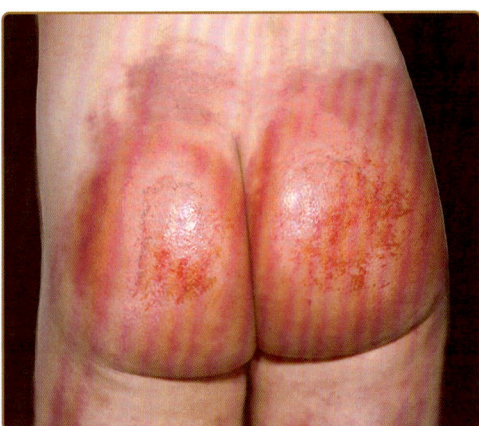

Figure 102-1 Purpura and erosions on the soft, padded areas of the buttock and thighs, representing very obvious abuse. (Used with permission from Paul Bellino, MD.)

Genitalia: Per the American Academy of Pediatrics, sexual abuse is the engaging of a child in sexual activities that the child cannot comprehend, for which the child is developmentally unprepared, and cannot give informed consent and that violate the social taboos of society.[15] Thus, as sexual abuse is not limited to physical abuse of genitalia, most victims of sexual abuse have no physical findings.[16,17] Although genital maltreatment (including touching, fondling, and penetration) can affect victims of all ages, the focus of sexual abuse in this chapter will be on its cutaneous manifestations in pediatric patients. Acute genital or anal injuries without plausible explanation and marked hymeneal opening enlargement with associated hymeneal disruption are very definitive signs of sexual abuse, yet these are not commonly present. The American Academy of Pediatrics Committee on Child Abuse and Neglect recommends that certain findings are consistent with, but not diagnostic of, abuse. These include chafing, abrasions, or bruising of the inner thighs and genitalia, scarring, tears or distortion of the hymen, a decreased amount or absent hymeneal tissue, scarring of the fossa navicularis, injury to or scarring of the posterior fourchette, scarring or tears of the labia minora, and enlargement of the hymeneal opening, even without disruption of the hymen.[15]

Genital warts pose a particularly difficult problem for practitioners. They certainly can be sexually transmitted to children, and the possibility of sexual abuse needs to be discussed with parents. However, there is much evidence that genital warts can be acquired perinatally from an infected mother, through autoinoculation from warts on other parts of the body, or through nonsexual contact with caretakers.[18] Children younger than 3 years of age at the onset of warts are least likely to have acquired their warts from sexual contact, whereas children with onset after 5 years of age have a much greater risk of having suffered sexual abuse. The ages in between represent a gray zone. Of note, human papillomavirus typing is not helpful.

DOMESTIC ABUSE

Unlike infants or debilitated adults, blows to a young adult may be to areas suggesting a defensive posture and might include purpura, sprains, dislocations, and fractures to the wrist or forearms, palms, and soles.

DISTRIBUTION

Injuries in particular distributions, namely those that are repeated, clustered, and/or patterned injuries are more concerning for intentional abuse. Repeated injuries pertain not only to multiple injuries in various stages of healing but also history of recurrent injuries of similar distribution. Regarding clustered injuries, while the rule of 3 or more individual injuries in the same body region is a classic guideline for raising concern for abuse, one study further identified concerning

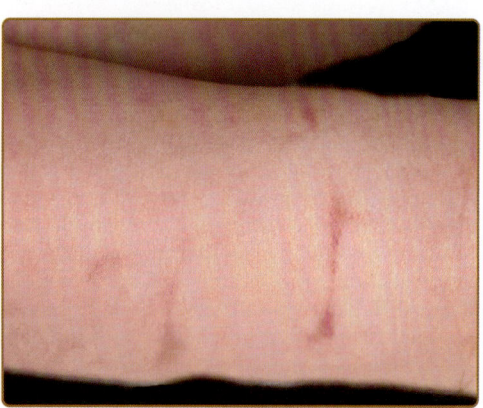

Figure 102-2 Linear purpura representing the interdigital spaces from a hand slap. Note the inferior triangular shape that corresponds to the finger web space. (Used with permission from Paul Bellino, MD.)

clustered injuries by age. Pre-mobile children should rarely have more than one isolated bruise, whereas infants who crawl/cruise infrequently have more than 2 bruises especially in the same body region, as compared with children who walk and have commonly greater than 5 or more bruises that may or may not be clustered based on location and activity.[22]

Certain patterned injury findings can reveal method of abuse and can provide a more specific clinical indicator of abuse. Inflicted bruises often leave patterned imprints of a hand, whip, or hard object. Linear purpura, with a small triangle at the base (Fig. 102-2) representing the interdigital and finger web spaces, occurs after a slap injury. Grab or pinch marks can be recognized by their location on soft padded areas and their unusual patterning. Circumferential purpura or hemosiderin pigmentation (Fig. 102-3) suggests a ligature injury, which would be difficult to explain as accidental. Tramline bruising, distinguished as 2 parallel linear bruises with appearance of preserved "normal skin" within the lines, results from trauma usually with a rectangular or round object (though an ovoid instrument can produce a variant finding). Tramline bruising results after a "high velocity" impact causes rupture of blood vasculature along the edges of the object with shunting of blood throughout the surface of contact with the skin. Withdrawal of the object allows blood from the periphery to return to the site of contact with preservation of vasculature of the center of the contact surface. Blood then extravasates from the damaged vasculature of the edges of impacted skin producing the parallel/symmetrical bruising pattern with often normal appearance of central impacted skin. Bite marks (Fig. 102-4) are always inflicted, although they are sometimes from children or pets. The shape and size of the marks can identify an adult mouth versus a bite from a child.

Inflicted burns can result from hot objects (such as iron, cigarette, spatula) applied to skin to cause shaped injuries. The most common agent involved in childhood burns (both accidental and inflicted) is hot liquid. Accidents such as inadvertently stepping into a hot tub or pulling a hot liquid off a table counter or stove leave irregular or geographic burn patterns that lack symmetry. By contrast, inflicted scalds tend to be symmetric, with sharply demarcated edges and an absence or paucity of splash marks characterized by tapered edges.

In one study, all the children whose bathtub burns were inflicted had associated features of abuse, including bruises, fractures, or evidence of neglect.[19] Stocking and glove burns result when the feet or hands are forcibly held under hot water. The uniformity of the burn indicates that the child was not able to reflexively withdraw from the scalding water as would happen with accidental immersion. A common pattern of inflicted immersion burn involves the buttocks, low back, and thighs. The child is flexed at the waist and dipped into the hot water, frequently as a punishment for a toilet training accident. The resultant pattern may give "zebra stripes" on the abdomen due to sparing of the flexural skin that is protected from the scald when bent forward. A "donut hole" pattern of sparing might

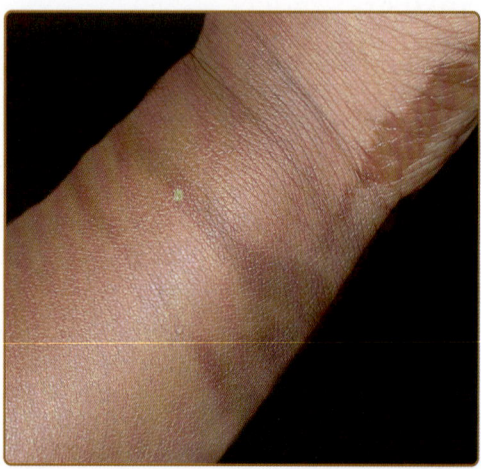

Figure 102-3 Linear, circumferential hyperpigmentation at the site of previous ligature. (Used with permission from Paul Bellino, MD.)

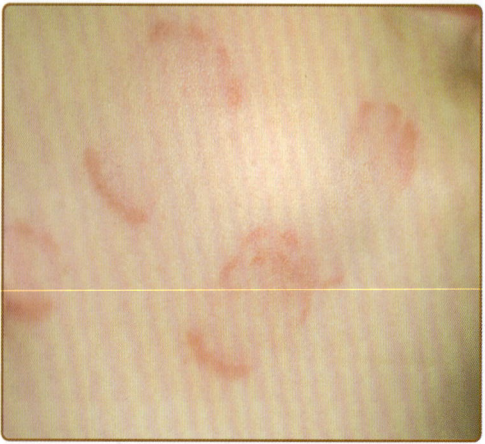

Figure 102-4 Human bite marks. (Used with permission from Paul Bellino, MD.)

be seen on the buttock if the child is pushed forcibly to the bottom of the tub that is cooler than the scalding water.[20] Inflicted splash burns are much more difficult to differentiate from accidents.

An inflicted contact burn can be recognized by the pattern that duplicates the object creating the injury. Accidental contact burns tend to be smaller, less severe, less patterned, and of irregular depth. When a patient is held against a hot object, the depth is more uniform, the pattern is more clearly defined, and the burn is more severe. Irons, curling irons, hot plates, and cigarettes are objects commonly used to inflict burns.[21] Some burns may, in fact, be accidental but represent inadequate supervision and neglect. This situation is also harmful and needs to be reported to the appropriate agencies.

ETIOLOGY AND PATHOGENESIS/RISK FACTORS

CHILD ABUSE

Victims and perpetrators span all racial, religious, and socioeconomic spectrums; however, identified factors placing children at higher risk for being victims of abuse are classified into characteristics of the patient, the provider, and the environment (society and community).[23] Typical children who suffer abuse have emotional, behavioral (including ADHD), or learning disabilities; have chronic illnesses (including failure to thrive and congenital anomalies) with special medical needs; may be premature at birth with low birth weight; have several siblings; resulted from unwanted pregnancy and/or deemed an unwanted child; live in single-parent households; or live at or below the poverty level. Girls are more likely than boys to suffer sexual abuse and the risk rises in preadolescence (Fig. 102-5). Perpetrators tend to have emotional or psychological problems, have frequently been victims of abuse themselves, abuse drugs or alcohol, are perpetrators of spousal abuse or have a history of marital discord, have marginal parental skills or knowledge, absentee mothers (extensively out of the home), and have poor self-esteem. Parents are the perpetrator 80% of the time[24]; only 10% child abuse is estimated as inflicted by strangers. Most common environmental factors seen in the setting of child abuse include poverty, social isolation, unrelated adult male in household, single-parent families, and significant family stressors. Although these profiles are helpful, it is important to remember that any child may be the victim of abuse.

ELDERLY ABUSE

Risk factors for abuse are listed in Table 102-2. Note that the risk factors have far more to do with the caretaker than the abused patient. In particular, the level of debility or health status of the patient does not predict abuse. Abuse most often occurs at the hands of caregivers or family members who have frequent close contact with patients and often may live with them. Historically, adult children of the abused patient have been the most common perpetrators, but most recent data show that spouses now account for the majority of abuse cases. Men are more likely to abuse than women. The abuser is often financially dependent on the victim, and they are usually in a shared living situation. However, financial abuse is more common among those who live alone.

DOMESTIC ABUSE

Women ages 19-29 years are the most common victims, with other risk factors being low income, mental health issues, alcohol or substance abuse by the victim or the perpetrator, pregnancy, large age difference between partners, separated or divorced status, and a family history or personal past history of abuse and violence. Women with educational or occupational levels above that of their partners may be at higher risk. Abusers

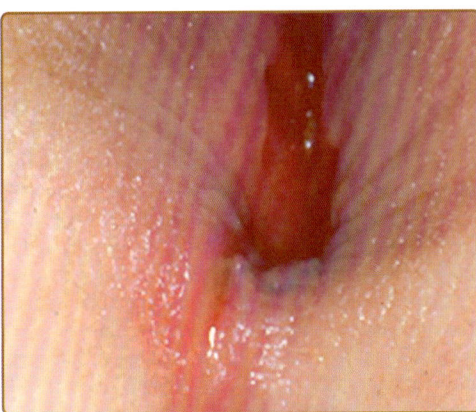

Figure 102-5 Sexual abuse. Perianal wound in a 3-year-old girl after anal penetration. (Used with permission from Dr. Francesca Navratil, Zurich, Switzerland.)

TABLE 102-2
Risk Factors for Elder Abuse

- Older age
- Lack of access to resources
- Low income
- Social isolation
- Minority status
- Low level of education
- Functional impairment
- Substance abuse by elder or caregiver
- Previous history of family violence
- History of psychological problems
- Caregiver stress
- Cognitive impairment

are typically underachievers with occupational status below their educational level.[11,12]

DIAGNOSIS

CHILD ABUSE

A careful history is needed to detect inconsistencies between the proposed injury and the physical examination. Identified red flags to trigger suspicion for abuse include unexplained delay in presentation, caregiver's history provided that is inconsistent or conflicting, denial of trauma despite concerning injury, trauma secondary to in-home resuscitation attempts, and severe injury for which blame is placed on pets or young children. As fall height and ground surface have been found to be predictors of severity of injury, short fall history in a child presenting with significant injuries should trigger suspicion for abuse.[25] The history should include as much detail as possible and inconsistencies in the parent's story clearly documented in the medical record.[26]

All historical information must be very well documented and preserved with the same care as any piece of forensic evidence. It is immensely important to enlist the help of an experienced abuse team in obtaining the history and completing an appropriately thorough physical examination.

It is essential to perform a total body, skin, and mucous membrane examination. It is also important to note the child's behavior and parent-child interactions. The color of all bruises should be noted and clearly documented. This may aid in determining the age of a bruise and may point out inconsistencies in the caretaker's history. It is helpful to include a ruled measuring scale in any photographs to help forensic identification at a later date. Most importantly, the child's spoken word is a valuable piece of evidence in establishing sexual abuse.

ELDERLY ABUSE

The US National Academy of Sciences has defined *elder abuse* as:

> (a) intentional actions that cause harm or create a serious risk of harm (whether or not harm is intended) to a vulnerable elder by a caregiver or other person who stands in a trust relationship to the elder, or (b) failure by a caregiver to satisfy the elder's basic needs or to protect the elder from harm.

Acts of commission and omission are thus included in the definition.

Unexplained repetitive injuries or explanations by caretakers that do not match the pattern of injury are concerning. Caretakers who act withdrawn, infantilize the patient, or insist on providing the medical history should alert the clinician.

It is important to interview by directing questions to the patient rather than the caregiver, and it is prudent to try to arrange a time to confer with and examine the patient alone. Repetitive followup visits help develop a rapport with the patient and allow serial observation of past and ongoing injuries. The assurance of confidentiality facilitates garnering sensitive information.

DOMESTIC ABUSE

Domestic violence is a pattern of coercive behaviors that may include repeated battering, psychological abuse, sexual abuse, social isolation, deprivation, and intimidation perpetrated by someone who is or was involved in an intimate relationship with the victim.

Whenever possible, the patient should be interviewed alone in the absence of her or his partner. A thorough examination should be done with a nurse chaperone, but not the partner, in the room. Repeat visits may be used to document new or progressing skin findings and to build trust with the patient. For various reasons, a victim may not want to reveal abuse. Implausible explanations for an injury or a delay in seeking medical attention may be clues of abuse. Signs of depression, excessive use of sedatives, chronic pain disorders, or vague stress-related symptoms may be subtle signs of abuse.[11]

SUPPORTIVE STUDIES— LABORATORY TESTING

The advised laboratory workup is patient presentation-dependent. Although there is an argument for obtaining basic bleeding studies (to include complete blood count with differential, platelet count, prothrombin and partial thromboplastin times) in all cases of suspected child abuse, the recommendation for other laboratory studies varies based on patient presentation.

Coagulation studies are helpful in identification of coagulopathy following trauma and can help to differentiate this from an underlying preceding coagulopathy. The above basic bleeding studies can be supplemented with additional coagulation studies, though hematology should be involved in opting for this more aggressive workup approach.[23,27]

For intraabdominal trauma, transaminase (alanine aminotransferase [ALT], aspartate aminotransferase [AST]) levels are elevated in those with hepatic damage whereas serum amylase and lipase are elevated in those with pancreatic injury.[28] Even in the absence of cutaneous findings to suggest intraabdominal trauma, transaminases can be elevated (greater than 80 U/L) correlating with hepatic injury in an abused child.[23] An observational study reported 17 of 54 children with no clinical findings to have intraabdominal injury, with 14 of the 17 injured to have elevated transaminases. Thus, not all patients with abdominal trauma have cutaneous manifestations nor is serologic testing perfectly sensitive to detect intraabdominal injury following abuse. Followup study performed noted transaminase elevation to be 83% specific and 84% sensitive for detection of such occult injury.[29]

Other serologies are ordered if suspecting specific injuries including serum electrolytes and osmolality for abusive head trauma; water intoxication or dehydration; as well as serum phosphate, calcium, and alkaline phosphatase in the setting of fractures to rule out bone disease as an underlying etiology. Workup for bone fragility is controversial, with no clear guidelines for screening; thus, it is proposed to consult with a bone metabolism expert should a child present with only fractures in the absence of cutaneous findings to suggest abuse.[23,30]

Urinalysis should be considered in patients with convincing history or examination suspicious for dehydration, abdominal trauma, or concerning urinary symptoms, such as hematuria (common finding following genitourinary or abdominal injury). If heme is found in the urine in the absence of red blood cells, further workup for rhabdomyolysis would then be warranted.

Toxicology testing can be performed but should be ordered based on patient presentation and clinical suspicion for the inappropriate administration of medications and street drugs. Regional poison control centers throughout the United States are always available for consultation and should be involved in unclear clinical cases and in critically ill patients.

SUPPORTIVE STUDIES—IMAGING

Imaging studies are case-dependent and should be tailored to the patient based on age, history, and examination.[31] Radiographic studies can aid in determining the extent of injury in intentional cases, but such studies can also help to provide an alternative etiology to injuries, especially fractures.[31-33]

FRACTURES

Fractures concerning for intentional trauma include: bilateral long bone acute fractures, metaphyseal corner fractures, long bone fracture in a non-ambulatory child, epiphyseal separations, rib/sternal/spinous process/scapular fractures, fractures of variable healing stages, digital fractures in children younger than 36 months, and vertebral subluxations/fractures without high force trauma, and severe skull fractures in children younger than 18 months. Despite being widely regarded as the superior study for detection of fractures in abused children,[23,31,34-36] skeletal surveys were found to rarely provide information supplemental to history and physical examination in newly diagnosed isolated skull fracture in infants, to help with determination of report to child protective services.[37]

HEAD INJURY

Neuroimaging has been proposed as indicated in all patients with suspected nonaccidental head trauma as well as all children younger than 6 months with any suspected injury.[23,34,38,39] Unenhanced CT of the head is the recommended imaging for initial workup and evaluation. Among cases of child abuse, in the absence of neurologic symptoms, patient age less than 1 year is the only key factor found to predict more thorough diagnostic evaluation. Considering history and examination to be poorly sensitive when compared with neuroimaging detected abnormalities, providers should have low threshold for neuroimaging in the setting of suspected child abuse,[40] as there are no specific physical findings to identify abusive head trauma. Although any physician can perform an eye examination, ophthalmology referral is recommended in the setting of concern for abusive head trauma, given the subjective nature of funduscopy and rendering a diagnosis of retinal hemorrhage.

VISCERAL TRAUMA

Esophageal, cardiac, pulmonary, or intraabdominal injury can be caused by many different methods of abuse with variable presenting signs and symptoms. Low threshold is warranted to perform such imaging, especially considering the need for early diagnosis of such organ injury with prompt intervention.

DIFFERENTIAL DIAGNOSIS

A broad knowledge of skin diseases provides a unique insight into those diagnoses that may mimic various forms of abuse, namely, child abuse (Tables 102-3 and 102-4) and sexual abuse (Table 102-5).

ELDERLY ABUSE

Diagnosis of abuse can be especially challenging in the elderly population because of bruising being so common in this population. Not only does the normal process of aging entail increased skin fragility, but this patient population is more likely to be on medications causing ease of bleeding, particularly blood thinners.

CLINICAL COURSE AND PROGNOSIS

Early recognition and prompt diagnosis allows for expeditious intervention to allow for appropriate medical treatment. Additionally, taking steps to provide protection from perpetrators helps to prevent recurrence and optimizes prognosis.

TABLE 102-3
Conditions Mistaken for Abusive Bruising

- True petechiae and purpura
- Disorders of coagulation
- Ehlers-Danlos syndrome
- Infections
  - Rocky Mountain spotted fever
  - Meningococcal infections
  - Group A streptococcal infections
- Palpable purpura of vasculitis
- Valsalva petechiae
- Lichen sclerosus
- Folk remedies
  - Cao gio: rubbing vigorously with a hard object such as a coin
  - Cupping: suction mark left by the cooling of a warm metal cup
- Nodular lesions mimicking deep bruises
- Neuroblastoma
- Vascular malformations
- Dermatomyositis-associated nodules
- Erythema nodosum
- Discolorations that look like bruises
- Phytophotodermatitis
- Maculae caeruleae from lice infestation
- Mongolian spots
- Dye from blue jeans
- Inflammatory conditions that mimic bruising
  - Urticaria/angioedema/urticarial vasculitis
  - Pernio
- Conditions that mimic whip marks
  - Incontinentia pigmenti
  - Striae
  - Phytophotodermatitis

TABLE 102-5
Conditions Mistaken for Sexual Abuse

- Lichen sclerosus
- Crohn disease
- Localized vulvar pemphigoid
- Langerhans cell histiocytosis
- Perianal streptococcal dermatitis
- Hemangiomas
- Urethral prolapse
- Entities that look like condylomata acuminata
  - Focal epithelial hyperplasia
  - Darier disease
  - Lymphangioma circumscriptum
  - Pigmented vulvar hamartomas
  - Pseudoverrucous papules
  - Epidermal nevus and inflammatory linear verrucous epidermal nevus
- Entities that look like herpes simplex
  - Localized varicella/zoster
  - Allergic contact dermatitis

CHILD ABUSE

Pediatric patients who suffer from abuse that was not initially promptly diagnosed with the first offense have up to 50% risk of a second event.[41-44] One retrospective study identified children in ED thought to have accidental traumatic injuries, reporting 13% of these patients to present for second physical abuse injury within 5 years of first event.[45] In the United States, deaths related to child abuse/neglect incidence is estimated to reach up to 2500 deaths annually (predominantly of infants less than 1 year of age).[6] The World Health Organization (WHO) proposed that 13% of the 1.2 million deaths worldwide of children younger than 15 years to be due to child abuse/neglect.[6]

TABLE 102-4
Conditions Mistaken for Nonaccidental Burns

- Phytophotodermatitis
- Folk remedies (Maquas, or moxibustion): burns delivered near diseased organs or therapeutic sites as in acupuncture
- Impetigo/ecthyma
- Epidermolysis bullosa
- Immunobullous diseases
- Sunburn/xeroderma pigmentosum
- Burns from objects heated by sun
- Electric burn from an enuresis blanket
- Chemical burn from use of undiluted acetic acid
- Chemical burn from Icy Hot balm
- Chemical burn from calcium chloride
- Diaper dermatitis
- Pernio
- Fixed drug eruption

MANAGEMENT

True abuse must be reported and a thorough evaluation conducted. It is essential that practitioners develop a relationship with the institution or individual in their area who is best able to manage these difficult cases. Ideally, there should be an abuse team consisting of a dermatologist, pediatrician, social worker, medical photographer, and, when needed, pediatric subspecialists such as orthopedists, hematologists, psychologists, and gynecologists. The need for specialization in this field is highlighted by the institution in the United States of pediatric subspecialty board certification in child abuse, beginning in 2010.

It is most helpful if one's relationship is forged with the abuse team before an abuse incident and a set protocol for dealing with alleged or suspected abuse is established in the practitioner's office. Hospitalization is indicated not only for medical stabilization to workup and manage acute injuries, but also in select patients to ensure safety from his or her perpetrator. Many countries including the United States require reporting any cases of suspected abuse to appropriate government authorities. Documentation is essential and should include a recount of the (preferably quoted) spoken word (by patient and by any other involved individuals, including providers and family members) as well as detailed physical examination findings with reliance on facts. Photographs are ideal for documentation of injuries.

CHILD ABUSE

Local emergency phone numbers for reporting abuse can be obtained from the Child Welfare Information Gateway or Childhelp National Headquarters.

ELDERLY ABUSE

Information on a particular state's laws can be obtained from the National Center on Elder Abuse. The nearest medical center's social service department is well equipped to offer guidance, but the agencies listed in Table 102-6 are also helpful resources.

DOMESTIC ABUSE

The social service department at the local medical center is a good resource for information and help on domestic violence. The National Domestic Violence hotline (800-799-7233) is a 24-hour resource for women who need to find a local shelter. Other helpful organizations can be contacted (Table 102-6).

TABLE 102-6
Helpful Agencies for Information on Abuse and Domestic Violence

- Child Welfare Information Gateway, 1250 Maryland Avenue, SW, Eighth Floor, Washington, DC 20024, Ph: (800) 394-3366, email: info@childwelfare.gov, http://www.childwelfare.gov/
- Childhelp National Headquarters, 15757 N. 78th Street, Suite B, Scottsdale, AZ 85260, Ph: (480) 922-8212, http://www.childhelpusa.org
- Domestic Violence International Resources, http://www.vachss.com/help_text/domestic_violence_intl.html
- International Network for the Prevention of Elder Abuse, http://www.inpea.net, e-mail contactus@inpea.net
- International Society for Prevention of Child Abuse and Neglect, 13123 E. 16th Ave, B390, Aurora, CO 80045, Ph: (303) 864-5220, Fax: (303) 864-5222, email: ispcan@ispcan.org, http://www.ispcan.org
- National Adult Protective Services Association, 920 S. Spring Street, Suite 1200, Springfield, IL 62704, Ph: (217) 523-4431, Fax: (217) 522-6650, http://www.apsnetwork.org
- National Center on Elder Abuse, c/o Center for Community Research and Services, University of Delaware, 297 Graham Hall, Newark, DE 19716, Ph: (302) 831-3525, Fax: (302) 831-42525, e-mail ncea-info@aoa.hhs.gov, http://www.elderabusecenter.org
- National Committee for the Prevention of Elder Abuse, 1612 K Street, NW, Suite 400, Washington, DC 20006, Ph: (202) 682-4140, Fax: (202) 223-2099, email: ncpea@verizon.net, http://www.preventelderabuse.org
- National Coalition Against Domestic Violence, 1120 Lincoln Street, Suite 1603, Denver, CO 80203, Ph: (303) 839-1852, Fax: (303) 831-9251, email mainoffice@ncadv.org, http://www.ncadv.org
- National Resource Center on Domestic Violence, 6400 Flank Drive, Suite 1300, Harrisburg, PA 17112, Ph: (800) 537-2238 ext. 5, Fax (717) 545-9456, http://www.nrcdv.org

REFERENCES

1. Vandeven AM, Newton AW. Update on child physical abuse, sexual abuse, and prevention. *Curr Opin Pediatr.* 2006;18(2):201-205.
2. Flaherty EG, Sege R. Barriers to physician identification and reporting of child abuse. *Pediatr Ann.* 2005;34(5):349-356.
3. Administration for Children and Families. *Child Maltreatment Annual Report.* http://www.acf.hhs.gov/programs/cb/pubs/cm10/cm10.pdf. Published 2010.
4. *Child Maltreatment Report.* http://www.acf.hhs.gov/sites/default/files/cb/cm11.pdf. Published 2011.
5. Sedlak AJ, Mettenberg J, Basena M, et al. *Fourth National Incidence Study of Child Abuse and Neglect (NIS–4): Report to Congress.* 2010, U.S. Department of Health and Human Services, Administration for Children and Families. Washington, DC.
6. Gilbert R, Widom CS, Browne K, et al. Burden and consequences of child maltreatment in high-income countries. *Lancet.* 2009;373(9657):68-81.
7. Finkelhor D, Turner HA, Shattuck A, et al. *Prevalence of Childhood Exposure to Violence, Crime, and Abuse: Results From the National Survey of Children's Exposure to Violence.* JAMA Pediatr. 2015;169(8):746-754.
8. National Research Council. Panel to Review Risk and Prevalence of Elder Abuse and Neglect. *Elder mistreatment: Abuse, Neglect, and Exploitation in an Aging America.* Washington, DC: National Academies Press; 2003.
9. Gorbien MJ, Eisenstein AR. Elder abuse and neglect: an overview. *Clin Geriatr Med.* 2005;21(2):279-292.
10. Abbey L. Elder abuse and neglect: when home is not safe. *Clin Geriatr Med.* 2009;25(1):47-60, vi.
11. Toohey JS. Domestic violence and rape. *Med Clin North Am.* 2008;92(5):1239-1252, xii.
12. Zolotor AJ, Denham AC, Weil A. Intimate partner violence. *Obstet Gynecol Clin North Am.* 2009;36(4):847-860, xi.
13. Tsokos M. Diagnostic criteria for cutaneous injuries in child abuse: classification, findings, and interpretation. *Forensic Sci Med Pathol.* 2015;11(2):235-242.
14. Maguire S, Mann MK, Sibert J, et al. Can you age bruises accurately in children? A systematic review. *Arch Dis Child.* 2005;90(2):187-189.
15. Kellogg N. American Academy of Pediatrics Committee on Child Abuse and Neglect. The evaluation of sexual abuse in children. *Pediatrics.* 2005;116(2):506-512.
16. Anderst J, Kellogg N, Jung I. Reports of repetitive penile-genital penetration often have no definitive evidence of penetration. *Pediatrics.* 2009;124(3):e403-e409.
17. Pillai M. Genital findings in prepubertal girls: what can be concluded from an examination? *J Pediatr Adolesc Gynecol.* 2008;21(4):177-185.
18. Cohen BA, Honig P, Androphy E. Anogenital warts in children. Clinical and virologic evaluation for sexual abuse. *Arch Dermatol.* 1990;126(12):1575-1580.
19. Yeoh C, Nixon JW, Dickson W, et al. Patterns of scald injuries. *Arch Dis Child.* 1994;71(2):156-158.
20. Kos L, Shwayder T. Cutaneous manifestations of child abuse. *Pediatr Dermatol.* 2006;23(4):311-320.
21. Swerdlin A, Berkowitz C, Craft N. Cutaneous signs of child abuse. *J Am Acad Dermatol.* 2007;57(3):371-392.
22. Kemp AM, et al. Patterns of bruising in preschool children—a longitudinal study. *Arch Dis Child.* 2015; 100(5): 426-31.
23. Christian CW. Committee on Child Abuse and Neglect, American Academy of Pediatrics. The evaluation of

suspected child physical abuse. *Pediatrics.* 2015;135(5): e1337-e1354.
24. Child Maltreatment 2007. U.S. Department of Health and Human Services, Administration on Children, Youth and Families, Washington, DC.
25. Hettler J, Greenes DS. Can the initial history predict whether a child with a head injury has been abused? *Pediatrics.* 2003;111(3):602-607.
26. Kellogg ND. American Academy of Pediatrics Committee on Child Abuse and Neglect. Evaluation of suspected child physical abuse. *Pediatrics.* 2007;119(6):1232-1241.
27. Minford AM, Richards EM. Excluding medical and haematological conditions as a cause of bruising in suspected non-accidental injury. *Arch Dis Child Educ Pract Ed.* 2010;95(1):2-8.
28. Cameron CM, Lazoritz S, Calhoun AD. Blunt abdominal injury: simultaneously occurring liver and pancreatic injury in child abuse. *Pediatr Emerg Care.* 1997;13(5):334-336.
29. Lindberg DM, Shapiro RA, Blood EA, et al. Utility of hepatic transaminases in children with concern for abuse. *Pediatrics.* 2013;131(2):268-275.
30. Jenny C. Committee on Child Abuse and Neglect. Evaluating infants and young children with multiple fractures. *Pediatrics.* 2006;118(3):1299-1303.
31. Section on Radiology; American Academy of Pediatrics. Diagnostic imaging of child abuse. *Pediatrics.* 2009;123(5):1430-1435.
32. Merten DF, Radkowski MA, Leonidas JC. The abused child: a radiological reappraisal. *Radiology.* 1983;146(2):377-381.
33. Ablin DS, Sane SM. Non-accidental injury: confusion with temporary brittle bone disease and mild osteogenesis imperfecta. *Pediatr Radiol.* 1997;27(2):111-113.
34. Meyer JS, Gunderman R, Coley BD, et al. ACR Appropriateness Criteria((R)) on suspected physical abuse-child. *J Am Coll Radiol.* 2011;8(2):87-94.
35. Offiah A, van Rijn RR, Perez-Rossello JM, et al. Skeletal imaging of child abuse (non-accidental injury). *Pediatr Radiol.* 2009;39(5):461-470.
36. British Society of Paediatric Radiology. *Standard for skeletal surveys in suspected non-accidental injury (NAI) in children.* www.bspr.org.uk/nai.htm. Published 2009.
37. Wood JN, Christian CW, Adams CM, et al. Skeletal surveys in infants with isolated skull fractures. *Pediatrics.* 2009;123(2):e247-e252.
38. Datta S, Stoodley N, Jayawant S, et al. Neuroradiological aspects of subdural haemorrhages. *Arch Dis Child.* 2005;90(9):947-951.
39. Rubin DM, Christian CW, Bilaniuk LT, et al. Occult head injury in high-risk abused children. *Pediatrics.* 2003;111(6, pt 1):1382-1386.
40. Laskey AL, Holsti M, Runyan DK, et al. Occult head trauma in young suspected victims of physical abuse. *J Pediatr.* 2004;144(6):719-722.
41. DePanfilis D, Zuravin SJ. Predicting child maltreatment recurrences during treatment. *Child Abuse Negl.* 1999;23(8):729-743.
42. Drake B, Jonson-Reid M, Way I, et al. Substantiation and recidivism. *Child Maltreat.* 2003;8(4):248-260.
43. Connell CM, Vanderploeg JJ, Katz KH, et al. Maltreatment following reunification: predictors of subsequent Child Protective Services contact after children return home. *Child Abuse Negl.* 2009;33(4):218-228.
44. Fluke JD, Shusterman GR, Hollinshead D, et al. *Rereporting and recurrence of child maltreatment: Findings from NCANDS.* ASPE Reports 2005. http://aspe.hhs.gov/hsp/05/child-maltreat-rereporting.
45. Friedman SB, Morse CW. Child abuse: a five-year follow-up of early case finding in the emergency department. *Pediatrics.* 1974;54(4):404-410.

Skin Changes Across the Span of Life

PART 19

第十九篇　皮肤在人一生中的变化

Chapter 103 :: Neonatal Dermatology
:: Raegan Hunt, Mary Wu Chang, & Kara N. Shah

第一百零三章

新生儿皮肤病学

中文导读

　　新生儿期定义为出生后的前30天。许多新生儿皮肤疾病是良性的和自限性的，但也可能发生严重的疾病，系统性疾病或相关遗传综合征的皮肤表现不应被忽视。

　　1. 新生儿皮肤　从生理学角度了解正常胚胎发育和新生儿皮肤生理，有助于了解出生后皮肤发生的适应性变化，以及指导足月和早产儿恰当的皮肤护理。作者介绍了表皮、胎毛、小汗腺、大汗腺、皮脂腺等皮肤附属器在胚胎时期的发育，以及皮脂的形成、组成及其抗菌、抗氧化和屏障功能等重要作用。特别关注了表皮屏障的发展，认为新生婴儿角质层的过度成熟是对空气的反应，这有助于表皮屏障功能的发展。

　　作者指出早产儿，是指妊娠37周之前出生的新生儿。特别是34周前出生的早产儿，表皮屏障功能明显下降，感染和出现败血症的风险增加。但关于应用以凡士林为基础的润肤剂治疗屏障功能的不完善的作用并不确定。

　　新生儿皮肤护理方面，作者讲述了欧洲专家小组提供的关于新生儿日常皮肤护理的建议。认为恰当的皮肤护理应包括避免过度沐浴，保持表皮屏障，减少接触潜在的刺激物或过敏原，以及清除排泄物，并进一步作了解析。此外，作者提出：局部外用物质引起全身毒性的风险增加，这在很大程度上是新生儿体表面积与体重的比值比较大的结果。这些不良影响在早产儿中会放大，因为，早产儿的体表面积与体重的比值要比足月新生儿更大。皮肤屏障功能障碍的新生儿，如先天性鱼鳞病，局部药物和化学物质的全身吸收风险更加增加。

　　2. 检查

　　（1）采集完整的病史。包括妊娠史、分

娩史以及家族史等；还应包括孕期的药物接触史和感染性疾病史，如水痘、风疹或性传播疾病等。此外，妊娠和分娩的其他并发症，以及胎盘剥脱时间等均是有用的临床信息。

（2）全面检查。作者认为，在良好的光源下对新生儿的皮肤进行全面检查是有价值的。特别是一些早期的皮损，变化非常细微。所有的先天性病变都需要彻底检查评估，以帮助排除相关综合征或系统疾病。当诊断不明确且结果将影响治疗时，应考虑活检。面部中线、头皮或脊柱的病变可能与中枢神经连接有关，在进行皮肤活检之前，应进行影像学检查以排除中枢神经病变。

3. 新生儿皮肤疾病　作者依次讲述了新生儿一过性皮肤病、胎记、新生儿发育异常导致的一些皮肤疾病、新生儿感染性皮肤疾病，最后，还讲述了新生儿皮炎、皮肤肿瘤及新生儿遗传性皮肤病等。

（1）新生儿一过性皮肤病：包括继发性头部血肿、Milia、皮脂腺增生、毒性新生儿红斑、短暂性新生儿黑色素疱病、热疹、吮吸水疱、斑驳痣及新生儿痤疮，讲述了这些疾病的大致病因及临床表现。

（2）分类讲述新生儿常见的胎记：与颜色相关的胎记包括皮肤黑素细胞增多症（蒙古斑）、咖啡牛奶斑、先天性黑素细胞痣（CMN）、色素嵌合体、色素减退痣、迷走痣等。特别提出，巨细胞CMN与黑色素瘤风险增加有关。

与血管相关的胎记包括单纯性胎记、婴儿血管瘤、血管畸形。重点讲述了单纯性胎记的发病率、发病部位、临床表现及转归。特别提出，虽然大多数单纯性胎记在出生后2年逐渐消失，但那些发生在枕部头皮的往往会持续存在。

还讲述了两个其他类型的胎记：皮脂腺痣和表皮痣。重点讲述了表皮痣的临床表现及治疗。

（3）发育异常：发育异常的皮肤和皮下组织和结构，从常见的、良性的、轻微的，如多生乳头，到主要的异常如皮肤再生发育不全，均可作为潜在严重异常的标记。

文章还讲述了新生儿中较少见的其他异常，包括鼻神经胶质瘤等，并分别简述了它们的形成原因和治疗手段。作者提出，了解哪些病变意味着可能有其他相关畸形的风险，对诊断和治疗很重要。对于鼻腔和面部中线的病变，在进行皮肤活检之前，需要进行放射学评估以排除颅内连接。

（4）新生儿感染：包括细菌感染、先天性病毒感染、新生儿单纯疱疹病毒感染及真菌感染。不到两个月的婴儿免疫系统不成熟，危及生命的败血症可以迅速地不知不觉地发展。需认真对待一些细微的迹象，如体温下降、喂养不良、肌张力差或其他非特异性体征等。作者具体阐述了这些感染性皮肤病的病因、临床表现、诊断及鉴别诊断及其治疗方法。

（5）红皮病：红皮病预示着一种严重的潜在疾病。许多遗传、感染、炎症、代谢和免疫紊乱都可出现红皮病，还有一些可能与新生儿期死亡有关。此外，红皮病容易导致潜在的危及生命的并发症，如败血症、脱水和电解质失衡。

炎性皮肤疾病可能出现在出生后的头几周，包括脂溢性皮炎、婴儿牛皮癣、青少年毛毛红斑糠疹、特应性或非特应性湿疹。它们与红皮病有关。

此外，几种先天代谢障碍，包括全新羧化酶合成酶缺乏和生物素酶缺乏，都可导致4种生物素依赖性羧化酶的缺乏(多重羧化酶缺乏)，可出现皮炎症状。

（6）两种常见的炎症性皮肤病：脂溢性皮炎和尿布皮炎。

脂溢性皮炎是一种婴儿期常见的炎症性皮肤病。最常见的表现是发生于头皮的油腻性黄色鳞屑并伴有轻微的红斑。作者进一步讲述了其病因、临床表现、诊断及鉴别诊断及其治疗方法。

尿布皮炎是婴幼儿常见的皮肤问题。

导致尿布皮炎发生的因素较多,主要因素是长时间暴露在潮湿环境中导致摩擦损伤的增加、屏障功能的降低和对刺激物的反应性增加。相关因素包括接触尿液和粪便、粪便蛋白水解酶和脂质消化酶、皮肤pH值的升高和念珠菌的重复感染。尿布皮炎的种类繁多,简单讲述了刺激物尿布皮炎、过敏性接触尿布皮炎、CANDIDAL尿布皮炎、假疣状丘疹和结节、JACQUET侵蚀性皮炎、肉芽肿GLU-TEALE INFANTUM等,并列表讲述了尿布皮炎的治疗。

(7)皮肤肿瘤:简述了婴儿肌纤维瘤病、婴儿纤维性错构瘤、幼儿数字纤维瘤、先天性平滑肌错构瘤,以及神经母细胞瘤、先天性白血病、朗格汉斯细胞组织细胞增生症、皮肤的肥大细胞增多症。

(8)出现在新生儿期的遗传性皮肤病:包括大疱性表皮松解症(EB)、先天性鱼鳞病、外胚层发育不良、色素失禁等。

(9)新生儿的其他皮肤病:包括新生儿皮下脂肪坏死、新生儿硬化症、早产皮肤松弛症(anetoderma of prematurity)、先天性毛细血管扩张症,并对它们进行了简单讲述。

〔刘芳芬〕

AT-A-GLANCE

- Many dermatologic diseases exhibit different manifestations in newborns, infants, and children, and a subset of skin conditions are only encountered in neonates.
- Certain neonatal skin conditions require special attention as they may be a sign of a serious health condition.
- The medical history and methods of clinical examination in neonates differ from the approaches used with older children and adults. It is very important to elicit a thorough maternal and obstetric history with an emphasis on maternal health and any complications during pregnancy or delivery.
- The neonate has increased risk for systemic toxicity from topically applied substances; the risk is even greater in premature infants.

Neonatal skin diseases are a fascinating and unique spectrum of dermatologic conditions. They encompass a broad range of diagnoses, including manifestations of neonatal or maternal infection, developmental defects, cutaneous features of genetic disorders, birthmarks, malignancy, complications of prematurity, and benign transient clinical findings. An understanding of benign cutaneous conditions of newborns and an ability to identify more worrisome presentations are essential to the care of the neonate.

Appropriate care of the neonatal patient requires a thorough understanding of the maternal health history, including maternal disease as well as pregnancy complications.

NEONATES

The neonatal period is defined as the first 30 days of life. Infancy is defined as beginning after the first 30 days of life. Although this chapter focuses on conditions presenting in the neonatal period, some conditions may occur in infancy as well. Even though many neonatal skin diseases are benign and self-limiting, serious disease may occur, and cutaneous manifestations of systemic disease or an associated genetic syndrome should not be overlooked.

Full-term infants are born between 37 and 42 weeks of gestation. Preterm or premature infants are born before 37 weeks of gestation.

NEONATAL SKIN

NEONATAL SKIN PHYSIOLOGY

The skin with its associated appendages provides several important functions. It serves as a barrier against microbes and environmental and other external toxins, provides thermoregulation, prevents transepidermal water loss, and aids in sensory perception. Knowledge of normal embryologic development and the physiology of neonatal skin is helpful for understanding the adaptive changes that occur after birth and for guiding appropriate skin care in both full-term and preterm neonates.

The epidermis begins to develop around 6 weeks of gestational age as a basal cell layer and a superficial periderm layer; the periderm does not contribute to the formation of the stratified squamous epithelium and is shed during the end of the second trimester.[1] Stratification of the fetal epidermis begins in the eighth week of gestation; terminal differentiation commences first in the skin appendages between the 11th and 15th weeks of gestation and then in the interfollicular epidermis; by 22 to 24 weeks of gestation the epidermis consists of 4 to 5 cell layers.[2,3] The dermal–epidermal junction is evident by 8 weeks of gestational age, and collagen fiber formation and organization of the papillary and reticular dermis occurs by 15 weeks of gestation; elastic fibers are noted at 22 to 24 weeks of gestation.[4,5] Hair follicles begin to develop around the 14th week of gestation; lanugo hair production begins around the 18th week of gestation and is complete by the 28th week of gestation.[6,7] Eccrine gland development is completed during the second trimester, although the eccrine glands are not functional until after birth. Apocrine gland formation occurs somewhat later in fetal development, and the apocrine glands are transiently functional during the third trimester of pregnancy. Sebaceous gland formation begins around the 16th week of gestation, and the sebaceous glands are functional shortly after formation; sebaceous gland products contribute significantly to the lipid composition of vernix caseosa.[8,9]

In utero, the skin of the fetus is protected by the vernix caseosa and is immersed in amniotic fluid. Vernix production correlates with epidermal maturation and the formation of the stratum corneum; production begins around the 36th week of gestation. Vernix caseosa is composed of water-containing corneocytes in a lipid matrix composed predominantly of nonpolar lipid such as sterol esters and triglycerides.[9,10] It provides antimicrobial, antioxidant, and barrier functions, and contains multiple antimicrobial peptides, including LL-37, cystatin A, and calgranulins.[11,12] After birth, the vernix is often manually removed and the skin exposed to room air, although some experts question the validity of this practice.

Of particular interest is the development of the epidermal barrier, including postnatal development of barrier function in term and preterm neonates.[13] After birth, the skin of the neonate undergoes a series of changes in adaptation to the extrauterine terrestrial environment. Additional maturation of the stratum corneum in neonates occurs in response to air, which contributes to the development of a functional epidermal barrier. It is generally accepted that full barrier function is achieved within 2 to 4 weeks of life in term neonates, and some experts believe that the barrier is fully developed at birth in this population.[14] In preterm infants, the epidermal barrier in immature. Barrier stabilization is a dynamic process dependent upon a balance between several biologic and environmental factors. Evaluation of parameters such as skin thickness, skin pH, transepidermal water loss (TEWL), and stratum corneum hydration indicate that neonatal skin undergoes continuous adjustment to the extrauterine environment. In full-term neonates, after drying of the skin in the first few hours after birth, TEWL is equivalent to that seen in adults, with the exception of some variability because for site and ambient temperature and/or humidity, including the diaper area, where TEWL vales are higher and contribute to impaired barrier function and risk for diaper dermatitis.[15,16]

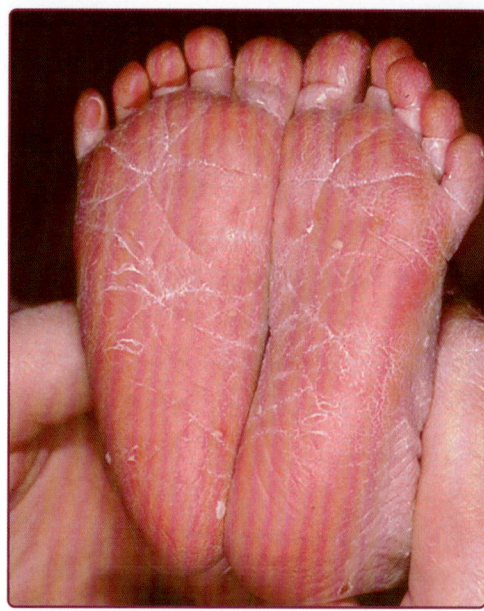

Figure 103-1 The feet of a postterm newborn. The dry, hyperlinear, and scaly skin is typical of babies born after 40 weeks of gestation. Incidentally, pustules of transient neonatal pustular melanosis are also seen.

One of the most visible early manifestations of the adaptive process is desquamation of the upper layers of the stratum corneum, which occurs in all infants. Postterm infants born after 40 weeks of gestation have decreased amounts of vernix caseosa on the skin and more notable desquamation (Fig. 103-1). During the first 3 months of life, the thickness of the stratum corneum decreases, and epidermal thickness increases, along with the formation of dermal papillae and epidermal ridges.[17]

Normal skin pH is acidic; the acidic pH of the stratum corneum results from multiple factors, including the production of free fatty acids from phospholipids and the presence of sweat and sebum.[18] In the term and preterm neonate, skin pH is more alkaline than that of older infants and adults, and it decreases gradually over the first few weeks of life.[19-21]

Sebum production is high in the neonate, and decreases over the first few months of life.[22] Eccrine sweating is present in term neonates, but delayed in preterm neonates.[23,24]

PREMATURITY

Premature neonates, particularly those born before 34 weeks of gestation, have markedly decreased epidermal barrier function. The functional maturation of the stratum corneum begins around 24 weeks of gestational age, and in preterm neonates born before 26 weeks of gestation, functional maturation of the epidermal barrier may take longer than 4 weeks.[25,26] TEWL is significantly increased in preterm and low-birthweight neonates, reflecting epidermal barrier immaturity, and TEWL increases with decreasing gestational age.[27] Use of radiant warmers and phototherapy also contribute to increased TEWL.[28,29] Impaired epidermal barrier function places the preterm infant at risk for electrolyte imbalances, poor thermoregulation, dehydration, increased absorption of topical agents, and infection.

Increased skin fragility is also noted in preterm infants. Epidermal and dermal injury may lead to significant cutaneous pain even with routine handling and nursing care. The premature infant is at risk for infection and sepsis from skin-associated organisms entering through breaks in the thin and fragile skin and via iatrogenic portals of entry such as indwelling venous catheters. Thermal regulation is dysfunctional because of a thin subcutaneous fat layer, decreased ability to sweat, poor autonomic control of cutaneous blood vessels, and a large surface-area-to-body-mass ratio. In the nursery, the premature infant is usually placed in a temperature- and humidity-controlled isolette until temperature and fluid regulation stabilize.

In the 1990s, researchers reported that application of petrolatum-based emollient therapy appeared to be beneficial by decreasing TEWL in hospitalized preterm infants.[30] Subsequently, many neonatal intensive care units began to implement the use of various emollients and skin-care regimens. However, while skin integrity consistently improved, a threefold increase in the incidence of systemic candidiasis was reported after emollient therapy was implemented in extremely low-birthweight (≤1000 g) premature infants in one neonatal intensive care unit.[31] Similarly, an outbreak of systemic candidiasis occurred in very-low-birthweight neonates (≤1500 g) using emollient therapy in a different neonatal intensive care unit.[32] A 2004 Cochrane review concluded that prophylactic application of topical ointments increased the risk for nosocomial infection and advised against their routine use in preterm infants. In contrast, randomized, controlled studies in a population of impoverished Bangladeshi preterm neonates have demonstrated decreased mortality rates when sunflower seed oil or Aquaphor ointment was applied by massage, compared to premature infants not receiving massage or emollients, suggesting that in certain populations, such as those without access to sophisticated neonatal intensive care practices, use of emollients may be beneficial in high-risk preterm infants.[33] A 2016 Cochrane review concluded that the use of topical emollients in preterm infants did not prevent invasive infection or death.[34] Until prospective, controlled trials are performed, neonates receiving petrolatum-based emollient therapy should be carefully monitored for infections, particularly those infants with birthweights less than 1500 g.

SKIN CARE IN THE NEONATE

Recommendations for routine skin care in the neonate, as provided by a panel of European experts, include bathing in water 2 to 3 times per week for no more than 5 to 10 minutes with use of a gentle soap-free liquid skin cleanser as opposed to a washcloth; application of an emollient after bathing is also recommended.[35] An appropriate skin-care regimen serves to minimize overbathing, maintain the epidermal barrier, minimize exposure to potential irritants or allergens, and remove fecal material.

Well-meaning parents often bathe their infants too frequently and use a multitude of products on their infant's skin. In addition to irritation and asteatosis, these practices may increase the risk of allergic contact dermatitis in infants. It has been estimated that the average newborn is exposed to approximately 10 skin care products in the first month of life, leading to exposure to more than 50 different chemicals, ranging from mildly toxic to toxic.[36] Parents should be taught that "less is best."[37] Use of a skin cleanser in healthy, term infants has been shown to have no effect on TEWL, skin surface pH, and stratum corneum hydration, as compared to bathing with water alone.[38] Skin care in full-term neonates from birth to 8 weeks of age with cleansing gel, gel plus cream, water alone, or water plus cream showed no significant differences in skin condition, microbial colonization, and sebum level.[39,40]

Neonates have an increased risk for systemic toxicity from topically applied substances. This is largely a result of the greater surface-area-to-body-mass ratio in the newborn. Preterm neonates have an even greater surface-area-to-body-mass ratio than term neonates. In addition, the metabolism, excretion, distribution, and protein binding of substances can differ significantly in neonates as compared to adults, which increases the risk of toxicity; these adverse effects may be magnified in the preterm neonate. Local or systemic toxicity can occur in the term or preterm neonate not only from topical medications, but also from soaps, lotions, and other cleansing solutions. Neonates with disorders of skin-barrier function, such as congenital ichthyosis, are at increased risk for systemic absorption of topical medications and chemicals.[41]

EXAMINATION TECHNIQUES

For the neonate, a complete medical history includes gestational and birth history as well as family history. Exposures during pregnancy, including medications, illicit drugs, and infectious diseases, such as varicella, rubella, or sexually transmitted diseases, are important to review in detail. Additionally, other complications of pregnancy and parturition and the appearance of the placenta offer useful clinical information.

Comprehensive examination of the skin of a neonate in good lighting is valuable, particularly as some skin findings are initially subtle. For example, a vasoconstricted macule or an erosion can be the presenting sign of an infantile hemangioma.[42] All congenital lesions (eg, pigmented lesions, vascular birthmarks, aplasia cutis, cutaneous nodules) warrant thorough evaluation to help exclude associated syndromes or internal disease. Biopsy should be considered when the diagnosis is unclear and the outcome will impact management. Midline face, scalp, or spine lesions may be associated with CNS connections and should be imaged to rule out CNS communication prior to performing a skin biopsy.

The newborn is completely dependent on caretakers, and the family structure and social support network should be considered when developing treatment plans. Some new parents may feel overwhelmed or unprepared to deal with a skin condition in their infant. At times, the treatment priorities of the parents may not seem to coincide with the best interests of the newborn at this early stage in their development. Medical and surgical decision making for affected infants is typically aimed at improving function in favor of cosmesis.

DISEASES OF NEONATES

TRANSIENT DERMATOSES OF THE NEONATE

Benign skin conditions encountered in newborns that tend to resolve by 30 days of age are considered to be transient. They are very common, and the majority do not require intervention. These conditions are discussed below, and Table 103-1 lists a selected differential diagnosis based on broad categories of skin lesions encountered in neonates and infants.

CAPUT SUCCEDANEUM AND CEPHALOHEMATOMA

Trauma during delivery may induce one of several injuries to the scalp of the neonate.[43] These range from common and usually benign conditions such as caput succedaneum and cephalohematoma to subgaleal hemorrhage, which is a serious, potentially life-threatening condition.

Caput succedaneum results from subcutaneous edema over the presenting part of the head owing to pressure against the cervix and is a common occurrence in newborns. Caput succedaneum is soft to palpation with ill-defined borders. Petechiae and ecchymosis also may be noted. The edema resolves spontaneously over 7 to 10 days.

Cephalohematoma results from rupture of the diploic and/or emissary veins and subsequent subperiosteal collection of blood. It is associated with birth trauma or the use of vacuum extraction vaginal delivery. Areas of hemorrhage respect the suture lines, are well-delimited, usually unilateral, and feel firm to palpation. An underlying skull fracture may be present. Cephalohematomas usually resolve without sequelae over several weeks, but calcification may occur.

Subgaleal hemorrhage is also associated with birth trauma and occurs when there is bleeding between the periosteum of the skull and the galea as a result of damage to the emissary veins. Extensive hemorrhage may occur with either subgaleal hemorrhage or cephalohematoma, and may lead to anemia and neonatal hyperbilirubinemia. With a subgaleal hemorrhage, bleeding can be catastrophic and result in hypovolemic shock or disseminated intravascular coagulation.

MILIA

Milia are pinpoint to 2-mm papules representing benign, superficial epidermal inclusion cysts. Usually few in number, they are seen most commonly on the

TABLE 103-1

Selected Differential Diagnosis of Neonates and Infants

- Pustules
    - Erythema toxicum neonatorum
    - Transient neonatal pustular melanosis
    - Congenital candidiasis
    - Pustular psoriasis
    - Langerhans cell histiocytosis
    - Neonatal cephalic pustulosis
    - Bacterial sepsis
    - Herpes simplex infection
- Blisters
    - Sucking blisters
    - Herpes simplex virus
    - Aplasia cutis congenita
    - Cutaneous mastocytosis
    - Epidermolysis bullosa
    - Neonatal pemphigus
    - Varicella
    - Impetigo
    - Incontinentia pigmenti
    - Epidermolytic ichthyosis
- The red scaly baby
    - Physiologic scaling and redness (postdates) infant
    - Psoriasis
    - Atopic dermatitis
    - Scabies
    - Seborrheic dermatitis
    - Immunodeficiency
    - Hypohidrotic ectodermal dysplasia
    - Netherton syndrome
    - Acrodermatitis enteropathica
- The collodion baby
    - Lamellar ichthyosis
    - Congenital ichthyosiform erythroderma
    - Gaucher syndrome
    - Trichothiodystrophy
    - Neutral lipid storage disorder
- The "blueberry muffin" baby
    - TORCH infections
    - Congenital leukemia
    - Congenital self-healing reticulohistiocytosis
    - Blue rubber bleb nevus syndrome
    - Twin–twin transfusion

TORCH, toxoplasmosis, other agents, especially syphilis, but also hepatitis B, coxsackievirus, Epstein-Barr virus, varicella-zoster virus, and human parvovirus, rubella, cytomegalovirus, herpes simplex virus.

face in newborns and may be present in the oral cavity as well, where they are called *Epstein pearls*. Congenital milia en plaque also has been reported.[44] Milia generally resolve spontaneously within a few weeks of life. When persistent and/or numerous, they may be seen in association with several rare genetic disorders, including oral-facial-digital syndrome, Bazex-Dupré-Christol syndrome, and Basan syndrome.

SEBACEOUS GLAND HYPERPLASIA

At least 50% of normal newborns have sebaceous gland hyperplasia (Fig. 103-2). Minute (<1 mm) yellow macules or papules are commonly seen at the opening of pilosebaceous follicles over the nose and central forehead of term newborns. This is a benign condition thought to occur secondary to maternal androgen stimulation of the sebaceous glands; it typically resolves spontaneously by 4 to 6 months of age.

ERYTHEMA TOXICUM NEONATORUM

Erythema toxicum neonatorum is an idiopathic, common skin condition seen in up to 75% of term newborns. It is rarely seen in premature infants. Blotchy erythematous patches 1 to 3 cm in diameter with a 1- to 4-mm central vesicle or pustule are characteristic of erythema toxicum neonatorum (Fig. 103-3). The eruption usually begins at 24 to 48 hours of age, but delayed eruption as late as 10 days of age has been documented.[45] These follicular-based lesions can be located anywhere but tend to spare the palms and soles. A smear of the central vesicle or pustule contents will reveal numerous eosinophils on Wright-stained preparations. A peripheral blood eosinophilia of up to 20% may be associated, particularly in infants with

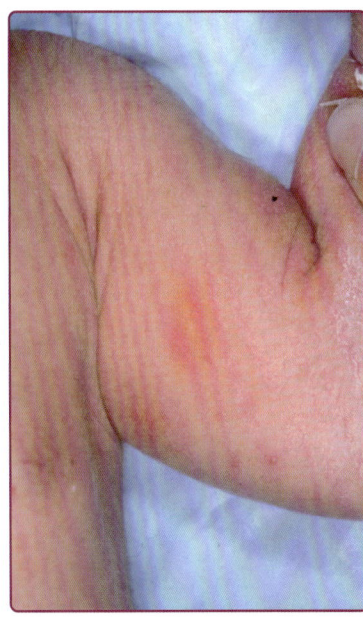

Figure 103-3 Erythema toxicum neonatorum. Erythematous macules, some with a tiny central papule or pustule, on the arm of a 1-day-old newborn.

numerous lesions. Erythema toxicum neonatorum is benign and clears spontaneously by 2 to 3 weeks of age without residua.

TRANSIENT NEONATAL PUSTULAR MELANOSIS

Transient neonatal pustular melanosis is an idiopathic pustular eruption of the newborn that resolves with hyperpigmented macules (Fig. 103-4). It is less common than erythema toxicum neonatorum and is more prevalent among newborns with darkly pigmented skin. Lesions are usually present at birth or shortly thereafter, but may appear as late as 3 weeks of age. The eruption is characterized by multiple superficial vesicles and pustules, with ruptured lesions evident as collarettes of scale. Hyperpigmented macules are also often present at birth or develop at the sites of resolving pustules or vesicles within several hours of birth or during the first days of life. Lesions can occur anywhere but are common on the forehead and mandibular area. The palms and soles may be involved. Smear of the vesicle or pustule contents will reveal a predominance of neutrophils with occasional eosinophils on Wright-stained preparations. The pustules usually disappear within 5 to 7 days; residual pigmented macules resolve over several weeks.

MILIARIA RUBRA AND CRYSTALLINA

Miliaria or "heat rash" is a common disorder of the eccrine glands that typically results from fever or overheating such as may occur when neonates are swaddled. Eccrine gland occlusion by sweat and possibly by the extracellular polysaccharides of *Staphylococcus*

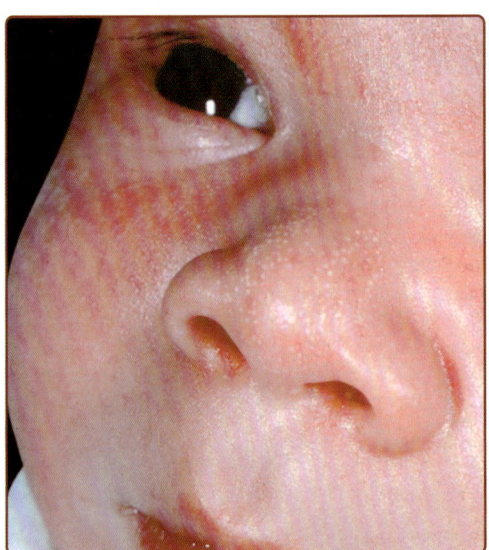

Figure 103-2 Sebaceous hyperplasia on the nose of a 1-day-old infant.

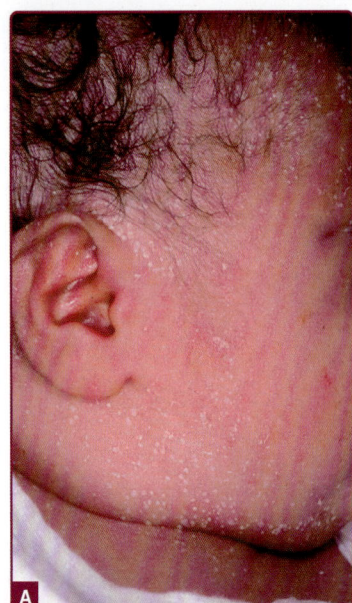

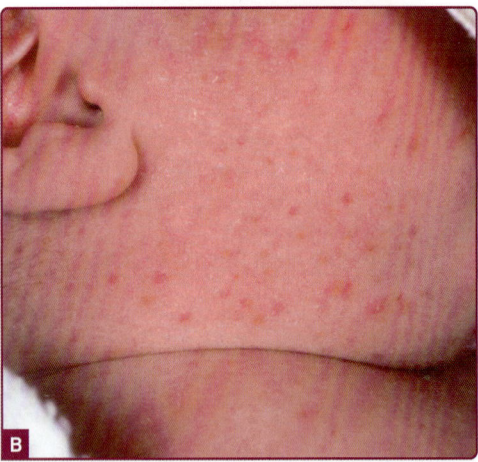

Figure 103-4 Transient neonatal pustular melanosis. **A,** A newborn with congenital, thin-walled pustules that rupture easily. **B,** Hyperpigmented macules appeared by 10 hours of age.

epidermidis leads to the development of minute superficial subcorneal vesicles (miliaria crystallina). A deeper level of occlusion within the epidermis with associated inflammation leads to miliaria rubra, which manifests as 1- to 3-mm erythematous papules and/or papulopustules. The condition resolves spontaneously once the inciting factors are addressed.

MOTTLING AND CUTIS MARMORATA

Mottling is a blotchy or lace-like pattern of dusky erythema over the extremities and trunk of neonates that occurs with exposure to cold environments. Virtually all babies demonstrate mottling at some time during the newborn period as a consequence of immature autonomic control of the cutaneous vascular plexus. This physiologic mottling disappears on rewarming, differentiating it from cutis marmorata telangiectatica congenita and livedo reticularis. Physiologic mottling resolves spontaneously by 6 months of age.

HARLEQUIN COLOR CHANGE

Harlequin color change is a rare vascular phenomenon that occurs in in full-term newborns, as well as in low-birthweight and premature infants, and in infants exposed to hypoxia or systemic treatment with prostaglandins. In harlequin color change, when the neonate is placed on one side, an erythematous flush with a sharp demarcation at the midline develops on the dependent side, and the upper half of the body becomes pale. The color change usually subsides within a few seconds of placing the baby in the supine position but may persist for as long as 20 minutes. Presentation may be localized to a single body area or may be more generalized. The exact mechanism of this unusual phenomenon is not known, but it may be a result of immaturity of autonomic vasomotor control.[46] Harlequin color change is seldom seen after 10 days of age, and if noted to be persistent or to develop at an older age, may be a manifestation of an underlying neurologic disorder.

SUCKING BLISTERS

Sucking blisters may be present at birth as the result of intrauterine sucking, but are more commonly seen during the first weeks of life. Sucking blisters are usually solitary, intact, oval or linear blisters, superficial erosions, or crusts, arising on noninflamed skin on the dorsal aspect of the forearms, wrists, or fingers; a callus may be noted on the upper lip. They resolve within a few days. If the affected extremity is brought up to the infant's mouth, the infant will often commence sucking at the site, confirming the diagnosis.

BENIGN NEONATAL CEPHALIC PUSTULOSIS

Neonatal acneiform facial eruptions usually develop within the first 30 days of life and are estimated to occur in 50% of newborns (Fig. 103-5). Neonatal cephalic pustulosis is most common, and has been attributed to overgrowth of *Malassezia* spp.[47,48] Most cases resolve spontaneously, but the eruption can be treated topically with ketoconazole. True infantile acne is less common and can be distinguished by later age of onset and the presence of comedones, acneiform cysts, and scars (Fig. 103-6).

BIRTHMARKS

Birthmarks are common in newborns, and range from common, benign conditions such as nevus simplex

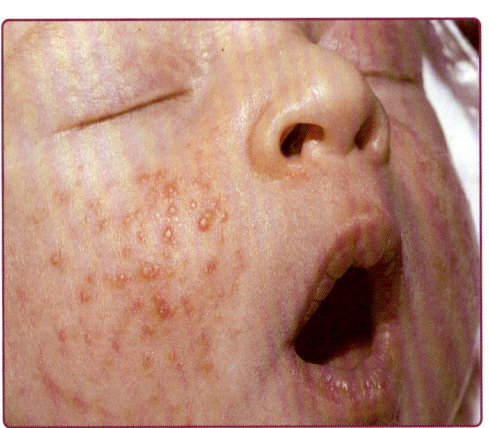

Figure 103-5 Benign neonatal cephalic pustulosis. Tiny papulopustules on the cheeks of a 3-week-old infant.

TABLE 103-2
Common Birthmarks in the Newborn

- Dermal melanocytosis (commonly called "Mongolian spots")
- Nevus simplex (salmon patch, "stork bite," "angel's kiss")
- Port-wine stain (capillary malformation)
- Infantile hemangioma
- Epidermal nevus and nevus sebaceus
- Congenital melanocytic nevi
- Nevus depigmentosus
- Café-au-lait spots

and dermal melanocytosis to more worrisome conditions such as large segmental hemangiomas and giant congenital melanocytic nevi. Although most birthmarks are of little medical or psychosocial consequence, the social and cultural impact of a disfiguring birthmark on both the patient and the parents should not be underestimated.[49] Table 103-2 lists common birthmarks.

PIGMENTARY BIRTHMARKS

Dermal Melanocytosis: Dermal melanocytosis (commonly called "Mongolian spots") is characterized by blue-gray patches typically located on the lumbosacral or buttock skin of infants. Collections of dermal melanocytes cause these common birthmarks, which are seen in 80% to 90% of infants of color and only 5% of white infants.[50,51]

Café-au-Lait Macules: Café-au-lait macules are well-demarcated tan macules or patches. Solitary café-au-lait macules are very common, however, the presence of multiple café-au-lait macules raises the possibility of neurofibromatosis type 1 (see Chap. 135). It is important to remember that findings of neurofibromatosis type 1 are progressive, so a potential

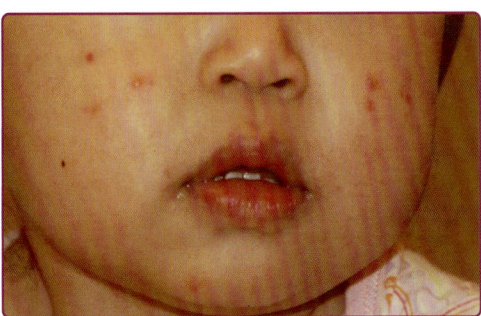

Figure 103-6 Infantile acne. True comedones and inflammatory papules are noted on the cheeks of a healthy 10-month-old girl.

neurofibromatosis type 1 diagnosis cannot be excluded based on neonatal examination of an infant with 1 or a few café-au-lait macules. Less-common genetic disorders are also associated with multiple café-au-lait macules. A large, geographic café-au-lait macule with a "coast-of-Maine" appearance is most likely to be an isolated skin finding but may be a marker for McCune-Albright syndrome.

Congenital Melanocytic Nevi: Melanocytic nevi that are present at birth or that appear within the first few months of life are "classic" congenital melanocytic nevi (CMN). Additionally, "late-onset" or "tardive" CMN may appear any time before age 2 years, and both are considered to be programmed from birth. CMN are typically barely elevated melanocytic papules or plaques that range in color from light brown to very dark brown or black. Some CMN have well-demarcated, geographic borders, and internal speckled patterns may be seen.

CMN enlarge proportionately as children grow. It is estimated that the size of CMN between infancy and adulthood will increase 1.7-fold on the head, whereas CMN on the lower extremities will increase 3.3-fold, and CMN of other sites will increase 2.8-fold. CMN are classified based on projected adult size into the following categories: small (<1.5 cm); medium (M1 1.5 to 10 cm, M2 >10 to 20 cm); large (L1 >20 to 30 cm, L2 >30 to 40 cm); and giant (G1 >40 to 60 cm, G2 >60 cm).[52]

Large and giant CMN are associated with an increased risk of melanoma. Additionally, individuals with large or giant CMN may be at risk for complications of neurocutaneous melanocytosis, particularly if the large or giant CMN has a posterior axial location or if more than 20 satellite nevi are present. Newborns with more than 2 medium-sized CMN are also at increased risk of neurocutaneous melanocytosis. Neurocutaneous melanocytosis results from abnormal melanocytic proliferations in the CNS, and can be complicated by obstructive hydrocephalus and primary CNS melanoma.

Pigmentary Mosaicism: Pigmentary mosaicism (patterned dyschromatosis) refers to areas of skin hypopigmentation or hyperpigmentation that are genetically determined by late somatic mosaic genetic mutations in skin cell progenitors. The dyschromia in pigmentary mosaicism tends not to cross the midline of the body. Altered pigmentation may be curvilinear along Blaschko lines, or may manifest with checkerboard, phylloid, or patchy patterns.[53] In most cases, pigmentary mosaicism is an isolated finding, but the practitioner should maintain high suspicion for associated disease in children with widespread skin dyschromia, associated neurologic, cardiac, or musculoskeletal disease, or in children who are delayed in accomplishing expected developmental milestones.[54]

Nevus Depigmentosus: Nevus depigmentosus is a well-demarcated hypopigmented patch present from birth, which may sometimes become more visible in the first year of life as the background skin pigmentation of the newborn gradually increases. Three or more nevus depigmentosus/hypomelanotic patches in a newborn should prompt evaluation for possible tuberous sclerosis complex.[55]

Nevus Anemicus: Nevus anemicus describes a hypopigmented patch that results from focal vasoconstriction. It is attributed to skin vessel hypersensitivity to catecholamines in the affected areas. Application of pressure with a glass slide (diascopy) across the edge of a nevus depigmentosus will blanch the normal skin surrounding the nevus depigmentosus by compressing local vessels and thus blur the border. Diascopy is helpful in distinguishing nevus anemicus from nevus depigmentosus (Table 103-3), as the border of a nevus depigmentosus remains crisp despite diascopy.

VASCULAR BIRTHMARKS

Vascular tumors and malformations may present during the neonatal period, and prompt diagnosis and differentiation of those that may be associated with systemic manifestations or complications allows for early intervention when needed.

Nevus Simplex: Nevus simplex represents a superficial vascular ectasia of the capillaries. It occurs most commonly on the glabella, upper eyelids, and nuchal area, and is colloquially termed "salmon patch," "stork bite," or "angel kiss." Less-common areas include the lower back and scalp. Nevus simplex appears with high frequency in all races, occurring in 70% of white infants and in 59% of black infants. Although the majority of nevus simplex birthmarks fade over the first 2 years of life, those on the occipital scalp tend to persist. Nevus simplex should be differentiated from other capillary malformations and their associations, including nevus flammeus (port-wine stain).[56,57] Vascular malformations are discussed in detail in Chap. 147.

Infantile Hemangiomas: Infantile hemangiomas are the most common tumors of infancy. They must be differentiated from vascular malformations and other vascular anomalies. Hemangiomas are discussed in detail in Chap. 118.

Vascular Malformations: Vascular malformations are a heterogeneous group of vascular dysplasias that encompass slow-flow malformations (eg, capillary, venous, and lymphatic malformations) and fast-flow malformations (eg, arteriovenous malformations and complex combined malformations). Vascular malformations are discussed in detail in Chap. 147.

OTHER BIRTHMARKS

Nevus Sebaceus: Nevus sebaceus is a benign skin hamartoma comprised of numerous sebaceous glands that most often appear as yellow-hued hairless plaque on the head of newborns. Around puberty, a nevus sebaceus may thicken and develop hyperkeratotic, verrucous features. Secondary benign neoplasms, including trichoblastoma or syringocystadenoma papilliferum, sometimes develop within a nevus sebaceus, and, uncommonly, basal cell carcinoma has been reported to arise within a nevus sebaceus.[58,59] Lesions can be monitored or excised if they are symptomatic or cause disfigurement. Widespread nevus sebaceous skin lesions may be associated with increased risk of abnormalities in the central nervous, eye, or skeletal systems (Schimmelpenning or nevus sebaceus syndrome).[60]

Epidermal Nevus: Epidermal nevi appear as curvilinear arrays of tan-brown hyperkeratotic papules and/or thin, elongated rough plaques that follow the lines of Blaschko. Epidermal nevi are difficult to treat. Surgical excision may result in large scars which, in some locations, can restrict range of motion. Laser treatment and local dermal shave excision are associated with focal scarring and a high recurrence risk. Infants with widespread epidermal nevi may be at risk for epidermal nevus syndrome, and should be evaluated for associated disease of the central nervous, ocular, and skeletal systems.[60]

DEVELOPMENTAL ABNORMALITIES

Developmental anomalies of the skin and subcutaneous tissues and structures range from common, benign, minor findings, such as the supernumerary nipple, to major anomalies, such as aplasia cutis congenita, which can be markers for potentially serious underlying anomalies.

TABLE 103-3
Pathology and Diascopy of Nevus Anemicus and Nevus Depigmentosus

	NEVUS ANEMICUS	NEVUS DEPIGMENTOSUS
Pathology	Focal vasoconstriction; skin vessel hypersensitivity to catecholamines	Hypomelanosis in affected site
Diascopy	Borders of lesion disappear as a result of the blanching effect	Borders of lesion remain crisp

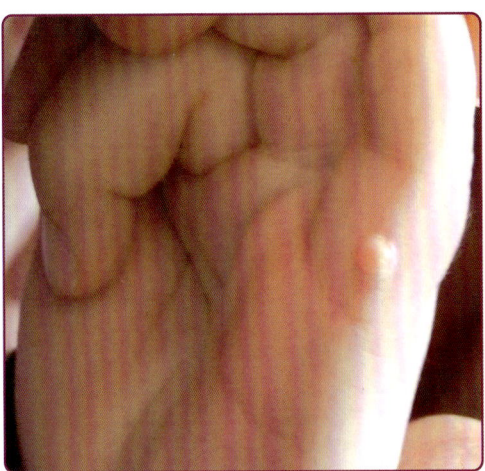

Figure 103-7 Supernumerary digit, a common minor malformation.

MINOR ANOMALIES

The supernumerary digit (Fig. 103-7), supernumerary nipple, and accessory tragus are common examples of minor anomalies of the skin and associated subcutaneous structures. Overall, single, minor congenital anomalies occur in approximately 15% of all newborns and have no functional significance. The occurrence of 2 minor congenital anomalies is less common; however, 3 or more minor congenital anomalies is unusual and warrants a complete thorough physical examination to rule out other congenital abnormalities.[61,62]

OTHER ANOMALIES

Other anomalies less frequently encountered in the neonate include dermoid cysts, aplasia cutis congenita, and branchial cleft cysts. Understanding which of these lesions imply possible risk of additional associated malformations is important for diagnosis and management.

The skin and the nervous system are both derived from the embryonic ectoderm. The neural ectoderm separates from the epithelial ectoderm during the third to fifth week of gestation, occurring simultaneously with the formation and closure of the neural tube. Hence, errors in neural tube development (ie, dysraphism [incomplete fusion]) can be associated with cutaneous anomalies. Midline facial lesions, such as dermoid cysts can be markers of cranial dysraphism, whereas cutaneous anomalies involving the lumbosacral midline may indicate underlying spinal dysraphism.

For midline nasal and facial lesions, radiologic evaluation is indicated to rule out intracranial connections before a skin biopsy is performed.[63] Radiologic imaging should also be performed in the presence of high-risk lumbosacral anomalies. The highest risk of occult spinal dysraphism occurs with the presence of 2 or more congenital midline lumbosacral skin lesions or if spinal cord dysfunction exists in the presence of 1 lumbar skin lesion.[64,65] In addition, lumbosacral lipoma, human tail, and dermal sinus (as isolated findings) are highly associated with occult spinal dysraphism, and MRI is indicated when these high-risk congenital lesions are present. An intermediate risk of occult spinal dysraphism is associated with atypical sacral dimple (≥5 mm diameter, or location ≥2.5 cm away from the anus), aplasia cutis congenita, overlying hamartoma, or deviated gluteal cleft. In the presence of any of these lesions, ultrasonography can be used to screen for occult spinal dysraphism if the infant is younger than 4 months of age. If the infant is older, MRI is needed to rule out dysraphism. Low-risk lesions that do not require imaging include small, focal infantile hemangioma, capillary malformation, mild focal hypertrichosis, congenital melanocytic nevus, dermal melanocytosis, or simple sacral dimple with a visible base (≤5 mm diameter and location ≤2.5 cm from the anus). Figure 103-8 summarizes these findings. Neurosurgical consultation is advised for infants with an intracranial or spinal anomaly.

DERMOID CYSTS

Dermoid cysts are congenital anomalies that typically arise along planes of embryonic fusion of the face and scalp. Dermoid cysts are not always apparent at birth; when appreciated, they present as a firm nodule that may adhere to the underlying periosteum. Nasal dermoid cysts may be associated with a dermal pit or sinus and carry a significant risk for intracranial extension.[66] Surgical excision is generally recommended; preoperative MRI should be considered to evaluate for deeper extension of midline dermoid cysts.[67]

NASAL GLIOMA

Nasal gliomas are composed of heterotopic neural tissue and present as firm, skin-colored to erythematous nodules on the nose (Fig. 103-9). They may distort the central facial structures. Referral to neurosurgery is indicated for surgical excision.

MENINGOCELE AND MYELOMENINGOCELE

A meningocele is formed when the meninges and cerebrospinal fluid herniate through a defect in the calvarium or vertebrae. A meningocele is a midline anomaly that may be associated with a persistent intracranial defect; as such, preoperative imaging is recommended prior to surgical excision and reconstruction. When neural tissue of the spinal cord is also present, the term *myelomeningocele* is used. Myelomeningocele is the most common presentation of spina bifida.

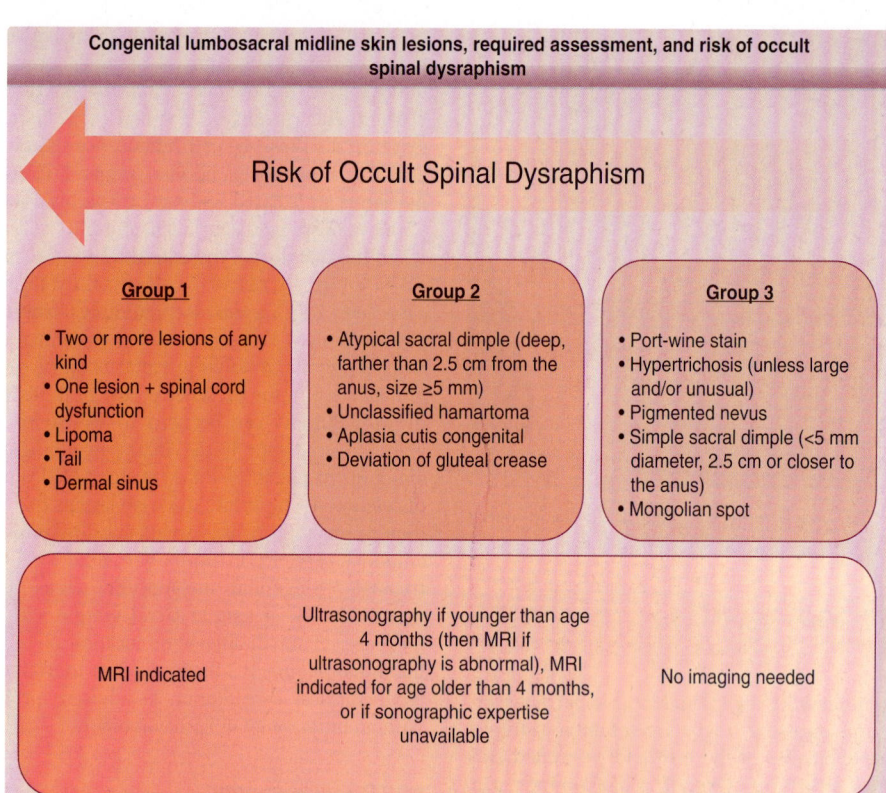

Figure 103-8 Congenital lumbosacral midline skin lesions, required assessment, and risk of occult spinal dysraphism. (Data from Guggisberg D, Hadj-Rabia S, Viney C, et al. Skin markers of occult spinal dysraphism in children: a review of 54 cases. *Arch Dermatol*. 2004;140(9):1109-1115.)

ENCEPHALOCELE

An encephalocele results from herniation of neural tissue along with the meninges and cerebrospinal fluid through a calvarial defect. As with meningoceles, preoperative imaging is recommended prior to surgical excision and reconstruction. Encephaloceles are often seen in association with other craniofacial defects, and neurodevelopmental sequelae may occur.

HUMAN TAIL

Human tails, pseudotails, and acrochordons are rare developmental anomalies. Human tails are vestigial appendages that may be composed of adipose tissue, blood vessels, muscle fibers, and nerves. Pseudotails resemble true human tails but are not related to the embryonic human tail; examples include sacrococcygeal teratomas and myelomeningoceles. True human tails, but not pseudotails, are associated with spinal dysraphism, and MRI is recommended.[68]

HYPERTRICHOSIS

Localized hypertrichosis overlying the lumbosacral, cervical, or thoracic spine may be associated with spinal dysraphism (Fig. 103-10), in particular when prominent ("faun tail").[69] Although there are only a few reported cases in the literature, the presence of a faun tail may be underestimated and mild presentations overlooked.

BRANCHIAL CLEFT ANOMALIES

Branchial cysts, clefts, and sinuses are common developmental remnants involving the neck. Presentation involves either a mass, a draining sinus, or recurrent infection.[70] Branchial cysts are the most common branchial cleft anomaly; the majority arise from the second branchial arch and present along the sternocleidomastoid muscle on the lateral aspect of the neck. The definitive treatment for branchial cleft anomalies is surgical excision.

THYROGLOSSAL DUCT CYST

Thyroglossal duct cysts are congenital neck anomalies that present as a midline mass arising anywhere from the suprasternal notch to the posterior tongue.[71] They arise from the developmental remnant of the migrational tract of the thyroid gland and, as such, may be associated with ectopic thyroid tissue. Surgical excision is the definitive treatment; preoperative verification of a normal thyroid gland is mandatory.

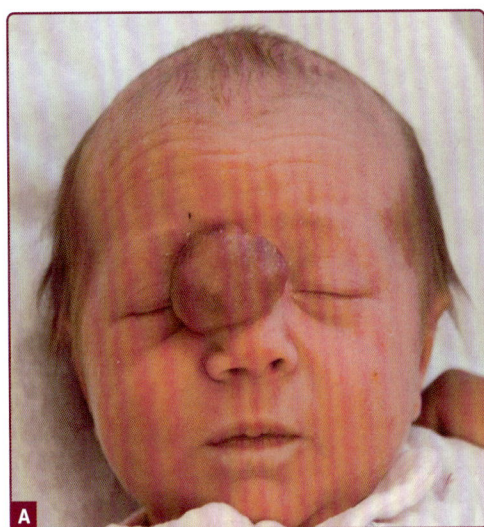
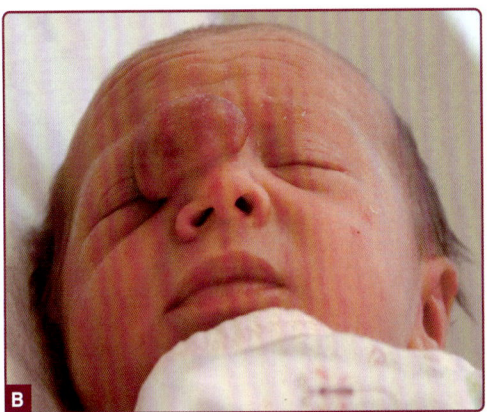
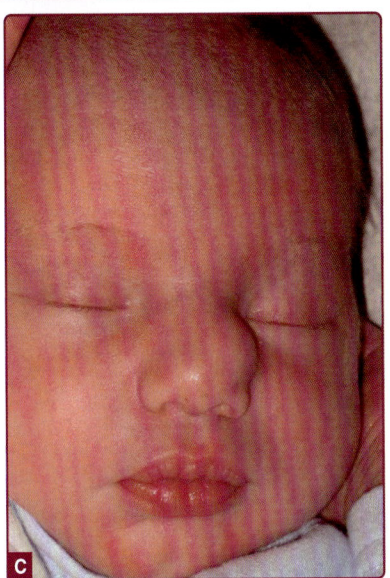

Figure 103-9 **A** and **B,** Nasal glioma initially thought to be a hemangioma of infancy. A firm, reddish, slightly pedunculated tumor was noted off of the midline of the nasal root. MRI showed no intracranial connection. **C,** Nasal glioma. Firm subcutaneous mass noted at birth.

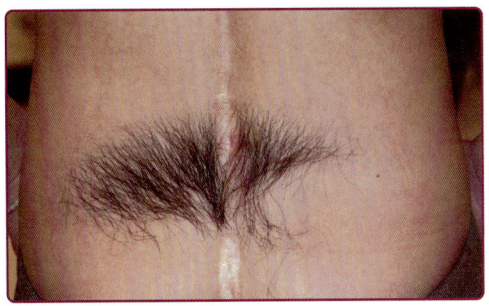

Figure 103-10 A large, wide tuft of thick terminal hair on the lumbosacral spine noted at birth. This infant had an underlying tethered cord (note midline scar from surgical repair).

URACHAL CYSTS AND POLYPS (OMPHALOMESENTERIC DUCT CYST)

Developmental anomalies of the umbilical cord represent failure of regression of the urachus (urachal cyst or fistula between the bladder and the umbilicus) or the omphalomesenteric duct (umbilical polyp or fistula between the ileum and the umbilicus). Urachal and omphalomesenteric remnants usually present with persistent drainage from the umbilicus or with an umbilical mass.[72] Surgical repair is indicated. In contrast, umbilical granulomas are common abnormalities of the umbilicus that present with persistent friable granulation tissue involving the umbilicus noted after separation of the umbilical cord. Treatment with silver nitrate chemical cautery is typically effective.

APLASIA CUTIS CONGENITA

Aplasia cutis congenita (ACC) describes localized areas of absence of the skin and sometimes the underlying subcutaneous tissues and bone. It most often involves the scalp, but may be noted elsewhere (Fig. 103-11). ACC is often an isolated finding, but a multitude of associated conditions have been described.[73] ACC has no single underlying cause and appears to be the end result of a number of distinct pathologic processes, including a forme fruste of a neural tube defect.

In the most common form of ACC, oval, sharply marginated atrophic macules are seen on the midline of the posterior scalp; they may be ulcerated or crusted or have a thin, shiny membranous covering (membranous aplasia cutis). They are usually solitary, but may be multiple. Aplasia cutis is always hairless, and when healed, lesions are usually atrophic scars, although keloidal scarring has been observed. Superficial lesions may involve only the epidermis and superficial dermis; in more-severe cases, a full-thickness tissue defect may be present, including involvement of the calvarium. Lesions may range from a few millimeters to many centimeters in diameter. Midline lesions should not be biopsied unless cranial imaging has been performed to exclude the possibility of an intracranial connection. After a careful examination

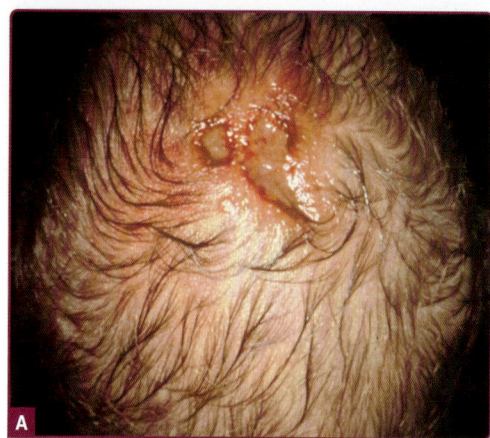 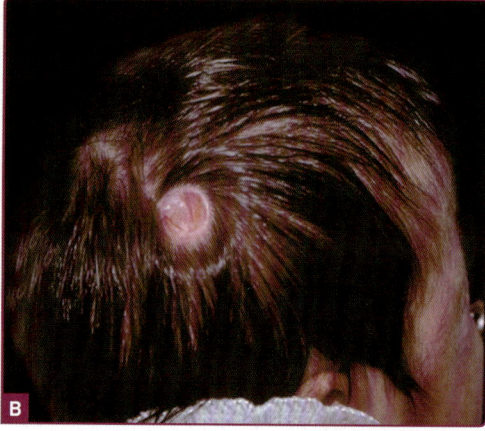

Figure 103-11 Two infants with aplasia cutis congenita. **A**, Scalp erosions grouped at the vertex scalp. Scraping or biopsy is contraindicated. **B**, An atrophic, well-circumscribed round patch with visible capillaries on the scalp of an infant. (Image A is from Bolognia JL, Jorizzo JL, Rapini RP, eds. *Dermatology*. 2nd ed. New York: Mosby Elsevier; 2008, with permission. Copyright © Elsevier.)

to rule out associated anomalies, ACC is treated conservatively with local wound care. Surgical revision of the scar later in childhood or adolescence can be done electively to improve cosmesis.

The "hair collar sign" is a ring of darker and/or coarser terminal hairs on the scalp, typically surrounding ACC, dermoid cyst, encephalocele, meningocele, or heterotopic brain tissue.[74] The hair collar sign itself is a marker of cranial dysraphism and its presence, like aplasia cutis, mandates careful examination of the infant.

INFECTIONS OF THE NEONATE

Infants younger than 2 months of age have immature immune systems. Life-threatening sepsis can develop quickly and insidiously. Subtle clues, such as a decrease in body temperature, poor feeding, poor muscular tone, or other nonspecific signs, are taken seriously by the pediatrician, and a "rule out sepsis" admission is initiated when clinical suspicion is high. In general, blood, cerebrospinal fluid, and urine cultures are obtained, and IV antibiotic therapy is started while culture results are pending. Table 103-4 lists cutaneous infections of the neonate. Bacterial skin infections that affect neonates, including staphylococcal scalded-skin syndrome, are further discussed in Chaps. 151 and 152, and viral infections that affect neonates, such as varicella and herpes simplex virus, are discussed in Chaps. 164 and 165.

CONGENITAL VIRAL INFECTION

Petechiae, purpura, jaundice, hepatomegaly, splenomegaly, microcephaly, encephalopathy, ocular abnormalities, anemia, thrombocytopenia, conjugated hyperbilirubinemia, or elevated serum hepatic transaminases prompt consideration of congenital viral infection, particularly if they arise in combination with "blueberry muffin" violaceous to purpuric nodules. These findings are concerning for possible congenital TORCH (toxoplasmosis; *other* which includes syphilis, enterovirus. and HIV; rubella; cytomegalovirus; herpes) infection.

NEONATAL HERPES SIMPLEX VIRUS INFECTION

It is estimated that untreated neonatal herpes simplex virus (HSV) infection has a 50% mortality rate, with 75% of survivors suffering neurologic sequelae. The greatest risk of neonatal herpes occurs when the delivery is vaginal and the mother has active, primary genital herpes (in contrast to recurrent herpes, in which the mother provides transplacental antibodies that offer some protection to the neonate). Chapter 164 discusses HSV in detail.

The vast majority of neonatal HSV cases are caused by HSV type 2. Herpes involves the skin, eye, or mouth in most infected neonates, but some patients with CNS

TABLE 103-4
Selected Cutaneous Infections in the Neonate

- Staphylococcal infections
  - Impetigo
  - Staphylococcal scalded-skin syndrome
  - Omphalitis
  - Breast abscess (usually caused by *Staphylococcus aureus* and Gram-negative organisms)
- Viral infections
  - Varicella
  - Herpes simplex virus
- Fungal/candidal infections
- Scabies

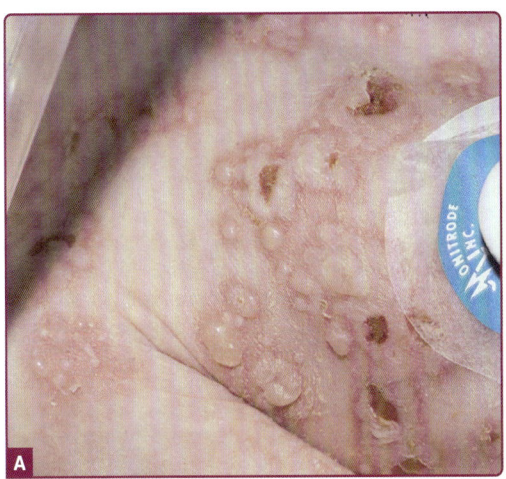 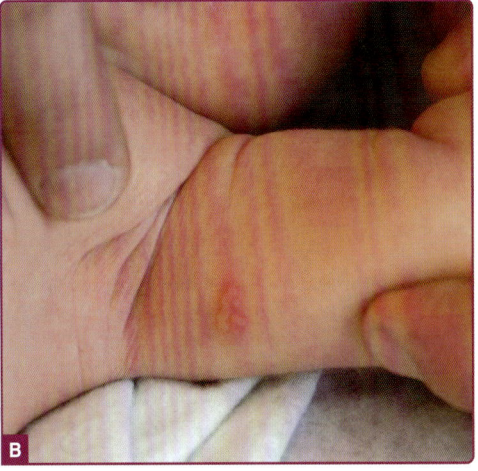

Figure 103-12 **A** and **B**, Herpes simplex infection in 2 infants. Grouped vesicles on an erythematous base. Pustules and erosions are also present. (**A** used with permission from Alvin H. Jacobs, MD.)

or disseminated disease never have skin lesions.[75] Herpetic skin lesions manifest as clusters of vesicles on an erythematous base (Fig 103-12). Vesicles that appear during the first 24 hours of life suggest in utero acquisition of HSV, but onset during the first week to 10 days of life is more common, representing exposure to the virus during the delivery.[75]

A high index of suspicion should be maintained even in the absence of maternal infection or history of genital herpes. Specimens should be obtained for direct fluorescent antibody assay and/or viral culture to detect HSV. A Tzanck smear prepared from a vesicle may provide supportive diagnostic information quickly. If available, a polymerase chain reaction test can be very helpful in rapid diagnosis. IV acyclovir should be instituted as soon as possible after specimens are collected to minimize the chance of virus replication in the CNS and systemic dissemination of HSV. Prompt recognition and early therapeutic intervention result in improved outcomes in HSV-infected infants.[75]

FUNGAL INFECTION

In full-term neonates, congenital cutaneous candidiasis typically presents with widespread erythematous macules, papules, and pustules associated with superficial desquamation, whereas preterm neonates with congenital cutaneous candidiasis may develop large, weeping erosions.[76] Angioinvasive fungal disease in the premature neonate often manifests as ulcerations or necrotic foci with eschar and surrounding erythema.

ERYTHRODERMA

Although uncommon in the neonate, erythroderma may signal a serious underlying condition. A number of genetic, infectious, inflammatory, metabolic, and immunologic disorders can present with erythroderma, and some are associated with possible death in the neonatal period. In addition, erythroderma predisposes to potentially life-threatening complications such as sepsis, dehydration, and electrolyte imbalance. In 1 retrospective case series of neonatal and infantile erythroderma, diagnostic prevalence was approximated as follows: immunodeficiency (30%), congenital ichthyosis (24%), Netherton syndrome (18%), eczematous or papulosquamous dermatitis (20%), and unknown (unspecified).[77]

Inflammatory dermatoses that may present in the first few weeks of life with generalized erythema and scaling include seborrheic dermatitis, infantile psoriasis, juvenile pityriasis rubra pilaris, and atopic or nonatopic eczema. Although seborrheic dermatitis typically presents with localized greasy scalp scaling, a more widespread inflammatory dermatitis is seen in some affected infants, typically with an onset in the first few weeks of life. Infantile psoriasis may present in the first few weeks of life as either a localized or a more widespread psoriasiform dermatitis; however, the characteristic clinical features of psoriasis may be lacking (see Chap. 28). Congenital psoriasis is an uncommon presentation that may not be associated with a family history of psoriasis.[78] In contrast, the presentation of atopic dermatitis is uncommon in the first few weeks of life, and onset of disease is usually delayed until after the first month of life (see Chap. 22). However, infantile eczema and psoriasis may coexist.[79] A family history of atopy or psoriasis and an assessment of areas of predilection and primary morphology may help to differentiate these disorders, although in some cases definitive diagnosis is only possible by observing over time.

Several inborn errors of metabolism, including holocarboxylase synthetase deficiency and biotinidase deficiency, both of which result in deficiency of the 4 biotin-dependent carboxylases (multiple carboxylase deficiency), can present with a desquamative dermatitis.[80] A collodion presentation with features of ichthyosis also has been reported.[81] Affected neonates typically also experience lethargy, seizures, and apnea; delayed presentation may be seen in those affected with late-onset biotinidase deficiency or late-onset multiple carboxylase deficiency in which symptoms may not develop until later in infancy or childhood.[82] In the United States, depending on the state where the infant was born, these disorders may be detected through the newborn screening program before significant symptoms arise.

Essential fatty acid deficiency is an uncommon acquired nutritional deficiency that may present with an exfoliative dermatitis.[83] Risk factors for essential fatty acid deficiency include malnutrition, which may result from the implementation of specialized infant formulas, improper infant feeding or fad diets, hyperalimentation, or disorders such as cystic fibrosis that result in malabsorption. Essential fatty acid deficiency may occur in association with other nutrient deficiencies, including zinc deficiency, in which case signs of acrodermatitis also may be noted.

Several neonatal infections may result in diffuse erythema with or without scaling or other primary lesions. In term and premature neonates, staphylococcal scalded skin syndrome may present with variable erythema, erosions, scaling, and desquamation; congenital presentation has rarely been reported because of presumed intrauterine infection.[84-87] Early congenital syphilis may present as a desquamative dermatitis or a more generalized vesiculobullous dermatitis.[88-90]

The congenital ichthyoses that may present with neonatal erythroderma include Netherton syndrome, autosomal recessive congenital ichthyosis (which commonly presents with a collodion membrane), Sjögren-Larsson syndrome, keratitis-ichthyosis-deafness syndrome, and neutral lipid storage disease (Chanarin-Dorfman syndrome).[91] Other genetic disorders that may sometimes present with erythroderma or a collodion membrane include X-linked hypohidrotic ectodermal dysplasia and type 2 Gaucher disease.[92,93]

Several primary immunodeficiency syndromes are associated with neonatal erythroderma, including Omenn syndrome, severe combined immunodeficiency syndrome (SCID), hyperimmunoglobulin E syndrome, and DiGeorge syndrome. SCID is a heterogeneous group of immunodeficiency disorders characterized by combined T-cell and B-cell dysfunction; there are at least 13 different genes associated with this phenotype.[94] The presence of a diffuse eczematous dermatitis is associated with SCID, and in at least a proportion of affected infants dermatitis results from maternal engraftment and cutaneous graft-versus-host disease; diagnosis can be facilitated by skin biopsy with appropriate ancillary genetic studies.[95,96] The prognosis for affected patients is poor because of the risk for severe infection, failure to thrive, immune dysregulation, and other complications; bone marrow transplantation before 3 to 4 months of age is generally recommended and ideally is performed before infectious complications arise. Many states include screening for SCID by the T-cell receptor excision circle (TREC) assay on the newborn screen.[97] Omenn syndrome is a rare form of SCID that results from autosomal recessive mutations in the *RAG-1* or *RAG-2* gene. In addition to an exfoliative erythroderma, the characteristic features include failure to thrive, chronic diarrhea, lymphadenopathy, and hepatosplenomegaly. In the absence of bone marrow transplantation, the prognosis is poor. Hyperimmunoglobulin E syndrome associated with mutations in the *STAT3* gene may present with a diffuse eczematous dermatitis in infancy; atopy, mucocutaneous candidiasis, and recurrent staphylococcal skin infections are typical features.[98] A characteristic clinical finding of hyperimmunoglobulin E syndrome in infancy is the development of a papulopustular dermatitis of the face and scalp.[99] DiGeorge syndrome results from a deletion of chromosome 22q11.21; the key features are thymic aplasia, cardiac anomalies involving the aortic arch, hypoparathyroidism, cleft palate, and dysmorphic features. An eczematous dermatitis has been reported in some infants with DiGeorge syndrome.[100,101]

Skin biopsy may be helpful in selected diagnoses, in particular Netherton syndrome and SCID.[102]

SEBORRHEIC DERMATITIS

Seborrheic dermatitis is a common and benign inflammatory dermatosis in infancy, and may be noted as early as the first few weeks of life. The most common presentation is the development of greasy yellow scale with mild underlying erythema on the scalp ("cradle cap"). In the diaper and intertriginous areas, scaling is less prominent and erythema more well-defined, and there is clinical overlap with infantile psoriasis ("sebopsoriasis"). Less-common areas of involvement include the face, in particular the eyebrows and nasolabial folds, and the torso, where the eruption manifests as variable erythema and greasy scaling; in darker-skinned infants, postinflammatory hypopigmentation may predominate. Impetiginization or secondary candidal infection may occur.

The pathophysiology of seborrheic dermatitis is hypothesized by some experts to involve an exaggerated immune response to skin colonization with *Malassezia* species.[103] Seborrheic dermatitis typically remits spontaneously within the first 1 to 2 years of life, although there may be an association with the development of adult seborrheic dermatitis and atopic dermatitis.[104,105]

For mild cases, application of baby oil or mineral oil to the affected areas of the scalp, followed by gentle combing and shampooing to remove scales, is sufficient. For more severe involvement, use of a topical antifungal shampoo or cream or a low-potency topical corticosteroid may be necessary.

Seborrheic dermatitis must be differentiated from other inflammatory skin disorders of infancy, including infantile psoriasis, atopic and nonatopic eczema, and Langerhans cell histiocytosis. Additionally, seborrheic dermatitis-like eruptions have been reported to occur in association with immunodeficiency, and nutritional and metabolic disease. Any history of failure to thrive, developmental delay, unexplained symptoms, or recurrent infection raises concern for possible associated systemic disease.

DIAPER DERMATITIS

Diaper dermatitis (Table 103-5) is a common skin problem in infants. Multiple factors contribute to the development of diaper dermatitis. Prolonged exposure to moisture results in increased frictional damage, decreased barrier function, and increased reactivity to irritants. Interrelated etiologic factors include contact with urine and feces, fecal proteolytic and lipolytic digestive enzymes, increased skin pH, and superinfection with *Candida*.[106] Less commonly, bacterial superinfection may complicate diaper dermatitis.

IRRITANT DIAPER DERMATITIS

Irritant contact dermatitis is the most common cause of diaper dermatitis. It is characterized by erythematous, moist, and sometimes scaly patches favoring the convex surfaces of the genitalia and buttocks. The skin folds are classically spared. Barrier diaper creams and frequent diaper changes are very helpful to treat this condition.

ALLERGIC CONTACT DIAPER DERMATITIS

Allergic contact dermatitis occurs in the diaper area as well. Common contact allergens for the diaper region include preservatives, fragrances, rubber additives, and disperse dyes in diapers or baby wipes.[107]

CANDIDAL DIAPER DERMATITIS

Candidiasis (see Chap. 161) is the second most common cause of diaper dermatitis and is characterized by bright red erythematous, moist papules, patches, and plaques that tend to involve body folds as well as convex surfaces. Satellite papules and pustules are frequently observed, and oral thrush may be present. *Candida* from intestinal flora may contaminate and exacerbate any type of diaper dermatitis present for longer than 3 days.[108]

PSEUDOVERRUCOUS PAPULES AND NODULES

Pseudoverrucous papules and nodules (Fig. 103-13) are flat-topped, skin-colored papules that develop in the diaper and perianal areas in patients of any age whose skin is chronically exposed to moisture, including children with prolonged urinary or fecal incontinence.[109]

JACQUET EROSIVE DERMATITIS

Jacquet erosive dermatitis is an uncommon, severe diaper dermatitis that is characterized by well-demarcated, punched-out ulcers and erosions.

TABLE 103-5
Lesions of the Diaper Area

	DIAPER DERMATITIS	CANDIDIASIS (CANDIDAL INTERTRIGO)	LANGERHANS CELL HISTIOCYTOSIS	PSORIASIS (NAPKIN PSORIASIS)[a]	SEBORRHEIC DERMATITIS[a]
Age	Any age	Any age	1 to 3 years	Usually 3 to 6 months	First few weeks to 3 months
Affected sites	Convexities of the genitalia affected, skin folds spared	Skin folds and convexities affected	Scalp, intertriginous skin folds	Trunk, limbs, face, skin folds, and diaper area may be affected	Scalp, intertriginous skin folds, face, torso
Appearance	Scaly erythematous patches	Bright red, erythematous, moist papules, patches, and plaques with satellite papules and pustules	Tan-to-pink papulovesicles, nodules, ulcerations, and petechiae	Well-defined erythema, white scales over trunk and body, but scaling usually absent in skin folds	Greasy yellow scales with mild erythema; in diaper areas, well-defined erythema, glistening appearance, scaling not prominent
Etiology	May be irritant or allergic in origin	*Candida* sp.	Reactive vs neoplastic (see Chap. 117)	Inflammatory disease, T-cell mediated	Exaggerated immune response to *Malassezia* sp.
Treatment	Barrier creams, frequent diaper changes (see Table 103-6)	Keep intertriginous areas dry, topical antifungal agents	(See Chap. 117)	Topical steroids, topical calcineurin inhibitors	Mineral or baby oil; antifungal shampoo; low-potency topical steroid

[a]Infantile psoriasis and seborrheic dermatitis may overlap ("sebopsoriasis").

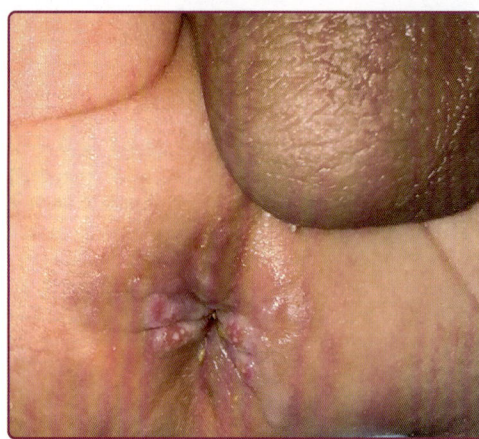

Figure 103-13 Pseudoverrucous papules and nodules in a newborn.

Prolonged contact with urine and feces under occlusion leads to this condition.[110] The availability of superabsorbent disposable diapers has made this diagnosis less common.

GRANULOMA GLUTEALE INFANTUM

Granuloma gluteale infantum is an uncommon diaper rash characterized by reddish purplish nodules of different sizes (0.5 to 3 cm) occurring on the convexities of the diaper area in 2- to 9-month-old infants. It arises within preexisting diaper dermatitis. Biopsy shows dense dermal infiltrates of lymphocytes, plasma cells, neutrophils, and eosinophils, but no true granulomas. It appears to be an unusual reaction to the usual irritant factors, *Candida* infection, and, in some cases, topical corticosteroid use in the diaper region.[110] Treatment consists of avoidance of irritants, use of a barrier ointment, and avoidance of topical corticosteroids. Resolution occurs over several months.

DERMATOSES NOT ETIOLOGICALLY RELATED TO DIAPER WEARING

Infantile seborrheic dermatitis, napkin psoriasis (Fig. 103-14), bullous impetigo, acrodermatitis enteropathica, scabies, herpes simplex infections, and Langerhans cell histiocytosis are conditions that may occur in the diaper region but are not primarily caused by the wearing of diapers. They should be considered in the differential diagnosis when evaluating diaper eruptions. Skin biopsy is indicated to rule out Langerhans cell histiocytosis (see Chap. 117) if nonhealing erosions or petechiae are seen in the diaper area (Fig. 103-15).

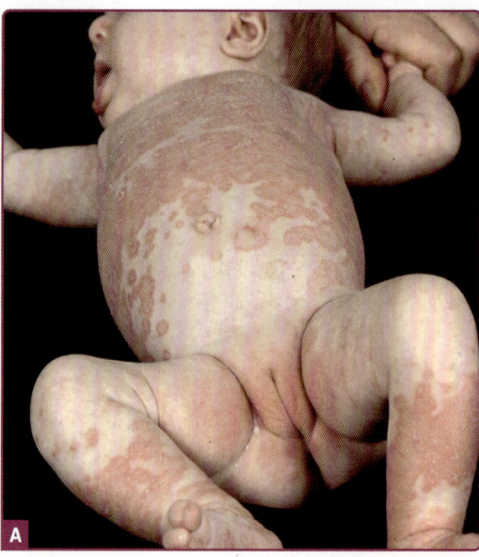

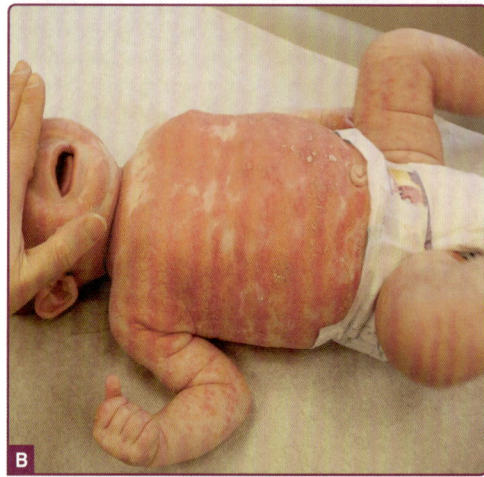

Figure 103-14 **A,** Infantile psoriasis with involvement in the diaper region. **B,** Infantile psoriasis. This generalized eruption responded well to topical steroids initially and topical tacrolimus later.

TREATMENT OF DIAPER DERMATITIS

Table 103-6 outlines the treatment of diaper dermatitis.[111]

HAMARTOMAS AND BENIGN TUMORS

INFANTILE MYOFIBROMATOSIS

Infantile myofibromas typically present as rubbery dermal and subcutaneous nodules. There can be a

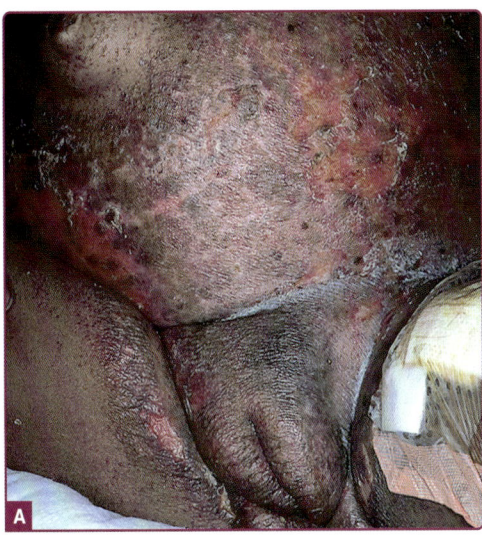 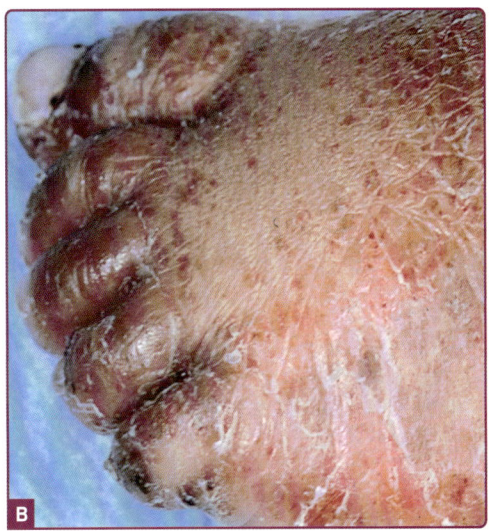

Figure 103-15 **A** and **B,** Langerhans cell histiocytosis with petechiae and erosions of the skin. This patient also had hepatosplenomegaly.

solitary myofibroma or multiple myofibromas (myofibromatosis). In addition to skin, infantile myofibromatosis can involve bone, the GI tract, heart, lungs, and kidneys.[112] Myofibromas limited to soft tissue typically resolve spontaneously within 1 to 2 years. Thus, clinical observation is warranted.

Excision is the mainstay of treatment, and recurrence rates are low.[113,114]

INFANTILE DIGITAL FIBROMA

Infantile digital fibromas are smooth pink nodules that appear on the phalanges of infants. Most commonly the fingers are involved, and the thumbs and great toes are classically spared. Approximately one-third of infantile digital fibromas are present at birth. Skin biopsy is diagnostic and shows bundles of myofibroblasts with round cytoplasmic inclusions that are highlighted by the Masson trichrome or phosphotungstic acid–hematoxylin stains. Infantile digital fibromas have a high recurrence rate after surgical excision and tend to resolve spontaneously over years. Conservative observation is typically recommended.[115]

FIBROUS HAMARTOMA OF INFANCY

Fibrous hamartoma of infancy is an uncommon infantile mass. Most cases appear as a solitary, painless, 0.5- to 10-cm skin nodule in the deep dermis or subcutis.

CONGENITAL SMOOTH MUSCLE HAMARTOMA

Congenital smooth muscle hamartomas (CSMHs) are benign dermal proliferations of hyperplastic smooth muscle. CSMHs most often appear as a solitary irregular dermal plaque on the trunk or proximal extremities. The overlying skin tends to be skin-toned to slightly hyperpigmented and may have associated hypertrichosis. Brisk rubbing of a CSMH results in transient piloerection and induration, which is termed the *pseudo-Darier sign*. The pseudo-Darier sign is elicited in approximately 80% of CSMHs and supports clinical diagnosis. CSMHs are benign and can be observed

TABLE 103-6
ABCs in the Treatment of Diaper Dermatitis

A = Air. The diaper should be left open as much as possible when the infant sleeps to allow drying of the skin.

B = Barrier ointments. Zinc oxide pastes, petrolatum, and other bland, unmedicated barrier preparations are mainstays of therapy. A continuous layer of barrier paste or ointment should be maintained, reapplying with every diaper change, if necessary. Baby powder on the diaper area offers no antimicrobial benefit to the infant and adds a risk of aspiration.

C = Cleansing and anticandidal treatment. Gentle cleansing with plain water, mineral oil, or unscented gentle cleanser is recommended. Avoidance of friction or rubbing is important. A topical anticandidal agent should be added for any signs of candidiasis. Oral nystatin is indicated if oral thrush is present.

D = Diapers. Diapers should be changed as frequently and as soon after soiling as possible, especially if cloth diapers are used.

E = Education of parents and caregivers.

Modified from Boiko S. Making rash decisions in the diaper area. *Pediatr Ann.* 2000;29(1):50-56.

with consideration of surgical excision for symptomatic or cosmetically concerning lesions.

NEOPLASTIC AND PROLIFERATIVE DISORDERS

NEUROBLASTOMA

Neuroblastoma is the second most common solid tumor of childhood, and approximately 25% of cases are congenital. Cutaneous metastatic neuroblastoma is included in the "blueberry muffin" baby differential diagnosis, owing to its purple-hued papules and nodules. Skin lesions of neuroblastoma may exhibit blanching, attributed to release of locally active catecholamines from the malignant cells, for up to 1 hour after stroking.[116] Skin biopsy is needed to determine the diagnosis of neuroblastoma and shows small, round cells with large atypical nuclei. The malignant cells may form pseudorosette structures. Immunohistochemistry for neuronal markers, particularly neuron-specific enolase, is helpful.

CONGENITAL LEUKEMIA

Congenital leukemia represents a small subset (<1%) of childhood leukemia. In the newborn, acute myeloid leukemia is more common than acute lymphocytic leukemia.[117] Signs of leukemia in newborn skin include ecchymoses, petechiae, and skin nodules. Multiple blue-to-purple skin nodules are found in approximately 60% of newborns with congenital leukemia, thus congenital leukemia is included in the differential diagnosis of the "blueberry muffin" baby. Skin biopsy shows sheets of atypical mononuclear cells infiltrating the dermis or subcutaneous fat. Complete blood counts and bone marrow biopsy help confirm the diagnosis.

LANGERHANS CELL HISTIOCYTOSIS

Langerhans cell histiocytosis (LCH) is an uncommon proliferative disorder of childhood. Approximately 5% of LCH cases are diagnosed in the newborn period. Cutaneous findings of LCH in the newborn include tan-to-pink papulovesicles, nodules, ulcerations, and petechiae that preferentially develop on the scalp and intertriginous skin folds. Cutaneous LCH may also manifest as a "blueberry muffin" baby, with blue-hued skin nodules. Red-brown skin nodules with or without ulceration are another possible presentation.

The skin lesions of congenital LCH may resolve spontaneously, which is likely responsible for the past nomenclature of congenital "self-healing" LCH. However, because of a risk for disease recurrence, even into childhood, continued monitoring for possible complications in other organ systems is required for all patients with LCH.[118] Skin biopsy of cutaneous lesions shows a histiocytic infiltrate that stains positive for CD1a and CD107 (Langerin).

CUTANEOUS MASTOCYTOSIS

Cutaneous mastocytosis refers to a spectrum of mast cell proliferative disorders that affect the skin. Infants with cutaneous mastocytosis may have a single tan-to-light brown ovoid plaque (solitary mastocytoma), many small red-brown macules and papules (urticaria pigmentosa, maculopapular cutaneous mast cell disease), or diffusely indurated, peau-de-orange textured skin (diffuse cutaneous mastocytosis). Telangiectasia macularis eruptive perstans, which manifests as small telangiectatic patches in older individuals, is an exceptionally rare form of mast cell disease in infants or children.

Of the mast cell disease spectrum entities, solitary mastocytoma and urticaria pigmentosa frequently appear in the first few months of life. Brisk stroking of affected skin will result in mast cell degranulation with a wheal and flare reaction. This useful clinical examination finding is termed *Darier sign*. Diagnosis can be made clinically in many cases, but if needed, skin biopsy demonstrates large numbers of mast cells in the dermis. Special stains, including toluidine blue, Giemsa, and c-kit (CD117), can highlight mast cell populations.

History of flushing, wheezing, vomiting, diarrhea, abdominal pain, bone pain, or shock should be elicited from patients with widespread cutaneous mast cell disease. In cases with extensive skin disease or a concerning review of symptoms, serum tryptase may be a useful clinical indicator. Based on extrapolation from adult systemic mastocytosis literature, some recommend bone marrow biopsy to rule out systemic mastocytosis in children with tryptase levels greater than 20 ng/mL, whereas others reserve bone marrow biopsy only with levels greater than 100 ng/mL. Recent work suggests that enlargement of the liver and/or spleen is a more sensitive indicator of systemic mast cell disease in children when compared to serum tryptase or history of severe mediator symptoms, and that serum tryptase levels tend to decrease over time in children.[119] In general, cutaneous mastocytosis is managed with oral antihistamines (H_1 and H_2). Parents should be counseled to avoid exposing affected children to common triggers of mast cell degranulation, which include anesthetics, other medications, and physical stimuli.

GENODERMATOSES PRESENTING IN THE NEONATAL PERIOD

Several genetic skin diseases may have the onset of characteristic cutaneous features in the neonatal period. The most common diagnoses include epidermolysis bullosa, congenital ichthyoses, and ectodermal dysplasia.

EPIDERMOLYSIS BULLOSA

Epidermolysis bullosa (EB) is a mechanobullous disease with variable presentation and prognosis (see Chap. 60). There are 4 main types: EB simplex, junctional EB, dystrophic EB, and Kindler syndrome; they are distinguished on the basis of the localization of the cleavage plane within the skin. EB should be suspected in the neonate with a bullous eruption; however, other etiologies, including infection, should also be considered.[120] Diagnosis relies on clinical examination and history, skin biopsy for transmission electron microscopy and immunoepitope mapping, and genetic testing. Prognosis for the milder forms of EB is excellent, whereas the more-severe forms (junctional EB and recessive dystrophic) are associated with significant morbidity and mortality.

CONGENITAL ICHTHYOSIS

The congenital ichthyoses or disorders of cornification are a heterogeneous group of inherited disorders which involve abnormal epidermal differentiation (see Chap. 47). The genetic basis for many of the congenital ichthyoses is known, and the current classification system differentiates syndromic from nonsyndromic forms of congenital ichthyosis.[121] Presentation in the neonatal period may include a collodion membrane, which is most commonly seen with the autosomal recessive congenital ichthyoses, such as lamellar ichthyosis and nonbullous congenital ichthyosiform erythroderma. The most extreme presentation of autosomal recessive congenital ichthyosis is harlequin ichthyosis, in which thick, plate-like hyperkeratotic scales cover the face, scalp and body, and ectropion and eclabium are present. Infants with harlequin ichthyosis may develop respiratory insufficiency and are at risk for dehydration, metabolic abnormalities, and sepsis.

ECTODERMAL DYSPLASIA

The ectodermal dysplasias are a large group of related disorders characterized by abnormalities in 1 or more ectodermal structures: the skin, hair, nails, teeth, and eccrine glands (see Chap. 131). As of this writing, there are more than 200 defined disorders, only a small proportion of which have a known genetic etiology.[122] Diagnosis of many of the forms of ectodermal dysplasia is not generally possible in the neonatal period and is delayed until features such as delayed dentition, alopecia, and nail dystrophy become more pronounced. The astute clinician, however, may suspect X-linked hypohidrotic ectodermal dysplasia, one of the more common forms of ectodermal dysplasias, by noting the characteristic facies, alopecia, and unexplained hyperpyrexia in a neonate or young infant. Other forms of ectodermal dysplasias that may present in the neonatal period include the spectrum of p63-related ectodermal dysplasias termed ankyloblepharon-ectrodactyly-clefting syndrome, which encompass the entities previously known as Hay-Wells syndrome, Rapp-Hodgkin syndrome, and ectodermal dysplasia-ectrodactyly-clefting syndrome.

INCONTINENTIA PIGMENTI

Incontinentia pigmenti is an X-linked disorder classified as a type of ectodermal dysplasia (see Chap. 131). Incontinentia pigmenti results from mutations in the nuclear factor κB essential modulator (*NEMO*) gene.[123] It is characterized by cutaneous manifestations, abnormalities of the hair, teeth and nails, ocular anomalies, and neurologic abnormalities.[124] The earliest clinical manifestations include a characteristic Blaschkoid vesicular eruption. Although more common in girls as a consequence of prenatal lethality in the majority of affected male fetuses, males may present with incontinentia pigmenti in a number of circumstances, including the presence of an XXY karyotype (Klinefelter syndrome), somatic mosaicism, or hypomorphic mutation.[125]

OTHER DERMATOSES OF THE NEONATE

SUBCUTANEOUS FAT NECROSIS OF THE NEWBORN

Subcutaneous fat necrosis of the newborn is characterized by firm, red to purple subcutaneous nodules or plaques on the back, cheeks, buttocks, arms, and thighs (Fig. 103-16; see Chap. 73). The lesions usually appear within the first 2 weeks of life and resolve spontaneously over several weeks.[126] Skin biopsy demonstrates lobular fat necrosis with needle-shaped clefts in lipocytes and mixed inflammation with lymphocytes, macrophages, and giant cells. Infants affected by subcutaneous fat necrosis of the newborn are at risk for hypercalcemia and should be monitored.

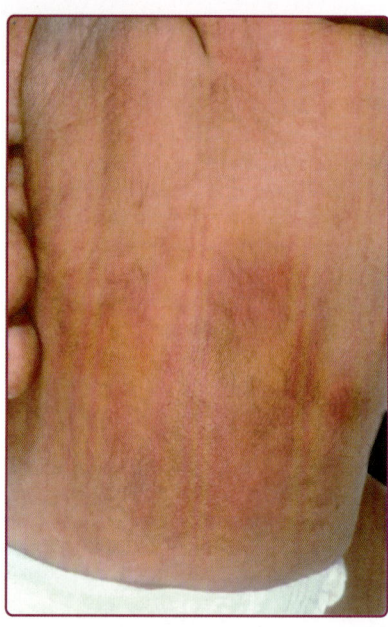

Figure 103-16 Subcutaneous fat necrosis of the newborn. This infant developed an erythematous firm mass on the back by 2 weeks of age and later developed hypercalcemia.

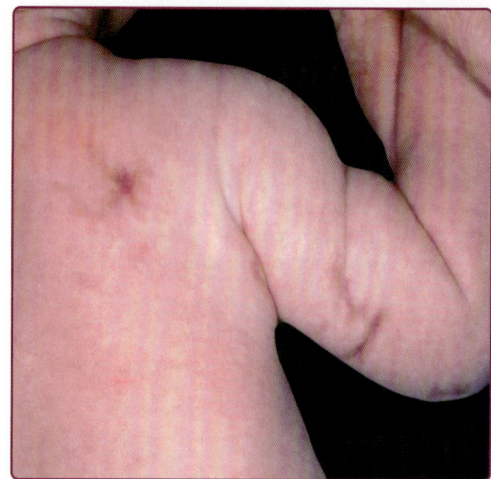

Figure 103-17 Cutis marmorata telangiectatica congenita. Note the atrophic, dusky, stellate patches with overlying telangiectasias.

SCLEREMA NEONATORUM

Sclerema neonatorum describes diffuse skin hardening in a sick, premature newborn. It is thought to be exceedingly uncommon with modern neonatal care. The onset is characteristically after 24 hours of age. Critically ill premature neonates with sepsis, hypoglycemia, acidosis, or other severe metabolic abnormalities are at most risk. The skin becomes hard and appears shiny. Biopsy shows needle-like crystals within lipocytes but no associated inflammatory infiltrate or fat necrosis, differentiating it from subcutaneous fat necrosis of the newborn. The etiology of sclerema neonatorum is unknown, and infant mortality is high.

ANETODERMA OF PREMATURITY

A specific form of iatrogenic anetoderma (see Chap. 70) has been described in premature infants (born at 24 to 30 weeks of gestation) with very-low birthweights and prolonged neonatal intensive care hospitalization.[127] A retrospective review of 11 cases noted the appearance of round, flat atrophic patches on the chest and abdomen (including the periumbilical region), developing between 6 weeks and 5 months of age. Among them, eight patients had lesions at sites where adhesive monitoring leads had been removed, and 5 patients had circular ecchymotic patches from removal of adhesive monitoring leads prior to the occurrence of the anetoderma. The anetoderma did not improve with time. Given the presumed relationship of the development of anetoderma and skin trauma from adhesive leads, avoidance of pressure (placing leads on the ventral chest when the infant slept on the back, for instance) may help reduce risk.[128]

CUTIS MARMORATA TELANGIECTATICA CONGENITA

Cutis marmorata telangiectatica congenita is characterized by persistent, reticulated atrophic violaceous vascular patches. It is sometimes associated with telangiectasias and ulceration (Fig. 103-17). It is a sporadic condition, and its etiology remains unknown. Theories of vascular malformation are currently favored. Diagnosis is usually evident on clinical examination. Most frequently, a lower extremity is involved, but location on the trunk or upper extremity is not uncommon. Limb asymmetry may be present. However, the majority of patients have a good prognosis, with half demonstrating improvement of the mottled appearance over the first 2 years.[129]

REFERENCES

1. Holbrook KA, Odland GF. The fine structure of developing human epidermis: light, scanning, and transmission electron microscopy of the periderm. *J Invest Dermatol.* 1975;65(1):16-38.
2. Akiyama M, Smith LT, Yoneda K, et al. Periderm cells form cornified cell envelope in their regression process during human epidermal development. *J Invest Dermatol.* 1999;112(6):903-909.

3. Dale BA, Holbrook KA, Kimball JR, et al. Expression of epidermal keratins and filaggrin during human fetal skin development. *J Cell Biol.* 1985;101(4):1257-1269.
4. Deutsch TA, Esterly NB. Elastic fibers in fetal dermis. *J Invest Dermatol.* 1975;65(3):320-323.
5. Smith LT, Holbrook KA, Madri JA. Collagen types I, III, and V in human embryonic and fetal skin. *Am J Anat.* 1986;175(4):507-521.
6. Holbrook KA, Odland GF. Structure of the human fetal hair canal and initial hair eruption. *J Invest Dermatol.* 1978;71(6):385-390.
7. Muller M, Jasmin JR, Monteil RA, et al. Embryology of the hair follicle. *Early Hum Dev.* 1991;26(3):159-166.
8. Fujita H, Asagami C, Murota S, et al. Ultrastructural study of embryonic sebaceous cells, especially of their serum droplet formation. *Acta Derm Venereol.* 1972;52(2):99-115.
9. Rissmann R, Groenink HW, Weerheim AM, et al. New insights into ultrastructure, lipid composition and organization of vernix caseosa. *J Invest Dermatol.* 2006;126(8):1823-1833.
10. Pickens WL, Warner RR, Boissy YL, et al. Characterization of vernix caseosa: water content, morphology, and elemental analysis. *J Invest Dermatol.* 2000;115(5):875-881.
11. Hoath SB, Pickens WL, Visscher MO. The biology of vernix caseosa. *Int J Cosmet Sci.* 2006;28(5):319-333.
12. Tollin M, Bergsson G, Kai-Larsen Y, et al. Vernix caseosa as a multi-component defence system based on polypeptides, lipids and their interactions. *Cell Mol Life Sci.* 2005;62(19-20):2390-2399.
13. Fluhr JW, Darlenski R, Taieb A, et al. Functional skin adaptation in infancy-almost complete but not fully competent. *Exp Dermatol.* 2010;19(6):483-492.
14. Fluhr JW, Darlenski R, Lachmann N, et al. Infant epidermal skin physiology: adaptation after birth. *Br J Dermatol.* 2012;166(3):483-490.
15. Rutter N, Hull D. Water loss from the skin of term and preterm babies. *Arch Dis Child.* 1979;54(11):858-868.
16. Visscher MO, Chatterjee R, Munson KA, et al. Changes in diapered and nondiapered infant skin over the first month of life. *Pediatr Dermatol.* 2000;17(1):45-51.
17. Miyauchi Y, Shimaoka Y, Fujimura T, et al. Developmental changes in neonatal and infant skin structures during the first 6 months: in vivo observation. *Pediatr Dermatol.* 2016;33(3):289-295.
18. Schmid-Wendtner MH, Korting HC. The pH of the skin surface and its impact on the barrier function. *Skin Pharmacol Physiol.* 2006;19(6):296-302.
19. Beare JM, Cheeseman EA, Gailey AA, et al. The effect of age on the pH of the skin surface in the first week of life. *Br J Dermatol.* 1960;72:62-66.
20. Hoeger PH, Enzmann CC. Skin physiology of the neonate and young infant: a prospective study of functional skin parameters during early infancy. *Pediatr Dermatol.* 2002;19(3):256-262.
21. Yosipovitch G, Maayan-Metzger A, Merlob P, et al. Skin barrier properties in different body areas in neonates. *Pediatrics.* 2000;106(1, pt 1):105-108.
22. Henderson CA, Taylor J, Cunliffe WJ. Sebum excretion rates in mothers and neonates. *Br J Dermatol.* 2000;142(1):110-111.
23. Harpin VA, Rutter N. Development of emotional sweating in the newborn infant. *Arch Dis Child.* 1982;57(9):691-695.
24. Harpin VA, Rutter N. Sweating in preterm babies. *J Pediatr.* 1982;100(4):614-619.
25. Evans NJ, Rutter N. Development of the epidermis in the newborn. *Biol Neonate.* 1986;49(2):74-80.
26. Kalia YN, Nonato LB, Lund CH, et al. Development of skin barrier function in premature infants. *J Invest Dermatol.* 1998;111(2):320-326.
27. Mathanda TR, M Bhat R, Hegde P, et al. Transepidermal water loss in neonates: baseline values using a closed-chamber system. *Pediatr Dermatol.* 2016;33(1):33-37.
28. Bertini G, Perugi S, Elia S, et al. Transepidermal water loss and cerebral hemodynamics in preterm infants: conventional versus LED phototherapy. *Eur J Pediatr.* 2008;167(1):37-42.
29. Maayan-Metzger A, Yosipovitch G, Hadad E, et al. Effect of radiant warmer on transepidermal water loss (TEWL) and skin hydration in preterm infants. *J Perinatol.* 2004;24(6):372-375.
30. Nopper AJ, Horii KA, Sookdeo-Drost S, et al. Topical ointment therapy benefits premature infants. *J Pediatr.* 1996;128(5, pt 1):660-669.
31. Campbell JR, Zaccaria E, Baker CJ. Systemic candidiasis in extremely low birth weight infants receiving topical petrolatum ointment for skin care: a case-control study. *Pediatrics.* 2000;105(5):1041-1045.
32. Edwards WH, Conner JM, Soll RF, et al. The effect of prophylactic ointment therapy on nosocomial sepsis rates and skin integrity in infants with birth weights of 501 to 1000 g. *Pediatrics.* 2004;113(5):1195-1203.
33. Darmstadt GL, Saha SK, Ahmed AS, et al. Effect of skin barrier therapy on neonatal mortality rates in preterm infants in Bangladesh: a randomized, controlled, clinical trial. *Pediatrics.* 2008;121(3):522-529.
34. Cleminson J, McGuire W. Topical emollient for preventing infection in preterm infants. *Cochrane Database Syst Rev.* 2016(1):CD001150.
35. Blume-Peytavi U, Cork MJ, Faergemann J, et al. Bathing and cleansing in newborns from day 1 to first year of life: recommendations from a European round table meeting. *J Eur Acad Dermatol Venereol.* 2009;23(7):751-759.
36. Cetta F, Lambert GH, Ros SP. Newborn chemical exposure from over-the-counter skin care products. *Clin Pediatr (Phila).* 1991;30(5):286-289.
37. Malloy-McDonald MB, Lambert GH. Neonatal skin care. *Compr Ther.* 1993;19(6):286-290.
38. Lavender T, Bedwell C, Roberts SA, et al. Randomized, controlled trial evaluating a baby wash product on skin barrier function in healthy, term neonates. *J Obstet Gynecol Neonatal Nurs.* 2013;42(2):203-214.
39. Garcia Bartels N, Mleczko A, Schink T, et al. Influence of bathing or washing on skin barrier function in newborns during the first four weeks of life. *Skin Pharmacol Physiol.* 2009;22(5):248-257.
40. Garcia Bartels N, Scheufele R, Prosch F, et al. Effect of standardized skin care regimens on neonatal skin barrier function in different body areas. *Pediatr Dermatol.* 2010;27(1):1-8.
41. Benis MM. Newborn percutaneous absorption: hazards and therapeutic uses. *Neonatal Netw.* 1999;18(8):63-69.
42. Liang MG, Frieden IJ. Perineal and lip ulcerations as the presenting manifestation of hemangioma of infancy. *Pediatrics.* 1997;99(2):256-259.
43. Parker LA. Part 1: early recognition and treatment of birth trauma: injuries to the head and face. *Adv Neonatal Care.* 2005;5(6):288-297; quiz 298-300.
44. Wang AR, Bercovitch L. Congenital milia en plaque. *Pediatr Dermatol.* 2016;33(4):e258-e259.

45. Chang MW, Jiang SB, Orlow SJ. Atypical erythema toxicum neonatorum of delayed onset in a term infant. *Pediatr Dermatol.* 1999;16(2):137-141.
46. Januario G, Salgado M. The Harlequin phenomenon. *J Eur Acad Dermatol Venereol.* 2011;25(12):1381-1384.
47. Niamba P, Weill FX, Sarlangue J, et al. Is common neonatal cephalic pustulosis (neonatal acne) triggered by *Malassezia sympodialis*? *Arch Dermatol.* 1998;134(8):995-998.
48. Bardazzi F, Patrizi A. Transient cephalic neonatal pustulosis. *Arch Dermatol.* 1997;133(4):528-530.
49. Shaw WC. Folklore surrounding facial deformity and the origins of facial prejudice. *Br J Plast Surg.* 1981;34(3):237-246.
50. Alper JC, Holmes LB. The incidence and significance of birthmarks in a cohort of 4,641 newborns. *Pediatr Dermatol.* 1983;1(1):58-68.
51. Jacobs AH, Walton RG. The incidence of birthmarks in the neonate. *Pediatrics.* 1976;58(2):218-222.
52. Krengel S, Scope A, Dusza SW, et al. New recommendations for the categorization of cutaneous features of congenital melanocytic nevi. *J Am Acad Dermatol.* 2013;68(3):441-451.
53. Happle R. Mosaicism in human skin. Understanding the patterns and mechanisms. *Arch Dermatol.* 1993;129(11):1460-1470.
54. Treat J. Patterned pigmentation in children. *Pediatr Clin North Am.* 2010;57(5):1121-1129.
55. Northrup H, Krueger DA, International Tuberous Sclerosis Complex Consensus Group. Tuberous sclerosis complex diagnostic criteria update: recommendations of the 2012 International Tuberous Sclerosis Complex Consensus Conference. *Pediatr Neurol.* 2013;49(4):243-254.
56. Happle R. Capillary malformations: a classification using specific names for specific skin disorders. *J Eur Acad Dermatol Venereol.* 2015;29(12):2295-2305.
57. Juern AM, Glick ZR, Drolet BA, et al. Nevus simplex: a reconsideration of nomenclature, sites of involvement, and disease associations. *J Am Acad Dermatol.* 2010;63(5):805-814.
58. Kaddu S, Schaeppi H, Kerl H, et al. Basaloid neoplasms in nevus sebaceus. *J Cutan Pathol.* 2000;27(7):327-337.
59. Cribier B, Scrivener Y, Grosshans E. Tumors arising in nevus sebaceus: a study of 596 cases. *J Am Acad Dermatol.* 2000;42(2, pt 1):263-268.
60. Asch S, Sugarman JL. Epidermal nevus syndromes. *Handb Clin Neurol.* 2015;132:291-316.
61. Leppig KA, Werler MM, Cann CI, et al. Predictive value of minor anomalies. I. Association with major malformations. *J Pediatr.* 1987;110(4):531-537.
62. Marden PM, Smith DW, McDonald MJ. Congenital anomalies in the newborn infant, including minor variations. A study of 4,412 babies by surface examination for anomalies and buccal smear for sex chromatin. *J Pediatr.* 1964;64:357-371.
63. Drolet B. Birthmarks to worry about. Cutaneous markers of dysraphism. *Dermatol Clin.* 1998;16(3):447-453.
64. Guggisberg D, Hadj-Rabia S, Viney C, et al. Skin markers of occult spinal dysraphism in children: a review of 54 cases. *Arch Dermatol.* 2004;140(9):1109-1115.
65. Sewell MJ, Chiu YE, Drolet BA. Neural tube dysraphism: review of cutaneous markers and imaging. *Pediatr Dermatol.* 2015;32(2):161-170.
66. Peter JC, Sinclair-Smith C, de Villiers JC. Midline dermal sinuses and cysts and their relationship to the central nervous system. *Eur J Pediatr Surg.* 1991;1(2):73-79.
67. Golden BA, Jaskolka MS, Ruiz RL. Craniofacial and orbital dermoids in children. *Oral Maxillofac Surg Clin North Am.* 2012;24(3):417-425.
68. Tubbs RS, Malefant J, Loukas M, et al. Enigmatic human tails: a review of their history, embryology, classification, and clinical manifestations. *Clin Anat.* 2016;29(4):430-438.
69. Gupta R, Singal A, Pandhi D. Faun tail naevus: a cutaneous marker of spinal dysraphism. *Indian Pediatr.* 2005;42(1):67-69.
70. Prosser JD, Myer CM 3rd. Branchial cleft anomalies and thymic cysts. *Otolaryngol Clin North Am.* 2015;48(1):1-14.
71. Chou J, Walters A, Hage R, et al. Thyroglossal duct cysts: anatomy, embryology and treatment. *Surg Radiol Anat.* 2013;35(10):875-881.
72. Carlisle EM, Mezhir JJ, Glynn L, et al. The umbilical mass: a rare neonatal anomaly. *Pediatr Surg Int.* 2007;23(8):821-824.
73. Frieden IJ. Aplasia cutis congenita: a clinical review and proposal for classification. *J Am Acad Dermatol.* 1986;14(4):646-660.
74. Stevens CA, Galen W. The hair collar sign. *Am J Med Genet A.* 2008;146A(4):484-487.
75. Kimberlin DW, Lin CY, Jacobs RF, et al. Natural history of neonatal herpes simplex virus infections in the acyclovir era. *Pediatrics.* 2001;108(2):223-229.
76. Darmstadt GL, Dinulos JG, Miller Z. Congenital cutaneous candidiasis: clinical presentation, pathogenesis, and management guidelines. *Pediatrics.* 2000;105(2):438-444.
77. Pruszkowski A, Bodemer C, Fraitag S, et al. Neonatal and infantile erythrodermas: a retrospective study of 51 patients. *Arch Dermatol.* 2000;136(7):875-880.
78. Lehman JS, Rahil AK. Congenital psoriasis: case report and literature review. *Pediatr Dermatol.* 2008;25(3):332-338.
79. Alexopoulos A, Kakourou T, Orfanou I, et al. Retrospective analysis of the relationship between infantile seborrheic dermatitis and atopic dermatitis. *Pediatr Dermatol.* 2014;31(2):125-130.
80. Mock DM. Skin manifestations of biotin deficiency. *Semin Dermatol.* 1991;10(4):296-302.
81. Arbuckle HA, Morelli J. Holocarboxylase synthetase deficiency presenting as ichthyosis. *Pediatr Dermatol.* 2006;23(2):142-144.
82. Baumgartner ER, Suormala T. Multiple carboxylase deficiency: inherited and acquired disorders of biotin metabolism. *Int J Vitam Nutr Res.* 1997;67(5):377-384.
83. Hansen AE, Haggard ME, Boelsche AN, et al. Essential fatty acids in infant nutrition. III. Clinical manifestations of linoleic acid deficiency. *J Nutr.* 1958;66(4):565-576.
84. Haveman LM, Fleer A, de Vries LS, et al. Congenital staphylococcal scalded skin syndrome in a premature infant. *Acta Paediatr.* 2004;93(12):1661-1662.
85. Kapoor V, Travadi J, Braye S. Staphylococcal scalded skin syndrome in an extremely premature neonate: a case report with a brief review of literature. *J Paediatr Child Health.* 2008;44(6):374-376.
86. Li MY, Hua Y, Wei GH, et al. Staphylococcal scalded skin syndrome in neonates: an 8-year retrospective study in a single institution. *Pediatr Dermatol.* 2014;31(1):43-47.
87. Lo WT, Wang CC, Chu ML. Intrauterine staphylococcal scalded skin syndrome: report of a case. *Pediatr Infect Dis J.* 2000;19(5):481-482.

88. Wood VD, Rana S. Congenital syphilis presenting as desquamative dermatitis. *J Fam Pract*. 1992;35(3):327-329.
89. Kim JK, Choi SR, Lee HJ, et al. Congenital syphilis presenting with a generalized bullous and pustular eruption in a premature newborn. *Ann Dermatol*. 2011;23(suppl 1):S127-S130.
90. Lee SH, Kim JH, Kim SC. Early congenital syphilis presenting with vesicobullous eruptions beyond palmoplantar regions. *Acta Derm Venereol*. 2014;94(3):321-322.
91. Craiglow BG. Ichthyosis in the newborn. *Semin Perinatol*. 2013;37(1):26-31.
92. Stone DL, Carey WF, Christodoulou J, et al. Type 2 Gaucher disease: the collodion baby phenotype revisited. *Arch Dis Child Fetal Neonatal Ed*. 2000;82(2):F163-F166.
93. Thomas C, Suranyi E, Pride H, et al. A child with hypohidrotic ectodermal dysplasia with features of a collodion membrane. *Pediatr Dermatol*. 2006;23(3):251-254.
94. Diamond CE, Sanchez MJ, LaBelle JL. Diagnostic criteria and evaluation of severe combined immunodeficiency in the neonate. *Pediatr Ann*. 2015;44(7):e181-e187.
95. Muller SM, Ege M, Pottharst A, et al. Transplacentally acquired maternal T lymphocytes in severe combined immunodeficiency: a study of 121 patients. *Blood*. 2001;98(6):1847-1851.
96. Denianke KS, Frieden IJ, Cowan MJ, et al. Cutaneous manifestations of maternal engraftment in patients with severe combined immunodeficiency: a clinicopathologic study. *Bone Marrow Transplant*. 2001;28(3):227-233.
97. Morinishi Y, Imai K, Nakagawa N, et al. Identification of severe combined immunodeficiency by T-cell receptor excision circles quantification using neonatal Guthrie cards. *J Pediatr*. 2009;155(6):829-833.
98. Minegishi Y, Saito M. Cutaneous manifestations of hyper IgE syndrome. *Allergol Int*. 2012;61(2):191-196.
99. Chamlin SL, McCalmont TH, Cunningham BB, et al. Cutaneous manifestations of hyper-IgE syndrome in infants and children. *J Pediatr*. 2002;141(4):572-575.
100. Markert ML, Alexieff MJ, Li J, et al. Complete DiGeorge syndrome: development of rash, lymphadenopathy, and oligoclonal T cells in 5 cases. *J Allergy Clin Immunol*. 2004;113(4):734-741.
101. Selim MA, Markert ML, Burchette JL, et al. The cutaneous manifestations of atypical complete DiGeorge syndrome: a histopathologic and immunohistochemical study. *J Cutan Pathol*. 2008;35(4):380-385.
102. Leclerc-Mercier S, Bodemer C, Bourdon-Lanoy E, et al. Early skin biopsy is helpful for the diagnosis and management of neonatal and infantile erythrodermas. *J Cutan Pathol*. 2010;37(2):249-255.
103. Ruiz-Maldonado R, Lopez-Matinez R, Perez Chavarria EL, et al. *Pityrosporum ovale* in infantile seborrheic dermatitis. *Pediatr Dermatol*. 1989;6(1):16-20.
104. Mimouni K, Mukamel M, Zeharia A, et al. Prognosis of infantile seborrheic dermatitis. *J Pediatr*. 1995;127(5):744-746.
105. Menni S, Piccinno R, Baietta S, et al. Infantile seborrheic dermatitis: seven-year follow-up and some prognostic criteria. *Pediatr Dermatol*. 1989;6(1):13-15.
106. Wolf R, Wolf D, Tuzun B, et al. Diaper dermatitis. *Clin Dermatol*. 2000;18(6):657-660.
107. Smith WJ, Jacob SE. The role of allergic contact dermatitis in diaper dermatitis. *Pediatr Dermatol*. 2009;26(3):369-370.
108. Weston WL, Lane AT, Weston JA. Diaper dermatitis: current concepts. *Pediatrics*. 1980;66(4):532-536.
109. Goldberg NS, Esterly NB, Rothman KF, et al. Perianal pseudoverrucous papules and nodules in children. *Arch Dermatol*. 1992;128(2):240-242.
110. De Zeeuw R, Van Praag MC, Oranje AP. Granuloma gluteale infantum: a case report. *Pediatr Dermatol*. 2000;17(2):141-143.
111. Boiko S. Making rash decisions in the diaper area. *Pediatr Ann*. 2000;29(1):50-56.
112. Stanford D, Rogers M. Dermatological presentations of infantile myofibromatosis: a review of 27 cases. *Australas J Dermatol*. 2000;41(3):156-161.
113. Kang G, Suh YL, Han J, et al. Fibrous hamartoma of infancy: an experience of a single institute. *J Korean Surg Soc*. 2011;81(1):61-65.
114. Saab ST, McClain CM, Coffin CM. Fibrous hamartoma of infancy: a clinicopathologic analysis of 60 cases. *Am J Surg Pathol*. 2014;38(3):394-401.
115. Heymann WR. Infantile digital fibromatosis. *J Am Acad Dermatol*. 2008;59(1):122-123.
116. Hawthorne HC Jr, Nelson JS, Witzleben CL, et al. Blanching subcutaneous nodules in neonatal neuroblastoma. *J Pediatr*. 1970;77(2):297-300.
117. van der Linden MH, Creemers S, Pieters R. Diagnosis and management of neonatal leukaemia. *Semin Fetal Neonatal Med*. 2012;17(4):192-195.
118. Simko SJ, Garmezy B, Abhyankar H, et al. Differentiating skin-limited and multisystem Langerhans cell histiocytosis. *J Pediatr*. 2014;165(5):990-996.
119. Carter MC, Clayton ST, Komarow HD, et al. Assessment of clinical findings, tryptase levels, and bone marrow histopathology in the management of pediatric mastocytosis. *J Allergy Clin Immunol*. 2015;136(6):1673-1679.e1-3.
120. Gonzalez ME. Evaluation and treatment of the newborn with epidermolysis bullosa. *Semin Perinatol*. 2013;37(1):32-39.
121. Oji V, Tadini G, Akiyama M, et al. Revised nomenclature and classification of inherited ichthyoses: results of the First Ichthyosis Consensus Conference in Soreze 2009. *J Am Acad Dermatol*. 2010;63(4):607-641.
122. Itin PH. Etiology and pathogenesis of ectodermal dysplasias. *Am J Med Genet A*. 2014;164A(10):2472-2477.
123. Smahi A, Courtois G, Vabres P, et al. Genomic rearrangement in NEMO impairs NF-kappaB activation and is a cause of incontinentia pigmenti. The International Incontinentia Pigmenti (IP) Consortium. *Nature*. 2000;405(6785):466-472.
124. Minic S, Trpinac D, Obradovic M. Incontinentia pigmenti diagnostic criteria update. *Clin Genet*. 2014;85(6):536-542.
125. Pacheco TR, Levy M, Collyer JC, et al. Incontinentia pigmenti in male patients. *J Am Acad Dermatol*. 2006;55(2):251-255.
126. Burden AD, Krafchik BR. Subcutaneous fat necrosis of the newborn: a review of 11 cases. *Pediatr Dermatol*. 1999;16(5):384-387.
127. Prizant TL, Lucky AW, Frieden IJ, et al. Spontaneous atrophic patches in extremely premature infants. Anetoderma of prematurity. *Arch Dermatol*. 1996;132(6):671-674.
128. Goujon E, Beer F, Gay S, et al. Anetoderma of prematurity: an iatrogenic consequence of neonatal intensive care. *Arch Dermatol*. 2010;146(5):565-567.
129. Amitai DB, Fichman S, Merlob P, et al. Cutis marmorata telangiectatica congenita: clinical findings in 85 patients. *Pediatr Dermatol*. 2000;17(2):100-104.

Chapter 104 :: Pediatric and Adolescent Dermatology :: Mary Wu Chang

第一百零四章
儿科和青少年皮肤病学

中文导读

本章按三个不同的年龄段分别讲述了婴儿、童年、青少年的用药特点、检查技巧和注意事项等，并分年龄段分别介绍了一些常见皮肤疾病。最后在讲述儿科专题时介绍了自闭症，讨论了儿童用药，以及儿童虐待等问题。

1．婴儿　评估方法应包括完整的病史和彻底的体查。婴儿的完整病史包括妊娠史和分娩史以及家族史。应询问孕妇妊娠期间的接触史，包括药物、非处方药物和感染性疾病（包括性传播疾病）等。作者认为，询问完整婴儿生长发育史和彻底体查是至关重要的，并列表提供了帮助儿科皮肤病评估的十条建议。

作者还提到了发生于婴儿时期的一些常见皮肤病，如胎记、脱发（休止期脱发、枕秃、皮脂腺痣、三角颞脱发、斑秃、头癣、拔毛癣）、尿布区域皮肤病（婴儿会阴突出、尿布皮炎）的病因及儿科临床表现。还提到了尿布皮炎的两个特殊型：红色粟疹和婴儿颗粒状角化病。

2．童年　针对童年时期的病患，评估方法除了包括完整的病史和彻底的体查，既往治疗经过和用药史也很有帮助。作者还细致地提供了让患儿更顺利接受检查的技巧和注意事项等。如果需要选择性活检或手术，应安排在第二次就诊时进行，而不是第一次就诊时进行，父母或孩子通常更容易接受。

接下来的检查内容部分，作者讲述了活检、手术、全身麻醉和镇静、皮肤斑贴试验等。在选择活检病例时，作者列表提供了一些"活检缺陷"的示例。还特别讲述了局麻活检的注意事项，应注意安全剂量，以及如何帮助缓解疼痛的具体方法包括选择麻药种类、注射前麻醉皮肤的其他方法，如冰敷或冷冻麻醉(如乙基氯)、在手术前和手术过程中可以用浸在蔗糖溶液中的奶嘴安抚婴儿、引导家长及患儿做好准备，比如"摆弄"他或她的脚趾、听音乐或看电影等。

3．青少年　青少年皮肤病的诊断与成人皮肤病学有重叠。但跟青少年患者有效地沟通需要各种面谈技巧和策略来提高依从性，作者提供了一些有效的沟通策略。

保密是向青少年患者提供有效医疗保健活动的一个必要组成部分。病人的隐私权应该得到尊重，但医生不应该对父母或监护人撒谎。此外，应告知青少年患者，虽然临床医生会尊重他们的保密约定，但不能保证无条件保密。

询问技巧包括首先问候青少年，其次是父母，单独与青少年患者进行部分询问有助于赢得患者的信任。使用第三人称的措辞和提问时给出选择，更容易有效地获取信息等。

本章还提到了一些发生于青少年的常见

皮肤问题，如粉刺、青少年痤疮、腋窝多汗症、室内晒黑等，并在用药及治疗上提供了选择方案。特别提出室内晒黑的学生可产生更严重的焦虑症状，以致更多的酒精、大麻和其他物质的使用，应对父母和我们的年轻人进行反对室内晒黑的教育，禁止未成年人使用日光浴床等。

4. 儿科专题

（1）自闭症谱系障碍，或称自闭症，是指一组复杂的大脑发育障碍这些障碍表现为不同程度上的社交困难、语言和非语言沟通困难和重复的行为来表现。ASD可能与智力障碍、注意力集中困难、感觉处理障碍、进食障碍、运动协调中断、睡眠障碍和胃肠道紊乱有关。ASD与皮肤科相关的疾病包括感官处理相关疾病（例如感官刺激功能障碍包括过敏症和低敏感性、触觉防御、无法容忍局部药物或润肤剂）和神经行为传播的皮肤病（如创伤、茧子和重复的刺激行为造成自残等）。并列表讲述了自闭症患儿常见的皮肤症状及照顾自闭症患儿的方法。之后，作者谈及自闭症患儿这一特殊群体相关的遗传性皮肤病及常见的皮肤病，还提供了这类患儿就诊时皮肤科医生可采取的处理方式。

（2）进一步讨论到儿童用药问题，分别讲述了局部用药和系统用药的要点。曾有一些局部外用药物引起儿童全身毒性的报告。虽然局部用药通常具有极佳的安全性和有效性，但必须认识到婴幼儿局部用药的毒性风险增加，因为与成人相比，表面面积与身体质量比增加。此外，与成人相比，婴儿和儿童有时会改变药物的代谢。此外，讲述了系统使用糖皮质激素、四环素等抗菌素的风险及注意事项等。

（3）最后，还讲到儿童虐待的问题。儿童虐待是指父母（或监护人）的虐待或忽视，导致对儿童潜在的、实际或威胁性的伤害。虐待儿童包括虐待行为和不作为行为。虐待儿童分为4类：①身体虐待（如殴打、摇晃或烧灼）；②性虐待（如强奸或抚摸）；③心理虐待（如恐吓或贬低）；④忽视（例如无法满足基本的身体、情感、教育或医疗需求）。通过举例说明了儿童虐待发生率就现在社会而言还是处于较多的状态。对于这类儿童，全身检查和客观记录，是至关重要的。并指出虐待的风险因素包括有特殊需要的儿童或慢性病、残疾以及增加照料者负担等。

〔刘芳芬〕

AT-A-GLANCE

- The infant or child is the patient, but working with the parents/caregivers and home situation is crucial in diagnosis and management.
- Obtaining a history, and methods of clinical examination in infants and children differ from the approaches chosen for adults. In adolescents, different skills are required to enhance communication and compliance.
- Many outpatient procedures in pediatric dermatology can be done with appropriate planning and age-appropriate techniques. Patch testing or biopsies should not be avoided simply because of a pediatric patient's age.
- The infant has increased risk for systemic toxicity from topically applied substances. Children with disorders of barrier function are at high risk of excess percutaneous absorption and toxicity as well.
- Drug labeling for pediatric patients is different from that in adults and most therapeutic agents are prescribed off-label.
- Autism spectrum disorders are now common. Dermatologists must be aware of special issues involved in caring for these patients.

Just as dermatology cannot be separated from internal medicine, pediatric dermatology is inseparable from general pediatrics. Most dermatologists have experience and training in internal medicine but less exposure to pediatrics, therefore an introduction to the special issues that can arise in pediatric dermatology is presented here. As it is impossible to discuss all of pediatric dermatology in a single chapter, the focus is instead on certain methods, diseases, and issues divided by age divisions: infants, children, and adolescents. This chapter discusses topics of special importance, such as pediatric medication use and biopsy pitfalls, and reviews methods to enhance success in outpatient procedures in pediatric dermatology.

Table 104-1 reviews 10 helpful tips in practicing pediatric dermatology. Successful care of the pediatric patient is best achieved via a partnership with the parents or caregivers, along with comanagement with the pediatrician or primary care physician. An awareness of the child's living situation is always relevant. For example, children living in 2 households because the parents are separated or divorced often do best with 2 sets of medications, 1 in each home, to enhance compliance. In the age of internet access, patients and caregivers will likely search online for medical information before or after the office encounter. They should be reminded that medical information on the internet is often inaccurate.[1] Instead, directing patients and families to specific internet websites, support groups, or pamphlets is valuable, but these resources should be reviewed before recommending them.

Parents are understandably very worried about their children and the office visit cannot be rushed. If conflicts arise in the office, discussions should be approached with the common goal of doing what is best for the child. At other times, the clinician must gently intervene and clarify when the parents' desire for treatment may not be in the best interest of the patient.

CONSIDERATIONS IN INFANTS

EVALUATION TECHNIQUES

A complete history for an infant includes gestational and birth history as well as family history. Exposures during pregnancy should be reviewed, including medications, illicit drugs, and infectious diseases, including sexually transmitted diseases. Inquiring about growth and development is crucial. Is the infant gaining weight along proper growth curves? Is the baby vigorous, with good tone, and feeding well with a good suck?

When examining an infant, it is crucial to be thorough. Whether the infant is examined in the lap of the parent or on the examination table, all surfaces, including the creases and valleys of body folds and the diaper region (including the genitalia), need close examination. The diaper area has its own unique set of problems and deserves examination at every visit. Even what is in the diaper (Fig. 104-1) can be useful information. An infant with atopic dermatitis and abnormal stools, for example, may have a food intolerance or allergy that must be addressed before dermatologic treatment will be successful. A vascular stain, vasoconstricted macule, or erosion can be the presenting sign of a hemangioma.[2] A stray hair may later strangulate an appendage and should be removed. Infants with digital tourniquet (pseudoainhum) and clitoral tourniquet have been described.[3,4] Cutaneous anomalies warrant closer inspection to rule out associated findings. Midline lesions on the face, scalp, or spine may have CNS connections and should not be biopsied without proper evaluation (Table 104-2).

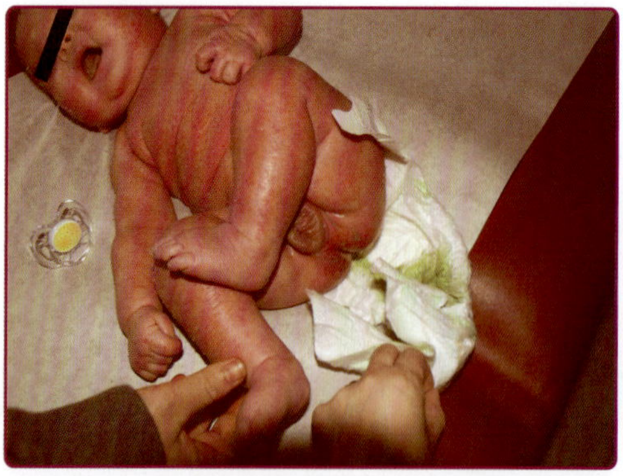

TABLE 104-1
Ten Helpful Tips in Pediatric Dermatology

1. The child is the patient, not the parents.
2. Biopsy when indicated, regardless of age. (Refer if necessary.)
3. What is the child's living situation? Does the child live in 2 homes? Are the parents going through a divorce?
4. Be aware of the parents' perspectives of the child. Was there difficulty in conceiving? Was the child premature? Was there significant early illness? Is there chronic illness?
5. A team approach with the pediatrician, neonatologist, or family physician is best. Comanagement with a psychiatrist may be indicated (isotretinoin issues or trichotillomania, for example).
6. A chronic condition or illness in a child affects the entire family.
7. Guide parents and patients to appropriate internet resources, but always review materials for accuracy beforehand.
8. Obtain consent from parents, and assent from children, for procedures and photos.
9. An adolescent's confidentiality must be maintained unless there is a danger of harm to the patient or others. Consider interviewing the patient alone without parents for a portion of the visit. Consider having a chaperone in the room for full skin examinations.
10. First, do no harm.

Figure 104-1 Four-month-old infant with extensive eczematous dermatitis and diaper dermatitis. Opening up the diaper reveals greenish liquid stools, very abnormal at this age. Referral for pediatric allergy testing and changing the diet was indicated in this case.

TABLE 104-2
Biopsy Pitfalls in Pediatric Dermatology

AGE GROUP	LESION AND SITE	DIAGNOSIS	DANGER	PROPER MANAGEMENT
Newborn to infant	Round or oval erosion or vesicle on the scalp, less commonly on the cheek or neck	Aplasia cutis congenita (see Chap. 103); differential diagnosis includes herpes simplex, fetal scalp electrode trauma	Possible intracranial connection, risk of meningitis with biopsy or scraping	Observation for spontaneous healing; consider ultrasonography or MRI if atypical
Infant	"Hair collar" sign surrounding congenital lesion on scalp or posterior axis midline lesion	Encephalocele, spina bifida occulta, meningomyelocele	Possible intracranial connection; risk of meningitis	Preoperative imaging; consider neurosurgical consultation
Infant	Tuft of hair over midline spine	Spina bifida occulta, meningomyelocele	Possible intracranial connection; risk of meningitis	Preoperative imaging; consider neurosurgical consultation
Infant	Preauricular "tag"	Accessory tragus	Risk of chondritis if removed by shave or snip excision or if ligated with suture	Appropriate closure when excised, if cartilaginous component is present
Infant, young child	Dome-shaped mass along midline scalp, glabella, side of forehead, or other embryonic fusion plane	Dermoid cyst	Intracranial connection in up to 25% for midline dermoids; risk is higher if sinus present; dermoids near the lateral eyebrows rarely have intracranial connections	Consider MRI and neurosurgical consultation
Infant, young child	Nasal midline mass	Nasal glioma, encephalocele, or other dysraphic state; differential diagnosis: "hypertelorism," deep infantile hemangioma	Intracranial connection in 100% of encephaloceles; gliomas may extend into oropharynx or have intranasal connections	Consider MRI and neuro-surgical consultation
Infant, young child	Vascular mass with greatly increased warmth, often with pulsation or bruit	Arteriovenous malformation; differential diagnosis: congenital or infantile hemangioma	Uncontrolled bleeding, problematic bony or soft-tissue hypertrophy	Consider Doppler studies, MRI, and surgical consultation

BIRTHMARKS

Although the term *birthmark* implies a skin lesion that is present at birth, some cutaneous changes with congenital origins only become visible later in infancy or childhood. For example, nevus depigmentosus in a very-pale-skinned newborn is commonly not discernable, but becomes apparent later in infancy or early childhood when the infant's normal pigmentation develops. Another birthmark that is present at birth but may not become visible until early childhood is epidermal nevus. These 2 birthmarks are examples of mosaicism (Figs. 104-2 and 104-3).

Solitary café-au-lait macules are extremely common and benign. However, the appearance of multiple café-au-lait macules during infancy and early childhood raises the possibility of neurofibromatosis Type 1 (see Chap. 135). Chapter 103 reviews birthmarks in detail.

HAIR LOSS

TELOGEN EFFLUVIUM

Telogen effluvium occurs frequently in young infants and is often overlooked. The hair loss may be gradual or sudden, and may occur as soon as the first few days after birth, with the telogen hairs shed by 3 to 4 months of age. No treatment is indicated as spontaneous resolution is the rule.

OCCIPITAL ALOPECIA

A transient circumscribed patch of nonscarring alopecia develops at the occiput in many infants. Thought to be

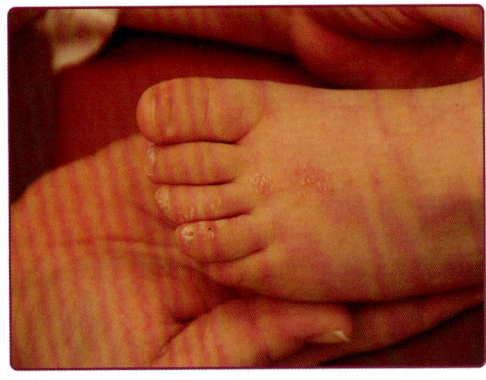

Figure 104-2 This 22-month-old child had a chronic, scaling, linear plaque extending onto 2 toes, representing linear epidermal nevus, an example of mosaicism.

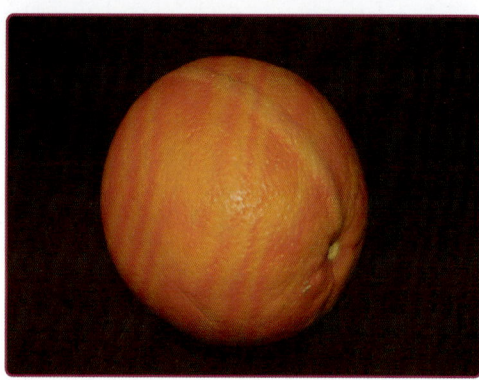

Figure 104-3 Mosaicism can be seen in nature, as demonstrated by the "birthmark" on this orange.

caused by a combination of physiologic telogen effluvium and localized pressure from lying in the supine position, occipital alopecia spontaneously resolves.

NEVUS SEBACEUS (ORGANOID NEVUS)

This hamartoma usually occurs on the head and neck as a waxy, yellowish plaque. On the scalp, it appears hairless owing to miniaturization of hairs. The typical yellow-orange color may not develop until later in childhood (Fig. 104-4).

TRIANGULAR TEMPORAL ALOPECIA

Triangular temporal alopecia is a form of nonscarring hair loss noted at 2 to 5 years of age as a triangular-shaped, oval-shaped, or lancet-shaped area of alopecia at the frontotemporal scalp. Often, a thin row of hair separates the affected area from the forehead. The terminal hairs are replaced by vellus hair. The condition is often mistaken for alopecia areata; however, distinguishing features include the typical location and shape, the presence of vellus hairs, and the absence of exclamation point hairs or histologic findings of alopecia areata. There is no known treatment, and the condition persists unchanged. However, triangular temporal alopecia is benign and will not expand.

ALOPECIA AREATA

Alopecia areata occurs in all ages (see Chap. 87). All variants of alopecia areata occur in infants and children, with similar disease presentation and treatment challenges as in adults. Onset at younger than 2 years of age is estimated to occur in 1% to 2% of alopecia areata patients; however, it may be underrecognized. Several cases of congenital alopecia areata have been documented. Early onset is considered to be a poor prognostic marker. Total alopecia during the first year of life after having hair at birth should be distinguished from genetic disorders, such as congenital atrichia with papular lesions and vitamin D resistance.

TINEA CAPITIS

Tinea capitis can occur at any age, including infancy. Hair loss associated with scaling, broken hairs, pustules, or black dots should prompt a potassium hydroxide scraping and/or fungal culture to confirm the diagnosis. Just as in older children, *Trichophyton tonsurans* is the most common dermatophyte, and oral griseofulvin is the treatment of choice.

Scrapings for potassium hydroxide examination and fungal culture should be obtained before administration of systemic antifungal therapy. In children, collection of specimens for tinea capitis may be accomplished by the use of a toothbrush, ring curette, moistened cotton swab, a scalpel, or by collection of infected hairs. If a child is not sitting still, the blunt side of a #15 scalpel can be used rather than the sharp blade side to collect scrapings. Alternatively, a media plate with nonslanted agar may be applied directly to the infected areas of the scalp to collect material.

TRICHOTILLOMANIA

Though alarming to parents, infant hair pulling usually has a good prognosis. It is often a self-soothing mechanism for infants, and may represent a different etiology than trichotillomania in adolescents and adults, which has a much poorer prognosis (Fig. 104-5).

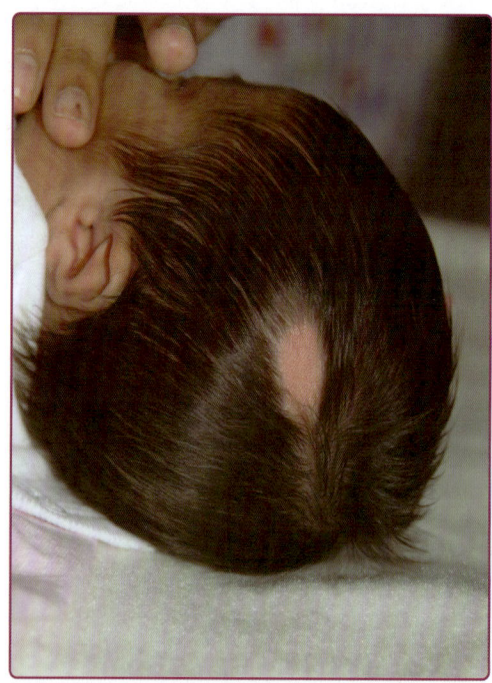

Figure 104-4 Nevus sebaceus (organoid nevus) appears hairless because of miniaturization of the hairs.

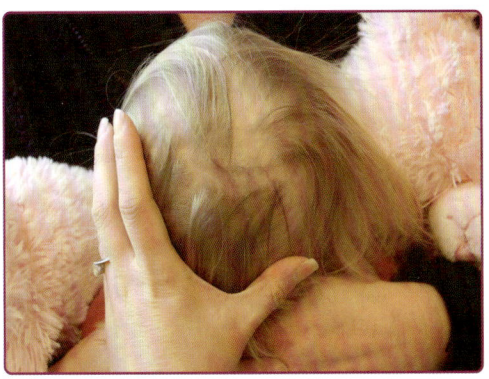

Figure 104-5 Irregular patches of alopecia developed in this healthy 2-year-old child. Broken hairs were noted. Trichotillomania was witnessed at home by the parents.

THE DIAPER REGION

INFANTILE PERINEAL PROTRUSION

Also known as *infantile pyramidal protrusion*, infantile perineal protrusion is a benign condition that occurs almost exclusively in female prepubertal girls. It appears as a pyramidal, soft-tissue, "tongue-like," smooth, or velvety pink protrusion. It is usually located in the midline just anterior to the anus. Infantile perineal protrusion is usually asymptomatic, but painful defecation has been reported. It occurs in 3 settings: constitutional, functional (after constipation, diarrhea, or other irritant exposure), or associated with lichen sclerosus et atrophicus. Often, infantile perineal protrusion is misdiagnosed as condyloma acuminatum, hemorrhoids, or as a sign of trauma. Conservative management is indicated. Spontaneous resolution, as well as resolution following a high-fiber diet to relieve constipation, has been noted.[5,6]

DIAPER DERMATITIS

Diaper dermatitis, like hand dermatitis, denotes a group of region-specific dermatoses. Diaper dermatitis is one of the most common dermatologic conditions in infants and children, noted in approximately 1 million pediatric outpatient visits each year.[7] With the advent of superabsorbent disposable diapers in the last decade, severe forms of diaper dermatitis have diminished in incidence. Irritant and candidal diaper dermatitis comprises the vast majority of diaper dermatitides in diaper-wearing individuals of all ages. Chap. 103 reviews diaper dermatitis and its variants. Additional considerations are presented below.

Miliaria Rubra ("Heat Rash"): Miliaria rubra tends to occur at sites where plastic components of the diaper cause occlusion of eccrine ducts of the skin. It is also seen in the folds of the neck and upper torso, and is particularly common when there is a rapid shift to warm weather, and the child is overdressed.

Infantile Granular Parakeratosis: Infantile granular parakeratosis represents an idiopathic form of retention keratosis in diaper-wearing infants. There are two clinical patterns: bilateral linear plaques in the inguinal folds and erythematous geometric plaques underlying pressure points from the diaper. A thick, flake-like scale is present in both forms and is characteristic. Therapeutic responsiveness to topical agents is ambiguous; however, spontaneous clearance after months to 1 year appears to be the rule.[8]

CONSIDERATIONS IN CHILDHOOD

EVALUATION TECHNIQUES

In addition to the themes discussed above for infants, further concepts are helpful when assessing children. Review of coexistent medical conditions and medications can lead to diagnostic clues. For example, perioral dermatitis (Fig. 104-6) can be triggered not only by topical corticosteroids, but also inhaled corticosteroids for asthma (particularly when a spacer with face mask is used), and by corticosteroid nasal sprays. Observing the play of a child allows for a quick assessment of the child's neurologic development. Interactions between caregivers and child are also informative. Early prolonged or intense eye contact with the young child should be avoided because this can be threatening to the child. If an elective biopsy or procedure is needed, it is often more acceptable for the parent or child if the procedure is scheduled for a second visit rather than for the initial visit.

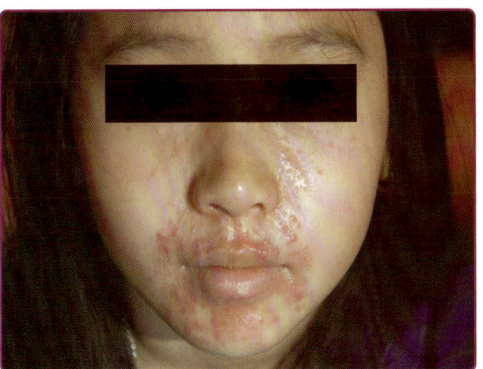

Figure 104-6 Perioral dermatitis is common in children and is exacerbated by topical corticosteroid use. Inhaled corticosteroids (for asthma) or nasal corticosteroid sprays (for allergic rhinitis) can also trigger perioral dermatitis. This condition responds well to discontinuing the corticosteroid exposure, and the use of topical metronidazole cream. Oral erythromycin is helpful in severe cases.

If a language barrier exists between the family and the physician, one should resist the urge to have the bilingual patient serve as interpreter for the parents/caregivers. This practice places an inappropriate burden of responsibility on the child and may increase fear and anxiety in the child. In addition, inaccurate transmission of information may occur.

Examination of young children may be performed with the child on the parent's lap or while playing with toys on the examination table. If needed, examination of the perineum and genitalia can be accomplished with the child in the knee-chest position on the examination table (Fig. 104-7) or the parent's lap. Alternatively, the child may sit on the parent's lap with legs held apart by the parent. Figure 104-8 illustrates anatomic terminology of the young female genitalia for accurate documentation, and can be helpful in conditions such as lichen sclerosus. Caution must be used in interpreting the genital examination in the young female so as not to underdiagnose or overdiagnose disease or abuse. For example, the presence of labia minora adhesions is not diagnostic of trauma or abuse because they occur in as many as one-third of girls who are not abused.[9] The diastasis ani is a normal structure that can be mistaken for perianal scarring.[10] The infantile perianal pyramidal protrusion may be mistaken for condyloma acuminata but is a harmless normal finding (see above).[5,6]

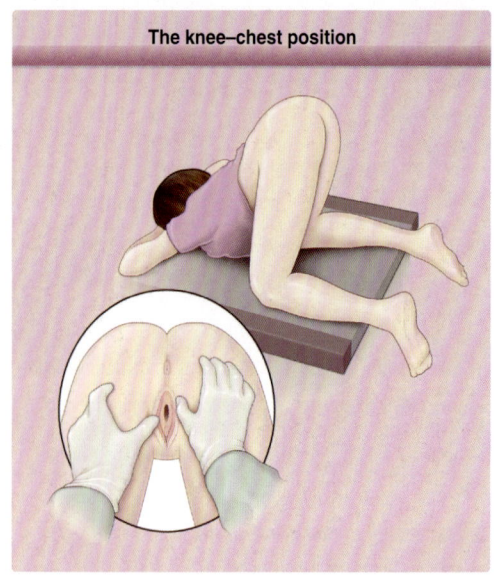

Figure 104-7 The knee–chest position allows visualization of the perineum and genitalia. (From Tintinalli JE, Stapczynski JS, Ma OJ, et al. *Tintinalli's Emergency Medicine: A Comprehensive Study Guide.* 7th ed. New York, NY: McGraw-Hill; 2010.)

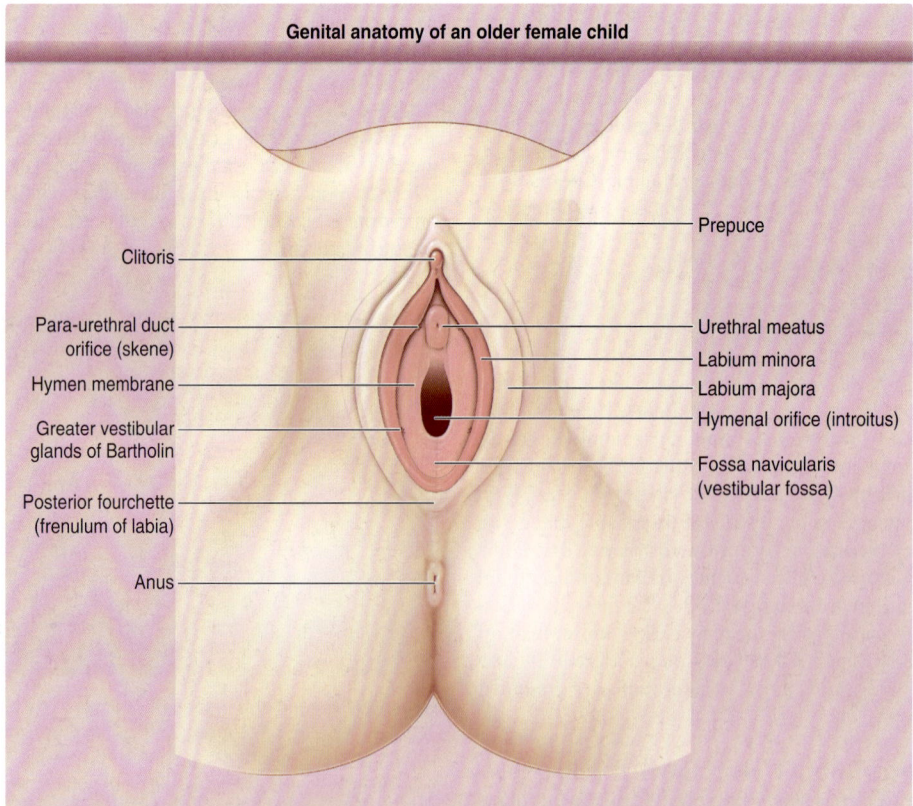

Figure 104-8 Genital anatomy of an older female child. (Redrawn from Finkel MA, DeJong AR. Medical findings in child abuse. In: Reece RM, ed. *Child Abuse: Medical Diagnosis and Management.* Philadelphia, PA: Lea & Febiger; 1994:185.)

PERFORMING PROCEDURES ON THE YOUNG CHILD

Historically, there has been a widespread reluctance to biopsy skin lesions in infants and children. This may lead to a delay in diagnosis of conditions such as childhood melanoma. In addition, many conditions in infants and children have a paucity of dermatopathologic information in the literature as a consequence of this reluctance. Parents may be anxious about causing pain or scarring, and children may be fearful because of their experience with immunizations, or an age-appropriate fear of bodily mutilation. However, with proper preparation of the parent and child, skin biopsies and other outpatient procedures are easily performed (Table 104-3). Note that there are certain situations in which a biopsy can be detrimental; Table 104-2 provides examples of these "biopsy pitfalls."

Eutectic mixtures of lidocaine and prilocaine (EMLA cream) or plain lidocaine cream are useful in minimizing the pain of intralesional injections or local anesthetic injections for biopsies. As EMLA use has become widespread, reports of toxicity in children have resulted, including methemoglobinemia and seizures. The maximum dose, body surface area exposed to drug, and application time should not be exceeded; these parameters are age dependent: 1 g for a 1- to 3-month-old, 2 g for a 3- to 12-month-old, 10 g for a 1- to 6-year-old, and 20 g for a 7- to 12-year-old child.[11] Note that increased absorption and toxicity can occur when applied on diseased skin, even with normal dosing. Other options to numb the skin prior to injections include the application of ice or anesthetic cryospray (eg, ethylchloride). Before and during procedures, young infants can be soothed with a pacifier dipped in a sucrose solution. A randomized, controlled, double-blinded study of 201 newborns found that orally administered glucose solution was superior to topical EMLA cream in reducing pain with venipuncture.[12] Infants may be swaddled with a blanket for comfort and immobilization. The young child can be effectively immobilized and comforted with a restraining "hug" by a parent or assistant. Distraction techniques are invaluable as well. For example, instructing the child to blow a colorful toy windmill, blow soap bubbles, or "wiggle" his or her toes during an injection or procedure helps to decrease pain. Older children may be effectively soothed by listening to music with headphones or by watching a movie during procedures.

Alkalinizing local anesthetics to a pH of 7.0 (0.1 mEq/mL sodium bicarbonate or a 1:10 bicarbonate-to-anesthetic ratio by volume) minimizes the pain of cutaneous infiltration without limiting anesthetic effects.[13] Alkalinization decreases the solution's shelf life to approximately 1 week[14] as a result of more rapid oxidation of epinephrine. Warming lidocaine also lessens the pain of injection.[13]

Gentle vibrational motions, applied with the surgeon's nondominant hand or a palm-sized vibrating device adjacent to the injection site while administering lidocaine, and infiltrating the anesthetic slowly are helpful to reduce the pain of anesthetic administration.

Instruments and materials laid out ahead of time ensure rapid performance of the procedure and are less frightening if kept out of sight by covering them with a drape. Needles, instruments, and blood-stained gauze should be kept out of view and out of reach of the patient.

Children sense their parents' anxiety and nervous energy. Parents who are overly anxious can be asked to sit farther away from the operating table, or sometimes are best positioned outside the procedure room.

Postoperative pain management is not necessary for the vast majority of biopsies and excisions in children. Acetaminophen, given on an as-needed basis, is usually sufficient.

TABLE 104-3
The ABCs of Successful Outpatient Procedures in Pediatric Dermatology

- **A: A**nesthesia techniques: EMLA or ice prior to injection, buffer the lidocaine, apply vibration next to injection site, and infuse slowly. **A**ppointment times in the morning are best for procedures on young children. If they are tired, they are less able to focus and cooperate.
- **B: B**lood: keep bloody gauze and instruments out of sight of patient and parents.
- **C: C**alm parents = calm child. **C**onsent by parents is required if the patient is a minor.
- **D: D**istraction techniques are essential: MP3 player, DVD player, *Where is Waldo?* books, and *I-Spy* books are all very helpful.
- **E: E**xpedite the procedure by preparing all instruments and materials before starting.
- **F: F**our hands (minimum) are needed—have at least 1 assistant to help, preferably not the parent.
- **G: G**o to a day surgery setting if the patient is unable to participate in local anesthesia because of age or abilities.
- **H: H**overing parents—keep parents seated and calm, with surgical site out of view.
- **I: I**nvest the time, do not rush.

GENERAL ANESTHESIA AND SEDATION

The use of general anesthesia for dermatologic procedures in healthy pediatric patients is very safe when properly performed. Fears of general anesthesia should not be a barrier to delivering necessary surgical or laser procedures to healthy children.[15]

However, for elective procedures, especially those requiring repeated or lengthy general anesthesia, the benefits of general anesthesia should be carefully weighed with the unknown risks to the developing brain in young children. Controversy exists whether repeated general anesthesia in infants and young children leads to increased risk of subsequent neurodevelopmental issues.

Obtaining an MRI study of infants and young children usually requires sedation or general anesthesia. MRI imaging typically requires the patient to lay motionless in a narrow dark space for 45 minutes or longer. Furthermore, the child must wear ear protection because the banging noises of the machine can reach sound levels of 118 to 125 decibels. Referral to a children's hospital or a radiology center that has a pediatric anesthesiologist is recommended to achieve a safe and accurate imaging study. For very young infants, sedation can sometimes be obviated by "feed and swaddle" techniques so that the infant patient sleeps deeply and remains motionless during the imaging procedure. However, this technique requires a center knowledgeable about imaging of infants.

PATCH TESTING IN CHILDREN

Allergic contact dermatitis (ACD) affects all ages (Fig. 104-9), but pediatric ACD is not well studied. In children, ACD tends to be misdiagnosed, underdiagnosed, and underreported. As a consequence, the epidemiology of ACD in children is not well understood. A recent multicenter pediatric contact dermatitis registry of 1142 children demonstrated that the prevalence of sensitization among patients with suspected ACD was up to 65%. The mean age of patch-tested children was 11 years. The top allergens were nickel (22%), fragrance mix 1 (11%), cobalt (9.1%), balsam of Peru (8%), neomycin (7%), propylene glycol (7%), cocamidopropyl betaine (6%), bacitracin (6%), formaldehyde (6%), and gold (6%).[16]

Strategies to ensure successful epicutaneous patch testing in young children need to be employed. Because of the mobility and flexibility of young children, it is helpful to have the young child stand up straight during application and marking of the patches. The use of Hypafix tape or other extra dressings or tape ensures the patches stay in place. Avoiding sports or gym class may be necessary to prevent sweating and movement of the patches. Additionally, the smaller surface area of the back in children may limit the number of patches placed.

ADOLESCENT DERMATOLOGY

Dermatologic diagnoses of adolescents overlap with those of general adult dermatology. However, caring effectively for the adolescent patient requires different interviewing skills and strategies to enhance compliance.

CONFIDENTIALITY

Confidentiality is a necessary component in providing effective health care to adolescents. Confidentiality

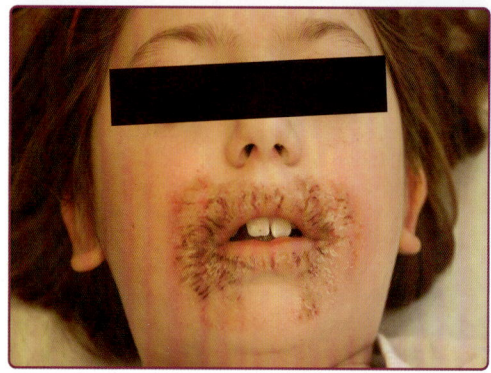

Figure 104-9 This healthy 8-year-old girl suffered from recurrent inflammatory, fissured, eczematous dermatitis on the face, and perianal region. Patch testing revealed methylisothiazolinone contact allergy. This preservative was contained in the wet wipes that were used to cleanse these regions. The eruption promptly cleared when the wipes were discontinued.[49]

laws vary from country to country; within the United States, they vary by state. Clinicians who treat adolescents should familiarize themselves with the state and local laws that affect the rights of minors to consent to health care services, as well as federal and state confidentiality laws.

The patient's right to privacy should be respected, but the clinician should never lie to the parent/guardian. Furthermore, adolescent patients should be informed that while clinicians will respect their confidentiality, unconditional confidentiality cannot be promised. In situations where there is the potential for harm to the minor or others, such as abuse, suicidal or homicidal ideation, the physician is required by law to report the situation to the local child protective services agency. Moreover, certain sexually transmitted infections must be reported to public health departments. Finally, as most adolescents are covered by their parent/guardian's health insurance policy, the resulting explanation of benefits often discloses information to the parent/guardian.

EVALUATION TECHNIQUES

Greeting the adolescent first and the parents second, and interviewing the adolescent patient alone for a portion of the visit help to earn the patient's trust.[17] The open-ended questioning style used for adults may fail with adolescents. Phrasings using the third person and giving choices when asking questions are more effective techniques to obtain information. For example, "Many women on oral contraceptives forget to take their pill once in a while. How often do you forget to take your birth control pills: often, sometimes, or almost never?" will yield a more accurate reply than, "Do you take your birth control pills every day?"

In adolescents, long-term consequences are often less valued than immediate outcomes. Goals should be concrete, short term, and relevant to the present. Rather than using goals related to more distant benefits, such as the reduction of potentially serious disease complications (eg, smoking causes increased risk of lung cancer), emphasis should be placed on immediate and concrete effects (eg, smoking causes your clothes, hair, and breath to smell bad and your teeth to turn yellow). Body image is a more powerful motivator, and messages such as "tanning salons cause premature wrinkles and ugly skin" are more effective than future health concerns (eg, "tanning salons increase your risk of skin cancer"). Any treatment that is disfiguring or has visible side effects will be met with resistance.[17]

Physical and psychosocial development may not be congruent. Adolescents should not be expected to shoulder all medical responsibilities for themselves, or for their younger siblings. The physician's role is not to befriend, nor is it to parent the adolescent patient; instead, it is to be a trusted, valuable authority.

ACNE AND THE ADOLESCENT

Acne vulgaris is an extremely common and variable disorder that can have far-reaching detrimental effects on self-image and self-esteem. Increased unemployment has been documented among patients with a history of severe acne.[18] A streamlined treatment plan (eg, a single-drug or two-drug regimen) will optimize compliance and cost-effectiveness. Chap. 78 discusses acne in detail.

Females with treatment-resistant acne, signs of virilization (including irregular menstrual cycles, hirsutism, and/or obesity) should have evaluation for androgen excess states including polycystic ovary syndrome. However, some females with polycystic ovary syndrome lack the classic clinical features; for example, they may be slender with no overt signs of virilization ("lean polycystic ovary syndrome"). Other patients have incomplete features and may be categorized as "provisional polycystic ovary syndrome."

Several oral contraceptives (Yaz, Yazmin, and Ortho Tri-Cyclen) have Food and Drug Administration (FDA) labeling for the treatment of acne and are an important therapeutic option for adolescent females with recalcitrant acne. The effectiveness of oral contraceptives often allows discontinuation of chronic oral antibiotic therapy. Patients should be counseled that adherence to 3 months of oral contraceptives is often needed to establish treatment efficacy for acne. Oral contraceptives with a higher androgenic component and lower estrogenic component may be less effective for acne management. Topical acne medications, such as retinoids, may need to be continued for best results.

Because of its antiandrogenic effects, spironolactone, a potassium-sparing diuretic, is a valuable adjunctive therapy for adolescent females with chronic acne, particularly in conjunction with an oral contraceptive. Because spironolactone is a teratogen, concurrent use of a contraceptive is recommended. In a healthy young patient without complicating factors, repeated monitoring for hyperkalemia while on spironolactone for acne management is probably unnecessary.[19] One caveat is that some oral contraceptives contain drospirenone, which has potassium-sparing effects. Thus, female acne patients receiving both spironolactone and drospirenone may need potassium monitoring.

Isotretinoin has been a valuable, unique, and effective agent for nodulocystic acne since 1982. Isotretinoin's teratogenicity is well known. The question of psychopathology induced by isotretinoin is more controversial. The FDA's Adverse Drug Event Reporting System has received reports of depression, suicide, and other psychiatric side effects (eg, aggression, psychosis) in patients using isotretinoin. The question of isotretinoin-induced depression is complicated by the high baseline incidence of depression and suicide in the adolescent population and by the depression and stress associated with severe acne.[20,21] Case reports, including positive cases of positive dechallenge and rechallenge, suggest that isotretinoin may induce depression and other psychiatric adverse effects, but larger retrospective and prospective studies do not demonstrate causation.[22] In some studies, depression scores improved when patients' acne improved with isotretinoin therapy.[23] Double-blind, placebo-controlled studies about isotretinoin and depression have not yet been done, and as of this writing, animal studies show conflicting results. Although a causal link has not been established between isotretinoin and depression/suicide at this time, it is likely that uncommon idiosyncratic psychiatric reactions to isotretinoin may occur in predisposed individuals. Pretreatment evaluation and, if cleared to proceed, subsequent comanagement by a psychiatrist or psychologist should be considered for vulnerable patients. If mood changes arise, the drug should be stopped until the patient is evaluated by the pediatrician or psychiatrist. If deemed appropriate, a rechallenge can be done cautiously.

A second unanswered question is whether the risk of inflammatory bowel disease increases with isotretinoin use. Studies show conflicting results thus far. It is possible that isotretinoin may trigger inflammatory bowel disease in predisposed individuals. Until we have better data, patients and parents should be counseled that a rare but potentially real risk might exist. If bowel symptoms develop, discontinuation of isotretinoin is advisable until the patient is evaluated by a gastroenterologist.[24,25]

Routine monthly laboratory monitoring during isotretinoin therapy is most important during the early months of therapy for healthy individuals receiving no other medications. If no abnormalities appear in the first 2 months, then reduced frequency of monitoring or forgoing laboratory monitoring is appropriate.[26] However, adolescents should be asked if they are taking medications or supplements, including nutritional, "energy," or "recovery" supplements. These supplements, as well as frequent or high-dose nonsteroidal antiinflammatory drug usage (eg, in athletes) may affect liver function, especially during isotretinoin therapy. More frequent laboratory monitoring of these patients may be needed if they decline to avoid supplements.

AXILLARY HYPERHIDROSIS

Idiopathic focal hyperhidrosis is a common condition that has been long been underrecognized. Axillary hyperhidrosis is the most common complaint, but palmar, plantar, and/or facial sites can be affected as well. It can be familial or sporadic. Although all ages may be affected, patients commonly present during adolescence when the condition becomes socially troubling and significantly impacts quality of life. The management of focal idiopathic hyperhidrosis is similar to that of adults. If topical and oral treatments (glycopyrrolate, oxybutynin) fail, injection of botulinum toxin A should be considered. Chap. 81 reviews hyperhidrosis.

INDOOR TANNING

The World Health Organization Cancer Group has classified tanning beds as "carcinogenic to humans." Extensive evidence has linked sunlamp or sun bed exposure to increased risk of melanoma and nonmelanoma skin cancers. Nevertheless, approximately 50,000 tanning salons exist in the United States and tanning bed use is increasing among adolescents and young adults. In addition to the desire for tanned skin and the socialization of the tanning salon, some individuals feel more relaxed, and have improved mood following tanning. Evidence is mounting that tanning bed use is physiologically and psychologically addictive. A study demonstrated that frequent tanners developed a preference for functional ultraviolet beds compared to otherwise identical sham light beds.[27] In addition, physiologic withdrawal symptoms arose in some subjects who were given naltrexone prior to their tanning sessions, suggesting that an opioid-mediated mechanism of dependency may exist in frequent tanners.[28]

Psychiatric studies, using modified tools originally used for substance abuse screening, confirm addictive behaviors of people who frequent tanning salons. Among 229 college students who had used indoor tanning facilities, 90 (39.3%) met *Diagnostic and Statistical Manual of Mental Disorders* IV-TR criteria and 70 (30.6%) met modified CAGE (cut down, annoyed, guilty, eye-opener) criteria for addiction to indoor tanning. In addition, these students also reported greater symptoms of anxiety and greater use of alcohol, marijuana, and other substances than those who did not meet these criteria.[29]

Currently, 13 states ban the use of tanning beds for all minors (persons younger than age 18 years), and at least 42 states regulate the use of tanning facilities by minors. The fight against indoor tanning is similar to the fight against the tobacco industry. Stronger legislation banning tanning bed use in minors, control of false safety claims in advertisements, and extensive education of parents and our youth are still needed.

SPECIAL TOPICS IN PEDIATRIC DERMATOLOGY

AUTISM SPECTRUM DISORDER

BACKGROUND

Autism spectrum disorder (ASD), or autism, refers to a group of complex disorders of brain development. These disorders are characterized, in varying degrees, by difficulties in social interaction and connection, verbal and nonverbal communication, and repetitive behaviors.[30,31] In 2013, the *Diagnostic and Statistical Manual of Mental Disorders* 5 merged autistic disorder, childhood disintegrative disorder, pervasive developmental disorder–not otherwise specified, and Asperger syndrome into 1 umbrella diagnosis of ASD. Instead of separate entities, they are considered to comprise the autism spectrum. ASDs range from mildly to profoundly disabling. ASD can be associated with intellectual disability, attention difficulties, sensory processing disorders, feeding disorders, disrupted motor coordination, sleep disorders, and GI disturbances. Some (but not all) persons with ASD excel in visual skills, music, math, and art.

Autism affects more than 3 million individuals in the United States and tens of millions worldwide. Autism occurs in all racial, ethnic, and socioeconomic groups. The Centers for Disease Control and Prevention estimates that 1 in 68 American children are on the autism spectrum—a 10-fold increase in prevalence in 40 years. This increase is only partly explained by improved diagnosis and awareness. Autism is 4 to 5 times more common among boys than girls. An estimated 1 in 42 boys and 1 in 189 girls are diagnosed with autism in the United States.[30,31]

There is no proven explanation for the rising prevalence of ASD, but the cause is likely multifactorial. Genetic predisposition exists for some individuals. Children with a sibling with autism are at higher risk of ASD, and individuals with certain genetic disorders are at much higher risk of ASD (Table 104-4). Pregnancy and environmental influences also play a role in the development of ASD. The theory that childhood immunizations cause autism, however, has been debunked.

While much of its genesis is not fully understood, ASD appears to originate in very early brain development: in utero, during, or immediately after birth.[31] The clearest signs of autism tend to emerge between 2 and 3 years of age, and, consequently, it is at this age that ASD is usually diagnosable. There is no medical diagnostic test for autism. The diagnosis depends on a constellation of developmental and clinical signs, many of which are nonspecific. Diagnosis often requires consultation

TABLE 104-4
Genodermatoses Associated with Autism Spectrum Disorder[32,33]

Genetic Condition
- *PTEN* hamartoma tumor syndromes
  - Cowden
  - Bannayan-Riley-Ruvalcaba
  - *PTEN*-related Proteus syndrome
  - Proteus-like syndrome

RAS Pathway Disorders
- Cardiofaciocutaneous syndrome
- Noonan syndrome
- Costello Syndrome
- Neurofibromatosis Type 1

Sex Chromosome Aneuploidies
- Turner syndrome (45XO)
- Klinefelter syndrome (47XXY)

Neurocutaneous Syndromes
- Tuberous sclerosis
- Neurofibromatosis 1
- Angelman syndrome
- Prader-Willi syndrome
- Segmental pigmentary disorder

TABLE 104-5
Common Skin Findings in Children with Autism Spectrum Disorder

Scars/callous formation
- Accidental (eg, hyposensitivity/low pain threshold)
- From wearing devices or equipment (eg, sound-blocking headphones)
- Past surgical procedures (comorbidities are common)
- Self-inflicted injury (eg, biting, rubbing, chewing, banging)

Xerosis and atopic dermatitis—intolerance of sensation of topical medications/emollients

Features of genodermatosis (if present)

---

with experts in developmental pediatrics, child neurology, and child psychology.

AUTISM AND THE DERMATOLOGIST

Features of ASD particularly relevant to the dermatologist include sensory processing disorders (eg, sensory dysfunction including both hypersensitivity and hyposensitivity to stimuli, tactile defensiveness, inability to tolerate topical medications or emollients), and overrepresentation of neurobehavioral dermatoses (eg, scars, callosities, and self-inflicted injury resulting from repetitive or ritualistic or stimulatory behaviors) (Table 104-5). Genodermatoses can be associated with autism (see Table 104-4), although many children do not have a diagnosable genetic condition. Nutritional disorders may develop (eg, scurvy), from either ritualized eating preferences of the child, or from imposed dietary manipulations with potential therapeutic benefits (gluten-free or casein-free diets, or ketogenic diets are often experimented with).[32,33]

A new medical consultation can be anxiety provoking for child with autism, the parent, and the physician. Some children are violent and/or self-injurious. "Antecedents," or stimuli that trigger outbursts or maladaptive behaviors should be shared with the physician before any examination occurs. Many children have much higher receptive language skills and lower verbal expressive skills. Some children prefer to be addressed directly in the examination room. Try to use the family's preferred mode of communication, such as signing, simple 1-word directives, Picture Exchange Communication System, or using an assistive technology device.

Families affected by ASD shoulder chronic stress from medical, financial, and emotional challenges, as well as acute stresses from unpredictable disruptions (eg, illness, sleep deprivation). Many, if not most, have had negative experiences with health care providers. Be gentle, quiet, flexible, nonjudgmental, and open to learning about what works for the family.

One mother of a teenage girl with severe nonverbal autism gives this advice:

> Thinking outside of the box is critical in treating autistic patients. Making special allowances will go a long way with parents, as most are trying their best with little to no support. An example might be allowing the child to have their favorite drink or snack while waiting, even if this is not usually allowed in the office. It can help keep the child calm and focused on eating rather than on the stress of being in a medical office. Allowing the child to rip paper might provide the same soothing effect. Try to complete the examination in small increments while taking the child's mind off the task at hand, using play or finding commonality in something they are interested in.

Acceptance of how these kids present is important. They understand when someone is looking negatively at them with disdain or annoyance. They understand when someone is fearful and aversive toward them.

Table 104-6 presents a treatment approach for dermatologists caring for individuals with ASD.

DRUG LABELING FOR PEDIATRIC PATIENTS

The lack of FDA labeling for pediatric use does not imply that a drug is contraindicated or disapproved; it simply means that insufficient data are available to grant approval status. Although attempts have been made to equate off-label prescribing with recklessness in the medical malpractice arena, the American Academy of Pediatrics has stated that failure to prescribe medications for off-label uses when the medication is appropriate under the standard of care may constitute malpractice.

The thalidomide tragedy led to more stringent regulation of drugs in the early 1960s, and manufacturers began omitting drug studies in infants and children. In the 1970s, pediatric dosage information in package

TABLE 104-6
An Approach to Caring for Children with Autism Spectrum Disorder

Characteristics of Autism
- While every child is different, the following are commonly seen:
- Emotional dysregulation is common in this population. Often, there are predictable precursors to behavioral issues called "antecedents" that trigger the maladaptive behavior. Knowing about the child's antecedents can help everyone avoid upset.
- Difficulties in social interaction and connection. Connection with full-time caregivers and close family is more readily evident, and can be inspiring.
- Self-stimulation behaviors or repetitive movements that may emerge when stressed; these behaviors can be calming to the patient:
  - Repetitive behaviors such as flapping, rocking, tapping, or flickering fingers in front of eyes
  - Playing with string, or shiny objects
  - Tearing paper
  - Spinning objects
- Hypersensitivity—Loud sounds (the child may prefer wearing protective headphones) or bright lights may be antecedents to maladaptive behaviors. Hearing certain sounds, or certain words, or even adults speaking to one another may provoke untoward responses. Tactile defensiveness.
- Hyposensitivity—High pain threshold in some individuals.
- Limited verbal or nonverbal communication, receptive and/or expressive.
- Ritualized environment—Strong desire to keep routines and things the same, in the same order and manner.

Do
- Put the family in a patient room to wait, instead of the waiting room.
- Consider booking the patient first or last on the schedule, and with extra time for the encounter.
- Ask the caregiver what works best for interactions and examinations, and what doesn't. Find out what self-soothing strategies the child employs to calm and organize.
- Consider lowering the lights. Many find bright lights difficult. Some may find the sounds of fluorescent lights annoying.
- Initially observe the child from a distance that is nonthreatening to the child.
- Use a quiet calm voice, not a loud, boisterous voice.
- Ask for permission before touching the child.
- Ask about the child's pain threshold. Is there increased or decreased pain sensitivity?
- Ask if the child tends to self-inflict injury (rubbing, biting, picking)?
- Ask about closing the office door. A lot of children have a hard time staying in the examination room and do not like any closed doors. Some doors need to have a way to be locked from the inside so the child does not bolt from the room.
- Consider using nonverbal communication. For example, some children will mimic your movements more readily than following verbal directions (eg, during a full skin examination, show how you turn your hands over, spreading fingers wide, or raise your arms above your head).
- Having a doll to point to (to convey where they are feeling hurt or uncomfortable) can be helpful.
- Be patient with the family and with yourself. Sometimes not everything will be accomplished in 1 office visit.

Don't
- Don't be afraid to ask the parent/caregiver what strategies work best for the child.
- Don't assume that general anesthesia is needed for every skin biopsy or procedure, because many will do extremely well with local anesthesia.
- Don't talk about the child as if the child is not there.
- Don't assume the child doesn't understand what you are saying, even if no acknowledgment is evident. Many children have better receptive skills than expressive communication skills.
- Don't assume every visit will unfold in the same way. The next visit may go surprisingly easily or pose unexpected challenges.

---

inserts tended to exclude children from therapeutic benefit. Performing research in healthy children is problematic because of ethical and logistic questions, medicolegal risk, and cost. It has been estimated that approximately 50% to 75% of drugs used in pediatrics have not been studied adequately to provide accurate labeling information, and the younger the patient, the more likely the lack of information.[34] Safety and effectiveness information for drug use in children younger than 2 years of age is particularly lacking. The absence of pediatric testing and labeling poses significant safety risks for children. Additionally, children may be denied the benefits from therapeutic advances because physicians choose to prescribe existing, less-effective medications in the face of insufficient pediatric information about new medications. In 1997, as part of the FDA Modernization Act, Congress enacted a law known as the *Pediatric Exclusivity Provision* that provides marketing incentives (ie, 6-month extension of patent protection) to manufacturers who conduct studies of drugs in children. This law was effective in generating pediatric studies on many drugs, and an increase in labeling information has occurred for some. Unfortunately, many studies have centered on children older than 6 years of age, and many drug studies were stimulated by market concerns rather than medical need.

Hopefully, with incentives such as the Pediatric Research Equity Act of 2003, significantly more pediatric drug research will proceed forward. Ideally in the future, physicians caring for children will no longer need to prescribe drugs "off label," and children will no longer be "therapeutic orphans."

TOPICAL MEDICATIONS

While topical medications often have excellent safety and efficacy profiles, one must be aware that infants and young children are at increased risk for toxicity from topically applied agents because of an increased surface-area-to-body-mass ratio compared to adults. In addition, at times infants and children have altered metabolism of drugs compared to adults. Patients with disorders of cornification (eg, lamellar ichthyosis) or other forms of skin barrier disruption (eg, Netherton syndrome) have a much higher risk of toxicity resulting from increased percutaneous absorption. Patients with Netherton syndrome who are treated with topical tacrolimus may develop immunosuppressive or toxic blood levels of tacrolimus, without clinical signs or symptoms of toxicity.[35] A heightened awareness of this problem is important because Netherton syndrome is often misdiagnosed as atopic dermatitis, and both conditions often improve with topical tacrolimus therapy. In addition, a patient with Netherton syndrome developed Cushing syndrome after application of hydrocortisone 1% ointment for longer than 1 year.[36] Table 104-7 lists examples of inadvertent percutaneous poisoning from topical agents.

SYSTEMIC MEDICATIONS

DRUG DOSAGES

Pediatric doses of systemic medications are calculated according to body weight (mg/kg) or body surface area to account for size variations between patients of the same age and to account for a child's growth. Prescriptions for liquid medications (syrups or suspensions) must indicate concentration (eg, milligrams per 5 mL) to avoid serious error. In addition, the appropriate measuring instrument should be dispensed, along with education on its use. Dosing cups (commonly included in nonprescription liquid medications) are a common cause of dosing errors. Dosing errors were almost 5 times more likely when parents used dosing cups rather than oral measuring syringes.[37] In addition, dosing cups tend to cause overdosing, up to 300% of the proper dose in another study.[38]

For guidelines on indications and dosing of antimicrobials and other medications, the reader is directed to excellent references including the *Red Book*,[39] published by the American Academy of Pediatrics, and *The Harriet Lane Handbook*.[40]

SYSTEMIC GLUCOCORTICOIDS

Hypothalamic–pituitary axis suppression, osteonecrosis, and other adverse effects of systemic glucocorticoid therapy affect patients of all ages and are reviewed in Chap. 184. The potential risk of growth suppression is unique to childhood. Exogenous glucocorticoids disrupt the secretion of growth hormone, causing abnormal spontaneous growth hormone secretion with reduced pulse amplitude of growth hormone release and reduced response to provocative stimuli.[41,42] There is also decreased local production of insulin-like growth factor 1. These and other effects of glucocorticoids act to cause delayed growth at the

TABLE 104-7
Topical Medications Reported to Cause Systemic Toxicity in Children

TOPICAL MEDICATION	COMPLICATION	REFERENCE
Tacrolimus 1% ointment	Three children with Netherton syndrome found to have blood levels of tacrolimus in the range of organ transplantation requirements	35
Hydrocortisone 1% ointment	Cushing syndrome developed in an 11-year-old boy with Netherton syndrome who received topical application to extensive areas for longer than 1 year	36
Benzocaine, 3% (Lanacane)	Methemoglobinemia in a 2-year-old child	50
Iodoquinol, clioquinol (Vioform)	Neurotoxicity when used as treatment for diaper dermatitis	51, 52
Lindane	Neurologic toxicity in children with disrupted epidermal barrier and/or excessive topical application or ingestion	53, 54
N,N-diethyl-m-toluamide (DEET)	Slurred speech, tremors, seizures, and death in children after repeated and extensive application of high concentrations of DEET	55
Povidone-iodine (Betadine)	Hypothyroidism in infants with spina bifida	56
Povidone-iodine (Betadine)	Decreased free thyroxine and elevated iodine levels in infants treated with diluted povidone-iodine during *Staphylococcus aureus* epidemic	57
Salicylic acid	A 7-year-old boy with ichthyosis vulgaris developed life-threatening salicylism with neurologic sequelae lasting 6 months	58
Saline, sodium chloride	Fatalities in infants and children following ancient Turkish custom of "salting"	59
Viscous lidocaine, 2%	Lidocaine overdose following frequent application to oral lesions	60

bony epiphyses, with the most noticeable reduction in growth velocity occurring during early childhood and adolescent growth spurts. There is a linear relation between the daily dose and growth suppression. Alternate-day dosing, with single morning doses, may decrease the risk of glucocorticoid growth suppression. Most children eventually will have adequate catchup growth with reduction of doses, alternate-day therapy, or cessation of therapy.[43] For the pediatric patient on long-term systemic steroid therapy, charting height and weight on a standardized growth curve is the best method for the pediatrician to screen for decreasing growth velocity.

Children taking immunosuppressive doses of systemic glucocorticoids should not be vaccinated with live-virus vaccines (eg, measles, oral polio, varicella). A dosage equivalent of 2 mg/kg/day or greater of prednisone or a total of 20 mg/day or greater for children weighing more than 10 kg, when given for more than 14 days, is sufficient to warrant withholding immunization with live-virus vaccines.[44] Systemic steroids should not be given to a healthy child if the child has had recent varicella exposure and is not varicella-immune, as varicella infection can be fatal in this situation. In addition, children with ocular herpes simplex and untreated tuberculosis should not be given systemic steroids, and patients with underlying diabetes, hypertension, peptic ulcer disease, renal insufficiency, or psychosis should be treated with great caution or with an alternative agent.[39]

ANTIMICROBIALS

Use of tetracycline family medications is contraindicated in children younger than 8 years of age because it causes brown discoloration of developing teeth and decreased bone growth. Ciprofloxacin and quinolone use in children younger than 18 years of age is restricted because the fluoroquinolones have been shown to cause cartilage damage in juvenile animal models at therapeutic doses. The mechanism is unknown. It is recommended that use of these medications be restricted to relatively serious infections for which no other oral agent is available or IV antibiotics would be impractical and for certain pathogenic infections or situations, such as multidrug resistance.[40]

Griseofulvin doses of 20 mg/kg/day of the (125 mg/5 mL) liquid and 15 mg/kg/day of the ultramicrosized tablets for 6 to 8 weeks have long been considered first-line therapy for tinea capitis. In 2007, terbinafine oral granules (sprinkled on nonacidic food) were approved for the treatment of tinea capitis in children 4 years of age and older. Currently, griseofulvin and terbinafine are the only FDA-approved agents for tinea capitis in children. Griseofulvin appears to be superior against *Microsporum canis*. Crushed generic terbinafine tablets (off-label) can be substituted for terbinafine granules if the granules are not readily available. Although further studies are needed, itraconazole also appears to be effective and to have a good safety profile. Fluconazole was not very effective against pediatric tinea capitis in a large, multicenter, double-blinded, randomized trial of 880 children.[45]

CHILD ABUSE AND NEGLECT (CHILD MALTREATMENT)

Child maltreatment is abuse or neglect by a parent (or caregiver) that results in potential, actual, or threats of harm to a child. Child maltreatment includes both acts of commission (abuse) and omission (neglect). Child maltreatment is divided into 4 categories: (a) physical abuse (eg, hitting, shaking, or burning); (b) sexual abuse (eg, rape or fondling); (c) psychological abuse (eg, terrorizing or belittling); and (d) neglect (eg, failure to meet basic physical, emotional, educational, or medical needs).

Unfortunately, child maltreatment is not rare. In the United States, 1 in 8 children are victims of maltreatment annually,[46] and the true prevalence is likely higher because of underreporting.

The Centers for Disease Control and Prevention reports that in 2014, approximately 1580 children died from abuse or neglect in the United States. The total lifetime cost of child abuse and neglect is $124 billion annually.[47]

Approximately 70% of documented child maltreatment deaths occur in children younger than age 3 years. Other risk factors for abuse include children with special needs or chronic illnesses, disabilities, and other factors that increase caregiver burden. Caregiver risk factors include stress, inadequate parenting skills, substance abuse, and depression. Other factors include poverty, unemployment, isolation from support, transient nonbiologic caregivers in the home, and intimate partner violence. Similarly, predisposing community factors include poverty, violence, and housing instability. However, it is important to note that abuse and neglect can occur in the absence of the above risk factors, and occurs within all socioeconomic classes.[46,47]

Ninety percent of all abused children are said to have suggestive or confirmative dermatologic findings.[48] In all situations, the immediate safety of the child must be ensured, removing the child from the home (eg, hospitalization) if necessary. Objective documentation of physical findings is vital. Ideally, because of the sensitive medical and legal aspects of this important problem, any case of suspected child abuse should be quickly referred to a team specializing in pediatric abuse. The appropriate evaluation should not be delayed in the absence of such a resource, however. Timely reporting to child protective services is required by law in all cases of suspected child maltreatment.

REFERENCES

1. Scullard P, Peacock C, Davies P. Googling children's health: reliability of medical advice on the internet. *Arch Dis Child.* 2010;95:580.
2. Liang MG, Frieden IJ. Perineal and lip ulcerations as the presenting manifestation of hemangioma of infancy. *Pediatrics.* 1997;99:256.
3. Poole SR. The infant with acute, unexplained, excessive crying. *Pediatrics.* 1991;88:450.
4. Press S, Schachner L, Paul P. Clitoris tourniquet syndrome. *Pediatrics.* 1980;66:781.
5. Kayashima K, Kitoh M, Ono T. Infantile perianal pyramidal protrusion. *Arch Dermatol.* 1996;132:1481.
6. Khachemoune A, Guldbakke KK, Ehrsam E. Infantile perineal protrusion. *J Am Acad Dermatol.* 2006;54:1046.
7. Ward DB, Fleischer AB Jr, Feldman SR, et al. Characterization of diaper dermatitis in the United States. *Arch Pediatr Adolesc Med.* 2000;14:943.
8. Chang MW, Kaufmann JM, Orlow SJ, et al. Infantile granular parakeratosis: recognition of two clinical patterns. *J Am Acad Dermatol.* 2004;50(5)(suppl):S93.
9. McCann J, Wells R, Simon M, et al. Genital findings in prepubertal girls selected for nonabuse: a descriptive study. *Pediatrics.* 1990;86:428.
10. Siegfried E. The spectrum of anogenital diseases in children. *Curr Probl Dermatol.* 1997;9:33.
11. EMLA cream [package insert]. Wilmington, DE: AstraZeneca; 2000. https://www.accessdata.fda.gov/drugsatfda_docs/label/2000/19941S11LBL.PDF
12. Gradin M, Eriksson M, Holmqvist G, et al. Pain reduction at venipuncture in newborns: Oral glucose compared with local anesthetic cream. *Pediatrics.* 2002;110:1053.
13. Mader TJ, Playe SJ, Garb JL. Reducing the pain of local anesthetic infiltration: warming and buffering have a synergistic effect. *Ann Emerg Med.* 1994;23:550.
14. Proudfoot J. Analgesia, anesthesia, and conscious sedation. *Emerg Med Clin North Am.* 1995;13:357.
15. Cunningham BB, Gigler V, Wang K, et al. General anesthesia for pediatric dermatologic procedures: risks and complications. *Arch Dermatol.* 2005;141:573.
16. Goldenberg A, Mousdicas N, Silverberg N, et al. Pediatric Contact Dermatitis Registry inaugural case data. *Dermatitis.* 2016;27:293.
17. Blair S, Bowes. Compliance issues in adolescence: practical strategies. *Aust Fam Physician.* 1995;24:2037.
18. Cunliffe WJ. Acne and unemployment. *Br J Dermatol.* 1986;115:386.
19. Plovanich M, Weng QY, Mostaghimi A. Low usefulness of potassium monitoring among healthy young women taking spironolactone for acne. *JAMA Dermatol.* 2015;151:941.
20. Wysowski DK, Pitts M, Beitz J. Depression and suicide in patients treated with isotretinoin. *N Engl J Med.* 2001;344:460.
21. Wysowski DK, Pitts M, Beitz J. An analysis of reports of depression and suicide in patients treated with isotretinoin. *J Am Acad Dermatol.* 2001;45:515.
22. Kontaxakis VP, Skourides D, Ferentinos P, et al. Isotretinoin and psychopathology: a review. *Ann Gen Psychiatry.* 2009;8:2.
23. Chia CY, Lane W, Chibnall J, et al. Isotretinoin therapy and mood changes in adolescents with moderate to severe acne: a cohort study. *Arch Dermatol.* 2005;141:557.
24. Crockett SD, Porter CQ, Martin CF, et al. Isotretinoin use and the risk of inflammatory bowel disease: a case-control study. *Am J Gastroenterol.* 2010;105:1986.
25. Shale M, Kaplan GG, Panaccione R, et al. Isotretinoin and intestinal inflammation: What gastroenterologists need to know. *Gut.* 2009;58:737.
26. Lee YH, Scharnitz TP, Muscat J, et al. Laboratory monitoring during isotretinoin therapy for acne: a systematic review and meta-analysis. *JAMA Dermatol.* 2016;152:35.
27. Feldman SR, Liguori A, Kucenic M, et al. Ultraviolet exposure is a reinforcing stimulus in frequent indoor tanners. *J Am Acad Dermatol.* 2004;51:45.
28. Kaur M, Liguori A, Lang W, et al. Induction of withdrawal-like symptoms in a small randomized, controlled trial of opioid blockade in frequent tanners. *J Am Acad Dermatol.* 2006;54:709.
29. Mosher CE, Danoff-Burg S. Addiction to indoor tanning: relation to anxiety, depression, and substance use. *Arch Dermatol.* 2010;145:412.
30. Christensen DL, Baio J, Van Naarden Braun K, et al. Prevalence and characteristics of autism spectrum disorder among children aged 8 years—Autism and Developmental Disabilities Monitoring Network, 11 sites, United States, 2012. *MMWR Surveill Summ.* 2016;65:1.
31. Schieve LA, Tian LH, Baio J, et al. Population attributable fractions for three perinatal risk factors for autism spectrum disorders, 2002 and 2008 Autism and Developmental Disabilities Monitoring Network. *Ann Epidemiol.* 2014;24:260.
32. Oza VS, Marco E, Frieden IJ. Improving the dermatologic care of individuals with autism: a review of relevant issues and a perspective. *Pediatr Dermatol.* 2015;32:447.
33. Accordino RE, Lucarelli J, Yan AC. Cutaneous disease in autism spectrum disorder: a review. *Pediatr Dermatol.* 2015;32:455.
34. Roberts R, Rodriguez W, Murphy D, et al. Pediatric drug labeling: improving the safety and efficacy of pediatric therapies. *JAMA.* 2003;290:905.
35. Allen A, Siegfried E, Silverman R, et al. Significant absorption of topical tacrolimus in 3 patients with Netherton syndrome. *Arch Dermatol.* 2001;137:747.
36. Halverstam CP, Vachharajani A, Mallory SB. Cushing syndrome from percutaneous absorption of 1% hydrocortisone ointment in Netherton syndrome. *Pediatr Dermatol.* 2007;24:42.
37. Yin HS, Dreyer BP, Ugboaja DC, et al. Liquid medication errors and dosing tools: a randomized controlled experiment. *Pediatrics.* 2016;138:e20160357.
38. Yin HS, Parker RM, Sanders LM, et al. Parents' medication administration errors: Role of dosing instruments and health literacy. *Arch Pediatr Adolesc Med.* 2010;164:181.
39. American Academy of Pediatrics. Section 4. Antimicrobial agents and related therapy. In: Kimberlin DW, Brady MT, Jackson MA, Long SS, eds. *Red Book 2015: Report of the Committee on Infectious Diseases.* 30th ed. Elk Grove Village, IL: American Academy of Pediatrics; 2015.
40. Engorn B, Flerlage J, eds. *The Harriet Lane Handbook,* 20th ed. Philadelphia, PA: Elsevier; 2014.
41. Book CG, Hindmarsh PC, Stanhope R. Growth and growth hormone secretion. *J Endocrinol.* 1988;119:179.
42. Fine RN. Corticosteroids and growth. *Kidney Int Suppl.* 1993;43:S59.
43. Lucky AW. Principles of the use of glucocorticosteroids in the growing child. *Pediatr Dermatol.* 1984;1:226.
44. American Academy of Pediatrics. Immunization in special clinical circumstances. In: Kimberlin DW, Brady MT, Jackson MA, Long SS, eds. *Red Book 2015: Report of the Committee on Infectious Diseases.* 30th ed. Elk Grove Village, IL: American Academy of Pediatrics; 2015.

45. Foster KW, Friedlander SF, Panzer H, et al. A randomized controlled trial assessing the efficacy of fluconazole in the treatment of pediatric tinea capitis. *J Am Acad Dermatol.* 2005;53:798.
46. Ferrara P, Guadagno C, Sbordone A, et al. Child abuse and neglect and its psycho-physical and social consequences: a review of the literature. *Curr Pediatr Rev.* 2016;12:301.
47. Saul J, Valle LA, Mercy JA, et al. CDC grand rounds: creating a healthier future through prevention of child maltreatment. *MMWR Morb Mortal Wkly Rep.* 2014;63:260.
48. Duarte AM, Pruksachatkunakorn C, Schachner LA. Life threatening dermatoses in pediatric dermatology. *Adv Dermatol.* 1995;10:329.
49. Chang MW, Nakrani R. Six children with allergic contact dermatitis to methylisothiazolinone in wet wipes (baby wipes). *Pediatrics.* 2014;133:e434.
50. Eldadah M, Fitzgerald M. Methemoglobinemia due to skin application of benzocaine. *Clin Pediatr (Phila).* 1993;32:687.
51. Singalavanija S, Frieden IJ. Diaper dermatitis. *Pediatr Rev.* 1995;16:142.
52. American Academy of Pediatrics Committee on Drugs. Clioquinol (iodochlorhydroxyquin, Vioform) and iodoquinol (diiodohydroxyquin): blindness and neuropathy. *Pediatrics.* 1990;86:797.
53. Davies JE, Dedhia HV, Morgade C, et al. Lindane poisonings. *Arch Dermatol.* 1983;199:142.
54. Friedman SJ. Lindane neurotoxic reaction in nonbullous congenital ichthyosiform erythroderma. *Arch Dermatol.* 1987;123:106.
55. Brown M, Hebert AA. Insect repellants: an overview. *J Am Acad Dermatol.* 1997;36:243.
56. Barakat M, Carson D, Hetherton AM, et al. Hypothyroidism secondary to topical iodine treatment in infants with spina bifida. *Acta Paediatr.* 1994;83:741.
57. Aihara M, Sakai M, Iwasaki M, et al. Prevention and control of nosocomial infection caused by methicillin-resistant *Staphylococcus aureus* in a premature infant ward: preventive effect of a povidone-iodine wipe of neonatal skin. *Postgrad Med J.* 1993;69(suppl 3):S117.
58. Germann R, Schindera I, Kuch M, et al. Life threatening salicylate poisoning caused by percutaneous absorption in severe ichthyosis vulgaris [in German]. *Hautarzt.* 1996;47:624.
59. Yercen N, Caglayan S, Yücel N, et al. Fatal hypernatremia in an infant due to salting of the skin. *Am J Dis Child.* 1993;147:716.
60. Gonzalez del Rey J, Wason S, Druckenbrod RW. Lidocaine overdose: another preventable case? *Pediatr Emerg Care.* 1994;10:344.

Chapter 105 :: Skin Changes and Diseases in Pregnancy
:: Lauren E. Wiznia & Miriam Keltz Pomeranz

第一百零五章
妊娠期的皮肤变化和疾病

中文导读

妊娠期内分泌、代谢和免疫环境的改变导致了多种皮肤生理和病理学改变。本章首先讲述了妊娠期间皮肤的生理学变化，包括色素沉着、腹白线变黑和黄褐斑等色素异常，黑素细胞痣的变化、膨胀纹、蜘蛛痣的出现等，表105-1提供了比较全面的生理变化，包括皮肤和附属器的。本章还提到瘙痒是妊娠期间常见的一种症状，可能是生理上的，但可能预示着先前存在的皮肤病或妊娠期特定皮肤病的发作。也从与胎儿妊娠风险有无相关性的两个方面详细讲述了多种皮肤疾病，包括妊娠类天疱疮、妊娠期肝内胆汁淤积症、妊娠期脓疱性银屑病、妊娠瘙痒性荨麻疹、妊娠期特应性皮炎等。

1. 与胎儿妊娠风险相关的皮肤疾病

（1）妊娠类天疱疮：妊娠类天疱疮（Pemphigoid gestationis，PG）是妊娠中后期和产后的一种严重瘙痒的水疱大疱性疾病。通常在妊娠的第二或第三个月开始，在正常或红斑皮肤上突然出现严重瘙痒性荨麻疹样皮损。作者依次讲述了PG的流行病学、临床特征、病因和发病机制、诊断及鉴别诊断、临床病程与预后、管理等。

文中提到：①PG与早产和低出生体重风险有关，这些胎儿发生并发症的风险与产妇疾病的严重程度相关。②母亲患有PG的新生儿可能会出现暂时性的大疱性皮损，通常不需要治疗。③如果母亲孕期长期接受大剂量的强的松龙治疗，需要评估婴儿的肾上腺功能。④单用皮质类固醇激素治疗疗效不满意，或者不能延长使用皮质类固醇激素治疗的，可以考虑血浆置换或静脉注射免疫球蛋白。

（2）妊娠期肝内胆汁淤积症：妊娠期肝内胆汁淤积症（Intrahepatic cholestasis of pregnancy，ICP）是一种罕见的可逆的胆汁淤积症，通常发生在妊娠晚期，此时血清雌激素浓度达到峰值。轻微的ICP病例，瘙痒不伴有黄疸，以前被称为妊娠瘙痒。作者依次讲述了ICP的流行病学、临床特征、病因和发病机制、诊断及鉴别诊断、临床病程与预后、管理等。

虽然ICP确切的发病机制尚不清楚，但激素、遗传、环境和营养因素的相互作用导致易感个体胆汁淤积是重要因素，并重点讲述了激素变化的重要作用。ICP的特点之一是症状和相关生化异常通常在分娩后2～4周内消失。因此，治疗的目的主要是降低血清胆汁酸水平，延长妊娠期，改善产妇症状和降低胎儿风险。

（3）妊娠期脓疱性银屑病：妊娠期脓疱

性银屑病（Pustular psoriasis of pregnancy）通常被认为是一种变异的脓疱性银屑病，但也有研究者认为妊娠期脓疱性银屑病是一个独立的疾病。作者依次讲述了妊娠期脓疱性银屑病的流行病学、临床特征、病因和发病机制、诊断及鉴别诊断、临床病程与预后、管理等。虽然妊娠期脓疱性银屑病的病因和发病机制不详，但不同于一般的脓疱性银屑病。它没有阳性的家族史，分娩时症状突然消失，再次妊娠有复发倾向，以及缺乏已知的脓疱性银屑病的触发因素，如感染、触发药物或系统性糖皮质激素的突然停用等。在讲述治疗进展时提到，系统性糖皮质激素是主要的传统治疗方法。现在，环孢素和英夫利昔单抗被认为是一线治疗用药。

2.与胎儿妊娠风险不相关的皮肤疾病

（1）妊娠多形疹（Polymorphic eruption of pregnancy，PEP）又称妊娠瘙痒性荨麻疹样丘疹和红斑（pruritic urticarial papules and plaques of Pregnancy，PUPPP），是一种常见的良性瘙痒性皮肤病，几乎只发生在妊娠晚期和产后初期。作者依次讲述了PEP的流行病学、临床特征、病因和发病机制、风险因素、诊断及鉴别诊断、临床病程与预后、管理等。

PEP发病机制不清楚，但本章讲述了PEP和多胎妊娠之间存在关联。临床诊断通常包括妊娠末期出现典型部位的皮损发作；组织病理学表现无特异性的，DIF显示在真表皮交界处或血管周围无颗粒状C3、IgM或IgA沉积，间接免疫荧光结果也为阴性。表105-4列出了PEP的鉴别诊断。

（2）妊娠特应性皮炎：妊娠特应性皮炎（Atopic eruption of pregnancy，AEP）是指一系列的妊娠期瘙痒性皮肤病，包括以前明确存在的妊娠痒疹和妊娠瘙痒性毛囊炎，以及妊娠中的湿疹。作者依次讲述了AEP的流行病学、临床特征、病因和发病机制、风险因素、诊断及鉴别诊断、临床病程与预后、管理等。讲述流行病学特点时，本章提到，AEP是妊娠期最常见的瘙痒性疾病。它往往比其他妊娠相关性皮肤病出现更早。临床特征部分提出AEP的显著特征包括在妊娠早期（妊娠晚期前）发病，以及个人和/或家族史。诊断主要靠临床特征，实验室检查及组织病理学检查缺乏特异性。鉴别诊断包括妊娠期的其他皮肤病，特别是ICP和PEP，孕妇发生的细菌性毛囊炎和过敏性接触性皮炎也应排除。AEP对治疗敏感，即使在皮损严重的情况下，产妇和胎儿的预后也很好。

〔刘芳芬〕

CHANGES COMMONLY ASSOCIATED WITH PREGNANCY

AT-A-GLANCE

- Cutaneous changes result from the altered endocrine, metabolic, and immunologic milieus that characterize pregnancy.
- Pigmentary disturbances, including hyperpigmentation, darkening of the linea alba, and melasma are the changes most commonly observed.
- Significant change in nevi size is not a feature of most pregnancies.
- Structural changes known to occur during pregnancy include, most commonly, striae distensae.
- Pruritus is a common complaint during pregnancy and may be related to flare of a preexisting dermatosis or onset of a specific dermatosis of pregnancy.

Pregnancy is characterized by altered endocrine, metabolic, and immunologic milieus. These dramatic alterations result in multiple cutaneous changes, both physiologic and pathologic. Table 105-1 provides a comprehensive list of physiologic alterations within the skin and appendages.[1-4]

Pigmentary disturbances are the most common of these physiologic changes. Hyperpigmentation of the areola, axillae, and genitalia are well documented in pregnancy. *Linea nigra* refers to the typically reversible darkening of the linea alba, a hypopigmented linear patch extending from the pubis symphysis to the sternal xiphoid process (Fig. 105-1). Melasma or chloasma comprises irregular, blotchy, facial hyperpigmentation that occurs in up to 70% of pregnant women (Fig. 105-2). It is aggravated by sun exposure and by oral contraceptive intake in nonpregnant women. Melasma may regress postpartum, but oftentimes persists, posing a therapeutic challenge.[1]

Changes in melanocytic nevi were historically deemed "normal" during pregnancy. However, few studies have objectively studied whether and how nevi evolve during pregnancy. Pennoyer and colleagues[5] photographically monitored 129 melanocytic nevi throughout the pregnancies of 22 healthy white women. Only 8 nevi (6.2%) changed in diameter from the first to third trimester, with a mean change in size of zero. The authors concluded that significant change in nevus size (excluding nevi on the pregnant abdomen) does not appear to be a feature of most pregnancies.[5] Dermoscopic changes of nevi in pregnancy have included widening in diameters and structure changes, that are seen, especially on the front of the body.[6] Until further controlled studies are performed, any pigmented lesion in a pregnant woman that undergoes change in morphology (size, color, or shape) or symptoms (begins to itch, bleed, or scale) should be considered for histopathologic review.

The most common structural change during pregnancy is striae distensae, also known as *striae gravidarum* or colloquially as *stretch marks* (Fig. 105-3). Sites of predilection for striae are those areas most prone to stretch, including the abdomen, hips, buttocks, and breasts. Factors such as family history, personal history, and race are the strongest predictors of an individual's risk of developing striae distensae, surpassing pregnancy weight gain or changes in body mass index.[7] These findings strongly support a genetic predisposition to this condition. Vascular changes are also common. Spider angiomas are the most common vascular lesion to develop.

Pruritus, a common complaint during pregnancy, may be physiologic, but may herald a flare of a preexisting dermatosis or onset of a specific dermatosis of pregnancy. The remainder of this chapter outlines the relatively rare conditions that may be specific to pregnancy. Table 105-2 provides an overview of these conditions.

DERMATOSES ASSOCIATED WITH FETAL RISK IN PREGNANCY

AT-A-GLANCE

- Pemphigoid gestationis is an immunologically mediated, intensely pruritic, vesiculobullous eruption of mid- to late pregnancy associated with fetal risk.
- Intrahepatic cholestasis of pregnancy represents a reversible form of cholestasis in late pregnancy associated with biochemical abnormalities and a risk of fetal complications but lacks primary cutaneous lesions. Symptoms remit within 2 to 4 weeks of delivery, but recurrences in subsequent pregnancies are common.
- Pustular psoriasis of pregnancy is a rare, acute, pustular eruption often accompanied by fever, leukocytosis, and an elevated erythrocyte sedimentation rate. This is generally regarded as a variant of psoriasis.

PEMPHIGOID (HERPES) GESTATIONIS

Pemphigoid (herpes) gestationis (PG) is an intensely pruritic, vesiculobullous eruption of mid- to late pregnancy and the immediate postpartum period. It classically begins during the second or third trimester, and is manifest by the abrupt appearance of severely pruritic urticarial lesions on a background of normal or erythematous skin. PG is associated with an increased incidence of small-for-gestational age births and premature delivery.

TABLE 105-1
Physiologic Skin Changes During Pregnancy

Pigmentary
- Hyperpigmentation (genitalia, axillae, recent scars)
- Secondary areolae
- Linea nigra
- Melasma (chloasma, mask of pregnancy)

Hair
- Hirsutism
- Thickening of scalp hair
- Postpartum telogen effluvium
- Postpartum androgenetic alopecia

Nail
- Subungual hyperkeratosis
- Distal onycholysis
- Transverse grooving
- Brittleness
- Accelerated growth

Glandular
- Increased eccrine function (except palms) (miliaria, dyshidrotic eczema, hyperhidrosis)
- Elevated thyroid activity with resultant relative iodine deficiency
- Increased sebaceous function (growth in Montgomery tubercles)
- Decreased apocrine function

Structural Changes
- Striae distensae (striae gravidarum)
- Molluscum fibrosum gravidarum (acrochordons)

Vascular
- Spider angiomas (spider nevi, nevi aranei)
- Palmar erythema
- Nonpitting edema (hands, ankles, feet, face)
- Varicosities
- Cutis marmorata
- Vasomotor instability
- Dermographism/pruritus
- Purpura
- Gingival hyperemia or hyperplasia
- Pyogenic granuloma (granuloma gravidarum, pregnancy epulis)
- Hemorrhoids
- Hemangiomas, hemangioendotheliomas, glomangiomas
- Unilateral nevoid telangiectasia (unilateral dermatomal superficial telangiectasia)

Mucosa
- Gingivitis (marginal gingivitis, papillomatous hypertrophy of the gums)
- Jacquemier-Chadwick sign (bluish discoloration of vagina and cervix)
- Goodell sign (cervical softening)

Adapted from Elling SV, Powell FC. Physiological changes in the skin during pregnancy. *Clin Dermatol.* 1997;15:35; Kroumpouzos G, Cohen LM. Dermatoses of pregnancy. *J Am Acad Dermatol.* 2001;45:1; and Muzaffar F, Hussain I, Haroon TS. Physiologic skin changes during pregnancy: a study of 140 cases. *Int J Dermatol.* 1998;77:429.

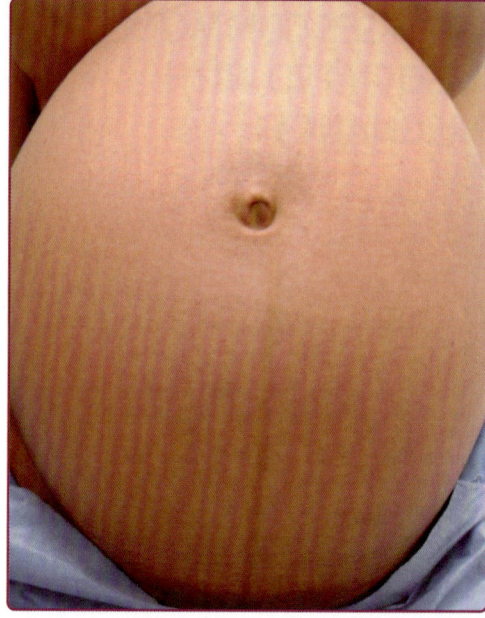

Figure 105-1 Linea nigra. A hyperpigmented line extends from the pubis symphysis to the xiphoid process of the sternum. Hyperpigmentation is often more pronounced inferior to the umbilicus.

EPIDEMIOLOGY

PG is rare, seen in 1 in 1700 to 1 in 50,000 pregnancies.

CLINICAL FEATURES

PG presents with urticarial followed by vesicular lesions on the trunk and extremities in mid-to-late pregnancy

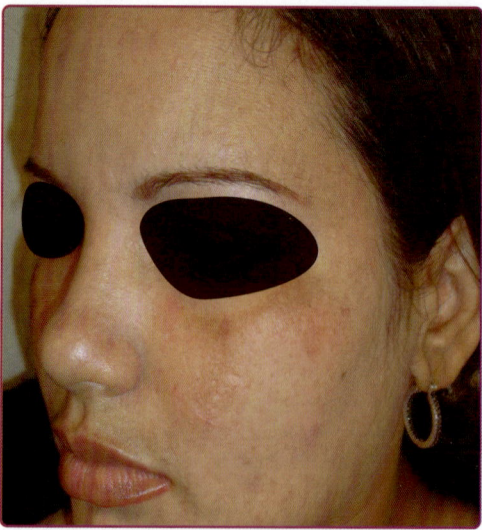

Figure 105-2 Melasma. Blotchy, mottled hyperpigmentation is evident on the malar cheek and upper cutaneous lip.

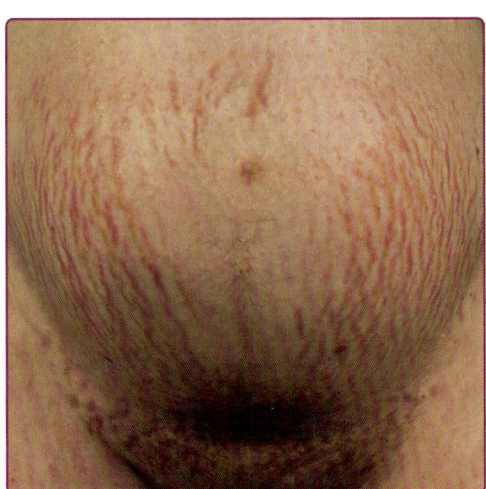

Figure 105-3 Striae distensae.

or the early postpartum period (Fig. 105-4). Unlike polymorphic eruption of pregnancy (see section "Dermatoses not Associated with Fetal Risk in Pregnancy"), PG includes periumbilical skin (Fig. 105-5).

ETIOLOGY AND PATHOGENESIS

PG is immunologically mediated, and linear deposition of C3, with or without immunoglobulin (Ig) G, is found at the dermal–epidermal junction by direct immunofluorescence (DIF).[8] In addition to occurring in pregnancy, PG can occur in abnormal pregnancies (hydatidiform mole, choriocarcinoma), implicating a role for paternally derived tissues in the pathogenesis of this condition.

DIAGNOSIS

Patients in whom PG is suspected usually require a biopsy for histology and DIF. Histopathologic examination reveals classic features of bullous pemphigoid. In the setting of pregnancy, DIF with C3 in a linear band at the dermal–epidermal junction is pathognomonic for PG.[8] Circulating autoantibodies are directed against the same target antigens as in bullous pemphigoid, more commonly against BP180 than BP230. Enzyme-linked immunosorbent assay (ELISA) or indirect immunofluorescence studies can be sent for the BP180 antigen. ELISA is as high as 96% specific and sensitive for PG.[9]

DIFFERENTIAL DIAGNOSIS

The differential diagnosis includes polymorphic eruption of pregnancy, drug eruptions, or urticaria (during the urticarial stage of pemphigoid gestationis). Even though DIF is the gold standard for diagnosis, the aforementioned ELISA and indirect immunofluorescence studies can be useful.

CLINICAL COURSE AND PROGNOSIS

PG is associated with premature delivery and a risk of low birth weight; the risk of these fetal complications correlates with maternal disease severity. Therefore, women with PG should be followed closely by their obstetrician.

Maternal prognosis is very good, with most cases resolving within a few months postpartum; however, it may take weeks, months, or even years until complete remission. Seventy-five percent of women flare postpartum and will require treatment. Exacerbations may occur postpartum with oral contraceptives and during the menstrual cycle.

Newborns of mothers with PG may develop bullous lesions that are transient and usually require no therapy. The development of these lesions is related to passive placental transfer of the anti–basement membrane zone antibody. If the mother has received long-term high doses of prednisolone, the infant should be evaluated for evidence of adrenal insufficiency.

MANAGEMENT

Treatment can be initiated with topical steroids and a systemic antihistamine. First-generation antihistamines are favored over second-generation antihistamines. Most patients require systemic corticosteroid treatment.[10] Many women will improve and may be tapered to lower doses or even to discontinuation of steroids. In cases that do not respond satisfactorily to prednisolone alone, or in cases where prolonged treatment with corticosteroids is contraindicated, plasmapheresis or IV immunoglobulin may be considered.[10,11]

INTRAHEPATIC CHOLESTASIS OF PREGNANCY

Intrahepatic cholestasis of pregnancy (ICP) is a rare, reversible cholestasis that typically occurs in late pregnancy, when serum concentrations of estrogen reach their peak. It was first recognized as a distinct clinical entity, separate from other forms of jaundice during pregnancy, by Svanborg and Ohlsson in 1939.[12] The terms *obstetric cholestasis*, *cholestasis of pregnancy*, *recurrent jaundice of pregnancy*, *cholestatic jaundice of pregnancy*, *idiopathic jaundice of pregnancy*, *prurigo gravidarum*, *pruritus gravidarum*, and *icterus gravidarum* all refer to this clinical entity. Mild cases of ICP, in which pruritus is not accompanied by jaundice, were previously referred to as prurigo gravidarum.

TABLE 105-2
A Summary of Dermatoses of Pregnancy

	MORPHOLOGY	DISTRIBUTION	USUAL ONSET	FETAL RISK	SYNONYM(S)
Pemphigoid (herpes) gestationis	Urticarial papules and plaques progress to vesicles and bullae	Begins on trunk, then progresses to generalized eruption Spares face, mucus membranes, palms, soles	Second or third trimester, or immediately postpartum	Small-for-gestational age births Preterm delivery Neonatal pemphigoid gestationis	Herpes gestationis
Intrahepatic cholestasis of pregnancy	Excoriations and excoriated papules ± jaundice	Generalized, including palms and soles	Third trimester	Preterm delivery Fetal distress Fetal death	Cholestasis of pregnancy Obstetric cholestasis Recurrent jaundice of pregnancy Cholestatic jaundice of pregnancy Idiopathic jaundice of pregnancy Prurigo gravidarum Icterus gravidarum
Pustular psoriasis of pregnancy	Erythematous patches with subcorneal pustules at their margins	Begins in flexures Generalizes demonstrating centrifugal spread	Third trimester	Placental insufficiency may lead to stillbirth or neonatal death	Impetigo herpetiformis
Pruritic urticarial papules and plaques of pregnancy	"Polymorphous" including urticarial papules and plaques ± vesicles	Begins within abdominal striae Spreads to remainder of trunk and then extremities Spares umbilicus	Third trimester or immediately postpartum	None	Polymorphic eruption of pregnancy Bourne toxemic rash of pregnancy Nurse's late onset prurigo of pregnancy Toxemic erythema of pregnancy (Holmes)
E-type atopic eruption of pregnancy	Eczematous patches and plaques	Face, neck, chest, flexural extremities	Before third trimester	None	Eczema in pregnancy[a]
P-type atopic eruption of pregnancy	Excoriated or crusted papules	Extremities, occasionally trunk	Before third trimester	None	Prurigo of pregnancy[a] Besnier prurigo gestationis Nurse's early onset prurigo of pregnancy Papular dermatitis of Spangler atopic eruption of pregnancy[a]

[a]A newly proposed classification by Ambros-Rudolph and associates[41] that combines the previously distinct entities prurigo of pregnancy and pruritic folliculitis of pregnancy into a single entity, atopic eruption of pregnancy, which also includes eczema in pregnancy.

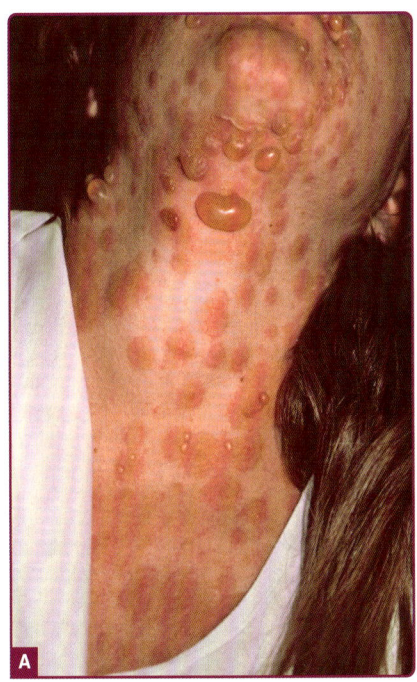
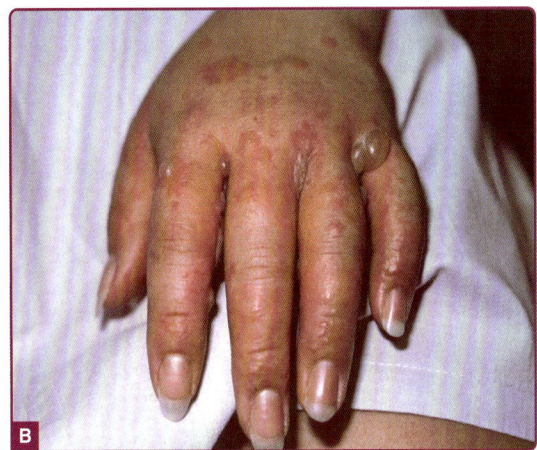

Figure 105-4 Pemphigoid gestationis. **A,** Urticarial plaques and tense bullae are seen on the face, neck, and chest. **B,** Similar lesions on the extremity. (Images from the Fitzsimmons Army Medical Center Dermatology Archive.)

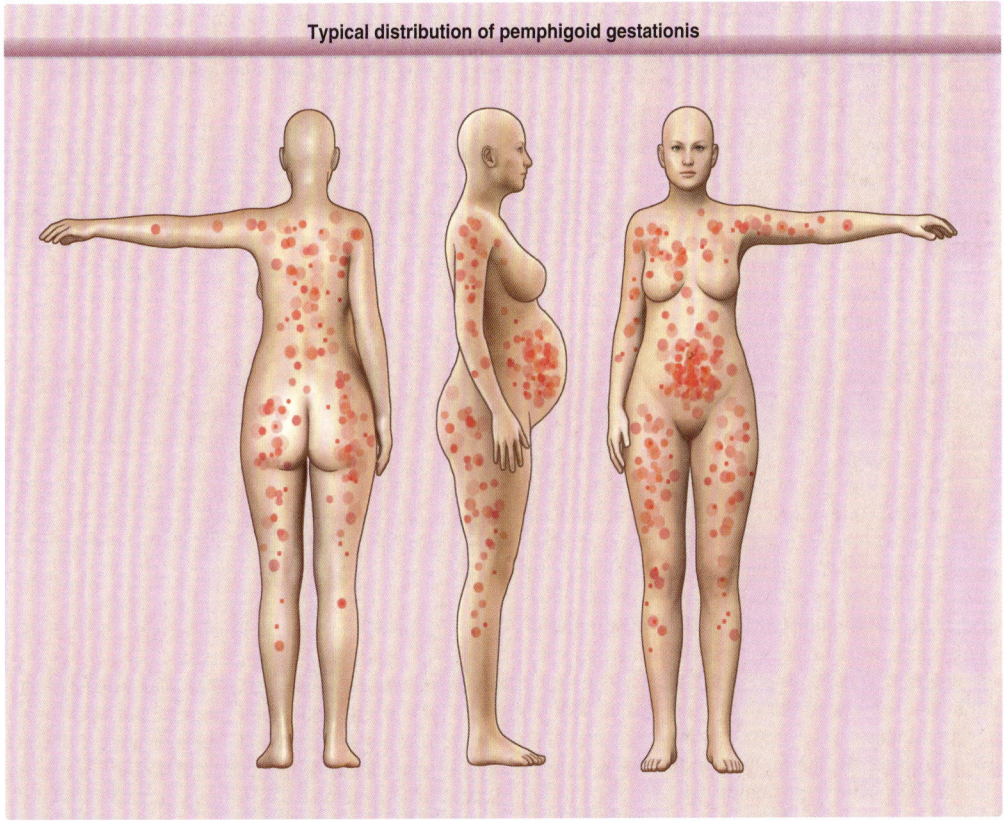

Figure 105-5 Pattern of rash in pemphigoid (herpes) gestationis.

EPIDEMIOLOGY

Jaundice develops in approximately 1 in 1500 pregnant women. With an estimated incidence of 70 cases per 10,000 pregnancies in the United States, ICP ranks second only to viral hepatitis in causing jaundice in pregnant women.[13] ICP is most common in Scandinavia and South America. The highest reported incidence rates are in Chile (14% to 16%), whereas much lower rates are seen among pregnant women in the United States (less than 0.1% to 0.7%), Canada (0.1%), Australia (0.2% to 1.5%), and Central Europe (0.1% to 1.5%).[13]

CLINICAL FEATURES

ICP is the only pregnancy dermatosis that presents without primary skin lesions. Patients classically present during the third trimester with moderate-to-severe pruritus, which may be either localized to the palms and soles or generalized. Pruritus begins during the first and second trimester in 10% and 25% of cases, respectively. Intense pruritus is often associated with secondary excoriations, although primary cutaneous lesions are invariably absent. Initially, patients may complain of nocturnal pruritus only, and symptoms are generally more severe at night throughout the course of ICP.

Constitutional symptoms such as fatigue, nausea, vomiting, or anorexia may accompany the pruritus. Progression to clinical jaundice, dark urine, or lightly colored stools occurs in approximately 1 in 5 patients. Pruritus generally precedes the onset of these symptoms by 1 to 4 weeks.[13]

Harmful effects on the fetus include an increase in premature births, intrapartum fetal distress, and fetal death.

ETIOLOGY AND PATHOGENESIS

Although the precise pathogenesis remains unclear, the interplay of hormonal, genetic, environmental, and alimentary factors is thought to induce a biochemical cholestasis in susceptible individuals. A prominent role for hormonal alterations is suggested by the following observations: (a) ICP is a disease of late pregnancy, corresponding to the period of highest placental hormone levels; (b) ICP spontaneously remits at delivery when hormone concentrations normalize; (c) twin and triplet pregnancies, which are characterized by greater rises in hormone concentrations, are linked to ICP; and, (d) ICP recurs during subsequent pregnancies in an estimated 45% to 70% of patients.[13]

Geographic variation and familial clustering indicate a genetic predisposition. ICP appears to be a polygenetic condition, with candidate genes including those mutated in a variety of other forms of inherited cholestasis: *ABCB4* (multidrug resistance gene3), *ABCB11* (bile salt export pump), and *ATP8B1* (*FIC1*). A recent decline in prevalence rates in Chile, reports of higher incidence rates during the winter months, and reports of relative reductions of selenium levels in some ICP patients all point toward etiologic roles for environmental and alimentary factors.[13,14] At least 1 study confirmed a higher risk of hepatitis C virus infection for women with ICP.[15]

DIAGNOSIS

Elevation in serum bile acids is the single most sensitive indicator of ICP. Total serum bile acid levels greater than 11 μM/L are consistent with ICP. In healthy pregnant women, total bile acids are slightly elevated above baseline and levels as high as 11 are accepted as normal in late pregnancy. Clearly defined biochemical indices of ICP have not yet been established. However, Brites and colleagues[16] identified the following common features of ICP: (a) serum total bile acid concentrations greater than 11 μM (reference range: 4.6 to 8.7 μM); (b) cholic acid-to-chenodeoxycholic acid ratio greater than 1.5 (reference range: 0.7 to 1.5) or cholic acid proportion of total bile acids greater than 42%; (c) glycine conjugates-to-taurine conjugates of bile acids ratio less than 1 (reference range: 0.9 to 2) or glycocholic acid concentration greater than 2 μM (reference range: 0.6 to 1.5 μM).[16] Degree of pruritus and disease severity generally correlate with bile acid concentrations.

Mild perturbations in liver function tests, including elevated transaminases, alkaline phosphatase, 5′-nucleotidase, cholesterol, triglycerides, phospholipids, and lipoprotein X are commonly found. Among these parameters, alanine transaminase is particularly sensitive, as an elevation in this enzyme is not a feature of healthy pregnancies but is commonly seen in ICP. γ-Glutamyl transferase, which is generally low in late gestation, is typically normal or slightly elevated in ICP. Direct (or conjugated) fractions of bilirubin are most commonly elevated in ICP. Albumin may be slightly reduced, whereas α_2-globulins and β-globulins are appreciably elevated. However, routine liver tests alone are not a sufficient basis for the diagnosis of ICP.[16]

Cutaneous biopsy does not aid in the diagnosis of ICP.

DIFFERENTIAL DIAGNOSIS

Distinction from other causes of pruritus in the pregnant woman can be challenging. The presence of primary lesions points away from a diagnosis of ICP, which lacks primary lesions. Other causes of liver derangement and jaundice, such as viral and nonviral hepatitis, medications, hepatobiliary obstruction, and other intrahepatic diseases (eg, primary biliary cirrhosis) must be ruled out. Finally, it must be remembered that hyperthyroidism, allergic reactions, polycythemia vera, lymphoma, pediculosis, and scabies may each manifest as generalized pruritus in pregnant (and nonpregnant) women.

CLINICAL COURSE AND PROGNOSIS

A hallmark of ICP is that symptoms and associated biochemical abnormalities typically resolve within 2 to 4 weeks of delivery. Recurrences during subsequent pregnancies occur in an estimated 45% to 70% of patients. Some women experience recurrent ICP after exposure to oral contraceptives or to contraceptive aids, such as synthetic estrogens and progestational agents.

Maternal outcomes are generally favorable, although women with severe cases are predisposed to postpartum hemorrhage secondary to vitamin K depletion. Additionally, affected women have a tendency toward the later development of cholelithiasis or gallbladder disease. Fetal risks in ICP include increased rates of prematurity, fetal distress, and fetal death. These complications generally correlate with higher bile acid levels and are attributed to acute placental anoxia and an increased incidence of meconium-stained amniotic fluid.

MANAGEMENT

Therapy aims to reduce serum bile acid levels and thereby prolong pregnancy, ameliorate maternal symptoms and reduce fetal risks. An interdisciplinary approach characterized by intense fetal surveillance is essential to the management of ICP.

Although in mild cases, relief can sometimes be achieved with bland emollients and topical antipruritic agents, ursodeoxycholic acid (UDCA), a naturally occurring hydrophilic bile acid, is the current treatment of choice. UDCA reduces maternal symptoms and fetal risk. UDCA exerts a hepatoprotective effect through augmentation of the excretion of hydrophobic bile acids, sulfated progesterone metabolites, and other hepatotoxic compounds. UDCA decreases bile acid levels in colostrum, cord blood, and amniotic fluid. The results of several small, randomized, placebo-controlled trials demonstrate that when administered at doses between 450 mg and 1200 mg daily, UDCA is well tolerated and highly effective in controlling the clinical and liver function abnormalities that define ICP.[17] Randomized, controlled trials comparing UDCA head-to-head with either dexamethasone[18] or cholestyramine[19] demonstrated the superior efficacy of UDCA.

There is mixed data in the literature on early delivery. A systematic review of unexplained term stillbirths associated with ICP-affected pregnancies that was completed to evaluate evidence supporting ICP as a medical indication for early delivery at less than 39 weeks of gestation found no evidence to support active management (early delivery) for ICP.[20] This article reported stillbirth rates in both groups—patients whose obstetric care did or did not include active management—similar to respective national stillbirth rate. A recent retrospective study reported that delivery at 36 weeks of gestation would reduce perinatal mortality risk as compared with expectant management.[21] Most authors recommend early induction of labor, commonly at 38 weeks of gestation or earlier.[13,21]

PUSTULAR PSORIASIS OF PREGNANCY (IMPETIGO HERPETIFORMIS)

Pustular psoriasis of pregnancy is generally regarded as a variant of pustular psoriasis attributable to hormonal alterations during pregnancy; however, some authors maintain that it is a distinct clinical entity.[22] Von Hebra first used the designation *impetigo herpetiformis* in 1872 to describe an acute pustular eruption with usual onset during the third trimester of pregnancy.

EPIDEMIOLOGY

Pustular psoriasis of pregnancy is very rare, with only approximately 350 cases described in the European and American literature as of 2000.[23]

CLINICAL FEATURES

Pustular psoriasis of pregnancy is characterized by an acute eruption occurring as early as the first trimester, but generally during the third trimester, of an otherwise uneventful pregnancy. The condition manifests as erythematous patches whose margins are studded with subcorneal pustules (Fig. 105-6). The eruption typically originates in flexural areas, spreads centrifugally and sometimes generalizes. Subungual lesions may result in onycholysis. Rarely, mucous membrane involvement may lead to painful erosions. The face, palms, and soles are commonly spared. The rash may be pruritic or painful.

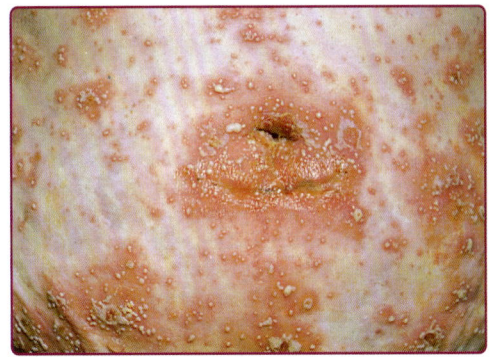

Figure 105-6 Pustular psoriasis of pregnancy. Erythematous patches are studded with subcorneal pustules.

Onset of the eruption is accompanied by constitutional symptoms such as fever, chills, malaise, diarrhea, nausea, and arthralgia.

Life-threatening maternal complications are infrequent but may result from profound hypocalcemia and bacterial sepsis. Rarely, tetany, delirium, and convulsions occur if hypocalcemia is severe.[1] The most feared complications are placental insufficiency and consequent stillbirth or neonatal death. For these reasons, early induction of labor is often contemplated.[22]

ETIOLOGY AND PATHOGENESIS

Although generally regarded as a form of pustular psoriasis, absence of a positive family history, abrupt resolution of symptoms at delivery, and a tendency to recur only during subsequent pregnancies distinguish this entity from generalized pustular psoriasis. Moreover, factors known to trigger pustular psoriatic flares, such as infection, exposure to certain culprit drugs, or abrupt discontinuation of systemic corticosteroids, are lacking in most patients with pustular psoriasis of pregnancy.[1]

DIAGNOSIS

Although the clinical picture is often typical, a biopsy is helpful to confirm this diagnosis. Histopathologic examination reveals classic features of pustular psoriasis. Initial laboratory evaluation should include complete blood count and comprehensive metabolic panel with particular attention to calcium level. The most common laboratory derangements include leukocytosis, neutrophilia, an elevated erythrocyte sedimentation rate, hypoferric anemia, and hypoalbuminemia. Less commonly, calcium, phosphate, and vitamin D levels are decreased. Serum parathyroid hormone levels are rarely decreased. Cultures of pustule contents and peripheral blood are negative unless secondarily infected.[1]

DIFFERENTIAL DIAGNOSIS

Table 105-3 outlines the differential diagnosis of pustular psoriasis of pregnancy.

CLINICAL COURSE AND PROGNOSIS

Pustular psoriasis of pregnancy classically presents during the third trimester, but there are reports of cases occurring as early as the first trimester, during the puerperium, in nonpregnant women taking oral contraceptives, and in postmenopausal women. Symptoms are invariably progressive throughout pregnancy. A cardinal feature of this disorder is the rapid resolution of symptoms after delivery. Recurrences in subsequent pregnancies are common and characteristically are more severe with onset earlier in gestation.[1] Several reports of subsequent menstrual exacerbation occurring either during or immediately preceding menses exist in the literature.[24]

More widespread disease generally portends a worse prognosis.

MANAGEMENT

Resolution after delivery is the norm. However, given its consistently progressive course, treatment is indicated to reduce the risk of fetal and maternal complications during pregnancy. Topical treatments, which include wet dressings and topical corticosteroids, are rarely effective as monotherapy. Narrowband ultraviolet B combined with topical steroids has been reported to be successful in rare cases as well.[25]

Systemic corticosteroids were historically the mainstay of therapy. Now, cyclosporine and infliximab are deemed first-line therapy.[26] Cyclosporine has been successfully used at doses between 5 mg/kg and 10 mg/kg daily.[27,28] Infliximab, a tumor necrosis factor-α blocking agent, has been successfully used without adverse effect on the fetus,[29] but with the caveat that live vaccines should be delayed in newborns of mothers treated with infliximab.[30] Although careful consideration of the benefits and risks of tumor necrosis factor blockade during pregnancy must be considered, these agents (including etanercept and adalimumab) may have a role in management.[26]

In all cases, fluid status and electrolytes should be monitored with rapid correction of imbalances. Fetal monitoring is essential as decelerations in fetal heart rate may be the earliest sign of fetal hypoxemia. Maternal cardiac and renal functions may be compromised with disease progression and therefore should also be monitored. Induction of labor is an option when symptoms do not remit despite supportive and pharmacologic therapy. The therapeutic armamentarium available after pregnancy termination or after delivery in a nonnursing mother can be extended to include oral psoralen and ultraviolet A, oral retinoids, and methotrexate.[31]

TABLE 105-3

Differential Diagnosis of Pustular Psoriasis of Pregnancy

Most Likely
- Pustular drug eruption (acute generalized exanthematous pustulosis)
- Pemphigoid gestationis

Consider
- Pemphigus vulgaris
- Dermatitis herpetiformis
- Subcorneal pustular dermatosis
- Pustular eruption in inflammatory bowel disease

Always Rule Out
- Infectious causes of pustular eruptions

DERMATOSES NOT ASSOCIATED WITH FETAL RISK IN PREGNANCY

> **AT-A-GLANCE**
>
> - Polymorphic eruption of pregnancy (previously pruritic urticarial papules and plaques of pregnancy) is a common, self-limited, intensely pruritic dermatosis that occurs almost exclusively in primigravidas during late pregnancy.
> - Atopic eruption of pregnancy (AEP) represents a relatively newly introduced term comprising pruritic folliculitis of pregnancy, prurigo of pregnancy, and eczema of pregnancy. Lesions typically appear before the third trimester and may resemble classic atopic dermatitis (AEP, E-type) or be papular (AEP, P-type).

POLYMORPHIC ERUPTION OF PREGNANCY (PRURITIC URTICARIAL PAPULES AND PLAQUES OF PREGNANCY)

Polymorphic eruption of pregnancy (PEP) is a common, benign, intensely pruritic dermatosis that occurs almost exclusively in primigravidas during the third trimester and immediate postpartum period. PEP (previously termed *pruritic urticarial papules and plaques of pregnancy*) is synonymous with Bourne's toxemic rash of pregnancy, Nurse's late onset prurigo of pregnancy, and toxic erythema of pregnancy.[32]

EPIDEMIOLOGY

The incidence of PEP ranges between 1 in 300 and 1 in 130 pregnancies.[33]

CLINICAL FEATURES

PEP typically occurs in primigravidas during the last trimester of pregnancy (mean onset: 35 weeks); however, cases of otherwise classic PEP have occurred earlier in pregnancy and in the immediate postpartum period. Polymorphous in nature, lesions may be urticarial (most commonly), vesicular, purpuric, polycyclic, targetoid, or eczematous in appearance (Fig. 105-7).[34] Typical lesions are 1- to 2-mm erythematous urticarial papules surrounded by a narrow pale halo. The eruption begins on the abdomen, classically within the striae gravidarum, and demonstrates periumbilical sparing (Fig. 105-8). Pruritus generally parallels the eruption and is localized to involved skin. Rapid spread to the thighs, buttocks, breasts, and arms

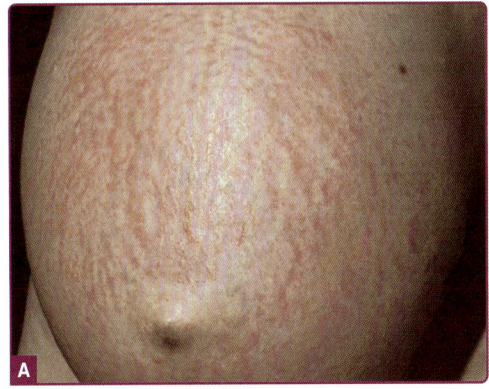
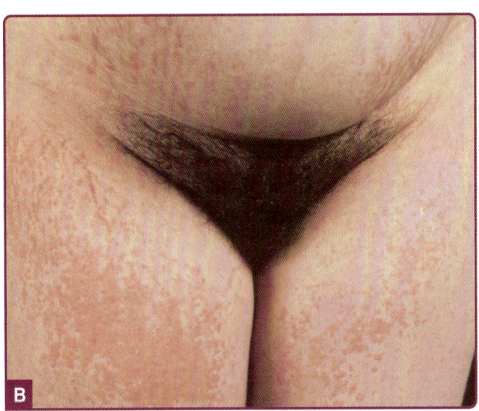
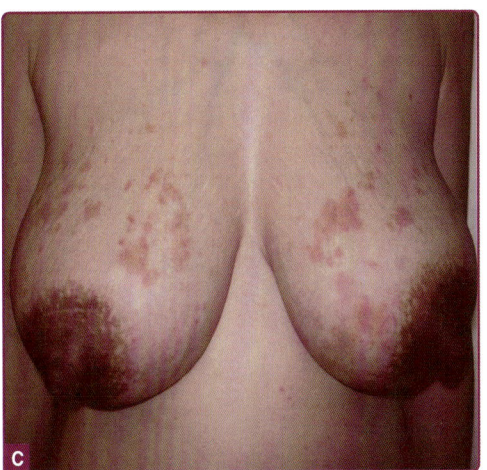

Figure 105-7 Pruritic urticarial papules and plaques of pregnancy. **A,** The earliest lesions are 1- to 2-mm, erythematous, urticarial papules localized within and around the striae distensae and sparing the umbilicus. **B,** The papules coalesce to form erythematous plaques that spread to involve the buttocks and thighs. **C,** Urticarial plaques on the breasts. Of note, the breasts also show a "secondary areola," the physiologic darkening, and reticular expansion of the areolar pigmentation. There are also striae distensae visible on the breast as well as Montgomery tubercles on the areolae.

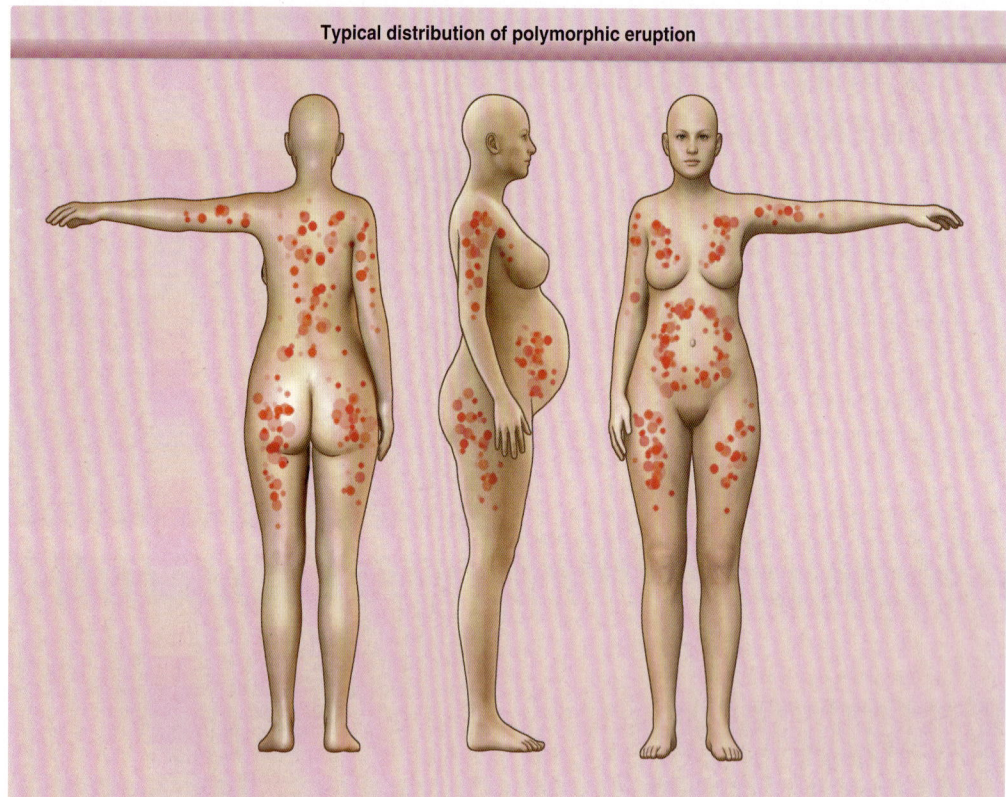

Figure 105-8 Pattern of rash in polymorphic eruption of pregnancy.

is the norm. Involvement of the palms, soles, or skin above the breast is exceptional.[1]

Severe pruritus may disturb sleep, but no other systemic symptoms are reported.

ETIOLOGY AND PATHOGENESIS

The pathogenesis remains unknown. Some postulate that increased abdominal cutaneous distension leads to altered collagen and/or elastic tissue, thereby triggering maternal immunoreactivity to previously non-antigenic stimuli.[33] Increased progesterone receptor immunoreactivity has been detected in lesional PEP, leading some to posit a role for progesterone activation of keratinocytes.[35]

RISK FACTORS

An association between PEP and multiple gestation is suggested by the higher-than-expected rates of twin and triplet pregnancies in most published series.[33,36,37] An unexplained association with male fetuses and delivery by cesarean section has been reported, although not consistently.[33,36,37] Reports linking PEP to increased maternal–fetal weight gain[33,38] are contested.

DIAGNOSIS

The diagnosis is generally made clinically when the patient presents with the eruption in typical locations at the end of pregnancy. Biopsy should be performed if PG is being considered in the differential diagnosis. Histopathologic findings, although nonspecific, generally include parakeratosis, spongiosis, and occasional exocytosis of eosinophils (eosinophilic spongiosis). The adjacent dermis may be edematous and contains a perivascular infiltrate of lymphocytes admixed with variable numbers of eosinophils and neutrophils. DIF studies reveal either granular or absent C3, IgM, or IgA deposits at the dermoepidermal junction or around blood vessels, and indirect immunofluorescence studies are negative.[1]

DIFFERENTIAL DIAGNOSIS

Table 105-4 outlines the differential diagnosis of PEP.

CLINICAL COURSE AND PROGNOSIS

PEP mostly affects primigravidas in the last trimester, although it may occur as early as the first trimes-

TABLE 105-4
Differential Diagnosis of Polymorphic Eruption of Pregnancy
Most Likely ■ Pemphigoid gestationis ■ Atopic eruption of pregnancy ■ Contact dermatitis
Consider ■ Drug eruption ■ Viral exanthem ■ Pityriasis rosea ■ Exfoliative or eczematous dermatitis
Always Rule Out ■ Scabies

ter. There are several reports of cases occurring in the immediate postpartum period as well. Duration of symptoms is typically brief, averaging 6 weeks. Severe symptoms rarely persist for more than 1 week. Spontaneous remission within days of delivery is the rule. Recurrences in subsequent pregnancies or with exposure to oral contraceptives are unusual. Fetal and maternal prognoses are unaltered.[1] There is a single report of involvement of a newborn.[39]

MANAGEMENT

Although harmless to the mother and fetus, pruritus is often intense and unremitting. Symptomatic relief of pruritus can usually be achieved with topical corticosteroids and/or oral antihistamines. A brief course of oral corticosteroids is rarely required, but effectively controls symptoms in most cases refractory to topical treatment. Early induction of labor was previously considered in instances in which severe pruritus is unrelenting, but has fallen out of favor given the lack of increased morbidity of the fetus or mother (other than relentless pruritus) and is generally considered unnecessary.[40] Reassurance regarding the self-limited nature of PEP can help to assuage anxiety.

ATOPIC ERUPTION OF PREGNANCY

Atopic eruption of pregnancy (AEP) is a benign pruritic condition of pregnancy characterized by an eczematous (AEP, E-type) and/or papular (AEP, P-type) eruption in individuals with a personal and/or familial atopic background and/or elevated serum IgE levels. AEP denotes the disease complex comprising the previously distinct entities prurigo of pregnancy and pruritic folliculitis of pregnancy, as well as eczema in pregnancy, which had not previously been considered a specific dermatosis of pregnancy.[41] Ambros-Rudolph and colleagues proposed this new nomenclature (AEP) in 2006. AEP includes Besnier's prurigo gestationis, Nurse's early-onset prurigo of pregnancy and papular dermatitis of Spangler.[40]

EPIDEMIOLOGY

AEP comprises approximately 50% of all pregnancy dermatoses, making it the most common pruritic disorder in pregnancy. It tends to present earlier in pregnancy than the other pregnancy-associated dermatoses.[41]

CLINICAL FEATURES

Whereas 20% of AEP patients present with a flare of preexisting atopic dermatitis, the remaining patients experience an atopic eruption for the first time ever (or after a long remission). A classic eczematous eruption primarily affecting flexural surfaces and the face occurs in two-thirds of affected individuals (AEP, E-type; Fig. 105-9). The remaining third present with papular lesions (AEP, P-type; Fig. 105-10) that would previously have been classified as prurigo of pregnancy. P-type lesions are discrete, pruritic, excoriated papules with a predilection for extensor surfaces (Fig. 105-11), with truncal involvement less common. Minor features of eczema, including xerosis or hyperlinear palms, may be noted in patients with either subtype. Distinguishing features of AEP include onset early in pregnancy (before the third trimester) and a personal and/or family history of atopy.[41]

ETIOLOGY AND PATHOGENESIS

AEP is thought to be triggered by pregnancy-related shifts in cytokine profile expression leading to preferential expression of T-helper 2 cytokines.[41]

RISK FACTORS

Risk factors for AEP include a personal and/or family history of atopy.[41]

DIAGNOSIS

The diagnosis is largely clinical as histopathologic features are nonspecific and direct and indirect immunofluorescence studies are negative.[1] Total serum IgE is elevated in 20% to 70% of individuals with AEP,[41] although the clinical relevance of testing for serum IgE is unclear. Serologic tests reveal no other abnormalities.

DIFFERENTIAL DIAGNOSIS

Other specific dermatoses of pregnancy, especially ICP and PEP, should be ruled out, as should microbial folliculitis and allergic contact dermatitis occurring in a pregnant woman.

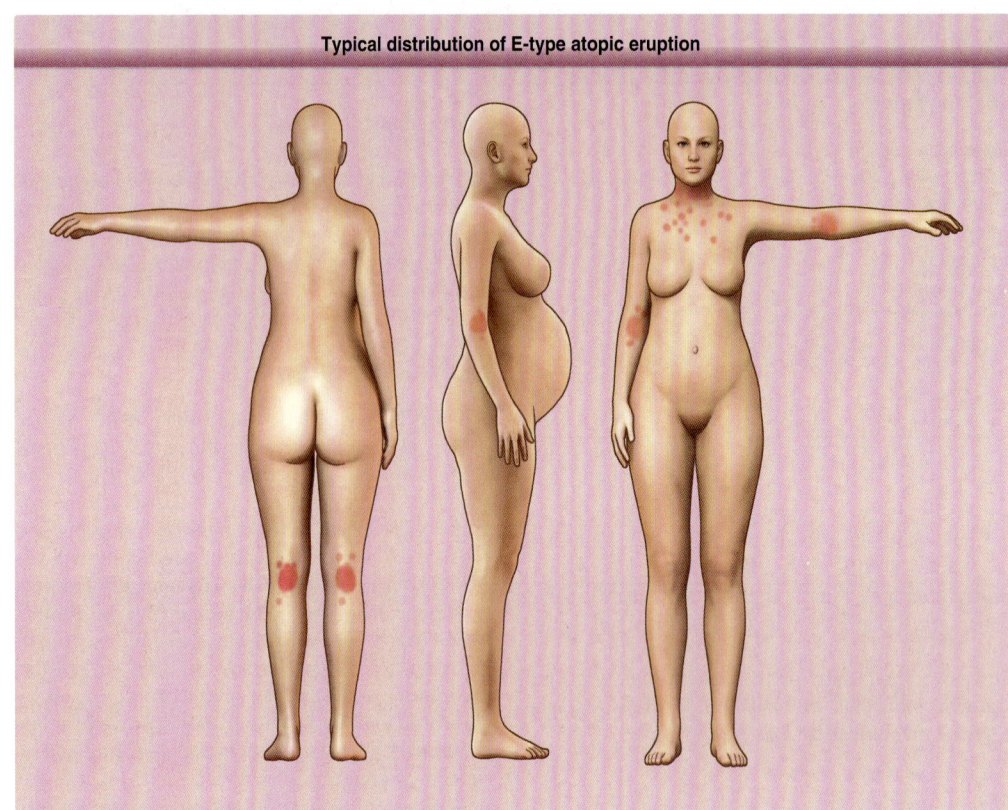

Figure 105-9 Pattern of rash for an eczematous eruption in atopic eruption of pregnancy.

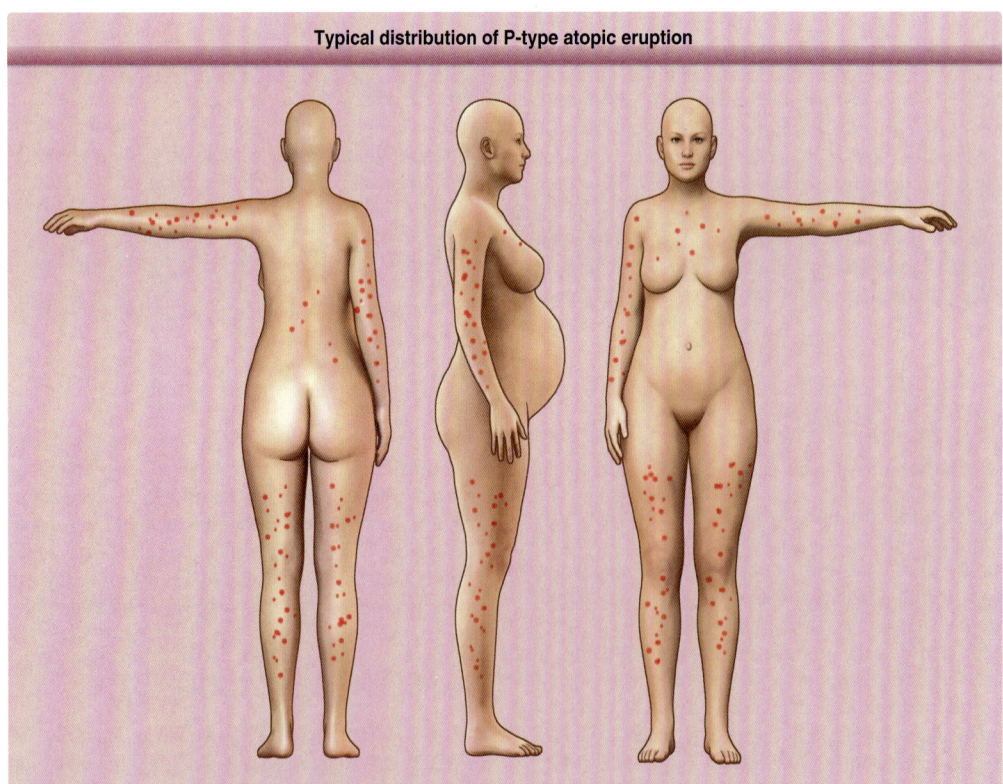

Figure 105-10 Pattern of rash for a papular eruption in atopic eruption of pregnancy.

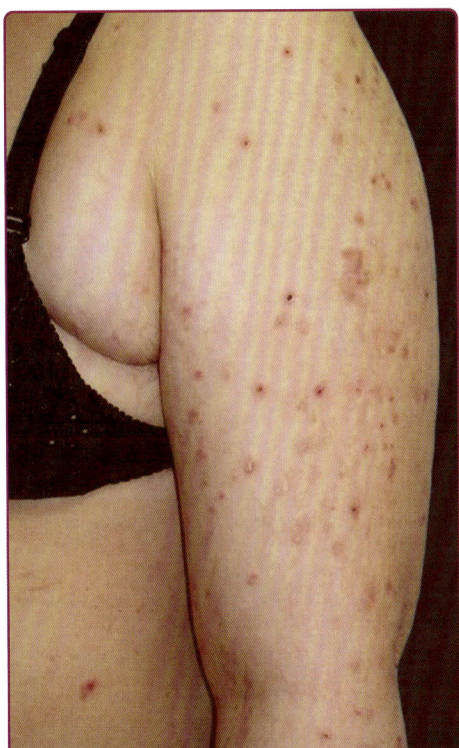

Figure 105-11 Atopic eruption of pregnancy, P-type (previously, prurigo of pregnancy). Multiple discrete, excoriated papules demonstrate a predilection for extensor surfaces.

CLINICAL COURSE AND PROGNOSIS

Onset is typically prior to the third trimester. Lesions respond quickly to therapy; however, recurrence with subsequent pregnancies is common, consistent with an atopic diathesis. Maternal and fetal prognoses are excellent, even in severe cases.[42] In a mother with a known history of atopy, the infant will be at increased risk for atopic dermatitis. In a mother with no prior history of eczematous eruptions, her risk of recurrence outside of pregnancy is unknown.[42]

MANAGEMENT

Treatment seeks to ameliorate pruritus and includes emollients, midpotency topical corticosteroids, and antihistamines. Benzoyl peroxide may be helpful for truncal, follicular lesions, and ultraviolet B phototherapy can be used in severe cases.[1,43,44]

ACKNOWLEDGMENTS

The authors thank Dr. Julie Karen, who contributed to the previous version of this chapter in the 8th edition.

REFERENCES

1. Kroumpouzos G, Cohen LM. Dermatoses of pregnancy. *J Am Acad Dermatol.* 2001;45:1-19; quiz 19-22.
2. Geraghty LN, Pomeranz MK. Physiologic changes and dermatoses of pregnancy. *Int J Dermatol.* 2011;50:771-782.
3. Muzaffar F, Hussain I, Haroon TS. Physiologic skin changes during pregnancy: a study of 140 cases. *Int J Dermatol.* 1998;37:429-431.
4. Elling SV, Powell FC. Physiological changes in the skin during pregnancy. *Clin Dermatol.* 1997;15:35-43.
5. Pennoyer JW, Grin CM, Driscoll MS, et al. Changes in size of melanocytic nevi during pregnancy. *J Am Acad Dermatol.* 1997;36:378-382.
6. Aktürk AS, Bilen N, Bayrämgürler D, et al. Dermoscopy is a suitable method for the observation of the pregnancy-related changes in melanocytic nevi. *J Eur Acad Dermatol Venereol.* 2007;21:1086-1090.
7. Salter SA, Kimball AB. Striae gravidarum. *Clin Dermatol.* 2006;24:97-100.
8. Tani N, Kimura Y, Koga H, et al. Clinical and immunological profiles of 25 patients with pemphigoid gestationis. *Br J Dermatol.* 2015;172:120-129.
9. Powell AM, Sakuma-Oyama Y, Oyama N, et al. Usefulness of BP180 NC16a enzyme-linked immunosorbent assay in the serodiagnosis of pemphigoid gestationis and in differentiating between pemphigoid gestationis and pruritic urticarial papules and plaques of pregnancy. *Arch Dermatol.* 2005;141: 705-710.
10. Jenkins RE, Hern S, Black MM. Clinical features and management of 87 patients with pemphigoid gestationis. *Clin Exp Dermatol.* 1999;24:255-259.
11. Gan DC, Welsh B, Webster M. Successful treatment of a severe persistent case of pemphigoid gestationis with antepartum and postpartum intravenous immunoglobulin followed by azathioprine. *Australas J Dermatol.* 2012;53:66-69.
12. Svanborg A, Ohlsson S. Recurrent jaundice of pregnancy; a clinical study of twenty-two cases. *Am J Med.* 1959;27:40-49.
13. Lammert F, Marschall HU, Glantz A, et al. Intrahepatic cholestasis of pregnancy: molecular pathogenesis, diagnosis and management. *J Hepatol.* 2000;33: 1012-1021.
14. Paus TC, Schneider G, Van De Vondel P, et al. Diagnosis and therapy of intrahepatic cholestasis of pregnancy. *Z Gastroenterol.* 2004;42:623-628.
15. Paternoster DM, Fabris F, Palù G, et al. Intra-hepatic cholestasis of pregnancy in hepatitis C virus infection. *Acta Obstet Gynecol Scand.* 2002;81:99-103.
16. Brites D, Rodrigues CM, van-Zeller H, et al. Relevance of serum bile acid profile in the diagnosis of intrahepatic cholestasis of pregnancy in an high incidence area: Portugal. *Eur J Obstet Gynecol Reprod Biol.* 1998;80:31-38.
17. Kroumpouzos G. Intrahepatic cholestasis of pregnancy: what's new. *J Eur Acad Dermatol Venereol.* 2002;16:316-318.
18. Glantz A, Marschall HU, Lammert F, et al. Intrahepatic cholestasis of pregnancy: a randomized controlled trial comparing dexamethasone and ursodeoxycholic acid. *Hepatology.* 2005;42:1399-1405.
19. Kondrackiene J, Beuers U, Zalinkevicius R, et al. Predictors of premature delivery in patients with intrahepatic cholestasis of pregnancy. *World J Gastroenterol.* 2007;13:6226-6230.

20. Henderson CE, Shah RR, Gottimukkala S, et al. Primum non nocere: how active management became modus operandi for intrahepatic cholestasis of pregnancy. *Am J Obstet Gynecol.* 2014;211:189-196.
21. Puljic A, Kim E, Page J, et al. The risk of infant and fetal death by each additional week of expectant management in intrahepatic cholestasis of pregnancy by gestational age. *Am J Obstet Gynecol.* 2015;212: 667.e1-667.e5.
22. Heymann WR. Dermatoses of pregnancy update. *J Am Acad Dermatol.* 2005;52:888-889.
23. Henson TH, Tuli M, Bushore D, et al. Recurrent pustular rash in a pregnant woman. *Arch Dermatol.* 2000;136:1055-1060.
24. Chaidemenos G, Lefaki I, Tsakiri A, et al. Impetigo herpetiformis: menstrual exacerbations for 7 years postpartum. *J Eur Acad Dermatol Venereol.* 2005;19: 466-469.
25. Vun YY, Jones B, Al-Mudhaffer M, et al. Generalized pustular psoriasis of pregnancy treated with narrowband UVB and topical steroids. *J Am Acad Dermatol.* 2006;54(2)(suppl):S28-S30.
26. Robinson A, Van Voorhees AS, Hsu S, et al. Treatment of pustular psoriasis: from the Medical Board of the National Psoriasis Foundation. *J Am Acad Dermatol.* 2012;67:279-288.
27. Imai N, Watanabe R, Fujiwara H, et al. Successful treatment of impetigo herpetiformis with oral cyclosporine during pregnancy. *Arch Dermatol.* 2002;138: 128-129.
28. Kapoor R, Kapoor JR. Cyclosporine resolves generalized pustular psoriasis of pregnancy. *Arch Dermatol.* 2006;142:1373-1375.
29. Puig L, Barco D, Alomar A. Treatment of psoriasis with anti-TNF drugs during pregnancy: case report and review of the literature. *Dermatology.* 2010;220:71-76.
30. Cheent K, Nolan J, Shariq S, et al. Case report: fatal case of disseminated BCG infection in an infant born to a mother taking infliximab for Crohn's disease. *J Crohns Colitis.* 2010;4:603-605.
31. Bukhari IA. Impetigo herpetiformis in a primigravida: successful treatment with etretinate. *J Drugs Dermatol.* 2004;3:449-451.
32. Ahmadi S, Powell FC. Pruritic urticarial papules and plaques of pregnancy: current status. *Australas J Dermatol.* 2005;46:53-58; quiz 59.
33. Vaughan Jones SA, Hern S, Nelson-Piercy C, et al. A prospective study of 200 women with dermatoses of pregnancy correlating clinical findings with hormonal and immunopathological profiles. *Br J Dermatol.* 1999;141:71-81.
34. Rudolph CM, Al-Fares S, Vaughan-Jones SA, et al. Polymorphic eruption of pregnancy: clinicopathology and potential trigger factors in 181 patients. *Br J Dermatol.* 2006;154:54-60.
35. Im S, Lee ES, Kim W, et al. Expression of progesterone receptor in human keratinocytes. *J Korean Med Sci.* 2000;15:647-654.
36. Elling SV, McKenna P, Powell FC. Pruritic urticarial papules and plaques of pregnancy in twin and triplet pregnancies. *J Eur Acad Dermatol Venereol.* 2000;14:378-381.
37. Regnier S, Fermand V, Levy P, et al. A case-control study of polymorphic eruption of pregnancy. *J Am Acad Dermatol.* 2008;58:63-67.
38. Cohen LM, Capeless EL, Krusinski PA, et al. Pruritic urticarial papules and plaques of pregnancy and its relationship to maternal-fetal weight gain and twin pregnancy. *Arch Dermatol.* 1989;125:1534-1536.
39. Uhlin SR. Pruritic urticarial papules and plaques of pregnancy. Involvement in mother and infant. *Arch Dermatol.* 1981;117:238-239.
40. Kroumpouzos G, Cohen LM. Specific dermatoses of pregnancy: an evidence-based systematic review. *Am J Obstet Gynecol.* 2003;188:1083-1092.
41. Ambros-Rudolph CM, Müllegger RR, Vaughan-Jones SA, et al. The specific dermatoses of pregnancy revisited and reclassified: results of a retrospective two-center study on 505 pregnant patients. *J Am Acad Dermatol.* 2006;54:395-404.
42. Roth MM, Cristodor P, Kroumpouzos G. Prurigo, pruritic folliculitis, and atopic eruption of pregnancy: facts and controversies. *Clin Dermatol.* 2016;34:392-400.
43. Holmes RC, Black MM. The specific dermatoses of pregnancy. *J Am Acad Dermatol.* 1983;8:405-412.
44. Reed J, George S. Pruritic folliculitis of pregnancy treated with narrowband (TL-01) ultraviolet B phototherapy. *Br J Dermatol.* 1999;141:177-179.

Chapter 106 :: Skin Aging
:: Michelle L. Kerns, Anna L. Chien, & Sewon Kang

第一百零六章

皮肤老化

中文导读

人类皮肤经历了两种不同类型的老化：内源性老化和外源性老化。本章主要分为6节：首先从氧化应激讲述皮肤衰老的发生机制；继而比较了内源性老化和外源性老化的发生机制、组织学改变和临床表现；重点讲述了光老化的发生机制和皮肤表现；还提到了皮肤老化的机制与雌激素水平相关。最后详细阐述了老化皮肤的组织结构变化，介绍了部分常见的老年皮肤疾病。

第一节综述了氧化应激与衰老的机制包括：有氧代谢产生的活性氧的清除能力下降，其氧化应激导致了内源性衰老。氧化损伤导致应激相关因子的上调，进而触发促进衰老过程的下游事件；氧化应激还改变端粒，当端粒达到"临界短"阈值时，根据细胞类型的不同，细胞会经历增殖性衰老或凋亡。并结合相关文献对上述衰老机制进行了深入论述。

第二节分别讲述了内源性老化和外源性老化的发生机制、组织学改变和临床表现，并在一定程度上进行了比较。作者还结合文献讲述了空气污染等环境因素对皮肤生理学影响的一些研究进展。

第三节介绍了光老化的概念，并讲述了地球表面紫外线辐射组成，及UVA和UVB对皮肤老化的影响。还进一步讨论了光老化机制。

第四节讲述了雌激素与皮肤老化的关系。雌激素是皮肤生理和伤口愈合的重要调节因子，列表讲述了雌激素对皮肤生理的影响。提到雌激素是通过特定的雌激素受体发挥作用的，雌激素受体信号是氧化还原平衡和氧化应激的关键调节剂，是皮肤老化的许多机制的中心。

在讲到雌激素水平变化对衰老的深远影响时，提到在绝经前的妇女中，雌激素的主要形式是雌二醇，它由卵巢产生，绝经后，雌二醇水平急剧下降，女性皮肤可能会迅速老化。最后，作者讲述了一些局部应用雌激素对人类皮肤的影响的相关研究进展。

第五节从表皮、真皮、皮肤附属器三个方面分别讲述了组织学结构和细胞水平的皮肤老化改变。

1. 表皮　随年龄增长，表皮的新陈代谢能力下降，与伤口修复能力下降相一致。组织学层面上，表皮整体变薄，其中棘细胞层受表皮萎缩影响最大，而角质层和颗粒层基本不受影响。作者特别提出，虽然角质层的平均厚度不随年龄而改变，但皮肤对外界刺激的敏感性增加。这里，作者提到老化皮肤的皮肤屏障受损后其修复能力下降与角质层脂质含量下降、表皮聚丝蛋白的减少等有关。

细胞水平上，作者详细讲述了表皮角

质形成细胞发生了许多与年龄相关的重要变化——细胞的异质性增加；表皮的其他常驻细胞如黑素细胞和朗格汉斯细胞等，也经历了与年龄相关的变化。作者还列表（表106-4）总结了不同年龄相关的表皮细胞类型的变化。

2．真皮　胶原蛋白是真皮和皮肤结构的主要成分。它与年龄相关的变化可能是许多皮肤老化特征的原因，包括皮肤变薄和伤口愈合受损等。

弹性蛋白，提供皮肤弹性，也随着年龄的增长而改变。文中提出，日光弹性纤维变性是光老化真皮最显著的组织学改变，其特征是正常弹性纤维被一团紊乱的弹性纤维取代，分布在真皮-表皮交界处附近。

老化还会影响皮肤的基质。基质由蛋白聚糖和糖胺聚糖组成，基质的减少导致蛋白质与水的相互作用减少，加重皮肤老化。作者还列表（表106-5）总结了皮肤真皮成分随年龄的相关变化。

3．皮肤附属器　分别讲述了头发、指甲、皮肤腺体和神经在皮肤老化过程中发生的细节性变化。

第六节分类阐述了良性皮肤肿瘤、恶性皮肤肿瘤、干燥、瘙痒、感染、老年性紫癜、大疱性类天疱疮等老年皮肤疾病。

1．良性皮肤肿瘤　良性皮肤肿瘤通常发生在老化的皮肤上。分别简单介绍了日光性色素痣、脂溢性角化病、老年血管瘤等疾病的临床表现及发病率、相关发病机理及治疗等。

2．恶性皮肤肿瘤　首先介绍了恶性皮肤肿瘤的发病率，以及紫外线辐射在恶性皮肤肿瘤发病中的作用。接着，依次讲述了默克尔细胞癌(MCC，见第113章)的临床症状、发病年龄、可能的发病机制等；介绍了血管肉瘤的临床特征、预后及治疗进展等；讲述了与人疱疹病毒-8有关的卡波西肉瘤(KS)，是一种淋巴血管增生性疾病，有4种变异的KS。文章回顾了CKS，并详细介绍了其发病人群、临床表现、危险因素及治疗手段等。作者提出CKS的疗效尚不肯定，仍需要标准化的治疗指南。

3．干燥　皮肤干燥，是一种老年人极其常见的皮肤疾病，其原因是多方面的。与干燥相关的皮肤病是乏脂性湿疹，治疗上以改变干燥环境和补充保湿霜为主。

4．瘙痒　瘙痒是老年人常见的主诉。作者提出，瘙痒可由干燥引起，但也可能是潜在系统性疾病或恶性肿瘤的征兆。瘙痒症与糖尿病、甲状腺疾病、肾和肝衰竭有关。恶性肿瘤也可表现为瘙痒。瘙痒也是骨髓增生性真性红细胞增多症的典型特征。疥疮和足癣等感染也是瘙痒的典型原因。对症治疗和解决任何潜在的发病因素是瘙痒治疗的主要方向。

5．感染　感染可使老年人产生皮肤损伤和系统性疾病。而老年人更容易感染侵袭性和危及生命的疾病。因此，在制定医疗干预措施时，必须了解老年人经常出现的细菌、寄生虫、真菌和病毒病原体的类型；并考虑到共病和使用多种药的可能性增加、药物代谢的差异、非典型症状和不良预后风险增加；感染的老年患者相对于年轻患者可能面临的特殊挑战。

接下来，就感染的不同病原体分类讲述了发生于老年人的数种感染性皮肤病，包括葡萄球菌感染的脓疱疮和毛囊炎，链球菌感染的蜂窝织炎、丹毒、坏死性筋膜炎等，特别强调了各种危险因素及有可能导致败血症和其他危及生命的严重并发症的危险因素。还简单介绍了疥疮、真菌感染的危险因素，以及疱疹病毒感染所致的带状疱疹和单纯疱疹的临床特征及治疗等。

6．其他　简要介绍了溃疡的形成与老年人创伤修复能力低下以及糖尿病和动脉粥样硬化性周围血管疾病等共病相关机制的研究。老年性紫癜与年龄有关的皮肤变薄和阳光导致的真皮结缔组织损伤导致支持不足和微血管脆弱性增加有关。较为详细地讲述了大疱的类天疱疮的临床表现、组织病理学改变，以及相关危险因素等。

文章的最后，指出皮肤药物不良反应在老年人中很常见。原因包括老年患者更容易发生药物诱导的自身免疫反应；老年人多患共病，多药联合使用；此外，随着年龄增长，对药物代谢和排泄能力降低。因此，建议老年人在处方新药物时应适当跟踪，并经常对药物进行评估。

〔刘芳芬〕

AT-A-GLANCE

- Intrinsic skin aging includes the inevitable physiologic changes of the skin that occur with time and are influenced by genetic and hormonal factors.
- Extrinsic skin aging is the preventable structural and functional changes of the skin that occur with exposure to environmental factors, the most important source being ultraviolet radiation.
- Intrinsic and extrinsic aging of the skin have distinct histologic and clinical manifestations.
- Oxidative damage is a common component of the multiple mechanisms of aging.
- Geriatric dermatoses include solar lentigines, seborrheic keratoses, senile angiomas, xerosis, asteatotic eczema, and pruritus.
- There is increased incidence of benign and malignant skin growths in the elderly population.
- Infections in the elderly often have distinctive causative organisms and increased morbidity and mortality relative to younger patients.

In Westernized countries, the chronologic age of older than 65 years is accepted as the definition of an elderly individual. By 2050, the elderly population is estimated to more than double in developing countries (World Health Organization. *Global Health and Aging.* 2011; http://www.who.int/ageing/publications/global_health/en/). This demographic transformation will present unique challenges to physicians across the medical specialties, including dermatology.

Aging is an inevitable and dynamic biologic process that is characterized by the progressive deterioration of many body systems and decline in physiologic reserve capacity. Given its location at the body's environmental interface, human skin undergoes 2 distinct types of aging: intrinsic and extrinsic. Intrinsically aged skin appears dry and pale with fine wrinkles and increased laxity; whereas, photoaged skin is darker, coarser, and often has mottled pigmentation (Fig. 106-1). Intrinsic aging encompasses a set of gradual physiologic changes that are a consequence of time and under genetic and hormonal control. Conversely, extrinsic aging, also termed *photoaging*, includes dramatic structural and functional changes that are caused by exogenous factors, the primary one being unprotected sun exposure.

OXIDATIVE STRESS AND AGING

One theory of aging involves cellular senescence or apoptosis secondary to oxidative damage.[1] The generation of reactive oxygen species is a normal consequence of aerobic metabolism. Accordingly, a complex antioxidant system of enzymatic and nonenzymatic effectors has evolved to counteract the endogenously and exogenously produced free radicals in the skin (Table 106-1). However, the skin's antioxidant defenses tend to weaken with age,[2] and the resultant oxidative stress contributes to intrinsic aging.

Oxidative damage leads to the upregulation of stress-related factors, which can then trigger downstream events enabling the aging process. For example, stress-induced factors, such as hypoxia-inducible factors and nuclear factor κB, induce the expression of cytokines. Some of these cytokines, like interleukin-1, interleukin-6, vascular endothelial growth factor and tumor necrosis factor-α, have been shown to be proinflammatory regulators of cell survival and modulators of matrix-degrading metalloproteins.[3-5] Additionally, oxidative damage to cellular proteins combined with the age-related deterioration of proteasome activity results in the accumulation of damaged proteins that interfere with normal cellular function.

Oxidative stress also modifies telomeres, the terminal portions of linear chromosomes that defend against degradation or fusion. Telomeres consist of hundreds of tandem DNA sequence repeats that are shortened with each somatic cell division. The shortening of telomeres is a result of the inability of DNA polymerase to replicate the final base pairs of a chromosome. When the telomeres reach a "critically short" threshold, the cell undergoes proliferative senescence or apoptosis, depending on the cell type. In addition to shortened telomeres secondary to serial cellular division, oxidative insult appears to trigger telomere signaling. Kosmadaki and Gilchrest have proposed a common final pathway for intrinsic and photoaging leading to the disruption of the normal loop structure at the end of telomeres. The exposure of the normally buried TTAGGG tandem repeat of the 3′ overhang strand then activates p53 signaling leading to downstream events that include proliferative senescence and apoptosis (Fig. 106-2).[6]

It has been suggested that cellular senescence is the cellular basis for aging.[7] After a finite number of cellular divisions, the cell cycle of a mammalian cell is

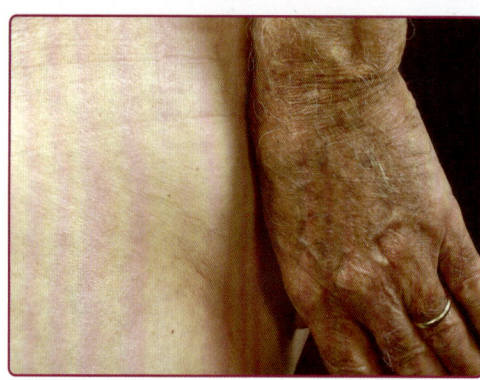

Figure 106-1 Difference between photoprotected and photoexposed skin.

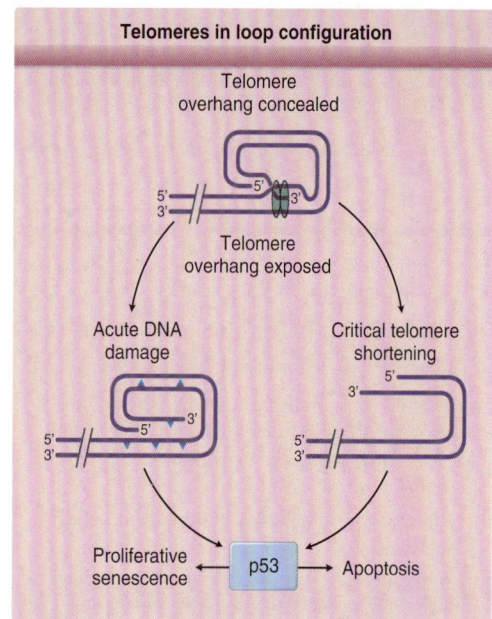

Figure 106-2 Schematic of cellular responses induced by exposure of the telomere repeat sequence. (From Yaar M. Clinical and histological features of intrinsic versus extrinsic skin aging. In: Gilchrest BA, Krutmann J, eds. *Skin Aging*. New York, NY: Springer; 2006:9-21, with permission. Copyright © 2006.)

irreversibly arrested and the cell has entered a state known as replicative senescence.[8] Cellular senescence has been described as a possible tumor-suppressor mechanism, which precludes the unregulated growth of cells that have acquired multiple genetic mutations over time. This apparent biologic trade off of increased life span and increased risk of malignant transformation is further underscored by the observation that improved DNA repair mechanisms correlate with longer life spans in mammalian species.[9]

INTRINSIC SKIN AGING

Intrinsic or chronologic skin aging refers to the seemingly unavoidable physiologic changes of the skin that occur with time and are influenced by genetic and hormonal factors. These alterations include decreased collagen production, reduced blood flow, lowered amounts of lipids, and the loss of rete ridges.[10] The result is dry, pale skin with fine wrinkles, less elasticity, and impaired reparative capacity (Fig. 106-3). Intrinsically aged skin is also characterized by the development of a range of benign neoplasms, resulting from impaired regulation of cellular proliferation.[11]

EXTRINSIC SKIN AGING

Extrinsic skin aging entails the physiologic and histologic changes caused by environmental factors. The most powerful source of extrinsic aging is ultraviolet radiation. The ultraviolet radiation–mediated structural and functional changes of the skin are known as photoaging, which is described in "Photoaging" section in more detail below. Other exogenous factors that contribute to extrinsic skin aging include cigarette

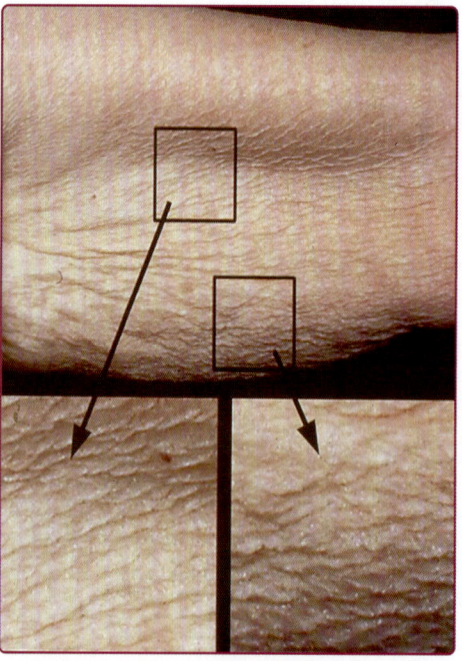

Figure 106-3 *Intrinsic aging (upper inner arm):* Intrinsic aging is characterized by fine wrinkling, increased skin laxity, and sagging.

TABLE 106-1 The Antioxidant Systems of the Skin	
ENZYMATIC	NONENZYMATIC
Glutathione peroxidase	Vitamin C (ascorbic acid)
Catalase	Vitamin E
Superoxide dismutase	Glutathione
	Thioredoxin system
	Carotenoids
	Flavonoids

smoking, diet, chemical exposure, trauma, and air pollutants (eg, particulate matter, CO_2, CO, SO_2, NO, and NO_2). In fact, an intense interest in the effects of air pollution on skin physiology has developed in recent years, giving rise to several mechanistic and epidemiologic studies.[12] The initial link between airborne particle exposure and extrinsic skin aging was established by a cross-sectional study in Germany that found an association between exposure to chronic traffic-related particulate matter and premature skin aging with pigment spot formation.[13] Indoor air pollution, such as cooking with fossil fuels, also has been associated with accelerated aging in Chinese populations.[14] Activation of the aryl hydrocarbon receptor by exogenous factors like tobacco smoke extract and airborne particulate matter has been identified as a potential contributor to extrinsic aging.[15,16] Ozone also causes skin inflammation and disrupts barrier function by inducing lipid peroxidation and protein oxidation in the stratum corneum.[16]

Unlike intrinsic aging, extrinsic aging is more amenable to intervention and preventive measures. Typical clinical features of extrinsically aged skin, which are mostly ultraviolet radiation–mediated, include deep wrinkles, laxity, coarseness, increased fragility, and multiple telangiectases. Moreover, photodamaged skin may appear darker and have mottled pigmentation (Fig. 106-4). Extrinsically aged skin has an increased tendency to develop benign and malignant growths.[11] Table 106-2 summarizes the histologic and clinical features that are typical of intrinsically and extrinsically aged skin.

TABLE 106-2
The Typical Histologic and Clinical Features of Intrinsic and Extrinsic Skin Aging

	INTRINSIC AGING	EXTRINSIC AGING
Histologic features	Epidermal thinning Loss of rete ridges Decreased number of collagen and elastin fibers	Solar elastosis Reduced number of fibroblasts Reduced amount of extracellular matrix
Clinical features	Xerosis Pallor Fine wrinkles Decreased elasticity Fragility	Xerosis Multiple telangiectases Deep wrinkles Decreased elasticity Fragility Dyspigmentation

PHOTOAGING

At the earth's surface, sunlight is composed of infrared, visible, and ultraviolet (UV) light, with most of the UV blocked by the earth's atmosphere. Of the UV radiation that reaches the earth's surface, more than 95% is UVA (320 to 400 nm) and approximately 5% is UVB (280 to 320 nm). Both UVA and UVB contribute to skin aging. UVB, which only penetrates into the epidermis and upper dermis, is a chief source of direct DNA damage, inflammation, and immunosuppression.[17] Conversely, UVA deeply penetrates the skin down to the lower dermis. UVA is considered a larger contributor to skin aging than UVB because of its greater depth of penetration and its higher percentage of surface sunlight.

In addition to the mechanisms of aging discussed before, photodamage contributes to extrinsic aging through other mechanisms. UV damage impacts collagen degradation and synthesis, as well as causes the production of elastotic material in the skin, both of which are further described in section "Dermis". Photodamaged skin is also associated with a higher frequency of mitochondrial DNA mutations that result in decreased mitochondrial function and the generation of reactive oxygen species.[16] The basement membrane at the dermal–epidermal junction is also damaged in sun-exposed skin. Following UV radiation exposure, the basement membrane becomes multilayered and partially disrupted. Additionally, matrix metalloproteinases (MMPs) and urinary plasminogen activator are increased in photodamaged skin.[18]

Recently, there has been a growing interest in the impact of non-UV solar radiation on skin physiology and aging. Approximately 50% of the total solar spectrum is visible light (400 to 700 nm), which is able to penetrate down to the hypodermis.[19] Visible light generates reactive oxygen species in human skin[20] and induces the formation of oxidized DNA bases.[21] Additionally, irradiation of human skin equivalents with visible light results in increased production of proinflammatory cytokines and MMP-1.[22] Nearly 45% of the

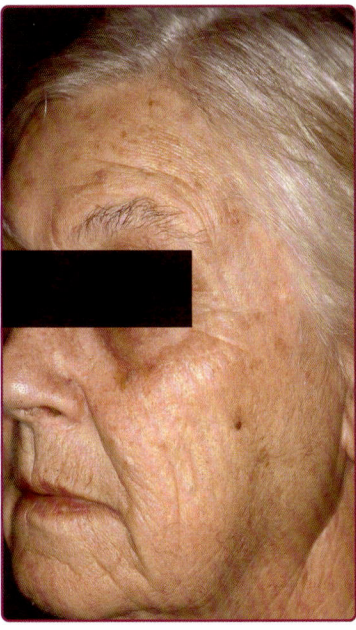

Figure 106-4 *Photoaging aging (face):* The photograph highlights salient features of photoaging including fine and coarse wrinkles, discrete tan-brown macules, mottled pigmentation, telangiectasias, loss of translucency and elasticity, xerosis, and sallow color.

solar spectrum reaching human skin is infrared, which is composed of infrared A (700 to 1400 nm), infrared B (1400 to 3000 nm), and infrared C (3000 nm to 1 mm). Infrared B and infrared C do not penetrate the skin well, but infrared A can reach down to the hypodermis, increase reactive oxygen species production, and impact mitochondrial integrity.[19]

ESTROGEN AND SKIN AGING

In addition to their reproductive roles, estrogens are important regulators of skin physiology and wound healing (Table 106-3). Estrogens exert their effects through specific estrogen receptors, which can act as ligand-activated transcription factors. Estrogen receptor signaling is a critical modulator of redox (reduction–oxidation) balance and oxidative stress, which is central to many of the mechanisms of skin aging. Recently, estrogens have been shown to have nongenomic effects that occur through estrogen receptor–independent mechanisms, including interactions with membrane-associated G-coupled protein receptors and subsequent activation of signal transduction pathways.[23] Both genomic and nongenomic effects of estrogen appear to be critical mediators of skin physiology and may impact skin aging.

As the population of menopausal women increases, the profound impact of changes in estrogen levels on aging grows in clinical relevance. In premenopausal women, the predominant form of estrogen is estradiol, which is produced by the ovaries. After menopause, the levels of estradiol drop dramatically and women may experience a rapid onset of skin aging. Postmenopausal changes that have been reported include decreased collagen content, thinner skin, reduced elasticity, dryness, and increased wrinkling. These changes reflect the loss of the protective effects of estrogen and can be ameliorated with estrogen replacement.[24]

Several studies have examined the effect of topical estrogens on human skin. Treatment of photoaged facial skin with a conjugated estrogen cream increased skin thickness and decreased fine wrinkles.[25] Several studies have found that topical administration of estradiol induces procollagen in sun-protected skin of postmenopausal women and age-matched men.[26,27] Despite the similar expression of estrogen receptors in photoaged and intrinsically aged skin, topical estradiol did not alter procollagen production in photoaged skin, suggesting that changes that result from long-term sun exposure impede the ability of topical estrogen to stimulate collagen synthesis. Furthermore, these findings indicate that the estradiol-mediated effect on collagen production is indirect, that is, independent of estrogen receptor signaling.

EPIDERMIS

The human epidermis undergoes several structural and functional age-related alterations. Between the third and eighth decades of life, the epidermal turnover rate decreases by 30% to 50%,[28] coinciding with a deterioration of wound repair capacity. During this time period, there is also an overall thinning of unexposed epidermis by 10% to 50%. The spinous cell layer appears to be the most greatly impacted by epidermal atrophy, whereas the stratum corneum and stratum granulosum are largely unaffected.[29] The most pronounced and consistent histologic change of aged skin is flattening of the dermal–epidermal junction and loss of rete ridges, resulting in decreased surface contact area and presumably less nutritional support of the avascular epidermis by the vascularized dermis.[11] These alterations account for the increased fragility of aged skin to minor trauma as well as propensity to blister.

Although the average thickness of the stratum corneum does not change with age, older skin has a greater susceptibility to irritant contact dermatitis and severe xerosis. Aged skin also has altered drug permeability with reduced absorption of hydrophilic substances observed in older skin relative to younger controls.[30] Taken together, these observations suggest a compromise of the aged epidermal permeability barrier. Indeed, intrinsically aged skin has impaired barrier recovery following challenge. This may be partly because of a global decline of stratum corneum lipids, leading to diminished lamellar bilayers in the stratum corneum interstices.[31] Moreover, between the ages of 50 and 80 years, abnormal stratum corneum acidification results in impaired lipid-processing enzymatic activity,[32] as well as abnormal permeability barrier homeostasis and stratum corneum integrity.[33] An age-related decrease in epidermal filaggrin also has been proposed to impact barrier function and to account for the increased dryness and scaliness of older skin.[34]

At the cellular level, a number of important age-related changes occur in epidermal keratinocytes. Cellular heterogeneity—for example, differences in cellular shape, size, and staining characteristics—results

TABLE 106-3
Impact of Estrogens on Skin Physiology

SKIN COMPONENT	EFFECT OF ESTROGENS
Epidermis	Increase in mitotic activity of epidermal cells Stimulation of epidermal melanocytes
Dermis	Increase in collagen synthesis, maturation, and turnover Morphologic improvement of collagen and elastic fibers
Glands	Reduction in activity of sebaceous and apocrine glands
Hair follicle	Influences hair follicle cycle May inhibit activity of follicular melanocytes

Data from Thornton MJ. The biological actions of estrogens on skin. *Exp Dermatol.* 2002;11(6):487-502.

TABLE 106-4
Age-Related Changes in the Various Epidermal Cell Types

CELL TYPE	STRUCTURAL CHANGES	FUNCTIONAL CHANGES
Epidermal keratinocytes	Epidermal dyscrasia	Reduced mitotic activity Increased migration time Increased senescence
Melanocytes	Atypia Decreased number of functional melanocytes Increased number in photodamaged skin	Decreased melanin production
Langerhans cells	Decreased number Fewer and shorter dendrites	Decreased antigen presentation capability

in epidermal dyscrasia, a mild actinic keratosis that is particularly accentuated in photoaged skin. Epidermal dyscrasia is associated with reduced mitotic activity, lengthened cell cycle, and increased migration time from the basal cell layer to the stratum corneum.[35] It has been shown in vitro that human keratinocytes approach replicative senescence after 50 to 100 doublings and arrest in G_1 phase.[36] Because senescent cells are resistant to apoptosis, they may accumulate DNA mutations and protein damage over time. The buildup of senescent keratinocytes over time may provide the mechanistic link between aging and epidermal carcinogenesis.[35]

In addition to keratinocytes, the other resident cells of the epidermis—melanocytes and Langerhans cells—experience age-associated changes. Although the density of melanocytes doubles in photodamaged skin, the number of functional melanocytes in the basal layer declines by up to 20% per decade.[37] This decrease of melanocytes is associated with a decrease in protective melanin, which in addition to the age-related impairment of DNA repair mechanisms, contributes to an elevated risk of skin cancer in the elderly. The incidence of melanocytic nevi also declines with age.[38] In aged epidermis, there is also a reduction of the number and the responsiveness of Langerhans cells,[39] the dendritic cells of the skin. Langerhans cells of older skin undergo structural changes, for example, fewer and shorter dendrites, and have diminished antigen presenting capacity,[40] which likely contributes to weakened cutaneous immunity in the elderly. Table 106-4 summarizes the age-related changes in the various epidermal cell types.

DERMIS

Age-related biochemical changes in collagen, the main component of the dermis and the structural scaffold of the skin, may account for many of the characteristics of older skin, including increased rigidity and impaired wound healing.[41] There is a reduction of collagen types I and III in intrinsically aged skin that is enhanced by photodamage.[42] There is a significant downregulation of collagen synthesis in the skin with age[43] and photodamage.[44] An age-dependent difference in the collagen-synthetic capacity of aging fibroblasts partially accounts for the lower collagen synthesis in intrinsically aged skin.[45] Collagen fragmentation also contributes to the downregulation of collagen synthesis in both intrinsically aged and photoaged skin. Collagen-degrading MMPs gradually increase with age.[43] Acute UV irradiation transiently upregulates 3 MMPs (MMP-1, MMP-3, and MMP-9) in the skin, with the epidermis being the major source.[46,47] In contrast, chronically photodamaged skin has been shown to constitutively express higher levels of 7 MMPs (MMP-1, MMP-2, MMP-3, MMP-9, MMP-11, MMP-17, and MMP-27), which are primarily derived from dermal fibroblasts.[48] The resulting fragmentation of collagen is unable to produce an amount of mechanical tension on the fibroblasts to stimulate collagen synthesis.[45] Thus, elevated MMP activity in the dermis of photodamaged skin creates a microenvironment of fragmented collagen that impairs fibroblast function leading to abnormal collagen homeostasis with increased degradation and decreased production of collagen.

Elastin, the dermal element that provides elasticity and resilience, is also altered with aging. Solar elastosis, the most striking histologic alteration of photodamaged dermis, is characterized by the replacement of normal elastic fibers with a disordered mass of elastotic material (ie, degraded elastic fibers, tropoelastin, and fibrillin) that is localized near the dermal–epidermal junction.[49] Even in sun-protected chronologically older (>70 years old) skin, elastin fibers are reduced in number and diameter, appear fragmented, and exhibit increased crosslinkage and calcification.[50,51] These structural abnormalities in elastin translate into impaired function, namely a fall off of elastic recovery and resilience in aged skin.

Aging also affects the ground substance of the skin, which is composed of proteoglycans and glycosaminoglycans leading to decreased interaction of proteins with water. Although glycosaminoglycans are increased in photoaged skin, their deposition in the abnormal elastotic material prevents the normal attraction of water molecules, resulting in tetrahedron water.[52,53] In contrast, in intrinsically aged skin there is a progressive decline of hyaluronic acid, possibly secondary to decreased secretion or extractability.[54,55] All of these changes in the ground substance of the skin may contribute to age-related declines in skin hydration and turgor. Table 106-5 summarizes the consequences of the age-dependent alterations of the dermal components.

SKIN APPENDAGES

HAIR

With aging, there are striking spatially dependent and hormonally influenced changes in overall hair density and texture. Elderly men commonly have a drop in the density of chest, axillary, and pubic hair, but an

TABLE 106-5

Age-Associated Changes in the Dermal Components of the Skin

DERMAL COMPONENT	STRUCTURAL CHANGES	FUNCTIONAL CHANGES
Collagen	Increased rigidity Reduction of types I and III collagen Increased fragmentation	Impaired wound healing Decreased mechanical stress on fibroblasts (→ decreased collagen synthesis)
Elastin	Reduced number and diameter of elastin fibers Solar elastosis (photodamage)	Decreased elasticity
Ground substance	Abnormal deposition of glycosaminoglycans preventing normal interaction with water Reduced hyaluronic acid	Decreased skin hydration

increase of hair in other body sites, especially the nostrils, external auditory meatus, and eyebrows. Elderly women typically experience a new growth of coarse hair on the chin and upper lip, likely resulting from the unopposed influence of testosterone secondary to falling estrogen levels.[11]

Both men and women are affected by age-related alopecia. Senescent alopecia is the age-related thinning of hair, whereas androgenetic alopecia (or male pattern hair loss) is a distinct entity that can occur at an earlier age and results from the effect of dihydrotestosterone on hair follicles.[56] Conversely, only a small portion of female pattern hair loss may actually be androgenic.[57]

By the age of 60 years, nearly half of the population has at least 50% gray scalp hair, with everyone experiencing some amount of graying.[58] Hair graying is a result of the progressive depletion of melanocytes specifically in the hair bulb. The reasons for the vulnerability of this specific melanocyte stem cell population is not completely understood, but may be related to the high lifetime proliferative rate and relative sensitivity to oxidative stressors.[59,60] Recently, a sublineage of hair shaft progenitors in the hair matrix that are differentiated from follicular epithelial cells expressing the transcription factor KROX2 have been identified and shown to be a source of stem cell factor, which is critical for the maintenance of differentiated follicular melanocytes and hair pigmentation.[61] Whether this stem cell factor–dependent niche for follicular melanocytes is impaired in aging remains to be seen.

NAILS

Until approximately the age of 25 years, the rate of linear nail growth steadily increases, then drops off.[62] The texture of the nails also changes with age. In elderly individuals, nails are typically more brittle. Older nails may also exhibit ridging as a consequence of variation in lipid composition.[63]

CUTANEOUS GLANDS AND NERVES

There are striking age-related alterations in all of the glands of the skin. Both the number and output of eccrine glands decline with age.[64] The resulting decrease in spontaneous sweating renders the elderly more vulnerable to heat stroke. There is also a reduction in the size and function of apocrine glands in older skin.[65] Although the size and number of sebaceous glands appear constant, there is a drop of sebum production that is likely associated with hormonal changes.[66]

With aging, tactile thresholds are increased.[67] The decrease in the size and density of Pacinian and Meissner corpuscles may account for this finding.[68,69] There is also an increase in thermal pain thresholds in the elderly.[70] An age-associated decline in the spatial acuity (ability to discriminate between 2 points, light touch, and vibration) of the skin also occurs.[71,72]

GERIATRIC DERMATOSES

BENIGN SKIN LESIONS

Benign proliferative growths commonly occur in aging skin. Solar lentigines, also known as senile lentigines and liver spots, are well-defined patches of hyperpigmentation that are associated with UV exposure and especially common in fair-skinned individuals (Fig. 106-5). The reported average prevalence of solar lentigines ranges from 10% to 90% in older subjects.[73] Solar lentigines do not require any treatment; however, lentigo maligna and lentigo maligna melanoma, which are more serious malignant conditions, should be excluded. The role of repeated UV exposure in the pathogenesis of solar lentigines is not completely

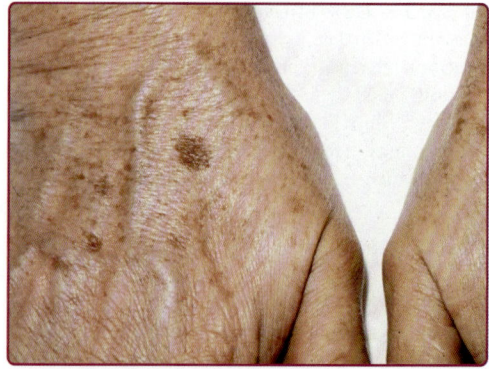

Figure 106-5 *Solar lentigo:* discrete tan, brown macules on photoexposed site. (Image from the Graham Library of Wake Forest Department of Dermatology, with permission.)

understood, but appears to involve increased melanin production and abnormal proliferation and differentiation of keratinocytes.[74]

Another common skin disorder in the elderly are seborrheic keratoses (Fig. 106-6A), which are benign papules or plaques that are highly variable in color, may have a waxy or wart-like appearance, and can arise as a single lesion or as multiple growths. Reported prevalences of seborrheic keratoses have ranged between 8% and 54% in elderly subjects.[73] Similar to senile lentigines, seborrheic keratoses have no malignant potential and do not require therapy beyond cosmetic reasons. Unlike senile lentigines, the development of seborrheic keratoses is independent of UV exposure and is likely a result of impaired focal epidermal homeostasis resulting in the clonal expansion of melanocytes and keratinocytes.[75] The pathogenesis of seborrheic keratoses is currently under investigation (see Chap. 108). Interestingly, keratinocyte-derived endothelin-1, which is a regulator of melanocyte function, has been implicated.[76]

Senile angiomas (Fig. 106-6B), also known as cherry angiomas, are another skin disorder that afflicts elderly subjects. They are small circular or oval red papules resulting from the proliferation of blood vessels that tend to increase in size and number with age and may bleed with minor trauma. The prevalence of senile angiomas has been reported as 50% to 75% in older individuals.[73] Treatment for senile angiomas is not needed unless for cosmetic reasons or repeated bleeding.

MALIGNANT SKIN LESIONS

The incidence of skin cancer, both melanoma and nonmelanoma skin cancers increases exponentially over a lifetime. In elderly populations, skin cancers represent approximately 40% of diagnosed malignant neoplasms. Older individuals with skin cancer are also at increased risk for poor outcomes. In particular, elderly males present with thicker melanomas and have increased mortality when compared to age-matched women and younger men.[77] The vast majority of skin cancer cases is basal cell cancer; however, squamous cell cancers are associated with greater nonmelanoma skin cancer–related morbidity and mortality.[78]

As one ages, the constant exposure to carcinogens, especially UV irradiation, leads to an accumulation of mutations. Compounding this risk is an age-related impairment of DNA repair capacity in response to UV exposure and decline in immune function.[79] There is a relationship between the risk of the type of skin cancer and the nature of the UV exposure. Squamous cell cancer and its precursor lesion, actinic keratosis, are associated with habitual sun exposure, whereas basal cell cancer and malignant melanoma correlate with a history of habitual or intense intermittent sun exposure.[80]

Merkel cell carcinoma (MCC, see Chap. 113) is a rare and aggressive type of cutaneous cancer that presents as a painless rapidly growing nodule that may be flesh-colored or bluish-red and typically occurs in sun-exposed areas of the body. Ninety percent of all cases of Merkel cell carcinoma occur in patients older than 50.[81] It is also associated with immunosuppression.[82] Merkel cell carcinoma is considered a neuroendocrine tumor of the skin that arises from a 2-step process: the integration of the Merkel polyomavirus genome into the host genome and development of T-antigen mutations that prevent autonomous replication of the viral genome. The result is an avoidance of DNA damage responses or recognition of the viral T-antigen by the immune system leading to tumor growth.[83] The clinical characteristics of Merkel cell carcinoma have been summarized in an acronym: AEIOU (*a*symptomatic/lack of tenderness, *e*xpanding rapidly, *i*mmune compromised, *o*lder than 50 years, and *U*V-exposed site on a person of fair skin).[84] These characteristics have been shown to be highly sensitive for Merkel cell carcinoma and can aid in the decision to biopsy and improve early detection of this aggressive cancer.

Angiosarcoma, a cancer of the inner lining of blood vessels, most commonly occurs in the elderly. It can affect any area of the body, but the majority present on the head and neck (Fig. 106-7). Rapidly proliferating and invasive anaplastic cells are characteristic of angiosarcoma. This aggressive and highly metastatic cancer is associated with a high mortality and often leads to death within 2 years of initial diagnosis.[85] These vascular tumors have been shown to express

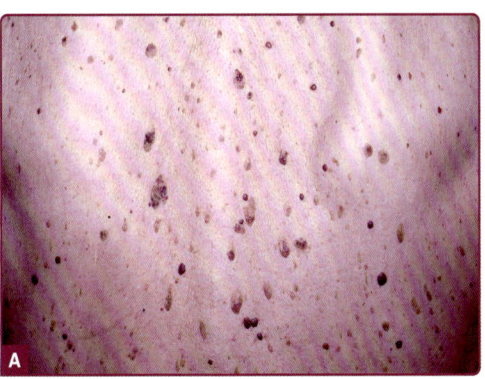

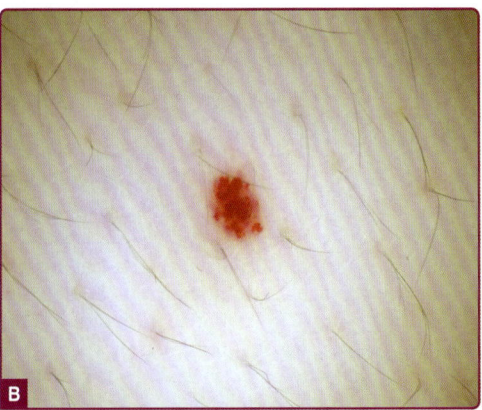

Figure 106-6 **A,** *Seborrheic keratoses:* brown, waxy, stuck-on papules and plaques and **B,** *Senile angioma:* erythematous to violaceous lobulated papules. (Image **B,** used with permission from Dr. Willy Huang.)

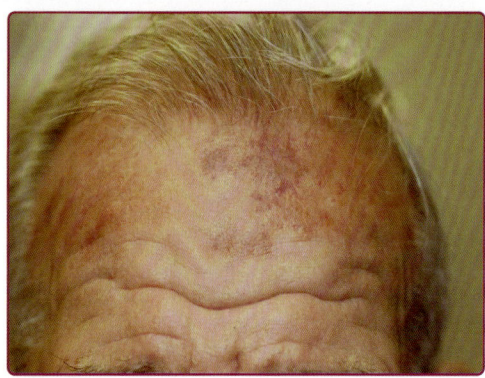

Figure 106-7 *Angiosarcoma:* Angiosarcomas in the elderly typically occur on head and neck, characterized by enlarging nonblanching violaceous patch or deeply violaceous nodule with ulceration and tenderness.

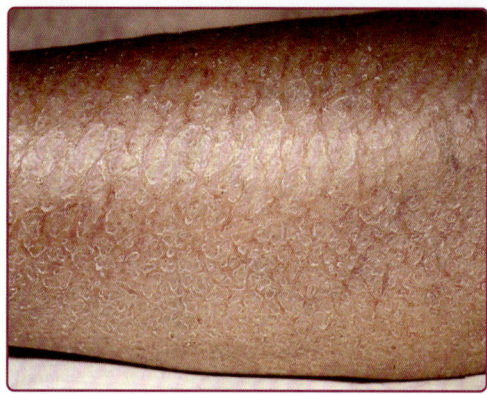

Figure 106-8 *Asteatotic eczema ("eczema craquelé"):* minimally erythematous scaly plaques with fissures on background of xerosis. (Image from the Graham Library of Wake Forest Department of Dermatology, with permission.)

high levels of vascular endothelial growth factor and vascular endothelial growth factor receptor-2, which have emerged as potential therapeutic targets.[86]

Kaposi sarcoma (KS) is a lymphoangioproliferative disease that is associated with human herpesvirus-8. There are 4 variants of KS: classic KS (CKS), AIDS-associated KS, iatrogenic posttransplantation KS, and endemic African KS. Only CKS is reviewed here. CKS primarily affects individuals of Eastern European Jewish or Mediterranean descent, and males more than females. CKS lesions are purple, red, or brown macules, plaques, and nodules that typically affect the face or lower extremities, often producing pain and debilitation. CKS lesions can also occur in the lungs, liver, and digestive tract, potentially causing life-threatening obstruction and bleeding. CKS is a rare disorder and its risk factors include increasing age, corticosteroid use, and diabetes. Treatment for localized disease entails observation, radiotherapy, surgery, or intralesional injections of vincristine or interferon alfa-2. However, the efficacy of the various therapies for CKS has not been validated, and standardized treatment guidelines are still needed.[87]

XEROSIS

Xerosis, or dry skin, is an extremely common skin disorder in the elderly and frequently affects the legs. The causes of xerosis are multifactorial. The age-associated reduction in the activity of sebaceous and sweat glands may contribute to its development. Alterations in lipid composition,[31] impaired filaggrin production,[34] and intrinsic changes in keratinization[88] are also potential etiologic factors. Xerosis is also associated with chronic renal failure, liver disorders, lower-leg atherosclerosis, autoimmune diseases, and hepatitis C virus infections.[73] Treatment options involve environmental changes and application of emollients.[88]

An associated skin condition is asteatotic eczema (Fig. 106-8), also known as winter itch, eczema craquelé, and desiccation dermatitis. Asteatotic eczema is xerosis complicated by dermatitis and is characterized by dry, extremely pruritic, fissured skin with scales. It typically presents in the elderly during the winter seasons and is often associated with low humidity in heated environments. Therapies are similar to those for xerosis, for example, behavior and environmental adaptions and topical emollients.[89]

PRURITUS

Pruritus, or itchy skin, is a common complaint of elderly patients that has a significant adverse effect on quality of life.[90] Pruritus can be caused by xerosis, but also can be a sign of an underlying systemic disease or malignancy. Pruritus has been associated with diabetes mellitus, thyroid disorders, and renal and liver failure. Malignant neoplasms, such as lymphoma or leukemia, can also present as pruritus. Pruritus is also a defining characteristic of the myeloproliferative neoplasm polycythemia vera. Infections such as scabies and tinea pedis are also typical causes of pruritus. Symptomatic treatment and addressing any underlying conditions are the mainstays of pruritus therapy.

INFECTIONS

There are many infections of medical significance that can produce both skin lesions and systemic disease in the elderly. Older individuals may be susceptible to aggressive and life-threatening infections that are rare in younger populations. In devising the appropriate medical intervention, it is important to be aware of the types of bacterial, parasitic, fungal, and viral pathogens that more frequently occur in the elderly. Given the increased likelihood of comorbidities and polypharmacy, differences in drug metabolism, atypical symptomology, and elevated risk of a poor outcome, the geriatric patient with an infection may present unique challenges relative to their younger counterparts.

BACTERIAL

Bacterial infections in elderly populations often have distinctive causative organisms and increased morbidity and mortality relative to younger patients. In elderly patients, infection with staphylococci is frequently the cause of impetigo (infection of the superficial layers of the epidermis) and folliculitis (inflammation of the hair follicles).[91] Cellulitis, an infection of the dermis and subcutaneous fat, is usually caused by streptococci or staphylococci and may present more subtly in elderly individuals. Risk factors for cellulitis, such as diabetes mellitus, immunodeficiency, lymphedema, and chronic venous insufficiency, are also more prevalent in the elderly. Older patients are particularly vulnerable to certain rare and aggressive forms of cellulitis. Orbital cellulitis can be caused by the contiguous spread of infections of the paranasal sinuses or metastatic spread from a systemic focus. In contrast to preseptal orbital cellulitis, orbital cellulitis involves the soft tissues posterior to the orbital septum. In the absence of adequate treatment, orbital cellulitis can lead to blindness and death from intracranial spread. In older individuals, the cause of orbital cellulitis is typically polymicrobial and may be a mix of aerobic and anaerobic bacteria. Elderly persons with diabetes are more likely to develop *Pseudomonas* cellulitis of the ear than are other populations.[91]

In addition to cellulitis, other rare cutaneous infections occur more frequently in the elderly. Erysipelas, a β-hemolytic streptococcal infection of the upper dermis that spreads to the lymphatics, is more common in older individuals and more likely to result in sepsis and other life-threatening complications. It can be distinguished from cellulitis by its demarcated borders. Necrotizing fasciitis, which is often caused by *Streptococcus*, is associated with increased morbidity and mortality in the elderly. Risk factors for necrotizing fasciitis, such as immunosuppression, diabetes, chronic systemic illnesses, and malignancies, are more prevalent in older individuals. The elderly population also has been identified as being at risk for carriage for methicillin-resistant *Staphylococcus aureus*,[92] which is often implicated in cases of necrotizing fasciitis.

PARASITIC[93]

Scabies is one of the most clinically significant parasitic infections in the geriatric population. Residents of nursing homes, like other communal living arrangements, are at increased risk for this highly contagious infestation. To complicate the clinical picture, the elderly, similar to other immunosuppressed groups, may present with less-severe pruritus and inflammation. Furthermore, given the common occurrence of xerosis in the elderly, pruritus in an older patient may fail to raise any alarm in the practitioner. Early detection and treatment with topical scabicides and oral ivermectin will help to limit the spread of the infestation. Another parasitic cause of pruritus in the elderly is pediculosis, or infestation with lice. Pediculosis can be treated with malathion, lindane, or permethrin. Less-frequent parasitic infections in the geriatric population include cutaneous larva migrans and cutaneous leishmaniasis.

FUNGAL[94]

There are several risk factors that predispose the geriatric population to cutaneous fungal infections, including age-associated decrease in immunity, vitamin deficiency, peripheral vascular disease, broad-spectrum antibiotic use for other infections, lymphoproliferative disorders, and malignancies. Dermatophytes, a type of fungi that requires keratin for growth, can cause superficial infections such as tinea capitis, tinea corporis, tinea pedis, and tinea unguium. Tinea pedis affects approximately 80% of patients older than 60 years age and in elderly persons with diabetes, it is often complicated by ulceration and cellulitis.[95] *Candida albicans*, a type of yeast that is part of the body's normal flora, is another frequent source of cutaneous infections in the elderly. *Pityrosporum ovale* may cause seborrheic dermatitis, tinea versicolor, and Pityrosporum folliculitis, conditions that frequently affect older patients. Antifungals are effective for the geriatric population, but have to be used with caution because of possible drug interactions and underlying disorders.

VIRAL[96]

Herpes zoster, commonly known as shingles, is a cutaneous viral disease that primarily affects elderly patients. It is characterized by painful vesicular rash in a dermatomal distribution and is often preceded by pain in the affected area. Herpes zoster is caused by the reactivation in adults of the varicella-zoster virus (VZV), which is the virus that causes chickenpox in children. Age-related changes in immunity may be responsible for the failed suppression of VZV in the elderly. Current treatment includes antivirals like acyclovir, famciclovir, and valacyclovir. There is also a live, attenuated VZV vaccine and a recently approved recombinant zoster vaccine available.[97] Pain can persist following an acute attack of herpes zoster. This is known as postherpetic neuralgia and is treated with topical anesthetics, analgesics, tricyclic antidepressants, and anticonvulsants. The VZV vaccine provides protection against herpes zoster for at least 3 years and reduce the incidence of postherpetic neuralgia by 66.5%.[98]

Infections caused by herpes simplex virus, which are characterized by vesicular eruptions in the genital and perioral regions, are also of clinical importance for the geriatric population. The vermilion border of the lip is the most frequent site of herpes simplex virus infection in older individuals. Recurrent herpes labialis in the geriatric patient can result in autoinoculation of the eye and genital area and subsequent spread of the disease. Similar to VZV infections, herpes simplex virus infections can be treated with antivirals including acyclovir, famciclovir, and valacyclovir.

ULCERS

Compromised wound repair capacity and comorbidities like diabetes mellitus and atherosclerotic peripheral vascular disease predispose the geriatric population to the development of chronic ulcers, particularly leg ulcers. Chronic venous insufficiency can lead to venous hypertension, resulting in the leakage of fibrinogen and other macromolecules into the dermis that can block the normal flow of oxygen, nutrients, growth factors, and cytokines, all of which are vital to tissue health and wound healing. Lipodermatosclerosis, a type of lower-extremity panniculitis, can develop and further impede wound repair. It is characterized by indurated skin with brownish-red pigmentation and is associated with tissue hypoxia, cytokine activation, and interstitial protein exudates.[99] The elderly are also more prone to develop decubitus ulcers than younger patients. This is because of age-related skin atrophy from constitutive elevation in MMPs and concomitant decline in collagen synthesis by dermal fibroblasts.[48] Furthermore, decline in physical mobility, urinary and fecal incontinence, and malnutrition all contribute to the ulcer formation in the elderly.[100]

SENILE PURPURA (BATEMAN PURPURA)

Senile purpura is the recurrent formation of ecchymoses on the sun-exposed extensor surfaces of the arms or hands of elderly patients. Age-related skin thinning and sun-induced damage of the connective tissue of the dermis results in inadequate support and increased fragility of the microvasculature. As a result, minor trauma of aged photodamaged skin can lead to vessel rupture and extravasation of blood into the dermal tissues.[38] This condition can be exacerbated with the use of aspirin and other anticoagulants, medications that are common in the elderly population. Blood is typically resorbed within 2 weeks, but postinflammatory hyperpigmentation may occur. Although benign and self-resolving, senile purpura is of great cosmetic concern with a significant impact on patient well-being.

BULLOUS PEMPHIGOID

Bullous pemphigoid is an autoimmune blistering disorder that primarily affects patients older than 60 years of age. The initial manifestation can be urticarial papules and plaques with significant pruritus that subsequently progress into large tense bullae. The formation of autoantibodies that target the basement membrane leads to the separation of the dermal–epidermal junction. Certain risk factors for bullous pemphigoid have been identified and include neurologic disorders (eg, dementia and Parkinson disease), psychiatric disorders, bedridden condition, and chronic polypharmacy.[101] Mortality in bullous pemphigoid cases is associated with increased disease severity and can occur as a result of therapies.[102]

DRUG ERUPTIONS

Adverse cutaneous drug reactions, such as morbilliform and urticarial eruptions, are frequent in the elderly and can have a significant impact on quality of life. Furthermore, older patients are more likely to develop drug-induced autoimmune reactions, like bullous pemphigoid (described before), lupus erythematosus, and pemphigus. One reason for increased risk of drug eruptions is polypharmacy. Additionally, renal, cardiac, and liver functions decline with age, which negatively impact drug metabolism and excretion. Thus, appropriate consideration and follow up when prescribing new medications, as well as frequent evaluation of existing medications is advised for the geriatric population.[103]

REFERENCES

1. Harman D. Free radical theory of aging: an update: increasing the functional life span. *Ann N Y Acad Sci.* 2006;1067:10-21.
2. Chung J, Cho S, Kang S. Why does the skin age? Intrinsic aging, photoaging, and their pathophysiology. In: Rigel DS, Weiss RA, Lim HW, Dover JS, eds. *Photoaging.* New York, NY: Marcel Dekker; 2004:1-13.
3. Ahmad A, Banerjee S, Wang Z, et al. Aging and inflammation: etiological culprits of cancer. *Curr Aging Sci.* 2009;2(3):174-186.
4. Ruland J, Mak TW. Transducing signals from antigen receptors to nuclear factor kappa B. *Immunol Rev.* 2003;193:93-100.
5. Kang S, Fisher GJ, Voorhees JJ. Photoaging: pathogenesis, prevention, and treatment. *Clin Geriatr Med.* 2001;17(4):643-659, v-vi.
6. Kosmadaki MG, Gilchrest BA. The role of telomeres in skin aging/photoaging. *Micron.* 2004;35(3):155-159.
7. Campisi J. Replicative senescence: an old lives' tale? *Cell.* 1996;84(4):497-500.
8. Hayflick L. The limited in vitro lifetime of human diploid cell strains. *Exp Cell Res.* 1965;37:614-636.
9. Hart RW, Setlow RB. Correlation between deoxyribonucleic acid excision-repair and life-span in a number of mammalian species. *Proc Natl Acad Sci U S A.* 1974;71(6):2169-2173.
10. Montagna W, Kirchner S, Carlisle K. Histology of sun-damaged human skin. *J Am Acad Dermatol.* 1989;21(5, pt 1):907-918.
11. Tobin DJ. Introduction to skin aging. *J Tissue Viability.* 2017;26(1):37-46.
12. Krutmann J, Berneburg M. Photodamage: pathophysiology-new concepts. *Eur J Dermatol.* 2002;12(6):XV-XVI.
13. Vierkotter A, Schikowski T, Ranft U, et al. Airborne particle exposure and extrinsic skin aging. *J Invest Dermatol.* 2010;130(12):2719-2726.
14. Li M, Vierkötter A, Schikowski T, et al. Epidemiological evidence that indoor air pollution from cooking with

solid fuels accelerates skin aging in Chinese women. *J Dermatol Sci.* 2015;79(2):148-154.
15. Ono Y, Torii K, Fritsche E, et al. Role of the aryl hydrocarbon receptor in tobacco smoke extract-induced matrix metalloproteinase-1 expression. *Exp Dermatol.* 2013;22(5):349-353.
16. Krutmann J, Liu W, Li L, et al. Pollution and skin: from epidemiological and mechanistic studies to clinical implications. *J Dermatol Sci.* 2014;76(3):163-168.
17. Kochevar I. Molecular and cellular effects of UV radiation relevant to chronic photodamage. In: Gilchrest BA, ed. *Photodamage.* Cambridge, MA: Blackwell Science, 1995.
18. Amano S. Possible Involvement of basement membrane damage in skin photoaging. *J Investig Dermatol Symp Proc.* 2009;14(1):2-7.
19. Dupont E, Gomez J, Bilodeau D. Beyond UV radiation: a skin under challenge. *Int J Cosmet Sci.* 2013;35(3):224-232.
20. Zastrow L, Groth N, Klein F, et al. The missing link—light-induced (280-1,600 nm) free radical formation in human skin. *Skin Pharmacol Physiol.* 2009;22(1):31-44.
21. Cadet J, Berger M, Douki T, et al. Effects of UV and visible radiation on DNA-final base damage. *Biol Chem.* 1997;378(11):1275-1286.
22. Liebel F, Kaur S, Ruvolo E, et al. Irradiation of skin with visible light induces reactive oxygen species and matrix-degrading enzymes. *J Invest Dermatol.* 2012;132(7):1901-1907.
23. Maran A, Zhang M, Kennedy AM, et al. ER-independent actions of estrogen and estrogen metabolites in bone cells. *J Musculoskelet Neuronal Interact.* 2003;3(4):367-369; discussion 381.
24. Thornton MJ. Estrogens and aging skin. *Dermatoendocrinol.* 2013;5(2):264-270.
25. Creidi P, Faivre B, Agache P, et al. Effect of a conjugated oestrogen (Premarin) cream on ageing facial skin. A comparative study with a placebo cream. *Maturitas.* 1994;19(3):211-223.
26. Son ED, Lee JY, Lee S, et al. Topical application of 17beta-estradiol increases extracellular matrix protein synthesis by stimulating TGF-beta signaling in aged human skin in vivo. *J Invest Dermatol.* 2005;124(6):1149-1161.
27. Rittié L, Kang S, Voorhees JJ, et al. Induction of collagen by estradiol: difference between sun-protected and photodamaged human skin in vivo. *Arch Dermatol.* 2008;144(9):1129-1140.
28. Grove GL, Kligman AM. Age-associated changes in human epidermal cell renewal. *J Gerontol.* 1983;38(2):137-142.
29. Moragas A, Castells C, Sans M. Mathematical morphologic analysis of aging-related epidermal changes. *Anal Quant Cytol Histol.* 1993;15(2):75-82.
30. Roskos KV, Bircher AJ, Maibach HI, et al. Pharmacodynamic measurements of methyl nicotinate percutaneous absorption: the effect of aging on microcirculation. *Br J Dermatol.* 1990;122(2):165-171.
31. Ghadially R, Brown BE, Sequeira-Martin SM, et al. The aged epidermal permeability barrier. Structural, functional, and lipid biochemical abnormalities in humans and a senescent murine model. *J Clin Invest.* 1995;95(5):2281-2290.
32. Choi EH, Man MQ, Xu P, et al. Stratum corneum acidification is impaired in moderately aged human and murine skin. *J Invest Dermatol.* 2007;127(12):2847-2856.
33. Hachem JP, Crumrine D, Fluhr J, et al. pH directly regulates epidermal permeability barrier homeostasis, and stratum corneum integrity/cohesion. *J Invest Dermatol.* 2003;121(2):345-353.
34. Tezuka T, Qing J, Saheki M, et al. Terminal differentiation of facial epidermis of the aged: immunohistochemical studies. *Dermatology.* 1994;188(1):21-24.
35. Wu J, Williams D, Walter GA, et al. Estrogen increases Nrf2 activity through activation of the PI3K pathway in MCF-7 breast cancer cells. *Exp Cell Res.* 2014;328(2):351-360.
36. Rheinwald JG, Hahn WC, Ramsey MR, et al. A two-stage, p16(INK4A)- and p53-dependent keratinocyte senescence mechanism that limits replicative potential independent of telomere status. *Mol Cell Biol.* 2002;22(14):5157-5172.
37. Lavker RM. Structural alterations in exposed and unexposed aged skin. *J Invest Dermatol.* 1979;73(1):59-66.
38. Fenske NA, Lober CW. Structural and functional changes of normal aging skin. *J Am Acad Dermatol.* 1986;15(4, pt 1):571-585.
39. Kurban RS, Bhawan J. Histologic changes in skin associated with aging. *J Dermatol Surg Oncol.* 1990;16(10):908-914.
40. Plowden J, Renshaw-Hoelscher M, Engleman C, et al. Innate immunity in aging: impact on macrophage function. *Aging Cell.* 2004;3(4):161-167.
41. Gerstein AD, Phillips TJ, Rogers GS, et al. Wound healing and aging. *Dermatol Clin.* 1993;11(4):749-757.
42. Fligiel SE, Varani J, Datta SC, et al. Collagen degradation in aged/photodamaged skin in vivo and after exposure to matrix metalloproteinase-1 in vitro. *J Invest Dermatol.* 2003;120(5):842-848.
43. Varani J, Warner RL, Gharaee-Kermani M, et al. Vitamin A antagonizes decreased cell growth and elevated collagen-degrading matrix metalloproteinases and stimulates collagen accumulation in naturally aged human skin. *J Invest Dermatol.* 2000;114(3):480-486.
44. Griffiths CE, Russman AN, Majmudar G, et al. Restoration of collagen formation in photodamaged human skin by Tretinoin (retinoic acid). *N Engl J Med.* 1993;329(8):530-535.
45. Varani J, Dame MK, Rittie L, et al. Decreased collagen production in chronologically aged skin: roles of Age-dependent alteration in fibroblast function and defective mechanical stimulation. *Am J Pathol.* 2006;168(6):1861-1868.
46. Fisher GJ, Datta SC, Talwar HS, et al. Molecular basis of sun-induced premature skin ageing and retinoid antagonism. *Nature.* 1996;379(6563):335-339.
47. Fisher GJ, Wang ZQ, Datta SC. Pathophysiology of premature skin aging induced by ultraviolet light. *N Engl J Med.* 1997;337(20):1419-1428.
48. Quan T, Little E, Quan H, et al. Elevated matrix metalloproteinases and collagen fragmentation in photodamaged skin: impact of altered extracellular matrix microenvironment on dermal fibroblast function. *J Invest Dermatol.* 2013;133(5):1362-1366.
49. Yaar M, Gilchrest BA. Photoageing: mechanism, prevention and therapy. *Br J Dermatol.* 2007;157(5):874-887.
50. Braverman IM, Fonferko E. Studies in cutaneous aging: I. The elastic fiber network. *J Invest Dermatol.* 1982;78(5):434-443.
51. Tsuji T, Hamada T. Age-related changes in human dermal elastic fibres. *Br J Dermatol.* 1981;105(1):57-63.
52. Gniadecka M, Nielsen OF, Wessel S, et al. Water and protein structure in photoaged and chronically aged skin. *J Invest Dermatol.* 1998;111(6):1129-1133.

53. Bernstein EF, Underhill CB, Hahn PJ, et al. Chronic sun exposure alters both the content and distribution of dermal glycosaminoglycans. *Br J Dermatol*. 1996;135(2):255-262.
54. Ghersetich I, Lotti T, Campanile G, et al. Hyaluronic acid in cutaneous intrinsic aging. *Int J Dermatol*. 1994;33(2):119-122.
55. Meyer LJ, Stern R. Age-dependent changes of hyaluronan in human skin. *J Invest Dermatol*. 1994;102(3):385-389.
56. Karnik P, Shah S, Dvorkin-Wininger Y, et al. Microarray analysis of androgenetic and senescent alopecia: comparison of gene expression shows two distinct profiles. *J Dermatol Sci*. 2013;72(2):183-186.
57. Olsen EA, Hordinsky M, Roberts JL, et al. Dermatologic Consortium for Women's Health. Female pattern hair loss. *J Am Acad Dermatol*. 2002;47(5):795.
58. Tobin DJ, Paus R. Graying: gerontobiology of the hair follicle pigmentary unit. *Exp Gerontol*. 2001;36(1):29-54.
59. Kauser S, Westgate GE, Green MR, et al. Human hair follicle and epidermal melanocytes exhibit striking differences in their aging profile which involves catalase. *J Invest Dermatol*. 2011;131(4):979-982.
60. Nishimura EK, Granter SR, Fisher DE. Mechanisms of hair graying: incomplete melanocyte stem cell maintenance in the niche. *Science*. 2005;307(5710):720-724.
61. Liao CP, Booker RC, Morrison SJ, et al. Identification of hair shaft progenitors that create a niche for hair pigmentation. *Genes Dev*. 2017;31(8):744-756.
62. Orentreich N, Markofsky J, Vogelman JH. The effect of aging on the rate of linear nail growth. *J Invest Dermatol*. 1979;73(1):126-130.
63. Helmdach M, Thielitz A, Röpke EM, et al. Age and sex variation in lipid composition of human fingernail plates. *Skin Pharmacol Appl Skin Physiol*. 2000;13(2):111-119.
64. Oberste-Lehn H. The number of sweat glands and aging in man. *Arch Klin Exp Dermatol*. 1966;227(1):342-346.
65. Rees J, Shuster S. Pubertal induction of sweat gland activity. *Clin Sci (Lond)*. 1981;60(6):689-692.
66. Jacobsen E, Billings JK, Frantz RA, et al. Age-related changes in sebaceous wax ester secretion rates in men and women. *J Invest Dermatol*. 1985;85(5):483-485.
67. Thornbury JM, Mistretta CM. Tactile sensitivity as a function of age. *J Gerontol*. 1981;36(1):34-39.
68. Schimrigk K, Rüttinger H. The touch corpuscles of the plantar surface of the big toe. Histological and histometrical investigations with respect to age. *Eur Neurol*. 1980;19(1):49-60.
69. Bolton CF, Winkelmann RK, Dyck PJ. A quantitative study of Meissner's corpuscles in man. *Neurology*. 1966;16(1):1-9.
70. Sherman ED, Robillard E. Sensitivity to pain in relationship to age. *J Am Geriatr Soc*. 1964;12:1037-1044.
71. Stevens JC, Cruz LA, Hoffman JM, et al. Taste sensitivity and aging: high incidence of decline revealed by repeated threshold measures. *Chem Senses*. 1995;20(4):451-459.
72. Shimokata H, Kuzuya F. Two-point discrimination test of the skin as an index of sensory aging. *Gerontology*. 1995;41(5):267-272.
73. Reszke R, Pełka D, Walasek A, et al. Skin disorders in elderly subjects. *Int J Dermatol*. 2015;54(9):e332-e338.
74. Aoki H, Moro O, Tagami H, et al. Gene Expression profiling analysis of solar lentigo in relation to immunohistochemical characteristics. *Br J Dermatol*. 2007;156(6):1214-1223.
75. Nakamura H, Hirota S, Adachi S, et al. Clonal nature of seborrheic keratosis demonstrated by using the polymorphism of the human androgen receptor locus as a marker. *J Invest Dermatol*. 2001;116(4):506-510.
76. Manaka I, Kadono S, Kawashima M, et al. The mechanism of hyperpigmentation in seborrhoeic keratosis involves the high expression of endothelin-converting enzyme-1alpha and TNF-alpha, which stimulate secretion of endothelin 1. *Br J Dermatol*. 2001;145(6):895-903.
77. Geller AC, Miller DR, Annas GD, et al. Melanoma incidence and mortality among US whites, 1969-1999. *JAMA*. 2002;288(14):1719-1720.
78. Syrigos KN, Tzannou I, Katirtzoglou N, et al. Skin cancer in the elderly. *In Vivo*. 2005;19(3):643-652.
79. Moriwaki S, Takahashi Y. Photoaging and DNA repair. *J Dermatol Sci*. 2008;50(3):169-176.
80. Armstrong BK, Kricker A. Epidemiology of sun exposure and skin cancer. *Cancer Surv*. 1996;26:133-153.
81. Feng H, Shuda M, Chang Y, et al. Clonal integration of a polyomavirus in human Merkel cell carcinoma. *Science*. 2008;319(5866):1096-1100.
82. Engels EA, Frisch M, Goedert JJ, et al. Merkel cell carcinoma and HIV infection. *Lancet*. 2002;359(9305):497-498.
83. Shuda M, Feng H, Kwun HJ, et al. T antigen mutations are a human tumor-specific signature for Merkel cell polyomavirus. *Proc Natl Acad Sci U S A*. 2008;105(42):16272-16277.
84. Heath M, Jaimes N, Lemos B, et al. Clinical characteristics of Merkel cell carcinoma at diagnosis in 195 patients: the AEIOU features. *J Am Acad Dermatol*. 2008;58(3):375-381.
85. Fedok FG, Levin RJ, Maloney ME, et al. Angiosarcoma: current review. *Am J Otolaryngol*. 1999;20(4):223-231.
86. Young RJ, Woll PJ, Staton CA, et al. Vascular-targeted agents for the treatment of angiosarcoma. *Cancer Chemother Pharmacol*. 2014;73(2):259-270.
87. Regnier-Rosencher E, Guillot B, Dupin N. Treatments for classic Kaposi sarcoma: a systematic review of the literature. *J Am Acad Dermatol*. 2013;68(2):313-331.
88. White-Chu EF, Reddy M. Dry skin in the elderly: complexities of a common problem. *Clin Dermatol*. 2011;29(1):37-42.
89. Gutman AB, Kligman AM, Sciacca J, et al. Soak and smear: a standard technique revisited. *Arch Dermatol*. 2005;141(12):1556-1559.
90. Kini SP, DeLong LK, Veledar E, et al. The impact of pruritus on quality of life: the skin equivalent of pain. *Arch Dermatol*. 2011;147(10):1153-1156.
91. Elgart ML. Skin infections and infestations in geriatric patients. *Clin Geriatr Med*. 2002;18(1):89-101, vi.
92. Eveillard M, Mortier E, Lancien E, et al. Consideration of age at admission for selective screening to identify methicillin-resistant *Staphylococcus aureus* carriers to control dissemination in a medical ward. *Am J Infect Control*. 2006;34(3):108-113.
93. Tan HH, Goh CL. Parasitic skin infections in the elderly: recognition and drug treatment. *Drugs Aging*. 2001;18(3):165-176.
94. Varade RS, Burkemper NM. Cutaneous fungal infections in the elderly. *Clin Geriatr Med*. 2013;29(2):461-478.
95. Martin ES, Elewski BE. Cutaneous fungal infections in the elderly. *Clin Geriatr Med*. 2002;18(1):59-75.

96. Bansal R, Tutrone WD, Weinberg JM. Viral skin infections in the elderly: diagnosis and management. *Drugs Aging.* 2002;19(7):503-514.
97. Oxman MN, Levin MJ, Johnson GR, et al. A vaccine to prevent herpes zoster and postherpetic neuralgia in older adults. *N Engl J Med.* 2005;352(22):2271-2284.
98. Shapiro M, Kvern B, Watson P, et al. Update on herpes zoster vaccination: a family practitioner's guide. *Can Fam Physician.* 2011;57(10):1127-1131.
99. Paquette D, Falanga V. Leg ulcers. *Clin Geriatr Med.* 2002;18(1):77-88, vi.
100. Baumgarten M, Margolis DJ, Localio AR, et al. Pressure ulcers among elderly patients early in the hospital stay. *J Gerontol A Biol Sci Med Sci.* 2006;61(7):749-754.
101. Bastuji-Garin S, Joly P, Lemordant P, et al. Risk factors for bullous pemphigoid in the elderly: a prospective case-control study. *J Invest Dermatol.* 2011;131(3):637-643.
102. Patton T, Korman N. Role of methotrexate in the treatment of bullous pemphigoid in the elderly. *Drugs Aging.* 2008;25(8):623-629.
103. Carneiro SC, Azevedo-e-Silva MC, Ramos-e-Silva M. Drug eruptions in the elderly. *Clin Dermatol.* 2011;29(1):43-48.

Chapter 107 :: Caring for LGBT Persons in Dermatology
:: Howa Yeung, Matthew D. Mansh, Suephy C. Chen, & Kenneth A. Katz

第一百零七章
关于LGBT人群的皮肤病学

中文导读

女同性恋、男同性恋、双性恋和变性人（LGBT）是一个涵盖性取向、性行为、性别认同和/或性别表达，以及不同健康需求的群体。本章共分为5节：讲述了与LGBT健康有关的术语和人口统计数据；讲述了男男性行为者（MSM）、女女性行为者（WSW）和变性人相关的皮肤病学问题；讲述了为LGBT群体提供具有文化竞争力（culturally competent）和以病人为中心的护理方法。

第一节介绍了与LGBT健康有关的部分术语和概念，并进一步阐述了性取向、性行为和性别认同这些不同的概念。女同性恋、男同性恋、双性恋和异性恋是指性取向，或一个人对他人情感和/或性吸引力的描述。作者提出，本章内容所使用的LGBT作为一个概括性术语，包括MSM和WSW，他们从事同性性行为；然而，一些男同性恋者或女同性恋者不一定被认定为LGBT。因为性取向并不决定性行为。MSM和WSW是描述同性性行为的术语，不考虑性取向，大多是研究人员用于描述与疾病风险相关的性行为（而不是性取向）。性别认同是指一个人内在的基本性别意识，如作为男人或女人。作者指出，这是一个不固定的概念，性别认同可能并不总是与生物性别相符，也不总是与一个人出生时根据其解剖结构而被分配的性别相符，并举例说明。最后，对LGBT人群的统计数据取决于人们评估的指标是性取向、性行为还是性别认同。因为按不同的指标进行评估，LGBT人群的统计数据差异很大。

第二节讲述了针对男男性行为者（MSM），美国疾病控制和预防中心和其他公共卫生机构关于艾滋病毒和性病筛查、与性健康相关的疫苗接种和艾滋病毒暴露前预防（PrEP）的建议，都有所不同（表107-3）。本章总结了4点：①需要更频繁地检查HIV和其他性传播疾病（一夫一妻关系中的MSM则不需要更频繁的筛查），建议对所有MSM进行乙型肝炎筛查，对HIV阳性的MSM还需进行丙型肝炎筛查；②推荐在MSM中通过肛门巴氏涂片（anal Papanicolaou smears）进行肛门癌筛查的数据不够充分；③MSM和26岁以下女性应接种人乳头瘤病毒（HPV）疫苗;对于非MSM，21岁之前建议接种HPV疫苗（但允许接种到26岁）；④HIV阴性的MSM感染艾滋病毒的风险较高，需进行预防性治疗。

第三节讲述了女女性行为者（WSW）关于性和皮肤健康的数据显示，WSW有从现有和以前的女性和/或男性伴侣处获得性传播疾病的风险，比如人乳头瘤病毒、单纯疱疹病毒、梅毒和艾滋病毒在女性性伴侣之间的传播。但文章指出，比较WSW和未与女性发生性关系的女性，发现HPV和HPV相关的癌前病变的患病率是相似的。艾滋病毒、梅毒、衣原体和淋病筛查指南，以及宫颈癌筛查和HPV疫苗接种指南，对WSW和没有与女性发生性关系的女性的要求没有区别。

第四节介绍了在变性人接受性别确认治疗（gender-affirming treatments）等健康管理方面，皮肤科医生发挥越来越大的作用。并分别讲述了皮肤科医生在参与管理变性人男性和变性人女性时的要点。

寻求男性化激素治疗的变性人男性可能会接受睾酮治疗，这会导致皮肤的改变，包括面部毛发和体毛增多，皮下脂肪的重新分布，以及汗液和气味的改变等。在皮肤相关疾病方面，作者首先讲述了痤疮，是使用睾酮治疗的常见副作用，使用维甲酸类药物治疗痤疮时应强调避孕，因为有些变性人男性保留了女性出生时的生殖器官，即使服用睾酮也能怀孕。其次讲述了雄激素性脱发，提出脱发程度与睾酮治疗的持续时间有关。由于米诺地尔治疗变性人男性使用睾酮引起的脱发还没有得到很好的研究，脱发严重的患者可以考虑进行毛发移植手术。

寻求女性化治疗的变性人女性可以接受雌激素和抗雄激素药物，预期效果包括乳房发育，减少体毛和面部毛发，皮下脂肪的重新分布，改变汗液和气味，阻止或逆转脱发，减少皮脂的产生，改善寻常痤疮，减少性别焦虑等。面部女性化和身体轮廓手术在变性人女性中很普遍。作者重点列举了数项手术带来的严重并发症，提出皮肤科医生应该提供安全、有效的局部注射治疗，特别是对那些喜欢非侵入性或非永久性治疗或不适合手术治疗的人群，可通过局部注射A型肉毒杆菌毒素、填充物等改善面部轮廓。

第五节提出：皮肤科医生应该努力为所有的病人提供具有文化竞争力的护理（culturally competent care）。对LGBT患者来说，具有文化竞争力的护理包括使用包容的语言，展示平等和尊重。以一种有效而敏感的方式获取有关性学解剖学、性别认同、性取向和性行为的相关信息，有助于提供适当的医疗服务，培养医患关系。文中进一步详细讲述了如何提供具有文化竞争力的护理方法和技巧等。

〔刘芳芬〕

AT-A-GLANCE

- Lesbian, gay, bisexual, and transgender persons face health disparities and experience unique health issues relevant to dermatologists.
- Dermatologists should follow guidelines for men who have sex with men from the Centers for Disease Control and Prevention and other public health agencies for HIV and other sexually transmitted diseases screening; HIV preexposure prophylaxis and HIV postexposure prophylaxis; and human papillomavirus, hepatitis A and B viruses, and meningococcal vaccination.
- Gender-affirming hormone treatments for transgender persons have distinct dermatologic effects.
- Eliciting a patient's sexual history and gender identity can facilitate diagnosis and management of dermatologically relevant diseases.

Lesbian, gay, bisexual, and transgender (LGBT) is an umbrella term referring to broad communities of individuals with diverse sexual orientations and behaviors, gender identities, and/or gender expressions, and distinct health needs.[1] Over 30 years into an ongoing HIV epidemic that disproportionately impacts LGBT persons, which dermatologists were among the first to recognize by helping to identify an epidemic of Kaposi sarcoma among gay men,[2] LGBT persons continue to face substantial health disparities related to both infectious and noninfectious diseases. These include higher rates of HIV and other sexually transmitted diseases (STDs), substance use, body image disorder, obesity, violence and victimization, mental health issues, and suicidality.[1,3] LGBT patients also encounter barriers in accessing health care that result from disparities in health insurance coverage, real or perceived discrimination by health care providers, and delayed or inappropriate care from providers unfamiliar with their specific health concerns.[4]

Improving the health of LGBT persons has become a priority, not only of clinicians, but also of educators,[5] researchers,[1] public health officials,[3] regulators,[4] and legislators.[6] Dermatologists should familiarize themselves with LGBT health issues, which have been rarely discussed in the dermatology literature, to provide patients with medically appropriate and patient-centered care.[7] For example, eliciting a patient's sexual history and gender identity can influence the assessment of the probability of diseases with higher prevalence among LGBT patients. Physicians can then recommend screening tests, vaccinations, and HIV prophylaxis appropriate for LGBT patients that might not apply to non-LGBT patients. This chapter reviews terminology and demographics related to LGBT health; health disparities faced by LGBT persons; dermatologic issues relevant to men who have sex with men (MSM), women who have sex with women (WSW), and transgender persons; and approaches to providing culturally competent and patient-centered care to LGBT persons.

TERMINOLOGY AND DEMOGRAPHICS

Terminology related to LGBT health is complex, evolves over time, and may not be accepted by all LGBT persons. Table 107-1 shows selected terminology and concepts.[8] Familiarity and openness with the use of appropriate and patient-preferred terminologies are essential in eliciting relevant sexual history and gender identity, discussing risk behaviors and contraception, and demonstrating respect and affirmation to patients.[4,5]

Sexual orientation, sexual behavior, and gender identity are separate concepts. Lesbian, gay, bisexual, and straight are terms that refer to sexual orientation, or one's characterization of emotional and/or sexual attraction to others. In this chapter, we use *LGBT* as an umbrella term to include MSM and WSW who engage in same-sex sexual behaviors; however, some MSM or WSW may not necessarily identify as LGBT. Sexual orientation does not dictate sexual behavior. For example, a self-identified straight person may engage in same-sex sexual behaviors, and a self-identified gay person may not be sexually active.[4,8]

MSM and WSW are terms that describe same-sex sexual behaviors, regardless of self-identified sexual orientation. Researchers and others use these terms to describe sexual behaviors (rather than sexual orientation) that can relate to disease risk, but people themselves rarely, if ever, identify as MSM or WSW. Homosexual is a term that used to refer to same-sex sexual behaviors, attraction, and/or identity; many LGBT persons consider it an outdated and derogatory term.[4,8]

Gender identity refers to one's basic internal sense of gender, such as being a man or a woman. It is fluid concept, with some persons identifying somewhere along the spectrum between man and woman, and others identifying as both, neither, or other genders. Gender identity may not always correspond to biologic sex, or the sex to which a person was assigned at birth based on their anatomy. For example, a transgender woman (also known as "male-to-female" transgender person or "trans woman") is a person whose sex assigned at birth was male but who identifies as a female. Some transgender persons experience gender dysphoria, defined as distress

TABLE 107-1
Selected Terminology and Concepts in LGBT Health[8]

CONCEPT	DEFINITION	EXAMPLES
Sex (sex assigned at birth, natal sex, biologic sex)	Sex assigned to a person at birth, commonly based on natal external genital anatomy, and less commonly by internal genital anatomy and/or chromosomal analysis	Male, female, intersex (differences of sex development such as congenital atypical chromosomal, gonadal, and/or anatomic sex)
Sexual orientation	A person's characterization of emotional and/or sexual attraction to others	Gay, lesbian, bisexual, straight
Gender identity	A person's basic internal sense of being a man, woman, or other gender	Man, woman, gender nonconforming
Gender expression	A person's method of communicating gender through appearance, personality, or behavior	Masculine, feminine, androgynous, gender nonconforming
Sexual behavior	Terms used by clinicians and researchers to describe same-sex sexual behaviors regardless of self-identified sexual orientation; rarely used by patients themselves	Men who have sex with men (MSM); women who have sex with women (WSW)
Transgender	An umbrella term describing persons whose gender identity or expression, to varying degrees, diverges from sex assigned at birth	Female-to-male (FTM) transgender person, transgender man; male-to-female (MTF) transgender person, transgender woman
Gender dysphoria	Distress from marked and persistent incongruence between one's gender identity and sex assigned at birth	
Gender affirmation /transition	Process of recognizing, accepting, and expressing one's gender identity, which may include behavioral, social, legal changes, medical or surgical treatments	

from a marked and persistent incongruence between one's assigned and experienced gender.[9] Some, but not all, transgender persons may seek medical or surgical gender-affirming treatments. Gender identity also does not dictate sexual orientation or sexual behavior.[4,8]

Demographics of LGBT persons depend on whether one is assessing sexual orientation, sexual behavior, or gender identity[10]:

- By sexual orientation, more than 8 million or an estimated 3.5% (range: 1.7% to 5.6%) of Americans identify as lesbian, gay, or bisexual.
- By sexual behavior, more than 19 million or an estimated 8.2% of Americans have ever engaged in same-sex sexual behaviors.
- By gender identity, approximately 700,000 or an estimated 0.3% of Americans identify as transgender.

MEN WHO HAVE SEX WITH MEN

MSM in the United States are disproportionately impacted by numerous dermatologically relevant conditions, including HIV, STDs, and other infectious and noninfectious diseases (Table 107-2). Recommendations from the Centers for Disease Control and Prevention and other public health agencies regarding HIV and STD screening, sexual health-related vaccinations, and HIV preexposure prophylaxis (PrEP) are different for MSM than for non-MSM men or for women regardless of sexual orientation (Table 107-3), as follows:

- More frequent screenings for HIV and additional STDs are indicated, including syphilis,[11] urethral and rectal gonorrhea and *Chlamydia*, and pharyngeal gonorrhea.[12] (MSM in mutually monogamous relationships might not require more frequent screening.) Hepatitis B screening is recommended for all MSM, and hepatitis C screening is recommended for HIV-positive MSM.[12]
- Data are insufficient to recommend anal cancer screening via anal Papanicolaou smears in MSM.[12]
- Human papillomavirus (HPV) vaccination is indicated for MSM and for women through age 26 years; for non-MSM men, HPV vaccination is indicated through age 21 years (but permissible through age 26 years).[13,14]
- PrEP is indicated for HIV-negative MSM who are at high risk of acquiring HIV (see Table 107-3).[15]

TABLE 107-2
Selected Dermatologically Relevant Conditions Important in Caring for Men Who Have Sex with Men

Viral Infections	
HIV	- 27,771 (70%) of 38,782 new HIV infections in the U.S. in 2016 occurred in MSM[33] - 10,477 (38%) of new HIV infections in MSM in the U.S. in 2016 occurred in Black/African-American MSM[33]
Genital herpes simplex virus (HSV)	- Seroprevalence of HSV Type 2 was 18.4% in 206 MSM, compared with 12.5% in 4,113 non-MSM ($P = 0.096$)[34]
Human papillomavirus (HPV)	- A systematic review and meta-analysis indicated that 74% of HIV-positive and 37% of HIV-negative MSM have anal infection of high-risk HPV (Types 16 and 18)[35] - Higher rates of anal intraepithelial neoplasia and anal cancer occur in MSM, particularly HIV-positive MSM[35]
Kaposi sarcoma	- Kaposi sarcoma may develop in HIV-positive MSM with a high CD4 count and viral suppression and in HIV-negative MSM, in addition to patients with AIDS[36,37]
Bacterial Infections	
Syphilis	- 16,155 (58%) of 27,814 primary and secondary syphilis cases reported in 2016 occurred in MSM[38]
Gonorrhea and *Chlamydia*	- Higher prevalence of *Chlamydia* and gonorrhea in MSM, with more oropharynx and rectal infections independent of urethral infections[38,39] - Lymphogranuloma venereum can cause classical genital ulcer disease and outbreaks of proctocolitis in MSM[40]
Community-associated methicillin-resistant *Staphylococcus aureus* (MRSA)	- Clusters of multidrug-resistant, community acquired MRSA skin and soft-tissue infections among MSM have occurred from the USA3000 clone[41]
Invasive meningococcal disease	- Outbreaks of *Neisseria* meningitis and invasive meningococcal disease with a high fatality rate have occurred in MSM living with and without HIV in urban cities in the United States and Europe[42,43]
Noninfectious Dermatoses	
Skin cancer risk factors	- Twice as many gay and bisexual men compared with straight men report a history of skin cancer[44] - Gay and bisexual men report using indoor tanning 2 to 6 times more often than straight men[44-46]
"Poppers" dermatitis	- Alkyl nitrites, commonly known as "poppers" and sold as "video head cleaners" and "room odorisers," are sometimes used by MSM to enhance sexual pleasure - Irritant or allergic contact dermatitis, chemical leukoderma in the perinasal and perioral region, acrocyanosis, and methemoglobinemia have been linked with poppers use[47,48]
Acne and depression	- Sexual minority adults with acne are 4.2 times more likely to report a history of depression and 8.1 times more likely to report suicidal ideation in the past 12 months as compared with heterosexual adults with acne[49]

TABLE 107-3

Screening, Vaccination, and HIV Preexposure and Postexposure Prophylaxis Indications and Recommendations for Men Who Have Sex with Men from the Centers for Disease Control and Prevention and Other Public Health Agencies[12,14,15,18]

SCREENING	INDICATIONS	RECOMMENDATIONS
HIV	Sexually active men who have sex with men (MSM), if HIV status is unknown or negative	Screen at least annually; every 3-6 months if risk behaviors persist or if the patient or his sexual partner(s) have multiple partners
Syphilis	Sexually active MSM	
Gonorrhea and *Chlamydia*		
Urethra	Any insertive oral or anal intercourse in the past year, regardless of reported condom use	Screen at least annually; every 3-6 months if risk behaviors persist or if the patient or his sexual partner(s) have multiple partners
Rectum	Any receptive anal intercourse in the past year, regardless of reported condom use	
Oropharynx	Any receptive oral intercourse in the past year, regardless of reported condom use[a]	
Hepatitis B virus	All MSM	One-time screening
Hepatitis C virus	HIV-positive MSM	Screen at least annually
Human papillomavirus (HPV), genital warts, herpes simplex virus (HSV), or anal cancer	Centers for Disease Control and Prevention (CDC) does not recommend routine screening	No recommended screening
VACCINATIONS	**INDICATIONS**	**RECOMMENDATIONS**
HPV (nonavalent or quadrivalent)	MSM through age 26 years, regardless of prior or current HPV infection status	Refer for vaccination
Hepatitis A virus and hepatitis B virus	MSM with no known prior viral hepatitis A or hepatitis B infection or vaccination	
Meningococcal	MSM in urban areas where state or local public health authorities have recommended vaccination (such as during serogroup C meningococcal disease outbreaks in New York, Chicago, and Los Angeles[50])[b]	
HIV PROPHYLAXIS	**INDICATIONS**	**RECOMMENDATIONS**
Preexposure prophylaxis (PrEP)	Adult man: • Without acute or established HIV infection • With any male sex partners in past 6 months • Not in a monogamous relationship with a recently tested, HIV-negative man AND at least 1 of the following: • Any anal sex without condoms (receptive or insertive) in past 6 months • A bacterial STI (syphilis, gonorrhea, or chlamydia) diagnosed or reported in past 6 months	Refer to primary care physician or infectious disease specialist for consideration of HIV PrEP, in addition to behavioral counseling on safer sex to decrease risk of HIV acquisition
Nonoccupational postexposure prophylaxis (nPEP)	Exposure to substantial risk for HIV acquisition within 72 hours from a source known to be HIV-positive; if source is of unknown HIV status, nPEP can be considered on case-by-case basis	Refer immediately for evaluation and treatment

[a]Centers for Disease Control and Prevention (CDC) recommends oropharyngeal testing for gonorrhea only, but many available tests screen for both gonorrhea and *Chlamydia*.
[b]CDC does not recommend routine meningococcal vaccination for all MSM; some state and local jurisdictions have recommended it, in response to outbreaks.

Nearly a quarter of HIV-negative MSM ages 18 to 59 years meet the specific indications.[16] PrEP with daily emtricitabine-tenofovir disoproxil fumarate can reduce HIV incidence in MSM (and transgender women) by up to 92%.[17]

Dermatologists should also be aware of nonoccupational HIV postexposure prophylaxis (nPEP), which is indicated in settings of substantial risk exposure to HIV transmission; for MSM, a relevant exposure would be unprotected receptive anal intercourse with an untreated HIV-positive person. A 28-day antiretroviral treatment course to prevent HIV acquisition must begin within 72 hours of exposure.[18]

WOMEN WHO HAVE SEX WITH WOMEN

Few data are available on the sexual and skin health of WSW.[11] WSW are at risk of acquiring STDs from current and prior female and/or male partners.[19] Transmissions of genital HPV, herpes simplex virus, syphilis, and HIV between female sexual partners have been described.[19] Seroprevalence of herpes simplex virus Type 2 is higher among women with same-sex partners in the past year (30%) or in their lifetime (36%) than women with no lifetime same-sex behaviors (24%).[20] Prevalence of HPV and HPV-related premalignant lesions is similar among WSW and women who do not have sex with women.[12] Guidelines for HIV, syphilis, *Chlamydia*, and gonorrhea screening, as well as cervical cancer screening and HPV vaccination, do not differ for WSW and women who do not have sex with women.[12]

TRANSGENDER PERSONS

Dermatologists may have increasing roles in the skin and sexual health of transgender persons. Some transgender persons undergo gender-affirming treatments, which may include psychological counseling, hormone therapy to alter secondary sex characteristics, and/or surgical interventions (eg, facial feminizing procedures, "top" surgery such as masculinizing chest surgery for transgender men or augmentation mammoplasty for transgender women, and "bottom" surgery such as hysterectomy and oophorectomy and/or phalloplasty for transgender men or orchiectomy and/or vaginoplasty for transgender women).[21] Dermatologists' involvement in in transgender health can include helping manage cutaneous adverse effects of hormonal treatments and surgical treatments, including keloids; performing safe and effective procedures that contribute to gender-affirming physical transformation through aesthetic procedures; and facilitating screening and preventive care.[22]

TRANSGENDER MEN

Transgender men seeking masculinizing hormone therapy may receive testosterone, which can cause cutaneous effects including increased facial and body hair, redistribution of subcutaneous fat, and changes in sweat and odor patterns.[21] Acne is a common adverse effect of testosterone and develops in 88% to 94% of transgender men within 4 to 6 months of testosterone initiation, typically with decreasing severity beyond 12 months of treatment.[23] Many cases can be managed effectively with topical acne treatments and/or oral antibiotics, without needing to adjust hormone therapy. Severe testosterone-induced acne in transgender men has been successfully treated with isotretinoin.[24] To receive isotretinoin in the United States, patients must register with the U.S. Food and Drug Administration's iPLEDGE system, a risk management program that aims to minimize fetal exposure to the teratogenic medicine.[25] Contraception counseling is important because transgender men who retain female natal reproductive organs can become pregnant, even while taking testosterone. Unfortunately, iPLEDGE requires transgender men to register in the program according to their sex assigned at birth (ie, female), which is unacceptable to some patients.[26] Physicians failing to register transgender men as female risk sanction from iPLEDGE, and transgender men refusing to register as female in iPLEDGE lack isotretinoin access. Some have advocated that iPLEDGE change this registration requirement.[26,27] When caring for transgender men taking testosterone who might become pregnant, recommended practices are to explain iPLEDGE program requirements and noncompliance risks to physicians; inform patients that dermatologists have made the Food and Drug Administration aware of this issue; express empathy with patients for having to register in iPLEDGE as female; and offer to order serum rather than urine pregnancy tests to decrease awkwardness in laboratory encounters.[27]

Male pattern alopecia is associated with duration of testosterone treatment: 33% develop mild alopecia and 31% develop moderate to severe alopecia with long-term use.[23] It may be considered desirable for some who consider it as a masculine feature, but undesirable for others. Minoxidil or finasteride for testosterone-induced alopecia in transgender men has not been well studied; hair transplantation may be considered for severe cases.[23]

TRANSGENDER WOMEN

Transgender women who seek feminizing hormone therapy may receive estrogens as well as antiandrogens, including medroxyprogesterone acetate, oral progesterone, spironolactone, finasteride, and dutasteride.[21] Desired effects include breast development, reduction of body and facial hair, redistribution of subcutaneous fat, change in sweat and odor pattern, arrest or reversal of hair loss, decreased sebum production, improvement in acne vulgaris, and reduction in gender dysphoria.[21] Facial hair growth and density is often resistant to hormonal therapy.[21] Topical eflornithine, electrolysis, photoepilation, or laser treatments may reduce the need for shaving or depilatory use.[21]

Facial feminization and body contouring procedures are prevalent among transgender women. Lack of treatment access has led many transgender women—up to 16% in San Francisco, 40% in Lima, and 68% in Thailand—to receive "silicone" or "filler" injections to buttocks, hips, breasts, face, and calves from unlicensed low-cost "pumpers."[21,28] While purportedly consisting of medical-grade silicone, various substances, including food- or industrial-grade silicone, paraffin, petroleum jelly, lanolin, beeswax, various oils, tire sealant, cement glue, or automobile transmission fluid, have been injected in volumes ranging from 2 ounces to 8 liters.[28] Serious complications, including foreign-body granulomatous dermatitis, bacterial or atypical mycobacterial infections, bleeding, pain, scarring, ulceration, fistula formation, gross disfiguration, lymphedema, silicone migration or embolism, sepsis, hypersensitivity pneumonitis, and death have occurred hours to decades later.[21,28] Treatment of silicone granulomas includes intralesional corticosteroid, topical imiquimod or tacrolimus, oral doxycycline or minocycline, isotretinoin, etanercept, carbon dioxide ablative laser, or surgical excision.[29] Transgender persons who inject "fillers" from unlicensed low-cost "pumpers" should be screened for hepatitis C.[21]

Dermatologists can make tremendous differences for transgender women by providing safe, effective gender-affirming injectable treatments, particularly for those who prefer noninvasive or nonpermanent treatments or are not surgical candidates.[22] Facial contouring may be achieved by botulinum toxin neuromodulation to lift, shape, or flatten the forehead and eyebrows, reduce appearance of periorbital rhytides, or reduce masseter hypertrophy for lower face contouring.[30] Soft-tissue augmentation can also add volume to the cheeks, lips, or chin.[30]

Transgender persons face a range of sexual health risks and should receive appropriate HIV and STD screening and prevention services, including vaccination, PrEP,[21] and nPEP, based on their sexual behaviors and the gender(s) of their sex partners.[21] In the United States, 28% of transgender women, and 56% of black transgender women tested HIV-positive.[31]

APPROACHES TO CARE

Like all clinicians, dermatologists should strive to provide culturally competent care for all patients. For LGBT patients, culturally competent care includes use of inclusive language and demonstration of equality and respect. Eliciting relevant information on sex anatomy, gender identity, sexual orientation and sexual behaviors in an effective and sensitive manner can facilitate the delivery of appropriate medical care and cultivate the physician–patient relationship.

Patients may or may not expect dermatologists to inquire about their sexual history or gender identity. When sexual health is relevant to one's skin and medical care, dermatologists can normalize the discussion by explaining that it is routine to ask patients with similar signs and/or symptoms about sexual history and/or gender identity. Depending on the context, persons accompanying the patient may be asked to leave the examination room before initiating that conversation. If discussing sexual history and/or gender identity is deemed acceptable to the patient, respectfully ask relevant questions, such as whether the patient is sexually active, and, if so, with men or women or both, followed by any appropriate questions relevant to establishing a diagnosis. Beyond making a diagnosis, sexual history or gender identity may be elicited if that information contributes, for example, to medical decision-making screening or vaccination recommendations, or PrEP or nPEP considerations. Clinicians should bear in mind that patients might not be comfortable disclosing sensitive information, especially during a first visit. Those who may be apprehensive in asking about sexual orientation and gender identity should know that the collection of these data is highly acceptable to LGBT and non-LGBT patients across diverse clinical settings in the United States.[32]

An inclusive care environment can also improve health care for LGBT persons.[4,5,21] Physicians and staff should appreciate the wide diversity of identities and experiences that patients may have; be aware of terminologies used by LGBT persons, asking respectfully for clarification when needed; respect each patient's preferences on name, pronoun and gender identity; avoid stereotypes about sexual orientation or gender identity based on appearance or other factors. When encountering patients whose name or gender identity might not match the sex or gender indicated on legal or insurance documents, patients should be asked how they would prefer to be addressed. Intake forms, electronic health records, and documentation should reflect such diversity and normalize disclosure of gender identity and sexual orientation. Information regarding patients' sex, gender, and sexuality should be kept confidential. Patients should be able to use restrooms of their choice; ideally, gender-neutral or unisex restrooms should be available. By incorporating patient-centered, culturally competent care into practice, dermatologists can contribute to improving the health of LGBT persons.

REFERENCES

1. The Institute of Medicine, Committee on Lesbian, Gay, Bisexual, and Transgender Health Issues and Research Gaps and Opportunities. *The Health of Lesbian, Gay, Bisexual, and Transgender People: Building a Foundation for Better Understanding*. Washington, DC: Institute of Medicine; 2011.
2. Bayer R, Oppenheimer GM. *AIDS Doctors: Voices from the Epidemic*. New York, NY: Oxford University Press; 2000.
3. U.S. Department of Human and Health Services, Office of Disease Prevention and Health Promotion. Lesbian, Gay, Bisexual and Transgender Health. 2014. https://www.healthypeople.gov/2020/topics-objectives/topic/lesbian-gay-bisexual-and-transgender-health. Accessed August 25, 2016.
4. The Joint Commission. *Advancing Effective Communication, Cultural Competence, and Patient- and Family-Centered Care for the Lesbian, Gay, Bisexual, and Transgender (LGBT) Community: A Field Guide*. Oak Brook, IL: The Joint Commission; 2011.
5. American Association of Medical Colleges. *Implementing Curricular and Institutional Climate Changes to Improve Health Care for Individuals Who Are LGBT, Gender Nonconforming, or Born with DSD: A Resource for Medical Educators*. Washington, DC: American Association of Medical Colleges; 2014.
6. LGBTQ Cultural Competency Continuing Education Amendment Act of 2015, 2015 DC B12-0168(2015).

http://lims.dccouncil.us/Download/33671/B21-0168-SignedAct.pdf. Accessed August 25, 2016.
7. Katz KA, Furnish TJ. Dermatology-related epidemiologic and clinical concerns of men who have sex with men, women who have sex with women, and transgender individuals. *Arch Dermatol*. 2005; 141(10):1303-1310.
8. National LGBT Health Education Center. Glossary of LGBT Terms for Health Care Teams. 2016. http://www.lgbthealtheducation.org/wp-content/uploads/LGBT-Glossary_March2016.pdf. Accessed August 20, 2016.
9. American Psychiatric Association. Gender Dysphoria. In: *Diagnostic and Statistical Manual of Mental Disorders*. 5th ed. Arlington, VA: American Psychiatric Association; 2013:451-459.
10. Gates GJ. How many people are lesbian, gay, bisexual and transgender? Los Angeles, CA: The Williams Institute, UCLA School of Law; 2011. http://williamsinstitute.law.ucla.edu/wp-content/uploads/Gates-How-Many-People-LGBT-Apr-2011.pdf. Accessed on February 4, 2016.
11. US Preventive Services Task Force (USPSTF). Screening for syphilis infection in nonpregnant adults and adolescents: US Preventive Services Task Force recommendation statement. *JAMA*. 2016;315(21):2321-2327.
12. Workowski KA, Bolan GA; Centers for Disease Control and Prevention. Sexually transmitted diseases treatment guidelines, 2015. *MMWR Recomm Rep*. 2015;64(RR-03):1-137. Available at: http://www.cdc.gov/std/tg2015/tg-2015-print.pdf. Accessed on July 17, 2016.
13. Giuliano AR, Palefsky JM, Goldstone S, et al. Efficacy of quadrivalent HPV vaccine against HPV Infection and disease in males. *N Engl J Med*. 2011;364(5):401-411.
14. Centers for Disease Control and Prevention. Recommended Immunization Schedule for Adults Aged 19 Years or Older by Medical Conditions and Other Indications, United States, 2018. https://www.cdc.gov/vaccines/schedules/hcp/imz/adult-conditions.html. Accessed May 8, 2018.
15. Centers for Disease Control and Prevention. Preexposure Prophylaxis for the Prevention of HIV Infection in the United States—2017 Update. 2017. https://www.cdc.gov/hiv/pdf/risk/prep/cdc-hiv-prep-guidelines-2017.pdf Accessed May 14, 2018.
16. Smith DK, Van Handel M, Wolitski RJ, et al. Vital signs: estimated percentages and numbers of adults with indications for preexposure prophylaxis to prevent HIV acquisition—United States, 2015. *MMWR Morb Mortal Wkly Rep*. 2015;64(46):1291-1295.
17. Grant RM, Lama JR, Anderson PL, et al. Preexposure chemoprophylaxis for HIV prevention in men who have sex with men. *N Engl J Med*. 2010;363(27):2587-2599.
18. Announcement: updated guidelines for antiretroviral postexposure prophylaxis after sexual, injection-drug use, or other nonoccupational exposure to HIV-United States, 2016. *MMWR Morb Mortal Wkly Rep*. 2016;65(17):458.
19. Gorgos LM, Marrazzo JM. Sexually transmitted infections among women who have sex with women. *Clin Infect Dis*. 2011;53(suppl 3):S84-S91.
20. Xu F, Sternberg MR, Markowitz LE. Women who have sex with women in the United States: prevalence, sexual behavior and prevalence of herpes simplex virus type 2 infection-results from national health and nutrition examination survey 2001-2006. *Sex Transm Dis*. 2010;37(7):407-413.
21. Deutsch MB, ed. *Guidelines for the Primary and Gender-Affirming Care of Transgender and Gender Nonbinary People*. 2nd ed. San Francisco, CA: UCSF Center of Excellence for Transgender Health, Department of Family and Community Medicine; 2016. http://www.transhealth.ucsf.edu/guidelines. Accessed August 11, 2016.
22. Ginsberg BA, Calderon M, Seminara NM, et al. A potential role for the dermatologist in the physical transformation of transgender people: a survey of attitudes and practices within the transgender community. *J Am Acad Dermatol*. 2016;74(2):303-308.
23. Irwig MS. Testosterone therapy for transgender men. *Lancet Diabetes Endocrinol*. 2017;5(4):301-311.
24. Turrion-Merino L, Urech-Garcia-de-la-Vega M, Miguel-Gomez L, et al. Severe acne in female-to-male transgender patients. *JAMA Dermatol*. 2015;151(11):1260-1261.
25. U.S. Food and Drug Administration. The iPLEDGE Program. Prescriber Isotretinoin Educational Kit. 2017. Available at: https://www.ipledgeprogram.com/iPledgeUI/rems/pdf/resources/Prescriber%20Isotretinoin%20Educational%20Kit.pdf. Accessed May 8, 2018.
26. Katz KA. Transgender patients, isotretinoin, and US Food and Drug Administration–mandated risk evaluation and mitigation strategies: a prescription for inclusion. *JAMA Dermatol*. 2016;152(5):513-514.
27. Yeung H, Chen SC, Katz KA, et al. Prescribing isotretinoin in the United States for transgender individuals: ethical considerations. *J Am Acad Dermatol*. 2016;75(3):648-651.
28. Wilson E, Rapues J, Jin H, et al. The use and correlates of illicit silicone or "fillers" in a population-based sample of transwomen, San Francisco, 2013. *J Sex Med*. 2014; 11(7):1717-1724.
29. Paul S, Goyal A, Duncan LM, et al. Granulomatous reaction to liquid injectable silicone for gluteal enhancement: review of management options and success of doxycycline. *Dermatol Ther*. 2015;28(2):98-101.
30. Ginsberg BA. Dermatology. In: Eckstrand KL, Ehrenfeld JM, eds. *Lesbian, Gay, Bisexual, and Transgender Healthcare: A Clinical Guide to Preventive, Primary, and Specialist Care*. Cham, Switzerland: Springer International Publishing; 2016:263-288.
31. Herbst JH, Jacobs ED, Finlayson TJ, et al. Estimating HIV prevalence and risk behaviors of transgender persons in the United States: a systematic review. *AIDS Behav*. 2008;12(1):1-17.
32. Cahill S, Singal R, Grasso C, et al. Do ask, do tell: high levels of acceptability by patients of routine collection of sexual orientation and gender identity data in four diverse American community health centers. *PLoS One*. 2014;9(9):e107104.
33. National Center for HIV/AIDS, Viral Hepatitis, STD, and TB Prevention, Centers for Disease Control and Prevention. Diagnoses of HIV Infection in the United States and Dependent Areas, 2016. Vol. 28. https://www.cdc.gov/hiv/pdf/library/reports/surveillance/cdc-hiv-surveillance-report-2016-vol-28.pdf Published November 2017. Accessed May 8, 2018.
34. Xu F, Sternberg MR, Markowitz LE. Men who have sex with men in the United States: demographic and behavioral characteristics and prevalence of HIV and HSV-2 infection: results from National Health and Nutrition Examination Survey 2001-2006. *Sex Transm Dis*. 2010;37(6):399-405.
35. Machalek DA, Poynten M, Jin F, et al. Anal human papillomavirus infection and associated neoplastic lesions

in men who have sex with men: a systematic review and meta-analysis. *Lancet Oncol*. 2012;13(5):487-500.
36. Lanternier F, Lebbe C, Schartz N, et al. Kaposi's sarcoma in HIV-negative men having sex with men. *AIDS*. 2008;22(10):1163-1168.
37. Maurer T, Ponte M, Leslie K. HIV-associated Kaposi's sarcoma with a high CD4 count and a low viral load. *N Engl J Med*. 2007;357(13):1352-1353.
38. Centers for Disease Control and Prevention. Sexually Transmitted Disease Surveillance 2016. https://www.cdc.gov/std/stats16/CDC_2016_STDS_Report-for508Web Sep21_2017_1644.pdf. Published September 2017. Accessed May 8, 2018.
39. Patton ME, Kidd S, Llata E, et al. Extragenital gonorrhea and chlamydia testing and infection among men who have sex with men—STD Surveillance Network, United States, 2010-2012. *Clin Infect Dis*. 2014; 58(11):1564-1570.
40. de Vries HJ, Zingoni A, Kreuter A, et al. 2013 European guideline on the management of lymphogranuloma venereum. *J Eur Acad Dermatol Venereol*. 2015;29(1):1-6.
41. David MZ, Daum RS. Community-associated methicillin-resistant *Staphylococcus aureus*: epidemiology and clinical consequences of an emerging epidemic. *Clin Microbiol Rev*. 2010;23(3):616-687.
42. Simon MS, Weiss D, Gulick RM. Invasive meningococcal disease in men who have sex with men. *Ann Intern Med*. 2013;159(4):300-301.
43. Janda WM, Bohnoff M, Morello JA, et al. Prevalence and site-pathogen studies of *Neisseria meningitidis* and *N gonorrhoeae* in homosexual men. *JAMA*. 1980;244(18):2060-2064.
44. Mansh M, Katz KA, Linos E, et al. Association of skin cancer and indoor tanning in sexual minority men and women. *JAMA Dermatol*. 2015;151(12):1308-1316.
45. Yeung H, Chen SC. Sexual orientation and indoor tanning device use: a population-based study. *JAMA Dermatol*. 2016;152(1):99-101.
46. Yeung H, Chen SC. Disparities in sunburns, photoprotection, indoor tanning, and skin cancer screening among U.S. men and women in same- and opposite-sex relationships [abstract]. *J Invest Dermatol*. 2015;135(suppl 1):S49.
47. Schauber J, Herzinger T. "Poppers" dermatitis. *Clin Exp Dermatol*. 2012;37(5):587-588.
48. Vine K, Meulener M, Shieh S, et al. Vitiliginous lesions induced by amyl nitrite exposure. *Cutis*. 2013; 91(3):129-136.
49. Gao Y, Wei EK, Arron ST, Linos E, Margolis DJ, Mansh MD. Acne, sexual orientation, and mental health among young adults in the United States: A population-based, cross-sectional study. *J Am Acad Dermatol*. 2017 Nov;77(5):971-973.
50. Kamiya H, MacNeil J, Blain A, et al. Meningococcal disease among men who have sex with men—United States, January 2012-June 2015. *MMWR Morb Mortal Wkly Rep*. 2015;64(44):1256-1257.

Neoplasia PART 20

第二十篇 皮肤肿瘤

Chapter 108 :: Benign Epithelial Tumors, Hamartomas, and Hyperplasias :: Jonathan D. Cuda, Sophia Rangwala, & Janis M. Taube

第一百零八章
良性上皮肿瘤、错构瘤和增生性病变

中文导读

本章分为6节：①脂溢性角化病；②线状苔藓；③透明细胞棘皮瘤；④耳轮结节性软骨皮炎；⑤表皮痣；⑥起源于表皮的囊肿。本章讨论了良性上皮肿瘤、错构瘤和皮肤增生的临床和病理特征。

第一节脂溢性角化症，介绍了其流行病学及临床特征、病因及发病机制、临床亚型、组织学变异及治疗。提到了其病因可能与遗传易感性和人乳头瘤病毒（HPV）感染有关。同时介绍了脂溢性角化症可发展为鳞状细胞癌，若快速生长、有症状或有变化的病变应活检以排除恶性肿瘤。

第二节线状苔藓，介绍了其病原学和流行病学、临床特征、鉴别诊断、组织病理学及治疗。提到了线状苔藓是一种突发性疾病，通常无症状和有自限性，不需要治疗，可局部使用类固醇或他克莫司和吡美莫司乳膏。

第三节透明细胞棘皮瘤，介绍了其病原学和流行病学、临床特征、鉴别诊断、组织病理学及治疗。提到了透明细胞棘皮瘤是一种良性上皮肿瘤，需要与小汗腺孢子瘤、化脓性肉芽肿、基底细胞癌、鳞状细胞癌等相鉴别，可采用冷冻疗法、刮除术、电干燥术、激光消融术和手术切除等方法治疗。

第四节耳轮结节性软骨皮炎，介绍了其病原学和流行病学、临床特征、鉴别诊断、组织病理学及治疗。提到了耳轮结节性软骨皮炎是一种慢性压痛性结节，被认为是一种胶原变性的疾病。需要与基底细胞癌、鳞状细胞癌、角化棘皮瘤、疣和痛风石等相鉴别。治疗

目的是减少疼痛和改善临床外观。

第五节表皮痣，介绍了表皮痣是一种良性的错构瘤性增生，详细介绍了线性角质形成细胞性表皮痣、皮脂腺痣、黑头粉刺痣、表皮痣综合征的临床特征、病因与发病机制、组织病理学、诊断、病程、并发症及治疗等。

第六节起源于表皮的囊肿，介绍了表皮样囊肿、毛鞘囊肿、粟丘疹、皮脂腺囊肿、皮样囊肿、鳃裂囊肿、耳前囊肿和窦道的病因和发病机制、临床特征、流行病学、组织病理学、治疗。

〔粟 娟〕

This chapter discusses clinical and pathologic features of benign epithelial tumors, hamartomas, and hyperplasias of the skin. A review of relevant systemic and syndromic associations is provided when applicable.

SEBORRHEIC KERATOSIS

AT-A-GLANCE

- Seborrheic keratosis is the most common benign epidermal tumor.
- They usually begin as well-circumscribed tan brown patches or thin plaques with pseudo-horn cysts (keratotic invaginations).
- Rapidly growing, symptomatic, or atypical lesions should be biopsied to rule out malignancy.
- Clinical and histologic variants include common seborrheic keratosis (SK), reticulated SK, stucco keratosis, melanoacanthoma, dermatosis papulosa nigra, clonal SK, and irritated SK.
- Hallmark histopathologic findings: acanthosis, papillomatosis, pseudo-horn cysts, and hyperkeratosis
- Multiple eruptive seborrheic keratoses may be indicative of internal malignancy (Leser-Trélat sign). Gastrointestinal malignancy is most common followed by lymphoproliferative disease.

EPIDEMIOLOGY AND CLINICAL FEATURES

Seborrheic keratoses (SKs) are the most common acquired benign epithelial tumor of the skin. They can occur anywhere on the cutaneous surface, with the exception of the palms and soles. They are common in middle-aged and older adults and have a range of clinical appearances. Differences in clinical morphology often correspond with different microscopic variations.

SKs begin as circumscribed tan brown patches or thin plaques. Over time, they may become more papular or verrucous with a greasy scale and a stuck-on appearance (Figs. 108-1 and 108-2). Hallmark histologic findings include hyperkeratosis, acanthosis, papillomatosis, and pseudohorn cysts.

Multiple SKs may be patterned along the lines of skin cleavage or Blaschko lines.[1,2] Eruptive lesions may be a sign of internal malignancy (Leser-Trélat sign).[3] The most common associated malignancy is gastrointestinal, followed by lymphoproliferative disease. Eruptive SKs have been reported in other clinical settings, including erythroderma and HIV infection.[4,5] Chemotherapeutic agents, such as cytarabine, may cause inflammation of preexisting SKs, which then become more clinically apparent ("pseudo-sign of Leser-Trélat").[6]

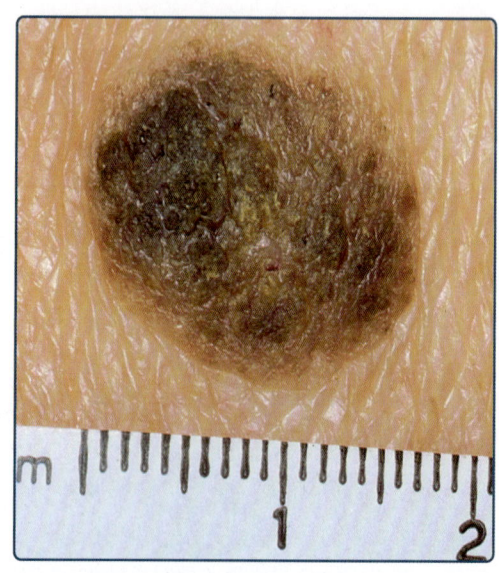

Figure 108-1 Seborrheic keratosis showing a rough surface and stuck-on appearance.

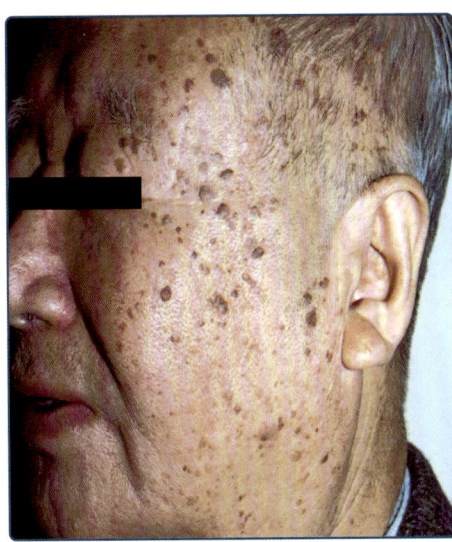

Figure 108-2 Multiple small seborrheic keratoses.

TABLE 108-1
Genetic Alterations Reported in Association with Seborrheic Keratosis[12]

GENETIC ALTERATION	PREVALENCE (%)
FGFR3 and PIK3CA	42
FGFR3	38
PIK3CA	15
FGFR3 and AKT	2
HRAS	2
PIK3CA and HRAS	1

hybridization or PCR analysis may be used to make the distinction in equivocal cases. In one study of genital SKs, 28 of 40 (70%) were positive for HPV.[15] The overwhelming majority contained HPV6, also the most common subtype detected in condylomata. HPV was detected in only 2 of 20 (10%) extragenital SKs. These findings highlight the morphologic plasticity of HPV-related keratoses on genital skin, ranging from SK-like histology to typical condyloma acuminatum.

On occasion, cutaneous malignancies arise from or adjacent to SKs, highlighting the importance of close examination and tissue biopsy of atypical, symptomatic, or changing lesions.[7,8]

ETIOLOGY AND PATHOGENESIS

Although the precise cause of SKs is unknown, most are sporadic. Interestingly, a family history of SKs is attainable in some instances, suggesting a genetic predisposition. Sun exposure may also contribute to their pathogenesis.[9] The monoclonal nature of these neoplasms was established in 2001.[10] By tracking polymorphisms in a human androgen receptor, researchers found that more than half of the 38 SKs sampled, regardless of subtype, were clonal in nature. Multiple oncogenic mutations have been reported in these keratinocyte-derived tumors (Table 108-1). The most frequently detected are activating mutations in the FGFR3 and PIK3CA genes.[11] Activating mutations of EGFR, HRAS, and KRAS likely also contribute to their pathogenesis, albeit at a lower frequency.[12] Hyperpigmentation of SKs is related to increased expression of tumor necrosis factor-α and endothelin-converting enzyme -1α, thereby stimulating secretion of endothelin 1, a potent melanogenic cytokine.[13]

There is not a clear etiologic relationship between human papillomavirus (HPV) infection and SKs. However, strains of HPV have been detected in SKs at both extragenital and genital sites.[14,15] There is some evidence to suggest a bystander effect, whereby lesions are colonized on their surface by regional HPV infection without an etiologic association.

SKs on genital skin may also share histologic characteristics with condyloma acuminata. Tissue in situ

CLINICOPATHOLOGIC VARIANTS

There are several variants of SK. Although distinction among variants is usually unnecessary, histologic variations often correlate with clinical features.

COMMON SEBORRHEIC KERATOSIS

Common SKs are classically described as verrucous stuck-on papules or plaques (see Figs. 108-1 and 108-2). They are characterized by an acanthotic proliferation of epidermal keratinocytes with hyperkeratosis, papillomatosis, and pseudohorn cysts (Fig. 108-3). An increased number of melanocytes and pigment may be present, resulting in a tan or dark brown coloration.

RETICULATED SEBORRHEIC KERATOSIS

Reticulated (adenoid) SKs clinically present as pigmented patches or thin papules. Histologically, these epidermal tumors are composed of interconnected delicate downgrowths of pigmented basilar epithelial cells with horn cysts (Fig. 108-4). In some instances, they may arise from a solar lentigo.

STUCCO KERATOSIS

Stucco keratoses present as multiple small 1- to 3-mm white to tan keratotic papules with predilection for

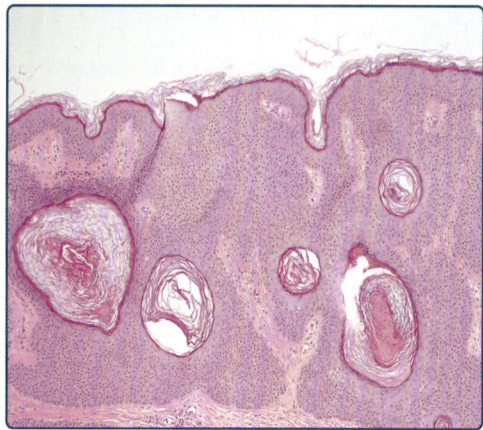

Figure 108-3 Seborrheic keratosis showing a papillomatous acanthotic epidermis consisting of small uniform basaloid keratinocytes with pseudohorn cysts.

the distal extremities, particularly the lower legs. Histologically, they show orthokeratosis, papillomatosis, and acanthosis with fusion of rete pegs.

MELANOACANTHOMA

Melanoacanthoma is considered a variant of pigmented SK. Clinically, this lesion may resemble melanoma and is commonly seen on the head and neck or trunk of older adults. It is characterized by an acanthotic proliferation of basaloid and spinous keratinocytes, often with horn cysts. Between keratinocytes, there are sporadically distributed pigmented dendritic melanocytes. Melanin-laden histiocytes are often present in the dermis.

DERMATOSIS PAPULOSA NIGRA

Dermatosis papulosa nigra most commonly presents as multiple small dark brown to black keratotic papules on the malar region of individuals with Fitzpatrick skin Type IV or greater (Fig. 108-5). They may also occur on the neck and upper chest. Histologically, they show orthokeratosis, acanthosis, papillomatosis, and interconnected rete with basal layer hyperpigmentation.

POLYPOID SEBORRHEIC KERATOSIS

Similar to skin tags, SKs may assume a polypoid configuration, particularly on the neck or intertriginous areas.

HISTOLOGIC VARIANTS

CLONAL SEBORRHEIC KERATOSIS

Clonal SK is a histologic term used to describe intraepithelial whorls of banal keratinocytes (Fig. 108-6).

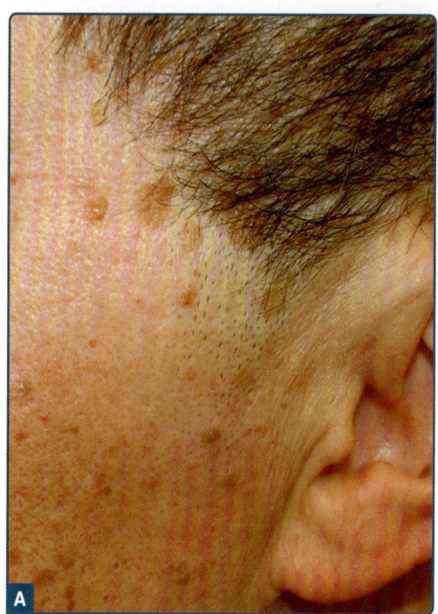

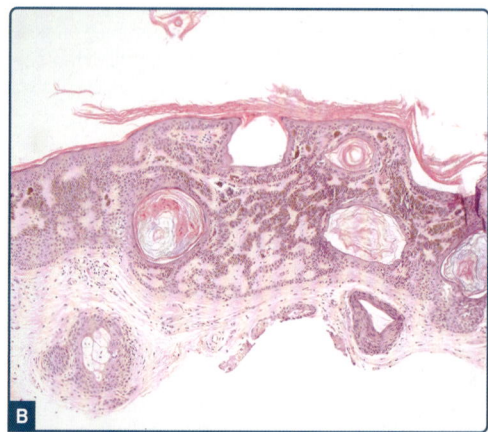

Figure 108-4 **A,** Multiple reticulated seborrheic keratoses. **B,** Reticulated seborrheic keratosis showing elongated interconnected downgrowths of pigmented basilar keratinocytes with horn cysts.

IRRITATED SEBORRHEIC KERATOSIS

SKs may become irritated by mechanical or chemical means, or spontaneous inflammation may occur. This variant of SK is characterized by a dense inflammatory infiltrate, typically lymphocytic and sometimes lichenoid. Small whorled collections of glassy keratinocytes or squamous eddies may be seen in this variant. Lesions with surrounding eczematous changes (Meyerson phenomenon) are also seen.[16]

MALIGNANT TRANSFORMATION OR COLLISION LESIONS

Varying degrees of squamous atypia may be seen in SKs. In most instances, the atypia is reactive because

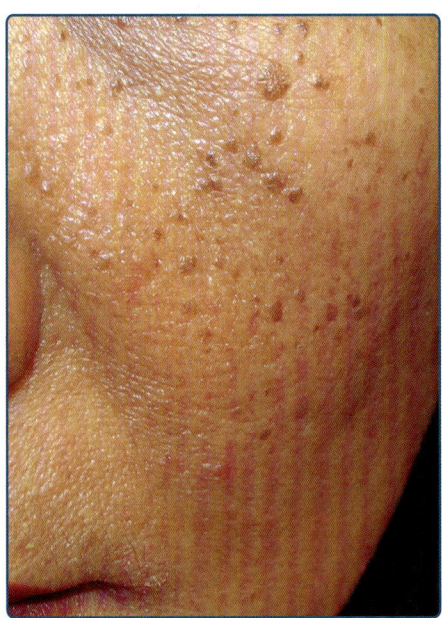

Figure 108-5 Dermatosis papulosa nigra.

TREATMENT

When evaluating SKs, care should be taken not to destroy lesions that may harbor malignancy. A history of rapid growth, symptomatology, color change, atypical morphology, or unusual location should prompt strong consideration for tissue biopsy and histologic examination.

For clearly benign lesions that are irritated or cosmetically undesirable, destructive techniques such as cryotherapy, electrodesiccation followed by curettage, or laser ablation have all been shown to be effective. There are reports of giant SKs effectively treated with either dermabrasion or topical fluorouracil.[17,18] Complications of these destructive measures include scarring, pigmentary alteration, incomplete removal, or recurrence. Multiple treatments may be required to ensure lesional eradication. Care should be taken to minimize the risk of scarring.

of intense inflammation or irritation. However, bowenoid transformation to squamous cell carcinoma (SCC) in situ may occur. Other cutaneous malignancies, including basal cell carcinoma (BCC), invasive SCC, and melanoma, rarely arise from or collide with SKs.[7,8] In a retrospective study of 813 lesions histologically diagnosed as SKs, 5.3% were associated with nonmelanoma skin cancer. In this study, the most common malignancy was SCC in situ followed by BCC and invasive SCC; no melanomas were observed in this study.[8] Rapidly growing, symptomatic, or changing lesions should be biopsied to exclude malignancy.

LICHEN STRIATUS

AT-A-GLANCE

- Lichen striatus is a rare, idiopathic, papular eruption that usually resolves in 1 to 2 years.
- It occurs most commonly on the limbs of children and adolescents with a female predilection.
- Eruption is characterized by the sudden onset of flat-topped, 1- to 3-mm, pink, tan, or hypopigmented papules in a linear or blaschkoid distribution.
- Differential diagnosis: lichen planus, "linear variants" of psoriasis, linear porokeratosis, lichen nitidus, "linear variants" of Darier disease, and inflammatory linear verrucous epidermal nevus

ETIOLOGY AND EPIDEMIOLOGY

Lichen striatus is a type of "BLAISE," described as *Blaschko linear acquired inflammatory skin eruption* (adult blaschkitis is another form), most commonly affects children and adolescents 5 to 15 years of age. The cause is unknown, and the disease is self-limiting. The limbs of females are most often affected, although involvement of the trunk and less frequently the face have been reported.[19] Nail changes are rare but can occur.[20] An association with atopic dermatitis has also been suggested.[21]

CLINICAL FEATURES

Lichen striatus is an eruption characterized by the sudden onset of flat-topped, 1- to 3-mm, pink, tan, or

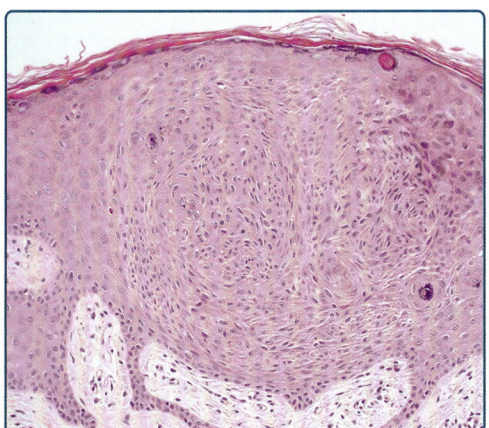

Figure 108-6 Clonal seborrheic keratosis with intraepidermal whorls of bland keratinocytes.

hypopigmented papules in a linear configuration or blaschkoid distribution (Fig. 108-7). The eruption is most commonly unilateral (Fig. 108-8), although bilateral eruptions sometimes occur. Nail changes include longitudinal ridging and nail plate thinning. The eruption is self-limited, with spontaneous regression within a few months to 2 years.

DIFFERENTIAL DIAGNOSIS

Lichen planus, psoriasis, linear porokeratosis, lichen nitidus, Darier disease, and inflammatory linear verrucous epidermal nevus (ILVEN) can have similar clinical morphology and distribution to lichen striatus.

HISTOPATHOLOGY

Lichen striatus is characterized by a lichenoid lymphocytic infiltrate with overlying epidermal acanthosis, dyskeratosis, hyperkeratosis, and focal parakeratosis. There is concomitant mild epidermal spongiosis with exocytosis of inflammatory cells. Intraepidermal Langerhans cell clusters may be seen. The dermal lymphocytic infiltrate may extend

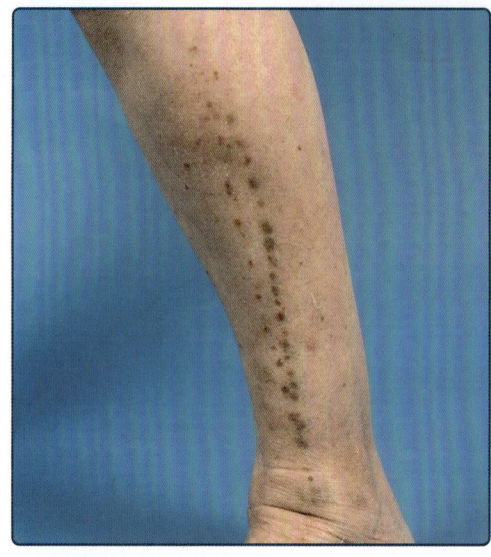

Figure 108-8 Lichen striatus. Linear configuration of slightly scaling papules in a blaschkoid distribution on the leg.

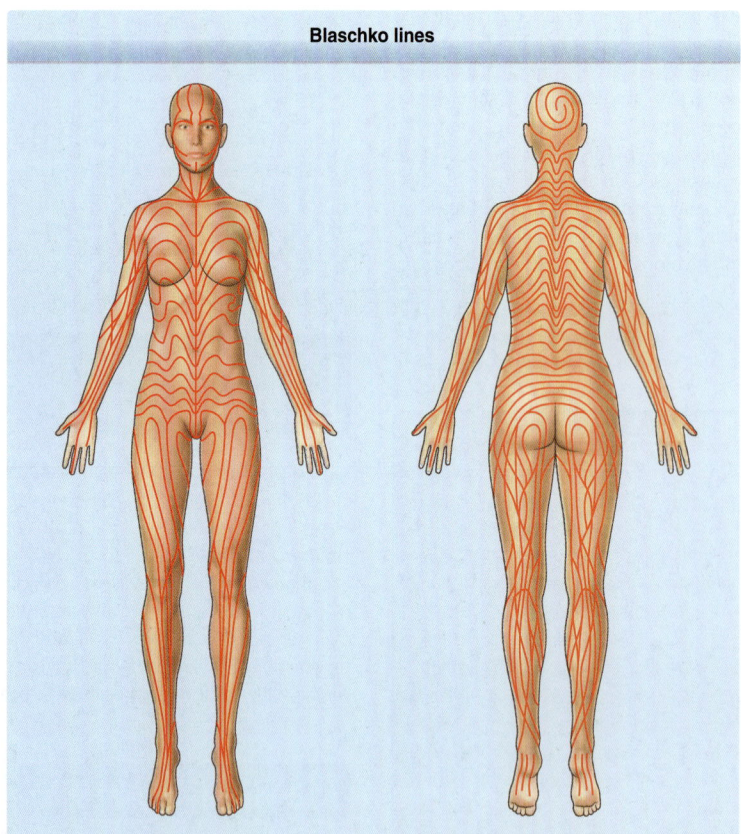

Figure 108-7 Blaschko lines. These lines represent pathways of epidermal cell migration and proliferation during fetal development and are the basis for the pattern distribution seen in cutaneous mosaicism.

into the deep dermis in a perivascular and periadnexal pattern, with characteristic accentuation around eccrine coils.

TREATMENT

Because the disease is usually asymptomatic and self-limited, treatment is not required. However, pruritic lesions may be offered symptomatic relief with topical steroids. Topical tacrolimus and pimecrolimus cream have also been reported to be effective.[22,23]

CLEAR CELL ACANTHOMA

AT-A-GLANCE

- Clear cell acanthoma is a tumor of epidermal origin.
- Solitary, shiny, erythematous or orange to brown, blanching, well-demarcated papule or nodule with collarette of scale
- Composed of distinctive, glycogen-rich keratinocytes
- Differential diagnosis: eccrine poroma, pyogenic granuloma, BCC, SCC, lichenoid keratosis

ETIOLOGY AND EPIDEMIOLOGY

Clear cell acanthoma is a benign epithelial tumor that occurs equally in men and women, with a predilection for the lower legs of middle-aged to older individuals. The cause of clear cell acanthoma is unknown. It was first described by Degos et al. in 1962 as a benign tumor of epithelial origin.[24] Interestingly, the cytokeratin expression profile of these lesions has revealed similar staining patterns to those commonly found in inflammatory dermatoses such as lichen planus, psoriasis, and discoid lupus.[25] The occasional association of clear cell acanthoma with other cutaneous inflammatory conditions also suggests a possible role for inflammation in their development.[26]

CLINICAL FEATURES

Clear cell acanthoma presents as a solitary, shiny, erythematous to brown, well-demarcated papule or nodule that blanches almost fully with pressure (Fig. 108-9A). There is a surrounding collarette of scale. Lesions range from 5 mm to 2 cm, although rarely giant variants can measure greater than 5 cm.[27] They are most commonly found on the lower part of the legs but can be seen on the trunk or face. Rarely, lesions are multiple. They show dermatoscopic features similar to psoriasis, with prominent vascular puncta.[28] Like psoriasis, they may bleed easily with trauma.

DIFFERENTIAL DIAGNOSIS

Eccrine poroma, pyogenic granuloma, BCC, SCC, and lichenoid keratosis are within the differential diagnosis for clear cell acanthoma.

HISTOPATHOLOGY

Clear cell acanthoma is characterized by a sharply demarcated zone of pale staining epidermal keratinocytes with psoriasiform epidermal hyperplasia and a parakeratotic scale (Fig. 108-9B). Keratinocyte pallor is because of heavy cytoplasmic glycogen, as evidenced by periodic acid–Schiff positivity, which can be digested with diastase. Neutrophils commonly migrate through the epidermis to accumulate in the surface scale. There are thinning of suprapapillary plates and sparing of adnexal epithelium. The papillary dermis shows mild edema with increased vessels and a mixed inflammatory infiltrate.

TREATMENT

Cryotherapy, curettage and electrodesiccation, laser ablation, and surgical excision have been used to successfully treat this lesion.

CHRONDRODERMATITIS NODULARIS HELICIS

AT-A-GLANCE

- A chronic tender solitary nodule, often ulcerated on the helix of the ear
- Histology: ulceration with underlying degeneration of dermal collagen, increased fibroblasts, and chronic inflammatory cell infiltrate; perichondrium and cartilage also with degenerative changes
- Differential diagnosis: BCC, SCC, keratoacanthoma, verruca, tophus
- Treatment: conservative treatment, including pressure-relieving pillows and steroid injection; curettage and cautery or surgical excision if necessary

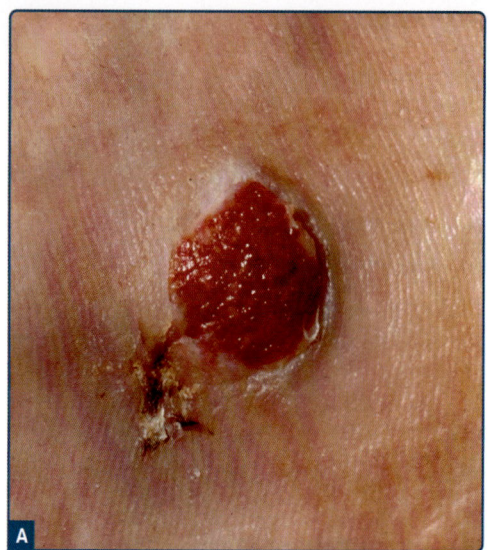

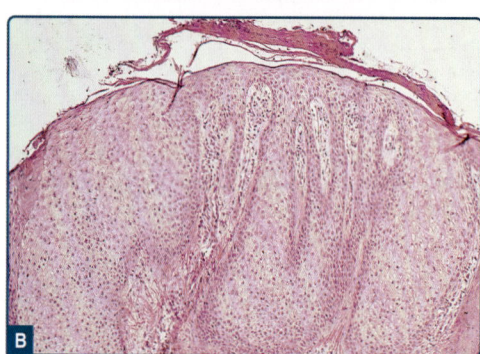

Figure 108-9 **A,** Clear cell acanthoma presenting as a flat red nodule on the sole. **B,** Histology showing a circumscribed sharply demarcated epidermal tumor composed of clear (glycogen rich) cells without cytologic atypia.

CLINICAL FEATURES

CNH is a chronic tender nodule that develops most commonly on the helix of the ear in men older than 50 years of age.[32] Lesions may also occur on the antihelix, particularly in women. CNH most often occurs on the helix as a small, 4 to 6 mm in diameter, nodular, tender lesion (Fig. 108-10A). Rarely, multiple lesions are present. Ulceration or scale crust are often evident. Lesions are persistent and do not typically regress spontaneously.

DIFFERENTIAL DIAGNOSIS

BCC, SCC, keratoacanthoma, warts, and tophi are within the differential diagnosis of CNH.

HISTOPATHOLOGY

There is often epidermal ulceration flanked by zones of epidermal hyperplasia. Beneath the ulcer, there are degenerative changes of dermal collagen with an increase in fibroblasts and capillary-sized blood vessels. A mild to moderate chronic inflammatory infiltrate is often present. Degenerative changes are also found within the underlying perichondrium and helical cartilage (Fig. 108-10B).

TREATMENT

Treatment is generally conservative aimed at reducing pain and improving clinical appearance. Pressure-relieving devices such as doughnut-shaped pillows can be effective. Other methods include intralesional steroids, laser therapy, curettage, and surgical excision if necessary.[33]

WARTY DYSKERATOMA

AT-A-GLANCE

- Solitary focus of acantholytic dyskeratosis
- Skin-colored, umbilicated papule on the head or neck of middle-aged and older individuals
- Histology: cup-shaped epidermal invagination with acantholysis and dyskeratosis filled with keratinaceous plug; may involve folliculosebaceous units
- Differential diagnosis: actinic keratosis, SCC
- Treatment: Excision is curative.

ETIOLOGY AND EPIDEMIOLOGY

Chondrodermatitis nodularis helicis (CNH) is thought to be a disease of collagen degeneration with subsequent transepidermal elimination.[29] Vascular insufficiency and local ischemia are thought to play inciting roles. Other possible associations include systemic microvascular disease and pressure related to cell phone use.[30,31] The presence of solar elastosis at the periphery of lesions and prevalence of CNH in lightly pigmented populations raises the possibility that chronic actinic damage may also play a role.[32]

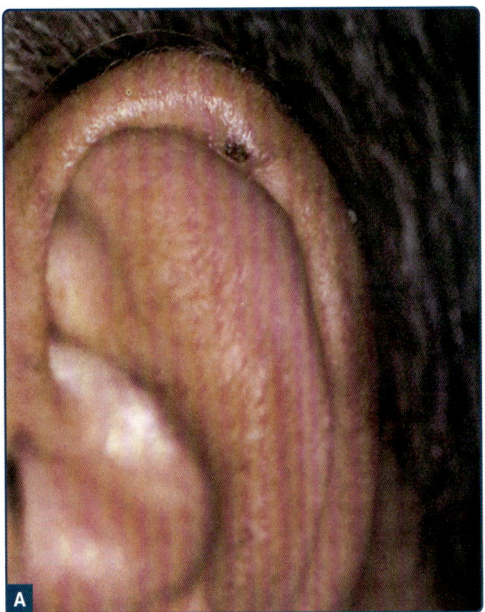

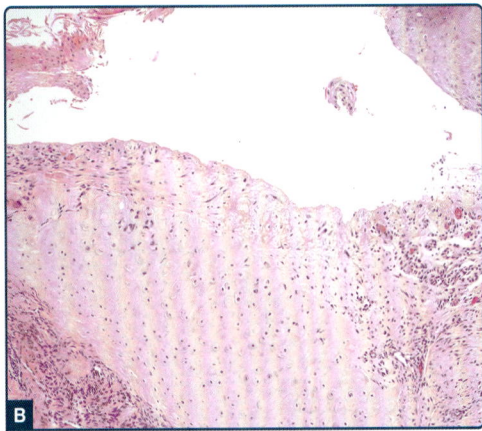

Figure 108-10. **A,** Chondrodermatitis nodularis helicis presenting as a painful nodule on the ear. **B,** Histology showing surface ulceration with fibrin, vascular proliferation, and cartilage with degenerative changes.

ACANTHOMA FISSURATUM (GRANULOMA FISSURATUM)

AT-A-GLANCE

- Fissured or ulcerated, firm, flesh-colored nodule, usually retroauricular, that appears in areas of friction, as with ill-fitting eyeglasses
- Histology: benign epidermal hyperplasia, hypergranulosis, and hyperparakeratosis; vascular telangiectasia, mild fibrosis, and chronic inflammatory cell infiltrate
- Differential diagnosis: BCC, SCC, CNH
- Treatment: Usually resolves after correction of the ill-fitting appliance.

EPIDERMAL NEVUS

INTRODUCTION

Epidermal nevi are benign hamartomatous proliferations of the epithelium and adnexae that present at birth or early childhood. Subtypes demonstrate varying degrees of proliferation of the squamous epithelium, sweat glands (sebaceous, apocrine, eccrine), smooth muscle, or hair follicle. Epidermal nevi are a product of cutaneous mosaicism, defined as a postzygotic genetic mutation or alteration occurring at the level of skin development.[34] This results in linear or whorled lesions that mirror the embryonic pathways of epidermal cell migration, termed the *lines of Blaschko* (Fig. 108-7). The blaschkoid distribution pattern has been described in multiple disease states, examples of which are listed in Table 108-2. Epidermal nevus syndromes are a heterogeneous group of disorders in which epidermal nevi are associated with extracutaneous anomalies and are thereby believed to represent a mosaic alteration occurring earlier in embryonic development.[35] In recent years, there have been major breakthroughs in our genetic understanding of these lesions.

KERATINOCYTIC EPIDERMAL NEVUS

AT-A-GLANCE

- The most common variant of epidermal nevi, usually presenting at birth or before adolescence
- Clinical examination: Verrucous papules coalesce to form linear or swirled plaques along the lines of Blaschko.
- Histology: epidermal acanthosis, papillomatosis, and hyperkeratosis
- Differential diagnosis: SK, verruca, nevus sebaceous, lichen striatus, linear psoriasis
- Treatment: Full-thickness excision is regarded as the most definitive.

EPIDEMIOLOGY

Keratinocytic epidermal nevi (linear epidermal nevi, linear verrucous epidermal nevi) are the most common variant of epidermal nevi. They occur in 1 in 1000 live births, without sexual predilection. Most cases are sporadic, but familial cases have been documented.[34]

CLINICAL FEATURES

Keratinocytic epidermal nevi are skin-colored to hyperpigmented verrucous or velvety papules that coalesce

TABLE 108-2
Skin Diseases that May Occur Along Blaschko Lines

Verrucous plaques	Keratinocytic epidermal nevi, nevus sebaceous, incontinentia pigmenti stage 2
Inflammatory plaques	ILVEN, lichen striatus, linear lichen planus, blaschkitis, linear psoriasis, linear porokeratosis, incontinentia pigmenti stages 1 and 2
Spiny or comedonal plaques	Nevus comedonicus, porokeratotic eccrine ostial and dermal duct nevus, linear lichen planopilaris
Atrophic plaques	Linear lichen sclerosus, linear atrophoderma of Moulin, Goltz syndrome (focal dermal hypoplasia), incontinentia pigmenti stage 4
Hyperpigmented patches	Linear and whorled nevoid hypermelanosis, incontinentia pigmenti stage 3
Hypopigmented patches	Linear nevoid hypopigmentation, hypomelanosis of Ito

ILVEN, inflammatory linear verrucous epidermal nevus.

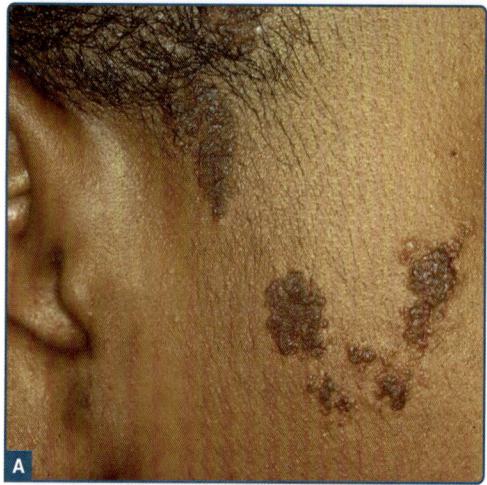
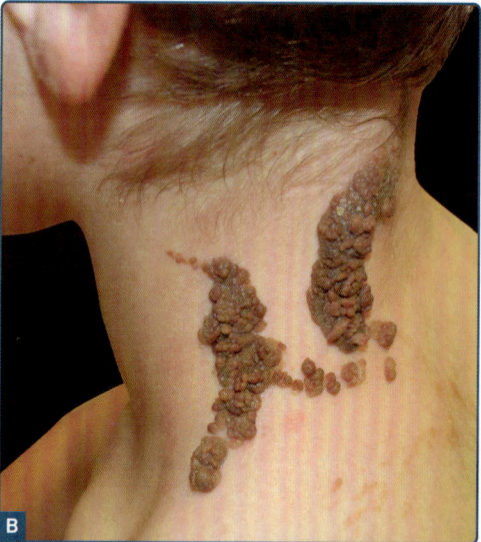

Figure 108-11 Keratinocytic epidermal nevus presenting as brown verrucous plaques arranged along Blaschko lines on the lateral cheek (**A**) and flexural neck (**B**). (Image **B** used with permission from Bernard Cohen, MD.)

to form plaques in a blaschkoid distribution. These lesions occur most commonly on the neck, trunk, and extremities and can appear more pronounced when present on flexural skin (Fig. 108-11). Eighty percent appear at birth or by the first year of life; the rest usually manifest by adolescence. The rare reports of adult onset may represent lesions that were present subclinically, with recent growth having resulted in clinical recognition.

A systematized epidermal nevus refers to a more extensively distributed variant of keratinocytic epidermal nevi. The unilateral subtype is termed nevus unius lateris (Fig. 108-12), but the bilateral subtype is known as ichthyosis hystrix.

ILVEN is a variant that clinically appears psoriasiform (erythematous with thick scale) and can be very pruritic (Fig. 108-13).[34,36] Keratinocytic epidermal nevi can also occur in the context of epidermal nevus syndromes (see section "Epidermal Nevus Syndromes").

ETIOLOGY AND PATHOGENESIS

Keratinocytic epidermal nevi are derived from pluripotent cells in the basal layer of the embryonic epidermis. Although keratinocytes are the predominant affected cell type, there is accompanying overgrowth of the papillary dermis as well. These lesions result from cutaneous mosaicism, particularly postzygotic activating mutations. Hafner and coworkers demonstrated that 40% of keratinocytic epidermal nevi harbor RAS mutations (usually *HRAS*), and another 40% have an *FGFR3* or *PIK3CA* mutation.[37-39] Up to 10% have a mutation in *KRT1* or *KRT10* and characteristically exhibit epidermolytic hyperkeratosis on pathology.[40]

DIAGNOSIS

These hamartomas are usually diagnosed clinically based on the combination of linear morphology, verrucous texture, and young age of the patient. If the diagnosis is in question, a skin biopsy can be done for histopathologic evaluation. Large or extensive epidermal nevi should trigger clinical workup to evaluate for involvement of other organ systems (see section "Epidermal Nevus Syndromes").

HISTOPATHOLOGY

The epidermis shows acanthosis, papillomatosis, and hyperkeratosis (Fig. 108-14). The epidermolytic variant demonstrates marked orthokeratosis with vacuolization and coarse keratohyalin granule deposition within the

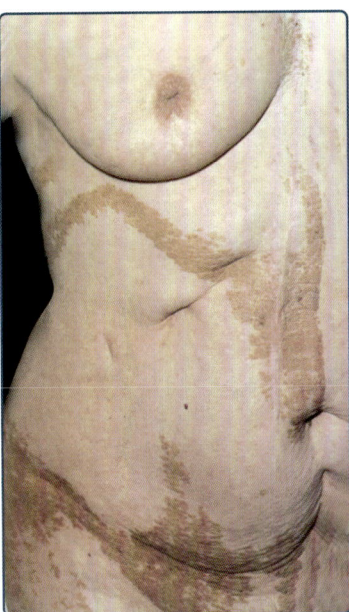

Figure 108-12 Nevus unius lateris, a more extensive variant of keratinocytic epidermal nevi that is limited to one side of the body.

bands of ortho- and parakeratosis in which the granular layer is generally absent under the areas of parakeratosis.

DIFFERENTIAL DIAGNOSIS

The individual papules that make up a plaque may clinically and pathologically resemble a SK or verruca if viewed in isolation. Very early and subtle lesions of keratinocytic epidermal nevi may be macular and can thus resemble linear and whorled nevoid hypermelanosis. Nevus sebaceous may mimic keratinocytic epidermal nevi on clinical examination, but helpful features include their propensity for the head and neck and the characteristic waxy yellow-orange coloration.

ILVEN can be clinically mistaken for lichen striatus, but the latter typically has an abrupt onset, is self-limited, and has a lichenoid reaction pattern on biopsy.[41] Unlike linear psoriasis, ILVEN tends to be treatment resistant.[42] Cases of linear psoriasis may also be accompanied by a family history of psoriasis, late onset, and features of traditional psoriasis elsewhere on examination. Histologically, linear psoriasis may have more confluent parakeratosis as would be seen in plaque psoriasis.

COURSE AND COMPLICATIONS

Although congenital lesions tend to be quiescent, those that present after birth can enlarge before stabilizing in size around puberty.[34] Intertriginous lesions may become macerated and secondarily infected, but the majority remain unaffected after adolescence. Rarely, cutaneous malignancies such as BCC or SCC have been reported to arise within keratinocytic epidermal nevi during adulthood.[43]

If histopathologic evaluation of an epidermal nevus reveals features of epidermolytic hyperkeratosis, the patient is at risk of having a child with epidermolytic ichthyosis if the postzygotic mutation for K1 or K10 is also present in gonadal tissue. Prenatal counseling is therefore important for this subset of patients.

granular layer, defined as epidermolytic hyperkeratosis. ILVEN displays chronic dermal inflammatory infiltrate, psoriasiform epidermal hyperplasia, and alternating

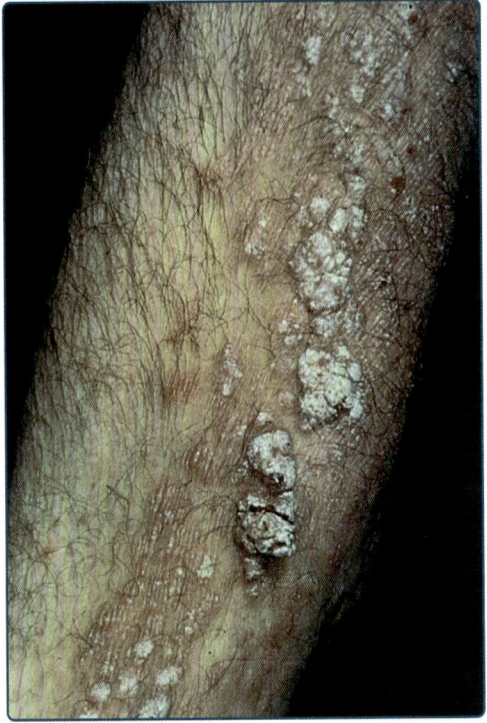

Figure 108-13 Inflammatory linear verrucous epidermal nevus, a rare variant characterized by recalcitrant pruritus, erythema, and scaling.

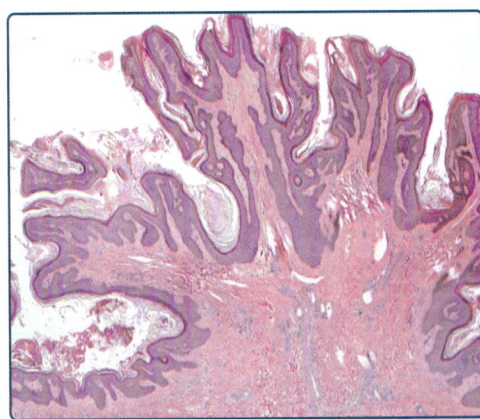

Figure 108-14 Keratinocytic epidermal nevus showing hyperkeratosis, acanthosis, and papillomatosis.

TREATMENT

If the patient desires removal, full-thickness surgical excision is considered the most definitive form of treatment. The low recurrence rate with this procedure is likely due to removal of the superficial dermal component of the lesion.[44] Destructive modalities such as laser ablation, electrofulguration, cryotherapy, and medium- to full-depth chemical peels may offer partial or full clearance. Like psoriasis, ILVEN may be treated with topical steroids, topical retinoids, or calcipotriene, but these medications usually provide little relief.[36]

NEVUS SEBACEOUS

AT-A-GLANCE

- Clinical examination: hairless waxy yellow linear plaque presenting on the head and neck between birth and adolescence
- Histology: epidermal hyperplasia, immature hair follicles, and increased sebaceous and/or apocrine glands
- Various benign and malignant neoplasms can arise within nevus sebaceous, such as trichoblastoma, syringocystadenoma papilliferum, or BCC.
- Differential diagnosis: epidermal nevus, syringocystadenoma papilliferum, SK, juvenile xanthogranuloma, cutaneous mastocytoma
- Treatment: Full-thickness excision should be considered on a case-by-case basis.
- Rapidly growing papules or nodules require pathologic evaluation to rule out malignancy.

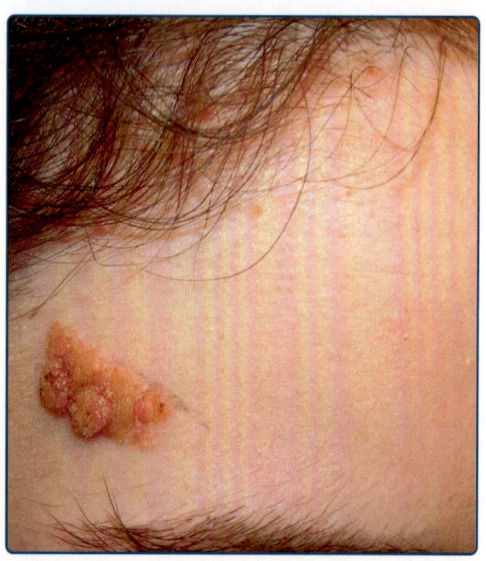

Figure 108-15 Nevus sebaceous appearing as a waxy yellow-orange linear verrucous plaque.

EPIDEMIOLOGY

Nevus sebaceous (nevus sebaceus of Jadassohn, organoid nevus) is a variant of epidermal nevus characterized by epidermal hyperplasia, immature hair follicles, and sweat gland overgrowth. These lesions occur in 0.1% to 0.3% of live births and have an equal male-female prevalence.[45] Cases are typically sporadic, but familial cases have been described.

CLINICAL FEATURES

Nevus sebaceous presents as hairless, yellow, waxy and verrucous plaques following a blaschkoid pattern (Fig. 108-15). These lesions can be subtle at birth, later becoming more elevated and verrucous under the hormonal influences of puberty.[46] They present most commonly on the scalp and can rarely occur elsewhere on the head and neck.

ETIOLOGY AND PATHOGENESIS

Like keratinocytic epidermal nevi, nevus sebaceous is a product of an activating postzygotic mutation. More than 90% are believed to harbor an *HRAS* mutation and less frequently a *KRAS* mutation.[47-49] The same genes appear to be affected in nevus sebaceous syndrome, also called Schimmelpenning syndrome (see section "Epidermal Nevus Syndrome").

DIAGNOSIS

Nevus sebaceous is usually diagnosed clinically based on the combination of linear morphology, waxy yellow coloration, location on the scalp, and young age of the patient. If the diagnosis is not certain, a skin biopsy can be performed.

HISTOPATHOLOGY

Histologic findings consist of epidermal hyperplasia, immature and vellus hair follicles, ectopic apocrine glands, and sebaceous glands located in the superficial dermis (Fig. 108-16). In prepubescent patients, the sebaceous glands usually appear immature and decreased in number.

DIFFERENTIAL DIAGNOSIS

Epidermal nevi are clinically similar to nevus sebaceous but tend to be uncommon on the scalp and face. A skin biopsy can be done to distinguish between these entities. Syringocystadenoma papilliferum is a rare benign tumor that is usually located on the scalp, either in isolation or within a nevus sebaceous. The papillomatous architecture resembles a nevus sebaceous on clinical examination but can be easily differentiated on histology. Less linear lesions of nevus sebaceous can mimic a SK in adults or a juvenile xanthogranuloma or solitary mastocytoma in children.

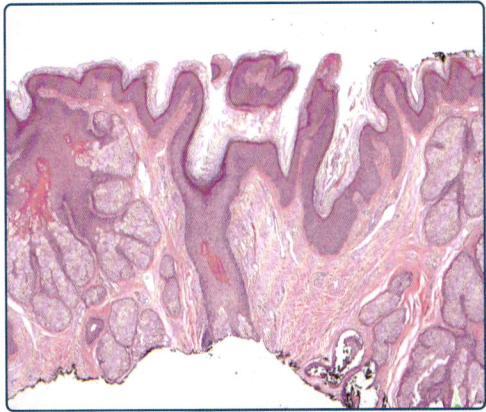

Figure 108-16 Nevus sebaceous showing hyperkeratosis, acanthosis, papillomatosis and increased sebaceous glands in the superficial dermis. A deeper sample may reveal the presence of ectopic apocrine glands.

Abrupt growth seen within a nevus sebaceous should alert the clinician to evaluate for a possible secondary malignancy.

COURSE AND COMPLICATIONS

After puberty, nevus sebaceous become more thickened and verrucous because of hormonal influences. About 25% of affected individuals will go on to develop benign or malignant (or both) secondary neoplasms within their nevus sebaceous.[45,46] Malignant growths are usually seen in older individuals but have occasionally been reported in children.[50]

The most common benign and malignant tumors found within nevus sebaceous are listed in Table 108-3.[50] Of those listed, the most common are trichoblastoma (7% of nevus sebaceous cases) and syringocystadenoma papilliferum (5%).[50] It was previously believed that individuals with nevus sebaceous were at a significantly elevated risk for BCC, but subsequent reviews have concluded that many diagnoses of trichoblastoma may have been overdiagnosed as BCC.[46,51] The risk for developing true BCCs is currently believed to be closer to 1%.[46,51]

TABLE 108-3

Neoplasms Associated with Nevus Sebaceous[a]

BENIGN NEOPLASMS	MALIGNANT NEOPLASMS
Trichoblastoma	Basal cell carcinoma
Syringocystadenoma papilliferum	Sebaceous carcinoma
Apocrine/eccrine adenoma	Squamous cell carcinoma
Trichilemmoma	Keratoacanthoma
Benign melanocytic nevus	Apocrine carcinoma
Sebaceoma	Eccrine porocarcinoma

[a]Within each column, the tumors are listed in decreasing order of frequency.

TREATMENT

Like other epidermal nevi, nevus sebaceous can be definitively treated with full-thickness surgical excision if there are cosmetic or psychosocial concerns. It is still debated whether these lesions' association with cutaneous malignancy warrant prophylactic removal, and if so, the appropriate timing for excision.[46,51] Watchful waiting is currently considered an acceptable option.[35] Alternatives to surgical excision include laser resurfacing and dermabrasion; however, these modalities only partially remove the lesion and do not curb the risk of future neoplasms.[52] Whenever a rapidly growing papule or nodule is observed within a nevus sebaceous, biopsy or excision should be conducted for pathologic evaluation.

NEVUS COMEDONICUS

AT-A-GLANCE

- Clinical examination: localized linear plaque composed of comedones and occasionally inflammatory acne lesions
- Histology: keratin-filled epidermal invaginations associated with atrophic pilosebaceous units
- Differential diagnosis: acne vulgaris, milia, acne neonatorum, nevus sebaceous, linear Darier disease
- Treatment: Full-thickness excision is regarded as the most definitive.

CLINICAL FEATURES

Nevus comedonicus (acneiform nevus) are rare hamartomas of the pilosebaceous unit that appear as localized plaques of comedonal acne at the time of birth or early childhood (Fig. 108-17). The lesions have an either clustered or linear distribution and most commonly occur on the face, chest, or upper arms. Although the noninflammatory variant is usually asymptomatic, the inflammatory form can result in significant suppuration and pain. Nevus comedonicus syndrome is the association of nevus comedonicus with noncutaneous findings such as skeletal defects, cerebral abnormalities, and cataracts.[53]

ETIOLOGY AND PATHOGENESIS

NEK9 kinase, a potential regulator of follicular homeostasis, has been postulated to be defective in nevus comedonicus.[49]

DIAGNOSIS

The diagnosis is usually made clinically.

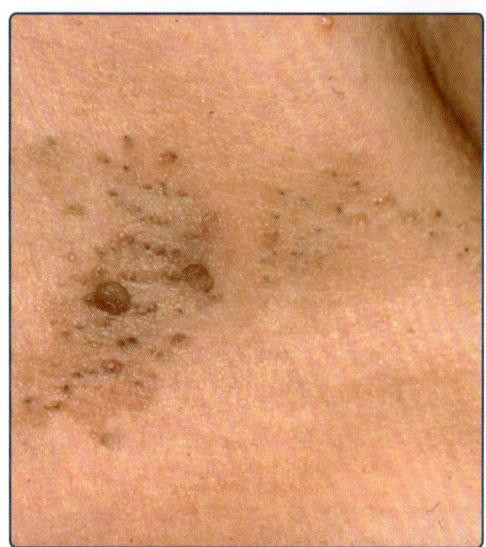

Figure 108-17 Nevus comedonicus presenting as a localized linear plaque composed of open and closed comedones. The two associated tan papules may correspond to areas of keratinocytic epidermal nevus-like changes.

EPIDERMAL NEVUS SYNDROME

AT-A-GLANCE

- *Epidermal nevus syndrome* is a term collectively describing several distinct syndromes that all demonstrate an epidermal nevus occurring in the context of other developmental abnormalities.
- Patients with extensive epidermal nevi and those with epidermal nevi and any systemic abnormalities should be screened for these syndromes.
- The most common extracutaneous features involve the ocular, neurologic, and skeletal systems.
- Management requires a multidisciplinary approach involving a dermatologist, pediatrician, ophthalmologist, neurologist, plastic surgeon, and orthopedic services.

HISTOPATHOLOGY

The hallmark histologic findings are keratin-filled epidermal invaginations in association with atrophic sebaceous glands or follicles.

DIFFERENTIAL DIAGNOSIS

The differential diagnosis includes acne vulgaris, milia, acne neonatorum, nevus sebaceous, and linear Darier disease.

COURSE AND COMPLICATIONS

Nevus comedonicus are persistent lesions. Some cases may develop inflammatory acne cysts, which can subsequently result in scarring. Malignant transformation of these lesions is extremely rare.[53] On initial clinical examination, the patient should be evaluated for features of nevus comedonicus syndrome. There seems to be no correlation between the size or extent of the lesion with risk for systemic anomalies.[53]

TREATMENT

Treatment can be reserved for cosmetically bothersome or symptomatic cases. Mild improvement can be achieved with emollients, keratolytics, topical steroids (for inflammatory lesions), and topical retinoids. Oral retinoids or destructive modalities have shown only limited efficacy, with best results being achieved with laser resurfacing. Full-thickness surgical excision is regarded as the most definitive option.

Epidermal nevus syndrome is loosely defined as the association of an epidermal nevus with any of various extracutaneous anomalies, most commonly of the ocular, neurologic, and skeletal systems (Table 108-4). These patients may exhibit other cutaneous abnormalities in addition to epidermal nevi. The above clinical phenotype is now known to encompass distinct diseases with differing genetic profiles of postzygotic mosaicism. Some of the well-characterized variants and their corresponding epidermal nevi are summarized in Table 108-5.[35,54-56]

Becker nevus syndrome is another well-known variant characterized by a segmental smooth muscle hamartoma in association with musculoskeletal defects such as ipsilateral breast hypoplasia.[35] Angora hair nevus syndrome consists of an epidermal hamartoma with long, fine white hair in addition to ocular, neurologic, and skeletal deficiencies.

DIAGNOSIS, COURSE AND COMPLICATIONS, AND TREATMENT

Patients with extensive epidermal nevi or those with concurrent systemic abnormalities should be promptly evaluated for an underlying epidermal nevus syndrome.[35] Evaluation and management of patients with an epidermal nevus syndrome requires a multidisciplinary approach involving a dermatologist, pediatrician, ophthalmologist, neurologist, plastic surgeon, and orthopedic services. These patients require a careful history with particular attention to developmental history, attainment of milestones, and abnormalities of the bones and eyes. Thorough mucocutaneous, neuro-

CYSTS OF EPIDERMAL ORIGIN

AT-A-GLANCE

- Many common cysts result from a plugged pilosebaceous unit.
  - Epidermoid cysts: derived from the infundibular portion of hair follicle and thus show flattened surface epithelium and keratohyaline granules
  - Trichilemmal cysts: lining resembles the isthmic portion of hair follicle and thus show a scalloped surface epithelium lacking a granular layer
  - Milia: thought to be the result of plugging of a vellus hair follicle or eccrine sweat duct; resemble small epidermal cysts
  - Steatocystoma: a sebaceous duct cyst characterized by a waxy, eosinophilic cuticle lining the cyst and characteristic sebaceous glands in the cyst walls
- Developmental cysts are much less common.
  - Dermoid cysts: collections of epidermis located along embryologic fusion planes, most commonly on the forehead, lateral eye, or neck
  - Branchial cysts: asymptomatic cysts caused by occlusion of branchial cleft sinuses that are located along the angle of the mandible if arising from the first branchial cleft and the middle to lower third of the anterior border of the sternocleidomastoid in cases arising from the second branchial cleft
  - Preauricular cysts or sinuses: epithelial invaginations located in the preauricular area that arise from the incomplete fusion of the first and second branchial arches in the preauricular area
- Removal of the entire cyst wall is required to prevent cyst recurrence.

TABLE 108-5
Variants of Epidermal Nevi and Their Associated Syndromes

EPIDERMAL NEVI TYPE	SYNDROMIC ASSOCIATIONS
Keratinocytic epidermal nevi (nonepidermolytic)	*HRAS/FGFR3* mutation: craniofacial, skeletal, and CNS anomalies (eg, mental retardation, seizures) Proteus syndrome (*AKT1* mutation): palmoplantar cerebriform hyperplasia, asymmetrical macrodactyly, soft tissue overgrowth; epidermal nevi characteristically soft and flat Type 2 segmental Cowden disease (*PTEN* mutation): focal segmental glomerulosclerosis, soft tissue overgrowth, colon polyps; epidermal nevi characteristically thick and papillomatous (also called linear Cowden nevi)
ILVEN	CHILD syndrome (*NSDHL* mutation): ipsilateral bone, visceral, and neurologic defects; epidermal nevi lateralized with flexural affinity
Nevus sebaceous	Schimmelpenning syndrome (*HRAS/KRAS* mutation): ocular (eg, lipodermoid, coloboma, cerebral, and skeletal anomalies Phakomatosis pigmentokeratotica (*HRAS* mutation): CNS anomalies; speckled lentiginous nevi and epidermal nevi following checkerboard pattern
Nevus comedonicus	Nevus comedonicus syndrome: ocular (eg, ipsilateral cataract, corneal erosion), skeletal, and CNS anomalies

CHILD, congenital hemidysplasia with ichthyosiform nevus and limb defects; CNS, central nervous system; ILVEN, inflammatory linear verrucous epidermal nevus.

logic, ophthalmologic, and orthopedic examinations are necessary, and a regular follow-up program should be planned for the patient.

TABLE 108-4
Systemic Manifestations Seen in Syndromes Associated with Epidermal Nevi

SYSTEM	SYSTEMIC MANIFESTATIONS
Skeletal	Craniofacial defects, frontal bossing, kyphoscoliosis, limb deformities, vertebral defects, hypophosphatemic rickets
Neurologic	Mental retardation, seizures, hemiparesis, sensory-motor neuropathy, cortical atrophy, hypoplasia of corpus callosum, spinal dysraphism
Ocular	Optic nerve deformities, corneal defects
Cutaneous	Lipomas, angiomas, soft tissue overgrowth

EPIDERMOID CYST

ETIOLOGY AND PATHOGENESIS

Epidermoid cysts (follicular cyst-infundibular type, keratin cyst, epidermal cyst, epidermal inclusion cyst, or epithelial cyst) are most commonly the result of plugged pilosebaceous units. The term *sebaceous cyst* is a misnomer and should be avoided because these cysts do not involve sebaceous glands, nor do they contain sebum. These cysts are lined by epithelium resembling the infundibulum of the hair follicle and express the same cytokeratin profile[57] and thus are thought to be derived from this structure. On non–hair-bearing sites such as the palms and soles, epidermoid cysts are thought to be the result of traumatic implantation of epidermal cells into deeper tissues or by cyst formation in an eccrine duct.[58,59] HPV types 57 and 60 DNA have been detected in palmoplantar epidermoid cysts.[60,61]

CLINICAL FEATURES

Epidermoid cysts are classically dermal or subcutaneous mobile nodules with a central punctum (Fig. 108-18). The punctum, when present, represents the plugged pilosebaceous unit from which foul-smelling cheesy debris may be expressed. They are most commonly found on the upper chest, upper back, neck, or head. The lesions thought to be traumatic in origin are most often seen on the palms, soles, or buttocks. Cysts are usually slow growing and asymptomatic. Cyst rupture is common. Although the clinical course of epidermoid cysts is benign, rarely, BCC, SCC, epithelioid carcinoma, and other malignancies have been reported to occur in conjunction with these cysts.[62-64]

EPIDEMIOLOGY

Epidermoid cysts are found most commonly in adults, both men and women. Genetic disorders, such as Gorlin syndrome (nevoid BCC syndrome), pachyonychia congenita type 2 (Jackson-Lawler type), and Gardner syndrome, may predispose individuals to having this type of cyst.

DIFFERENTIAL DIAGNOSIS

Steatocystomas, pilar cysts, and lipomas can all mimic epidermoid cysts. However, clinically, steatocystomas usually express a liquid rather than a cheesy material. Pilar cysts are most commonly on the scalp, and lipomas are softer and deeper and lack a punctum. Histopathology also distinguishes among these lesions.

HISTOPATHOLOGY

An epidermoid cyst has a stratified, squamous lining with an intact granular layer (Fig. 108-19). These cysts contain orthokeratotic debris. When released into the dermis and surrounding tissues, the keratin can incite a foreign-body reaction of multinucleated giant cells and histiocytes.

TREATMENT

Complete excision or destruction of the cyst lining is the definitive treatment and is required to prevent cyst recurrence. If a cyst becomes inflamed, painful, or purulent, incision and drainage should be performed, and infection must be considered. Common microbes associated with cyst infection include *Staphylococcus aureus*, group A streptococcus, *Escherichia coli*, *Peptostreptococcus* spp., and *Bacteroides* spp. Polymicrobial infection is most common. Wound cultures with directed therapy may be indicated based on the clinical presentation of the lesion. If the cyst has ruptured or has become infected, excision of the lesion should be deferred until the inflammation has decreased, which will decrease the likelihood of wound dehiscence. For small, inflamed, symptomatic lesions, intralesional steroids may be considered.

TRICHILEMMAL CYST (PILAR CYST)

ETIOLOGY AND PATHOGENESIS

Pilar cysts arise from the epithelium located between the orifice of the sebaceous gland and the arrector pili muscle. This squamous epithelium undergoes rapid keratinization, resulting in a cyst wall without a granular layer.

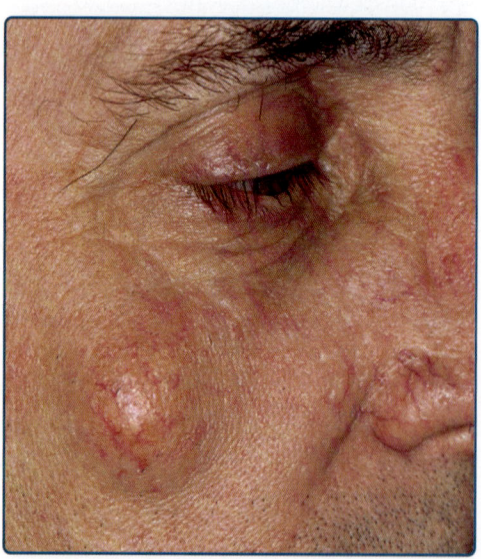

Figure 108-18 Epidermoid cyst presenting as a dome-shaped protuberance of the cheek.

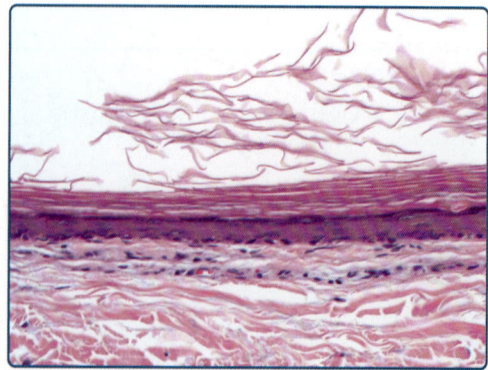

Figure 108-19 Epidermoid cyst lined by stratified epithelium with a granular layer. Within the cyst, the keratinous material is arranged in laminated layers.

CLINICAL FEATURES

Pilar cysts are mobile, firm, well-circumscribed nodules located overwhelmingly in the scalp (Fig. 108-20). These lesions can also be found on the face, head, and neck. Although these lesions largely remain asymptomatic, rupture and infection can occur. Most patients have more than one lesion, with 10% of people having more than 10 lesions. Rapid growth is abnormal and can be a sign of infection or malignant transformation.[65]

EPIDEMIOLOGY

Trichilemmal cysts can be found in 5% to 10% of the population, most commonly in middle-aged women.

DIFFERENTIAL DIAGNOSIS

See section "Differential Diagnosis" under Epidermoid Cyst.

HISTOPATHOLOGY

Trichilemmal cysts arise from the outer root sheath of the hair follicle, and thus are characterized by the absence of a granular layer and eosinophilic keratin contents (Fig. 108-21). If abundant folds and lobules of squamous epithelium are seen in the walls of the lesion, it is most likely a proliferating trichilemmal cyst. Extensive cellular atypia and invasion of the cyst lining into the surrounding tissue are indicative of a malignant proliferating pilar tumor.

TREATMENT

The treatment is the same as with epidermoid cysts. Because the cyst wall of these tumors is typically less adherent to the surrounding stroma than epidermoid cysts, it is possible to extract the lesion through a small incision made with a dermal punch trephine.

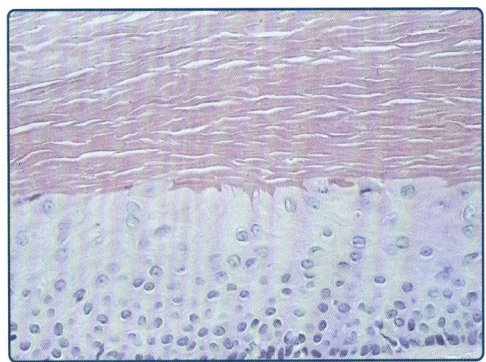

Figure 108-21 Trichilemmal cysts showing an epithelial lining that lacks a granular layer.

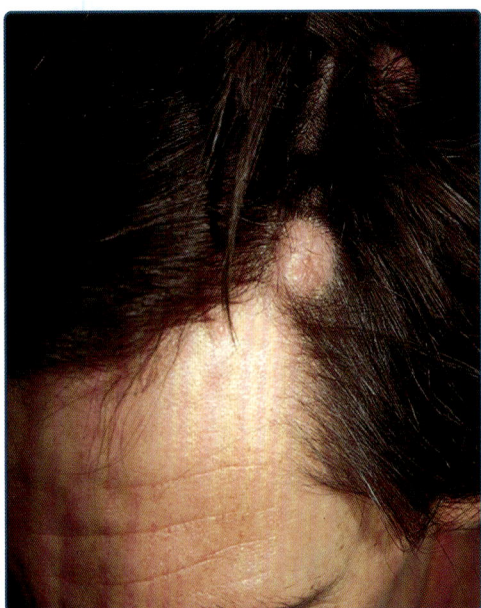

Figure 108-20 A trichilemmal (pilar) cyst on the scalp.

MILIUM

ETIOLOGY AND PATHOGENESIS

Milia are thought to result from pilosebaceous or eccrine sweat duct plugging. These superficial lesions can be primary or secondary, with the latter resulting from injury to the basement membrane of the skin. Secondary lesions are common in patients with burns, in subepidermal blistering diseases such as epidermolysis bullosa and porphyria, after dermabrasion or ablative laser resurfacing, or in conjunction with topical therapy such as glucocorticoid therapy or 5-fluorouracil treatment.[66-69]

CLINICAL FEATURES

Milia are 1- to 2-mm, white, domed papules commonly located on the cheeks and eyelids of adults (Fig. 108-22). In infants, milia are common on the face and the mucosa. Epstein pearls are milia on the palate. Eruptive milia have been reported, though this is a rare occurrence.[69] Milia en plaque is a plaque-type, inflammatory variant of milia that is commonly located on the ear.[70] Acquired milia can be located anywhere the predisposing trauma or other factors have occurred.

EPIDEMIOLOGY

Milia are common congenital and acquired lesions in both infants and adults. Men and women are affected equally.

DIFFERENTIAL DIAGNOSIS

Closed comedones may appear clinically similarly in isolation, but comedones are more likely to contain a mixture of bacteria, keratinaceous debris, and hair shaft fragments.

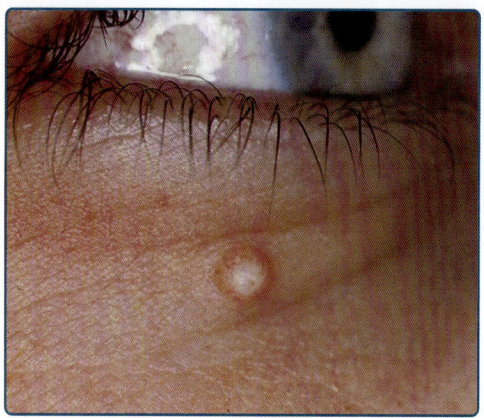

Figure 108-22 Primary milium. A 3-mm, hard, seedlike white papule.

HISTOPATHOLOGY

Milia are minute epidermoid cysts, lined by stratified squamous epithelium and filled with keratin. Occasionally, a connection to eccrine ducts or vellus hair follicles may be observed. Bacteria are not usually present.

TREATMENT

Congenital milia tend to spontaneously resolve. Acquired milia can resolve spontaneously as well but can also be removed by disrupting the overlying epidermis with light electro-desiccation or incision followed by expression of the keratin contents.

STEATOCYSTOMA

ETIOLOGY AND PATHOGENESIS

Steatocystoma multiplex (sebocystomatosis, epidermal polycystic disease) can be a sporadic or autosomal-dominant disorder. These lesions can also be found in syndromes such as Alagille syndrome and pachyonychia congenita type II. In the latter, lesions are associated with mutations in K17. Sporadic solitary lesions are termed *steatocystoma simplex*.

CLINICAL FEATURES

These lesions present as asymptomatic, yellow or skin-colored dermal papules or cysts located most commonly on the trunk, upper arms, scrotum, or chest (Fig. 108-23). Oily material can be expressed from these lesions when incised. These lesions can become infected and suppurate, resulting in sinus formation and scarring.

EPIDEMIOLOGY

It is relatively rare, and the true incidence is unknown. The average age of onset is 26 years old, with no sex predilection.[71]

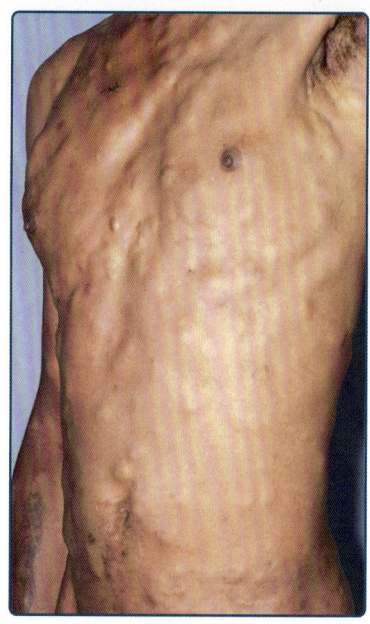

Figure 108-23 Steatocystoma multiplex. Multiple skin-colored cystic lesions on the trunk.

DIFFERENTIAL DIAGNOSIS

Eruptive vellus hair cysts can mimic steatocystoma multiplex clinically. They may have a tuft of hairs protruding from the cyst centrally, with findings of vellus hairs in the lumen with follicles in the wall. Epidermal inclusion cysts also have to be excluded. The pathogenesis of steatocystoma, epidermal inclusion cysts, and eruptive vellus hair cysts may be similar.[72]

HISTOPATHOLOGY

The cyst walls of steatocystoma multiplex are composed of stratified, squamous epithelium with an absent granular layer and an eosinophilic cuticle on the luminal side. Sebaceous glands are characteristically located in the cyst wall, and keratin, oil, and hairs are typically found in the lumen.

TREATMENT

Simple excision or drainage with manual removal of the cyst wall may facilitate the clinical resolution of lesions.[73,74] Inflamed lesions have been reported to respond to intralesional steroids, carbon dioxide laser, oral retinoids, or cryotherapy.[75]

DERMOID CYST

ETIOLOGY AND PATHOGENESIS

Dermoid cysts are epithelial-lined cysts containing various appendageal structures resulting from retained epithelium along embryonic fusion planes. These cysts are either congenital or develop in childhood.

CLINICAL FEATURES

Dermoid cysts are smooth, can occur in the midline, and commonly possess a deep sinus tract that connects to the epidermis. They can measure between 1 cm and 4 cm and are most commonly located on the forehead, lateral eye, or neck.[76,77] A superficial dermoid cyst located on the dorsal nose is referred to as fistula of the dorsum of the nose and is characterized by a central tuft of hair or communication intracranially. Dermoid cysts can be located deep in the subcutaneous tissue, intracranially, or intraorbitally.[78] Infections, rupture, and abscess formation from the manipulation of these cysts can potentially lead to serious complications.

EPIDEMIOLOGY

The prevalence is equal in men and women.

DIFFERENTIAL DIAGNOSIS

The differential diagnosis of dermoid cysts includes gliomas, encephaloceles, hemangiomas, soft tissue sarcomas, and other epidermal cysts such as branchial cleft cysts and thyroglossal duct cysts.

HISTOPATHOLOGY

Cysts are lined by stratified squamous epithelium and typically contain keratin and hairs. Adnexal structures are characteristically present in the cyst walls and may include pilosebaceous units, apocrine or eccrine glands, smooth muscle bundles, or goblet cells.

TREATMENT

Imaging studies that help to characterize the extent of the tumor are necessary before excision is undertaken. Consultation with neurosurgery, otolaryngology, or plastic surgery may be indicated.

BRANCHIAL CYST (BRANCHIAL CLEFT CYST)

ETIOLOGY AND PATHOGENESIS

Sequestration of first or second branchial cleft membranes results in these cysts, sinuses, or tags.

CLINICAL FEATURES

These asymptomatic lesions are often located along the angle of the mandible if arising from the first branchial cleft and the middle to lower third of the anterior border of the sternocleidomastoid in cases arising from the second branchial cleft. They may present after an upper respiratory infection as a painful mass. These lesions tend to drain internally, but communication with the epidermis can occur. Branchial cysts may become complicated by infection.

EPIDEMIOLOGY

Branchial cleft cysts are largely sporadic, but autosomal-dominant cases have been reported. There is no gender predominance. Ten percent of lesions are bilateral.

DIFFERENTIAL DIAGNOSIS

Branchial cleft cysts are can be distinguished from bronchogenic cysts by their lateral location and by histologic features, namely the presence of lymphoid follicles and the lack of smooth muscle in the cyst walls.

HISTOPATHOLOGY

Branchial cleft cysts are lined with epithelium containing a lymphocytic infiltrate and lymphoid follicles are common. Mucous glands may be found in the walls, and in these cases, the cyst contents are often mucinous.

TREATMENT

Excision is the treatment of choice. Infected cysts may require incision and drainage or antibiotic therapy.

PREAURICULAR CYST AND SINUS (CONGENITAL AURICULAR FISTULA, EAR PITS)

ETIOLOGY AND PATHOGENESIS

Preauricular cysts or sinuses are congenital epithelial invaginations. They are thought to reflect a local defect in embryonic fusion planes. They are often sporadic but may also be inherited as an autosomal-dominant trait with variable expression. They have been associated with branchial cleft anomalies and hearing and renal abnormalities.[79]

CLINICAL FEATURES

Ear pits are located in the preauricular area near the ascending limb of the helix. They can be unilateral or bilateral and are more common on the right side.

EPIDEMIOLOGY

They occur in approximately 1% of infants, with a higher incidence in certain African regions.[79]

HISTOPATHOLOGY

Ear pits are lined by stratified squamous epithelium and often show overlying hyperkeratosis.

TREATMENT

Assessment for hearing loss or associated syndromes should be completed. Simple excision may be performed if eradication of the pit is desired.

ACKNOWLEDGMENTS

This chapter was revised and updated from the former version written by Valencia D. Thomas, Nicholas R. Snavely, Ken K. Lee, and Neil A. Swanson, and we thank them for their contribution.

REFERENCES

1. Li X, Zhu W. A case of seborrheic keratosis distributed along skin cleavage lines. *J Dermatol*. 1998;25(4):272-274.
2. Mabuchi T, Akasaka E, Kondoh A, et al. Seborrheic keratosis that follows Blaschko's lines. *J Dermatol*. 2008;35(5):301-303.
3. Schwartz RA. Sign of Leser-Trelat. *J Am Acad Dermatol*. 1996;35(1):88-95.
4. Schwengle LE, Rampen FH. Eruptive seborrheic keratoses associated with erythrodermic pityriasis rubra pilaris. Possible role of retinoid therapy. *Acta Derm Venereol*. 1988;68(5):443-445.
5. Inamadar AC, Palit A. Eruptive seborrhoeic keratosis in human immunodeficiency virus infection: a coincidence or "the sign of Leser-Trelat"? *Br J Dermatol*. 2003;149(2):435-436.
6. Patton T, Zirwas M, Nieland-Fisher N, et al. Inflammation of seborrheic keratoses caused by cytarabine: a pseudo sign of Leser-Trelat. *J Drugs Dermatol*. 2004;3(5):565-566.
7. Cascajo CD, Reichel M, Sanchez JL. Malignant neoplasms associated with seborrheic keratoses. An analysis of 54 cases. *Am J Dermatopathol*. 1996;18(3):278-282.
8. Vun Y, De'Ambrosis B, Spelman L, et al. Seborrhoeic keratosis and malignancy: collision tumour or malignant transformation? *Australas J Dermatol*. 2006;47(2):106-108.
9. Yeatman JM, Kilkenny M, Marks R. The prevalence of seborrhoeic keratoses in an Australian population: does exposure to sunlight play a part in their frequency? *Br J Dermatol*. 1997;137(3):411-414.
10. Nakamura H, Hirota S, Adachi S, et al. Clonal nature of seborrheic keratosis demonstrated by using the polymorphism of the human androgen receptor locus as a marker. *J Invest Dermatol*. 2001;116(4):506-510.
11. Hafner C, Lopez-Knowles E, Luis NM, et al. Oncogenic PIK3CA mutations occur in epidermal nevi and seborrheic keratoses with a characteristic mutation pattern. *Proc Natl Acad Sci U S A*. 2007;104(33):13450-13454.
12. Hafner C, Toll A, Fernández-Casado A, et al. Multiple oncogenic mutations and clonal relationship in spatially distinct benign human epidermal tumors. *Proc Natl Acad Sci U S A*. 2010;107(48):20780-5.
13. Manaka L, Kadono S, Kawashima M, et al. The mechanism of hyperpigmentation in seborrhoeic keratosis involves the high expression of endothelin-converting enzyme-1alpha and TNF-alpha, which stimulate secretion of endothelin 1. *Br J Dermatol*. 2001;145(6):895-903.
14. Li YH, Chen G, Dong XP, et al. Detection of epidermodysplasia verruciformis-associated human papillomavirus DNA in nongenital seborrhoeic keratosis. *Br J Dermatol*. 2004;151(5):1060-1065.
15. Tardio JC, Bancalari E, Moreno A, et al. Genital seborrheic keratoses are human papillomavirus-related lesions. A linear array genotyping test study. *APMIS*. 2012;120(6):477-483.
16. Meyerson LB. A peculiar papulosquamous eruption involving pigmented nevi. *Arch Dermatol*. 1971;103(5):510-512.
17. Tsuji T, Morita A. Giant seborrheic keratosis on the frontal scalp treated with topical fluorouracil. *J Dermatol*. 1995;22(1):74-75.
18. Pepper E. Dermabrasion for the treatment of a giant seborrheic keratosis. *J Dermatol Surg Oncol*. 1985;11(6):646-647.
19. Valerio E, Giordano C, Mameli S, et al. Facial lichen striatus. *Arch Dis Child*. 2016;101(12):1148.
20. Tosti A, Peluso AM, Misciali C, et al. Nail lichen striatus: clinical features and long-term follow-up of five patients. *J Am Acad Dermatol*. 1997;36(6 Pt 1):908-913.
21. Patrizi A, Neri I, Fiorentini C, et al. Lichen striatus: clinical and laboratory features of 115 children. *Pediatr Dermatol*. 2004;21(3):197-204.
22. Kus S, Ince U. Lichen striatus in an adult patient treated with pimecrolimus. *J Eur Acad Dermatol Venereol*. 2006;20(3):360-361.
23. Sorgentini C, Allevato MA, Dahbar M, et al. Lichen striatus in an adult: successful treatment with tacrolimus. *Br J Dermatol*. 2004;150(4):776-777.
24. Degos R, Delort J, Civatte J, et al. Epidermal tumor with an unusual appearance: clear cell acanthoma. *Ann Dermatol Syphiligr (Paris)*. 1962;89:361-371.
25. Ohnishi T, Watanabe S. Immunohistochemical characterization of keratin expression in clear cell acanthoma. *Br J Dermatol*. 1995;133(2):186-193.
26. Finch TM, Tan CY. Clear cell acanthoma developing on a psoriatic plaque: further evidence of an inflammatory aetiology? *Br J Dermatol*. 2000;142(4):842-844.
27. Murphy R, Kesseler ME, Slater DN. Giant clear cell acanthoma. *Br J Dermatol*. 2000;143(5):1114-1115.

28. Blum A, Metzler G, Bauer J, et al. The dermatoscopic pattern of clear-cell acanthoma resembles psoriasis vulgaris. *Dermatology*. 2001;203(1):50-52.
29. Santa Cruz DJ. Chondrodermatitis nodularis helicis: a transepidermal perforating disorder. *J Cutan Pathol*. 1980;7(2):70-76.
30. Magro CM, Frambach GE, Crowson AN. Chondrodermatitis nodularis helicis as a marker of internal disease [corrected] associated with microvascular injury. *J Cutan Pathol*. 2005;32(5):329-333.
31. Elgart ML. Cell phone chondrodermatitis. *Arch Dermatol*. 2000;136(12):1568.
32. Goette DK. Chondrodermatitis nodularis chronica helicis: a perforating necrobiotic granuloma. *J Am Acad Dermatol*. 1980;2(2):148-154.
33. Shah S, Fiala KH. Chondrodermatitis nodularis helicis: a review of current therapies. *Dermatol Ther*. 2017;30(1).
34. Brandling-Bennett HA, Morel KD. Epidermal nevi. *Pediatr Clin North Am*. 2010;57(5):1177-1198.
35. Happle R. The group of epidermal nevus syndromes Part I. Well defined phenotypes. *J Am Acad Dermatol*. 2010;63(1):1-22; quiz 23-24.
36. Khachemoune A, Janjua SA, Guldbakke KK. Inflammatory linear verrucous epidermal nevus: a case report and short review of the literature. *Cutis*. 2006;78(4):261-267.
37. Hafner C, Toll A, Gantner S, et al. Keratinocytic epidermal nevi are associated with mosaic RAS mutations. *J Med Genet*. 2012;49(4):249-253.
38. Hafner C, van Oers JM, Vogt T, et al. Mosaicism of activating FGFR3 mutations in human skin causes epidermal nevi. *J Clin Invest*. 2006;116(8):2201-2207.
39. Toll A, Fernandez LC, Pons T, et al. Somatic embryonic FGFR2 mutations in keratinocytic epidermal nevi. *J Invest Dermatol*. 2016;136(8):1718-1721.
40. Paller AS, Syder AJ, Chan YM, et al. Genetic and clinical mosaicism in a type of epidermal nevus. *N Engl J Med*. 1994;331(21):1408-1415.
41. Muller CS, Schmaltz R, Vogt T, et al. Lichen striatus and blaschkitis: reappraisal of the concept of blaschkolinear dermatoses. *Br J Dermatol*. 2011;164(2):257-262.
42. Happle R. Linear psoriasis and ILVEN: is lumping or splitting appropriate? *Dermatology*. 2006;212(2):101-102.
43. Messerschmidt A, Wolter M, Ter-Nedden J, et al. Multiple basal cell carcinomas arising in an epidermal nevus. *J Dtsch Dermatol Ges*. 2016;14(11):1133-1135.
44. Kim R, Marmon S, Kaplan J, et al. Verrucous epidermal nevus. *Dermatol Online J*. 2013;19(12):20707.
45. Aslam A, Salam A, Griffiths CE, et al. Naevus sebaceus: a mosaic RASopathy. *Clin Exp Dermatol*. 2014;39(1):1-6.
46. Moody MN, Landau JM, Goldberg LH. Nevus sebaceous revisited. *Pediatr Dermatol*. 2012;29(1):15-23.
47. Groesser L, Herschberger E, Ruetten A, et al. Postzygotic HRAS and KRAS mutations cause nevus sebaceous and Schimmelpenning syndrome. *Nat Genet*. 2012;44(7):783-787.
48. Happle R. Nevus sebaceus is a mosaic RASopathy. *J Invest Dermatol*. 2013;133(3):597-600.
49. Levinsohn JL, Tian LC, Boyden LM, et al. Whole-exome sequencing reveals somatic mutations in HRAS and KRAS, which cause nevus sebaceus. *J Invest Dermatol*. 2013;133(3):827-830.
50. Idriss MH, Elston DM. Secondary neoplasms associated with nevus sebaceus of Jadassohn: a study of 707 cases. *J Am Acad Dermatol*. 2014;70(2):332-337.
51. Rosen H, Schmidt B, Lam HP, et al. Management of nevus sebaceous and the risk of Basal cell carcinoma: an 18-year review. *Pediatr Dermatol*. 2009;26(6):676-681.
52. Patel P, Malik K, Khachemoune A. Sebaceus and Becker's nevus: overview of their presentation, pathogenesis, associations, and treatment. *Am J Clin Dermatol*. 2015;16(3):197-204.
53. Ferrari B, Taliercio V, Restrepo P, et al. Nevus comedonicus: a case series. *Pediatr Dermatol*. 2015;32(2):216-219.
54. Lindhurst MJ, Sapp JC, Teer JK, et al. A mosaic activating mutation in AKT1 associated with the Proteus syndrome. *N Engl J Med*. 2011;365(7):611-619.
55. Happle R. Type 2 segmental Cowden disease vs. proteus syndrome. *Br J Dermatol*. 2007;156(5):1089-1090.
56. Martinez-Lopez A, Blasco-Morente G, Perez-Lopez I, et al. CLOVES syndrome: review of a PIK3CA-related overgrowth spectrum (PROS). *Clin Genet*. 2017;91(1):14-21.
57. Ohnishi T, Watanabe S. Immunohistochemical analysis of cytokeratin expression in multiple eccrine hidrocystoma. *J Cutan Pathol*. 1999;26(2):91-94.
58. Baker BR, Mitchell DF. The Pathogenesis of Epidermoid Implantation Cysts. *Oral Surg Oral Med Oral Pathol*. 1965;19:494-501.
59. Smirniotopoulos JG, Chiechi MV. Teratomas, dermoids, and epidermoids of the head and neck. *Radiographics*. 1995;15(6):1437-1455.
60. Lee S, Lee W, Chung S, et al. Detection of human papillomavirus 60 in epidermal cysts of nonpalmoplantar location. *Am J Dermatopathol*. 2003;25(3):243-247.
61. Kashima M, Takahama H, Baba T, et al. Detection of human papillomavirus type 57 in the tissue of a plantar epidermoid cyst. *Dermatology*. 2003;207(2):185-187.
62. Delacretaz J. Keratotic basal-cell carcinoma arising from an epidermoid cyst. *J Dermatol Surg Oncol*. 1977;3(3):310-311.
63. Shelley WB, Wood MG. Occult Bowen's disease in keratinous cysts. *Br J Dermatol*. 1981;105(1):105-108.
64. Lopez-Rios F, Rodriguez-Peralto JL, Castano E, et al. Squamous cell carcinoma arising in a cutaneous epidermal cyst: case report and literature review. *Am J Dermatopathol*. 1999;21(2):174-177.
65. Leppard BJ, Sanderson KV. The natural history of trichilemmal cysts. *Br J Dermatol*. 1976;94(4):379-390.
66. Hisa T, Goto Y, Taniguchi S, et al. Post-bullous milia. *Australas J Dermatol*. 1996;37(3):153-154.
67. Iacobelli D, Hashimoto K, Kato I, et al. Clobetasol-induced milia. *J Am Acad Dermatol*. 1989;21(2 Pt 1):215-217.
68. Tsuji T, Kadoya A, Tanaka R, et al. Milia induced by corticosteroids. *Arch Dermatol*. 1986;122(2):139-140.
69. Diba VC, Al-Izzi M, Green T. A case of eruptive milia. *Clin Exp Dermatol*. 2005;30(6):677-678.
70. Stefanidou MP, Panayotides JG, Tosca AD. Milia en plaque: a case report and review of the literature. *Dermatol Surg*. 2002;28(3):291-295.
71. Cho S, Chang SE, Choi JH, et al. Clinical and histologic features of 64 cases of steatocystoma multiplex. *J Dermatol*. 2002;29(3):152-156.
72. Yamada A, Saga K, Jimbow K. Acquired multiple pilosebaceous cysts on the face having the histopathological features of steatocystoma multiplex and eruptive vellus hair cysts. *Int J Dermatol*. 2005;44(10):861-863.
73. Keefe M, Leppard BJ, Royle G. Successful treatment of steatocystoma multiplex by simple surgery. *Br J Dermatol*. 1992;127(1):41-44.
74. Krahenbuhl A, Eichmann A, Pfaltz M. CO2 laser therapy for steatocystoma multiplex. *Dermatologica*.

1991;183(4):294-296.
75. Apaydin R, Bilen N, Bayramgurler D, et al. Steatocystoma multiplex suppurativum: oral isotretinoin treatment combined with cryotherapy. *Australas J Dermatol*. 2000;41(2):98-100.
76. Pryor SG, Lewis JE, Weaver AL, et al. Pediatric dermoid cysts of the head and neck. *Otolaryngol Head Neck Surg*. 2005;132(6):938-942.
77. Weedon D, Strutton G. *Skin Pathology*. 2nd ed. London: Churchill Livingstone; 2002.
78. Golden BA, Zide MF. Cutaneous cysts of the head and neck. *J Oral Maxillofac Surg*. 2005;63(11):1613-1619.
79. Scheinfeld NS, Silverberg NB, Weinberg JM, et al. The preauricular sinus: a review of its clinical presentation, treatment, and associations. *Pediatr Dermatol*. 2004;21(3):191-196.

Chapter 109 :: Appendage Tumors of the Skin
:: Ruth K. Foreman & Lyn McDivitt Duncan

第一百零九章
皮肤附属器肿瘤

中文导读

皮肤附属器肿瘤包括良性肿瘤和恶性肿瘤，传统上根据其向皮肤正常附属器的分化程度进行分类：小汗腺、大汗腺、毛囊和皮脂腺。本章介绍了一系列常见和/或有临床意义的附属器肿瘤，共分为4节：①向小汗腺分化的肿瘤；②向顶泌汗腺方向分化的肿瘤；③向毛囊分化的肿瘤；④向皮脂腺分化的肿瘤。

第一节向小汗腺分化的肿瘤，介绍了良性肿瘤中的汗腺腺瘤、汗孔瘤、皮肤圆柱瘤、螺旋腺瘤、汗管瘤的流行病学及临床特征、病因及发病机制、组织病理学、鉴别诊断、临床病程和预后及临床管理。恶性肿瘤中介绍了汗腺癌、汗孔癌、圆柱癌/螺旋癌、指趾乳头状腺癌、微囊性附属器癌的流行病学及临床特征、病因及发病机制、组织病理学、鉴别诊断、临床病程和预后及临床管理。

第二节向顶泌汗腺方向分化的肿瘤，介绍了良性肿瘤中的汗腺囊瘤、大汗腺混合瘤、乳头状汗管囊腺瘤、管状腺瘤、大汗腺乳头状汗腺瘤、乳头腺瘤的流行病学及临床特征、病因及发病机制、组织病理学、鉴别诊断、临床病程和预后及临床管理。恶性肿瘤中介绍了腺样囊性癌、大汗腺癌、黏液性癌的流行病学及临床特征、病因及发病机制、组织病理学、鉴别诊断、临床病程和预后及临床管理。

第三节向毛囊分化的肿瘤，介绍了毛囊瘤、基底细胞瘤、毛母细胞瘤、毛发上皮瘤和纤维增生性毛囊上皮瘤、毛盘瘤/纤维毛囊瘤、毛母质瘤、毛母质癌、毛鞘瘤、毛囊漏斗肿瘤、毛鞘棘皮瘤、增生性毛发瘤、毛发腺瘤、扩张孔的流行病学及临床特征、病因及发病机制、组织病理学、鉴别诊断、临床病程和预后及临床管理。

第四节向皮脂腺分化的肿瘤，介绍了良性肿瘤中的皮脂腺瘤、皮脂瘤/皮脂腺上皮瘤及恶性肿瘤中的皮脂腺癌的流行病学及临床特征、病因及发病机制、组织病理学、鉴别诊断、临床病程和预后及临床管理。

〔粟 娟〕

AT-A-GLANCE

- Cutaneous appendage tumors are classified into eccrine, apocrine, follicular, and sebaceous entities, and can be benign or malignant.
- Clinically, appendage tumors are dermally based, usually with minimal epidermal change, and histopathologic evaluation is necessary to make a diagnosis.
- Certain appendage tumors can serve as markers for genetic diseases and syndromes.

Cutaneous appendage (adnexal) tumors encompass both benign and malignant neoplasms and have been traditionally classified by their line of differentiation toward normal adnexal structures of the skin: eccrine, apocrine, follicular, and sebaceous (Table 109-1).[1-3] Many specific types of appendage tumors have been described, and rather than providing an exhaustive list, this chapter focuses on the more common and/or clinically significant tumors. In general, with some exceptions, appendage tumors are relatively rare. Benign appendage tumors have no potential to metastasize, whereas malignant appendage tumors do. There is also a subset of tumors that may be locally aggressive but are not associated with metastasis. Appendage tumors may occur sporadically or may serve as markers of rare genetic syndromes, including Muir-Torre syndrome, Cowden syndrome, Birt-Hogg-Dubé syndrome, and Brooke-Spiegler syndrome. We describe the clinical and histopathologic features with an emphasis on differential diagnosis and tumor biology.

The clinical presentation of appendage tumors is most commonly that of solitary or multiple dermal papule(s) or nodule(s), with minimal overlying epidermal changes. The tumors may appear skin-colored, pink, or with a bluish hue. The presence of a hair follicle orifice or other central punctum may be seen. Some appendage tumors have specific site or age predilections, which may help in the differential diagnosis. Although the patient's age, gender, site of presentation, and clinical morphology may lead one to suspect an appendage tumor, biopsy with subsequent histopathology is usually required for diagnosis. Careful review of routinely processed hematoxylin-and-eosin–stained slides is often the most important part in making the diagnosis of an appendage tumor. An adequate sample is necessary given the heterogeneity of many tumors and the histologic overlap between appendage neoplasms. Furthermore, analysis of the architecture is often necessary in diagnosing appendage tumors, especially when distinguishing between benign and malignant neoplasms. Immunohistochemistry is used sparingly, only in certain instances, and often as a panel, as the cell types that compose these neoplasms are closely related and often express the same markers. Molecular testing (including cytogenetics, fluorescence in situ hybridization, and sequence analysis), is currently used primarily for research purposes, but its use in diagnosis may be become more important in the future. Some tumors are associated with specific genetic abnormalities that may assist in identifying tumors in the setting of a clinical syndrome.[4] Table 109-2 lists appendage neoplasms that are associated with genetic syndromes.

Eccrine and apocrine tumors display a range of secretory and ductal differentiation, follicular tumors show differentiation toward different components of the hair follicle, and sebaceous neoplasms display sebaceous differentiation.[1-3] Although eccrine, apocrine, and sebaceous tumors may all display ductal differentiation, this is most commonly observed in eccrine tumors, perhaps because the normal eccrine duct is much longer, extending from the eccrine coil to the epidermis, in contrast to the apocrine and sebaceous ducts which are rather short and merely connect these adnexal units to the adjacent hair follicle. The folliculosebaceous apocrine unit develops separately from the eccrine unit during embryonic development (see Chaps. 6 and 7 for detailed descriptions of the biology of normal sweat glands and hair follicles). While this may imply that eccrine neoplasms share no features of follicular, sebaceous, or apocrine differentiation, this is not always true, and some appendage tumors can show mixed differentiation and metaplasia.

In some cases, the histopathologic diagnosis of appendage tumors is straightforward, but many factors can make it difficult to precisely classify them[5]: (a) their relative rarity means that clinicians are not always familiar with them; (b) histopathologically similar appendage tumors may have many synonyms, being reported by distinct observers who have used divergent descriptive terminology; (c) tumor heterogeneity/mixed differentiation of some tumors can make it impossible to assign a tumor to a specific line of differentiation; (d) small biopsies can hamper the ability to visualize the majority of the tumor; and (e) there is significant histopathologic and immunophenotypic overlap, making it difficult, in some cases, to place the tumor in a specific diagnostic category. Because appendage tumors are neoplasms that form as aberrant proliferations derived from normal adnexal structures, there is understandably a spectrum of tumors, including a subset that will be impossible to definitively classify. Fortunately, most can be specifically diagnosed according to the patterns of appendage differentiation displayed by the neoplasm.

The histopathologic diagnosis of appendage tumors is important not only to distinguish the benign from the malignant, but also to identify those that are associated with genetic syndromes that have significant clinical implications for the patient, even if the tumor itself is benign. In addition to arriving at a specific diagnosis, the aim of histopathologic evaluation is to identify the line(s) of differentiation and determine whether the tumor is benign or malignant, and either low or high grade. This can help to further guide treatment.

TABLE 109-1
Classification of Cutaneous Appendage Tumors

DIFFERENTIATION	BENIGN	MALIGNANT
Eccrine 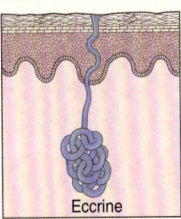	- Hidradenoma - Poroma - Cylindroma - Spiradenoma - Syringoma	- Hidradenocarcinoma - Porocarcinoma - Cylindrocarcinoma/spiradenocarcinoma - Digital papillary adenocarcinoma - Microcystic adnexal carcinoma
Apocrine 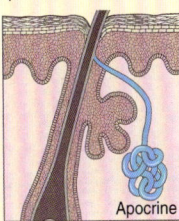	- Hidrocystoma - Apocrine mixed tumor - Syringocystadenoma papilliferum - Tubular adenoma - Hidradenoma papilliferum - Nipple adenoma	- Adenoid cystic carcinoma - Apocrine adenocarcinoma - Mucinous carcinoma
Follicular 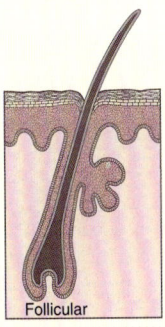		
Pan-follicular	- Trichofolliculoma	
Follicular germinative cells		- Basal cell carcinoma (see Chap. 111)
Follicular germinative and follicular stromal cells	- Trichoblastoma - Trichoepithelioma - Desmoplastic trichoepithelioma	
Follicular mesenchymal differentiation	- Trichodiscoma (fibrofolliculoma)	
Matrical	- Pilomatricoma (pilomatrixoma)	- Pilomatrical carcinoma
Bulb/stem outer root sheath differentiation	- Trichilemmoma	
Isthmic outer root sheath	- Tumor of follicular infundibulum - Pilar sheath acanthoma - Proliferating pilar tumor	
Infundibular	- Trichoadenoma - Dilated pore (of Winer)	
Sebaceous 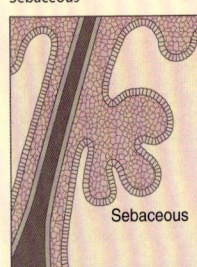	- Sebaceous adenoma - Sebaceoma/sebaceous epithelioma	- Sebaceous carcinoma

TABLE 109-2
Genetic Syndromes Associated with Appendage Neoplasms

GENETIC SYNDROME	APPENDAGE NEOPLASM (S)	GENE (S)	LOCATION
Brooke-Spiegler	Cylindroma, Spiradenoma, Cylindrocarcinoma/Spiradenocarcinoma	CYLD1	16q12-13
Multiple familial trichoepitheliomas	Multiple trichoepitheliomas, Cylindroma	CYLD1	16q12-13
Rombo	Multiple trichoepitheliomas	Unknown	Unknown
Bazex-Dupré-Christol	Multiple trichoepitheliomas	Unknown	Xq24-q27
Schöpf-Schulz-Passarge	Multiple hidrocystomas	WNT10A	2q35
Goltz-Gorlin	Multiple hidrocystomas	PORCN	Xp11
Birt-Hogg-Dubé	Trichodiscoma/fibrofolliculoma	FLCN (folliculin)	17p11
Gardner	Pilomatricoma	CTNNB1 (β-catenin)	3p21
Myotonic muscular dystrophy	Pilomatricoma	DMPK or CNBP	19q13, 3q21
Rubinstein-Taybi	Pilomatricoma	CREBBP, EP300	16p13, 22q13
Cowden	Trichilemmoma (with mucosal involvement)	PTEN	10q23
Keratitis, ichthyosis, and deafness (KID)	Proliferating pilar tumor	GJB2 (connexin 26)	13q12
Muir-Torre	Sebaceous adenoma (especially at sites other than head and neck), sebaceoma, sebaceous carcinoma	MLH1, MSH2, MSH6, PMS2	3p21, 2p21, 2p16, 7p22

Benign appendage tumors can be carefully monitored clinically, surgically excised or treated with ablative therapies, such as electrodessication and cryotherapy. Malignant tumors are usually surgically excised, typically by conventional or Mohs micrographic techniques.

TUMORS WITH ECCRINE DIFFERENTIATION

Normal eccrine glands are found everywhere in the body, but are present in larger numbers on the palms and soles. The normal eccrine unit is composed of a secretory coil located in the deep reticular dermis, and a duct that connects the secretory coil to the overlying epidermis and provides an exit path for eccrine secretions to the skin surface. The ductal portion is divided into the straight dermal portion and the spiraled, intraepidermal portion termed the acrosyringium.[1,2] (See Chap. 6 for a full discussion of normal sweat glands.) The secretory coil is composed of eccrine glands with luminal cells surrounded by myoepithelial cells, whereas the ductal structure is manifest by cuboidal epithelial cells. Eccrine tumors show a range of differentiation from the clear cell patterns derived from the secretory component to more keratinized structures derived from the ductal portion, often with obvious duct formation. These tumors also characteristically are surrounded by eosinophilic stromal deposits of basement membrane-like material. Table 109-3 lists appendage tumors with eccrine differentiation.

BENIGN

HIDRADENOMA

Hidradenoma has historically been referred to by multiple names, including nodular hidradenoma, eccrine acrospiroma, and clear-cell hidradenoma. The largest initial series of hidradenomas was published by Johnson and Helwig in 1969, which detailed clinical and histologic features of 319 tumors.[6]

Epidemiology and Clinical Features: Hidradenomas are relatively common, benign appendage neoplasms that occur in patients over a wide age range, with an average age in the fifth decade.[1,6] They present in women and men, and while hidradenomas can occur at all anatomic sites, the head and neck region and trunk are involved in approximately 50%

TABLE 109-3
Eccrine Appendage Neoplasms

BENIGN	MALIGNANT
Hidradenoma	Hidradenocarcinoma
Poroma	Porocarcinoma
Cylindroma	Cylindrocarcinoma
Spiradenoma	Spiradenocarcinoma
Syringoma	Digital papillary adenocarcinoma
	Microcystic adnexal carcinoma

of cases.[1,6] Hidradenoma presents as a solitary dermal nodule that can be solid and/or cystic, and ranges from flesh-colored to red to bluish in color (Fig. 109-1A). Hidradenomas are reported to be between 0.5 and 10.5 cm, with a median of 1 cm.[6]

Etiology and Pathogenesis: Recent studies have found that 50% of hidradenomas carry a t(11;19) translocation resulting in a fusion between the *MECT1* (*TORC1, CRTC1*) gene at chromosome 19p13 and the *MAML2* gene located at chromosome 11q21.[7,8] This is the same translocation identified in salivary gland mucoepidermoid carcinomas and is hypothesized to promote tumorigenesis by inducing *cAMP/CREB* target genes.

Histopathology: Microscopically, hidradenoma is a circumscribed, unencapsulated dermal neoplasm that displays solid and solid/cystic growth patterns with ductal differentiation (see Fig. 109-1B, C). Numerous cells types can be observed within hidradenomas, including clear, epidermoid (squamoid), mucinous, oncocytic, and eosinophilic polyhedral cells.[1,6] Sclerotic or hyalinized stroma also can be seen, but is usually focal. Atypical hidradenomas have been documented and, as their name implies, show focal areas of atypia, including lack of circumscription, nuclear pleomorphism, focal necrosis, and increased mitotic activity.[9]

Differential Diagnosis: The clinical differential diagnosis of hidradenoma includes cysts and other dermal cutaneous neoplasms. Histologically, hidradenoma with prominent squamous differentiation can be confused with conventional squamous cell carcinoma, although squamous cell carcinoma does not display ductal differentiation. Ductal differentiation and sclerotic stroma can be confused with invasive adenocarcinoma, although they are usually focally present within hidradenomas. Hidradenoma with prominent clear cells can imitate metastatic renal cell carcinoma.

Clinical Course and Prognosis: Hidradenoma is a benign neoplasm. Local recurrence is approximately 10% if not completely excised,[2] and more frequently occurs in atypical hidradenomas.[9] Malignant transformation to hidradenocarcinoma is a rare event, but can occur (see the section "Hidradenocarcinoma").

Management: Complete excision with clear margins is recommended, given the risk of recurrence.

POROMA

Poroma is a benign eccrine neoplasm initially described by Pinkus and colleagues in 1956,[10] and is further subclassified into a group of 4 entities: poroma, hidroacanthoma simplex, dermal duct tumor, and poroid hidradenoma.[1,2]

Epidemiology and Clinical Features: Poroma affects middle-aged to elderly patients, with an average age of 55 to 57 years, and with an equal sex predilection. Hidroacanthoma simplex more

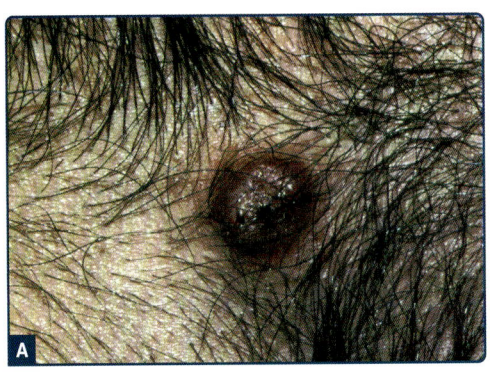
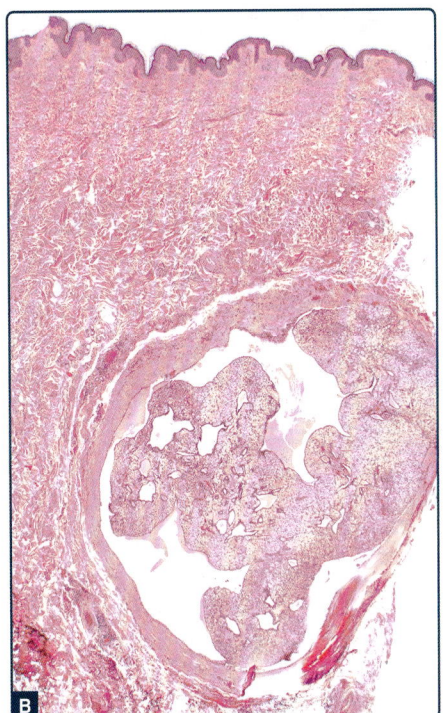
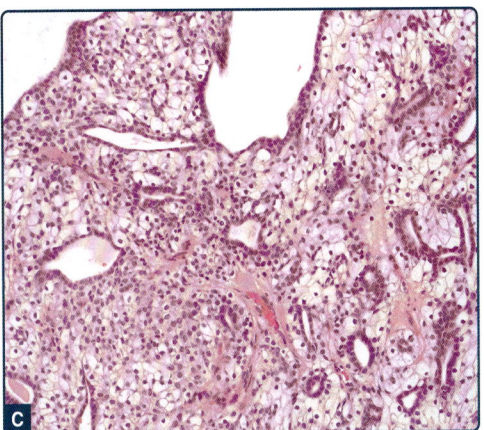

Figure 109-1 **A,** Hidradenoma is a solitary, indistinct dermal nodule. **B,** The tumor is a circumscribed, nonencapsulated, solid and cystic dermal neoplasm. **C,** Hidradenoma is composed of clear cells and cells with ductal and glandular differentiation. (Image **A,** used with permission from Dr. Ernesto Gonzalez, MD, Boston, MA, USA.)

commonly affects patients in their sixth decade. Classic poroma presents as a single, flesh-colored to red papule or nodule, sometimes surrounded by an epidermal rim (Fig. 109-2A). It occurs most commonly on acral surfaces, but also has been documented at other anatomic sites. Hidroacanthoma simplex presents as a verrucous or flat plaque most commonly on the trunk. Dermal duct tumor is a flesh-colored dermal papule and also occurs commonly on the trunk. Poroid hidradenoma presents as a dermal or subcutaneous nodule with pink, red, or blue coloration and is frequently found on the trunk. By dermoscopy, poromas can show a leaf-and-flower–like vascular pattern with interlacing white cords.[11]

Histopathology: Microscopically, classic poromas are relatively well-circumscribed endophytic proliferations of cuboidal cells with basophilic round nuclei and eosinophilic cytoplasm with extension from the epidermis into the dermis (see Fig. 109-2B). Ductal differentiation is variably present and is lined by an eosinophilic cuticle (see Fig. 109-2C). Epithelial membrane antigen (EMA) and carcinoembryonic antigen (CEA) immunostains can be used to highlight duct formation within the tumor. The other poroma variants are categorized based on their location in the skin. Hidroacanthoma simplex is located intraepidermally. Dermal duct tumor is composed of intradermal clusters with duct formation (see Fig. 109-2D, E). Poroid hidradenoma is an intradermal proliferation with both solid and cystic areas.

Differential Diagnosis: The histologic differential diagnosis of poroma can include seborrheic kera-

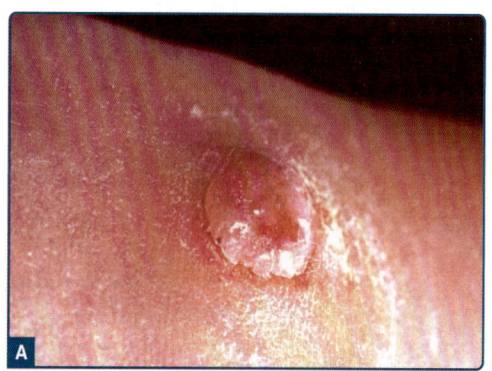
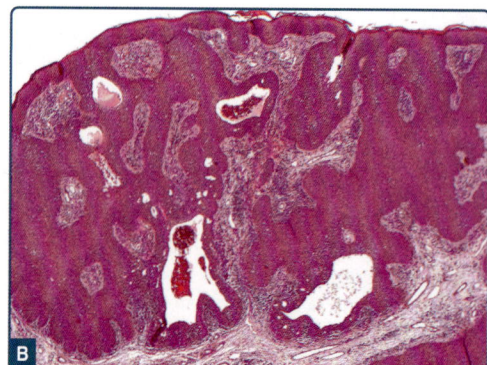
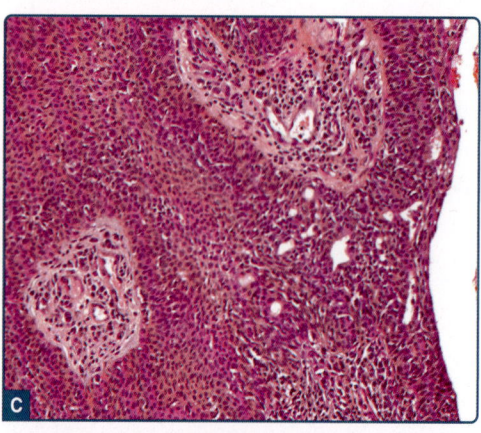
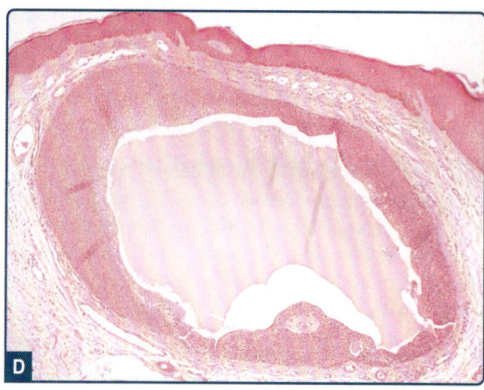
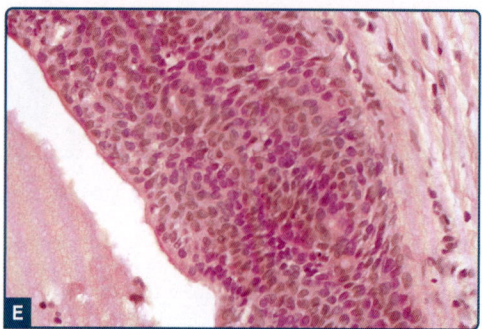

Figure 109-2 **A,** Eccrine poroma is an erythematous dermal nodule with an epidermal rim that often occurs on acral surfaces. **B,** The tumor is an endophytic proliferation of cuboidal epithelium. **C,** Eccrine poroma extends from the epidermis into the dermis and is composed of epithelial cells with eosinophilic cytoplasm, uniformly sized round nuclei, and occasional small clear spaces representing duct formation. **D,** Dermal duct tumor is a variant of eccrine poroma that is predominantly intradermal and composed of a cyst lined by multiple layers of cuboidal epithelium. **E,** Small clear spaces represent ductal differentiation. (Image **A,** used with permission from Dr. Ernesto Gonzalez, MD, Boston, MA, USA.)

tosis. Trichilemmoma can be considered if there are prominent clear cells. Hidradenoma is in the histologic differential diagnosis of poroid hidradenoma.

Clinical Course and Prognosis: Poromas are benign tumors, but malignant transformation to porocarcinoma can occur. (See the section "Porocarcinoma").

Management: Simple excision is curative, but they also can be treated with electrodessication.[11]

CYLINDROMA

Cylindromas are benign neoplasms of uncertain origin. While they have been historically classified as eccrine tumors,[12] more recent immunohistochemical studies showing expression of follicular stem cell markers in cylindromas suggest a folliculosebaceous-apocrine origin for these tumors.[13,14] Some also consider cylindroma and spiradenoma to be related entities that occur on a histologic spectrum.[1,15]

Epidemiology and Clinical Features:
Cylindromas occur in adult patients, with a female predilection.[2,16] Cylindromas typically present singly as a smooth, flesh-colored to red nodule in the head and neck region in adults (Fig. 109-3A). Multiple lesions are seen in patients with Brooke-Spiegler and multiple familial trichoepitheliomas syndromes (see Table 109-2).[17] Multiple lesions can coalesce into a single, large mass.

Etiology and Pathogenesis: As mentioned before, multiple cylindromas manifest in Brooke-Spiegler syndrome, an autosomal dominant condition caused by mutations in the *CYLD* tumor-suppressor gene located on chromosome 16q.[17,18] In addition to multiple cylindromas, patients with Brooke-Spiegler syndrome also present with spiradenomas and trichoepitheliomas.[18] *CYLD* encodes an ubiquitin hydrolase and mutations in the gene lead to misregulation of nuclear factor-κB signaling.[17,18] Sporadic cylindromas have been shown to harbor *MYB-NFIB* gene fusions, similar to adenoid cystic carcinoma.[19] Interestingly, familial cylindromas with *CYLD* mutations do not contain these translocations. *MYB* expression is increased in many sporadic, as well as inherited, cylindromas, and is thought to drive proliferation in the tumors.[20]

Histopathology: Cylindroma has a characteristic histologic appearance with islands of basaloid cells arranged in a "jigsaw puzzle"–like arrangement in the dermis surrounded by eosinophilic basement

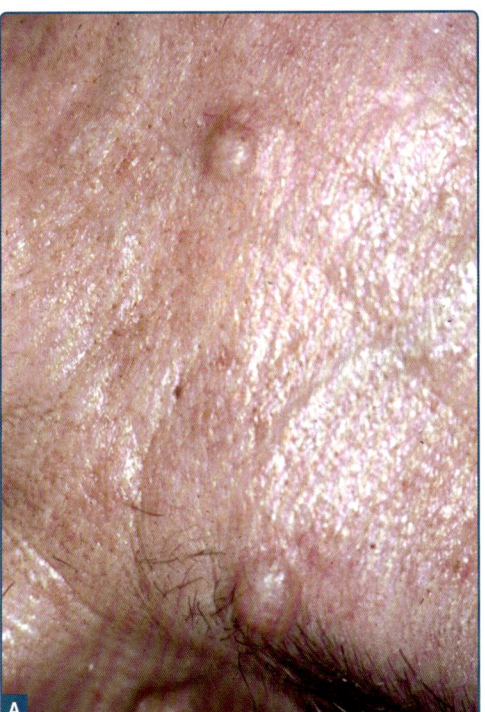
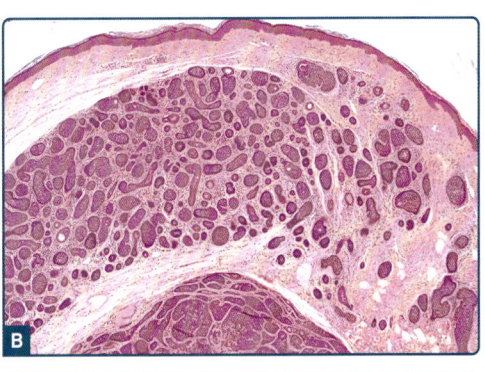
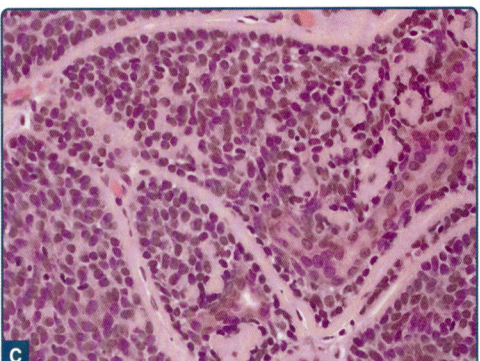

Figure 109-3 **A,** Cylindroma is a smooth, flesh-colored papule, often presenting on the head and neck. **B,** The tumor is a dermally based proliferation of islands of basaloid epithelium, arranged in a pattern similar to that seen in a jigsaw puzzle. **C,** An eosinophilic zone of basement membrane material separates the interlocking nests of tumor cells. Within the tumor nests, central cells have vesicular nuclei and eosinophilic cytoplasm, while peripheral cells have round basophilic nuclei with scant cytoplasm. (Image **A,** used with permission from Dr. Ernesto Gonzalez, MD, Boston, MA, USA.)

membrane material (see Fig. 109-3B). Within the islands there are centrally located larger cells and peripheral, smaller cells with palisading (see Fig. 109-3C). Extension into the subcutaneous fat is sometimes seen.

Clinical Course and Prognosis: Cylindroma is a benign tumor. Malignant transformation is rare, but has been documented in both sporadic and inherited cylindromas (see the section "Cylindrocarcinoma/Spiradenocarcinoma").

Management: Surgical excision is the treatment of choice for cylindromas.[16] For solitary lesions this is straightforward, but for patients with multiple lesions, this can be a complex undertaking. Complete scalp excision was used in the past, but is no longer favored as it is not curative and has high morbidity.[17] Tumor enucleation with secondary intention healing and other scalp-sparing surgical techniques are currently employed. Some studies have looked at the use of aspirin, both topical and systemic, in the treatment of patients with multiple cylindromas, but the outcomes were not favorable.[17]

SPIRADENOMA

Spiradenomas are benign neoplasms of uncertain origin. It was originally hypothesized that spiradenomas derive from the intradermal portion of the eccrine duct.[21] However, recent immunohistochemical studies show that spiradenomas express follicular stem cell markers, suggesting a folliculosebaceous-apocrine origin.[13,14] To some, cylindroma and spiradenoma are related entities that occur on a morphologic spectrum.[1,15]

Epidemiology and Clinical Features: Spiradenoma presents as a single, pink, gray, or blue, dermal nodule located on the trunk in young to middle-aged adults (Fig. 109-4A). Rarely, multiple spiradenomas occur in patients with Brooke-Spiegler syndrome (see Table 109-2).[18]

Histopathology: Histologically, spiradenoma has a characteristic appearance and is a multinodular, unencapsulated dermal neoplasm composed of basaloid cells arranged in cords in a trabecular pattern (see Fig. 109-4B). Two cell types are seen in spiradenomas: (a) small basaloid cells with hyperchromatic nuclei and scant cytoplasm located at the periphery of the nodules, and (b) larger basaloid cells with vesicular nuclei and pale cytoplasm located in the center of the nodules (see Fig. 109-4C). Scattered lymphocytes are seen throughout the tumor and deposits of periodic acid–Schiff (PAS)-positive hyaline basement membrane material are present in the tumor lobules.

Clinical Course and Prognosis: Malignant transformation of spiradenoma is described in rare cases (see the section "Cylindrocarcinoma/Spiradenocarcinoma").

Management: Surgical excision with clear margins is the treatment of choice for spiradenomas.

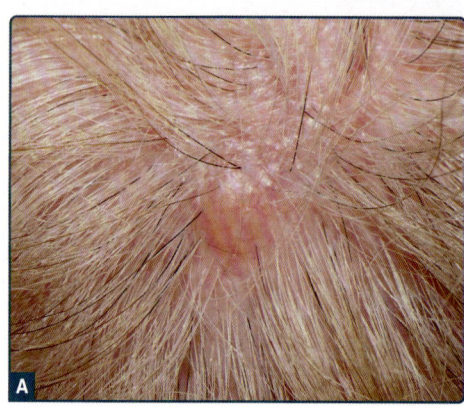
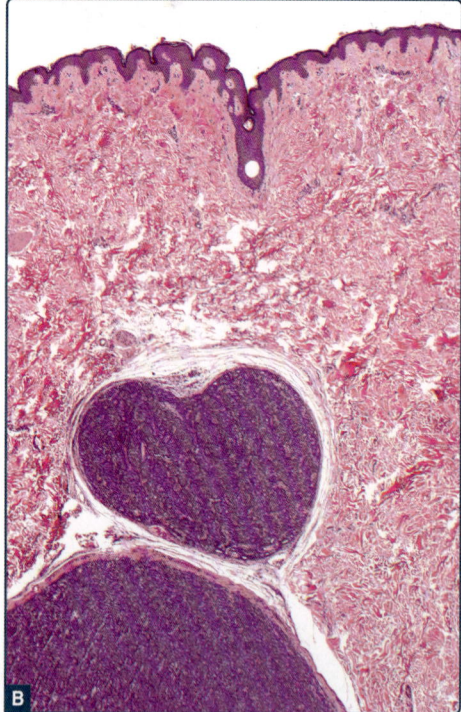
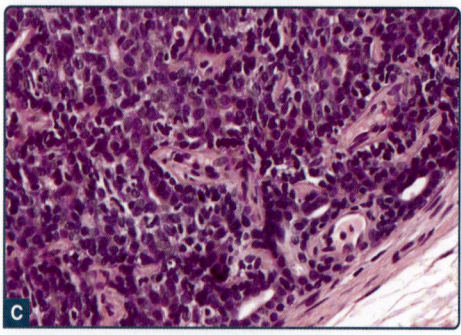

Figure 109-4 **A,** Spiradenoma is a flesh-colored nodule. **B,** It is usually a multinodular nonencapsulated dermal tumor wherein the basaloid nodules resemble blue balls in the dermis. **C,** The central tumor cells have vesicular nuclei and eosinophilic cytoplasm, and the peripheral cells have smaller, round, basophilic nuclei with scant cytoplasm. (Image **A,** used with permission from Dr. Ryan Trowbridge MD, Boston, MA, USA.)

SYRINGOMA

Epidemiology and Clinical Features: Syringoma is a benign appendage tumor typically seen in adolescent and young, adult females.[22] Syringomas often present as multiple, 1- to 3-mm, flesh-colored, sometimes yellow, papules commonly on the face in a periorbital distribution (Fig. 109-5A). They can also present on the scalp, vulva, penis, chest, and axillae. An eruptive form, often affecting the chest and trunk, can be seen. Syringomas have been reported in association with Down syndrome.[22]

Etiology and Pathogenesis: Syringomas are thought to derive from the intraepidermal eccrine ducts.

Histopathology: Microscopically, syringomas are well-circumscribed and composed of epithelial cells arranged in cords, nests, and small ductal structures within a sclerotic stroma in the upper dermis (see Fig. 109-5B). The ductal structures classically have a "tadpole"-shaped or "comma"-shaped tail (see Fig. 109-5C). The lumina of the cells can contain PAS-positive material.

Differential Diagnosis: Clinically, milia, xanthelasma, and angiofibroma are in the differential diagnosis with syringoma.[22] Histologically, the diagnosis of syringoma is usually straightforward, but must be distinguished from microcystic adnexal carcinoma. This distinction can be challenging in superficial biopsies, as the hallmark of microcystic adnexal carcinoma is banal cytomorphology with a deeply invasive growth pattern. Clinicopathologic correlation can aid in the diagnosis in some cases.[5]

Management: As syringomas are benign neoplasms, treatment is focused on cosmesis. Destructive methods, such as laser, chemical peels, and electrodessication, and surgical excision have been used with varying results, and can have adverse side effects, such as scarring.[22] Medical therapies, such as retinoids, have been employed in small cases series without significant effectiveness.[22]

MALIGNANT

HIDRADENOCARCINOMA

Hidradenocarcinoma is a rare adnexal neoplasm that is the malignant counterpart of hidradenoma. Other terms used in the literature for hidradenocarcinoma include clear-cell eccrine hidradenocarcinoma, clear-cell hidradenocarcinoma, and cutaneous mucoepidermoid carcinoma.[23] Published reports of hidradenocarcinoma are predominantly from case reports and small case series.

Epidemiology and Clinical Features: Hidradenocarcinoma presents in adult patients with an average age in the sixth decade.[23,24] Tumors are often seen in the head and neck region, but any part of the body can be involved. Hidradenocarcinoma presents as a solitary mass averaging 2 to 2.5 cm.

Histopathology: Histologically, hidradenocarcinoma has a similar composition of cell types as hidradenoma, including clear, eosinophilic polyhedral, epidermoid (squamoid), oncocytic, and mucinous, but with malignant cytomorphology and architecture. Hidradenocarcinomas are reported to show deep extension, large areas of comedo necrosis, infiltrative growth, nuclear pleomorphism, and 4 or more mitoses per 10 high-power fields.[24] These features can help

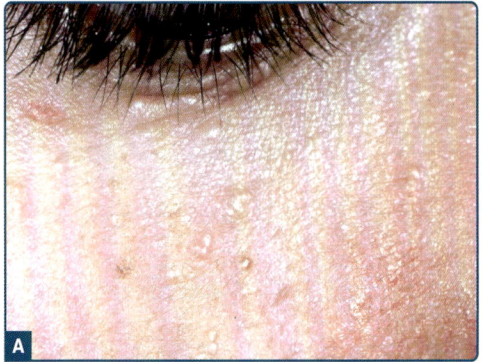
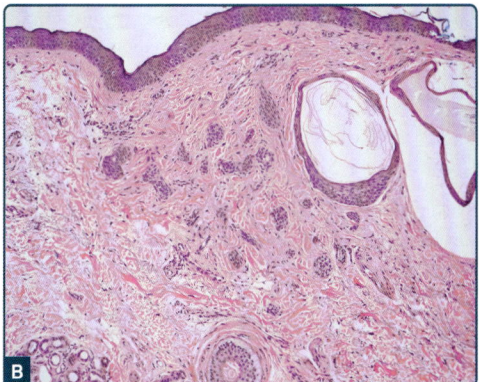
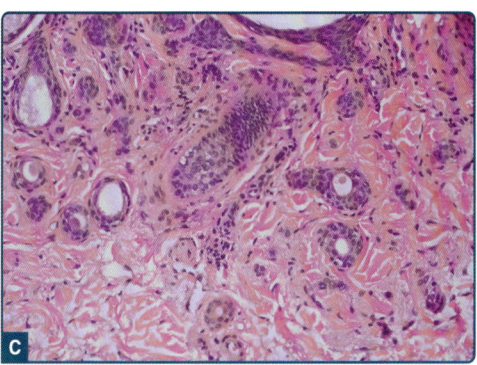

Figure 109-5 **A,** Syringoma presents as multiple, small, flesh-colored papules, often in a periorbital distribution. **B,** The tumor is composed of a dermal proliferation of cords and nests of tumor cells in the upper dermis. **C,** Small ductal structures are present in a sclerotic stroma forming tadpole-shaped and comma-shaped epithelial structures. (Image **A,** used with permission from Dr. Ernesto Gonzalez, MD, Boston, MA, USA.)

distinguish hidradenocarcinoma from an atypical hidradenoma. Residual benign hidradenoma is seen in association with hidradenocarcinoma in approximately one-third of cases.[1]

Etiology and Pathogenesis: One case of hidradenocarcinoma with *HER2/neu* gene amplification has been described,[25] but the *HER2/neu* gene amplification has not been demonstrated in subsequently tested cases.[24] The t(11;19) translocation resulting in *MECT1 (TORC1, CRTC1)-MAML2* gene fusion has been rarely detected in hidradenocarcinomas, this translocation occurs at a lower rate than hidradenomas.[26]

Differential Diagnosis: Atypical hidradenomas can be difficult to distinguish from hidradenocarcinoma in small biopsy specimens. Pattern of growth, cytology, presence of necrosis, and mitotic activity can help to differentiate the 2 entities (see "Histopathology" before).[24]

Clinical Course and Prognosis: Local recurrence and locoregional and distant metastases are not uncommon in hidradenocarcinoma.[23]

Management: Hidradenocarcinoma is treated mainly with wide local excision. There are case reports of patients with metastatic hidradenocarcinoma treated with chemotherapy, but it is unclear if this can be extrapolated to all patients.[23] Similarly, sentinel lymph node sampling has been proposed for hidradenocarcinoma, but currently has no proven therapeutic or survival benefits.[23]

POROCARCINOMA

Porocarcinoma was first described by Coburn and Smith in 1956,[27] and again in 1963 as a single case report.[28] A metaanalysis of 105 cases was reported in 1992,[29] followed by the largest single series of 69 cases in 2001.[30]

Epidemiology and Clinical Features: Porocarcinoma typically affects adult patients in their sixth and seventh decades, although there is a wide age range.[29,30] Some reports have found it occurs more frequently in males,[29] whereas others have found a female predilection.[30] Porocarcinoma presents as a nodular or verrucous growth, most frequently affecting the lower extremities. The trunk and head are also common sites of involvement. A clinical history of recent ulceration or rapid growth from an existing lesion is sometimes reported.

Etiology and Pathogenesis: Porocarcinoma is thought to derive from the acrosyringium. Next-generation sequencing of porocarcinoma has found mutations in *HRAS* and *EGFR* genes, as well as mutations in common tumor-suppressor genes, such as *TP53*.[31]

Histopathology: Histologically, porocarcinoma is composed of malignant basaloid epithelial cells with attachment to the epidermis. The presence of ductal formation is variable, and although the majority of tumors do display duct formation, more poorly differentiated tumors may not. Both in situ and invasive forms of porocarcinoma have been described. Invasive porocarcinoma can show an infiltrative or pushing border. Approximately 20% of porocarcinomas arise in association with a benign poroma.[30] Duct formation should be distinguished from cellular dropout and can be highlighted by PAS staining or by EMA or CEA immunohistochemistry. Clear-cell change and squamous differentiation can be seen in porocarcinoma.

Differential Diagnosis: Distinguishing porocarcinoma from squamous cell carcinoma histologically can be difficult, especially in poorly differentiated tumors or in tumors with significant squamous differentiation. Demonstration of ductal differentiation is important in this distinction and can be augmented by EMA or CEA immunohistochemistry. One study found that immunohistochemistry for cytokeratin 19 (CK19) can be useful in distinguishing porocarcinoma (positive staining for CK19) from squamous cell carcinoma (negative for CK19), with a specificity of 82% and sensitivity of 67%.[32] It is important to note, however, that porocarcinomas can show focal, positive CK19 staining and that 18% of squamous cell carcinomas also showed focal, positive staining for CK19 (Table 109-4). A more recent report using CD117 (cKIT) immunohistochemistry showed positive staining in 100% of porocarcinomas, with approximately 20% of squamous cell carcinomas displaying only focal staining.[33]

TABLE 109-4
Summary of Immunohistochemical Stains in the Distinction between Squamous Cell Carcinoma and Select Appendage Neoplasms

	SCC	POROCARCINOMA	PROLIFERATING PILAR TUMOR	DESMOPLASTIC TRICHILEMMOMA
CEA	+	+ (highlights ducts)	ND	ND
CK19	−	+	ND	ND
CD34	−	ND	+	+
AE13	−	ND	+	ND
AE14	−	ND	+	ND

−, Negative; +, positive; ND, no robust data; SCC, squamous cell carcinoma.

Clinical Course and Prognosis: Porocarcinoma has a propensity for recurrence and regional lymph node metastasis (at a rate of approximately 20% each) and distant metastatic disease occurs in approximately 10% of cases.[29,30,34] High mitotic activity (>14 mitoses per high-power field), tumor thickness greater than 7 mm, and lymphovascular invasion are histologic features associated with a poorer prognosis.[30]

Management: Treatment is focused on surgical excision, by both conventional and Mohs micrographic techniques.[34] Overall, current chemotherapeutic regimens appear to have little therapeutic value in metastatic disease.[35]

CYLINDROCARCINOMA/SPIRADENOCARCINOMA

Malignant neoplasms arising from cylindromas and spiradenomas are rare, with case reports and small case series published in the literature.[36-38] These neoplasms have been referred to by numerous names, including malignant spiradenoma, malignant cylindroma, carcinoma ex spiradenoma, and carcinoma ex cylindroma. As discussed in the "Spiradenoma" and "Cylindroma" sections before, many consider these entities to be related and to exist on a morphologic spectrum. Given their similarities and their rarity, we consider them in a single section.

Epidemiology and Clinical Features: Malignant transformation of cylindroma and spiradenoma can occur sporadically in solitary lesions or as part of the Brook-Spiegler syndrome (see Table 109-2). They arise in elderly adults without apparent sex predilection. Cylindrocarcinoma and spiradenocarcinoma present as solitary nodules, and can be quite large in size, measuring up to 17.5 cm with a median size of 4 cm.[37] There are reports of recent increases in size in preexisting tumors, as well as ulceration, which could suggest malignant transformation of existing benign neoplasms. Regions in the head and neck are the most frequently affected sites, with lower-extremity and trunk involvement also reported.[36-38]

Histopathology: Histopathologic diagnosis requires adequate sampling and recognition of a benign cylindroma or spiradenoma component within the tumor. Transition between the benign and malignant components can be gradual or abrupt.[37,38] Malignant transformation is typified by high mitotic rate, nuclear pleomorphism, sheet-like and/or infiltrative growth patterns, and necrosis. Adenocarcinoma in situ has been described and manifests as proliferations of atypical cells with a preserved myoepithelial cell layer.[37] Adenocarcinoma in situ can be difficult to distinguish from benign cylindroma and spiradenoma. A wide range of morphologies is seen in cylindrocarcinoma and spiradenocarcinoma. A study of 24 cylindrospiradenocarcinomas reported 4 main patterns seen in these tumors[37]:

1. Salivary gland–type basal cell adenocarcinoma–like pattern, low grade;
2. Salivary gland–type basal cell adenocarcinoma–like pattern, high grade;
3. Invasive adenocarcinoma, not otherwise specified; and
4. Sarcomatoid carcinoma.

As the name implies, the salivary gland–type basal cell adenocarcinoma–like pattern closely resembles basal cell adenocarcinoma of the salivary gland with either low-grade or high-grade morphology. The adenocarcinoma, not otherwise specified (or NOS), pattern is poorly differentiated and does not resemble any particular tumor. The sarcomatoid pattern shows biphasic morphologies, with both epithelial and sarcomatous components. The sarcomatous component typically resembles an unspecified pleomorphic sarcoma.

Differential Diagnosis: Depending on the morphology of the tumor cells, the histologic differential diagnosis can include squamous cell carcinoma and metastasis from salivary gland or breast tissue. In cases of in situ adenocarcinoma, a benign cylindroma or spiradenoma is in the differential diagnosis.

Clinical Course and Prognosis: Cylindrocarcinoma and spiradenocarcinoma have been documented to metastasize and associated deaths are reported, although with varying frequency.[39] Poor prognosis seems to be associated with high-grade morphology, either salivary gland–type basal cell adenocarcinoma-like, high grade, or adenocarcinoma pattern.[37] Similarly, patients with Brooke-Spiegler syndrome who undergo malignant transformation appear to have poor overall outcomes.[17]

Management: Surgical excision remains the mainstay treatment of cylindrocarcinoma and spiradenocarcinoma.[38] The role of chemotherapy and radiation therapy is unclear and not currently recommended.

DIGITAL PAPILLARY ADENOCARCINOMA

An initial case series of digital papillary adenocarcinoma from the Armed Forces Institute of Pathology files was published in 1987 and included 57 cases, with tumors classified as either adenomas or adenocarcinomas.[40] A followup study of that same cohort revealed that tumors originally classified as adenomas had recurred or developed metastases.[41] Based on these findings, the authors proposed that all such lesions be classified as adenocarcinoma regardless of their histologic features. An additional series of 31 cases was published more recently in 2012, and included immunohistochemical findings.[42]

Epidemiology and Clinical Features: Digital papillary adenocarcinoma predominantly affects males in middle age and presents as a solitary 1- to 4-cm mass. It often presents on the distal aspect of a finger or, sometimes, a toe. The palms and soles are rarely affected. Digital papillary adenocarcinoma is slow growing and is often present for years prior to excision. Rarely, patients are found to have metastatic disease at the time of clinical presentation.[42]

Histopathology: Microscopically, digital papillary adenocarcinoma is a multinodular, poorly circumscribed dermal tumor. Extension into the subcutis is not uncommon. Tumors contain solid and cystic areas with papillary projections. The papillary structures include both true papillae with fibrovascular cores, as well as pseudopapillary structures without fibrovascular cores. Areas of ductal differentiation and cribriform growth can be seen. By immunohistochemistry, myoepithelial cells are present to varying degrees within the tumor and their presence does not portend improved patient outcomes.[42]

Differential Diagnosis: The clinical differential diagnosis for digital papillary adenocarcinoma includes a cyst, giant cell tumor, and vascular tumor. Histologically, the differential diagnosis of digital papillary adenocarcinoma includes hidradenoma, tubular adenoma, and metastatic disease from thyroid, breast, and GI primaries.[39]

Clinical Course and Prognosis: Tumors have the propensity to recur and have late metastases, with lung being the most common site of metastatic disease.[41,42]

Management: Wide excision or digital amputation of the primary lesion is recommended. Close clinical followup is recommended as metastases have been reported up to 20 years following initial presentation.[41,42]

MICROCYSTIC ADNEXAL CARCINOMA

Microcystic adnexal carcinoma is a rare, malignant adnexal tumor originally described in 1982.[43] Synonyms for microcystic adnexal carcinoma include sclerosing sweat duct carcinoma and malignant syringoma.

Epidemiology and Clinical Features: Microcystic adnexal carcinoma affects adult patients over a wide age range with an equal sex distribution.[44,45] It clinically presents as a firm, indurated plaque, typically affecting the central face, and classically described in perioral or periocular areas.

Etiology and Pathogenesis: There are reports of microcystic adnexal carcinoma occurring following radiation therapy.[44,45] Additionally, in the United States, microcystic adnexal carcinoma often presents on the left side of the face, suggesting a role for ultraviolet exposure in tumor development.[44,45] Originally believed to be of eccrine derivation, follicular differentiation can be observed within microcystic adnexal carcinoma, and suggests either metaplasia within the tumor or a possible folliculosebaceous origin.

Histopathology: Microscopically, microcystic adnexal carcinoma displays an infiltrative growth pattern with frequent extension beyond the dermis into subcutaneous tissues (Fig. 109-6A, B). The tumor is

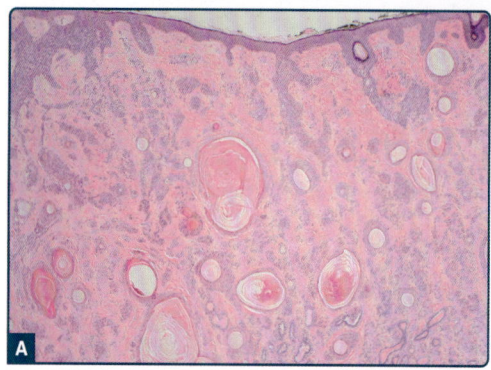
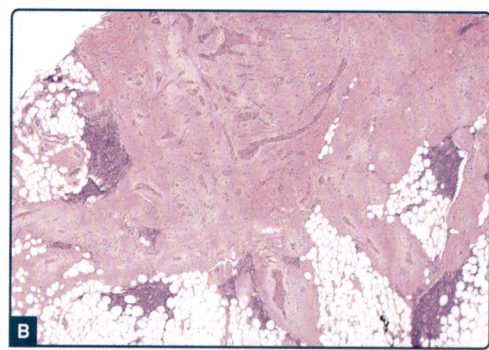
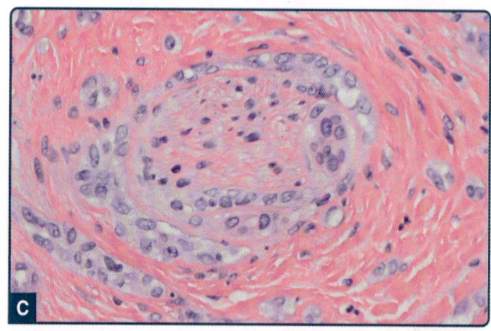
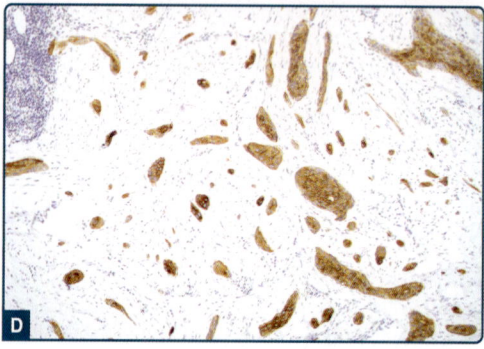

Figure 109-6 **A,** Microcystic adnexal carcinoma is an infiltrative tumor composed of cords and cysts of varying sizes and shapes. **B,** The tumor extends through the dermis to involve the subcutaneous fat. **C,** Perineural invasion is often seen. **D,** The tumor cells may be positive for CK7.

composed of strands, cords, and cysts of epithelial tumor cells embedded in a sclerotic stroma. There is often zonation within the tumor, with keratocysts observed mainly in the superficial dermis, strands and cords of tumor cells in the mid dermis, and duct-like structures in the deep dermis and subcutaneous tissues. Cytologically, microcystic adnexal carcinoma is deceptively bland, and superficial biopsies do not convey the infiltrative growth pattern. Perineural invasion is a frequent finding (Fig. 109-6C).

Tumor cells stain for cytokeratins and ductal formation is positive for EMA and CEA immunostaining (see Fig. 109-6D). Immunohistochemistry is of relatively little use in making a definitive diagnosis of microcystic adnexal carcinoma. Numerous studies have tried to use an immunohistochemical approach to distinguish microcystic adnexal carcinoma from its histologic mimics, and have produced variable results, especially when considering small biopsy specimens (see "Differential Diagnosis" below).[1,5,45] Accurate diagnosis relies most heavily on reviewing hematoxylin-and-eosin–stained slides of an adequately deep biopsy.

Differential Diagnosis: Clinically and histologically, morpheaform basal cell carcinoma mimics microcystic adnexal carcinoma, although basal cell carcinoma lacks ductal differentiation. Immunohistochemistry for cytokeratin 15 (CK15) and CEA (or EMA, highlighting duct formation) may be helpful in distinguishing microcystic adnexal carcinoma from morpheaform basal cell carcinoma, with positivity for CK15 and the presence of ductal structures supporting a diagnosis of microcystic adnexal carcinoma (Table 109-5).[46] Desmoplastic trichoepithelioma is also in the histologic differential diagnosis of microcystic adnexal carcinoma, as both can have superficial dermal keratocysts. Desmoplastic trichoepithelioma, however, does not display the infiltrative growth pattern of microcystic adnexal carcinoma. Immunohistochemistry is not particularly useful in distinguishing between microcystic adnexal carcinoma and desmoplastic trichoepithelioma.[5] Syringoma can have a similar histologic appearance to microcystic adnexal carcinoma, but does not display a deep, infiltrative pattern of growth.

Clinical Course and Prognosis: Microcystic adnexal carcinoma is a slow-growing tumor, but is locally aggressive with significant morbidity, possibly because of the frequent perineural involvement associated with this tumor. Metastatic disease is exceedingly rare.[44,45]

Management: Microcystic adnexal carcinoma is treated with surgical excision, with reports suggesting that Mohs micrographic surgery has lower recurrence rates than conventional surgical techniques.[44,45] Radiation therapy is not recommended as a first-line treatment of microcystic adnexal carcinoma, but can be considered in patients who are poor surgical candidates.[44] Chemotherapy has no role in treating microcystic adnexal carcinoma. For patients with recurrent disease in the periocular area, a study showed that review of paraffin sections (either by slow Mohs or traditional surgical excision) can be of benefit in detecting residual, small tumor foci.[47]

TUMORS WITH APOCRINE DIFFERENTIATION

Normal apocrine glands develop in association with the hair follicle and have a more limited anatomic distribution than eccrine glands, being found in the axillary, groin, and perineal regions. (See Chap. 6 for a full discussion of normal sweat glands.) Apocrine glands are composed of a secretory coil, located in the deep dermis or subcutis, and a ductal portion. The secretory portion is composed of glands lined by cuboidal epithelium with intracytoplasmic zymogen granules and characteristic decapitation secretion with apical "snouting." These luminal cells are surrounded by myoepithelial cells. Tumors with apocrine differentiation are classically composed of cells that show this decapitation secretion. Table 109-6 lists appendage tumors with apocrine differentiation.

BENIGN

HIDROCYSTOMA

Hidrocystomas are described in both apocrine and eccrine forms and have been referred to by numerous

TABLE 109-5

Summary of Immunohistochemical Stains in the Distinction Between Basal Cell Carcinoma, Microcystic Adnexal Carcinoma, and Adenoid Cystic Carcinoma

	BCC	MAC	ADCC
CK7	+/−	−	+
CK15	−	+	+
S100	−	ND	+ (myoepithelial cells)
CD117 (cKIT)	−	ND	+

−, Negative; +, positive; AdCC, adenoid cystic carcinoma; BCC, basal cell carcinoma; MAC, microcystic adnexal carcinoma; ND, no data.

TABLE 109-6

Apocrine Appendage Neoplasms

BENIGN	MALIGNANT
Hidrocystoma	Adenoid cystic carcinoma
Tubular adenoma (tubular apocrine adenoma/papillary eccrine adenoma)	Apocrine adenocarcinoma (including cribriform carcinoma)
Syringocystadenoma papilliferum	Mucinous carcinoma
Apocrine mixed tumor	
Hidradenoma papilliferum	
Nipple adenoma	

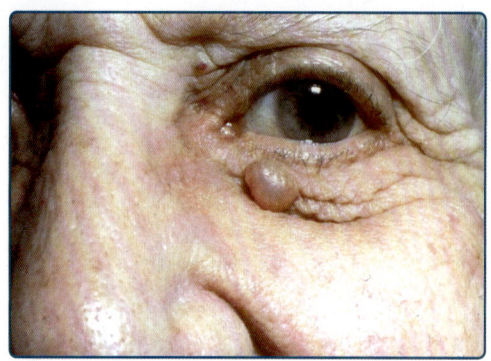

Figure 109-7 Hidrocystoma is a translucent papule, frequently seen in a periorbital distribution. (Image used with permission from Dr. Ernesto Gonzalez, MD, Boston, MA, USA.)

names, including apocrine cystadenoma, apocrine gland cyst, and eccrine cyst.[1]

Epidemiology and Clinical Features: Hidrocystomas present in adults of middle age with a slight predilection for females.[48] A hidrocystoma presents as a tan to bluish-black, translucent papule, often in the periorbital area of the face (Fig. 109-7). Other locations, including the axilla and groin, can be affected. Multiple lesions are sometimes seen.

Etiology and Pathogenesis: Apocrine hidrocystomas are considered adenomas arising from the apocrine secretory coil. Eccrine hidrocystomas are considered retention cysts of the eccrine duct.[1] Multiple hidrocystomas are associated with Schöpf-Schulz-Passarge syndrome and Goltz-Gorlin syndrome (see Table 109-2).[48] Schöpf-Schulz-Passarge syndrome is an autosomal recessive condition with ectodermal dysplasia, manifesting as multiple hidrocystomas (often involving the bilateral eyelid margins), palmoplantar keratoderma, nail dystrophy, hypodontia, and hypotrichosis.[48] Goltz-Gorlin syndrome is a sporadic condition with microcephaly, facial hypoplasia, multiple hidrocystomas, papillomas (of the lip, tongue, anus, and axilla), mental retardation, and skeletal abnormalities.[48] A relationship between multiple eccrine hidrocystomas and hyperthyroidism and warm temperatures has been suggested.[48]

Histopathology: Microscopically, hidrocystomas are epithelial-lined unilocular or multilocular cysts, present in the dermis. The epithelium is typically bilayered with an outer myoepithelial cell layer. Apocrine hidrocystomas display characteristic decapitation secretion. Flattening of the epithelium can occur, and sometimes makes the distinction between apocrine and eccrine differentiation difficult. There are claims that apocrine epithelium stains positively for HMFG (human milk fat globule)-1 and GCDFP (gross cystic disease fluid protein)-15 immunohistochemical stains, while eccrine epithelium is negative for these markers.[1] More complex epithelial proliferations, such as micropapillary projections, have been noted in apocrine hidrocystomas.

Differential Diagnosis: The clinical differential diagnosis includes epidermoid cyst, basal cell carcinoma, and, sometimes melanoma, depending on the color of the lesion. Histologically, dacryops, a cyst of the lacrimal gland, can resemble hidrocystoma, but dacryops can be distinguished by the presence of lacrimal gland tissue.[1]

Clinical Course and Prognosis: Hidrocystomas are benign adnexal lesions.

Management: As hidrocystomas are benign, treatment is focused on cosmesis. Solitary lesions can be punctured or surgically excised. The presence of multiple hidrocystomas is more difficult to treat, with numerous treatment strategies described in the literature, including botulinum toxin, electrodessication and curettage, laser treatment, and topical atropine.[48]

APOCRINE MIXED TUMOR

Mixed tumor of the skin, also referred to historically as chondroid syringoma, is a benign myoepithelial neoplasm with tubuloductal/glandular differentiation. It can be classified as either apocrine or eccrine, although the apocrine variant is more commonly seen than the eccrine variant.[1] As follicular and sebaceous differentiation can be observed in apocrine mixed tumors (as befitting the embryologic origin of the folliculosebaceous-apocrine unit), some authors prefer the term *mixed tumor of the pilosebaceous–apocrine complex*.[49] Apocrine mixed tumor is morphologically identical to pleomorphic adenoma of the salivary gland.

Epidemiology and Clinical Features: Apocrine mixed tumor is seen in middle-aged adult patients with a male predominance.[49] Eccrine mixed tumor also affects adult patients, but has a slight female predominance.[50] Cutaneous mixed tumor typically arises in the head and neck area as a firm, flesh-colored, slow-growing nodule. Subcutaneous lesions can also present on the extremities.

Etiology and Pathogenesis: As it is a homolog of pleomorphic adenoma, mixed tumors show *PLAG1* gene rearrangements as well as PLAG1 protein expression by immunohistochemistry.[51]

Histopathology: Histologically, mixed tumors are unencapsulated, multinodular, dermal neoplasms with frequent infiltration into the surrounding tissue (Fig. 109-8A). The tumor is composed of epithelial, myoepithelial, and stromal elements, which are present in varying amounts (Fig. 109-8B). The epithelial component, by definition, is gland forming, even if focal (Fig. 109-8C). The glandular epithelium in apocrine mixed tumors displays decapitation secretion (Fig. 109-8D); in the eccrine variant, this feature is absent. Follicular and sebaceous differentiation can be observed in apocrine mixed tumors.[49] Heterologous differentiation of the stromal component can be seen, often as cartilaginous, osseous, or adipocytic differentiation.

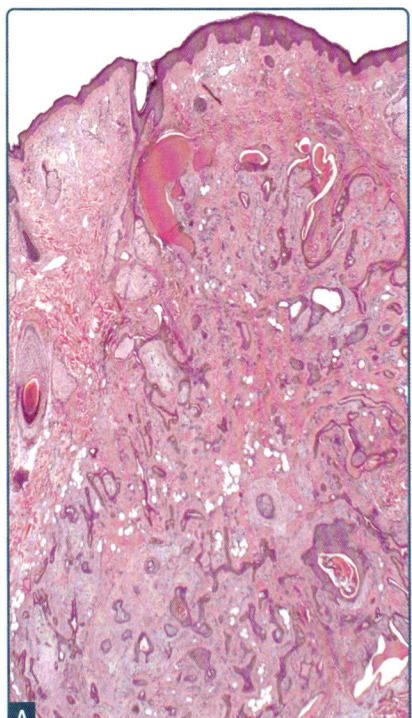
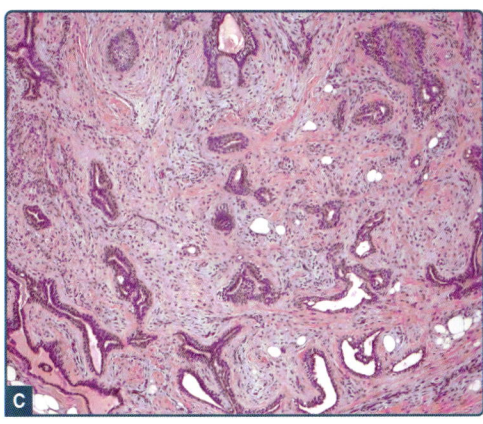
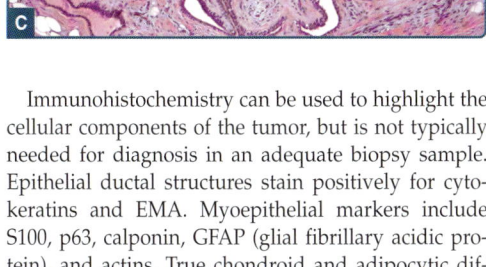
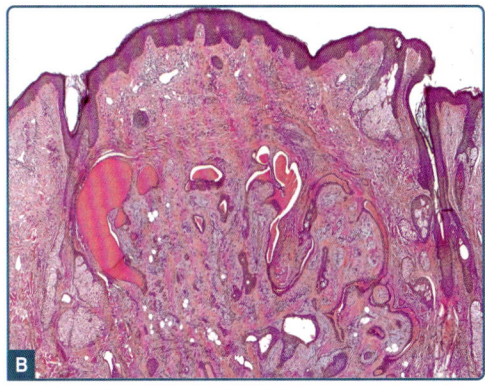
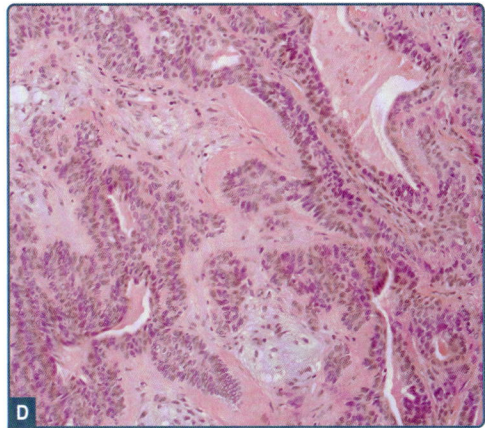

Figure 109-8 **A,** Apocrine mixed tumor occurs as a dermal nodule often with an infiltrative growth pattern. **B,** There is a proliferation of epithelial and myoepithelial cells with characteristic basophilic stromal changes. **C,** Glandular differentiation is seen with surrounding basophilic myxochondroid stroma. **D,** Areas with glandular differentiation often show decapitation secretion characteristic of apocrine tumors.

Immunohistochemistry can be used to highlight the cellular components of the tumor, but is not typically needed for diagnosis in an adequate biopsy sample. Epithelial ductal structures stain positively for cytokeratins and EMA. Myoepithelial markers include S100, p63, calponin, GFAP (glial fibrillary acidic protein), and actins. True chondroid and adipocytic differentiation will be positive for S100.

Differential Diagnosis: In the head and neck region, extension from or recurrence resulting from an incompletely excised salivary gland pleomorphic adenoma must be ruled out before making a diagnosis of mixed tumor.[51] Mixed tumor typically has a characteristic histologic appearance, but if tubuloductal differentiation is focal, a myoepithelial neoplasm could be considered.[51] Likewise, if there is significant metaplasia, including follicular, chondroid, or adipocytic, additional neoplasms, such as trichoblastoma, chondroma, or adenolipoma, could be included in the histologic differential diagnosis.

Clinical Course and Prognosis: Mixed tumors of the skin are benign and typically follow an indolent clinical course. Malignant transformation is extremely rare.

Management: Complete surgical excision is recommended to prevent recurrence, which can occur in up to 18% of benign myoepithelial neoplasms.[51]

SYRINGOCYSTADENOMA PAPILLIFERUM

Epidemiology and Clinical Features: Syringocystadenoma papilliferum is a rare, benign neoplasm that presents in children and young adults.[52]

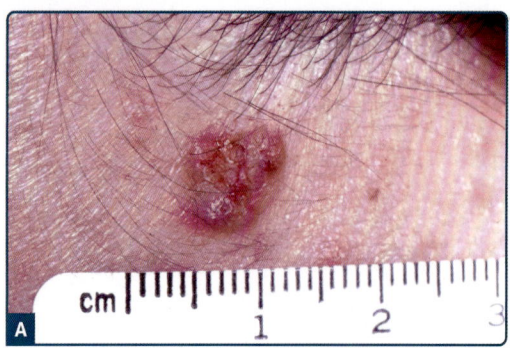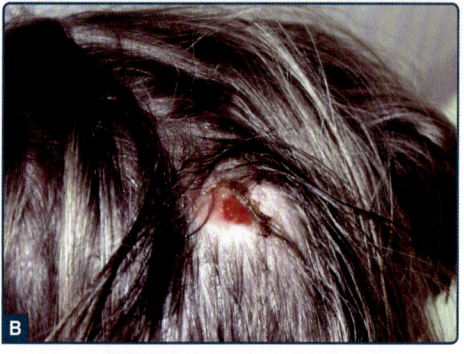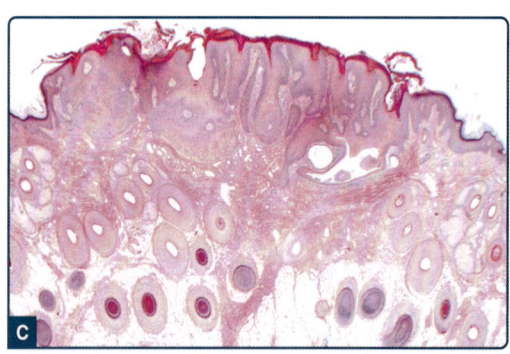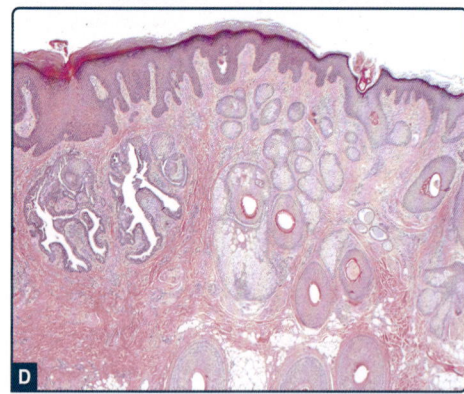

Figure 109-9 **A,** Syringocystadenoma papilliferum can present as a crusted verrucous plaque on the scalp. **B,** Serous drainage is not an uncommon finding. **C,** The tumor occurs as an invagination of papillomatous projections in the epidermis. **D,** On the left side of this image a papillary projection is seen, composed of an inner layer of columnar epithelium with decapitation secretion and an outer layer of myoepithelial cells. (Clinical images **A** and **B,** Used with permission from Dr. Ernesto Gonzalez, MD, Boston, MA, USA.)

Syringocystadenoma papilliferum presents as a single, brown to red plaque, typically on the scalp, and can have a wart-like appearance (Fig. 109-9A). Serosanguinous drainage and ulceration are not uncommon (Fig. 109-9B). Alternatively, it can also present as small papules, be distributed linearly, and occur in association with nevus sebaceus. Syringocystadenoma papilliferum can occur in other areas of the head and neck, and have rarely been reported at other sites, including the trunk and extremities.

Etiology and Pathogenesis: Some cases of syringocystadenoma papilliferum have shown deletion at 9p22 (*PTCH*) or at 9p21 (*p16*).[53] Mutations in *BRAF* (V600E), *NRAS*, and *HRAS* also have been reported in syringocystadenoma papilliferum.[54] The role these genetic alterations play, if any, in tumor pathogenesis remains unclear.

Histopathology: Syringocystadenoma papilliferum has a characteristic histologic appearance and is composed of an invagination of papillations that connect to the surface squamous epithelium (see Fig. 109-9C). The epithelium covering the papillae consists of 2 layers. The lining layer is columnar to cuboidal, often with conspicuous decapitation secretion, and the outer layer is composed of basal/myoepithelial cells (see Fig. 109-9D). The fibrous cores of the papillae frequently contain a plasma cell infiltrate. The epithelial cells express cytokeratins, including CK7, as well as EMA and CEA. The inner, myoepithelial layer is positive for smooth muscle actin.

Clinical Course and Prognosis: Syringocystadenoma papilliferum is a benign adnexal neoplasm. Very rare cases of adenocarcinoma (syringocystadenocarcinoma papilliferum) are reported arising from syringocystadenoma papilliferum, mainly in older adults with a history of rapid growth of a preexisting nodule.[55,56] Histologically, syringocystadenocarcinoma papilliferum has a malignant appearance, with epithelial multilayering, an infiltrative growth pattern, nuclear atypia, and high mitotic activity.[56]

Management: Surgical excision of syringocystadenoma papilliferum is recommended even though malignant transformation is rare. Syringocystadenocarcinoma papilliferum is treated surgically, either by conventional or Mohs micrographic techniques.

TUBULAR ADENOMA

Tubular apocrine adenoma, also referred to as tubulopapillary hidradenoma and tubular syringoadenoma, was first reported by Landry and Winkelmann in 1972.[57] Papillary eccrine adenoma was reported by

Rulon and Helwig in 1977.[58] There can be morphologic overlap between the lesions, with some preferring to separate the 2 entities, and others considering them 1 entity that exists on a morphologic spectrum.[1] Because they are rare, we discuss them in 1 section.

Epidemiology and Clinical Features: Tubular adenomas affect adult patients with a mean age in the fifth decade.[1] Tubular adenoma presents as a single, flesh-colored nodule between 1 and 3 cm in size. Tubular apocrine adenomas are described as typically occurring on the scalp, whereas papillary eccrine adenomas often present on the distal extremities.

Etiology and Pathogenesis: Tubular adenomas are rare, benign appendage neoplasms with apocrine and/or eccrine differentiation.

Histopathology: Microscopically, tubular adenoma is a relatively well-circumscribed, unencapsulated dermal nodule composed of tubules embedded in a fibrotic stroma. The epithelium lining the tubules is composed of single to multiple layers of cuboidal cells with an outer layer of myoepithelial cells. The luminal cells stain for cytokeratins, such as CK7, CEA, and EMA. Myoepithelial markers (calponin, p63, smooth muscle actin) stain the myoepithelial cell layer. Of note, myoepithelial markers can be lost with distension of the tubules and should not be interpreted as invasive carcinoma.[1] Complex architecture within the tubules, such as micropapillae and cribriforming, can be seen.

Differential Diagnosis: Histologically, tubular adenoma can sometimes display overlapping features with syringocystadenoma papilliferum.

Clinical Course and Prognosis: Tubular adenomas are benign and have an indolent clinical course.

Management: Treatment focuses on surgical methods of excision, including Mohs micrographic surgery.

HIDRADENOMA PAPILLIFERUM

Epidemiology and Clinical Features: Hidradenoma papilliferum occurs in the anogenital region in females and is typically located on the vulva.[59] It presents clinically as a flesh-colored to red nodule, often less than 1 cm in size.

Etiology and Pathogenesis: Hidradenoma papilliferum is considered an adenoma of the mammary-like anogenital glands and is morphologically similar to mammary intraductal papilloma.[59] A recent study showed that hidradenoma papilliferum contains activating mutations in *PIK3CA*, similar to those found in mammary ductal papillomas, further highlighting the similarities between these 2 entities.[60]

Histopathology: Histologically, hidradenoma papilliferum is a well-circumscribed, unencapsulated, solid-cystic dermal nodule (Fig. 109-10A).[59] Hidradenoma papilliferum displays a complex pattern of interconnected tubules and glands, often arranged in a labyrinth-like appearance. Papillae formation is common. The bilayered epithelium lining the tubules and papillary structures is composed of a luminal layer of cuboidal to columnar cells surrounded by a layer of myoepithelial cells (Fig. 109-10B). Decapitation secretion is frequently seen in the luminal layer. Oxyphilic metaplasia is not an uncommon finding. Other morphologic changes, such as sclerosing adenosis–like changes and ductal hyperplasia, also can be seen. Mitotic figures can be observed and the overall proliferative index can be variable. Adjacent remnants of mammary-like anogenital glands are seen in approximately one-third of hidradenoma papilliferum cases.[59] Connection to the overlying epidermis is rare, but when seen, is often accompanied by a plasma cell-rich infiltrate.

The luminal epithelial cells stain for cytokeratins (CK5/CK6, AE1/AE3) and GCDFP-15, as well as estrogen receptors.[1] The myoepithelial cells stain for typical myoepithelial markers, including S100, actins, calponin, and p63.

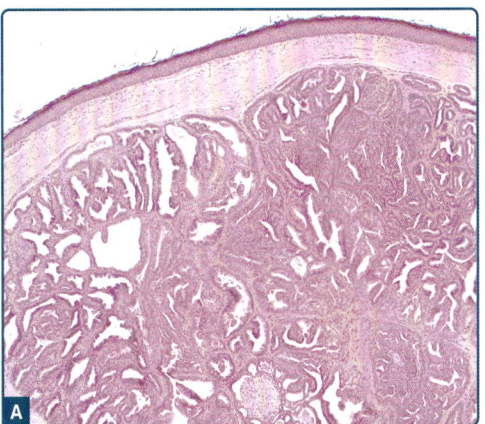

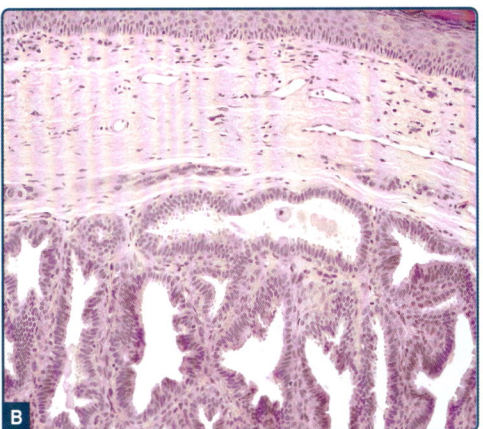

Figure 109-10 **A,** Hidradenoma papilliferum occurs as a well-circumscribed solid and cystic dermally based nodule, with interconnected glands that form labyrinth-like arrangements of tumor cells. **B,** The projections are composed of cuboidal and columnar epithelium with decapitation secretion and a basal layer of myoepithelial cells.

Differential Diagnosis: Hidradenoma papilliferum is often confused clinically with a cyst. Histologically, if there is connection with the epidermis, syringocystadenoma papilliferum can be considered in the differential diagnosis.

Clinical Course and Prognosis: Hidradenoma papilliferum is benign, but there are rare reports of ductal carcinoma in situ arising in hidradenoma papilliferum, manifested by increased cellularity, nuclear atypia, and abnormal mitotic figures.[1] Adenocarcinoma arising in hidradenoma papilliferum (hidradenocarcinoma papilliferum) is a controversial diagnosis.[1] Loss of the myoepithelial cell layer should allow differentiation between ductal carcinoma in situ (with a retained myoepithelial layer) and invasive adenocarcinoma. Extremely rare cases of extramammary Paget disease associated with hidradenoma papilliferum have been reported.[1]

Management: Surgical excision is the treatment of choice for hidradenoma papilliferum.

NIPPLE ADENOMA

Nipple adenoma is a benign proliferation in the breast. It has been described using many names, including florid papillomatosis, erosive adenomatosis, and papillary adenoma, among others, likely reflecting the differing clinical and histologic appearances this entity can have.[61,62]

Epidemiology and Clinical Features: Nipple adenoma affects females in their fourth and fifth decades and presents unilaterally as a serous or bloody nipple discharge, as well as crusting or ulceration of the nipple.[61,62] A dermal nodule is identified in some cases.

Etiology and Pathogenesis: Nipple adenoma is a benign proliferation of the lactiferous ducts in the nipple.

Histopathology: Microscopically, nipple adenoma appears as an endophytic, well-circumscribed proliferation of glandular structures.[61] The glands, or tubules, are lined by a bilayered epithelium, with an inner (luminal) apocrine secretory epithelium and an outer myoepithelial layer. Solid, papillary, and cystic areas can be seen. Sclerosis can impart the appearance of an irregular border or infiltration. Epidermal erosion or ulceration with an associated inflammatory infiltrate is not uncommon. Cytologically, the tumor cells are banal. Focal necrosis can be seen, but should not be florid in nipple adenoma.[61]

Differential Diagnosis: Depending on the clinical presentation, the clinical differential diagnosis includes Paget disease, mammary carcinoma, and eczema. Microscopically, the presence of sclerosis can simulate an invasive carcinoma, but the lack of atypia and the presence of myoepithelial cells (confirmed by immunohistochemistry) allows for a diagnosis of nipple adenoma.[61] Focal necrosis may raise the possibility of mammary ductal carcinoma in situ; however, cytological atypia should be absent in nipple adenoma.[61]

Clinical Course and Prognosis: Nipple adenoma is a benign proliferation, although coincidental mammary carcinoma has been reported.[61,62]

Management: Surgical excision is the treatment of choice to evaluate the entirety of the lesion. Recurrence can occur following incomplete excision.[62]

MALIGNANT

ADENOID CYSTIC CARCINOMA

Adenoid cystic carcinoma is a malignant adnexal neoplasm that rarely occurs as a primary skin disease, and more frequently arises in salivary gland tissues.

Epidemiology and Clinical Features: Primary cutaneous adenoid cystic carcinoma occurs in adults over a wide age range, with a median age in the sixth decade, and a slight female predominance.[63,64] It presents as a slow-growing nodule, averaging between 2 and 3 cm in size, on the head and neck, and, frequently, on the scalp. Adenoid cystic carcinoma can sometimes present on the trunk or extremities.

Etiology and Pathogenesis: Salivary gland adenoid cystic carcinoma has been shown to harbor a t(6;9)(q22-23;p23-24) translocation, resulting in a *MYB-NFIB* gene fusion.[65] This is considered a driving oncogenic event in the development of salivary gland adenoid cystic carcinoma. A recent study showed that the majority of primary cutaneous adenoid cystic carcinomas either harbored the *MYB-NFIB* fusion gene or showed overexpression of MYB by immunohistochemistry, suggesting a shared pathway in the development of salivary and primary cutaneous adenoid cystic carcinoma.[65]

Histopathology: Adenoid cystic carcinoma has a classic histologic appearance and is composed of dermal islands of basaloid cells arranged in a cribriform pattern with "punched-out" pseudocysts filled with mucin (Fig. 109-11A, B). The mucin is sialomucin, detected by an Alcian blue stain (pH 2.5).[63] The islands of basaloid cells are present in a hyalinized stroma and eosinophilic basement membrane material within the clusters of cells is often seen. Tubular and solid growth patterns also can be evident. Histologic grading for adenoid cystic carcinoma is defined as: grade 1, tubular and cribriform patterns; grade 2, less than 30% solid pattern; and grade 3, more than 30% solid pattern.[66] Perineural invasion is seen in a majority of cases.

True ductal differentiation can be seen in adenoid cystic carcinoma and highlighted by immunohistochemistry for EMA and CEA.[63,64] Adenoid cystic carcinoma tumor cells are reported to be positive for

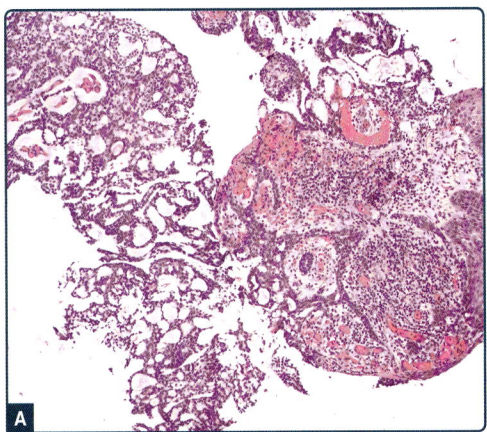

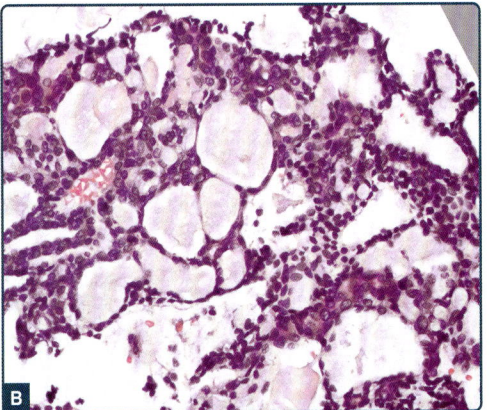

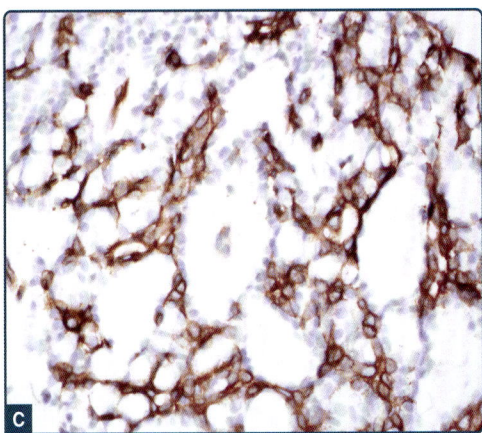

Figure 109-11 **A,** Adenoid cystic carcinoma is composed of dermal islands of basaloid cells. **B,** The tumor cells have a characteristic cribriform arrangement, with punched out pseudocysts filled with mucin. **C,** The tumor cells usually stain positively for CD117 (cKIT).

cytokeratins (including CK7), CD117 (cKIT), CK15, and SOX-10 (see Fig. 109-11C).[63-65,67] There is a myoepithelial component in adenoid cystic carcinoma, with those cells staining for typical myoepithelial markers, including smooth muscle actin, S100, and p63.[63,65]

Differential Diagnosis: Because primary cutaneous adenoid cystic carcinoma frequently occurs in the head and neck region, a salivary gland metastasis must be excluded, especially given the relative rarity of primary cutaneous adenoid cystic carcinoma compared to its salivary gland counterpart. There is significant histologic overlap between primary cutaneous and salivary gland adenoid cystic carcinoma, but reports suggest using differing immunohistochemical profiles to distinguish between them. CK15 and CK7 positivity are reported to favor primary cutaneous adenoid cystic carcinoma; CK15, however, has a high specificity and low sensitivity, whereas CK7 lacks specificity.[65] Prior reports of using CK5/CK6 and p63 to distinguish between primary cutaneous and salivary gland adenoid cystic carcinoma could not be validated in subsequent studies.[65]

Also in the histologic differential diagnosis of adenoid cystic carcinoma is basal cell carcinoma, which should be negative for CD117, EMA, CEA, or S100 immunostains (see Table 109-5).[63]

Clinical Course and Prognosis: Primary cutaneous adenoid cystic carcinoma follows an indolent clinical course, but recurrence is a frequent event, perhaps secondary to the high rates of perineural invasion.[63,64] Metastases are a rare event, but have been documented.[63-65] The prognosis for primary cutaneous adenoid cystic carcinoma is better than its salivary gland counterpart, which has an overall poor long-term survival rate. Unlike in the salivary gland, where histologic grade influences prognosis, no significant difference in recurrence has been seen between low-grade and high-grade cutaneous adenoid cystic carcinomas.[63]

Management: Wide local surgical excision is the treatment of choice, given the tendency to recur. Chemotherapy has been used to treat metastatic pulmonary disease.[64]

APOCRINE ADENOCARCINOMA

Cutaneous apocrine adenocarcinoma is a rare, malignant appendage neoplasm with apocrine differentiation.

Epidemiology and Clinical Features: Cutaneous apocrine adenocarcinoma affects elderly adults, typically in their sixth decade of life. It presents as a dermal nodule, ranging in size from 0.5 to 7.5 cm.[68] Cutaneous apocrine adenocarcinoma presents in areas of the body with a high distribution of apocrine glands, with the most frequent site being the axilla. Involvement of the anogenital region and scalp by apocrine adenocarcinoma also has been reported.

Etiology and Pathogenesis: Cutaneous apocrine adenocarcinoma is hypothesized to arise from normal or modified apocrine glands.

Histopathology: Histologically, cutaneous apocrine adenocarcinoma is a dermal tumor that displays apocrine differentiation with decapitation secretion and overt malignant features, including atypical architecture and cytological atypia. The tumor has irregular or infiltrative borders with frequent extension into the subcutaneous fat.[68] Tubular, tubulopapillary, and solid growth patterns can be seen and there is heterogeneity between tumors. An in situ component is often identified and can help to distinguish primary disease from a metastasis.

By immunohistochemistry, apocrine adenocarcinoma expresses cytokeratins (including CK7 and CK5/CK6), as well as GCDFP-15, CEA, EMA, ER (estrogen receptor), PR (progesterone receptor), and androgen receptor.[68]

Differential Diagnosis: Given the relative frequency of mammary adenocarcinoma, metastasis of a breast primary to the skin must be excluded to make the diagnosis of cutaneous apocrine adenocarcinoma. This requires predominantly clinicopathologic correlation, although identification of an in situ component can aid in the diagnosis of primary disease. A more recent study suggests using an immunohistochemical panel, including adipophilin, ER, PR, HER2 (human epidermal growth factor 2), CK5/CK6, and mammaglobin to distinguish cutaneous apocrine carcinoma (adipophilin−, ER+, PR+/−, HER2−, CK5/CK6+, mammaglobin+) from mammary apocrine carcinoma (adipophilin+, ER−, PR−, HER2 3+).[69]

Clinical Course and Prognosis: As cutaneous apocrine carcinoma is rare, prognostic factors are difficult to assess. In their series, Robson and colleagues, classified tumors similarly to mammary carcinomas using the modified Bloom-Richardson method, assigning scores based on histologic criteria.[68] Patients with high-grade tumors (grade 3) had statistically significant poorer survival rates than those with lower-grade tumors (grades 1 and 2). Aggressive behavior, including local recurrence, lymph node metastasis, and distant metastases, has been reported in cases of cutaneous apocrine adenocarcinoma. Patients with metastatic disease (locoregional and distant) have a poor prognosis with reduced survival rates.[70]

Management: Cutaneous apocrine adenocarcinoma is treated surgically by wide excision. Given the risk of metastatic disease and its associated poorer prognosis, some advocate for sentinel lymph node biopsy at the time of excision.[70]

Primary Cutaneous Cribriform Carcinoma: There is a more recently described variant of cutaneous apocrine carcinoma, primary cutaneous cribriform carcinoma.[71,72] Cutaneous cribriform carcinoma is a rare appendage tumor that affects adults and commonly presents on the limbs. Histologically, it is a relatively well-circumscribed, dermal neoplasm composed of connected, solid aggregates of basaloid cells with characteristic "punched out" cribriform spaces. These tumors have an indolent behavior with no recurrences or metastases reported as of this writing.

MUCINOUS CARCINOMA

Epidemiology and Clinical Features: Primary cutaneous mucinous carcinoma is a rare, malignant appendage neoplasm that primarily affects adult women in their sixth decade.[73] It presents as a solitary, flesh-colored nodule, often on the head, and can involve the scalp, eyelids, and face.

Histopathology: Mucinous carcinoma is classically composed of nests of epithelial cells floating within pools of mucin, although heterogeneity between tumors can be observed, including the presence of in situ and invasive ductal components.

Differential Diagnosis: Primary cutaneous mucinous carcinoma is a diagnosis of exclusion and the possibility of metastatic mucinous carcinoma, including from the breast or GI tract, must be evaluated. Clinical history, imaging, and site of involvement are crucial aspects in the workup of the patient. Immunohistochemistry plays a limited role, including in the evaluation of metastatic disease, but CK20 and CDX-2 can be helpful in evaluating for metastatic disease from a colonic primary.[5,73]

Clinical Course and Prognosis: Local recurrence of primary cutaneous mucinous carcinoma is a common occurrence at a reported rate between 30% and 43%, but clinically aggressive behavior is extremely rare.[74]

Management: Treatment of primary cutaneous mucinous carcinoma is surgical excision.

TUMORS WITH FOLLICULAR DIFFERENTIATION

The hair follicle is a complex miniorgan that cycles through different phases, including anagen, telogen, and catagen. (See Chap. 7 for a detailed discussion on normal hair follicles.) A mature hair follicle is composed of different horizontal portions: bulb, stem, isthmus, and infundibulum. Additionally, there is an inner root sheath and an outer root sheath that encompasses the hair shaft. Follicular neoplasms show differentiation toward these different portions of the hair follicle, as well as follicular mesenchyme and developmental stages of hair growth.[3,75] Table 109-7 lists appendage tumors with follicular differentiation. Differentiation toward follicular germinative cells recapitulates embryonic follicular hair germ and shows basaloid differentiation with peripheral palisading. Differentiation toward the perifollicular sheath (or mesenchyme) is typified by thin collagen fibrils, mucinous matrix, fibroblasts, and blood vessels. Differentiation toward the hair bulb displays matrical cell differentiation. Differentiation toward the outer root sheath shows clear cells, whereas differentiation toward the inner root sheath shows eosinophilic cells. Infundibular differentiation is similar to normal epidermal differentiation with basal, spinous, granular, and corneal layers represented.

TABLE 109-7
Classification of Follicular Appendage Neoplasms

TYPE (LINEAGE) OF FOLLICULAR DIFFERENTIATION	BENIGN	MALIGNANT
Pan-follicular	Trichofolliculoma	
Germinative cells		Basal cell carcinoma
Biphasic (Epithelial-Mesenchymal)	Trichoblastoma Trichoepithelioma Desmoplastic trichoepithelioma	
Mesenchymal	Trichodiscoma/Fibrofolliculoma	
Matrical	Pilomatricoma	Pilomatrical carcinoma
Outer root sheath at the level of bulb/stem	Trichilemmoma (including desmoplastic)	Trichilemmal carcinoma
Outer root sheath at the level of the isthmus	Tumor of follicular infundibulum Pilar sheath acanthoma Proliferating pilar tumor	
Infundibulum	Trichoadenoma Dilated pore (of Winer)	

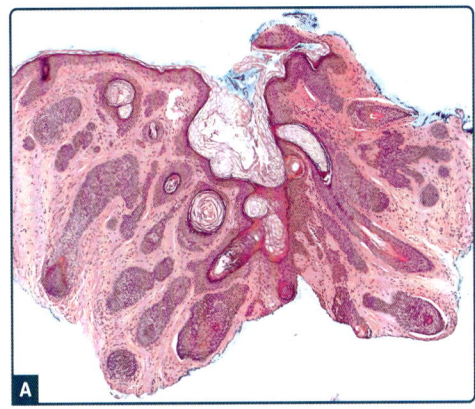

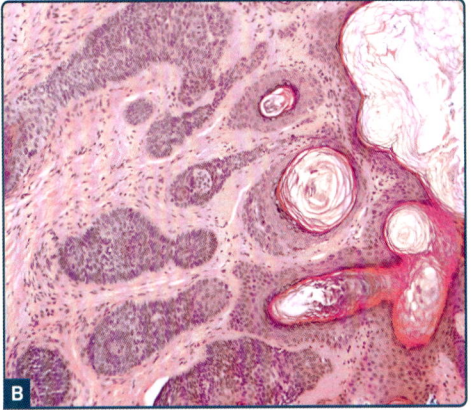

Figure 109-12 **A,** Trichofolliculoma is characterized by numerous small hair follicles radiating from a central pore. **B,** The follicles vary in stages of differentiation.

NEOPLASM WITH PAN-FOLLICULAR DIFFERENTIATION

TRICHOFOLLICULOMA

Epidemiology and Clinical Features: Trichofolliculoma is a rare, benign entity that typically presents as a single, flesh-colored papule in the head and neck region in adults.[76] The nose is the most commonly affected site. Classically, a central dell with protruding vellus hairs is seen.

Etiology and Pathogenesis: Trichofolliculoma is a benign follicular hamartoma that shows differentiation toward all portions of the hair follicle.[1,3]

Histopathology: Trichofolliculoma displays characteristic histopathologic findings, with a central dilated or cystic infundibulum and secondary hair follicles radiating into the dermis (Fig. 109-12A).[3,75,76] The secondary hair follicles are surrounded by connective tissue. The hair follicles can display different stages of differentiation, from immature hair germ to mature hair follicles to vellus hairs (Fig. 109-12B). Similarly, the abundance of connective tissue can vary between lesions. Sebaceous differentiation can be observed.

Differential Diagnosis: The histologic differential diagnosis for trichofolliculoma can include folliculosebaceous cystic hamartoma, especially if there is sebaceous differentiation. In contrast to trichofolliculoma, folliculosebaceous cystic hamartoma typically has mesenchymal differentiation (eg, into adipose tissue) and prominent sebaceous differentiation.

Clinical Course and Prognosis: Trichofolliculoma is a benign entity.

Management: The treatment of choice for trichofolliculoma is surgical excision, with an emphasis on cosmesis.

NEOPLASM OF FOLLICULAR GERMINATIVE CELLS

BASAL CELL CARCINOMA

Basal cell carcinoma is a malignant neoplasm of follicular germinative differentiation and is discussed in detail in Chap. 111.

BIPHASIC (EPITHELIAL–MESENCHYMAL) NEOPLASMS OF FOLLICULAR GERMINATIVE AND FOLLICULAR STROMAL CELLS

TRICHOBLASTOMA

Trichoblastoma is a benign neoplasm, showing differentiation toward both follicular germinative and follicular stromal cells. Trichoepithelioma (cribriform trichoblastoma) and desmoplastic trichoepithelioma (columnar trichoblastoma) are considered variants of trichoblastoma (see the section "Trichoepithelioma").[1,75]

Epidemiology and Clinical Features: Trichoblastoma (Fig. 109-13A) affects adults and presents as a flesh-colored to red, dermal nodule on the head and neck, with reported involvement of the trunk and extremities as well.[1,3]

Etiology and Pathogenesis: Trichoblastoma shows differentiation toward both follicular germinative and follicular stromal cells.

Histopathology: Microscopically, trichoblastoma is a well-circumscribed dermal tumor composed of nests of basaloid cells in a cellular stroma (see Fig. 109-13B). The basaloid nests can be arranged in a variety of patterns, including nodular and trabecular. The stromal component consists of collagen fibrils and fibroblasts. Clefting within the stroma is common (but not between the basaloid nests and the stroma, as in basal cell carcinoma; see Fig. 109-13C). Abortive follicular structures, so-called papillary mesenchymal bodies, can be seen, as can more advanced follicular differentiation.

Cutaneous lymphadenoma is considered the adamantoid form of trichoblastoma, and is composed of nests of basaloid germinative cells with peripheral palisading and epithelioid cells with pale cytoplasm in the center of the nests. The tumor is infiltrated by small lymphocytes.

Differential Diagnosis: The main differential diagnosis for trichoblastoma is basal cell carcinoma. Trichoblastoma should show little cytologic atypia, a low mitotic rate, absent necrosis (although single-cell apoptosis can be seen), and clefting within the stroma. Basal cell carcinoma often displays cytologic atypia, frequent mitoses, necrosis, stromal mucinosis, and clefting between the epithelial nests and the tumor stroma. However, there can be overlap, and distinction on small biopsies can be difficult.

Studies have reported the usefulness of immunohistochemistry in distinguishing basal cell carcinoma from trichoblastoma. CK20+ Merkel cells tend to be absent in basal cell carcinoma, but are commonly found in trichoblastoma.[77] Another study showed that CD10 stains the stromal cells in trichoblastoma, but highlights the epithelial cells in basal cell carcinoma.[78] CK17 staining has been reported to distinguish basal cell carcinoma from lymphadenoma, with strong, diffuse staining in basal cell carcinoma, and weak, peripheral staining in lymphadenoma.[79] Drebin shows strong expression in basal cell carcinoma, with weak staining in both trichoblastoma and trichoepithelioma.[80] (Table 109-8 summarizes these immunohistochemical findings.)

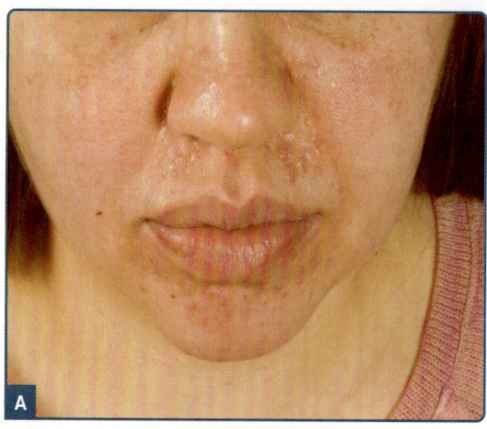
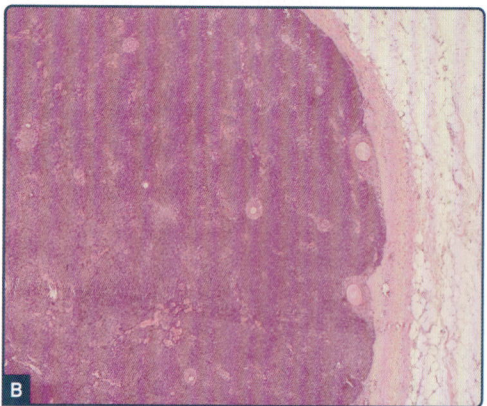
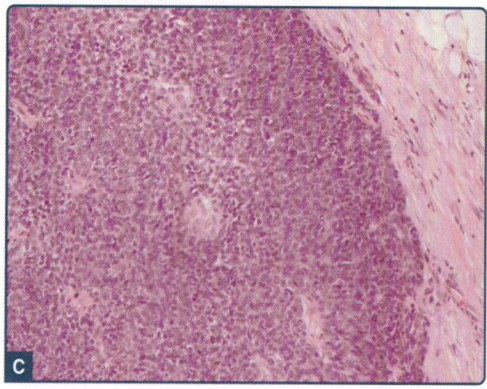

Figure 109-13 **A,** Trichoblastoma present as red to flesh-colored dermal nodules, often on the face. **B,** The tumor is a circumscribed dermal nodule composed predominantly of basaloid cells. **C,** The basaloid epithelioid structures may resemble basal cell carcinoma; however, the characteristic mucin-containing clefts separating basal cell carcinoma from the stroma are not a feature of trichoblastoma.

TABLE 109-8
Summary of Immunohistochemical Stains in the Distinction between Basal Cell Carcinoma, Trichoblastoma, and Trichoepithelioma

	BCC	TRICHOBLASTOMA	TRICHOEPITHELIOMA	DESMOPLASTIC TRICHOEPITHELIOMA
CK15	−	ND	+	+
BerEP4	+	+/−	−	+/−
CK20	−	+ (Merkel cells)	+ (Merkel cells)	+ (Merkel cells)
CD10	+ (epithelial cells)	+ (stromal cells)	ND	ND
CD34	− (stromal cells)	ND	+ (stromal cells)	− (stromal cells)
Drebin	+	−	ND	ND
PHLDA1	−	ND	+	+

−, Negative; +, positive; BCC, basal cell carcinoma; ND, no data.

Clinical Course and Prognosis: Malignant transformation from trichoblastoma to trichoblastic carcinoma or sarcoma is extremely rare.[81]

Management: Although it is a benign neoplasm, complete surgical excision of trichoblastoma is recommended, given the low risk of malignant transformation and the difficulty in distinguishing it from basal cell carcinoma on small biopsies.

TRICHOEPITHELIOMA AND DESMOPLASTIC TRICHOEPITHELIOMA

Trichoepithelioma is considered the cribriform variant of trichoblastoma with infundibulocystic differentiation. Solitary (sporadic), multiple, and desmoplastic types occur.[3,75] Desmoplastic trichoepithelioma is also known as the columnar variant of trichoblastoma.[1]

Epidemiology and Clinical Features: Both solitary and desmoplastic trichoepitheliomas affect middle-aged adults with a female predilection.[82,83] Multiple trichoepitheliomas typically affect a younger patient population in their 20s.[18] Solitary trichoepithelioma presents as a single, flesh-colored papule on the face, measuring approximately 5 mm in size, and is often located on the nose or cheek. Desmoplastic trichoepithelioma presents as a single, white to yellow, firm papule or plaque with a central depression. Desmoplastic trichoepithelioma is frequently found on the face, with the cheek and nose the most common locations. Multiple trichoepitheliomas present as multiple small papules on the face, often involving the nasolabial folds and sometimes occurring in an X-like pattern.

Etiology and Pathogenesis: Multiple trichoepitheliomas are observed with an autosomal dominant inheritance pattern and are associated with mutations in the *CYLD* gene on chromosome 16, similar to Brooke-Spiegler syndrome (see Table 109-2).[18] Multiple trichoepitheliomas are also seen in Rombo syndrome and Bazex-Dupré-Christol syndrome,[75] where patients have atrophoderma, milia, basal cell carcinomas, and hypotrichosis. Deletions of the *PTCH1* gene locus at 9q22 have been found in some trichoepitheliomas.[84]

Histopathology: Trichoepithelioma is a well-circumscribed, dermal tumor composed of basaloid germinative epithelial cells arranged in a cribriform pattern within a fibrous stroma (Fig. 109-14A). Retiform and small nodular patterns also can be seen. Desmoplastic trichoepithelioma is located in the upper dermis and composed of strands and small nests of basaloid cells in a sclerotic stroma. Like other variants of trichoblastoma, varying degrees of follicular differentiation can be seen in trichoepitheliomas. Papillary mesenchymal bodies are a characteristic finding (Fig. 109-14B). Infundibulocystic changes can be seen in both trichoepithelioma and desmoplastic trichoepithelioma.

Differential Diagnosis: If it has a classic appearance, the diagnosis of trichoepithelioma can be suggested clinically, prior to histologic evaluation. For trichoepithelioma, the main differential diagnosis is a basal cell carcinoma (see Fig. 109-14C), and like trichoblastoma, can be difficult to discern on small biopsies. Similarly, for desmoplastic trichoepithelioma, the differential diagnosis includes basal cell carcinoma, microcystic adnexal carcinoma, and, sometimes, syringoma.

Trichoepithelioma and desmoplastic trichoepithelioma, in contrast to basal cell carcinoma, tend to have symmetric growth, lack of invasion into the surrounding dermis, follicular-type stroma, and clefting within the stroma. Expression of PHLDA1 has been suggested as an immunohistochemical tool to distinguish basal cell carcinoma (PHLDA1−) from trichoepithelioma and desmoplastic trichoepithelioma (PHLDA1+).[85-87] CK20+ Merkel cells are also more prevalent in desmoplastic trichoepithelioma than in basal cell carcinoma or microcystic adnexal carcinoma (see Fig. 109-14D).[88] Although androgen receptor (AR) expression has been suggested as a way to differentiate desmoplastic trichoepithelioma (AR−) from basal cell carcinoma (AR+),[89] subsequent studies

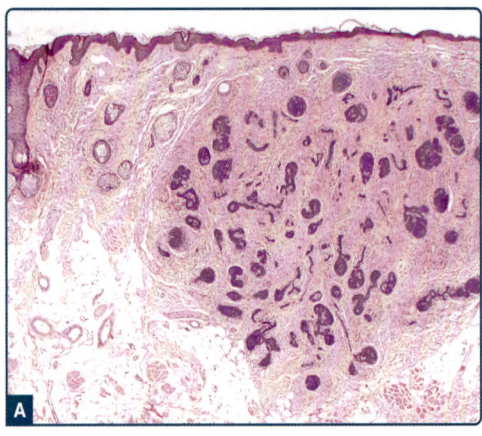 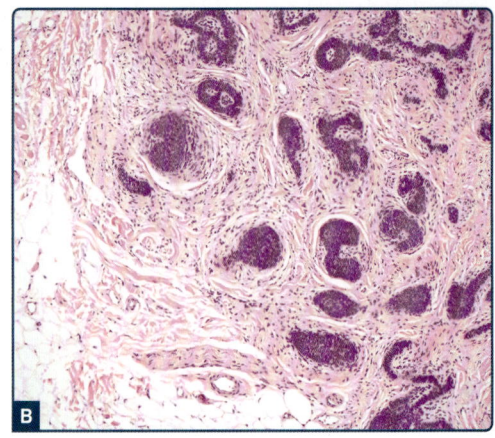
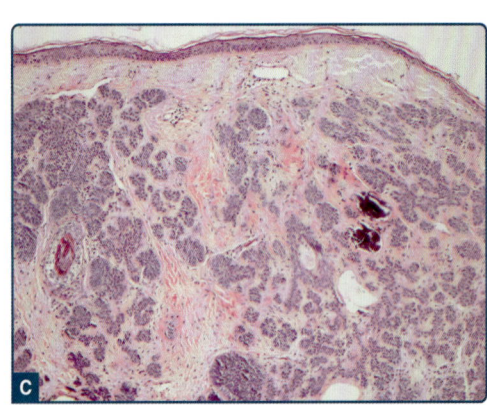 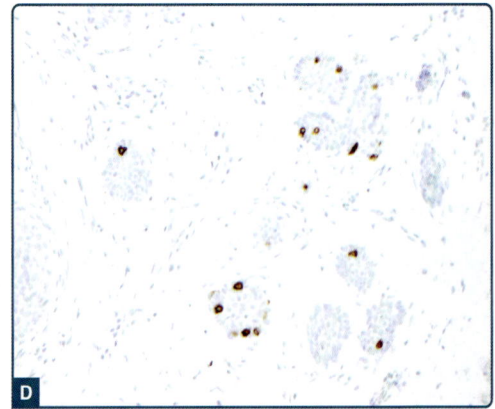

Figure 109-14 **A,** Trichoepithelioma is a well-circumscribed, superficial, dermal tumor. **B,** The tumor is composed of basaloid germinative epithelial cells that form papillary mesenchymal bodies, which are composed of a cup-shaped arrangement of basaloid epithelium with a central cellular fibroblastic core. **C,** In tumors with a predominance of basaloid cells the differential diagnosis includes basal cell carcinoma. **D,** CK20+ Merkel cells are often present.

have been less supportive.[90] Trichoepithelioma may have staining of the tumor cells and the surrounding stromal cells for CD34[91]; the tumor is usually without staining for BerEP4. In contrast, basal cell carcinoma is usually BerEP4+ without CD34+ surrounding stromal cells.[91] Desmoplastic trichoepithelioma, conversely, can show positive staining for BerEP4 and the peritumoral stromal cells are negative for CD34 staining.[5] (Table 109-8 summarizes these immunohistochemical findings.)

Clinical Course and Prognosis: Trichoepithelioma and desmoplastic trichoepithelioma are benign appendage neoplasms.

Management: Surgical excision, including by Mohs micrographic surgery, can be considered for solitary lesions, especially if the histologic diagnosis is in doubt. Treatment of multiple facial trichoepitheliomas is focused on cosmesis and can be challenging. Ablative methods, such as electrosurgery, cryosurgery, and laser treatment have been employed in the treatment of multiple trichoepitheliomas, as have topical treatments, such as imiquimod.[82]

NEOPLASMS WITH FOLLICULAR MESENCHYMAL DIFFERENTIATION

TRICHODISCOMA/ FIBROFOLLICULOMA

Historically, trichodiscoma and fibrofolliculoma were considered separate entities. They are now thought to be a single entity that exists on a morphologic spectrum, in part because they can coexist in the same patient, and because individual lesions can contain features characteristic of each entity.[1,75,92] We include trichodiscoma/fibrofolliculoma in the follicular neoplasm section, given the abundant follicular-type mesenchyme present in the tumor. Others, however, regard trichodiscoma/fibrofolliculoma as a sebaceous neoplasm, as it shows differentiation toward the mantle.[1,92] The mantle is an immature sebaceous gland with shrunken lobules that corresponds to the state of the gland between infancy and puberty when circulating androgens are absent.

Epidemiology and Clinical Features:
Trichodiscoma/fibrofolliculoma occurs in adult patients over a wide age range.[92] It presents as a firm, white to flesh-colored papule, measuring between 1 and 3 mm in size. Trichodiscoma/fibrofolliculoma is typically observed on the face, but they can be present on the trunk. Multiple lesions are associated with Birt-Hogg-Dubé syndrome (see "Etiology and Pathogenesis" below).

Etiology and Pathogenesis:
Multiple trichodiscomas/fibrofolliculomas are manifestations of Birt-Hogg-Dubé syndrome, an autosomal dominant syndrome caused by mutations in the *folliculin (FLCN)* gene on chromosome 17 (see Table 109-2).[93] Patients with Birt-Hogg-Dubé syndrome have an increased risk of renal tumors, lung cysts, and recurrent pneumothoraces.[93]

Histopathology:
Trichodiscomas classically are dermal neoplasms composed predominantly of fibrous stromal elements with islands of mature sebaceous lobules at the periphery. Fibrofolliculomas classically are described with a central follicular infundibulum in the dermis with radially oriented thin epithelial cords, which may or may not contain mature sebocytes (Fig. 109-15A, B). As previously mentioned, lesions may contain one or both histologic patterns with morphologic variability.[92] The stromal cells show positivity for CD34 and Nestin by immunohistochemistry, while the cellular cords are positive for CK15, suggesting the neoplastic cells are derived from the follicular bulge stem cell.[92]

Differential Diagnosis:
When stromal differentiation predominates, neural tumors enter into the histologic differential diagnosis, but can be easily distinguished by S100 immunohistochemistry, which is negative in trichodiscoma/fibrofolliculoma.

Clinical Course and Prognosis:
Trichodiscoma/fibrofolliculoma is benign, but given its association with Birt-Hogg-Dubé syndrome, genetic screening should be considered for patients with the neoplasm.

Management:
Laser ablation of multiple trichodiscomas/fibrofolliculomas results in short-term improvement with eventual regrowth.[93]

NEOPLASMS WITH MATRICAL DIFFERENTIATION

PILOMATRICOMA (PILOMATRIXOMA)

Pilomatricoma (or pilomatrixoma) is a benign neoplasm with follicular differentiation. It was initially

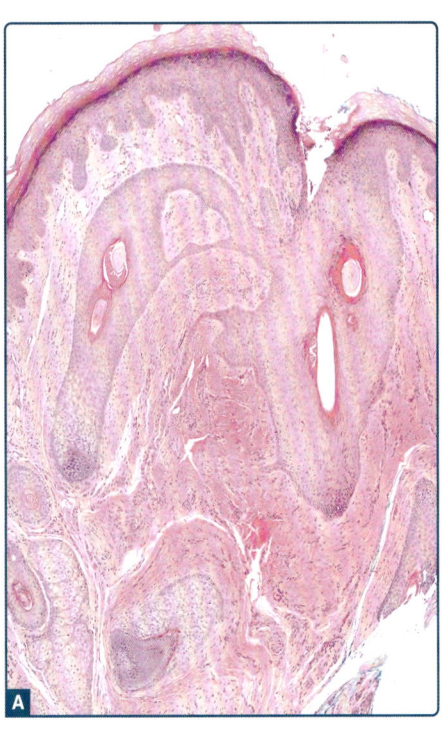 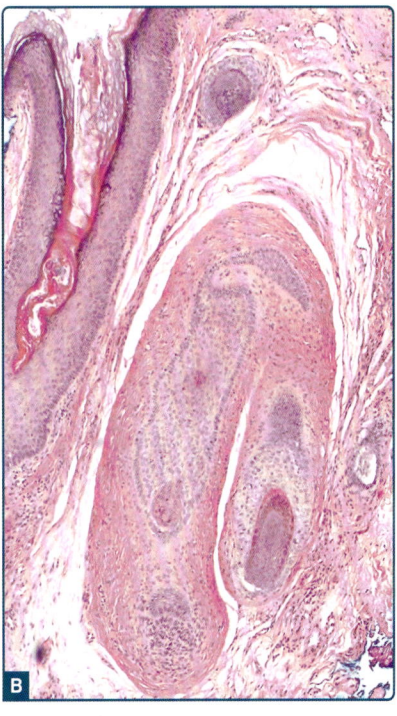

Figure 109-15 **A,** Fibrofolliculoma is composed of pilar and stromal elements. **B,** Irregularly shaped follicles with delicate fronds extend into a densely fibrotic perifollicular stroma.

described as "calcifying epithelioma of Malherbe" in 1880 and was thought to arise from sebaceous glands.[94-96]

Epidemiology and Clinical Features: Pilomatricoma (Fig. 109-16A) affects a wide age range, but is most common in children and young adults, and is the most common appendage tumor in children.[94-96] One series reported a bimodal age distribution in the first and sixth decades.[94] Some studies report a female predilection.[94,96] It presents clinically as a firm, asymptomatic, slow-growing nodule between 1 and 1.5 cm in size. The head and neck region is the most common site of involvement, followed by the upper extremities.[94-96]

Etiology and Pathogenesis: Pilomatricoma displays differentiation toward the follicular matrix. Pilomatricoma can be associated with a variety of genetic syndromes, including Gardner syndrome, myotonic muscular dystrophy, and Rubinstein-Taybi syndrome (see Table 109-2).[75] Most pilomatricomas harbor mutations in the gene encoding the β-catenin protein, *CTNNB1*, implicating WNT signaling in tumor pathogenesis.[97]

Histopathology: Pilomatricoma has a characteristic histologic appearance and is a well-circumscribed dermal nodule with peripheral, nucleated basaloid cells and central, enucleated eosinophilic "ghost" cells (see Fig. 109-16B, C). The basaloid cells have hyperchromatic, round nuclei and scant cytoplasm and resemble the matrical cells of the normal hair follicle. Tumors are initially cystic with relatively few numbers of ghost cells, but with increasing age of the lesion, ghost cells increase in number until they predominate. Calcification of pilomatricomas is not uncommon (see Fig. 109-16D).

Differential Diagnosis: Pilomatricoma can clinically resemble a cyst. Given its characteristic histologic appearance, pilomatricoma is rarely confused with other entities in an adequate biopsy specimen.

Clinical Course and Prognosis: Pilomatricoma is a benign neoplasm with rare malignant transformation (see "Pilomatrical Carcinoma" below). Local recurrences following surgery are also uncommon.[94,95]

Management: Wide local surgical excision is the treatment of choice for pilomatricoma.

PILOMATRICAL CARCINOMA

Pilomatrical carcinoma is a rare, malignant appendage neoplasm. It also has been referred to as pilomatrix carcinoma, malignant pilomatricoma, and matrical carcinoma.[98]

Epidemiology and Clinical Features: Pilomatrical carcinoma occurs in middle-aged to elderly patients, most often presenting in white males.[98] Pilomatrical carcinoma presents as a dermal nodule, frequently arising in the head and neck

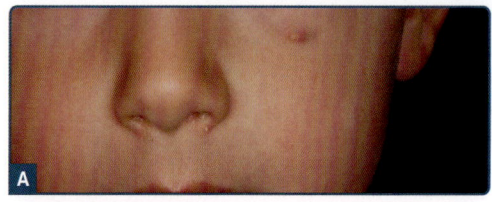
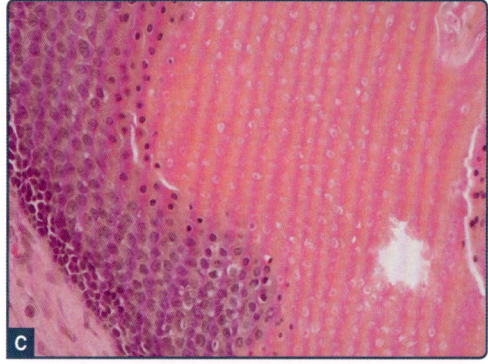
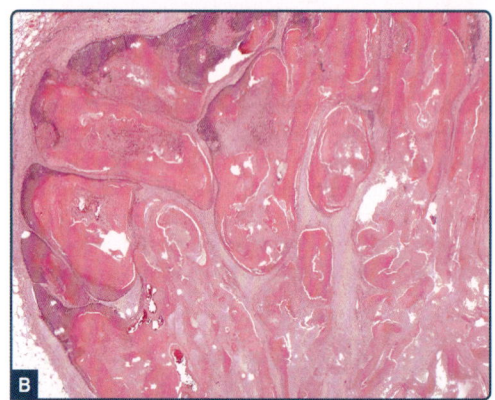
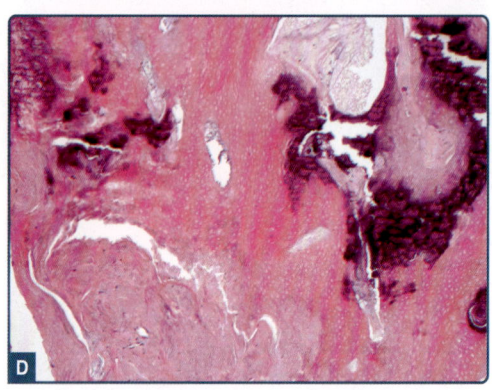

Figure 109-16 **A,** Pilomatricoma is a circumscribed dermal nodule, with (**B**) peripheral nucleated basaloid cells and central eosinophilic shadow cells (ghost cells). **C,** The basaloid cells have round nuclei resembling pilar matrical cells, whereas shadow cells are composed of eosinophilic cellular material with a faint outline of nuclear membrane. **D,** In some cases basaloid cells are inconspicuous and there is prominent calcification, in which event, the tumor also has been known as calcifying epithelioma of Malherbe.

region. "Rapid growth" is cited as a common reason for biopsy.

Etiology and Pathogenesis: Histologic evaluation can reveal areas of benign pilomatricoma with transition to malignancy; however, pilomatrical carcinoma rarely develops at the site of a previously biopsied or excised pilomatricoma.[98] Both benign pilomatricoma and malignant pilomatrical carcinoma harbor mutations in the gene encoding β-catenin, suggesting at least some role for the WNT signaling pathway in the tumorigenesis of matrical follicular tumors, but also implying that additional mutations be acquired to achieve malignant transformation.[98]

Histopathology: Histologically, pilomatrical carcinoma is a poorly circumscribed, nodular, dermal tumor, with infiltrative borders and central necrosis.[98] A desmoplastic stroma surrounds the tumor. The tumor is composed of pleomorphic, basaloid cells with frequent mitoses. "Ghost" cells can be present, but do not predominate. Lymphovascular invasion is not common.

Differential Diagnosis: Clinically, the differential diagnosis of a rapidly growing dermal nodule is broad and includes other malignant appendage neoplasms, cutaneous metastases, soft-tissue tumors, and benign cysts. Histologically, follicular matrical differentiation should be conspicuous and cytological pleomorphism, infiltrative growth, and necrosis all favor malignancy.

Clinical Course and Prognosis: Local recurrence is common and is a risk factor for locoregional metastasis.[98] Distant metastatic disease and death have been reported in association with pilomatrical carcinoma.[98]

Management: Wide local excision is the current recommended treatment for pilomatrical carcinoma, with close clinical followup given the risk of recurrence and metastasis.[98] Limited data is available for using radiation therapy either as the sole therapy or as adjuvant therapy.[98] Chemotherapy currently plays no role in the treatment of pilomatrical carcinoma.

NEOPLASMS WITH BULB/STEM OUTER ROOT SHEATH DIFFERENTIATION

TRICHILEMMOMA

Epidemiology and Clinical Features: Trichilemmoma is a benign neoplasm that presents in adults over a wide age range.[99] Clinically, it can present singly or as multiple lesions. Trichilemmomas are flesh-colored papules and can have a verrucous surface. They typically present on the head and neck and have a predilection for the nose. Multiple trichilemmomas, including involvement of the oral mucosa, are associated with Cowden syndrome (multiple hamartoma syndrome).[100] Desmoplastic trichilemmoma is a histologic variant.

Etiology and Pathogenesis: Trichilemmoma is a follicular neoplasm with differentiation toward the outer root sheath at the level of the hair bulb and stem ("trichilemmal"). Some consider trichilemmoma to be a viral wart, but studies looking at the presence of human papillomavirus DNA in trichilemmomas have produced conflicting results.[1,75] Multiple trichilemmomas with involvement of mucocutaneous sites are associated with Cowden syndrome (multiple hamartoma syndrome), an autosomal dominant syndrome caused by mutations in the tumor-suppressor gene *PTEN* (see Table 109-2).[100] Patients with Cowden syndrome have hamartomas affecting multiple organ systems, including the skin, breast, thyroid, endometrium, and GI tract, and have an increased risk of malignancy in those affected organs, especially the breast. Other clinical manifestations of Cowden syndrome include oral papillomatosis and acral and palmoplantar keratosis.[100] Expression of PTEN protein, as measured by immunohistochemistry, is lost in most Cowden syndrome–associated trichilemmomas, but is retained in sporadic trichilemmomas.[100] A recent study found *HRAS* activating mutations in 60% of sporadic trichilemmomas.[101]

Histopathology: Microscopically, trichilemmoma is a well-circumscribed tumor with endophytic lobules extending from the epidermis into the dermis (Fig. 109-17A).[99] Surface verrucous changes are often present. The lobules are composed of pale, eosinophilic keratinocytes with peripheral palisading and are surrounded by a thick, PAS-positive, hyaline membrane (Fig. 109-17B).

Desmoplastic trichilemmoma is a histologic variant and is composed of central strands of pale eosinophilic keratinocytes in a fibrotic stroma (Fig. 109-18A). The periphery of desmoplastic trichilemmoma typically has a more classic, circumscribed appearance with a PAS-positive hyaline membrane (Fig. 109-18B).

Differential Diagnosis: Clinically, trichilemmoma can resemble a wart or basal cell carcinoma. Histologically, the diagnosis of trichilemmoma is straightforward, unless a partial biopsy is received, and then the differential can include wart, seborrheic keratosis, clear-cell poroma, and clear-cell acanthoma.

Infiltrative carcinoma, including squamous cell carcinoma and basal cell carcinoma, is in the histologic differential diagnosis of desmoplastic trichilemmoma. Trichilemmoma, including the desmoplastic variant, is positive for CD34 (see Fig. 109-18C), and should not show cytologic atypia, as would be seen in a carcinoma (see Table 109-4).[2,75] Areas of conventional trichilemmoma with clear cells and surrounding hyaline membrane can aid in the diagnosis.

Clinical Course and Prognosis: Trichilemmoma is a benign follicular neoplasm. Trichilemmal carcinoma is considered the malignant counterpart,

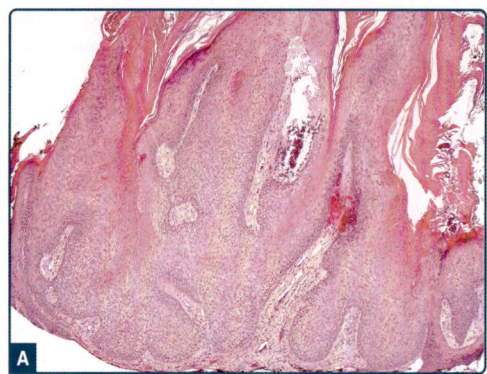
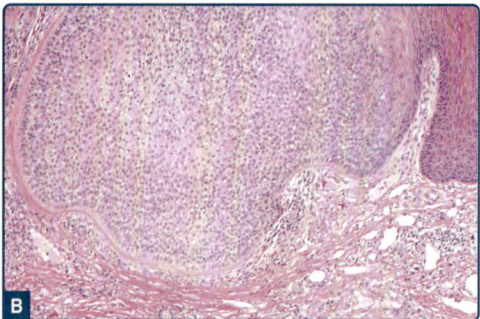

Figure 109-17 A, Trichilemmoma is an endophytic proliferation of epithelial cells with clear cytoplasm resembling the hair follicle outer root sheath; the surface may have a verrucous appearance. **B,** There is a palisaded proliferation of basaloid cells, surrounded by a variably dense eosinophilic hyaline membrane; the clear cells have round to oval nuclei without cellular atypia.

and appears to be a rare entity.[102] Trichilemmal carcinoma was originally described by Headington in 1976, and some now question whether entities originally diagnosed as trichilemmal carcinomas are instead clear-cell squamous carcinomas or even desmoplastic trichilemmomas.[1,102]

Management: Trichilemmomas are benign neoplasms and can be treated with surgical excision. Cases of desmoplastic trichilemmomas treated with Mohs micrographic surgery have been reported.[103] Trichilemmoma also can be treated by laser ablation. Trichilemmal carcinoma is treated by surgical excision using either conventional or Mohs micrographic techniques.[104]

NEOPLASMS WITH ISTHMIC OUTER ROOT SHEATH DIFFERENTIATION

TUMOR OF FOLLICULAR INFUNDIBULUM

Tumor of follicular infundibulum is a rare, benign appendage neoplasm originally described by Mehregan and Butler in 1961.[105]

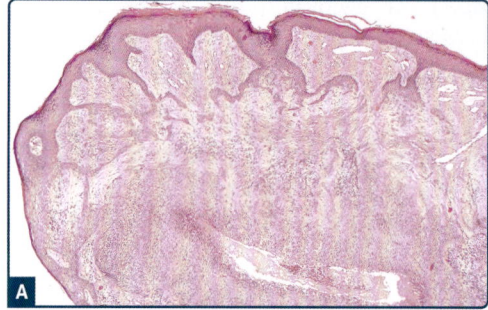
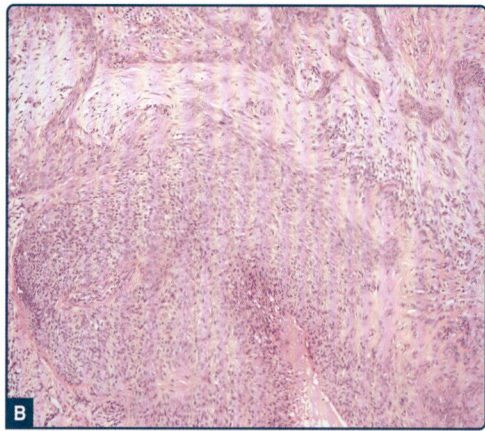
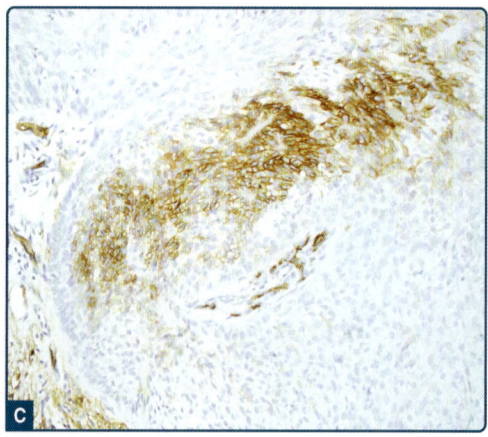

Figure 109-18 A, Desmoplastic trichilemmoma has features similar to trichilemmoma but with a central zone of stromal sclerosis entrapping cords of epithelium. **B,** The top of this image shows areas of desmoplastic change with cords of tumor cells; the bottom of this image shows clear cells and a thick hyaline membrane characteristic of trichilemmoma. **C,** The tumor cells may stain positively for CD34.

Epidemiology and Clinical Features: Tumor of follicular infundibulum presents in adult patients with an average age in the sixth decade. There is no apparent sex predilection, with different reports showing varying results.[1,106] Tumor of follicular infundibulum often presents as a solitary keratotic papule on the head and neck.[106] Multiple tumors of follicular infundibulum can present as hypopigmented macules, also located on the head and neck.

Etiology and Pathogenesis: Despite its name, tumor of follicular infundibulum displays follicular isthmic differentiation, rather than infundibular, and its pathogenesis is still unclear. Although most regard tumor of follicular infundibulum as a benign appendage neoplasm, some regard it as a type of basal cell carcinoma.[106]

Histopathology: Microscopically, tumor of follicular infundibulum is composed of strands of eosinophilic, isthmic keratinocytes that extend from the epidermis into the superficial dermis in a reticular pattern. Special stains reveal a "brush-like" network of elastic fibers that surround the base of the tumor.[75,106] Tumor cells are negative for BerEP4 and show scattered CK20+ Merkel cells, in contrast to basal cell carcinoma.[106] Rarely, tumor of follicular infundibulum can be associated with other entities, such as basal cell carcinoma, squamous cell carcinoma, and melanoma in situ.[106]

Differential Diagnosis: The clinical differential diagnosis includes basal cell carcinoma and seborrheic keratosis.

Clinical Course and Prognosis: Tumor of follicular infundibulum is a benign entity, but can be associated with malignancies. Transformation to basal cell carcinoma also has been reported in a patient with numerous tumors of follicular infundibulum.[107]

Management: Follicular infundibulum tumor treatments include topical steroids, retinoids, cryotherapy, curettage, and surgery, with all showing limited results, especially in patients with multiple tumors.[108]

PILAR SHEATH ACANTHOMA

Pilar sheath acanthoma is a rare, benign appendage neoplasm that was first described in 1978.[109]

Epidemiology and Clinical Features: Pilar sheath acanthoma affects adult patients over a wide age range without apparent sex predilection.[110] Clinically, it presents as a single, flesh-colored nodule with a central keratotic plug, often on the upper lip or central face.

Etiology and Pathogenesis: Pilar sheath acanthoma shows differentiation toward both infundibular and isthmic portions of the normal hair follicle.[75]

Histopathology: Microscopically, pilar sheath acanthoma is a well-circumscribed cystic epithelial proliferation with superficial/central infundibulocystic differentiation and peripheral isthmic differentiation. Lobules composed of eosinophilic, pale keratinocytes (showing isthmic differentiation at the level of the outer root sheath) emanate radially from the central cystic cavity. Horn cysts, sebocytes, and sebaceous ducts can be observed within the lobules.

Differential Diagnosis: Histologically, dilated pore and trichofolliculoma are in the differential diagnosis of pilar sheath acanthoma.[75,110] The radial projections are more lobular in pilar sheath acanthoma, as compared to dilated pore, and the radial projections in trichofolliculoma contain vellus hairs. Dilated pore does not show isthmic differentiation.

Clinical Course and Prognosis: Pilar sheath acanthoma is a benign entity.

Management: Surgical excision of pilar sheath acanthoma can be performed for cosmetic purposes.

PROLIFERATING PILAR TUMOR

Proliferating pilar tumor was first described by Jones in 1966 as "proliferating epidermoid cyst."[111] Other names used for this entity include proliferating pilar cyst, proliferating trichilemmal cyst, pilar tumor of the scalp, and invasive hair matrix tumor.[112,113]

Epidemiology and Clinical Features: Proliferating pilar tumor occurs in adult patients typically in their sixth decade or older; there is a marked female predilection.[112,113] The tumor presents as a dermal nodule on the scalp with a mean size of 3 cm, but sizes up to 25 cm have been documented.[112] Tumors can present singly or as multiple lesions.

Etiology and Pathogenesis: Proliferating pilar tumor is a follicular neoplasm with differentiation toward the outer root sheath at the level of the isthmus. Consequently, it displays characteristic trichilemmal keratinization with abrupt transition from squamous epithelium to glassy, compact keratin without a granular cell layer. Proliferating pilar tumor is thought to derive from existing pilar (trichilemmal) cysts.[113] Proliferating pilar tumors have been reported in patients with keratitis, ichthyosis, and deafness (KID) syndrome, which is caused by mutations in the gene encoding connexin-26 (see Table 109-2).[114,115]

Histopathology: Microscopically, proliferating pilar tumors are well-circumscribed dermal neoplasms with a lobular architecture (Fig. 109-19A). They are composed of eosinophilic keratinocytes with central trichilemmal keratinization and peripheral palisading. Squamous eddies and calcifications within the neoplasm are common findings (Fig. 109-19C). The basement membrane surrounding the tumor can be eosinophilic and prominent.

Differential Diagnosis: The clinical differential diagnosis includes a cyst, either epidermoid or pilar. Histologically, proliferating pilar tumor can be difficult to distinguish from squamous cell carcinoma, especially in areas of solid growth or in limited biopsies (see Fig. 109-19B). Identification of squamous eddies, trichilemmal keratinization, or possibly the remnant of a pilar cyst can be instrumental in the distinction between proliferating pilar tumor and squamous cell carcinoma. Immunohistochemistry has been proposed to distinguish proliferating pilar tumor and squamous cell carcinoma. Proliferating pilar tumor cells show

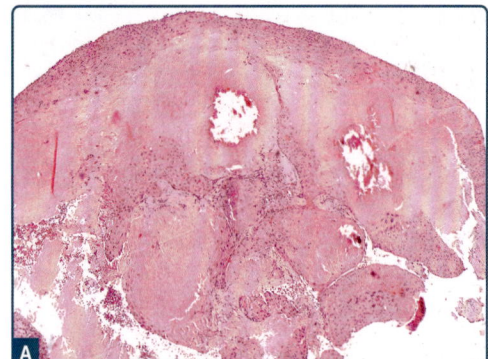
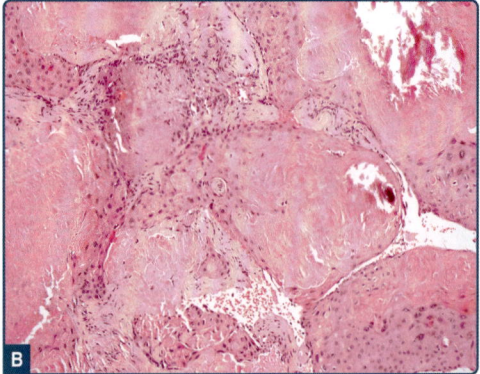
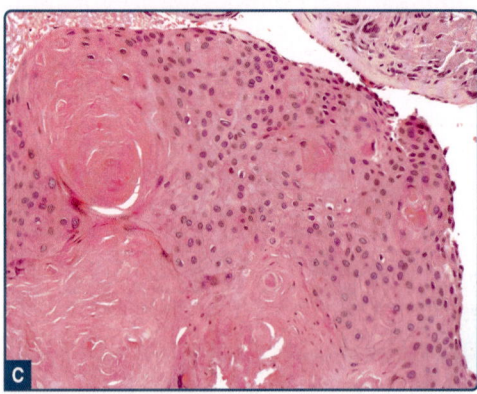

Figure 109-19 **A,** Proliferating pilar tumor occurs as a lobular proliferation of keratinocytes with pilar keratinization. **B,** The tumor forms multiple whorled nodules of keratinizing epithelium that may resemble well differentiated carcinoma. **C,** Squamous eddies resemble those observed in irritated seborrheic keratosis and inverted follicular keratosis and may be prominent.

positive staining for AE13, AE14, and CD34, whereas squamous cell carcinoma tumor cells show negative staining for these markers (see Table 109-4).[5,112]

Clinical Course and Prognosis: The majority of proliferating pilar tumors follow a benign clinical course, but malignant transformation and even metastatic disease have been described. In a study by Ye and colleagues, a 3-tier grading system of benign, low-grade malignant, and high-grade malignant proliferating pilar tumors was proposed based on histologic features and with followup clinical data.[112] Benign proliferating pilar tumors showed good circumscription, minimal cytologic atypia, and had no known recurrences. Low-grade malignant proliferating pilar tumors showed invasion into surrounding tissues, had moderate cytologic atypia and did not have local disease recurrence. High-grade malignant proliferating pilar tumors were invasive, displayed anaplastic cytologic atypia, and on clinical followup had recurrences and cases of metastatic disease. Overall, the recurrence rate for all proliferating pilar tumors is 3.7% and the rate of metastasis is 1.2%.[112,113] The metastatic rate for high-grade proliferating pilar tumors, however, is estimated at 25%, based on small series.[113]

Management: Treatment for proliferating pilar tumor is complete surgical excision.[113] Both conventional and Mohs micrographic surgical techniques have been utilized. Chemotherapy and radiotherapy in patients with malignant proliferating pilar tumor has been of limited therapeutic benefit.[113]

NEOPLASMS WITH INFUNDIBULAR DIFFERENTIATION

TRICHOADENOMA

Trichoadenoma was first described in the German literature by Nikolowski in 1958.[116] The first series published in the English literature was in 1977.[117]

Epidemiology and Clinical Features: Trichoadenoma presents in adult patients as a flesh-colored papule on the face or buttock, without apparent gender predilection.[75,118]

Etiology and Pathogenesis: Trichoadenoma is a benign follicular neoplasm with differentiation toward the infundibulum.

Histopathology: Trichoadenoma is a well-circumscribed, dermal nodule composed of infundibulocystic structures (keratin cysts) within a fibrotic stroma. Scattered cords and strands of epithelial cells can be seen.

Differential Diagnosis: The histologic features are typically characteristic for trichoadenoma. Other neoplasms with infundibulocystic structures include trichoepithelioma, desmoplastic trichoepithelioma, and microcystic adnexal carcinoma. Distinction between trichoadenoma and these other neoplasms is generally straightforward in an adequate biopsy.

Clinical Course and Prognosis: Trichoadenoma is a benign neoplasm.

Management: Excision of trichoadenoma can be performed for cosmetic purposes.

DILATED PORE (OF WINER)

Winer originally described the dilated pore in a series of 10 cases in 1954.[119]

Epidemiology and Clinical Features: Dilated pore presents in adult patients as a single papule most frequently on the head and neck, but involvement on the back also has been noted.[1,75,120] Keratinaceous material can sometimes be expressed from the lesion.

Etiology and Pathogenesis: Some have regarded dilated pore as a variant of infundibular cyst, while others consider it as a unique follicular neoplasm.[1,75,120] Dilated pore shows differentiation toward the follicular infundibulum.

Histopathology: Histologically, dilated pore shows a dilated infundibulum oriented perpendicularly to the epidermal surface. Epithelial projections resembling rete ridges radiate from the central pore. There is epithelial atrophy at the ostium of the pore and it is filled with lamellar orthokeratosis.

Differential Diagnosis: Clinically and histologically, a dilated pore can mimic a comedo. Also in the histologically differential diagnosis is a pilar sheath acanthoma. Dilated pore shows infundibular differentiation, rather than isthmic differentiation with eosinophilic or clear cytoplasm seen in pilar sheath acanthoma. The epithelial projections in dilated pore are less bulbous than those in pilar sheath acanthoma.

Clinical Course and Prognosis: Dilated pore is a benign entity.

Management: Dilated pore can be treated cosmetically by excision.

TUMORS WITH SEBACEOUS DIFFERENTIATION

Normal sebaceous glands develop from the hair sheath and are located throughout the body, except the palms and soles. They are most abundant in the head and neck. (See Chap. 6 for a thorough discussion of normal sebaceous glands.) Sebaceous neoplasms show sebaceous differentiation and are typified by mature sebocytes with characteristic vacuolated cytoplasm and scalloped nuclei. Table 109-9 lists appendage tumors with sebaceous differentiation.

TABLE 109-9
Sebaceous Appendage Neoplasms

BENIGN	MALIGNANT
Sebaceous adenoma	Sebaceous carcinoma
Sebaceoma	

BENIGN

SEBACEOUS ADENOMA

Sebaceous adenomas are benign neoplasms with sebaceous differentiation.

Epidemiology and Clinical Features: Sebaceous adenomas (Fig. 109-20A) typically occur in the head and neck region of adult patients and present as single or multiple tan, pink, or yellow papules, typically around 0.5 cm.[3,121]

Etiology and Pathogenesis: Sebaceous adenomas, as well as other sebaceous neoplasms, are associated with Muir-Torre syndrome, a variant of Lynch (hereditary nonpolyposis colorectal carcinoma) syndrome (see Table 109-2).[122] It is an autosomal dominant cancer predisposition syndrome caused by mutations in genes encoding DNA mismatch repair proteins (MLH1, MSH2, MSH6, and PMS2). Visceral malignancies, such as colon and endometrial cancer, are also associated with the syndrome. In addition to DNA mismatch repair pathways, WNT/β-catenin, Hedgehog, and p53 signaling pathways have been implicated in the development of sebaceous neoplasms.[1,121]

Histopathology: Histologically, sebaceous adenomas display a lobular architecture with central mature sebocytes with vacuolated cytoplasm and peripheral basaloid germinative cells (see Fig. 109-20B). Connection to the epidermis is often seen. Basaloid germinative cells comprise less than 50% of the tumor volume in sebaceous adenomas (see Fig. 109-20B).

Differential Diagnosis: Clinically, sebaceous adenoma may be confused with basal cell carcinoma. Histologically, the identification of mature sebocytes, basaloid epithelial cells, and lobular architecture in an adequate biopsy make the diagnosis straightforward, although clear-cell neoplasms, such as metastatic renal cell carcinoma and clear-cell squamous cell carcinoma, may enter into the differential diagnosis.

Clinical Course and Prognosis: Sebaceous adenomas are benign, but can be associated with Muir-Torre syndrome. In fact, sebaceous adenomas found at sites other than the head and neck have been found to be more highly associated with Muir-Torre syndrome.[122]

Management: Although they are benign, modest, complete excision of sebaceous adenomas is recommended.[121] Patients with sebaceous adenomas should be screened for Muir-Torre syndrome, as they can be the presenting feature.[122,123] This can be performed, at least initially, by immunohistochemistry for the mismatch repair proteins on the biopsy material. Loss of expression correlates with microsatellite instability and suggests involvement by Muir-Torre syndrome.[122] DNA microsatellite analysis also can be

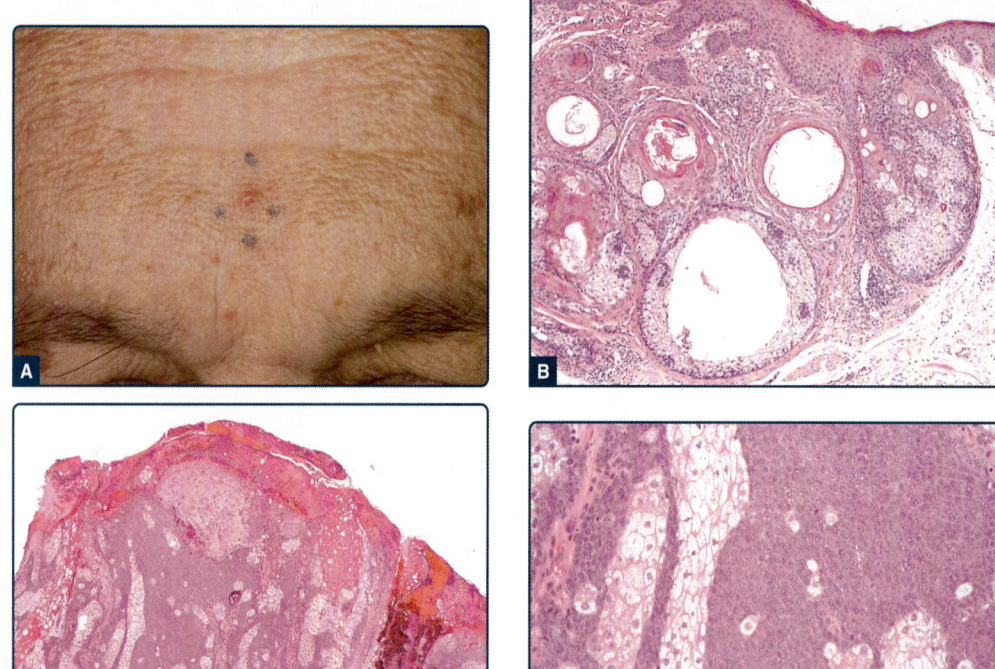

Figure 109-20 **A,** Sebaceous adenoma presents as a pink or orange-yellow papule, often in the head and neck region. **B,** Sebaceous adenoma is a lobular proliferation of basaloid epithelial cells and mature sebaceous elements that extends from the epidermis into the dermis. **C,** There is a prominent basaloid component, however it comprises less than half of the tumor cells. **D,** The sebaceous and basaloid cells have uniform round nuclei without significant atypia or mitotic activity.

performed on sebaceous neoplasms to assess for the presence of microsatellite instability.

SEBACEOMA/SEBACEOUS EPITHELIOMA

Epidemiology and Clinical Features:
Sebaceoma presents as an orange-yellow papule, ranging between 0.5 and 1 cm in the head and neck region of adult patients in their fifth and sixth decades.[3,121]

Etiology and Pathogenesis:
Sebaceomas are benign sebaceous neoplasms and are associated with Muir-Torre syndrome, although the association occurs with less frequency than with sebaceous adenomas (see Table 109-2).[122]

Histopathology:
Histologically, sebaceoma is a well-circumscribed dermal nodule composed of greater than 50% basaloid germinative cells (Fig. 109-21A to C). Mature sebocytes can be conspicuous (but less than 50% of the neoplasm) or focal/rare. Cytologic atypia is rare and focal when present (Fig. 109-21D).

Differential Diagnosis:
In small and/or superficial biopsies, the distinction between sebaceoma and sebaceous carcinoma may be difficult, and a differential diagnosis may be made. Difficulty in making the diagnosis of sebaceoma can occur when mature sebaceous differentiation is scant, with basal cell carcinoma entering the histologic differential diagnosis. Immunohistochemical stains for BerEP4 and EMA have been proposed to distinguish between basal cell carcinoma (BerEP4+, EMA−) and sebaceoma (BerEP4−, EMA+), keeping in mind that EMA staining can be weak to absent in the basaloid germinative cells of sebaceoma.[124] Immunohistochemical staining for adipophilin in a vesicular cytoplasmic pattern may confirm the presence of sebaceous differentiation (see Fig. 109-21E). (Table 109-10 summarizes the immunohistochemical stains used to distinguish between sebaceous neoplasms and basal cell carcinoma and squamous cell carcinoma.)

Clinical Course and Prognosis:
Sebaceomas are benign neoplasms without an aggressive clinical course.

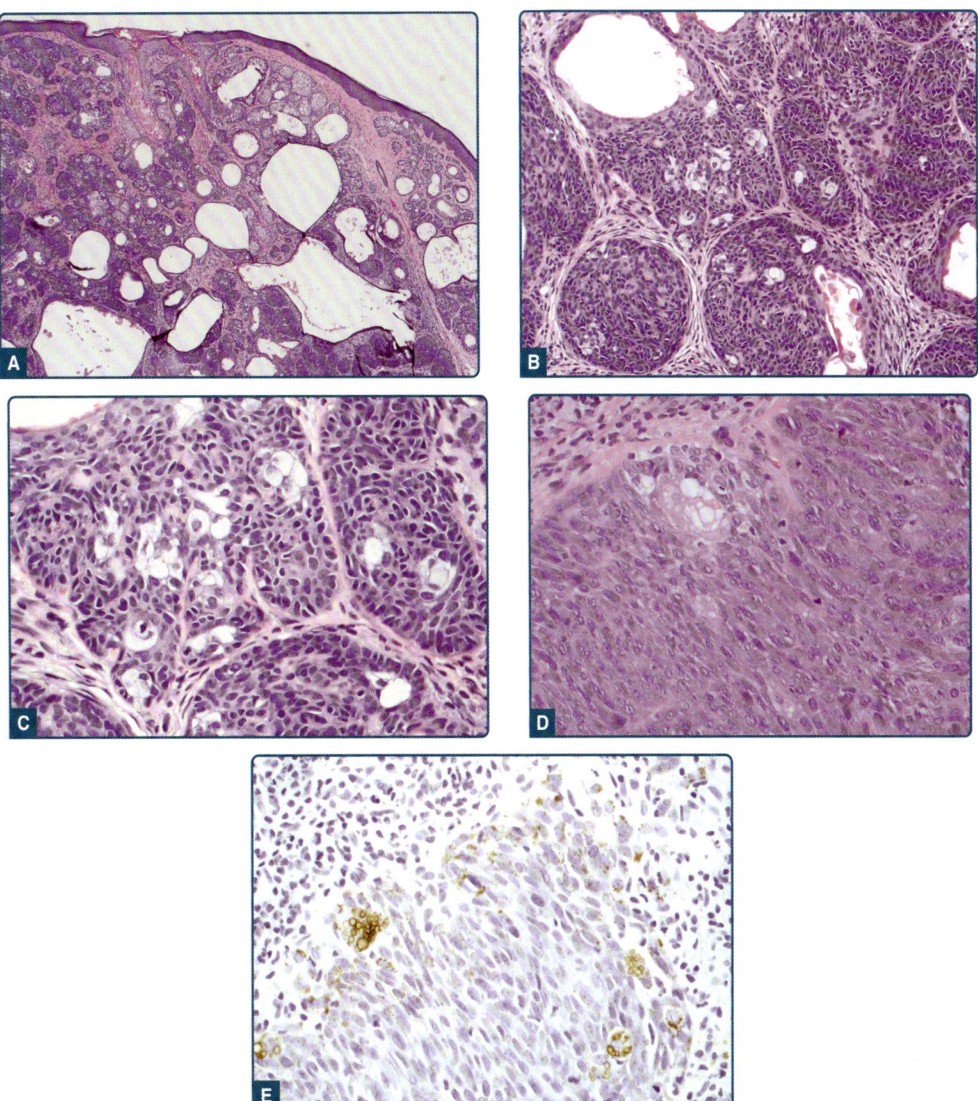

Figure 109-21 **A,** Sebaceoma occurs as a dermal nodule that usually shows connection to the epidermis. **B,** Less than half of the tumor is composed of mature sebaceous cells. **C,** The basaloid germinative cells have small round nuclei and are intermixed with small nests of mature sebocytes with prominent multivacuolated cytoplasm. **D,** In some cases there may be focal cytological atypia with nuclear pleomorphism. **E,** Immunohistochemistry for adipophilin reveals intracytoplasmic droplets of lipid.

Management: Sebaceomas are treated with surgical excision.[121,122] Screening of patients with sebaceoma(s) for Muir-Torre syndrome should be performed given their association with the syndrome.[122]

MALIGNANT

SEBACEOUS CARCINOMA

Sebaceous carcinoma is a rare, malignant sebaceous neoplasm traditionally separated into ocular (involving the orbit, conjunctiva, and eyelid) and extraocular counterparts, in part because the prognosis was considered worse for ocular sebaceous carcinoma in comparison to extraocular sites. A more recent retrospective study analyzing data from the National Cancer Institute's Surveillance, Epidemiology, and End Results (SEER) database suggest similar overall survival rates, although the regional metastatic rate is higher for orbital sebaceous carcinoma.[125,126] Categorization does appear to be important, however, as sebaceous carcinoma occurring in extraocular sites is more frequently associated with Muir-Torre syndrome (see Table 109-2).[127]

Epidemiology and Clinical Features: Both ocular and extraocular sebaceous carcinoma present in elderly patients.[126] Although previous reports suggest an increased incidence in females, the SEER study found a nearly equal incidence in men (54%)

TABLE 109-10

Summary of Immunohistochemical Stains in the Distinction between Sebaceous Neoplasms and Basal Cell Carcinoma and Squamous Cell Carcinoma

	SEBACEOMA	SEBACEOUS CARCINOMA	BCC	SCC
EMA	+	+	−	+
CK7	+	+	+/−	+/−
BerEP4	−	+/−	+	−
Adipophilin	+ (vesicular)	+ (vesicular)	−	−
Androgen receptor	+	+	−	−
Factor XIIIa (clone AC-1A1)	+ (nuclear)	+	−	−

−, Negative; +, positive; BCC, basal cell carcinoma; SCC, squamous cell carcinoma.

and women (46%).[125] Clinically, sebaceous carcinoma presents as a painless, slow-growing nodule (Fig. 109-22A, B). Ocular sebaceous carcinoma occurs more frequently than extraocular sebaceous carcinoma, but the most common extraocular site is the head and neck region (face, lip, ear).[125]

Etiology and Pathogenesis: Ocular sebaceous carcinoma arises in association with the sebaceous glands of the eyelid (the Meibomian glands and glands of Zeis).[126] Sebaceous carcinoma, especially the extraocular form, is associated with Muir-Torre syndrome, indicating a role for DNA repair mechanisms in its pathogenesis.[121,122,126] HER2/neu amplification has been identified in ocular sebaceous carcinoma.[128] A more recent study shows mutations in sebaceous carcinomas that converge on the PI3K (phosphatidylinositol 3′-kinase) signaling pathway.[129]

Histopathology: Histologically, sebaceous carcinoma is composed of poorly differentiated basaloid cells growing in sheets with an infiltrative growth pattern. The cells are cytologically malignant with atypia and frequent mitoses. Mature sebocytes are variably present and may be focal. Epidermal involvement with pagetoid spread is more common in ocular sebaceous carcinoma (see Fig. 109-22C, D).[121,126]

Differential Diagnosis: Benign lesions, such as chalazion and blepharitis, as well as malignancies, such as basal cell carcinoma, are in the clinical differential diagnosis.[126] Histologically, other poorly differentiated carcinomas, such as basal cell carcinoma, squamous cell carcinoma, and metastatic carcinoma, can enter into the differential diagnosis if sebaceous differentiation is not conspicuous. Melanoma in situ can be

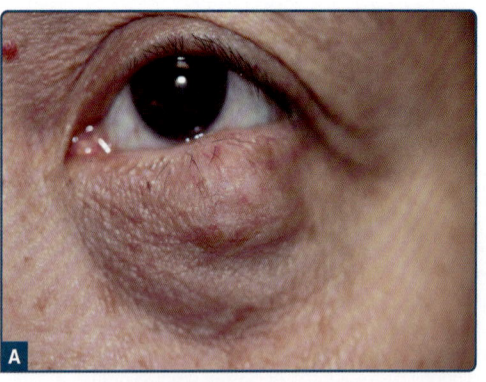
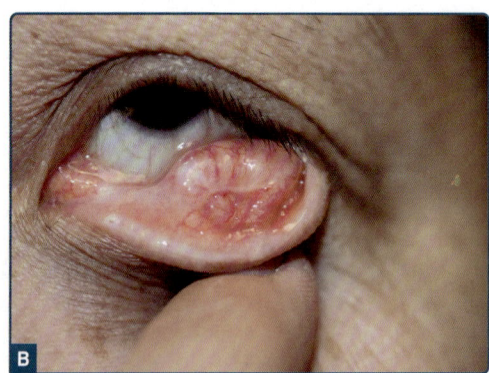
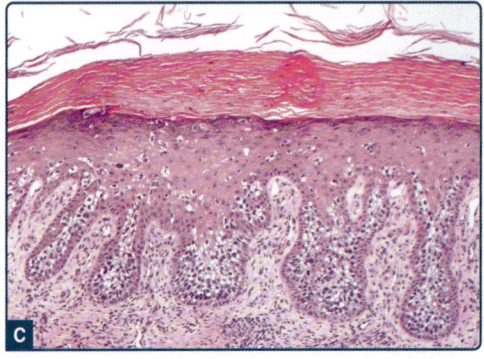
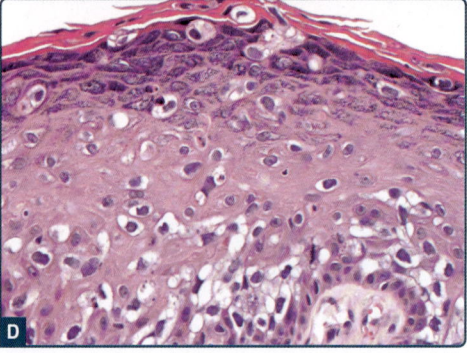

Figure 109-22 **A,** Sebaceous carcinoma can present as a discrete nodule and can clinically mimic a chalazion; however, accompanying lash loss is seen in sebaceous carcinoma. **B,** Everting the eyelid reveals a yellow-white nodule. **C,** Sebaceous carcinoma in situ occurs as an intraepidermal proliferation of cytologically atypical cells with varying degrees of sebaceous differentiation. **D,** Pagetoid growth pattern maybe prominent. (Clinical images **A** and **B,** Used with permission from Drs. Nahyoung Grace Lee, MD, and Fouad R. Zakka, MD, Boston, MA, USA.)

in the differential diagnosis of sebaceous carcinoma in situ. Immunohistochemistry has been proposed as a method to distinguish sebaceous carcinoma from its mimics. Sebaceous carcinomas have been shown to have positive staining for adipophilin and androgen receptor, while squamous cell carcinoma and basal cell carcinoma are negative.[5,130,131] Positive adipophilin staining should be membranous and vesicular, rather than the granular staining that can be seen in clear cell carcinomas.[5] EMA is positive in both sebaceous carcinoma and squamous cell carcinoma, but negative in basal cell carcinoma.[5,130] While some have found BerEP4 to be a marker to distinguish between basal cell carcinoma (BerEP4+) and sebaceous carcinoma (BerEP4−), others have found positive BerEP4 staining in up to 80% of sebaceous carcinomas.[5] Recently, nuclear factor XIIIa staining was found to highly sensitive for sebaceous differentiation compared to clear-cell carcinomas.[132,133] Sebaceous carcinoma is negative for melanocytic markers. (Table 109-10 summarizes these immunohistochemical findings.)

Clinical Course and Prognosis: Sebaceous carcinoma was historically thought to have a very poor prognosis.[121] The more recent SEER study suggests a less-aggressive course, with a 92% 5-year and a 79% 10-year age-matched relative survival rates.[125] Metastatic disease is not uncommon, with a reported range of regional metastases between 2.4% and 28%.[126] Poor clinical prognostic factors include delayed diagnosis and size of tumor greater than 1 cm.[126] Poor histologic factors include poor differentiation, pagetoid spread, multicentricity, size greater than 1 cm, and lymphovascular or perineural invasion.[126]

Management: Sebaceous carcinoma is treated with wide excision, using both conventional and Mohs micrographic surgical techniques.[121,122,126] Adjuvant radiation is used if regional lymph node metastases are detected at the time of diagnosis. Use of radiation as the sole treatment has increased rates of recurrence, but can be considered for poor surgical candidates.[126] Radiation also has been used for recurrences and for palliation.[126] Data on the role of sentinel lymph node biopsy are currently limited, but it is recommended for ocular sebaceous carcinomas greater than 1 cm.[126] Chemotherapy plays a limited role in the treatment of sebaceous carcinoma. Patients diagnosed with sebaceous carcinoma should be screened for Muir-Torre syndrome, particularly if they are younger than 50 years old and/or the tumor arises in a site other than the head and neck.[122,126]

REFERENCES

1. Kazakov DV, Kacerovska D, Michal M, et al. *Cutaneous Adnexal Tumors*. Philadelphia, PA: Lippincott Williams and Wilkins; 2012.
2. Obaidat NA, Alsaad KO, Ghazarian D. Skin adnexal neoplasms—part 2: an approach to tumours of cutaneous sweat glands. *J Clin Pathol*. 2007;60(2): 145-159.
3. Alsaad KO, Obaidat NA, Ghazarian D. Skin adnexal neoplasms—part 1: an approach to tumours of the pilosebaceous unit. *J Clin Pathol*. 2007;60(2): 129-144.
4. Kraft S, Granter SR. Molecular pathology of skin neoplasms of the head and neck. *Arch Pathol Lab Med*. 2014;138(6):759-787.
5. Danialan R, Mutyambizi K, Aung P, et al. Challenges in the diagnosis of cutaneous adnexal tumours. *J Clin Pathol*. 2015;68(12):992-1002.
6. Johnson BL, Helwig EB. Eccrine acrospiroma. A clinicopathologic study. *Cancer*. 1969;23(3):641-657.
7. Behboudi A, Winnes M, Gorunova L, et al. Clear cell hidradenoma of the skin-a third tumor type with a t(11;19)—associated TORC1-MAML2 gene fusion. *Genes Chromosomes Cancer*. 2005;43(2):202-205.
8. Winnes M, Molne L, Suurkula M, et al. Frequent fusion of the CRTCI and MAML2 genes in clear cell variants of cutaneous hidradenomas. *Genes Chromosomes Cancer*. 2007;46(6):559-563.
9. Mambo NC. The significance of atypical nuclear changes in benign eccrine acrospiromas: a clinical and pathological study of 18 cases. *J Cutan Pathol*. 1984;11(1):35-44.
10. Pinkus H, Rogin J, Goldman P. Eccrine poroma: tumors exhibiting features of the epidermal sweat duct unit. *AMA Arch Derm*. 1956;74(5):511-521.
11. Sawaya JL, Khachemoune A. Poroma: a review of eccrine, apocrine, and malignant forms. *Int J Dermatol*. 2014;53(9):1053-1061.
12. Crain RC, Helwig EB. Dermal cylindroma (dermal eccrine cylindroma). *Am J Clin Pathol*. 1961;35: 504-515.
13. Mahalingam M, Srivastava A, Hoang MP. Expression of stem-cell markers (cytokeratin 15 and nestin) in primary adnexal neoplasms—clues to etiopathogenesis. *Am J Dermatopathol*. 2010;32(8):774-779.
14. Sellheyer K. Spiradenoma and cylindroma originate from the hair follicle bulge and not from the eccrine sweat gland: an immunohistochemical study with CD200 and other stem cell markers. *J Cutan Pathol*. 2015;42(2):90-101.
15. Michal M, Lamovec J, Mukenšnabl P, et al. Spiradenocylindromas of the skin: tumors with morphological features of spiradenoma and cylindroma in the same lesion: report of 12 cases. *Pathol Int*. 1999;49(5):419-425.
16. Jordao C, de Magalhaes TC, Cuzzi T, et al. Cylindroma: an update. *Int J Dermatol*. 2015;54(3):275-278.
17. Rajan N, Ashworth A. Inherited cylindromas: lessons from a rare tumour. *Lancet Oncol*. 2015;16(9):e460-e469.
18. Kazakov DV. Brooke-Spiegler syndrome and phenotypic variants: an update. *Head Neck Pathol*. 2016;10(2):125-130.
19. Fehr A, Kovacs A, Loning T, et al. The MYB-NFIB gene fusion-a novel genetic link between adenoid cystic carcinoma and dermal cylindroma. *J Pathol*. 2011;224(3):322-327.
20. Rajan N, Andersson MK, Sinclair N, et al. Overexpression of MYB drives proliferation of CYLD-defective cylindroma cells. *J Pathol*. 2016;239(2):197-205.
21. Kersting DW, Helwig EB. Eccrine spiradenoma. *AMA Arch Derm*. 1956;73(3):199-227.
22. Williams K, Shinkai K. Evaluation and management of the patient with multiple syringomas: a systematic review of the literature. *J Am Acad Dermatol*. 2016;74(6):1234-1240.e9.

23. Gauerke S, Driscoll JJ. Hidradenocarcinomas: a brief review and future directions. *Arch Pathol Lab Med*. 2010;134(5):781-785.
24. Nazarian RM, Kapur P, Rakheja D, et al. Atypical and malignant hidradenomas: a histological and immunohistochemical study. *Mod Pathol*. 2009;22(4):600-610.
25. Nash JW, Barrett TL, Kies M, et al. Metastatic hidradenocarcinoma with demonstration of Her-2/neu gene amplification by fluorescence in situ hybridization: Potential treatment implications. *J Cutan Pathol*. 2007;34(1):49-54.
26. Kazakov DV, Ivan D, Kutzner H, et al. Cutaneous hidradenocarcinoma: a clinicopathological, immunohistochemical, and molecular biologic study of 14 cases, including Her2/neu gene expression/amplification, TP53 gene mutation analysis, and t(11;19) translocation. *Am J Dermatopathol*. 2009;31(3):236-247.
27. Coburn JG, Smith JL. Hidroacanthoma simplex; an assessment of a selected group of intraepidermal basal cell epitheliomata and of their malignant homologues. *Br J Dermatol*. 1956;68(12):400-418.
28. Pinkus H, Mehregan AH. Epidermotropic eccrine carcinoma: a case combining features of eccrine poroma and Paget's dermatosis. *Arch Dermatol*. 1963;88:597-606.
29. Snow SN, Reizner GT. Eccrine porocarcinoma of the face. *J Am Acad Dermatol*. 1992;27(2, pt 2):306-311.
30. Robson A, Greene J, Ansari N, et al. Eccrine porocarcinoma (malignant eccrine poroma): a clinicopathologic study of 69 cases. *Am J Surg Pathol*. 2001;25(6):710-720.
31. Harms PW, Hovelson DH, Cani AK, et al. Porocarcinomas harbor recurrent HRAS-activating mutations and tumor suppressor inactivating mutations. *Hum Pathol*. 2016;51:25-31.
32. Mahalingam M, Richards JE, Selim MA, et al. An immunohistochemical comparison of cytokeratin 7, cytokeratin 15, cytokeratin 19, CAM 5.2, carcinoembryonic antigen, and nestin in differentiating porocarcinoma from squamous cell carcinoma. *Hum Pathol*. 2012;43(8):1265-1272.
33. Goto K, Takai T, Fukumoto T, et al. CD117 (KIT) is a useful immunohistochemical marker for differentiating porocarcinoma from squamous cell carcinoma. *J Cutan Pathol*. 2016;43(3):219-226.
34. Brown CW Jr, Dy LC. Eccrine porocarcinoma. *Dermatol Ther*. 2008;21(6):433-438.
35. De Iuliis F, Amoroso L, Taglieri L, et al. Chemotherapy of rare skin adnexal tumors: a review of literature. *Anticancer Res*. 2014;34(10):5263-5268.
36. Granter SR, Seeger K, Calonje E, et al. Malignant eccrine spiradenoma (spiradenocarcinoma): a clinicopathologic study of 12 cases. *Am J Dermatopathol*. 2000;22(2):97-103.
37. Kazakov DV, Zelger B, Rutten A, et al. Morphologic diversity of malignant neoplasms arising in preexisting spiradenoma, cylindroma, and spiradenocylindroma based on the study of 24 cases, sporadic or occurring in the setting of Brooke-Spiegler syndrome. *Am J Surg Pathol*. 2009;33(5):705-719.
38. Dai B, Kong YY, Cai X, et al. Spiradenocarcinoma, cylindrocarcinoma and spiradenocylindrocarcinoma: a clinicopathological study of nine cases. *Histopathology*. 2014;65(5):658-666.
39. Cardoso JC, Calonje E. Malignant sweat gland tumours: an update. *Histopathology*. 2015;67(5):589-606.
40. Kao GF, Helwig EB, Graham JH. Aggressive digital papillary adenoma and adenocarcinoma. A clinicopathological study of 57 patients, with histochemical, immunopathological, and ultrastructural observations. *J Cutan Pathol*. 1987;14(3):129-146.
41. Duke WH, Sherrod TT, Lupton GP. Aggressive digital papillary adenocarcinoma (aggressive digital papillary adenoma and adenocarcinoma revisited). *Am J Surg Pathol*. 2000;24(6):775-784.
42. Suchak R, Wang W, Prieto VG, et al. Cutaneous digital papillary adenocarcinoma: a clinicopathologic study of 31 cases of a rare neoplasm with new observations. *Am J Surg Pathol*. 2012;36(12):1883-1891.
43. Goldstein DJ, Barr RJ, Santa Cruz DJ. Microcystic adnexal carcinoma: a distinct clinicopathologic entity. *Cancer*. 1982;50(3):566-572.
44. Wetter R, Goldstein GD. Microcystic adnexal carcinoma: a diagnostic and therapeutic challenge. *Dermatol Ther*. 2008;21(6):452-458.
45. Gordon S, Fischer C, Martin A, et al. Microcystic adnexal carcinoma: a review of the literature. *Dermatol Surg*. 2017;43(8):1012-1016.
46. Hoang MP, Dresser KA, Kapur P, et al. Microcystic adnexal carcinoma: an immunohistochemical reappraisal. *Mod Pathol*. 2008;21(10):178-185.
47. Palamaras I, McKenna JD, Robson A, et al. Microcystic adnexal carcinoma: a case series treated with Mohs micrographic surgery and identification of patients in whom paraffin sections may be preferable. *Dermatol Surg*. 2010;36(4):446-452.
48. Sarabi K, Khachemoune A. Hidrocystomas—a brief review. *MedGenMed*. 2006;8(3):57.
49. Kazakov DV, Belousova IE, Bisceglia M, et al. Apocrine mixed tumor of the skin ("mixed tumor of the folliculosebaceous-apocrine complex"). Spectrum of differentiations and metaplastic changes in the epithelial, myoepithelial, and stromal components based on a histopathologic study of 244 cases. *J Am Acad Dermatol*. 2007;57(3):467-483.
50. Kazakov DV, Kacerovska D, Hantschke M, et al. Cutaneous mixed tumor, eccrine variant: a clinicopathologic and immunohistochemical study of 50 cases, with emphasis on unusual histopathologic features. *Am J Dermatopathol*. 2011;33(6):557-568.
51. Jo VY. Myoepithelial tumors: an update. *Surg Pathol Clin*. 2015;8(3):445-466.
52. Mammino JJ, Vidmar DA. Syringocystadenoma papilliferum. *Int J Dermatol*. 1991;30(11):763-766.
53. Boni R, Xin H, Hohl D, et al. Syringocystadenoma papilliferum: a study of potential tumor suppressor genes. *Am J Dermatopathol*. 2001;23(2):87-89.
54. Levinsohn JL, Sugarman JL, Bilguvar K, et al. Somatic V600E BRAF mutation in linear and sporadic syringocystadenoma papilliferum. *J Invest Dermatol*. 2015;135(10):2536-2538.
55. Zhang YH, Wang W-L, Rapini RP, et al. Syringocystadenocarcinoma papilliferum with transition to areas of squamous differentiation. *Am J Dermatopathol*. 2012;34(4):428-433.
56. Kazakov DV, Requena L, Kutzner H, et al. Morphologic diversity of syringocystadenocarcinoma papilliferum based on a clinicopathologic study of 6 cases and review of the literature. *Am J Dermatopathol*. 2010;32(4):340-347.
57. Landry M, Winkelmann RK. An unusual tubular apocrine adenoma. *Arch Dermatol*. 1972;105(6):869-879.
58. Rulon DB, Helwig EB. Papillary eccrine adenoma. *Arch Dermatol*. 1977;113(5):596-598.

59. Konstantinova AM, Michal M, Kacerovska D, et al. Hidradenoma papilliferum: a clinicopathologic study of 264 tumors from 261 patients, with emphasis on mammary-type alterations. *Am J Dermatopathol*. 2016;38(8):598-607.
60. Liau J-Y, Lan J, Hong J-B, et al. Frequent PIK3CA activating mutations in hidradenoma papilliferums. *Hum Pathol*. 2016;55:57-62.
61. Dillon DA, Lester SC. Lesions of the nipple. *Surg Pathol Clin*. 2009;2(2):391-412.
62. Salemis NS. Florid papillomatosis of the nipple: a rare presentation and review of the literature. *Breast Dis*. 2015;35(2):153-156.
63. Ramakrishnan R, Chaudhry IH, Ramdial P, et al. Primary cutaneous adenoid cystic carcinoma: a clinicopathologic and immunohistochemical study of 27 cases. *Am J Surg Pathol*. 2013;37(10):1603-1611.
64. Naylor E, Sarkar P, Perlis CS, et al. Primary cutaneous adenoid cystic carcinoma. *J Am Acad Dermatol*. 2008;58(4):636-641.
65. North JP, McCalmont TH, Fehr A, et al. Detection of MYB alterations and other immunohistochemical markers in primary cutaneous adenoid cystic carcinoma. *Am J Surg Pathol*. 2015;39(10):1347-1356.
66. Batsakis JG, Luna MA, El-Naggar A. Histopathologic grading of salivary gland neoplasms: III. Adenoid cystic carcinomas. *Ann Otol Rhinol Laryngol*. 1990;99(12):1007-1009.
67. Mino M, Pilch BZ, Faquin WC. Expression of KIT (CD117) in neoplasms of the head and neck: an ancillary marker for adenoid cystic carcinoma. *Mod Pathol*. 2003;16(12):1224-1231.
68. Robson A, Lazar AJF, Ben Nagi J, et al. Primary cutaneous apocrine carcinoma: a clinico-pathologic analysis of 24 cases. *Am J Surg Pathol*. 2008;32(5):682-690.
69. Piris A, Peng Y, Boussahmain C, et al. Cutaneous and mammary apocrine carcinomas have different immunoprofiles. *Hum Pathol*. 2014;45(2):320-326.
70. Hollowell KL, Agle SC, Zervos EE, et al. Cutaneous apocrine adenocarcinoma: defining epidemiology, outcomes, and optimal therapy for a rare neoplasm. *J Surg Oncol*. 2012;105(4):415-419.
71. Rutten A, Kutzner H, Mentzel T, et al. Primary cutaneous cribriform apocrine carcinoma: a clinicopathologic and immunohistochemical study of 26 cases of an under-recognized cutaneous adnexal neoplasm. *J Am Acad Dermatol*. 2009;61(4):644-651.
72. Arps DP, Chan MP, Patel RM, et al. Primary cutaneous cribriform carcinoma: report of six cases with clinicopathologic data and immunohistochemical profile. *J Cutan Pathol*. 2015;42(6):379-387.
73. Kazakov DV, Suster S, LeBoit PE, et al. Mucinous carcinoma of the skin, primary, and secondary: a clinicopathologic study of 63 cases with emphasis on the morphologic spectrum of primary cutaneous forms: homologies with mucinous lesions in the breast. *Am J Surg Pathol*. 2005;29(6):764-782.
74. Jih MH, Friedman PM, Kimyai-Asadi A, et al. A rare case of fatal primary cutaneous mucinous carcinoma of the scalp with multiple in-transit and pulmonary metastases. *J Am Acad Dermatol*. 2005;52(5)(suppl 1):S76-S80.
75. Tellechea O, Reis JP, Gameiro AR, et al. Benign follicular tumors. *An Bras Dermatol*. 2006;90(6):780-798.
76. Misago N, Kimura T, Toda S, et al. A revaluation of trichofolliculoma: the histopathological and immunohistochemical features. *Am J Dermatopathol*. 2010;32(1):35-43.
77. Schulz T, Hartschuh W. Merkel cells are absent in basal cell carcinomas but frequently found in trichoblastomas. An immunohistochemical study. *J Cutan Pathol*. 1997;24(1):14-24.
78. Cordoba A, Guerrero D, Larrinaga B, et al. Bcl-2 and CD10 expression in the differential diagnosis of trichoblastoma, basal cell carcinoma, and basal cell carcinoma with follicular differentiation. *Int J Dermatol*. 2009;48(7):713-717.
79. Goyal A, Solus JF, Chan MP, et al. Cytokeratin 17 is highly sensitive in discriminating cutaneous lymphadenoma (a distinct trichoblastoma variant) from basal cell carcinoma. *J Cutan Pathol*. 2016;43(5):422-429.
80. Mizutani Y, Iwamoto I, Kanoh H, et al. Expression of drebrin, an actin binding protein, in basal cell carcinoma, trichoblastoma and trichoepithelioma. *Histol Histopathol*. 2014;29(6):757-766.
81. Rosso R, Lucioni M, Savio T, et al. Trichoblastic sarcoma: a high-grade stromal tumor arising in trichoblastoma. *Am J Dermatopathol*. 2007;29(1):79-83.
82. du Toit JP, Derm FC, Schneider JW, et al. The clinicopathological spectrum of trichoepitheliomas: a retrospective descriptive study. *Int J Dermatol*. 2016;55(3):270-277.
83. Mamelak AJ, Goldberg LH, Katz TM, et al. Desmoplastic trichoepithelioma. *J Am Acad Dermatol*. 2010;62(1):102-106.
84. Matt D, Xin H, Vortmeyer AO, et al. Sporadic trichoepithelioma demonstrates deletions at 9q22.3. *Arch Dermatol*. 2000;136(5):657-660.
85. Sellheyer K, Krahl D. PHLDA1 (TDAG51) is a follicular stem cell marker and differentiates between morphoeic basal cell carcinoma and desmoplastic trichoepithelioma. *Br J Dermatol*. 2011;164(1):141-147.
86. Sellheyer K, Nelson P. Follicular stem cell marker PHLDA1 (TDAG51) is superior to cytokeratin-20 in differentiating between trichoepithelioma and basal cell carcinoma in small biopsy specimens. *J Cutan Pathol*. 2011;38(7):542-550.
87. Yeh I, McCalmont TH, LeBoit PE. Differential expression of PHLDA1 (TDAG51) in basal cell carcinoma and trichoepithelioma. *Br J Dermatol*. 2012;167(5):1106-1110.
88. Abesamis-Cubillan E, El-Shabrawi-Caelen L, LeBoit PE. Merkel cells and sclerosing epithelial neoplasms. *Am J Dermatopathol*. 2000;22(4):311-315.
89. Arits AH, Van Marion AM, Lohman BG, et al. Differentiation between basal cell carcinoma and trichoepithelioma by immunohistochemical staining of the androgen receptor: an overview. *Eur J Dermatol*. 2011;21(6):870-873.
90. Astarci HM, Gurbuz GA, Sengul D, et al. Significance of androgen receptor and CD10 expression in cutaneous basal cell carcinoma and trichoepithelioma. *Oncol Lett*. 2015;10(6):3466-3470.
91. Tebcherani AJ, de Andrade HF, Sotto MN. Diagnostic utility of immunohistochemistry in distinguishing trichoepithelioma and basal cell carcinoma: evaluation using tissue microarray samples. *Mod Pathol*. 2012;25(10):1345-1353.
92. Lopez-Garcia DR, Teague D, Landis ET, et al. Morphological diversity of trichodiscomas and fibrofolliculomas. *Am J Dermatopathol*. 2014;36(9):734-740.
93. Toro J. Birt-Hogg-Dubé Syndrome. In: Adam MP, Ardinger HH, Pagon RA, et al, eds. GeneReviews [Internet]. Seattle, WA: University of Washington, Seattle; 1993-2018 February 27, 2006 (updated August 7, 2014). https://www.ncbi.nlm.nih.gov/books/NBK1522/#bhd.Summary.

94. Julian CG, Bowers PW. A clinical review of 209 pilomatricomas. *J Am Acad Dermatol*. 1998;39(2):191-195.
95. Lan M-Y, Lan M-C, Ho C-Y, et al. Pilomatricoma of the head and neck: a retrospective review of 179 cases. *Arch Otolaryngol Head Neck Surg*. 2003;129(12):1327-1330.
96. Moehlenbeck FW. Pilomatrixoma (calcifying epithelioma): a statistical study. *Arch Dermatol*. 1973;108(4):532-534.
97. Chan EF, Gat U, McNiff JM, et al. A common human skin tumour is caused by activating mutations in beta-catenin. *Nat Genet*. 1999;21(4):410-413.
98. Herrmann JL, Allan A, Trapp KM, et al. Pilomatrix carcinoma: 13 new cases and review of the literature with emphasis on predictors of metastasis. *J Am Acad Dermatol*. 2014;71(1):38-43.e2.
99. Brownstein MH, Shapiro L. Trichilemmoma. Analysis of 40 new cases. *Arch Dermatol*. 1973;107(6):866-869.
100. Al-Zaid T, Ditelberg JS, Prieto VG, et al. Trichilemmomas show loss of PTEN in Cowden syndrome but only rarely in sporadic tumors. *J Cutan Pathol*. 2012;39(5):493-499.
101. Tsai J-H, Huang W-C, Jhuang J-Y, et al. Frequent activating HRAS mutations in trichilemmoma. *Br J Dermatol*. 2014;171(5):1073-1077.
102. Dalton SR, LeBoit PE. Squamous cell carcinoma with clear cells: how often is there evidence of tricholemmal differentiation? *Am J Dermatopathol*. 2008;30(4):333-339.
103. Afshar M, Lee RA, Jiang SIB. Desmoplastic trichilemmoma—a report of successful treatment with Mohs micrographic surgery and a review and update of the literature. *Dermatol Surg*. 2012;38(11):1867-1871.
104. Hamman MS, Brian Jiang SI. Management of trichilemmal carcinoma: an update and comprehensive review of the literature. *Dermatol Surg*. 2014;40(7):711-717.
105. Mehregan AH, Butler JD. A tumor of follicular infundibulum. Report of a case. *Arch Dermatol*. 1961;83:924-927.
106. Alomari A, Subtil A, Owen CE, et al. Solitary and multiple tumors of follicular infundibulum: a review of 168 cases with emphasis on staining patterns and clinical variants. *J Cutan Pathol*. 2013;40(6):532-537.
107. Schnitzler L, Civatte J, Robin F, et al. Multiple tumors of the follicular infundibulum with basocellular degeneration. Apropos of a case [in French]. *Ann Dermatol Venereol*. 1987;114(4):551-556.
108. Cheng AC, Chang YL, Wu YY, et al. Multiple tumors of the follicular infundibulum. *Dermatol Surg*. 2004;30(9):1246-1248.
109. Mehregan AH, Brownstein MH. Pilar sheath acanthoma. *Arch Dermatol*. 1978;114(10):1495-1497.
110. Choi YS, Park SH, Bang D. Pilar sheath acanthoma—report of a case with review of the literature. *Yonsei Med J*. 1989;30(4):392-395.
111. Jones EW. Proliferating epidermoid cysts. *Arch Dermatol*. 1966;94(1):11-19.
112. Ye J, Nappi O, Swanson PE, et al. Proliferating pilar tumors: a clinicopathologic study of 76 cases with a proposal for definition of benign and malignant variants. *Am J Clin Pathol*. 2004;122(4):566-574.
113. Satyaprakash AK, Sheehan DJ, Sangueza OP. Proliferating trichilemmal tumors: a review of the literature. *Dermatol Surg*. 2007;33(9):1102-1108.
114. Nyquist GG, Mumm C, Grau R, et al. Malignant proliferating pilar tumors arising in KID syndrome: a report of two patients. *Am J Med Genet A*. 2007;143A(7):734-741.
115. Kim K-H, Kim J-S, Piao Y-J, et al. Keratitis, ichthyosis and deafness syndrome with development of multiple hair follicle tumours. *Br J Dermatol*. 2002;147(1):139-143.
116. Nikolowski W. Trichoadenoma (organoid follicular hamartoma) [in German]. *Arch Klin Exp Dermatol*. 1958;207(1):34-45.
117. Rahbari H, Mehregan A, Pinkus H. Trichoadenoma of Nikolowski. *J Cutan Pathol*. 1977;4(2):90-98.
118. Shimanovich I, Krahl D, Rose C. Trichoadenoma of Nikolowski is a distinct neoplasm within the spectrum of follicular tumors. *J Am Acad Dermatol*. 2010;62(2):277-283.
119. Winer LH. The dilated pore, a tricho-epithelioma. *J Invest Dermatol*. 1954;23(3):181-188.
120. Steffen C. Winer's dilated pore: the infundibuloma. *Am J Dermatopathol*. 2001;23(3):246-253.
121. Shalin SC, Lyle S, Calonje E, et al. Sebaceous neoplasia and the Muir-Torre syndrome: important connections with clinical implications. *Histopathology*. 2010;56(1):133-147.
122. John AM, Schwartz RA. Muir-Torre syndrome (MTS): an update and approach to diagnosis and management. *J Am Acad Dermatol*. 2016;74(3):558-566.
123. Jessup CJ, Redston M, Tilton E, et al. Importance of universal mismatch repair protein immunohistochemistry in patients with sebaceous neoplasia as an initial screening tool for Muir-Torre syndrome. *Hum Pathol*. 2016;49:1-9.
124. Fan YS, Carr RA, Sanders DS, et al. Characteristic Ber-EP4 and EMA expression in sebaceoma is immunohistochemically distinct from basal cell carcinoma. *Histopathology*. 2007;51(1):80-86.
125. Dasgupta T, Wilson LD, Yu JB. A retrospective review of 1349 cases of sebaceous carcinoma. *Cancer*. 2009;115(1):158-165.
126. Kyllo RL, Brady KL, Hurst EA. Sebaceous carcinoma: review of the literature. *Dermatol Surg*. 2015;41(1):1-15.
127. Dores GM, Curtis RE, Toro JR, et al. Incidence of cutaneous sebaceous carcinoma and risk of associated neoplasms: insight into Muir-Torre syndrome. *Cancer*. 2008;113(12):3372-3381.
128. Kwon MJ, Shin HS, Nam ES, et al. Comparison of HER2 gene amplification and KRAS alteration in eyelid sebaceous carcinomas with that in other eyelid tumors. *Pathol Res Pract*. 2015;211(5):349-355.
129. Tetzlaff MT, Singh RR, Seviour EG, et al. Next-generation sequencing identifies high frequency of mutations in potentially clinically actionable genes in sebaceous carcinoma. *J Pathol*. 2016;240(1):84-95.
130. Plaza JA, Mackinnon A, Carrillo L, et al. Role of immunohistochemistry in the diagnosis of sebaceous carcinoma: a clinicopathologic and immunohistochemical study. *Am J Dermatopathol*. 2015;37(11):809-821.
131. Ansai S, Takeichi H, Arase S, et al. Sebaceous carcinoma: an immunohistochemical reappraisal. *Am J Dermatopathol*. 2011;33(6):579-587.
132. Uhlenhake EE, Clark LN, Smoller BR, et al. Nuclear factor XIIIa staining (clone AC-1A1 mouse monoclonal) is a sensitive and specific marker to discriminate sebaceous proliferations from other cutaneous clear cell neoplasms. *J Cutan Pathol*. 2016;43(8):649-656.
133. Clark LN, Elwood HR, Uhlenhake EE, et al. Nuclear factor XIIIa staining (clone AC-1A1 mouse monoclonal) is a highly sensitive marker of sebaceous differentiation in normal and neoplastic sebocytes. *J Cutan Pathol*. 2016;43(8):657-662.

Chapter 110 :: Epithelial Precancerous Lesions
:: Markus V. Heppt, Gabriel Schlager, & Carola Berking

第一百一十章
上皮癌前病变

中文导读

本章介绍了一系列上皮癌前病变，共分为6节：①光化性角化病；②鲍温病；③病毒相关性上皮癌前病变；④口腔潜在恶性疾病；⑤砷角化病；⑥其他。

第一节光化性角化病，介绍了其流行病学及临床特征、临床亚型、分级、病因及发病机制、诊断、鉴别诊断、临床病程和预后、治疗及预防，其中特别介绍该病可进展为侵袭性鳞状细胞癌或者部分可自然消退。

第二节鲍温病，介绍了其流行病学及临床特征、病因及发病机制、诊断与鉴别诊断、临床病程和预后、治疗，其中特别提出该病可能在临床和组织病理学上很难与其他皮肤病相区别。

第三节病毒相关性上皮癌前病变，主要介绍了鲍温样丘疹病、疣状表皮发育不良的流行病学及临床特征、病因及治疗，简单提及了肛门-生殖道癌前病变。

第四节口腔潜在恶性疾病，重点介绍了口腔黏膜白斑和口腔红斑的流行病学及临床特征、病因及发病机制、诊断与鉴别诊断、临床病程和预后、治疗。

第五节砷角化病，介绍了其病因、临床特征、组织病理学、治疗及预防。

第六节其他，提及了上皮癌前病变还包括热性角化病、碳氢化合物角化病、慢性放射性角化病及慢性瘢痕角化病。

〔粟 娟〕

ACTINIC KERATOSES

AT-A-GLANCE

- Precursor lesions of cutaneous squamous cell carcinoma (SCC).
- Long-term and cumulative ultraviolet (UV) radiation exposure is the most important etiologic factor in the development of actinic keratoses.
- Risk factors include fair skin, age, cumulative UV radiation exposure, immunosuppression, prior history of non-melanoma skin cancer.
- The overall risk of progression to invasive SCC is estimated as 5% to 10%.
- Treatment is recommended to reduce the risk of SCC formation and to improve patients' quality of life.
- Treatment modalities include cryosurgery, shave excision, curettage, dermabrasion, ablative lasers, topical drugs (diclofenac + hyaluronic acid, 5-fluorouracil ± salicylic acid, imiquimod, ingenol mebutate), chemical peelings, and photodynamic therapy.

Actinic keratoses (AKs, also known as solar keratoses or senile keratoses) are cutaneous lesions that consist of proliferations of atypical epidermal keratinocytes that may progress to invasive squamous cell carcinoma (SCC). The concept of a precancerous keratosis was first presented by Dubreuilh in the late 1800s. AKs were first identified and named keratoma senilis by Freudenthal in 1926. In 1958, Pinkus further characterized these lesions and coined the term *actinic keratosis*. It literally means a condition (*-osis*) of excessive horny (*kerat-*) tissue induced by a ray of light (*aktis*), presumably ultraviolet (UV) light. AKs have historically been considered precancerous or premalignant lesions with a potential for developing into SCCs. However, there is a debate at what grade of atypia AKs should be considered carcinoma in situ because not all AKs progress to SCCs and some lesions may spontaneously regress. Attempts have been made to coin AK as "keratinocytic intraepidermal neoplasia" grades I to III according to the degree of atypia.[1] This concept is analogous to the grading of other precancerous lesions such as the classification of cervical intraepithelial neoplasia or vulvar intraepithelial neoplasia (VIN) as precursor lesions of cervical and vulvar carcinoma, respectively.

Regardless of the clinical course of single lesions, AKs are a strong indicator of chronic exposure to UV radiation with actinic skin damage and identify patients who are at high risk to develop nonmelanoma skin cancer. In an increasingly aging society with generations that poorly used sun protection measures and sunscreen, AKs are nowadays rated among the most common reasons to consult a dermatologist in regions with predominantly white populations such as the United States, Australia, and Europe.[2] The high prevalence and the uncertainty of the clinical course of the precancerous lesions make AKs an important challenge for patients and physicians, and an economic burden for health-care providers.

EPIDEMIOLOGY

In European countries, such as Spain and Austria, the prevalence of AKs in adult dermatology outpatients was reported to be approximately 30% in 2011. In the Netherlands, a total of 23.5% of the general population older than 50 years of age was estimated to be affected in 2011.[3] Similar numbers were reported in the United States, where AK is the most common diagnosis among dermatology patients 45 years of age and older. The disease is estimated to account for more than 5 million physician visits in the United States per year. The highest prevalence of AK was shown in Australia, it being up to 59% in the general population older than age 40 years in the 1980s. In contrast, only 0.52% of dermatology patients in China were diagnosed with AK from 2008-2012. The prevalence in other geographical regions is widely unknown.

Various risk factors for the development of AKs exist. The most important ones include skin phenotype, cumulative UV exposure, age, and gender. AKs occur most commonly in individuals with fair skin, red or blond hair, and blue eyes (Fitzpatrick type 1). People with darker skin (Fitzpatrick types 2 to 6), brown eyes, and dark hair are less likely to develop AKs.[3] The risk of AK is strongly associated with high cumulative UV exposure. Workers with a long history of outdoor occupation, such as farmers, construction workers, or fishermen, have an up to 2.5-fold increased risk compared to indoor workers.[4,5] This also accounts for individuals with predominantly outdoor hobbies.[4,5] Evidence that sun exposure plays a role in the development of AKs is reflected by their distribution on the body. They typically develop on sun-exposed areas, such as the balding scalp, head, neck, forearms, dorsal hands, and in women, additionally the dorsal legs (Fig. 110-1).

Age is another major risk factor. The number of sunburns during childhood is associated with a higher likelihood of developing AKs in the future.[5] Therefore, the age at which a person received the greatest amount and intensity of sun exposure appears to be important. The risk of AK steadily increases with lifetime exposure to UV radiation, as seen in the significantly higher prevalence of AK in elderly people.[2,3] In Austria, for instance, 1.1% of female and 2.4% of male dermatology outpatients from 30 to 39 years of age are affected by AKs, compared to 68.1% of females and 89.7% of males older than 90 years of age.[2] The prevalence increases with age in both sexes. However, men are more likely to develop AK than women. This presumably reflects greater cumulative sun exposure in males than in females, and less protection on the bald scalp.[3,5,6]

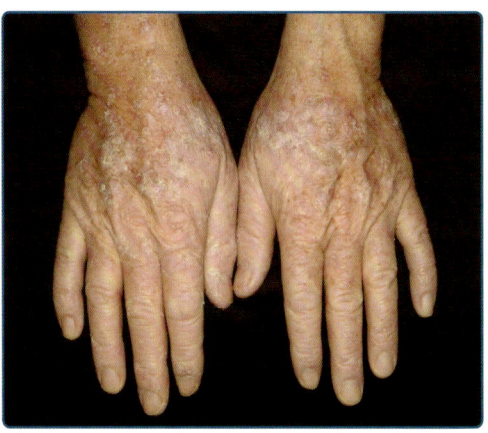

Figure 110-1 Multiple scaly and erythematous plaques on the dorsal hands of a 71-year-old male patient with a history of significant ultraviolet exposure. The lesions were grade II to grade III actinic keratoses.

Immunosuppressed patients, such as organ transplant recipients, are at increased risk of developing AKs. In addition, immunosuppression is associated with both developing AKs earlier in life and with a more rapid malignant transformation.[7] Furthermore, persons with certain genetic syndromes, namely albinism and xeroderma pigmentosum, are more likely to develop AKs. There are case reports of patients with Rothmund or Kindler syndrome who developed AKs early in life.

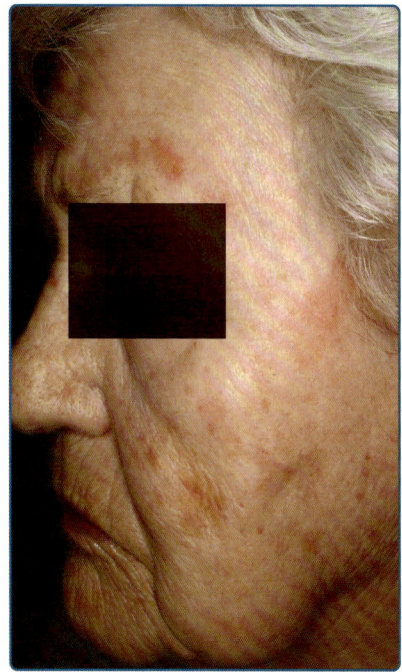

Figure 110-2 Mild actinic keratoses on the face of a fair-skinned woman (grade I). The lesions appear as erythematous patches with a rough texture on palpation. Note other signs of actinic skin damage such as perioral wrinkling and the presence of solar lentigines.

CLINICAL FEATURES

The typical patient with AKs is an older, fair-skinned, light-eyed individual, who has a history of significant sun exposure, who burns and freckles rather than tans, and who has significant solar elastosis on examination. AKs can be seen in younger individuals if they had sustained sufficient sun exposure over their lives. Eighty percent of AKs are found on chronically sun-exposed sites of the body, such as the bald scalp, face, ears, neck, forearms, and dorsal hands. They are mostly asymptomatic, but may come along with pruritus, burning or stinging pain, bleeding, and crusting.

CLINICAL SUBTYPES

The typical AK lesion, sometimes called the erythematous AK, presents most commonly as a 2- to 6-mm, erythematous, flat, rough, gritty or scaly papule (Fig. 110-2). It is usually more easily felt than seen. AKs can vary in size and sometimes reach to several centimeters in diameter. They are most often found against a background of photodamaged skin (dermatoheliosis), with solar elastosis, dyspigmentation, yellow discoloration, ephelides and lentigines, telangiectasias, and sagging skin notably prominent. At times, the number and confluence of AKs are so great that the patient appears to have a rash.

In some cases, multiple AKs may affect a large area of the sun-exposed skin. In addition, alongside clinically detectable AKs, multiple subclinical lesions may be present (Fig. 110-3). This concept is known as *field cancerization* and is crucial for the therapeutic approach. Various definitions of field cancerization have been proposed including (a) more than 2 AKs within 1 skin area with signs of solar damage, (b) at least 3 AKs within 25 cm^2 of skin, or (c) more than 5 AKs in 1 body region or field and contiguous areas of chronic actinic sun damage and hyperkeratosis.[8]

In addition to the typical erythematous AK, there are several other clinical subtypes. Some AKs have a pigmented brownish appearance and may be difficult to distinguish from other dermatoses of the elderly, such as seborrheic keratosis. If such lesions are ill defined, some authors have proposed the term *spreading pigmented actinic keratosis*. A hypertrophic AK presents as a thicker, scaly, rough papule or plaque that is skin-colored, gray-white, or erythematous (Fig. 110-4). It can be found on any chronically sun-exposed body site, but has a propensity for dorsal hands, arms, and scalp. A typical erythematous AK can progress into an hypertrophic AK. It can be difficult to distinguish an hypertrophic AK from an SCC, clinically necessitating a biopsy. Biopsies must be taken to a level deep enough to ensure that the dermal extent of the keratinocytic proliferation can be evaluated in order to obtain an unequivocal histopathologic diagnosis. Induration,

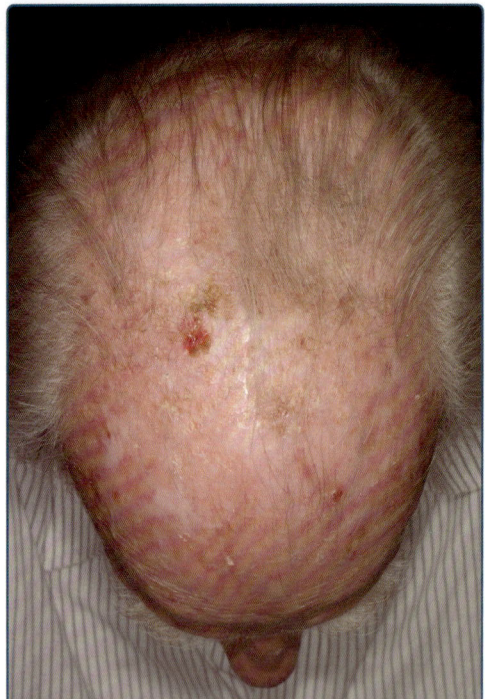

Figure 110-3 Field cancerization. There are several ill-defined erythematous and scaly plaques, crusts, and ulcerations affecting a large area ("field") of the balding scalp. Further alterations, such as mottled hypopigmentation and hyperpigmentation, are present and indicate actinic damage.

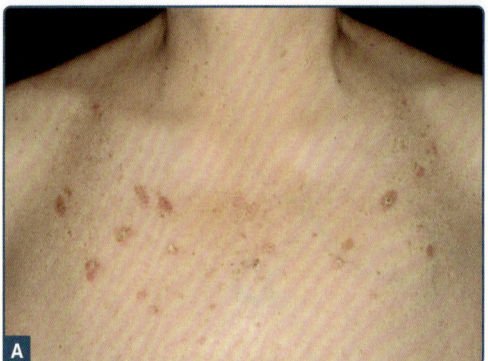
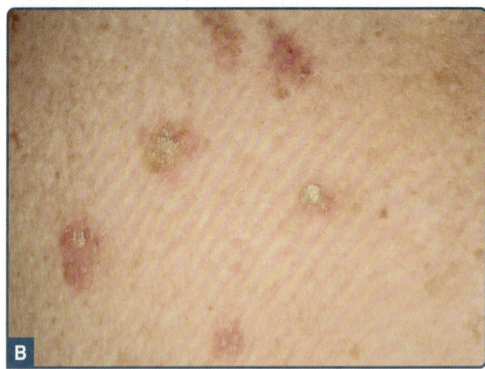

Figure 110-4 **A,** Multiple well-defined hypertrophic actinic keratoses on the decollete of a middle-aged female. **B,** A higher magnification reveals the rough and hyperkeratotic texture of some lesions.

inflammation, pain, and ulceration are the main clues to the transition of AK to SCC.

Cutaneous horn, also known as cornu cutaneum, refers to a reaction pattern and not a particular lesion. In reference to AKs, a cutaneous horn is a type of hypertrophic AK that presents with a conical hypertrophic protuberance emanating from a skin-colored to erythematous papular base (Fig. 110-5). Classical definitions of a cutaneous horn maintain that the height is at least one-half of the largest diameter. Approximately 21% of all cutaneous horns represent AKs. The pathology underlying a cutaneous horn can be a number of different lesions, such as AK, SCC, seborrheic keratosis, filiform verruca vulgaris, trichilemmoma, and keratoacanthoma.

Actinic cheilitis represents confluent AKs on the lips, most often the lower lip. Persons with this condition have red, scaly, chapped lips, and at times erosions or fissures may be present (Fig. 110-6). The vermilion border of the lip is often indistinct, and focal hyperkeratosis and leukoplakia also may be seen. Individuals with this condition often complain of persistent dryness and cracking of the lips. The diagnosis of actinic cheilitis should always be suspected in patients with photodamaged skin and such complaints. Biopsy is then necessary to confirm the diagnosis. Persistent ulcerations or indurated areas on the lip are suspicious for SCC.

CLASSIFICATION

The widely accepted Olsen classification suggests 3 grades of clinical severity of AK.[8,9] It is based on the palpable thickness of AK lesions. According to this classification, grade 1 includes lesions that are mild, slightly palpable, and are better seen than felt. Grade 2 represents lesions that are moderately thick and easily seen and felt. Grade 3 lesions are severe, very thick and/or obvious AKs (Table 110-1).[9]

On a histologic level, a recommended scheme for grading AK severity is the Roewert-Huber classification.[8,10] This scheme distinguishes 3 types of AK based on the extent of atypical keratinocytes in the epidermis. In type AK I, atypical keratinocytes are restricted to the lower third of the epidermis and are only found within the basal and suprabasal layers. In type AK II, atypical keratinocytes are found within the lower two-thirds of the epidermis, alternating with zones of normal epidermis. In the upper papillary dermis buds of keratinocytes can be found. In type AK III, atypical keratinocytes extend to the lower two-thirds of the full thickness of the epidermis. They can also involve the epithelia of the hair follicle, infundibula, and acrosyringium. As in type AK II, buds of keratinocytes can be found in the upper papillary dermis. If a biopsied AK lesion shows different histologic types, the classification suggests that the highest type defines the

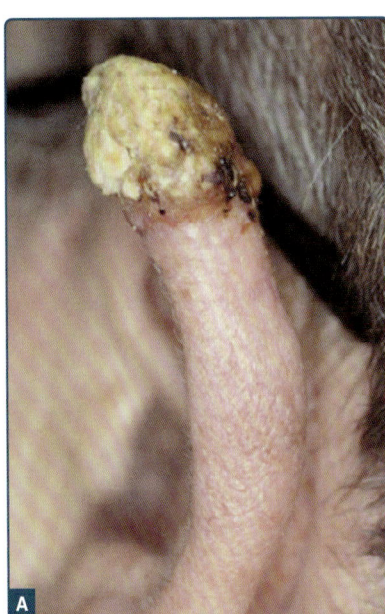

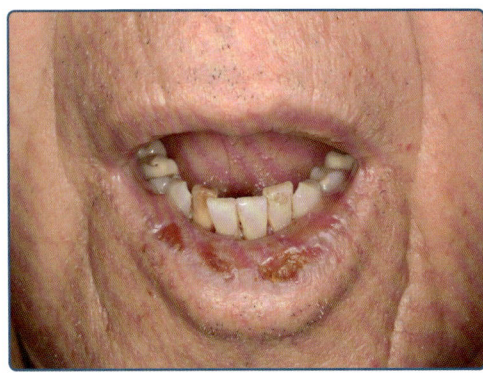

Figure 110-6 Actinic cheilitis. Reddish to yellow crusts and erosions on the lower lip are typical features of actinic damage along the vermilion border. The patient complained of a persistent dryness of the lip.

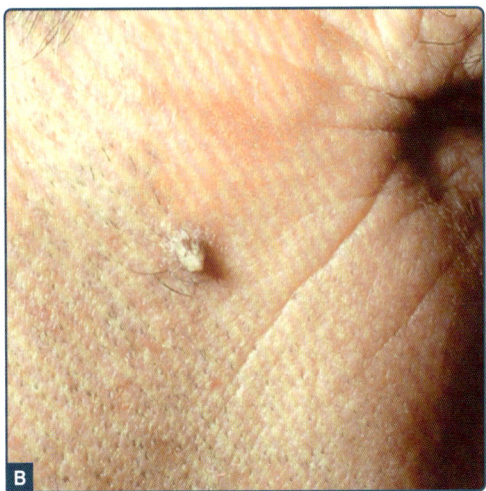

Figure 110-5 **A,** Cutaneous horn of the ear. Only biopsy will confirm whether this is an actinic keratosis or a squamous cell carcinoma. **B,** Cutaneous horn of the cheek.

lesion. Histologically, type I and type II AK represent the same severity grade as the former term "early in situ SCC." Type AK III has been proposed to be equivalent to the previous term "in situ SCC".[10]

In daily practice, AK is a clinical diagnosis. However, it was shown that the clinical classification following Olsen and the histologic classification of Roewert-Huber do not match in all cases. In a systematic study of 892 AK lesions, a correlation between both classification systems was found in 480 lesions (54%) only. Whereas 21 out of 259 lesions (8%) that were clinically graded as mild (Olsen grade 1) were histologically severe (Roewert-Huber type AK III), 36 out of 101 lesions (36%) that were clinically severe (Olsen grade 3) were histologically mild (Roewert-Huber type AK I).[11]

ETIOLOGY AND PATHOGENESIS

ETIOLOGIC FACTORS

Fair skin and exposure to UV radiation are the most important contributing factors for the formation of AKs. The majority of lesions develop in areas with chronic exposure to sunlight, such as the balding scalp, nose, ears, lips, and dorsal hands and forearms. A high extent of cumulative UV exposure, frequent sunburns in patient history, poor use of sun protection, and outdoor activities or occupations have been consistently

TABLE 110-1
Classification of Actinic Keratosis

Clinical Classification (Olsen et al.[9])
Grade 1 (Mild)
- Slight palpability
- AK better felt than seen

Grade 2 (Moderate)
- Moderately thick AK
- Easily seen and felt

Grade 3 (Severe)
- Very thick or obvious AK

Histologic Classification (Roewert-Huber et al.[10])
Early in situ SCC (type AK I)
- Involvement of basal and suprabasal layers of the epidermis
- Nuclei hyperchromatic and variable in size
- Loss of nuclear polarity

Early in situ SCC (type AK II)
- Involvement of the lower two-thirds of the epidermis
- Alternation with zones of normal epidermis
- Buds of keratinocytes in the upper papillary dermis

In situ SCC (type AK III)
- Involvement of more than two-thirds of the full epidermal thickness
- Involvement of hair follicle, infundibula, and acrosyringium
- Buds of keratinocytes in the upper papillary dermis

associated with AK formation. Other risk factors include male sex, advancing age, and immunosuppression. It is currently under debate whether infection with human papillomavirus (HPV; particularly HPV types 5, 8, 21, and 38) contributes to the development of AK. Although HPV was detected in several epithelial tumors of the skin, it is uncertain if there is a causal relationship or only random coincidence as a result of the high prevalence of HPV infection. Rare exogenous risk factors comprise ionizing radiation and radiant heat. Rare endogenous predisposing conditions are genetic disorders with impaired DNA damage repair mechanisms after exposure to UV like xeroderma pigmentosum, Bloom syndrome, and Rothmund-Thompson syndrome.

PATHOGENESIS

Chronic UVB radiation induces genetic alterations of the keratinocytes residing at the basal layer of the epidermis. On a molecular level, UV light induces the formation of cyclobutane pyrimidine dimers which modify the structure of the DNA (photomutagenesis). Inactivating mutations of the tumor-suppressor gene *p53* occur as early and common events (Fig. 110-7). *p53* has a critical role in cell-cycle progression and DNA damage repair. If the gene is inactivated, *p53*-mutant keratinocytes show unrestricted cell growth and acquire cellular and morphologic atypia. Somatic UV signature mutations of *p53* are present in more than 50% of all AKs and SCCs. In contrast, activating mutations of the oncogene H-ras lead to constitutive activation of the extracellular signal-regulated kinase signaling pathway and uncontrolled proliferation of affected cells. Other UV-induced mutations may affect the genes *p16*, *K-ras*, telomerase, *CDKN2A*, nuclear factor κB, or tumor necrosis factor α.[11] Photodamaged transformed keratinocytes escape apoptosis and immunosurveillance and proliferate into clinically and histologically evident premalignant lesions.

Notch 1 regulates numerous processes in keratinocytes such as proliferation, differentiation, and apoptosis. Proper expression of Notch 1 within the epidermis appears to be tumor suppressive and to prevent the progression to invasive SCC, which may show decreased levels of the protein. In addition to epidermal tissue alterations, there is growing evidence that mesenchymal factors within the dermis such as the Notch/CSL signaling pathway have a significant role in the establishment of epithelial lesions.[12]

DIAGNOSIS

The diagnosis of AK is usually made clinically by touch and visual inspection recognizing the typical clinical features. Some lesions present as visually discreet macules or patches that are diagnosed best by feeling their rough texture. If the diagnosis is uncertain or if SCC cannot be excluded clinically, a histologic examination is obligatory. Common indications for a biopsy are rapidly enlarging lesions, bleeding or ulceration, evidence of inflammation, strong induration, lesions extending beyond 1 cm of size, or resistance to treatment.

HISTOPATHOLOGY

A punch or shave biopsy should be performed to confirm the diagnosis. The depth of the biopsy needs to reach the mid-reticular dermis to allow for the assessment of invasiveness of a given lesion. Initially, a compact packing of basal and suprabasal atypic keratinocytes with hyperchromatic and pleomorphic nuclei can be seen. Atypic mitotic figures, apoptotic cells and dyskeratosis may be present. The architecture is increasingly lost in the basal layers, but not the full thickness of the epidermis (Fig. 110-8). The alternation of hyperorthokeratosis and hyperparakeratosis is common in later stages, a feature that is referred to as "flag sign" or "pink and blue." Per definition, the lesion is confined to the epidermis. The underlying dermis often shows solar elastosis and a superficial inflammatory infiltrate. Immunohistochemically, AK lesions show increased expression of p53, proliferating cell nuclear antigen, Ki-67 (MiB-1), and cyclin E. Histologic variants comprise lichenoid, bowenoid, and, rarely, acantholytic forms.

DERMOSCOPY

If it is difficult to recognize the clinical features by naked eye, dermoscopic evaluation may help to facilitate the correct diagnosis. Common features of nonpigmented lesions are scales that appear as whitish or yellowish crystalline structures and a reddish pseudonetwork with erythema and wavy configuration of telangiectasias between enlarged hair follicles. The follicles may show a perifollicular halo, resulting in a "strawberry pattern." Hyperkeratotic AK lesions on the face may have prominent keratotic plugs within the hair follicles (targetoid-like pattern). The rosette sign consists of white dots localized inside the follicular openings, which may reflect alternating orthokeratosis and parakeratosis. Pigmented lesions may show brown dots and globules surrounding the follicular openings.

DIFFERENTIAL DIAGNOSIS

There are various dermatoses that may be difficult to differentiate from AKs. Spreading pigmented AK may mimic seborrheic keratosis or facial lentigo maligna. In contrast to spreading pigmented AKs, seborrheic keratoses have a velvety to finely verrucous surface that usually feels soft and greasy on palpation. In addition, seborrheic keratoses are also found on the trunk and other body surfaces that are rarely exposed to sunlight.

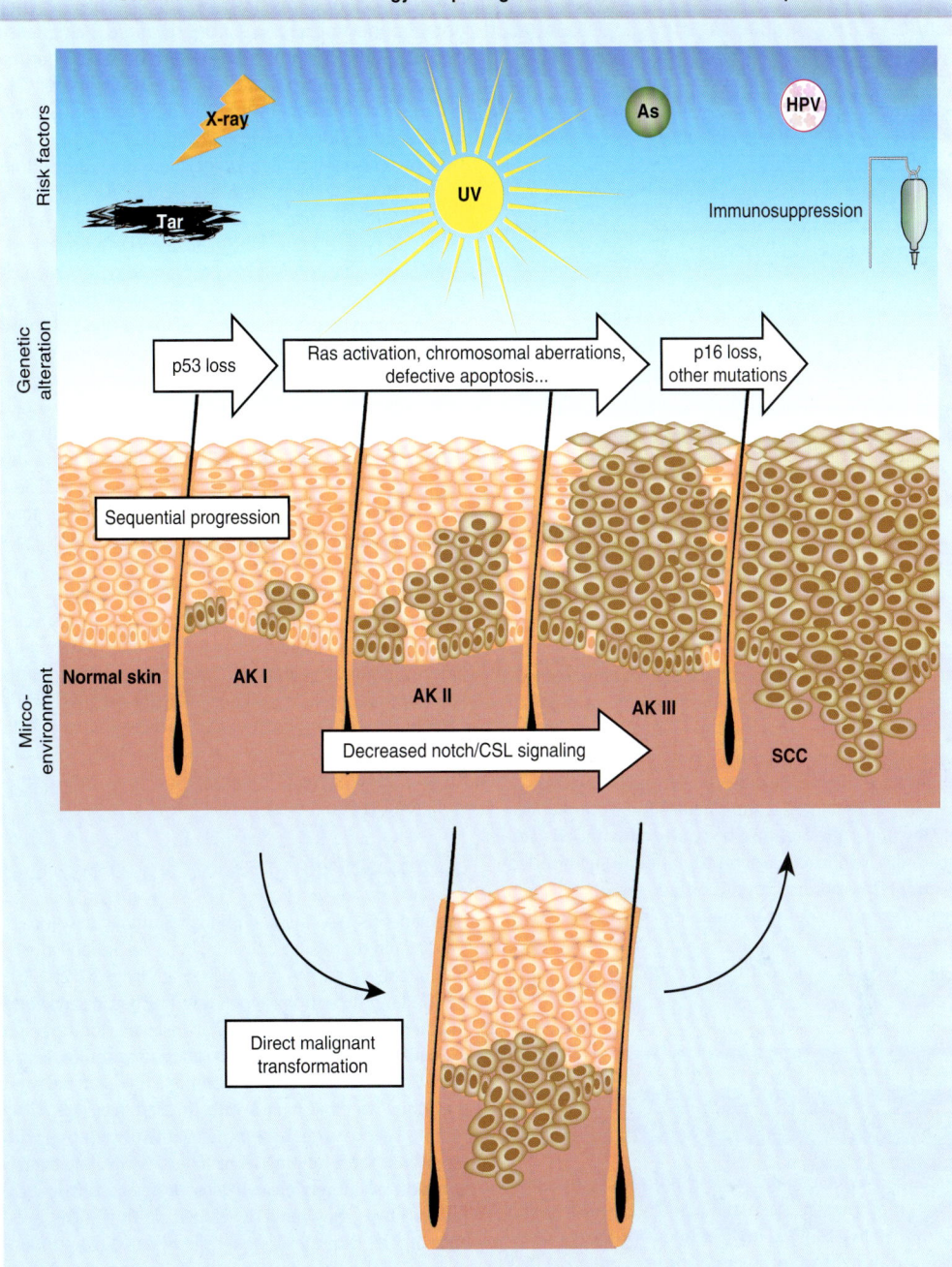

Figure 110-7 Schematic overview on the etiology and pathogenesis of actinic keratosis (AK) development. The most important etiologic factors are fair skin, ultraviolet (UV) radiation, immunosuppression, human papillomavirus (HPV) infection or exposure to tar, arsenic, and X-rays. The classic pathway (*upper panel*) assumes a stepwise progression from early lesions confined to the basal layers of the epidermis (AK I) toward intermediate (AK II) and late AK lesions (AK III), which may progress to invasive squamous cell carcinoma (SCC). A common and early molecular event is loss or inactivation of the tumor-suppressor gene *p53*. Recent evidence suggests decreased Notch signaling in underlying dermis may contribute to the formation and progression of AK. The alternative pathway (*lower panel*) assumes that any AK, including low-grade lesions, bears the potential to directly progress to invasive SCC. Abbreviation: As, arsenic; HPV, human papillomavirus.

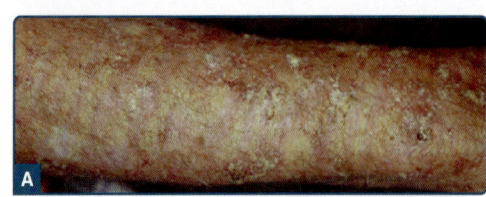
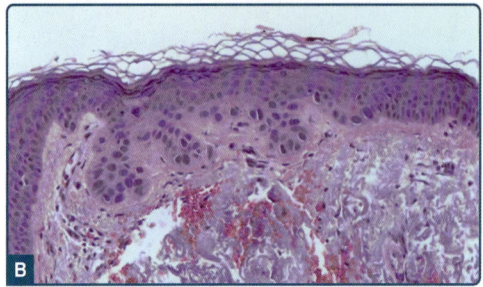

Figure 110-8 A, Severe solar damage of the dorsal arm demonstrating hypertrophic actinic keratoses. **B,** Histopathologic preparation of actinic keratosis demonstrates atypical cells along the basal layer with sparing of adnexal epithelium and a sparse lymphocytic infiltrate with marked actinic elastosis in the upper dermis underlying the lesion.

Dermoscopy can help to distinguish pigmented AK from facial lentigo maligna. Dermoscopic findings of pigmented AK are white and evident follicles, scales, and red color. Intense pigmentation and gray rhomboidal lines are diagnostic clues for lentigo maligna.[13] In rare cases, disseminated superficial actinic porokeratoses may affect the face and be confused with AK. The flat lesions are normally asymptomatic and surrounded by a ridge-like border. Besides other precancerous (eg, arsenical keratosis) or malignant (eg, SCC) lesions, differential diagnoses include melanocytic nevi, senile lentigo, and cutaneous lupus erythematosus.

CLINICAL COURSE AND PROGNOSIS

Established AKs usually take a chronic course and lesions may persist, spontaneously regress, or progress to invasive SCCs. The likelihood for these events was investigated in a panel of studies, but revealed inconsistent and varying results. Most investigations show major methodologic limitations with a follow up period of less than 12 months and are of low quality. Thus, reliable estimates for the clinical course and prognosis of AK lesions remain uncertain to date.

PROGRESSION TO INVASIVE SQUAMOUS CELL CARCINOMA

Although atypical keratinocytes may penetrate the basement membrane and become invasive, the annual progression rate of a single lesion to SCC is supposedly below 1%, ranging from 0 to 0.53% in individuals without a history of nonmelanoma skin cancer and without immunosuppression. Currently, there is an intense debate on how the progression from AK to SCC occurs. One model assumes that low-grade AKs successively progress toward high-grade AKs and ultimately invade the epidermal–dermal junction (classic pathway of progression). However, there is evidence that not all SCCs develop from high-grade AKs, but that the majority of invasive carcinomas have their origin from AK type I. These findings suggest that each AK per se bears the potential to progress into SCC regardless of the grade of histologic atypia, and that a direct cancerous invasive transformation of basaloid atypical keratinocytes is the most common mechanism of disease progression (differentiated pathway of progression). Overall, it is estimated that only 5% to 10% of all AKs progress to invasive SCC (see Fig. 110-7). The risk for progression of AK to SCC reported in the literature varies from less than 1% to 20%. The risk for SCC formation increases with the duration of presence, total lesion count (>5), and individual patient characteristics, such as suppressed immune status. Conversely, more than 60% of cutaneous SCCs are believed to develop from preexisting AKs. Several histopathologic studies examined invasive SCC specimens and determined the percentage of associated or contiguous AKs. Premalignant AK-like areas were detected at the periphery or within the invasive parts of SCC in 60% to 100% of cases.[14-19] A lesion may become tender or painful and show signs of inflammation prior to progression, requiring a biopsy to rule out SCC formation.

REGRESSION

Spontaneous resolution without treatment may occur. The annual regression rates for single AK lesions identified in cohort studies generally range from 20% to 30% with a large variation, depending on the presence and maintenance of risk factors. For instance, limiting sun exposure and the use of sunscreen may promote regression. The resolution rates of complete fields on face and scalp are lower and have been estimated to be 0 to 7.2%.[8] Lesions that have regressed can eventually relapse, with recurrence rates ranging from 15% to 53%.[8] However, it is often not entirely clear if these lesions are true local relapses or if they have developed de novo. The presence of AKs indicates long-term sun damage and identifies individuals who are at high risk for developing actinic skin lesions. Thus, AKs are sometimes considered a chronic skin condition where lesions come and go.

TREATMENT

It is not possible to reliably predict which lesions will persist, regress, or become SCCs based on clinical and histologic features. Thus, despite the relatively low risk of transformation and high rates of spontaneous resolution, early and consequent therapy is warranted. Furthermore, treatment can help minimize symptoms like scaling, pain, or pruritus, improve the cosmetic appearance and ultimately improve the quality of lives of the patients. A plethora of treatment options exists and more agents and procedures are constantly being launched and approved by regulatory agencies. Treatment modalities for AKs can be broadly divided into lesion-targeted therapies and field-targeted therapies (Table 110-2).

LESION-TARGETED THERAPIES

The majority of lesion-targeted therapies are mechanically destructive, such as cryosurgery, surgical approaches, or ablative lasers. Other lesion-directed approaches include medical treatment with 5-fluorouracil (5-FU) plus salicylic acid and lesion-directed photodynamic therapy (PDT).

Cryosurgery: Liquid nitrogen cryosurgery is a commonly performed destructive procedure that is typically administered with a spray device, cotton swab, or probe. The freezing procedure leads to the formation of extracellular and intracellular ice crystals. With subsequent thawing, destruction of atypical keratinocytes occurs through cell dehydration and rupture of cell membranes and organelles. Cryosurgery is easy to administer, cheap, and efficient in clearing single lesions. More benefits include the lack of need for local anesthesia and simple posttreatment care. Frequent short-term complications are procedure-related discomfort with pain and hemorrhage, accompanied by, in many cases, the formation of a blister. Further drawbacks include the danger of nerve damage, pigmentary changes resulting from the destruction of adjacent melanocytes, and scarring. The application procedure of cryosurgery for AK is little standardized with varying durations of freeze–thaw cycles, number of freeze–thaw repetitions, or duration of freezing. Cryosurgery is suitable to treat a limited number of clinically perceptible or symptomatic lesions.

Surgical Approaches: Surgical approaches generally have the advantage of obtaining specimens for further histopathologic assessment. Conventional surgical excision is not a routine procedure for AK. It can be considered for clinically atypical lesions that warrant further histologic evaluation or to rule out invasive SCCs. Shave excisions are commonly performed for single hyperkeratotic lesions. However, the pathologic evaluation after shave excision may be problematic if the biopsy is taken too superficially to determine if the lesion is confined to the epidermis or invasive. Curettage takes advantage of a curette to mechanically scrape away the atypical keratinocytes. It may either be applied as single technique or in combination with shave excision, electrodessication,

TABLE 110-2
Treatment of Actinic Keratoses

	ADVANTAGES	DISADVANTAGES
Lesion-Targeted Therapies		
Liquid nitrogen cryosurgery	▪ Short treatment duration (sec-min) ▪ No need for local anesthesia	▪ Little standardized ▪ Frequent blister formation ▪ Hypopigmentation
Surgical approaches (conventional excision, shave excision with/without electrodessication)	▪ Histopathologic assessment ▪ Low recurrence rates	▪ Local anesthesia needed ▪ Surgery-related complications ▪ Hypopigmentation/hyperpigmentation ▪ Scarring
Ablative lasers	▪ Short treatment duration	▪ Dyspigmentation ▪ Risk of scarring ▪ High equipment costs
Topical therapy (5-fluorouracil plus salicylic acid)	▪ Easy application by the patient ▪ No need for local anesthesia	▪ Long treatment duration (6-12 weeks) ▪ Local inflammation
Lesion-directed photodynamic therapy (PDT) ("patch" PDT)	▪ No need for local anesthesia ▪ Cosmetic outcome	▪ Local pain and adverse events (eg, erythema, edema, erosion) ▪ Lamp device needed
Field-Targeted Therapies		
Topical/Medical		
5-fluorouracil Imiquimod Diclofenac-Na Ingenol mebutate	▪ Application by the patient ▪ Cosmetic outcome	▪ Potential of contact hypersensitivity ▪ Treatment duration (3-90 days) ▪ Local adverse events (eg, erythema, edema, erosion) ▪ Rarely systemic adverse events
Procedural		
Conventional PDT (with blue light or red light)	▪ Cosmetic outcome	▪ Local adverse events (eg, erythema, edema) ▪ Local pain/burning sensation ▪ Lamp device needed
Natural daylight PDT	▪ Cosmetic outcome	▪ Local adverse events (eg, erythema, edema) ▪ Dependent on weather condition (<10°C [50°F], no rain)

or cryosurgery. It is useful for single, hypertrophic AKs on the extremities, and is technically easy to perform in an office-based setting. Yet, the quality of specimens obtained with curettage is usually poor and histologic evaluation may be equivocal. Some studies suggest that surgical therapies show lower rates of recurrence than other destructive treatments. Nevertheless, disadvantages of all surgical procedures include the need for local anesthesia, potentially prolonged wound healing, infection, bleeding, dyspigmentation, scarring, and rather poor cosmetic outcomes.

Laser Therapies: Laser devices are increasingly used for the treatment of AKs. Most experience and evidence has been collected for ablative resurfacing with the carbon dioxide (CO_2) and erbium:yttrium aluminium garnet (Er:YAG)-laser. Both devices ablate the epidermis at varying depths, allowing for reepithelialization with adnexal or lesion-adjacent keratinocytes that are less actinically damaged. The CO_2 laser has a higher penetration depth than the Er:YAG laser and may offer advantages when treating thicker and hyperkeratotic lesions. Adverse events comprise hypopigmentation and atrophic scarring. Although lesion clearance rates were promising in a panel of studies, AKs can relapse after laser treatment. Laser resurfacing is probably best reserved for use by specially trained and experienced physicians and for patients with more cosmetic concerns. The efficacy of nonablative fractional photothermolysis is currently unclear and well-designed trials are lacking.

Lesion-Directed Photodynamic Therapy:
PDT is increasingly used for the treatment of both single AK lesions and field cancerization with superb cosmetic outcomes. It is based on the topical application of a photosensitizing agent followed by exposure to a specific wavelength of light. 5-Aminolevulinic acid (ALA) and methyl aminolevulinate (MAL) are the 2 substances that are used in PDT for AKs. They are absorbed by the epidermis and preferentially accumulate in atypical cells where they are further processed to protoporphyrin IX. Subsequent exposure to a specific wavelength light source activates protoporphyrin IX, resulting in a phototoxic reaction with release of reactive oxygen species and, ultimately, in destruction of target cells by necrosis and apoptosis.

Although PDT is predominantly perceived as field therapy (see section "Field-targeted Therapies"), 5-ALA can be applied with a patch to isolated lesions to spare and protect healthy skin. This targeted application of the photosensitizer can help minimize local adverse events like erythema, crusting, blister formation and is usually well tolerated by patients. The efficacy of the patch PDT is high and results in excellent cosmetic outcomes. In particular, hypopigmentation which is observed in many cases with destructive lesion-directed approaches is not seen with this technique.

FIELD-TARGETED THERAPIES

Field-centered approaches do not target at single lesions, but treat entire actinically damaged areas ("fields"). This strategy is applicable if several ill-defined AK lesions exist within 1 field or if subclinical lesions are suspected and field cancerization is present. Field therapies can be further categorized into topical and procedural treatments (see Table 110-2).

Topical Treatment: A variety of topical agents exist for the treatment of AKs such as diclofenac, 5-FU, imiquimod, and ingenol mebutate (Table 110-3).

Diclofenac is an inhibitor of cyclooxygenase and belongs to the nonsteroidal antiinflammatory drugs. Topical therapy with 3% diclofenac in 2.5% hyaluronic acid gel is a widely used effective treatment option for patients with multiple AKs or field cancerization.[20] It was shown to be protective against the appearance of new AKs, as it also acts against subclinical lesions.[21] Diclofenac is well tolerated, but may lead to local adverse events, such as erythema, scaling, burning sensation or pruritus. The recommended treatment duration of 90 days with twice daily application is relatively long. This may have a negative impact on practicability and patient adherence.[22]

5-FU is a pyrimidine analog and acts as an antimetabolite and via inhibition of the thymidylate synthetase as a cytostatic drug. In a cream formulation, 5-FU is a well-established topical treatment option for AK. 5-FU is available in numerous preparations, most commonly as 0.5% cream once daily or 5% cream twice

TABLE 110-3
Topical Treatments for Actinic Keratoses

DRUG	PREPARATION	DOSAGE/APPLICATION
Diclofenac-Na	3% gel	Twice daily for 90 days
5-Fluorouracil (5-FU)	0.5% cream	Once daily for up to 4 weeks
	1% cream	Twice daily for 2-6 weeks
	4% cream	Once daily for 4 weeks
	5% cream	Twice daily for 2-4 weeks
	2% solution	Twice daily for 2-4 weeks
	5% solution	Twice daily for 2-4 weeks
5-FU plus salicylic acid (SA)	0.5% (5-FU) and 10% (SA) solution	Once daily up to 12 weeks
Imiquimod	5% cream	Three times per week for 4 weeks
	3.75% cream	Once daily for 2 weeks
	2.5% cream	Once daily for 2 weeks
Ingenol mebutate	0.015% gel	Once daily for 3 days
	0.05% gel	Once daily for 2 days

daily. Both are effective and similarly safe, but patients may prefer the 0.5% preparation as it is applied only once daily.[23] Typical adverse events are erythema, erosion and discomfort at the site of application. Treatment duration is usually 2 to 4 weeks.

Another formulation is a combination of 0.5% 5-FU with 10% salicylic acid.[24,25] It is applied once daily for up to 12 weeks on an area not larger than 25 cm^2. It may be more suited for hypertrophic lesions than 5-FU alone because salicylic acid has a keratolytic effect and improves the penetration of 5-FU.

Imiquimod is a Toll-like receptor 7 agonist and activates innate immune cells to produce interferon-α and other cytokines. Topical imiquimod is an effective treatment option for AK and available as 2.5%, 3.75%, and 5% cream.[26,27] Application frequency depends on which concentration is used. Imiquimod at 2.5% and 3.75% concentration is usually applied once daily for 14 consecutive days. The 5% formulation is applied 3 times per week during a 4-week period. Adverse events are usually limited to the site of application including local irritation, pain, pruritus and swelling. In some cases, systemic events, like cardiovascular disorders, myalgia, arthralgia, and flu-like symptoms, may occur. In the light of long-term experience and better tolerability, 3.75% imiquimod is commonly preferred for the treatment of single AK lesions as well as for field-directed therapy.[8] In immunosuppressed patients, 5% imiquimod cream was shown to be safe.

Ingenol mebutate is a hydrophobic triterpene ester that is extracted from the sap of the plant *Euphorbia peplus*. It is effective against AK by chemoablative and immunostimulatory properties.[28,29] Ingenol mebutate is available as a 0.015% gel for scalp and face and a 0.05% gel for the trunk and extremities. In contrast to other topical treatments for AK, 0.015% and 0.05% ingenol mebutate are only applied for 3 and 2 consecutive days, respectively. Local adverse events are virtually obligatory and are irritation, pruritus, and inflammatory changes, including erythema, blister, edema, erosion, scaling, and crusting. All these reactions appear early and usually subside within 14 days.[30] However, because of the short treatment duration and good efficacy, ingenol mebutate was shown to increase treatment satisfaction and the quality of life of patients.[31]

Cryopeeling: This procedure refers to the extensive application of liquid nitrogen not only to single lesions, but to a complete field of manifest and subclinical AK. Cryopeeling is relatively easy to apply and was found effective for hypertrophic AK. Compared to conventional cryosurgery, it may help to reduce recurrence rates, although it bears a higher risk for hypopigmentation of treated areas.

Chemical Peelings: Medium-depth chemical peels using Jessner solution and 35% trichloroacetic acid, 70% glycolic acid, or solid CO_2 are moderately effective in treating diffuse nonhypertrophic AKs, especially when a series of such peelings is repeated over time. They cause skin damage in the superficial papillary dermis and induce a wound reaction with exfoliation of the atypical keratinocytes and reepithelialization. Common side effects are stinging, burning sensation, erythema, and scaling.

Deep chemical peelings using phenol or higher concentrations of trichloroacetic acid are more effective in treating hyperkeratotic AK or AK with appendageal epithelial atypia. However, they are rarely used because of the potential cardiac and renal toxicity of phenol and a higher risk of scarring, infection, and hypopigmentation.

Dermabrasion: Dermabrasion (also known as surgical skin planing) is an older technique that is nowadays rarely used for AK treatment. It is based on physical ablation of lesions with superficial abrasion of the epidermis at the level of the epidermis. Devices for dermabrasion are either drywall sanding sheets or diamond fraises that are powered or handheld. The procedure is painful and should be performed under sedation or general anesthesia. It may be applied for field therapy for an actinically damaged bald scalp or forehead.

Field-Targeted Photodynamic Therapy: Field-targeted PDT is usually performed with 5-ALA cream or MAL nanoemulsion as photosensitizing substances in combination with visible light (ie, blue, green or red light). Randomized, placebo-controlled studies demonstrated the efficacy of both ALA-PDT and MAL-PDT. They are equally effective, with lesion clearance rates ranging from 70% to 90%. A common adverse event is local discomfort ranging from burning or stinging to intolerable pain during exposure to the light source. Allergic reactions to ALA and MAL have been rarely reported. One to 2 days after treatment, local erythema, edema, blistering, sterile pustule formation, and crusting are commonly observed as clinical correlates for the phototoxic reaction. The cosmetic outcome of PDT is excellent and the term *photorejuvenation* has been coined. The effect is characterized by collagen remodeling and a decrease of small wrinkles, telangiectasias, and lentigines.

An alternative to conventional PDT is the so-called natural daylight PDT, using much shorter incubation times of MAL/ALA and exposing the affected skin to sunlight instead of artificial visible light. Within 30 minutes after topical application of MAL/ALA patients are advised to stay outdoors for 2 hours. Natural daylight PDT is significantly less painful than conventional PDT, while the other local side effects are comparable. For the treatment of mild to moderate AKs, the effectiveness of natural daylight PDT was noninferior to conventional PDT in several trials.

APPROACH TO INDIVIDUAL MANAGEMENT

As described above, there are a number of effective lesion-targeted and field treatments available to choose from to decrease the burden of AKs. The individual patient's needs and expectations, the physician's skills, the mechanisms of action of the various treatments and their side-effect profiles, and the costs of the agents and procedures should all be considered when choosing a treatment strategy. To help physicians in their choice several national and international guidelines for the management of AKs have been proposed.[8,32]

PREVENTION

Measures of primary prevention are primarily based on the avoidance of exposure to UV, because it is the main risk factor for the development of AKs. Educational and preventive efforts should be directed toward all patients, including children and high-risk populations such as organ transplant recipients or outdoor workers. Minimizing UV radiation is the single most effective means of decreasing the risk of AKs. Because complete avoidance of the sun is impractical, the next best preventive measures are to avoid exposure to intense midday sun; consistently apply and reapply broad-spectrum sunscreens; wear UV-protective clothing, hats, and sunglasses; install UV-protective windows where indicated; and make sure to take an oral vitamin D supplement if necessary to avoid vitamin D insufficiency or deficiency. Tanning beds should be avoided. Newborns should not be exposed to sun.

USE OF SUNSCREENS

Numerous randomized studies show that the use of sunscreen can decrease the incidence and prevalence of AKs, reduce the number of AK lesions, and increase their rate of regression. There is also evidence that sunscreen use can prevent certain types of skin cancer, mostly SCC. Broad-spectrum sunscreen against UVB and UVA radiation with a minimum sun protection factor of 30 should be applied to areas that cannot be protected by physical measures like UV-protective clothes or UV avoidance. It is important to apply sunscreen in sufficient amounts at least 20 minutes before going outside and to reapply it every 2 to 3 hours especially when excessive sweating or swimming.

CHEMOPREVENTION

Some agents or dietary interventions can prevent or delay the development of AKs in high-risk populations. There is limited evidence that adhering to a low-fat diet may decrease the incidence of AKs and nonmelanoma skin cancer. Nutritional supplements, like vitamin A, selenium, and carotenes, are currently not recommended for prevention. Topical imiquimod also has been safely used in organ transplant recipients to prevent development of cutaneous SCC.

Retinoids: There is a debate on whether the application of topical retinoids is effective in the prevention of AKs because prevention trials have yielded discordant results. Unlike the controversy with topical retinoids, there is strong evidence for the use of systemic retinoids in preventing nonmelanoma skin cancer and AKs, especially in high-risk populations, such as organ transplant recipients, patients with xeroderma pigmentosum, and other chronically immunosuppressed patients.[33] However, systemic retinoids are only effective while taking them. Their use is also limited by the frequent occurrence of systemic toxicities, including hypercholesterolemia, hypertriglyceridemia, mucocutaneous xerosis, musculoskeletal abnormalities, and alteration in liver function. Thus, when considering the use of systemic retinoids as chemoprevention one must weigh the risks and benefits.

Nicotinamide: Oral nicotinamide (vitamin B_3) was reported safe and effective in reducing the rates of new nonmelanoma skin cancer and AK in high-risk patients in a recent phase III trial. Specifically, the number of AKs was reduced by 13% in patients who took 500 mg of nicotinamide twice daily for 12 months compared to placebo.[34] However, the beneficial effects disappeared when the treatment was discontinued. Furthermore, it is unclear if nicotinamide is associated with an increased risk for infectious adverse events.

BOWEN DISEASE

AT-A-GLANCE

- Bowen disease (BD) is squamous cell carcinoma (SCC) in situ.
- It can progress to Bowen carcinoma (invasive SCC) in up to 5% of cases.
- Etiologic factors include UV radiation, arsenic, previous therapy with psoralen and UVA radiation, immunosuppression, exposure to ionizing radiation, and infection with human papillomavirus.
- Clinical variants are pigmented, intertriginous, periungual, and subungual BD.
- Histopathologic features include full-thickness epidermal atypia with large, round cells and possible adnexal involvement.
- Therapeutic options include surgical, topical, and ablative interventions.
- Surgical treatment methods include excision and Mohs micrographic surgery, which permit histopathologic evaluation to exclude invasive SCC.
- Topical therapy may be used in areas that are difficult to treat with other methods.

Bowen disease (BD) is a distinct type of SCC in situ and was originally described in 1912 by John T. Bowen, a Boston dermatologist. It may affect both skin and mucous membranes and has the potential to progress to Bowen carcinoma, that is, an invasive SCC.

EPIDEMIOLOGY

The exact incidence of BD in the United States is unknown. The incidence was estimated at 142 per 100,000 persons in Hawaii. BD usually occurs in adults, and is typically seen in individuals older than age 60 years. It affects both sexes with a preponderance in men.[35] BD mostly affects sun-exposed areas, such as head and neck, as well as the upper and lower limbs. Men are more likely to have BD on the balding scalp, ear, and anterior trunk. In contrast, women commonly have BD on the cheeks and lower legs. Immunocompromised patients are more likely to develop BD at a younger age. It also affects more often the trunk, limbs, and neck, and recurrence rates are higher compared to immunocompetent patients.[35]

CLINICAL FEATURES

BD lesions grow slowly and may be accompanied by pruritus, but are usually asymptomatic. Lesions typically present as erythematous plaques with irregular, clearly demarcated borders. The surface may be scaling, crusting, or hyperkeratotic (Fig. 110-9A). Over time, lesions may grow in size and measure up to several centimeters. The flat plaque may transform to a nodular or verrucous form. BD usually appears pink or reddish, whereas crusty or hyperkeratotic lesions may take a gray or brownish color. In very few cases, lesions are pigmented. Lesions of BD are usually solitary, but may be multiple in up to 20% of individuals. Sites of predilection include sun-exposed areas such as the head and neck and lower legs, although any site of the body may be affected.

There are a few clinical variants of BD. In the periungual region BD may appear as an erythematous, scaly, thin plaque around the cuticular margin or as a verrucous plaque. It may lead to nail discoloration, onycholysis, or destruction of the nail plate (see Fig. 110-9B). In intertriginous areas, BD can present as an oozing, erythematous, or pigmented patch or plaque. BD of the mucosal surfaces may appear as verrucous or polypoid papules and plaques, erythroplakia, or a velvety erythematous plaque. These variants are discussed in the sections on precancerous lesions of the oral cavity

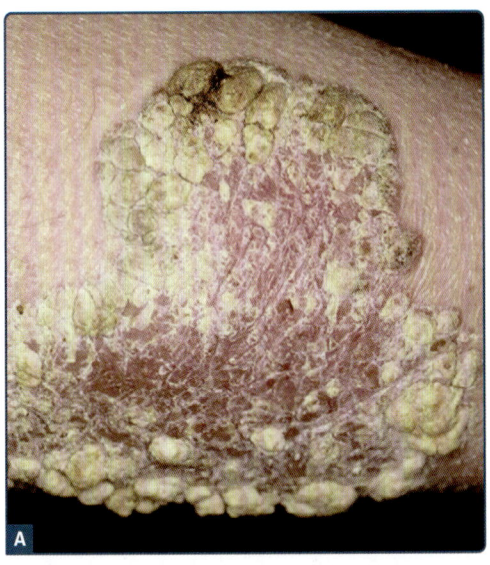

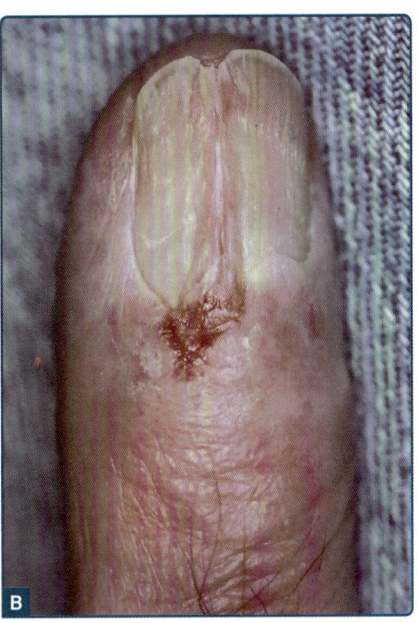

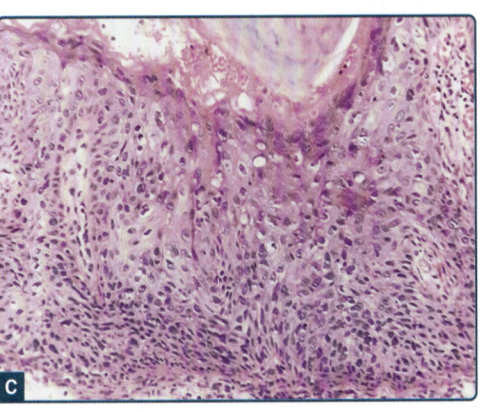

Figure 110-9 **A,** Large plaque of Bowen disease of the leg. **B,** Bowen disease of the nail unit resulting in onycholysis. **C,** Typical histopathologic features of Bowen disease include full-thickness epidermal atypia with loss of the stratified architecture. Involvement of adnexal structures is commonly seen.

(see section "Potentially Malignant Disorders of the Oral Cavity,") and the lower anogenital tract (see section "Precancerous Lesions of the Lower Anogenital Tract"), respectively.

ETIOLOGY AND PATHOGENESIS

The most important etiologic factors for the development of BD include a long history of significant UV exposure and infection with HPV. BD has been described with increased frequency in patients undergoing psoralen plus UVA therapy. In contrast, it is rarely seen in stronger-pigmented individuals. Up to 30% of extragenital BD lesions have been found to harbor HPV DNA. Several HPV subtypes, such as HPV types 16, 18, 31, 34, 35, 54, 58, 61, 62, and 73 have been detected in BD lesions.[36] Infection with high-risk HPV subtypes such as HPV 16 may be responsible for BD lesions on hands or fingers after anodigital infection in patients that simultaneously have anal and genital lesions. However, the prevalence of HPV-associated BD lesions is higher on sun-protected than on sun-exposed body areas.[37] Organ transplant recipients, HIV patients and other patients with long-term immunosuppression are at higher risk of developing BD. Other etiologic factors include arsenic exposure and ionizing radiation.

DIAGNOSIS

The clinical picture together with the typical history of a slowly growing, mostly asymptomatic lesion that remains resistant to topical corticosteroid treatment is highly suspicious for BD. However, final diagnosis requires biopsy and histologic examination.

On a histologic level, BD lesions display full-thickness epidermal atypia with loss of the stratified epidermal architecture that is clearly demarcated from the surrounding physiologic structures (see Fig. 110-9C). Abnormal mitoses, acanthosis, and hyperkeratosis are further characteristics. Toward the upper epidermal layers parakeratosis is usually present. The degree of cytologic atypia may be variable. Typical are hyperchromatic, pleomorphic, and enlarged nuclei. The cells show a pale staining and eosinophilic cytoplasm. Vacuoles may be present within the keratinocytes. Atypical cells can be seen throughout the epidermal thickness alongside with mitotic figures and apoptotic cells. Intraepidermal portions of adnexal structures, such as the pilosebaceous units, may be affected as well.[14] As the basement membrane remains intact, atypia does not affect subepidermal structures. The upper dermis is usually infiltrated by numerous inflammatory cells, including lymphocytes, plasma cells, and histiocytes.

Several histopathologic subtypes, such as psoriasiform, atrophic, acantholytic, and epidermolytic BD can be distinguished. Psoriasiform BD displays parakeratosis and marked acanthosis with broad, sometimes fused, epidermal rete ridges. Atrophic BD is characterized by a thinned epidermis. Acantholytic BD shows acantholysis in the epidermis. Epidermolytic BD has changes of incidental epidermolytic hyperkeratosis present. The phenomenon of intraepidermal epithelioma of Borst-Jadassohn—namely, nesting of the atypical cells within the epidermis, or so-called pagetoid BD—can also be seen. Furthermore, verrucous-hyperkeratotic and papillomatous variants have been described.

DIFFERENTIAL DIAGNOSIS

Clinically and histologically, BD may be difficult to distinguish from other dermatoses (Tables 110-4 and 110-5).

CLINICAL DIFFERENTIAL DIAGNOSIS

Superficial basal cell carcinoma may mimic BD but can be distinguished by its elevated, subtle and translucent

TABLE 110-4
Clinical Differential Diagnosis of Bowen Disease

- Erythematous Bowen disease
  - Superficial basal cell carcinoma
  - Dermatitis, eczema
  - Psoriasis
  - Seborrheic dermatitis
  - Lichen planus
  - Benign lichenoid keratosis
  - Irritated or inflamed seborrheic keratosis
  - Actinic keratosis
  - Squamous cell carcinoma
  - Amelanotic melanoma
- Hyperkeratotic Bowen disease
  - Verruca vulgaris
  - Seborrheic keratosis
  - Discoid lupus erythematosus
  - Hypertrophic lichen planus
  - Squamous cell carcinoma
- Pigmented Bowen disease
  - Melanoma
  - Bowenoid papulosis
- Intertriginous Bowen disease
  - Inverse psoriasis
  - Seborrheic dermatitis
  - Candidiasis
  - Paget disease
  - Hailey-Hailey disease
- Subungual or periungual Bowen disease
  - Nail dystrophy
  - Onychomycosis
  - Squamous cell carcinoma
  - Amelanotic melanoma

TABLE 110-5
Histopathologic Differential Diagnosis of Bowen Disease

- Paget disease
- Pagetoid melanoma in situ
- Intraepidermal eccrine carcinoma
- Intraepidermal Merkel cell carcinoma
- Intraepidermal sebaceous carcinoma
- Bowenoid papulosis
- Hidroacanthoma simplex
- Podophyllin-induced changes in a wart

border. Patches of psoriasis, atopic dermatitis or lichen planus are typically accompanied by itching and located on their sites of predilection together with other lesions. In addition, they usually respond to topical corticosteroid therapy. Hyperkeratotic or verrucous lesions of BD can be misinterpreted as viral warts, seborrheic keratosis, and SCC. For both pigmented and unpigmented BD lesions, it is important to consider melanoma and amelanotic melanoma as differential diagnoses, respectively. Because of their very similar histologic picture, the clinical setting is crucial in differentiating BD from sexually transmitted bowenoid papulosis.

HISTOPATHOLOGIC DIFFERENTIAL DIAGNOSIS

BD may be confused with (extramammary) Paget disease. Both entities show atypical cells with pleomorphic, hyperchromatic nucleus, clear cytoplasm, and mitotic figures. While BD affects the full-thickness of the epidermis, Paget cells typically form nest-like or glandular-like patterns with a central lumen that are most abundant in the basal layers. Immunohistochemistry is essential for diagnosis, as Paget cells stain positive for carcinoembryonic antigen, mucin, Alcian blue, aldehyde fuchsin, and periodic acid-Schiff and are diastase resistant. In addition, unlike BD, Paget disease overexpresses low-weight cytokeratins, such as cytokeratin 7, and gross cystic disease fluid protein 15 (GCDFP-15).[38,39]

Similar to BD, AK type III (bowenoid AK) displays cell atypia throughout the entire thickness of the epidermis. In contrast to BD, they do not have a clear border, but show a diffuse transition into the surrounding epidermis. In addition, mitotic figures are less prominent. Finally, lumican, a small leucine-rich proteoglycan, is expressed in most BD lesions, but not in AK.[40] In hidroacanthoma simplex, Lumican staining is also observed, but atypical mitoses cannot be seen.[15]

Pagetoid melanoma in situ can be difficult at times to distinguish histopathologically from BD. In BD, the intercellular desmosomal bridges should be identifiable between the atypical keratinocytes. Additionally, melanocyte-specific immunoperoxidase staining gives positive results in melanoma cells, but negative results in BD and Paget disease cells. The other rare pagetoid neoplasms are usually recognizable, but erroneous diagnoses can be made by the unwary.

Bowenoid papulosis may lack the full-thickness epidermal atypia present in BD, but the clinical setting is paramount. Podophyllin applied topically to skin lesions induces metaphase arrest, leading to bizarre keratinocyte formation, architectural disturbance, vacuolation, and sometimes a pattern of pseudoepitheliomatous hyperplasia that can be mistaken for BD. These changes typically resolve after a few days to a week.

CLINICAL COURSE AND PROGNOSIS

In general, recurrence of BD is rare and estimated to be approximately 6% within 5 years after sufficient treatment. The theory that persistent BD within the deep portion of the follicle is mainly responsible for recurrence could not be confirmed.[14] In fact, recurrent BD may be more likely caused by subclinical lateral spread, as excision with narrower lateral margin is associated with a higher risk of recurrence.[16]

The overall risk that untreated BD will progress to invasive carcinoma is estimated at approximately 5%. Immunocompromised individuals, such as organ transplant recipients, are at particular risk of recurrence, multiple BD lesions and transformation into invasive SCC.[7,35]

Once BD occurs, the risk of developing subsequent nonmelanoma skin cancer is particularly higher. There is no evidence, however, that BD is associated with a higher risk for internal malignancies. One exception is in cases of BD related to previous arsenic exposure, where the occurrence of an internal malignancy is possible. Also, BD involving the vulvar region in females and the perianal region in males may be associated with an increased risk of uterine, cervical, vaginal, and anal cancer, most likely as a consequence of HPV infection.[36]

TREATMENT

There are various treatment approaches for BD. Such therapies can be divided into 3 main categories: surgical or destructive therapies, topical therapies, and radiation therapy (Table 110-6). The evidence on efficacy and safety is strongly limited and mostly restricted to PDT.[17] However, this does not necessarily imply that other treatments lack efficacy. The choice on which treatment is best rather depends on several individual aspects, such as availability, patient or clinician's preference, affected body area, and treatment costs. Surgical and destructive therapies include excision, Mohs micrographic surgery, curettage with or without electrosurgery, chemoablation with trichloroacetic acid, and cryosurgery. These interventions are widely available and relatively cheap, and surgical approaches permit histopathologic evalua-

TABLE 110-6
Treatment of Bowen Disease

		ADVANTAGE	DISADVANTAGE
Surgical and Destructive Therapies			
	• Excision • Mohs micrographic surgery • Curettage with or without electrosurgery • Cryosurgery	• Histopathologic assessment (not for cryosurgery) • Short treatment duration	• Surgery-related complications • Scarring • Cryosurgery: hypopigmentation, blister formation
Topical Therapies			
	• 5-Fluorouracil	• Application by the patient • Cosmetic outcome • No need for local anesthesia	• Long treatment duration • Local adverse events (eg, erythema, edema, erosion) • Toxic for eyes
Nonsurgical Ablative Therapies			
	• Photodynamic therapy (PDT) • Laser ablation • Chemoablation (trichloroacetic acid) • Radiation therapy	• Cosmetic outcome (PDT)	• Local adverse events • Dyspigmentation • Chronic radiation dermatitis

TABLE 110-7
Association of Human Papillomavirus Types with Epithelial Precancerous Lesions

PRECANCEROUS LESION	ASSOCIATED HUMAN PAPILLOMAVIRUS TYPES[a]
Bowenoid papulosis (BP)	**16, 18**, 31-35, 39, 42, 48, 51-54
Epidermodysplasia verruciformis (EV)	2, **3, 5, 8**, 9, 12, 14, 15, 17, 19, 25, 26, 38, 47, 50
Anal and perianal intraepithelial lesions (AIN, PaIN)	**16, 18, 31, 33**
Vulvar intraepithelial lesions (VIN)	**16, 18, 31, 33**
Penile intraepithelial lesions (PIN)	**16, 18, 31, 33**
Digital/periungual Bowen disease	**16**

[a]The most common associations are highlighted in bold.

tion. They are simple, rapid, and suitable for small BD lesions on easily accessible body areas. In particular for BD affecting the periungual region, local excision or Mohs micrographic surgery are commonly used. The most preferred topical therapies are 5-FU and 5% imiquimod cream, but others, such as ingenol mebutate, have been tried as well.[18] Like surgical interventions, they are effective and widely available and therefore suitable for the outpatient setting. In addition, they can be used in individuals who refuse surgery, have significant comorbidities or impaired healing capability. Nonsurgical ablative therapies include PDT, laser ablation, and radiation therapy. There is good evidence for the use of PDT with MAL and ALA. One major advantage of PDT is an excellent cosmetic outcome. Combination therapies using PDT, CO_2-laser, surgery, imiquimod 5% cream, and radiation have been described.[19,41,42] If previous nonsurgical therapies have failed, BD warrants surgical intervention to exclude invasiveness and involvement of large surface areas.

VIRAL-ASSOCIATED EPITHELIAL PRECANCEROUS LESIONS

It has been suggested that some epithelial precancerous lesions are associated with HPV infection. HPVs are double-stranded DNA viruses belonging to the Papillomaviridae family. More than 100 different types have been identified so far. According to their oncogenic potential, one distinguishes high-risk types from low-risk types. They can further be subdivided according to their tissue tropism into cutaneous and mucosal categories. Chapter 167 discusses HPV infections and HPV-associated diseases in more detail. The conditions bowenoid papulosis (BP), epidermodysplasia verruciformis (EV), and precancerous lesions of the lower anogenital tract (anal intraepithelial neoplasia [AIN], perianal intraepithelial neoplasia [PaIN], VIN, penile intraepithelial neoplasia [PIN]) are reviewed here (Table 110-7).

BOWENOID PAPULOSIS

AT-A-GLANCE

- Synonyms: Bowenoid papulosis (BP) of the genitalia, pigmented penile papules with carcinoma in situ changes, genital keratinocytic dysplasia, penile carcinoma in situ associated with human papillomavirus (HPV) infection.

- BP is a precancerous condition of the genitalia caused by infection with high-risk HPV, most commonly with types 16, 18, and 33.

- BP most commonly affects young to middle-aged males.

- BP typically presents with multiple red to brownish flat papules on the penis or vulva.

- BP rarely transforms into Bowen disease or invasive squamous cell carcinoma.

- Treatment options include topical imiquimod, curettage, excision, and laser vaporization.

- Vaccination may help to reduce the prevalence of BP among young adults.

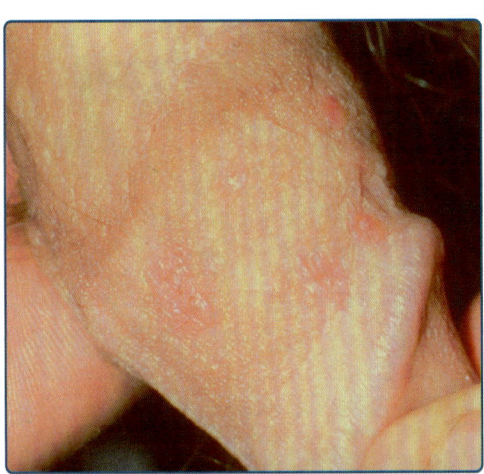

Figure 110-10 Bowenoid papulosis of the penis. Multiple erythematous to brownish papules can be seen on the dorsum of the penis of this sexually active young male. (Used with permission from James E. Fitzpatrick, MD.)

Genital lesions that histopathologically resembled SCC in situ were first described by Lloyd in 1970 as multicentric pigmented BD of the groin. In 1977, Kopf and Bart described multiple bowenoid papules of the penis, which were thereafte referred to as BP. Its association with high-risk HPV, most commonly with HPV types 16 and 18, was discovered only later. To date, numerous other mucosal HPV types have been associated with the condition, including types 31 to 35, 39, 42, 48, and 51 to 54.

BP typically presents with multiple flat verrucous papules and plaques with a red-to-brownish color (Fig. 110-10). It is most common among young to middle-aged sexually active individuals with a male predominance. Lesions are multiple, pigmented. and typically located on the glans penis, prepuce, and penis shaft in males, and around the labia minora and majora in females. Depending on sexual practices lesions may be found in the perineal and anal area. Involvement of other sites such as oral cavity, neck, and periungual area is rarely seen. BP lesions may be confused with genital warts, lichen planus, condylomata acuminata, erythroplasia, molluscum contagiosum, and seborrheic keratoses. The multiplicity of the lesions is an important distinctive feature of BP compared to BD. Patients often report condylomata acuminata in their history.

Histopathologically, BP is characterized by the presence of SCC in situ–like changes. The epidermis is usually hyperplastic and shows acanthosis, hyperorthokeratosis, and focal parakeratosis. Keratinocytes show signs of cellular atypia and disordered maturation. Dyskeratotic and pyknotic keratinocytes with scattered mitotic figures are commonly seen. HPV infection and identification of high-risk types can be achieved with polymerase chain reaction from lesional material.

BP is perceived as transitional state between genital warts and in situ SCC. It has a variable, but mostly benign, clinical course, ranging from spontaneous regression to persistence of lesions to, rarely, transformation into BD and invasive SCC. It is estimated that the risk of malignant transformation is rather low, ranging from less than 1% to 2.6%. BP is highly contagious and patients with BP and their sexual partners should be followed and examined periodically, because of the increased risk of developing SCC or cervical or vulvar neoplasia. Patients with persistent disease should probably undergo testing for altered immune status.

Despite the low risk for malignant transformation, treatment of BP is recommended. It typically responds well to local therapy, although recurrences are common. Therapeutic options include local destructive measures such as curettage with or without electrosurgery, CO_2-laser, neodymium:YAG laser, cryosurgery, and excision. Topical tretinoin, topical 5-FU, and topical cidofovir have been used in anecdotally reported cases with mixed results. Imiquimod 5% cream 3 times per week for up to 12 weeks showed high lesion clearance rates in several studies and is a valid treatment option in clinical practice. Also, the efficacy of PDT in the treatment of BP has been demonstrated. Whether HPV-specific vaccination for types 6, 11, 16, and 18 can help reduce the prevalence and incidence of BP in which HPV types 16 and 18 have frequently been identified is currently under investigation.

EPIDERMODYSPLASIA VERRUCIFORMIS

AT-A-GLANCE

- Epidermodysplasia verruciformis (EV) is an inherited skin condition with a high local susceptibility to infection with human papillomavirus (HPV), most commonly with HPV types 5 and 8.
- Sporadic and familial cases of EV may occur.
- Loss-of-function mutations of the genes *EVER1* and *EVER2* are associated with EV.
- The clinical presentation is with either widespread, flat, wart-like papules and plaques, or hypopigmented scaly patches in childhood.
- Patients with EV are at high risk to develop actinic keratosis, Bowen disease, or invasive squamous cell carcinoma in the further course of the disease.
- Late-onset EV may occur in patients with cellular immunodeficiency (HIV, organ transplant recipients).
- Sun avoidance, sun-protective measures, regular dermatologic follow up, and screening of family members for the disease are recommended.

EV is a rare inherited skin condition that is characterized by a high susceptibility to infection with some types of HPV, in particular types 5 and 8 (termed

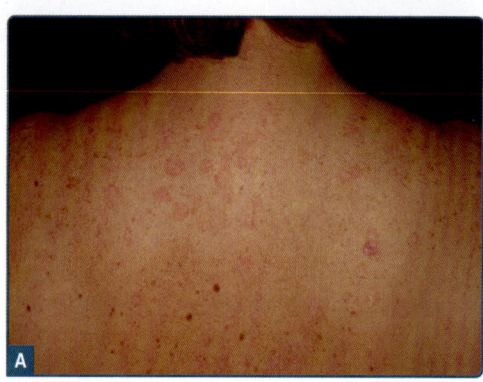 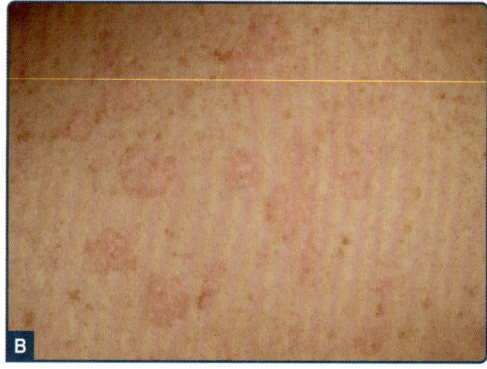

Figure 110-11 **A,** Scaly and erythematous plaques on the back of a female patient with epidermodysplasia verruciformis. **B,** The plaques are slightly elevated above skin surface level and may show areas of ill-defined hypopigmentation. These lesions may be confused with tinea corporis or tinea versicolor.

EV-HPV). In addition to the host genetic background and HPV infection, UV exposure and immunosuppression contribute to the pathogenesis of the disease.[43]

The exact prevalence of EV is not known. Sporadic and familial cases of EV have been reported in the literature. It is probably inherited as an autosomal recessive or X-chromosomal recessive disorder with 2 gene loci: EV1 (located on chromosome 17q25.3) and EV2 (located on chromosome 2p21-24). The genes *TMC6* (*EVER1*) and *TMC8* (*EVER2*) have been identified within the locus EV1.[44,45] Even though loss-of-function mutations of both genes have been linked with EV, approximately 25% of all patients do not show mutations in either gene. The *EVER* genes belong to a transmembrane-like channel protein family and are thought to be involved in zinc homeostasis of the endoplasmic reticulum and transcriptional regulation within the nucleus of keratinocytes. Cells deficient for *EVER1* or *EVER2* are unable to prevent the replication of certain HPV types, mostly beta-HPV. Thus, EV patients develop a selective immunodeficiency for HPV infection. Most commonly, HPV 5 and HPV 8 can be found in EV, but also HPV types 9, 12, 14, 15, 17, 19, 25, 36, 38, 47, and 50 have been reported.

Patients with EV develop skin lesions early in life as infection with HPV typically occurs during infancy. Skin findings comprise 2 different morphologies. First, numerous thin, pink, flat-topped papules and plaques that resemble flat warts (verrucae planae) may be seen. Therefore, these papules are sometimes referred to as *EV-plane warts*. Sites of predilection for these warts are knees, elbows, and trunk. Second, patients can present with widespread scaly, erythematous, or hypopigmented macules and flat papules that appear similar to tinea versicolor (Fig. 110-11). The mucosal membranes are usually not affected. Histopathologically, the EV-plane warts share features with plane warts not associated with EV. Dyskeratosis and pyknosis are observed more commonly in EV. However, the diagnosis is made based on a combination of the clinical image, histopathologic findings, plus viral and genetic testing.

The clinical course of EV is not entirely known and variable. It is estimated that more than 60% of patients affected by EV develop cutaneous malignancies in the wart-like lesions, most often in the fourth to fifth decades of life and usually on sun-exposed or acral areas of the skin. Patients may develop AK, BD, and invasive SCC. Some patients with immunodeficiency, such as organ transplant recipients and HIV-positive patients, can have a late-onset of EV (called *acquired EV*). Thus, older patients suspected of having EV should also be tested for HIV and other conditions with impaired cell-mediated immunity.

No specific or successful treatments exist for EV lesions. Mixed results have been achieved with topical 5% imiquimod cream and retinoids. Patients with EV should undergo a regular and thorough follow up to detect precancerous and invasive lesions as early as possible. UV radiation should be avoided because it increases the risk of malignant transformation. Single EV-plane warts can be treated successfully with excision, curettage, cryosurgery, or ablative lasers.

PRECANCEROUS LESIONS OF THE LOWER ANOGENITAL TRACT

ANAL INTRAEPITHELIAL NEOPLASIA

AT-A-GLANCE

- Synonyms: anal squamous intraepithelial neoplasia or anal dysplasia.
- Anal intraepithelial neoplasia (AIN) is associated with high-grade human papillomavirus (HPV) types, most commonly with types 16, 18, 31, and 33.
- AIN shows biologic and clinical analogy to cervical intraepithelial neoplasia.

(Continued)

AT-A-GLANCE (Continued)

- Major risk factors for AIN are HPV infection, high-risk sexual behavior (anal intercourse), HIV infection with low levels of CD4+ T cells, smoking, immunosuppression, a history of genital warts, and a history of cervical cancer in females.
- AIN is commonly localized within the transitional zone of squamous epithelium of the anus and columnar epithelium of the rectum, which is highly susceptible to HPV infection (dentate line).
- AIN is usually asymptomatic, but may occasionally cause local symptoms like pruritus, pain, bleeding, tenesmus, or rectal discharge.
- The diagnosis of AIN is made by anal cytology, high-resolution anoscopy, and histopathologic examination of biopsy specimens.
- AIN 1 is a low-grade squamous intraepithelial lesion (LSIL) with a low risk of progression to anal cancer.
- AIN 2 and AIN 3 are precursor high-grade squamous intraepithelial lesions (HSILs) of anal squamous cell carcinoma and histopathologically display moderate and severe dysplasia, respectively.
- It is currently under debate whether screening for AIN should be performed in high-risk populations.
- HPV vaccination with a quadruple vaccine against HPV types 6, 11, 16, and 18 may reduce the incidence of AIN.
- Patients with HSIL (AIN 2 or AIN 3) should receive treatment; treatment is optional for LSIL (AIN 1).
- Therapy options include topical treatment with trichloroacetic acid, infrared coagulation, 5-FU, intraanal imiquimod, or electrocauterization.

PERIANAL INTRAEPITHELIAL NEOPLASIA

AT-A-GLANCE

- Synonyms: genital Bowen disease (GBD).
- Perianal intraepithelial neoplasia (PaIN) is less likely than AIN to be associated with human papillomavirus than anal intraepithelial neoplasia.
- Only 5% of patients with PaIN may progress to invasive squamous cell carcinoma.
- PaIN may present with a variety of clinical patterns, including well-demarcated erythematous, or variably pigmented plaques.
- Dermatologists play a role in high-risk patients by examining the perianal skin and clinically diagnosing PaIN.
- Treatment options for PaIN include wide local excision, Mohs micrographic surgery, and various topical agents.

VULVAR INTRAEPITHELIAL NEOPLASIA

AT-A-GLANCE

- The term *vulvar intraepithelial neoplasia* (VIN) should be restricted to high-grade precancerous lesions of the vulva (formerly VIN 2 and VIN 3) that may progress to vulvar squamous cell carcinoma.
- VIN grade 1 (formerly VIN 1) is similar to vulvar condyloma acuminatum with a low oncogenic potential and not considered VIN in the nomenclature of the Vulvar Oncology Subcommittee of the International Society for the Study of Vulvar Diseases (ISSVD).
- VIN is primarily a disease of younger, sexually active females (75% of all cases) with rising incidence and prevalence.
- Three categories of VIN are distinguished: (a) usual type, (b) differentiated (simplex) type, and (c) unclassified type.
  - VIN usual type is associated with high-risk human papillomavirus (HPV) (types 16, 18, 31), occurs in younger premenopausal females, and presents with multifocal and multicentric lesions; in up to 50% of cases associations with cervical intraepithelial neoplasia can be found.
  - VIN differentiated type is less common than usual type and usually not associated with HPV; it affects postmenopausal females with a unifocal presentation and has a significant association with lichen sclerosus.

(Continued)

AT-A-GLANCE (Continued)

- Risk factors for VIN (usual type) are smoking, sexual promiscuity, HPV infection, and immunosuppression.
- The clinical presentation of VIN ranges from reddish patches to gray-white plaques and verrucous wart-like papules.
- The differential diagnosis of VIN includes lichen sclerosus, lichen planus, condyloma acuminatum, and other vulvar neoplasias like SCC and melanoma.
- VIN is asymptomatic in many cases, but may cause vulvodynia, vulvar pain and burning sensation, dysuria, or pruritus.
- The diagnosis of VIN is made by physical examination, biopsy, and optionally colposcopy.
- Treatment modalities include surgical excision and ablative laser therapy for single lesions, while topical treatment with 5-FU or imiquimod is more suited for multicentric VIN.
- A diagnosis of VIN mandates referral to a gynecologist to look for synchronous vaginal and cervical intraepithelial neoplasia.
- Quadrivalent HPV vaccination (HPV types 6, 11, 16, 18) may reduce the risk for VIN usual type in young females.

PENILE INTRAEPITHELIAL NEOPLASIA

AT-A-GLANCE

- Penile intraepithelial neoplasia (PIN) is an umbrella term for precursor lesions of the male genital to penile squamous cell carcinoma (SCC).
- Two clinical variants of PIN are the genital Bowen disease (GBD) and erythroplasia of Queyrat (EQ) (Fig. 110-12).
- PIN and penile SCC mainly affect older, uncircumcised males.
- Risk factors for PIN are poor genital hygiene, smegma retention, phimosis, chronic inflammatory and infectious conditions of the penis, lichen sclerosus, lichen planus, immunosuppression (HIV infection, organ transplant recipients), smoking, and preceding psoralen plus ultraviolet A or ultraviolet exposure.
- Approximately 40% to 45% of PIN cases are associated with HPV, mainly with high-risk types such as types 16, 18, 31, and 33; low-risk types 6 and 11 may be present in low-grade PIN.
- PIN associated with HPV infection are supposedly more aggressive and may develop to warty and basaloid subtypes of penile SCC.
- PIN without HPV infection is morphologically associated with the usual or differentiated type of penile SCC.
- EQ is a common type of PIN usually associated with HPV 8 and HPV 16 infection; it presents as a well-demarcated, glistening, erythematous, velvety plaque or plaques on the mucosal surfaces of the penis (Fig. 110-12A).
- The GBD variant of PIN is less common than the EQ variant; it presents as a well-demarcated, erythematous to variably pigmented plaque on the shaft of the penis (Fig. 110-12B).
- Both variants have histopathologic features of SCC in situ; EQ shows prominent epithelial hypoplasia and plasma cells in the dermal infiltrate.
- The EQ variant of PIN has a higher risk of progression to invasive SCC (~30%) than the GBD variant (3% to 6%).
- Treatment options include local excision, cryosurgery, ablative lasers (CO_2-laser), imiquimod, or topical cidofovir.
- Preventive measures comprise circumcision, proper hygiene, stopping smoking, and avoiding genital UV exposure.
- It is currently under investigation if immunization of young males with HPV vaccines can reduce the risk of PIN; however, HPV-unrelated lesions are not affected by this approach.

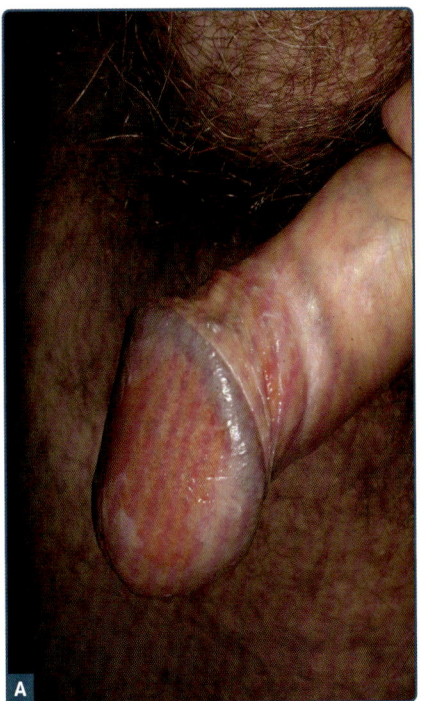
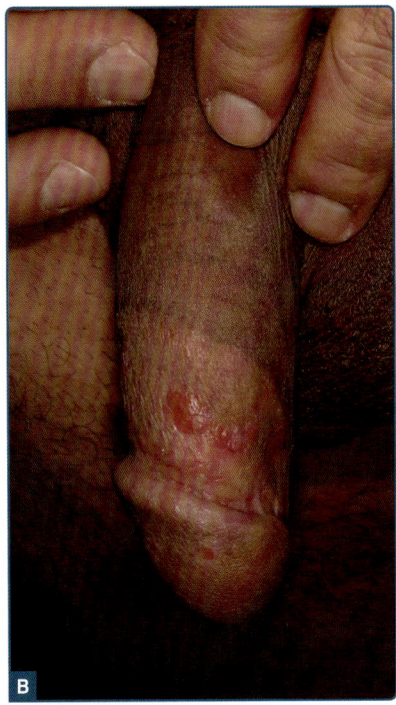
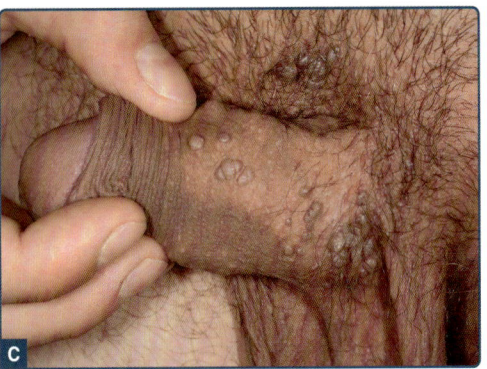

Figure 110-12 Penile intraepithelial neoplasia (PIN) in a male patient. **A,** The erythroplasia of Queyrat (EQ) variant clinically presents with well-demarcated, erythematous plaques on the mucosal surface of the penis. **B,** In contrast, the genital Bowen disease (GBD) variant shows variably pigmented and erythematous papules, mainly located on the shaft of the penis. This condition is at times difficult to distinguish from typical condylomata acuminata (**C**).

POTENTIALLY MALIGNANT DISORDERS OF THE ORAL CAVITY

In a World Health Organization (WHO) workshop held in 2005, the terminology, definitions, and classification of oral lesions with a predisposition to malignant transformation were discussed.[46] The term *potentially malignant* was preferred over *premalignant* or *precancerous*. In addition, it was recommended that the traditional distinction between potentially malignant lesions and potentially malignant conditions be abandoned and that the term *potentially malignant disorders* be used instead. Here, the focus will be on oral leukoplakia and erythroplakia.

LEUKOPLAKIA

Leukoplakia is a clinical term that refers to a predominantly white lesion of the oral mucosa that cannot be rubbed off or characterized by any other definable lesion or known disease. Leukoplakia is the most common potential malignant lesion of the oral mucosa, with the potential to become oral SCC. It is in the same clinical spectrum of disease as oral erythroplakia, but leukoplakia is more common and the likelihood of malignant transformation is lower.

> ### AT-A-GLANCE
>
> - Leukoplakia is a clinical diagnosis of exclusion for a fixed white lesion in the oral cavity that does not resolve spontaneously.
> - Oral leukoplakia is the most common potentially malignant lesion of the oral mucosa, with the potential to become oral squamous cell carcinoma (SCC).
> - The prevalence is 0.2% to 3.4%.
> - Approximately 50% of oral SCCs are associated with potentially malignant lesions.
> - Leukoplakia and erythroplakia are markers for increased risk for additional oral or upper aerodigestive tract malignancies.
> - Risk factors for leukoplakia are the use of any tobacco product, alcohol abuse, history of previous or premalignant lesions, and infection with certain human papillomavirus subtypes.
> - No consensus exists on how best to treat leukoplakia.

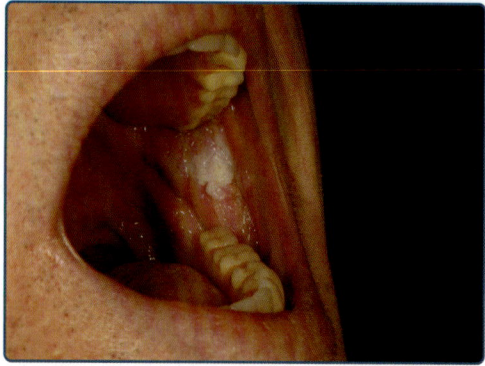

Figure 110-13 Oral leukoplakia of the left cheek in a 65-year-old male with chronic HIV infection and a history of smoking. Note the irregular and verrucous surface (non-homogeneous variant).

EPIDEMIOLOGY

The prevalence of leukoplakia varies significantly by geographical region and demographic group. Estimates for global prevalence vary from 0.5% to 3.4%. Individuals 40 years of age and older are at higher risk. Males are affected more often than females with an estimated male-to-female ratio of 2:1. This may be explained by a higher exposure to certain risk factors. For instance, leukoplakia is 6 times more common among smokers than among nonsmokers.

CLINICAL FINDINGS

Leukoplakia is clinically divided into a homogeneous and nonhomogeneous form. Homogeneous leukoplakia has been defined as a mostly white, flat, uniform lesion. It may have shallow cracks and a smooth, wrinkled, or corrugated surface (Fig. 110-13). Nonhomogeneous leukoplakia is defined as a mostly white or white-reddish lesion ("erythroleukoplakia") that may be irregular and flat, nodular, ulcerative, or verrucous. Nonhomogeneous leukoplakia has a significant higher risk of malignancy than does homogeneous leukoplakia. Proliferative verrucous leukoplakia represents a rare form, which is most often found in patients who do not use tobacco products. It has a high rate of malignant transformation and recurrence after treatment.

ETIOLOGY AND PATHOGENESIS

Etiologic factors for leukoplakia include chronic chemotoxic exposure, mechanical trauma, and HPV infection. Tobacco is probably the strongest risk factor for the development of leukoplakia. It was shown that most patients with leukoplakia consumed tobacco, either as smoke or by chewing. In addition, tobacco-related white lesions of the oral mucosa may disappear once the tobacco use has been discontinued. The combination of tobacco use and alcohol consumption has a strong synergistic effect in the development of leukoplakia. However, alcohol consumption was also identified as an independent risk factor, regardless of beverage type or drinking pattern. Typical causes for chronic mechanical trauma of the oral mucosa are ill-fitting prosthesis, chronic cheek biting, and reduced dental status with poor oral hygiene.

HPV represents another etiologic factor for leukoplakia. It was detected in up to 22% of leukoplakia lesions and its prevalence compared to normal mucosa is significantly higher. High-risk oncogenic subtypes, such as HPV types 16 and 18, were isolated more frequently than low-risk HPV (type 6 or type 11). For this reason, HPV is widely believed to be an independent risk factor in the development of leukoplakia, or at least an intensifier of other carcinogenic effects. However, the specific role of HPV in carcinogenesis remains controversial, as no correlation between mucosal dysplasia and HPV infection was found. Persons with a previous malignancy or premalignancy of the upper aerodigestive tract are at greater risk for the development of leukoplakia.

DIAGNOSIS AND DIFFERENTIAL DIAGNOSIS

Leukoplakia is a clinical diagnosis. Whitish lesions in the oral mucosa that cannot be rubbed off are suspicious for leukoplakia. If causative agents, such as tobacco or mechanical irritation, are detected, it is recommended to eliminate these factors for a period of 2 to 6 weeks. If regression does not occur during this observational period, biopsy and histologic examination should be performed. If upon initial examination

TABLE 110-8
Clinical Differential Diagnosis of Oral Leukoplakia

- Tobacco-associated lesion
- *Candida*-associated lesion
- Leukoedema
- Lichen planus
- Lupus erythematosus
- Linea alba
- Habitual cheek biting
- Frictional lesion
- Aspirin burn
- Oral white sponge nevus
- Oral hairy leukoplakia
- Verrucous carcinoma
- Squamous cell carcinoma

TABLE 110-9
Risk Factors for the Conversion of Oral Leukoplakia into Oral Squamous Cell Carcinoma

Main risk factors
- Presence of epithelial dysplasia
- Nonhomogeneous clinical subtype
- Large size
- Location on the tongue or the floor of the mouth

Other risk factors
- Female gender
- Long duration of oral leukoplakia
- Leukoplakia in nonsmokers

Adapted and modified from van der Waal.[47,52]

no causative agent can be identified, biopsy should be performed directly. This is particularly important for symptomatic leukoplakia. In this case, malignant transformation into invasive SCC should be ruled out.[46] Further important differential diagnoses include Epstein-Barr virus–induced hairy leukoplakia in HIV patients, lichen planus, and lupus erythematosus, among others (Table 110-8).

HISTOPATHOLOGY

On a histologic level, characteristic findings are hyperkeratosis, epithelial hyperplasia, and dysplasia. The latter includes atypical mitosis, polymorphic cells, as well as hyperchromatic and polymorphic nuclei. Epithelial hyperplasia and hyperkeratosis give the lesion the characteristic whitish appearance. The degree of dysplasia varies from lesions showing only hyperkeratosis with no dysplasia toward lesions with moderate dysplasia and those with severe dysplasia resembling SCC in situ. There are different growing patterns, which include clinically flat, papillary endophytic and papillary exophytic, verrucous proliferation. Transformation into invasive SCC occurs as dysplastic cells break through the basement membrane.

CLINICAL COURSE AND PROGNOSIS

Once a definitive diagnosis of leukoplakia has been made, the risk of malignant transformation should be evaluated. The rate of all clinical subtypes of leukoplakia is estimated to be approximately 2% to 3% per year.[46,47] Table 110-9 lists the numerous identified risk factors for malignant transformation. Of these factors, epithelial dysplasia and nonhomogeneous clinical subtype are the most important indicators for malignant transformation. However, it should be recognized that not all dysplastic lesions progress to malignancy. Some remain clinically unchanged and others may regress spontaneously or after elimination of the causative agent, such as cessation of smoking. In addition, malignant transformation may also occur in nondysplastic leukoplakia.

TREATMENT AND PREVENTION

There is a chance of spontaneous remission of leukoplakia. However, the risk of malignant transformation warrants treatment if remission does not occur within a short period of observation. In general, any possible causative agent or risk factor such as consumption of tobacco products, alcohol, bethel nuts, or chronic mechanical trauma should be omitted. There are numerous therapeutic approaches for leukoplakia, but evidence remains strongly limited and recurrence rates for all interventions are high. Usually, surgical excision is the first treatment of choice. In contrast to other therapies, surgery allows histologic workup and unexpected carcinomas may be identified.[48] However, adequate surgical excision may be limited as field cancerization may be present and normal-appearing surrounding mucosa may harbor clones of cancer stigmatized cells. In the case of recurrence after surgical excision, cryotherapy or CO_2-laser represent useful treatment options. Other therapies include PDT, herbal extracts, beta-carotene supplements, antiinflammatory drugs, and vitamin A, among others.[49-51] Independent of the treatment, the patient should be followed closely.

ERYTHROPLAKIA

Erythroplakia (or erythroplasia) is a clinical term used to describe a red macule or patch on a mucosal surface that cannot be categorized as any other known disease entity caused by inflammatory, vascular, or traumatic factors. It is commonly seen in association with leukoplakia, a condition termed *erythroleukoplakia*.

AT-A-GLANCE

- Erythroplakia is a clinical diagnosis of exclusion for a persistent fixed red patch in the oral cavity.
- It is the least common of all oral potentially malignant lesions but has the greatest potential to harbor or become oral squamous cell carcinoma.
- Risk factors are use of tobacco products and alcohol consumption.
- Early and effective treatment is important.

TABLE 110-10
Clinical Differential Diagnosis of Oral Erythroplakia

- Erythematous candidiasis
- Atrophic lichen planus
- Lupus erythematosus
- Pemphigus
- Cicatricial pemphigoid
- Kaposi sarcoma
- Chronic contact or allergic contact dermatitis
- Chronic mechanical trauma
- Thermal or mechanical injury
- Squamous cell carcinoma
- Amelanotic melanoma

EPIDEMIOLOGY

Erythroplakia is rare and the least-frequent potentially malignant lesion in the oral cavity. The prevalence depends on the geographical area and varies between 0.02% and 0.83%. Erythroplakia mainly occurs in middle-aged individuals. Males are affected more often than females, which may be explained by a higher exposure to certain risk factors, such as tobacco consumption. Erythroplakia has been well described in the chutta smokers (reverse cigar smokers) of India.

CLINICAL FINDINGS

Erythroplakia usually presents as an asymptomatic, solitary, subtle, erythematous macule or patch. It is sharply demarcated from the surrounding pink mucosa, and its surface is most often smooth and homogeneous in color. However, some lesions may have a pebbled or stippled surface and feel soft and velvety on palpation. Induration is highly suspicious for transformation into invasive SCC. The most common areas in the oral cavity are the soft palate, the floor of the mouth, and the buccal mucosa. Most often it is less than 1.5 cm in its widest diameter, but lesions up to 4 cm in diameter have been described.

ETIOLOGY AND PATHOGENESIS

The underlying etiology of erythroplakia is unknown. Risk factors are equal to those of other potentially malignant lesions in the oral cavity: consumption of tobacco products, alcohol and chewing nuts that contain carcinogenic substances, such as areca nuts. Genetic analyses have shown a high mutation rate of the tumor-suppressor gene *p53* in erythroplakia lesions, reflecting their high potential to malignant transformation.

DIAGNOSIS

Erythroplakia is a diagnosis of exclusion. Table 110-10 outlines differential diagnoses. On a histologic level, erythroplakia typically displays moderate to severe dysplasia. Frequently, SCC in situ and focal areas of invasive SCC are present.

CLINICAL COURSE AND PROGNOSIS

Of all potentially malignant lesions in the oral cavity, erythroplakia is considered to be the most dangerous and carries the greatest risk of progressing to or harboring invasive carcinoma. In erythroleukoplakia, the red patches are most prone for malignant transformation. After excision, lesions that exceed 80 mm^2 have a significant higher risk of recurrence.

TREATMENT

The high potential for malignant transformation warrants early treatment. Surgery or excision with CO_2-laser is the treatment of choice. Any risk factors, such as consumption of tobacco or alcohol, should be avoided.

ARSENICAL KERATOSES

AT-A-GLANCE

- Arsenical keratoses (ArKs) result from chronic exposure to arsenic.
- ArKs have the potential to become squamous cell carcinoma (SCC), although reliable estimates of progression rates are unknown.
- Clinical appearance comprises punctuate, keratotic, yellow papules overlying pressure points on palms and soles.
- Further arsenic-related skin diseases are superficial basal cell carcinoma, SCC, Bowen disease, and diffuse hyperpigmentation.
- No standard recommendations for treatment exist and most lesions are followed clinically or treated symptomatically.

Arsenical keratoses (ArKs) result from chronic intake or intoxication with arsenic. Arsenic is a ubiquitous element that has no color, taste, or odor. It has the

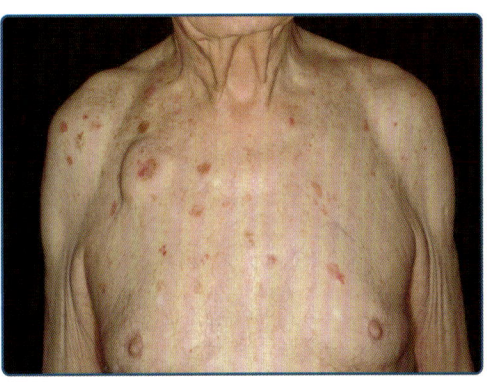

Figure 110-14 Disseminated arsenic keratoses in a male patient who had been exposed to arsenic therapeutically for many years in the past to treat his psoriasis. The lesions were found on the entire skin including trunk, arms, and legs. Keratoses of the chest are shown.

potential to cause characteristic acute and chronic symptoms in persons exposed to it. Arsenic exposures are typically obscure and medicinal, occupational, and environmental sources still exist. ArKs are considered precancerous lesions because they have the potential to progress into invasive SCC.

ArKs are localized most commonly on the palms and soles. Clinically, they appear as gray-to-yellow keratotic papules. If lesions are large, they may acquire a verruciform look (Fig. 110-14). Further signs of a chronic exposure to arsenic are diffuse hyperpigmentation and the presence of superficial basal cell carcinoma or BD. Histopathologically, ArKs resemble hypertrophic AKs with a more cellular atypia and prominent vacuolization of keratinocytes. The diagnosis may be difficult. Taking a thorough history is an important clue and the first step toward the correct diagnosis. ArKs may be confused with vulgar warts, hypertrophic lichen planus, keratosis palmaris, and plantaris dissipata or diffusa, or AKs in sun-exposed areas. Although ArKs and arsenic-induced skin disorders tend to persist for many years, progression to invasive SCC is believed to be a relatively rare event. However, reliable estimates for progression rates are lacking as a consequence of the rarity of the disease. Some evidence exists that invasive SCCs that arise from ArKs are more locally aggressive and have a greater chance of metastasis than SCCs arising from AKs.

If ArKs are suspected, a thorough skin examination and physical examination are obligatory. The sources of exposure to arsenic should be identified and discontinued. The exact incidence of internal malignancies associated with chronic arsenism is unknown, so there is no standard protocol for the evaluation of potential internal malignancies. Exhaustive evaluations to detect such malignancies have not been recommended. Biannual detailed history taking and physical examination, yearly chest radiography, and selective testing when clinically indicated are probably reasonable recommendations.

Single lesions can be treated with surgical excision, cryosurgery, or curettage. Ablative resurfacing with the CO_2-laser and Er:YAG-laser were successfully applied in some cases. If diffuse hyperkeratosis or disseminated ArK lesions are present, topical and systemic retinoids are a valuable option, although lesion clearance is generally lower compared to treatment of AKs. Patients with verified ArKs should be followed-up and monitored regularly, possibly every 6 to 12 months.

THERMAL KERATOSES

AT-A-GLANCE

- Precancerous lesions that result from long-term exposure to infrared radiation; can progress to squamous cell carcinoma (SCC).
- Sources of infrared radiation include open fires, railway engines, wood-burning stoves, heating pads and blankets, and laptop computers.
- Precursor lesion is erythema ab igne; biopsy should be performed on any hyperkeratotic papule or plaque within such a patch.
- Risk of progression of thermal keratosis to SCC is unknown.

HYDROCARBON KERATOSES

AT-A-GLANCE

- Synonyms: pitch keratoses, tar keratoses, tar warts.
- Precancerous lesions resulting from prolonged exposure to tar.
- Tar contains highly cancerogenic polycyclic aromatic hydrocarbons such as benzpyrene, dibenzanthracene, or methylcholanthrene.
- May be present in patients with occupational exposure to tar; occupations at risk include tar distiller, shale extractor, roofer, asphalt worker, road paver, highway maintenance worker, brick mason, diesel engineer, and chimney sweep.
- Ultraviolet exposure is a cofactor in the establishment of tar keratosis.
- Hydrocarbon keratosis can progress to squamous cell carcinoma (SCC), but the rate of progression and risk are unknown.
- Latency periods between exposure and development of hydrocarbon keratosis or SCC range from 2.5 years to 45 years.
- Lesions typically present as hyperkeratotic papules with a verruciform surface; sites of predilection are face, neck, forearms, and scrotal skin.

(Continued)

AT-A-GLANCE (Continued)

- Other skin findings include patchy hyperpigmentation, acne, and telangiectasias.
- Therapeutic options include excision, curettage, and ablative lasers (CO_2, Er:YAG).

CHRONIC RADIATION KERATOSES

AT-A-GLANCE

- Chronic radiation keratoses are precancerous lesions that may arise at irradiated sites years after such exposure and may progress to squamous cell carcinoma.
- Ionizing radiation sources include X-rays, grenz rays, and contaminated gold rings.
- Common sites are the palms, soles, and mucosal surfaces.
- They most commonly present as hyperkeratotic papules or plaques within areas of chronic radiation dermatitis and occasionally on clinically normal skin.
- Latency for the development of lesions can be up to 50 years after exposure.
- Patients with ionizing radiation exposure and chronic radiation keratoses are also at risk for internal malignancies.

CHRONIC SCAR KERATOSES

AT-A-GLANCE

- Synonym: cicatrix keratoses.
- Chronic scar keratoses are precancerous lesions that arise in longstanding scars from various causes.
- Common conditions comprise burn scars, chronic wounds, sinuses, and leg ulcers.
- Approximately 2% of burn scars will undergo malignant changes.
- Marjolin ulcer is an umbrella term covering malignant changes within a scar from any cause.
- Acute Marjolin ulcer develops within 1 year of the time of injury; chronic Marjolin ulcer develops more than 1 year after an injury.

- Most invasive carcinomas are squamous cell carcinomas (SCCs), but basal cell carcinomas, melanomas, sarcomas, and malignant fibrous histiocytomas also have been described.
- SCCs deriving from scar keratoses show an aggressive growth pattern with a high propensity to metastasize.
- Sites of predilection are the extremities and overlying joints.
- Any persistent lesion, erosion, or ulceration within a scar requires biopsy.
- Prevention includes wound care, early skin grafting, avoidance of contractures, and early excision of any tissue showing degenerative changes.

ACKNOWLEDGMENTS

We thank Saskia A. Graf for her support with Fig. 110-1 and Karynne O. Duncan, John K. Geisse, and David J. Leffell who are the authors of the previous version of this chapter.

REFERENCES

1. Cockerell CJ. Histopathology of incipient intraepidermal squamous cell carcinoma ("actinic keratosis"). *J Am Acad Dermatol*. 2000;42(1, pt 2):11-17.
2. Eder J, Prillinger K, Korn A, et al. Prevalence of actinic keratosis among dermatology outpatients in Austria. *Br J Dermatol*. 2014;171(6):1415-1421.
3. Flohil SC, van der Leest RJ, Dowlatshahi EA, et al. Prevalence of actinic keratosis and its risk factors in the general population: the Rotterdam Study. *J Invest Dermatol*. 2013;133(8):1971-1978.
4. Trakatelli M, Barkitzi K, Apap C, et al. Skin cancer risk in outdoor workers: a European multicenter case-control study. *J Eur Acad Dermatol Venereol*. 2016;30(suppl 3):5-11.
5. Traianou A, Ulrich M, Apalla Z, et al. Risk factors for actinic keratosis in eight European centres: a case-control study. *Br J Dermatol*. 2012;167(suppl 2):36-42.
6. Memon AA, Tomenson JA, Bothwell J, et al. Prevalence of solar damage and actinic keratosis in a Merseyside population. *Br J Dermatol*. 2000;142(6):1154-1159.
7. Iannacone MR, Sinnya S, Pandeya N, et al. Prevalence of skin cancer and related skin tumors in high-risk kidney and liver transplant recipients in Queensland, Australia. *J Invest Dermatol*. 2016;136(7):1382-1386.
8. Werner RN, Stockfleth E, Connolly SM, et al. Evidence- and consensus-based (S3) guidelines for the treatment of actinic keratosis—International League of Dermatological Societies in cooperation with the European Dermatology Forum—short version. *J Eur Acad Dermatol Venereol*. 2015;29(11):2069-2079.

9. Olsen EA, Abernethy ML, Kulp-Shorten C, et al. A double-blind, vehicle-controlled study evaluating masoprocol cream in the treatment of actinic keratoses on the head and neck. *J Am Acad Dermatol*. 1991;24(5, pt 1):738-743.
10. Rowert-Huber J, Patel MJ, Forschner T, et al. Actinic keratosis is an early in situ squamous cell carcinoma: a proposal for reclassification. *Br J Dermatol*. 2007;156(suppl 3):8-12.
11. Schmitz L, Kahl P, Majores M, et al. Actinic keratosis: correlation between clinical and histological classification systems. *J Eur Acad Dermatol Venereol*. 2016;30(8):1303-1307.
12. Hu B, Castillo E, Harewood L, et al. Multifocal epithelial tumors and field cancerization from loss of mesenchymal CSL signaling. *Cell*. 2012;149(6):1207-1220.
13. Lallas A, Tschandl P, Kyrgidis A, et al. Dermoscopic clues to differentiate facial lentigo maligna from pigmented actinic keratosis. *Br J Dermatol*. 2016;174(5):1079-1085.
14. Christensen SR, McNiff JM, Cool AJ, et al. Histopathologic assessment of depth of follicular invasion of squamous cell carcinoma (SCC) in situ (SCCis): implications for treatment approach. *J Am Acad Dermatol*. 2016;74(2):356-362.
15. Niiyama S, Oharaseki T, Mukai H: Giant hidroacanthoma simplex mimicking Bowen's disease. *Case Rep Dermatol*. 2015;7(3):241-244.
16. Westers-Attema A, van den Heijkant F, Lohman BG, et al. Bowen's disease: a six-year retrospective study of treatment with emphasis on resection margins. *Acta Derm Venereol*. 2014;94(4):431-435.
17. Bath-Hextall FJ, Matin RN, Wilkinson D, et al. Interventions for cutaneous Bowen's disease. *Cochrane Database Syst Rev*. 2013;(6):CD007281.
18. Lee JH, Lee JH, Bae JM, et al. Successful treatment of Bowen's disease with ingenol mebutate 0.05% gel. *J Dermatol*. 2015;42(9):920-921.
19. Cai H, Wang YX, Zheng JC, et al. Photodynamic therapy in combination with CO_2 laser for the treatment of Bowen's disease. *Lasers Med Sci*. 2015;30(5):1505-1510.
20. Pflugfelder A, Welter AK, Leiter U, et al. Open label randomized study comparing 3 months vs. 6 months treatment of actinic keratoses with 3% diclofenac in 2.5% hyaluronic acid gel: a trial of the German Dermatologic Cooperative Oncology Group. *J Eur Acad Dermatol Venereol*. 2012;26(1):48-53.
21. Malvehy J, Roldan-Marin R, Iglesias-Garcia P, et al. Monitoring treatment of field cancerisation with 3% diclofenac sodium 2.5% hyaluronic acid by reflectance confocal microscopy: a histologic correlation. *Acta Derm Venereol*. 2015;95(1):45-50.
22. Shergill B, Zokaie S, Carr AJ. Non-adherence to topical treatments for actinic keratosis. *Patient Prefer Adherence*. 2013;8:35-41.
23. Pomerantz H, Hogan D, Eilers D, et al. Long-term efficacy of topical fluorouracil cream, 5%, for treating actinic keratosis: a randomized clinical trial. *JAMA Dermatol*. 2015;151(9):952-960.
24. Stockfleth E, Kerl H, Zwingers T, et al. Low-dose 5-fluorouracil in combination with salicylic acid as a new lesion-directed option to treat topically actinic keratoses: histological and clinical study results. *Br J Dermatol*. 2011;165(5):1101-1108.
25. Herranz P, Morton C, Dirschka T, et al. Low-dose 0.5% 5-fluorouracil/10% salicylic acid topical solution in the treatment of actinic keratoses. *J Cutan Med Surg*. 2016;20(6):555-561.
26. Swanson N, Abramovits W, Berman B, et al. Imiquimod 2.5% and 3.75% for the treatment of actinic keratoses: results of two placebo-controlled studies of daily application to the face and balding scalp for two 2-week cycles. *J Am Acad Dermatol*. 2010;62(4):582-590.
27. Gebauer K, Shumack S, Cowen PS. Effect of dosing frequency on the safety and efficacy of imiquimod 5% cream for treatment of actinic keratosis on the forearms and hands: a phase II, randomized placebo-controlled trial. *Br J Dermatol*. 2009;161(4):897-903.
28. Lebwohl M, Swanson N, Anderson LL, et al. Ingenol mebutate gel for actinic keratosis. *N Engl J Med*. 2012;366(11):1010-1019.
29. Garbe C, Basset-Seguin N, Poulin Y, et al. Efficacy and safety of follow-up field treatment of actinic keratosis with ingenol mebutate 0.015% gel: a randomized, controlled 12-month study. *Br J Dermatol*. 2016;174(3):505-513.
30. Samorano LP, Torezan LA, Sanches JA. Evaluation of the tolerability and safety of a 0.015% ingenol mebutate gel compared to 5% 5-fluorouracil cream for the treatment of facial actinic keratosis: a prospective randomized trial. *J Eur Acad Dermatol Venereol*. 2015;29(9):1822-1827.
31. Augustin M, Tu JH, Knudsen KM, et al. Ingenol mebutate gel for actinic keratosis: the link between quality of life, treatment satisfaction, and clinical outcomes. *J Am Acad Dermatol*. 2015;72(5):816-821.
32. Peris K, Calzavara-Pinton PG, Neri L, et al. Italian expert consensus for the management of actinic keratosis in immunocompetent patients. *J Eur Acad Dermatol Venereol*. 2016;30(7):1077-1084.
33. Ianhez M, Fleury LF Jr, Miot HA, Bagatin E. Retinoids for prevention and treatment of actinic keratosis. *An Bras Dermatol*. 2013;88(4):585-593.
34. Chen AC, Martin AJ, Choy B, et al. A phase 3 randomized trial of nicotinamide for skin-cancer chemoprevention. *N Engl J Med*. 2015;373(17):1618-1626.
35. Drake AL, Walling HW. Variations in presentation of squamous cell carcinoma in situ (Bowen's disease) in immunocompromised patients. *J Am Acad Dermatol*. 2008;59(1):68-71.
36. Murao K, Yoshioka R, Kubo Y. Human papillomavirus infection in Bowen disease: negative p53 expression, not p16(INK4a) overexpression, is correlated with human papillomavirus-associated Bowen disease. *J Dermatol*. 2014;41(10):878-884.
37. Svajdler M Jr, Mezencev R, Kaspirkova J, et al. Human papillomavirus infection and p16 expression in extragenital/extraungual Bowen disease in immunocompromised patients. *Am J Dermatopathol*. 2016;38(10):751-757.
38. Shu B, Shen XX, Chen P, et al. Primary invasive extramammary Paget disease on penoscrotum: a clinicopathological analysis of 41 cases. *Hum Pathol*. 2016;47(1):70-77.
39. Lopes Filho LL, Lopes IM, Lopes LR, et al. Mammary and extramammary Paget's disease. *An Bras Dermatol*. 2015;90(2):225-231.
40. Takayama R, Ishiwata T, Ansai S, et al. Lumican as a novel marker for differential diagnosis of Bowen disease and actinic keratosis. *Am J Dermatopathol*. 2013;35(8):827-832.
41. MacFarlane DF, El Tal AK. Cryoimmunotherapy: superficial basal cell cancer and squamous cell carcinoma in situ treated with liquid nitrogen followed by imiquimod. *Arch Dermatol*. 2011;147(11):1326-1327.

42. Sotiriou E, Lallas A, Apalla Z, et al. Treatment of giant Bowen's disease with sequential use of photodynamic therapy and imiquimod cream. *Photodermatol Photoimmunol Photomed*. 2011;27(3):164-166.
43. Burger B, Itin PH. Epidermodysplasia verruciformis. *Curr Probl Dermatol*. 2014;45:123-131.
44. Ramoz N, Rueda LA, Bouadjar B, et al. Mutations in two adjacent novel genes are associated with epidermodysplasia verruciformis. *Nat Genet*. 2002;32(4):579-581.
45. Ramoz N, Taieb A, Rueda LA, et al. Evidence for a nonallelic heterogeneity of epidermodysplasia verruciformis with two susceptibility loci mapped to chromosome regions 2p21-p24 and 17q25. *J Invest Dermatol*. 2000;114(6):1148-1153.
46. van der Waal I. Oral leukoplakia, the ongoing discussion on definition and terminology. *Med Oral Patol Oral Cir Bucal*. 2015;20(6):e685-e692.
47. van der Waal I. Oral potentially malignant disorders: is malignant transformation predictable and preventable? *Med Oral Patol Oral Cir Bucal*. 2014;19(4):e386-e390.
48. Holmstrup P, Dabelsteen E. Oral leukoplakia-to treat or not to treat. *Oral Dis*. 2016;22(6):494-497.
49. Kumar A, Cascarini L, McCaul JA, et al. How should we manage oral leukoplakia? *Br J Oral Maxillofac Surg*. 2013;51(5):377-383.
50. Vohra F, Al-Kheraif AA, Qadri T, et al. Efficacy of photodynamic therapy in the management of oral premalignant lesions. A systematic review. *Photodiagnosis Photodyn Ther*. 2015;12(1):150-159.
51. Lodi G, Franchini R, Warnakulasuriya S, et al. Interventions for treating oral leukoplakia to prevent oral cancer. *Cochrane Database Syst Rev*. 2016;7:CD001829.
52. van der Waal I. Potentially malignant disorders of the oral and oropharyngeal mucosa; terminology, classification and present concepts of management. *Oral Oncol*. 2009;45(4-5):317-323.

Chapter 111 :: Basal Cell Carcinoma and Basal Cell Nevus Syndrome
:: Jean Y. Tang, Ervin H. Epstein, Jr., & Anthony E. Oro

第一百一十一章
基底细胞癌和基底细胞痣综合征

中文导读

本章介绍了两种基底细胞的疾病，分为2节：①基底细胞癌；②基底细胞痣综合征。

第一节基底细胞癌，介绍了其流行病学、病因及发病机制、临床和组织学表现、诊断及亚型、治疗及特殊问题的管理、病程及预后，其中特别提到的特殊问题包括了神经周围侵犯、局部晚期基底细胞癌、转移性基底细胞癌和刺猬信号通路拮抗剂。

第二节基底细胞痣综合征，介绍了其流行病学、病因及发病机制、临床和组织学表现、诊断及鉴别诊断、并发症、预后和临床病程、治疗。

〔粟 娟〕

BASAL CELL CARCINOMA

AT-A-GLANCE

- Basal cell carcinomas (BCCs) are the most common cancers in humans. All BCCs have mutations activating the Hedgehog signaling pathway.
- BCCs are caused by exposure to ultraviolet light and are associated with *PTCH1* gene mutation in most cases.
- BCCs are locally destructive and rarely metastatic.
- BCCs are primarily treated by surgical excision, electrodesiccation and curettage, Mohs micrographic surgery, and topical agents.

EPIDEMIOLOGY

Basal cell carcinoma (BCC) is the most common cancer in humans. It is estimated that more than 3 million new cases occur each year in the United States.[1] The malignancy accounts for approximately 75% of all nonmelanoma skin cancers (NMSCs) and almost 25% of all cancers diagnosed in the United States.[2] Epidemiological data indicate that the overall incidence is increasing worldwide significantly by 3% to 10% per year.[3]

BCC is more common in older individuals but is becoming increasingly frequent in people younger than 50 years of age. Christenson and coworkers noted a disproportionate increase in BCC in women younger than age 40 years.[3] Men are affected slightly more often than are women. Tumors were more frequent in patients older than 60 years of age, and 57% were in men. The vast majority of BCCs were located on the head and neck.[2]

BCC tumors most typically develop on sun-exposed skin of lighter skinned individuals. Incidence rates of BCC in Asians living in Singapore increased from 1968 to 2006, especially among the older, fair-skinned Chinese patients.[4] BCC is rare in dark skin because of the inherent photoprotection of melanin and melanosomal dispersion. An estimated 1.8% of BCCs occur in blacks, and BCC is approximately 19 times more common in whites than blacks.[5]

Risk factors for BCC have been well characterized and include ultraviolet radiation (UVR) exposure, light hair and eye color, northern European ancestry, and inability to tan.[2]

ETIOLOGY AND PATHOGENESIS

The pathogenesis of BCC involves exposure to UVR, particularly the ultraviolet (UV) B spectrum (290–320 nm) that induces mutations in tumor suppressor genes.[6] UVB radiation damages DNA, leading to genetic alterations and neoplasms. UV-induced mutations in the *p53* tumor suppressor gene have been found in about 50% of BCC cases.[7,8]

Malignant activation of the sonic hedgehog (SHH) signaling pathway, a developmental signaling pathway, is the pivotal abnormality in all BCCs.[7] Common mutations that activate the aberrant HH signaling pathway are loss of PTCH1 or Suppressor of Fused (SUFU) and activation of Smoothened (SMO) (Fig. 111-1, discussed more in the basal cell nevus syndrome [BCNS] section of this chapter). Approximately 90% of sporadic BCCs have identifiable mutations in at least one allele of *PTCH1*, and an additional 10% have activating mutations in the downstream SMO protein.[9] The most frequently identified mutations in PTCH1 and SMO are of a type consistent with UV-induced damage.[10,11]

Based on genetic profiling of 293 BCCs, the majority of BCCs were found to have mutations in HH pathway genes: *PTCH1* (73%), *SMO* (20%), and *SUFU* (8%) (Table 111-1). Sporadic BCCs also commonly harbor mutations in TP53 (61%) (see Table 111-1).[12]

The contribution of high-intensity sunlight exposure to BCC development in the general population is well established.[13] A latency period of 20 to 50 years is typical between the time of UV damage and the clinical onset of BCC. Therefore, in most cases, BCC develops on sun-exposed skin in older adults, most commonly on the head and neck.[13] Other factors that appear to be involved in the pathogenesis include mutations

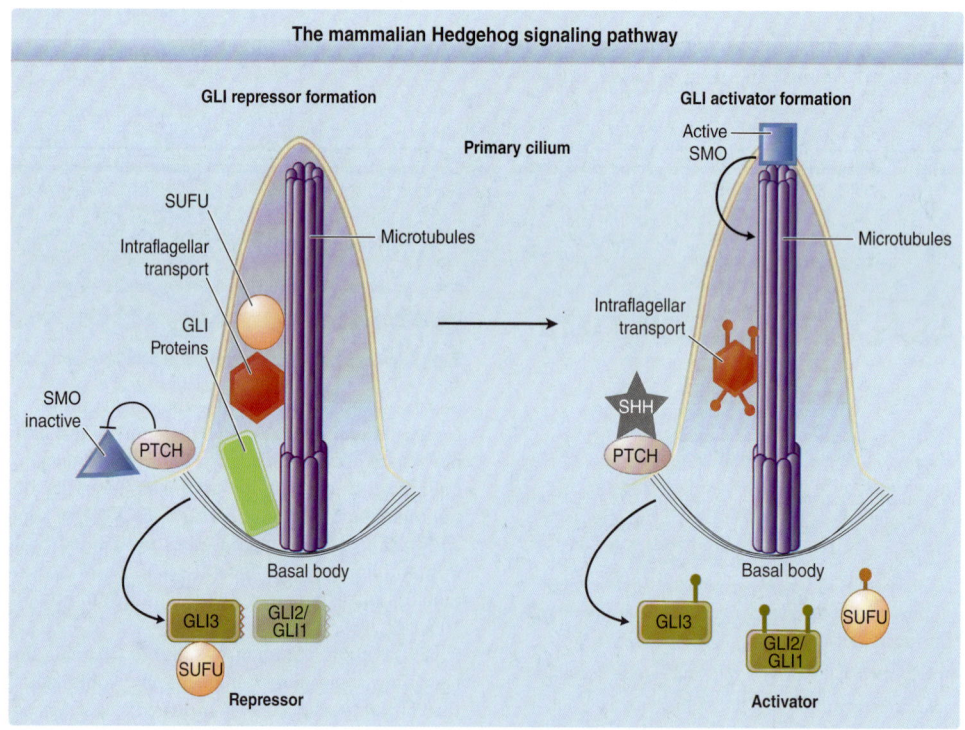

Figure 111-1 The mammalian Hedgehog signaling pathway. PTCH1 is the receptor for the growth factor Hedgehog and inhibits the function of Smoothened (SMO) by sequestering it in an inactive state outside of the microtubule-based organelle, the primary cilium. Sonic Hedgehog (SHH) inhibits PTCH1, allowing activation of SMO in the cilium. SMO inhibits Suppressor of Fused (SUFU), which in turn inhibits the GLI transcription factors GLI1, GLI2, GLI3. Intraflagellar transport proteins help mediate GLI processing.

TABLE 111-1
Most Common Genes Mutated in Sporadic Basal Cell Carcinoma

GENE	PREVALENCE (%)
PTCH1 (tumor suppressor gene, part of the Hedgehog signaling pathway)	73
SMO (oncogene, part of the Hedgehog signaling pathway)	20
SUFU (tumor suppressor gene, part of the Hedgehog signaling pathway)	8
TP53 (also known as p53)	61

in regulatory genes. exposure to ionizing radiation,[14] and alterations in immunosurveillance.[15,16] A recent genome-wide association study (GWAS) identified 14 new single nucleotide polymorphisms and new candidate genes and noncoding RNAs involved in telomere maintenance, immune regulation, and tumour progression, providing deeper insight into the pathogenesis of BCC.[17]

CLINICAL AND HISTOLOGIC MANIFESTATIONS

The presence of any nonhealing lesion should raise the suspicion of skin cancer. BCC usually develops on sun-exposed areas of the head and neck but can occur anywhere on the body. Commonly seen features include translucency, ulceration, telangiectasias, and the presence of a rolled border. Characteristics may vary for different clinical subtypes, which include nodular, superficial, morpheaform, and pigmented BCCs and fibroepithelioma of Pinkus (FEP).[18] The anatomic location of BCC may favor the development of a particular subtype.

The histopathologic features vary somewhat with subtype, but most BCCs share some common histologic characteristics. The malignant basal cells have large nuclei and relatively little cytoplasm. Although the nuclei are large, they may not appear atypical. Usually, mitotic figures are absent. Frequently, slit-like retraction of stroma from tumor islands is present, creating peritumoral lacunae that are helpful in histopathologic diagnosis.[19] The most common form of BCC is nodular followed by superficial and then morpheaform. Also, nodular and morpheaform are most commonly found on the head and neck, and superficial is most often found on the trunk region.[19]

DIAGNOSIS

Diagnosis of BCC is accomplished by accurate interpretation of the skin biopsy results (Table 111-2). The preferred biopsy methods are shave biopsy, which is often sufficient, and punch biopsy. A punch biopsy may be useful for flat lesions of morpheaform BCC or for recurrent BCC occurring in a scar. When biopsying a lesion, adequate tissue should be taken. Small, fragmented tissue samples may make diagnosis difficult, potentially compromising the ability to accurately assess BCC subtype and thickness, which can affect treatment choice.

BASAL CELL CARCINOMA SUBTYPES

NODULAR BASAL CELL CARCINOMA

Nodular BCC is the most common clinical subtype of BCC (Fig. 111-2).[20,21] It occurs most often on the sun-exposed areas of the head and neck and appears as a translucent papule or nodule. There are usually telangiectasias and often a rolled border. Larger lesions with central necrosis are referred to by the historical term *rodent ulcer* (Fig. 111-3). The differential diagnosis of nodular BCC includes traumatized intradermal nevus, irritated seborrheic keratosis, and amelanotic melanoma. Nodular BCCs are characterized by nodules of large basophilic cells and stromal retraction. The term *micronodular BCC* is used to describe tumors with multiple microscopic nodules smaller than 15 μm.

PIGMENTED BASAL CELL CARCINOMA

Pigmented BCC is a subtype of nodular BCC that exhibits increased melanization. Pigmented BCC appears as a hyperpigmented, translucent papule. The differential diagnosis includes nodular melanoma and seborrheic keratosis. Approximately 75% of BCCs contain melanocytes, but only 25% contain large amounts of melanin. The melanocytes are interspersed between tumor cells and contain numerous melanin granules in their cytoplasm and dendrites. Although the tumor cells contain little melanin, numerous melanophages populate the stroma surrounding the tumor.[19]

SUPERFICIAL BASAL CELL CARCINOMA

Superficial BCC occurs most commonly on the trunk and appears as an often well-demarcated erythematous patch (Fig. 111-4).[20,21] The differential diagnosis includes SCC, lichenoid keratosis, and nummular dermatitis. An isolated patch of "eczema" that does not respond to treatment should raise suspicion for superficial BCC. Superficial BCC is characterized microscopically by buds of malignant cells extending into the dermis from the basal layer of the epidermis. The peripheral layer shows palisading cells. There may

TABLE 111-2
Common Basal Cell Carcinoma Subtypes with Corresponding Kodachrome

TYPE OF BASAL CELL CARCINOMA (BCC)	CLINICAL DESCRIPTION	CLINICAL PHOTOGRAPHS	HISTOLOGIC DESCRIPTION	HISTOLOGY
Nodular BCC	Translucent papule or nodule, with telangiectasis and rolled border; may ulcerate		Nodules of basophilic nests with stromal retraction	
Pigmented BCC	Hyperpigmented translucent papule		Nodules of basophilic nests with melanocytes interspersed between tumor cells; melanophages within stroma	
Superficial BCC	Well-demarcated, erythematous patch		Buds of malignant cells extending into the dermis from the basal layer of the epidermis. Minimal dermal involvement.	
Morpheaform (sclerosing, infiltrative) BCC	Scarlike in appearance; ivory-white		Strands of tumor cells within a dense fibrous stroma	

be epidermal atrophy, and dermal invasion is usually minimal. There may be a chronic inflammatory infiltrate in the upper dermis. This histologic subtype is encountered most often on the trunk and extremities but may also appear on the head and neck.

MORPHEAFORM (SCLEROSING, INFILTRATIVE) BASAL CELL CARCINOMA

Morpheaform BCC is an aggressive growth variant of BCC with a distinct clinical and histologic appearance. Lesions of morpheaform BCC may have an ivory-white appearance and may resemble a scar or a small lesion of morphea (Fig. 111-5). Thus, the appearance of scar tissue in the absence of trauma or previous surgical procedure or the appearance of atypical-appearing scar tissue at the site of a previously treated skin lesion should alert the clinician to the possibility of morpheaform BCC and the need for biopsy. Morpheaform BCC consists of strands of tumor cells embedded within a dense fibrous stroma.[19] Tumor cells are closely packed columns, and in some cases, only one to two cells thick enmeshed in a densely collagenized fibrous stroma. Strands of tumor extend deeply into the dermis. The

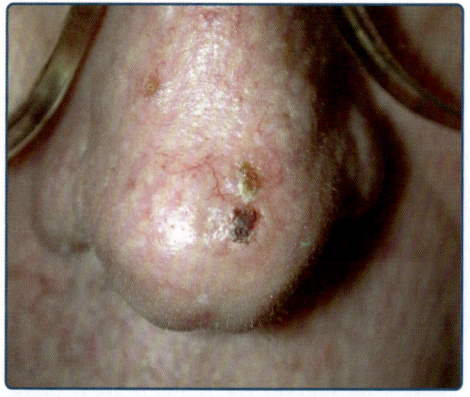

Figure 111-2 Basal cell carcinoma, nodular type.

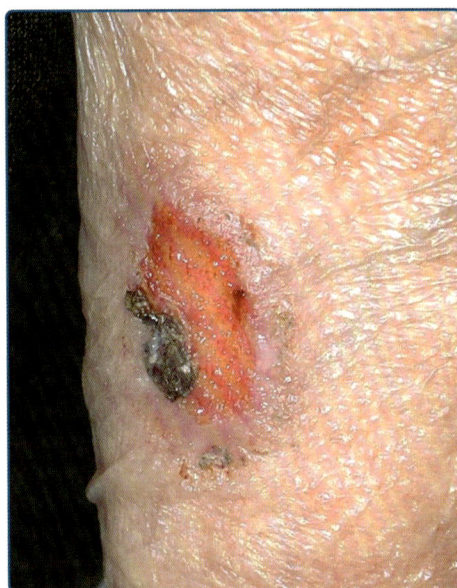

Figure 111-3 Basal cell carcinoma, rodent ulcer type.

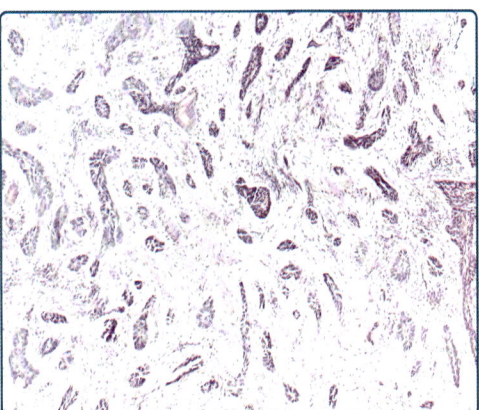

Figure 111-5 Basal cell carcinoma.

cancer is often larger than the clinical appearance indicates. Recurrent BCC may also demonstrate infiltrating bands and nests of cancer cells embedded within the dense fibrous stroma of scar.

BASOSQUAMOUS CARCINOMA

Basosquamous carcinoma is a form of aggressive growth BCC. It can be confused with squamous cell carcinoma (SCC) and promotes controversy considering its precise histologic classification as it shows both basal cell and SCC differentiation in a continuous fashion. Histologically, basosquamous carcinoma shows infiltrating jagged tongues of tumor cells admixed with other areas that show squamous intercellular bridge formation and cytoplasmic keratinization.

FIBROEPITHELIOMA OF PINKUS

FEP classically presents as a pink papule, usually on the lower back. It may be difficult to distinguish from an acrochordon or skin tag. In FEP, long strands of interwoven basiloma cells are embedded in fibrous stroma with abundant collagen.[18]

TREATMENT

Management of BCC is guided by anatomic location and histological features. Approaches include standard surgical excision or destruction by various other physical modalities, Mohs micrographic surgery (MMS), and topical chemotherapy. The Cochrane Collaboration found surgery and radiotherapy to appear the most effective treatments for BCC, with the best overall results being obtained with surgery.[22] Table 111-3 outlines situations when therapies other than surgery should be considered.

The best chance to achieve cure is through adequate initial treatment because recurrent tumors are more likely to be relatively resistant to further treatments and to cause further local destruction. An algorithmic approach to management is summarized in Fig. 111-6. Although most trials have only evaluated BCCs in low-risk locations, surgery and radiotherapy appear to be the most effective treatments with surgery showing the lowest failure rates. Although cosmetic outcomes appear good with PDT (see later), long-term follow-up data are needed. Overall, removal of the tumor with clear margins remains the gold standard for treating BCC.

MOHS MICROGRAPHIC SURGERY

MMS offers superior histologic analysis of tumor margins while permitting maximal conservation of tissue compared with standard excisional surgery.[23,24] Rowe

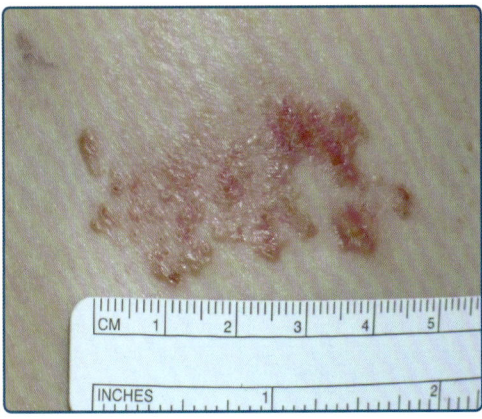

Figure 111-4 Superficial basal cell carcinoma. The well-demarcated plaque with a rolled edge characteristically occurs on the trunk.

and coworkers report a recurrence rate of 1% for primary BCCs treated by MMS. This was superior to the rate for other modalities, including standard excision (10%), curettage and desiccation (C&D) (7.7%), radiation therapy (XRT) (8.7%), and cryotherapy (7.5%).[24] Leibovitch and coworkers found that after 5 years, MMS-treated BCCs recurred in 1.4% of primary and 4% of recurrent tumors. This low 5-year recurrence rate of BCC with MMS emphasizes the importance of margin-controlled excision over other modalities.[25] MMS is the treatment of choice for morpheaform, poorly delineated, incompletely removed, and otherwise high-risk primary BCCs as per National Comprehensive Cancer Network Guidelines.[26] It is the preferred treatment for recurrent BCC and for any BCC that occurs at a site where tissue conservation is desired. MMS is particularly useful in treating BCCs at high-risk anatomic sites, including the embryonic fusion planes represented by the nasofacial junction and retroauricular sulcus. Based on the fact that MMS provides the lowest recurrence rates, it is the treatment of first choice for primary facial BCCs with an aggressive histopathological subtype and for recurrent facial BCCs.[27] MMS has shown greater efficacy than surgical excision for the treatment of recurrent facial BCCs.[28] Recurrent BCCs treated by MMS reappeared at a rate of 5.6%, which was again superior to the rate for other modalities, including excision (17.6%), XRT (9.8%), and C&D (40%).[29] Mosterd and coworkers also found that treatment with MMS leads to a significantly lower number of recurrences than treatment with surgical excision in recurrent facial BCCs.[23] From a patient perspective, one needs to consider whether MMS is necessary in older patients with limited life expectancy or other serious medical comorbidities versus patient preference.[30,31]

STANDARD EXCISION

Compared with nonexcisional techniques, standard surgical excision offers the advantage of histologic evaluation of the removed specimen; however, depending on the sectioning method used (eg, breadloafing), areas of margin involvement can be missed during routine histologic evaluation.[32] The authors of a recent Cochrane review by Bath-Hextall and coworkers in 2007 concluded that based on the available published work, surgery is the standard treatment of choice for BCC.[22] Although standard excision is appropriate for many BCCs, cure rates for standard excisional surgery are inferior to those for MMS in cases of primary morpheaform BCCs, recurrent BCCs, and tumors located in high-risk anatomic sites.[25] This is discussed further in Chap. 204 and 206.

CURETTAGE AND DESICCATION

C&D is one of the most frequently used treatment modalities for BCC.[33] That C&D is operator dependent was shown by Kopf and coworkers, who identified a significant difference in cure rate between patients treated by private practitioners (94.3%) and those treated by residents (81.2%). High 5-year cure rates of up to 98.8% have been obtained after C&D of primary, nonfibrosing BCCs of medium- and high-risk areas of

TABLE 111-3
When to Consider Nonsurgical Treatment

TYPE OF BASAL CELL CARCINOMA (BCC)	FDA-APPROVED THERAPIES	OTHER THERAPIES
Metastatic BCC	Vismodegib	Platinum-based chemotherapy
Locally advanced BCC (defined as BCC that is unable to be treated with surgery or radiation without significant morbidity)	Vismodegib, sonidegib	Platinum-based chemotherapy

FDA, Food and Drug Administration.

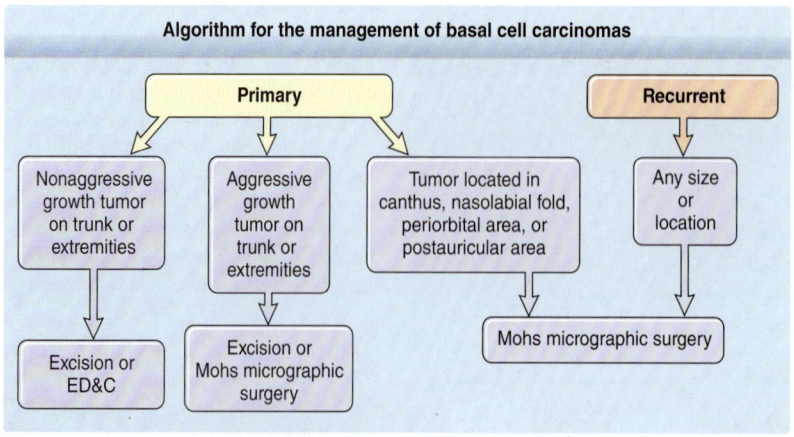

Figure 111-6 Algorithm for the management of basal cell carcinomas. ED&C, electrodesiccation and curettage.

the face when performed by a skilled operator.[34] Cure rates decreased as a function of primary lesion size: for lesions smaller than 1.0 cm, the cure rate was 98.8%; for lesions between 1.0 cm and 2.0 cm, 95.5%; and for lesions larger than 2.0 cm, 84%. Therefore, C&D is not recommended for large primary BCCs nor for morpheaform or recurrent BCCs.[35] For appropriately selected lesions and locations, C&D remains an efficacious and cost-effective treatment modality.

CRYOSURGERY

Cryosurgery is another destructive modality that has been used in the treatment of BCC. Two freeze–thaw cycles with a tissue temperature of −50°C (−58°F) are required to destroy BCC. In addition, a margin of clinically normal tissue must be destroyed to eradicate subclinical extension. A systematic review of recurrence rates published between 1970 and 1997 indicated that cryotherapy in the treatment of primary BCC resulted in a 5-year recurrence rate from 4% to 17%.[35] Kuflik and Gage reported 99% cure rates in 628 patients followed for 5 years.[36] Possible complications of cryosurgery include hypertrophic scarring and postinflammatory pigmentary changes.[37] Any recent change in a cryosurgery scar after normal healing is completed should raise the suspicion of recurrent BCC.

TOPICAL TREATMENT

(Discussed more in Chap. 192).

Imiquimod: Imiquimod (5% cream) has been used in the treatment of skin cancers.[38,39] Approved in 2004 by the U.S. Food and Drug Administration (FDA) for the topical treatment of biopsy-confirmed, small (<2 cm), primary superficial BCC, imiquimod is a Toll-like receptor 7 agonist believed to induce interferon-α, tumor necrosis factor-α, and other cytokines to boost T helper 1 type immunity. In two double-blind, randomized, vehicle-controlled trials, clinical and histological clearance rates for dosing five and seven times per week were 75% and 73%, respectively, for superficial BCC.[38-40] In another study, 10 of 19 nodular BCCs (approximately 53%) cleared after treatment with imiquimod.[40] In general, adverse side effects are limited to local skin reactions; however, researchers have noted the significant correlation between the severity of the local skin reaction (erythema, erosion, and crusting) and the histologic clearance rate. Imiquimod is FDA approved for only for superficial BCCs limited to small tumors in low-risk locations in patients.[41] The safety and effectiveness of imiquimod for other types of BCC have not been established, with up to 25% of treated patients failing therapy.

5-Fluorouracil: 5-Fluorouracil (5-FU), a topically applied chemotherapeutic agent used in the treatment of actinic keratoses, has also been used to treat superficial BCCs. In one series, Epstein showed a 5-year recurrence rate of 21% for thin BCCs after 5-FU treatment, which was reduced to 6% when curettage was performed initially.[42] Gross and coworkers observed a 90% histologic clearance rate 3 weeks after 5-FU treatment but with no long-term follow-up.[43] The use of 5-FU to treat BCC should be considered carefully and should include an evaluation of the risk of recurrence and treatment failure.

PHOTODYNAMIC THERAPY

Photodynamic therapy (PDT) (discussed more in Chap. 199) involves the activation of a photosensitizing drug by visible light to produce activated oxygen species that destroy the constituent cancer cells. Exogenous δ-aminolevulinic acid increases intracellular production of the endogenous photosensitizer protoporphyrin type IX, which preferentially accumulates in tumor cells.[44] Basset-Seguin and coworkers reported complete response rates for superficial BCCs from 85% to 93% at 3 months and a response rate on par with cryosurgery at 60 months (75% vs. 74%).[44] Marmur and coworkers reviewed PDT for NMSC and reported recurrence rates ranging from 0% to 31% for BCC.[45] The long-term cure rates for superficial BCC with PDT remains around 75%, and because of the appreciable nonresponse and recurrence rates, patients should be monitored closely during the first 2 to 3 years after PDT, which is when most lesion recurrences are seen.[45,46] The Cochrane Collaboration found that cosmetic outcome for PDT was significantly better than surgery.[22] However, there were also comparatively high failure rates associated with PDT when compared with surgery, radiotherapy, and cryotherapy. For superficial BCC, one randomized trial showed that 5-FU and imiquimod were superior to PDT. There was no difference between 5-FU and imiquimod at 3- and 12-month follow-up.[47]

RADIATION THERAPY

XRT (discussed more in Chap. 200) may be useful in cases of primary BCC or in cases in which postsurgical margins are positive for cancer. Advantages include minimal patient discomfort and avoidance of an invasive procedure for a patient unwilling or unable to undergo surgery. XRT may be a very useful modality as adjunct treatment for BCC when margins are positive after excision or for extensive perineural or large nerve involvement.[28] Good control rates of 93% to 97% have been reported; however, long-term randomized results suggest XRT remains inferior to surgery both in recurrence rate and cosmesis. The 4-year failure rate was 0.7% in the surgery group compared with 7.5% in the radiotherapy group.[48]

SPECIAL MANAGEMENT ISSUES

Perineural Invasion: In one series, Niazi and Lamberty identified perineural invasion (PNI) in fewer than 0.2% of cases. Defined as the observation of malignant cells in the perineural space of nerves, when PNI is detected, every effort should be made to clear the tumor, preferably by MMS.[49] Patients with gross PNI manifested by neurologic symptoms would benefit from preoperative magnetic resonance imaging to assess extent of tumor spread. Perineural spread may manifest as pain, paresthesias, weakness, or paralysis.

Locally Advanced Basal Cell Carcinoma:
The greatest danger of BCC results from local invasion. In general, BCC is a slow-growing tumor that invades locally rather than metastasizes.[50] If left untreated, the tumor will progress to invade subcutaneous tissue, muscle, and even bone. Anatomic fusion planes appear to provide a low-resistance path for tumor progression. Metastases are rare and are correlated to the size (>7.5 cm) and a long delay in seeking treatment for the tumor.[51] The term *locally advanced BCCs* is applied to BCCs that cannot be adequately excised without significant functional impairment or tumors that cannot be treated with radiotherapy.[52] Inhibitors of the Hedgehog signaling pathway (vismodegib, sonidegib) have been FDA approved for the treatment of locally advanced BCCs.[52-54]

Metastatic Basal Cell Carcinoma:
Metastasis of BCC occurs only rarely, with rates varying from 0.0028% to 0.55%.[55] If nodal disease is suspected on surgical examination, lymph node biopsy and imaging studies, as well as evaluation by medical and surgical oncologists, are indicated.[56] The most common sites of metastasis are the regional lymph nodes, lungs, and bone.[51] Aggressive histologic characteristics, including morpheaform features, squamous metaplasia, and PNI, have been identified as risk factors for metastasis.[55] The median survival period of patients with metastatic BCC is 10 months.[51] Platinum-based chemotherapy has been used with modest results in treatment of metastatic BCC; however, rapid clinical response was reported using a combination of cisplatin and paclitaxel.[57] Complete response to carboplatin and paclitaxel has been reported in case series.

Hedgehog Inhibitors:
Studies have now identified a natural antagonist of the Hedgehog signaling pathway derived from the *Veratrum californicum* plant called *cyclopamine*. This substance binds and antagonizes SMO and has been shown to be effective in animal models of BCCs. Other small-molecule Hedgehog pathway antagonists with similar properties have been identified and are currently being tested for their clinical efficacy.[58] In a phase 1 trial of the first of these specific Hedgehog inhibitors, vismodegib, 33 patients with locally advanced or metastatic BCCs showed significant shrinkage of metastatic and advanced cutaneous BCCs with relatively mild systemic toxicity.[53]

Vismodegib was approved by the FDA in 2012 for patients with locally advanced or metastatic BCC.[52] In 104 patients enrolled in the ERIVANCE multicenter clinical response trial, vismodegib (150 mg/day) led to an objective response rate (complete plus partial response) of 33.3% in patients with metastatic disease and 47.6% in patients with the locally advanced form. The median duration of response in patients with metastatic disease was 7.6 months and in patients with locally advanced BCC was 9.5 months.[52]

Sonidegib, another inhibitor of SMO in the SHH pathway, has similar efficacy and is approved for locally advanced BCCs.[54] Unfortunately, as has been the case with several other such molecularly targeted anticancer drugs, about 30% of treated tumors either do not respond or develop resistance to treatment and relapse through mutations in SMO or a combination of SUFU inactivation and GLI2 amplification.[12,59] Mutations in SMO (the drug target) have been identified in 50% of resistant tumors; these mutations maintain Hedgehog signaling in the presence of SMO inhibitors.[60-62]

COURSE AND PROGNOSIS

With appropriate treatment, the prognosis for most patients with BCC is excellent. Control rates as high as 99% have been achieved by MMS. Although tumor control rates for primary tumors are high, patients must be monitored for recurrence and development of new primary BCCs. The risk for development of a second primary BCC ranges from 36% to 50%.[63] Periodic full-body skin examinations and counseling about sun protection are recommended for any patient with a history of BCC. This is especially important because patients with a history of BCC are at increased risk for melanoma. The prognosis for patients with recurrent BCC is favorable, although recurrent tumors are more likely to appear again and to behave aggressively. Patients with a history of recurrent disease must be monitored more frequently for the development of further recurrences and new primary tumors. An estimated 40% to 50% of patients with primary BCC will develop at least one or more further BCCs within 5 years.[2] For the rare patient with metastatic disease, the prognosis is poor, with a mean survival time of 8 to 10 months without treatment from the time of diagnosis. Recent clinical trials have highlighted a potential role of nicotinamide 500 mg twice a day[64] and of the nonsteroidal antiinflammatory drug celecoxib[65] in producing some decrease in BCC risk.

BASAL CELL NEVUS SYNDROME

- Patients with basal cell nevus syndrome (BCNS, Gorlin syndrome) inherit an inactivating mutation in the *PTCH1* gene.
- BCNS is a rare autosomal-dominant disorder with phenotypic abnormalities that include developmental anomalies and postnatal tumors, especially BCCs.

- In BCNS, the three most characteristic abnormalities are tumors such as medulloblastomas or BCCs, pits of the palms and soles, and odontogenic cysts of the jaw.
- Inhibitors of the Hedgehog signaling pathway (SMO inhibitors such as vismodegib, sonidegib) are FDA approved for advanced or metastatic BCCs.

Basal cell nevus syndrome, also known as *nevoid basal cell carcinoma syndrome* and *Gorlin syndrome* (Online Mendelian Inheritance in Man [OMIM] #109400), is a rare autosomal-dominant disorder associated with a panoply of phenotypic abnormalities that can be divided into developmental anomalies and postnatal tumors, especially BCCs.[66] Although individual aspects had been reported previously, their syndromic association was first appreciated widely in the late 1950s.[67,68]

EPIDEMIOLOGY

The prevalence of BCNS is variously estimated to be 1 in 31,000 to 1 in 60,000 persons.[69-71] The syndrome affects both sexes and occurs in a wide variety of cultural groups and therefore does not have a predilection for a particular skin type. The condition appears to have complete penetrance but variable expressivity of traits, such that their clinical presentation among families is nonuniform. Furthermore, as with many dominantly inherited conditions, new mutations are common. As a result, in many cases, patients may have no apparent affected ancestors or siblings.

ETIOLOGY AND PATHOGENESIS

GENETIC ABNORMALITY

Almost all known BCNS patients thus far carry mutations in the *PATCHED1* (*PTCH1*, UniGene Hs.494538) gene residing on the long arm of chromosome 9.[72,73] PTCH1 plays a central role in the Hedgehog signaling pathway that is essential for the establishment of normal body and limb patterning.[74] The *PTCH1* locus behaves like a classic tumor suppressor gene (see Fig. 111-1). The appearance of BCCs in small numbers at an older age in sporadic cases and in larger numbers at a younger age in patients with BCNS is reminiscent of differences in sporadic and hereditary cases of retinoblastoma.[75] BCNS, like other tumor susceptibility syndromes, is inherited in an autosomal-dominant manner, with inheritance of a loss-of-function allele followed by somatic loss of the remaining copy before tumor formation.

Identification of the gene mutation responsible for BCNS facilitated a molecular verification of the tumor suppressor prediction.[72,73] In BCNS, patients inherit one defective *PTCH1* allele, but their tumors contain an additional somatic mutation. As with some other tumor suppressor genes, *PTCH1* mutations have also been found in older adults with sporadic BCCs and other sporadic tumors known to be overrepresented in patients with BCNS (eg, medulloblastomas and meningiomas), which supports the idea that two somatic "hits" are required in sporadic tumors.

In contrast, the two-hit genetic model proposed for *PTCH1*-dependent tumor development may not fully explain the developmental abnormalities seen in BCNS, which occur earlier. *PTCH1* heterozygote mice display many of the developmental abnormalities seen in patients with BCNS despite a wild-type copy of the nonaffected allele.[76-78] This argues that certain tissues (skeleton, limb, neural tube) require higher levels of PTCH1 to regulate tissue development and that heterozygotes cannot compensate for loss of the other allele (haploinsufficiency).

Are *PTCH1* mutations the only cause of BCNS? Despite direct sequencing of *PTCH1* exons in patients, somatic mutations are found in fewer than half of BCCs and germline mutations in fewer than 100% of BCNS patients.[79,80] On the one hand, this suggests that mutations in other unidentified genes may underlie the disease. On the other hand, early linkage studies found strong association with the *PTCH1* locus. Moreover, although mutations are not found in PTCH1 exons in some patients, Hedgehog signaling pathway abnormalities are still present in these tumors. One family with BCNS and atypical features (medulloblastoma and plantar pits but no BCCs) was found to have germline mutations in SUFU, a tumor suppressor gene and negative regulator of SHH signaling (see Fig. 111-1).[81,82] This suggests that mutations may be found in other members of the signaling pathway in rare cases.

PTCH1 FUNCTION

PTCH1 protein plays a critical role in the hedgehog signaling pathway (see Fig. 111-1). Genetic and biochemical studies in *Drosophila* and mammals indicate that PTCH1 protein inhibits this signaling pathway by inhibiting the function of the central G protein–coupled receptor SMO and that the extracellular ligand hedgehog abrogates this inhibition. Signaling by SMO results in the activation of the GLI family of zinc finger proteins that mediate all the transcriptional effects of Hedgehog signaling. Three GLI proteins mediate activation and suppression of Hedgehog target genes, with GLI1 and GLI2 acting as activators and GLI2 and GLI3 as suppressors. SMO signaling tips the balance toward activation and away from target gene suppression. In mammals, GLI activity is controlled by the novel cytoplasmic protein SUFU, which promotes the transcriptional repression and inhibits activation.[83] SMO inhibits SUFU activity, thus releasing GLI proteins to become transcriptional activators. When

Hedgehog binds to PTCH1, PTCH1 inhibition of SMO is relieved, and the pathway is activated. Thus, loss of PTCH1 function allows unregulated SMO activity and initiates tumor formation.

How PTCH1 functions as a tumor suppressor is still under investigation. A significant aspect of PTCH1 function is inhibition of SMO, although how PTCH1 accomplishes this is unknown. PTCH1 acts in an enzymatic manner as only a few molecules are necessary able to inhibit SMO by severalfold.[84] Moreover, PTCH1 and SMO are thought to exist in distinct endosomes and thought not to physically interact. Components of the Hedgehog pathway are localized to a novel microtubule-based organelle called the primary cilium (see Fig. 111-1). Mutations that affect the structure and function of the cilium, known collectively as the human ciliopathies, are also known to disrupt maximal Hedgehog signaling and have some similarities to BCNS. SMO accumulation through the actions of intraflagellar transport proteins within this organelle is correlated with pathway activation. PTCH1 is localized at the base of the organelle and appears to prevent SMO entry. Loss of PTCH1 or mutations that allow SMO to move into the cilium result in increased pathway activity.[85]

MUTATIONS IN SONIC HEDGEHOG PATHWAY IN BASAL CELL CARCINOMAS

Supporting the central role of SHH target gene induction in BCC pathogenesis is the finding of mutations in members of the SHH pathway in both BCNS patients and in sporadic BCCs. Identified mutations involving PTCH1 are by far the most common in BCNS tumors.[9] The particular type of mutation found in PTCH is consistent with mutation caused by UV light, which provides additional evidence for PTCH and sunlight in cancer development.[86]

Mutations of SMO protein have been identified in approximately 10% of BCCs, and these mutations appear to render SMO protein resistant to PTCH1 inhibition.[87] Indeed, experimental transfection of cells with mutant SMO sequences can transform them to a malignant phenotype. This finding that BCCs may have upregulation of Hedgehog target gene expression caused by mutations in either PTCH1 or SMO argues that it is the upregulation of Hedgehog signaling rather than the specific mutation that is crucial to BCC formation. Consistent with this is the finding that mutations in the gene encoding SUFU have been reported to underlie formation of medulloblastomas and BCNS.[81,88]

CLINICAL FINDINGS

CUTANEOUS LESIONS

Hedgehog signaling plays a critical role in the expansion of progenitor cells in a wide variety of tissues in both invertebrate and vertebrate organisms. PTCH1 normally is expressed both during development and in adults, which suggests an ongoing postnatal role. Patients with BCNS show multiple abnormalities, none of which is unique to this syndrome.[70,79,80] The three abnormalities considered to be most characteristic of the syndrome are tumors such as medulloblastomas or BCCs, pits of the palms and soles, and keratocystic odontogenic tumors (odontogenic cysts) of the jaw.

Individual BCCs from patients with BCNS cannot be distinguished from those in sporadic cases, which is not surprising in view of the similar pathogenesis in familial and sporadic cases. What is distinguishing is their appearance in large numbers starting at an early age. They may be banal appearing and confused grossly with nevocytic nevi, hence the name *basal cell nevus*. They may also have a translucent, papulonodular appearance more characteristic of sporadic BCCs and may invade locally. In rare cases, they may even metastasize, causing the patient's death. Although the ratio of sun-protected to sun-exposed BCCs may be higher in BCNS than in sporadic cases, sunlight and ionizing radiation (thus making ionizing radiation a very poor choice for treatment of most BCCs in BCNS patients) clearly accelerate BCC formation in BCNS patients, and darkly pigmented BCNS patients may have few to no BCCs (Figs. 111-7 and 111-8).

Palmoplantar pits are small defects in the stratum corneum and may be pink or, if dirt has accumulated, dark in color (Fig. 111-9). They appear early in life and can be a valuable aid in diagnosis in addition to jaw cysts or medulloblastoma. Their basis is poorly understood, but they are thought to be caused by aborted attempts to generate hair follicles

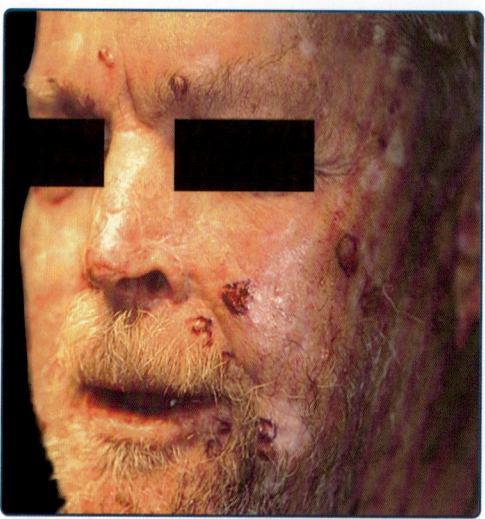

Figure 111-7 Face of a man with severe scarring from growth and treatment of multiple basal cell carcinomas (BCCs). Note multiple outlined new BCCs despite extensive and frequent surgery.

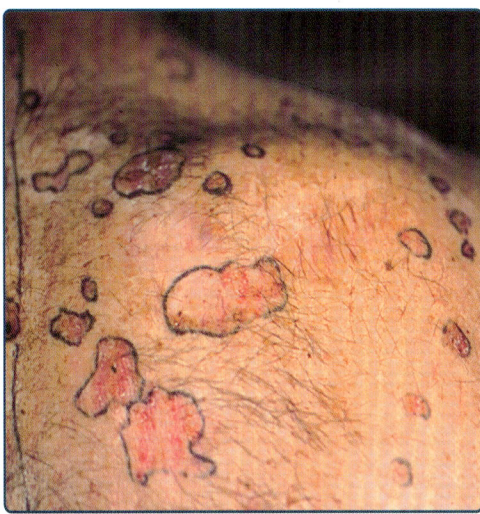

Figure 111-8 Upper back of man with basal cell nevus syndrome with innumerable basal cell carcinomas, some of which are nodular and most of which are flat, erythematous patches.

in the palms. They are also seen in mouse PTCH1 heterozygotes.[89]

RELATED PHYSICAL FINDINGS

Tissue overgrowth, which is also a feature of Hedgehog signaling pathway activation in *Drosophila*, often is manifested by an overall body size larger than that of other family members. Limbs may be particularly long, giving a marfanoid appearance (see Fig. 111-10), and a large head circumference (at least in probands) and frontal bossing are often described.

Jaw cysts often are the first detectable abnormality[70,79,80] (Fig. 111-11). They may be asymptomatic and therefore diagnosed only radiologically. However, they also may erode enough bone to cause pain, swelling, and loss of teeth. They occur more often in the mandibular jaw than in the maxillary jaw.[90] These jaw cysts presumably form from inappropriate SHH induction of dental epithelium and can recur often and be the most debilitating aspect of the syndrome.[91]

DIAGNOSIS

Because the individual abnormalities are not unique to patients with BCNS, it is possible to diagnose BCNS clinically only when multiple typical defects are present. The severity of abnormalities may differ markedly among members of a single kindred, and diagnostic certainty may be difficult for specific individuals even if they belong to a kindred with known BCNS.[92] Generally, the diagnosis is suggested to the dermatologist when multiple BCCs arise in a patient at an unexpectedly early age and in unexpectedly large numbers, with the average age of onset in the early 20s.

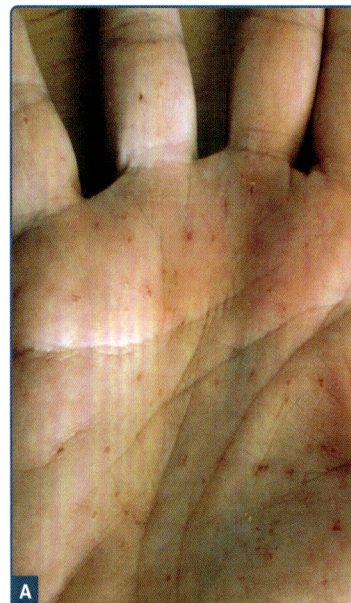

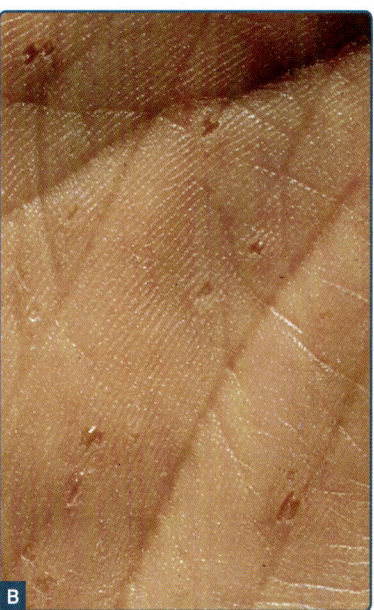

Figure 111-9 **A,** Unusually florid palmar pits in a patient with basal cell nevus syndrome (BCNS). **B,** Larger magnification showing that these lesions in BCNS are really punched-out pits.

Further evaluation should include (1) questions about whether other family members have had abnormalities consistent with BCNS (although perhaps 30% of patients with BCNS have no affected ancestors) and whether the patient is taller and heavier than his or her relatives; (2) examination for palmoplantar pits and skin cysts and assessment of body and head size; and (3) radiologic evaluation for jaw cysts (which often appear around the start of the second decade), calcification of the falx (which occurs in nearly all adults with BCNS and may be present

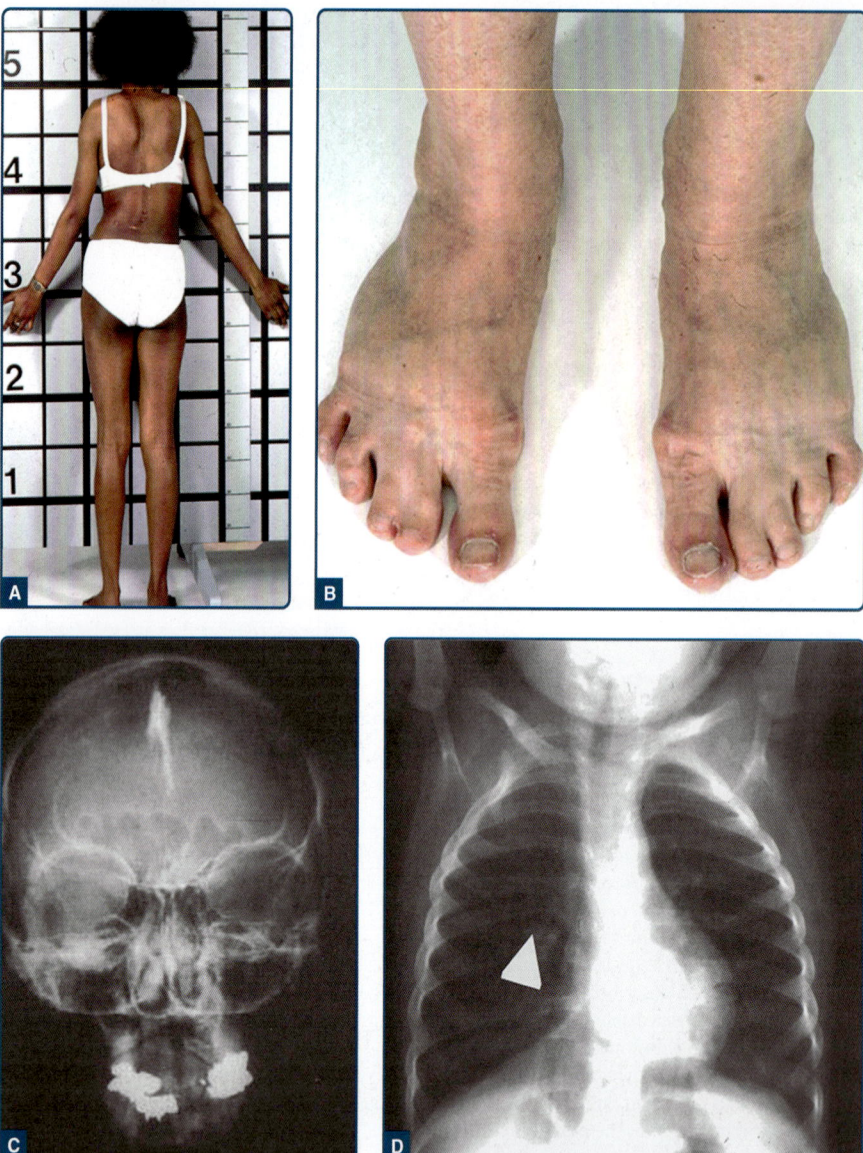

Figure 111-10 Skeletal and radiographic findings in basal cell nevus syndrome. **A,** Unusually large body habitus and extremities. **B,** Syndactyly in the digits. **C,** Calcification of the falx cerebri. **D,** Rib development abnormalities, including rib fusion (*arrowhead*).

in early childhood in patients with BCNS, thus suggesting the diagnosis of BCNS in those patients with early-onset medulloblastomas), and abnormalities of the ribs, spine, and phalanges (flame-shaped lucencies), each of which is present in one-third to one-half of BCNS patients.[70,71,79,80] Kimonis and colleagues proposed a set of major and minor criteria for presumptive diagnosis of BCNS (Table 111-4), which has since been modified.[79] For cases in which the diagnosis is in doubt or for genotyping of other family members, identification of *PTCH1* gene mutations is now available commercially through GeneDX (Gaithersburg, MD).

DIFFERENTIAL DIAGNOSIS

Other syndromes exist that are characterized by the development of multiple BCCs. These include Bazex syndrome (OMIM 301845),[93] Rombo syndrome (OMIM 180730),[94] and a syndrome observed in a family with BCCs, milia, and coarse, sparse hair.[95] Hair abnormalities are present in all three syndromes, which is a finding of interest in view of the often-repeated suggestion that BCCs arise from hair follicles rather than from interfollicular epidermis. The exact nosologic relationships among these three

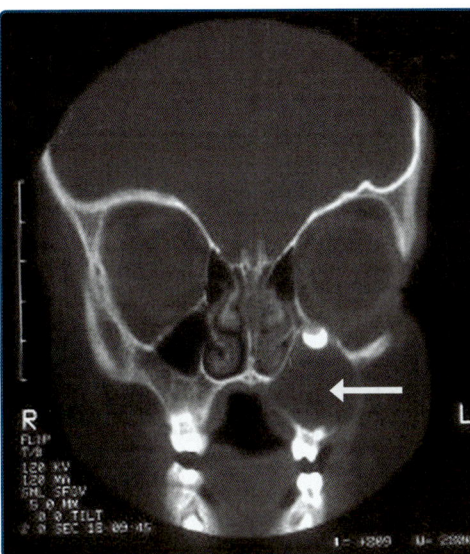

Figure 111-11 Radiographic findings of odontogenic keratocyst (*arrow*).

palmar pits and milia. Recent molecular characterization of MHIBCC suggest that loss of SUFU underlies many of these cases, consistent with the well-differentiated nature of the tumors.[98,99] GBFH is acquired and associated with autoimmune disease, which suggests an immunologic stimulation of the hedgehog pathway.

Patients with long-term arsenic ingestion may have multiple BCCs. Their dyschromia and lack of other phenotypic abnormalities differentiate them from BCNS patients. Patients with xeroderma pigmentosum develop multiple BCCs but are readily differentiated from BCNS patients by their severe photosensitivity and other phenotypic abnormalities (see Chap. 130).

The most challenging patients are those who have a marked propensity to develop multiple BCCs throughout life, sometimes sporadically or in rare cases after therapeutic irradiation (eg, for Hodgkin disease) without showing any of the other signs of BCNS. These patients resemble BCNS patients with many BCCs, but do not have mutations in *PTCH1* alleles and are called High-Frequency (HF-BCC) patients.[100,101]

syndromes are uncertain, but patients with BCNS have normal hair, and all three syndromes seem quite different from BCNS.

Two other syndromes that have been described include multiple hereditary infundibulocystic basal cell carcinoma (MHIBCC)[96] and generalized basaloid follicular hamartoma (GBFH).[97] Both demonstrate histologic variants of BCCs, with more hamartomatous lesions, and are characterized by

TABLE 111-4
Diagnostic Criteria for Basal Cell Nevus Syndrome (BCNS, Gorlin Syndrome)

Major Criteria
1. Basal cell carcinoma before age 20 yr
2. Odontogenic keratocysts before age 15 yr
3. Three or more palmar or plantar pits
4. Bilamellar calcification of the falx cerebri (if younger than 20 yr)
5. Fused, bifid, or markedly splayed ribs
6. First-degree relative with BCNS
7. *PTCH* gene mutation in normal tissue

Minor Criteria
1. Macrocephaly determined after adjustment for height
2. Congenital malformations: cleft lip or palate, frontal bossing, "coarse face," moderate or severe hypertelorism
3. Skeletal abnormalities: Sprengel deformity, marked pectus deformity, or marked syndactyly of the digits
4. Radiologic abnormalities: bridging of the sella turcica; rib anomalies such as bifid or splayed ribs; vertebral anomalies such as hemivertebrae, fusion, or elongation of the vertebral bodies; modeling defects of the hands and feet; or flame-shaped lucencies of the hands or feet
5. Ovarian fibroma
6. Medulloblastoma

COMPLICATIONS, PROGNOSIS, AND CLINICAL COURSE

Although disease pathogenesis involves abnormalities in SHH signaling, the wide variability in clinical course among families and even between generations of the same family make prediction of the clinical course difficult. If BCNS is suspected or confirmed, physicians should also screen for the most frequent sequelae of the disease during childhood or adolescence (Table 111-5). No large-scale survival studies have been performed to determine whether BCNS patients die earlier because of their disease.[79,102] The major complications are developmental delay, physical impairment in children, and the childhood tumors that arise, such as medulloblastoma. The latter often occur within the first 5 years of life and are frequently the initial sign of BCNS. Complications arising from medulloblastoma treatment (radiation, shunt placement) are relatively common, and multidisciplinary teams of physicians are required to optimally treat these patients.

In the skin, BCCs that arise are locally aggressive but very rarely metastasize.[103] No reports document an increased risk for metastatic BCCs, which suggests that the basic character of the tumor is similar to that seen in sporadic BCC cases. However, because of the high numbers and wide distribution of the tumor, even in the absence of sun exposure, involvement of key epithelial surfaces or membranes is likely and can be disfiguring for the patient.

TABLE 111-5
Approach to the Patient with Known or Suspected Basal Cell Nevus Syndrome (BCNS)
Pediatric Patients
• Baseline MRI of brain; repeat yearly (if asymptomatic) until age 8 yr
• Baseline dermatologic examination; repeat yearly until first BCC develops and then every 6 months (or more frequently as needed) throughout life
• Digital Panorex of jaw at age 3 or 4 hr (or as soon as tolerated) and then yearly until the first jaw cyst develops. Repeat yearly (or more frequently as needed) until age 21 yr
• Pelvic ultrasonography in girls at menarche (or earlier if symptomatic)
• Molecular diagnosis (if desired) for patients with family history and known mutation
• Baseline scoliosis assessment at one year of age and then annually for progression if present
• Routine developmental screening and referral for all children who do not meet developmental milestones
Adult Patients
• Baseline MRI of brain (if not done at age 8 yr or later)
• Dermatologic examination at 4 mo (or more frequently if new lesions present at each examination)
• Digital Panorex of jaw twice yearly until cyst free for 2 years and then yearly or less frequently (depending on patient's concern about radiation)
• Prenatal or preconception counseling if desired

BCC, basal cell carcinoma; MRI, magnetic resonance imaging.
Data from Kimonis VE, Goldstein AM, Pastakia B, et al. Clinical manifestations in 105 persons with nevoid basal cell carcinoma syndrome. *Am J Med Genet.* 1997;69(3):299-308.

TREATMENT

Therapy must be directed at the individual lesions as they arise, and the most important aspects of management are frequent examination, counseling about avoidance of sun exposure, and early treatment of small tumors. In animal models of BCNS, small, clinically undetectable tumors arise throughout the skin. This suggests that many more tumors form than are detectable visibly by the clinician.[89,104] This has several therapeutic ramifications. One is that clinicians caring for patients with BCNS should become confident in their clinical acumen so that they can diagnose and treat tiny BCCs without histopathologic confirmation. This would eliminate multiple scar-inducing biopsies in addition to potentially disfiguring treatments. Another is that invasive treatments should be focused on lesions that are potentially the most harmful, such as those invading mucous membranes or adjacent structures. Repetitive surgical treatments run the risk of severe disfigurement for the patient. Finally, clear surgical margins may be difficult to achieve when using Mohs surgery, so aggressive pursuit of a clear margin needs to be balanced against other factors in treating these patients.

Nonsurgical approaches to BCC treatment should be used aggressively in patients with BCNS when possible. Because the key is to convince the patient to accept frequent treatments, minimization of discomfort and scarring is a major goal. Approaches that may be of benefit are topical treatment with 5-FU (with or without occlusion, depending on the degree of inflammation produced),[105] the Toll-like receptor agonist imiquimod,[106] and PDT.[107] Oral therapy with retinoids also may be of value but often only at a dosage that generally causes severe side effects. There are several agents for BCC prevention in BCNS patients, including PDT, celecoxib, topical retinoids, and topical 5-FU, each with some suggestion of efficacy. The most effective agent appears to be oral vismodegib 150 mg/day, which dramatically shrank existing BCCs and prevented new BCCs (30 BCC/year in placebo vs 1 BCC/year on drug) in a 3-year randomized, double-blinded controlled trial in patients with BCNS.[108,109] Unfortunately, the mild to moderate side effects of muscle cramps, taste loss, and hair loss precluded most patients with BCNS from taking vismodegib long term (>3 years).[107,109] In contrast to advanced and metastatic BCCs, resistance to SMO inhibitors is rare in patients with BCNS; few SMO mutations have been detected in tumors, and BCCs shrink when systemic HH inhibitor treatment is resumed.[12,108]

The X-irradiation of BCCs has been advocated in otherwise normal patients who are not surgical candidates. However, excessive radiation should be avoided if possible because enhanced radiation-induced carcinogenesis (eg, in the skin of the portals of irradiation for childhood medulloblastomas) is characteristic of BCNS. Patients with BCNS who receive radiation have developed an unusually large number of basal cell tumors in the irradiated area a short time after exposure.

Genetic counseling is appropriate. With the availability of direct sequencing of the PTCH1 locus, genotyping for prenatal diagnosis is potentially achievable for interested families. Because PTCH1 is transmitted with complete penetrance, half of the children of affected individuals are expected to develop BCNS.

ACKNOWLEDGMENTS

The authors acknowledge the contributions of John A. Carucci, David J. Leffell, and Julia S. Pettersen, the former authors of this chapter.

REFERENCES

1. Asgari MM, Moffet HH, Ray GT, et al. Trends in basal cell carcinoma incidence and identification of high-risk subgroups, 1998-2012. *JAMA Dermatol.* 2015;151(9):976-981.
2. Rubin AI, Chen EH, Ratner D. Basal-cell carcinoma. *N Engl J Med.* 2005;353:2262-2269.
3. Christenson LJ, Borrowman TA, Vachon CM, et al. Incidence of basal cell and squamous cell carcinomas

4. Sng J, Koh D, Siong WC, et al. Skin cancer trends among Asians living in Singapore from 1968 to 2006. *J Am Acad Dermatol*. 2009;61(3):426-432.
5. Gloster HM Jr, Neal K. Skin cancer in skin of color. *J Am Acad Dermatol*. 2006;55(5):741-760; quiz 761-764.
6. Gailani MR, Leffell DJ, Ziegler A, et al. Relationship between sunlight exposure and a key genetic alteration in basal cell carcinoma. *J Natl Cancer Inst*. 1996;88(6):349-354.
7. Epstein EH. Basal cell carcinomas: attack of the hedgehog. *Nat Rev Cancer*. 2008;8(10):743-754.
8. Benjamin CL, Ananthaswamy HN. p53 and the pathogenesis of skin cancer. *Toxicol Appl Pharmacol*. 2007;224(3):241-248.
9. Reifenberger J, Wolter M, Knobbe CB, et al. Somatic mutations in the PTCH, SMOH, SUFUH and TP53 genes in sporadic basal cell carcinomas. *Br J Dermatol*. 2005;152(1):43-51.
10. Lindström E, Shimokawa T, Toftgård R, et al. PTCH mutations: distribution and analyses. *Hum Mutat*. 2006;27(3):215-219.
11. Heitzer E, Lassacher A, Quehenberger F, et al. UV fingerprints predominate in the PTCH mutation spectra of basal cell carcinomas independent of clinical phenotype. *J Invest Dermatol*. 2007;127(12):2872-2881.
12. Bonilla X, Parmentier L, King B, et al. Genomic analysis identifies new drivers and progression pathways in skin basal cell carcinoma. *Nat Genet*. 2016;48(4):398-406.
13. Pelucchi C, Di Landro A, Naldi L, et al. Risk factors for histological types and anatomic sites of cutaneous basal-cell carcinoma: an Italian case-control study. *J Invest Dermatol*. 2007;127(4):935-944.
14. Karagas MR, Nelson HH, Zens MS, et al. Squamous cell and basal cell carcinoma of the skin in relation to radiation therapy and potential modification of risk by sun exposure. *Epidemiology*. 2007;18(6):776-784.
15. Berg D, Otley CC. Skin cancer in organ transplant recipients: epidemiology, pathogenesis, and management. *J Am Acad Dermatol*. 2002;47(1):p. 1-17; quiz 18-20.
16. Brewer JD, Colegio OR, Phillips PK, et al. Incidence of and risk factors for skin cancer after heart transplant. *Arch Dermatol*. 2009;145(12):1391-1396.
17. Chahal HS, Wu W, Ransohoff KJ, et al. Genome-wide association study identifies 14 novel risk alleles associated with basal cell carcinoma. *Nat Commun*. 2016;7:12510.
18. Pinkus H. Epithelial and fibroepithelial tumors. *Arch Dermatol*. 1965;91:24-37.
19. Scrivener Y, Grosshans E, Cribier B. Variations of basal cell carcinomas according to gender, age, location and histopathological subtype. *Br J Dermatol*. 2002;147(1):41-47.
20. Raasch BA, Buettner PG, Garbe C. Basal cell carcinoma: histological classification and body-site distribution. *Br J Dermatol*. 2006;155(2):401-407.
21. McCormack CJ, Kelly JW, Dorevitch AP. Differences in age and body site distribution of the histological subtypes of basal cell carcinoma. A possible indicator of differing causes. *Arch Dermatol*. 1997;133(5):593-596.
22. Bath-Hextall FJ, Perkins W, Bong J, et al. Interventions for basal cell carcinoma of the skin. *Cochrane Database Syst Rev*. 2007;(1):CD003412.
23. Mosterd K, Krekels GA, Nieman FH, et al. Surgical excision versus Mohs' micrographic surgery for primary and recurrent basal-cell carcinoma of the face: a prospective randomised controlled trial with 5-years' follow-up. *Lancet Oncol*. 2008;9(12):1149-1156.
24. Rowe DE, Carroll RJ, Day CL Jr. Long-term recurrence rates in previously untreated (primary) basal cell carcinoma: implications for patient follow-up. *J Dermatol Surg Oncol*. 1989;15(3):315-328.
25. Leibovitch I, Huilgol SC, Selva D, et al. Basal cell carcinoma treated with Mohs surgery in Australia II. Outcome at 5-year follow-up. *J Am Acad Dermatol*. 2005;53(3):452-457.
26. NCCN.org. *NCCN Clinical Practice Guidelines in Oncology (NCCN Guidelines) Basal Cell and Squamous Cell Skin Cancers*. Version 2.2014.
27. Smeets NW, Kuijpers DI, Nelemans P, et al. Mohs' micrographic surgery for treatment of basal cell carcinoma of the face—results of a retrospective study and review of the literature. *Br J Dermatol*. 2004;151(1):141-147.
28. Ceilley RI, Del Rosso JQ. Current modalities and new advances in the treatment of basal cell carcinoma. *Int J Dermatol*. 2006;45(5):489-498.
29. Rowe DE, Carroll RJ, Day CL Jr. Mohs surgery is the treatment of choice for recurrent (previously treated) basal cell carcinoma. *J Dermatol Surg Oncol*. 1989;15(4):424-431.
30. Linos E, Parvataneni R, Stuart SE, et al. Treatment of nonfatal conditions at the end of life: nonmelanoma skin cancer. *JAMA Intern Med*. 2013;173(11):1006-1012.
31. Asgari MM, Bertenthal D, Sen S, et al. Patient satisfaction after treatment of nonmelanoma skin cancer. *Dermatol Surg*. 2009;35(7):1041-1049.
32. Fernandes JD, de Lorenzo Messina MC, de Almeida Pimentel ER, et al. Presence of residual basal cell carcinoma in re-excised specimens is more probable when deep and lateral margins were positive. *J Eur Acad Dermatol Venereol*. 2008;22(6):704-706.
33. Kopf AW, Bart RS, Schrager D, et al. Curettage-electrodesiccation treatment of basal cell carcinomas. *Arch Dermatol*. 1977;113(4):439-443.
34. Rodriguez-Vigil T, Vazquez-Lopez F, Perez-Oliva N. Recurrence rates of primary basal cell carcinoma in facial risk areas treated with curettage and electrodesiccation. *J Am Acad Dermatol*. 2007. 56(1):91-95.
35. Thissen MR, Neumann MH, Schouten LJ. A systematic review of treatment modalities for primary basal cell carcinomas. *Arch Dermatol*. 1999;135(10):1177-1183.
36. Kuflik EG, Gage AA. The five-year cure rate achieved by cryosurgery for skin cancer. *J Am Acad Dermatol*. 1991;24(6 Pt 1):1002-1004.
37. Thissen MR, Nieman FH, Ideler AH, et al. Cosmetic results of cryosurgery versus surgical excision for primary uncomplicated basal cell carcinomas of the head and neck. *Dermatol Surg*. 2000;26(8):759-764.
38. Geisse J, Caro I, Lindholm J, et al. Imiquimod 5% cream for the treatment of superficial basal cell carcinoma: results from two phase III, randomized, vehicle-controlled studies. *J Am Acad Dermatol*. 2004;50(5):722-733.
39. Geisse JK, Rich P, Pandya A, et al. Imiquimod 5% cream for the treatment of superficial basal cell carcinoma: a double-blind, randomized, vehicle-controlled study. *J Am Acad Dermatol*. 2002;47(3):390-398.
40. Peri K, Campione E, Micantonio T, et al. Imiquimod treatment of superficial and nodular basal cell carcinoma: 12-week open-label trial. *Dermatol Surg*. 2005;31(3):318-323.

41. Murphy ME, Brodland DG, Zitelli JA. Definitive surgical treatment of 24 skin cancers not cured by prior imiquimod therapy: a case series. *Dermatol Surg*. 2008;34(9):1258-1263.
42. Epstein E. Fluorouracil paste treatment of thin basal cell carcinomas. *Arch Dermatol*. 1985;121(2):207-213.
43. Gross K, Kircik L, Kricorian G. 5% 5-Fluorouracil cream for the treatment of small superficial Basal cell carcinoma: efficacy, tolerability, cosmetic outcome, and patient satisfaction. *Dermatol Surg*. 2007; 33(4):433-439; discussion 440.
44. Basset-Seguin N, Ibbotson SH, Emtestam L, et al. Topical methyl aminolaevulinate photodynamic therapy versus cryotherapy for superficial basal cell carcinoma: a 5 year randomized trial. *Eur J Dermatol*. 2008;18(5):547-553.
45. Marmur ES, Schmults CD, Goldberg DJ. A review of laser and photodynamic therapy for the treatment of nonmelanoma skin cancer. *Dermatol Surg*. 2004; 30(2 Pt 2):264-271.
46. Szeimies RM. Methyl aminolevulinate-photodynamic therapy for basal cell carcinoma. *Dermatol Clin*. 2007; 25(1):89-94.
47. Arits AH, Mosterd K, Essers BA, et al. Photodynamic therapy versus topical imiquimod versus topical fluorouracil for treatment of superficial basal-cell carcinoma: a single blind, non-inferiority, randomised controlled trial. *Lancet Oncol*. 2013;14(7):647-654.
48. Avril MF, Auperin A, Margulis A, et al. Basal cell carcinoma of the face: surgery or radiotherapy? Results of a randomized study. *Br J Cancer*. 1997;76(1):100-106.
49. Dunn M, Morgan MB, Beer TW. Perineural invasion: identification, significance, and a standardized definition. *Dermatol Surg*. 2009;35(2):214-221.
50. Sherman JE, Talmor M. Slow progression and sequential documentation of a giant basal cell carcinoma of the face. *Surgery*. 2001;130(1):90-92.
51. Wysong A, Aasi SZ, Tang JY. Update on metastatic basal cell carcinoma: a summary of published cases from 1981 through 2011. *JAMA Dermatol*. 2013;149(5): 615-616.
52. Sekulic A, Migden MR, Lewis K, et al. Pivotal ERIVANCE basal cell carcinoma (BCC) study: 12-month update of efficacy and safety of vismodegib in advanced BCC. *J Am Acad Dermatol*. 2015;72(6):1021-6;e8.
53. Von Hoff DD, LoRusso PM, Rudin CM, et al. Inhibition of the hedgehog pathway in advanced basal-cell carcinoma. *N Engl J Med*. 2009;361(12):1164-1172.
54. Migden MR, Guminski A, Gutzmer R, et al. Treatment with two different doses of sonidegib in patients with locally advanced or metastatic basal cell carcinoma (BOLT): a multicentre, randomised, double-blind phase 2 trial. *Lancet Oncol*. 2015;16(6):716-728.
55. von Domarus H, Stevens PJ. Metastatic basal cell carcinoma. Report of five cases and review of 170 cases in the literature. *J Am Acad Dermatol*. 1984; 10(6):1043-1060.
56. Elghissassi I, Mikou A, Inrhaoun H, et al. Metastatic basal cell carcinoma to the bone and bone marrow. *Int J Dermatol*. 2009;48(5):481-483.
57. Carneiro BA, Watkin WG, Mehta UK, et al. Metastatic basal cell carcinoma: complete response to chemotherapy and associated pure red cell aplasia. *Cancer Invest*. 2006;24(4):396-400.
58. Williams JA, Guicherit OM, Zaharian BI, et al. Identification of a small molecule inhibitor of the hedgehog signaling pathway: effects on basal cell carcinoma-like lesions. *Proc Natl Acad Sci UA*. 2003;100(8): 4616-4621.
59. Rudin CM, Hann CL, Laterra J, et al. Treatment of medulloblastoma with hedgehog pathway inhibitor GDC-0449. *N Engl J Med*. 2009;361(12):1173-1178.
60. Atwood SX, Sarin KY, Whitson RJ, et al. Smoothened variants explain the majority of drug resistance in basal cell carcinoma. *Cancer Cell*. 2015;27(3): 342-353.
61. Atwood SX, Chang AL, Oro AE. Hedgehog pathway inhibition and the race against tumor evolution. *J Cell Biol*. 2012;199(2):193-197.
62. Sharpe HJ, Pau G, Dijkgraaf GJ, et al. Genomic analysis of smoothened inhibitor resistance in basal cell carcinoma. *Cancer Cell*. 2015;27(3):327-341.
63. Madan V, Lear JT, Szeimies RM. Non-melanoma skin cancer. *Lancet*. 2010;375(9715):673-685.
64. Chen AC, Martin AJ, Damian DL. Nicotinamide for skin-cancer chemoprevention. *N Engl J Med*. 2016; 374(8):790.
65. Elmets CA, Viner JL, Pentland AP, et al. Chemoprevention of nonmelanoma skin cancer with celecoxib: a randomized, double-blind, placebo-controlled trial. *J Natl Cancer Inst*. 2010;102(24):1835-1844.
66. Gorlin RJ. Nevoid basal-cell carcinoma syndrome. *Medicine (Baltimore)*. 1987;66(2):98-113.
67. Gorlin RJ, Goltz RW. Multiple nevoid basal-cell epithelioma, jaw cysts and bifid rib. A syndrome. *N Engl J Med*. 1960;262:908-912.
68. Howell JB, Caro MR. The basal-cell nevus: its relationship to multiple cutaneous cancers and associated anomalies of development. *AMA Arch Derm*. 1959;79(1):67-77; discussion 77-80.
69. Farndon PA, Morris DJ, Hardy C, et al. Analysis of 133 meioses places the genes for nevoid basal cell carcinoma (Gorlin) syndrome and Fanconi anemia group C in a 2.6-cM interval and contributes to the fine map of 9q22.3. *Genomics*. 1994;23(2): 486-489.
70. Shanley S, Ratcliffe J, Hockey A, et al. Nevoid basal cell carcinoma syndrome: review of 118 affected individuals. *Am J Med Genet*. 1994;50(3):282-290.
71. Evans DG, Ladusans EJ, Rimmer S, et al. Complications of the naevoid basal cell carcinoma syndrome: results of a population based study. *J Med Genet*. 1993;30(6):460-464.
72. Hahn H, Wicking C, Zaphiropoulous PG, et al. Mutations of the human homolog of Drosophila patched in the nevoid basal cell carcinoma syndrome. *Cell*. 1996;85:841-851.
73. Johnson RL, Rothman AL, Xie J, et al. Human homolog of patched, a candidate gene for the basal cell nevus syndrome. *Science*. 1996;272(5268): 1668-1671.
74. Ingham PW. Hedgehog signalling. *Curr Biol*. 2008; 18(6):R238-R241.
75. Howell JB. Nevoid basal cell carcinoma syndrome. Profile of genetic and environmental factors in oncogenesis. *J Am Acad Dermatol*. 1984;11(1):98-104.
76. Goodrich LV, Milenković L, Higgins KM, et al. Altered neural cell fates and medulloblastoma in mouse patched mutants. *Science*. 1997;277(5329): 1109-1113.
77. Hahn H, Wicking C, Zaphiropoulous PG, et al. Mutations of the human homolog of Drosophila patched

in the nevoid basal cell carcinoma syndrome. *Cell*. 1996;85(6):841-851.
78. Hahn H, Wojnowski L, Zimmer AM, et al. Rhabdomyosarcomas and radiation hypersensitivity in a mouse model of Gorlin syndrome. *Nat Med*. 1998;4(5):619-622.
79. Kimonis VE, Goldstein AM, Pastakia B, et al. Clinical manifestations in 105 persons with nevoid basal cell carcinoma syndrome. *Am J Med Genet*. 1997;69(3):299-308.
80. Pruvost-Balland C, Gorry P, Boutet N, et al. Etude clinique et recherche de mutations germinales du gene PTCH1 dans le syndrome des harmatomaes basocellulaires. *Ann Dermatol Venereol*. 2006;113:117-123.
81. Pastorino L, Ghiorzo P, Nasti S, et al. Identification of a SUFU germline mutation in a family with Gorlin syndrome. *Am J Med Genet A*. 2009;149A(7):1539-1543.
82. Smith MJ, Beetz C, Williams SG, et al. Germline mutations in SUFU cause Gorlin syndrome–associated childhood medulloblastoma and redefine the risk associated with PTCH1 mutations. *J Clin Oncol*. 2014;32(36):4155-4161.
83. Oro AE. Mammalian variations on a theme: a Smo and Sufu surprise. *Dev Cell*. 2006;10(2):156-158.
84. Taipale J, Cooper MK, Maiti T, et al. Patched acts catalytically to suppress the activity of Smoothened. *Nature*. 2002;418(6900):892-897.
85. Rohatgi R, Milenkovic L, Scott MP. Patched1 regulates hedgehog signaling at the primary cilium. *Science*. 2007;317(5836):372-376.
86. Ling G, Ahmadian A, Persson A, et al. PATCHED and p53 gene alterations in sporadic and hereditary basal cell cancer. *Oncogene*. 2001;20(53):7770-7778.
87. Xie J, Murone M, Luoh SM, et al. Activating Smoothened mutations in sporadic basal-cell carcinoma. *Nature*. 1998;391(6662):90-92.
88. Taylor MD, Liu L, Raffel C, et al. Mutations in SUFU predispose to medulloblastoma. *Nat Genet*. 2002;31(3):306-310.
89. Aszterbaum M, Epstein J, Oro A, et al. Ultraviolet and ionizing radiation enhance the growth of BCCs and trichoblastomas in patched heterozygous knockout mice. *Nat Med*. 1999;5(11):1285-1291.
90. Sun LS, Li XF, Li TJ. PTCH1 and SMO gene alterations in keratocystic odontogenic tumors. *J Dent Res*. 2008;87(6):575-579.
91. Shear M. The aggressive nature of the odontogenic keratocyst: is it a benign cystic neoplasm? Part 2. Proliferation and genetic studies. *Oral Oncol*. 2002;38(4):323-331.
92. Wicking C, Shanley S, Smyth I, et al. Most germline mutations in the nevoid basal cell carcinoma syndrome lead to a premature termination of the PATCHED protein, and no genotype-phenotype correlations are evident. *Am J Hum Genet*. 1997;60(1):21-26.
93. Goeteyn M, Geerts ML, Kint A, et al. The Bazex-Dupre-Christol syndrome. *Arch Dermatol*. 1994;130(3):337-342.
94. Ashinoff R, Jacobson M, Belsito DV. Rombo syndrome: a second case report and review. *J Am Acad Dermatol*. 1993;28(6):1011-1014.
95. Oley CA, Sharpe H, Chenevix-Trench G. Basal cell carcinomas, coarse sparse hair, and milia. *Am J Med Genet*. 1992;43(5):799-804.
96. Requena L, Fariña MC, Robledo M, et al. Multiple hereditary infundibulocystic basal cell carcinomas: a genodermatosis different from nevoid basal cell carcinoma syndrome. *Arch Dermatol*. 1999;135(10):1227-1235.
97. Jih DM, Shapiro M, James WD, et al. Familial basaloid follicular hamartoma: lesional characterization and review of the literature. *Am J Dermatopathol*. 2003;25(2):130-137.
98. Schulman JM, Oh DH, Sanborn JZ, et al. Multiple hereditary infundibulocystic basal cell carcinoma syndrome associated with a germline SUFU mutation. *JAMA Dermatol*. 2016;152(3):323-327.
99. Mann K, Magee J, Guillaud-Bataille M, et al. Multiple skin hamartomata: a possible novel clinical presentation of SUFU neoplasia syndrome. *Fam Cancer*. 2015;14(1):151-155.
100. Cho HG, Kuo KY, Epstein E, et al. Inherited cancer susceptibility mutations in individuals who develop high frequency of basal cell carcinomas [abstract]. Portland, OR, Society of Investigative Dermatology, April 26-29, 2017.
101. Cho HG, Kuo KY, Li S, et al. Frequent basal cell cancer development is a clinical marker for inherited cancer susceptibility. *JCI Insight*. 2018;3(15):e122744.
102. Kimonis VE, Mehta SG, Digiovanna JJ, et al. Radiological features in 82 patients with nevoid basal cell carcinoma (NBCC or Gorlin) syndrome. *Genet Med*. 2004;6(6):495-502.
103. Ionescu DN, Arida M, Jukic DM. Metastatic basal cell carcinoma: four case reports, review of literature, and immunohistochemical evaluation. *Arch Pathol Lab Med*. 2006;130(1):45-51.
104. Oro AE, Higgins KM. Hair cycle regulation of Hedgehog signal reception. *Dev Biol*. 2003;255(2):238-248.
105. Reymann F. Treatment of basal cell carcinoma of the skin with 5-fluorouracil ointment. A 10-year follow-up study. *Dermatologica*. 1979;158(5):368-372.
106. Stockfleth E, Ulrich C, Hauschild A, et al. Successful treatment of basal cell carcinomas in a nevoid basal cell carcinoma syndrome with topical 5% imiquimod. *Eur J Dermatol*. 2002;12(6):569-572.
107. Wilson BD, Mang TS, Stoll H, et al. Photodynamic therapy for the treatment of basal cell carcinoma. *Arch Dermatol*. 1992;128(12):1597-1601.
108. Tang JY, Mackay-Wiggan JM, Aszterbaum M, et al. Inhibiting the hedgehog pathway in patients with the basal-cell nevus syndrome. *N Engl J Med*. 2012;366(23):2180-2188.
109. Tang JY, Ally MS, Chanana AM, et al. Inhibiting the hedgehog pathway in patients with basal-cell nevus syndrome: final results from the 36-month trial. *Lancet Oncol*. 2016;17(12):1720-1731.

Chapter 112 :: Squamous Cell Carcinoma and Keratoacanthoma
:: Anke S. Lonsdorf & Eva N. Hadaschik

第一百一十二章
鳞状细胞癌和角化棘皮瘤

中文导读

本章介绍了鳞状细胞癌的相关知识，分为8节：①流行病学和人口学；②病因和发病机制；③临床表现；④诊断；⑤分级；⑥鉴别诊断；⑦临床管理；⑧预防。

第一节流行病学和人口学，介绍了鳞状细胞癌的发病率、死亡率、地理因素、年龄、性别、及人种的特征。

第二节病因和发病机制，介绍了前驱病变、危险因素，详细介绍了危险因素包括紫外线辐射、遗传易感性、物理和化学致癌物、免疫抑制、药物、病毒感染、皮肤慢性炎症和慢性损伤、分子层面的因素。

第三节临床表现，介绍了经典表现及特殊部位的表现，其中包括口腔、唇、疣状鳞状细胞癌、角化棘皮瘤等的表现，认为角化棘皮瘤为鳞状细胞癌的一种特殊表现。

第四节诊断，介绍了标准的鳞状细胞癌组织病理学报告应包括的具体内容：组织病理学中的一般问题、基本组织病理学特征、亚型与鉴别诊断。

第五节分级，介绍了组织学分级对于复发和转移的风险是非常重要的，目前沿用的是美国癌症联合委员会(AJCC)的分类和1932年Broders提出的基于细胞分化程度的鳞癌组织学分级。

第六节鉴别诊断，介绍了根据鳞状细胞癌的部位和类型，需要排除不同的鉴别诊断。

第七节临床管理，介绍了原发病灶的治疗方式是局部复发风险的主要决定因素，主要手段包括手术和非手术干预。介绍了早期治愈率高，预后良好。确诊时局部晚期鳞癌和一线手术治疗后进展性疾病的患者的预后一般较差。总体预后包括局部复发、转移、鳞癌的高危病变及预后危险因素、院后护理、继发性皮肤肿瘤。

第八节预防，介绍了鳞状细胞癌在很大程度上是可以预防的。避免阳光照射和密切监测高危人群的皮肤病是预防鳞癌的关键因素。

〔粟 娟〕

AT-A-GLANCE

- Squamous cell carcinoma (SCC) is the second most common skin cancer, after basal cell carcinoma, in immunocompetent white individuals, and the most common skin cancer in immunosuppressed organ transplantation recipients worldwide.

- SCC development in the skin is considered a multistep process, most invasive SCCs develop from preinvasive lesions or in situ tumors such as actinic keratosis or Bowen disease.

- Risk factors for SCC include ultraviolet (UV) radiation, genetic predisposition, physical and chemical carcinogens, immunosuppression, drugs, viral infection, chronic inflammation, and chronic injury of the skin.

- Diagnosis of SCC is established histologically. Histologic subtypes include spindle-cell, acantholytic, verrucous, and desmoplastic SCCs, and keratoacanthoma.

- High-risk features for local recurrence and the development of metastatic disease include >2 mm thickness; Clark level higher than IV; perineural invasion; lip or ear as primary site; poorly or undifferentiated tumor.

- The primary mode of therapy for localized SCC is complete surgical excision, preferentially microscopically controlled surgery (Mohs surgery). Nonsurgical interventions include topical therapy, and for locally advanced, unresectable or metastatic SCC, radiation therapy and systemic treatment with chemotherapy or targeted therapy.

- Primary prevention for the development of SCC is based on decreasing UV radiation exposure and concomitant risk factors, and the effective treatment of precursor lesions. Systemic retinoids, niacinamide, as well as change of the immunosuppressive regimen in solid-organ transplantation recipients may be options for the secondary prevention of SCC in high-risk patients.

EPIDEMIOLOGY AND DEMOGRAPHICS

An accurate incidence of squamous cell carcinoma (SCC) is unknown, but the cancer is among the most common and costly malignancies in populations of European ancestry.[1] The morbidity and mortality of SCC seem to be rather underestimated public health issues,[2] and the health burden is considerable, particularly when considering high-risk populations, such as immunosuppressed patients, in which a 65-fold to 250-fold increased incidence of SCC has been reported.[3,4]

INCIDENCE

The accurate incidence of SCC is unknown as the majority of cancer registries in most countries do not generally document nonmelanoma skin cancers (NMSCs) and statistics frequently fail to include any subsequent tumors after the first SCC and to discriminate between cutaneous and mucosal SCC. However, assuming that 20% of NMSCs are SCCs,[5,6] the estimated annual incidence of SCC in the United States is 700,000 cases. Therefore, SCC is, after basal cell carcinoma (BCC), the second most common skin cancer in immunocompetent white individuals and the most common skin cancer in immunosuppressed organ transplantation recipients worldwide.[7] The incidence of SCC is steadily rising, with reported increases of 50% to 200% over the past 3 decades; this rise is largely attributed to a greater lifetime ultraviolet radiation (UVR) exposure as a result of greater longevity, ozone depletion, and increased voluntary exposure to UVR.[8]

MORBIDITY AND MORTALITY

The vast majority of SCC patients present with early-stage disease, and prognosis is excellent in the majority of cases. Most SCCs are readily treated and cured with surgery. However, after a diagnosis of SCC, patients have an increased risk of developing secondary NMSC.

The risk of developing metastasis from SCC is generally low, with a 5-year metastatic rate of 5%.[9] Metastases are predominantly nodal.[10] However, depending on patient and tumor characteristics, certain subgroups of patients are at significantly higher risk for metastasis, with metastatic rates of up to 30% in some subgroups (see 'Prognosis').[9] Outcome is particularly poor for metastatic disease, and SCC accounts for the vast majority of deaths attributed to NMSC.[5]

GEOGRAPHIC FACTORS

Geographic variation in the incidence of SCC is largely attributed to ambient UV irradiation as suggested by the reported inverse association with latitude.[5,7] Ethnicity and skin type have an effect on incidence rates and therefore reported incidence rates worldwide may somewhat reflect the geographical distribution of ethnicity and skin type; however, within countries, the closer to the equator the higher the incidence of SCC in white individuals with similar gradients for both genders and all ages.[5,7] With a reported rate of 387 per 100,000 person-years, Australians, exposed to very high, long-term UVR levels, are more likely to develop SCC than other populations in countries with more intermittent UVR exposure such as the United Kingdom.[7,11] Altitude also has an effect on SCC incidence; Switzerland has the highest altitude of all mainland Europe and reportedly the highest SCC incidence rates, as well as showing the fastest increase.[7]

AGE

SCC incidence increases with age and mostly affects individuals 60 years of age and older.[12] As the cumulative lifetime exposure to UVR is thought to be the predominant etiologic risk factor for skin carcinogenesis, the age shift in the population along with lifestyle changes (ie, increased voluntary exposure to UVR) during the past decades have been suggested to be major causes of the overall increase in total numbers of SCC in most countries.[5]

SEX

The incidence of SCC is higher in men than in women[5] and is attributed to a greater lifetime UVR exposure in men. However, studies on the role of functional polymorphisms in UV-induced immunosuppression pathways have suggested the existence of a gender-based differential genetic susceptibility to UV-induced immunosuppression and the risk for SCC.[13]

RACE

Sun-sensitive individuals with red hair, blue eyes, and fair complexion are at higher risk for developing SCC than individuals with darker pigmentation. Even though SCC is the most common skin cancer phenotype in American blacks, the incidence of SCC is decreased by 30-fold compared to whites, with SCC typically arising on non–sun-exposed skin at sites of predisposing skin conditions.[14] Albinism is associated with a high risk for SCC, even in black individuals, which provides further evidence for the relationships between skin carcinogenesis and sun-exposure and the protective effect of eumelanin in the skin.[15]

ETIOLOGY AND PATHOGENESIS

Figure 112-1 is a schematic of SCC etiology/pathophysiology. Table 112-1 outlines the syndromes and genes associated with a predisposition for SCC and/or keratoacanthoma (KA).

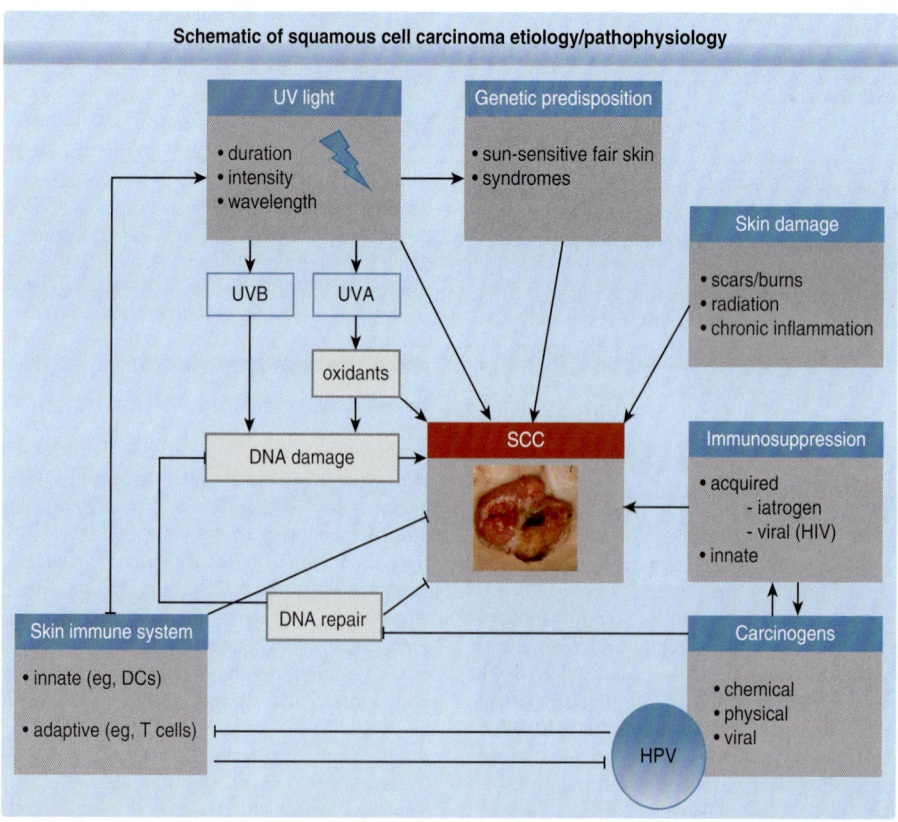

Figure 112-1 Schematic of squamous cell carcinoma (SCC) etiology/pathophysiology.

TABLE 112-1
Syndromes and Genes Associated with a Predisposition for Squamous Cell Carcinoma and/or Keratoacanthoma

DISEASE/SYNDROME	GENE(S)	MAIN FUNCTION
Squamous Cell Carcinoma		
Bloom syndrome	BLM/RECQL3	Maintenance of chromosomal stability
Dyskeratosis congenita (Zinsser-Cole-Engman syndrome)	DKC1, TERC, TINF2, NHP2/NOLA2	Telomere homeostasis and trafficking of telomerase
Epidermodysplasia verruciformis (EV)	EVER1/TMC6, EVER2/TMC8	Regulation of zinc homeostasis, signal transduction in endoplasmic reticulum
Epidermolysis bullosa (EB) (a) Dystrophic EB (DEB) (b) Junctional EB (JEB)	(a) COL7A1 (b) LAMA3, LAMB3, LAMC2, COL17A1	(a) Anchoring of basement membrane to dermis (b) Anchoring of epidermis to basement membrane, connective tissue
Fanconi anemia	FANCA, FANCB, FANCC, FANCD1/BRCA2, FANCD2, FANCE, FANCF, FANCG/XRCC9, FANCI, FANCJ/BACH1, FANCL/PHF9, FANCM, FANCN/PALB2, FANCO/RAD51C, FANKP/SLX4, FANCQ/ERCC4, FANCS	DNA crosslink repair
Oculocutaneous albinism (OCA)	TYR, OCA2, MATP/OCA4, TYRP1, Locus 4q24, SLC24A5, C10Orf11	Melanin synthesis
Other syndromes associated with albinism/decreased pigmentation of the skin: (a) Chediak-Higashi syndrome (b) Elejalde disease (c) Griscelli syndrome (d) Hermansky-Pudlak syndrome	(a) LYST (b) MYO5A (c) MYO5A, RAB27A, MLPH (d) HPS1, HPS3, HPS4, HPS5, HPS6, HPS7/DTNBP1, HPS8/BLOC1S3	(a) Regulation of lysosomal transport (b) Transport of pigment granule (c) Transport of pigment granule (d) Melanosomal and lysosomal storage
Rothmund-Thomson syndrome	RECQL4, C16orf57	Maintenance of chromosomal stability
Werner syndrome	WRN/RECQL2	Maintenance of chromosomal stability
Xeroderma pigmentosum (XP)	XPA, XPB/ERCC3, XPC, XPD/ERCC2, XPE/DDB2, XPF/ERCC4, XPG/ERCC5, XPG	Nucleotide excision repair
XP variant	POLH/XPV	Error-prone DNA polymerase
Keratoacanthoma		
Muir-Torre syndrome	MSH1, MSH2	DNA mismatch repair
Multiple self-healing squamous epithelioma (Ferguson–Smith syndrome)	TGFBR1	Transforming growth factor β–receptor 1 signaling

Information adapted from the National Cancer Institute Database, available at http://www.cancer.gov.

PRECURSOR LESIONS

SCCs are thought to typically arise from basal keratinocytes of the interfollicular epidermis. SCC development in the skin is considered a multistep process, and most invasive SCCs develop from preinvasive lesions or in situ tumors, such as actinic keratosis (AK) or Bowen disease (see Chap. 110).[16] Although the cumulative risk depends on the number of lesions and the length of time they persist, estimates of the annual rate per AK of progression into invasive disease range from 0.025% to 20%.[17,18] The estimated cumulative lifetime risk among patients with multiple AK is approximately 6% to 10%.[19]

Other noninvasive, precancerous conditions that may evolve into SCC include bowenoid papulosis and erythroplasia of Queyrat.

KA is a squamous neoplasm characterized by a rapid growth phase and subsequent slow spontaneous regression and is controversially discussed in the classical sequence of skin carcinogenesis.[20]

RISK FACTORS

The risk for SCC development is attributed to genotypic, phenotypic, and environmental factors. UVR is classified by the IARC (International Agency for Research on Cancer) as a class I carcinogen, sufficient for the initiation, promotion, and progression of squamous carcinogenesis of the skin,[21] and the most important environmental risk factor for SCC. Other major risk factors predisposing for SCC include exposure to physical and chemical carcinogens, genetic predisposition and immunosuppression (Table 112-2).

ULTRAVIOLET RADIATION

Exposure to UVR (both UVB and UVA) has been recognized as the most important environmental risk factor for the development of SCC with a strong dose–response association,[5,22] as suggested by the preferential localization of AK and SCC on sun-exposed and chronically photodamaged sites and in sun-sensitive

TABLE 112-2
Risk Factors for the Development of Squamous Cell Carcinoma

RISK FACTOR	EXAMPLES
Carcinoma in situ and precursor lesions	- Actinic keratoses - Bowen disease - Erythroplasia of Queyrat - Bowenoid papulosis
Physical and chemical carcinogens	- Ultraviolet (UV) radiation (UVA and UVB) - Ionizing irradiation - Arsenic - Polycyclic aromatic hydrocarbons
Genetic predisposition	- Skin phenotype (sun-sensitive, fair skin complexion) - Oculocutaneous albinism - Xeroderma pigmentosum (XP) - Epidermodysplasia verruciformis (EV) - Recessive dystrophic epidermolysis bullosa (RDEB)
Immunosuppression	- Iatrogenic immunosuppression (eg, solid-organ transplantation recipients, patients with autoimmune or rheumatoid disease) - Hematopoietic stem cell transplantation - Infection with HIV/AIDS - Chronic lymphatic leukemia (CLL)
Drugs	- Immunosuppressive drugs (eg, azathioprine, cyclosporine) - Photosensitizing drugs (eg, doxycycline, fluoroquinolone, triazole antifungals) - Targeted therapies (eg, BRAF [v-raf murine sarcoma viral oncogene homolog B] inhibitors vemurafenib and dabrafenib; tyrosine kinase inhibitor sorafenib; hedgehog pathway inhibitor vismodegib)
Chronic inflammation and chronic injury of the skin	- Chronic ulcers - Burn scars - Discoid lupus erythematodes - Lichen ruber mucosae - Lichen sclerosus - Lupus vulgaris - Infection with human papillomavirus (HPV) - RDEB

phenotypes (ie, patients with fair complexions) with increasing age and high cumulative UV irradiation.

UVB-induced mutagenesis of the skin gives rise to specific UV signature mutations (ie, characteristic C-T and CC-TT dipyrimidine transitions), which constitute the majority of mutations found in SCC.[23] Genotoxicity of UVA radiation seems mostly to indirectly add to the risk, primarily by photooxidative stress-mediated mechanisms such as the induction of reactive oxygen species in the skin.[24,25]

In addition to the mutagenic effects, UVR is thought to promote SCC development by its immunosuppressive and immunomodulatory properties, such as depletion of Langerhans cells from the epidermis, improper antigen presentation in skin-draining lymph nodes, and hindered tumor surveillance by the expansion of tumor antigen-specific regulatory T cells and a shift toward T-helper cell type 2 responses in UV-irradiated skin.[13]

GENETIC PREDISPOSITION

Genetic factors may critically potentiate the risk conveyed by environmental risk factors such as UVR. Clinical skin phenotype is defined by constitutive and facultative pigmentation, which are controlled by more than 150 genes.[23] Light skin complexion (as in skin photo types I and II) and the underlying genetic variations in the melanocortin-1 receptor, predispose for UV sensitivity of the skin and are associated with a high incidence of SCC.[26] Single-nucleotide polymorphisms in pigmentation genes, such as *tyrosinase (TYR)* required for melanization in melanosomes, are significantly associated with SCC risk.[13,27,28]

Oculocutaneous albinism, which is characterized by impaired melanin biosynthesis, is the most common inherited pigmentary disorder of the skin and is associated with an increased risk of developing SCC, particularly in sun-exposed skin areas.[15] Black albinos in sub-Saharan Africa are at approximately a 1000-fold higher risk of developing SCC of the skin than the general population.[15]

The incidence of SCC is also highly elevated in other genetic skin disorders.[10] Patients with recessive dystrophic epidermolysis bullosa (RDEB), a skin fragility disorder caused by mutations in the *COL7A1* gene encoding collagen VII, are at high risk for developing aggressive SCC. In the most-severe form of RDEB, the cumulative risk of SCC is greater than 90% by age 55 years and 80% of RDEB patients die from metastasis within 5 years after their first SCC.[29]

A genetic predisposition to SCC is well recognized in certain family cancer syndromes, and inherited defects in DNA repair and genomic stability, such as aberrations in nucleotide excision repair genes *XPA-G* and *XP-V* (xeroderma pigmentosum), *PTEN* (Cowden syndrome), *FANCA-N* (Fanconi anemia), *TP53* (Li-Fraumeni syndrome), *RECQL4* (Rothmund-Thomson syndrome), *WRN* (Werner syndrome), telomere maintenance (dyskeratosis congenita), and mammalian mismatch repair (Muir-Torre syndrome).[23]

A 40-year followup found that patients with xeroderma pigmentosum before age 20 years had a more than 10,000-fold increase in NMSC, especially at UV-exposed sites.[30]

PHYSICAL AND CHEMICAL CARCINOGENS

Historically, the exposure to occupational and environmental carcinogenic agents has been a major cause of SCC.[9] Arsenic, used in various medications, tainted wine, and unprocessed well water may stimulate skin carcinogenesis.[31] Cutting oils constitute a risk of SCC development in certain industrial occupations and the high incidence of SCC on the scrotum of chimney sweeps is attributed to chronic exposure to ash and polycyclic aromatic hydrocarbons derived from carbon compounds such as coal tar.[9]

In addition to the significant contribution of UVR, ionizing irradiation also is implicated in the pathogenesis of SCC, based on studies on ionizing irradiation being used for the treatment of acne, hemangiomas, and other skin conditions, and workers in certain medical or industrial fields who may be exposed to ionizing irradiation. The latency period for SCC development in patients with chronic radiation dermatitis is typically long (approximately 30 years).[32] The risk for SCC is reported to be directly related to the cumulative dose of ionizing radiation.[9]

IMMUNOSUPPRESSION

Innate and acquired immunosuppression dramatically increases the risk of developing SCC.[33] Immunosuppression is reported as a risk factor for high tumor burden,[34] metastatic disease,[35] and disease-specific death from SCC.[36]

Long-term immunosuppressed patients, such as in solid-organ transplantation recipients (OTRs),[33] hematopoietic stem-cell transplant recipients,[37] and patients with HIV or a history of autoimmune or rheumatoid disease,[38] are at increased risk for SCC of the skin. In OTRs, the most frequent malignancy is skin cancers, 95% of which are NMSC, mostly SCC.[33] The ratio of SCC to basal cell carcinoma (BCC) reverses in immunosuppressed patients, with SCC being the most frequent NMSC; in the general population, BCC occurs 6 times more frequently than SCC.[3,33] SCC in OTRs occur predominantly in sun-exposed skin in areas of field cancerization and appear an average of 2 to 4 years after transplantation.[39] OTRs have been reported to have an up to 65-fold increase in the incidence of SCC,[3] an increased risk for high tumor burden[34] and developing multiple and aggressive, high-risk histologic subtypes of SCC, and a poorer outcome in advanced disease compared with the general population.[22,39] The incidence of SCC in OTRs in the United States and western Europe increases from 10% to 27% at 10 years after transplantation to 40% to 60% at 20 years after transplantation, compared to the highest incidence in Australia, which is 80% at 20 years after transplantation.[40] Type, duration, and intensity of the immunosuppressive regimen, as well as the age at transplantation, cumulative exposure to UVR, and skin type affect the risk for posttransplantation skin cancer.[40,41] Heart and lung transplantation recipients have a higher risk of SCC development than renal transplantation or liver transplantation recipients because of generally more intensive immunosuppressive regimens and older age at time of transplantation.[41] Revision of the immunosuppressive regimen, strict sun-protection measures, the early treatment of preinvasive and invasive NMSC, and close dermatologic surveillance is crucial in the management of high-risk immunosuppressed patients.[41]

DRUGS

The chronic use of photosensitizing drugs (eg, antibiotics, fluoroquinolone, triazole antifungals) and long-term therapy with psoralen plus UVA radiation for chronic inflammatory skin diseases increases the risk for SCC, particularly in patients with sun-sensitive skin types[42,43] and immunosuppressed patients such as OTRs.[41]

Substance-specific effects of immunosuppressive drugs are reported to affect the skin cancer risk independent of host immunity. Interference with cellular DNA repair, induction of oxidative stress, and upregulation of the $p53$ oncogene are reported mechanisms by which commonly used immunosuppressants may contribute to the elevated risk for SCC. Azathioprine, in particular, may drive photocarcinogenesis in the skin by synergizing with mutagenic UV(A)-induced DNA-damage and DNA repair.[44,45]

Conversely, a multicenter, randomized, controlled trial indicated that the mammalian target of rapamycin (mTOR) inhibitor sirolimus decreases the risk of developing secondary posttransplantation SCC and delays the occurrence of lesions in kidney transplantation recipients compared to cyclosporine-based immunosuppressive therapy.[46] Although the exact mechanisms for the antineoplastic properties of mTOR inhibitors in SCCs are unknown, mTOR inhibitors are reported to interrupt the phosphatidylinositide 3′-kinase (PI3K)–AKT pathway, which plays a critical role in the regulation of cell proliferation, survival, mobility, and angiogenesis, and may attenuate the pathway downstream of epidermal growth factor receptor (EGFR) signaling, which is frequently dysregulated in SCC.[23]

Although the conversion to a sirolimus-based immunosuppressive regimen may be limited by adverse side effects in some patients, it provides a strategy for the secondary skin cancer prevention in high-risk patients, such as OTRs.[46]

Drugs influencing the cell cycle, including v-raf murine sarcoma viral oncogene homolog B (BRAF)-inhibitors such as vemurafenib and dabrafenib, approved for the treatment of metastatic melanoma, and the kinase inhibitor sorafenib, are associated with the induction of rapidly developing well-differentiated SCC and/or eruptive KA as a side effect in up to 25% of patients.[47] A contribution of beta-human papillomavirus (HPV) infection and additional preexisting UV-induced somatic genetic alterations to the rapid-onset of SCC during BRAF-inhibition therapy has been suggested.[48,49] Likewise, the hedgehog pathway inhibitor vismodegib, approved for the targeted therapy for unresectable BCC, is reported to increase the risk for SCC with a hazard ratio of 8.12, accounting for age and basal cell nevus syndrome status,[50] highlighting the importance of continued skin surveillance after initiation of these therapies.

VIRAL INFECTION

Even though the exact role for HPVs in SCC pathogenesis remains poorly defined, HPVs have proposed to be a possible cocarcinogen in the development of SCC with environmental factors such as UVR. Epidemiologic studies suggest a link between these 2 factors in skin carcinogenesis[51,52] as a high prevalence of HPV DNA has been reported in sun-exposed skin in immunocompetent individuals.[51] Also, HPV prevalence and viral load are reportedly higher in AK compared to invasive SCC and normal-appearing skin, and HPVs, particularly of genus type beta, are believed to play a role in the initiation of SCC but may not be necessary for tumor maintenance.[53,54]

The oncogenic potential of HPV infection in SCC has been studied in epidermodysplasia verruciformis, an autosomal-recessive genodermatosis characterized by a high susceptibility for infection with predominantly beta-genus HPV-5 and HPV-8, and at high risk for developing SCC in chronically HPV-infected skin, particularly in sun-exposed areas.[51,55]

While the significance of specific types of alpha-genus HPV is well recognized in cervical and anogenital SCC, no specific cutaneous HPV subtypes have been clearly identified to be associated with cutaneous SCC because of the very high frequency of multiple infections.[1,52] Unlike the mucosal cancer–associated alpha-genus HPV, cutaneous beta-HPV is unable to integrate into the cellular DNA and is thought to convey its oncogenic potential indirectly by disturbing cellular DNA repair or apoptosis mechanisms, resulting in higher susceptibility for UV-induced damage in keratinocytes.[56-58] The oncogenicity of beta-HPV is largely attributed to a synergistic role between UV-induced DNA damage and the oncogenic potential of the viral proteins E6 and E7 to impair the tumor-suppressor function of p53 in keratinocytes (see section "Molecular Aspects").[53] The E6 proteins of certain HPV types of the beta genus are thought to prevent UV-induced apoptosis by degrading the proapoptotic protein Bak,[57,59] and some of the beta-HPV E6 proteins extend the life span of keratinocytes by activation of telomerase.[60] Conversely, UV light may have a transient immunosuppressive effect on skin predisposing for HPV infection and HPV viral immune evasion.[54] An increase in HPV prevalence was found in SCC from immunosuppressed patients compared with immunocompetent patients.[55]

KA, as a highly differentiated subtype of SCC has been proposed to represent a midpoint between a viral acanthoma and SCC.[61]

Even though its etiologic role remains to be elucidated, MCPyV polyoma virus, originally discovered in Merkel cell carcinoma, is reported to be associated with SCC arising in patients treated with BRAF inhibitors for metastatic melanoma.[62,63]

CHRONIC INFLAMMATION AND CHRONIC INJURY OF THE SKIN

SCCs are more likely to develop in chronically diseased or injured skin, including skin affected by chronic ulcers, burn scars, and radiation dermatitis. Chronic inflammatory disorders of the skin and mucosal tissue may also predispose for SCC development; these diseases include discoid lupus erythematodes, lichen ruber mucosae, lichen sclerosus, and dystrophic epidermolysis bullosa.[9] SCCs in RDEB most commonly occur in chronic, nonhealing ulcers with minimal UV exposure and chronic injury-driven stiffening of the dermal tumor microenvironment is a major contributing factor for rapid carcinoma progression in RDEB.[64]

MOLECULAR ASPECTS

The sequence of events in which normal keratinocytes transform into SCCs, referred to as *skin carcinogenesis*, is thought to be a multistep process of progressive and accumulating genetic and epigenetic alterations in key signaling pathways regulating cell survival, cell cycle, and genome maintenance.[16,65] The genomic instability and very high burden of mutations in SCC, which is significantly greater than in other solid tumors, impedes the identification of critical driver mutations, and it is increasingly apparent that multiple genes and pathways may be involved (reviewed in Harwood et al[23]).

TP53

Mutations in the tumor-suppressor gene p53 (*TP53*) are the most prominent and best studied aberrations in skin cancers,[20] and are likely to be a cause of the marked genomic instability observed in SCCs.[16] *TP53* exerts a central tumor-suppressor function in the response to UV damage through mechanisms such as induction of apoptosis and cell-cycle arrest. The protective role of p53 and the significance of p53-dependent apoptosis in response to UV-damage is emphasized by the high susceptibility of p53-deficient mice to UV-induced SCCs.[66]

Supporting the contribution of cumulative UV exposure in the pathogenesis of SCCs, clones of mutated *TP53* are highly prevalent in AK and in fields of chronically sun-damaged skin, and their expansion seems to be driven by continuing UVB exposure.[23] The loss of p53 provides a survival advantage for UV-damaged keratinocytes as the induction of apoptosis following UV-mediated DNA damage is hampered.[67] In this concept, UVR acts as a major initiator and promoter of skin carcinogenesis by inducing the accumulation of genetic alterations, such as p53 mutations in the skin, that allow for uncontrolled proliferation of keratinocytes and create a selective growth advantage as compared to normal cells. The loss of the second p53 allele is commonly found at later stages of SCC development and may be a critical event for the transition from AK and in situ carcinomas to invasive SCC.[23]

Of note, the E6 and E7 viral proteins of certain HPV types dysregulate the UV-activated cell-cycle checkpoints by inhibiting p53-mediated transcription of genes, which suggests a synergistic role between UV-induced DNA damage and the oncogenic potential of HPV.[68]

THE *RAS* PROTOONCOGENE AND EPIDERMAL GROWTH FACTOR RECEPTOR SIGNALING

The protooncogene *RAS* has been implicated in the initiation of SCC in murine chemical carcinogenesis models.[69] Data from the Catalog of Somatic Mutations in Cancer (COSMIC) indicates that 21% of SCCs harbor activating mutations in a least 1 of the 3 Ras genes (9% Hras, 7% Nras, 5% Kras).[70] UV-induced mutations in Ras genes also are found in AK and postulated to play a role during early stages of human UV-induced SCC development.[16,71] In an experimental setting, oncogenic *RAS* was insufficient to drive SCC formation in human keratinocytes alone, but did trigger epidermal tumorigenesis in the presence of additional blockade of nuclear factor κB, which is important for growth inhibition in keratinocytes.[72]

Interestingly, an increase in RAS mutations has been detected in rapidly developing, well-differentiated SCCs arising in patients receiving the BRAF-inhibitor vemurafenib for the treatment of advanced melanoma.[73]

Although the frequency of RAS mutations in most sporadic human SCCs is relatively low, an increase in levels of activated RAS in non-RAS mutant tumors and a consecutive upregulation of the downstream mitogen-activated protein kinase and the mTOR signaling pathways has been observed in human SCC.[72] It is postulated that in non-*RAS* mutant SCC the aberrant expression of the EGFR may contribute to the downstream activation of mitogen-activated protein kinase and mTOR signaling pathways.[23] EGFR (HER-1) is a member of the human epidermal growth receptor family of receptor tyrosine kinases on the surface of keratinocytes and persistently activated in SCC.[74] Although there is a high level of EGFR expression in SCC, the overall incidence of EGFR mutations is low and advanced SCC often shows a dysregulated EGFR expression in the absence of EGFR or RAS mutation.[74-76] Treatment with sirolimus, the mTOR inhibitor, is associated with a reduced rate of secondary SCCs in OTRs,[46] possibly in part by attenuating the downstream EGFR pathway, EGFR blockade, by employing either small molecules (eg, erlotinib) or antibodies (eg, cetuximab), may represent a therapeutic option for advanced or metastatic SCC.[77,78]

CLINICAL PRESENTATION

CLASSICAL PRESENTATION

The clinical presentation of SCC is variable and depends on the histologic subtype and location of the tumor. Typically, SCCs arise on sun-exposed areas, especially the face, head, and neck region, and the forearms and dorsum of the hands.[9] In UV-exposed skin, SCCs usually develop on a background of AK or Bowen disease as precursor lesions (see Chap. 110). Field cancerization with numerous precursor lesions on UV-damaged skin (Fig. 112-2) constitutes a high risk for progression to SCC; de novo formation on undamaged skin rarely occurs. The typical clinical finding of SCC includes slowly enlarging, firm, skin-colored to erythematous plaques or nodules (Fig. 112-2) with marked hyperkeratosis. Ulceration, exophytic (Fig. 112-3), or infiltrative growth patterns are seen.

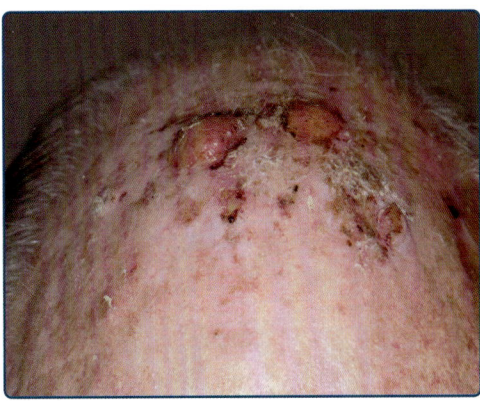

Figure 112-2 Classical clinical presentation of cutaneous squamous cell carcinoma (SCC). Two nodular SCCs and several actinic keratoses as precursor lesions are present on the forehead in the setting of field cancerization on heavily sun-damaged skin.

SPECIAL LOCATIONS

ORAL SQUAMOUS CELL CARCINOMA

Oral SCC may arise on apparently normal mucosa but are usually preceded by leukoplakia, erythroplakia, or leukoerythroplakia, which are localization-specific precursor lesions.[79] The typical clinical presentation of oral SCC is tumors with whitish surface or ulcers with elevated indurated borders. Exophytic or endophytic growth patterns with subsequent ulcer formation occur.

SQUAMOUS CELL CARCINOMA OF THE LOWER LIP

SCC of the lip occurs on the lower lip (Fig. 112-4) more often than on the upper lip, because the lower lip, along with the nose and cheeks, is regarded as one of the typical "sun terraces."[80] Because SCCs on the lip and ear show higher rates of metastasis, tumors at these locations require special attention.

VERRUCOUS SQUAMOUS CELL CARCINOMA

Verrucous SCC clinically presents as a slowly growing ulcerated plaque or an exophytic cauliflower-like slowly growing tumor. Typical locations of verrucous SCC include the oral cavity (oral florid papillomatosis), the genitoanal region (often referred to as *giant condyloma acuminatum Buschke-Löwenstein*), plantar skin (in this location it is commonly named *epithelioma cuniculatum*), and amputation stumps. Verrucous SCC is less common than other forms of invasive SCC.[81]

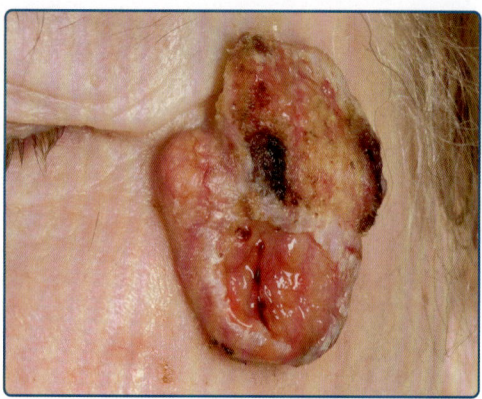

Figure 112-3 Large, exophytic squamous cell carcinoma with erosion on the left cheek.

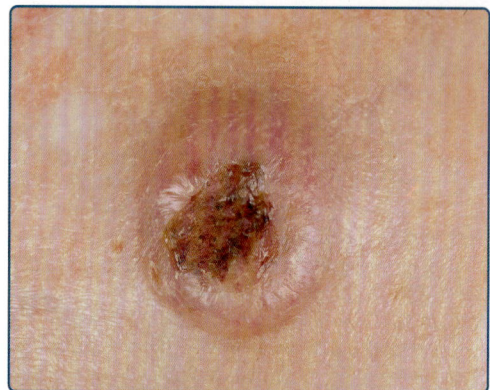

Figure 112-5 Typical clinical presentation of a keratoacanthoma on the forehead as a sharply circumscribed symmetric nodule with the characteristic horn-filled crater in the middle.

KERATOACANTHOMA

KA commonly is regarded as a subtype of highly differentiated SCC with typical clinical and histopathologic features. KA usually erupts rapidly within a few weeks and has the ability to spontaneously regress. KA clinically presents as a sharply circumscribed firm nodule with a central horn-filled crater that typically arises on the head and sun-exposed areas of the extremities (Fig. 112-5). There are several distinct clinical variants, including grouped KA, subungual KA, intraoral KA, giant KA, KA centrifugum marginatum, multiple KA of the Ferguson-Smith type, eruptive KA of Grzybowski, and KA associated with Muir-Torre syndrome.

DIAGNOSIS

The standard histopathology report of SCC should include the following: histologic subtype (acantholytic, spindle cell, verrucous, or desmoplastic type); grade of differentiation (G1 to G4); maximum vertical tumor diameter in millimeters; extent of dermal invasion (Clark level); and presence or absence of perineural, vascular, or lymphatic invasion. To facilitate correct management of SCC, information about whether the margins are free or do not have the minimum distance required between the tumor and the resection margin also should be included in the histopathology report (Table 112-3).

TABLE 112-3
Basic Features of Histopathology Report of Cutaneous Squamous Cell Carcinoma Diagnosis

Histopathology Report	
Histologic subtype	Common Verrucous Desmoplastic Acantholytic Spindle-cell Other
Grading	Well differentiated Moderately differentiated Poorly differentiated Undifferentiated Cannot be assessed
Maximum tumor thickness	_____ mm
Clark level	>IV <IV
Perineural invasion	No Yes
Vascular/lymphatic invasion	No Yes
Complete excision	No Yes
Minimum lateral margin	_____ mm
Minimum deep margin	_____ mm

Modified from Bonerandi JJ, Beauvillain C, Caquant L, et al. Guidelines for the diagnosis and treatment of cutaneous squamous cell carcinoma and precursor lesions. *J Eur Acad Dermatol Venereol*. 2011;25(suppl 5):1-51.

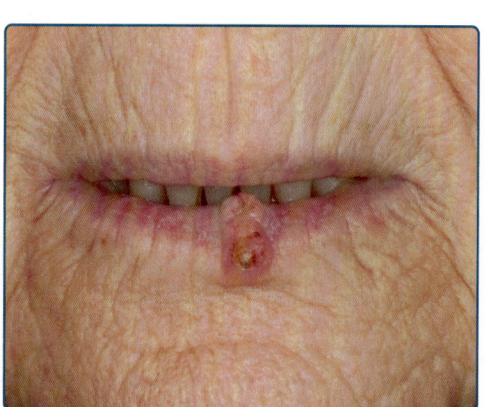

Figure 112-4 Hyperkeratotic squamous cell carcinoma located centrally on the lower lip.

GENERAL CONSIDERATIONS IN HISTOPATHOLOGY

The hallmark of invasive SCC is the growth of atypical keratinocytes beyond the basement membrane into the dermis. The diagnosis of SCC is established histologically. All clinically suspicious lesions should be subjected to a skin biopsy or excision biopsy followed by histologic examination. Depending on the size of the tumor, its localization, and treatment options, different biopsy techniques are available, including incisional biopsy, punch biopsy, shave biopsy, or an excisional biopsy of the entire lesion. The diagnosis is confirmed by histologic examination using routine hematoxylin and eosin stains and additional immunohistochemical markers, such as cytokeratins or molecular markers in the case of uncertain diagnosis, especially in tumors with little or no keratinization.

BASIC HISTOPATHOLOGIC FEATURES OF SQUAMOUS CELL CARCINOMA

The typical histopathologic picture of SCC shows atypical keratinocytes originating in the epidermis and infiltrating into the dermis (Fig. 112-6). The degree of differentiation is variable among SCCs. It ranges from well-differentiated SCC with minimal pleomorphism, prominent keratinization as represented morphologically by parakeratosis, individual cell dyskeratosis, and horn pearl formation (Fig. 112-7A) to poorly differentiated SCCs showing pleomorphic nuclei with a high degree of atypia, frequent mitoses, and very few areas of keratinization.

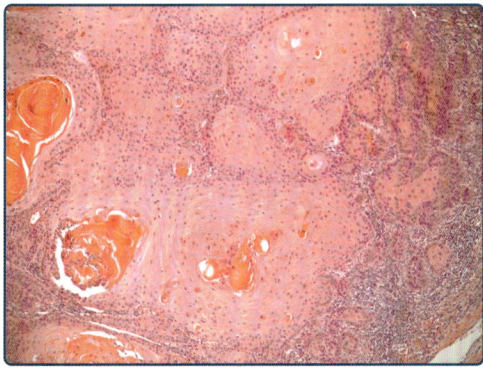

Figure 112-6 Typical histopathologic picture of a well-differentiated squamous cell carcinoma (grade 1) with atypical keratinocytes originating in the epidermis and infiltrating into the dermis with minimal pleomorphism and prominent keratinization (hematoxylin and eosin stain, ×50 magnification).

HISTOPATHOLOGIC VARIANTS OF SQUAMOUS CELL CARCINOMA WITH DIFFERENTIAL DIAGNOSIS

In addition to the typical histopathologic picture of SCC described above, there are distinct histologic subtypes, some of which account for classification of the tumor as high risk. To facilitate the prognostic classification and correct management of SCC, the following well-established histologic subtypes should be distinguished:

SPINDLE-CELL SQUAMOUS CELL CARCINOMA

Spindle-cell SCC is a relatively rare form of SCC. It is characterized by spindled morphology of the atypical keratinocytes and lack of keratinization (see Fig. 112-7B). It typically arises in sun-exposed areas of skin of elderly patients, and sometimes in the setting of radiation therapy. The histologic differential diagnoses include other spindle-cell neoplasms like atypical fibroxanthoma, spindle-cell melanoma, and sarcoma. Immunohistochemical staining, including cytokeratins, often is necessary to confirm the diagnosis.[82]

ACANTHOLYTIC (ADENOID) SQUAMOUS CELL CARCINOMA

Acantholytic SCC comprises less than 5% of all SCCs and bears an increased propensity for metastasis as shown in 1 study that reported metastatic disease in 19% of acantholytic SCCs.[83] The main histologic characteristic of acantholytic SCC is extensive acantholysis of the atypical keratinocytes leading to pseudoglandular structures within the tumor area (see Fig. 112-7C).

VERRUCOUS SQUAMOUS CELL CARCINOMA

Verrucous SCC is a well-differentiated variant of SCC that slowly grows and is locally destructive, but with only low metastatic potential.[81] For the histopathologic diagnosis of verrucous SCC, a large, deep incisional biopsy is necessary. The superficial parts resemble verrucae with parakeratosis, acanthosis, and a prominent stratum granulosum. In the deeper parts, monomorphic well-differentiated keratinocytes with small nuclei form broad, deep, downward proliferations of light eosinophilic tumor cells. The tumor areas show noninvasive pushing borders, and even in the deeper areas, nuclear atypia is rare. Keratinization, individual cell dyskeratosis, and horn pearl formation are absent.

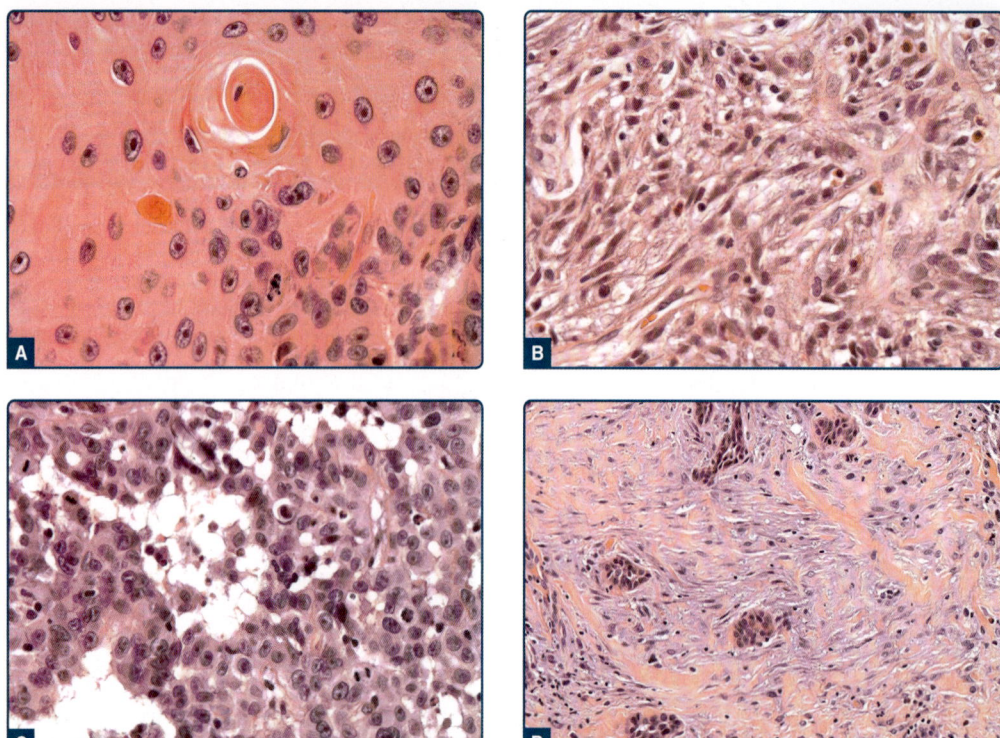

Figure 112-7 Histopathologic variants of squamous cell carcinoma (SCC). **A,** Well-differentiated SCC with minimal pleomorphism and individual cell dyskeratosis with horn pearl formation (hematoxylin and eosin stain [H&E], ×400 magnification). **B,** Spindle-cell SCC revealing spindled morphology of the atypical keratinocytes and lack of keratinization (H&E, ×400 magnification). **C,** Acantholytic SCC with extensive acantholysis of the atypical keratinocytes leading to pseudoglandular structures within the tumor (H&E, ×400 magnification). **D,** Desmoplastic SCC showing infiltrative growth pattern with abundant mucinous stroma surrounding the tumor cells (H&E, ×200 magnification).

DESMOPLASTIC SQUAMOUS CELL CARCINOMA

Desmoplastic SCC is a distinct variant of SCC that shows a highly infiltrative growth pattern with abundant mucinous stroma surrounding the tumor cells (see Fig. 112-7D). Desmoplastic SCC often is associated with perineural (Fig. 112-8) or perivascular infiltration, and reveals a high rate of recurrence and metastases.[84]

KERATOACANTHOMA

KA is commonly regarded as a highly differentiated variant of SCC with distinct clinical and histomorphologic characteristics. KA has an overall symmetric aspect at scanning magnification (Fig. 112-9). Cytomorphologically, KAs are built of large strands of monomorphic keratinocytes with eosinophilic cytoplasm and small nuclei; a surrounding inflammatory infiltrate containing lymphocytes, eosinophils, and neutrophils is commonly observed (Fig. 112-9, insert). The final histomorphologic diagnosis needs the entire lesion because there is a characteristic growth pattern and the histopathologic diagnosis of KA relies mainly on the silhouette of the tumor as assessed at scanning magnification.

The histopathologic features of KA vary depending on the evolutionary stage of the tumor: The epithelium of early lesions is markedly hyperplastic and the central keratotic plug is not as pronounced as in later stages. Fully developed lesions are characterized by a large central core of keratin surrounded by a well-differentiated proliferation of squamous epithelium (Fig. 112-9). In regressing lesions, the epithelium is rather hypoplastic; epithelial hyperplasia and atypical cells are no longer present, but the central crater can still be recognized.

GRADING

In addition to the subtyping of cutaneous SCC, histologic grading of SCC is very important with respect to recurrences and risk of metastasis. The classification system of the American Joint Committee on Cancer (AJCC) includes histologic grading in consideration of so-called high-risk features for staging. Histologic grading of SCC based on the degree of cellular differentiation was introduced in 1932 by Broders and is still commonly used today.[85] Tumors are graded on a scale of 1 to 4 based on increasing percentages of undifferentiated cells: G1 = well differentiated; G2 =

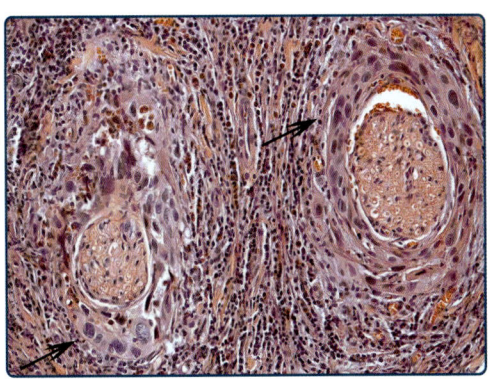

Figure 112-8 Histopathologic picture of perineural invasion of squamous cell carcinoma showing the atypical keratinocytes (*black arrows*) growing around a central nerve fiber (hematoxylin and eosin staining, ×200 magnification).

moderately differentiated; G3 = poorly differentiated; G4 = undifferentiated grade; and Gx = grade cannot be assessed.

STAGING

If a SCC is suspected, a complete examination of the entire skin should be performed followed by assessment for nodal involvement of the regional lymph nodes by palpation and/or ultrasound examination.

The current classification and staging of cutaneous SCC is based on the most recent TNM (tumor, node, metastasis) system of the Union International Contre le Cancer (UICC, 2009)[86] and the AJCC (2010).[87] *T1* defines "low-risk" tumors smaller than 2 cm in diameter in greatest dimension and fewer than 2 high-risk features (high-risk features include >2 mm thickness, Clark level >IV, perineural invasion, primary site being the lip or ear, and poorly or undifferentiated tumor). *T2* includes "high-risk" tumors larger than 2 cm in diameter in greatest dimension and tumors of any size with 2 or more high-risk features. *T3* is used for tumors that invade muscle, bone, or cartilage of maxilla, mandible or orbit, and *T4* includes tumors that invade the skull base or axial skeleton (Table 112-4).

Lymph node involvement of cutaneous SCC significantly increases the risk of recurrence and mortality, especially in high-risk tumors. If evaluation for nodal involvement of the regional lymph nodes by palpation and/or ultrasound examination is suspicious, histologic confirmation should be sought by fine-needle aspiration or lymph node biopsy. The TNM/UICC classifies lymph node involvement in 3 groups (N1, N2, N3) depending on size and number of involved nodes, whereas the AJCC uses 5 categories (N1, N2a, N2b, N2c, N3) based on number, localization and size (see Table 112-4).

Concerning distant metastases, both TNM/UICC and AJCC distinguish no distant metastases (M0) from distant metastases (M1) (see Table 112-4).

TABLE 112-4

Staging of Primary Tumor (T) of the TNM Staging Classification for Cutaneous Squamous Cell Carcinoma According to the American Joint Committee on Cancer (2010)

Tx	Primary tumor cannot be assessed
T0	No evidence of primary tumor
Tis	Carcinoma in situ
T1	Tumor ≤2 cm or less in greatest dimension with fewer than 2 high-risk features[a]
T2	Tumor >2 cm in greatest dimension or tumor any size with 2 or more high-risk features[a]
T3	Tumor with invasion of maxilla, mandible, orbit, or temporal bone
T4	Tumor with invasion of skeleton (axial, appendicular) or perineural invasion of skull base
Nx	Regional lymph nodes cannot be assessed
N0	No regional lymph node metastases
N1	Metastasis in a single ipsilateral lymph node, 3 cm or less in greatest dimension
N2a	Metastasis in a single ipsilateral lymph node, more than 3 cm but not more than 6 cm in greatest dimension
N2b	Metastasis in multiple ipsilateral lymph nodes, none more than 6 cm in greatest dimension
N2c	Metastasis in bilateral or contralateral lymph nodes, none more than 6 cm in greatest dimension
N3	Metastasis in a lymph node, more than 6 cm in greatest dimension
M0	No distant metastases
M1	Distant metastases

[a]High-risk features include >2 mm thickness, Clark level >IV, perineural invasion, primary site being the lip or ear, and poorly or undifferentiated tumor.

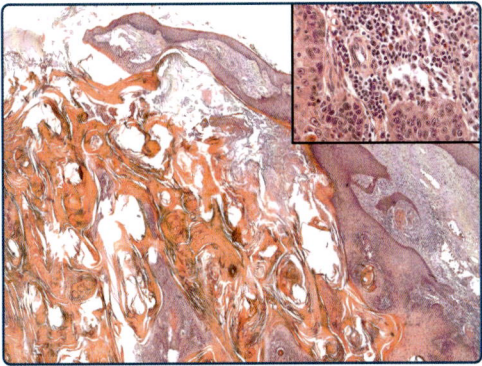

Figure 112-9 Histopathologic picture of keratoacanthoma as a fully developed lesion with a central core of keratin surrounded by a well-differentiated proliferation of squamous epithelium (hematoxylin and eosin staining [H&E], ×25 magnification). The insert shows the surrounding inflammatory infiltrate containing lymphocytes, eosinophils, and neutrophils (H&E, ×400 magnification).

DIFFERENTIAL DIAGNOSES

Depending on the localization and type of SCC there are different differential diagnoses to be ruled out, including SCC with a classical clinical presentation of hyperkeratotic seborrheic keratoses; viral acanthoma; viral warts; and acanthoma fissuratum. For SCCs with ulcerative or infiltrative growth, scars, chronic discoid lupus erythematodes, lichen planus, and morpheaform BCC are to be considered. SCCs at special locations require exclusion of site-specific differential diagnoses such as chondrodermatitis nodularis chronica helicis for SCC on the ear.

MANAGEMENT

As the treatment modality for the primary lesion is a major determinant for the risk of local recurrence, the ideal management of SCC is predicated on local tumor control along with maximal preservation of function and cosmetics. In cases of clinical uncertainty about invasiveness, surgical resection or a biopsy followed by histologic evaluation is recommended before employing any therapeutic intervention other than surgery.[77]

SURGERY

Surgical excision, preferably microscopically controlled surgery (Mohs surgery), is regarded as the primary mode of therapy for localized SCC and has a cure rate of 95%.[78,88,89] Full histopathologic characterization of the tumor and its margins allows for the adequate management of the patient[77,88] and is particularly important for recurring and deeply infiltrating tumors, that is, tumors with histologic risk factors such as perineural invasion, tumors in immunosuppressed patients, and at sites where tissue preservation is essential (ie, eyelid, nasal tip, ear). Conventional standard excision with 4- to 6-mm margins may be acceptable as primary treatment of local, low-risk SCCs.[78]

SCC may give rise to local in-transit metastasis, which may be removed by wide surgical excision or treated by irradiation of a wide field around the primary lesion. Treatment of nodal metastasis may involve lymph node dissection, radiation, or a combination of both.

NONSURGICAL INTERVENTION

TOPICAL THERAPY

Topical therapeutic treatments such as topical imiquimod, topical or intralesional 5-fluorouracil, cryotherapy, and photodynamic therapy for SCC have been reported.[90-92] As evidence for the efficacy of these treatments is lacking and limited to case reports, topical therapy is generally not regarded an appropriate treatment modality for invasive SCC.

RADIATION THERAPY

While surgery is regarded the primary mode of local therapy for the vast majority of SCCs, patient preference and other factors, such as problematic locations for surgery, may lead to the selection of radiation therapy as the treatment modality. In any case, appropriate confirmation of the diagnosis by histologic evaluation is mandatory prior to radiotherapy. Radiation therapy may serve as an alternative to surgery in the primary treatment of superficially invasive, small SCCs in low-risk areas, and may be discussed for inoperable, local in-transit metastasis, and in the adjuvant setting for patients with potentially aggressive local tumors, such as histopathologically confirmed, extensive, perineural involvement.[77] Patients treated with Mohs surgery (microscopically controlled surgery) should be considered for postoperative adjuvant radiation if clear margins cannot be achieved.[77,78]

ELECTIVE PROPHYLACTIC LYMPH NODE DISSECTION AND SENTINEL LYMPH NODE BIOPSY

Sentinel lymph node biopsy and elective prophylactic lymph node dissection have been proposed in SCC patients at high risk for metastatic disease, but there is no conclusive evidence of its prognostic or therapeutic value.[77,93]

SYSTEMIC TREATMENT OF LOCALLY ADVANCED AND METASTATIC SQUAMOUS CELL CARCINOMA

Locally advanced, unresectable or metastatic SCC is a therapeutic challenge because of the scarce amount of available prospective data on systemic therapy. In addition, only approximately 30% of patients are reported as responsive to any type of standard treatment.[94] In patients undergoing iatrogenic immunosuppression, such as OTRs, dose reduction of the immunosuppressive agents and minimizing the doses of calcineurin inhibitors and/or antimetabolites in favor of mTOR inhibitors should be the goal.[41,78]

CHEMOTHERAPY

Although there are limited data on the efficacy of chemotherapy for metastatic SCC, standard options in metastatic or unresectable SCC include systemic platinum-based chemotherapeutic regimens, 5-fluorouracil/capecitabine, or monotherapy/chemotherapy with methotrexate.[77,78,88,89] However, besides a limited effect on overall survival, currently available therapy for locally advanced or metastatic disease is frequently restricted by comorbidities and advanced age of the patient.

TARGETED THERAPY

Using therapeutic strategies targeting the EGFR either by small molecules (ie, erlotinib and gefitinib) or antibodies (ie, cetuximab and panitumumab) may be nonsurgical, off-label options for advanced SCC beyond radiotherapy and conventional chemotherapy. A prospective Phase II trial has demonstrated the efficacy of monotherapy with cetuximab as a first-line treatment of unresectable SCC (a 29% response rate).[95] Although mostly in case reports, the use of cetuximab also has been reported in SCC in neoadjuvant and adjuvant therapy settings and as radiosensitizer combined with radiation therapy.[23]

Recent evidence suggest that, immune inhibitory pathways such as the programmed death protein 1 (PD-1)/PD-1 ligand pathway may control skin carcinogenesis. Although not yet explored sufficiently in either an independent or a combined therapeutic setting, preclinical studies reveal that the overexpression of the PD-1 ligand in keratinocytes of transgenic mice results in accelerated SCC formation,[96] and therapeutic checkpoint blockade of the immune inhibitory PD-1 pathway has resulted in a notable antitumor response in a case of unresectable SCC.[97]

PROGNOSIS

The majority of SCCs are low risk and present with early stage disease, resulting in a high cure rate and excellent prognosis.

Prognosis for locally advanced SCC at the time of diagnosis and patients with progressive disease after first-line surgical therapy is generally poor.[94] A retrospective study of patients with unresectable SCC reported a poor overall survival of only 10.9 months and unresponsiveness to the majority of available treatments.[94]

A poorer outcome of immunosuppressed patients with advanced disease compared with the general population has been reported.[22,39] Immunosuppression is a risk factor for a greater tumor burden, more aggressive tumor behavior, metastatic disease,[35,98] and disease-specific death from SCC.[36] SCCs in immunosuppressed patients are designated as high-risk tumors per the National Comprehensive Cancer Network (NCCN). SCC accounts for more than 60% of deaths from all skin malignancies in OTRs with a death rate of approximately 5%.[7,41]

LOCAL RECURRENCE

Table 112-5 outlines the NCCN's guidelines regarding risk factors for local recurrence. Local recurrence may result from a failure to completely treat the primary tumor or from local metastasis. Local recurrence at the site of the primary lesion often precedes metastasis and is frequently found to be the first indicator of aggressive biologic behavior in SCC.[9,99] Local recurrence rates are considerably lower with microscopically controlled surgery (Mohs surgery) as compared to other local treatment modalities.[99,100]

METASTASIS

Table 112-5 outlines the NCCN's guidelines regarding risk factors for metastases. The risk of developing metastasis from SCC is generally low, with a 5-year metastatic rate of 5%, and 85% of metastatic cases are nodal disease.[9,10] However, depending on patient and tumor characteristics, certain subgroups of patients are at significantly higher risk for metastasis, with metastatic rates of up to 30%.[9] The incidence of metastatic SCC in OTRs is significantly higher than in the general population (8% vs. 0.5% to 5%), with metastasis developing rapidly after diagnosis of the primary tumor in a mean of only 1.4 years and a poor prognosis.[22]

HIGH-RISK LESIONS AND PROGNOSTIC RISK FACTORS FOR SQUAMOUS CELL CARCINOMA

Histopathologic and clinical features, as well as host-dependent factors, considerably influence the metastatic potential and prognosis of SCC.

A metaanalysis and systematic review on all published data found that tumor depth (ie, Breslow thickness exceeding 2 mm and invasion beyond subcutaneous fat) is associated with the highest relative risk of local recurrence and metastasis of SCC.[35] A tumor diameter exceeding 20 mm is associated with the highest relative risk for disease-specific death of SCC (relative risk 19.10, confidence interval 95%). Additional risk factors for local recurrence and/or metastasis are clinical and histopathologic features. A prospective study investigated potential risk factors for metastasis or local recurrence of SCC in a large cohort of patients and found that only SCCs thicker than 2 mm are associated with a significant risk of metastasis. Tumors larger than 6 mm are associated with a high risk of metastasis and local recurrence. Desmoplastic growth is an independent risk factor for local recurrence. Additional key prognostic factors for metastasis besides increased horizontal size are immunosuppression and localization at the ear.[101] Another prospective study found that lesion size equal to or greater than 4 cm and histologic evidence of perineural invasion and deep invasion beyond subcutaneous structures were the factors most significantly associated with disease-specific mortality in cutaneous SCC.[102]

TABLE 112-5

NCCN Clinical Practice Guidelines in Oncology (NCCN Guidelines®): Risk Factors for Local Recurrence or Metastases

NCCN Guidelines Version 2.2019 — Squamous Cell Skin Cancer

RISK FACTORS FOR LOCAL RECURRENCE OR METASTASES

H&P	Low Risk	High Risk
Location/size[1]	Area L <20 mm	Area L ≥20 mm
	Area M <10 mm[4]	Area M ≥10 mm
		Area H[5]
Borders	Well-defined	Poorly defined
Primary vs. recurrent	Primary	Recurrent
Immunosuppression	(−)	(+)
Site of prior RT or chronic inflammatory process	(−)	(+)
Rapidly growing tumor	(−)	(+)
Neurologic symptoms	(−)	(+)
Pathology (See SCC-A)		
Degree of differentiation	Well or moderately differentiated	Poorly differentiated
Acantholytic (adenoid), adenosquamous (showing mucin production), desmoplastic, or metaplastic (carcinosarcomatous) subtypes	(−)	(+)
Depth[2,3]: Thickness or level of invasion	≤6 mm and no invasion beyond subcutaneous fat	>6 mm or invasion beyond subcutaneous fat
Perineural, lymphatic, or vascular involvement	(−)	(+)

[1] Must include peripheral rim of erythema.
[2] If clinical evaluation of incisional biopsy suggests that microstaging is inadequate, consider narrow margin excisional biopsy.
[3] Deep invasion is defined as invasion beyond the subcutaneous fat OR >6 mm (as measured from the granular layer of adjacent normal epidermis to the base of the tumor, consistent with AJCC 8th edition).
[4] Location independent of size may constitute high risk.
[5] Area H constitutes high risk based on location, independent of size, narrow excision margins due to anatomic and functional constraints are associated with increased recurrence rates with standard histologic processing. Complete margin assessment such as with Mohs micrographic surgery is recommended for optimal tumor clearance and maximal tissue conservation. For tumors <6 mm in size, without other high risk features, other treatment modalities may be considered if at least 4-mm clinically tumor-free margins can be obtained without significant anatomic or functional distortions.

Area H = "mask areas" of face (central face, eyelids, eyebrows, periorbital, nose, lips [cutaneous and vermilion], chin, mandible, preauricular and postauricular skin/sulci, temple, ear), genitalia, hands, and feet.
Area M = cheeks, forehead, scalp, neck, and pretibia.
Area L = trunk and extremities (excluding pretibia, hands, feet, nail units, and ankles).

Note: All recommendations are category 2A unless otherwise indicated.
Clinical Trials: NCCN believes that the best management of any patient with cancer is in a clinical trial. Participation in clinical trials is especially encouraged.

SCC-B

Reproduced with permission from the NCCN Clinical Practice Guidelines in Oncology (NCCN Guidelines®) for Squamous Cell Skin Cancer V.2.2019. © 2018 National Comprehensive Cancer Network, Inc. All rights reserved. The NCCN Guidelines® and illustrations herein may not be reproduced in any form for any purpose without the express written permission of NCCN. To view the most recent and complete version of the NCCN Guidelines, go online to NCCN.org. The NCCN Guidelines are a work in progress that may be refined as often as new significant data becomes available.
NCCN makes no warranties of any kind whatsoever regarding their content, use or application and disclaims any responsibility for their application or use in any way.

AFTERCARE

As standardized followup schedules for patients with SCC generally do not exist, it is recommended to follow patients closely based on risk assessment for the development of new lesions, local recurrence, and metastatic spread.[77] The significant tumor burden and high incidence of SCC in immunosuppressed patients such as OTRs highlight the importance of dermatologic surveillance, skin cancer prevention strategies, and the timely treatment of precancerous and in situ lesions in this high-risk population.

Early detection and treatment improves survival of patients with recurrent and progressive disease. Of locally recurring and metastatic SCCs, 70% to 80% are detected within 2 years after primary diagnosis.

SECONDARY SKIN CANCER

After diagnosis of SCC, all patients should be considered to be at risk for the development of additional secondary SCC as well as BCC. Overall, the 3-year cumulative risk of a subsequent SCC after an index SCC is 18%, at least a 10-fold increase in incidence compared with the incidence of first tumors in a comparable general population.[103]

Compared to the general population, immunosuppressed OTRs are at particularly high risk of developing subsequent secondary SCC after the initial diagnosis of NMSC, with 25% of patients developing another NMSC within 13 months, and 50% developing another cancer within 3.5 years.[8]

PREVENTION

NMSCs, including SCC, are largely preventable.[9] Prevention can be emphasized through education for skin cancer risk factors, effective UV protection measures, and regular self-examination. Sun avoidance and close dermatologic surveillance of high-risk individuals are key factors for the prevention of SCC.

SUN PROTECTION

In general, sun avoidance and sun protection (protective clothing, sunscreens) are cost-effective measures to prevent the development of cutaneous SCC.[104] The preventive effect of sunscreens with high sun protection factor and broad UVA/UVB coverage is well established and there is evidence that sun protection throughout life can prevent the development of both SCC precursor lesions and invasive SCC.[105]

TREATMENT OF PRECURSOR LESIONS

Effective treatment of AK and Bowen disease or areas of field cancerization in photodamaged skin is expected to reduce the incidence of SCC, because cutaneous SCC develop from these precursor lesions. Several treatment options are available and need to be chosen and adapted to the individual patient's situation (see Chap. 110). Regular complete skin examination incorporated in a structured dermatooncologic concept of primary and secondary prevention represents an important measure in the prevention of the development of SCC.

OTHER PREVENTIVE MEASURES

Chemoprevention of skin tumors represents an innovative new preventive concept. The general idea of chemoprevention is to prevent progression of clinically undiscovered precursor lesions into invasive carcinoma, reducing, in particular, the risk of the occurrence of secondary tumors for patients at risk.

NIACINAMIDE

Niacinamide (vitamin B_3) is suitable for chemoprevention of NMSC, as supported by animal studies and data from a large, randomized Phase III clinical study.[106] Compared with placebo, the administration of niacinamide 500 mg twice daily resulted in a 23% lower rate of newly formed NMSC (similar for SCC and BCC) during an intervention period of 12 months.[106] In addition, the safety profile was favorable. Niacinamide constitutes a part of nicotinamide adenine dinucleotide, which, in turn, is an essential cofactor for the production of nicotinamide adenine trinucleotide. Consequently, niacinamide can prevent nicotinamide adenine trinucleotide deficiency, which occurs in the epidermis under the action of UV light and prevents repair of DNA damage. Consequently, vitamin B_3 protects keratinocytes against UV-induced cellular nicotinamide adenine trinucleotide loss,[107] promotes epidermal differentiation in photodamaged skin, and inhibits UV-induced immunosuppression and photocarcinogenesis as shown in different mouse models.[108-110]

VITAMIN A

Systemic retinoids have a transient preventive effect for secondary SCC in both immunocompetent and immunosuppressed patients.[111-113] Some years ago, data from small, randomized trials, especially in OTRs[114] and other high-risk patients,[115] suggested a role for prophylactic administration of systemic retinoids for chemoprevention of NMSC. One study assessed the prevention of new skin cancers in xeroderma pigmentosum patients using vitamin A derivatives.[115] Vitamin A derivatives are associated with promotion of normal differentiation. Five xeroderma pigmentosum patients with a high frequency of new primary skin cancers were selected. Their cancers were cataloged and surgically removed over a period of 2 years. Patients were then treated for 2 years with high-dose oral 13-*cis* retinoic acid (isotretinoin). During the treatment interval there was a 63% reduction in frequency of new skin cancers. Although there were numerous side effects, this treatment was the first demonstration of effective chemoprevention of cancer in humans.[115] A future indication of retinoids as a chemopreventive agent may include patients on BRAF inhibitors who are at risk of developing multiple cutaneous SCC. However, significant side effects, mainly affecting quality of life, but also including teratogenesis in female patients of child-bearing age, need to be taken considered.

CHANGE OF IMMUNOSUPPRESSIVE REGIMEN IN SOLID ORGAN TRANSPLANTATION RECIPIENTS

For an OTR, a change of the immunosuppressive regimen may be an important preventive measure, especially if the immunosuppressed OTR has a life-threatening SCC or multiple, rapidly developing tumors.[41] In this situation, either a dose reduction of the immunosuppressive agent and/or a change from calcineurin inhibitors or antimetabolites to mTOR inhibitors is recommended.[46]

REFERENCES

1. Housman TS, Feldman SR, Williford PM, et al. Skin cancer is among the most costly of all cancers to treat for the Medicare population. *J Am Acad Dermatol*. 2003;48(3):425-429.
2. Carucci JA. Press for an underestimated nemesis. *JAMA Dermatol*. 2013;149(10):1147-1148.
3. Berg D, Otley CC. Skin cancer in organ transplant recipients: epidemiology, pathogenesis, and management. *J Am Acad Dermatol*. 2002;47(1):1-17; quiz 18-20.
4. Lindelof B, Sigurgeirsson B, Gabel H, et al. Incidence of skin cancer in 5356 patients following organ transplantation. *Br J Dermatol*. 2000;143(3):513-519.
5. Madan V, Lear JT, Szeimies RM. Non-melanoma skin cancer. *Lancet*. 2010;375(9715):673-685.
6. Rogers HW, Weinstock MA, Harris AR, et al. Incidence estimate of nonmelanoma skin cancer in the United States, 2006. *Arch Dermatol*. 2010;146(3):283-287.
7. Lomas A, Leonardi-Bee J, Bath-Hextall F. A systematic review of worldwide incidence of nonmelanoma skin cancer. *Br J Dermatol*. 2012;166(5):1069-1080.
8. Karia PS, Han J, Schmults CD. Cutaneous squamous cell carcinoma: estimated incidence of disease, nodal metastasis, and deaths from disease in the United States, 2012. *J Am Acad Dermatol*. 2013;68(6):957-966.
9. Alam M, Ratner D. Cutaneous squamous-cell carcinoma. *N Engl J Med*. 2001;344(13):975-983.
10. Kivisaari A, Kahari VM. Squamous cell carcinoma of the skin: Emerging need for novel biomarkers. *World J Clin Oncol*. 2013;4(4):85-90.
11. Staples MP, Elwood M, Burton RC, et al. Non-melanoma skin cancer in Australia: the 2002 national survey and trends since 1985. *Med J Aust*. 2006;184(1):6-10.
12. Diffey BL, Langtry JA. Skin cancer incidence and the ageing population. *Br J Dermatol*. 2005;153(3):679-680.
13. Welsh MM, Karagas MR, Kuriger JK, et al. Genetic determinants of UV-susceptibility in non-melanoma skin cancer. *PLoS One*. 2011;6(7):e20019.
14. Mora RG, Perniciaro C. Cancer of the skin in blacks. I. A review of 163 black patients with cutaneous squamous cell carcinoma. *J Am Acad Dermatol*. 1981;5(5):535-543.
15. Lekalakala PT, Khammissa RA, Kramer B, et al. Oculocutaneous albinism and squamous cell carcinoma of the skin of the head and neck in sub-Saharan Africa. *J Skin Cancer*. 2015;2015:167847.
16. Ratushny V, Gober MD, Hick R, et al. From keratinocyte to cancer: the pathogenesis and modeling of cutaneous squamous cell carcinoma. *J Clin Invest*. 2012;122(2):464-472.
17. Callen JP, Bickers DR, Moy RL. Actinic keratoses. *J Am Acad Dermatol*. 1997;36(4):650-653.
18. Glogau RG. The risk of progression to invasive disease. *J Am Acad Dermatol*. 2000;42(1, pt 2):23-24.
19. Salasche SJ. Epidemiology of actinic keratoses and squamous cell carcinoma. *J Am Acad Dermatol*. 2000;42(1, pt 2):4-7.
20. Boukamp P. Non-melanoma skin cancer: what drives tumor development and progression? *Carcinogenesis*. 2005;26(10):1657-1667.
21. IARC Working Group on the Evaluation of Carcinogenic Risks in Humans. Monographs on the evaluation of carcinogenic risks in humans. A review of human carcinogens: radiation. *IARC Monogr Eval Carcinog Risks Hum*. 2012;100D.
22. Martinez JC, Otley CC, Stasko T, et al. Defining the clinical course of metastatic skin cancer in organ transplant recipients: a multicenter collaborative study. *Arch Dermatol*. 2003;139(3):301-306. Available at http://monographs.iarc.fr/ENG/Monographs/vol100D/index.php.
23. Harwood CA, Proby CM, Inman GJ, et al. The promise of genomics and the development of targeted therapies for cutaneous squamous cell carcinoma. *Acta Derm Venereol*. 2016;96(1):3-16.
24. Nishigori C, Hattori Y, Toyokuni S. Role of reactive oxygen species in skin carcinogenesis. *Antioxid Redox Signal*. 2004;6(3):561-570.
25. Hussein MR. Ultraviolet radiation and skin cancer: molecular mechanisms. *J Cutan Pathol*. 2005;32(3):191-205.
26. Box NF, Duffy DL, Irving RE, et al. Melanocortin-1 receptor genotype is a risk factor for basal and squamous cell carcinoma. *J Invest Dermatol*. 2001;116(2):224-229.
27. Asgari MM, Wang W, Ioannidis NM, et al. Identification of susceptibility loci for cutaneous squamous cell carcinoma. *J Invest Dermatol*. 2016;136(5):930-937.
28. Nan H, Kraft P, Hunter DJ, et al. Genetic variants in pigmentation genes, pigmentary phenotypes, and risk of skin cancer in Caucasians. *Int J Cancer*. 2009;125(4):909-917.
29. Fine JD, Johnson LB, Weiner M, et al. Epidermolysis bullosa and the risk of life-threatening cancers: the National EB Registry experience, 1986-2006. *J Am Acad Dermatol*. 2009;60(2):203-211.
30. Bradford PT, Goldstein AM, Tamura D, et al. Cancer and neurologic degeneration in xeroderma pigmentosum: long term follow-up characterises the role of DNA repair. *J Med Genet*. 2011;48(3):168-176.
31. Yu HS, Liao WT, Chai CY. Arsenic carcinogenesis in the skin. *J Biomed Sci*. 2006;13(5):657-666.
32. Davis MM, Hanke CW, Zollinger TW, et al. Skin cancer in patients with chronic radiation dermatitis. *J Am Acad Dermatol*. 1989;20(4):608-616.
33. Euvrard S, Kanitakis J, Claudy A. Skin cancers after organ transplantation. *N Engl J Med*. 2003;348(17):1681-1691.
34. Harwood CA, Mesher D, McGregor JM, et al. A surveillance model for skin cancer in organ transplant recipients: a 22-year prospective study in an ethnically diverse population. *Am J Transplant*. 2013;13(1):119-129.
35. Thompson AK, Kelley BF, Prokop LJ, et al. Risk factors for cutaneous squamous cell carcinoma recurrence, metastasis, and disease-specific death: a systematic review and meta-analysis. *JAMA Dermatol*. 2016;152(4):419-428.
36. Karia PS, Jambusaria-Pahlajani A, Harrington DP, et al. Evaluation of American Joint Committee on Cancer, International Union Against Cancer, and Brigham and Women's Hospital tumor staging for cutaneous squamous cell carcinoma. *J Clin Oncol*. 2014;32(4):327-334.
37. Omland SH, Gniadecki R, Haedersdal M, et al. Skin cancer risk in hematopoietic stem-cell transplant recipients compared with background population and renal transplant recipients: a population-based cohort study. *JAMA Dermatol*. 2016;152(2):177-183.
38. Scott FI, Mamtani R, Brensinger CM, et al. Risk of non-melanoma skin cancer associated with the use of immunosuppressant and biologic agents in patients with a history of autoimmune disease and nonmelanoma skin cancer. *JAMA Dermatol*. 2016;152(2):164-172.
39. Jensen P, Hansen S, Moller B, et al. Skin cancer in kidney and heart transplant recipients and different

40. Zwald FO, Brown M. Skin cancer in solid organ transplant recipients: advances in therapy and management: part I. Epidemiology of skin cancer in solid organ transplant recipients. *J Am Acad Dermatol*. 2011;65(2):253-261; quiz 262.
41. Zwald FO, Brown M. Skin cancer in solid organ transplant recipients: advances in therapy and management: part II. Management of skin cancer in solid organ transplant recipients. *J Am Acad Dermatol*. 2011; 65(2):263-279; quiz 280.
42. Karagas MR, Stukel TA, Umland V, et al. Reported use of photosensitizing medications and basal cell and squamous cell carcinoma of the skin: results of a population-based case-control study. *J Invest Dermatol*. 2007;127(12):2901-2903.
43. Lindelof B, Sigurgeirsson B, Tegner E, et al. PUVA and cancer: a large-scale epidemiological study. *Lancet*. 1991;338(8759):91-93.
44. O'Donovan P, Perrett CM, Zhang X, et al. Azathioprine and UVA light generate mutagenic oxidative DNA damage. *Science*. 2005;309(5742):1871-1874.
45. Brem R, Li F, Montaner B, et al. DNA breakage and cell cycle checkpoint abrogation induced by a therapeutic thiopurine and UVA radiation. *Oncogene*. 2010;29(27):3953-3963.
46. Euvrard S, Morelon E, Rostaing L, et al. Sirolimus and secondary skin-cancer prevention in kidney transplantation. *N Engl J Med*. 2012;367(4):329-339.
47. Kwiek B, Schwartz RA. Keratoacanthoma (KA): an update and review. *J Am Acad Dermatol*. 2016;74(6): 1220-1233.
48. Cohen DN, Lawson SK, Shaver AC, et al. Contribution of beta-HPV infection and UV damage to rapid-onset cutaneous squamous cell carcinoma during BRAF-inhibition therapy. *Clin Cancer Res*. 2015;21(11): 2624-2634.
49. Arnault JP, Mateus C, Escudier B, et al. Skin tumors induced by sorafenib; paradoxic RAS-RAF pathway activation and oncogenic mutations of *HRAS*, *TP53*, and *TGFBR1*. *Clin Cancer Res*. 2012;18(1):263-272.
50. Mohan SV, Chang J, Li S, et al. Increased risk of cutaneous squamous cell carcinoma after vismodegib therapy for basal cell carcinoma. *JAMA Dermatol*. 2016;152(5):527-532.
51. Asgari MM, Kiviat NB, Critchlow CW, et al. Detection of human papillomavirus DNA in cutaneous squamous cell carcinoma among immunocompetent individuals. *J Invest Dermatol*. 2008;128(6):1409-1417.
52. Karagas MR, Nelson HH, Sehr P, et al. Human papillomavirus infection and incidence of squamous cell and basal cell carcinomas of the skin. *J Natl Cancer Inst*. 2006;98(6):389-395.
53. Chockalingam R, Downing C, Tyring SK. Cutaneous squamous cell carcinomas in organ transplant recipients. *J Clin Med*. 2015;4(6):1229-1239.
54. Wang J, Aldabagh B, Yu J, et al. Role of human papillomavirus in cutaneous squamous cell carcinoma: a meta-analysis. *J Am Acad Dermatol*. 2014;70(4):621-629.
55. Harwood CA, McGregor JM, Proby CM, et al. Human papillomavirus and the development of non-melanoma skin cancer. *J Clin Pathol*. 1999;52(4):249-253.
56. Akgul B, Cooke JC, Storey A. HPV-associated skin disease. *J Pathol*. 2006;208(2):165-175.
57. Jackson S, Storey A. E6 proteins from diverse cutaneous HPV types inhibit apoptosis in response to UV damage. *Oncogene*. 2000;19(4):592-598.
58. Jackson S, Harwood C, Thomas M, et al. Role of Bak in UV-induced apoptosis in skin cancer and abrogation by HPV E6 proteins. *Genes Dev*. 2000;14(23):3065-3073.
59. Howley PM, Pfister HJ. Beta genus papillomaviruses and skin cancer. *Virology*. 2015;479-480:290-296.
60. Gabet AS, Accardi R, Bellopede A, et al. Impairment of the telomere/telomerase system and genomic instability are associated with keratinocyte immortalization induced by the skin human papillomavirus type 38. *FASEB J*. 2008;22(2):622-632.
61. LeBoit PE. Can we understand keratoacanthoma? *Am J Dermatopathol*. 2002;24(2):166-168.
62. Falchook GS, Rady P, Hymes S, et al. Merkel cell polyomavirus and HPV-17 associated with cutaneous squamous cell carcinoma arising in a patient with melanoma treated with the BRAF inhibitor dabrafenib. *JAMA Dermatol*. 2013;149(3):322-326.
63. Falchook GS, Rady P, Konopinski JC, et al. Merkel cell polyomavirus and human papilloma virus in proliferative skin lesions arising in patients treated with BRAF inhibitors. *Arch Dermatol Res*. 2016;308(5):357-365.
64. Mittapalli VR, Madl J, Loffek S, et al. Injury-driven stiffening of the dermis expedites skin carcinoma progression. *Cancer Res*. 2016;76(4):940-951.
65. Vogelstein B, Papadopoulos N, Velculescu VE, et al. Cancer genome landscapes. *Science*. 2013;339(6127): 1546-1558.
66. Jiang W, Ananthaswamy HN, Muller HK, et al. p53 protects against skin cancer induction by UV-B radiation. *Oncogene*. 1999;18(29):4247-4253.
67. Ziegler A, Jonason AS, Leffell DJ, et al. Sunburn and p53 in the onset of skin cancer. *Nature*. 1994;372(6508): 773-776.
68. Dong W, Arpin C, Accardi R, et al. Loss of p53 or p73 in human papillomavirus type 38 E6 and E7 transgenic mice partially restores the UV-activated cell cycle checkpoints. *Oncogene*. 2008;27(20):2923-2928.
69. Balmain A, Ramsden M, Bowden GT, et al. Activation of the mouse cellular Harvey-ras gene in chemically induced benign skin papillomas. *Nature*. 1984;307(5952):658-660.
70. Bamford S, Dawson E, Forbes S, et al. The COSMIC (Catalogue of Somatic Mutations in Cancer) database and website. *Br J Cancer*. 2004;91(2):355-358.
71. Tsai KY, Tsao H. The genetics of skin cancer. *Am J Med Genet C Semin Med Genet*. 2004;131C(1):82-92.
72. Dajee M, Lazarov M, Zhang JY, et al. NF-kappaB blockade and oncogenic Ras trigger invasive human epidermal neoplasia. *Nature*. 2003;421(6923):639-643.
73. Su F, Viros A, Milagre C, et al. RAS mutations in cutaneous squamous-cell carcinomas in patients treated with BRAF inhibitors. *N Engl J Med*. 2012;366(3): 207-215.
74. Uribe P, Gonzalez S. Epidermal growth factor receptor (EGFR) and squamous cell carcinoma of the skin: molecular bases for EGFR-targeted therapy. *Pathol Res Pract*. 2011;207(6):337-342.
75. Ridd K, Bastian BC. Somatic mutation of epidermal growth factor receptor in a small subset of cutaneous squamous cell carcinoma. *J Invest Dermatol*. 2010; 130(3):901-903.
76. Mauerer A, Herschberger E, Dietmaier W, et al. Low incidence of EGFR and HRAS mutations in cutaneous squamous cell carcinomas of a German cohort. *Exp Dermatol*. 2011;20(10):848-850.
77. Stratigos A, Garbe C, Lebbe C, et al. Diagnosis and treatment of invasive squamous cell carcinoma of

78. National Comprehensive Cancer Network. NCCN Guidelines Version 1.2016. Squamous Cell Skin Cancer. http://www.nccn.org. 2016.
79. Chi AC, Day TA, Neville BW. Oral cavity and oropharyngeal squamous cell carcinoma—an update. *CA Cancer J Clin*. 2015;65(5):401-421.
80. Biasoli ER, Valente VB, Mantovan B, et al. Lip cancer: a clinicopathological study and treatment outcomes in a 25-year experience. *J Oral Maxillofac Surg*. 2016;74(7):1360-1367.
81. Rinker MH, Fenske NA, Scalf LA, et al. Histologic variants of squamous cell carcinoma of the skin. *Cancer Control*. 2001;8(4):354-363.
82. Kanner WA, Brill LB 2nd, Patterson JW, et al. CD10, p63 and CD99 expression in the differential diagnosis of atypical fibroxanthoma, spindle cell squamous cell carcinoma and desmoplastic melanoma. *J Cutan Pathol*. 2010;37(7):744-750.
83. Nappi O, Wick MR, Pettinato G, et al. Pseudovascular adenoid squamous cell carcinoma of the skin. A neoplasm that may be mistaken for angiosarcoma. *Am J Surg Pathol*. 1992;16(5):429-438.
84. Breuninger H, Schaumburg-Lever G, Holzschuh J, et al. Desmoplastic squamous cell carcinoma of skin and vermilion surface: a highly malignant subtype of skin cancer. *Cancer*. 1997;79(5):915-919.
85. Goyanna R, Torres ET, Broders AC. Histological grading of malignant tumors; Broder's method [in undetermined language]. *Hospital (Rio J)*. 1951;39(6):791-818.
86. Greene FL, Sobin LH. A worldwide approach to the TNM staging system: collaborative efforts of the AJCC and UICC. *J Surg Oncol*. 2009;99(5):269-272.
87. Edge SB, Compton CC. The American Joint Committee on Cancer: the 7th edition of the AJCC cancer staging manual and the future of TNM. *Ann Surg Oncol*. 2010;17(6):1471-1474.
88. Breuninger H, Eigentler T, Bootz F, et al. Brief S2k guidelines—cutaneous squamous cell carcinoma. *J Dtsch Dermatol Ges*. 2013;11(suppl 3):37-45, 39-47.
89. Bonerandi JJ, Beauvillain C, Caquant L, et al. Guidelines for the diagnosis and treatment of cutaneous squamous cell carcinoma and precursor lesions. *J Eur Acad Dermatol Venereol*. 2011;25(suppl 5):1-51.
90. Oster-Schmidt C. Two cases of squamous cell carcinoma treated with topical imiquimod 5%. *J Eur Acad Dermatol Venereol*. 2004;18(1):93-95.
91. Morse LG, Kendrick C, Hooper D, et al. Treatment of squamous cell carcinoma with intralesional 5-fluorouracil. *Dermatol Surg*. 2003;29(11):1150-1153; discussion 1153.
92. Marmur ES, Schmults CD, Goldberg DJ. A review of laser and photodynamic therapy for the treatment of nonmelanoma skin cancer. *Dermatol Surg*. 2004;30(2, pt 2):264-271.
93. Krediet JT, Beyer M, Lenz K, et al. Sentinel lymph node biopsy and risk factors for predicting metastasis in cutaneous squamous cell carcinoma. *Br J Dermatol*. 2015;172(4):1029-1036.
94. Jarkowski A 3rd, Hare R, Loud P, et al. Systemic therapy in advanced cutaneous squamous cell carcinoma (CSCC): the Roswell Park experience and a review of the literature. *Am J Clin Oncol*. 2016;39(6):545-548.
95. Maubec E, Petrow P, Scheer-Senyarich I, et al. Phase II study of cetuximab as first-line single-drug therapy in patients with unresectable squamous cell carcinoma of the skin. *J Clin Oncol*. 2011;29(25):3419-3426.
96. Ritprajak P, Azuma M. Intrinsic and extrinsic control of expression of the immunoregulatory molecule PD-L1 in epithelial cells and squamous cell carcinoma. *Oral Oncol*. 2015;51(3):221-228.
97. Chang AL, Kim J, Luciano R, et al. A case report of unresectable cutaneous squamous cell carcinoma responsive to pembrolizumab, a programmed cell death protein 1 inhibitor. *JAMA Dermatol*. 2016;152(1):106-108.
98. Lott DG, Manz R, Koch C, et al. Aggressive behavior of nonmelanotic skin cancers in solid organ transplant recipients. *Transplantation*. 2010;90(6):683-687.
99. Rowe DE, Carroll RJ, Day CL Jr. Prognostic factors for local recurrence, metastasis, and survival rates in squamous cell carcinoma of the skin, ear, and lip. Implications for treatment modality selection. *J Am Acad Dermatol*. 1992;26(6):976-990.
100. Rapini RP. Comparison of methods for checking surgical margins. *J Am Acad Dermatol*. 1990;23(2, pt 1):288-294.
101. Brantsch KD, Meisner C, Schonfisch B, et al. Analysis of risk factors determining prognosis of cutaneous squamous-cell carcinoma: a prospective study. *Lancet Oncol*. 2008;9(8):713-720.
102. Clayman GL, Lee JJ, Holsinger FC, et al. Mortality risk from squamous cell skin cancer. *J Clin Oncol*. 2005;23(4):759-765.
103. Marcil I, Stern RS. Risk of developing a subsequent nonmelanoma skin cancer in patients with a history of nonmelanoma skin cancer: a critical review of the literature and meta-analysis. *Arch Dermatol*. 2000;136(12):1524-1530.
104. Lautenschlager S, Wulf HC, Pittelkow MR. Photoprotection. *Lancet*. 2007;370(9586):528-537.
105. Gordon LG, Scuffham PA, van der Pols JC, et al. Regular sunscreen use is a cost-effective approach to skin cancer prevention in subtropical settings. *J Invest Dermatol*. 2009;129(12):2766-2771.
106. Chen AC, Martin AJ, Choy B, et al. A phase 3 randomized trial of nicotinamide for skin-cancer chemoprevention. *N Engl J Med*. 2015;373(17):1618-1626.
107. Surjana D, Halliday GM, Damian DL. Nicotinamide enhances repair of ultraviolet radiation-induced DNA damage in human keratinocytes and ex vivo skin. *Carcinogenesis*. 2013;34(5):1144-1149.
108. Oblong JE. The evolving role of the NAD+/nicotinamide metabolome in skin homeostasis, cellular bioenergetics, and aging. *DNA Repair (Amst)*. 2014;23:59-63.
109. Gensler HL. Prevention of photoimmunosuppression and photocarcinogenesis by topical nicotinamide. *Nutr Cancer*. 1997;29(2):157-162.
110. Kuchel JM, Barnetson RS, Halliday GM. Cyclobutane pyrimidine dimer formation is a molecular trigger for solar-simulated ultraviolet radiation-induced suppression of memory immunity in humans. *Photochem Photobiol Sci*. 2005;4(8):577-582.
111. Shimizu M, Suzui M, Deguchi A, et al. Effects of acyclic retinoid on growth, cell cycle control, epidermal growth factor receptor signaling, and gene expression in human squamous cell carcinoma cells. *Clin Cancer Res*. 2004;10(3):1130-1140.
112. Amini S, Viera MH, Valins W, et al. Nonsurgical innovations in the treatment of nonmelanoma skin cancer. *J Clin Aesthet Dermatol*. 2010;3(6):20-34.

113. Bavinck JN, Tieben LM, Van der Woude FJ, et al. Prevention of skin cancer and reduction of keratotic skin lesions during acitretin therapy in renal transplant recipients: a double-blind, placebo-controlled study. *J Clin Oncol*. 1995;13(8):1933-1938.
114. Chen K, Craig JC, Shumack S. Oral retinoids for the prevention of skin cancers in solid organ transplant recipients: a systematic review of randomized controlled trials. *Br J Dermatol*. 2005;152(3):518-523.
115. Kraemer KH, DiGiovanna JJ, Moshell AN, et al. Prevention of skin cancer in xeroderma pigmentosum with the use of oral isotretinoin. *N Engl J Med*. 1988;318(25):1633-1637.

Chapter 113 :: Merkel Cell Carcinoma
:: Aubriana McEvoy & Paul Nghiem

第一百一十三章

梅克尔细胞癌

中文导读

梅克尔细胞癌(MCC)是一种越来越常见的神经内分泌皮肤癌，与紫外线照射、高龄、免疫抑制和梅克尔细胞多瘤病毒有关。本章分为9节：①历史视角；②流行病学；③临床表现；④临床病程和并发症；⑤病因和发病机制；⑥诊断；⑦鉴别诊断；⑧分期与预后；⑨临床管理。

第一节历史视角，介绍了梅克尔细胞发现的历程，并提出了MCC更可能来自表皮前体细胞的观点，正常的Merkel细胞和MCC之间表型具有高度的相似性。

第二节流行病学，介绍了从1986—2006年间，报告的MCC发病率增加了两倍，原因之一可能是提高了这种肿瘤的准确诊断，第二个可能原因是MCC危险因素的增加。

第三节临床表现，介绍了MCC的皮肤表现和皮肤外表现，皮肤表现中提出了AEIOU缩写，容易误诊为囊肿或痤疮样病变。

第四节临床病程和并发症，介绍了90%以上MCC患者在病理确诊之前误诊为其他疾病，并存在局部区域和远处复发的几种模式。

第五节病因和发病机制，介绍了其高危因素包括年龄大于65岁、日照、免疫抑制，同时详细介绍了梅克尔细胞多瘤病毒在MCC中的作用。

第六节诊断，介绍了诊断方法包括病理组织学特点、苏木精伊红染色及免疫组化染色。

第七节鉴别诊断，通过表113-2概述了MCC的鉴别诊断。

第八节分期与预后，介绍了根据美国癌症联合委员会(AJCC)的第8版MCC分期系统进行分期，同时介绍了与预后相关的组织学特点，包括淋巴血管侵犯、肿瘤生长模式、梅克尔细胞多瘤病毒癌蛋白表达、P63、CD8浸润。

第九节临床管理，介绍了多种治疗方式的优缺点、临床监测的影像学监测及血清学监测、最佳治疗方案。

〔粟 娟〕

AT-A-GLANCE

- The risk of death from Merkel cell carcinoma (MCC) is 2 to 3 times higher than from melanoma.
- Reported incidence of MCC quadrupled from 1986 to 2006.
- Risk factors for MCC include advanced age, immune suppression, and fair skin.
- Merkel cell polyomavirus (MCPyV) is integrated in 80% of MCC cases.
- Consider MCC in the differential diagnosis of any rapidly growing, nontender nodule on a sun-exposed area.
- Management is challenging as therapy is unique and controversial.
- Sentinel lymph node biopsy, surgery, and radiation are indicated in many cases.
- Imaging (CT, MRI, positron emission tomography) has poor sensitivity and specificity in early stages of MCC, but can be useful in assessment of and surveillance for metastatic disease.
- MCC is an especially radiosensitive tumor. Adjuvant radiation therapy is highly effective, and overaggressive surgery should be avoided. Radiation monotherapy is an important and effective option for managing disease in patients who are not candidates for surgery.
- Immune therapies, including checkpoint inhibition and T-cell therapies are now the treatment of choice for advanced disease.
- Chemotherapy has very limited utility in treating MCC, and adjuvant chemotherapy is not beneficial. Adjuvant immune therapy is an area of new research.
- Optimal care includes multidisciplinary coordination between dermatologists, surgeons, radiologists, and medical oncologists with reference to the National Comprehensive Cancer Network (NCCN) guidelines.

Merkel cell carcinoma (MCC) is an increasingly common neuroendocrine skin cancer that is associated with ultraviolet (UV) light exposure, advanced age, immune suppression, and the Merkel cell polyomavirus (MCPyV). The reported incidence of MCC has more than tripled in the past 20 years[1] to approximately 1500 U.S. cases/year,[2] and is expected to grow with the aging population. Although it is 40 times less common than malignant melanoma, it carries a markedly poorer prognosis, with disease-associated mortality at 5 years of 46%[3] as compared with 9% for invasive melanoma.[4] Management of MCC is controversial as optimal therapy is rapidly evolving with promising immune therapy options.

HISTORICAL PERSPECTIVE

MCC is a relatively recently described entity, although the Merkel cell was identified more than 100 years ago. In 1875, human Merkel cells were first described by Friedrich S. Merkel (1845-1919). He named these cells *Tastzellen* (touch cells) assuming that they had a sensory touch function within the skin because of their association with nerves. In 2009, a series of studies using mouse models resolved several longstanding debates by conclusively establishing that (a) Merkel cells are essential for light touch responses,[5] (b) Merkel cells have an epidermal origin,[5,6] and (c) Merkel cells do not divide, but are renewed by a reservoir of epidermal progenitor cells.[6]

In 1972, Toker described 5 cases of "trabecular cell carcinoma of the skin," consistent with what we now call MCC. In 1978, Tang and Toker found that cells from these tumors contained dense core granules on electron microscopy that were typical of Merkel cells and other neuroendocrine cells. In 1980, the name *Merkel cell carcinoma* was first applied to this tumor because of the characteristic ultrastructural features it shares with normal Merkel cells. In 1992, it was found that antibodies to cytokeratin-20 stain normal skin Merkel cells as well as the vast majority of MCC tumors. This critical finding enables specific and relatively easy diagnosis of MCC to be made through immunohistochemistry. Since that time, electron microscopy is no longer used to make this diagnosis. Of note, it is unlikely that MCC is derived from normal Merkel cells within the skin (these cells are postmitotic and it has proven impossible to coax them to divide). Even though it is more likely that MCC derives from epidermal precursor cells, the phenotypic similarities between the normal Merkel cells and MCC are striking and informative.

EPIDEMIOLOGY

Between 1986 and 2006, the reported incidence of MCC quadrupled from 0.15 per 100,000[1] to 0.6 per 100,000 persons.[7] This increase in reported incidence is more rapid than any other type of skin cancer, and can be attributed to two factors. One factor is an increase in the accurate diagnosis of this malignancy through the routine use of cytokeratin-20 immunohistochemistry and the improved recognition of this malignancy by dermatopathologists. In the past, MCCs were often mischaracterized as lymphoma, melanoma, or undifferentiated carcinoma in the era before immunohistochemistry. A second likely factor is an increase in the prevalence of MCC risk factors: a growing population older than age 65 years with extensive sun exposure history, and more individuals living with prolonged immune suppression. Risk factors for MCC are discussed in section "Etiology and Pathogenesis".

There are approximately 2500 MCC cases per year in the United States.[2] It is far more common in white individuals than in black individuals, which is consistent with a known role for UV radiation in

MCC pathogenesis. Specifically, the MCC rates for white individuals have been reported as 0.23 per 100,000 as compared to 0.01 per 100,000 for black individuals.[8] Although not specifically reported, rates in Latino and Asian populations are likely intermediate between those in populations of black and white individuals. MCC is more common in men than in women (2:1 ratio).[9] Furthermore, men also tend to have a worse prognosis than women, with reported 10-year disease-associated survival rates of 51% for men and 65% for women.[7]

CLINICAL PRESENTATION

CUTANEOUS FINDINGS

In a 2008 systematic analysis of 195 MCC patients, clinical features of MCC were characterized.[10] The most significant features can be summarized in an acronym: AEIOU (asymptomatic/lack of tenderness, expanding rapidly, immune suppression, older than age 50 years, and UV-exposed site on a person with fair skin; Table 113-1). This study found that 89% of MCC cases exhibited at least 3 of the 5 features listed below in Table 113-1. If a lesion exhibits at least 3 of these features, suspicion of MCC should increase, and biopsy of the lesion is indicated. In particular, a lesion that is red or purple, rapidly growing, and nontender should be concerning.

Strikingly, in more than one-half of MCC cases, the clinician listed a benign diagnosis as the initial clinical impression. In particular, a cyst or acneiform lesion were the most common diagnoses (Table 113-2 and Figs. 113-1A and 113-1B), and nonmelanoma skin cancer was also a relatively frequent presumptive diagnosis (Fig. 113-1C).

NONCUTANEOUS FINDINGS

MCC may present with regional lymph node or distant metastatic disease, with or without a known primary cutaneous lesion. Reports indicate that MCC patients presenting without an identifiable primary lesion—"unknown primary"—have better outcomes than similarly staged patients with known primary tumors.[11] It is possible that primary lesion regression is immune mediated, and that the immune system of a patient with an unknown primary lesion is able to recognize and respond to the disease. This underlines the importance of developments in immune therapy such as T-cell therapy and checkpoint therapy as systemic treatment options.

Recurrent or metastatic MCC is generally detectable via positron emission tomography–CT scan and/or clinical examination, and frequently includes noncutaneous sites. One study demonstrated that about half of patients with local or nodal disease at presentation recurred after primary treatment. For patients who experienced a recurrence, the site of first recurrence was: local (21% of first recurrences), nodal (27% of first recurrences presented as regional lymphadenopathy), and distant (52% of first recurrences occurred at sites beyond the regional draining lymph nodes).[12] In the past, MCC metastases to the viscera indicated incurable disease. However, immune therapy trials have reported a high percentage of positive, durable responses of advanced MCC as detailed in section "Immune Therapy".

CLINICAL COURSE AND COMPLICATIONS

In more than 90% of cases, MCC is an unanticipated diagnosis before the pathology results become known. Most commonly, the lesion in question was thought to be a cyst or acneiform lesion. Although most patients and many physicians are not familiar with this disease or its specific management, MCC can be lethal and it is important to initiate therapy promptly. In one Australian study, a high fraction of patients (45%) developed progressive disease while waiting for adjuvant radiation therapy to begin (median wait time: 41 days).[13]

TABLE 113-2
Differential Diagnosis of Merkel Cell Carcinoma

Most Likely
- Cyst
- Basal cell carcinoma
- Squamous cell carcinoma (see Fig. 113-1C)
- Amelanotic melanoma
- Cutaneous lymphoma
- Adnexal tumor

Consider
- Metastasis
- Dermatofibrosarcoma protuberans
- Keratoacanthoma
- Neuroblastoma

TABLE 113-1
Clinical Features of Merkel Cell Carcinoma

- **A**symptomatic (nontender, firm, red, purple, or skin-colored papule or nodule; ulceration is rare; see Figs. 113-1A and 113-1B)
- **E**xpanding rapidly (significant growth noted within 1-3 months of diagnosis, but most lesions are <2 cm at time of diagnosis)
- **I**mmune suppression (eg, HIV/AIDS, chronic lymphocytic leukemia, solid organ transplant)
- **O**lder than 50 years of age
- **U**ltraviolet-exposed site on a person with fair skin (most likely presentation, but can also occur in sun-protected areas; see Fig. 113-2)

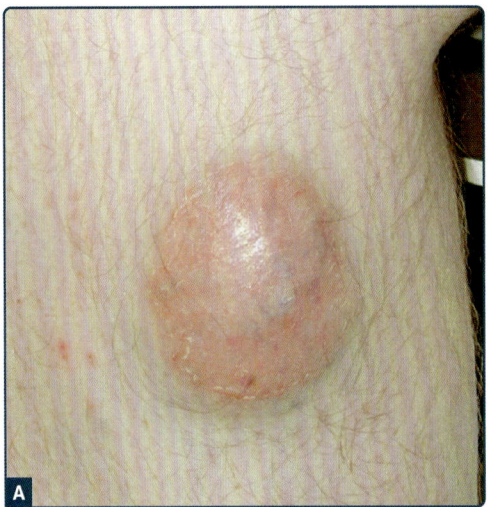
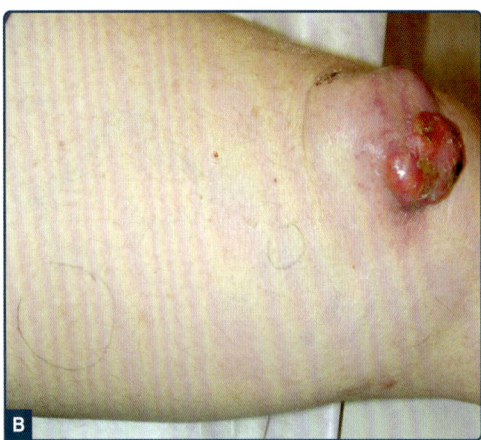
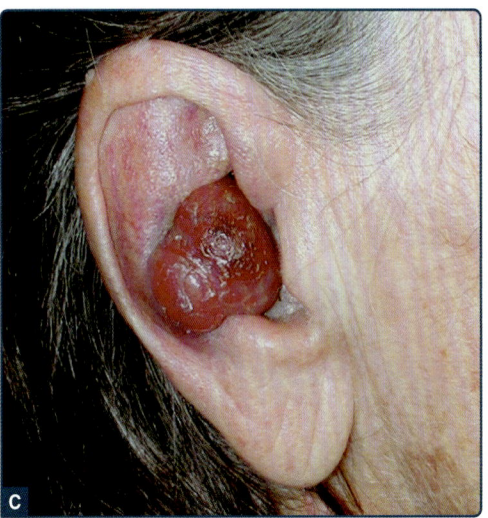

Figure 113-1 Clinical appearance of Merkel cell carcinoma (MCC). **A,** MCC frequently has a "cyst-like" appearance. This is reflected in the differential diagnoses given by clinicians at the time of the biopsy, with cyst/acneiform lesion being the most common clinical impression. **B,** MCC on the knee of a 70-year-old woman with chronic lymphocytic leukemia. For 6 months this lesion was thought to be a "cyst"; consequently, diagnosis and treatment were delayed. Pen marks indicate palpable satellite metastases that developed several months after the primary lesion, presumably tracking via lymphatics. **C,** MCC on the ear of an 87-year-old woman. The lesion grew rapidly and was nontender. After approximately 3 months, it was biopsied by a clinician who listed squamous cell carcinoma as the presumptive diagnosis.

The patterns of MCC local, regional, and distant recurrences differ from melanoma. Among patients who experience a recurrence of their MCC, approximately 80% recur within 2 years of diagnosis.[14] MCC patients who have had no recurrences for 3 to 5 years, have a greatly reduced risk of recurrence.

The complications for those who do not experience a metastasis depend very much on the therapy they received. We believe that treatment with surgical excision, radiation therapy, and possibly systemic therapy as outlined in this chapter has relatively minimal complication rates and the best possible chance of cure based on current literature. Furthermore, for those who receive very aggressive surgical excision, amputation, or chemotherapy for low-risk disease, complication rates tend to be higher without improved outcomes.

ETIOLOGY AND PATHOGENESIS

There are several known risk factors for MCC that have led to an increase in the incidence of this disease.

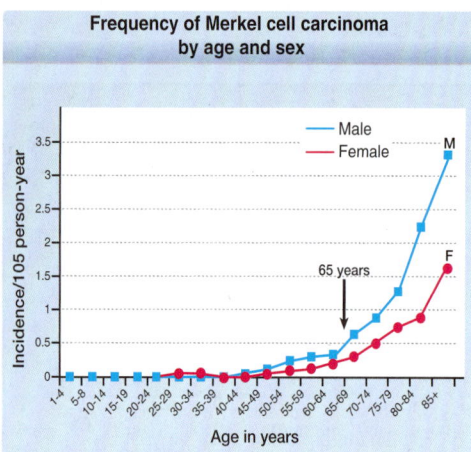

Figure 113-2 Frequency of Merkel cell carcinoma by age and sex. The most significant risk factor for Merkel cell carcinoma is age. M, male (■); F, female (●). (Reprinted from Agelli M, Clegg LX. Epidemiology of primary Merkel cell carcinoma in the United States. *J Am Acad Dermatol.* 2003;49:832, with permission. Copyright © American Academy of Dermatology.)

RISK FACTORS

AGE GREATER THAN 65 YEARS

The median age for diagnosis of MCC is 70 years, and there is a 5- to 10-fold increase in incidence after age 70 years, compared with age younger than 60 years (Fig. 113-2). Furthermore, only approximately 10% of MCC cases present in patients younger than age 50 years, and it is extremely rare in childhood.[10]

SUN EXPOSURE

Sunlight, prolonged UV exposure, and photochemotherapy are all associated with an increased risk of MCC. As Fig. 113-3 illustrates, the majority of MCC tumors present on sun-exposed skin.[10] However, it is clear that sun exposure is not required for MCC to develop. MCC cases can occur on sun-protected skin, including buttocks and the inguinal/groin/genital regions, as well as portions of the scalp that are covered by hair.

IMMUNE SUPPRESSION

MCC is strongly associated with immune suppression. Approximately 8% of MCC patients are profoundly immune suppressed, which is a 16-fold overrepresentation compared with what is expected.[10] Multiple forms of immune suppression are associated with an increased risk for MCC, including HIV/AIDS,[15] non-Hodgkin lymphoma including chronic lymphocytic leukemia,[10] immune suppressive regimens associated with solid-organ transplantation, and chronic treatment of autoimmune disease.[9]

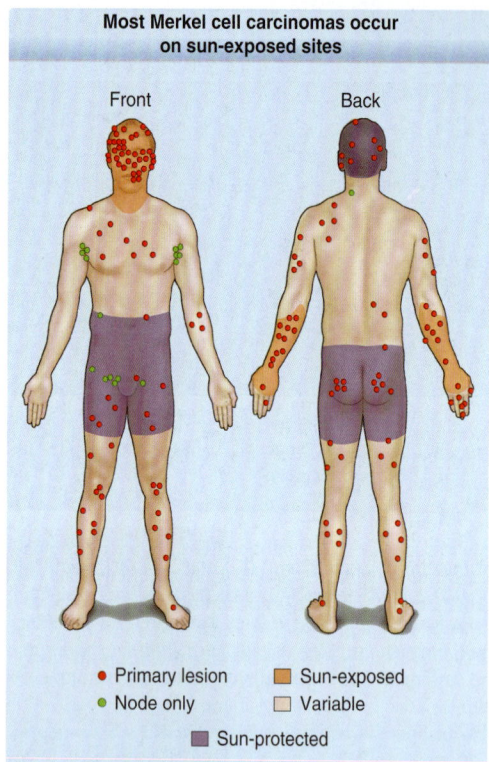

Figure 113-3 Merkel cell carcinomas (MCCs) occur frequently, but not exclusively, on sun-exposed sites. This diagram shows the locations of tumor presentation for 195 MCC patients. For the 168 patients with a known primary lesion, 96 of them (57%) presented with a primary tumor located on the heavily sun-exposed face, neck, or arm (*brown shading*). 62 patients (37%) of patients presented with MCC in partially sun-protected skin (*skin tone*), and 10 patients (~6%) presented with tumors in completely sun-protected skin areas (*purple shading*). (Adapted from Heath M, Jaimes N, Lemos B, et al. Clinical characteristics of Merkel cell carcinoma at diagnosis in 195 patients: the AEIOU features. *J Am Acad Dermatol.* 2008;58:375-381.)

Additionally, there are 19 reported cases of complete spontaneous regression in the MCC literature—a far greater number than expected for its rarity—suggesting immune recognition and clearance of MCC.[8,16]

MERKEL CELL POLYOMAVIRUS

In 2008, the MCPyV was discovered by extensive sequencing of MCC tumor RNA. MCPyV was reported to be present in 80% of MCC tumors compared to only 7% of skin controls.[17] Numerous groups across several continents (more than 25 literature citations) have verified a strong association between MCPyV and MCC.

MCPyV is a small, circular, double-stranded DNA virus related to other known polyomaviruses (including SV40, BK, JC, KI, and WU). MCPyV is unique among the human polyomaviruses as it is the only one proven to integrate into and be causal for human cancer.[17] Monoclonal integration of MCPyV into MCC tumors suggests that the virus is present prior to or very early in tumorigenesis.

In an analysis of exome sequencing of 49 MCCs, each tumor was grouped into 1 of 2 mutational profiles: one group of MCC tumors with relatively low mutational burden (relatively few single-nucleotide variants, *MCC-LO*, on the left side of Fig. 113-4), and the other group included tumors with relatively high mutational burden (*MCC-HI*, on the far right of Fig. 113-4).[18] Analysis demonstrated strong relationships between the mutational burden and presence of either MCPyV integration or UV-induced mutations. A vast majority of the MCC-LO tumors contained MCPyV (virus-positive), whereas virtually all of the MCC-HI tumors were virus-negative. Furthermore, the mutations in the MCC-HI tumors were almost entirely UV-induced. Simply put, it appears that generation of a MCC tumor requires either integration of the Merkel polyomavirus, or extensive UV-induced mutations—even a higher number than for melanoma (*SKCM* in Fig. 113-4).

A large fraction of the population has been exposed to the MCPyV. Accurate data about prior exposure to polyomaviruses can be derived by determining the prevalence of MCPyV capsid antibodies, which are easily differentiated from other polyomaviruses. The capsid proteins are very specific to MCPyV. By the age of 5 years, the prevalence of individuals who produce antibodies to the MCPyV capsid protein is approximately 35%; it increases to 50% by the age of 15 years.[19] Interestingly, among MCC patients, the prevalence of individuals that produce capsid antibodies is significantly higher (88%) than age-matched and sex-matched controls (53%).[20]

Despite the nearly ubiquitous exposure to this virus in the general population, the incidence of MCC is very low. For MCPyV to cause cancer, the virus must integrate into the host's DNA and evade the host's immune system. A key portion of the MCPyV—the "oncoprotein" or T-antigen—is present in approximately 80% of all MCC tumors. This protein is critical for most MCC tumors to grow.

Antibodies to the MCPyV oncoprotein can be detected and measured using a clinically available serology test. Determining the oncoprotein antibody status is clinically useful for newly diagnosed MCC patients, whether or not they are antibody producers. For patients who produce oncoprotein antibodies, tracking their antibody titer can be used to detect early MCC recurrence. Patients who do not produce detectable oncoprotein antibodies are at higher risk of recurrence and will need to be followed more closely with surveillance, consisting of clinical and radiologic examinations (more details in section "Surveillance").

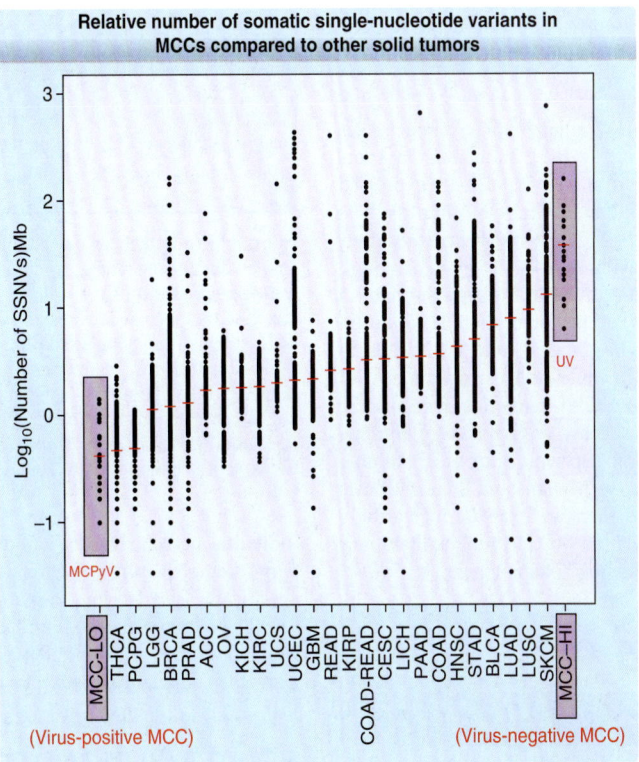

Figure 113-4 Relative number of somatic single-nucleotide variants (SSNVs) in MCCs compared to other solid tumors sequenced by The Cancer Genome Atlas. The red lines reflect the median number of SSNVs in each group. (Reproduced from Goh G, Walradt T, Markarov V, et al: Mutational landscape of MCPyV-positive and MCPyV-negative Merkel cell carcinomas with implications for immunotherapy. *Oncotarget.* 2016;7(3):3403-3415, with permission.)

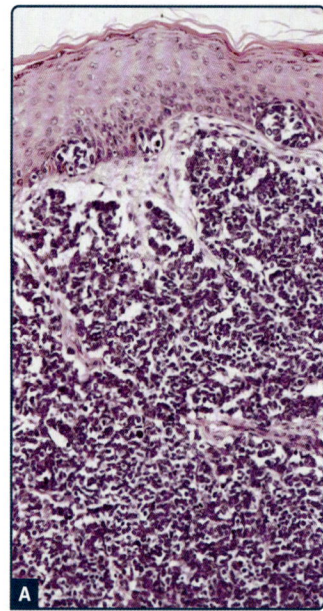

Figure 113-5 Merkel cell carcinoma (MCC) carcinogenesis: 2 distinct mechanisms. Virus-negative MCCs harbor extremely large numbers of UV-induced mutations, which can serve as neoantigens for tumor recognition by the immune system. Merkel polyomavirus-positive MCCs persistently express viral proteins that drive the cancer cells to divide. These viral oncoproteins can be used to track disease progression (via antibodies in the blood that indicate tumor recurrence) and serve as nonself proteins that can be recognized by the immune system.

The MCPyV and UV radiation play distinct roles in MCC tumorigenesis. In the 80% of MCC tumors that contain MCPyV, viral oncoproteins are expressed through clonal integration of viral DNA into the host genome. In the 20% of MCCs that are virus-negative, UV-induced mutations are present at extremely high levels (on average, several times higher even than in malignant melanoma). A portion of these UV-induced mutations represent neoantigens that are visible to the immune system. In either case, expression of viral oncoproteins or UV-induced neoantigens means the tumor must develop effective mechanisms of immune evasion for the tumor to survive. Figure 113-5 summarizes these oncogenic mechanisms and their relevance to the immune-based therapies that are increasingly available to treat advanced MCC. (Immune therapy is discussed further in section "Management".)

DIAGNOSIS

PATHOLOGY

As Figure 113-6A shows, the classic histologic features of MCC include sheets of small basophilic cells with scant cytoplasm, fine chromatin, and no nucleoli. There are numerous mitotic figures and occasional

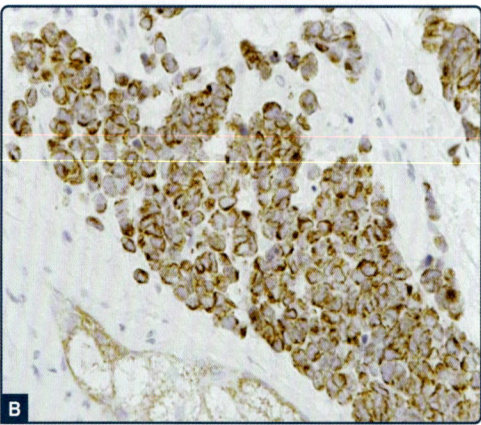

Figure 113-6 Merkel cell carcinoma pathology. **A,** Hematoxylin and eosin. There is diffuse dermal as well as intraepidermal involvement with Merkel cell carcinoma. This case was seen in consultation, with an initial diagnosis of cutaneous T-cell lymphoma. **B,** Cytokeratin-20. Showing the pathognomonic "perinuclear pattern" of cytokeratins (CAM5.2). (Reprinted from Nghiem P, Mckee P, Haynes H. Merkel cell [cutaneous neuroendocrine] carcinoma. In: Sober A, Haluska F, eds. *Skin Cancer, Atlas of Clinical Oncology*. Atlanta, GA:, American Cancer Society; 2001, with permission.)

individual necrotic cells. Lymphovascular invasion is a very common feature and often can be found when it is specifically searched for, even in a "negative" margin. This helps to explain the high local recurrence rate in MCC for narrow or even relatively wide margin excision when adjuvant radiation therapy is not given.

HEMATOXYLIN AND EOSIN STAIN

Three histologic patterns have been described up to now and none is clearly associated with a better or worse prognosis. The most common type is the "intermediate type." This type features uniform small cells with minimal cytoplasm, pale nuclei, and a dispersed chromatin appearance. On hematoxylin and eosin staining, the differential diagnosis for this presentation is that of the small, blue-cell tumors, including melanoma and lymphoma. The second most common pattern is the "small cell type." This takes its name from small-cell lung carcinoma, which is the principal differential diagnosis for this pattern. It shows irregular, hyperchromatic cells with scant cytoplasm and malignant cells that are arranged in linear patterns infiltrating stromal structures. The least common, but perhaps most histologically distinctive type, is the "trabecular" type. This is the pattern originally described by Toker in 1972. It has a lattice-like, or network appearance, and the differential diagnosis includes metastatic carcinoid tumor.

IMMUNOHISTOCHEMICAL STAINS

The use of antibody-based stains has greatly facilitated the ease and specificity of MCC diagnosis (Table 113-3). The single most useful of these stains is cytokeratin-20.

CYTOKERATIN-20

This intermediate filament protein is expressed in MCC as well as in adenocarcinomas of the colon, stomach, and pancreas. However, within the skin, the expression of cytokeratin-20 is limited to Merkel cells. A "perinuclear dot" pattern of cytokeratin is essentially pathognomonic for MCC (see Fig. 113-6B). However, 10% to 20% of MCCs are cytokeratin-20–negative.

ANTIBODIES TO CAM5.2

CAM5.2, a cocktail of antibodies that detects multiple human cytokeratin epitopes, typically reacts with both MCC and small-cell lung carcinoma. Although it is useful as an initial screening tool to detect tumors of squamous origin, its lack of selectivity relative to cytokeratin-20 means that it cannot be used to definitively diagnose MCC.

THYROID TRANSCRIPTION FACTOR-1

Thyroid transcription factor-1 is negative in MCC and positive in small-cell lung cancer. Consequently, it is useful for the differential diagnosis between these 2 tumors that can look identical by routine histology.

CYTOKERATIN-7

Cytokeratin-7 has the same staining pattern as thyroid transcription factor-1, that is, typically negative in MCC and positive in small-cell lung carcinoma. It is also expressed in epithelial cells of the lung, ovary, and breast.

MERKEL CELL POLYOMAVIRUS ONCOPROTEIN

MCC tumor tissue may be tested for the MCPyV oncoprotein using the CM2B4 antibody. The CM2B4 antibody is specific for MCC, rather than other tumors, and is an excellent tool for determining if an MCC is virally induced or not. MCC tumors induced only by UV radiation (no virus) would be negative for CM2B4, and approximately 20% of MCCs would thus be negative for this antibody. The relationship between CM2B4 antibody presence and prognosis is controversial, but viral positivity is likely associated with moderately decreased risk of MCC recurrence.

DIFFERENTIAL DIAGNOSIS

Table 113-2 outlines the differential diagnosis of MCC.

STAGING AND PROGNOSIS

Survival after a diagnosis of MCC is highly dependent on the stage at presentation, and decreases markedly with nodal involvement and metastatic disease.

TABLE 113-3
Immunohistochemistry Panel

	CYTOKERATIN-20	CYTOKERATIN-7 AND THYROID TRANSCRIPTION FACTOR-1	LEUKOCYTE COMMON ANTIGEN	S-100	ONCOPROTEIN ANTIBODY CM2B4
Merkel cell carcinoma	+	−	−	−	+ (In Merkel cell polyomavirus-induced Merkel cell carcinomas)
Small-cell lung carcinoma	−	+	−	−	−
Lymphoma	−	−	+	−	−
Melanoma	−	−	−	+	−

In 2010, the American Joint Committee on Cancer (AJCC) adopted the 7th edition staging system for MCC that replaced 5 existing—and conflicting—staging systems.[19] The AJCC's 8th edition staging system for MCC was adopted in 2018. As with other staging systems, the 8th edition system uses the TNM (tumor, node, metastasis) staging system, with information from clinical examinations, imaging studies, and pathologic evaluation of the primary tumor, lymph nodes, and metastatic lesions. A major change with this new staging system is that patients with clinically apparent lymph node involvement are split into 2 groups based on whether or not they have a detectable/known primary lesion. Those without a known primary lesion have significantly better survival and are now included in stage IIIA, while those with a known primary lesion are stage IIIB.[20] Table 113-4 summarizes this staging system.

MCC-specific survival and progression-free survival are important analyses for estimating prognosis by stage. An online resource, http://www.merkelcell.org, is devoted to aiding patients and physicians by presenting current data, including stage-specific prognostic information, and referral center availability. Figure 113-7 details overall survival by stage.

SENTINEL LYMPH NODE BIOPSY

In addition to its established role in managing higher risk melanoma, several studies have indicated that sentinel lymph node biopsy (SLNB) is also a sensitive test for detecting MCC spread to the lymph nodes.[21-23] Interestingly, MCC is far more likely to have occult lymph node involvement (approximately 30% for the average 1.7-cm MCC) than melanoma (~1% for melanomas with the average Breslow thickness of 0.63 mm).[23,24] SLNB (typically involving 1 to 3 nodes) clearly has less morbidity than an elective lymph node

TABLE 113-4
Outline of American Joint Committee on Cancer 8th Edition Staging System for Merkel Cell Carcinoma

STAGE		PRIMARY TUMOR	LYMPH NODE	METASTASIS
0		In situ (within epidermis only)	No regional lymph node metastasis	No distant metastasis
I	Clinical[a]	≤2 cm maximum tumor dimension	Nodes negative by clinical examination (no pathologic examination performed)	No distant metastasis
I	Pathologic[b]	≤2 cm maximum tumor dimension	Nodes negative by pathologic examination	No distant metastasis
IIA	Clinical	>2 cm tumor dimension	Nodes negative by clinical examination (no pathologic examination performed)	No distant metastasis
IIA	Pathologic	>2 cm tumor dimension	Nodes negative by pathologic examination	No distant metastasis
IIB	Clinical	Primary tumor invades bone, muscle, fascia, or cartilage	Nodes negative by clinical examination (no pathologic examination performed)	No distant metastasis
IIB	Pathologic	Primary tumor invades bone, muscle, fascia, or cartilage	Nodes negative by pathologic examination	No distant metastasis
III	Clinical	Any size/depth tumor	Nodes positive by clinical examination (no pathologic examination performed)	No distant metastasis
IIIA	Pathologic	Any size/depth tumor	Nodes positive by pathologic examination only (nodal disease not apparent on clinical examination)	No distant metastasis
		Not detected ("unknown primary")	Nodes positive by clinical examination, and confirmed via pathologic examination	No distant metastasis
IIIB	Pathologic	Any size/depth tumor	Nodes positive by clinical examination, and confirmed via pathologic examination OR in-transit metastasis[c]	No distant metastasis
IV	Clinical	Any	+/− Regional nodal involvement	Distant metastasis detected via clinical examination
IV	Pathologic	Any	+/− Regional nodal involvement	Distant metastasis confirmed via pathologic examination

[a]Clinical detection of nodal or metastatic disease may be via inspection, palpation, and/or imaging
[b]Pathologic detection/confirmation of nodal disease may be via sentinel lymph node biopsy, lymphadenectomy, or fine-needle biopsy; and pathologic confirmation of metastatic disease may be via biopsy of the suspected metastasis
[c]In transit metastasis: a tumor distinct from the primary lesion and located either (a) between the primary lesion and the draining regional lymph nodes or (b) distal to the primary lesion
Note: In this staging system updated for 2017, it is necessary to specify whether staging was determined by clinical evaluation or microscopic/pathologic evaluation.
Adapted by Aubriana McEvoy and Dr. Paul Nghiem with permission of Springer: Harms KL, Healy MA, Nghiem P, et al. Analysis of prognostic factors from 9387 Merkel cell carcinoma cases forms the basis for the new 8th edition AJCC staging system. *Ann Surg Oncol.* 2016;23(11):3564-3571. Copyright © Society of Surgical Oncology 2016. See www.merkelcell.org/staging for more information.

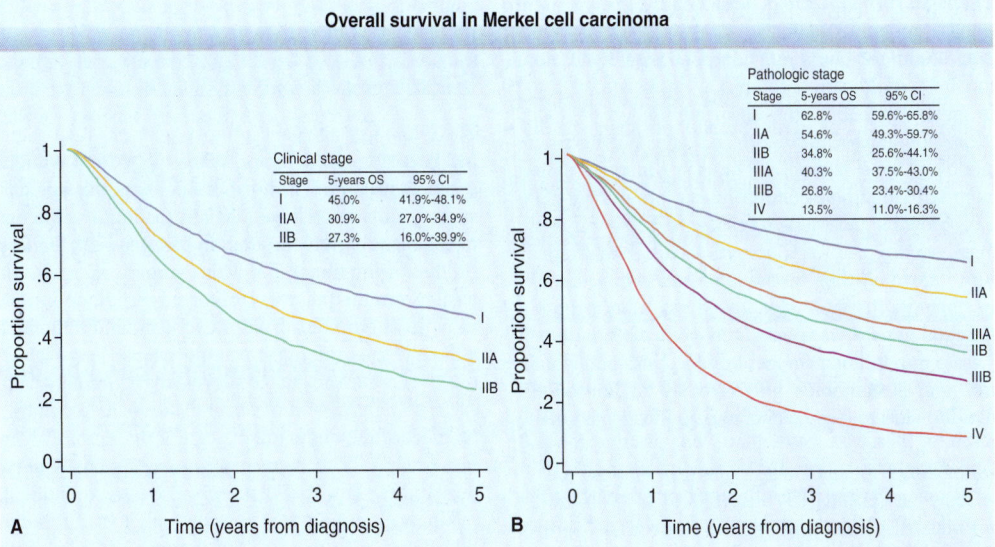

Figure 113-7 Overall survival in Merkel cell carcinoma (MCC). Prognosis of MCC depends on stage at diagnosis. This figure shows overall survival curves for 9387 Merkel cell carcinoma patients by "Clinical Stage" (see Fig. 113-6A) and "Pathologic Stage" (see Fig. 113-6B). Particularly for low-risk (stage I) MCC, most deaths are not from MCC in this older population. (Reprinted with permission of Springer: Harms KL, Healy MA, Nghiem P, et al. Analysis of prognostic factors from 9387 Merkel cell carcinoma cases forms the basis for the new 8th edition AJCC staging system. *Ann Surg Oncol*. 2016;23(11): 3564-3571. Copyright © Society of Surgical Oncology 2016.)

dissection (typically involving more than 20 nodes). Ideally, an SLNB should be performed at the time of the wide resection, as opposed to after the wide excision when local lymphatics have been disturbed.

The SLNB is critical for detecting microscopic lymph node disease, which is not apparent on clinical examination. It has been demonstrated that one-third of patients with local-only disease based on clinical examination, in fact, have occult nodal disease that very much affects their subsequent survival (see Fig. 113-7).[23] Specifically, one-third of patients would be understaged by clinical examination only, and would shift to stage III disease with microscopic evaluation. Identification of microscopic nodal disease also importantly alters therapy for the node bed, as discussed in subsequent sections.

RADIOLOGIC IMAGING

In the era of immune therapy, there is a potentially stronger rationale for more frequent imaging studies. New therapies are sometimes curative and are more likely to be effective in earlier stages of MCC, which correspond to lower disease burdens. Thus, baseline scans are indicated in most patients except those with very-low-risk disease (eg, primary ≤1 cm and negative SLNB), or those who would not be candidates for systemic treatment because of advanced age or comorbidities. Although in some situations, positron emission tomography/CT may have better sensitivity and is often performed at diagnosis for baseline imaging, CT scans are typically performed for ongoing surveillance because of cost.

PROGNOSTIC FINDINGS ON HISTOLOGY

There are 6 histologic findings that may be associated with MCC outcomes. Each histologic feature and its correlation to survival is discussed below.

LYMPHOVASCULAR INVASION

Lymphovascular invasion can be defined as tumor emboli within vascular spaces. One study found that the tumors of MCC patients with detectable lymphovascular invasion had a worse overall survival as compared to those with tumors without lymphovascular invasion (hazard ratio: 3.84; $P = 0.007$).[25] However, the clinical correlation of lymphovascular invasion evaluation awaits independent validation.

TUMOR GROWTH PATTERN

MCC growth pattern is described as nodular (well-circumscribed interface between tumor and surrounding tissue) or infiltrative (rows, trabeculae, or single cells that penetrate the dermis). Tumors that exhibited both features were considered infiltrative. An infiltrative tumor growth pattern was associated with poor outcomes as compared to MCC tumors with a nodular growth pattern (hazard ratio: 6.85; $P = 0.001$).[25] Tumor growth pattern and its association with outcomes has not been independently validated and clinically utility is controversial.

MERKEL CELL POLYOMAVIRUS ONCOPROTEIN EXPRESSION

The monoclonal antibody, CM2B4, recognizes the large T-antigen of MCPyV in MCC tissue specimens. As discussed in section "Merkel Cell Polyomavirus" above, MCC tumors can be classified into 1 of 2 subgroups depending on their MCPyV involvement. Although controversial, MCPyV positivity tends to be associated with better outcomes.[26]

P63

Transformation-related/tumor protein 63 can be identified in approximately one-third to one-half of MCC cases. In 2 studies, cases that were positive for p63 demonstrated a more aggressive clinical course than those that were negative, although the strength of the association has been questioned.[27] Clinical significance is controversial.

CD8 INFILTRATION

One 2013 study investigated whether specific mechanisms of T-cell migration may be commonly disrupted in MCC tumors with poor CD8 lymphocyte infiltration. Intratumoral vascular E-selectin, critical for T-cell entry into skin, was downregulated in the majority (52%) of MCCs and its loss was associated with poor intratumoral CD8 lymphocyte infiltration ($p < 0.05$; n = 45). Importantly, survival was improved in MCC patients whose tumors had higher vascular E-selectin expression ($p < 0.05$). These data suggest that one mechanism of immune evasion in MCC may be restriction of T-cell entry into the tumor.[28] Further investigation demonstrated a reliable method for evaluating CD8 lymphocyte infiltration via paraffin-embedded tissue examination, and that infiltration is independently associated with improved MCC-specific survival.[29,30]

MANAGEMENT

In the past 10 years, the optimal therapy for MCC has evolved with exciting advances in treatment options. Furthermore, the expanding availability of clinical trials is allowing for more data collection to support optimization of treatment. These developments have provided an especially improved outlook for stage IV patients, whose disease was previously only viewed as treatable with palliation.

The best summary of consensus treatment of MCC is available through the National Comprehensive Cancer Network (http://www.nccn.org) and is updated annually (these guidelines and other useful information can also be found at http://www.merkelcell.org/usefulInfo/). The best outcome for MCC is clearly obtained when multidisciplinary management is carried out by an experienced team. Each major treatment modality is summarized next.

SURGERY AT THE PRIMARY SITE

The initial management in most cases of MCC is surgical excision of the tumor. When carried out without subsequent adjuvant radiation, patients treated with surgery only may have a relatively high recurrence rate depending on the margins chosen and the risk profile for the tumor. For Mohs surgical excision, the local recurrence rate was 16% for surgery alone and 0% in patients who also had adjuvant radiation therapy, although this difference was not statistically significant.[31] There are no data to suggest that extremely wide excision margins improve overall survival. Depending on the location of the tumor, significant morbidity can result when 2- to 3-cm margins are taken. Numerous studies show that if surgery is the sole treatment, recurrence rates are significantly higher than if radiation therapy is added to the regimen. Excision with narrow but clear margins (carried out at the time of SLNB) followed by adjuvant radiation therapy is a reasonable approach to management in many cases. Overly aggressive surgery, including amputation, or very wide margins in cosmetically sensitive areas, decreases quality of life, increases morbidity, delays time to initiation of adjuvant radiation, and does not appear to improve survival or local control rates.

SURGERY AT THE DRAINING NODE BED

Completion lymphadenectomy is typically carried out if there is clinically apparent involvement of the draining node bed. However, the role of completion lymphadenectomy in MCC is controversial. For example, a 2010 study suggests that patients with nodal MCC disease who underwent complete lymphadenectomy had comparable outcomes as those patients who only underwent radiation therapy to the nodal bed.[32] These 2 options have similar and excellent control rates for node-positive disease. Although either surgery or radiation can be chosen, depending on the clinical situation, it is clear that for microscopic nodal disease, only 1 of these 2 modalities should be performed. This is because regional control rates were 100% for each modality and the combination of radiation and surgery to the lymph node bed greatly increases risk of chronic lymphedema.

RADIATION THERAPY

MCC is an unusually radiosensitive tumor.[33-36] There are several case series of successful treatment of MCC with radiation as monotherapy. One study of 43 patients with MCC, for whom surgical excision was not possible, demonstrated an excellent infield control rate (75%) after treatment with radiation therapy alone.[32] In a separate cohort, there were no recurrences among 9 patients treated with radiation monotherapy.[37] Figure 113-8 shows one of our cases treated with radiation monotherapy. In most of these cases, the lesion was thought to be inoperable and radiation was given for palliation, but typically resulted in long-lasting local control.

More commonly, radiation is used as an adjuvant treatment to surgery. Adjuvant radiation is critical if surgical margins are positive or if microscopic margins are relatively narrow (<0.5 cm). There is a statistically significant improved local and nodal rate of control of MCC if radiation is added.[38] A cancer registry-based study also indicates improved survival in patients with adjuvant radiation therapy.[39] The typical doses of radiation for MCC are 50 Gy to 56 Gy for a primary site with negative excision margins. Detailed dosing regimens can be found in the National Comprehensive Cancer Network's MCC guidelines. Radiation doses are typically given in 2-Gy fractions, 5 times per week over 4 to 6 weeks. Acute side effects from radiation therapy include erythema at the site and mild-to-moderate fatigue that peaks toward the end of radiation and usually resolves within 1 to 2 months of completing a 5-week course. Chronic radiation skin changes include temporary or permanent alopecia within the irradiated field, epidermal atrophy, loss of adnexal structures leading to skin or mucosal dryness, and risk of subsequent secondary skin cancers in the irradiated region in patients with a life expectancy of greater than 20 years after the radiation treatment. Perhaps the most significant potential side effect is lymphedema. This is more commonly an issue in lower extremities, when radiation therapy is given to the inguinal lymph nodes, especially after surgery also has been done in that region. Early referral to a physical therapist trained in lymphedema management is indicated to minimize the severity and incidence of this potential complication in higher risk cases.

Single-fraction radiotherapy is a viable option for treatment and palliation in some cases of MCC. In one 2015 study, 26 patients received single-fraction radiotherapy (8 Gy) to 93 MCC tumors. The responses were generally excellent, demonstrating infield control and durable responses with minimal toxicity.[33] Single-fraction radiotherapy may represent a convenient and appealing alternative to systemic chemotherapy for palliation, for which most patients with 1 or few metastatic MCC lesions are eligible.

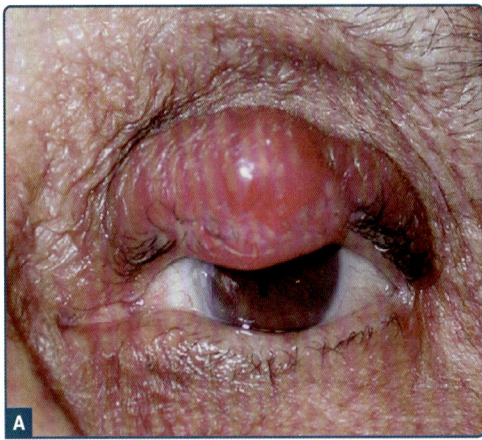
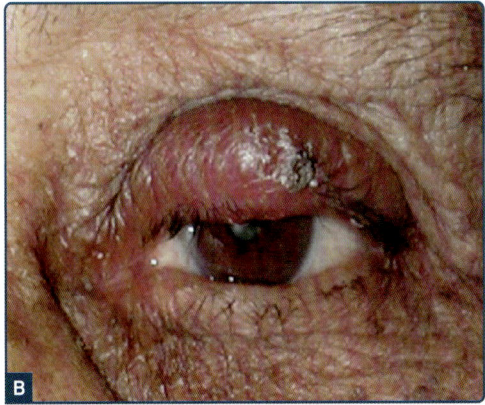
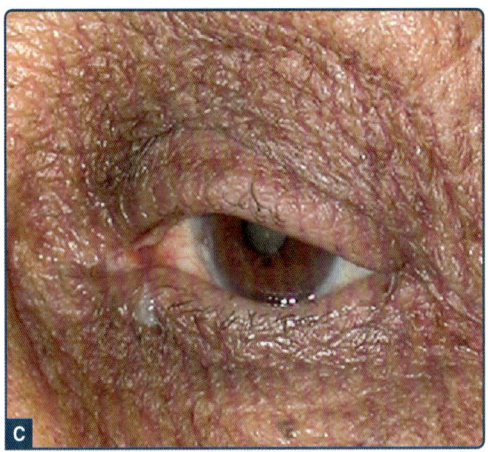

Figure 113-8 **A,** Merkel cell carcinoma on the eyelid arising 3 months before biopsy. The lesion was initially presumed to be a chalazion or cyst. **B,** Using a thin lead shield to protect the globe, the eyelid, the surrounding tissues, and the draining lymph node bed were treated with radiation monotherapy. **C,** The patient remained recurrence-free at 4.5 years after diagnosis, and thus had a greater than 97% chance of cure.

IMMUNE THERAPY

As detailed in section "Etiology and Pathogenesis" above, MCC virus-positive and virus-negative subtypes are both immunogenic, and certain immune evasion mechanisms are now targetable for MCC therapy. Immune therapies are rapidly evolving and, in a subset of patients, are associated with a durable, if not curative, response, even in tumors resistant to standard chemotherapy.

Multiple inhibitors of immune checkpoints, such as programmed death ligand 1 or its receptor, programmed death 1, are the subjects of clinical trials.

In a Phase II clinical trial published in 2016, pembrolizumab, an anti–programmed death 1 antibody, elicited a complete or partial response in more than half of MCC patients treated.[34] Several other clinical trials have demonstrated promising results, and National Comprehensive Cancer Network guidelines indicate that patient participation in clinical trials is recommended, whenever possible.

CHEMOTHERAPY

The most commonly used chemotherapeutic regimen for MCC is the combination of etoposide and either cisplatin (perhaps more clinically effective) or carboplatin (less nephrotoxic). Chemotherapy is often useful in palliation for symptomatic disease that is otherwise inoperable. MCC patients receiving chemotherapy for the first time usually have a significant response with shrinkage of the tumor. Unfortunately, in almost all cases, the tumor grows back and is resistant to chemotherapy, even if entirely different agents are used on a subsequent round of chemotherapy. After careful analysis of the literature, we currently do not recommend adjuvant chemotherapy for patients whose MCC has been treated with surgery, radiation therapy, or both. There are 6 reasons why we do not recommend adjuvant chemotherapy:

1. *Mortality:* There is a 4% to 7% acute death rate from adjuvant chemotherapy in MCC partly because these patients are often elderly.[12,35]
2. *Morbidity:* Neutropenia is reported to occur in 60% of patients with fever, and sepsis in 40%.[36]
3. *Decreased quality of life:* This can be quite severe in this older population, including fatigue, hair loss, nausea, and vomiting.
4. *Resistance to chemotherapy:* MCC that recurs after chemotherapy is less responsive to later palliative chemotherapy.

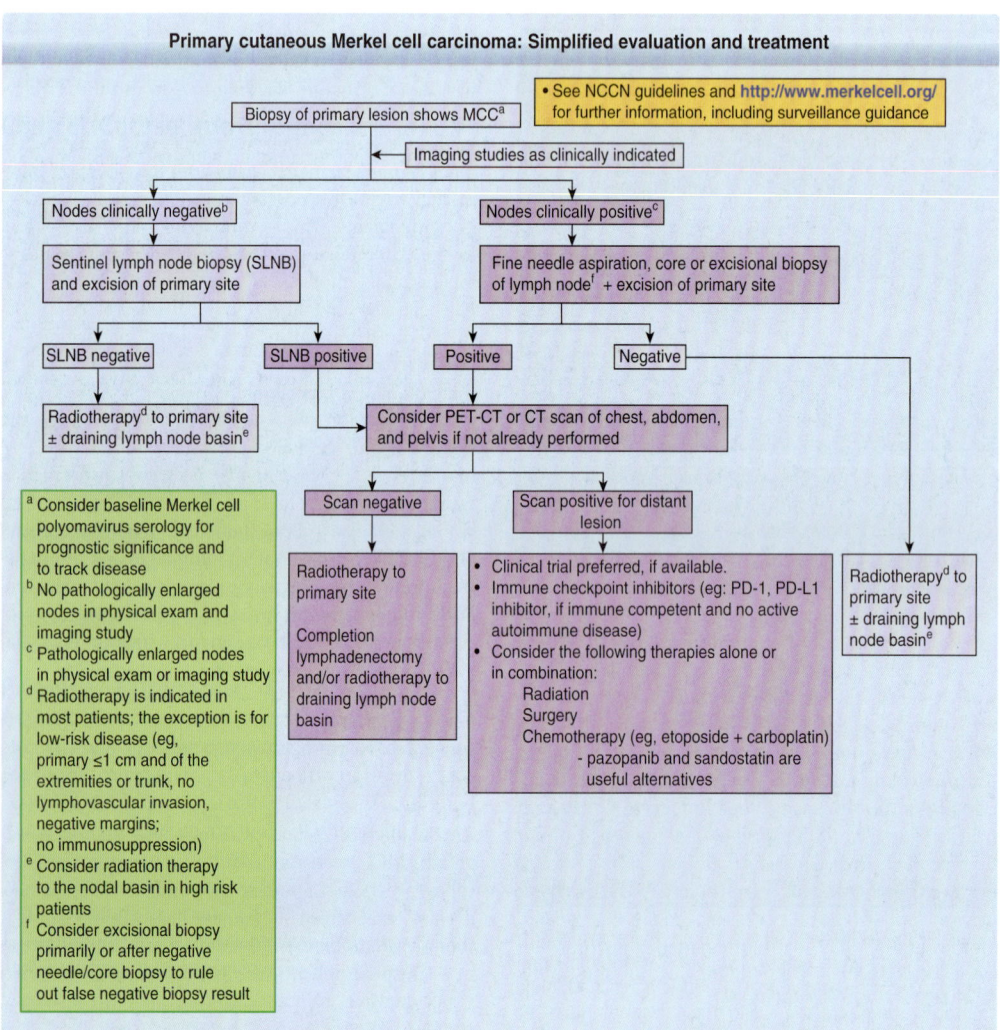

Figure 113-9 Simplified evaluation and treatment diagram for primary cutaneous Merkel cell carcinoma (MCC). NCCN, National Comprehensive Cancer Network; PD-1, programmed death 1; PD-L1, programmed death ligand 1; PET, positron emission tomography; SLNB, sentinel lymph node biopsy.

5. *Immunity:* Chemotherapy suppresses immune function, and this is known in general to be very important in preventing and controlling MCC.
6. *Outcomes are not improved:* A large analysis of 6908 patients from the National Cancer Database demonstrated no survival benefit among node-positive patients who received chemotherapy as compared to those who did not. Even though this was a not randomized study, the results certainly do not suggest a clinically meaningful benefit for adjuvant chemotherapy.[40]

SURVEILLANCE

Currently, there is a paucity of data on which to develop national guidelines for surveillance of MCC patients. Current guidelines include relatively general recommendations for clinical examination every 3 to 6 months for the first 2 years after diagnosis, and every 6 to 12 months thereafter. Imaging studies are recommended "as clinically indicated."[41] Disease-specific and progression-free survival data available at www.merkelcell.org/prognosis can be useful for guiding surveillance/imaging decisions. Given the lower risk of progression in early stage disease, surveillance can be tapered more rapidly (by year 3 or 4), than for patients with higher-risk disease at presentation. Additionally, in patients who produce antibodies to the Merkel polyomavirus oncoprotein, surveillance via serology may be an approach to monitoring disease burden with less cost and less exposure to radiation (see "Merkel Cell Polyomavirus" above for more details).[26]

OPTIMAL TREATMENT

In general, optimal treatment of MCC should involve obtaining pathologically clear margins by surgery, typically with 1- to 2-cm margins if possible, depending on the site. Narrower margins or even positive margins can often be effectively treated by local radiation, typically extending 3 to 5 cm beyond the tumor bed. We also recommend treating the draining lymph node bed, likely with radiation therapy, for patients with high-risk disease including a positive SLNB, immune suppression, or a tumor greater than 2 cm in diameter. Although still controversial, we currently do not recommend adjuvant radiation therapy for MCC patients with all of the following 5 good prognostic features: (a) primary tumor diameter ≤1 cm; (b) microscopic margins that are confidently negative following surgery; (c) no lymphovascular invasion noted in the tumor; (d) no profound immune suppression (eg, HIV, chronic lymphocytic leukemia); and (e) SLNB that was negative with proper immunohistochemistry studies.

Figure 113-9 provides a flow chart for evaluation and treatment of primary MCC.

REFERENCES

1. Hodgson NC. Merkel cell carcinoma: changing incidence trends. *J Surg Oncol.* 2005;89:1-4.
2. Paulson KG, Park SY, Vandeven NA et al. Merkel cell carcinoma: Current US incidence and projected increases based on changing demographics. *J Am Acad Dermatol.* 2018;78(3):457-463;e452.
3. Lemos BD, Storer BE, Iyer JG, et al. Pathologic nodal evaluation improves prognostic accuracy in Merkel cell carcinoma: analysis of 5823 cases as the basis of the first consensus staging system. *J Am Acad Dermatol.* 2010;63:751-761.
4. U.S. National Cancer Institute Surveillance, Epidemiology, and End Results (SEER) Program. *SEER Cancer Statistics Review, 1973-1993.* Bethesda, MD: National Institutes of Health; 1993. Available at: https://seer.cancer.gov/archive/csr/1973_1993/
5. Maricich SM, Wellnitz SA, Nelson AM, et al. Merkel cells are essential for light-touch responses. *Science.* 2009;324:1580-1582.
6. Van Keymeulen A, Mascre G, Youseff KK, et al. Epidermal progenitors give rise to Merkel cells during embryonic development and adult homeostasis. *J Cell Biol.* 2009;187:91-100.
7. Albores-Saavedra J, Batich K, Chable-Montero F, et al. Merkel cell carcinoma demographics, morphology, and survival based on 3870 cases: a population based study. *J Cutan Pathol.* 2010;37:20-27.
8. Miller RW, Rabkin CS. Merkel cell carcinoma and melanoma: etiological similarities and differences. *Cancer Epidemiol Biomarkers Prev.* 1999;8:153-158.
9. Agelli M, Clegg LX. Epidemiology of primary Merkel cell carcinoma in the United States. *J Am Acad Dermatol.* 2003;49:832-841.
10. Heath M, Jaimes N, Lemos B, et al. Clinical characteristics of Merkel cell carcinoma at diagnosis in 195 patients: the AEIOU features. *J Am Acad Dermatol.* 2008;58:375-381.
11. Kotteas EA, Pavlidis N. Neuroendocrine Merkel cell nodal carcinoma of unknown primary site: management and outcomes of a rare entity. *Crit Rev Oncol Hematol.* 2015;94:116-121.
12. Santamaria-Barria JA, Boland GM, Yeap BY, et al. Merkel cell carcinoma: 30-year experience from a single institution. *Ann Surg Oncol.* 2013;20(4):1365-1373.
13. Tsang G, O'Brien P, Robertson R, et al. All delays before radiotherapy risk progression of Merkel cell carcinoma. *Australas Radiol.* 2004;48:371-375.
14. Allen PJ, Bowne WB, Jaques DP, et al. Merkel cell carcinoma: prognosis and treatment of patients from a single institution. *J Clin Oncol.* 2005;23:2300-2309.
15. Engels EA, Frisch M, Goedert JJ, et al. Merkel cell carcinoma and HIV infection. *Lancet.* 2002;359: 497-498.
16. Pan D, Narayan D, Ariyan S. Merkel cell carcinoma: five case reports using sentinel lymph node biopsy and a review of 110 new cases. *Plast Reconstr Surg.* 2002;110:1259-1265.
17. Feng H, Shuda M, Chang Y, et al. Clonal integration of a polyomavirus in human Merkel cell carcinoma. *Science.* 2008;319:1096-1100.
18. Goh G, Walradt T, Markarov V, et al. Mutational landscape of MCPyV-positive and MCPyV-negative Merkel cell carcinomas with implications for immunotherapy. *Oncotarget.* 2016;7:3403-3415.

19. Edge SB, Compton CC. The American Joint Committee on Cancer: the 7th edition of the AJCC cancer staging manual and the future of TNM. *Ann Surg Oncol*. 2010;17:1471-1474.
20. Harms KL, Healy MA, Nghiem P, et al. Analysis of prognostic factors from 9387 Merkel cell carcinoma cases forms the basis for the new 8th edition AJCC staging system. *Ann Surg Oncol*. 2016;23(11):3564-3571.
21. Messina JL, Reintgen DS, Cruse CW, et al. Selective lymphadenectomy in patients with Merkel cell (cutaneous neuroendocrine) carcinoma. *Ann Surg Oncol*. 1997;4:389-395.
22. Hill AD, Brady MS, Coit DG. Intraoperative lymphatic mapping and sentinel lymph node biopsy for Merkel cell carcinoma. *Br J Surg*. 1999;86:518-521.
23. Gupta SG, Wang LC, Peñas PF, et al. Sentinel lymph node biopsy for evaluation and treatment of patients with Merkel cell carcinoma: the Dana-Farber experience and metaanalysis of the literature. *Arch Dermatol*. 2006;142:685-690.
24. Lens MB, Dawes M, Newton-Bishop JA, et al. Tumour thickness as a predictor of occult lymph node metastases in patients with stage I and II melanoma undergoing sentinel lymph node biopsy. *Br J Surg*. 2002;89:1223-1227.
25. Andea AA, Coit DG, Amin B, et al. Merkel cell carcinoma: histologic features and prognosis. *Cancer*. 2008;113:2549-2558.
26. Paulson KG, Carter JJ, Johnson LG, et al. Antibodies to Merkel cell polyomavirus T antigen oncoproteins reflect tumor burden in Merkel cell carcinoma patients. *Cancer Res*. 2010;70:8388-8397.
27. Stetsenko GY, Malekirad J, Paulson KG, et al. p63 expression in Merkel cell carcinoma predicts poorer survival yet may have limited clinical utility. *Am J Clin Pathol*. 2013;140:838-844.
28. Afanasiev OK, Nagase K, Simonson W, et al. Vascular E-selectin expression correlates with CD8 lymphocyte infiltration and improved outcome in Merkel cell carcinoma. *J Invest Dermatol*. 2013;133:2065-2073.
29. Paulson KG, Iyer JG, Tegeder AR, et al. Transcriptome-wide studies of Merkel cell carcinoma and validation of intratumoral CD8+ lymphocyte invasion as an independent predictor of survival. *J Clin Oncol*. 2011;29:1539-1546.
30. Paulson KG, Iyer JG, Simonson WT, et al. CD8+ lymphocyte intratumoral infiltration as a stage-independent predictor of Merkel cell carcinoma survival: a population-based study. *Am J Clin Pathol*. 2014;142:452-458.
31. Boyer JD, Zitelli JA, Brodland DG, et al. Local control of primary Merkel cell carcinoma: review of 45 cases treated with Mohs micrographic surgery with and without adjuvant radiation. *J Am Acad Dermatol*. 2002;47:885-892.
32. Fang LC, Lemos B, Douglas J, et al. Radiation monotherapy as regional treatment for lymph node-positive Merkel cell carcinoma. *Cancer*. 2010;116:1783-1790.
33. Iyer JG, Parvathaneni U, Gooley T, et al. Single-fraction radiation therapy in patients with metastatic Merkel cell carcinoma. *Cancer Med*. 2015;4:1161-1170.
34. Nghiem PT, Bhatia S, Lipson EJ, et al. PD-1 blockade with pembrolizumab in advanced Merkel-cell carcinoma. *N Engl J Med*. 2016;374:2542-2552.
35. Tai PT, Yu E, Winquist E, et al. Chemotherapy in neuroendocrine/Merkel cell carcinoma of the skin: case series and review of 204 cases. *J Clin Oncol*. 2000;18:2493-2499.
36. Poulsen M, Rischin D, Walpole E, et al. Analysis of toxicity of Merkel cell carcinoma of the skin treated with synchronous carboplatin/etoposide and radiation: a Trans-Tasman Radiation Oncology Group study. *Int J Radiat Oncol Biol Phys*. 2001;51:156-163.
37. Mortier L, Mirabel X, Fournier C, et al. Radiotherapy alone for primary Merkel cell carcinoma. *Arch Dermatol*. 2003;139:1587-1590.
38. Longo MI, Nghiem P. Merkel cell carcinoma treatment with radiation: a good case despite no prospective studies. *Arch Dermatol*. 2003;139:1641-1643.
39. Mojica P, Smith D, Ellenhorn JD. Adjuvant radiation therapy is associated with improved survival in Merkel cell carcinoma of the skin. *J Clin Oncol*. 2007;25:1043-1047.
40. Bhatia S, Storer BE, Iyer JG, et al. Adjuvant radiation therapy and chemotherapy in Merkel cell carcinoma: survival analyses of 6908 cases from the national cancer data base. *J Natl Cancer Inst*. 2016;108(9).
41. Bichakjian CK, Olencki T, Alam M, et al. Merkel cell carcinoma, version 1.2014. *J Natl Compr Canc Netw*. 2014;12:410-424.

Chapter 114 :: Paget's Disease
:: Conroy Chow, Isaac M. Neuhaus, & Roy C. Grekin

第一百一十四章
佩吉特病

中文导读

Paget's病包括乳房Paget's病（MPD）和乳房外Paget's病（EMPD），虽然临床和组织学上相似，但发病机制和与潜在恶性肿瘤相关的频率不同。本章分为8节：①历史视角；②流行病学；③临床特征；④病因和发病机制；⑤诊断；⑥鉴别诊断；⑦临床病程和并发症；⑧临床管理。

第一节历史视角，首先介绍了18世纪70年代首次报道了乳房Paget's病与乳腺癌相关。接着介绍了在18世纪80年代末，首次将阴囊和阴茎上的一种疾病描述为EMPD，其组织病理学与MPD相似。

第二节流行病学，介绍了MPD的发病高峰年龄与乳腺癌的相关性及EMPD的发病率。

第三节临床特征，介绍了MPD的皮肤表现主要累及乳头和/或乳晕的单侧，出现红斑或斑块，EMPD表现为边界清楚、湿润、红斑、鳞屑性斑块，通常累及大汗腺丰富的皮肤。同时介绍了MPD要注意潜在乳房肿块，EMPD要注意膀胱、尿道、前列腺肿瘤及结直肠癌等。

第四节病因及发病机制，首先介绍了MPD发病的两种理论即嗜表皮理论和转化理论。原发性EMPD起源于大汗腺的表皮内部分或表皮中的恶性细胞，而继发性EMPD起源于潜在的附件癌或内脏恶性肿瘤。

第五节诊断，介绍了其组织病理学特征，并且推荐所有患者都应该进行系统的全面检查和全身皮肤检查，包括触诊淋巴结。MPD和EMPD的完整检查还应包括排除潜在恶性肿瘤。

第六节鉴别诊断，在表114-1概述了EMPD和MPD的鉴别诊断。

第七节临床病程和并发症，介绍了影响EMPD和MPD预后的因素，MPD患者的预后取决于临床可触及的乳腺肿块和淋巴结转移的存在与否。原发性EMPD的预后佳，继发性EMPD的预后通常比原发性EMPD的差，并取决于潜在癌症的发生。

第八节临床管理，介绍了MPD和EMPD的治疗方法及监测手段。

〔粟 娟〕

AT-A-GLANCE

- Uncommon intraepithelial adenocarcinoma occurring in apocrine gland-bearing skin in patients older than age 50 years.
- Erythematous, scaly plaque frequently misdiagnosed as inflammatory or infectious dermatitis.
- Most commonly affected sites: unilateral nipple/areola (mammary Paget's disease [MPD]); vulva, perianal skin, scrotum, and penis (extramammary Paget's disease [EMPD]).
- Nearly all cases of MPD are associated with underlying breast carcinoma; EMPD is associated with underlying cancer in a minority (20% to 30%) of cases.

DEFINITIONS

Mammary Paget's disease (MPD; also called Paget's disease of the breast) is an intraepidermal adenocarcinoma of the nipple and/or areola, typically associated with underlying breast carcinoma. Extramammary Paget's disease (EMPD) is a clinically distinct condition that affects extramammary sites, such as the vulva, penis, scrotum, perineum, and anus. Even though both MPD and EMPD may appear similar clinically and histologically, they differ in their pathogenesis and frequency of associations with underlying malignancies.

HISTORICAL PERSPECTIVE

In 1874, Sir James Paget first reported MPD in a series of 15 women with chronic dermatitis of the nipple and areola who were subsequently diagnosed with underlying breast carcinoma.[1] In 1889, English dermatologist Henry Racliffe Crocker first described EMPD as a condition on the scrotum and penis with histopathology similar to MPD.[2]

EPIDEMIOLOGY

MPD represents approximately 1% to 3% of breast cancers.[3] The peak incidence is between 50 and 60 years of age, with most reported cases occurring in women. In various studies, between 82% and 100% of MPD cases are associated with an underlying in situ or invasive ductal carcinoma.[3]

EMPD is a rare malignancy of the anogenital region, with various studies citing incidence rates ranging from 0.6 per 1,000,000 person-years to 0.11 per 100,000 person-years.[4,5] The majority of cases occur in the sixth through eighth decades of life, with women more commonly affected than men.[6-8] In contrast to MPD, most cases of EMPD are not associated with an underlying adnexal carcinoma or visceral malignancy, with most studies reporting approximately a 20% to 30% risk.[7]

CLINICAL FEATURES

HISTORY

Both MPD and EMPD present with a longstanding history of erythematous, scaly, or velvety patches or plaques on the breast and anogenital skin, respectively. The most commonly reported symptom is pruritus. Other symptoms may include pain, bleeding, a burning sensation, and serosanguinous discharge. Because of the rather nondescript appearance, there is often a several-month delay in diagnosis as initial treatment frequently involves topical steroids (for presumed inflammatory dermatitis) or antifungal agents (for presumed infectious dermatitis).

CUTANEOUS FINDINGS

MPD frequently presents as a unilateral, erythematous, scaly plaque involving the nipple and/or the areola (Fig. 114-1). The associated pruritus may lead to lichenification and excoriations. Ulceration, weeping, and crusting are often present. Nipple erosion and discharge may occur. Retraction of the nipple and areola may be seen in advanced disease.

Lesions of EMPD are clinically similar to MPD and often present as well-defined, moist, erythematous, scaly plaques, usually involving apocrine gland-bearing skin (eg, in the genitoperineal region and axilla). Hypopigmentation and hyperpigmentation may occur. Lichenification and excoriations of the involved area are commonly found because of pruritus. The vulva is the most commonly affected area, representing 65% of EMPD cases but less than 2% of all vulvar neoplasms.[3,9] EMPD in other sites, such as the perineum, scrotum (Fig. 114-2), perianal skin (Fig. 114-3), and penis, is less common. In rare cases, ectopic EMPD has been reported in areas that are relatively free of apocrine glands, such as the chest, abdomen, thigh, eyelids, face, and external auditory canal.[10-14]

Table 114-1 outlines the differential diagnoses of MPD and EMPD.

NONCUTANEOUS FINDINGS

Patients may present with symptoms and physical findings of an underlying carcinoma or metastatic disease. Complete physical examination including thorough full-body skin examination is required in all cases of MPD and EMPD, as approximately one-half of patients presenting with MPD are found concurrently to have a palpable underlying breast mass.[15,16] Of these patients, one-half to two-thirds have axillary lymph node metastases.[16]

Given the less-established association with underlying carcinoma in EMPD as compared to MPD, a

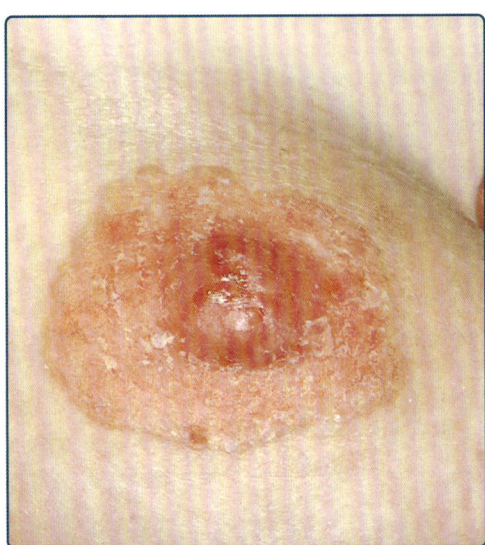

Figure 114-1 Paget's disease of the nipple. Erythematous and scaly plaque involving the nipple and areola.

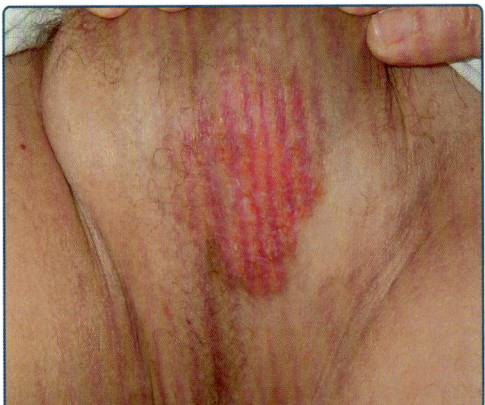

Figure 114-2 Scrotal extramammary Paget's disease. Moist, eroded, oozing plaque on the scrotum of an older man.

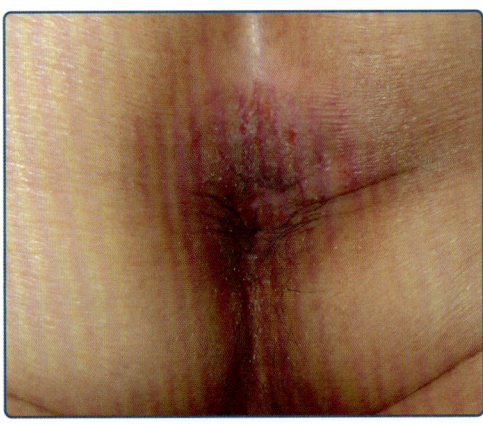

Figure 114-3 Perianal extramammary Paget's disease presenting as moist, superficially eroded plaque.

palpable mass or lymph node is much less frequently found on physical examination in EMPD. EMPD of the external male and female genitalia may be associated with tumors of the bladder and urethra and of the prostate in men.[17] Perianal EMPD may be associated with colorectal cancer.[17]

Failure to identify and adequately treat MPD and EMPD can lead to progression and metastasis, with a poor prognosis.

ETIOLOGY AND PATHOGENESIS

MAMMARY PAGET'S DISEASE

Historically, 2 contrasting theories, known as the *epidermotropic* and *transformation* theories, attempted to explain the pathogenesis of MPD.

In the epidermotropic theory, malignant Paget cells arise from an underlying breast adenocarcinoma and directly extend into the epidermis via the lactiferous ducts and ductules (epidermotropism).[9] These malignant cells then invade the epidermis of the nipple and areola, leading to the clinical manifestations detailed above. In multiple reports, immunohistochemical studies showed significant similarities between the Paget cells and the underlying breast carcinoma in a majority of cases, further suggesting that MPD arose from intraepidermal extension of the ductal carcinoma.[9,18,19] In contrast, epidermal keratinocytes expressed a different immunohistochemical staining pattern.

In one study, overexpression of the heregulin receptor HER2/neu (also known as cluster of differentiation 340 [CD340], c-erbB-2, and human epidermal growth factor receptor 2) was identified in 80% of MPD cases. In all these cases, there was complete concordance between HER2/neu overexpression in both the Paget cells and the underlying ductal carcinoma.[20] Normal epidermis does not show overexpression of HER2/neu. Another study suggested that movement of Paget cells is induced by the action of the heregulin-alpha motility factor, which is produced by normal epidermal keratinocytes, on HER2/neu receptors on the Paget cells, leading to chemotaxis to the overlying nipple epidermis.[21] These studies suggest that a common mutation or progenitor cell leads to the development of both MPD and the underlying breast carcinoma.

The transformation theory suggests that epidermal keratinocytes on the nipple transform or degenerate into malignant Paget cells that are distinct from any underlying breast carcinoma.[15,22] Therefore, MPD originates as an in situ carcinoma that may subsequently progress.

The epidermotropic theory is supported by the presence of an underlying breast carcinoma in nearly all cases of MPD, but the transformation theory is supported by the small fraction of cases without an under-

TABLE 114-1
Differential Diagnosis of Mammary and Extramammary Paget's Disease

	MOST COMMON	CONSIDER	ALWAYS RULE OUT
Mammary Paget's disease	Nipple dermatitis	Hailey-Hailey disease	Bowen disease
	Erosive adenomatosis	Pemphigus	Melanoma
	Contact dermatitis	Lichen simplex chronicus	
	Dermatophyte infection		
Extramammary Paget's disease	Candidiasis	Lichen sclerosus et atrophicus	Bowen disease
	Tinea cruris	Pemphigus	Erythroplasia of Queyrat
	Inverse psoriasis	Lichen simplex chronicus	Melanoma
	Contact dermatitis	Lichen planus	
	Intertrigo	Symmetrical drug-related intertriginous and flexural exanthema	

lying ductal carcinoma.[15] Although both theories are possible, the literature currently favors the epidermotropic theory for the very reason that almost all cases of MPD are associated with underlying breast carcinoma.

EXTRAMAMMARY PAGET'S DISEASE

Unlike MPD, which, in most cases, has a documented underlying carcinoma, EMPD more commonly occurs in the absence of underlying malignancy and accounts for the majority of EMPD cases. Known as primary EMPD, this form of EMPD represents malignant cells that are believed to originate from the intraepidermal parts of apocrine glands or from pluripotent cells in the epidermis.[7] Primary EMPD is thought to start as an in situ carcinoma that can progress by invading the dermis and subsequently metastasizing via lymphatic spread.[7] In contrast, secondary EMPD arises from an underlying adnexal carcinoma or internal malignancy in approximately 20% to 30% of cases. These cases are caused by epidermotropic spread of malignant cells from the underlying tumor.[7] Common visceral malignancies associated with EMPD are carcinomas of the colon, rectum, bladder, urethra, cervix, and prostate.[9]

DIAGNOSIS

Diagnosis of MPD and EMPD requires a high index of suspicion, with full-thickness punch, wedge, or excisional biopsy of the skin for histopathologic confirmation. A complete review of systems and full-body skin examination, including palpation of lymph nodes, should be performed in all patients. A complete workup for both MPD and EMPD should also include a thorough search for underlying malignancy.

MAMMARY PAGET'S DISEASE

Punch, wedge, or excisional biopsy of lesional skin is necessary to confirm the diagnosis by histopathology. A few studies in the past suggested a role for nipple scrapings for cytologic evaluation, but this method has not gained widespread acceptance because of the potential for false-positives and false-negatives results that occur from processing artifact.[23,24]

Bilateral mammography is required in all cases, with biopsy of any detectable breast mass. Various studies have shown approximately 35% to 65% of patients with biopsy-proven MPD show findings on mammography that are concerning for underlying breast carcinoma.[25,26] However, because nearly all patients with MPD have underlying breast carcinoma, a negative mammogram does rule out this possibility.

Although the likelihood of an invasive breast carcinoma is low (~5%) in patients without a clinically palpable breast mass and with a negative mammogram, ductal carcinoma in situ may be present and not detected by mammography.[27] In one particular study, 68% of patients without a palpable breast mass and with negative mammography were found to have ductal carcinoma in situ.[27]

Because of the limitations of mammography, a few newer studies have suggested use of MRI in patients with biopsy-proven MPD and negative mammogram to help identify occult breast malignancy.[25,28] However, despite the increased sensitivity of MRI compared to mammography, this imaging modality has limitations because there remains a small possibility of an underlying cancer that was not visualized with MRI (potential for a false negative). In addition, because MRI is very sensitive but not very specific, it may detect findings that lead to unnecessary diagnostic testing, so patients should be counseled to the possibility of a false-positive result.

EXTRAMAMMARY PAGET'S DISEASE

As in MPD, histopathologic confirmation from a punch or excisional biopsy of lesional skin is necessary. As a consequence of the low incidence of EMPD, there is currently no standardized diagnostic algorithm once EMPD is diagnosed, but workup (Table 114-2) is directed to the possibility of an underlying GI or genitourinary neoplasm. Colonoscopy, cystoscopy, and, in female patients, pelvic examination with Papanicolaou test and colposcopy should all be considered as first-line studies to evaluate underlying malignancy.

Further imaging studies should be guided by the results of the initial studies, sex of the patient, and anatomic areas of involvement. Other imaging studies to consider, as clinically indicated, include pelvic ultrasound, positron emission tomography, chest radiography, MRI, mammography, and intravenous pyelogram.

The clinical utility of other laboratory tests and imaging remain unclear. In 2 reports, patients with significantly elevated serum carcinoembryonic antigen (CEA) levels had a greater risk of death from EMPD compared to patients with normal serum CEA, and the level of CEA paralleled disease course.[8,29] Other studies suggest that positron emission tomography (PET)-CT scans may be useful for cases of invasive EMPD to evaluate for lymph node involvement and metastases.[29-31] However, even PET-CT scans may not detect microscopic metastases.

The role of sentinel lymph node biopsy (SLNB) for patients with EMPD is discussed in section "Management Extramammary Paget's Disease".

PATHOLOGY

The intraepidermal adenocarcinoma of EMPD and MPD has a similar histologic appearance. There are groups, clusters, or single cells within the epidermis that show nuclear enlargement with atypia, prominent nucleoli, and well-defined ample cytoplasm (Fig. 114-4).[32] Intercellular bridges are absent. The cells may be in all levels of the epidermis, and compress, but preserve, the basal layer without junctional nest formation. The cells may extend into the contiguous epithelium of hair follicles and sweat gland ducts. Acanthosis, hyperkeratosis, and parakeratosis are often present. These cells have a "pagetoid" appearance and simulate other intraepidermal malignancies, such as melanoma, pagetoid squamous cell carcinoma, mycosis fungoides, cutaneous adnexal carcinomas (eg, sebaceous carcinoma, porocarcinoma, and others), Merkel cell carcinoma, Langerhans cell histiocytosis, and other epidermotropic cutaneous metastases. The cells of MPD and EMPD can be pigmented, which does not necessarily indicate that they are melanocytic.

Paget cells have intracellular mucopolysaccharides, with EMPD having a greater amount of mucin compared to MPD. As a result, cells stain positive for periodic acid-Schiff, mucicarmine, Alcian blue, and colloidal iron, and are diastase resistant. There may be focal "skip areas" that are devoid of mucin, resulting in sections of negative staining.

Immunohistochemistry is invaluable in confirming the diagnosis (Table 114-3). Low-molecular-weight cytokeratin stains cytokeratin 7 (CK7) and anticytokeratin (CAM 5.2) are sensitive markers for both MPD and EMPD (Fig. 114-5), as they stain Paget cells but do not typically react with epidermal or mucosal keratinocytes, helping to distinguish MPD and EMPD from pagetoid squamous cell carcinoma.[33] These cytokeratin stains are not completely specific, however; for example, both Toker and Merkel cells also exhibit CK7 positivity. The cells of MPD and EMPD also commonly stain with CEA and epithelial membrane antigen, but these stains also are not specific for these entities.[33] HER2/neu has been used in select studies and is more often positive in MPD than in EMPD.[34] S100, Melan-A (also known as MART-1), and HMB-45 are useful markers to exclude melanoma and are typically negative in MPD and EMPD. Cytokeratin 20 (CK20) positivity has been

TABLE 114-2
Suggested Laboratory Workup for Extramammary Paget's Disease[a]

- Sigmoidoscopy
- Cystoscopy
- Papanicolaou test
- Colposcopy
- Pelvic ultrasound
- Positron emission tomography
- Chest radiography
- MRI
- Mammogram
- Intravenous pyelogram
- Serum carcinoembryonic antigen
- Positron emission tomography–CT scans

[a]These should be guided by the results of the initial studies, sex of the patient, and anatomic areas involved.

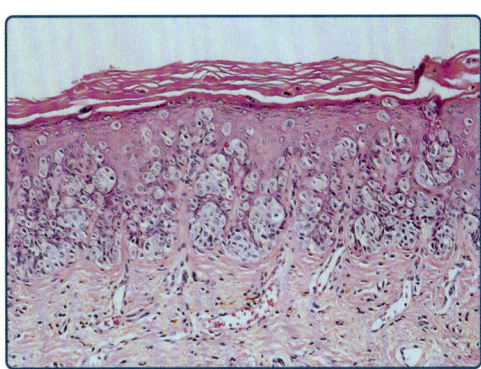

Figure 114-4 Paget's disease, hematoxylin and eosin stain. Paget cells have distinctive pale-staining cytoplasm and are usually randomly dispersed throughout the epidermis.

TABLE 114-3
Immunohistochemistry Markers for Mammary and Extramammary Paget's Disease

	S100	CK7	CAM 5.2	CEA	CK20	EMA	GCDFP-15	MUC1	MUC2	HER2/NEU
MPD	−	+	+	+	−	+		+		+
1° EMPD	−	+	+	+	−	+	+	+	−	+/−
2° EMPD	−	+			+		−		+[a]	

[a]Positivity in underlying colorectal adenocarcinoma.

1°, primary; 2°, secondary; CAM 5.2, anticytokeratin; CEA, carcinoembryonic antigen; CK, cytokeratin; EMA, epithelial membrane antigen; EMPD, extramammary Paget's disease; GCDFP-15, gross cystic disease fluid protein-15; HER2, human epidermal growth factor receptor 2 (also known as cluster of differentiation 340 [CD340], c-erbB-2, and neu); MPD, mammary Paget's disease; MUC, mucin core protein.

found more frequently in cases of secondary EMPD with underlying carcinoma as compared to cases of primary EMPD (CK7+/CK20−).[35] Gross cystic disease fluid protein-15 (GCDFP-15) is a marker for apocrine epithelium and is more commonly positive in primary EMPD and negative in cases of secondary EMPD with an associated malignancy.[36]

Mucin core protein (MUC) expression is useful in the diagnosis of MPD and EMPD.[37] MUC1 positivity is noted in both MPD and EMPD. MUC2 expression is generally negative in primary EMPD but may be expressed in cases of secondary EMPD with an associated underlying colorectal adenocarcinoma.[38] MUC5AC is more frequently positive in invasive and metastatic EMPD than in noninvasive EMPD.[39]

A study investigating a relationship between expression of androgen receptor on Paget cells in EMPD and 5α-reductase levels showed an elevated 5α-reductase level more frequently in invasive (81%) compared with purely intraepidermal (45%) cases of EMPD.[40] For invasive cases, men had a significantly higher level of androgen receptor and 5α-reductase positivity than women (70% vs 17%), suggesting the possibility of autocrine synthesis of androgens in EMPD and gender-specific microenvironments that may contribute to invasiveness of the disease.[40] In a related study, Ki-67 and cyclin D1 were expressed more frequently in cases of invasive EMPD than in intraepidermal EMPD. When both Ki-67 and cyclin D1 were expressed, the likelihood of invasive disease was higher than when either was expressed alone.[41] This study raised the question of whether androgens may be associated with cell-cycle regulation and invasiveness of EMPD.[41]

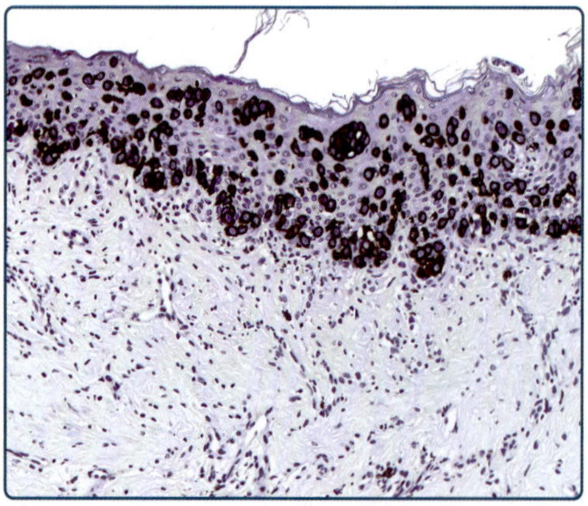

DIFFERENTIAL DIAGNOSIS

Table 114-1 outlines the differential diagnosis of EMPD and MPD.

CLINICAL COURSE AND PROGNOSIS

The prognosis in patients with MPD depends on the presence or absence of a clinically palpable breast mass and nodal metastases. Patients with MPD who present with a palpable breast mass tend to have more advanced disease than patients without a palpable breast mass. In these 2 groups, the rates of metastases to the lymph nodes were 57% to 63% (with a palpable breast mass) versus 11% to 21% (without a palpable breast mass).[42-44] In addition, patients with MPD who also present with a palpable mass were more likely to have invasive, rather than in situ, and multifocal ductal carcinoma.[44] The median survival of patients with a palpable breast mass was 42 months compared to 126 months for patients without a palpable breast mass, and the 5-year overall survival rates of patients with a palpable breast mass were 35% to 43% versus 75% to 93% for patients without a palpable breast mass.[43,45]

As a result of the limited number of longitudinal studies, heterogeneity in disease stage, and variability in management of MPD, recurrence rates are extremely variable across studies. One study found about one-third of the underlying breast carcinomas were located more than 2 cm beyond the areolar margin. Thus, with limited excision of the

Figure 114-5 Anticytokeratin (CAM 5.2) is a sensitive marker for both mammary and extramammary Paget's disease on histopathology. (Image used with permission from Thaddeus Mully, MD, UCSF.)

MPD and the underlying breast carcinoma, rather than mastectomy, a significant number of underlying breast carcinomas may be inadequately treated, which may help explain why some studies show higher recurrence rates.[43] See "Management: Mammary Paget's Disease" below for a full discussion of treatment of MPD.

The prognosis for primary EMPD is excellent with appropriate treatment, with 5-year overall survival rates ranging between 72% and 91% across several studies.[4,5,8] Risk factors that appear to carry a worse prognosis include lymphovascular invasion and increasing depth of tumor invasion, with one study suggesting that a dermal invasion greater than 1 mm confers a worse prognosis.[7] The presence of lymph node metastases markedly reduces overall survival and indicates a very poor prognosis, with 5-year survival rates ranging from 0 to approximately 20% in case series.[8,17] Two studies noted that patients with elevated serum CEA levels were more likely to have a worse prognosis, with 1 study noting that all the patients with elevated CEA levels had metastatic disease, but not all patients with metastatic disease had elevated CEA levels.[8,29] The usefulness of measuring CEA levels in the serum at this time is unclear; however, this particular study suggested that, for the subset of patients with a history of metastatic disease and elevated serum CEA, trending the serum CEA values over time may be useful in surveillance of the disease.[29] Nevertheless, regular surveillance for early detection of local recurrence is critical given the multifocal pattern often present in EMPD.

The prognosis for secondary EMPD caused by an underlying adnexal carcinoma or visceral malignancy is generally worse than for primary EMPD and depends on the prognosis of the underlying cancer.[17]

MANAGEMENT

MAMMARY PAGET'S DISEASE

Figure 114-6 outlines an approach to treatment of MPD. Historically, the standard of care for MPD has been mastectomy, but emerging evidence suggests that select cases of MPD may be treated with breast-conserving therapy (BCT) plus radiotherapy with excellent results and low rates of recurrences.[45-47] However, standardized, evidence-based treatment recommendations for MPD are not available because of the lack of studies directly comparing outcomes for mastectomy versus BCT plus radiotherapy. Most of the current treatment recommendations are based on small studies with variable treatment techniques and followup periods, making comparisons among different studies difficult.

For patients with MPD with a clinically palpable breast mass, most studies recommend mastectomy versus BCT (resection of the nipple and areola with wide local excision of the breast mass) followed by whole-breast radiotherapy.[43,45-47] In patients with an underlying invasive ductal carcinoma, SLNB is typically recommended at the time of excision if no clinically palpable pathologic nodes are identified. However, for patients with underlying invasive ductal carcinoma and clinically pathologic lymph nodes, biopsy of the lymph nodes should be performed prior to surgery. If lymph node biopsy confirms metastatic disease, axillary lymph node dissection should be considered. If pathology is negative for metastatic disease on lymph node biopsy, SLNB should be considered at the time of wide local excision.

In patients with MPD with negative mammography and without a palpable breast mass, most studies rec-

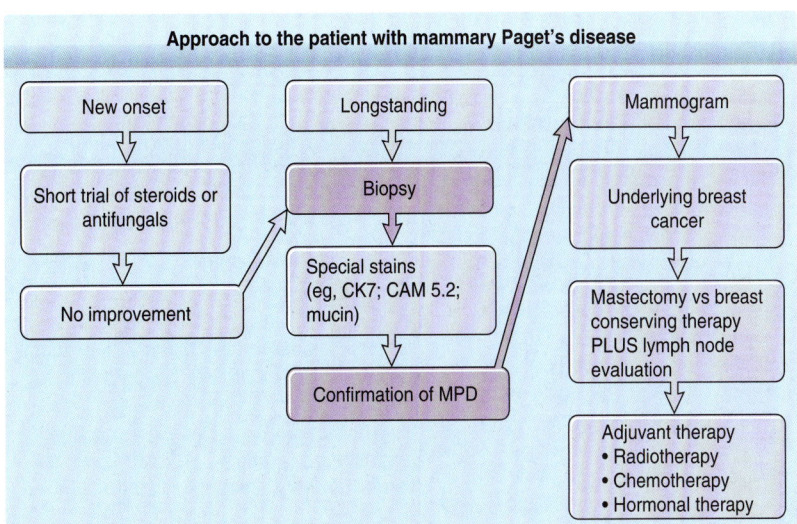

Figure 114-6 Approach to the patient with mammary Paget's disease (MPD). CAM 5.2, anticytokeratin stain; CK7, cytokeratin 7 stain.

ommend mastectomy versus BCT followed by whole-breast radiotherapy.[43,45-47] Most of these patients have ductal carcinoma in situ, rather than invasive ductal carcinoma, so many studies do not routinely recommend SLNB in these patients. However, 1 study found that approximately 20% of patients without an associated breast mass had metastases to the axillary lymph nodes and suggested consideration of SLNB even in cases of ductal carcinoma in situ.[43] Another study in patients with MPD without any identified underlying breast carcinoma found that 11% had metastases to the axilla and, thus, recommended SLNB for all patients.[48] Because all diagnoses of MPD require management by a surgical oncologist with expertise in breast cancer, a thorough discussion regarding the pros and cons of these various surgical approaches is warranted before proceeding with treatment.

EXTRAMAMMARY PAGET'S DISEASE

Figure 114-7 outlines an approach to treatment of EMPD. EMPD has been treated with a variety of modalities. The condition is most frequently managed with surgery, but other treatments have a role for poor surgical candidates and as adjuvant therapy.

SURGERY

Surgery is generally considered the standard treatment for EMPD. However, local recurrences are common, even when wide excision margins are used, with studies reporting rates ranging from approximately 30% to 60%.[7,49] Invasive disease has a higher recurrence rate than in situ disease, with one study reporting rates of 67% and 35%, respectively.[7,49] The high recurrence rates are likely the result of the clinical characteristics of EMPD: the ill-defined clinical margins, multifocal nature of the tumor, and involvement of clinically normal-appearing adjacent skin.[6] More extensive procedures are associated with lower rates of recurrence, but also may be more technically difficult and disfiguring for patients. In one study, patients with primary vulvar EMPD treated with radical vulvectomy, radical hemivulvectomy, and wide local excision had recurrence rates of 15%, 20%, and 43%, respectively.[7]

A few studies have attempted to decrease recurrences of EMPD using adjuvant techniques for surgery. Intraoperative frozen-section analysis reduced recurrences in some studies but not in others.[50,51] Multiple scouting biopsies performed prior to surgery have been reported

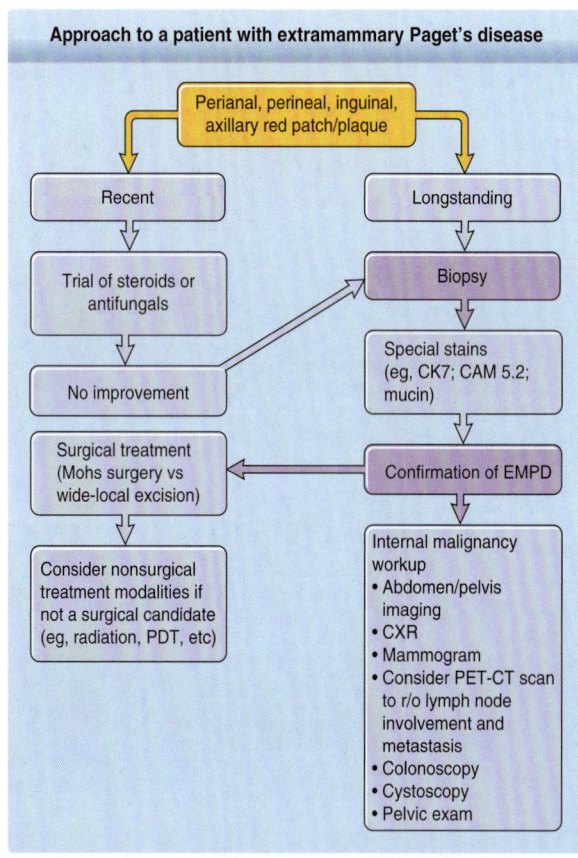

Figure 114-7 Approach to a patient with extramammary Paget's disease (EMPD). CAM 5.2, anticytokeratin stain; CK7, cytokeratin 7 stain; CXR, chest radiography; PDT, photodynamic therapy; PET-CT, positron emission tomography–computed tomography; r/o, rule out.

to be helpful in delineating the extent of disease and surgical planning.[52,53] Intraoperative CK7 immunostaining during Mohs micrographic surgery also has been reported to be helpful in delineating tumor margins.[53]

SLNB has been described in the treatment of EMPD.[54] This technique has been limited to a small number of reported patients, and most cases of EMPD have in situ disease. However, SLNB may prove beneficial for the prognosis and management of patients with increased risk of metastatic disease, such as those with invasive disease or elevated serum CEA levels.[55] A study involving patients with in situ, microinvasive (to the papillary dermis), or deeply invasive (to the reticular dermis or deeper) EMPD found that the incidence of sentinel lymph node metastasis was 16.9%. Stratified by depth of invasion, the rates were 0% for intraepidermal lesions, 4.1% for microinvasive disease, and 42.8% for deeply invasive disease.[56] Thus, some advocate the use of SLNB and/or regional lymph node dissection in all high-risk EMPD cases, despite negative findings on PET-CT, as micrometastases are undetectable with this form of imaging.[29]

With the high rates of local recurrence and the significant morbidity associated with radical and repeated surgical procedures, Mohs micrographic surgery has been used to improve cure rates and for tissue sparing of critical genitourinary anatomic structures.[6,7,57] The recurrence rate with Mohs micrographic surgery has ranged from 16% to 28% for primary EMPD in recent studies, and 50% for recurrent EMPD.[6,57] It was also reported that 97% of the cases treated with Mohs micrographic surgery required margins of 5 cm from the clinical margin for tumor clearance.[57] The same study found that surgical margins of 2 cm would clear only 59% of the cases, which is consistent with reported recurrence rates of approximately 40% with wide local excision. This further suggests a potential benefit of frozen horizontal sectioning for complete peripheral and deep margin mapping to reduce the possibility of residual tumor.

RADIOTHERAPY

Radiotherapy may be indicated in patients who are poor surgical candidates or are concerned with the risk of compromising genitourinary function as a consequence of the extensive surgery required for curative treatment.[7] Although initial studies indicated poor success with radiotherapy as a primary treatment modality, subsequent case series reported acceptable outcomes, with recurrence rates of less than 35%.[58-60] Even though these results may appear more favorable than some of the surgical modalities, it is important to note that the sample sizes in these reports were several patients, making generalizations difficult. In addition, one of the studies reported no recurrences in a subset of 7 patients with intraepidermal disease but had a recurrence in 1 of 2 patients with invasive disease.[59]

Moreover, radiotherapy is beneficial for local recurrences after surgery or as an adjuvant therapy in those patients with a high risk of recurrence.[61,62] No randomized controlled studies comparing surgery to radiotherapy have been performed as of this writing.

TOPICAL CHEMOTHERAPY AND IMMUNOMODULATOR

Topical 5-fluorouracil (5-FU) and imiquimod have been used to treat EMPD with varying degrees of success.

5-FU has been used as a neoadjuvant modality prior to surgery to delineate clinical margins and for early postoperative detection of recurrence.[63,64] However, topical 5-FU has not proven to be a reliably curative agent in the treatment of EMPD because of the limited penetration of the drug and the inability to reach the deeper epidermal layers and adnexal structures that are frequently involved in EMPD.[7,64]

Imiquimod has been reported to result in clinical and histologic clearance in a few case series involving primary and recurrent EMPD.[65,66] In one study of 8 patients with recurrent primary intraepidermal EMPD, 6 patients initially experienced complete clinical and histologic response, but 4 patients subsequently developed recurrences during the followup period (median: 35 months).[67] All the patients with recurrences did not have progression to invasive disease, declined further surgery for their recurrences, and chose to retreat with imiquimod.[67]

As a result of the limited number of patients treated with these topical agents, the ideal duration and frequency of application is unknown. Further studies and long-term followup in a larger cohort are necessary.

PHOTODYNAMIC THERAPY

Photodynamic therapy has been used as an adjuvant to chemoradiotherapy, neoadjuvant prior to surgery, and as a primary modality with reasonable success.[7] However, as in the case of other topical treatment modalities, the ideal duration and frequency of application is unknown. Further studies and long-term followup in a larger cohort are necessary.

SYSTEMIC CHEMOTHERAPY

Systemic chemotherapy has been used to treat patients with invasive and metastatic disease and may be considered in rare cases in which surgery and radiotherapy are contraindicated. Limited reports of systemic chemotherapy for the treatment of EMPD have been described, including a combination of low-dose 5-FU and cisplatin[68]; a combination of 5-FU, carboplatin/cisplatin, mitomycin C, epirubicin, and vincristine[69,70]; docetaxel[71-73]; and combination trastuzumab, docetaxel, and carboplatin followed by lapatinib.[74]

REFERENCES

1. Paget J. On disease of the mammary areola preceding cancer of the mammary gland. *St Bartholomew Hosp Res Lond*. 1874;10:87-89.

2. Crocker HR. Paget's disease affecting the scrotum and penis. *Trans Pathol Soc London*. 1889;40:187-191.
3. Caliskan M, Gatti G, Sosnovskikh I, et al. Paget's disease of the breast: the experience of the European Institute of Oncology and review of the literature. *Breast Cancer Res Treat*. 2008;112(3):513-521.
4. van der Zwan JM, Siesling S, Blokx WA, et al. Invasive extramammary Paget's disease and the risk for secondary tumours in Europe. *Eur J Surg Oncol*. 2012;38(3):214-221.
5. Siesling S, Elferink MA, van Dijck JA, et al. Epidemiology and treatment of extramammary Paget disease in the Netherlands. *Eur J Surg Oncol*. 2007;33(8):951-955.
6. Zollo JD, Zeitouni NC. The Roswell Park Cancer Institute experience with extramammary Paget's disease. *Br J Dermatol*. 2000;142(1):59-65.
7. Shepherd V, Davidson EJ, Davies-Humphreys J. Extramammary Paget's disease. *BJOG*. 2005;112(3):273-279.
8. Hatta N, Yamada M, Hirano T, et al. Extramammary Paget's disease: treatment, prognostic factors and outcome in 76 patients. *Br J Dermatol*. 2008;158(2):313-318.
9. Lopes Filho LL, Lopes IM, Lopes LR, et al. Mammary and extramammary Paget's disease. *An Bras Dermatol*. 2015;90(2):225-231.
10. Saida T, Iwata M. "Ectopic" extramammary Paget's disease affecting the lower anterior aspect of the chest. *J Am Acad Dermatol*. 1987;17(5, pt 2):910-913.
11. Nagai Y, Ishibuchi H, Takahashi M, et al. Extramammary Paget's disease with bowenoid histologic features accompanied by an ectopic lesion on the upper abdomen. *J Dermatol*. 2005;32(8):670-673.
12. Cohen MA, Hanly A, Poulos E, et al. Extramammary Paget's disease presenting on the face. *Dermatol Surg*. 2004;30(10):1361-1363.
13. Chilukuri S, Page R, Reed JA, et al. Ectopic extramammary Paget's disease arising on the cheek. *Dermatol Surg*. 2002;28(5):430-433.
14. Gonzalez-Castro J, Iranzo P, Palou J, et al. Extramammary Paget's disease involving the external ear. *Br J Dermatol*. 1998;138(5):914-915.
15. Günhan-Bilgen I, Oktay A. Paget's disease of the breast: clinical, mammographic, sonographic and pathologic findings in 52 cases. *Eur J Radiol*. 2006;60(2):256-263.
16. Sakorafas GH, Blanchard K, Sarr MG, et al. Paget's disease of the breast. *Cancer Treat Rev*. 2001;27(1):9-18.
17. Lloyd J, Flanagan AM. Mammary and extramammary Paget's disease. *J Clin Pathol*. 2000;53(10):742-749.
18. Fu W, Lobocki CA, Silberberg BK, et al. Molecular markers in Paget disease of the breast. *J Surg Oncol*. 2001;77(3):171-178.
19. Cohen C, Guarner J, DeRose PB. Mammary Paget's disease and associated carcinoma. An immunohistochemical study. *Arch Pathol Lab Med*. 1993;117:291-294.
20. Anderson JM, Ariga R, Govil H, et al. Assessment of Her-2/Neu status by immunohistochemistry and fluorescence in situ hybridization in mammary Paget disease and underlying carcinoma. *Appl Immunohistochem Mol Morphol*. 2003;11(2):120-124.
21. Schelfhout VR, Coene ED, Delaey B, et al. Pathogenesis of Paget's disease: epidermal heregulin-alpha, motility factor, and the HER receptor family. *J Natl Cancer Inst*. 2000;92(8):622-628.
22. Lagios MD, Westdahl PR, Rose MR, et al. Paget's disease of the nipple. Alternative management in cases without or with minimal extent of underlying breast carcinoma. *Cancer*. 1984;54:545-551.
23. Gupta RK, Simpson J, Dowle C. The role of cytology in the diagnosis of Paget's disease of the nipple. *Pathology*. 1996;28(3):248-250.
24. Lucarotti ME, Dunn JM, Webb AJ. Scrape cytology in the diagnosis of Paget's disease of the breast. *Cytopathology*. 1994;5(5):301-305.
25. Morrogh M, Morris EA, Liberman L, et al. MRI identifies otherwise occult disease in select patients with Paget disease of the nipple. *J Am Coll Surg*. 2008;206(2):316-321.
26. Ikeda DM, Helvie MA, Frank TS, et al. Paget disease of the nipple: radiologic-pathologic correlation. *Radiology*. 1993;189(1):89-94.
27. Zakaria S, Pantvaidya G, Ghosh K, et al. Paget's disease of the breast: accuracy of preoperative assessment. *Breast Cancer Res Treat*. 2007;102(2):137-142.
28. Frei KA, Bonel HM, Pelte MF, et al. Paget disease of the breast: findings at magnetic resonance imaging and histopathologic correlation. *Invest Radiol*. 2005;40(6):363-367.
29. Zhu Y, Ye DW, Yao XD, et al. Clinicopathological characteristics, management and outcome of metastatic penoscrotal extramammary Paget's disease. *Br J Dermatol*. 2009;161(3):577-582.
30. Cho SB, Yun M, Lee MG, et al. Variable patterns of positron emission tomography in the assessment of patients with extramammary Paget's disease. *J Am Acad Dermatol*. 2005;52(2):353-355.
31. Aoyagi S, Sato-Matsumura KC, Shimizu H. Staging and assessment of lymph node involvement by 18F-fluorodeoxyglucose-positron emission tomography in invasive extramammary Paget's disease. *Dermatol Surg*. 2005;31(5):595-598.
32. Requena L, Kutzner H, Hurt MA, et al. Malignant tumours with apocrine and eccrine differentiation. In: LeBoit PE, Burg G, Weedon D, et al, eds. *World Health Organization Classification of Tumours of Skin*. Lyon, France: IARC Press; 2006:125-138.
33. Lau J, Kohler S. Keratin profile of intraepidermal cells in Paget's disease, extramammary Paget's disease, and pagetoid squamous cell carcinoma in situ. *J Cutan Pathol*. 2003;30(7):449-454.
34. Plaza JA, Torres-Cabala C, Ivan D, et al. HER-2/neu expression in extramammary Paget disease: a clinicopathologic and immunohistochemistry study of 47 cases with and without underlying malignancy. *J Cutan Pathol*. 2009;36(7):729-733.
35. Ohnishi T, Watanabe S. The use of cytokeratins 7 and 20 in the diagnosis of primary and secondary extramammary Paget's disease. *Br J Dermatol*. 2000;142(2):243-247.
36. Kohler S, Smoller BR. Gross cystic disease fluid protein-15 reactivity in extramammary Paget's disease with and without associated internal malignancy. *Am J Dermatopathol*. 1996;18(2):118-123.
37. Yoshii N, Kitajima S, Yonezawa S, et al. Expression of mucin core proteins in extramammary Paget's disease. *Pathol Int*. 2002;52(5-6):390-399.
38. Kuan SF, Montag AG, Hart J, et al. Differential expression of mucin genes in mammary and extramammary Paget's disease. *Am J Surg Pathol*. 2001;25(12):1469-1477.
39. Hata H, Abe R, Hoshina D, et al. MUC5AC expression correlates with invasiveness and progression of extramammary Paget's disease. *J Eur Acad Dermatol Venereol*. 2014;28(6):727-732.
40. Kasashima S, Ozaki S, Kawashima A, et al. Androgen receptor and 5alpha-reductase immunohistochemical profiles in extramammary Paget disease. *Br J Dermatol*. 2010;162(5):1098-1102.

41. Aoyagi S, Akiyama M, Shimizu H. High expression of Ki-67 and cyclin D1 in invasive extramammary Paget's disease. *J Dermatol Sci*. 2008;50(3):177-184.
42. Fu W, Mittel VK, Young SC. Paget disease of the breast: analysis of 41 patients. *Am J Clin Oncol*. 2001;24(4):397-400.
43. Kollmorgen DR, Varanasi JS, Edge SB, et al. Paget's disease of the breast: a 33-year experience. *J Am Coll Surg*. 1998;187(2):171-177.
44. Yim JH, Wick MR, Philpott GW, et al. Underlying pathology in mammary Paget's disease. *Ann Surg Oncol*. 1997;4(4):287-292.
45. Marshall JK, Griffith KA, Haffty BG, et al. Conservative management of Paget disease of the breast with radiotherapy: 10- and 15-year results. *Cancer*. 2003;97(9):2142-2149.
46. Bijker N, Rutgers EJ, Duchateau L, et al. Breast-conserving therapy for Paget disease of the nipple: a prospective European Organization for Research and Treatment of Cancer study of 61 patients. *Cancer*. 2001;91(3):472-477.
47. Pierce LJ, Haffty BG, Solin LJ, et al. The conservative management of Paget's disease of the breast with radiotherapy. *Cancer*. 1997;80(6):1065-1072.
48. Sukumvanich P, Bentrem DJ, Cody HS 3rd, et al. The role of sentinel lymph node biopsy in Paget's disease of the breast. *Ann Surg Oncol*. 2007;14(3):1020-1023.
49. Fanning J, Lambert HC, Hale TM, et al. Paget's disease of the vulva: prevalence of associated vulvar adenocarcinoma, invasive Paget's disease, and recurrence after surgical excision. *Am J Obstet Gynecol*. 1999;180(1, pt 1):24-27.
50. Kodama S, Kaneko T, Saito M, et al. A clinicopathologic study of 30 patients with Paget's disease of the vulva. *Gynecol Oncol*. 1995;56(1):63-70.
51. Fishman DA, Chambers SK, Schwartz PE, et al. Extramammary Paget's disease of the vulva. *Gynecol Oncol*. 1995;56(2):266-270.
52. Appert DL, Otley CC, Phillips PK, et al. Role of multiple scouting biopsies before Mohs micrographic surgery for extramammary Paget's disease. *Dermatol Surg*. 2005;31(11, pt 1):1417-1422.
53. O'Connor WJ, Lim KK, Zalla MJ, et al. Comparison of Mohs micrographic surgery and wide excision for extramammary Paget's disease. *Dermatol Surg*. 2003;29(7):723-727.
54. Hatta N, Morita R, Yamada M, et al. Sentinel lymph node biopsy in patients with extramammary Paget's disease. *Dermatol Surg*. 2004;30(10):1329-1334.
55. Tsutsumida A, Yamamoto Y, Minakawa H, et al. Indications for lymph node dissection in the treatment of extramammary Paget's disease. *Dermatol Surg*. 2003;29(1):21-24.
56. Ogata D, Kiyohara Y, Yoshikawa S, et al. Usefulness of sentinel lymph node biopsy for prognostic prediction in extramammary Paget's disease. *Eur J Dermatol*. 2016;26(3):254-259.
57. Hendi A, Brodland DG, Zitelli JA. Extramammary Paget's disease: surgical treatment with Mohs micrographic surgery. *J Am Acad Dermatol*. 2004;51(5):767-773.
58. Brierley JD, Stockdale AD. Radiotherapy: an effective treatment for extramammary Paget's disease. *Clin Oncol (R Coll Radiol)*. 1991;3(1):3-5.
59. Besa P, Rich TA, Delclos L, et al. Extramammary Paget's disease of the perineal skin: role of radiotherapy. *Int J Radiat Oncol Biol Phys*. 1992;24(1):73-78.
60. Moreno-Arias GA, Conill C, Castells-Mas A, et al. Radiotherapy for genital extramammary Paget's disease in situ. *Dermatol Surg*. 2001;27(6):587-590.
61. Luk NM, Yu KH, Yeung WK, et al. Extramammary Paget's disease: outcome of radiotherapy with curative intent. *Clin Exp Dermatol*. 2003;28(4):360-363.
62. Guerrieri M, Back MF. Extramammary Paget's disease: role of radiation therapy. *Australas Radiol*. 2002;46(2):204-208.
63. Bewley AP, Bracka A, Staughton RC, et al. Extramammary Paget's disease of the scrotum: treatment with topical 5-fluorouracil and plastic surgery. *Br J Dermatol*. 1994;131(3):445-446.
64. Del Castillo LF, Garcia C, Schoendorff C, et al. Spontaneous apparent clinical resolution with histologic persistence of a case of extramammary Paget's disease: response to topical 5-fluorouracil. *Cutis*. 2000;65(5):331-333.
65. Sendagorta E, Herranz P, Feito M, et al. Successful treatment of three cases of primary extramammary Paget's disease of the vulva with imiquimod-proposal of a therapeutic schedule. *J Eur Acad Dermatol Venereol*. 2010;24(4):490-492.
66. Marchitelli C, Peremateu MS, Sluga MC, et al. Treatment of primary vulvar paget disease with 5% imiquimod cream. *J Low Genit Tract Dis*. 2014;18(4):347-350.
67. Cowan RA, Black DR, Hoang LN, et al. A pilot study of topical imiquimod therapy for the treatment of recurrent extramammary Paget's disease. *Gynecol Oncol*. 2016;142(1):139-143.
68. Kariya K, Tsuji T, Schwartz RA. Trial of low-dose 5-fluorouracil/cisplatin therapy for advanced extramammary Paget's disease. *Dermatol Surg*. 2004;30(2, pt 2):341-344.
69. Mochitomi Y, Sakamoto R, Gushi A, et al. Extramammary Paget's disease/carcinoma successfully treated with a combination chemotherapy: report of two cases. *J Dermatol*. 2005;32(8):632-637.
70. Oashi K, Tsutsumida A, Namikawa K, et al. Combination chemotherapy for metastatic extramammary Paget disease. *Br J Dermatol*. 2014;170(6):1354-1357.
71. Yoshino K, Fujisawa Y, Kiyohara Y, et al. Usefulness of docetaxel as first-line chemotherapy for metastatic extramammary Paget's disease. *J Dermatol*. 2016;43(6):633-637.
72. Fujisawa Y, Umebayashi Y, Otsuka F. Metastatic extramammary Paget's disease successfully controlled with tumour dormancy therapy using docetaxel. *Br J Dermatol*. 2006;154(2):375-376.
73. Oguchi S, Kaneko M, Uhara H, et al. Docetaxel induced durable response in advanced extramammary Paget's disease: a case report. *J Dermatol*. 2002;29(1):33-37.
74. Shin DS, Sherry T, Kallen ME, et al. Human epidermal growth factor receptor 2 (HER-2/neu)-directed therapy for rare metastatic epithelial tumors with HER-2 amplification. *Case Rep Oncol*. 2016;9(2):298-304.

Chapter 115 :: Melanocytic Nevi
:: Jonathan D. Cuda, Robert F. Moore, & Klaus J. Busam

第一百一十五章

黑素细胞痣

中文导读

黑素细胞痣为黑素细胞的良性肿瘤，其特征是在表皮、真皮或其他组织的巢穴中存在普通黑素细胞，形成这些痣的黑素细胞被称为痣细胞。本章分为10节：①先天性黑素细胞痣；②斑痣；③常见获得性黑素细胞痣；④蓝痣；⑤色素性梭形细胞痣；⑥Spitz痣；⑦淋巴结痣；⑧单纯性黑子；⑨日光性黑子；⑩发育不良痣。分别从流行病学、临床特征、危险因素、病因和发病机制、诊断、鉴别诊断、临床病程和预后、临床管理等多个方面介绍了这些类型的黑素细胞痣。

〔粟 娟〕

INTRODUCTION

This chapter discusses melanocytic nevi, defined as benign neoplasms of melanocytes, most of which manifest themselves as cutaneous pigmented lesions. They are characterized by the presence of banal melanocytic cells in nests (defined as three or more melanocytes in direct contact [also known as *thèque*]), within the epidermis, dermis, or in other tissues. The melanocytic cells forming these nevi are referred to as *nevomelanocytes*. The term *melanocytic hyperplasia* is a descriptive term used to indicate increased melanocytes confined to the basal layer of the epidermis in the absence of nest formation.

Simplistically, melanocytic nevi can be divided into those that arise from junctional melanocytes (often termed *acquired nevi*) and those that arise from neural-crest derived melanocytic precursors that migrate along neurovascular bundles, stop before they reach the epidermis, and proliferate at those sites. The latter are termed *congenital melanocytic nevi* (CMNs).

Dysplastic nevi are defined as those that display atypical architectural and cytologic features. Historically, the nomenclature associated with these lesions includes B-K moles (recognizing the first two families described with such lesions whose surnames began with the letters B and K),[1] familial atypical multiple mole and melanoma syndrome,[2] atypical mole syndrome,[3] Clark nevus,[4] atypical moles, and nevus with architectural disorder and (varying degrees of) cytologic atypia.[5] Although the nomenclature for these lesions remains contentious, the term *dysplastic nevus* (DN) is most frequently utilized[5,6] and is the term that will be used in this chapter. It is also important to note that in practice, the terms *dysplastic* and *atypical* are sometimes used as a modifier for other melanocytic neoplasias (eg, Spitz nevi) or hyperplasias to indicate a variation from a typical pattern or to recognize an increased concern for malignant biologic potential.

The nevi described in this chapter include CMNs, nevus spilus, common acquired melanocytic nevi, blue nevi, Spitz nevi, pigmented spindle cell nevi

(PSCN), dysplastic nevi, and nodal nevi. Benign melanocytic hyperplasias include lentigo simplex and solar lentigo.

CONGENITAL MELANOCYTIC NEVI

AT-A-GLANCE

- Pigmented neoplasms of melanocytes that are evident at birth or shortly thereafter.
- Lesions may be small, medium-sized, or large and cover substantial body surface area.
- Large or giant lesions have a significant risk for melanoma development. Cranial or midline congenital melanocytic nevi and those with satellite lesions have an increased risk of leptomeningeal involvement.
- Histology shows extensive nevomelanocytic infiltration of the dermis, accentuation along the adventitia of skin adnexa and nerves, single-filing between collagen bundles, often with involvement of subcutaneous tissues.

EPIDEMIOLOGY

CMNs are found in approximately 1% to 3% of neonates across ethnicities.[7] The majority of lesions are small to medium in size and are present at birth; however, there are also congenital nevi (>1.5 cm) that appear for the first time between 1 month and 2 years of life (termed *tardive congenital nevi*). A significant gender predilection has not been demonstrated. CMNs occur most commonly on the trunk and extremities, although scalp and facial involvement are seen. Giant CMNs are uncommon. CMNs that attain 99 mm or more in diameter occur in approximately 1 of every 20,000 newborns, and those with a garment distribution affect 1 of every 500,000 newborns.[8]

CLINICAL FEATURES

Nevi of congenital onset have traditionally been grouped based on diameter into small, medium, and large sizes. The size limits of each type are arbitrary because the diameter of these lesions lies on a continuum. There is some rationale for standardizing congenital nevi by size because there is increased risk of melanoma associated with large and giant CMNs.[9,10] The most accepted system is based on the expected size of the nevus in adult life[11] because CMNs have been shown to grow in proportion with the affected anatomic region.[12] Small CMNs are less than 1.5 cm in diameter (projected adult size), medium ones are divided into two groups—M1, 1.5 to 10 cm and M2, >10 to 20 cm—as are large ones—L1, >20 to 30 cm and L2, >30 to 40 cm. Last, giant CMNs are categorized as G1, >40 to 60 cm and G2, >60 cm (Fig. 115-1). This classification scheme also rates the number of satellite nevi (S1: <20, S2: >20–50, S3: >50).

CUTANEOUS FINDINGS

Although CMNs are on average larger than acquired nevi, there is no specific size limitation that can be used to reliably predict whether a given nevus is congenital or acquired. Pigmented lesions attaining a diameter of 1.5 cm or more are likely to be CMN, dysplastic nevi, or melanoma.

Most CMNs present as flat brown patches or plaques with smooth or slightly uneven borders. Many show hypertrichosis compared to surrounding unaffected skin. Hair growth may be present at birth or commence in the years thereafter. Most congenital nevi begin with even pigmentation, but some variability of pigmentation and irregularity of surface texture eventuates in most medium- and large-sized lesions over time. Lesions may have a pebbly, rugose, verrucous, or lobular appearance.

Dermoscopic features are variable and include a reticular, globular, homogeneous, and cobblestone pattern or a combination thereof. Dermoscopic findings in dysplastic nevi sometimes overlap with those of CMN. In one study, most of the features related to dysplastic nevi, including atypical dots and globules, focal hypopigmentation, and perifollicular hypopigmentation, were observed in CMN.[13] Therefore, eliciting a history with regards to the time of lesion onset is important. In large CMN, there can be significant variability in pigmentation and structure, and melanomas

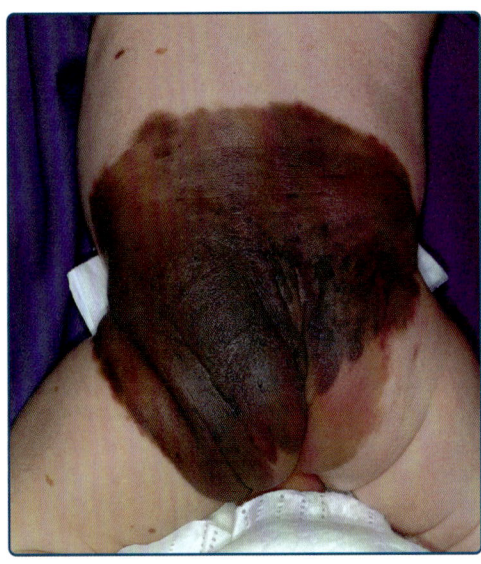

Figure 115-1 Giant congenital pigmented nevus in the bathing trunk distribution. Note the satellite nevi.

may develop in the deep components, potentially limiting the utility of dermoscopy in such lesions.

Some CMNs show an atypical clinical appearance, including significant color variegation and irregularities in outline and surface contour. Color variations include dark brown, black, or hues of blue. These features often correlate with atypical histopathologic findings. Loss of pigmentation, halo depigmentation, and regression can also occur.

RELATED PHYSICAL CONDITIONS

One of the most important related physical conditions in patients with CMNs on the head, neck, or posterior midline is neurocutaneous melanosis (NCM). In this condition, the cells of the congenital nevus involve the meninges or even the parenchymal cells of the brain. Most patients with NCM have many cutaneous congenital nevi, either in the form of a giant nevus with many satellites or in the form of many medium-sized lesions.

Symptomatic NCM presents with seizures and hydrocephalus in the first few years of life when melanocytes are diffusely distributed along the meninges. There may be neurologic deficits and vomiting from increased intracranial pressure. When an intracranial mass is present, symptoms may present later in life.[14] The prognosis is poor if neurologic symptoms develop. Patients often die within 3 years of symptom onset.

COMPLICATIONS

The most important complication of congenital nevi is that they can give rise to melanoma. The overall incidence of this complication is approximately 1% to 2%.[9] The risk of melanoma appears to be proportionate to the number of melanocytes that comprise the nevus. This in turn is closely related to its size. Thus, small- and medium-sized lesions have a low risk of developing melanoma, but large- and giant-sized lesions have greater risk. Additionally, satellite nevi are associated with increased risk of melanoma. In one systematic literature review, melanoma arising from CMN exceeded 40 cm in 74% of 52 cases studied and 94% of those had satellite nevi.[15] The lifetime risk of melanoma development in lesions exceeding 40 cm (projected adult size) with satellite nevi has been estimated at 10% to 15%.[9]

Although melanoma arising from CMN may occur at the dermal–epidermal junction (DEJ) (as they do in acquired nevi), they show a tendency to arise in deeper dermal and subcutaneous components of the nevus. These tumors are highly aggressive in part because of their greater Breslow thickness at presentation. They present with the sudden appearance of a dermal or subcutaneous nodule. Sometimes lymph node metastasis precedes clinical detection of the primary melanoma. Other clinical features that should raise concern for melanoma include very dark pigmentation, ulceration, bleeding, or onset of other sensory symptoms. There is no ethnic predilection for melanoma developing in CMN.

For cranial, midline, or CMN with multiple satellite lesions, there is a risk of leptomeningeal involvement (NCM). Symptomatic NCM carries a poor prognosis, even in the absence of malignant degeneration (central nervous system [CNS] melanoma). A recent literature review revealed that 37% of 178 melanomas arising in patients with congenital nevi were primary CNS melanomas rather than of cutaneous origin, and most of these (53.9%) developed in patients with multiple medium-sized CMNs.[16]

Proliferative nodules also constitute a significant complication of congenital nevi because they need to be removed. They typically present as a lightly pigmented or flesh-colored nodule developing in a preexisting congenital nevus. Although they almost always behave in a benign fashion, histopathologic examination of a lesion that is clinically indistinguishable from a proliferative nodule may show the findings of a clear-cut melanoma.

RISK FACTORS

There are rare reports of familial clustering of congenital nevi (Fig. 115-2).[17] Patients with neurofibromatosis type 1 appear to have an increased incidence of giant CMNs.[18]

ETIOLOGY AND PATHOGENESIS

CMN result from postzygotic somatic mutations of proteins involved in the mitogen-activated protein kinase (MAPK) pathway within the embryonic melanocyte. These primarily include mutations of *NRAS*, resulting in abnormal accumulation of melanocytic cells along migration pathways during normal development. Whereas *NRAS* mutations are most prevalent in large- and giant-sized CMNs, small- and medium-sized lesions have been reported to have either *NRAS* mutations or in a small number of cases, activating mutations in *BRAF*.

It should be noted that the proportion of cases with *NRAS* or *BRAF* mutations vary between studies in the literature, which probably reflects the different methodologies used (ie, whether CMN was defined as historically being present at birth, the exact measurements that were used, whether both genes were sequenced, and so on).[19] In one study of 32 congenital nevi confirmed to be present at birth, the authors found that 81% of cases had mutations in *NRAS*, but no *BRAF* mutations were detected; furthermore, 7 of the 10 proliferating nodules that developed within the congenital nevi also harbored mutations in *NRAS* rather than *BRAF*. In contrast, 20 of 28 nevi studied that had a congenital pattern histologically but were not confirmed to be present since birth harbored *BRAF*

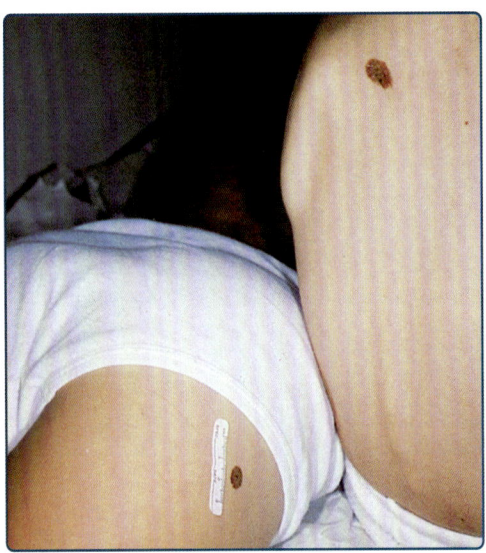

Figure 115-2 Familial aggregation of small congenital nevomelanocytic nevi. Note the small congenital nevus on the thigh of a 3-year-old Caucasian boy and on the back of his 5-year-old brother.

mutations (similar to acquired nevi); only 7 had mutations of *NRAS*.[20]

Clinical findings such as a congenital divided nevus of the eyelid can give us insight into when these mutational events may occur (Fig. 115-3). The palpebral buds develop during the 7th week of gestation and the upper and lower eyelids fuse by week 9 or 10. The eyelids then begin to separate during the 20th week, and complete separation commences between weeks 28 and 30.[21] Because of the contiguous nature of the lesion on the upper and lower eyelids, it may be presumed that the nevus cells migrated into this location sometime during or after eyelid fusion but before the eyelids separated.

DIAGNOSIS

The diagnosis of a congenital nevus is usually straightforward. The more challenging problem is whether the nevus contains any areas that necessitate biopsy. For patients with congenital nevi on the head or axial midline, an important question is whether there is subjacent NCM. This is best addressed by imaging studies (see later).

PATHOLOGY

Although there are histopathologic features that are suggestive of a congenital nevus, there are no criteria with absolute sensitivity and specificity for predicting whether a lesion is of congenital onset.

Prototypical large- or medium-sized CMNs involve the entire skin from the junctional zone to the subcutis (Fig. 115-4). Small, round melanocytes are present in subcutaneous septae and to a lesser extent in lobules, with progressively (slightly) larger cells in the upper levels of the dermis and along the junctional zone. Some lesions are densely cellular, and there is a propensity for the cells to surround neurovascular bundles, appendageal structures, and folliculosebaceous units. Subendothelial protrusion by nevomelanocytes within lymphovascular spaces is sometimes prominent. The junctional zone may be involved by cells distributed singly and in small nests. These are often separated from the upper dermal part of the lesion by a zone of uninvolved papillary dermis. The junctional cells are usually larger than those beneath them, and basilar hyperpigmentation is common. A rim of pigmented melanocytes is often present along the upper border of the dermal component, which often extends along the innermost perifollicular melanocytes.

In some large and in most small congenital nevi, the subcutis is not involved. In such cases, at the base of the lesion, melanocytes splay between collagen bundles in cords and strands within the deep or mid reticular dermis.

Congenital nevi that undergo neurotization show areas where schwannian differentiation occurs. Instead of small round melanocytes, one sees small S-shaped spindle cells. These can form thin, wavy fascicles with clefts in between them containing mucin. Admixed adipocytes are commonly seen. Collections of neuroid cells can form pseudomeissnerian corpuscles, a palisaded arrangement of cells around a cellular mass of homogeneous material, simulating native Wagner-Meissner corpuscles. In highly neurotized lesions, one may not be able to morphologically distinguish between nevus and neurofibroma. Neural differentiation is sometimes responsible for the lobulation and redundancy of tissue corresponding clinically with soft rugose areas of the nevus.

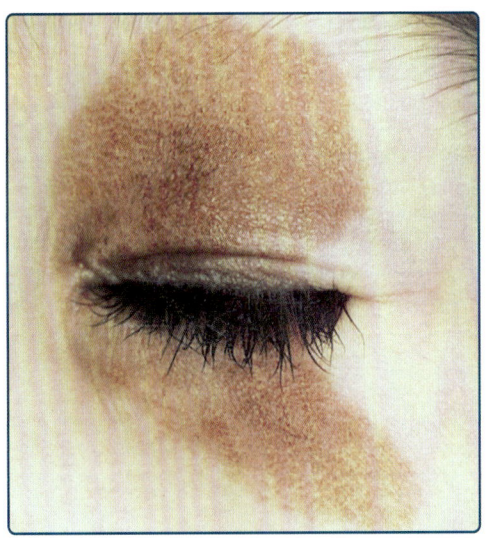

Figure 115-3 Congenital divided nevomelanocytic nevus of the eyelid. The nevus is contiguous when the eyelids are closed, suggesting that the lesion was formed in the developing fetus before the eyelids split (ie, before 24 weeks).

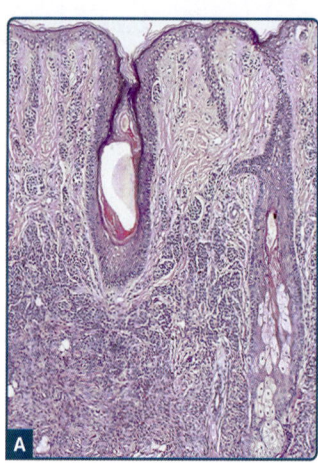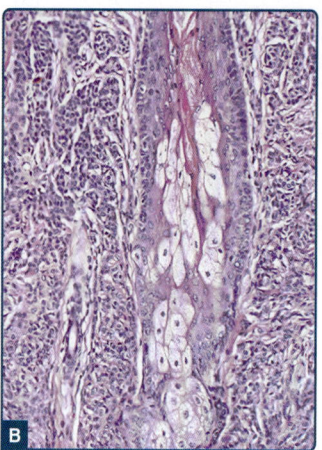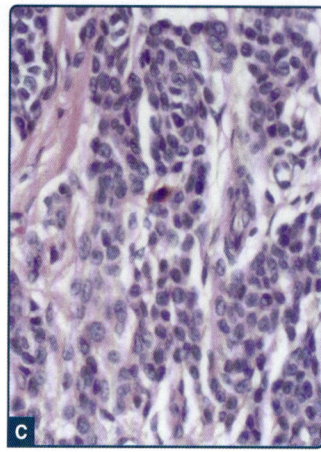

Figure 115-4 Histopathologic features of congenital nevomelanocytic nevus. Nevomelanocytes in the low-magnification image (**A**) reveal dense accumulation in the lower two-thirds of the dermis; at medium magnification (**B**), these cells encroach on dermal adnexal structures (follicular, sebaceous, and eccrine); and higher magnification (**C**) reveals dense collections of small nevomelanocytic cells.

Other histologic variations seen include cells with a combined epithelioid cell (Spitz) phenotype, which are often admixed with more conventional round cell and neuroid elements. CMNs may also have elements of blue nevus (either common or cellular type) with heavily pigmented spindle-shaped melanocytic cells or show features of inverted type-A or deep penetrating nevus. In a recent series of 197 congenital nevi in children younger than 3 years of age, 74% of patients studied had atypical histopathologic features. These included cytologic atypia (mostly mild or moderate), architectural disorder (mostly mild or moderate), and pagetoid scatter; no cases of melanoma were identified in these patients with a mean follow-up period of 7.3 years.[22]

Proliferative nodules feature large, round hypercellular aggregates of melanocytes that appear discrete on scanning magnification but tend to blend in with the background nevus cells. True to their name, they often contain mitotic figures. The melanocytes in these nodules may have a range of appearances, including cells with small to moderately enlarged nuclei, cells with epithelioid cytology, spindled cells, and blue nevus–like features. Proliferative nodules tend to have lower mitotic counts than melanoma and are less likely to show ulceration or the cytogenetic or epigenetic aberrations detected in melanoma.[23,24]

SPECIAL TESTS

Imaging studies to detect NCM include magnetic resonance imaging of the brain or spinal cord concordant with the anatomic location of the nevus.

DIFFERENTIAL DIAGNOSIS

See Table 115-1.

CLINICAL COURSE AND PROGNOSIS

CMNs have a dynamic evolution during body growth. CMNs at birth usually distort the skin surface at least slightly when assessed by oblique lighting and may become more elevated over time. Surface pigmentation also may change. Lightly pigmented CMNs may become more darkly pigmented, and darkly pigmented CMNs eventually may become less pigmented. CMNs may also develop a halo of depigmentation, potentially heralding spontaneous regression. Relatively hairless CMNs at birth may develop long, dark, coarse hair or may maintain a relatively normal hair density. CMNs generally expand in direct proportion to growth of a given anatomic region.[12] Proliferative nodules present as flesh-colored or lightly pigmented nodules that develop and then stabilize. CMNs in fully grown individuals should remain stable. The prognosis is excellent unless complicated by NCM or melanoma.

MANAGEMENT

TREATMENT

The treatment of CMN depends on the perceived risk of melanoma plus cosmetic and functional considerations. The risk of developing melanoma is related to its size, and melanoma may arise in large CMNs even in the first few years of life. Therefore, debulking of large nevi and excision of smaller or medium-sized ones is desirable when feasible. This can be done for large nevi in serial stages.

It is probably prudent to delay treatment until after the first 6 months of life to reduce surgical and anesthetic risks. Management of patients with large and

TABLE 115-1
Differential Diagnosis of Congenital Melanocytic Nevus
- Café-au-lait macule
- Nevus spilus
- Lentigo simplex
- Nevus of Ota/Ito
- Dermal melanocytosis (Mongolian spot)
- Becker melanosis
- Arrector pili (smooth muscle) hamartoma
- Epidermal nevus
- Nevus sebaceous
- Solitary mastocytoma

giant CMNs must be individualized. Extensive involvement of the body surface, with little or no normal skin available for graft sites, may necessitate abandoning efforts at prophylactic excision and accepting lifelong surveillance to detect the earliest signs of malignant change. It may be impossible to remove every nevomelanocyte in large CMN, particularly when there is involvement of vital structures or deep anatomic zones. The treatment goal is to remove as much of the nevus as possible while preserving function and improving cosmetic appearance.

Other indications for surgical excision include symptomatology (ie, chronic pruritus, pain, ulceration). Unlike surgical excision, dermabrasion, lasers, and other modes of destructive therapy do not address the malignant potential of CMN; nevomelanocytes will still be left behind in the dermis, and the cosmetic results associated with destructive therapy are not always predictable.

Although atypical-appearing CMN should be considered for immediate excision, careful surveillance without excision may be an option for clinically benign lesions depending on gross appearance, size, location, cosmetic and functional deficits (or improvement) resulting from excision, and general health issues. Given the risk of general anesthesia, for lesions perceived to be at low risk during the first decade of life, it is appropriate to consider waiting until the child is old enough to tolerate local anesthesia.

All CMNs should be documented at birth, preferably in the form of high-quality photographs that can be used to aid follow-up by parents and physicians. Follow-up is complicated by the natural evolutionary changes that take place in a nevus during body growth (ie, surface, size, color, and hair), and periodic updates of photographs may be warranted. Suspicious changes in color, surface, or size require urgent evaluation.

PREVENTION AND COUNSELING

There is no known preventive approach to avoid the development of CMNs. UV radiation (UVR)–induced mutations play no role in the initial development of lesions already present at birth. The issues around body image and social adjustment raised by large and giant congenital nevi may benefit from counseling and support groups, including Nevus Network (www.nevusnetwork.org) and Nevus Outreach, Inc. (www.nevus.org).

NEVUS SPILUS

AT-A-GLANCE

- Nevus spilus (derived from Greek *spilos*, meaning *spot*)—spotted nevus
- Synonyms: speckled lentiginous nevus, zosteriform lentiginous nevus
- Pigmented neoplasm of melanocytes that develops during infancy or early childhood.
- Lesion presents with two components, a light brown patch (café-au-lait) containing speckled dark macules or papules.
- Risk for melanoma is low but may occur.
- Histology shows localized collections of nevus elements forming in the background of mild melanocytic hyperplasia.

EPIDEMIOLOGY

Nevus spilus occurs in approximately 1% to 2% of the population. They are present either at birth or in the first years of life and have therefore been regarded as a variant of congenital nevus. There does not appear to be gender or ethnic predilection.

CLINICAL FEATURES

Darkly pigmented flat macules or papules are usually present within the nevus spilus on presentation. New pigmented elements may evolve within the lesion over time.

CUTANEOUS FINDINGS

The background pigmentation of a nevus spilus is circumscribed and similar in appearance to a café-au-lait macule in hue, with even light pigmentation. There are scattered superimposed more darkly pigmented macules or papules. The tan macular background pigmentation can range in size from less than 1 cm to larger than 10 cm in diameter (Fig. 115-5).

Lesions are most commonly found on the trunk and extremities, although any cutaneous site may be affected. Multiple lesions may be present and have a segmental distribution. There are rare reports of a

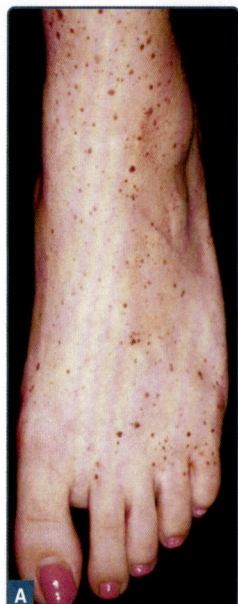

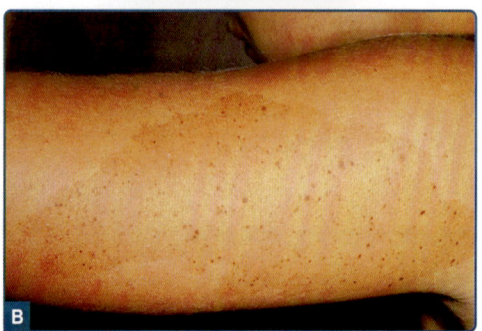

Figure 115-5 Nevus spilus. **A,** Nevus spilus appearing first at age 3 years on the ankle and foot of a 25-year-old white woman. **B,** Congenital nevus spilus on the arm of a 10-year-old white boy.

is typically seen in phakomatosis pigmentokeratotica. Phakomatosis spilorosea constitutes presentation of both nevus flammeus and nevus spilus with or without nevus anemicus. Systemic disease may or may not be present, which include vascular anomalies, ocular abnormalities, limb hemihypertrophy, or development of multiple granular cell tumors. Phakomatosis pigmentokeratotica includes nevus spilus plus organoid nevus with or without systemic symptoms, which include neurologic deficits and skeletal abnormalities.

COMPLICATIONS

The main concern that prompts a biopsy is a changing lesion, where one may see enlargement of dark macules or papules within the nevus spilus. One can see larger, irregularly shaped macules, sometimes with a central papule in so-called *dysplastic nevus spilus*. In such cases, the lesion can show any of the changes seen in dysplastic nevi. Rare cases of melanoma arise in nevus spilus and are recognizable as larger, irregularly shaped areas with variegated pigmentation. It is likely the risk of melanoma increases to some degree with the size of the nevus spilus, particularly with larger segmental lesions greater than 40 cm.[30]

RISK FACTORS

There are no known risk factors for nevus spilus, aside from the association with phakomatosis spilorosea and pigmentokeratotica.

ETIOLOGY AND PATHOGENESIS

Nevus spilus is believed to develop secondary to a postzygotic mutational event initiating a clonal field of melanocytes susceptible of creating multiple melanocytic tumors within. These arise likely secondary to additional mutational or epigenetic events. Sarin and coworkers identified an activating HRAS mutation (c.37G->C, p.Gly13Arg) in eight of eight nevi spili studied, implicating this gene locus as the predominant causative mutation in sporadic nevi spili.[31] The same author previously described a nevus spilus giving rise to agminated Spitz nevi with the same mutation.[32]

Kinsler and coworkers performed next-generation sequencing on three nevi spili with a distinct phenotype, large background café-au-lait–type patches with superimposed multiple medium or large pigmented patches indistinguishable from CMN.[33] This phenotype was termed *nevus spilus-type congenital melanocytic nevus*. In contrast to the activating HRAS mutations seen in small sporadic nevi spili,[30] nevus spilus–type CMNs displayed activating mutations of NRAS in all three patients (two with c.183A->Cp.Q61H, one with c.37G->Cp.G13R). Targeted exon capture of two

divided nevus spilus of the eyelid[25] as well as a report of one in the oral cavity.[26]

Dermoscopy reveals dark speckled foci with a reticuloglobular pattern in a background light brown and reticular pattern. Mixed patterns may occur that include combinations of homogeneous, reticular, globular, granular, and spitzoid patterns.[27] Dermoscopy and reflectance confocal microscopy have been used for early detection of melanoma, a rare complication of nevus spilus.[28]

RELATED PHYSICAL CONDITIONS

Nevus spilus has been associated with other anomalies of vascular, CNS, or connective tissue origin. It has been proposed by Vidaurri-de la Cruz and Happle that two distinct forms of nevus spilus exist, those with macular and those with papular speckles.[29] Whereas macular varieties are more commonly associated with phakomatosis spilorosea (previously classified as pigmentovascularis type III), the papular variant

skin samples from an additional patient also showed the same NRAS mutation (p.Q61H) in both the background pigmentation and the superimposed nevus.[33]

DIAGNOSIS

The diagnosis of nevus spilus is usually straightforward. Small lesions are sometimes mistaken for dysplastic nevi and large lesions for conventional CMN.

PATHOLOGY

Histologic sections reveal that the tan background corresponds to a diffuse area where there is slight epidermal hyperplasia with basilar hyperpigmentation, from no perceptible increase in melanocytes to a slight increase in singular melanocytes along the basal layer. The dark spots correspond to small lentiginous junctional and compound nevi featuring increased numbers of single melanocytes and small nests along the DEJ and small, round melanocytes in the superficial dermis, in cases of compound nevi. Rarely agminated nevi within a nevus spilus may have the phenotype of a blue nevus (pigmented dendritic melanocytes) or Spitz nevus (epithelioid and spindled melanocytes).

SPECIAL TESTS

There are no other diagnostic tests at present.

DIFFERENTIAL DIAGNOSIS

See Table 115-2.

CLINICAL COURSE AND PROGNOSIS

Nevus spilus is a benign lesion that may develop more spotted nevoid elements over time. After developing, they are presumed to persist throughout life, although it is possible that some elements within the nevus spilus or rarely the entire nevus spilus itself could regress with time. The prognosis is excellent with the exception of rare cases complicated by melanoma.

TABLE 115-2
Differential Diagnosis of Nevus Spilus

- Agminated nevomelanocytic nevi
- Agminated lentigines
- Becker melanosis
- Congenital nevomelanocytic nevus with heterogeneous pigmentation
- Café-au-lait macule

MANAGEMENT

TREATMENT

No standard guidelines exist for the management of patients with nevus spilus. Clinical appearance (typical or atypical), history of stability or instability of pigmented elements, congenital or noncongenital onset, perceived risk of developing melanoma, and cosmetic concerns are considerations when determining whether to excise or recommend periodic clinical evaluation for life. Documentation with high-quality photographs can be used to aid follow-up by parents and physicians. Atypical-appearing new or unstable elements in nevus spilus should be evaluated by histopathologic examination to exclude melanoma.

PREVENTION AND COUNSELING

There are no preventive measures for nevus spilus. UV protection is theoretically prudent in light of the propensity for melanocytic neoplasms to develop within nevi spili, as well as the rare reported cases complicated by melanoma.

COMMON ACQUIRED MELANOCYTIC NEVUS

AT-A-GLANCE

- Synonyms: nevocellular nevus, common nevus, melanocytic nevus
- Lesions are pigmented or skin-colored macules or papules which tend to be uniform in appearance and relatively small in size.
- They primarily develop during childhood or early adulthood.
- Increased numbers of acquired nevi impart an increased risk for melanoma development.
- Common nevi are subcategorized based on location of cells: cells in the epidermis (junctional), dermis (intradermal), or both areas (compound). Pathologically, the cells mature becoming smaller in size within the deeper dermis and express melanocytic antigen HMB-45 at lower levels.

EPIDEMIOLOGY

Common acquired melanocytic nevi develop after birth, slowly enlarge symmetrically, stabilize, and regress after a period of time. The number of nevi peaks in the third decade of life and declines thereafter. A number of studies have quantified the number of acquired nevi in different age groups. In a study of 432 European with white skin between the ages of 4 days and 96 years, nevi that were 3 mm in diameter or larger were detected in females and males, respectively, at median numbers of 0 and 2 in the first decade, 10 and 16 in the second decade, 16 and 24 in the third decade, 10 and 19 in the fourth decade, 12 and 15 in the fifth decade, 4 and 12 in the sixth decade, and 2.0 and 3.5 in the seventh through the ninth decades.[34] Numbers of nevi vary among study populations, but a similar age-related trend has been documented in most other large epidemiologic studies.

The prevalence of acquired nevi also varies according to ethnicity. In a longitudinal study of children in Colorado, non-Hispanic white children showed significantly more nevi than all other ethnic groups, developing an average of four to six new nevi per year from ages 3 to 8 years.[35] Nevi tend to be increased in individuals with light skin tone and those who have a tendency to sunburn.

CLINICAL FEATURES

Acquired common nevi develop over the first 3 decades of life and can persist in a stable state for decades, and many regress thereafter. In later adult years, nevus counts are significantly less and the rate of new or growing nevi declines, but melanoma incidence increases. Therefore, a new, growing, or changing pigmented lesion in an adult assumes a greater risk of being melanoma.

CUTANEOUS FINDINGS

The majority of common acquired nevi are less than 6 mm in diameter. Individual lesions have a homogeneous surface and coloration pattern, are round to oval in shape, and have sharply demarcated borders (Fig. 115-6). Most are skin colored, pink, or brown. Very dark brown or black nevi are unusual for people with light skin tones and should be viewed with suspicion. On the other hand, darkly colored nevi are common in those with dark skin tones. Blue, gray, red, and white areas are not typical for common acquired nevi and should raise concern for melanoma.

Lesions that are papillomatous or dome shaped tend to be lighter in color and display a more dominant intradermal component, but flat lesions tend to show more pigmentation and a more robust junctional component. Similar to congenital nevi, acquired nevi sometimes show hypertrichosis compared with the surrounding skin.

Common acquired nevi occur anywhere on the skin surface. However, compared with light-skinned individuals, those with dark skin more commonly develop nevi on the palms, soles, nail apparatus, and mucous membranes. Nevi on the palms and soles tend to be flat and may not distort the skin surface because of the thickness of the stratum corneum. Nevi of the nail apparatus commonly present as a linear longitudinal streak of dark

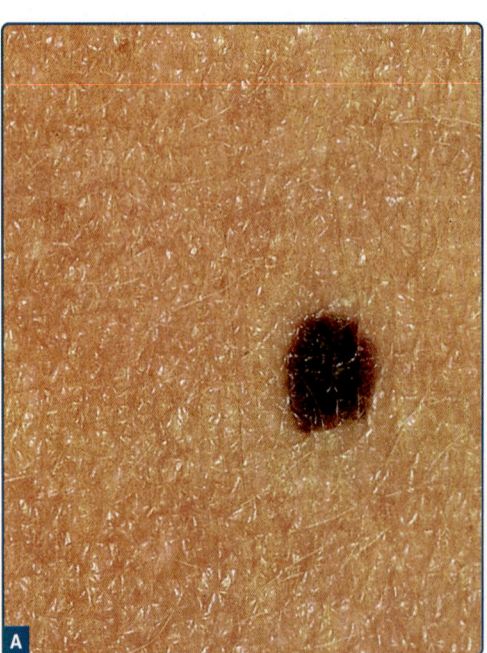
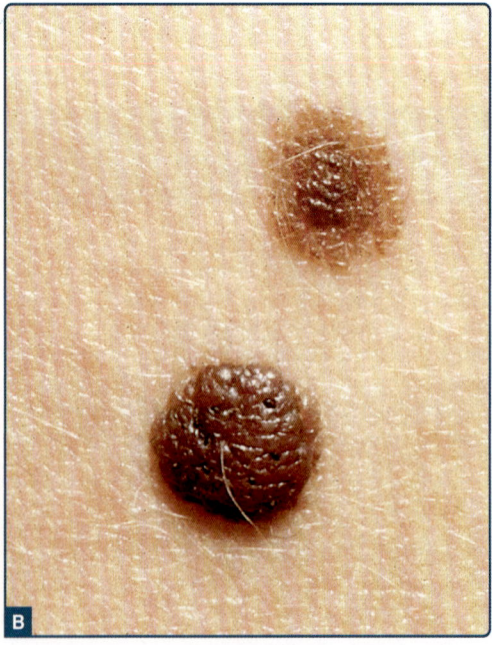

Figure 115-6 Typical acquired nevomelanocytic nevi. **A,** Junctional nevus. A uniformly dark brown macule, round in shape, with a smooth, regular border. **B,** Two compound nevi. A uniformly pigmented papule and domed nodule. The upper lesion is flatter and tan with slight central elevation. The lower lesion is older and is uniformly elevated because of an increased intradermal component.

or light-brown pigment from the nail matrix extending to the distal edge of the nail plate. Extension of pigment onto the proximal nail fold or beyond the distal nail groove should be considered suspicious for melanoma.

Dermoscopy can reveal a number of patterns, but a reticular or globular pattern is commonly seen in acquired nevi. Nevi on the palms and soles can show a parallel-furrow pattern, lattice-like, or fibrillar pattern. Nonuniform patterns and parallel-ridge patterns are worrisome for melanoma. Nail matrix nevi show regular lines on a brown background. A recent comparative analysis of the dermoscopic features of benign nail matrix nevi in adults and children revealed that those in children more often showed atypical melanoma-associated dermoscopic features.[36]

Halo nevi are usually asymptomatic, often multiple, and most commonly affect the trunk of teenagers (Fig. 115-7). The halo phenomenon signifies self-immunologic regression of a preexisting melanocytic nevus. Lesions present with a central pink or brown nevus centrally, surrounded by a symmetric round or oval halo of depigmented skin. The central nevus may be small and typical of common acquired nevi or be large in dysplastic or congenital nevi. The radial zone of depigmented skin around the nevus ranges from less than 5 mm to 5 cm. Over time, the central nevus may lose its pigmentation and disappear followed by gradual repigmentation of the entire area.

Other names for the halo phenomenon include *leukoderma acquisitum centrifugum*, *Sutton nevus*, *leukopigmentary nevus*, *perinevoid vitiligo*, and *perinevoid leukoderma*. An atypical gross appearance of the central lesion or an asymmetric halo of depigmentation, particularly in adults, should raise suspicion for a DN or melanoma.

The Meyerson's nevus presents as an asymptomatic or slightly pruritic, red, and slightly scaly eczematous halo around a central nevus. Lesions occur most often on the trunk and proximal extremities and may be multiple. Unlike halo nevi, the skin does not depigment, and regression of the nevus does not occur. Eczematous changes often self-resolve over the course of months.

The spontaneous and concurrent development of multiple nevi, often similar in appearance, is termed eruptive nevi. This phenomenon has been described in the context of blistering diseases of the skin (immunobullous as well as erythema multiforme–Stevens-Johnson syndrome–toxic epidermal necrolysis spectrum), immunosuppression, neoplasia, and drugs (particularly chemotherapeutic and immune-modulating agents). Eruptive nevi may be of the common acquired type, Spitz, or blue nevus varieties.

RELATED PHYSICAL CONDITIONS

There is a general increased risk of melanoma in patients with multiple nevi. This risk is further increased in the setting of multiple atypical nevi or a personal or family history of melanoma. In patients with eruptive nevi, there may be findings of bullous disease or immunosuppression. Halo nevi, particularly when multiple, may be associated with concurrent or subsequent development of vitiligo or other autoimmune disease.[37] Halo nevi are also more frequent in patients with Turner syndrome.[38]

COMPLICATIONS

Several studies demonstrate that increased numbers of nevi indicate an increased risk for melanoma development. In one large meta-analysis, the relative risk for people with high nevus counts (101–120 nevi) was 6.89 compared with those with low nevus counts (0–15 nevi).[39] In addition, those with five atypical nevi had a relative risk of 6.52 compared with those with no atypical nevi.[39] Other risk factors such as skin color, freckling, and patterns of sun exposure may be multiplicative to the number of nevi in increasing melanoma risk.

Most melanoma arise from normal skin and thus increased number of nevi are associated with a general melanoma risk. However, approximately 20% of melanomas are reported to have associated nevus elements

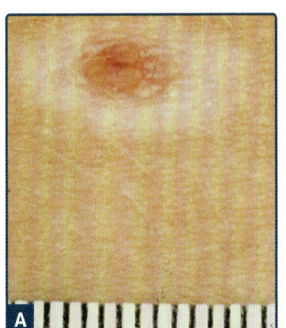 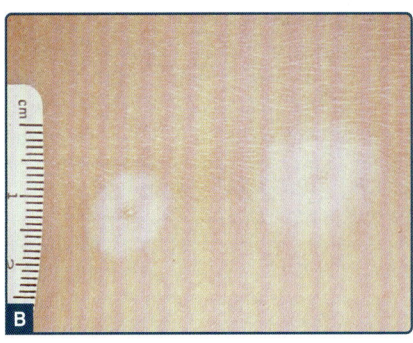 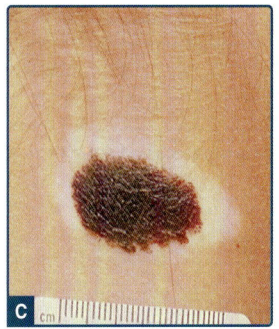

Figure 115-7 Halo nevomelanocytic nevus. **A,** Acquired halo nevus on the chest of a 16-year-old Caucasian boy whose maternal grandmother had melanoma. **B,** Acquired halo nevi on the back of a 6-year-old Caucasian boy. Scale in millimeters. **C,** Halo congenital nevomelanocytic nevus on the neck of a 4-year-old girl. This child also had scattered areas of vitiligo-like depigmentation in other sites. A 3-year follow-up after excision of the nevus revealed almost total repigmentation of the widely scattered previously depigmented areas.

suggesting a precursor pathway. In one study of 131 melanomas, a history of frequent sunburns predicted the greatest risk for nevus-associated melanoma.[40]

RISK FACTORS

Environmental exposure to UV radiation appears to be the most critical risk factor for the development of acquired nevi. In a US population-based longitudinal study of nevi in children (n = 443), spending 5 to 6 hours per week outside between 10 AM and 4 PM, painful sunburn(s), decreased UV barrier protection, and male gender were significantly associated with increased number of nevi.[41] Intermittent intense sun exposure appears to impose greatest risk for nevus development. A randomized trial assessing sunscreen use on nevi development in white school-aged children also demonstrated a significant reduction in the number of nevi on intermittently sun-exposed body sites compared with control participants.[42]

Genetic factors appear to play a role in their development. The size, frequency, and distribution patterns of acquired nevi tend to aggregate in families. This observation is also well documented for atypical nevi in the setting of DN and melanoma syndromes (see dysplastic nevi).

ETIOLOGY AND PATHOGENESIS

Common acquired nevi are clonal neoplasms, the majority of which demonstrate activating *BRAF* mutations. It is likely that this mutation is an early or initiating event in melanocytic neoplasia. All cells within common nevi have been shown to be fully clonal and contain the same heterozygous *BRAF* mutation by droplet digital polymerase chain reaction.[43]

Eruptive nevi occur in the setting of immunosuppression or chemotherapy. *BRAF* mutations have been identified in eruptive melanocytic nevi associated with 6-mercaptopurine therapy.[44] However in one case, eruptive nevi of the Spitz type showed absence of *BRAF* and *HRAS* mutations in 39 nevi analyzed.[45] This is not surprising because of the diverse molecular pathways that have been implicated in Spitz nevus development (see Spitz nevi).

Halo nevi are nevi in which the body attempts an immune-mediated attack on nevus cells orchestrated by effector CD8+ cytotoxic T-lymphocytes. In this phenomenon, increased levels of interferon—γ-inducible chemokine pair CXCL10–CXCR3 have been demonstrated, similar to that seen in vitiligo.[46] The precise trigger for this immunologic phenomenon in the absence of disease remains unclear. In patients with Turner syndrome, there was a significantly higher association of HLA-CW6 in those who developed halo nevi, suggesting a genetic predisposition.[38]

DIAGNOSIS

The diagnosis of common acquired nevi is usually made by clinical inspection, assessing that the lesion is relatively small, symmetrical, has even borders, is not ulcerated, and has a limited variety of colors and normal pigment network.

PATHOLOGY

The common junctional nevus is circumscribed and mostly nested at the basal layer of the epidermis (Figs. 115-8 and 115-9). Junctional melanocytes have pale or pigmented cytoplasm and small, monomorphous nuclei with inconspicuous nucleoli. In some common junctional nevi, the nests of melanocytes are positioned toward the bases of rete ridges, but in others, the rete ridge pattern is unrelated. Epidermal melanocytes between junctional nests are disposed as single typical cells along the basal layer, with overall numbers equal to or slightly greater than that in adjacent skin. The epidermis is often hyperpigmented with lentiginous architecture (elongated and club-shaped rete pegs).

In compound nevi (see Fig. 115-9), the epidermis may be normal or hyperplastic, with an appearance similar to seborrheic keratosis complete with horn cysts or epidermal verrucous hyperplasia similar to epidermal nevus. The dermal component of compound and intradermal nevi has an orderly progression from top to bottom, with larger epithelioid cells above (within the epidermis and superficial dermis) blending into a pattern of smaller round and spindled cells in the deeper dermis. This orderly progression of larger, more epithelioid cells in the superficial aspect of the nevus to smaller cells in its deep aspect is known as maturation.

In the epidermis and superficial dermis, nevomelanocytes frequently contain melanin pigment. With descent into the dermis (see Fig. 115-9), nevus cells become smaller and lose their pigmentation. Nevomelanocytes in the dermis have a monotonous similarity to one another within the same anatomic level and an overall symmetry of architecture from top to bottom and side to side.

Multinucleated nevomelanocytes occur occasionally within the superficial and mid-dermal portions of the nevus. Nevomelanocytes in the deep dermis may be disposed as spindle cells within a collagenous framework that is loose, pale, and wavy in formations similar to a neurofibroma or sometimes disposed in concentrically arranged whorls resembling Meissner tactile corpuscles. The term *neural nevus* is used when the vast majority of the nevus demonstrates a neural phenotype.

Sometimes dermal nevus cells aggregate around epithelial adnexal structures or lie as cords and strands in the superficial reticular dermis, making these "congenital pattern nevi" or "congenital-like nevi." Such histologic features are not limited to nevi that were present since birth.

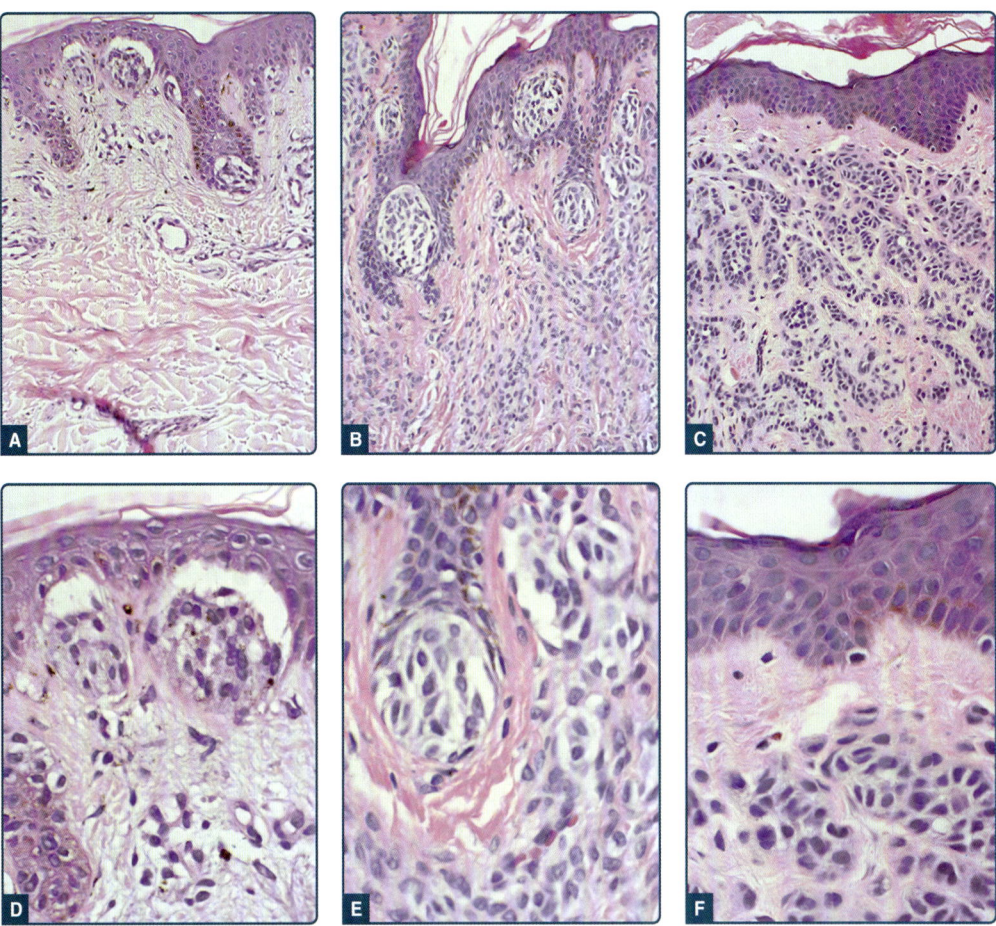

Figure 115-8 Histopathologic features of acquired nevi. Junctional nevus (**A**) and higher magnification (**D**). Compound nevus (**B**) and higher magnification (**E**). Intradermal nevus (**C**) and higher magnification (**F**). Well-formed nests of nevomelanocytes are present in the junctional and compound nevi. Sheets and cords of nevocytes are present in the dermis of the compound and intradermal nevi. A grenz zone free of nevomelanocytes is present just below the epidermis in the intradermal nevus (**C** and **F**).

Other findings identified in nevi include fibrous, mucinous, and fatty degeneration.

Inflammatory cellular infiltrates in typical, stable acquired nevi are usually scanty or absent. Melanin-laden macrophages are usually apparent in the superficial papillary dermis of nevi; their number usually proportional to the degree of melanin production. Asymmetry between the junctional and dermal elements, poor circumscription, and lamellar fibroplasia (features frequently seen in dysplastic nevi) are usually not prominent in common acquired nevi.

Histopathologic artifacts include shrinkage clefts, which may resemble lymphatics or vascular spaces, may be prominent in the midportion of nevi and in areas with hemorrhage. Separation of sheets of nevomelanocytes into parallel rows may be caused by improper cutting. Local anesthesia injection directly into the nevus also may be associated with artifactual changes.

The *balloon cell nevus* is a histopathologic variant of common acquired nevus, composed of peculiar foam cells comprising a portion or all of a given lesion. In addition to clear cells with a single central basophilic nucleus, multinucleated balloon cells may be seen. Electron microscopy suggests that vacuolization of nevomelanocytes in balloon cell nevi is a degenerative change, with melanosome swelling, microvacuole formation in nevus granules, and loss of particulate martrix.[47] In contrast to balloon cell melanoma, a maturation pattern is evident, and no cytologic atypia or significant mitotic activity is present.

The *combined nevus* refers to the intermingling of two different nevus types in one lesion. Most such lesions are composed of either an acquired or congenital nevus and blue nevus.

Recurrent melanocytic nevus is the name given to recurrent lesions after incomplete removal of a benign nevus. A markedly atypical clinical and histopathologic appearance may accompany this recurrence, making these lesions worrisome for possible melanoma. Clinically, the recurrent nevus is confined to the scar but may be markedly irregular in appearance. Recurrent nevi

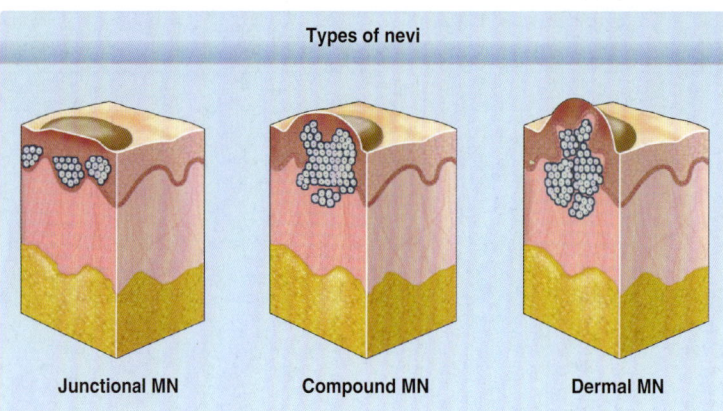

Figure 115-9 Types of nevi. MN, melanocytic nevi.

demonstrate melanocytic hyperplasia in a lentiginous and junctional pattern (often to a greater extent than the original nevus). Junctional melanocytes are frequently hyperpigmented and may display moderate cytologic atypia, significant architectural disorganization, and pagetoid growth, raising concern for melanoma. However, such features do not extend beyond the scar, and banal-appearing nevus cells may be seen within the underlying dermis. It is important to review the original histopathologic specimen to ensure that the findings can be solely attributed to nevus regeneration when making determinations for reexcision.

No distinguishing histopathologic features have been described for eruptive nevi.

In halo nevi, the usual histopathologic findings are a central nevus associated with an obscuring dermal lymphohistiocytic infiltrate and a surrounding depigmented zone totally or almost devoid of epidermal melanocytes. Immunohistochemical staining with melanocytic markers such as Melan-A or Sox-10 may help to identify residual epidermal melanocytes or residual dermal melanocytes obscured by the inflammatory infiltrate. Lymphocytes in halo nevi are mostly of the CD8[+] subset.

Normal-growing nevi in childhood and adolescence may show histologically alarming features, including more prominent epithelioid cell change of melanocytes and architectural variability of junctional melanocytic nests. Rare mitotic figures may also be evident.

Site-related changes also influence the histopathology of common acquired nevi. These are known as *special site nevi* because of their unconventional histopathologic appearances. Special site locations include the scalp, ear, nipple, abdominal milk line, umbilicus, anogenital region, and acral surfaces. At these locations, there is often more architectural variability of junctional nests, some of which may be larger and discohesive. Limited pagetoid scatter can be seen in the central portions of some lesions, particularly on acral surfaces or in areas with frequent friction. Anogenital nevi commonly share architectural features with dysplastic nevi, including lamellar fibroplasia, bridging of rete by junctional nests, and lymphocytic infiltrates.

Worrisome features for possible melanoma include pagetoid upward migration of cells in the epidermis, cytologic atypia of melanocytes (including irregularity of size and shape of cells and nuclear hyperchromasia), failure of the cells to "mature" in the deeper dermis, persistence of pigment production in the deep dermis, lack of symmetry, increased or deep dermal mitotic figures, focal areas of necrosis, and desmoplasia or fibroplasia.

SPECIAL TESTS

Special tests are not usually required in the gross and microscopic assessment of melanocytic or nevomelanocytic nevi. However, for patients who have eruptive nevi, given the association with immunosuppression, immunologic tests may be in order. Immunohistochemical profiles may be of value for difficult to diagnose lesions. Low Ki67 activity and loss of HMB45 in deeper dermal cells may help support a benign diagnosis. Compared with melanoma, common acquired nevi are genomically stable.[48] Fluorescence in situ hybridization (café-au-lait) or comparative genomic hybridization (CGH) analysis may be useful in discriminating a nevus from nevoid melanoma.

DIFFERENTIAL DIAGNOSIS

See Table 115-3.

CLINICAL COURSE AND PROGNOSIS

There may be relatively sudden changes in nevi that are unrelated to malignant transformation. Any single nevus that is noted to suddenly change or become symptomatic independently should be cause for concern. Causes of sudden changes in a nevus (color,

TABLE 115-3
Differential Diagnosis of Common Acquired Nevomelanocytic Nevus

Pigmented Lesions
- Solar lentigo
- Lentigo simplex
- Café-au-lait macule
- Blue nevus
- Pigmented fibrous histiocytoma (dermatofibroma)
- Kaposi sarcoma
- Pigmented basal cell carcinoma
- Pigmented actinic keratoses
- Mastocytoma
- Seborrheic keratoses
- Epidermal nevus
- Subungual hematoma
- Supernumerary nipple
- Pigmented spindle cell nevus
- Spitz nevus
- Sclerosing hemangioma
- Pyogenic granuloma
- Dysplastic (atypical) melanocytic nevus
- Cutaneous melanoma
- Nonpigmented or pink lesion
- Basal cell carcinoma
- Fibrous papule
- Verruca vulgaris
- Molluscum contagiosum
- Dermal mucinosis
- Spitz nevus (epithelioid cell nevus)
- Appendageal tumors
- Clear cell acanthoma
- Large cell acanthoma
- Other lesions with halo phenomenon
- Congenital nevomelanocytic nevus
- Melanoma
- Histiocytoma
- Molluscum contagiosum
- Flat wart
- Acrochordon
- Basal cell epithelioma
- Neurofibroma
- Congenital dermal melanocytosis (mongolian spot)
- Blue nevus
- Lichen planus
- Sarcoidosis
- Psoriasis
- Angioma
- Angiokeratoma

surface, or size, with or without pain, itching, ulceration, or bleeding) over days or weeks include cystic dilation of a hair follicle, folliculitis, abscess, trauma, hemorrhage, and, in the case of a pedunculated nevus, strangulation and thrombosis. These benign causes of sudden change may require close observation for several weeks until resolution occurs or removal for histopathologic examination.

The vast majority of acquired nevi are harmless. New nevi may continue to appear and disappear throughout life, but most develop during childhood and early adulthood. New or growing nevi in older individuals are more worrisome. Melanoma risk appears to be related to the number and size of nevi; patients with numerous nevi, dysplastic nevi, and a personal or family history of melanoma should be closely monitored with periodic surveillance examinations for life.

MANAGEMENT

TREATMENT

The vast majority of acquired common nevi require no treatment. Indications for removal of benign-appearing lesions may include cosmetic concerns or continual irritation. Lesions with worrisome clinical features need to be excised for histopathologic examination. Dermoscopy may be used to differentiate benign from potentially malignant features. Photographic surveillance can play a critical role in identifying change, or lack of change, in suspicious nevi.

Although a benign-appearing nevus associated with halo depigmentation does not require excision, it is reasonable to recommend periodic examination of affected individuals for dysplastic nevi, vitiligo, and melanoma. Atypical-appearing central nevi, presence of an asymmetric halo, eccentric placement of a melanocytic lesion within a halo, or in the setting of dysplastic nevi or melanoma (personal or family history) suggest the need for histopathologic examination for melanoma. Cover-ups or sunscreens should be recommended for sun-exposed areas of depigmentation to prevent acute burn, chronic actinic damage, and UVR-induced carcinogenesis.

Complete removal of nevi is best accomplished by excision. Leaving a partially excised nevus, regardless of the initial pathology, is fraught with potentially concerning consequences of repigmentation, regrowth, or both (see *recurrent melanocytic nevus*). Incisional biopsy is necessary at times, particularly for lesions that cannot be excised easily but require histopathologic diagnosis. Destructive modes of therapy (electrodesiccation, cryotherapy, dermabrasion, and laser) should be avoided. These destructive modes of therapy preclude histopathologic assessment of the treated nevi. They have the disadvantage of not providing tissue for histopathology. Although dermabrasion may eliminate pigmentation of nevi, residual nevomelanocytes in the dermis are to be expected, cosmetic outcome is often unpredictable, and recurrence with worrisome clinical features may complicate future management.

PREVENTION AND COUNSELING

There appears to be a direct relationship between the number of acquired nevi and sun exposure and a decrease with sunscreen use. Patients should be encouraged to minimize UVR overexposure without impeding day-to-day activities. Sensible UVR exposure includes confining outdoor activities to the early morning or late afternoon or evening and avoiding the most intense UVR exposure occurring 2 hours on either side of noon. Cover-up clothing that blocks light transmission should be worn during intense UVR exposure. Clothing is often easier to put on than sunscreen and does not rapidly wear off with swimming or sweating. Effective sunscreens should be used as part of a comprehensive sun-protection program. Vitamin D supplementation should be recommended for patients who diligently practice UVR avoidance and protection.

BLUE NEVUS

AT-A-GLANCE

- A group of lesions composed of deeply pigmented spindle or epithelioid melanocytes in the dermis; includes common blue, cellular blue, combined blue, and atypical cellular blue lesions
- Lesions appear as blue, blue-gray, or blue-black papules, nodules, or plaques.
- Lesions are generally acquired but may be congenital.
- Cellular blue nevi may have an elevated risk for development of melanoma.
- Related lesions include nevus of Ota/Ito, Mongolian spot, dermal dendritic hamartoma.
- Initiating mutations in GNAQ or GNA11 are present in most blue nevi.

EPIDEMIOLOGY

Blue nevi are present in approximately 1% to 2% of white adults and in 3% to 5% of Japanese adults. Women are more often affected than men. The vast majority of blue nevi present in the second decade of life and are single, small, deep-blue macules or papules less than 1 cm in diameter. Common blue nevi arise most often in adolescence and cellular blue nevi before age 40 years. Congenital onset or those that appear in the first few years of life are less common.

CLINICAL FEATURES

The most frequent sites for blue nevi are on the dorsal hands and feet, scalp, and buttocks or sacral skin. The blue hue seen in many lesions comes from the *Tyndall effect*, the result of the refraction of light reflected from the nevus by the overlying dermis.

Blue nevi have been reported to rarely occur in the oral mucosa, uterine cervix, vagina, spermatic cord, prostate, and lymph nodes, and several clinical variants have been described: eruptive, plaquelike, linear, agminate, disseminated, satellite, familial, and targetoid.[49]

CUTANEOUS FINDINGS

Most blue nevi are blue, blue-gray, or blue-black smooth surfaced papules or nodules (Fig. 115-10). Common blue nevi are deeply pigmented small lesions, usually less than 1 cm in diameter. Cellular blue nevi have a similar color but are often larger plaques or nodules greater than 1 cm.

Blue nevi tend to be firm, reflecting their dermal location and often fibrotic stroma. *Hypomelanotic blue nevus* is a rare variant in which not much melanin pigment is produced. The resultant lesions are flattish skin-colored firm papules or plaques.

Many group the dermal melanocytoses, conditions in which there are pigmented dendritic melanocytes, in the blue nevus family. Nevus of Ota and Ito share similar underlying defects to blue nevi and are also commonly acquired (in early childhood, often before age 1 year or around puberty) but are far more extensive, encompassing a portion of the trigeminal (ophthalmic and maxillary) and brachial (posterior supraclavicular and lateral cutaneous) nerve distributions, respectively. Dermal melanocyte hamartoma presents at birth as coalescing macules, resulting in diffuse blue-gray pigmentation. Mongolian spot is usually present at birth or within the first few weeks of life and centered over the lumbosacral area. Mongolian spots typically regress in early childhood but may persist in approximately 10% of cases. Nevus of Ota/Ito typically persist into adulthood. Acquired adult variants of dermal melanocytosis rarely occur.

RELATED PHYSICAL CONDITIONS

Multiple blue nevi and epithelioid blue nevi may be associated with lentigines, cardiac myxoma, and mucocutaneous myxomas (Carney complex/LAMB syndrome [*l*entigines, *a*trial myxomas, *m*ucocutaneous myxomas, and *b*lue nevi]). Extensive dermal melanocytosis may be associated with phakomatosis pigmentovascularis.

COMPLICATIONS

Malignant blue nevus (melanoma) may arise de novo but more often arises in contiguity with a cellular blue nevus. Rarely, there is malignant transformation of a dermal melanocytosis.[50] This event may present as an expanding dermal or subcutaneous nodule with or without ulceration.

RISK FACTORS

Other than Carney complex/LAMB syndrome and phakomatosis pigmentovascularis, there are no known risk factors for blue nevi. The risk of UVR in the development of blue nevi is unknown.

ETIOLOGY AND PATHOGENESIS

Most blue nevi have initiating mutations in *GNAQ* and to a lesser extent *GNA11*. These mutations result in loss of GTPase activity and constitutive activation of the MAPK pathway, resulting in increased cellular proliferation. Although the frequency of these mutations varies among studies, mutation in the *GNAQ* gene has been identified in up to 87% of blue nevi, almost all of them in codon 209.[51]

The distribution of blue nevi is thought to parallel sites of colonization by active non-neoplastic pigmented bipolar dermal melanocytes during embryogenesis.[19] These cells typically migrate and disappear during embryonic life, but occasionally incidental pigmented dendritic cells can be seen in biopsies from the scalp, upper face, dorsal hands or feet, and sacrum.

GNAQ mutations have been reported in nevus of Ota,[52] and more recently mosaic activating mutations in *GNA11* and *GNAQ* were discovered in the pigmented lesions of phakomatosis pigmentovascularis with extensive dermal melanocytosis.[53] Thus, the

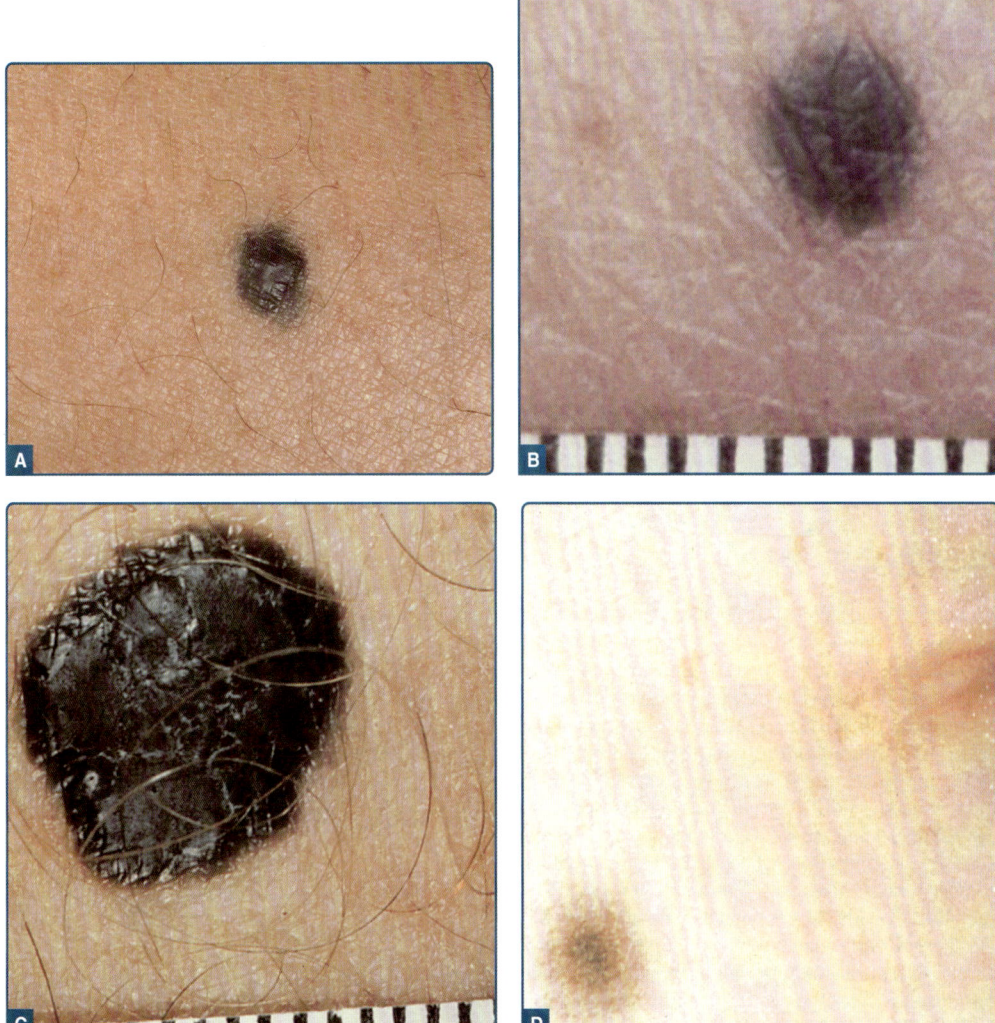

Figure 115-10 Blue nevus. **A,** Common blue nevus appearing as an acquired blue–gray papule on an adult male. **B,** Common blue nevus appearing as an acquired blue-gray papule on the buttock of a 62-year-old white man. **C,** Cellular blue nevus appearing as a congenital blue papule on the low back of a 30-year-old white man. **D,** Combined common blue nevus–nevomelanocytic nevus appearing as a brown papule with a blue-gray center on the cheek of a 12-year-old white boy, beginning as a pinpoint dot at age 1 year and enlarging slowly over time. Scale in millimeters. (Part A used with permission from Logical Images, Inc., Rochester, NY.)

molecular mutational profile of dermal melanocytoses appears to parallel that of blue nevi.

In contrast, neither *GNAQ* nor *GNA11* mutations have been documented in deep penetrating nevi; rather, *HRAS* mutations were seen in 6% of lesions in one study, implicating that these lesions may be more related to Spitz nevi.[51] Recently, deep penetrating nevi have been found to harbor activating mutations in both the MAPK and β-catenin pathways.[54] There is also a subgroup of lesions with mixed morphologic features of blue nevus and Spitz nevus. Evidence mounts that such "Blitz" nevi are best classified as blue melanocytic neoplasms because of their high frequency (57%) of *GNAQ* and *GNA11* mutations.[55]

Pigmented epithelioid melanocytoma is indistinguishable from epithelioid blue nevus of Carney complex. In the sporadic setting, it is considered an intermediate-grade melanocytic tumor that demonstrates a propensity to spread to regional lymph nodes but has a favorable long-term clinical course.[56] Those that occur in the setting of Carney complex behave in an entirely benign fashion. In both settings, such lesions are linked to mutations of protein kinase A regulatory subunit type 1 α (*PRKAR1α*) gene.[57] Protein kinase C alpha isoform (PRKCA) fusion genes have also been recently reported in pigmented epithelioid melanocytoma.[58]

DIAGNOSIS

The diagnosis of blue nevus is sometimes made clinically when a small, very dark or blue lesion is found in a typical location for a common blue nevus. For larger lesions and those in less typical locations, it is customary to confirm the diagnosis by biopsy.

PATHOLOGY

All types of blue nevus have components that include some of the following: deeply pigmented dendritic melanocytes, spindled and less pigmented melanocytes, oval melanocytes, melanophages, and fibrotic stroma (Fig. 115-11). Nevus cells may show perivascular or periadnexal accentuation. Almost all blue nevi lack a junctional component. Very occasionally, one can see single dendritic melanocytes in increased number along the DEJ (so-called compound blue nevus). Another exception is combined blue nevus, in which another form of nevus is contiguous and a junctional component occurs (eg, common or congenital nevus).

The stereotypic common blue nevus is an inverted dermal wedge-shaped mass in which pigmented dendritic melanocytes are admixed with melanophages within a fibrotic stroma.

The prototypical cellular blue nevus has vertically oriented dumbbell-shaped masses of melanocytes that protrude into the subcutis. The superficial dermis often contains a fibrotic stroma in which there are dendritic melanocytes and melanophages, but the definitional component is the presence of larger streaming aggregates of oval melanocytes. These cells usually have only scant melanin. Multinucleated melanocytes are sometimes present within aggregates. The presence of cells with large central nucleoli, more than a few mitotic figures per section, atypical mitotic figures, necrosis, or lymphocytic infiltrates evokes concern for melanoma.

Sparsely scattered mid and deep dermal dendritic melanocytes oriented parallel to the skin surface typify the dermal melanocytoses.

The cells of blue nevus are usually positive with S100 immunohistochemistry, stain strongly with Melan-A/Mart-1, and are positive for HMB-45. They have a low proliferation rate.

Deep penetrating nevi may clinically simulate a blue nevus but can be distinguished histopathologically. They are named for their tendency to extend through most of the thickness of the dermis, and some lesions reach the superficial subcutis. They are usually wedge shaped, with the apex sometimes surrounding a folliculosebaceous unit. They are composed of nests of large, oval melanocytes with abundant, pale vacuolated cytoplasm with dusty melanin and moderately enlarged nuclei. Mitoses are few, although two or three can occur in a single section. Combined deep penetrating nevi have a component of common nevus or congenital-like nevus to the side, above, or both. The criteria for distinguishing deep penetrating nevi from intermediate-grade lesions, in which metastases are rare, and higher grade lesions are still being developed.

Benign epithelioid blue nevi of Carney complex are histologically indistinguishable from pigmented epithelioid melanocytoma, which occurs in the sporadic setting.[56] It is characterized by a mostly dermal nodular and sheetlike proliferation of enlarged epithelioid melanocytes with round nuclei, conspicuous nucleoli, and heavily pigmented cytoplasm. Numerous admixed melanophages are present. Some melanocytes show a spindled morphology, particularly at the periphery of the lesion. Occasional mitotic figures may be evident in some lesions. No morphologic criteria have been determined to reliably predict metastatic potential in sporadically occurring pigmented epithelioid melanocytoma.

SPECIAL TESTS

Imaging tests of the heart may be required if there is concern for Carney complex/myxoma syndrome/LAMB syndrome. Mutation analysis can be helpful diagnostically for distinguishing cellular blue nevi or atypical blue nevi from blue nevus–like melanoma.

DIFFERENTIAL DIAGNOSIS

See Table 115-4.

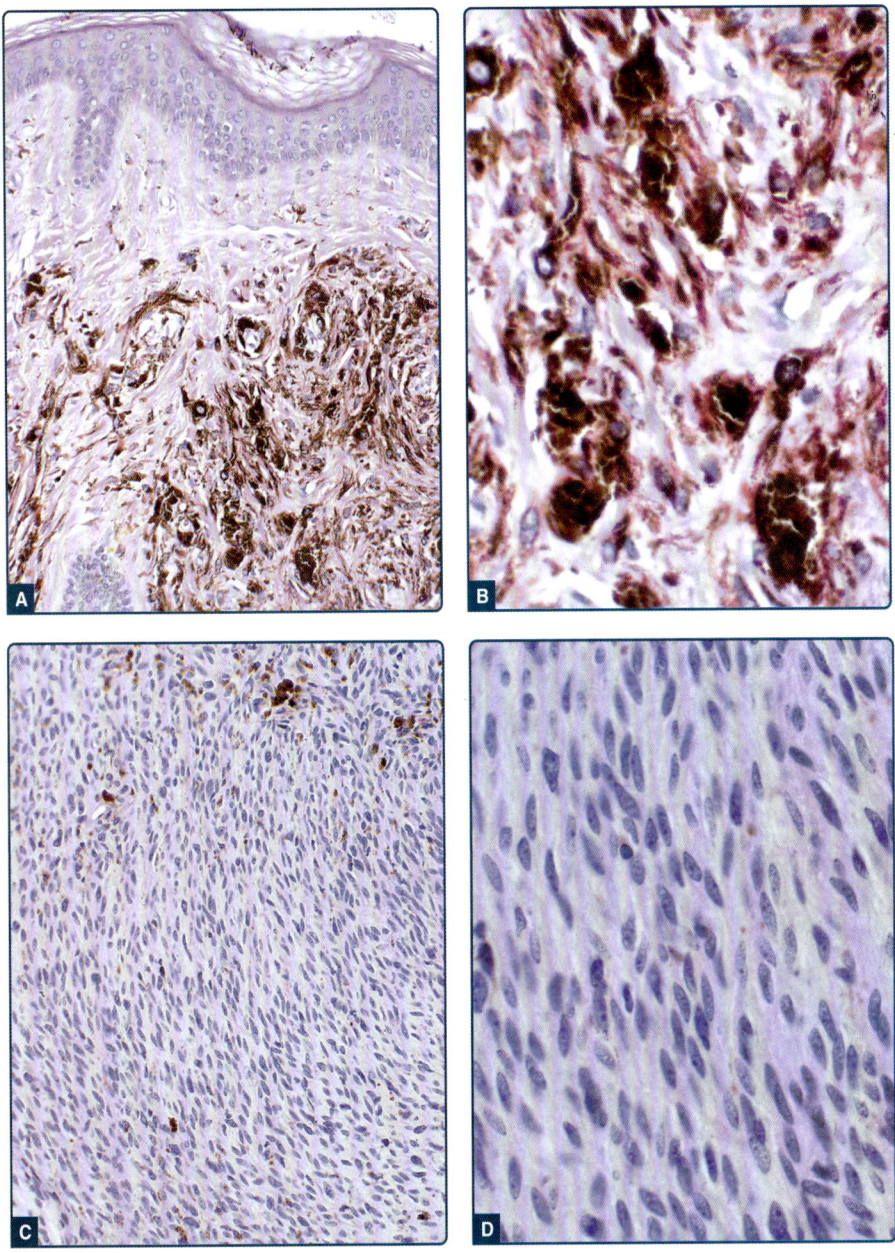

Figure 115-11 Histopathologic features of common and cellular blue nevi. Common blue nevus (**A**) and higher magnification of the dermal component (**B**) revealing heavily pigmented, elongated melanocytes. Cellular blue nevus (**C**) and higher magnification (**D**) revealing sheets of melanocytes with ovoid nuclei.

TABLE 115-4
Differential Diagnosis of Blue Nevus

- Pigmented spindle cell nevus
- Tattoo (traumatic, radiation port marker)
- Primary or metastatic melanoma
- Glomus tumor
- Pyogenic granuloma
- Sclerosing hemangioma
- Dermatofibroma
- Ochronosis

CLINICAL COURSE AND PROGNOSIS

Blue nevi are benign lesions, and their only adverse prognostic event is the development of melanoma within one. This more frequently occurs in cellular blue nevi. Melanomas associated with or mimicking cellular blue nevi have been demonstrated to have a propensity for the scalp and a high frequency of *GNA11* mutations with loss of BAP1 expression.[59]

MANAGEMENT

TREATMENT

Stable common blue nevi usually do not require therapy. However, clinical change of a blue nevus, such as sudden appearance of a new nodule, enlargement of an existing nevus, or a large or atypical clinical appearance should prompt histopathologic examination. Cellular blue nevi, particularly in adults, should be evaluated for excision because of the small risk of malignant transformation. Excision should include subcutaneous fat to ensure removal of the deeper melanocytic components that are often present in cellular blue nevi.

The prognosis for deep penetrating nevi is excellent, although there may be a very low conversion rate to deep penetrating-like melanoma for lesions that are not completely removed. What this rate is and how much higher it is than for other forms of nevus are unknown. Some dermatopathologists advocate complete removal of deep penetrating nevi, but others regard clinical removal as sufficient.

Pigmented epithelioid melanocytoma occurring in the sporadic setting are typically treated similar to melanoma, with wide excision and sentinel lymph node biopsy.

PREVENTION AND COUNSELING

There are no known preventative measures. As with other nevi, it is reasonable to minimize excessive UVR exposure.

PIGMENTED SPINDLE CELL NEVUS

AT-A-GLANCE

- Synonym: Reed nevus
- Acquired, benign melanocytic tumor composed of heavily pigmented spindle-shaped melanocytes in nests confined primarily to the epidermis
- Lesions are jet black often with "starburst" appearance on dermoscopy.
- They may develop quickly and then stabilize.
- Malignant degeneration is thought to be rare.

EPIDEMIOLOGY

The pigmented spindle cell nevus (PSCN) presents most commonly in the third decade of life. The mean age at presentation has been reported to be 25.3 years, ranging from 2.5 to 56.0 years of age.[60] Similar age ranges have been reported in other studies.[61] Female patients outnumber male patients with reported ratios of up to 2:1.[60,62] The majority of these lesions are found on the extremities with reported frequencies of 67.0%,[60] 69.6%,[62] and 75.0%.[61] There is a preference for the lower extremity, particularly the thigh.[61]

CLINICAL FEATURES

PSCN was first described by Reed in 1975.[63] Many authors consider it a variant of Spitz nevus, but others define it as a distinct entity. At presentation, patients often note that the lesion has increased in size, prompting biopsy.[61,62] If allowed to fully develop, they are thought to generally remain stable over time.

CUTANEOUS FINDINGS

PSCN classically presents as a sharply circumscribed darkly pigmented papule, usually less than 7 mm in diameter. They are jet-black but may have shades of blue, gray, or brown (Fig. 115-12). Dermoscopically, most have streaks or pseudopods, giving the lesion a starburst appearance; others may have a globular pattern with reticular depigmentation.[64]

RELATED PHYSICAL CONDITIONS

There are no known associations.

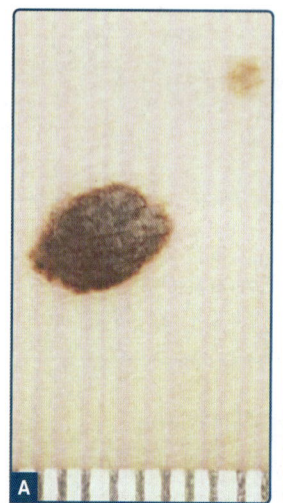

Figure 115-12 Pigmented spindle cell nevus. **A,** Very dark brown plaque appearing over several weeks on the posterior thigh of a 22-year-old white woman. **B,** Very dark-bluish plaque appearing de novo 3 months previously on the back of an 8-month-old white (Hispanic) boy. Scale in millimeters.

COMPLICATIONS

There are no reported complications, but misinterpretation as a melanoma may result in overtreatment.

RISK FACTORS

There are no known risk factors.

ETIOLOGY AND PATHOGENESIS

Although *BRAF* mutation and gene fusions have been detected, these changes are also present in other types of acquired and Spitz nevi, respectively. No known specific mutation has been identified for PSCN.

DIAGNOSIS

The diagnosis may be suspected given the clinical scenario and supportive dermoscopic features. However, the diagnosis should be confirmed by biopsy.

PATHOLOGY

The PSCN is a sharply circumscribed lesion composed of fascicles of uniform pigment-synthesizing melanocytes with spindled appearance along the junction and to a lesser extent the superficial dermis (Fig. 115-13). Melanocytes have uniform nuclei and small nucleoli. Occasionally, there is an admixture of epithelioid appearing cells. Pagetoid cells may be seen but are usually limited to the central portion of the nevus. Extension of the spindle cells along skin adnexal structures is relatively common. There are invariably pigment-laden macrophages in the papillary dermis with a mild perivascular infiltrate of lymphocytes. Atypical variants of PSCN exist in which there are architectural alterations and striking cellular atypia, raising a differential diagnosis of melanoma.[62]

SPECIAL TESTS

In cases with atypical histologic features, immunohistochemical markers (Ki-67, cyclin-D1, survivin) and FISH have shown utility in distinguishing PSCN from melanoma.[65]

DIFFERENTIAL DIAGNOSIS

See Table 115-5.

CLINICAL COURSE AND PROGNOSIS

PSCN is considered benign. No local recurrence or distant spread was noted for 38 patients followed for an average of 14 months.[60] In another study, 57 patients were followed for an average of 6 years, and again no local recurrence or metastasis was noted.[61]

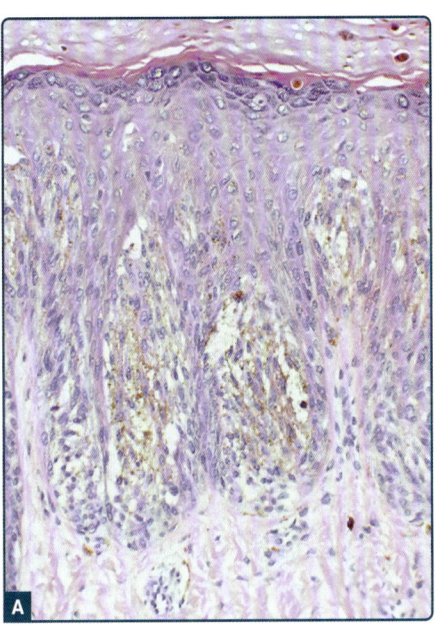 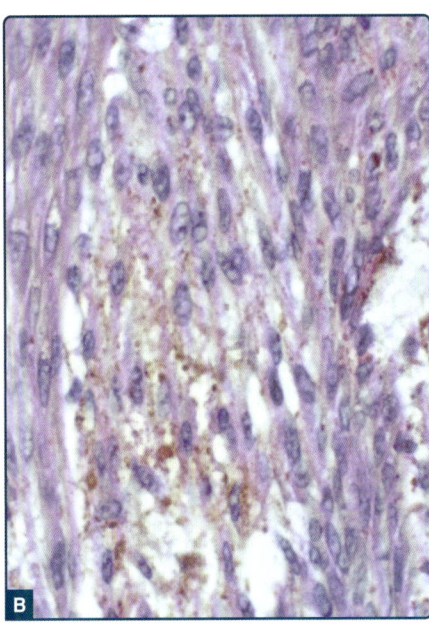

Figure 115-13 Histopathologic features of pigmented spindle cell nevus (**A**) and higher magnification of the intraepidermal component (**B**) revealing pigmented spindle-shaped cells.

TABLE 115-5
Differential Diagnosis of Pigmented Spindle Cell Nevus
- Spitz tumor
- Blue nevus
- Hematoma
- Dysplastic junctional nevus
- Hypermelanotic nevomelanocytic nevus
- Combined nevomelanocytic/blue nevus
- Melanoma

MANAGEMENT

TREATMENT

Given the difficulties in the histopathologic differentiation from melanoma in some cases, these lesions should be considered for excision to attain histologically free margins.

PREVENTION AND COUNSELING

There are no known preventative measures. The role of UVR exposure in the development of PSCN is unknown.

SPITZ NEVUS

AT-A-GLANCE

- Spitz nevi represent a spectrum of unique, usually acquired lesions, exhibiting epithelioid and often spindle-shaped melanocytic cells with abundant eosinophilic cytoplasm, large nuclei, and often prominent nucleoli. The often develop in the epidermis and dermis or may be purely intradermal and even desmoplastic. Atypical variants exist.
- Clinically, they often present as red, dome-shaped papules. Some have varying degrees of pigmentation.
- Spitz nevi are thought to develop quickly and then stabilize. Their clinical presentation and histopathology can cause diagnostic confusion for melanoma.
- Synonyms: spindle and epithelioid cell nevus

EPIDEMIOLOGY

The annual incidence rate of Spitz nevi is approximately 1.4 to 1.6 cases per 100,000 individuals.[66] In a series reported by Weedon and Little, 70% of 211 Spitz nevi occurred in patients younger than 20 years of age.[67] This higher pediatric prevalence of Spitz nevi is confirmed in most large epidemiologic studies. There appears to be no gender predilection for Spitz nevi in children. Whites are more commonly affected than other ethnicities.

CLINICAL FEATURES

Spitz nevi typically begin with an initial phase of growth, with either gradual or relatively rapid enlargement followed by a stable quiescent period. The presence of a new or growing lesion in the pediatric population often prompts tissue biopsy.

CUTANEOUS FINDINGS

The most common variety of Spitz nevus is solitary, asymptomatic, pink or red, hairless, firm, and dome shaped (Fig. 115-14). Some Spitz nevi may resemble a keloid or pyogenic granuloma when eroded. The surface is commonly smooth, and the borders may fade into surrounding skin. Verrucous, scaly, stippled, and crusted lesions may occur. Spitz nevi are usually asymptomatic, but pruritus, tenderness, or bleeding is sometimes noted. The halo phenomenon may occur in Spitz nevi as they do in common acquired nevi.

Spitz nevi can also present as widespread eruptive lesions or in a grouped manner as multiple agminated lesions consisting of red, red-brown, brown, or dark-brown papules or nodules, with a fine stippled surface. Agminated Spitz nevi often occur in the early years of life within a background of congenital (sometimes acquired) macular pigmentation (nevus spilus) or occasionally within a hypopigmented plaque. Spitz nevi may also develop as single or multiple lesions in a large CMN.

The diameter of Spitz nevi ranges from several millimeters to several centimeters. They have a predilection for the head and neck and extremities, although truncal lesions are not uncommon. Spitz nevi tend to spare the palms, soles, and mucous membranes.

RELATED PHYSICAL FINDINGS

Multiple epithelioid Spitz nevi with loss of BAP-1 expression may occur as part of a familial cancer syndrome.[68,69]

COMPLICATIONS

Misinterpretation of benign or malignant behavior of the lesion could result in unnecessary or insufficient treatment, respectively. Spitz nevi rarely acquire more mutational aberrations over time and thus may attain metastatic (atypical Spitz tumor) or malignant potential (Spitzoid melanoma).

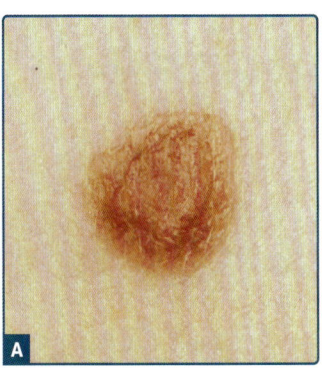 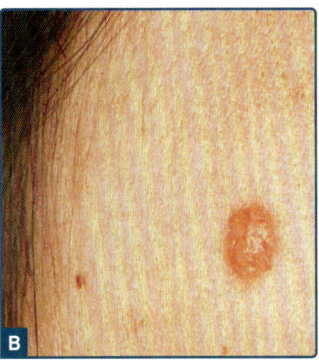 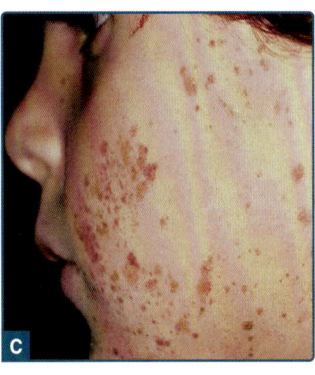

Figure 115-14 Spitz nevi. **A,** Pink plaque, which appeared de novo over an 8-week period, becoming more elevated with time, in the preauricular area of a 4-year-old white boy. **B,** Dome-shaped pink papule, which appeared de novo over a 2-week interval 4 months before, on the forehead of a 5-year-old white boy. **C,** Agminated Spitz tumors. Numerous grouped pink papules and plaques, appearing at age 6 months, on the face of a 4-year-old white boy.

ETIOLOGY AND PATHOGENESIS

Unlike common acquired nevi, congenital nevi, and melanoma, which frequently harbor *BRAF* or *NRAS* mutations, Spitz tumors often either harbor *HRAS* mutations or demonstrate genomic rearrangements involving kinase genes (*ALK, ROS1, NTRK1, BRAF, RET, MET*).[70] The combination of *BAP1* loss and *BRAF* mutation has been shown to be characteristic of a subset of atypical Spitz tumors that display distinct histopathologic features.[69] Such lesions often occur sporadically via somatic mutation, although a subset of *BAP1*-deficient melanocytic neoplasms arises in the setting of a familial germline mutation, resulting in *BAP1*-associated cancer susceptibility syndrome. Affected individuals are at increased risk for cutaneous and uveal melanoma, mesothelioma, renal cell carcinoma, cholangiocarcinoma, and other malignancies.[71]

DIAGNOSIS

PATHOLOGY

Spitz nevi are characterized by melanocytic cells with large epithelioid nuclei, often with prominent nucleoli and surrounded by a rim of eosinophilic cytoplasm with "ground-glass" appearance (Fig. 115-15). These lesions are well-circumscribed and symmetric from side to side and from top to bottom. In contrast to melanoma, the melanocytic cells in Spitz nevi show progressive maturation with increasing depth, becoming smaller with the overall distribution of cells in the dermis being wedge shaped, with narrowing of the wedge toward the subcutaneous fat. Purely junctional and dermal lesions also occur.

When there is a junctional component, there is often epidermal hyperplasia. Small intraepidermal eosinophilic globules (Kamino bodies), which are positive for periodic acid–Schiff and diastase resistant (resembling colloid bodies), may be seen. Melanocytic elements are usually well nested, although there may be permeation of the epidermis by single cells or small groups of cells. Pagetoid cells are more commonly encountered in the center of the lesion. There are often artifactual clefts between melanocytic nests and the epidermis. Ovoid junctional nests often show vertical streaming of the constituent cells.

In most cases, dermal inflammation is mild and confined to a sparse perivascular lymphocytic infiltrate. However, more intense infiltrates including a halo may occur. Atypical features including nuclear pleomorphism, increased or atypical or deep mitoses, asymmetry, and lack of maturation should raise concern for an atypical Spitz tumor or melanoma.

SPECIAL TESTING

Immunohistochemical studies may be helpful when the differential diagnosis includes Spitzoid melanoma. In most Spitz nevi, there is full or partial retention of p16 staining, but Spitzoid melanomas tend to lose p16 expression. Ki-67 proliferation marker is low in nevi but elevated in melanoma. In difficult cases, CGH or FISH studies may help better define the biologic potential of a given lesion.

DIFFERENTIAL DIAGNOSIS

See Table 115-6.

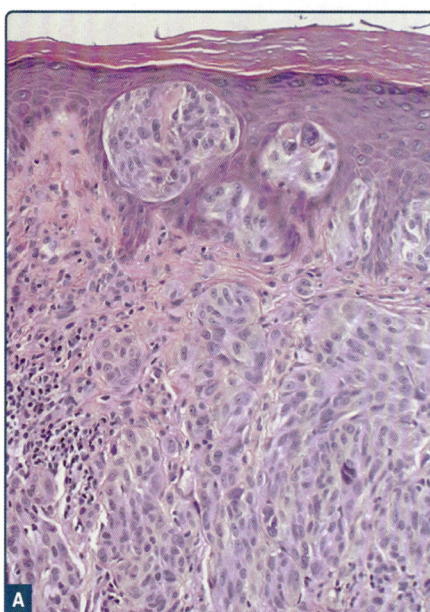 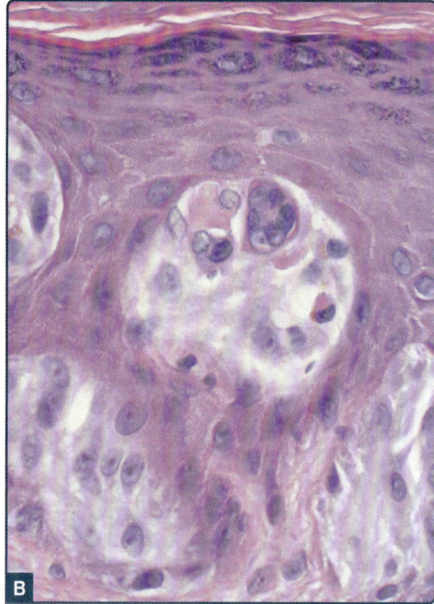

Figure 115-15 Histopathologic features of Spitz tumor (**A**) and higher magnification of the intraepidermal component revealing eosinophilic globules (Kamino bodies) adjacent to junctional nests (**B**).

CLINICAL COURSE AND PROGNOSIS

The natural history of the Spitz nevus is that most have an initial growth phase and then remain stable over time. However, a small subset may show atypical histopathologic features corresponding with accrual of additional genomic aberrations (atypical Spitz tumor or Spitzoid melanoma). Spitz tumors in the adult population should be viewed with suspicion, particularly if they are new or changing.

MANAGEMENT

TREATMENT

Complete excision with histologically clear margins is generally sufficient treatment for benign Spitz nevi. Given the difficulty of confidently excluding the possibility of melanoma in certain cases, such as those with atypical histopathologic features, an even wider margin of normal skin may be prudent for worrisome lesions. The role of sentinel lymph node biopsies for atypical Spitz tumors is controversial because tumor cells may be present in the regional lymph nodes but not have the biologic significance or poor prognosis associated with metastatic melanoma. Management of patients who have numerous Spitz nevi requires individual judgment and periodic surveillance for new or unstable lesions.

PREVENTION

There are no known preventative measures for the development of Spitz nevus.

TABLE 115-6
Differential Diagnosis of Spitz Nevi

Nonpigmented or Red
- Amelanotic melanoma
- Juvenile xanthogranuloma
- Hemangioma
- Pyogenic granuloma
- Molluscum contagiosum
- Intradermal nevus
- Solitary mastocytoma
- Granuloma
- Clear cell acanthoma
- Insect bite reaction
- Dermatofibroma
- Appendageal tumor
- Keloid

Pigmented
- Blue nevus
- Deep penetrating nevus
- Hypermelanotic intradermal nevus
- Melanoma
- Hematoma

Warty Variants
- Verruca vulgaris
- Seborrheic keratoses
- Epidermal nevus
- Epidermolytic acanthoma

NODAL NEVI

AT-A-GLANCE

- Benign melanocytic neoplasia present in a lymph node. Nevomelanocytes are characteristically located in the capsule.
- They are generally asymptomatic and found incidentally as a result of lymph node removal.
- Cells may be deposited passively into the node from a cutaneous melanocytic lesion. It is also possible that abnormal migration pathways result in the nevomelanocytes taking up residence in lymph nodes during embryonic development.
- The presence of melanocytic cells in nodal tissue may create difficulties for pathologists evaluating sentinel node biopsies in patients with cutaneous melanoma.

EPIDEMIOLOGY

Nevomelanocytes can be identified in lymph nodes with a frequency ranging from 0.3% to 7.3% in lymphadenectomies not related to melanoma and up to 22% in regional nodes removed because of melanoma.[72] A significant association has also been noted for the presence of cutaneous nevomelanocytic nevi in the zones of skin drained by lymph nodes that were found to include nevomelanocytes.[73] This association was strongest with congenital nevi. In most cases, nodal nevomelanocytes phenotypically resemble common acquired nevomelanocytic nevi, but nevi with congenital features, blue nevi, cellular blue, and Spitz nevi have all also been reported to involve regional lymph nodes.[74]

CLINICAL FEATURES

HISTORY

Generally, nodal nevi are identified in lymph nodes that are removed for other reasons, usually melanoma or breast cancer, but these benign cells are also identified in nodes removed for other reasons. Patients do not note symptoms related to nodal nevi.

CUTANEOUS FINDINGS

Melanocytic neoplasia in the form of melanoma or melanocytic nevi may be present at the cutaneous site corresponding to the draining lymph node basin.

RELATED PHYSICAL FINDINGS

Lymph nodes harboring benign nodal nevi are most commonly seen in patients undergoing lymphadenectomy for melanoma but are also seen in lymphadenectomy specimens for breast carcinoma and other causes.

COMPLICATIONS

Complications, such as scarring or lymphedema, may be the consequence of lymphadenectomy. Misinterpretation of benign nodal deposits as malignant could result in unnecessary regional lymph node dissection and treatment with systemic agents. Misinterpretation of malignant melanocytes as benign in lymph nodes may lead to under treatment.

ETIOLOGY AND PATHOGENESIS

There are two prevailing theories as to the mechanism by which nevomelanocytes appear in regional lymph nodes.

The first theory is that during development, melanoblasts get trapped in developing nodal tissues. Some support for this theory could be based on the fact that nodal nevi can be found in association with CMN. This observation suggests that there is an opportunity for nevomelanocytes to be deposited during development. Furthermore, blue nevus cells can be found in tissues such as prostate, cervix, vagina, spermatic cord, and seminal vesicles.[74] Thus, aberrant migration and differentiation of melanocytic cells does occur.

The second theory suggests that there may be passive transfer from the cutaneous lesion to the lymph node. Substances such as carbon, tattoo ink, and radioactive colloid are readily transferred to the draining lymph node. It is reasonable to assume that loosely adherent nevomelanocytes could also traverse the same path. In fact, nevomelanocytes have been noted in lymph channels.[74] In the lymph node, nevomelanocytes are generally identified in the capsule, but they can also be found in the parenchyma.[72] It is not known how nevomelanocytes get into the capsule, but it is reasonable to assume that these cells migrate from the parenchyma into the capsule. It is important to note that melanoma cells can also be found in the capsule, so it is rational to assume that entry into the capsule is not limited to a developmental event. The fact that nevomelanocytes in regional lymph nodes are highly correlated with the presence of nevomelanocytic nevi in the skin supports the concept that these cells may arrive in lymph nodes via dissemination from benign cutaneous lesions.[75]

TABLE 115-7
Differential Diagnosis of Nodal Nevi
- Melanoma
- Cells from another neoplastic source
- Foreign body deposit (tattoo ink, carbon)

DIAGNOSIS

PATHOLOGY

Pathology often reveals nevomelanocytes largely confined to the nodal capsule or trabeculae. However, cells may also be noted in the parenchyma. Nodal nevi should lack cellular atypia and mitotic activity.

SPECIAL TESTING

The use of standard immunohistochemical tests may help identify the location and cellular features of nevomelanocytes in lymph node tissue sections. Weak or negative staining for HMB-45, lack of proliferative markers (Ki67), and strong p16 expression support a benign diagnosis.[76,77] A recent study determined that fatty acid synthase and acetyl-CoA carboxylase are not expressed in intracapular nodal nevi but are expressed in metastatic melanoma.[78]

DIFFERENTIAL DIAGNOSIS

See Table 115-7.

CLINICAL COURSE AND PROGNOSIS

If the lymph node deposits are determined to be benign, no further treatment is warranted.

TREATMENT

None required for benign nodal nevi.

LENTIGO SIMPLEX

AT-A-GLANCE

- Clinically, lesions are hyperpigmented macules, occurring alone, in focal clusters (agminated), or have a generalized distribution. They occur on the skin, conjunctivae and mucous membranes.

(Continued)

AT-A-GLANCE *(Continued)*

- They commonly develop in early childhood.
- Multiple lentigines may be associated with somatic abnormalities.
- Synonyms: simple lentigo, melanotic macule, lentiginosis. Other names for agminated lentigines include unilateral lentigines, partial unilateral lentiginosis, lentiginous mosaicism, and segmental lentiginosis.
- Other lesions in which epidermal melanocytic hyperplasia may be noted, where overlap may exist with simple lentigines, include café-au-lait macules, melanoacanthoma, labial melanotic macule, melasma, and inflammatory/cytokine-induced proliferation.

EPIDEMIOLOGY

Lentigo simplex is a very common melanocytic lesion, present either at birth or developing later in childhood or adulthood. Although acral lentigo is more prevalent in blacks, lentigo simplex does not have a racial or gender predilection. The incidence of agminated and generalized lentiginosis is rare.

CLINICAL FEATURES

Lentigo simplex occurs on the skin, conjunctivae, and mucocutaneous surfaces. They may develop as early as the first decade of life (juvenile lentigo) and arise on both sun-exposed and sun-protected sites. Lentigines may develop in a unilateral, agminated (partial or segmental lentigines), or generalized distribution (lentigines profuse) and may occur as an isolated phenomenon or in associated with a number of inherited disorders, including LEOPARD (lentigines, electrocardiographic conduction abnormalities, ocular hypertelorism, pulmonary valve stenosis, abnormalities of genitalia, growth retardation, and sensorineural deafness) syndrome, Carney syndrome, Peutz-Jeghers syndrome, Laugier-Hunziker syndrome (idiopathic lenticular mucocutaneous pigmentation), and centrofacial lentiginosis.

CUTANEOUS FINDINGS

Lentigo simplex are usually sharply circumscribed macules, measuring 1 to 5 mm in size, with uniform light brown to black pigmentation. If partial or generalized lentiginosis is present, the specific pattern and clinical course of lesions may be suggestive of a specific inherited syndrome.

In LEOPARD syndrome, lentigines are often absent during the first years of life; patients subsequently may develop hundreds of lentigines during childhood,

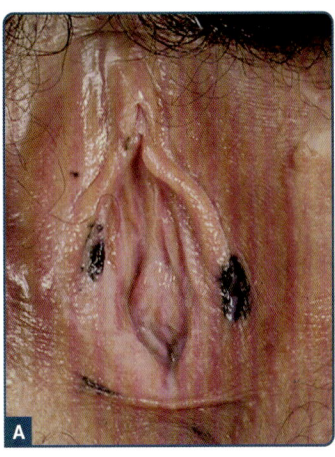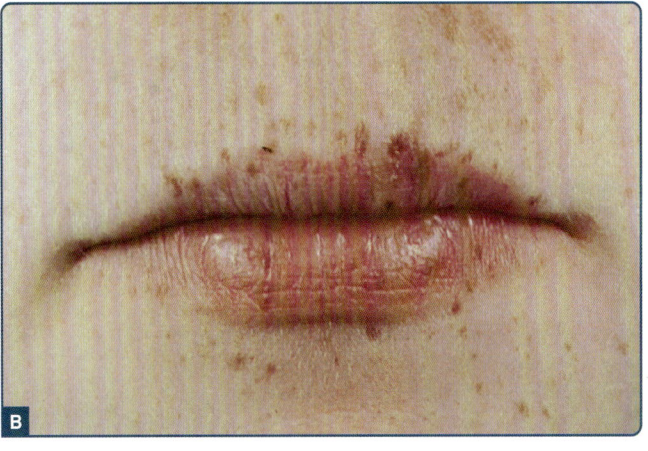

Figure 115-16 Lentigo simplex. **A,** Acquired darkly pigmented lentigines on the vulva of a 13-year-old white girl who has *l*entigines, *a*trial myxomas, *m*ucocutaneous myxomas, and *b*lue nevi (LAMB, myxoma syndrome, Carney complex). **B,** Multiple lentigines on the lips of the same patient. This patient died in her mid-20s of a malignant schwannoma.

including on the genitalia, conjunctiva, oral cavity, palms, and soles.

In Peutz-Jeghers syndrome, lentigines are commonly present on the buccal mucosa, lips, perioral skin, and ventral surfaces of the hands and feet. Although cutaneous lesions may fade at puberty, oral lentigines usually persist into adulthood.

In centrofacial lentiginosis, lentigines are characteristically distributed in a horizontal band across the face.

In Laugier-Hunziker syndrome, lentigines predominantly occur on the lips, hard and soft palates, fingers, nail matrix and palms, and infrequently at other sites, including conjunctivae and genitalia.

In LAMB (lentigines, atrial myxoma, mucocutaneous myxomas and blue nevi) syndrome, lentigines mainly occur on the face, trunk, and genitalia as tan to black macules (Fig. 115-16).

Agminated lentigines are congenital or develop shortly after birth and often are confined to a localized area of the skin, often in a segmental distribution and frequently demonstrate a curvilinear or swirled pattern (Fig. 115-17).

RELATED PHYSICAL FINDINGS

In addition to several inherited syndromes, lentigines may be associated with Addison disease; topical immunosuppressive calcineurin inhibitors, such as tacrolimus; and type 1 hereditary punctate palmoplantar keratoderma.[79,80] Eruptive acral lentigines have been reported with synchronous malignancies, including gastric adenocarcinoma, mammary carcinoma, large-cell lymphoma, non-Hogkin lymphoma, melanoma, and AIDS.[81-84]

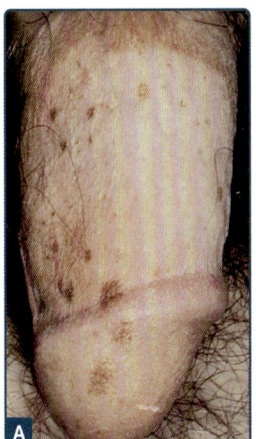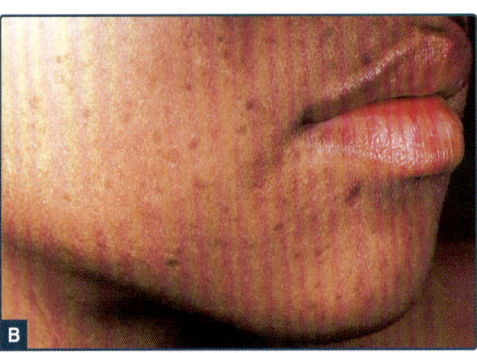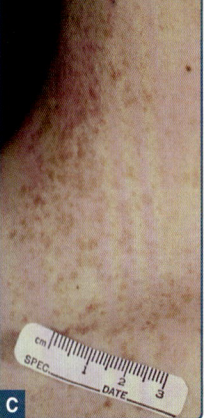

Figure 115-17 Agminated lentigines. **A,** Grouping of small light brown macules, present since age 14 years, on the right side of the shaft and glans penis of a 17-year-old healthy white male patient. **B,** Grouping of small, light brown macules, present for at least 6 years, on the right cheek of a healthy 10-year-old African American male patient. **C,** Grouping of small, light-brown macules, present since age 2 years, on the right neck and supraclavicular area of a 13-year-old healthy white female patient.

COMPLICATIONS

Complications may arise from associated syndromes; however, lentigines are benign without any direct complications.

ETIOLOGY AND PATHOGENESIS

The mechanisms underlying lentigo simplex formation are not well understood. An increased density of melanocytes suggests that melanocyte homeostasis is disrupted in lentigo simplex. Additionally, the presence of melanin macroglobules in melanocytes suggests that melanization is dysregulated and may contribute to the formation of lentigines. The presence of lentigines in association with various inherited syndromes underscores the likelihood that lentigo development may be influenced by a variety of different genetic and developmental factors.

Interestingly, lentigo simplex does not harbor characteristic mutations found in solar lentigo, psoralen UVA (PUVA) lentigines, and common acquired nevi. In a study by Hafner and coworkers, lentiginous junctional nevi, compound, and intradermal nevi harbored $BRAF^{V600E}$ mutations in 17%, 55%, and 78% of cases, respectively, but lentigo simplex was shown to lack $BRAF^{V600E}$ mutation.[85] Likewise, lentigo simplex lacks $FGFR3$ and $PIK3CA$ mutations, which are frequently present in solar lentigo and PUVA lentigines.[85,86]

DIAGNOSIS

PATHOLOGY

Histologic sections of lentigo simplex show slight to moderate elongation of rete ridges, basilar melanocytic hyperplasia, and increased pigmentation within the epidermis and melanophages in the papillary dermis. Melanocytes lack atypia. Rarely, giant pigment granules (melanin macroglobules) may be present. Frequently, a lymphohistiocytic infiltrate is present within the superficial dermis. Commonly, a junctional nevus and lentigo may coexist (lentiginous junctional nevus). Solar lentigo characteristically shows greater elongation of rete ridges and prominent solar elastosis with the papillary dermis.

LABORATORY TESTING

Immunohistochemistry to highlight melanocyte density with the epidermis (MITF, Mart-1, Sox10) is typically not necessary for histologic diagnosis.

DIFFERENTIAL DIAGNOSIS

See Table 115-8.

TABLE 115-8
Differential Diagnosis of Lentigo Simplex

Solitary
- Solar lentigo
- Ephelis
- Junctional nevomelanocytic nevus
- Dysplastic (atypical) melanocytic nevus
- Café-au-lait macule
- Melanoma (lentigo maligna)

Grouped
- Agminated nevomelanocytic nevi or lentigines
- Nevus spilus

CLINICAL COURSE AND PROGNOSIS

Generally, when present, lentigo simplex are relatively stable. During pregnancy, lentigines may become more conspicuous. There is not an association with progression to nevomelanocytic nevus or increased risk of malignant transformation to melanoma.

MANAGEMENT

TREATMENT

Treatment is not necessary for lentigo simplex. Cosmetic removal has been completed with cryotherapy or other approaches, including Q-switched laser.

PREVENTION

There are no known preventive measures for lentigo simplex. Avoidance of sun exposure and UVR does not reduce the risk of development of lentigo simplex.

SOLAR LENTIGO

AT-A-GLANCE

- Solar lentigines are hyperpigmented macules that occur on photodamaged skin, singly or as multiple lesions.
- They predominantly develop in older individuals. Children with xeroderma pigmentosum develop solar lentigines during the first year of life because of increased susceptibility to UV radiation.
- Histology shows elongation of rete ridges with budlike processes, hyperpigmentation, normal or slightly increased melanocytes, and dermal solar elastosis.

- Solar lentigines are benign. Development is associated with increased risk of UV-related cutaneous malignancies, including squamous cell carcinoma, basal cell carcinoma, and melanoma.
- Synonyms: actinic lentigo, sun-induced freckle, liver spot, lentigo senilis, senile lentigo

CLINICAL FEATURES

Solar lentigines are acquired hyperpigmented lesions that generally arise on sun-exposed sites on light-skinned individuals. They most commonly occur on the face and dorsal surfaces of the forearm and hand.

EPIDEMIOLOGY

The prevalence of solar lentigines is strongly associated with older age and photodamage. They mainly arise on sun-exposed skin of those with white skin and Asians. More than 90% of those with white skin develop a solar lentigo by the age of 50 years.[87] Multiple lentigines on the face appear to be associated with dark skin (types III and IV).[88,89] In addition to age and sun exposure, they are associated with history of facial ephelides (freckles), tanning capacity, and concurrent use of oral contraceptive therapy.[88]

Chronic psoralen photochemotherapy may induce lentigines, termed PUVA lentigines. A study of 1380 adults undergoing PUVA treatment for psoriasis observed buttock lentigines in 53% of patients, arising an average of 5.7 years after initiating treatment (Fig. 115-18).[90] PUVA lentigines are associated with total number of treatments, male gender, fair-skin, and older age.[90] Additionally, lentigines are associated with UVA exposure from artificial sunbed use.[91]

CUTANEOUS FINDINGS

Solar lentigines arise on skin exposed to natural sunlight or artificial sources of UV radiation. They have well-defined, irregular borders, with a tendency to coalesce at sites of severe sun damage where multiple lesions may be present (Fig. 115-19). They range in size from less than 1 mm to several centimeters in greatest dimension. Lesions are light to dark brown in color. Ink spot lentigo (reticulated black solar lentigo) is a variant with black pigmentation.

Unlike solar lentigo, PUVA lentigines commonly develop on sun-protected sites, including the buttocks and genitalia (see Fig. 115-18), in addition to sun-exposed areas. They often have brown-black pigmentation and are irregular.

An ephelis (freckle) is a small, uniformly pigmented macule that may be clinically distinct from a solar lentigo. Freckles are most common on the central face. Typically, they develop in early childhood, increase in adulthood, and may regress in the elderly or in the absence of continued sun-exposure.

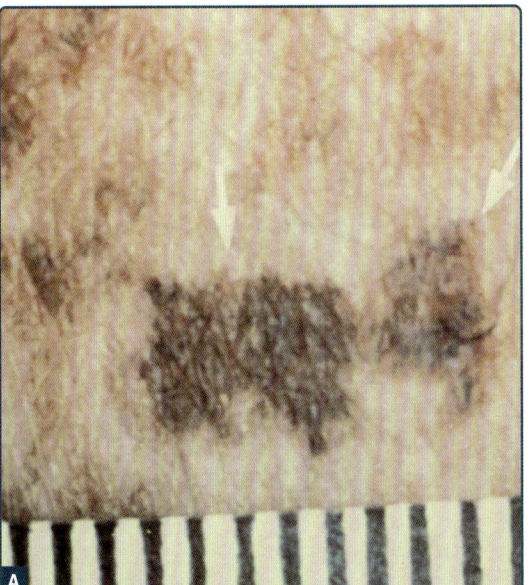 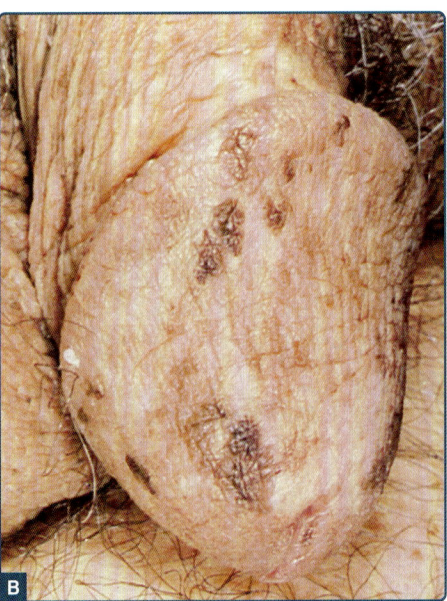

Figure 115-18 Photochemotherapy (psoralen and ultraviolet A light [PUVA])-induced lentigines (*arrow*) on the buttock (**A**) and penis (**B**) of a 57-year-old white man who had received PUVA for psoriasis several times per week for 5 years. The PUVA lentigines appeared between 1 and 2 years after PUVA therapy was begun. The current recommendation is to shield the male genitalia during PUVA therapy to prevent squamous cell carcinoma of the penis and scrotum.

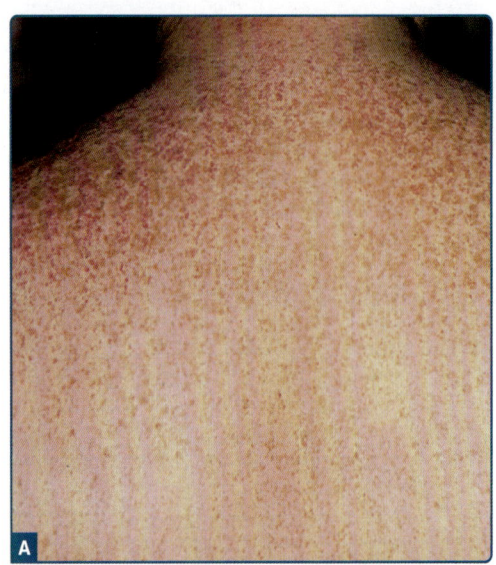
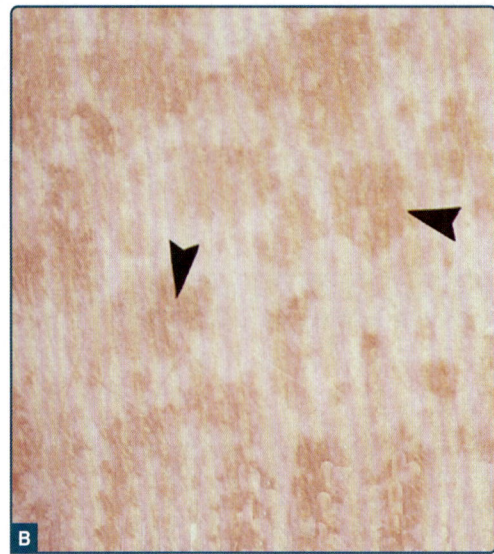
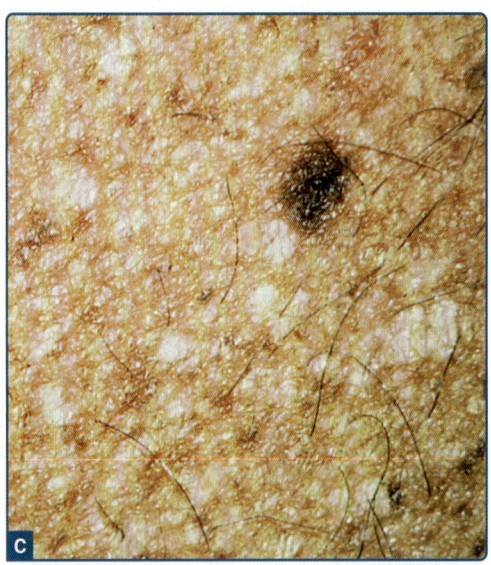

Figure 115-19 Solar lentigo. **A,** Uncountable solar lentigines on the back of a 30-year-old white man, appearing initially during early childhood after multiple sunburns. **B,** High magnification of lentigines in (**A**) showing light-brown macules with markedly irregular outlines (*arrowheads*). **C,** Solar lentigines on sun-damaged dorsal hand skin (hypopigmentation, wrinkling, and telangiectasia) of an older white man.

RELATED PHYSICAL FINDINGS

Given that solar lentigines occur on photodamaged skin, they are associated with actinic keratosis, squamous cell carcinoma, basal cell carcinoma, and melanoma. Type 2 diabetes has been shown to be independently associated with solar lentigo.[92]

COMPLICATIONS

Although solar lentigines may sometimes show melanocytic atypia on sun-damaged skin, they are benign. However, in lesions where significant atypia is present, distinction between atypical solar lentigo and melanoma in situ, lentigo maligna type may be challenging.

ETIOLOGY AND PATHOGENESIS

Solar lentigines arise from proliferation of basal melanocytes and increased melanin production. The relationship between UVR and development of lentigines is well-recognized. The cumulative effects of photodamage produce genetic and epigenetic changes in gene expression within both keratinocytes and melanocytes. Interestingly, keratinocytes are more sensitive to UVR than melanocytes.[93,94]

In response to UVR exposure, keratinocytes upregulate multiple ligands and produce reactive oxygen species (ROS), ultimately leading to MC1R and subsequently MITF activation in melanocytes through direct cell-to-cell communication and paracrine signaling.[95] MITF is a key transcription factor for melanin production in melanocytes.

Studies have reported the association of solar lentigo with loss of function MC1R alleles, MC1R promoter polymorphisms, and SLC45A2 allele variants.[96-98] Hafner and coworkers observed FGFR3 and PIK3CA mutations in 17% and 7% of solar lentigos, respectively. Kadono and coworkers demonstrated increased expression of endothelin B receptor and endothelin 1 in solar lentigo, which are key factors for melanocyte development and melanogenesis.[99] Additionally, fibroblast-derived growth factors, including keratinocyte growth factor, hepatocyte growth factor, and stem cell factor, may contribute to formation of solar lentigo.[100,101] T1799A *BRAF* mutation are detected in 33% of PUVA lentigines.[102]

DIAGNOSIS

PATHOLOGY

Histologic sections of solar lentigo show elongated rete ridges, extending into the papillary dermis with club-shaped or budlike endings. The epidermis between the rete ridges may be atrophic and have minimal overlying hyperkeratosis. The rete ridges may branch and become fused, creating a reticular pattern, caused by epidermal proliferation. Within the lesion, melanocytes may be normal in number or slightly increased and are hyperactive with markedly increased melanin production. Both within the lesion and background adjacent skin, melanocytes may have mild nuclear atypia, likely because of actinic changes. Occasionally, small horn cysts form, resulting in histologic overlap with seborrheic keratosis. The dermis characteristically shows solar elastosis. A scant to moderate perivascular chronic inflammatory infiltrate is usually present within the dermis, along with melanin-laden macrophages.

PUVA lentigines show a variety of histologic features, ranging from predominantly basal cell hyperpigmentation with normal melanocyte count to markedly elongated rete ridges with melanocyte hyperplasia. In a subset of cases, melanocytes show cellular atypia, including nuclear pleomorphism, pseudoinclusions, multinucleation, irregular nuclear contours and melanin macroglobules.[103]

In electron microscopy studies of solar lentigo, melanosome complexes were greatly enlarged within keratinocytes compared with background adjacent skin.[104] PUVA lentigines had more dendrites and more active melanogenesis.[103]

LABORATORY TESTING

Immunohistochemistry to highlight melanocyte density is generally not required for histologic diagnosis.

DIFFERENTIAL DIAGNOSIS

See Table 115-9.

CLINICAL COURSE AND PROGNOSIS

Over time, solar lentigines may enlarge or darken, persist as a stable lesion, or regress. They may evolve into lichenoid keratoses.[105] Subsequent resolution of the lichenoid keratosis ultimately may cause complete resolution of the prior lentigo. Recent molecular studies support this pathway of solar lentigo regression. Benign lichenoid keratoses have been shown to harbor *FGFR3*, *PIK3CA*, and *RAS* mutations, which are known to be involved in the pathogenesis of solar lentigo.[106]

Some authors have suggested that solar lentigo may evolve into large cell acanthoma or that large cell acanthoma is a variant with cellular hypertrophy.[107] Although the lesions share similar morphological features, differences in immunophenotype, including keratin 10 and BCL-2 expression, have been observed. Higher expression of keratin 10 and lower expression of BCL-2 suggests large cell acanthoma to have advanced maturation compared with solar lentigo.[107]

PUVA lentigines may persist years after treatment discontinuation.[90] Long-term follow-up of a large cohort of patients treated with PUVA demonstrated increased risk of melanoma, which emerged 15 years after initial therapy and continued to increase as time progressed.[108] Solar lentigines are similarly associated with increased risk of cutaneous malignancies.

MANAGEMENT

TREATMENT

Solar lentigines are benign lesions that do not require therapy. If desired, cosmetic removal may be completed with cryotherapy or other techniques, including Q-switched laser.

TABLE 115-9
Differential Diagnosis of Solar Lentigo

- Reticulated seborrheic keratoses
- Lentigo simplex
- Ephelis
- Junctional nevomelanocytic nevus
- Pigmented actinic keratoses
- Large cell acanthoma
- Lentigo maligna

PREVENTION

Avoidance of UVR exposure may decrease the risk of developing additional solar lentigines.

DYSPLASTIC MELANOCYTIC NEVI

AT-A-GLANCE

- Commonly occur in Caucasians; prevalence varies by population
- Flat or raised with smooth or "pebbly" surface, irregular shape, indistinct borders, variable pigmentation, and measure at least 5 mm in diameter
- Identify population at risk for melanoma
- Most frequent on sun-exposed areas, especially intermittently exposed, including the upper back
- Associated with large numbers of common acquired nevi
- May persist or involute; subset undergoes malignant transformation to melanoma
- Histologic features include lentiginous melanocytic hyperplasia with architectural and cytologic atypia and stromal response.

EPIDEMIOLOGY

Dysplastic nevi are common melanocytic lesions, predominantly occurring in Caucasians. The prevalence of dysplastic nevi varies by population. Individuals from melanoma-prone families have the highest incidence of dysplastic nevi. In a study by Rhodes and coworkers, dysplastic nevi were present in 30.4% of patients with melanoma compared with 1.8% of the control group.[109] Studies involving populations of northern European descent have reported variable ranges for clinically atypical nevi from 7% to 18%, with histologic-proven dysplastic nevi estimated near 10%.[6] Some support a more accurate frequency to be between 2% to 8% in this population. Dysplastic nevi are uncommon in Japanese.[110] Individuals with dysplastic nevus syndrome (DNS) may develop more than 100 clinically atypical nevi by adolescence.

CLINICAL FINDINGS

CUTANEOUS FINDINGS

Clinically, dysplastic nevi often measure at least 5 mm in diameter and characteristically have irregular, indistinct borders and variable pigmentation (Fig. 115-20). Color is typically a mixture of tan and brown, with some lesions showing pink-red coloration. Black pigmentation is more commonly associated with melanoma.[111] Rarely, nonpigmented dysplastic nevi may develop. Additionally, dysplastic nevi frequently have a flat macular component, which corresponds to a 'shoulder' or junctional component of a compound lesion. Absence of a macular component and lesional symmetry are clinically suggestive of benignity. A study by Barnhill and Roush found that nevus size and irregular borders are the most significant clinical features that had the highest correlation to histologically proven dysplastic nevi.[112] Notably, nevi that are clinically atypical may be recognized on microscopy as benign. Moreover, site-specific changes should be well-known to dermatopathologists. For instance, acral and flexural site nevi may display atypia both clinically and histologically but lack diagnostic criteria for frank dysplasia on histologic examination.

Dysplastic nevi are often slightly raised and have a "pebbly" or smooth texture. They predominate on intermediate sun-exposed skin sites, such as the trunk and especially the upper back (Fig. 115-21). To a lesser extent, they occur on sun-protected sites, such as the chest and buttocks, and less commonly the scalp. Skin creases are usually unaffected. Patients may have solitary or numerous dysplastic nevi. Agminated lesions are rarely described.

In DNS, more than 100 nevi may develop. In affected individuals, large numbers of common acquired nevi develop during childhood and subsequently acquire dysplastic features at or around puberty. Patients tend to develop melanoma at an earlier age, often in the mid-30s, and may have multiple sites of malignancy. The trunk is the most common site of malignant transformation in DNS.

RELATED PHYSICAL FINDINGS

Patients with DN may develop melanoma. A subset of melanoma cases directly progress from dysplastic nevi, and histologic evidence of an associated nevus may be apparent on microscopy. However, the majority of melanomas arise from normal skin. Several physical and environmental factors, independent of dysplastic nevi, are known to increase the risk of melanoma, including cutaneous phenotype, solar injury, and presence of ephelides (freckles). Cases of eruptive dysplastic nevi have been described in patients with AIDS, renal transplantation, chronic myeloid leukemia, and after chemotherapy for pre–B-cell acute leukemia.[113-115] Individuals with dysplastic nevi have higher numbers of common acquired nevi.

COMPLICATIONS

Melanoma is the most clinically concerning complication, associated with dysplastic nevi. Its relative risk increases with the number of dysplastic nevi

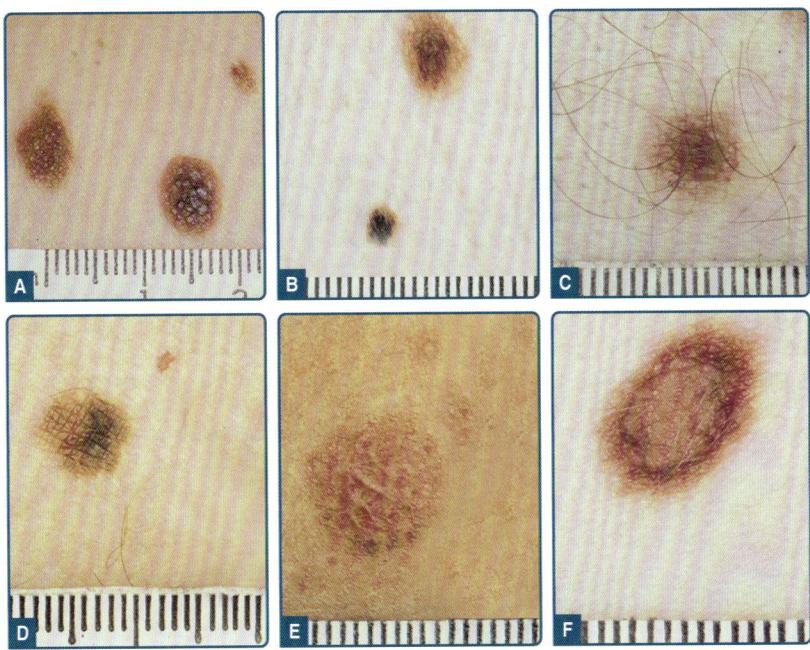

Figure 115-20 **A–F,** Atypical nevi typically have a diameter (diameter in one dimension at least 5 mm and a prominent flat component) and two of three other features (irregular asymmetric outline, indistinct borders, and variable pigmentation).

on an individual and the presence of personal or family history of melanoma. A large meta-analysis found that sporadic dysplastic nevi are associated with a 10-fold increased risk for melanoma.[39] If family history of melanoma is present in at least two relatives, there is an associated 200-fold increased risk of melanoma.[116]

ETIOLOGY AND PATHOGENESIS

The pathogenesis of dysplastic nevi is not well understood. DNS can be sporadic or inherited as an autosomal-dominant trait with variable expressiv-

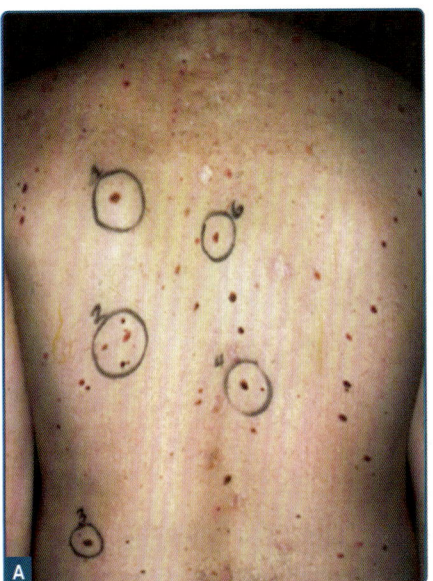
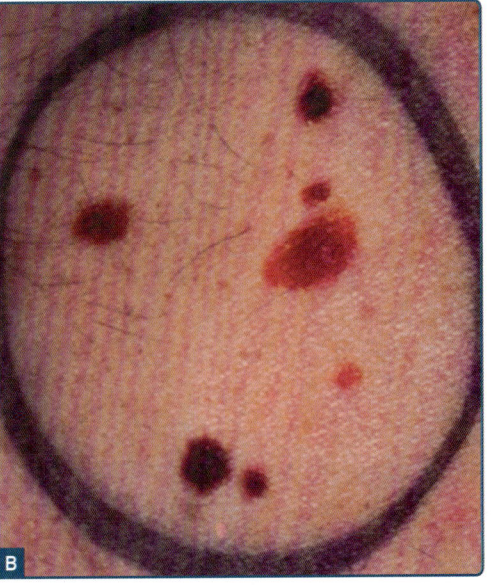

Figure 115-21 **A,** A back view showing the distribution of dysplastic nevus (DN) and lesion-to-lesion variability, with an increased number of common acquired nevi also. **B,** A closer view of a cluster of lesions marked as #2 on the back. The lesions are of different sizes, colors, and shapes with differing amounts of asymmetry and indistinct borders. The largest lesion meets all of the criteria for a clinical DN.

ity and incomplete penetrance.[117] Recently, genetic variants in *CDK6* and *XRCC1* were found to be associated with dysplastic nevi in melanoma-prone families, independent of melanoma status. Mutations on 9p21-22 (*CDKN2A*) are present in approximately 40% of cases of DNS and are associated with melanoma; however, they are not frequently detected in dysplastic nevi.[118,119] *CDKN2A* encodes tumor suppressor gene products p16INK4a and p14ARK. Microsatellite instability at chromosome 1p and 9p is frequently identified in dysplastic nevi and melanoma.[120] Similar to common acquired nevi, dysplastic nevi have a similar rate of *BRAF* mutation and can show loss of PTEN expression and altered p53 expression.[121,122] Studies have demonstrated that dysplastic nevi may have higher levels of reactive oxidative species and a higher proliferative rate than common nevi, but less than melanoma.[123]

Additionally, UVR exposure is important for the development of dysplastic nevi. Dysplastic nevi are more likely to develop on sun-exposed sites compared with doubly covered locations such as the buttocks. Sun exposure and sunburns, especially before the age of 20 years, have been shown to be associated with dysplastic nevi.[124] In melanoma-prone families, sun-protective measures in childhood reduce the number of nevi that occur. Additionally, the dysplastic and common nevi are more likely to involute in this population with adherence to sun-protective measures.[118]

DIAGNOSIS

PATHOLOGY

The histological features of dysplastic nevi characteristically show an intraepidermal lentiginous melanocytic hyperplasia with cytologic and architectural atypia and dermal stromal response (Fig. 115-22). Melanocytes are irregular in shape and distribution. In a common acquired nevus, nests of melanocytes are confined to the tips of the rete ridges. Dysplastic nevi show melanocytes distributed singly and in nests located at the tips and sides and between rete ridges. Pagetoid spread, especially atypical melanocytes at the level of the granular layer, are more commonly seen in severely dysplastic nevi and melanoma. Additional features of architectural atypia include bridging of melanocytic nests at the tips of the rete ridges, and a "shouldering" junctional component of atypical melanocytes, extending at least three rete ridges beyond a dermal nevomelanocytic component. Confluence of atypical melanocytes along the epidermis is suggestive of melanoma in situ. The epidermis usually shows elongated rete ridges and a normal epidermal thickness. Although effacement of the rete ridges and attenuation of the epidermis, may occur, regressive features are more common in melanoma. A range of cytologic atypia is present in melanocytes, including dusty cytoplasm, nuclear enlargement, nuclear membrane irregularity, prominent nucleoli, and nuclear pleomorphism. If present, the dermal nevomelanocytic component is usually bland. Dermal fibroplasia is commonly seen directly under the epidermal component in the papillary dermis. A superficial lymphocytic infiltrate and melanin-laden macrophages may be present in the papillary dermis.

The overall degree of dysplasia should be scored by a dermatopathologist. Studies examining diagnostic accuracy and reproducibility for melanocytic lesions, including dysplastic nevi, have demonstrated variable results. Multiple studies have moderate to good interobserver agreement, but others have yielded limited to fair concordance.[125-128] A recent well-designed study demonstrated poor interobserver accuracy and reproducibility.[129] It should be noted that although

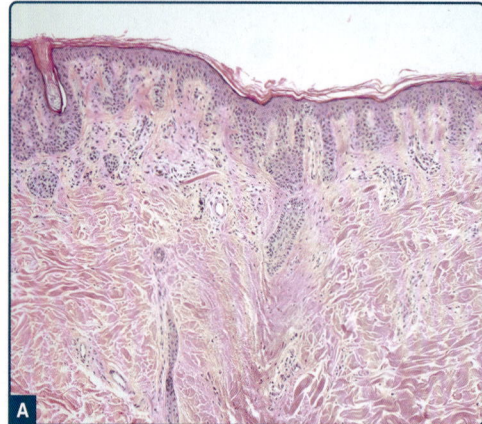 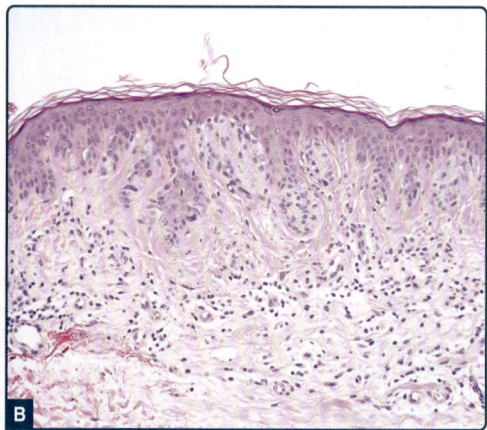

Figure 115-22 Dysplastic nevus. **A,** Compound dysplastic nevus with architecturally disordered junctional nests extending well beyond the dermal component (100× magnification). **B,** Junctional melanocytic nests are situated along the tips and sides of rete and display random cytologic atypia. There is underlying papillary dermal fibroplasia, lymphocytic infiltrate, and pigment incontinence (200× magnification).

grading systems have been proposed by multiple groups, consensus amongst dermatopathologists is lacking. Site- and gender-specific differences in DN are well described.[111] Additionally, margin status should be noted, particularly in cases of moderate and severe dysplasia.

SPECIAL TESTING

Dermoscopy (dermatoscopy or epiluminescence microscopy) is recommended during the evaluation of melanocytic neoplasia. Dermoscopy increases the diagnostic accuracy of melanoma detection.[130]

Digital imaging may be beneficial for clinical and histologic evaluation of pigmented lesions. Total-body photography, or mole mapping, is recommended for patients with multiple pigmented lesions or DNS. Total body photography has been shown to detect melanomas at earlier stages and reduce biopsies of benign lesions.[131] Other noninvasive and objective imaging techniques are being developing and include Raman spectroscopy, confocal microscopy, and multispectral imaging.

Recent work has focused on the development of a clinically validated molecular test to classify challenging melanocytic lesions as benign or malignant. Several panels have shown some promise differentiating benign nevi from melanoma with respectable sensitivity and specificity. Gene expression profiling may have additional utility in predicting responses to specific treatments or understanding treatment resistance. Further validation of gene-expression signatures in diagnostically challenging melanocytic lesions is critical.

DIFFERENTIAL DIAGNOSIS

See Table 115-10.

CLINICAL COURSE AND PROGNOSIS

The majority of dysplastic nevi do not progress to melanoma. Most studies support that only about 20% of melanoma arise from dysplastic nevi.[132,133] The risk of developing melanoma is dependent on a combination of factors, including number of dysplastic nevi, personal history of melanoma or nonmelanoma skin cancer, family history of melanoma, and UVR exposure. Given that early diagnosis of melanoma improves prognosis, periodic dermatologic follow-up is recommended and should be based on the perceived risk of malignancy and competency in self-examination. For high-risk patients, intensive surveillance is initially recommended at 4- to 6-month intervals. For patients with a family history of melanoma and multiple dysplastic nevi, annual surveillance may be appropriate. Surveillance should be initiated at 10 years of age for high-risk individuals with a family history of melanoma in at least two family members and a history of dysplastic nevi in the patient or a family member. Of patients who subsequently develop melanoma, those followed in pigmented lesion clinics usually are diagnosed and treated at earlier stages.[131] If performed, the patient should receive a copy of his or her total-body photography. Sun-protective measures, self-examination, and family screening are recommended.

MANAGEMENT

TREATMENT

Biopsy should be performed of clinically suspicious, changing, or symptomatic lesions. If melanoma is of significant concern, excision is appropriate. For patients with DNS, wholesale removal of dysplastic nevi does not significantly reduce the lifetime risk of melanoma. Lesions suspicious for melanoma should be identified as early as possible and completely excised. Reexcision may be necessary to obtain a 5-mm margin if a dysplastic nevi with severe atypia is identified on histology.

Patients should be educated on the warning signs of melanoma, including changing pigmented lesions and the ABCD rule (asymmetry, border irregularity, color variation, diameter >6 mm). Sun-protective measures, such as use of sun-protective clothing, sunglasses, sunscreens, and avoidance of overexposure, should be recommended.

PREVENTION

Sun-protective measures reduce the incidence of dysplastic and common acquired nevi.

ACKNOWLEDGMENTS

We acknowledge and extend our thanks to the contributions contained herein by Dr. Philip LeBoit as well as the prior authors of the corresponding chapters in the eighth edition. The former authors are James M. Grichnik, Arthur R. Rhodes, and Arthur J. Sober ("Benign Neoplasias and Hyperplasias of Melanocytes") and James M. Grichnik and Margaret A. Tucker ("Atypical [Dysplastic] Melanocytic Nevi").

TABLE 115-10
Differential Diagnosis of Dysplastic Nevi

- Common acquired nevus
- Congenital or congenital-type nevus
- Combined nevus
- Spitz nevus or /Spitz variant
- Pigmented spindle cell nevus
- Recurrent nevus
- Melanoma

REFERENCES

1. Clark WH Jr, Reimer RR, Greene M, et al. Origin of familial malignant melanomas from heritable melanocytic lesions. "The B-K mole syndrome." *Arch Dermatol*. 1978;114(5):732-738.
2. Lynch HT, Frichot BC 3rd, Lynch JF. Familial atypical multiple mole-melanoma syndrome. *J Med Genet*. 1978;15(5):352-356.
3. Slade J, Marghoob AA, Salopek TG, et al. Atypical mole syndrome: risk factor for cutaneous malignant melanoma and implications for management. *J Am Acad Dermatol*. 1995;32(3):479-494.
4. Ackerman AB, Magana-Garcia M. Naming acquired melanocytic nevi. Unna's, Miescher's, Spitz's Clark's. *Am J Dermatopathol*. 1990;12(2):193-209.
5. Shapiro M, Chren MM, Levy RM, et al. Variability in nomenclature used for nevi with architectural disorder and cytologic atypia (microscopically dysplastic nevi) by dermatologists and dermatopathologists. *J Cutan Pathol*. 2004;31(8):523-530.
6. Naeyaert JM, Brochez L. Clinical practice. Dysplastic nevi. *N Engl J Med*. 2003;349(23):2233-2240.
7. Kanada KN, Merin MR, Munden A, et al. A prospective study of cutaneous findings in newborns in the United States: correlation with race, ethnicity, and gestational status using updated classification and nomenclature. *J Pediatr*. 2012;161(2):240-245.
8. Castilla EE, da Graca Dutra M, Orioli-Parreiras IM. Epidemiology of congenital pigmented naevi: I. Incidence rates and relative frequencies. *Br J Dermatol*. 1981;104(3):307-315.
9. Kinsler VA, O'Hare P, Bulstrode N, et al. Melanoma in congenital melanocytic naevi. *Br J Dermatol*. 2017; 176(5):1131-1143.
10. Turkeltaub AE, Pezzi TA, Pezzi CM, et al. Characteristics, treatment, and survival of invasive malignant melanoma (MM) in giant pigmented nevi (GPN) in adults: 976 cases from the National Cancer Data Base (NCDB). *J Am Acad Dermatol*. 2016;74(6):1128-1134.
11. Krengel S, Scope A, Dusza SW, et al. New recommendations for the categorization of cutaneous features of congenital melanocytic nevi. *J Am Acad Dermatol*. 2013;68(3):441-451.
12. Rhodes AR, Albert LS, Weinstock MA. Congenital nevomelanocytic nevi: proportionate area expansion during infancy and early childhood. *J Am Acad Dermatol*. 1996;34(1):51-62.
13. Cengiz FP, Emiroglu N, Ozkaya DB, et al. Dermoscopic features of small, medium, and large-sized congenital melanocytic nevi. *Ann Dermatol*. 2017;29(1): 26-32.
14. Monica I, Kumar LP, Uppin MS, et al. Neurocutaneous melanocytosis presenting in a teenager: a case report and review of the literature. *J Cancer Res Ther*. 2015;11(3):649.
15. Vourc'h-Jourdain M, Martin L, Barbarot S. aRED Large congenital melanocytic nevi: therapeutic management and melanoma risk: a systematic review. *J Am Acad Dermatol*. 2013;68(3):493-498, e491-414.
16. Neuhold JC, Friesenhahn J, Gerdes N, et al. Case reports of fatal or metastasizing melanoma in children and adolescents: a systematic analysis of the literature. *Pediatr Dermatol*. 2015;32(1):13-22.
17. de Wijn RS, Zaal LH, Hennekam RC, et al. Familial clustering of giant congenital melanocytic nevi. *J Plast Reconstr Aesthet Surg*. 2010;63(6):906-913.
18. Silfen R, Skoll PJ, Hudson DA. Congenital giant hairy nevi and neurofibromatosis: the significance of their common origin. *Plast Reconstr Surg*. 2002; 110(5):1364-1365.
19. Roh MR, Eliades P, Gupta S, et al. Genetics of melanocytic nevi. *Pigment Cell Melanoma Res*. 2015;28(6): 661-672.
20. Bauer J, Curtin JA, Pinkel D, et al. Congenital melanocytic nevi frequently harbor NRAS mutations but no BRAF mutations. *J Invest Dermatol*. 2007;127(1): 179-182.
21. Desai SC, Walen S, Holds JB, et al. Divided nevus of the eyelid: review of embryology, pathology and treatment. *Am J Otolaryngol*. 2013;34(3):223-229.
22. Simons EA, Huang JT, Schmidt B. Congenital melanocytic nevi in young children: Histopathologic features and clinical outcomes. *J Am Acad Dermatol*. 2017; 76(5):941-947.
23. Yelamos O, Arva NC, Obregon R, et al. A comparative study of proliferative nodules and lethal melanomas in congenital nevi from children. *Am J Surg Pathol*. 2015;39(3):405-415.
24. Busam KJ, Shah KN, Gerami P, et al. Reduced H3K27me3 expression is common in nodular melanomas of childhood associated with congenital melanocytic nevi but not in proliferative nodules. *Am J Surg Pathol*. 2017;41(3):396-404.
25. Sato S, Kato H, Hidano A. Divided nevus spilus and divided form of spotted grouped pigmented nevus. *J Cutan Pathol*. 1979;6(6):507-512.
26. Torres KG, Carle L, Royer M. Nevus spilus (speckled lentiginous nevus) in the oral cavity: report of a case and review of the literature. *Am J Dermatopathol*. 2017;39(1):e8-e12.
27. Kaminska-Winciorek G. Dermoscopy of nevus spilus. *Dermatol Surg*. 2013;39(10):1550-1554.
28. Tavoloni Braga JC, Gomes E, Macedo MP, et al. Early detection of melanoma arising within nevus spilus. *J Am Acad Dermatol*. 2014;70(2):e31-32.
29. Vidaurri-de la Cruz H, Happle R. Two distinct types of speckled lentiginous nevi characterized by macular versus papular speckles. *Dermatology*. 2006; 212(1):53-58.
30. Boot-Bloemen MCT, de Kort WJA, van der Spek-Keijser LMT, et al. Melanoma in segmental naevus spilus: a case series and literature review. *Acta Derm Venereol*. 2017;97(6):749-750.
31. Sarin KY, McNiff JM, Kwok S, et al. Activating HRAS mutation in nevus spilus. *J Invest Dermatol*. 2014;134(6):1766-1768.
32. Sarin KY, Sun BK, Bangs CD, et al. Activating HRAS mutation in agminated Spitz nevi arising in a nevus spilus. *JAMA Dermatol*. 2013;149(9):1077-1081.
33. Kinsler VA, Krengel S, Riviere JB, et al. Next-generation sequencing of nevus spilus-type congenital melanocytic nevus: exquisite genotype-phenotype correlation in mosaic RASopathies. *J Invest Dermatol*. 2014;134(10):2658-2660.
34. MacKie RM, English J, Aitchison TC, et al. The number and distribution of benign pigmented moles (melanocytic naevi) in a healthy British population. *Br J Dermatol*. 1985;113(2):167-174.
35. Crane LA, Mokrohisky ST, Dellavalle RP, et al. Melanocytic nevus development in Colorado children born in 1998: a longitudinal study. *Arch Dermatol*. 2009;145(2):148-156.
36. Ohn J, Choe YS, Mun JH. Dermoscopic features of nail matrix nevus (NMN) in adults and children: a

comparative analysis. *J Am Acad Dermatol*. 2016; 75(3):535-540.
37. Patrizi A, Bentivogli M, Raone B, et al. Association of halo nevus/i and vitiligo in childhood: a retrospective observational study. *J Eur Acad Dermatol Venereol*. 2013;27(2):e148-152.
38. Brazzelli V, Larizza D, Martinetti M, et al. Halo nevus, rather than vitiligo, is a typical dermatologic finding of Turner's syndrome: clinical, genetic, and immunogenetic study in 72 patients. *J Am Acad Dermatol*. 2004;51(3):354-358.
39. Gandini S, Sera F, Cattaruzza MS, et al. Meta-analysis of risk factors for cutaneous melanoma: I. Common and atypical naevi. *Eur J Cancer*. 2005;41(1):28-44.
40. Carli P, Massi D, Santucci M, et al. Cutaneous melanoma histologically associated with a nevus and melanoma de novo have a different profile of risk: results from a case-control study. *J Am Acad Dermatol*. 1999;40(4):549-557.
41. Oliveria SA, Satagopan JM, Geller AC, et al. Study of Nevi in Children (SONIC): baseline findings and predictors of nevus count. *Am J Epidemiol*. 2009;169(1):41-53.
42. Crane LA, Mokrohisky ST, Dellavalle RP, et al. Melanocytic nevus development in Colorado children born in 1998: a longitudinal study. *Arch Dermatol*. 2009;145(2):148-156.
43. Yeh I, von Deimling A, Bastian BC. Clonal BRAF mutations in melanocytic nevi and initiating role of BRAF in melanocytic neoplasia. *J Natl Cancer Inst*. 2013;105(12):917-919.
44. Sekulic A, Colgan MB, Davis MD, et al. Activating BRAF mutations in eruptive melanocytic naevi. *Br J Dermatol*. 2010;163(5):1095-1098.
45. Gantner S, Wiesner T, Cerroni L, et al. Absence of BRAF and HRAS mutations in eruptive Spitz naevi. *Br J Dermatol*. 2011;164(4):873-877.
46. Yang Y, Li S, Zhu G, et al. A similar local immune and oxidative stress phenotype in vitiligo and halo nevus. *J Dermatol Sci*. 2017;87(1):50-59.
47. Okun MR, Donnellan B, Edelstein L. An ultrastructural study of balloon cell nevus. Relationship of mast cells to nevus cells. *Cancer*. 1974;34(3):615-625.
48. Bastian BC, Olshen AB, LeBoit PE, et al. Classifying melanocytic tumors based on DNA copy number changes. *Am J Pathol*. 2003;163(5):1765-1770.
49. Phadke PA, Zembowicz A. Blue nevi and related tumors. *Clin Lab Med*. 2011;31(2):345-358.
50. Tse JY, Walls BE, Pomerantz H, et al. Melanoma arising in a nevus of Ito: novel genetic mutations and a review of the literature on cutaneous malignant transformation of dermal melanocytosis. *J Cutan Pathol*. 2016;43(1):57-63.
51. Bender RP, McGinniss MJ, Esmay P, et al. Identification of HRAS mutations and absence of GNAQ or GNA11 mutations in deep penetrating nevi. *Mod Pathol*. 2013;26(10):1320-1328.
52. Van Raamsdonk CD, Bezrookove V, Green G, et al. Frequent somatic mutations of GNAQ in uveal melanoma and blue naevi. *Nature*. 2009;457(7229):599-602.
53. Thomas AC, Zeng Z, Riviere JB, et al. Mosaic activating mutations in GNA11 and GNAQ are associated with phakomatosis pigmentovascularis and extensive dermal melanocytosis. *J Invest Dermatol*. 2016;136(4):770-778.
54. Yeh I, Lang UE, Durieux E, et al. Combined activation of MAP kinase pathway and beta-catenin signaling cause deep penetrating nevi. *Nat Commun*. 2017;8(1):644.
55. Isales MC, Haugh AM, Bubley J, et al. Genomic assessment of blitz nevi suggests classification as a subset of blue nevus rather than Spitz nevus: clinical, histopathologic, and molecular analysis of 18 cases. *Am J Dermatopathol*. 2017.
56. Mandal RV, Murali R, Lundquist KF, et al. Pigmented epithelioid melanocytoma: favorable outcome after 5-year follow-up. *Am J Surg Pathol*. 2009;33(12): 1778-1782.
57. Zembowicz A, Knoepp SM, Bei T, et al. Loss of expression of protein kinase a regulatory subunit 1alpha in pigmented epithelioid melanocytoma but not in melanoma or other melanocytic lesions. *Am J Surg Pathol*. 2007;31(11):1764-1775.
58. Cohen JN, Joseph NM, North JP, et al. Genomic Analysis of Pigmented Epithelioid Melanocytomas Reveals Recurrent Alterations in PRKAR1A, and PRKCA Genes. *Am J Surg Pathol*. 2017;41(10):1333-1346.
59. Costa S, Byrne M, Pissaloux D, et al. Melanomas associated with blue nevi or mimicking cellular blue nevi: clinical, pathologic, and molecular study of 11 cases displaying a high frequency of GNA11 mutations, BAP1 expression loss, and a predilection for the scalp. *Am J Surg Pathol*. 2016;40(3):368-377.
60. Sagebiel RW, Chinn EK, Egbert BM. Pigmented spindle cell nevus. Clinical and histologic review of 90 cases. *Am J Surg Pathol*. 1984;8(9):645-653.
61. Sau P, Graham JH, Helwig EB. Pigmented spindle cell nevus: a clinicopathologic analysis of ninety-five cases. *J Am Acad Dermatol*. 1993;28(4):565-571.
62. Barnhill RL, Barnhill MA, Berwick M, et al. The histologic spectrum of pigmented spindle cell nevus: a review of 120 cases with emphasis on atypical variants. *Hum Pathol*. 1991;22(1):52-58.
63. Reed RJ, Ichinose H, Clark WH Jr, et al. Common and uncommon melanocytic nevi and borderline melanomas. *Semin Oncol*. 1975;2(2):119-147.
64. Lallas A, Apalla Z, Ioannides D, et al. Update on dermoscopy of Spitz/Reed naevi and management guidelines by the International Dermoscopy Society. *Br J Dermatol*. 2017;177(3):645-655.
65. Diaz A, Valera A, Carrera C, et al. Pigmented spindle cell nevus: clues for differentiating it from spindle cell malignant melanoma. A comprehensive survey including clinicopathologic, immunohistochemical, and FISH studies. *Am J Surg Pathol*. 2011;35(11):1733-1742.
66. Sepehr A, Chao E, Trefrey B, et al. Long-term outcome of Spitz-type melanocytic tumors. *Arch Dermatol*. 2011;147(10):1173-1179.
67. Weedon D, Little JH. Spindle and epithelioid cell nevi in children and adults. A review of 211 cases of the Spitz nevus. *Cancer*. 1977;40(1):217-225.
68. Busam KJ, Wanna M, Wiesner T. Multiple epithelioid Spitz nevi or tumors with loss of BAP1 expression: a clue to a hereditary tumor syndrome. *JAMA Dermatol*. 2013;149(3):335-339.
69. Wiesner T, Murali R, Fried I, et al. A distinct subset of atypical Spitz tumors is characterized by BRAF mutation and loss of BAP1 expression. *Am J Surg Pathol*. 2012;36(6):818-830.
70. Wiesner T, Kutzner H, Cerroni L, et al. Genomic aberrations in spitzoid melanocytic tumours and their implications for diagnosis, prognosis and therapy. *Pathology*. 2016;48(2):113-131.
71. Marusic Z, Buljan M, Busam KJ. Histomorphologic spectrum of BAP1 negative melanocytic neoplasms in a family with BAP1-associated cancer susceptibility syndrome. *J Cutan Pathol*. 2015;42(6):406-412.

72. Biddle DA, Evans HL, Kemp BL, et al. Intraparenchymal nevus cell aggregates in lymph nodes: a possible diagnostic pitfall with malignant melanoma and carcinoma. *Am J Surg Pathol*. 2003;27(5):673-681.
73. Fontaine D, Parkhill W, Greer W, et al. Nevus cells in lymph nodes: an association with congenital cutaneous nevi. *Am J Dermatopathol*. 2002;24(1):1-5.
74. Patterson JW. Nevus cell aggregates in lymph nodes. *Am J Clin Pathol*. 2004;121(1):13-15.
75. Howell BG, Lipa JE, Ghazarian DM. Intracapsular melanoma: a new pitfall for sentinel lymph node biopsy. *J Clin Pathol*. 2006;59(8):891-892.
76. Piana S, Tagliavini E, Ragazzi M, et al. Lymph node melanocytic nevi: pathogenesis and differential diagnoses, with special reference to p16 reactivity. *Pathol Res Pract*. 2015;211(5):381-388.
77. Mihic-Probst D, Saremaslani P, Komminoth P, et al. Immunostaining for the tumour suppressor gene p16 product is a useful marker to differentiate melanoma metastasis from lymph-node nevus. *Virchows Arch*. 2003;443(6):745-751.
78. Saab J, Santos-Zabala ML, Loda M, et al. Fatty acid synthase and acetyl-CoA carboxylase are expressed in nodal metastatic melanoma but not in benign intracapsular nodal nevi. *Am J Dermatopathol*. 2018;40(4):259-264.
79. Erkek E, Erdogan S, Tuncez F, et al. Type I hereditary punctate keratoderma associated with widespread lentigo simplex and successfully treated with low-dose oral acitretin. *Arch Dermatol*. 2006;142(8):1076-1077.
80. Castelo-Soccio L, Di Marcantonio D, Shah P, et al. Induced lentiginosis with use of topical calcineurin inhibitors. *Arch Dermatol*. 2012;148(6):766-768.
81. Mohizea SA, Al-Balbeesi A. Acral lentigines, is it a paraneoplastic syndrome? *Int J Health Sci (Qassim)*. 2009;3(1):89-92.
82. Wolf R, Lipozencic J, Segal Z, et al. Eruptive acral lentigines—a new paraneoplastic sign? *Acta Dermatovenerol Croat*. 2008;16(3):130-132.
83. Wolf R, Orion E, Davidovici B. Acral lentigines: a new paraneoplastic syndrome. *Int J Dermatol*. 2008;47(2):168-170.
84. Gallais V, Lacour JP, Perrin C, et al. Acral hyperpigmented macules and longitudinal melanonychia in AIDS patients. *Br J Dermatol*. 1992;126(4):387-391.
85. Hafner C, Stoehr R, van Oers JM, et al. The absence of BRAF, FGFR3, and PIK3CA mutations differentiates lentigo simplex from melanocytic nevus and solar lentigo. *J Invest Dermatol*. 2009;129(11):2730-2735.
86. Hafner C, Stoehr R, van Oers JM, et al. FGFR3 and PIK3CA mutations are involved in the molecular pathogenesis of solar lentigo. *Br J Dermatol*. 2009;160(3):546-551.
87. Ortonne JP. Pigmentary changes of the ageing skin. *Br J Dermatol*. 1990;122(suppl 35):21-28.
88. Ezzedine K, Mauger E, Latreille J, et al. Freckles and solar lentigines have different risk factors in Caucasian women. *J Eur Acad Dermatol Venereol*. 2013;27(3):e345-356.
89. Monestier S, Gaudy C, Gouvernet J, et al. Multiple senile lentigos of the face, a skin ageing pattern resulting from a life excess of intermittent sun exposure in dark-skinned Caucasians: a case-control study. *Br J Dermatol*. 2006;154(3):438-444.
90. Rhodes AR, Stern RS, Melski JW. The PUVA lentigo: an analysis of predisposing factors. *J Invest Dermatol*. 1983;81(5):459-463.
91. Kadunce DP, Piepkorn MW, Zone JJ. Persistent melanocytic lesions associated with cosmetic tanning bed use: "sunbed lentigines." *J Am Acad Dermatol*. 1990;23(5 Pt 2):1029-1031.
92. Moazzami B, Razavi N, Babaei M, et al. The association between solar lentigines and type-2 diabetes. *Caspian J Intern Med*. 2017;8(4):317-320.
93. Cui R, Widlund HR, Feige E, et al. Central role of p53 in the suntan response and pathologic hyperpigmentation. *Cell*. 2007;128(5):853-864.
94. Gordon PR, Mansur CP, Gilchrest BA. Regulation of human melanocyte growth, dendricity, and melanization by keratinocyte derived factors. *J Invest Dermatol*. 1989;92(4):565-572.
95. Praetorius C, Sturm RA, Steingrimsson E. Sun-induced freckling: ephelides and solar lentigines. *Pigment Cell Melanoma Res*. 2014;27(3):339-350.
96. Vierkotter A, Kramer U, Sugiri D, et al. Development of lentigines in German and Japanese women correlates with variants in the SLC45A2 gene. *J Invest Dermatol*. 2012;132(3 Pt 1):733-736.
97. Motokawa T, Kato T, Hashimoto Y, et al. Polymorphism patterns in the promoter region of the MC1R gene are associated with development of freckles and solar lentigines. *J Invest Dermatol*. 2008;128(6):1588-1591.
98. Motokawa T, Kato T, Hashimoto Y, et al. Effect of Val92Met and Arg163Gln variants of the MC1R gene on freckles and solar lentigines in Japanese. *Pigment Cell Res*. 2007;20(2):140-143.
99. Kadono S, Manaka I, Kawashima M, et al. The role of the epidermal endothelin cascade in the hyperpigmentation mechanism of lentigo senilis. *J Invest Dermatol*. 2001;116(4):571-577.
100. Chen N, Hu Y, Li WH, et al. The role of keratinocyte growth factor in melanogenesis: a possible mechanism for the initiation of solar lentigines. *Exp Dermatol*. 2010;19(10):865-872.
101. Kovacs D, Cardinali G, Aspite N, et al. Role of fibroblast-derived growth factors in regulating hyperpigmentation of solar lentigo. *Br J Dermatol*. 2010;163(5):1020-1027.
102. Lassacher A, Worda M, Kaddu S, et al. T1799A BRAF mutation is common in PUVA lentigines. *J Invest Dermatol*. 2006;126(8):1915-1917.
103. Nakagawa H, Rhodes AR, Momtaz TK, et al. Morphologic alterations of epidermal melanocytes and melanosomes in PUVA lentigines: a comparative ultrastructural investigation of lentigines induced by PUVA and sunlight. *J Invest Dermatol*. 1984;82(1):101-107.
104. Montagna W, Hu F, Carlisle K. A reinvestigation of solar lentigines. *Arch Dermatol*. 1980;116(10):1151-1154.
105. Goldenhersh MA, Barnhill RL, Rosenbaum HM, et al. Documented evolution of a solar lentigo into a solitary lichen planus-like keratosis. *J Cutan Pathol*. 1986;13(4):308-311.
106. Groesser L, Herschberger E, Landthaler M, et al. FGFR3, PIK3CA and RAS mutations in benign lichenoid keratosis. *Br J Dermatol*. 2012;166(4):784-788.
107. Fraga GR, Amin SM. Large cell acanthoma: a variant of solar lentigo with cellular hypertrophy. *J Cutan Pathol*. 2014;41(9):733-739.
108. Stern RS, PUVA Follow up Study. The risk of melanoma in association with long-term exposure to PUVA. *J Am Acad Dermatol*. 2001;44(5):755-761.
109. Rhodes AR, Seki Y, Fitzpatrick TB, et al. Melanosomal alterations in dysplastic melanocytic nevi. A quantitative, ultrastructural investigation. *Cancer*. 1988;61(2):358-369.

110. Hara K, Nitta Y, Ikeya T. Dysplastic nevus syndrome among Japanese. A case study and review of the Japanese literature. *Am J Dermatopathol*. 1992;14(1):24-31.
111. Elder DE. Precursors to melanoma and their mimics: nevi of special sites. *Mod Pathol*. 2006;19(suppl 2):S4-S20.
112. Barnhill RL, Roush GC. Correlation of clinical and histopathologic features in clinically atypical melanocytic nevi. *Cancer*. 1991;67(12):3157-3164.
113. Lozeau DF, Farber MJ, Lee JB. A nongrading histologic approach to Clark (dysplastic) nevi: a potential to decrease the excision rate. *J Am Acad Dermatol*. 2016;74(1):68-74.
114. Reutter JC, Long EM, Morrell DS, et al. Eruptive postchemotherapy in situ melanomas and dysplastic nevi. *Pediatr Dermatol*. 2007;24(2):135-137.
115. Duvic M, Lowe L, Rapini RP, et al. Eruptive dysplastic nevi associated with human immunodeficiency virus infection. *Arch Dermatol*. 1989;125(3):397-401.
116. Halpern AC, Guerry Dt, Elder DE, et al. A cohort study of melanoma in patients with dysplastic nevi. *J Invest Dermatol*. 1993;100(3):346S-349S.
117. Celebi JT, Ward KM, Wanner M, et al. Evaluation of germline CDKN2A, ARF, CDK4, PTEN, and BRAF alterations in atypical mole syndrome. *Clin Exp Dermatol*. 2005;30(1):68-70.
118. Tucker MA, Fraser MC, Goldstein AM, et al. A natural history of melanomas and dysplastic nevi: an atlas of lesions in melanoma-prone families. *Cancer*. 2002;94(12):3192-3209.
119. Piepkorn M. Whither the atypical (dysplastic) nevus? *Am J Clin Pathol*. 2001;115(2):177-179.
120. Hussein MR, Sun M, Tuthill RJ, et al. Comprehensive analysis of 112 melanocytic skin lesions demonstrates microsatellite instability in melanomas and dysplastic nevi, but not in benign nevi. *J Cutan Pathol*. 2001;28(7):343-350.
121. Uribe P, Andrade L, Gonzalez S. Lack of association between BRAF mutation and MAPK ERK activation in melanocytic nevi. *J Invest Dermatol*. 2006;126(1):161-166.
122. Tsao H, Mihm MC, Jr, Sheehan C. PTEN expression in normal skin, acquired melanocytic nevi, and cutaneous melanoma. *J Am Acad Dermatol*. 2003;49(5):865-872.
123. Duffy K, Grossman D. The dysplastic nevus: from historical perspective to management in the modern era: part II. Molecular aspects and clinical management. *J Am Acad Dermatol*. 2012;67(1):19 e11-12; quiz 31-32.
124. Titus-Ernstoff L, Ernstoff MS, Duray PH, et al. A relation between childhood sun exposure and dysplastic nevus syndrome among patients with nonfamilial melanoma. *Epidemiology*. 1991;2(3):210-214.
125. Clemente C, Cochran AJ, Elder DE, et al. Histopathologic diagnosis of dysplastic nevi: concordance among pathologists convened by the World Health Organization Melanoma Programme. *Hum Pathol*. 1991;22(4):313-319.
126. Piepkorn MW, Barnhill RL, Cannon-Albright LA, et al. A multiobserver, population-based analysis of histologic dysplasia in melanocytic nevi. *J Am Acad Dermatol*. 1994;30(5 Pt 1):707-714.
127. Nobre AB, Pineiro-Maceira J, Luiz RR. Analysis of interobserver reproducibility in grading histological patterns of dysplastic nevi. *An Bras Dermatol*. 2013;88(1):23-31.
128. de Wit PE, van't Hof-Grootenboer B, Ruiter DJ, et al. Validity of the histopathological criteria used for diagnosing dysplastic naevi. An interobserver study by the pathology subgroup of the EORTC Malignant Melanoma Cooperative Group. *Eur J Cancer*. 1993;29A(6):831-839.
129. Elmore JG, Barnhill RL, Elder DE, et al. Pathologists' diagnosis of invasive melanoma and melanocytic proliferations: observer accuracy and reproducibility study. *BMJ*. 2017;357:j2813.
130. Vestergaard ME, Macaskill P, Holt PE, et al. Dermoscopy compared with naked eye examination for the diagnosis of primary melanoma: a meta-analysis of studies performed in a clinical setting. *Br J Dermatol*. 2008;159(3):669-676.
131. Banky JP, Kelly JW, English DR, et al. Incidence of new and changed nevi and melanomas detected using baseline images and dermoscopy in patients at high risk for melanoma. *Arch Dermatol*. 2005;141(8):998-1006.
132. Ko JS, Matharoo-Ball B, Billings SD, et al. Diagnostic distinction of malignant melanoma and benign nevi by a gene expression signature and correlation to clinical outcomes. *Cancer Epidemiol Biomarkers Prev*. 2017;26(7):1107-1113.
133. Duffy K, Grossman D. The dysplastic nevus: from historical perspective to management in the modern era: part I. Historical, histologic, and clinical aspects. *J Am Acad Dermatol*. 2012;67(1):1 e1-16; quiz 17-18.

Chapter 116 :: Melanoma
:: Jessica C. Hassel & Alexander H. Enk

第一百一十六章
黑色素瘤

中文导读

　　黑色素瘤是一种起源于黑素细胞的恶性肿瘤，最常见为皮肤黑色素瘤，也可见于黏膜、葡萄膜、脑膜等部位。其中还有10%的黑色素瘤"原发灶未知"。本章分为7节：①历史视角；②流行病学；③临床特征；④病因和发病机制；⑤诊断；⑥临床病程和预后；⑦临床管理。

　　第一节介绍了黑色素瘤发现的最早证据来自于2400年前秘鲁的木乃伊骨骼，但对其最早的描述来自公元前5世纪的希波克拉底的著作。

　　第二节介绍了黑色素瘤的发病率在全球范围内显著增加，但与死亡人数并无相关，发病率随着年龄的增长而上升，55岁至74岁间达到最高水平。

　　第三节介绍了皮肤黑色素瘤的不同亚型、皮肤外黑色素瘤以及黑色素瘤引起的并发症。

　　第四节介绍了阳光曝晒和遗传是最重要的两个因素，痣的数量、雀斑的存在、晒伤史、发色和肤色是评估黑色素瘤风险的最佳指标。同时介绍了癌基因激活、肿瘤抑制基因丢失或染色体不稳定性增加等基因异常是遗传性黑色素瘤发病的主要机制。

　　第五节介绍了早期发现是改善黑色素瘤预后的关键，提到了体格检查、皮肤镜、组织病理学及一些实验室检查、影像学检查等用于黑色素瘤的诊断。此外特别介绍了前哨淋巴结的活检。

　　第六节介绍了不同分期的黑色素瘤的临床特征与预后，并重点介绍了影响临床预后的因素。

　　第七节介绍了原发性黑色素瘤的外科治疗、区域转移瘤的外科治疗、辅助治疗、卫星灶或移行转移瘤的处理、葡萄膜黑色素瘤合并肝转移的局部肝治疗、不能完全切除的转移性肿瘤的治疗、未来治疗的方向及随访要求。

〔粟　娟〕

AT-A-GLANCE

- Rising incidence worldwide in countries with white inhabitants, with highest incidence rates in Australia (35 new cases per year per 100,000 population), followed by North America (21.8 new cases per 100,000 population) and Europe (13.5 new cases per 100,000 population).

- Risk factors include history of sunburns and/or heavy sun exposure, blue or green eyes, blonde or red hair, fair complexion, >100 typical nevi, any atypical nevi, prior personal or family history of melanoma, or *p16* mutation.

- Mean age of diagnosis is 63 years, with 15% being younger than 45 years.

- Most common location is the back for men, and lower extremities followed by trunk for women, but can occur anywhere on the skin surface.

- Features used for melanoma recognition: A (*a*symmetry), B (*b*order), C (*c*olor), D (*d*iameter, >5 mm in most common use), and E (*e*volution).

- Follows a highly variable course and represents a heterogeneous disorder; surgically curable if diagnosed and treated in early phase, but potentially lethal with increased risk when diagnosed and treated late.

- In the last decades, completely new and effective treatment options for metastatic melanoma approved with immunotherapies such as the immune checkpoint blockade (anti-CTLA4, anti-PD-1 antibodies) and targeted therapies like BRAF/MEK inhibitors leading to a median overall survival of 2 years in stage IV melanoma and the chance for a long-term tumor control.

INTRODUCTION

DEFINITIONS

Melanoma (a word derived from the greek *melas* [dark] and *oma* [tumor]) is a malignant tumor arising from melanocytic cells and hence can occur anywhere where these cells are found. The most frequent type is cutaneous melanoma but melanomas develop also at the mucosal, the uveal, or even the meningeal membrane. Ten percent of melanomas are detected by lymph node metastases with so-called "unknown primary" and are likely to develop in the lymph node from preexisting nodal nevi.[1]

HISTORICAL PERSPECTIVE

Cancer is a disease that probably accompanied human life from the very beginning. The earliest physical evidence of melanoma comes from diffuse melanotic metastases found in skeletons of Pre-Colombian mummies from Chancay and Chingas in Peru, dated to be about 2400 years old (radiocarbon). However, the first descriptions of the disease can be found in the writings of Hippocrates of Cos in the 5th century BC.[2]

Until a few years ago, the only cure was by surgery in the early stages. The first documented operation of a melanoma was done by the Scottish surgeon John Hunter in 1787. The preserved tumor is still housed in the Hunterian Museum at Lincolns Inn Fields in London.[2] Until recently, in the unresectable metastatic setting, no treatment was available that could prolong patients' survival. This was revolutionized in the last decade by the approval of immunotherapies, the so-called immune checkpoint blockers, and targeted treatments to the frequently found *BRAF* mutations.

EPIDEMIOLOGY

The incidence of melanoma has increased significantly worldwide over the last several decades. It is mainly a tumor of people with fair skin from more developed regions. There is a low annual incidence in the whole world population of 3.0 new cases per 100,000 population—thus, it is not one of the top 10 cancers worldwide.[3] The highest incidence of melanoma is reported for Australia/New Zealand with about 35 new cases per year and 100,000 population, followed by Northern Europe and Northern America (Fig. 116-1). In the year 2016, an estimated 76,380 new cases of melanoma will be diagnosed in the United States of America translating to an annual incidence of 21.8 new cases per 100,000 population.[4] In Europe, incidence rates are lower, with an annual incidence of 13.5 new cases per 100,000 population and large differences between European countries, with the highest incidence in Switzerland for men and in Denmark for women.[5] Central and Eastern European countries have the lowest reported incidence rates in Europe. In the United States, incidence rises about 2.6% per year, leading to an increase of 33% for men and 23% for women between 2002 and 2006.[6] Across all cancers, melanoma incidence is the most rapidly increasing in men and is only second to lung cancer in women. Invasive melanoma of the skin is the fourth most frequent site for cancer to occur in men and the sixth most frequent site in women. By 2015, it is estimated that 1 in 50 Americans will develop melanoma in their lifetime.[6]

The median age for a melanoma diagnosis is 63 years with 15% being younger than 45 years. Incidence rises with age to a maximum between 55 and 74 years. Mortality data parallel incidence data, with a median age at death of 69 years.[4] Even though melanoma accounts for only 4% of all skin cancer diagnoses each year in the United States, it is responsible for 75% of skin cancer deaths. Currently, one US citizen dies from a melanoma every hour. However, even though melanoma incidence is rising rapidly with a tripling from

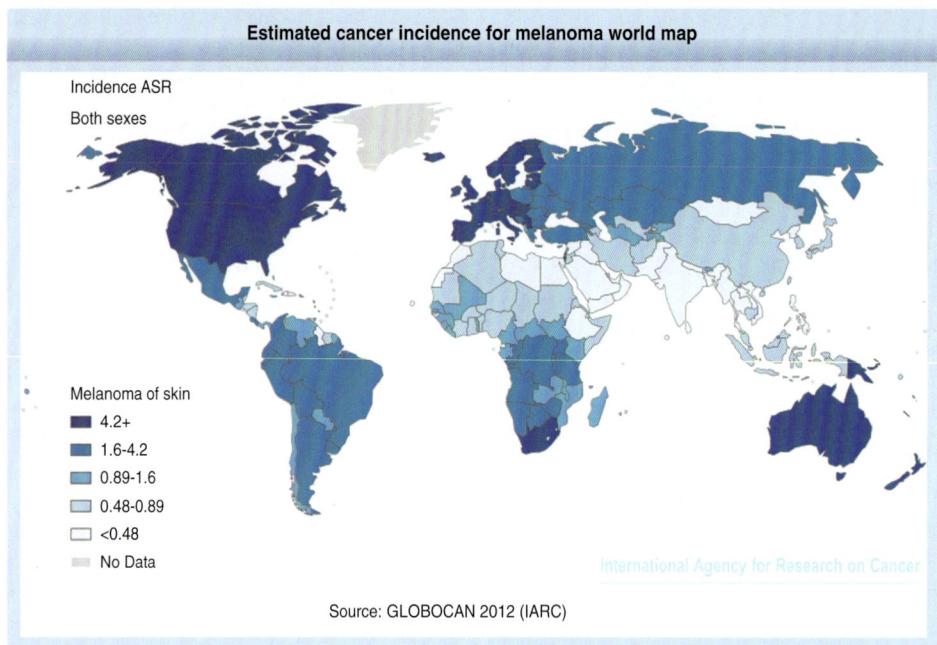

Figure 116-1 Estimated cancer incidence for melanoma world map. ASR = age-standardized rate. (Reproduced with permission from Ferlay J, Soerjomataram I, Ervik M, et al. GLOBOCAN 2012 v1.0, Cancer Incidence and Mortality Worldwide: IARC CancerBase No. 11 [Internet]. Lyon, France: International Agency for Research on Cancer; 2013. Available from: http://globocan.iarc.fr, accessed 13 September 2016.)

1980 to 2003, it is not associated with a corresponding increase in melanoma deaths. This is probably based on earlier detection and hence better prognosis of the melanoma.[6]

CLINICAL FEATURES

CUTANEOUS FINDINGS

The different subtypes of cutaneous melanoma can be distinguished clinically. However, these subtypes are not of prognostic significance itself, for example, a nodular or amelanotic melanoma might have a poorer prognosis compared to a superficial spreading melanoma but this is most likely based on a higher tumor thickness because of a later diagnosis.[7] However, clinical heterogeneity of melanomas might be explained by genetically distinct types of melanoma with different susceptibility to ultraviolet light.[8]

SUPERFICIAL SPREADING MELANOMA (SSM)

SSM is the most common subtype, accounting for approximately 70% of all cutaneous melanomas. It is diagnosed most commonly on intermittently sun-exposed areas, most frequently the lower extremity of women, and the upper back of men. Its classic clinical appearance best fits into the ABCD criteria (see section "Making a Diagnosis"), with irregular borders and irregular pigmentation, but it may present subtly as a discrete focal area of darkening within a preexisting nevus. The range of appearance of SSM is broad (Figs. 116-2A,B, and Fig. 116-3). Although varying shades of brown typify most melanocytic lesions, striking aspects of dark brown to black, blue-gray, red, and gray-white (which may represent regression) may be found in melanoma. SSM is the subtype of melanoma most commonly associated with preexisting nevi. The history of SSM is often of a lesion slowly changing over months to years. It may be mistaken for an atypical nevus or seborrheic keratosis.

NODULAR MELANOMA (NM)

NM is the second most common melanoma subtype and accounts for approximately 15% to 30% of all melanomas. The trunk is the most common site. NM is remarkable for rapid evolution, often arising over several weeks to months. NM more often lacks an apparent radial growth phase. It is more common for NM to begin de novo than to arise in a preexisting nevus. NM typically appears as a uniformly dark blue-black or bluish-red raised lesion, but 5% are amelanotic (Fig. 116-2C,D). Early lesions often lack

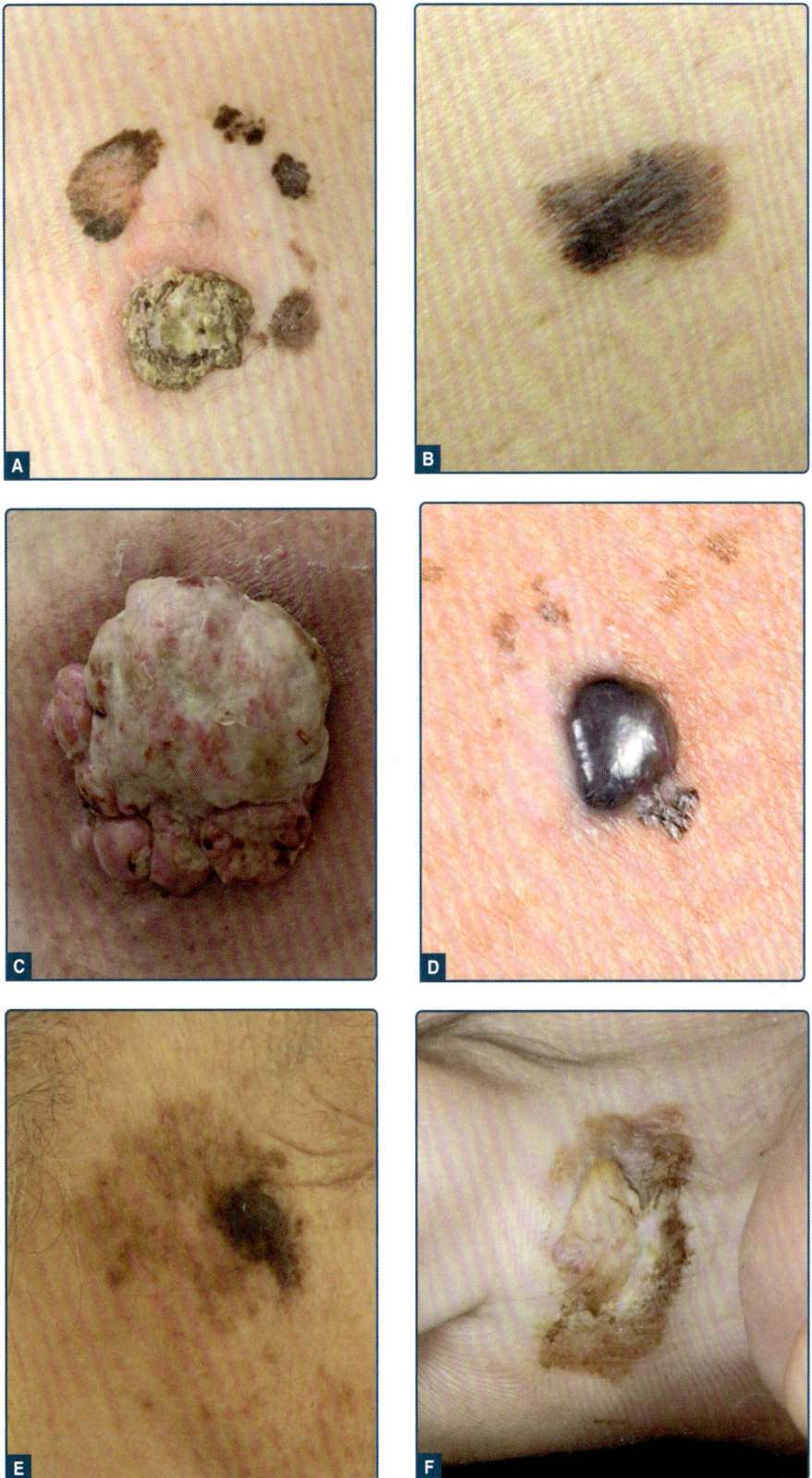

Figure 116-2 Clinical subtypes of melanoma: **A, B,** Superficial spreading melanoma, in **A** with extensive signs of regression (whole center of the lesion); **C,** ulcerated amelanotic nodular melanoma; **D,** pigmented nodular melanoma; **E,** lentigo maligna melanoma; **F,** acral lentiginous melanoma; **G,** subungual melanoma with melanonychia striata; **H,** ulcerated desmoplastic melanoma.

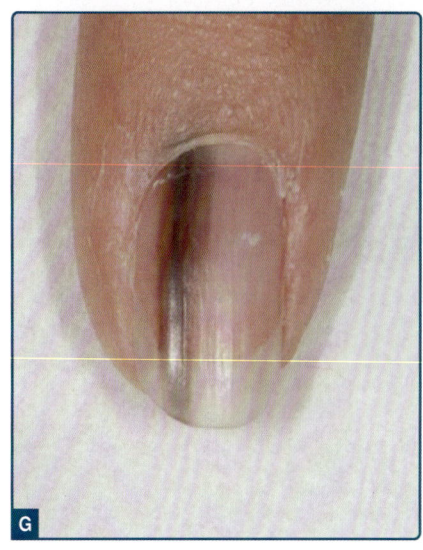
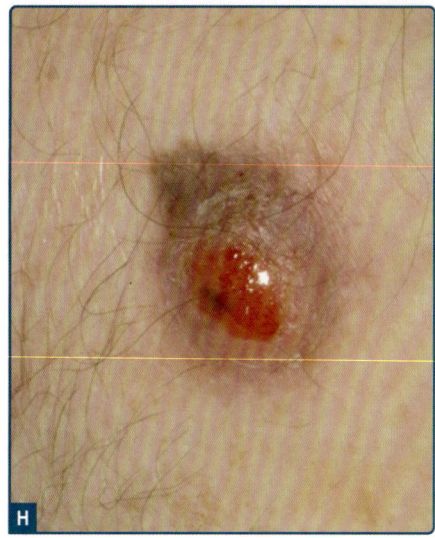

Figure 116-2 (*Continued*)

asymmetry, have regular borders, and are a uniform color. Amelanotic lesions may be mistaken for basal cell carcinoma, pyogenic granuloma, or hemangioma, whereas pigmented lesions may be mistaken for blue nevi or pigmented basal cell carcinomas. SSM and NM have the highest rate of mutations in the *BRAF* gene, with up to 56% of the melanomas harboring this alteration.[8] There is also an association with multiple melanocytic nevi.

LENTIGO MALIGNA (LM) AND LENTIGO MALIGNA MELANOMA (LMM)

LM is a melanoma in situ with a prolonged radial growth phase that eventually becomes invasive and is then called LMM. LMM constitutes 10% to 15% of cutaneous melanomas. LM and LMM are diagnosed most commonly in the seventh to eighth decades in an older

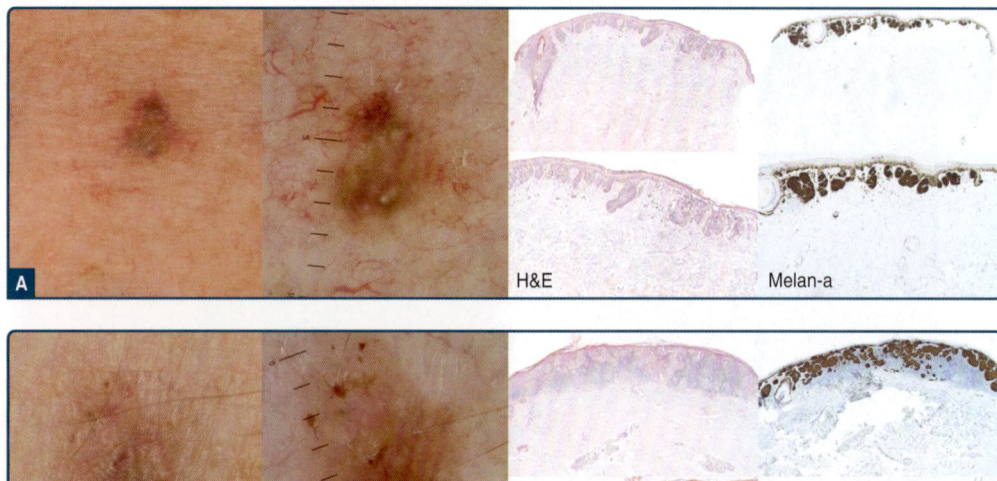

Figure 116-3 Clinical, dermoscopic and histologic presentation of 2 superficial spreading melanomas (**A, B**).

population than other types of melanoma—uncommon before the age 40. The most common location is on the chronically sun-exposed face, on the cheeks and nose in particular; the neck, scalp, and ears in men. Its pathogenesis is thought to be related to cumulative sun exposure rather than intermittent exposure. Clinical appearance is an initially flat, slowly enlarging, brown, frecklelike macule with irregular shape and differing shades of brown and tan, usually arising in a background of photodamage (Fig. 116-2E). Both LM and LMM often have clinically ill-defined borders, which may be obscured by background actinic damage consisting of lentigines, pigmented actinic keratoses, or ephelides. LM and LMM are associated with significantly higher rates of extensive subclinical lateral growth, resulting in higher recurrence rates with standard recommended margins and failure to completely excise the lesion. LM and LMM have the least common association with nevi, at 3% of cases, but the highest rate of association with desmoplastic melanoma (DM, see below). Molecularly, melanomas occurring in sun-damaged skin carry c-KIT aberrations (mutations and copy number changes) more frequently than BRAF mutations, with up to 28% versus 6%.[9]

ACRAL LENTIGINOUS MELANOMA (ALM)

ALM is a subtype of melanoma with distinct differences in frequencies seen between ethnic groups. ALM constitutes only 2% to 8% of melanomas in whites but represents the most common form in darker-pigmented individuals (60% to 72% in African Americans and 29% to 46% in Asians). Although the proportion of ALM seen in darker-pigmented individuals is higher, the incidence of ALM is similar between whites and other ethnicities. ALM is diagnosed more often in an older population, with the median age of onset of 65. The most common site for ALM is the sole, with the palm and subungual locations following (Fig. 116-2F). The clinical appearance of ALM is mainly brown to black, but red with variegations in color and irregular borders can occur. Often ALM are misdiagnosed first as a plantar wart or hematoma, leading to a more advanced lesion upon diagnosis associated with poorer outcomes. ALM is not thought to be associated with sun exposure.

Subungual melanoma, considered a variant of ALM, generally arises from the nail matrix, most commonly on the great toe or thumb (Fig. 116-2G). It appears as a brown to black discoloration or growth in the nail bed (Table 116-1). A widening, dark, or irregularly pigmented longitudinal nail streak (melanonychia striata) with or without nail dystrophy and nail plate elevation may be seen. Hutchinson sign, the finding of pigmentation on the proximal nail fold, may be noted with subungual melanoma. Benign lesions that mimic subungual melanoma include benign longitudinal melanonychia, subungual hematoma, pyogenic granuloma, or even onychomycosis with pigmentation or hemorrhage.

TABLE 116-1
When to Consider Malignancy in Pigmented Nail Lesions

- Lesion is isolated on a single digit
- Occurrence in the fourth to sixth decade
- Abrupt pigmentation in a previously normal nail plate
- Pigmentation appears darker, larger, or blurred towards the nail matrix (proximally)
- Acquired pigmentation of the thumb, index finger, or large toe
- Pigmentation occurring after a history of trauma, after ruling out subungual hematoma
- Individual with a history of melanoma
- Pigmentation associated with nail dystrophy, or absence of nail plate
- Pigmentation extending to the periungual skin (Hutchinson sign)

Braun R, Baran R, Frederique A, et al. Diagnosis and management of nail pigmentations. *J Am Acad Dermatol*. 2007;56(5):835-847.

In acral melanoma, the most frequent targetable mutation is the BRAF mutation (21%), followed by a c-KIT mutation (13%)[10]—c-KIT aberrations including copy number changes are higher, with up to 36% but with questionable clinical significance.[9]

DESMOPLASTIC MELANOMA (DM)

DM most commonly develops in the sixth or seventh decade on sun-exposed head and neck regions. The lesions typically have a firm, sclerotic, or indurated quality, and one-half are amelanotic (Fig. 116-2H). Approximately half of the lesions arise in association with the LM histologic subtype. Although often deeply invasive at the time of diagnosis with a tendency to perineural growth, DM is associated with higher local recurrence but lower nodal metastatic rates than other subtypes of melanoma when matched for depth of invasion. Results from a small study that involved 10 samples that investigated gene expression profiling demonstrated a molecular distinction between DM and nondesmoplastic melanoma.[11] DMs reveal a high mutation burden most likely induced by UV radiation. BRAF and NRAS mutations are not found; instead, other genetic alteration known to activate the MAPK signaling cascade were identified, for example, mutations in neurofibromin (NF1) in more than 90% of cases.[12,13]

MUCOSAL MELANOMA

Melanoma can infrequently (1.3% of melanomas) arise on mucosal surfaces on the head and neck (conjunctival, intranasal, sinus, and oral cavities), genital, anorectal, or even urethral mucosa (Fig. 116-4).[14] With the exception of the conjunctiva, patients present most often with delayed detection and a deeply pigmented, irregular lesion, often tumorous with signs of bleeding. As most of these lesions present initially with a radial growth phase manifesting a macular pigmentation, any suspicious area in these sites should be biopsied. Lesions of the conjunctiva are visible and appear

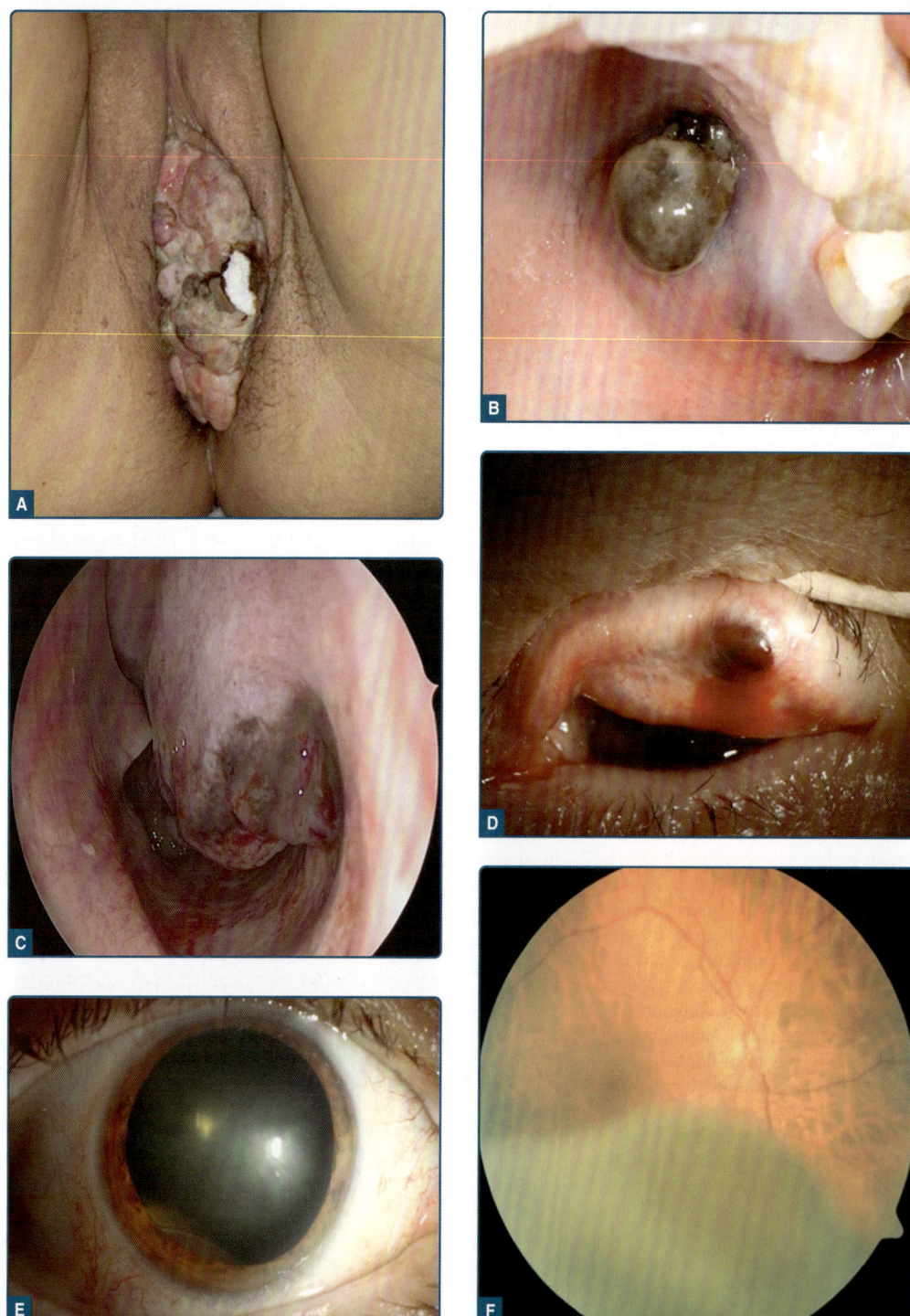

Figure 116-4 Mucosal melanomas: **A,** Introitus vaginae; **B,** gingiva; **C,** intranasal; **D,** conjunctiva; **E, F** uveal melanoma. (**A-C,** With friendly permission to publish from J. Thierauf, Department of ENT, University Hospital Heidelberg; **D-F,** Permission to publish from A. Scheuerle, Department of Ophthalmology, University Hospital Heidelberg.)

increased in patients with atypical nevi.[15] Mucosal melanomas are more frequent in women, especially based on the genital tract melanomas. Melanomas on vulva and vagina account for about 50% of the mucosal melanomas among women. In both genders, the nasal cavity was otherwise the most frequent location for mucosal melanomas. Anorectal melanomas account for only 16.5% of mucosal melanomas.[14]

Mucosal melanoma differs from cutaneous melanoma on the molecular level. Besides NF1, the most frequently occurring driver mutations are RAS alterations, consisting of *NRAS* and *KRAS* mutations with a frequency between 5% and 30% that lead to an activation of the MAPK pathway similar to BRAF mutations. Less than 10% of mucosal melanomas harbor *BRAF* mutations.[16-18] Only in mucosal melanomas of vulvovaginal origin, the mutation frequency is higher, with up to 26% for BRAF and lower for RAS.[19] More frequent than in cutaneous melanoma, mutations of the receptor tyrosine kinase c-kit can be found with varying frequencies in between 5% and 20% of mucosal melanomas.[9,16,17] Here, frequency again seems to be higher in tumors of vulvovaginal or anorectal origin, compared with other sites.[19,20] This mutation is targetable with multi-kinase inhibitors such as imatinib[21]; however, the mutation status of the tumors showed no association with patients' survival outcomes.[17]

NEVOID MELANOMA

Nevoid melanoma describes a heterogeneous group of rare lesions that histologically resemble benign nevi by their symmetry and apparent maturation with descent in the dermis, thus with greater potential for misdiagnosis. Clues to their histologic diagnosis include marked hyperchromasia of the nuclei of the tumor cells, the presence of mitoses, and expansive growth of the dermal cells. Clinically, this may correspond to a tan papule or nodule, more often >1 cm in diameter on a young adult.[22]

SPITZOID MELANOMA

Spitzoid melanoma is a subtype of melanoma that clinically and histologically resembles a Spitz nevus, but tends to be larger and have asymmetry and irregular coloration. Features that favor the diagnosis of a Spitzoid melanoma over a benign Spitz nevus are large size (greater than 1 cm in greatest dimension); lesions with a thick invasive component (>2 mm Breslow thickness); lesions with numerous mitoses (especially any atypical forms), many cytologically atypical cells, and lesions that have a clinically concerning course such as very rapid growth in size or satellitosis. Clinical and histologic distinction between the two is often extremely difficult, and tumors with overlapping features of Spitz nevi and melanoma are classified as atypical Spitz tumors of uncertain biologic behavior (AST).[23]

Whereas common acquired nevi and melanoma often harbor *BRAF* mutations, *NRAS* mutations, or inactivation of NF1, Spitz tumors show *HRAS* mutations, inactivation of *BAP1*, or genomic rearrangements involving kinases like ALK, ROS1 and others. Additional genomic aberrations may abrogate various tumor-suppressive mechanisms and lead to atypia and malignant transformation. Comparative genomic hybridization (CGH) is generally able to differentiate Spitz tumors of benign or malignant behavior and may help classify the histologically ambiguous tumors, that is, the AST.[24]

OTHER RARE TYPES

Several other rare and unusual types of melanoma are beyond the scope of this chapter, but previously reported in a comprehensive review, which include metaplastic melanoma, balloon cell melanoma, signet-ring cell melanoma, myxoid melanoma, rhabdoid melanoma, animal-type melanoma, and malignant blue nevus.[22,25]

NONCUTANEOUS FINDINGS

Although most melanomas develop on the skin, there are rarer types of noncutaneous melanomas arising from extracutaneous melanocytes, for example, in the choroidea. In addition, mucosal melanomas (see before) are defined as noncutaneous melanomas as they can occur at mucosa of the ear, nose, and throat (ENT) region, intestine, or urinary tract. Melanomas of unknown primary that most often are diagnosed with lymph node metastases might develop from nodal nevi.[1] As nodal nevi only occur in skin draining lymph nodes, the precursor lesion here might be nevus cells that escaped from melanocytic nevi of the skin.[26,27]

UVEAL MELANOMAS

Uveal melanomas account for about 5% of all melanomas and develop mainly in the choroid, followed by ciliary body and iris of the eye.[28] Nevertheless, uveal melanoma is the most common primary intraocular malignancy. The median age at diagnosis is 58 years. Risk factors include the presence of a choroidal nevus, a nevus of Ota, and dysplastic nevus syndrome. There is an 8 times higher incidence rate in whites as compared to the black population, leading to the hypothesis that UV exposure increases the risk for uveal melanoma, but this has not been definitely proven.[14] Clinically most patients present with painless loss or distortion of vision or the tumor is diagnosed in asymptomatic patients in routine ophthalmic screening. The risk of metastases could be linked to chromosomal aberrations. Patients with monosomy 3 (about 50% of patients) had a much poorer clinical outcome, with a disease-specific mortality of 75.1% for patients with monosomy 3 and 13.2% for patients with disomy 3 after 5 years, respectively.[29] Patients usually die from liver metastases, the primary metastatic site in uveal melanoma probably based on the microenvironment in the liver that seems to support growth of the metastases there, for example, by secretion of the hepatocyte growth factor (HGF).[30]

COMPLICATIONS

If complications occur with melanoma, they are usually based on *metastatic disease* within organs leading to symptoms associated with the affected organ.

These include pain (any metastases), convulsion (brain metastases), instabilities (bone metastases), etc and later on all the symptoms associated with progression of the disease and death in the palliative setting.

Relatively frequent *cutaneous changes* associated with melanoma are localized or diffuse hypo- or hyperpigmentation. The development of a melanoma-associated vitiligo as an accompanying autoimmune disease against melanocytes is reported to occur in up to 4% of patients and is associated with a better prognosis.[31] Vitiligo has become especially frequent in patients treated with immune checkpoint blockers, and is also correlated with a better treatment response.[32] In highly advanced patients, a diffuse cutaneous melanosis can occur that is characterized by a slate-grey pigmentation over the entire skin surface, mucosal membranes, and internal organs, with accentuation in photo-exposed areas. Such cases are often associated with melanuria, a darkening of the urine. Histopathologically, melanin deposits in the connective tissue and within macrophages in a perivascular distribution can be found. These most likely come from ischemic metastases distributed through the body via the blood.[31]

Rare complications based on *paraneoplastic mechanisms* described like dermatomyositis (Chap. 62)[31] and autoimmune retinopathies also occur.[33] Melanoma-associated retinopathies (MAR) present after the melanoma has been diagnosed as metastatic and are more frequent in men. Patients may develop vision problems years later, leading to latency from melanoma diagnosis to recognition of MAR on average after 3.6 years. Pathophysiologically, antiretinal antibodies against different structures like the bipolar cells, transducing, rhodopsin, and others can be found.

ETIOLOGY AND PATHOGENESIS

There are several risk factors for melanoma, with sun exposure and genetics being the 2 most important ones. Risk prediction models reveal in detail that the number of nevi, presence of freckles, history of sunburn, hair color, and skin color are the best measures to estimate melanoma risk.[34,35] All these factors are influenced by the genetic background leading to a certain photosensitivity.

SUN EXPOSURE

There is clear convincing evidence that sun exposure, and more specifically ultraviolet (UV) exposure, is a major environmental cause of melanoma, especially in high-risk populations. However, certainly not all melanomas are sun related. Bastian and others suggested a molecular classification for melanoma based on the hypothesis that clinical heterogeneity is explained by genetically distinct types of melanoma with different susceptibility to ultraviolet light.[8]

Epidemiologic studies suggest that periodic, intense sun exposure (particularly during the critical time period of childhood and adolescence) rather than long, continued, heavy sun exposure is most important in melanoma causation, termed the *intermittent exposure* hypothesis. Sunburn history, notably blistering and peeling burns, serves as a surrogate measure of intermittent intense sun exposure. In most melanoma risk prediction models, the history of sunburns is an important risk factor, not just in childhood,[34-36] that is, the more sunburns in a lifetime, the higher the melanoma risk. One blistering sunburn in childhood more than doubles a person's chances of developing melanoma later in life.[37]

The anatomic distribution of melanoma by body site demonstrates that intermittently exposed skin areas have the highest rates of developing melanoma. In men, the trunk, particularly the upper back, is the most common site for melanoma. In women, the lower legs, followed by the trunk, are the most common sites.[38] These intermittently exposed areas are the most common areas to develop melanoma in younger persons. In older persons, there is a greater incidence of melanomas located on chronically exposed areas with maximal cumulative sun exposure. The face is the most common location for melanoma in older persons, with the addition of the neck, scalp, and ears as well, in older men.[39]

Several forms of artificial light have been associated with the development of melanoma, particularly psoralen and UVA light (PUVA) and UVB as well as tanning booths. The so-called *PUVA Follow-up Study* demonstrated increased rates of melanoma after PUVA exposure, with an incidence rate ratio of 9.3 approximately 20 years after PUVA therapy; these rates increase over time and are higher in patients exposed to high cumulative doses of PUVA.[40] However, in 2 European cohorts of PUVA-treated patients, there was no increased risk for melanoma detected in contrast to nonmelanoma skin cancers such as squamous and basal cell carcinomas.[41] There is also rising concern over tanning beds and melanoma risk, especially because exposure to the artificial UV radiation is intermittent in nature. Any exposure to artificial tanning devices significantly increases the risk of cutaneous melanoma, and longer duration of bed use, younger age at first exposure, and higher frequency of use are associated with a significantly elevated risk (odds ratio 1.69).[42] Moreover, indoor tanning also has been associated with accelerated skin aging and ocular melanoma.[43]

Pathophysiologically, DNA-damaging, carcinogenic, inflammatory, and immunosuppressive properties of UV radiation contribute to initiation, progression, and metastasis of primary melanoma.[37,44] UV-A (320 to 400 nm) and UV-B (280 to 320 nm) have a significant impact, with UV-B directly damaging the DNA and UV-A mainly by the production of reactive oxygen species (ROS). The final proof of the carcinogenic property of UV on melanoma development was given by a large Australian clinical trial. In 1992, a total of 1621 randomly selected residents from Queensland between

25 and 75 years of age were randomly assigned to daily or discretionary sunscreen use to head and arms until 2006. Ten years after trial cessation, the rate of primary melanomas was halved in the daily sunscreen group, with 11 new primary melanomas instead of 22 in the discretionary sunscreen group.[45]

SKIN PHENOTYPE

Light skin pigmentation, blond or red hair, blue or green eyes, prominent freckling tendency, and tendency to sunburn with Fitzpatrick skin phototype I–II are phenotypic features associated with an increased risk of melanoma of 2- to 3-fold.[34,46] Melanoma occurs much less frequently in Type V–VI skin, suggesting that skin pigment plays a protective role. This is explained of course by different photosensitivity and ability to tan.

MELANOCYTIC NEVI

There is an increased risk of melanoma associated with nevi, both in a quantitative (ie, number of nevi) and qualitative (ie, typical vs atypical nevi) manner.[34,47] Adults with more than 100 clinically typical-appearing nevi, children with more than 50 typical-appearing nevi, and any patient with atypical nevi are at risk. The presence of a solitary dysplastic nevus doubles the risk of melanoma, while having 10 or more atypical nevi is associated with a 12-fold elevation of risk.[48] Nevi more often serve as a genetic marker of increased risk rather than a premalignant lesion, as most melanomas arise de novo. In a study of 1606 patients with melanoma, only 26% of the melanomas were histologically associated with nevi (43% of these atypical nevi, 57% other nevi).[49] However, sun exposure plays an important role to acquire melanocytic nevi, particularly in early childhood. Hence, the amount of melanocytic nevi as a risk factor for melanoma development is influenced by genetic as well as environmental factors.[47]

There is a recognized risk of melanoma development in large congenital nevi, which varies depending on the size of the lesion.[50,51] Many series define large congenital nevi as greater than 20 cm in diameter in adulthood, and lifetime risks for developing melanoma are generally accepted to be in the 2% to 10% range. In a large review of more than 2500 patients with a large congenital melanocytic nevus, 2% developed a melanoma at a median age of 12.6 years (range birth to 58 years). In 74% of patients, the melanocytic nevus was greater than 40 cm in diameter, and 94% had satellite nevi.[51] Patients with large congenital nevi located on the posterior axis (paraspinal, head, and neck regions) or in conjunction with multiple satellite lesions are at risk for neurocutaneous melanosis, with an increased risk of developing melanoma in the CNS. Melanomas developing on large congenital nevi are usually detected late and hence have a bad prognosis, with more than 50% of them being fatal.[51] For small- to medium-sized congenital nevi, the melanoma risk is similar to any other area of skin.[50] Thus, prophylactic excision of small- and medium-sized congenital nevi is usually unwarranted.

TABLE 116-2
Genes Associated with Melanoma

| CDKN2A |
| p16 |
| CDK4 |
| POT1 |
| TERT |
| BAP1 |
| BRAF |
| NRAS |
| HRAS |
| NF1 |
| c-KIT |

FAMILY HISTORY

Patients with familial melanoma are estimated to account for approximately 5% to 12% of all patients with melanoma.[46] Having one first-degree relative with melanoma doubles the risk of melanoma, whereas having 3 or more first-degree relatives with melanoma increases the risk 35- to 70-fold.[52] Some of this risk may be attributed to shared risk factors such as skin phenotype, multiple nevi, and excessive sun exposure. The association between familial melanoma and multiple atypical nevi has historically been given various names, including *B-K mole* syndrome*, *familial atypical multiple mole-melanoma syndrome*, and *dysplastic nevus syndrome*. Patients with familial melanoma typically have earlier-onset melanoma and multiple primaries as well as atypical nevi. In addition, patients with familial melanoma have an increased risk of internal cancers, such as pancreatic cancer or CNS tumors.[46]

Different genes are responsible for the development of inherited melanoma (Table 116-2) and genetic alterations typically increase cancer risk via 3 major mechanisms: the activation of oncogenes, the loss of tumor suppressor genes, or increased chromosomal instability. Inherited mutations in *CDKN2A*, *CDK4*, *POT1*, and *TERT* confer a 60% to 90% lifetime risk of melanoma.

CDKN2A-CDK4-TP53 PATHWAY MUTATIONS

Germline mutations in the chromosome 9p21 tumor suppressor gene, cyclin-dependent kinase inhibitor 2A (*CDKN2A*), account for approximately 40% of hereditary melanoma cases (≥3 melanomas in one lineage). In countries with high levels of UV exposure, the lifetime melanoma risk in carriers of the *CDKN2A* mutation

---

*B-K=initials of the first 2 described related patients.

is 76% (United States) and 91% (Australia), whereas the risk is lower in countries with low levels of UV exposure (58%, United Kingdom).[46] Individuals with germline *CDKN2A* mutations also exhibit a higher risk of pancreatic cancer; an estimated 15% of individuals with a mutant allele will develop pancreatic cancer in their lifetime.[53] Bona fide deleterious point mutations in *CDKN2A* are relatively uncommon in primary melanoma tumors although homozygous deletions of this gene may obscure the true rate of somatic loss in melanoma. *CDKN2A* encodes 2 gene products: p16 (also known as *INK4a*, inhibitor of kinase 4a) and p14[ARF] (alternative reading frame). p16 is a cell-cycle regulator that binds and inhibits cyclin-dependent kinases Cdk4 or Cdk6, thereby inhibiting progression of cells through the G1 phase of the cell cycle (Fig. 116-5). If p16 function is absent or inactivated by mutation, unrestrained Cdk4 activity phosphorylates the retinoblastoma protein, thereby releasing the transcription factor E2-F and inducing S-phase entry. This sequence culminates in enhanced cellular proliferation, which, in the absence of checkpoint regulation, results in unrestrained growth and neoplasia.

The binding partner of the p16 protein is Cdk4. Only a handful of families worldwide thus far have been reported to carry hereditary mutations in *CDK4*, while somatic mutations in this gene also have been detected in some melanoma cell lines. Functional studies suggest that mutations in Cdk4 render the cyclin-dependent protein kinase resistant to p16 inhibition, resulting in a phenotype identical to that from p16 loss.

The p14[ARF] protein from *CDKN2A* inhibits a cellular oncogene Hdm2, which in turn accelerates the destruction of the p53 tumor-suppressor gene.[54] Complete loss of *CDKN2A* also leads to abrogation of p14[ARF] and loss of p53 function. Thus, this single locus can inactivate both the retinoblastoma protein and p53 pathways and probably explains the low rate of direct *TP53* mutagenesis in melanoma.

GENES INVOLVED IN TELOMERE MAINTENANCE

POT1 and TERT mutations are prevalent in 9% of patients with hereditary melanoma and, when normally functioning, contribute to protection of exposed chromosomal ends.[46] Increased TERT activity may allow unlimited cell division and subsequently promote cancer progression.

DIAGNOSIS

Early detection is the key to improving prognosis in melanoma, as the risk of metastases increases with infiltration depth of the primary. Although melanoma may have a characteristic appearance, there is no single clinical feature that ensures or excludes a diagnosis of melanoma. Change in color and increase in size (or a new lesion) are the 2 most common early characteristics noticed by patients that may be useful in discriminating between melanoma and other benign lesions.[55]

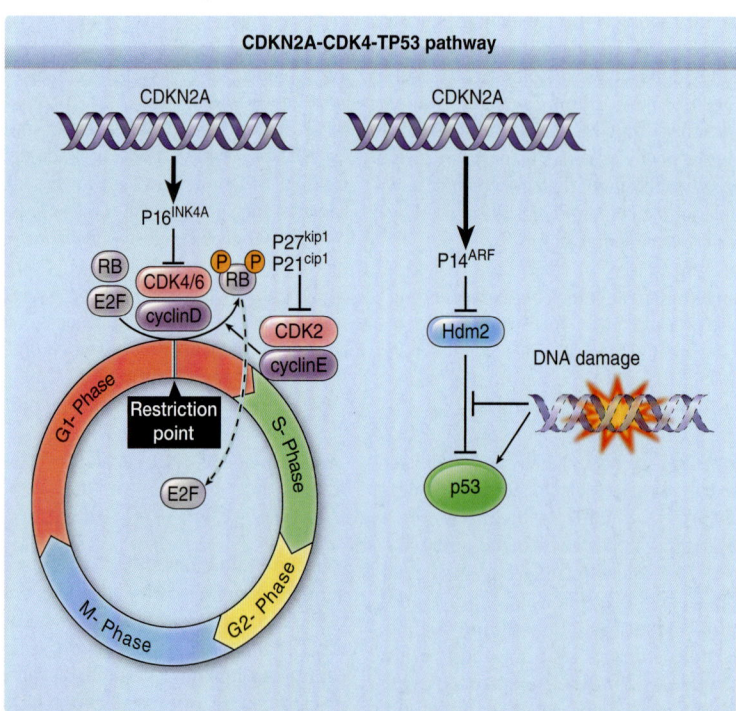

Figure 116-5 Mutations in the tumor suppressor gene *CDKN2A* account for approximately 40% of hereditary melanoma cases and lead to a loss of cell cycle control (**A**) and antiapoptosis (**B**).

PHYSICAL EXAMINATION

The skin examination should be conducted under optimal lighting and encompass the entire skin integument, including the scalp, external ocular/conjunctivae, oral mucosa, groin, buttocks, and palms/soles/web spaces. Melanomas in hidden anatomic sites are associated with thicker tumors at diagnosis, often as a result of later detection.[56] Clinical diagnosis of melanoma can be made in about 80% to 90% of cases. The well-known *ABCDE acronym* for melanoma detection continues to be a useful tool for the lay public and physicians.[57,58] *A* stands for asymmetry (one half is not identical to the other half), *B* for border (irregular, notched, scalloped, ragged, or poorly defined borders as opposed to smooth and straight edges), *C* for color (having varying shades from one area to another), *D* for diameter (ie, greater than 5 mm), and *E* for evolution (changes in the lesion over time). Lesions having these characteristics may potentially represent melanoma. Studies have found the sensitivity of the ABCDE checklist (Table 116-3) to be very high, but the specificity much lower.[59]

Another diagnostic aid that is useful in detecting melanoma is the "ugly duckling" sign.[60] A pigmented lesion that is different from other pigmented lesions on a particular individual should be approached with a high index of suspicion. This is based on the premise that within an individual, nevi should globally share a common appearance or family resemblance. Even in an individual with multiple atypical nevi, the nevi should be morphologically similar.

DERMOSCOPY

Dermoscopy (also known as *epiluminescence microscopy, dermatoscopy, incident light microscopy,* and *surface microscopy*) is a noninvasive technique in which a handheld device is used to examine a lesion through a film of liquid (eg, immersion oil), using nonpolarized light (contact dermoscopy), or the lesion is examined under polarized light without a contact medium (noncontact dermoscopy). In experienced hands, it may improve both the sensitivity and specificity for the clinical diagnosis of melanoma and other pigmented and nonpigmented lesions.[61,62] Morphologic features (Table 116-4) that are otherwise not visible to the naked eye are observed using this technique that allows visualization of microstructures of the epidermis, the dermoepidermal junction, and the papillary dermis (Fig.116-3).

Different diagnostic algorithms using dermoscopic findings have been developed for melanoma, including the ABCD rule, the 7-point checklist, pattern analysis, Menzies method, modified ABC-point list, and CASH (color, architecture, symmetry, and homogeneity).[63-66] Several studies have compared these methods to determine the most effective method for dermoscopic detection of melanoma.[63,64] Pattern analysis, which provides an overall impression of multiple dermoscopic patterns without rigid rules, based primarily on a subjective, simultaneous evaluation of a number of different criteria, is the most widely used method among experienced users of dermoscopy for evaluating pigmented lesions.[67]

Digital dermoscopy or digital epiluminescent microscopy permits computerized digital dermoscopic images to be retrieved and examined at a later date so that comparisons can be made and changes detected over time. There are also a number of commercially available automated computer image analysis programs, devices that incorporate image analysis algorithms to digital dermoscopic images, providing objective measurement of changes over time. Sequential digital dermoscopy was shown to improve early diagnosis of melanoma compared to standard dermoscopy.[68,69]

The use of body or lesional photography can help to monitor minor changes in melanocytic lesions, particularly in patients with many nevi. Finally, confocal scanning laser microscopy and multispectral digital dermoscopy are among a number of new imaging techniques being evaluated for early detection of melanomas.[70,71]

HISTOLOGY

Patients with lesions clinically suspicious for melanoma should, whenever possible, undergo prompt excisional biopsy with narrow margins. A wider margin should be avoided to permit the most accurate

TABLE 116-4
Dermoscopic Features of Melanoma

- Atypical pigment network
- Negative network
- Atypical dots or globules
- Irregular streaks
- Regression structures
- Blue-white veil
- Shiny white lines
- Atypical blotch
- Polymorphous vessels

Data from Wolner Z, Yelamos O, Liopyris K, et al. Enhancing skin cancer diagnosis with dermoscopy. *Dermatol Clin.* 2017;35(4):417-37.

TABLE 116-3
ABCDE Checklist[a]

- A = Asymmetry
- B = Border
- C = Color
- D = Diameter
- E = Evolution

[a]Does not apply to nodular or desmoplastic melanoma.

subsequent SLNB if indicated.[72] However, if the lesion is large and/or located on anatomic areas such as the palm/sole, digit, face, or ear, an incisional skin biopsy may be performed in the most elevated or darkest area of the lesion, with a strong appreciation that the clinically most suspicious area may not always correlate with the thickest portion of the lesion. There is no evidence that biopsy or incision of a primary melanoma leads to "seeding" of tissue and adversely affects survival.[73] Excisional biopsy performed after incisional biopsy of melanoma with ≥50% of the lesion remaining resulted in significant upstaging in 21% of patients, and change in SLNB consideration in 10% of patients in one large study.[74] Hence, a wider margin should be taken after complete excision with narrow margins and histologic evaluation of the whole lesion.

Excisional biopsy, if possible, is important because symmetry of the whole lesion is one major criterion in differentiating a benign melanocytic nevus from melanoma. The histologic diagnosis of melanoma is based on the assessment of a constellation of findings, including both architectural and cytologic features. No single feature is diagnostic. The major architectural features of melanoma include asymmetry, poor circumscription (cells at the edge of the lesion tend to be small, single, and scattered rather than nested), and large size (>5 to 6 mm). Nests of melanocytes in the lower epidermis and dermis tend to vary in size and shape, and to become confluent. There is a lack of maturation of nests with descent into the dermis. In addition, single melanocytes dominate over nests and show an aberrant distribution (Fig. 116-3).[75] The presence of melanocytes above the basal layer (pagetoid spread), usually considered diagnostic of melanoma in situ, should be assessed cautiously in the context of other findings, as pagetoid spread may be seen in benign lesions including Spitz nevi and nevi in special anatomic regions (vulvar nevi, acral nevi). The different subtypes of melanoma may also have histopathologic differences (Fig. 116-6), especially DM, which is composed of strands of elongated, spindle-shaped cells that often infiltrate deeply in a sarcomatoid pattern.

Immunohistochemistry may be useful for the diagnosis of melanoma, especially in poorly differentiated neoplasms with little or no pigment (ie, amelanotic melanomas), spindle cell tumors, or tumors with pagetoid spread that are not obviously melanoma. S100 and Sox10 proteins are expressed by almost all melanomas,

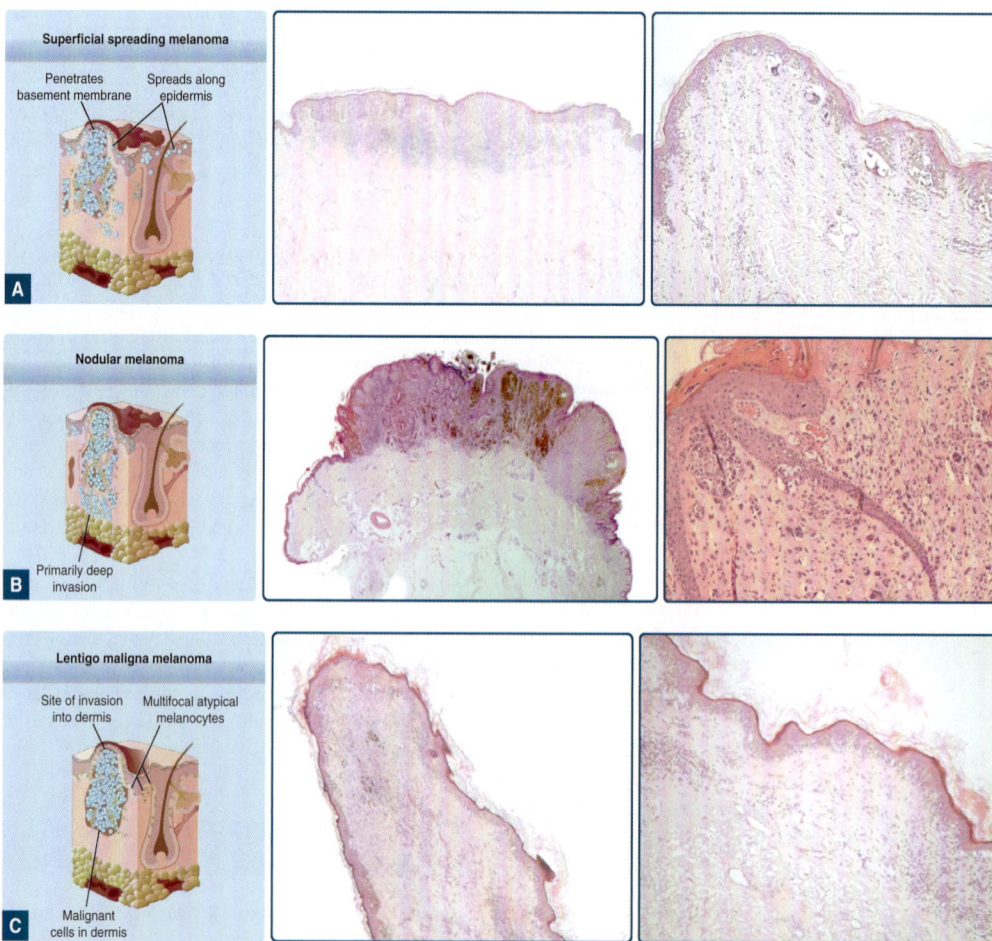

Figure 116-6 Histologic appearance (schematic, histopathologic overview, and close-up) of superficial spreading melanoma (**A**), nodular melanoma (**B**), and lentigo maligna melanoma (**C**).

but also by melanocytic nevi, and other tumor types, including cutaneous neural tumors. HMB-45 is a monoclonal antibody with high specificity for melanoma cells. Melan-A and MART-1 (melanoma antigen recognized by T cells) are the names given independently to the same gene encoding a melanocytic differentiation antigen expressed in the skin and retina. Melan-A is broadly expressed in benign and malignant melanocytic lesions. It is more sensitive than HMB-45 and more specific than S100 for melanoma. Search for the microphthalmia-associated transcription factor (MiTF) may be useful, especially in amelanotic melanomas, as it is a marker in the nucleus, whereas all other markers are mainly intracytoplasmic.[76] Immunohistochemically, DMs commonly express only S100 and Sox10[77] and lack other melanocytic markers like HMB-45, Melan-A, and MiTF.

In nevoid melanomas staining for the proliferation rate, for example, with Ki-67, might be helpful to uncover malignancy.

In addition to diagnosis, histology gives further clinically important information on the infiltration depth (Breslow thickness) and ulceration status—features needed for AJCC (American Academy of Dermatology) classification and prognostic evaluation.[78] Further diagnostic investigations are stage dependent as the risk to metastasize increases with tumor stage.[78]

LABORATORY TESTING

As early as in 1954, increased levels of lactate dehydrogenase (LDH) were detected in the serum of melanoma patients.[79] Ever since, the value of LDH as a tumor marker for melanoma has been discussed. S100B in the serum is a bit more specific than LDH but lacks sensitivity. For that reason, S100B can be detected and monitored in clinical followup as an additional marker to detect progression of the disease.[80] Hence, blood investigations to measure for tumor markers play a minor role in the diagnosis of melanoma, but are mainly used to monitor the clinical course. Testing of the nonspecific tumor marker LDH is indicated only for patients with distant metastatic disease as it is needed for AJCC classification and prognostic evaluation.[78,81]

Other tumor markers like melanoma-inhibiting activity (MIA), tumor-associated antigen 90 immune complex (TA90IC), and YKL-40 are under investigation and not used in routine clinical practice. It is not clear as of this writing if they add a benefit to S100B and LDH.[79]

IMAGING

REGIONAL SKIN AND LYMPH NODE ULTRASOUND

Patients should be evaluated for regional spread by careful palpation of lymph nodes first, particularly the primary echelon nodal basin(s). The concepts of aberrant lymphatic drainage pathways to unexpected nodal basins and interval nodes located between the primary site and the expected regional nodal basin have taught physicians to search for clinically detectable nodal disease in unexpected locations.[82] Skin and lymph node ultrasonography is perhaps the most sensitive noninvasive method to detect small nodal metastases and is much more sensitive than clinical examination.[83] Lymph node metastases are characterized by a ballooned shape, loss of central echo, and peripheral perfusion.[84] If a lymph node or a dermal/subcutaneous nodule in the regional area of the primary is found, an excisional biopsy should be performed if possible.

TOMOGRAPHY

Routine imaging and hematologic tests in asymptomatic patients rarely identifies occult systemic disease.[85] Tomographic investigations like computed tomography (CT), magnet resonance imaging (MRI) and positron emission tomography (PET) are generally not recommended at the stage of primary melanoma.[86,87] The rate of false positive findings is far too high (8%-15%), for example, unspecific lung lesions,[88] which leads to additional cost of followup studies and possibly invasive procedures, as well as increased patient anxiety. Unfortunately, there are no data demonstrating improved survival rates if metastases are detected when clinically asymptomatic versus early symptomatic stage IV disease. However, especially in high-risk melanomas (>4 mm Breslow thickness), the risk for hematologic spread increases, and tomographic imaging can be justified. Distant metastases are more likely in patients with regional metastases. However, in a retrospective analysis of 185 patients with a positive sentinel lymph node (SLN), only 1 patient (0.5%) had detectable metastatic disease on the imaging. Hence, imaging with CT, MRI, or PET is indicated only in high-risk and known metastatic melanoma and recommended to be performed as clinically indicated. This further emphasizes the importance of a thorough melanoma-focused review of systems and physical examination.

SENTINEL LYMPH NODE BIOPSY (SLNB)

The SLN is per definition the first draining lymph node in the lymphatic draining system of the primary tumor. SLNB is a powerful staging and prognostic tool which may be used to detect occult micrometastases in regional lymph nodes,[89] and represents the best baseline staging test for detection of occult nodal metastasis in the subset of melanoma patients where it is indicated. SLNB is far more sensitive and accurate at detecting microscopic metastases than PET scan, CT scans, or ultrasonographic imaging combined with lymph node fine-needle aspiration.[85] In a meta-analysis of 34 studies, a Breslow thickness of <1 mm was associated with a positive SLN in 5.6% of patients.[90] This rate was higher (19.5%) in patients younger than 40 years and a tumor with 0.75 to 1 mm thickness as well as in ulcerated primary melanomas and melanomas with detectable mitoses.[91-93] For patients with lesions of a Breslow thickness between 1 and 4 mm Breslow, 25.2% had a positive SLN, whereas those with lesions >4 mm in thickness had a 50% likelihood of SLN positivity.[92,94] Based on this risk stratification, SLNB is recommended in patients with a melanoma ≥1 mm Breslow thickness.[89,90] In addition, it can be offered for patients with thinner melanomas (0.8-1 mm) or even <0.8 mm if additional risk factors such as high mitotic index or lymphovascular invasion exists, especially in the setting of young age.[91]

In current practice, technetium-99–labeled radiocolloid solution, often complemented with vital blue dye, allows for detection of the SLN >98% of the time in skilled hands.[95] Ideally, the procedure should be performed at the same time as wide local excision (WLE) of the primary melanoma for greatest accuracy. SLNB may not be accurate if performed after WLE in areas of ambiguous or surgically altered lymphatic drainage or following a local skin flap due to radiocolloid and dye injection location away from the true primary site.[96] Once removed, the SLN(s) must be assessed with serial sectioning, using standard hematoxylin and eosin (H&E) techniques often combined with immunohistochemical stains such as S100, HMB-45, and/or Melan-A. The use of immunostains increases sensitivity for melanoma and has resulted in the upstaging of up to 10% to 20% of patients.[97] In melanoma, even single melanoma cells in the immunostains of the sentinel define the lymph node as sentinel positive (N1a). In 2006, Morton et al published the third interim analysis of the multicenter sentinel lymphadenectomy trial (MSLT)–I, the first prospective randomized controlled clinical trial of SLNB in melanoma.[98] In this analysis, 1269 clinically node-negative patients with newly diagnosed melanoma 1.2 to 3.5 mm in depth were randomized to wide excision and nodal basin observation versus wide excision and SLNB. Patients with a positive SLN received an immediate complete lymph node dissection (CLND), and patients in the observation arm also received CLND if they developed regional lymph node metastasis. SLN status was demonstrated to be a powerful predictor of survival, as those with a negative SLN had a 5-year survival of 90.2%, versus 72.3% 5-year survival for those with a positive SLN. Recently, results of the DECOG-SLT trial have been published. In this German trial, almost 500 patients with a positive SLN with an at least 1-mm metastasis were randomized to obtain CLND or observation. This led to an improvement in local recurrence rate but did not lead to a survival benefit.[99] Final analysis of both trials confirm these results with no significant benefit of an immediate CLND. Hence, this procedure is not recommended any more in patients with only microscopic nodal disease. However, Sentinel positive patients might be selected for adjuvant therapy.

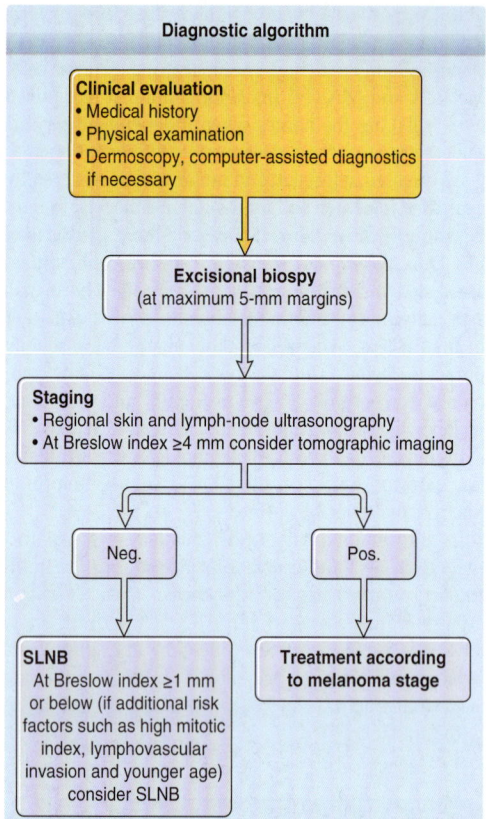

Figure 116-7 Diagnostic algorithm.

DIAGNOSTIC ALGORITHM

See Fig. 116-7.

DIFFERENTIAL DIAGNOSIS

See Table 116-5.

TABLE 116-5
Differential Diagnosis of Melanoma

- Atypical nevus: ABCD criteria help to differentiate
- Seborrheic keratosis: no pigment net in dermoscopy
- Basal cell carcinoma, especially if pigmented: more black than brown, prominent vasculature
- Hemangioma: can be difficult to distinguish from amelanotic melanoma
- Pyogenic granuloma: especially difficult to distinguish from amelanotic acral melanoma
- Solar lentigo, pigmented actinic keratosis, flat seborrheic keratosis: can mimic lentigo maligna melanoma
- Plantar wart: might be hard to distinguish from acral melanoma
- Hematoma: especially acral or subungual hematoma
- Longitudinal melanonychia: look for Hutchinson sign

CLINICAL COURSE AND PROGNOSIS

Melanoma can progress to different stages of the disease, starting with the primary (stage I/II), regional metastases (stage III) and distant metastases (stage IV) (Fig. 116-8). In general, prognosis and survival rates worsen with increasing stage. At initial presentation, approximately 85% of patients have localized disease, 10% have regional metastatic disease, and 5% have distant metastatic disease already.[78]

STAGES I AND II MELANOMA

In general, the 5- to 10-year survival for patients with localized thin primary melanoma <1 mm in Breslow depth is more than 90%. Melanoma typically recurs in a predictable fashion, first in a local and regional distribution, then to distant sites. It is also recognized that melanoma may bypass the regional nodes with direct hematogenous dissemination. The majority of recurrences manifest in the first 5 years after diagnosis and treatment, depending on tumor thickness and other prognostic features of the primary lesion. However, melanoma can recur at any time, and the incidence of late recurrence 10 or more years after initial diagnosis is approximately 1% to 5%.[100]

STAGE III MELANOMA

Stage III melanoma represents a broad range of patients with a diverse clinical outcome, from patients with microscopic nodal disease (IIIA) to patients with bulky clinical nodes or in-transit metastases (IIIC) (Fig. 116-8). The general overall 5-year survival range of 38% to 78% is wide, primarily related to several variables such as the number of positive lymph nodes (most important); tumor burden within a lymph node (microscopic vs macroscopic); age; and ulceration status as well as Breslow thickness of the primary melanoma (Table 116-6).[78] There is a significant decline in survival in melanoma patients who present with clinically evident macroscopic nodal disease versus those with microscopic nodal disease identified via SLNB.

STAGE IV MELANOMA

Melanoma is known for its propensity to metastasize to virtually any organ and also for its highly variable clinical course. Melanoma metastasizes to nonvisceral sites: distant skin/subcutaneous tissue and distant lymph nodes in approximately half of the stage IV cases (42% to 57%) (Fig. 116-8). The most

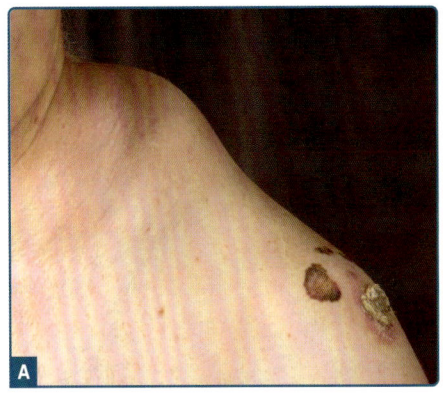
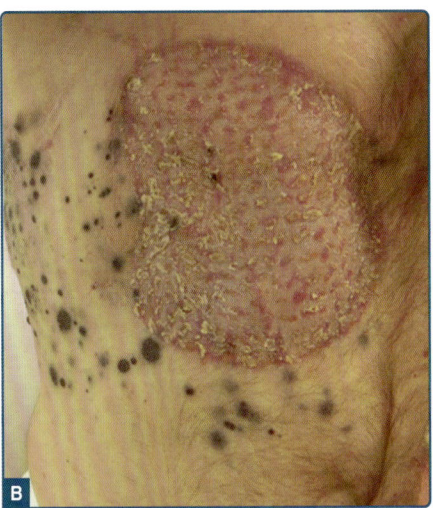
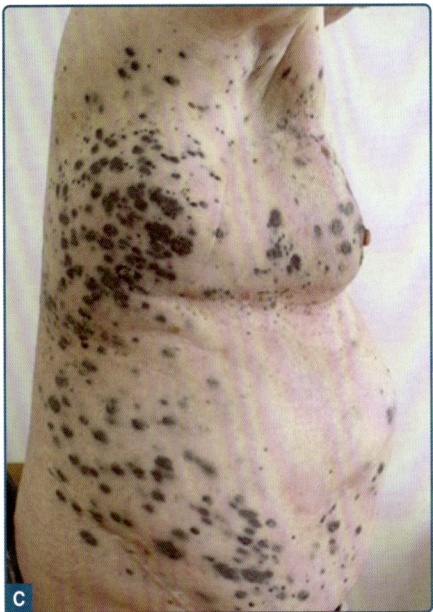

Figure 116-8 **A,** Patient with stage III disease (primary melanoma with bulky lymph node metastases). **B,** Patient with in-transit metastases. **C,** Patient with stage IV disease and extensive cutaneous metastases.

TABLE 116-6
Melanoma TNM Classifications (AJCC 2017)

T CLASSIFICATION	THICKNESS (mm)	ULCERATION STATUS
T1	≤1.0	a: <0.8 mm without ulceration
		b: <0.8 mm with ulceration or 0.8-1 mm (with or without ulceration)
T2	1.01-2.0	a: without ulceration
		b: with ulceration
T3	2.01-4.0	a: without ulceration
		b: with ulceration
T4	>4.0	a: without ulceration
		b: with ulceration

N CLASSIFICATION	NUMBER OF METASTATIC NODES	NODAL METASTATIC MASS
n1	1	a: clinically occult
		b: clinically apparent
		c: pure in-transit met(s)/satellite(s) without metastatic nodes
N2	2-3	a: only occult metastases
		b: at least one clinically apparent metastasis
		c: in-transit met(s)/satellite(s) with 1 metastatic node (clinically occult or apparent)
N3	≥4	a: only clinically occult metastases
		b: at least one clinically apparent metastasis
		c: in-transit met(s)/satellite(s) with at least 2 metastatic nodes (clinically occult or apparent)

M CLASSIFICATION	SITE	SERUM LACTATE DEHYDROGENASE
m1a	Distant skin or soft tissue including muscles, or nodal metastases	M1a(0): Normal M1a(1): Elevated
M1b	Lung metastases (with or without M1a involvement)	M1b(0): Normal M1b(1): Elevated
M1c	All other visceral metastases without CNS metastases (with or without M1a or M1b involvement)	M1c(0): Normal M1c(1): Elevated
M1d	CNS metastasis (with or without M1a, M1b, or M1c involvement)	M1d(0): Normal M1d(1): Elevated

common visceral sites are the lungs (18%-36%), liver (14%-20%), brain (12%-20%), bone (11%-17%), and GI tract (1%-7%). Once metastases to distant sites have been detected, median survival without any treatment is approximately 6 to 9 months. With the help of targeted and immunotherapies this can be increased to 2 years, and even long-term tumor control can be achieved.[101,102]

METASTATIC MELANOMA OF UNKNOWN PRIMARY (MUP)

Metastatic melanoma of unknown primary (MUP) is defined as the presence of histologically confirmed melanoma in a lymph node, visceral site, or distant skin/subcutaneous tissues without a history or evidence of a primary cutaneous, mucosal, or ocular melanoma. This situation occurs in 2% to 5% of all cases of melanoma. Approximately 60% of these involve the lymph nodes and might have developed from nodal nevi.[1] The remaining involve distant sites, typically skin/subcutaneous tissue, and less commonly lung, brain, or GI tract. MUP has similar survival rates compared to equivalently staged cutaneous melanomas of known primary origin. MUP metastatic to lymph nodes had 5- and 10-year survival rates of 46% and 41%, which is comparable to the equivalent stage III melanoma of known primary.[103] Melanoma of unknown primary metastatic to viscera had a median survival of 6 months.[104]

Evaluation of melanoma of unknown primary should involve a complete skin examination looking for a primary site. Wood lamp may be used to identify subclinical hypopigmented areas, which may suggest a regressed primary lesion. In melanoma of unknown primary metastatic to a lymph node, particular attention should be focused on the skin areas that drain to the nodal basin involved. A complete history of previously excised skin lesions should be reviewed. The patient should be referred for proctoscopic, gynecologic, ocular, and nasal mucosal examinations, when warranted. However, only rarely a primary tumor is detectable, and hence more invasive procedures like gastroscopy/colonoscopy should be avoided without any clinical hints for a melanoma at these locations. Staging workup and treatment should be performed as for the equivalent clinical stage of known primary.

THE AJCC CLASSIFICATION

Accurate staging forms the basis for prognosis and treatment, which is invaluable for the majority of patients in their informed decision-making process. The American Joint Committee on Cancer (AJCC) published a revised staging system for melanoma in 2017

TABLE 116-7
Stage Groupings for Cutaneous Melanoma

	CLINICAL STAGING[a]			PATHOLOGIC STAGING[b]		
	T	N	M	T	N	M
0	Tis	N0	M0	Tis	N0	M0
IA	T1a	N0	M0	T1a/b	N0	M0
IB	T1b	N0	M0	T2a	N0	M0
	T2a	N0	M0			
IIA	T2b	N0	M0	T2b	N0	M0
	T3a	N0	M0	T3a	N0	M0
IIB	T3b	N0	M0	T3b	N0	M0
	T4a	N0	M0	T4a	N0	M0
IIC	T4b	N0	M0	T4b	N0	M0
III[c]	Any T	N1	M0			
		N2				
		N3				
IIIA				T1a/b–	N1a or N2a	M0
				T2a	N1a or N2a	M0
IIIB				T0	N1b/c	M0
				T1a/b–T2a	N1b/c or N2b	M0
				T2b/T3a	N1a-N2b	M0
IIIC				T0	N2b/c or N3b/c	M0
				T1a–T3a	N2c or N3a/b/c	M0
				T3b/T4a	Any N	M0
				T4b	N1a-N2c	M0
IIID				T4b	N3a/b/c	M0
IV	Any T	Any N	Any M1	Any T	Any N	Any M1

[a]Clinical staging includes microstaging of the primary melanoma and clinical/radiologic evaluation for metastases. By convention, it should be used after complete excision of the primary melanoma with clinical assessment for regional and distant metastases.

[b]Pathologic staging includes microstaging of the primary melanoma and pathologic information about the regional lymph nodes after partial or complete lymphadenectomy. Pathologic stage 0 or stage IA patients are the exception; they do not require pathologic evaluation of their lymph nodes.

[c]There are no stage III subgroups for clinical staging.

M, metastasis classification; N, node status; T, tumor size.

From Amin MB et al. *AJCC Cancer Staging Manual*, 8th ed. 2016.

(Tables 116-6 and 116-7).[78,105,106] The 2017 melanoma staging system was obtained from a data set of >46,000 melanoma patients from 10 centers worldwide. This represents the largest body of AJCC melanoma data analyzed in an evidence-based approach and incorporates many patients more accurately staged using SLNB. The *t*umor size, *n*ode status, *m*etastasis classification (TNM) system continues to form the backbone of the staging system, in which T describes the extent or thickness of the primary tumor, N the extent of lymph node metastases, and M the extent of distant metastases. Table 116-6 presents the TNM categories, and Table 116-7 lists the Stage groupings.

CLINICAL PROGNOSTIC FACTORS

GENDER AND AGE

A large number of studies have reported that women have better survival rates than men, even after adjustment for tumor thickness and anatomic site.[107] In addition, increasing patient age portends a worse prognosis with respect to overall survival rates. Males more than 60 years of age have the highest mortality rates from melanoma. Older patients have thicker primaries and a higher proportion of ulcerated melanomas, but even after adjusting for these factors, age appears to be an independent prognostic factor.[108,109] It has been postulated that age may serve as a surrogate for declining host immune defense mechanisms.

PROGNOSTIC FACTORS OF THE PRIMARY MELANOMA

TUMOR THICKNESS (BRESLOW INDEX)

The single most important prognostic factor for survival and clinical management in localized stage I and II cutaneous melanoma is tumor thickness.[78] As originally described by Breslow, thickness is measured from the top of the granular layer of the epidermis to the greatest depth of tumor invasion using an ocular micrometer measured in millimeters. Survival decreases with increasing Breslow thickness. Clark level is an alternate, less accurate method of measuring tumor thickness by the anatomic level of invasion. Clark level of invasion is no longer used in routine staging of melanoma.

ULCERATION

Ulceration correlates with tumor thickness; it occurs infrequently in thin melanomas (6% for melanomas <1 mm) and frequently in thick melanomas (63% for melanomas >4 mm). However, patients with an ulcerated melanoma do much worse than patients with a non-ulcerated melanoma with the same Breslow thickness.[110] Ulceration is an independent prognostic factor for localized melanoma.[78] The presence of ulceration in the primary confers a higher risk of developing advanced disease and lower survival rate and upstages all patients with localized and regional disease (ie, stages I to III [Table 116-6]). The worse prognosis of ulcerated melanoma might be due to the fact that ulceration may be indicative of a melanoma with different biologic potential.[111] Ulcerated melanomas tend to have increased vascularity and lymphatic and angiogenic metastatic rates, immunosuppressive features, and a gene profile that differs from nonulcerated melanoma. In 2 large European Organization for Research and Treatment of Cancer (EORTC) trials with adjuvant interferon, ulceration was found to be an independent predictive factor for the beneficial effect of the immunotherapy.[111-113] The same was seen for ipilimumab adjuvant in stage III disease.[111]

MITOTIC RATE

Several studies reported the importance of tumor mitotic rate as an independent predictor of survival, with an increasing mitotic rate correlating with decreasing survival.[114] Among patients with clinically localized melanoma, a mitotic rate of 1/mm^2 or greater was described as the second most powerful predictor of survival, after tumor thickness.[78] In the 2009 revised AJCC staging system, the mitotic rate had replaced Clark level of invasion in defining T1b melanomas because when ulceration, tumor thickness, and mitotic rate are accounted for, Clark level was no longer an independent predictor of survival. Mitotic rate may also correlate with SLNB positivity, especially in younger patients.[115] However, in the new classification system based on >46,000 patients the mitotic rate was not an independent prognostic factor any more and hence, does not define clinical staging (Tables 116-6 and 116-7).

ANGIOLYMPHATIC INVASION

Vascular involvement denotes the invasion of tumor cells into the microvasculature in the dermis. Some reports note that vascular invasion significantly increases the risk of relapse, lymph node involvement, distant metastases, and death.[108,115]

MICROSCOPIC SATELLITES

The presence of microscopic satellitosis, in particular, has been consistently reported to correlate with a poorer outcome, and this has been retained in the current AJCC melanoma staging system (Tables 116-6 and 116-7).[78,105] Patients with any satellite metastases, including microsatellite metastases, are considered to have stage III disease even in the absence of nodal metastases (N1c, satellite metastases without nodal metastases).

TUMOR INFILTRATING LYMPHOCYTES (TILs)

TILs in primary melanomas are thought to represent the host antitumor immune response. In the radial growth phase, a brisk host response is commonly present, and this feature may be associated with the appearance of areas of partial regression (Fig. 116-2A).[116] However, signs of regression itself play no role for the risk of nodal involvement nor in survival of patients with melanoma.[107] In contrast to this, TIL in the vertical growth phase of the melanoma are less frequent and might be relevant for prognosis of the patient. They have been characterized as brisk (a dense band of lymphocytes among tumor cells across the entire base or throughout the tumor), nonbrisk, or absent, and a direct relationship between the TIL grade and prolonged survival was observed.[116] In 2 large studies, up to 3330 and 1241 primary melanomas were investigated for TIL infiltration. TILs were classified as absent in 21% and 31%, nonbrisk in 64% and 27%, and brisk in 15% and 42%, respectively.[117,118] Patients with a higher TIL grade of the primary melanoma were associated with a lower risk of melanoma-specific death, independent of tumor characteristics by AJCC tumor stage.[117] Patients with brisk TIL had improved recurrence-free and overall survival compared to patients with non-brisk and absent TILs.[118]

PROGNOSTIC FACTORS IN REGIONAL METASTASES

The status of the regional lymph nodes is the most powerful prognostic factor for survival in melanoma, with regional lymph node metastasis portending a worse prognosis. The number of lymph nodes involved (independent of tumor deposit size) is the most significant risk factor in patients with stage III melanoma.[78] The second most important risk factor is tumor burden, stratified into micro-metastatic disease (determined by SLNB) or macro-metastatic disease (clinically palpable nodes). In clinically node-negative stage I or II patients, SLN status is the most significant prognostic factor with respect to disease-free and disease-specific survival.[98,119] As such, consideration of SLNB to search for micro-metastatic disease has become the standard of care for most clinically node-negative patients with melanomas 1 mm and greater in thickness, and for a subset of thinner melanomas, with additional risk factors such as high mitotic rate and lymphovascular invasion, especially in younger patients. SLNB is a powerful tool for accurately staging clinically node-negative patients and as such, use of this technique continues to play a central role in the AJCC staging classification system for melanoma.[78] Ulceration of the primary lesion indicates a worse prognosis in regional stage III disease. Mitotic rate of the primary lesion strongly correlates with a worse prognosis for microscopic regional stage III disease. Satellite metastases, both clinical and microscopic, around a primary melanoma and in-transit metastases between the primary and its nodal basin represent intra-lymphatic disease (N1c, N2c, N3c) and portend the worst prognosis for regional metastases (stage IIIB/C disease) with a 5-year survival rate less than 50%.[78]

PROGNOSTIC FACTORS IN DISTANT METASTASES

The presence of distant metastases is associated with the worst prognosis, with mean survival rates measured in months rather than years—at least till a few years ago. Site of metastasis continues to be an important prognostic factor in the AJCC melanoma staging; with visceral metastases having a relatively poorer prognosis than nonvisceral (skin, subcutaneous tissue, and distant lymph nodes) sites.[78] Other variables of prognostic significance are the number of metastatic sites and surgical resectability. Solitary metastases resected after radiologic demonstration of stability over 3 to 6 months have been associated with prolonged survival in some patients, but no strong evidence exists that asymptomatic detection is associated with significant overall survival as of this writing.[120] Elevated serum LDH levels are associated with a worse prognosis, regardless of the site of metastatic disease (Table 116-6).

MANAGEMENT

SURGICAL TREATMENT OF PRIMARY MELANOMA

The standard of therapy for primary cutaneous melanoma is wide local excision (WLE). The purpose of the wider excision is to prevent local recurrence due to subclinical persistent disease—whether there is a minor influence on overall survival is not clear as of this writing.[121,122] The risk of satellite metastases is directly related to primary melanoma thickness.[123] Hence, current recommendations on the clinical margins differ depending on the Breslow thickness of the primary and are based on several large randomized trials comparing different-sized margins.[121] For melanoma in situ, a 0.5- to 1-cm margin, for melanoma <1 mm Breslow depth a 1-cm margin, for melanoma 1 to 2 mm thick a 1- to 2-cm margin, and for melanoma >2 mm thick a 2-cm margin is recommended. Wider excisions with up to 5-cm margins have not shown a benefit for local recurrence rate.[124]

Ultimately, each patient should be evaluated individually, taking into account current surgical guidelines as well as anatomic site (ie, location near a vital structure), the possibility of primary closure versus need for skin graft, and the presence or lack of adverse prognostic factors from micro-staging. Melanoma excision at special sites, such as the digits, soles, ears, vagina, or anus, also requires separate surgical and functional considerations. When anatomically in a difficult location, for example, lentigo maligna on the face or acral melanoma on the hands/feet, an excision with histopathologically confirmed free margins can be done instead after informed consent of the patient.[125] Still, the fundamental oncologic principle should always be tumor clearance first, reconstruction second.

SURGICAL TREATMENT OF REGIONAL METASTASES

MICROSCOPIC NODAL DISEASE

Elective lymph node dissection (ELND) is the removal of regional lymph nodes draining the site of a primary cutaneous melanoma in the absence of any palpable or clinically evident metastatic disease. Historically, before the advent of SLNB, ELND was advocated for melanomas at higher risk of regional spread to eradicate occult micro-metastases in a potentially curative manner. Multiple prospective randomized controlled trials failed to demonstrate a significant benefit from ELND for melanoma.[126] Thus, there is no role for ELND today, especially in light of the development and availability of SLNB.

As mentioned previously, the SLNB procedure is a powerful staging tool that identifies micro-metastatic nodal disease.[127] After positive SLNB, up to 15% to 20% of patients have evidence of non-SLN metastases found during CLND.[128-130] For the entire group, patients in the randomized MSLT-I trial who received an SLNB did not have an improved melanoma specific survival when compared to patients who did not receive an SLNB, and thus SLNB cannot be classified as therapeutic as of this writing based on interim data. Importantly, the study is underpowered to answer that question, with approximately 80% of subjects not harboring nodal deposits. Nevertheless, in the group of patients with melanoma metastatic to the lymph nodes, the 5-year survival was significantly higher among patients with a positive SLNB and immediate CLND compared to patients in the observation followed by CLND for clinical nodal disease arm (72% vs 52%).[98] Critics accurately point to the fact that this trial component was not randomized and data are not mature.

In the DECOG-SLT trial where patients with a positive SLN were randomized to CLND or observation (followed by CLND in the case of local recurrence) no benefit in overall survival was found for the CLND group.[99] Three-year overall survival was 81.2% in the CLND group and 81.7% in the observation group (hazard ratio [HR] 0.96; $P = .87$). The only difference detected between the groups was the rate in regional lymph node recurrences, with 8.3% in the CLND arm and 14.6% in the observation arm ($P = .029$). This finding did not translate into a benefit in recurrence-free survival, with a 3-year recurrence-free survival of 66.8% in the CLND arm and 67.4% in the observation arm ($P = .75$). Hence, CLND is not recommended any more for patients with a positive Sentinel node. Recent data from the MSLT-II trial with a similar scientific objective of assessing the impact of SLNB on survival support this recommendation.

MACROSCOPIC NODAL DISEASE

The current standard of therapy for macroscopic (stage IIIB or IIIC) melanoma in lymph nodes is CLND of the involved regional basin. Uncontrolled nodal disease is a cause of melanoma-related morbidity with a significant high negative impact on quality of life. CLND for regional metastatic melanoma has been associated with long-term survival in a proportion of patients.[131]

ADJUVANT TREATMENT

Adjuvant therapy is treatment for patients with surgically resected disease who are at high risk for relapse, such as those with thick primary melanomas or nodal disease. For decades, treatment with interferon-α was the only adjuvant option outside clinical trials for these patients. Recently, the immune checkpoint blockers used to treat stage IV disease like the anticytotoxic T-lymphocyte–associated protein 4 (CTLA-4) antibody ipilimumab and the anti-PD-1 antibodies nivolumab and pembrolizumab have been studied in the adjuvant setting for stage III disease, leading to FDA approval of ipilimumab and nivolumab already.[111]

INTERFERON-α

Interferons (IFNs) are cytokines that are usually released by cells in response to the presence of several pathogens such as viruses, bacteria, parasites, and also tumor cells. Typically, IFNs lead to a protection of neighboring cells from virus infection. But they have various other functions like the activation of natural killer cells and macrophages and enhancing immune recognition by upregulation of MHC class I and II molecules. In addition, IFN-α has direct antineoplastic activity leading to the inhibition of tumor cell proliferation likely via activation of STAT1[132-134] and a possible antimetastatic effect.[135] However, in the treatment of melanoma, IFN-α only has moderate activity and the survival advantage associated with this treatment is unclear. Two different dosage regimens were routinely used: high-dose (HDI) and low-dose interferon (LDI) treatment. The high-dose regimen consists of 20 million units per square meter of body surface area per day given intravenously 5 days a week for 4 weeks (induction phase), followed by 10 million units per square meter per day given subcutaneously 3 times a week for 48 weeks (maintenance phase). The low-dose regimen uses 3 million units 3 times a week given subcutaneously for 1.5 years. In a Cochrane data review, 18 randomized controlled trials were included, with a total of 10,499 patients.[136] This analysis showed that adjuvant interferon was associated with significantly improved disease-free survival (HR 0.83; $P < .00001$) and overall survival (OS) (HR 0.91; $P = .003$). The authors state that considering a 5-year OS rate for TNM stage II to III is 60%, the number needed to treat to prevent 1 death is 35. However, the patients treated with IFN have very different prognoses worsening from stage I to III. Unfortunately, even though so many patients were included, subgroup analysis failed to answer the question of whether some treatment features like dosage or treatment duration might have an impact on interferon efficacy or whether subgroups (eg, stage II vs stage III) might benefit.

In another meta-analyses of more than 6000 patients, survival benefit was 7% for progression-free survival (PFS) and 3% for OS after 5 years with no significant differences between HDI and LDI treatment.[137] A subgroup analysis of 2 EORTC trials revealed that patients with an ulcerated primary melanoma and/or a positive SLN might benefit more from IFN.[112] The effect on ulcerated primary melanoma is currently being validated by another prospective EORTC trial (NCT01502696) in SLN-negative melanoma patients. For patients with a positive SLN, the Sunbelt Melanoma Trial showed that they do not benefit from HDI treatment after CLND.[138] However, patient numbers were too small to answer this question.

There are significant toxicities associated with IFN treatment, the most frequent being flulike symptoms in almost all patients (ie, fatigue, anorexia, weight loss, myalgias, fever, nausea, and headache). Other side effects include depression, hepatotoxicity (elevated transaminases), and myelosuppression.[132] The toxicities may require dose modification, especially in HDI treatment, and if the patient makes it through the first 3 months of therapy, most are able to complete at least 80% of the scheduled dosing and are able to finish treatment.[139] Interestingly, the appearance of autoantibodies or clinical manifestations of autoimmunity such as vitiligo during treatment with IFN may be associated with a significant improvement in relapse-free survival and overall survival in melanoma patients undergoing adjuvant IFN.[140]

Importantly, HDI treatment is not recommended any more as more effective treatments are now approved for stage III disease.

IMMUNE CHECKPOINT BLOCKERS

For patients with stage III disease in the USA, treatment with the anti-CTLA-4 antibody ipilimumab is FDA approved. CTLA-4 (or CD152) is a so-called immune checkpoint molecule that is expressed on the surface of activated T cells and leads to their deactivation on binding to CD80 or CD86 on the surface of antigen-presenting cells. This mechanism seems to be in place to downregulate an immune response after activation and thereby prevent autoimmunity. In a randomized double-blind phase 3 trial, 951 stage III melanoma patients were included after complete resection of nodal metastases of at least 1 mm diameter to receive either 10 mg/kg ipilimumab or placebo every 3 weeks for 4 doses and then every 3 months for up to

3 years.¹¹¹ Ipilimumab treatment led to an improvement of the median recurrence-free survival by 9 months from 17.1 months in the placebo group to 26.1 months in the ipilimumab group. Three-year recurrence-free survival was 34.8% in the placebo group and 46.5% in the ipilimumab group. Whether this approach leads to a benefit in overall survival is still under analysis. In addition, the ipilimumab treatment is also being compared to HDI in clinical trials to assess relative effectivity.

Side effects with ipilimumab are mainly of autoimmune nature and can be severe but are manageable (see below). However, treatment with less toxic immune checkpoint blockers nivolumab or pembrolizumab directed against programmed cell death protein 1 (PD-1) have just been reported to be even more effective with a better tolerability -reducing the relative risk for recurrence by half (Checkmate 238, Keynote-054).

ADJUVANT RADIOTHERAPY

Adjuvant radiotherapy after CLND can help to control metastases in the nodal basin of stage III melanoma patients. Recommendations are based on retrospective analyses focusing on the likelihood of nodal recurrence as a function of different risk factors.[141-143] These investigations revealed 3 main risk factors for relapse: ≥3 lymph node metastases, lymph nodes with extracapsular spread, or lymph nodes >3 cm in diameter. In addition, adjuvant radiotherapy should be considered in the case of nodal recurrence. A small randomized controlled trial with patients at high risk for lymph node relapse judged on these criteria confirmed data from the retrospective analyses and demonstrated a significantly higher loco-regional control rate for patients with adjuvant radiotherapy but no effect on relapse-free or overall survival.[144] If this stays right under adjuvant immunotherapies with immune checkpoint blockers needs to be verified.

MANAGEMENT OF SATELLITE OR IN-TRANSIT METASTASES

In general, regional in-transit or satellite disease should be surgically excised whenever possible with curative intent. However, if multiple lesions make surgery unreasonable, other treatment options should be considered. In locally limited disease, radiation can be a good option, especially in multiple small metastases.[145] Additional application of hyperthermia can increase the ratio for complete responses.[146] Small and superficial metastases respond very well to intralesional interleukin-2. For bigger metastases, intralesional injections with the oncolytic virus Talimogene Laherparepvec (T-VEC) or electrochemotherapy (ECT) are therapeutic options. In a meta-analysis, 47 trials on skin-directed treatment approaches were compared.[147] In these trials, 915 patients with 4313 metastases received different treatments such as ECT, photodynamic therapy, radiotherapy, intralesional, or topical treatments. Patients showed an overall response rate of 60.2%, a complete remission rate of 35.5%, and a recurrence rate of 9.2%. If local treatments do not lead to local control, patients with extensive disease in the extremities can benefit from locally applied chemotherapy by isolated limb perfusion. All systemic treatment options are also available for nonresectable stage III disease.

INTRALESIONAL INTERLEUKIN-2

This is a very effective approach especially for small and superficial metastases, with a response rate of more than 80% if applied 2 to 3 times a week over multiple weeks (Fig. 116-9). Unexpectedly long survival times and good responses to subsequent chemotherapies were noted in a retrospective analysis, suggesting that a systemic effect may accompany such intralesional administration.[148] In a systemic review, 140 patients with 2182 metastases from 6 publications were evaluated and showed a complete response rate of 50%.[149] Treatment is tolerated well, with local pain and swelling and mild flu-like symptoms as main side effects.

TALIMOGENE LAHERPAREPVEC (T-VEC)

Intralesional application of an oncolytic virus is a new treatment option for patients with unresectable stage III or stage IV M1a disease. T-VEC is a transgenic herpes virus (Type 1) that is selectively replicated in the tumor and produces granulocyte macrophage colony-stimulating factor (GM-CSF) to augment local and potentially distant immune responses. In a randomized phase 3 trial versus GM-CSF monotherapy, the best durable response with T-VEC was found in patients with stage IIIB/C or M1a disease without systemic pretreatment.[150] Also, this treatment is tolerated relatively well, with fatigue and fever being the most frequent side effects.

ELECTROCHEMOTHERAPY (ECT)

ECT is an effective and tolerable treatment option for patients with in-transit metastases, but needs special technical equipment. ECT is a combination of a local or systemic chemotherapy (usually bleomycin or cisplatin) with intralesionally applied electrical pulses. As these lead to painful muscle contractions the procedure should be done in general anaesthesia or local anaesthesia with sedation and is hence usually done in the operating room. Theoretically, the electric pulses increase the permeability of the tumor cell membranes (electroporation) and thereby sensitize them to the chemotherapy. In a systematic review and meta-analysis, data from 44 trials with altogether

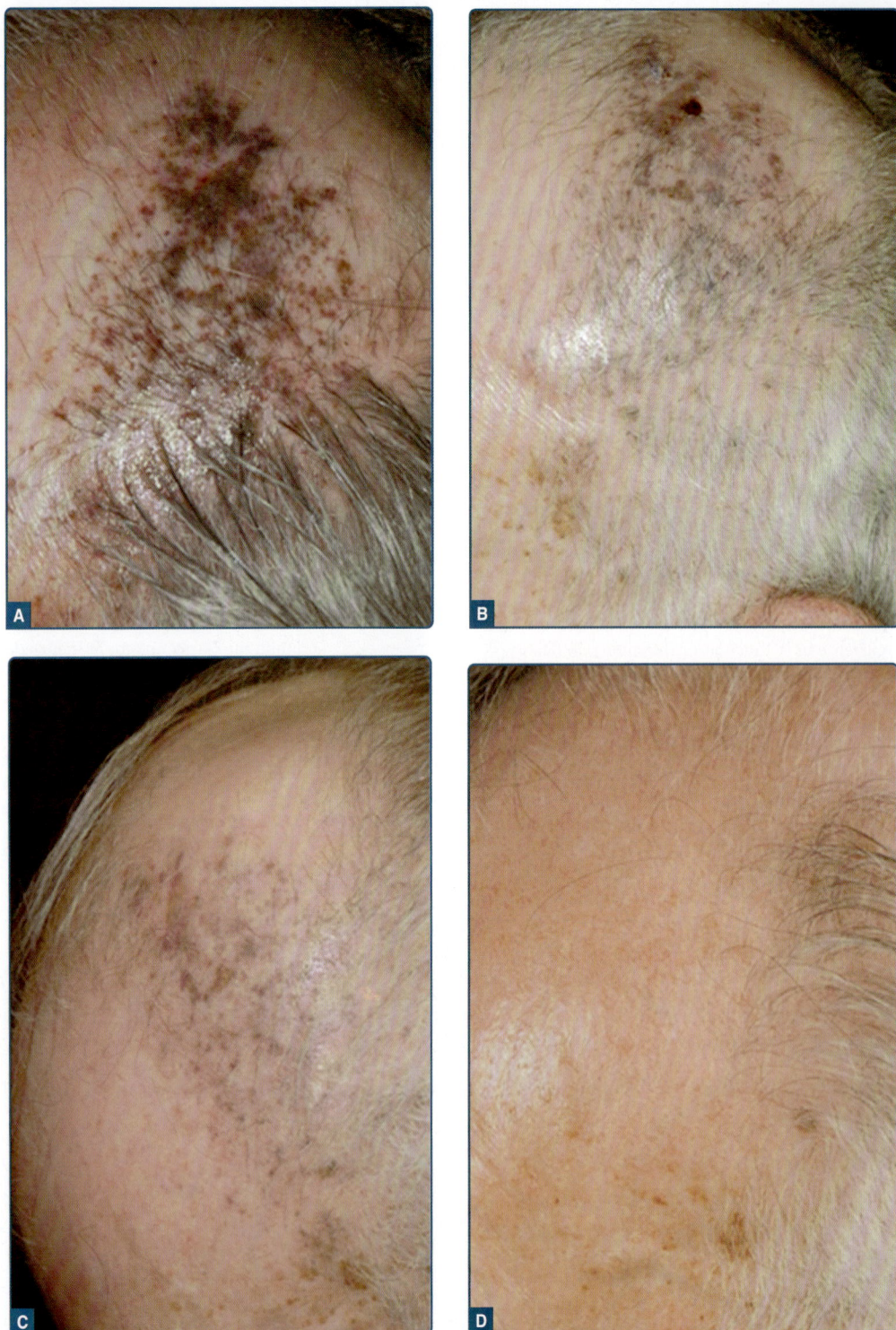

Figure 116-9 Treatment of satellite metastases with intralesional interleukin-2: **A,** before treatment; **B,** after 6 weeks of treatment; **C,** 4 weeks later without any further treatment; **D,** 2 years later without any further treatment.

431 patients and 1894 metastases were pooled.[151] The response rate of single metastases was 80.6%, complete remissions were observed in 56.8%. Even though intralesional injections of the chemotherapy were associated with a higher response rate compared to systemic chemotherapy, because of practical reasons systemic chemotherapy is preferred in routine clinical practice.

ISOLATED LIMB PERFUSION (ILP)

Isolated limb perfusion (ILP) may be considered for loco-regional disease control limited to an extremity. ILP is a form of regional chemotherapy that delivers higher doses of chemotherapeutic agents to the limb with less systemic toxicities. The technique involves perfusing an isolated extremity under hyperthermic conditions with cytotoxic agents, conventionally melphalan. ILP with melphalan is an effective form of regional therapy in some cases with an associated considerable morbidity, producing partial or complete regional responses in up to 80%.[152] The benefit is aimed at loco-regional control, not overall survival. The ILP procedure may be associated with serious local morbidities, including significant tissue damage or compartment syndrome. Elderly age and serious medical comorbidities are generally considered exclusion criteria. Isolated limb infusion (ILI) is a, simpler, less-invasive technique. Early studies of ILI with melphalan and actinomycin D demonstrate efficacy comparable to that of ILP with melphalan.[153] ILI may be considered for patients ineligible for ILP.

LOCAL HEPATIC THERAPY FOR UVEAL MELANOMA WITH LIVER METASTASES

As uveal melanomas metastasize preferentially into the liver, local treatments to the liver can be a treatment option. Different procedures have been established from surgery or ablation of isolated metastases to chemoperfusion/embolization or radio-embolization. In a phase 3 trial, hepatic intraarterial infusion of fotemustine was compared with fotemustine applied intravenously. The trial was stopped early, as interim analysis revealed that the local application of fotemustine did not improve overall survival compared to the IV arm despite having a better response rate and better PFS.[154] In another randomized phase 3 trial of percutaneous hepatic perfusion with melphalan (chemosaturation) versus best available care, a highly significant difference was found concerning hepatic PFS (7.0 vs 1.6 months; $P < .0001$) and overall PFS (5.4 vs 1.6 months; $P < .0001$). However, overall survival again was not significantly different—though this might be influenced by the cross-over design of the trial.[155] All procedures can achieve responses but have not been shown to prolong survival of the patients. Additionally, the procedure is laborious and has a significant risk of complications. As such, randomized controlled trials are rarely performed.

TREATMENT OF UNRESECTABLE METASTATIC DISEASE

Until a few years ago, treatment of stage IV melanoma was purely palliative with the intention to potentially increase length of survival and palliation of symptoms. Recently, significant progress was achieved and treatment modalities are available now that substantially improve patient survival from a median of 6 to 9 months to 2 years with the chance to achieve long-term tumor control.[101,102,156]

SURGERY AND RADIOTHERAPY

Even though hematologic spread should be defined as unresectable in general, surgical excision of isolated visceral metastases (ie, metastasectomy) can be considered and may be performed with long-term disease-free intervals in some patients. In addition, surgery also may be palliative, for example, to treat isolated brain metastases or relieve obstruction from GI metastases. Surgical excision of skin/subcutis or distant lymph node metastases may result in improved loco-regional control and decreased morbidity.[157] Radiotherapy is an option and preferably used to treat brain metastases, especially using stereotactic radiation for limited brain disease. Palliative radiation may be indicated for spinal cord compression and painful bone metastases.

IMMUNOTHERAPIES

The importance of the immune system in cancer control was nicely shown in a mouse experiment where sarcomas can be induced by chemical carcinogenesis with 3′-methylcholanthrene (MCA).[158] Mice with clinically stable tumors were either injected with depleting antibodies against T cells (CD4/CD8/IFN-γ) or a control antibody. Mice receiving the control antibody remained stable but mice with a T-cell depletion developed growing sarcomas in 60% of cases. Hence, tumors can be controlled by the immune system. This is suggested to work via the so-called Cancer-Immunity-Cycle[159] where the release of cancer cell antigens by cancer cell death leads to presentation of the antigens by dendritic cells. These prime and activate T cells in the lymph nodes, which then traffic through the blood vessels to the tumor and infiltrate it. Finally, recognition of cancer cells by these T cells lead to cancer killing and elimination.

A known phenomenon in primary melanomas is the tendency for regression (Fig. 116-2). When observed in melanoma metastases it is often associated with a favorable outcome.[160] This has been linked to an effective immune defense, and the number of TILs in the primary melanoma could be correlated with patients' survival.[117,118] In addition, it is well known that immunosuppressed patients, for example, transplant recipients have an increased risk for developing melanoma and show an aggressive clinical course of the disease.[161] Hence, treatments that stimulate the immune response and aim to overcome immune escape mechanisms of the tumor have a potential to effectively fight cancer.

Historically, several approaches have been studied starting with William Coley, an American surgeon, who tried to elicit a therapeutic immune response through injection of bacterial broth (later called Coley toxin) into soft-tissue tumors. In the following decades cytokines like interleukin-2 and interferon-α have been used in the clinic. In addition, multiple attempts have been made to develop a therapeutic vaccine—all with limited success.[162] The scientific turning point for cancer immunotherapy came with the understanding that T-cell immune responses are controlled through on and off switches, the so-called immune checkpoints that protect the body from possibly damaging immune responses.

Immune Checkpoint Blockade: T-cell activation relies on 2 stimulating signals mediated via several surface receptors: one is the T-cell receptor (TCR) recognition of antigens associated with MHC antigen–presenting molecules, the second is binding of a costimulatory molecule like CD28, CD27, GITR, OX40, or ICOS. On activation, T cells express coinhibitory receptors like CTLA-4, PD-1, TIM-3, and LAG-3, the so-called immune checkpoints that lead to downregulation of the T-cell response and T-cell anergy. Ipilimumab is a monoclonal blocking antibody against CTLA-4 and hence stops inhibition of the T-cell response (Fig. 116-10). Ipilimumab is particularly remarkable because it was the first drug to show a significant benefit for OS in patients with stage IV melanoma.[163] In addition, despite a response rate of only about 10%, more than 20% of patients reach a long-term tumor control of more than 3 years.[156]

These results were improved even further by the use of blocking antibodies against PD-1, namely, nivolumab and pembrolizumab. PD-1 on the surface of activated T cells binds to PD-L1 and PD-L2, which are expressed in peripheral tissues and different cancer types, including melanoma. The PD-1/PD-L1 pathway plays a critical role in tumor escape as binding leads to downregulation of tumor-associated T cells. In some tumors, surface expression of PD-L1 has been reported to be an independent predictor of adverse clinical outcome,[164] although it appears to be a positive prognostic feature in patients with melanoma.[165-167]

In melanoma, PD-1 blockage leads to significant tumor reduction in 30% to 40% of patients and was shown to prolong PFS and OS with a 2-year OS of roughly 60%.[102,168] Patients with a PD-L1 tumor expression of at least 5% might have a better objective response to the treatment (odds ratio 2.52) ranging from 46% for PD-L1-positive and 27% for PD-L1-negative tumors.[164] Two-year OS rates differ too, with 57.2% of patients alive with a PD-L1-positive tumor and 32.6% with a PD-L1-negative tumor in the Keynote 001 trial.[169] Hence, patients with a PD-L1-negative tumor can still respond to treatment. This might be partly based on the fact that PD-L1 expression is focal and dynamic, leading to potential sampling error on smaller biopsies. Additionally, numerous immunohistochemical assays with potentially different scoring systems of positivity as well as sensitivity for PD-L1 detection are currently being used to test specimens. For patients with melanoma, testing for PD-L1 expression is not required for anti-PD-1 administration, as it is for some other tumor types.

The combination of both ipilimumab and nivolumab lead to remarkable responses in melanoma in the Checkmate 067 trial. Response rates of 58% and

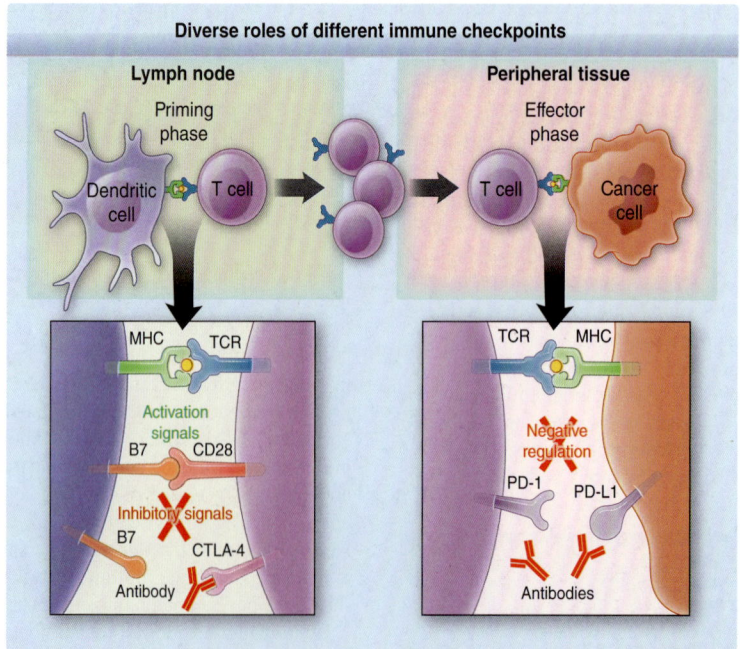

Figure 116-10 Mechanism of action of immune checkpoint blockage: The anti-CTLA-4 antibodies block the downregulation of T cells in their priming phase in the lymph nodes whereas the anti-PD-1 antibodies block the downregulation of activated T cells in their effector phase in the tumor microenvironment.

a median PFS of 11.5 months were seen with the combination compared to a 19.0% response rate and a median PFS of 2.9 months with ipilimumab monotherapy.[170] In addition, responses to the combination immunotherapy seem to occur faster, including potentially in patients with highly advanced disease. Concerning OS, median OS had not been reached yet for the ipilimumab plus nivolumab combination at a minimum followup of 36 months, it was 37.5 months in the nivolumab and 19.9 months in the ipilimumab monotherapy group. The overall survival rate at 3 years was 58% for ipilimumab plus nivolumab, 52% for nivolumab, and 34% for ipilimumab.[171] Unfortunately, in the treatment of metastasized ocular melanoma immunotherapies have been of limited success with no responses and a median OS of 6.8 months in a Phase II trial.[172] Responses to PD-1 directed treatment are rarely observed. Reported response rates range from 3% to 30% and may be higher in patients with extrahepatic disease.[173-175]

Side effects from these treatments can be severe to life-threatening. These consist of mainly autoimmune effects, so-called immune-related adverse events (irAEs), against different organs secondary to immune stimulation. The most frequent side effects affect the skin, the liver, the GI tract, and the endocrine system (hypophysis, thyroid) (Table 116-8).[176] The dermatitis is typically mild in degree. IrAEs affecting other organ systems such as colitis, however, can be severe and require high-dose immunosuppressant treatment to prevent complications like bowel perforations.

Even though the character of these side effects is similar between the anti-CTLA-4 antibodies, the PD-1 antibodies, and a combination of both, the frequency differs considerably. Side effects can be nicely compared within the CheckMate 067 trial.[170] Here, severe side effects (grade 3 or higher according to the common toxicity criteria for adverse events [CTC-AE]) occurred in only 16% of patients receiving treatment with nivolumab, 27% in those receiving ipilimumab, and 55% of those receiving nivolumab plus ipilimumab. In addition to experiencing a higher frequency of side effects with combination therapy, patients receiving combination treatment tended to have several organs affected, for example, one patient experiencing colitis, hepatitis, thyroiditis, and pancreatitis. An increasing familiarity with this new class of side effects led to the development of special treatment algorithms that can be used to effectively treat patients experiencing irAEs (see Fig. 116-11). In general, side effects should be treated quickly, with the choice of the immunosuppressive treatment dependent on the severity of symptoms. The relationship between the side effects and response to therapy is still under discussion, though a number of reports have suggested that there might be a relationship with an improved clinical outcome.[32,177-181]

Adoptive T-Cell Therapy: Adoptive T-cell therapy (ACT), in particular, autologous in vitro expanded TIL therapy, is another promising approach in immunotherapy of cancer but is only established in a few cancer centers worldwide. TILs from melanoma metastases are expanded under GMP conditions and reinfused into the patient after lymphoablative chemotherapy followed by high-dose interleukin-2 treatment. Several clinical trials demonstrated durable clinical responses for more than 50% of patients.[182,183] However, not much is known on the nature of expanded T cells. Recent findings suggest that a crucial component of the therapeutic T-cell response targets patient- and tumor-specific neoantigens resulting from somatic mutations and that only a minority of TILs respond to defined melanoma-associated antigens like differentiation (MART-a, gp100, tyrosinase) or cancer/testis antigens (MAGE, NY-Eso).[184] Newer approaches attempt to genetically modify the T cells with expression of TCRs or chimeric antigen receptors (CARs) against known antigens before re-infusion.

TABLE 116-8
Common Side Effects from Immune Checkpoint Blocker Treatment (Treatment-Related Adverse Events from CheckMate 067 Trial)

IMMUNE CHECKPOINT BLOCKER	IPILIMUMAB		NIVOLUMAB		IPILIMUMAB + NIVOLUMAB	
SEVERITY (CTC-AE) OF EVENT	ANY	3 OR 4	ANY	3 OR 4	ANY	3 OR 4
All treatment-related events (in %)	86	27	82	16	96	55
GI (lower tract: Diarrhea, Colitis)	37	12	22	3	48	15
GI (upper tract: Nausea, decreased appetite)	29	1	24	0	44	3.5
Dermatologic (Rash, Pruritus)	55	3	44	2	60	6
Hepatic (elevated transaminases)	7	2	7	3	32	20
Endocrine (Hypo-/hyperthyroidism)	12	3	16	2	32	6
Pulmonary (Pneumonitis)	2	<1	2	<1	7	1
Renal (elevated creatinine)	3	<1	1	<1	6	2
Fatigue	28	1	34	1	35	4
Arthralgia	6	0	8	0	11	<1

Severity	Examinations	Management
CTC Grade 1	**Monitor clinical course** • Blood draws (especially in hepatitis, thyroiditis, pancreatitis, nephritis) • Exclude other cause (eg, stool test on pathogens in colitis, CMV/EBV reactivation in hepatitis)	**Symptomatic treatment** eg, • Topical steroids for exanthema • Loperamide for diarrhea
CTC Grade 2	**Monitor clinical course** as Grade 1 plus • Consider colonoscopy in colitis • Consider bronchoscopy in pneumonitis • Consider renal biopsy in nephritis • Consider liver biopsy in hepatitis	**Oral corticosteroid treatment** • Interrupt treatment with immune checkpoint blocker • 1 mg/kg prednisolone (or equivalent) orally once a day
CTC Grade 3/4	**Hospital admission** • As Grade 2 but examinations strongly recommended if possible on day of admission • Don't delay corticosteroid treatment • Daily monitoring for symptoms and blood values where applicable	**IV corticosteroid treatment** • Discontinue treatment with immune checkpoint blocker • 2 mg/kg methylprednisolone (or equivalent) IV once a day • If no improvement within 2 days add another immunosuppressive agent, eg, mycophenolate mofetil 3 g orally daily (hepatitis) or infliximab 5 mg/kg IV (colitis)

Figure 116-11 Algorithm to treat side effects from immune checkpoint blockers.

High-Dose Interleukin-2 (IL-2): Before the era of immune checkpoint inhibition, high-dose bolus IL-2 was the only FDA-approved immunologic treatment for metastatic melanoma that was recognized to produce rare but durable complete responses. It has been shown as a single agent to induce a 16% overall response rate with durable response in up to 5% to 8% of patients.[185] High-dose IL-2 is associated with significant toxicity, for example, a capillary-leak syndrome. Following FDA approval of immune checkpoint blocking agents, IL-2 is generally not used systemically in routine clinical use.

TARGETED THERAPIES

Melanoma is characterized by a high genetic instability that leads to a high mutation rate and molecular heterogeneity attributed to the mutagenic effects of UV irradiation. In a 2002 genomewide screen, *BRAF* point mutations were discovered at high frequency in melanomas relative to other cancers such as those of the thyroid and colon.[186] Most oncogenic *BRAF* mutations cause valine-to-glutamic acid substitutions at codon 600 (V600E) that constitutively activate the kinase domain and thereby the mitogen-activated protein kinase (MAPK) signaling pathway. Further sequencing studies identified numerous novel melanoma genes involved in regulation of the MAPK and other signaling pathways. BRAF and NRAS mutations are found in two-thirds of melanomas (other genetic alterations include amplification of AKT3 and loss of PTEN), leading to an activation of the phosphatidylinositol 3-kinase (PI3K) pathway. In addition, these pathways can be hyperactivated by overexpression or mutation of growth factor receptors such as c-Kit, Met and EGF-R or inactivating mutation in neurofibromin 1 (NF1).[187]

BRAF/MEK Inhibition: The BRAF V600 mutation is most common in melanomas of sun-exposed skin[8] and can be detected in about 50% of melanomas. The first BRAF inhibitor used was sorafenib which is an orally available unspecific RAF inhibitor that inhibits B-raf and C-raf in addition to other kinases. Sorafenib demonstrated little activity in patients with unresectable stage III or stage IV melanoma.[187,188] The observed clinical benefit was substantially different with the development of the selective BRAF inhibitors such as vemurafenib and dabrafenib (Fig. 116-12), both of which are FDA approved. Approximately 50% of patients with a BRAF V600-mutated melanoma respond, and those who do tend to demonstrate incredibly fast responses.[189,190] Treatment prolongs survival, with a median PFS of 7 to 8 months and a median OS of 16 to 18 months.[101,191] Because patients do tend to respond quickly, these agents can specifically benefit those with a high tumor load (Fig. 116-13) and provide symptom relief. Unfortunately, most patients develop later resistance to the treatment.[192] Mutational analysis of resistant metastases revealed several genes known to reactivate the MAPK pathway by bypassing BRAF. These include somatic mutations in *NRAS*, amplifications of BRAF and mutation in *MAP2K1/K2*, *MITF*, and *NF1*. Additional alterations with less clear of a relationship to resistance were observed in the PI3K pathway,

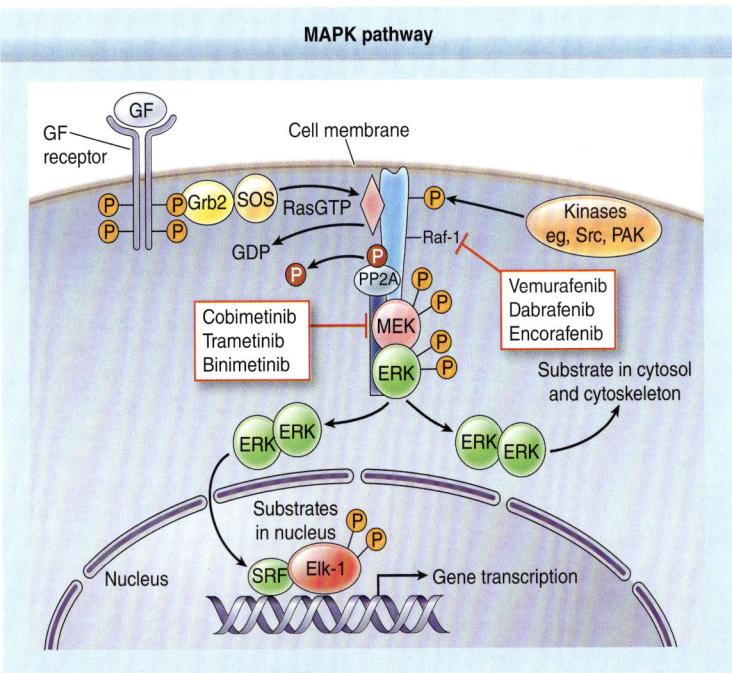

Figure 116-12 The BRAF and MEK inhibitors block the activity of the respective kinases in the MAPK signaling pathway and hence block cell proliferation and facilitate apoptosis.

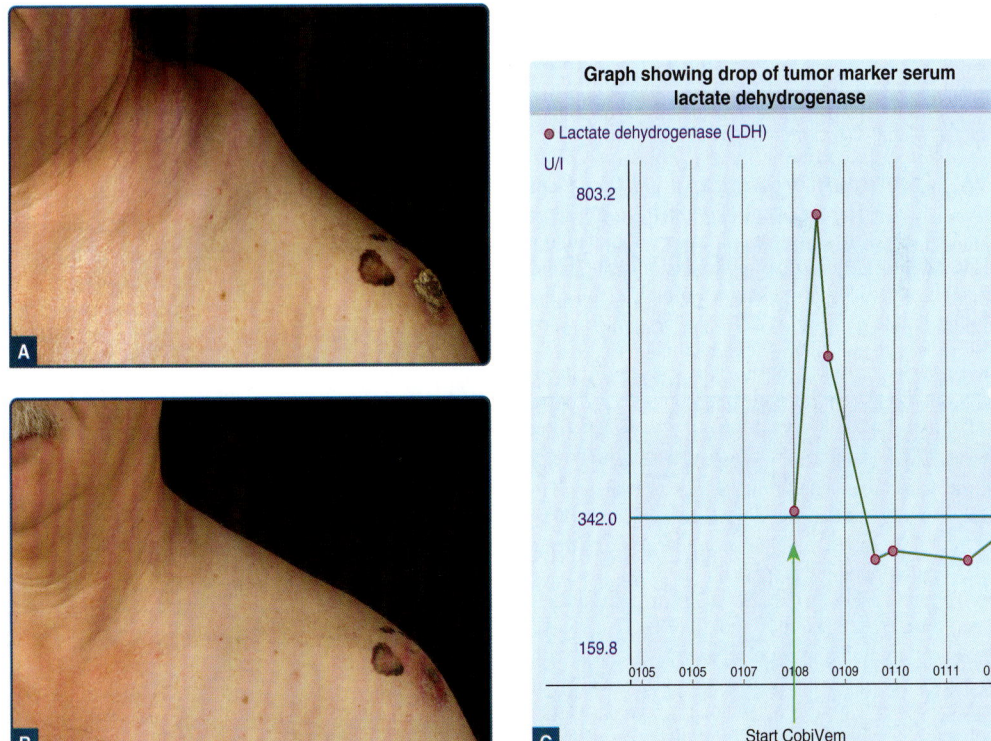

Figure 116-13 A 62-year-old patient with a superficial spreading melanoma on the left shoulder that metastasized to the regional lymph nodes already and was unresectable at the time of diagnosis (**A**). As a BRAF V600E mutation was detected, he received a combination treatment with the BRAF inhibitor dabrafenib and the MEK inhibitor trametinib. After 2 months of treatment, the lymph node conglomerates decreased in size significantly (**B**), accompanied by a drop of the tumor marker serum lactate dehydrogenase (**C**).

including *PIK3CA/R1*, *PTEN*, and *HOXD8* or *RAC1*. Reactivation of the MAPK pathway is the most frequent mechanism of acquired therapeutic resistance; thus, BRAF inhibitors have been combined with MEK inhibitors such as trametinib and cobimetinib. Combination treatment leads to even higher response rates of up to 70%, a median PFS of 10 to 11 months, and a median OS of about 2 years. Hence, combination treatment with a BRAF and a MEK inhibitor is standard of care for patients with *BRAF* mutant melanoma in addition to the immunotherapeutic options.

Treatment is generally well tolerated, with fatigue, nausea, diarrhea, arthralgia, and skin side effects as most common.[101] Skin side effects include exanthemas, hyperkeratosis, verrucous lesions, and secondary malignancies (cutaneous squamous cell carcinoma and even melanoma). The squamous lesions are explained by a paradoxical activation of MAPK signaling during treatment with BRAF inhibitors in BRAF wildtype keratinocytes. In most of the lesions, an *RAS* mutation can be found.[193,194] Such lesions are less frequent in the combination of BRAF and MEK inhibition.

Some side effects are not class but substance specific such as photosensitivity by vemurafenib and fever by dabrafenib. MEK inhibitors can worsen a preexisting heart insufficiency and lead to eye side effects like retinal vein occlusions and retinopathies. Hence, patients need surveillance by a cardiologist and an ophthalmologist under treatment.

In patients with NRAS mutations, the MEK inhibitor binimetinib was tested in a phase 3 trial against dacarbazine. It revealed limited efficacy, with an overall response rate of 15% and a median PFS of 2.8 months,[195] and hence will at best be a treatment after failure of immunotherapy.

c-KIT Inhibition: Melanomas from acral and mucosal sites are genetically distinct from other melanomas.[8] Most melanomas from acral and mucosal sites do not demonstrate mutations in *BRAF*, but a subset have activating mutations or amplification of the tyrosine kinase receptor *KIT*. These oncogenic lesions occur mostly in the juxtamembrane domain (*KIT* exons 11, 13, and 17)—a region that is frequently targeted in other cancers, including GI stromal tumors. Early studies with the tyrosine kinase inhibitor imatinib have demonstrated significant responses in patients with metastatic melanoma harboring activating mutations in c-KIT.[196,197] In several Phase II trials, imatinib and other KIT inhibitors such as nilotinib were tested in patients with KIT mutations and amplifications. Responses were observed in 16% to 23% of patients.[198,199] In both studies, certain mutations in exon 11 and 13 of c-KIT (particularly L576P mutation in exon 11) were associated with the highest response rate. Thus, sensitivity to KIT inhibition exists in metastatic melanoma but it is confined to a subset of this already small subpopulation of patients.

CHEMOTHERAPIES

The alkylating agent dacarbazine (DTIC) is the only FDA-approved chemotherapy for metastatic melanoma and is generally tolerated very well. However, response rates are only in the 10% range, with a median response duration of 4 to 6 months.[200] There is no difference in terms of response rates and duration of response between the various dosing schedules used. The major side effects are nausea and vomiting, which can be controlled by antiemetics. Temozolomide (TMZ) is an alkylating agent with the same active metabolite as DTIC, but it is absorbed orally and can be taken as a capsule. TMZ has been shown in a randomized Phase III study to have efficacy equal to DTIC.[201] Combination chemotherapies, for example, carboplatin/paclitaxel, might reveal higher response rates but have no survival benefit compared with monochemotherapy.[187,202] Toxicity is generally remarkably higher.

With the approval of immune checkpoint blocker and BRAF/MEK inhibitors, the use of chemotherapies has faded into the background. They might be used in a later line though it is important to keep in mind that an advantage in patient survival has not been shown. No randomized clinical trial exists where chemotherapy was compared to best supportive care.

TREATMENT ALGORITHM

See Fig. 116-14.

FUTURE DIRECTIONS

First results are available for the combination of targeted therapies with immune checkpoint blockade. The combination is enticing as the fast response to targeted therapies might be combined with a higher rate of long-term remissions, especially in patients with highly advanced disease. Combination of vemurafenib and ipilimumab demonstrated apparent success in a case series.[203] However, a significant hepatotoxicity was seen in a Phase I trial testing this combination.[204] Combination of BRAF/MEK inhibitors with PD-1/PD-L1–directed therapy seems to be less toxic.[205] Randomized phase 3 trials are recruiting patients, and data are pending.

Other combination strategies combine different immunotherapeutic approaches, for example, the combination of the PD-1 antibody pembrolizumab with the oncolytic virus T-VEC (Masterkey-265; NCT02263508)[206] or the indolamin-2,3-dioxygenase (IDO) inhibitor indoximod (NCT02073123) (Table 116-9). IDO is a negative immune modulator that may be expressed by antigen-presenting cells in the tumor microenvironment. Other inhibitory checkpoint molecules that could be targeted to modulate the immune response include LAG-3 and TIM-3, both of which are being targeted in early clinical trials for a number of indications. In addition, costimulatory TCR signals could be elicited, eg, by targeting CD137, OX40, CD27 or GITR. The complexity of the immune system and tumor microenvironment gives an idea of possible future treatment

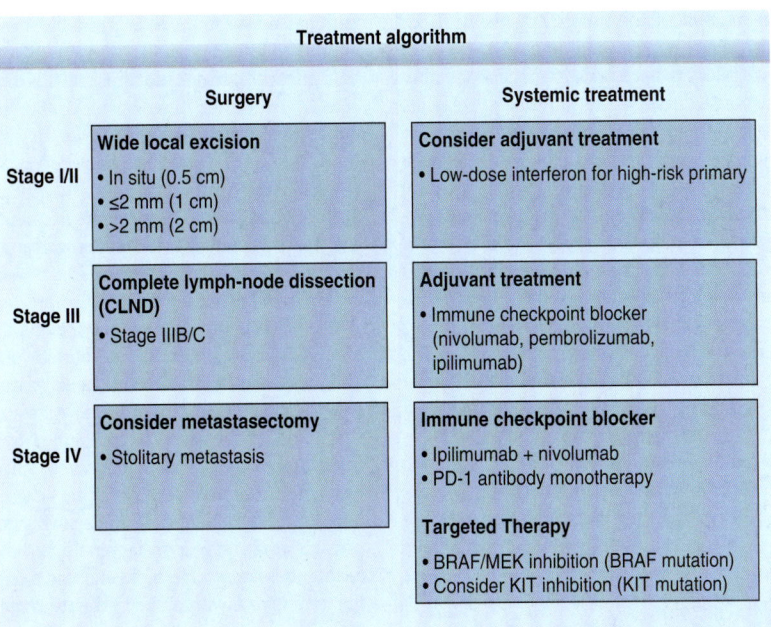

Figure 116-14 Treatment algorithm.

strategies and the challenge will be to find the best suitable targets and combinations.

The best treatment option might differ considerably between patients eg, it is known already that tumor characteristics like the mutational load (number of mutations) correlates with response to treatment with immune checkpoint blockers.[207,208] This is probably based on an increased chance for the immune system

TABLE 116-9			
New Developments in Immunotherapy of Stage IV Melanoma			
SUBSTANCE	TARGET	CLINICAL TRIALS	NCT NUMBER
Epacadostat	IDO inhibitor	Phase 3, in combination with pembrolizumab	NCT02752074
Indoximod	IDO inhibitor	Phase I/2 in combination with either ipilimumab, nivolumab or pembrolizumab	NCT02073123
Immune Checkpoint Blockers			
IMP321	LAG-3Ig Fusion Protein	Phase I, in combination with pembrolizumab	NCT02676869
Costimulatory TCR Signals			
BMS-663513	CD137 (4-1BB) antibody	Phase II, monotherapy	NCT00612664
Varlilumab	CD27 antibody	Phase I/2, in combination with ipilimumab +/- CDX-1401 (NY-ESO vaccine)	NCT02413827
TRX518-001	GITR antibody	Phase I, monotherapy	NCT01239134
Other Costimulatory Signals			
APX005M	CD40 antibody	Phase I/2 in combination with pembrolizumab	NCT02706353
Vaccinations			
Lipo-Merit	RNA vaccine encoding for 4 shared tumor antigens	Phase I, first in human	NCT02410733
IVAC Mutanome	Individual RNA vaccine encoding neoantigens	Phase I, first in human	NCT02035956
Other Mechanisms			
RFT-5-dgA	Immunotoxin against CD25+ T cells	Phase II, monotherapy	NCT00314093
IMCgp100	Bispecific soluble gp100-specific TCR fused to anti-CD3protein	Phase1b/2 monotherapy and combination with either durvalumab (PD-L1 Ab) or tremilimumab (CTLA-4 Ab)	NCT02535078
		Phase I in uveal melanoma	NCT02570308

to detect neo-antigens of the tumor by specific T-cell clones and hence a cancer-specific immune attack. In addition, other patient characteristics such as composition and responsiveness of the immune system are likely to influence treatment efficacy. Hence, it is very likely that several individual patient characteristics beyond the BRAF status will direct treatment choice to an individualized treatment in the near future—including analysis of tumor mutations, expression of immunoactive proteins such as PD-L1, and studies on the composition and geography of tumor-infiltrating immune cells. The understanding of the tumor immune defense can lead to new therapeutic strategies, for example, vaccination approaches not only against tumor-associated antigens[209] but individualized vaccines targeting the tumor mutanome of the patient.

In addition to combination with other systemic treatments, combination of immune checkpoint blockers with radiotherapy likely enhances tumor immune response by release of tumor antigens and proinflammatory cytokines as well as enhanced antigen presentation by upregulation of MHC molecule expression.[210] After radiation of single metastases, responses have been seen in metastases outside the radiation field, so-called abscopal responses.[211] Clinical trials will be necessary to evaluate fully the efficacy of this combination.

PREVENTION/SCREENING

Public awareness and knowledge of melanoma and UV exposure is improving, but still a substantial gap exists between knowledge and behavior. Primary prevention strategy should focus on safe sun exposure, including limited UV exposure and sunburn prevention, especially in childhood and adolescence when the risk is greatest. Avoidance of peak sunlight hours and use of wide-brimmed hats, clothing, and sunscreen are recommended. In addition, early detection by regular self-skin examinations, skin awareness, and knowledge of the early signs and symptoms of melanomas should also be emphasized to patient, partners, and family members. The goal of secondary prevention is early diagnosis, which greatly reduces melanoma-related morbidity and mortality.

FOLLOWUP

Patients with melanoma are at risk for local, regional, and distant recurrence, with the level of risk dependent on the stage at initial diagnosis and workup. Followup visits are an opportunity to review how to perform monthly skin and lymph node self-examinations, address any psychosocial emotional distress issues, obtain a melanoma-focused review of systems, and provide continuing patient education regarding early detection signs and symptoms and sun-protection/prevention strategies. Regular followup is indicated for all patients with melanoma. Current NCCN and national melanoma center guidelines call for at least annual followup visits for life, with followup intervals generally ranging from every 3 to 6 months for 1 to 3 years after diagnosis and annually thereafter, depending primarily on stage of disease.[212] Patients with other risk factors, such as a positive family history of melanoma, numerous nevi, or difficulty with self-examination, may require more frequent followup. A referral to a genetics counselor is warranted if there is a strong family history of melanoma, or a family history of pancreatic cancer.

The followup visit should consist of a thorough complete skin examination for additional primary lesions and cutaneous/subcutaneous metastases, particularly in the regional distribution of the primary, palpation of lymph nodes preferably accompanied by lymph node ultrasound with particular attention to the regional nodal basin, and thorough history taking. The review of systems is the foundation for detecting symptomatology possibly attributable to melanoma, and directs additional testing or imaging. The yield and value of routine imaging to restage asymptomatic patients as part of standard melanoma followup are low and, thus, internationally recommendation concerning followup procedures based on imaging and hematologic tests differ substantially.

ACKNOWLEGDMENTS

This chapter was revised and updated from the former version, composed by Evans C. Bailey, Arthur J. Sober, Hensin Tsao, Martin C. Mihm Jr, and Timothy M. Johnson, and we thank them for their contribution. We thank Nina Reuter, Media Center, University Hospital Heidelberg for photograph search.

REFERENCES

1. Shain AH, Bastian BC. From melanocytes to melanomas. *Nat Rev Cancer*. 2016;16(6):345-358.
2. Rebecca VW, Sondak VK, Smalley KSM. A brief history of melanoma: from mummies to mutations. *Melanoma Res*. 2012;22(2):114-122.
3. Ferlay J, Soerjomataram I, Ervik M, et al. GLOBOCAN 2012 v1.0, Cancer Incidence and Mortality Worldwide: IARC CancerBase No. 11 [Internet]. Lyon, France: International Agency for Research on Cancer; 2013. http://globocan.iarc.fr. Accessed day/month/year.
4. Howlader N, Noone AM, Krapcho M, et al. SEER Cancer Statistics Review, 1975-2013, National Cancer Institute. Bethesda, MD, http://seer.cancer.gov/csr/1975_2013/, based on November 2015 SEER data submission, posted to the SEER web site, April 2016.
5. Svedman FC, Pillas D, Taylor A, et al. Stage-specific survival and recurrence in patients with cutaneous malignant melanoma in Europe—a systematic review of the literature. *Clin Epidemiol*. 2016;8:109-122.
6. Arrangoiz R, Dorantes J, Cordera F, et al. Melanoma review: epidemiology, risk factors, diagnosis and staging. *J Cancer Treat Res*. 2016;4(1):1-15.
7. Thomas NE, Kricker A, Waxweiler WT, et al; Genes, Environment, and Melanoma (GEM) Study Group.

Comparison of clinicopathologic features and survival of histopathologically amelanotic and pigmented melanomas: a population-based study. *JAMA Dermatol.* 2014;150(12):1306-1314.
8. Curtin JA, Fridlyand J, Kageshita T, et al. Distinct sets of genetic alterations in melanoma. *N Engl J Med.* 2005;353(20):2135-2147.
9. Curtin JA, Busam K, Pinkel D, et al. Somatic activation of KIT in distinct subtypes of melanoma. *J Clin Oncol.* 2006;24(26):4340-4346.
10. Torres-Cabala CA, Wang WL, Trent J, et al. Correlation between KIT expression and KIT mutation in melanoma: a study of 173 cases with emphasis on the acral-lentiginous/mucosal type. *Mod Pathol.* 2009;22(11):1446-1456.
11. Busam KJ, Zhao H, Coit DG, et al. Distinction of desmoplastic melanoma from non-desmoplastic melanoma by gene expression profiling. *J Invest Dermatol.* 2005;124(2):412-418.
12. Shain AH, Garrido M, Botton T, et al. Exome sequencing of desmoplastic melanoma identifies recurrent NFKBIE promoter mutations and diverse activating mutations in the MAPK pathway. *Nat Genet.* 2015;47(10):1194-1199.
13. Wiesner T, Kiuru M, Scott SN, et al. NF1 Mutations are common in desmoplastic melanoma. *Am J Surg Pathol.* 2015;39(10):1357-1362.
14. McLaughlin CC, Wu XC, Jemal A, et al. Incidence of noncutaneous melanomas in the U.S. *Cancer.* 2005;103(5):1000-1007.
15. Rodriguez-Sains RS. Pigmented conjunctival neoplasms. *Orbit.* 2002;21(3):231-238.
16. Cosgarea I, Ugurel S, Sucker A, et al. Targeted next generation sequencing of mucosal melanomas identifies frequent NF1 and RAS mutations. *Oncotarget.* 2017;8(25):40683-40692.
17. Amit M, Tam S, Abdelmeguid AS, et al. Mutation status among patients with sinonasal mucosal melanoma and its impact on survival. *Br J Cancer.* 2017;116(12):1564-1571.
18. Öztürk Sari Ş, Yilmaz İ, Taşkin OÇ, et al. BRAF, NRAS, KIT, TERT, GNAQ/GNA11 mutation profile analysis of head and neck mucosal melanomas: a study of 42 cases. *Pathology.* 2017;49(1):55-61.
19. Hou JY, Baptiste C, Hombalegowda RB, et al. Vulvar and vaginal melanoma: a unique subclass of mucosal melanoma based on a comprehensive molecular analysis of 51 cases compared with 2253 cases of nongynecologic melanoma. *Cancer.* 2017;123(8):1333-1344.
20. Yang HM, Hsiao SJ, Schaeffer DF, et al. Identification of recurrent mutational events in anorectal melanoma. *Mod Pathol.* 2017;30(2):286-296.
21. Kim KB, Alrwas A. Treatment of KIT-mutated metastatic mucosal melanoma. *Chin Clin Oncol.* 2014;3(3):35.
22. Magro CM, Crowson AN, Mihm MC. Unusual variants of malignant melanoma. *Mod Pathol.* 2006;19(suppl 2):S41-S70.
23. Ludgate MW, Fullen DR, Lee J, et al. The atypical Spitz tumor of uncertain biologic potential: a series of 67 patients from a single institution. *Cancer.* 2009;115(3):631-641.
24. Wiesner T, Kutzner H, Cerroni L, et al. Genomic aberrations in spitzoid melanocytic tumours and their implications for diagnosis, prognosis and therapy. *Pathology.* 2016;48(2):113-131.
25. Ludgate MW, Fullen DR, Lee J, et al. Animal-type melanoma: a clinical and histopathological study of 22 cases from a single institution. *Br J Dermatol.* 2010;162(1):129-136.
26. Dutton-Regester K, Kakavand H, Aoude LG, et al. Melanomas of unknown primary have a mutation profile consistent with cutaneous sun-exposed melanoma. *Pigment Cell Melanoma Res.* 2013;26(6):852-860.
27. Carson KF, Wen DR, Li PX, et al. Nodal nevi and cutaneous melanomas. *Am J Surg Pathol.* 1996;20(7):834-840.
28. Chattopadhyay C, Kim DW, Gombos DS, et al. Uveal melanoma: from diagnosis to treatment and the science in between. *Cancer.* 2016;122(15):2299-2312.
29. Thomas S, Pütter C, Weber S, et al. Prognostic significance of chromosome 3 alterations determined by microsatellite analysis in uveal melanoma: a long-term follow-up study. *Br J Cancer.* 2012;106(6):1171-1176.
30. Woodward JK, Elshaw SR, Murray AK, et al. Stimulation and inhibition of uveal melanoma invasion by HGF, GRO, IL-1alpha and TGF-beta. *Invest Ophthalmol Vis Sci.* 2002;43(10):3144-3152.
31. Vyas R, Selph J, Gerstenblith MR. Cutaneous manifestations associated with melanoma. *Semin Oncol.* 2016;43(3):384-389.
32. Hua C, Boussemart L, Mateus C, et al. Association of vitiligo with tumor response in patients with metastatic melanoma treated with pembrolizumab. *JAMA Dermatol.* 2016;152(1):45-51.
33. Grewal DS, Fishman GA, Jampol LM. Autoimmune retinopathy and antiretinal antibodies: a review. *Retina.* 2014;34(5):827-845.
34. Usher-Smith JA, Emery J, Kassianos AP, et al. Risk prediction models for melanoma: a systematic review. *Cancer Epidemiol Biomarkers Prev.* 2014;23(8):1450-1463.
35. Vuong K, McGeechan K, Armstrong BK, et al. Risk prediction models for incident primary cutaneous melanoma: a systematic review. *JAMA Dermatol.* 2014;150(4):434-444.
36. Elwood JM, Jopson J. Melanoma and sun exposure: an overview of published studies. *Int J Cancer.* 1997;73(2):198-203.
37. Volkovova K, Bilanicova D, Bartonova A, et al. Associations between environmental factors and incidence of cutaneous melanoma. *Environ Health.* 2012;11(suppl 1):S12.
38. Gillgren P, Brattström G, Djureen Mårtensson E, et al. A new computerized methodology to analyse tumour site in relation to phenotypic traits and epidemiological characteristics of cutaneous malignant melanoma. *Br J Dermatol.* 2002;146(6):1023-1030.
39. Elwood JM, Gallagher RP. Body site distribution of cutaneous malignant melanoma in relationship to patterns of sun exposure. *Int J Cancer.* 1998;78(3):276-280.
40. Stern RS. The risk of melanoma in association with long-term exposure to PUVA. *J Am Acad Dermatol.* 2001;44(5):755-761.
41. Pouplard C, Brenaut E, Horreau C, et al. Risk of cancer in psoriasis: a systematic review and meta-analysis of epidemiological studies. *J Eur Acad Dermatol Venereol.* 2013;27(suppl 3):36-46.
42. Gallagher RP, Spinelli JJ, Lee TK. Tanning beds, sunlamps, and risk of cutaneous malignant melanoma. *Cancer Epidemiol Biomarkers Prev.* 2005;14(3):562-566.
43. Le Clair MZ, Cockburn MG. Tanning bed use and melanoma: establishing risk and improving prevention interventions. *Prev Med Rep.* 2016;3:139-144.

44. Bald T, Quast T, Landsberg J, et al. Ultraviolet-radiation-induced inflammation promotes angiotropism and metastasis in melanoma. *Nature.* 2014; 507(7490):109-113.
45. Green AC, Williams GM, Logan V, et al. Reduced melanoma after regular sunscreen use: randomized trial follow-up. *J Clin Oncol.* 2011;29(3):257-263.
46. Ransohoff KJ, Jaju PD, Tang JY, et al. Familial skin cancer syndromes: increased melanoma risk. *J Am Acad Dermatol.* 2016;74(3):423-434.
47. Bauer J, Garbe C. Acquired melanocytic nevi as risk factor for melanoma development. A comprehensive review of epidemiological data. *Pigment Cell Res.* 2003;16(3):297-306.
48. Tucker MA, Halpern A, Holly EA, et al. Clinically recognized dysplastic nevi. A central risk factor for cutaneous melanoma. *JAMA.* 1997;277(18):1439-1444.
49. Bevona C, Goggins W, Quinn T, et al. Cutaneous melanomas associated with nevi. *Arch Dermatol.* 2003;139(12):1620-1624.
50. Tromberg J, Bauer B, Benvenuto-Andrade C, et al. Congenital melanocytic nevi needing treatment. *Dermatol Ther.* 2005;18(2):136-150.
51. Vourc'h-Jourdain M, Martin L, Barbarot S, et al. Large congenital melanocytic nevi: therapeutic management and melanoma risk: a systematic review. *J Am Acad Dermatol.* 2013;68(3):493-498,e1-e14.
52. Niendorf KB, Tsao H. Cutaneous melanoma: family screening and genetic testing. *Dermatol Ther.* 2006; 19(1):1-8.
53. Hansen CB, Wadge LM, Lowstuter K, et al. Clinical germline genetic testing for melanoma. *Lancet Oncol.* 2004;5(5):314-319.
54. Sharpless E, Chin L. The INK4a/ARF locus and melanoma. *Oncogene.* 2003;22(20):3092-3098.
55. Liu W, Hill D, Gibbs AF, et al. What features do patients notice that help to distinguish between benign pigmented lesions and melanomas? The ABCD(E) rule versus the seven-point checklist. *Melanoma Res.* 2005;15(6):549-554.
56. Nagore E, Oliver V, Moreno-Picot S, et al. Primary cutaneous melanoma in hidden sites is associated with thicker tumours—A study of 829 patients. *Eur J Cancer.* 2001;37(1):79-82.
57. Friedman RJ, Rigel DS, Kopf AW. Early detection of malignant melanoma: the role of physician examination and self-examination of the skin. *CA Cancer J Clin.* 1985;35(3):130-151.
58. Abbasi NR, Shaw HM, Rigel DS, et al. Early diagnosis of cutaneous melanoma: revisiting the ABCD criteria. *JAMA.* 2004;292(22):2771-2776.
59. Whited JD, Grichnik JM. The rational clinical examination. Does this patient have a mole or a melanoma? *JAMA.* 1998;279(9):696-701.
60. Gachon J, Beaulieu P, Sei JF, et al. First prospective study of the recognition process of melanoma in dermatological practice. *Arch Dermatol.* 2005;141(4):434-438.
61. Vestergaard ME, Macaskill P, Holt PE, et al. Dermoscopy compared with naked eye examination for the diagnosis of primary melanoma: a meta-analysis of studies performed in a clinical setting. *Br J Dermatol.* 2008;159(3):669-676.
62. Bafounta ML, Beauchet A, Aegerter P, et al. Is dermoscopy (epiluminescence microscopy) useful for the diagnosis of melanoma? Results of a meta-analysis using techniques adapted to the evaluation of diagnostic tests. *Arch Dermatol.* 2001;137(10):1343-1350.
63. Annessi G, Bono R, Sampogna F, et al. Sensitivity, specificity, and diagnostic accuracy of three dermoscopic algorithmic methods in the diagnosis of doubtful melanocytic lesions: the importance of light brown structureless areas in differentiating atypical melanocytic nevi from thin melanomas. *J Am Acad Dermatol.* 2007;56(5):759-767.
64. Dolianitis C, Kelly J, Wolfe R, et al. Comparative performance of 4 dermoscopic algorithms by nonexperts for the diagnosis of melanocytic lesions. *Arch Dermatol.* 2005;141(8):1008-1014.
65. Blum A, Rassner G, Garbe C. Modified ABC-point list of dermoscopy: a simplified and highly accurate dermoscopic algorithm for the diagnosis of cutaneous melanocytic lesions. *J Am Acad Dermatol.* 2003;48(5):672-678.
66. Henning JS, Dusza SW, Wang SQ, et al. The CASH (color, architecture, symmetry, and homogeneity) algorithm for dermoscopy. *J Am Acad Dermatol.* 2007;56(1):45-52.
67. Noor O 2nd, Nanda A, Rao BK. A dermoscopy survey to assess who is using it and why it is or is not being used. *Int J Dermatol.* 2009;48(9):951-952.
68. Haenssle HA, Krueger U, Vente C, et al. Results from an observational trial: digital epiluminescence microscopy follow-up of atypical nevi increases the sensitivity and the chance of success of conventional dermoscopy in detecting melanoma. *J Invest Dermatol.* 2006;126(5):980-985.
69. Kittler H, Guitera P, Riedl E, et al. Identification of clinically featureless incipient melanoma using sequential dermoscopy imaging. *Arch Dermatol.* 2006;142(9): 1113-1139.
70. Goodson AG, Grossman D. Strategies for early melanoma detection: approaches to the patient with nevi. *J Am Acad Dermatol.* 2009;60(5):719-735.
71. Lien MH, Sondak VK. Diagnostic techniques for primary cutaneous melanoma [review]. *G Ital Dermatol Venereol.* 2009;144(2):187-194.
72. Tran KT, Wright NA, Cockerell CJ. Biopsy of the pigmented lesion—when and how. *J Am Acad Dermatol.* 2008;59(5):852-871.
73. Martin RC 2nd, Scoggins CR, Ross MI, et al. Is incisional biopsy of melanoma harmful? *Am J Surg.* 2005;190(6):913-917.
74. Karimipour DJ, Schwartz JL, Wang TS, et al. Microstaging accuracy after subtotal incisional biopsy of cutaneous melanoma. *J Am Acad Dermatol.* 2005; 52(5):798-802.
75. Smoller BR. Histologic criteria for diagnosing primary cutaneous malignant melanoma. *Mod Pathol.* 2006;19(suppl 2):S34-S40.
76. Davis IJ, Kim JJ, Ozsolak F. Oncogenic MITF dysregulation in clear cell sarcoma: defining the MiT family of human cancers. *Cancer Cell.* 2006;9(6):473-484.
77. Ramos-Herberth FI, Karamchandani J, Kim J, et al. SOX10 immunostaining distinguishes desmoplastic melanoma from excision scar. *J Cutan Pathol.* 2010;37(9):944-952.
78. Balch CM, Gershenwald JE, Soong SJ, et al. Final version of 2009 AJCC melanoma staging and classification. *J Clin Oncol.* 2009;27(36):6199-6206.
79. Gogas H, Eggermont AM, Hauschild A, et al. Biomarkers in melanoma. *Ann Oncol.* 2009;20(suppl 6):vi8-vi13.
80. Mocellin S, Zavagno G, Nitti D. The prognostic value of serum S100B in patients with cutaneous melanoma: a meta-analysis. *Int J Cancer.* 2008;123(10):2370-2376.

81. Wang TS, Johnson TM, Cascade PN, et al. Evaluation of staging chest radiographs and serum lactate dehydrogenase for localized melanoma. *J Am Acad Dermatol.* 2004;51(3):399-405.
82. Uren RF, Howman-Giles R, Thompson JF. Patterns of lymphatic drainage from the skin in patients with melanoma. *J Nucl Med.* 2003;44(4):570-582.
83. Bafounta ML, Beauchet A, Chagnon S, et al. Ultrasonography or palpation for detection of melanoma nodal invasion: a meta-analysis. *Lancet Oncol.* 2004;5(11):673-680.
84. Voit C, Van Akkooi AC, Schäfer-Hesterberg G, et al. Ultrasound morphology criteria predict metastatic disease of the sentinel nodes in patients with melanoma. *J Clin Oncol.* 2010;28(5):847-852.
85. Sabel MS, Wong SL. Review of evidence-based support for pretreatment imaging in melanoma. *J Natl Compr Canc Netw.* 2009;7(3):281-289.
86. Sawyer A, McGoldrick RB, Mackey SP, et al. Does staging computed tomography change management in thick malignant melanoma? *J Plast Reconstr Aesthet Surg.* 2009;62(4):453-456.
87. Vereecken P, Laporte M, Petein M, et al. Evaluation of extensive initial staging procedure in intermediate/high-risk melanoma patients. *J Eur Acad Dermatol Venereol.* 2005;19(1):66-73.
88. Johnson TM, Bradford CR, Gruber SB, et al. Staging workup, sentinel node biopsy, and follow-up tests for melanoma: update of current concepts. *Arch Dermatol.* 2004;140(1):107-113.
89. Valsecchi ME, Silbermins D, de Rosa N, et al. Lymphatic mapping and sentinel lymph node biopsy in patients with melanoma: a meta-analysis. *J Clin Oncol.* 2011;29(11):1479-1487.
90. Warycha M, Zakrzewski J, Ni Q, et al. Metaanalysis of sentinel lymph node positivity in thin melanoma (≤1 mm). *Cancer.* 2009;115(4):869-879.
91. Kretschmer L, Starz H, Thoms KM, et al. Age as a key factor influencing metastasizing patterns and disease-specific survival after sentinel lymph node biopsy for cutaneous melanoma. *Int J Cancer.* 2011;129(6):1435-1442.
92. Kunte C, Geimer T, Baumert J, et al. Prognostic factors associated with sentinel lymph node positivity and effect of sentinel status on survival: an analysis of 1049 patients with cutaneous melanoma. *Melanoma Res.* 2010;20(4):330-337.
93. McMasters KM, Reintgen DS, Ross MI, et al. Factors that predict the presence of sentinel lymph node metastasis in patients with melanoma. *Surgery.* 2001;130(2):151-156.
94. Gutzmer R, Satzger I, Thoms KM, et al. Sentinel lymph node status is the most important prognostic factor for thick (> or = 4 mm) melanomas. *J Dtsch Dermatol Ges.* 2008;6(3):198-203.
95. Morton DL, Wen DR, Wong JH, et al. Technical details of intraoperative lymphatic mapping for early stage melanoma. *Arch Surg.* 1992;127(4):392-399.
96. McCready DR, Ghazarian DM, Hershkop MS, et al. Sentinel lymph-node biopsy after previous wide local excision for melanoma. *Can J Surg.* 2001;44(6):432-434.
97. Thompson JF, Shaw HM, Hersey P, et al. The history and future of melanoma staging. *J Surg Oncol.* 2004;86(4):224-235.
98. Morton DL, Thompson JF, Cochran AJ, et al. Sentinel-node biopsy or nodal observation in melanoma. *N Engl J Med.* 2006;355(13):1307-1317.
99. Leiter U, Stadler R, Mauch C, et al. German Dermatologic Cooperative Oncology Group (DeCOG): complete lymph node dissection versus no dissection in patients with sentinel lymph node biopsy positive melanoma (DeCOG-SLT): a multicentre, randomised, phase 3 trial. *Lancet Oncol.* 2016;17(6):757-767.
100. Crowley NJ, Seigler HF. Late recurrence of malignant melanoma. Analysis of 168 patients. *Ann Surg.* 1990;212(2):173-177.
101. Long GV, Stroyakovskiy D, Gogas H, et al. Dabrafenib and trametinib versus dabrafenib and placebo for Val600 BRAF-mutant melanoma: a multicentre, double-blind, phase 3 randomised controlled trial. *Lancet.* 2015;386(9992):444-451.
102. Robert C, Ribas A, Hamid O, et al. Three-year overall survival for patients with advanced melanoma treated with pembrolizumab in Keynote-001 [abstract 9503]. *J Clin Oncol.* 2016;34(suppl).
103. Chang P, Knapper WH. Metastatic melanoma of unknown primary. *Cancer.* 1982;49(6):1106-1111.
104. Schlagenhauff B, Stroebel W, Ellwanger U, et al. Metastatic melanoma of unknown primary origin shows prognostic similarities to regional metastatic melanoma: recommendations for initial staging examinations. *Cancer.* 1997;80(1):60-65.
105. Edge SB, Compton CC. The American Joint Committee on Cancer: the 7th edition of the AJCC cancer staging manual and the future of TNM. *Ann Surg Oncol.* 2010;17(6):1471-1474.
106. Gershenwald JE, Scolyer RA, Hess KR, et al. Melanoma staging: evidence-based changes in the American Joint Committee on Cancer eighth edition cancer staging manual. *CA Cancer J Clin.* 2017;67(6):472-492.
107. Tas F, Erturk K. Presence of histological regression as a prognostic factor in cutaneous melanoma patients. *Melanoma Res.* 2016;26(5):492-496.
108. Stucky CC, Gray RJ, Dueck AC, et al. Risk factors associated with local and in-transit recurrence of cutaneous melanoma. *Am J Surg.* 2010;200(6):770-774.
109. Homsi J, Kashani-Sabet M, Messina JL, et al. Cutaneous melanoma: prognostic factors. *Cancer Control.* 2005;12(4):223-229.
110. Balch CM, Soong SJ, Gershenwald JE, et al. Prognostic factors analysis of 17,600 melanoma patients: validation of the American Joint Committee on Cancer melanoma staging system. *J Clin Oncol.* 2001;19(16):3622-3634.
111. Eggermont AM, Chiarion-Sileni V, Grob JJ, et al. Adjuvant ipilimumab versus placebo after complete resection of high-risk stage III melanoma (EORTC 18071): a randomised, double-blind, phase 3 trial. *Lancet Oncol.* 2015;16(5):522-530.
112. Eggermont AM, Suciu S, Rutkowski P, et al. EORTC Melanoma group: long term follow up of the EORTC 18952 trial of adjuvant therapy in resected stage IIB-III cutaneous melanoma patients comparing intermediate doses of interferon-alpha-2b (IFN) with observation: ulceration of primary is key determinant for IFN-sensitivity. *Eur J Cancer.* 2016;55:111-121.
113. Eggermont AM, Spatz A, Lazar V, et al. Is ulceration in cutaneous melanoma just a prognostic and predictive factor or is ulcerated melanoma a distinct biologic entity? *Curr Opin Oncol.* 2012;24(2):137-140.
114. Azzola MF, Shaw HM, Thompson JF, et al. Tumor mitotic rate is a more powerful prognostic indicator than ulceration in patients with primary cutaneous melanoma: an analysis of 3661 patients from a single center. *Cancer.* 2003;97(6):1488-1498.

115. Paek SC, Griffith KA, Johnson TM, et al. The impact of factors beyond Breslow depth on predicting sentinel lymph node positivity in melanoma. *Cancer.* 2007;109(1):100-108.
116. Elder DE, Gimotty PA, Guerry D. Cutaneous melanoma: estimating survival and recurrence risk based on histopathologic features. *Dermatol Ther.* 2005; 18(5):369-385.
117. Thomas NE, Busam KJ, From L, et al. Tumor-infiltrating lymphocyte grade in primary melanomas is independently associated with melanoma-specific survival in the population-based genes, environment and melanoma study. *J Clin Oncol.* 2013;31(33):4252-4259.
118. Weiss SA, Han SW, Lui K, et al. Immunologic heterogeneity of tumor infiltrating lymphocyte composition in primary melanoma. *Hum Pathol.* 2016;57:116-125.
119. Gershenwald JE, Thompson W, Mansfield PF, et al. Multi-institutional melanoma lymphatic mapping experience: the prognostic value of sentinel lymph node status in 612 stage I or II melanoma patients. *J Clin Oncol.* 1999;17(3):976-983.
120. Tsao H, Feldman M, Fullerton JE, et al. Early detection of asymptomatic pulmonary melanoma metastases by routine chest radiographs is not associated with improved survival. *Arch Dermatol.* 2004;140(1):67-70.
121. Sladden MJ, Balch C, Barzilai DA, et al. Surgical excision margins for primary cutaneous melanoma. *Cochrane Database Syst Rev.* 2009;(4):CD004835.
122. Hayes AJ, Maynard L, Coombes G, et al; UK Melanoma Study Group; British Association of Plastic, Reconstructive and Aesthetic Surgeons; Scottish Cancer Therapy Network; wide versus narrow excision margins for high-risk, primary cutaneous melanomas: long-term follow-up of survival in a randomised trial. *Lancet Oncol.* 2016;17(2):184-192.
123. Veronesi U, Cascinelli N. Narrow excision (1-cm margin). A safe procedure for thin cutaneous melanoma. *Arch Surg.* 1991;126(4):438-441.
124. Cohn-Cedermark G, Rutqvist LE, Andersson R, et al. Long term results of a randomized study by the Swedish Melanoma Study Group on 2-cm versus 5-cm resection margins for patients with cutaneous melanoma with a tumor thickness of 0.8-2.0 mm. *Cancer.* 2000;89(7):1495-1501.
125. McLeod M, Choudhary S, Giannakakis G, et al. Surgical treatments for lentigo maligna: a review. *Dermatol Surg.* 2011;37(9):1210-1228.
126. Lens MB, Dawes M, Goodacre T, et al. Elective lymph node dissection in patients with melanoma: systematic review and meta-analysis of randomized controlled trials. *Arch Surg.* 2002;137(4):458-461.
127. Morton DL, Cochran AJ, Thompson JF, et al. Sentinel node biopsy for early-stage melanoma: accuracy and morbidity in MSLT-I, an international multicenter trial. *Ann Surg.* 2005;242(3):302-311.
128. Sabel MS, Griffith K, Sondak VK, et al. Predictors of nonsentinel lymph node positivity in patients with a positive sentinel node for melanoma. *J Am Coll Surg.* 2005;201(1):37-47.
129. Ghaferi AA, Wong SL, Johnson TM, et al. Prognostic significance of a positive nonsentinel lymph node in cutaneous melanoma. *Ann Surg Oncol.* 2009;16(11):2978-2984.
130. Sabel MS, Griffith KA, Arora A, et al. Inguinal node dissection for melanoma in the era of sentinel lymph node biopsy. *Surgery.* 2007;141(6):728-735.
131. Young SE, Martinez SR, Faries MB, et al. Can surgical therapy alone achieve long-term cure of melanoma metastatic to regional nodes? *Cancer J.* 2006;12(3):207-211.
132. Bender C, Hassel JC, Enk A. Immunotherapy of melanoma. *Oncol Res Treat.* 2016;39(6):369-376.
133. Hassel JC, Winnemöller D, Schartl M, et al. STAT5 contributes to antiapoptosis in melanoma. *Melanoma Res.* 2008;18(6):378-385.
134. Wellbrock C, Weisser C, Hassel JC, et al. STAT5 contributes to interferon resistance of melanoma cells. *Curr Biol.* 2005;15(18):1629-1639.
135. Ortiz A, Fuchs SY. Anti-metastatic functions of type 1 interferons: Foundation for the Adjuvant Therapy of Cancer. *Cytokine.* 2016;S1043-4666(16)30010-2.
136. Mocellin S, Lens MB, Pasquali S, et al. Interferon alpha for the adjuvant treatment of cutaneous melanoma. *Cochrane Database Syst Rev.* 2013;18(6):CD008955.
137. Wheatley K, Ives N, Eggermont A, et al. Interferon-alpha as adjuvant therapy for melanoma: an individual patient data meta-analysis of randomized trials [abstract 8526]. *J Clin Oncol.* 2007;25(suppl).
138. McMasters KM, Egger ME, Edwards MJ, et al. Final results of the sunbelt melanoma trial: a multi-institutional prospective randomized phase III study evaluating the role of adjuvant high-dose interferon alfa-2b and completion lymph node dissection for patients staged by sentinel lymph node biopsy. *J Clin Oncol.* 2016;34(10):1079-1086.
139. Kirkwood JM, Ibrahim JG, Sondak VK, et al. High- and low-dose interferon alfa-2b in high-risk melanoma: first analysis of intergroup trial E1690/S9111/C9190. *J Clin Oncol.* 2000;18(12):2444-2458.
140. Gogas H, Ioannovich J, Dafni U, et al. Prognostic significance of autoimmunity during treatment of melanoma with interferon. *N Engl J Med.* 2006;354(7):709-718.
141. Agrawal S, Kane JM 3rd, Guadagnolo BA, et al. The benefits of adjuvant radiation therapy after therapeutic lymphadenectomy for clinically advanced, high-risk, lymph node-metastatic melanoma. *Cancer.* 2009;115(24):5836-5844.
142. Bibault JE, Dewas S, Mirabel X, et al. Adjuvant radiation therapy in metastatic lymph nodes from melanoma. *Radiat Oncol.* 2011;6(Web Page):12.
143. Strojan P, Jancar B, Cemazar M, et al. Melanoma metastases to the neck nodes: role of adjuvant irradiation. *Int J Radiat Oncol Biol Phys.* 2010;77(4):1039-1045.
144. Burmeister BH, Henderson MA, Ainslie J, et al. Adjuvant radiotherapy versus observation alone for patients at risk of lymph-node field relapse after therapeutic lymphadenectomy for melanoma: a randomised trial. *Lancet Oncol.* 2012;13(6):589-597.
145. Chadha M, Hilaris B, Nori D, et al. Role of brachytherapy in malignant melanoma: a preliminary report. *J Surg Oncol.* 1990;43(4):223-227.
146. Overgaard J, Gonzalez Gonzalez D, Hulshof MC, et al. Hyperthermia as an adjuvant to radiation therapy of recurrent or metastatic malignant melanoma. A multicentre randomized trial by the European Society for Hyperthermic Oncology. *Int J Hyperthermia.* 2009; 25(Web Page):323-334.
147. Spratt DE, Gordon Spratt EA, Wu S, et al. Efficacy of skin-directed therapy for cutaneous metastases from advanced cancer: a meta-analysis. *J Clin Oncol.* 2014;32(28):3144-3155.
148. Weide B, Eigentler TK, Pflugfelder A, et al. Survival after intratumoral interleukin-2 treatment of 72 melanoma patients and response upon the first chemotherapy during follow-up. *Cancer Immunol Immunother.* 2011;60(4):487-493.

149. Byers BA, Temple-Oberle CF, Hurdle V, et al. Treatment of in-transit melanoma with intra-lesional interleukin-2: a systematic review. *J Surg Oncol.* 2014;110(6):770-775.
150. Andtbacka RH, Kaufman HL, Collichio F, et al. Talimogene laherparepvec improves durable response rate in patients with advanced melanoma. *J Clin Oncol.* 2015;33(25):2780-2788.
151. Mali B, Jarm T, Snoj M, et al. Antitumor effectiveness of electrochemotherapy: a systematic review and meta-analysis. *Eur J Surg Oncol.* 2013;39(1):4-16.
152. Grunhagen DJ, de Wilt JH, van Geel AN, et al. Isolated limb perfusion for melanoma patients—a review of its indications and the role of tumour necrosis factor-alpha. *Eur J Surg Oncol.* 2006;32(4):371-380.
153. Thompson JF, Kam PC. Isolated limb infusion for melanoma: a simple but effective alternative to isolated limb perfusion. *J Surg Oncol.* 2004;88(1):1-3.
154. Leyvraz S, Piperno-Neumann S, Suciu S, et al. Hepatic intra-arterial versus intravenous fotemustine in patients with liver metastases from uveal melanoma (EORTC 18021): a multicentric randomized trial. *Ann Oncol.* 2014;25(3):742-746.
155. Hughes MS, Zager J, Faries M, et al. Results of a randomized controlled multicenter phase III trial of percutaneous hepatic perfusion compared with best available care for patients with melanoma liver metastases. *Ann Surg Oncol.* 2016;23(4):1309-1319.
156. Schadendorf D, Hodi FS, Robert C, et al. Pooled analysis of long-term survival data from phase II and phase III trials of ipilimumab in unresectable or metastatic melanoma. *J Clin Oncol.* 2015;33(17):1889-1894.
157. Tagawa ST, Cheung E, Banta W, et al. Survival analysis after resection of metastatic disease followed by peptide vaccines in patients with Stage IV melanoma. *Cancer.* 2006;106(6):1353-1357.
158. Koebel CM, Vermi W, Swann JB, et al. Adaptive immunity maintains occult cancer in an equilibrium state. *Nature.* 2007;450(7171):903-907.
159. Chen DS, Mellman I. Oncology meets immunology: the cancer-immunity cycle. *Immunity.* 2013;39(1):1-10.
160. Kalialis LV, Drzewiecki KT, Klyver H. Spontaneous regression of metastases from melanoma: review of the literature. *Melanoma Res.* 2009;19(5):275-282.
161. Robbins HA, Clarke CA, Arron ST, et al. Melanoma risk and survival among organ transplant recipients. *J Invest Dermatol.* 2015;135(11):2657-2665.
162. Hoos A. Development of immuno-oncology drugs- from CTLA4 to PD1 to the next generations. *Nat Rev Drug Discov.* 2016;15(4):235-247.
163. Hodi FS, O'Day SJ, McDermott DF, et al. Improved survival with ipilimumab in patients with metastatic melanoma. *N Engl J Med.* 2010;363(8):711-723.
164. Gandini S, Massi D, Mandalà M. PD-L1 expression in cancer patients receiving anti PD-1/PD-L1 antibodies: a systematic review and meta-analysis. *Crit Rev Oncol Hematol.* 2016;100:88-98.
165. Taube JM, Anders RA, Young GD, et al. Colocalization of inflammatory response with B7-h1 expression in human melanocytic lesions supports an adaptive resistance mechanism of immune escape. *Sci Transl Med.* 2012;4(127):127ra37.
166. Obeid JM, Erdag G, Smolkin ME, et al. PD-L1, PD-L2 and PD-1 expression in metastatic melanoma: correlation with tumor-infiltrating immune cells and clinical outcome. *Oncoimmunology.* 2016;5(11):e1235107.
167. Danilova L, Wang H, Sunshine J, et al. Association of PD-1/PD-L axis expression with cytolytic activity, mutational load, and prognosis in melanoma and other solid tumors. *Proc Natl Acad Sci U S A.* 2016;113(48):e7769-e7777.
168. Robert C, Long GV, Brady B, et al. Nivolumab in previously untreated melanoma without BRAF mutation. *N Engl J Med.* 2015;372(4):320-330.
169. Daud A, Hamid O, Robert C, et al. Relationship between PD-L1 expression and efficacy in 655 patients with melanoma treated with pembrolizumab (MK-3475). Society for Melanoma Research Annual Meeting; San Francisco, CA; November 18-21, 2015.
170. Larkin J, Chiarion-Sileni V, Gonzalez R, et al. Combined nivolumab and ipilimumab or monotherapy in untreated melanoma. *N Engl J Med.* 2015;373(13):1270-1271.
171. Wolchok JD, Rollin L, Larkin J. Nivolumab and ipilimumab in advanced melanoma. *N Engl J Med.* 2017;377(25):2503-2504.
172. Zimmer L, Vaubel J, Mohr P, et al. Phase II DeCOG-study of ipilimumab in pretreated and treatment-naïve patients with metastatic uveal melanoma. *PLoS One.* 2015;10(3):e0118564.
173. Algazi AP, Tsai KK, Shoushtari AN, et al. Clinical outcomes in metastatic uveal melanoma treated with PD-1 and PD-L1 antibodies. *Cancer.* 2016;122(21):3344-3353.
174. Karydis I, Chan PY, Wheater M, et al. Clinical activity and safety of pembrolizumab in ipilimumab pre-treated patients with uveal melanoma. *Oncoimmunology.* 2016;5(5):e1143997.
175. Kottschade LA, McWilliams RR, Markovic SN, et al. The use of pembrolizumab for the treatment of metastatic uveal melanoma. *Melanoma Res.* 2016;26(3):300-303.
176. Hassel JC, Heinzerling L, Aberle J, et al. Combined immune checkpoint blockade (anti-PD-1/anti-CTLA-4): evaluation and management of adverse drug reactions. *Cancer Treat Rev.* 2017;57:36-49.
177. Sanlorenzo M, Vujic I, Daud A, et al. Pembrolizumab cutaneous adverse events and their association with disease progression. *JAMA Dermatol.* 2015;151(11):1206-1212.
178. Weber JS, Hodi FS, Wolchok JD, et al. Safety profile of nivolumab monotherapy: a pooled analysis of patients with advanced melanoma. *J Clin Oncol.* 2017;35(7):785-792.
179. Dick J, Lang N, Slynko A, et al. Use of LDH and autoimmune side effects to predict response to ipilimumab treatment. *Immunotherapy.* 2016;8(9):1033-1044.
180. Buder-Bakhaya K, Benesova K, Schulz C, et al. Characterization of arthralgia induced by PD-1 antibody treatment in patients with metastasized cutaneous malignancies. *Cancer Immunol Immunother.* 2017;41(10):1381-1389.
181. Kaunitz GJ, Loss M, Rizvi H, et al. Cutaneous eruptions in patients receiving immune checkpoint blockade: clinicopathologic analysis of the nonlichenoid histologic pattern. *Am J Surg Pathol.* 2017;41(10):1381-1389.
182. Dudley ME, Yang JC, Sherry R, et al. Adoptive cell therapy for patients with metastatic melanoma: evaluation of intensive myeloablative chemoradiation preparative regimens. *J Clin Oncol.* 2008;26(32):5233-5239.

183. Besser MJ, Shapira-Frommer R, Treves AJ, et al. Clinical responses in a phase II study using adoptive transfer of short-term cultured tumor infiltration lymphocytes in metastatic melanoma patients. *Clin Cancer Res.* 2010;16(9):2646-2655.
184. Lu YC, Yao X, Crystal JS, et al. Efficient identification of mutated cancer antigens recognized by T cells associated with durable tumor regressions. *Clin Cancer Res.* 2014;20(13):3401-3410.
185. Atkins MB, Lotze MT, Dutcher JP, et al. High-dose recombinant interleukin 2 therapy for patients with metastatic melanoma: analysis of 270 patients treated between 1985 and 1993. *J Clin Oncol.* 1999;17(7):2105-2116.
186. Lo JA, Fisher DE. The melanoma revolution: from UV carcinogenesis to a new era in therapeutics. *Science.* 2014;346(6212):945-949.
187. Hauschild A, Agarwala SS, Trefzer U, et al. Results of a phase III, randomized, placebo-controlled study of sorafenib in combination with carboplatin and paclitaxel as second-line treatment in patients with unresectable stage III or stage IV melanoma. *J Clin Oncol.* 2009;27(17):2823-2830.
188. Egberts F, Gutzmer R, Ugurel S, et al. Sorafenib and pegylated interferon-α2b in advanced metastatic melanoma: a multicenter phase II DeCOG trial. *Ann Oncol.* 2011;22(7):1667-1674.
189. Chapman PB, Hauschild A, Robert C, et al. BRIM-3 Study Group: improved survival with vemurafenib in melanoma with BRAF V600E mutation. *N Engl J Med.* 2011;364(26):2507-2516.
190. Hauschild A, Grob JJ, Demidov LV, et al. Dabrafenib in BRAF-mutated metastatic melanoma: a multicentre, open-label, phase 3 randomised controlled trial. *Lancet.* 2012;380(9839):358-365.
191. Sosman JA, Kim KB, Schuchter L, et al. Survival in BRAF V600-mutant advanced melanoma treated with vemurafenib. *N Engl J Med.* 2012;366:707-714.
192. Van Allen EM, Wagle N, Sucker A, et al. Dermatologic Cooperative Oncology Group of Germany (DeCOG): the genetic landscape of clinical resistance to RAF inhibition in metastatic melanoma. *Cancer Discov.* 2014;4(1):94-109.
193. Su F, Viros A, Milagre C, et al. RAS mutations in cutaneous squamous-cell carcinomas in patients treated with BRAF inhibitors. *N Engl J Med.* 2012;366(3):207-215.
194. Hassel JC, Groesser L, Herschberger E, et al. RAS mutations in benign epithelial tumors associated with BRAF inhibitor treatment of melanoma. *J Invest Dermatol.* 2015;135(2):636-639.
195. Dummer R, Schadendorf D, Ascierto PA, et al. Results of NEMO: a phase II trial of binimetinib vs dacarbazine in NRAS-mutant cutaneous melanoma [abstract 9500]. *J Clin Oncol.* 2016;34(suppl).
196. Lutzky J, Bauer J, Bastian BC. Dose-dependent, complete response to imatinib of a metastatic mucosal melanoma with a K642E KIT mutation. *Pigment Cell Melanoma Res.* 2008;21(4):492-493.
197. Hodi FS, Friedlander P, Corless CL, et al. Major response to imatinib mesylate in KIT-mutated melanoma. *J Clin Oncol.* 2008;26(12):2046-2051.
198. Guo J, Si L, Kong Y. Phase II, open-label, single-arm trial of imatinib mesylate in patients with metastatic melanoma harboring c-Kit mutation or amplification. *J Clin Oncol.* 2011;29(21):2904-2909.
199. Lee SJ, Kim TM, Kim YJ, et al. Phase II trial of nilotinib in patients with metastatic malignant melanoma harboring KIT gene aberration: a multicenter trial of Korean Cancer Study Group (UN10-06). *Oncologist.* 2015;20(11):1312-1319.
200. Tarhini AA, Agarwala SS. Cutaneous melanoma: available therapy for metastatic disease. *Dermatol Ther.* 2006;19(1):19-25.
201. Middleton MR, Grob JJ, Aaronson N, et al. Randomized phase III study of temozolomide versus dacarbazine in the treatment of patients with advanced metastatic malignant melanoma. *J Clin Oncol.* 2000;18(1):158-166.
202. Eigentler TK, Caroli UM, Radny P, et al. Palliative therapy of disseminated malignant melanoma: a systematic review of 41 randomised clinical trials. *Lancet Oncol.* 2003;4(12):748-759.
203. Hassel JC, Lee SB, Meiss F, et al. Vemurafenib and ipilimumab: a promising combination? Results of a case series. *Oncoimmunology.* 2015;5(4):e1101207.
204. Ribas A, Hodi FS, Callahan M, et al. Hepatotoxicity with combination of vemurafenib and ipilimumab. *N Engl J Med.* 2013;368(14):1365-1366.
205. Ribas A, Hodi FS, Lawrence DP, et al. Pembrolizumab (pembro) in combination with dabrafenib (D) and trametinib (T) for BRAF-mutant advanced melanoma: phase 1 KEYNOTE-022 study [abstract 3014]. *J Clin Oncol.* 2016;34(suppl).
206. Ribas A, Dummer R, Puzanov I, et al. Oncolytic virotherapy promotes intratumoral T cell infiltration and improves anti-PD-1 immunotherapy. *Cell.* 2017;170(6):1109.e10-1119.e10.
207. Van Allen EM, Miao D, Schilling B, et al. Genomic correlates of response to CTLA-4 blockade in metastatic melanoma. *Science.* 2015;350(6257):207-211.
208. Snyder A, Makarov V, Merghoub T, et al. Genetic basis for clinical response to CTLA-4 blockade in melanoma. *N Engl J Med.* 2014;371(23):2189-2199.
209. Kranz LM, Diken M, Haas H, et al. Systemic RNA delivery to dendritic cells exploits antiviral defence for cancer immunotherapy. *Nature.* 2016;534(7607):396-401.
210. Shahabi V, Postow MA, Tuck D, et al. Immune-priming of the tumor microenvironment by radiotherapy: rationale for combination with immunotherapy to improve anticancer efficacy. *Am J Clin Oncol.* 2015;38(1):90-97.
211. Postow MA, Callahan MK, Barker CA, et al. Immunologic correlates of the abscopal effect in a patient with melanoma. *N Engl J Med.* 2012;366(10):925-931.
212. Coit DG, Andtbacka R, Bichakjian CK, et al. Melanoma. *J Natl Compr Canc Netw.* 2009;7(3):250-275.

Chapter 117 :: Histiocytosis
:: Astrid Schmieder, Sergij Goerdt, & Jochen Utikal

第一百一十七章

组织细胞增生症

中文导读

朗格汉斯细胞组织细胞（LCHs）增生症和非朗格汉斯细胞组织细胞（N-LCHs）增生症是一组罕见的肿瘤和反应性疾病，其特征是髓系细胞在不同器官部位的增殖，且好发于皮肤。本章从历史视角、流行病学、临床特征、诊断、鉴别诊断、临床病程和预后等方面分别介绍了朗格汉斯细胞组织细胞增生症和非朗格汉斯细胞组织细胞增生症。

〔粟 娟〕

CUTANEOUS CLINICAL FEATURES OF HISTIOCYTOSIS

AT-A-GLANCE

- *Langerhans cell histiocytosis*: Translucent, rose-yellowish, crusted papules or papulovesicles, eczematous lesions, hemorrhagic papules and nodules, petechiae, noduloulcerative mucosal lesions, and nail involvement
- *Rosai-Dorfman disease*: Lymphadenopathy, cutaneous nodules, and plaques
- *Hemophagocytic lymphohistiocytosis*: Various cutaneous manifestations such as erythroderma, generalized purpuric macules and papules, and morbilliform eruptions
- *Juvenile xanthogranuloma*: Solitary as well as multiple (oligolesional) papules or nodules—early lesions show a reddish-brown color; mature lesions have a reddish-yellow appearance
- *Benign cephalic histiocytosis*: Like juvenile xanthogranuloma; ultrastructural presence of worm-like bodies

- *Generalized eruptive histiocytoma of childhood*: Widespread, erythematous, essentially symmetrical papules
- *Adult xanthogranuloma*: Oligolesional, yellow-orange papules that usually appear on the face, neck, and lower arms
- *Papular xanthoma*: Solitary yellowish papule
- *Generalized eruptive histiocytoma*: Multiple asymptomatic and symmetrically distributed brownish erythematous papules, particularly involving the axial regions such as the trunk, face, and proximal extremities, frequently flares
- *Xanthoma disseminatum*: Small, yellow-red to brown papules and nodules that are discrete and are disseminated with a predilection for the flexural and intertriginous areas, as well as for mucous membranes

- *Multicentric reticulohistiocytosis*: Firm, yellow-brownish papules or nodules that reach a size of several centimeters and progress slowly in size; lesions over the joints of fingers and wrists are typical; often involvement of mucosae and conjunctivae
- *Erdheim-Chester disease*: Xanthelasma and xanthoma are present in one-sixth of cases; long bone and other extracutaneous involvement
- *Necrobiotic xanthogranuloma*: Yellowish plaques and nodules that can ulcerate
- *Hereditary progressive mucinous histiocytosis*: Skin-colored to red-brown papules that usually develop in the first decade on the nose, hands, forearms, and thighs that can later develop into persistent and progressive erythematous papules
- *Progressive nodular histiocytosis*: Generalized, discrete yellow to red-brown papules and nodules measuring a few centimeters in size with prominent facial involvement

Langerhans cell histiocytoses (LCHs) and non–Langerhans cell histiocytoses (N-LCHs) present a rare group of neoplastic and reactive diseases characterized by the proliferation of myeloid cells in various organ sites with a predilection to the skin. As shown in Table 117-1, they are categorized in different subgroups.

TABLE 117-1
Classification of Langerhans and Non–Langerhans Cell Histiocytosis

Langerhans Cell Histiocytosis
1. Single system
2. Multisystem

Non–Langerhans Cell Histiocytosis
1. Systemic non–Langerhans cell histiocytosis
   - Rosai-Dorfman disease
   - Hemophagocytic lymphohistiocytosis
2. Cutaneous non–Langerhans cell histiocytosis
   - Juvenile xanthogranuloma
     - Juvenile xanthogranuloma
     - Benign cephalic histiocytosis
     - Generalized eruptive histiocytoma of childhood
   - Adult xanthogranuloma
     - Oligolesional
       - Adult xanthogranuloma
       - Papular xanthoma
     - Disseminated
       - Generalized eruptive histiocytoma
       - Xanthoma disseminatum
       - Multicentric reticulohistiocytosis
       - Erdheim-Chester disease
   - Necrobiotic xanthogranuloma
   - Spindle-cell non–Langerhans cell histiocytosis
     - Hereditary progressive mucinous histiocytosis
     - Progressive nodular histiocytosis

LANGERHANS CELL HISTIOCYTOSIS

AT-A-GLANCE

- New definition of Langerhans cell histiocytosis (LCH) as rare, inflammatory neoplasia of myeloid-dendritic (mostly clonal) cells with heterogeneous clinical manifestation
- Histopathology:
  - Infiltration of the organs with immature, morphologically rounded myeloid dendritic cells with bean-shaped nuclei; shared characteristics of cell surface antigens (CD1a/S100B/CD207-positive) with mature skin Langerhans cells
  - 60% of LCH biopsy specimens bear the V600E mutation in cell-growth-directing oncogene *BRAF* (v-Raf murine sarcoma viral oncogene homolog B)
  - Highly variable clinical manifestations ranging from single, osteolytic bone lesions to an aggressive, life-threatening multisystem disease affecting risk organs such as the spleen, the liver, and the hematopoietic system
  - Skin involvement in 39% (crucial for early diagnosis)
- New (clinical) classification according to the extent of organ involvement:
  - Single-organ system LCH
  - Multisystem LCH
- Treatment:
  - Close monitoring for single-organ system LCH ("watch and wait")
  - Topical or systemic treatments include topical nitrogen mustard, narrowband ultraviolet light-B, photochemotherapy, methotrexate, 6-mercaptopurine, and chemotherapy, depending on the extent of the disease

HISTORICAL PERSPECTIVE

LCH is newly defined as a rare, heterogeneous neoplasm of dendritic cells. Characteristically, CD1a/S100B/CD207-positive mononuclear cells with bean-shaped nuclei infiltrate single-organ systems, most commonly the bone, but also the skin, or multiple-organ systems.

A long-term controversy regarding the neoplastic nature of this disease exists as there are some arguments in support of a reactive condition resulting from an immunologic dysregulation such as a regulatory T-cell expansion found in LCH and the lack of mutations in tumor-suppressor genes.[1] Another argument is the broad spectrum of clinical manifestations of LCH, ranging from a self-healing single bone lesion to aggressive multiorgan involvement with a lethal outcome. Thus, in the past, patients were divided into 4 main clinical types: Hashimoto-Pritzker disease, eosinophilic granuloma, Hand-Schüller-Christian disease, and Letterer-Siwe disease (Table 117-2 outlines the traditional classification of LCH).

Hashimoto-Pritzker disease, first described in 1973, is the benign clinical variant typically presenting with multiple firm red-brown nodules with an elevated border or papulovesicular and papulocrusted lesions mostly on the scalp and face in the first few months and years of life, with no signs of systemic involvement. These lesions usually heal within 2 to 3 months and occasionally leave whitish atrophic scars.

Eosinophilic granuloma is also a mainly benign isolated or multifocal osteolytic bone LCH, which sometimes affects the skin and mucous membranes. Consequently, skin lesions often resemble those seen in Hand-Schüller-Christian (HSC) disease with nodulo-ulcerative lesions in the mouth and yellowish-brown papules and plaques on the scalp or in the perineal or perivulvar region. The first publication by Thomas Smith describing this disease can be found in the 1865 edition of the *American Journal of Pathology*.

HSC disease is the chronic variant of a multisystem LCH mostly found in children 2 to 5 years old, but the age-range is wide. It was first described by Alfred Hand in 1893, followed by Arthur Schüller in 1915 and Henry Christian in 1920. It is characterized by the triad of diabetes insipidus, bone lesions, and exophthalmos and affects the skin in approximately 30% of cases. Patients frequently complain about a chronic otitis media that is the result of an involvement of the mastoid or the petrous temporal bones. Cutaneous lesions can resemble seborrheic dermatitis with small reddish-brown crusted papules, but also vesicles and pustules on the scalp and face and in intertriginous areas. Also, nodulo-ulcerative lesions can develop in mucous membranes, especially in the gingiva and the perioral and genital areas. Xanthomatous yellowish-brown or yellowish-red papules and plaques also have been described.

Letterer-Siwe disease is the most aggressive acute LCH multisystem variant with apparent systemic symptoms such as fever, hepatosplenomegaly, polylymphadenopathy, anemia, arthralgia, malaise, and weight loss. Letterer first described the disease in 1924, followed by Siwe in 1933. Frequently affected organs are the lung, the bone marrow, and the brain. Skin lesions are common and consist of yellow-brown, sometimes translucent papules, which can have a hemorrhagic aspect and ulcerate similar to the ones seen in HSC disease. Also, purpura is frequently found and is a poor prognostic sign. Untreated, Letterer-Siwe disease is lethal.

TABLE 117-2
Variants of Langerhans Cell Histiocytosis (LCH)[a]

	AGE AT ONSET	CLINICAL CHARACTERISTICS	COURSE OF DISEASE	PROGNOSIS
Hashimoto-Pritzker disease	First months to years of age	Multiple firm, red-brown nodules with an elevated border; papulovesicular and crusted lesions on scalp and face	Self-healing with resolution in 2-3 months and occasional atrophic scarring	No systemic involvement; excellent prognosis
Eosinophilic granuloma[b] (unifocal LCH)	Most commonly childhood	Skin not always involved; when present, lesions are nodulo-ulcerative on mouth, yellowish-brown papules and plaques on scalp or perineal or perivulvar region; swelling over bony lesions	Benign isolated or multifocal osteolytic bone LCH	No systemic involvement; good prognosis; may have complications with tissue destruction
Hand-Schüller-Christian disease[b]	2-5 years old (age range is wide)	Triad of diabetes insipidus, bone lesions, and exophthalmos; seborrheic dermatitis-like lesions, with small reddish-brown crusted papules, vesicles, and pustules on scalp, face, and intertriginous areas. Nodulo-ulcerative lesions may affect the gingiva, perioral, and genital area; xanthomatous plaques may be present	Chronic, progressive, multifocal form of LCH with systemic involvement	Progressive; prognosis poorer at extremes of age and with extrapulmonary involvement
Letterer-Siwe disease[b]	Mostly younger than 2 years of age	Lung, bone marrow, and brain commonly affected; cutaneous lesions consist of yellow-brown to translucent papules, occasionally with a hemorrhagic or ulcerative aspect; purpura is a poor prognostic sign	Most aggressive, multisystem variant	Lethal, if untreated

[a]This table represents the traditional classification of LCH for reader reference; newer classifications (see Fig. 117-1) have greater implications for treatment and prognosis.
[b]These variants fall under a single nosologic entity called histiocytosis X.

Although these LCH types show a distinct clinical course, the cellular infiltrate in the affected organs is the same. Thus, in 1953, Lichtenstein proposed to combine eosinophilic granuloma, HSC, and Letterer-Siwe disease into a single nosologic entity called *histiocytosis X*. In 1973, Nezelof termed the lesional cell as a "Langerhans-like" cell based on the presence of Birbeck granules found with the help of the electron microscope. In 1987, the Histiocyte Society published the classification of the histiocytic disorders, which finally consolidated the strenghtened position that all the above-mentioned diseases are part of a single entity. Since then there has been a vivid dispute about whether LCH should be classified as a neoplastic or a reactive disease. This was finally resolved in 2010 with the discovery of the *BRAF-V600E* somatic point mutation in approximately 60% of patients with LCH,[2] which led to the conclusion that LCH is a clonal neoplastic disorder. The resolution of this controversy is important as it will significantly accelerate research in this field and progress in treatment.

EPIDEMIOLOGY

Because LCH is a rare neoplastic disease, exact epidemiologic data is missing. In children younger than 15 years of age, the annual incidence is approximately 0.7 to 4.1 cases per 1 million population with a median age at diagnosis of 30.2 months to 5.9 years.[3] In adults, the incidence is lower with only 1 to 2 cases per 1 million adults of all ethnicities per year reported. A lower incidence has been observed in black patients, whereas the Hispanic population shows a slightly higher incidence. Other risk factors include living in crowded conditions and lower education level as well as exposure to metal, granite, wood dust, or solvents in parents, a family history of thyroid disease and cancer, and perinatal infections, but these risk factors should be interpreted with caution.[3,4]

ETIOLOGY AND PATHOGENESIS

From an etiologic point of view, LCH is an inflammatory myeloid neoplasm characterized by infiltrations of different organ systems with CD1a/S100B/CD207-positive mononuclear cells, which morphologically and immunohistochemically resemble specialized dendritic cells of the skin known as Langerhans cells. Gene expression arrays revealed that these cells are different from resident mature Langerhans cells of the skin as they express immature myeloid markers and are more closely related to a myeloid-derived precursor dendritic cell.[5] Also, approximately 60% of LCH-cells bear a V600E mutation in the *BRAF* (v-Raf murine sarcoma viral oncogene homolog B) oncogene, and 33% of BRAF wild-type lesions harbor mutations in the *MAP2K1* (mitogen-activated protein kinase kinase1) gene leading to universal MEK (mitogen activated protein/extracellular signal-related kinase kinase) and ERK (extracellular signal-regulated kinase) activation (Fig. 117-1A). Based on these results the "Misguided Myeloid Dendritic Cell Precursor Model," in which precursor bone marrow–derived myeloid dendritic cells acquire a pathologic ERK activation and express antigens typically found in mature Langerhans cells such as CD207 and CD1a (Fig. 117-1B), has been proposed. These cells secrete factors such as osteopontin, vanin, and different proinflammatory factors, as well as transforming growth factor-β and attract, among other inflammatory cells such as macrophages and eosinophils, activated T cells, especially activated regulatory FOXP3/CTLA4, and SPP-positive T cells.[5] The severity and the extent of the organ involvement is supposed to depend on the stage of differentiation in which ERK gets activated: whereas an activation in a hematopoietic stem cell or an undifferentiated myeloid dendritic cell leads to multisystem disease, ERK activation in more differentiated myeloid precursors only results in multifocal or unifocal disease.[1] More studies are needed to gain further insights into the pathogenesis of LCH as there are still many open questions, including: Why is it that in adult pulmonary LCH, unlike in the other organs, the infiltrating mononuclear cells seem to be mostly nonclonal mature dendritic cells? Another interesting question is whether a high expression of PD-L1 (programmed death ligand 1) immune checkpoint protein in LCH could serve as a new therapeutic target[6]; as of this writing, it is still too early to tell.

CLINICAL FEATURES

CLASSIFICATION

The traditional classification of LCH in Hashimoto-Pritzker disease, eosinophilic granuloma, HSC, and Letterer-Siwe disease has been abandoned because the disease spectrum is broader than that of the traditional classification and many patients do not fit into these clinical subtypes. Also, the clinical course can change with time. The new classification considers the extent of organ involvement as this has significant implications for treatment and prognosis (see Fig. 117-1). In addition, LCH might best be described as a continuum as illustrated in Figure 117-2. Patients are divided into:

- Single-system LCH: Approximately 55% to 65% of the LCH patients present with single-system LCH, in which only 1 organ system is involved. Organ systems most commonly affected are bone, skin, lymph nodes, lungs, and the CNS.[7]
- Multisystem LCH: In multisystem LCH, more than 1 organ system is affected by the disease. It is important to distinguish whether high-risk organs are involved.

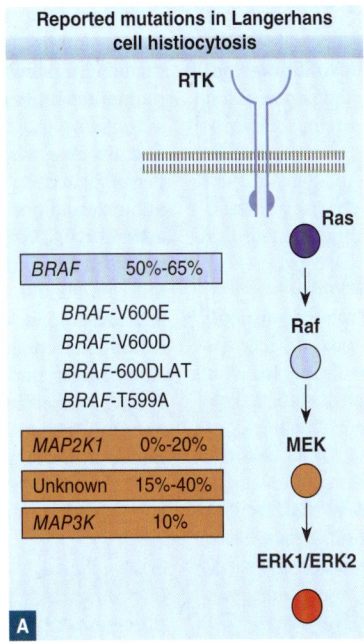
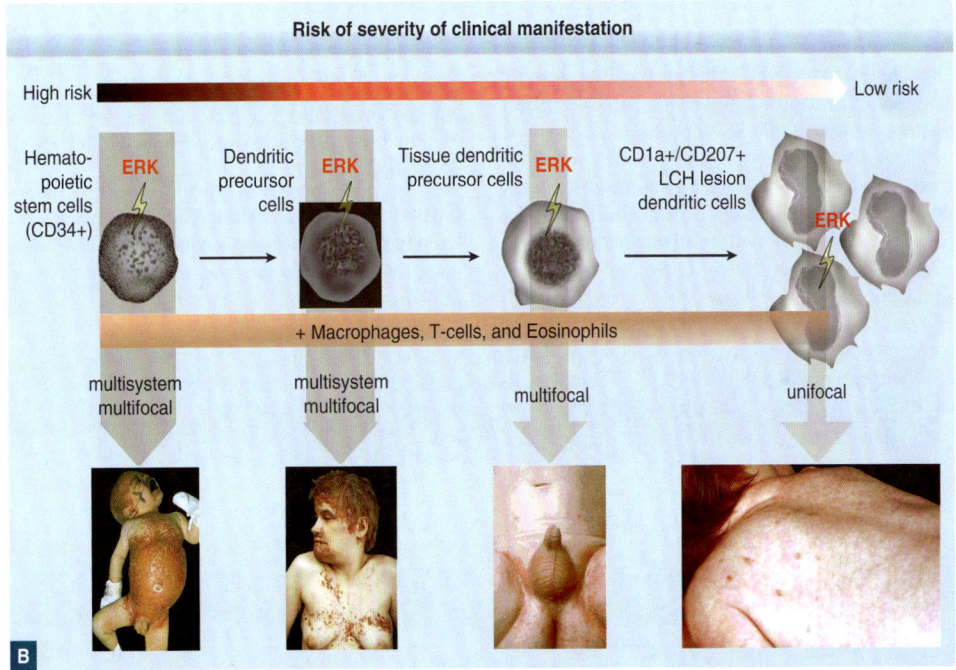

Figure 117-1 **A,** Reported mutations in Langerhans cell histiocytosis (LCH). This figure illustrates the frequency of identified mutations in LCH, leading to a downstream activation of the transcription factor ERK (extracellular signal-regulated kinase). In 50% to 65% of LCH cases, a mutation in the *BRAF* (v-Raf murine sarcoma viral oncogene homolog B) gene was found. The *BRAF-V600E* mutation was by far the most common mutation found, but *BRAF-V600D*, *BRAF-600DLAT*, and *BRAF-T599A* mutations also have been described. MAP2K1, mitogen-activated protein kinase kinase 1; MAP3K, mitogen-activated protein kinase kinase kinase; MEK, mitogen-activated protein/extracellular signal-related kinase kinase; RTK, receptor tyrosine kinase. **B,** The "Misguided Myeloid Dendritic Cell Model." Based on the "Misguided Myeloid Dendritic Cell Model," the clinical manifestation depends on the stage of differentiation of the hematopoietic cell in which the ERK activation takes place. ERK activation in the hematopoietic stem cell and the dendritic precursor cell leads to an extensive LCH, whereas ERK activation in the tissue dendritic precursor cell and the CD1a+/CD207+ LCH lesion dendritic cell leads to a single-system LCH.

At-risk organs include the hematopoietic system, the liver, and the spleen. The lung is no longer regarded as a high-risk organ, as recent studies could not confirm lung involvement as a negative prognostic factor. Table 117-1 provides an overview of the currently accepted classification.

CUTANEOUS FINDINGS

Cutaneous findings in LCH can be identified in more than one-third of LCH. It is the second most common organ involved after bone lesions and can be the earliest sign of disease. Only 12% of children with single-system disease and 53% of patients affected by multisystem LCH show a skin involvement.[7] Consequently, age is an important risk factor as children younger than the age of 1 year more frequently show a true skin-only LCH, while those older than the age of 18 months have a higher risk for multisystem LCH. The role of the dermatologist in making an early diagnosis is, therefore, crucial.

Patients can present with a broad variety of skin manifestations. The most typical ones are small, translucent rose-yellowish crusted papules or papulovesicles on the trunk, in the intertriginous areas and the scalp, associated with eczematous scaling which resembles "candida intertrigo" or "seborrheic dermatitis" (Figs. 117-3, 117-4, and 117-5). Lesions can also present as hemorrhagic papules and nodules associated with petechiae reminiscent of vascular lesions or "varicella-like eruptions" (Fig. 117-6). Vesicles, pustules, and nail involvement have been described. Nail involvement can present as paronychia, nailfold destruction, onycholysis, subungual hyperkeratosis, longitudinal grooving, and pigmented and purpuric striae of the nail bed. Mucosal lesions most commonly are nodulo-ulcerative and involve the perioral, the perigenital, and the perianal areas as well as the gingiva. Mucosal lesions and external otitis media seem to be associated with a higher risk for multisystem LCH.[7] Purpura with nail involvement might be a poor prognostic sign, but this should be evaluated in larger clinical trials. This broad variety of skin and mucosal manifestations frequently leads to a delayed diagnosis as skin lesions are misinterpreted as eczema, miliaria, scabies, varicella, seborrheic dermatitis, folliculitis, or candidiasis. LCH should be kept in mind as a rare, but important, differential diagnosis when the above-mentioned lesions are seen, especially if they are resistant to therapy and are spreading.

NONCUTANEOUS FINDINGS

The most common noncutaneous organ involved in LCH is bone (77% of cases), followed by lymph nodes (19%), liver (16%), spleen (13%), lung (10%), and the CNS (6%). In aggressive manifestations of the disease, patients present with a variety of clinical symptoms such as malaise, fever, nausea, weight loss, myalgia and arthralgia, and memory problems.

Bone Lesions: Although LCH can affect any bone in the body, it most frequently affects the skull,

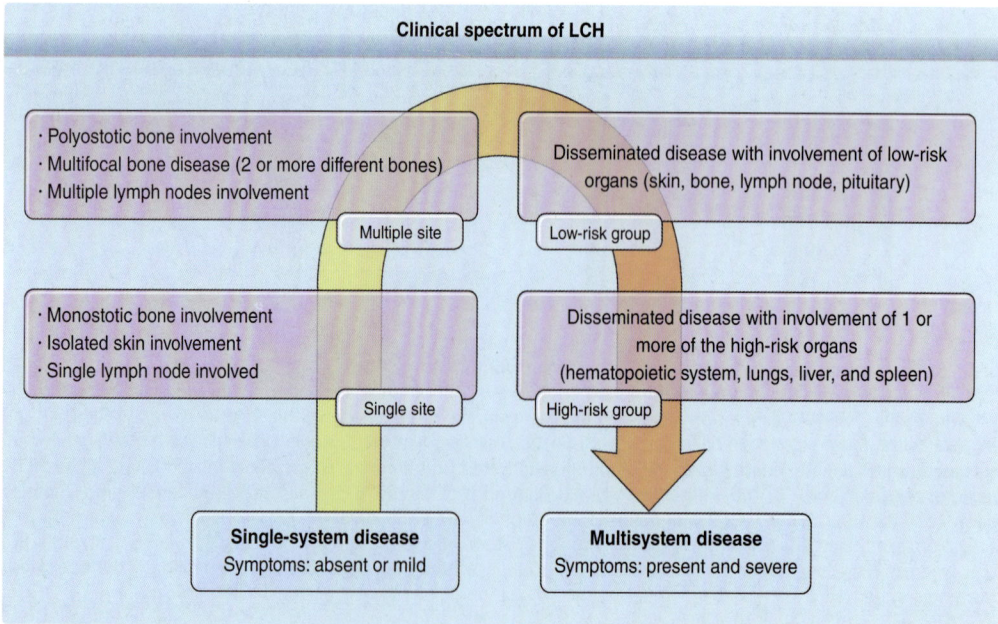

Figure 117-2 Clinical spectrum of Langerhans cell histiocytosis (LCH). Any single patient affected by LCH can be situated in a given point on the arrow.

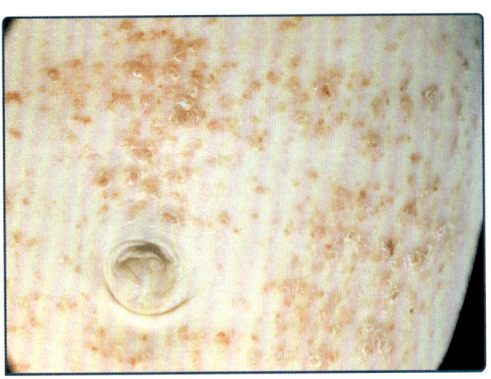

Figure 117-3 Rose-yellowish papules on the abdominal area of an infant suffering from extensive Langerhans cell histiocytosis.

jaw, femur, rib, vertebra, and humerus. Patients complain about tender masses, and the radiologic workup shows lytic areas in affected bones with a "punched out" appearance. Particularly in children, the cervical vertebrae are commonly involved, which can lead to vertebra plana. In adults, an asymmetric collapse of the vertebrae is more common, which can provoke neurologic defects. Involvement of the jaw can cause loose teeth. Vertebral collapse can be one of the most prominent diagnostic hints for LCH. Involvement of the base of the skull might result in hearing loss, recurrent otitis externa, diabetes insipidus, or cranial nerve

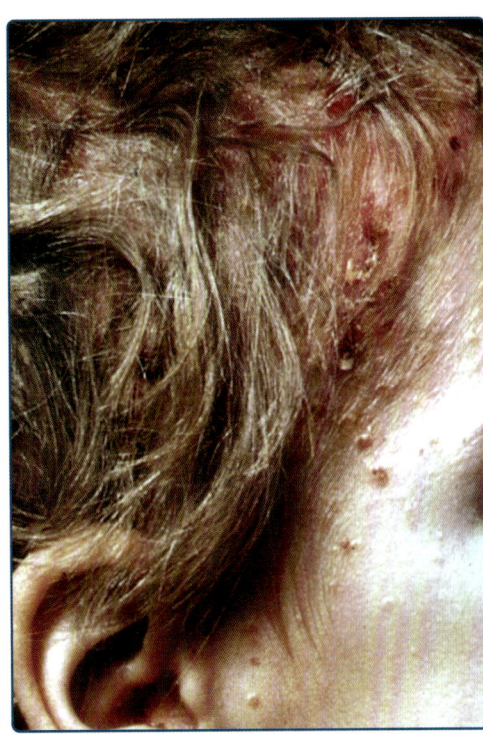

Figure 117-5 "Seborrheic dermatitis"–like eruptions on the scalp of an infant with Langerhans cell histiocytosis.

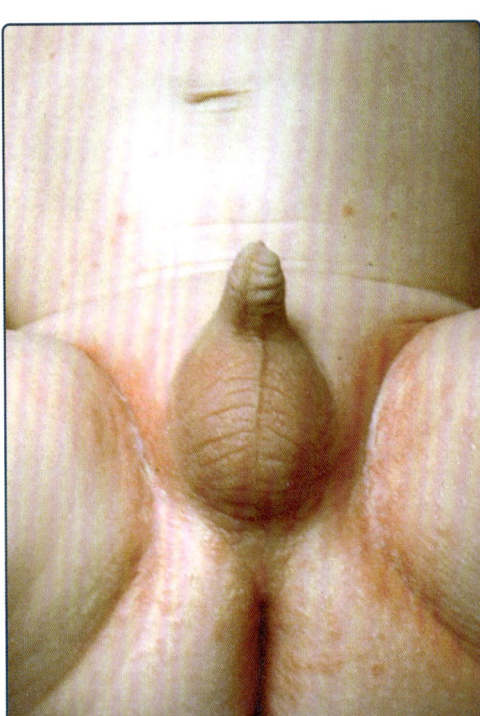

Figure 117-4 "*Candida* intertrigo"–like eruptions in the genital area of an infant with Langerhans cell histiocytosis.

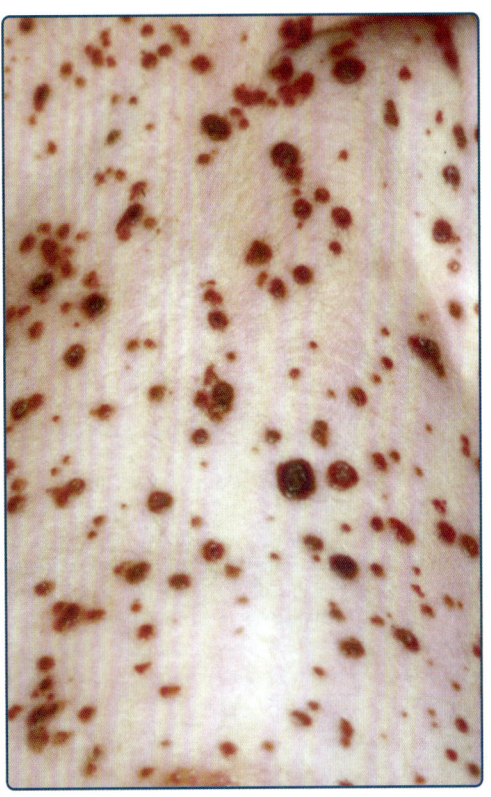

Figure 117-6 Hemorrhagic papules and nodules on the abdominal area of a patient who has Langerhans cell histiocytosis.

palsies. Lesions of the facial bones and anterior or middle cranial fossae classify as "CNS-risk" lesions as they are associated with a 3-fold increased risk for developing CNS diseases such as diabetes insipidus, which at diagnosis is mostly an irreversible condition.

Lymph Nodes: Cervical lymph nodes are the most frequently affected by LCH, but LCH can also involve lymph nodes of the mediastinum, which could be misdiagnosed as lymphoma, and can cause asthma-like symptoms because of airway system compression. A biopsy for proper diagnosis is mandatory.

Bone Marrow: Bone marrow involvement frequently affects young children when other risk organs, such as liver and spleen, are involved. In the past, bone marrow involvement was suspected only if significant anemia, thrombocytopenia, or neutropenia was present. A recent study found CD1a+ cells in the bone marrow in single-system LCH even if no hematologic abnormalities could be detected. When thrombocytopenia and anemia, especially in combination with hypoalbuminemia, are present, LCH was associated with a poor outcome.[8]

Liver and Spleen: Cholestasis and sclerosing cholangitis induced by hepatic involvement of LCH are among the most serious complications of LCH. In most cases, sclerosing cholangitis will not respond to chemotherapy and liver transplantation remains the only possible treatment option. Clinically, patients present with hepatosplenomegaly and elevated liver enzymes such as elevated liver transaminases, γ-glutamyltransferase, and/or alkaline phosphatase. Also, hypoalbuminemia with ascites and clotting deficiencies can appear. Involvement of the spleen with massive splenomegaly can significantly worsen the clinical outcome because of hypersplenism with resulting cytopenias and respiratory compromise.

Lungs: Involvement of the lungs is more frequently seen in adults than in children, and smoking has been identified as a major risk factor. LCH induces a cystic and/or nodular destruction of lung tissue of the upper and middle lung fields and can result in a spontaneous pneumothorax, tachypnea, and/or dyspnea,[9] ultimately leading to severe pulmonary insufficiency.

Central Nervous System: LCH can directly affect any part of the brain. A risk factor for CNS involvement (25% risk) is LCH lesions of the facial bones or bones of the anterior or middle cranial fossae ("CNS-risk" lesions). The most common manifestations of CNS involvement include endocrine abnormalities resulting from large pituitary tumors, most frequently diabetes insipidus, and neurodegenerative symptoms such as ataxia, dysarthria, cognitive dysfunction, and behavior changes. Radiologic changes can precede these symptoms by many years. Interestingly, histologically in neurodegenerative lesions, no CD1a+ cells are found; instead, lymphocytes and activated microglia cells are found, which leads to the speculation that it could be a paraneoplastic inflammatory response.

Endocrinopathies: Diabetes insipidus is the most common endocrinopathy encountered in LCH. Patients present with polyuria, polydipsia, and nocturia. This is a sign of damage to the antidiuretic hormone-secreting cells of the posterior pituitary. In approximately 4% of patients, idiopathic diabetes insipidus can precede the diagnosis of LCH.[10] In patients with diagnosed LCH, the risk of developing diabetes insipidus is approximately 24%. In most cases, diabetes insipidus persists despite treatment.

Other endocrine abnormalities associated with the anterior pituitary, such as hypogonadism, growth failure, thyroid hormone dysfunctions, and abnormalities in glucose metabolism, can manifest. Therefore, a complete endocrine work-up is recommended.

Gastrointestinal System: Patients with GI involvement can present clinically with diarrhea, hematochezia, perianal fistulas, and/or malabsorption, but this organ system is rarely affected. If patients present with GI symptoms, multiple biopsies are required, as in most cases GI involvement is patchy.

DIAGNOSIS

The diagnosis of LCH is based on clinicopathologic and radiologic features of affected organs.

TABLE 117-3

Recommended Baseline Laboratory Tests and Imaging Studies of Patients Suffering from Langerhans Cell Histiocytosis

Full blood count
- Hemoglobin, white blood cell and differential count, and platelet count

Blood chemistry
- Total protein, albumin, bilirubin, alanine aminotransferase (serum glutamic-pyruvic transaminase), aspartate aminotransferase (serum glutamic-oxaloacetic transaminase), alkaline phosphatase, γ-glutamyl transpeptidase
- Blood urea nitrogen, creatinine, electrolytes
- Ferritin
- Fasting glucose level
- Serum protein electrophoresis

Coagulation studies
- International normalized ratio/prothrombin time, activated partial thromboplastin time/partial thromboplastin time, fibrinogen

Early morning urine sample
- Specific gravity and osmolarity

Abdominal ultrasound

Chest radiography

Bone scans, skeletal survey, or fluorodeoxyglucose positron emission tomography

Adapted from the recommendations of the Histiocyte Society (https://histiocytesociety.org/).

COMPLETE HISTORY

Nature and duration of symptoms should be assessed. In addition based on the recommendations of the Histiocyte Society, a complete history should include questions regarding pain, swelling, skin rash, otorrhea, irritability, fever, loss of appetite, diarrhea, weight loss, growth failure, polydipsia, polyuria, changes in activity level, dyspnea, smoke exposure, and behavioral and neurologic changes.

COMPLETE PHYSICAL EXAMINATION

Temperature, height, and weight should be measured. In addition, the Histiocyte Society recommends assessment of pubertal status; for thorough skin and mucous membrane evaluation, for presence of jaundice, pallor, edema, lymphadenopathy, ear discharge, orbital abnormalities, abnormal mucosal lesions, abnormal dentation, and soft-tissue swelling, as well as evaluation of any tachypnea, intercostal retractions, and ascites; and evaluation of liver and spleen size evaluation. Also, a complete neurologic evaluation is mandatory.

LABORATORY TESTING AND IMAGING STUDIES

Table 117-3 lists the recommended laboratory investigations and imaging studies for patients suffering from LCH. Table 117-4 identifies the recommendations for specific clinical scenarios.

HISTOPATHOLOGY

A histopathologic diagnosis is by far the most reliable and accurate diagnostic tool for a definitive diagnosis of LCH and should always be performed if it doesn't put the patient at an increased risk. Histopathologically, typical findings in a skin biopsy show a dense and band-like infiltration of the papillary dermis with LCH cells (Fig. 117-7). These cells are oval shaped with an eosinophilic cytoplasm and typically display an irregular, vesicular, and infolded (kidney-shaped) nucleus (Fig. 117-8). In some cases, longitudinal nuclear grooves, which confer onto these cells a coffee bean-like appearance, can be seen. Conspicuously, LCH cells are 4 to 5 times larger than lymphocytes and are admixed with variable numbers of neutrophils, eosinophils, lymphocytes, plasma cells, and histiocytes, especially in early lesions. In later lesions, foamy histiocytes and a prominent fibrosis of the dermis prevail. LCH cells often show a marked epidermotropism with the formation of intraepidermal microabscesses and a periappendageal distribution (Figs. 117-7 and 117-9). The epidermotropism can be so marked that the dermoepidermal junction gets obscured and the epidermis gets thinned and even destroyed. Also, edema in the papillary dermis and multinucleated giant cells can be found on occasion. Typical immunohistochemical markers of LCH cells are CD1a (Fig. 117-9), S100B, CD207 (Langerin), and fascin. Stabilin-1 and CD34 are not expressed (Table 117-5). A typical finding in LCH cells is the presence of Birbeck granules in the cytoplasm, as identified by electron microscopy. They are organelles, which resemble a tennis racquet and have a zipper-like appearance along the "handle" (Fig. 117-10). In the past, the detection of Birbeck granules by electron microscopy was the diagnostic gold standard for LCH. Nowadays however, immunohistochemical staining with CD207, an antibody that recognizes a C-type lectin associated with Birbeck granules, is the most sensitive marker. Electron microscopy is no longer needed for a specific diagnosis.

TABLE 117-4

Specific Clinical Scenarios and Recommended Additional Laboratory, Imaging, and Specialized Clinical Assessments

Skin lesions
- Skin biopsy

Bicytopenia, pancytopenia, or persistent unexplained single cytopenia
- Bone marrow aspirate and trephine biopsy to exclude causes other than Langerhans cell histiocytosis (LCH)

Liver dysfunction
- Liver biopsy only recommended if there is clinically significant liver involvement and the result will alter treatment (ie, to differentiate between active LCH and sclerosing cholangitis)

Lung involvement
- Lung high-resolution computed tomography
- Lung function test

Abnormal lung CT and findings not characteristic for LCH or suspicious for atypical infection
- Bronchoalveolar lavage (BAL): >5% CD1a+ cells in BAL fluid is diagnostic in nonsmokers
- Lung biopsy (if BAL is not diagnostic)

Suspected craniofacial bone lesions, including maxilla and mandible
- MRI of head

Suspected vertebral lesions
- MRI of spine

Visual or neurologic abnormalities
- MRI of head
- Neurology assessment
- Neuropsychometric assessment

Suspected endocrine abnormality (eg, growth failure, polyuria, polydipsia, hypothalamic syndromes, precocious or delayed puberty)
- Endocrine assessment (including water deprivation test and dynamic tests of the anterior pituitary and thyroid)
- MRI of the head

Aural discharge or suspected hearing impairment/mastoid involvement
- Formal hearing assessment
- MRI of head
- High-resolution CT of temporal bone

Unexplained chronic diarrhea, failure to thrive, or evidence of malabsorption
- Endoscopy and biopsy

Adapted from the recommendations of the Histiocyte Society (https://histiocytesociety.org/).

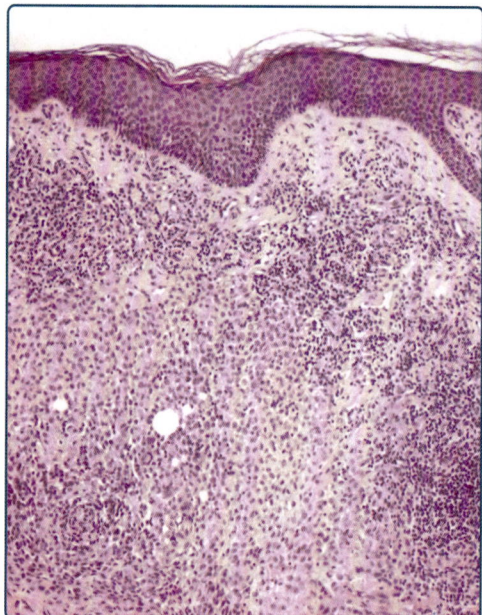

Figure 117-7 Histology of Langerhans cell histiocytosis (LCH) showing a dense mononuclear infiltrate of the dermis with oval to rounded LCH cell and lymphocytes as well as some eosinophils with epidermal involvement.

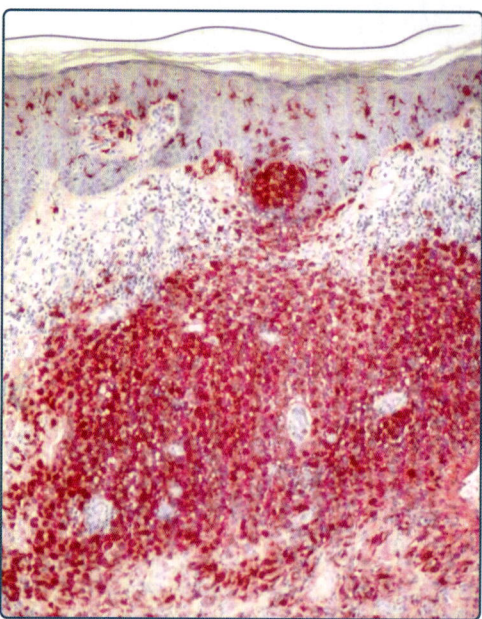

Figure 117-9 Histology of Langerhans cell histiocytosis (LCH). The LCH cells stain for CD1a (red) and show a marked epidermotropism.

DIFFERENTIAL DIAGNOSIS

Table 117-6 lists possible differential diagnoses for different clinical manifestations of LCH in the skin.

CLINICAL COURSE AND PROGNOSIS

LCH is a heterogeneous disease. Patients can present with lesions confined to a single-organ system with an indolent self-healing course or with multiple lesions in different organs—especially in at-risk organs—with a fatal outcome. Consequently, risk stratification is crucial to delivering the optimal treatment regimen to each patient. The prognosis depends on a variety of factors. A recent multicenter LCH Phase III trial investigated a 12-month treatment with vinblastine and prednisolone demonstrating 5-year survival rates of 95%, 83%, and 57%, respectively, in patients who showed a complete resolution of disease, intermediate response to treatment, and progression of the disease after the 6-week induction phase.[11] Therefore, one of the most important predictors of outcome in patients with multiorgan

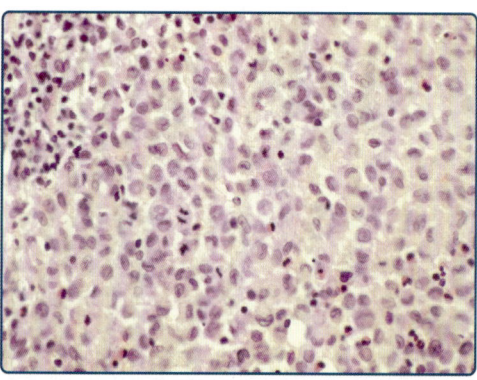

Figure 117-8 Histology of Langerhans cell histiocytosis (LCH). LCH cells have a kidney-shaped nucleus.

TABLE 117-5
Marker Expression of Langerhans and Non–Langerhans Cell Histiocytosis

Langerhans cell histiocytosis
- Positive: CD1a, CD2, CD11b, CD11c, CD13, CD66c, CD68, CD207 (Langerin), CD300LF, S100B, fascin
- Negative: stabilin-1

Non–Langerhans cell histiocytosis
1. Systemic non–Langerhans cell histiocytosis
    - Positive: CD68
    - Negative: *CD1a*
2. Cutaneous non–Langerhans cell histiocytosis:
    - Positive: CD68, stabilin-1
    - Negative: *S100B, CD1a*

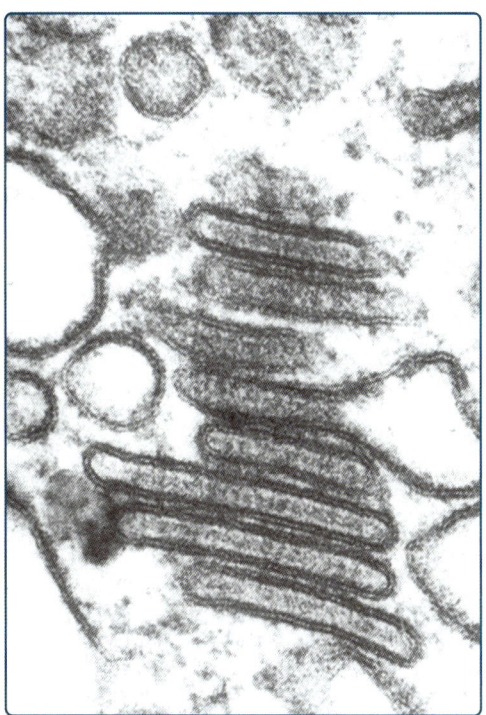

Figure 117-10 Electron microscope picture of a Langerhans cell histiocytosis cell shows typical Birbeck granules.

involvement is how the disease responds to systemic treatment in the first 6 weeks.[11] Other predictors previously associated with a poor outcome, such as age younger than 2 years or lung involvement, are now no longer regarded as risk factors for a poor outcome. Involvement of at-risk organs such as the liver, the spleen, and the bone marrow is also associated with a poor outcome. Enlargement of the liver by more than 3 cm below the costal margins at the midclavicular line; hyperbilirubinemia greater than 3 times normal; hypoalbuminemia less than 30 g/dL; γ-glutamyl transpeptidase increased by more than 2 times normal; alanine aminotransferase and aspartate aminotransferase greater than 3 times normal; ascites; edema; or an intrahepatic nodular mass are signs for liver involvement and need to be confirmed by ultrasound and, if possible, by biopsy. Involvement of the spleen should be suspected if the organ can be palpated by more than 3 cm below the costal margin at the midclavicular line. Hematopoietic involvement can be divided into a mild form with hemoglobin between 10 and 7 g/dL, not the result of other causes, and/or a thrombocytopenia with platelets between 20,000 and 100,000/mm^3, and a severe form with hemoglobin below 7 g/dL and platelets less than 20,000/mm^3.[12] To date, no data has demonstrated diabetes insipidus to be a predictor of poor outcome. Small numbers of lesions, a prompt resolution of lesions, and single-organ involvement are usually associated with a good outcome.

The prognosis is, however, not only dependent on the disease itself, but also on associated findings. LCH patients tend to suffer from intercurrent infections, mostly mild ones, such as candidiasis and dermatophytosis, but they are also prone to more severe systemic infections, which can lead to sepsis and death. Also, LCH is associated with other malignancies, which may precede, occur concurrently with, or follow the diagnosis of LCH. Described associated malignant neoplasms are solid tumors (lung tumors, celiomesenteric neuroblastoma), malignant lymphomas, and leukemias, in particular, acute lymphoblastic leukemia and myeloid leukemias. Some of these malignancies may be related to alkylating chemotherapeutic regimens and radiotherapy used for LCH. These possible complications and/or associations should be considered at every clinical visit.

MANAGEMENT

Treatment strategies depend on the extent and localization of the disease and the age of the patient. Patients with more limited disease confined to bone or skin are usually not treated systemically, except for "special site" lesions such as the odontoid peg, vertebral lesions with intraspinal soft-tissue extension, and anatomically functionally critical sites. All treatment recommendations are based on the recommendations of the Histiocyte Society. Systemic treatment also can be considered for multifocal bone lesions and "CNS-risk" lesions. In children with LCH confined to the skin, a watch-and-wait strategy is the best approach. Topical treatment can be tried with corticosteroid ointments, but topical steroids have shown little efficacy. A skin rash that does not respond to topical steroids is considered a clue for LCH. Other topical treatment options include imiquimod and tacrolimus as well as intralesional corticosteroid injections, CO_2 laser therapy, or excision of single LCH nodules. Nitrogen mustard ointment can be applied to treat skin lesions in adults. Several case reports exist that show a significant improvement after narrowband ultraviolet B irradiation in adults and children. This treatment might work well with papules and eczematous lesions, but not when nodules are present. Photochemotherapy is effective in some adult patients. In case of ineffective local therapy, systemic glucocorticoids, thalidomide, or antimitotic drugs, such as low-dose methotrexate, can be tried. Thalidomide can ameliorate skin lesions, but the treatment is associated with neurologic toxicity and fatigue. Thalidomide should not be used in women with child-bearing potential if the skin is the only organ affected. There is 1 case report in which a patient went into complete remission after oral isotretinoin therapy (1.5 mg/day for 8 months). Table 117-7 outlines some treatment options.

TABLE 117-6
Differential Diagnosis of Langerhans Cell Histiocytosis (Lesion Specific)

	TYPE OF LESION			
	PAPULAR	**VESICOPUSTULAR**	**XANTHOMATOUS**	**NODULOULCERATIVE**
Most likely	Seborrheic dermatitis	Scabies	Papular xanthoma	Juvenile xanthogranuloma
	Lichen nitidus	Miliaria	Xanthoma disseminatum	Urticaria pigmentosa
	Generalized eruptive histiocytosis	Varicella	Juvenile xanthogranuloma	Diffuse neonatal hemangiomatosis
	Benign cephalic histiocytosis	Intertrigo	Urticaria pigmentosa	Blueberry muffin baby
	Darier disease	Candidiasis		Hidradenitis
	Lichen planus	Rosacea Folliculitis decalvans		Tuberculosis
Consider	Leukemia	Dermatitis	Hyperlipidemic xanthomatosis	Leukemia
	Pityriasis lichenoides chronica	Pityriasis lichenoides et varioliformis acuta	Granuloma annulare disseminatum	Pyoderma gangrenosum
	Hidradenitis suppurativa	Granuloma faciale		Cherry angioma
	Psoriasis, guttate	Perioral dermatitis		
	Tinea corporis, tinea capitis	Lupus miliaris faciei		

Also for single-bone lesions a watch-and-wait strategy can be used. Other options include simple curettage, complete excision of small lesions (lesions <2 cm diameter) and intralesional steroid injections of steroids (see Table 117-7).

Thanks to the efforts of the Histiocyte Society, which was founded 1985, the scientific evidence for the treatment of LCH multisystem disease is far better than that for single-system LCH based on the reported results of multicenter trials (LCH-I, LCH-II, LCH-III).

Based on the results of the most recent LCH-III trial, patients should be treated systemically for 12 months because patients treated for only 6 months have an increased frequency of early relapse. The treatment protocol consists of a 6-week induction chemotherapy phase with vinblastine (6 mg/m^2 weekly intravenous bolus) combined with prednisolone (40 mg/m^2/day orally for 4 weeks and then tapered over 2 weeks) and a subsequent therapy with vinblastine/prednisolone with or without mercaptopurine, depending on the treatment response after 6 weeks and the involvement of at-risk organs (Fig. 117-11). With this treatment regimen, 86% of patients without risk-organ involvement and 66% with risk-organ involvement show a response to therapy after 6 weeks—an important prognostic factor for outcome. Still, 50% of patients in this study did not respond to treatment,[11] illustrating the need for additional therapeutic strategies. Other chemotherapeutic agents used as salvage strategies with proven efficacy for multisystem LCH, albeit with serious side effects, are cytarabine, cladribine, and clofarabine. Allogeneic bone marrow transplantation has been attempted in 87 patients with high-risk LCH. Among patients transplanted, 77% survived after 3 years following myeloablative and reduced-intensity conditioning regimens.[13] Based on recent research results, which provided evidence for a strong ERK activation arising from somatic mutations in the mitogen-activated protein kinase (MAPK) signaling pathway in LCH, novel therapeutic options include BRAF and MAPK inhibitors. Although limited data exist for these treatment regimens, first reports are promising.[14,15] Also, a high programmed death ligand 1 expression in LCH has been described,[6] which suggests that anti–programmed death 1 and anti–programmed death ligand 1 treatments might be successful.

TABLE 117-7
Treatment Options for Patients Suffering from Single-System Langerhans Cell Histiocytosis

SKIN	BONE
▪ Observation	▪ Observation
▪ Nitrogen mustard	▪ Biopsy or curettage
▪ Tacrolimus	▪ Surgery
▪ Imiquimod	▪ Steroid injections
▪ Intralesional steroids	▪ Vinblastine/prednisolone (multiple bone lesions or "special site" lesions)
▪ Narrowband ultraviolet B	
▪ Photochemotherapy	
▪ CO_2 laser	
▪ Methotrexate	
▪ Systemic steroids	
▪ Thalidomide	
▪ Isotretinoin	
▪ Excision (single lesions)	

NON–LANGERHANS CELL HISTIOCYTOSIS

AT-A-GLANCE

- Non–Langerhans cell histiocytosis (N-LCH) represents a group of different disorders characterized by the proliferation of histiocytes that do not meet criteria to be diagnosed as Langerhans cells
- N-LCH are immunohistochemically positive for CD68 and negative for S100B and CD1a
- Stabilin-1 (formerly MS-1 antigen or MS-1-HMWP) can discriminate N-LCH from LCH and other granulomatous diseases
- Systemic manifestations, such as diabetes insipidus, or ocular involvement, as well as an association with malignancies can occur in N-LCH
- Local skin manifestations of the disease can be treated by excision, laser therapy, or intralesional steroid injection. Radiotherapy also is used for the treatment of skin lesions and cerebral lesions. For the treatment of patients with visceral lesions, systemic glucocorticoids and chemotherapy, and in some cases targeted therapies, such as imatinib mesylate or BRAF and MEK inhibitors, are useful.

N-LCH is a group of different disorders characterized by the proliferation of histiocytes other than Langerhans cells. N-LCH can be classified as systemic or cutaneous N-LCH (see Table 117-1). Cutaneous N-LCH can be subclassified as juvenile, adult, and necrobiotic xanthogranulomas, as well as spindle-cell N-LCH.

ETIOLOGY AND PATHOGENESIS

Systemic forms of N-LCH are regarded as an accumulation of classically activated macrophages (Mφ1). In contrast, the lesions of cutaneous N-LCH are characterized by the presence of alternatively activated macrophages (Mφ2).

In forms with single lesions, local trauma might play a pathogenetic role. In diffuse forms an association with malignancies and autoimmune diseases suggests an immunologic cause.

Mφ1 are known to develop in response to proinflammatory stimuli such as T-helper (Th) 1 cytokines (interferon-γ or bacterial products [lipopolysaccharides]). They are characterized by secretion of proinflammatory cytokines, such as interleukin (IL)-1, IL-6, IL-1, and tumor necrosis factor-α, and possess a strong oxidative burst and a profound antimicrobial activity.

In contrast to systemic N-LCHs, the lesions of cutaneous N-LCHs show alternatively activated effector macrophages (Mφ2). Mφ2 are induced by Th2 cytokines, including IL-4, IL-10, IL-13, and transforming growth factor-β, or by antiinflammatory mediators such as glucocorticoids. They express antiinflammatory cytokines such as IL-1R antagonist and IL-10, chemokine receptor antagonists such as AMAC-1, broad-spectrum receptors of innate immunity, such as macrophage mannose receptor and the haptoglobin receptor CD163.

N-LCHs are positive for CD68 but negative for CD1a. Stabilin-1 (formerly MS-1 antigen or MS-1-HMWP) is expressed on some N-LCH. Because of its specific expression in N-LCH, it can be used as one marker to discriminate N-LCH from LCH or granulomatous diseases (see Table 117-5).

ROSAI-DORFMAN DISEASE (SINUS HISTIOCYTOSIS WITH MASSIVE LYMPHADENOPATHY)

PATHOPHYSIOLOGIC ASPECTS AND CLINICAL FEATURES

In 1969, sinus histiocytosis with massive lymphadenopathy was described by Juan Rosai and Ronald Dorfman. Rosai-Dorfman disease (RDD) is an idiopathic disease, but its occurrence has frequently been observed after infectious disease. A possible viral etiology, such as Epstein-Barr virus, human herpesvirus 6, parvovirus B19, and polyomavirus, has been suggested by several authors.[16,17] Lymphadenopathy is the main clinical manifestation. The neck lymph nodes are the most common place of histiocyte accumulation, although accumulation outside of lymph nodes may occur. Here, the skin (Fig. 117-12) and other organs, such as the breast, kidney, thyroid, testis, and CNS, may be affected.[17] Similar to other regional tumors, the symptoms of this disease vary with the site of accumulation. Despite the rarity of RDD, the co-occurrence with LCH, lymphomas, or autoimmune disorders has been reported.[17] Because of the expression of S100B by histiocytes, S100B can be used as a serum marker to monitor disease progression or therapy response.

HISTOPATHOLOGIC FINDINGS

RDD cells are characteristically S100B+ (Fig. 117-13A) and CD1a−. The RDD cells are also positive for CD68,

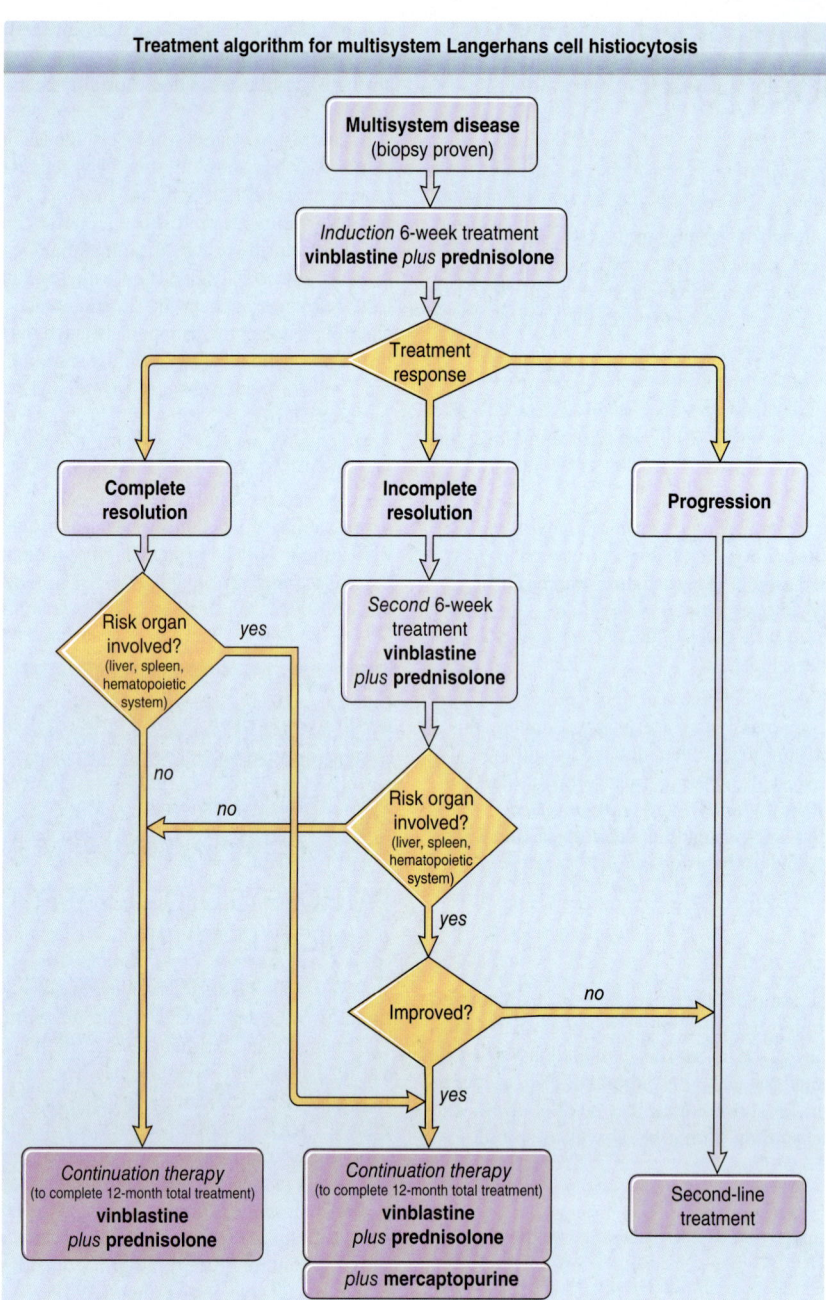

Figure 117-11 Treatment algorithm for multisystem Langerhans cell histiocytosis.

CD163, α_1-antitrypsin, α_1-antichymotrypsin, fascin, HAM-56 (human alveolar macrophage 56), and stabilin-1 (Fig. 117-13B). The hallmark of RDD is emperipolesis, in which different types of bone marrow cells, such as lymphocytes or neutrophils, are found in the cytoplasm of histiocytes with a background of mature lymphocytes and plasma cells.[17]

DIFFERENTIAL DIAGNOSIS

Because enlarged and massive unilateral or bilateral lymph nodes are a frequent manifestation in isolated or multiple regions, lymphoma or abscesses may be clinically suspected. Extranodal RDD can also mimic other diseases, such as meningioma.[17]

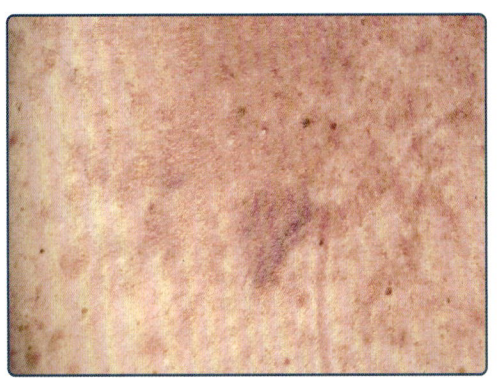

Figure 117-12 Rosai-Dorfman disease.

CLINICAL COURSE AND PROGNOSIS

Spontaneous resolution in patients with RDD was reported. There are reports that surgical resection as well as radiotherapy for affected lymph nodes or skin lesions has resulted in the complete disappearance of RDD. Oral prednisone can have a remarkably favorable response, mainly in patients with lymph node involvement. However, intralesional corticosteroid or oral prednisone does not always result in resolution of cutaneous lesions. Treatment with chemotherapeutic agents has been disappointing in general. There are reports, however, that some patients could benefit from a combination of methotrexate/6-mercaptopurine/vinblastine/6-thioguanine.[17] Tyrosine kinase inhibitors such as imatinib mesylate are effective in some patients with RDD.[18]

HEMOPHAGOCYTIC LYMPHOHISTIOCYTOSIS

CLINICAL FEATURES

Hemophagocytic lymphohistiocytosis (HLH) was first described in 1952 by Farquhar and Claireaux and is a rare disease. The 70% of HLH cases are children younger than the age of 1 year. HLH is characterized by persistent fever, splenomegaly with cytopenia, hypertriglyceridemia, and hypofibrinogenemia. The infiltration of histiocytes is usually observed in reticuloendothelial systems, including the bone marrow and CNS. Various cutaneous manifestations, such as erythroderma, generalized purpuric macules and papules, and morbilliform eruptions, have been described in up to 65% of HLH patients. HLH is classified as one of the cytokine storm syndromes because high amounts of inflammatory cytokines are secreted.

There are 2 major forms: primary and secondary. Primary HLH includes familial HLH and several primary immunodeficiencies, which exhibit genetic inheritance and usually occur in infancy. Several genetic defects in primary HLH—particularly familial HLH genes such as *HPLH1*, perforin, *UNC13D*, *STX11*, and *STXBP2*—have been identified. Secondary HLH is associated with infections (eg, Epstein-Barr virus), autoimmune disorders (eg, juvenile idiopathic arthritis), and malignancies (mainly non-Hodgkin lymphoma). Increased levels of various cytokines and soluble IL-2 receptor are biologic markers of HLH.[19]

DIFFERENTIAL DIAGNOSIS

The differential diagnosis of HLH includes autoimmune lymphoproliferative syndrome, Griscelli syndrome, macrophage activation syndrome, and other primary immunodeficiencies that present with HLH, such as X-linked lymphoproliferative disease.[19]

CLINICAL COURSE AND PROGNOSIS

The prognosis is guarded with an overall mortality of 50%. It is a poor prognostic factor if HLH is associated

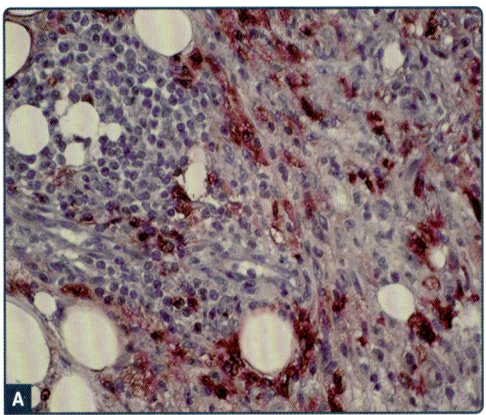

S100B

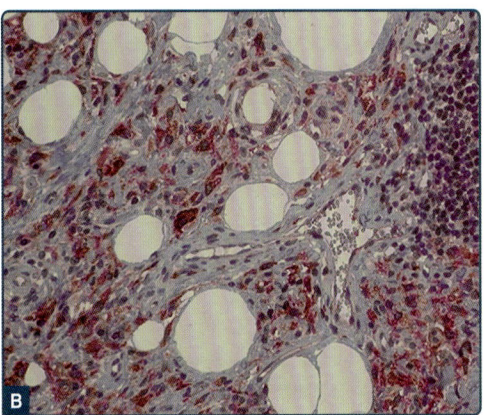

Stabilin 1

Figure 117-13 Photomicrographs of a lesion of Rosai-Dorfman disease. Histiocytes are positive for S100B (**A**) and stabilin-1 (**B**).

with malignancy.[20] In some individuals, secondary HLH may be self-limited.

Therapeutic options include high-dose corticosteroids, cyclosporine, etoposide, methotrexate, and vincristine. Use of intravenous immunoglobulin also has been described. An aggressive therapeutic approach is warranted in most cases, including immunochemotherapy and hematopoietic stem cell transplantation.[19]

JUVENILE XANTHOGRANULOMA

CLINICAL FEATURES

Juvenile xanthogranuloma (JXG) was first described in 1905 by Adamson. It is a benign, self-healing skin disorder that primarily affects infants younger than 1 year of age, but also can be found in older children. At birth, 5% to 17% of children already have cutaneous lesions. In 40% to 70% of children who are affected by JXG, the disorder presents during the first year of life.

JXG usually manifests with both solitary and multiple (oligolesional) papules or nodules that are usually located on the face, neck, and upper trunk, and on other body parts, including lungs, bone, heart, and GI tract. Early lesions show a reddish-brown color (Fig. 117-14A). Mature lesions have a reddish-yellow appearance (Fig. 117-14B). Telangiectasia can be present. Ocular lesions occur in up to 10% of children with JXG and may affect their vision. JXG is often accompanied with other disorders, such as neurofibromatosis Type 1 and juvenile chronic myelogenous leukemia.[21]

HISTOPATHOLOGIC FINDINGS

In early lesions, microscopic examination shows monomorphous, non–lipid-containing histiocytic infiltrates in the dermis (Fig. 117-15A). In contrast mature lesions are characterized by foam cells, Touton giant cells, and foreign-body giant cells in the superficial dermis and on the border of infiltrates (Fig. 117-15B). Also, fibrosis can be appreciated. Lesional histiocytes are positive for stabilin-1. Cells stain for macrophage markers such as CD163, CD11b, CD11c, CD36, CD68, factor XIIIa, and vimentin. S100B and CD1a are not expressed.

DIFFERENTIAL DIAGNOSIS

JXG can be distinguished from LCH by the expression of stabilin-1 and the absence of CD1a and CD207. Other differential diagnoses include, for example, molluscum contagiosum, hemangioma, and neurofibroma (Table 117-8).

CLINICAL COURSE AND PROGNOSIS

JXG usually resolves spontaneously over 1 to 5 years. Ocular lesions, however, rarely improve spontaneously and require treatment. Treatments include surgical excision, CO_2 laser treatment, intralesional steroid injection, cryotherapy, and low-dose radiotherapy. In the case of a resistant or recurring lesion, chemotherapy should be considered.[21]

BENIGN CEPHALIC HISTIOCYTOSIS

CLINICAL FEATURES

Benign cephalic histiocytosis was reported initially by Gianotti in 1971 and was separated from JXG. Because of the ultrastructural presence of worm-like bodies, it also has been called "histiocytosis with intracytoplasmic worm-like bodies." However, these bodies can be found in other forms of N-LCH. An overlap with other forms of N-LCH, especially with JXG, has been reported.

Benign cephalic histiocytosis usually presents with small, yellow-red or yellow-brown, asymptomatic papules, located on the head and neck of young children with a tendency toward spontaneous remission.[22]

HISTOPATHOLOGIC FINDINGS

Histologic examination of skin samples reveals an infiltrate of histiocytes, which closely approach the epidermis, accompanied by scattered lymphocytes and eosinophils. The histiocytes express the typical macrophage marker CD68, whereas immunostaining for Langerhans cell markers such as CD1a and CD207 is negative.[22] Ultrastructural presence of worm-like bodies is typical.

DIFFERENTIAL DIAGNOSIS

It is difficult to separate benign cephalic histiocytosis from other forms of N-LCH, especially JXG. Therefore, it can be discussed as a variant of JXG.

CLINICAL COURSE AND PROGNOSIS

Benign cephalic histiocytosis usually resolves spontaneously. Therapeutic options include CO_2 laser therapies.

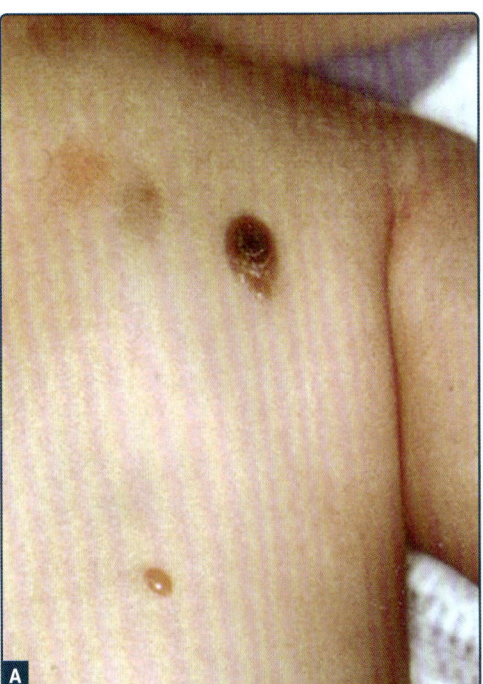
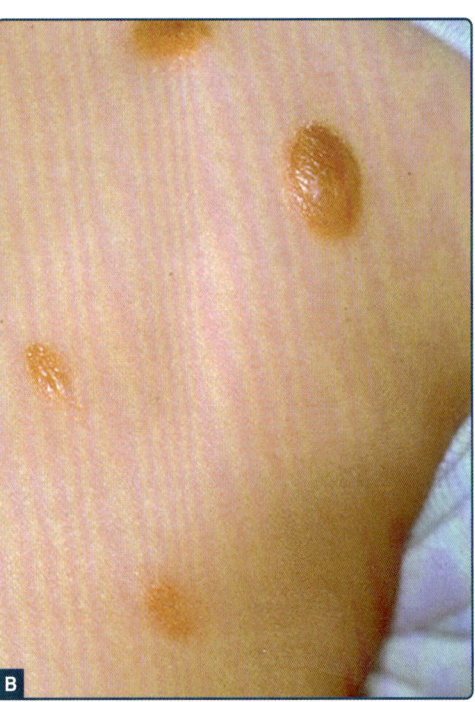

Figure 117-14 Juvenile xanthogranuloma. **A,** Early stage presents with reddish papules. **B,** Mature stage shows a reddish-yellow shade of color.

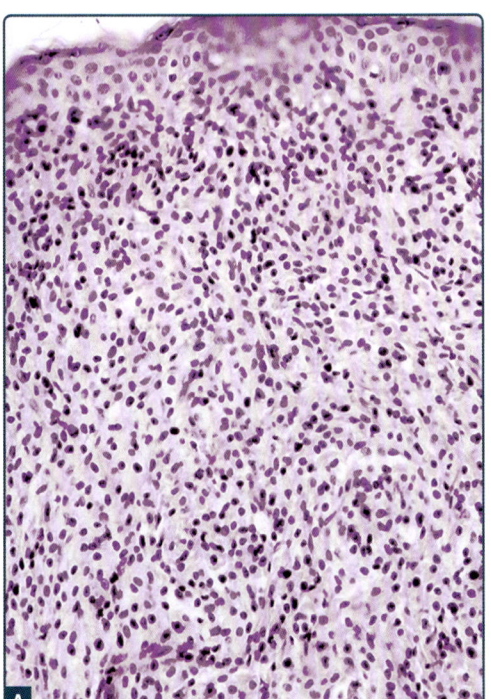
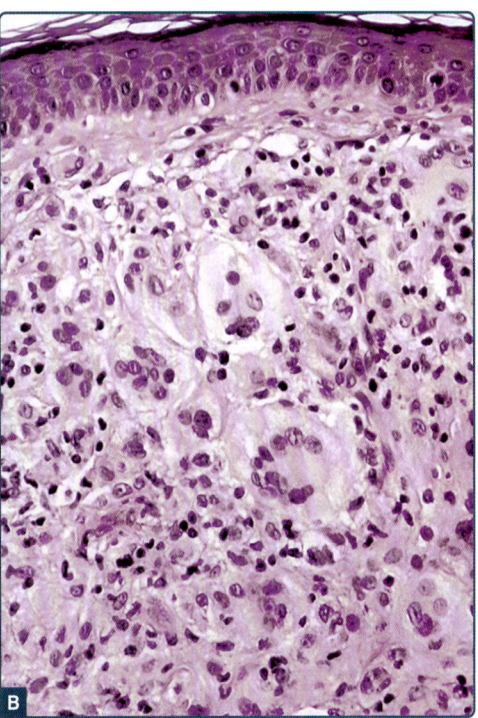

Figure 117-15 Photomicrographs of lesions of juvenile xanthogranuloma. **A,** The early stage is characterized by small, mostly mononuclear histiocytes with a small cytoplasm and less lipid reaching the epidermis without any Grenz zone. **B,** The mature stage shows big, cytoplasm-rich, lipidized histiocytes, big foam cells, and typical Touton giant cells.

TABLE 117-8
Differential Diagnosis of Juvenile Xanthogranuloma

- Xanthoma
- Neurofibroma
- Hemangioma
- Molluscum contagiosum
- Spitz nevus
- Papular mastocytosis
- Sarcoidosis
- Dermatofibroma
- Cutaneous leukemia
- Other forms of non–Langerhans cell histiocytosis and Langerhans cell histiocytosis

GENERALIZED ERUPTIVE HISTIOCYTOMA OF CHILDHOOD

CLINICAL FEATURES

Generalized eruptive histiocytoma (GEH) (also known as "eruptive histiocytoma" or "generalized eruptive histiocytosis") was initially reported by Winkelmann and Muller in 1963. This rare disease is characterized by widespread, erythematous, essentially symmetrical papules, particularly involving proximal extremities as well as the trunk. Unlike in JXG, brownish papules and nodules do not develop; mucosal membranes, however, can be affected. Cutaneous lesions resolve spontaneously with remaining hyperpigmented maculae. There is also a report associating GEH with rheumatic fever. GEH can be seen as a variant of JXG.

ADULT XANTHOGRANULOMA

CLINICAL FEATURES

Adult xanthogranuloma was originally described by Gartmann and Tritsch in 1963. Both solitary and oligolesional yellow-orange papules usually appear on the face, neck, and lower arms. In contrast to JXG, adult xanthogranuloma does not show a spontaneous remission. No association with systemic diseases such as neurofibromatosis or leukemia has been reported. Histologic findings of adult and juvenile forms of the disease are almost identical. Usually in adult xanthogranuloma there are more giant cells. Therapeutic options include excisions of lesions or CO_2 laser therapies.

PAPULAR XANTHOMA

CLINICAL FEATURES

Papular xanthoma was reported for the first time in 1981 by Winkelmann. It is a rare disease in normolipemic patients who present clinically. It appears mainly as a solitary yellowish papule, and seems to appear more often in males. It shows a biphasic occurrence in young adolescents and in persons of middle age. A congenital form has been reported. Mucous membranes were affected in some cases but there is no systemic involvement. A plaque-like form of papular xanthoma can be seen as a variant.[23,24]

HISTOPATHOLOGIC FINDINGS

Histology shows a normal epidermis and a dense infiltration of xanthomatized macrophages interspersed by numerous Touton-type giant cells. Immunohistochemically mononucleated and multinucleated macrophages are positive for KiM1p. Only giant cells are positive for CD68. Up to 50% of the xanthomatized cells are positive for the lectin peanut agglutinin. Stainings for factor XIIIa and CD1a are negative.

DIFFERENTIAL DIAGNOSIS

Differential diagnoses include xanthoma, atheroma, keloid, histiocytoma, Spitz nevus, clear cell acanthoma, and other benign and malignant cutaneous tumors.

CLINICAL COURSE AND PROGNOSIS

Papular xanthoma usually resolves spontaneously. Therapeutic options include surgical excision and CO_2 laser therapy.[22,23]

GENERALIZED ERUPTIVE HISTIOCYTOMA

CLINICAL FEATURES

GEH was first described by Winkelmann and Muller in 1963. There are fewer than 50 case reports worldwide and it affects mainly adults.[25] GEH is characterized by multiple asymptomatic and symmetrically distributed brownish erythematous papules that involve the axial regions—trunk, face, and proximal extremities—that frequently evolve to flares. The big flexures are spared (Fig. 117-16). Mucous membranes were reported to be affected in some cases.[26] Although the disorder usually follows a benign clinical course, there are 2 reports of an atypical form associated with acute monocytic leukemia.

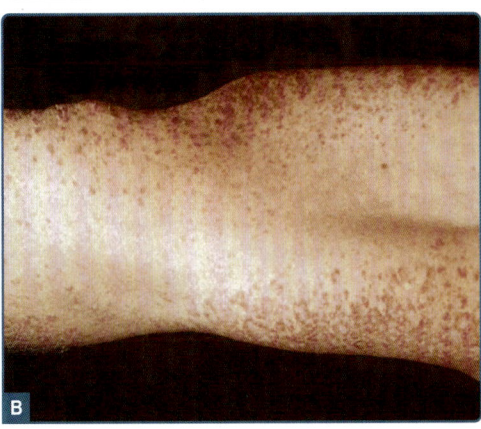

Figure 117-16 Generalized eruptive histiocytoma. Note that the big flexures are spared, as seen in part B of the figure.

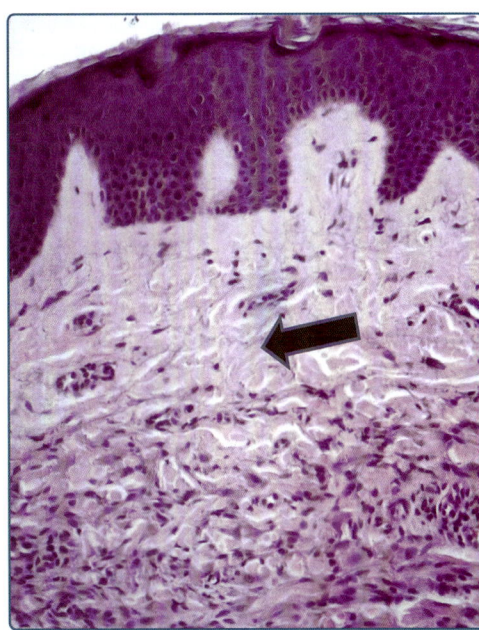

Figure 117-17 Photomicrographs of a lesion of generalized eruptive histiocytoma. In the papillary dermis an infiltration of mostly small, nonlipidized cells and of few lymphocytes underneath a Grenz zone (*arrow*) can be seen. This is a typical sign for generalized eruptive histiocytoma. Giant cells are missing.

CLINICAL COURSE AND PROGNOSIS

GEH usually resolves spontaneously. Therapeutic options include surgical excision and CO_2 laser therapy. Systemic psoralen and ultraviolet A therapy was reported to produce rapid regression of the skin lesions. Given the potential development of acute monocytic leukemia, close follow-up of patients with GEH is recommended.[25,26]

XANTHOMA DISSEMINATUM

CLINICAL FEATURES

Xanthoma disseminatum was described by Montgomery in 1938. It preferentially affects male children. The disease is characterized by the sudden appearance of small, yellow-red to brown papules and nodules that are discrete and disseminated with a predilection for the flexural and intertriginous areas as well as mucous membranes (Fig. 117-18). Involvement of mucosae and a variety of internal organs can result in significant morbidity and mortality. Systemic associations include central diabetes insipidus owing to involvement of the pituitary stalk and paraproteinemias, such as multiple myeloma.[27]

HISTOPATHOLOGIC FINDINGS

Skin biopsies show a normal epidermis. The papillary dermis is infiltrated by mostly small, nonlipidized cells and few lymphocytes underneath a Grenz zone, which is characteristic for GEH (Fig. 117-17). Giant cells are missing. Macrophages are positive for CD68 and stabilin-1, and negative for CD1a, CD34, and S100B.

DIFFERENTIAL DIAGNOSIS

Differential diagnosis includes LCH, other forms of N-LCH, and urticaria pigmentosa. Other N-LCHs are easily distinguished by histology.

Variants of xanthoma disseminatum include disseminated xanthosiderohistiocytosis, which was described by Halprin and Lorincz in 1960 and is associated with multiple myeloma. In 1998, Ferrando described a case of systemic xanthohistiocytoma that can be also seen as a variant of xanthoma disseminatum.

HISTOPATHOLOGIC FINDINGS

Histopathologic examination of early lesions of xanthoma disseminatum shows a predominance of scalloped histiocytes, whereas more established lesions consist mainly of foamy histiocytes with few scalloped cells. In the most established or mature lesions, a mixture of scalloped cells, foam cells, lymphocytes, and Touton giant cells is seen. These cells are positive for stabilin-1, HAM-56, HHF35, KP1, KiM1P, factor XIIIa, and vimentin, and negative for S100B and CD1a (Fig. 117-19).[27]

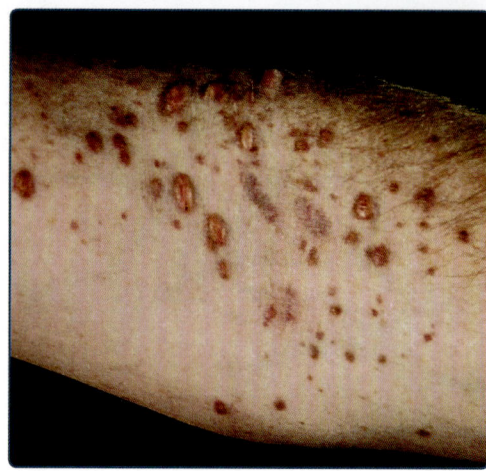

Figure 117-18 Xanthoma disseminatum.

DIFFERENTIAL DIAGNOSIS

The main differential diagnosis includes eruptive xanthomas, other N-LCH, and LCH.

CLINICAL COURSE AND PROGNOSIS

Xanthoma disseminatum is a slowly progressing disease. Cutaneous lesions can be treated, for example, by CO_2 laser therapy. Lesions are not very radiosensitive. Several medications, including statins, fibrates, glitazones, prednisolone, azathioprine, cyclophosphamide, and thalidomide, have been tried with variable results. A successful therapeutic approach seems to be the administration of 2-chlorodeoxyadenosine.[27,28]

MULTICENTRIC RETICULOHISTIOCYTOSIS

CLINICAL FEATURES

Multicentric reticulohistiocytosis (MRH) was first reported by Weber and Freudenthal in 1937. The term was coined by Goltz and Laymon in 1954. It is a rare, multisystem inflammatory disease that usually appears around the age of 50 years, but there are a few reports of its occurrence during childhood. It is twice as common in females. Cutaneous lesions are firm, yellow-brownish papules or nodules that reach a size of several centimeters and progress slowly in size. The occurrence of lesions over the joints of fingers and wrist is typical (Figs. 117-20 and 117-21). Leonine facies can occur via confluence of facial lesions. Involvement of mucosae and conjunctivae can be appreciated in every second patient. MRH can affect any organ. However, the most common clinical manifestations are cutaneous eruptions and symmetric inflammatory polyarthritis. Internal organs, such as the lungs (resulting in pleural effusion) and heart (pericardial effusion and congestive heart failure), have been described as affected by MRH. In addition, mesenteric lymphadenopathy and urogenital lesions have been reported.[29] Constitutional symptoms such as fever, weight loss, and malaise can be observed.[30] A malignancy rate of 33 (25%) in 133 cases of MRH has been reported in the literature. The malignancies were most commonly hematologic, breast, or stomach carcinomas.[31]

HISTOPATHOLOGIC FINDINGS

Histology reveals mid-dermal infiltrates of mononuclear histiocytes and multinucleated histiocytes with a ground-glass appearance and a variable number of vacuolated, spindle-shaped, and xanthomatized mononuclear histiocytes. In the case of MRH, immunohistochemical analyses are usually positive for CD45, CD68 and HLA-DR (human leukocyte antigen-D related), but are negative for S100B, CD1a, or HHF-35 actin.[29,30]

DIFFERENTIAL DIAGNOSIS

Differential diagnosis includes François syndrome (dermochondrocorneal dystrophy), Morbus Farber (lipogranulomatosis disseminata) as well as different metabolic diseases such as gout.

CLINICAL COURSE AND PROGNOSIS

The disease can be self-limited. However, severe joint destruction usually results. Surgical excision, pulsed-dye laser, oral corticosteroids, methotrexate, cyclophosphamide, and tocilizumab have shown success in

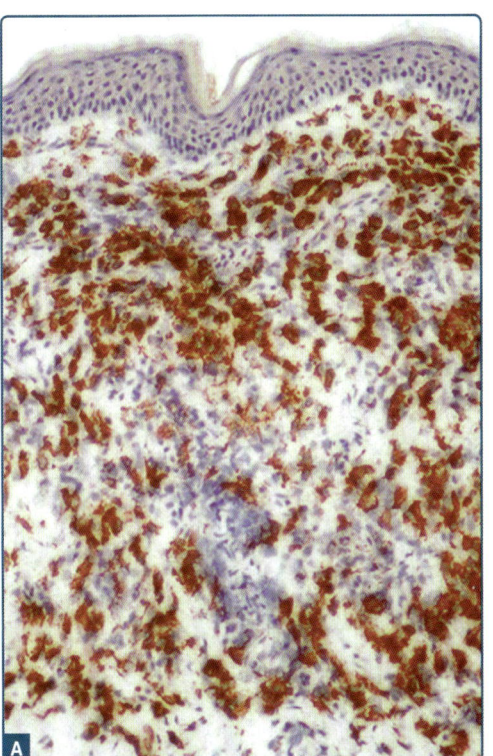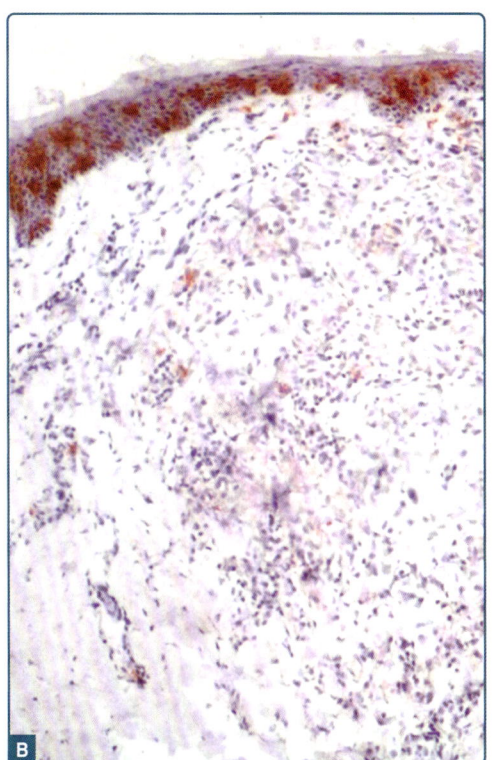

Figure 117-19 Photomicrographs of an early-stage lesion of xanthoma disseminatum. **A,** Stabilin-1 shows strong expression in lesional histiocytes. **B,** CD1a staining is limited mainly to the epidermal Langerhans cells.

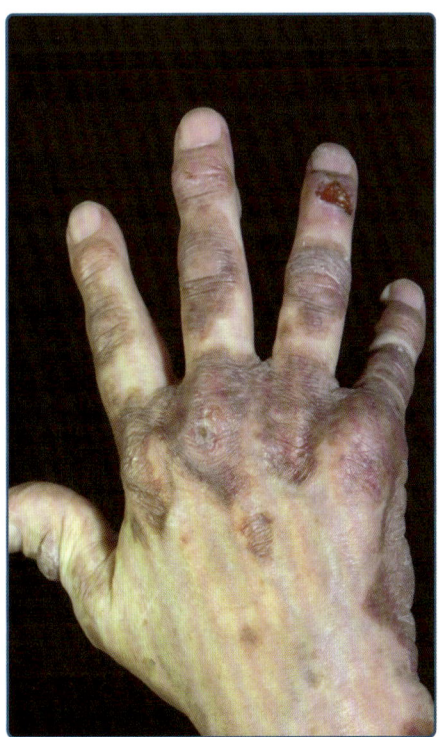

Figure 117-20 Multicentric reticulohistiocytosis.

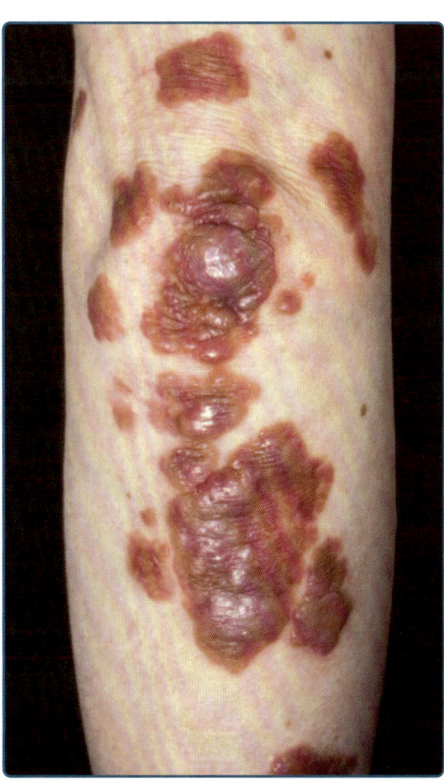

Figure 117-21 Multicentric reticulohistiocytosis.

treating extensive MRH lesions. A systematic review of 17 cases of MRH treated with tumor necrosis factor antagonists showed an efficacy of anti–tumor necrosis factor treatment in MRH.[30]

ERDHEIM-CHESTER DISEASE

CLINICAL FEATURES

The first report of the disease was by Chester who cooperated with Erdheim in 1930. In 1972, Jaffe reported on a similar case and named the disease Erdheim-Chester disease.

Erdheim-Chester disease is a rare disease with onset in middle age. Long bone involvement is almost universal in Erdheim-Chester disease patients, and is bilateral and symmetrical in nature. It encompasses a spectrum of disorders, ranging from asymptomatic bone lesions to multisystem, life-threatening variants.

More than 50% of cases have some sort of extraskeletal involvement. This can include kidney, skin, brain, and lung involvement; less frequently, retro-orbital tissue, pituitary gland, and heart involvement is observed.[32,33] On the skin, xanthelasma and xanthoma are present in one-sixth of cases. Yellow-brown papular and widespread infiltrated lesions have been described in some patients. Newer studies demonstrate that approximately 50% of Erdheim-Chester disease patients have *BRAF* mutations in early multipotent myelomonocytic precursors or in tissue-resident histiocytes. Rarely, other genes involved in the MAPK signaling pathway also mutate.[32]

HISTOPATHOLOGIC FINDINGS

Tissue samples show a xanthomatous or xanthogranulomatous infiltration by lipid-laden or foamy histiocytes that are usually surrounded by fibrosis, especially in longer-standing lesions. Bone biopsies show infiltration of lipid-laden macrophages, multinucleated giant cells, inflammatory infiltrates of lymphocytes, and histiocytes as well as a generalized sclerosis of the long bones.

DIFFERENTIAL DIAGNOSIS

Differential diagnosis mainly includes LCH.

CLINICAL COURSE AND PROGNOSIS

Interferon-α is the first-line treatment in Erdheim-Chester disease, as it has been clearly demonstrated to increase overall survival. Anakinra and infliximab have also led to encouraging results and should be considered when treatment with interferon-α fails. More recently, BRAF inhibitors have been shown to be efficient in all treated cases.[33]

NECROBIOTIC XANTHOGRANULOMA

CLINICAL FEATURES

Necrobiotic xanthogranuloma was first reported by Kossard and Winkelmann in 1980. However, a necrobiosis with xanthogranulomas associated with paraproteinemia was already observed in the 1960s. It is a multisystem disease that affects older adults and it manifests as yellowish plaques and nodules that can ulcerate. Necrobiotic xanthogranuloma is predominantly located on the trunk, the extremities, and the face (periorbital lesions). Extracutaneous involvement also has been described, such as of the eyes, heart, skeletal muscle, larynx, spleen, and ovaries. A systemic association in the form of serum monoclonal gammopathy usually of immunoglobulin G κ and λ type is seen in 80% of necrobiotic xanthogranuloma patients. There is an increased risk for concomitant hematologic and lymphoproliferative malignancies.[34]

HISTOPATHOLOGIC FINDINGS

Necrobiotic xanthogranuloma is characterized by typical necrobiotic areas surrounded by granulomas composed of lymphocytes, Touton giant cells, foamy histiocytes and foreign body-type multinucleated giant cells in the dermis as well as subcutis. As with other N-LCHs, there is no expression of CD1a antigen or CD207. There are no Birbeck granules.

DIFFERENTIAL DIAGNOSIS

Necrobiosis lipoidica, subcutaneous granuloma annulare, and noduli rheumatica can be considered as differential diagnoses. In cases with only a modest necrobiosis, xanthoma that is associated with paraproteinemia and lymphomas should be considered. In cases with periorbital skin lesions, xanthelasma can be a differential diagnosis.

CLINICAL COURSE AND PROGNOSIS

The prognosis is poor with several treatments showing variable results. Neither treatment nor nontreatment of monoclonal gammopathy with alkylating agents necessarily influences the activity of the skin disease. There are no randomized controlled trials and studies on long-term outcomes do not exist. Treatment options are mainly described in case reports and include topical and systemic corticosteroids, thalidomide, high-dose intravenous immunoglobulin, chlorambucil, cyclophosphamide, fludarabine, rituximab, melphalan, infliximab, interferon-α, cladribine, hydroxychloroquine, azathioprine, and methotrexate. In addition, laser therapy, radiotherapy, surgery, psoralen and ultraviolet A, plasmapheresis, and extracorporeal photopheresis are described (systematically reviewed in Miguel et al[35]).

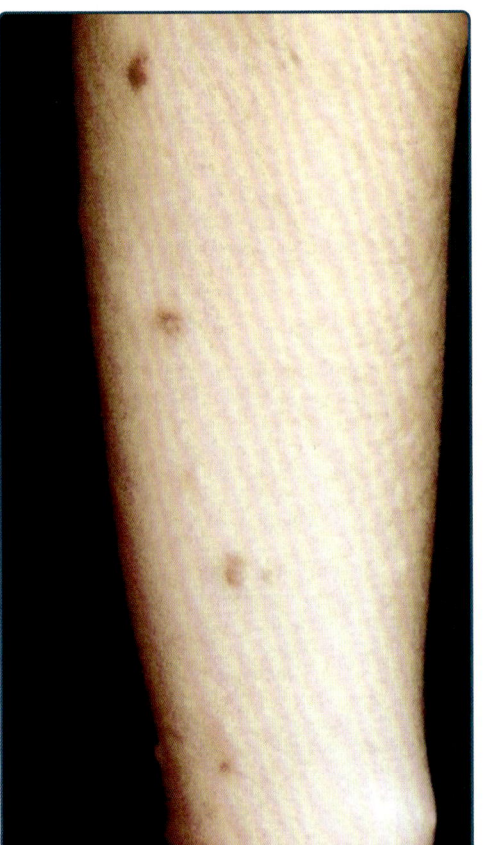

Figure 117-22 Hereditary progressive mucinous histiocytosis.

DIFFERENTIAL DIAGNOSIS

Acral persistent papular mucinosis, scleromyxedema, granuloma annulare, dermatofibroma, and GEH can be distinguished by histology.

CLINICAL COURSE AND PROGNOSIS

Ablative laser therapy for single lesions is an option.

PROGRESSIVE NODULAR HISTIOCYTOSIS

CLINICAL FEATURES

Progressive nodular histiocytosis was described by Taunton and colleagues in 1978. The disease is characterized by generalized, discrete yellow to red-brown papules and nodules measuring a few centimeters in size. A prominent facial involvement has been described. Other organs are not affected. There is an association with chronic myeloid leukemia as well as with tumors of the hypothalamus.[37]

HISTOPATHOLOGIC FINDINGS

The dermis contains abundant spindle-shaped histiocytes, some with foamy cytoplasm. Cells are positive for CD68, CD163, vimentin, and fascin, while negative for CD1a and S100B.

HEREDITARY PROGRESSIVE MUCINOUS HISTIOCYTOSIS

CLINICAL FEATURES

Hereditary progressive mucinous histiocytosis was described by Bork and Hoede in 1988. It is a rare, potentially autosomal dominant inherited disease. Progressive eruptions of self-resolving skin-colored to red-brown papules usually develop in the first decade on the nose, hands, forearms, and thighs (Fig. 117-22). These lesions can later develop into persistent and progressive erythematous papules. Visceral involvement has not yet been reported.

HISTOPATHOLOGIC FINDINGS

Collections of epithelioid S100B/CD1a− and CD68 as well as weak stabilin-1+ histiocytes and telangiectatic vessels in the upper dermis of early lesions can be seen. In the mid-dermis of early and well-developed lesions, nodular aggregates of tightly packed spindle-shaped cells are present. Moderate to extensive mucin production was demonstrated in epithelioid histiocytes and spindle-shaped cells (Fig. 117-23).[36]

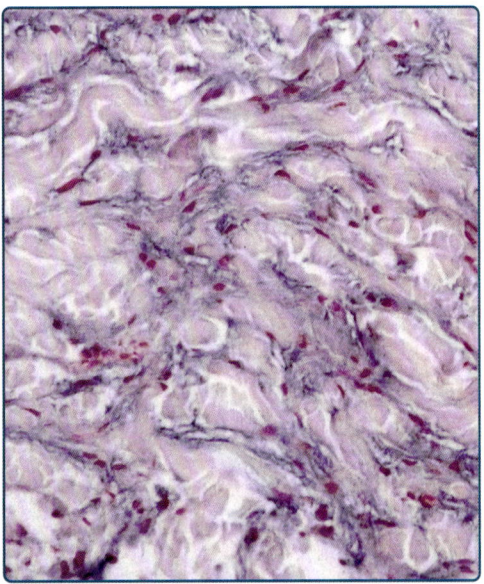

Figure 117-23 Photomicrographs of a lesion of hereditary progressive mucinous histiocytosis. Production of mucin by histiocytes in the dermis is a typical feature of the disease.

DIFFERENTIAL DIAGNOSIS

MRH, which usually shows an involvement of other organ sites, is a differential diagnosis.

CLINICAL COURSE AND PROGNOSIS

Surgical ablation, for example, with a CO_2 laser, of all visible lesions is a therapeutic option.

REFERENCES

1. Zinn DJ, Chakraborty R, Allen CE. Langerhans cell histiocytosis: emerging insights and clinical implications. *Oncology (Williston Park)*. 2016;30:122-132, 139.
2. Badalian-Very G, Vergilio JA, Degar BA, et al. Recurrent BRAF mutations in Langerhans cell histiocytosis. *Blood*. 2010;116:1919-1923.
3. Ribeiro KB, Degar B, Antoneli CB, et al. Ethnicity, race, and socioeconomic status influence incidence of Langerhans cell histiocytosis. *Pediatr Blood Cancer*. 2015;62:982-987.
4. Venkatramani R, Rosenberg S, Indramohan G, et al. An exploratory epidemiological study of Langerhans cell histiocytosis. *Pediatr Blood Cancer*. 2012;59:1324-1326.
5. Allen CE, Li L, Peters TL, et al. Cell-specific gene expression in Langerhans cell histiocytosis lesions reveals a distinct profile compared with epidermal Langerhans cells. *J Immunol*. 2010;184:4557-4567.
6. Gatalica Z, Bilalovic N, Palazzo JP, et al. Disseminated histiocytoses biomarkers beyond BRAFV600E: frequent expression of PD-L1. *Oncotarget*. 2015;6:19819-19825.
7. Morren MA, Vanden Broecke K, Vangeebergen L, et al. Diverse cutaneous presentations of Langerhans cell histiocytosis in children: a retrospective cohort study. *Pediatr Blood Cancer*. 2016;63:486-492.
8. Braier JL, Rosso D, Latella A, et al. Importance of multi-lineage hematologic involvement and hypoalbuminemia at diagnosis in patients with "risk-organ" multi-system Langerhans cell histiocytosis. *J Pediatr Hematol Oncol*. 2010;32:e122-e125.
9. Abbritti M, Mazzei MA, Bargagli E, et al. Utility of spiral CAT scan in the follow-up of patients with pulmonary Langerhans cell histiocytosis. *Eur J Radiol*. 2012;81:1907-1912.
10. Richards GE, Thomsett MJ, Boston BA, et al. Natural history of idiopathic diabetes insipidus. *J Pediatr*. 2011;159:566-570.
11. Gadner H, Minkov M, Grois N, et al. Therapy prolongation improves outcome in multisystem Langerhans cell histiocytosis. *Blood*. 2013;121:5006-5014.
12. Haupt R, Minkov M, Astigarraga I, et al. Langerhans cell histiocytosis (LCH): guidelines for diagnosis, clinical work-up, and treatment for patients till the age of 18 years. *Pediatr Blood Cancer*. 2013;60:175-184.
13. Veys PA, Nanduri V, Baker KS, et al. Haematopoietic stem cell transplantation for refractory Langerhans cell histiocytosis: outcome by intensity of conditioning. *Br J Haematol*. 2015;169:711-718.
14. Heritier S, Jehanne M, Leverger G, et al. Vemurafenib use in an infant for high-risk Langerhans cell histiocytosis. *JAMA Oncol*. 2015;1:836-838.
15. Haroche J, Cohen-Aubart F, Emile JF, et al. Dramatic efficacy of vemurafenib in both multisystemic and refractory Erdheim-Chester disease and Langerhans cell histiocytosis harboring the BRAF V600E mutation. *Blood*. 2013;121:1495-1500.
16. Al-Daraji W, Anandan A, Klassen-Fischer M, et al. Soft tissue Rosai-Dorfman disease: 29 new lesions in 18 patients, with detection of polyomavirus antigen in 3 abdominal cases. *Ann Diagn Pathol*. 2010;14:309-316.
17. Maia RC, de Meis E, Romano S, et al. Rosai-Dorfman disease: a report of eight cases in a tertiary care center and a review of the literature. *Braz J Med Biol Res*. 2015;48:6-12.
18. Dalia S, Sagatys E, Sokol L, et al. Rosai-Dorfman disease: tumor biology, clinical features, pathology, and treatment. *Cancer Control*. 2014;21:322-327.
19. Ishii E. Hemophagocytic lymphohistiocytosis in children: pathogenesis and treatment. *Front Pediatr*. 2016;4:47.
20. Parikh SA, Kapoor P, Letendre L, et al. Prognostic factors and outcomes of adults with hemophagocytic lymphohistiocytosis. *Mayo Clin Proc*. 2014;89:484-492.
21. Kim MS, Kim SA, Sa HS. Old-age-onset subconjunctival juvenile xanthogranuloma without limbal involvement. *BMC Ophthalmol*. 2014;14:24.
22. Lange M, Izycka-Swieszewska E, Michajlowski I, et al. Benign cephalic histiocytosis. *Cutis*. 2015;95:E15-E17.
23. Emberger M, Zelger BW, Laimer M, et al. Plaque-like papular xanthoma, an unusual, localized variant of non-Langerhans cell disease. *Eur J Dermatol*. 2013;23:278-279.
24. Coutinho I, Moreira S, Ramos L, et al. Plaque-like papular xanthoma: a new variant of non-Langerhans cell disease. *J Eur Acad Dermatol Venereol*. 2016;30:332-333.
25. Hansel G, Schonlebe J, Tchernev G, et al. Generalized eruptive histiocytoma in adult patient. *J Biol Regul Homeost Agents*. 2015;29:15-17.
26. Cardoso F, Serafini NB, Reis BD, et al. Generalized eruptive histiocytoma: a rare disease in an elderly patient. *An Bras Dermatol*. 2013;88:105-108.
27. Krishna CV, Parmar NV, Ganguly S, et al. Xanthoma disseminatum with extensive koebnerization associated with familial hypertriglyceridemia. *JAAD Case Rep*. 2016;2:253-256.
28. Khezri F, Gibson LE, Tefferi A. Xanthoma disseminatum: effective therapy with 2-chlorodeoxyadenosine in a case series. *Arch Dermatol*. 2011;147:459-464.
29. Tariq S, Hugenberg ST, Hirano-Ali SA, et al. Multicentric reticulohistiocytosis (MRH): case report with review of literature between 1991 and 2014 with in depth analysis of various treatment regimens and outcomes. *Springerplus*. 2016;5:180.
30. Zhao H, Wu C, Wu M, et al. Tumor necrosis factor antagonists in the treatment of multicentric reticulohistiocytosis: current clinical evidence. *Mol Med Rep*. 2016;14:209-217.
31. Han L, Huang Q, Liao KH, et al. Multicentric reticulohistiocytosis associated with liver carcinoma: report of a case. *Case Rep Dermatol*. 2012;4:163-169.
32. Cives M, Simone V, Rizzo FM, et al. Erdheim-Chester disease: a systematic review. *Crit Rev Oncol Hematol*. 2015;95:1-11.
33. Campochiaro C, Tomelleri A, Cavalli G, et al. Erdheim-Chester disease. *Eur J Intern Med*. 2015;26:223-229.
34. Girisha BS, Holla AP, Fernandes M, et al. Necrobiotic xanthogranuloma. *J Cutan Aesthet Surg*. 2012;5:43-45.
35. Miguel D, Lukacs J, Illing T, et al. Treatment of necrobiotic xanthogranuloma—a systematic review. *J Eur Acad Dermatol Venereol*. 2017;31(2):221-235.

36. Nguyen NV, Prok L, Burgos A, et al. Hereditary progressive mucinous histiocytosis: new insights into a rare disease. *Pediatr Dermatol*. 2015;32:e273-e276.

37. Hilker O, Kovneristy A, Varga R, et al. Progressive nodular histiocytosis. *J Dtsch Dermatol Ges*. 2013;11:301-307.

Chapter 118 :: Vascular Tumors
:: Kelly M. MacArthur & Katherine Püttgen

第一百一十八章

血管性肿瘤

中文导读

血管异常的分类一直存在问题，术语和命名法存在相互矛盾，最广泛接受和最全面的是2014年更新的国际血管异常研究学会（ISSVA）的分类，该分类包括临床、影像学、组织学和遗传特征，将血管异常大致分为血管畸形和血管肿瘤。血管畸形是血管形态发生的异常，而婴儿血管瘤和其他血管肿瘤是增殖性的。目前ISSVA分类中的血管肿瘤分为良性、局部侵袭性或交界性以及恶性；根据组织学、生物学、临床表现、行为、预后和治疗，每种肿瘤都有其独特的特征。本章分2节：①婴儿血管瘤；②其他血管瘤。

第一节介绍了婴儿血管瘤的流行病学、临床特征、病因和发病机制、诊断、临床病程和预后、临床管理，其中重点介绍了β受体阻滞药和皮质类固醇的治疗。

第二节介绍了先天性血管瘤、丛状血管瘤、卡波西样血管内皮瘤、梭形细胞血管瘤、化脓性肉芽肿、多灶性淋巴管瘤伴血小板减少症、乳头状淋巴管内血管内皮细胞瘤、网状血管内皮瘤、先天性小汗腺血管瘤样错构瘤等的临床特点。

〔粟　娟〕

Vascular anomalies commonly present as birthmarks.[1] Their classification has historically been problematic, with contradictory and confusing terminology and nomenclature. Although several classification schemes exist, the most widely accepted and comprehensive is the International Society for the Study of Vascular Anomalies (ISSVA) classification, updated in 2014, to incorporate clinical, imaging, histologic and (where known) genetic characteristics.[1,2] Vascular anomalies are broadly divided into vascular malformations and vascular tumors.[3] Vascular malformations (see Chap. 147) are errors of vascular morphogenesis whereas infantile hemangiomas and other vascular tumors are proliferative. Vascular tumors in the current ISSVA classification are subdivided into (a) benign, (b) locally aggressive or borderline, and (c) malignant; each has unique features based upon histology, biology, clinical appearance, behavior, prognosis, and treatment (Table 118-1).

There are several types of vascular tumors, many of which occur in childhood. These tumors also have confusing nosology,[4] with descriptive but imprecise terminology such as *strawberry*, *capillary*, and *cavernous*. The nonspecific term *hemangioma* should be avoided as a standalone term without a qualifying descriptor (eg, infantile, rapidly involuting congenital, lobular capillary, spindle cell).

INFANTILE HEMANGIOMAS

AT-A-GLANCE

- Infantile hemangiomas are the most common tumor of infancy.
- Infantile hemangiomas in high-risk anatomic sites are likely to require further workup and treatment.
- Segmental infantile hemangiomas are associated with greater morbidity than localized infantile hemangiomas.
- Kasabach-Merritt syndrome does not occur with infantile hemangiomas.

EPIDEMIOLOGY

Infantile hemangiomas (IHs) are the most common benign tumors of childhood, occurring in approximately 4% to 5% of children.[4-7] IHs are distinguished from other vascular tumors and malformations by their unique growth pattern (rapid proliferative phase with subsequent slower involution.) They are more common in girls (2 to 3:1 ratio), in white, non-Hispanic infants,[6,8,9] and infants with low birth weight, and affect up to 30% of premature infants,[5,10] especially those weighing less than 2500 g.[8,11] Low birth weight appears to be the most significant risk factor for IH development, conferring greater risk than prematurity alone, with a 40% risk increase for every 500 g decrease in birth weight,[11] which complements earlier data showing that nearly 1 in 4 infants whose birth weight is less than 1000 g develops IH. Prenatal risk factors include advanced maternal age (older than 30 years of age), preeclampsia, placenta previa, and other placental anomalies.[8,12] Preterm infants are more likely to have multiple IHs. IH in the setting of prematurity is less-strongly associated with female predominance.[8,13] Complicated IHs are more common in girls; the cause is unknown.[14] Chorionic villus sampling is no longer accepted as a significant risk factor.[8,11,13]

CLINICAL FEATURES

CUTANEOUS FINDINGS

A clinical history of a life cycle marked by characteristic proliferation and involution is critical in the diagnosis of IH (Table 118-2).[15]

Growth Characteristics—Proliferation: Absence at birth or presence of a nascent IH, often an area of pallor, telangiectasias, or duskiness is characteristic. A fully formed soft-tissue mass at birth is almost certainly another vascular anomaly or other disease process. Most IHs occur on the head and neck, but IHs can be found at any cutaneous or mucosal site and can, less commonly, involve internal organs (see section "Noncutaneous Findings and Complications").

Almost all IHs with a superficial component become apparent in the first month of life, and most will at least double in size within the first 2 months of life. The early proliferative phase is associated with rapid nonlinear growth with the peak IH growth period occurring between 5.5 weeks and 7.5 weeks of age.[16] While 80% of growth has occurred by 3 months of age, 80% of IHs have completed all growth by 5 months of age (Fig. 118-1).[17] The late proliferative stage of ongoing slower growth that occurs after peak rapid growth typically ends by 9 months of age; only 3% of IHs have clinically documented growth beyond this age.[17]

TABLE 118-1
International Society for the Study of Vascular Anomalies Classification

VASCULAR ANOMALIES				
VASCULAR TUMORS			VASCULAR MALFORMATIONS	
BENIGN	LOCALLY AGGRESSIVE	MALIGNANT	SIMPLE	COMBINED
Infantile hemangioma	Kaposiform hemangioendothelioma	Angiosarcoma	Capillary malformation (C)	CVM, CLM
Congenital hemangioma	Retiform hemangioendothelioma	Epithelioid hemangioendothelioma	Lymphatic malformation (LM)	LVM, CLVM
Tufted hemangioma	PILA, Dabska tumor		Venous malformation (VM)	CAVM
Spindle-cell hemangioma	Composite hemangioendothelioma		Arteriovenous malformation (AVM)	CLAVM
Epithelioid hemangioma	Kaposi sarcoma		Arteriovenous fistula	
Pyogenic granuloma				

CAVM, capillary arteriovenous malformation; CLAVM, capillary lymphatic arteriovenous malformation; CLM, capillary lymphatic malformation; CLVM, capillary lymphatic venous malformation; CVM, capillary venous malformation; LVM, venous malformation; PILA, papillary intralymphatic angioendothelioma. Abbreviated ISSVA classification for Vascular Anomalies by International Society for the Study of Vascular Anomalies is licensed under a Creative Commons Attribution 4.0 International License.

TABLE 118-2
History

- Birth history
  - Was the child of low birth weight and/or premature?
  - Part of a multiple gestational birth?
  - Placental abnormalities?
- Overall health and past medical history
  - Is the child feeding well and gaining weight appropriately?
  - Have there been any hospitalizations or major illnesses?
- History of "birthmark"
  - Was it visible at the time of birth?
  - Has it changed since birth?
  - Growth: Is the birthmark growing proportionately or disproportionately with child's somatic growth? Is it still growing, stable, or shrinking in size? (Serial photographs are helpful.)
  - Any complications such as ulceration, pain or bleeding?
  - Any prior treatments?
- Family history
  - Is there a family history of infantile hemangiomas or other vascular birthmarks?

Deep IHs are more likely to have a longer proliferative phase. Large, segmental and parotid gland IHs may also continue to enlarge slowly for months to, rarely, years, which is longer than other IHs.[17-19]

Growth Characteristics—Involution: The rapid and late proliferative growth phases are followed by a slower involution phase that is more variable in length, lasting for months to years (Fig. 118-2). Evidence of involution, often referred to as *graying*, involves change to a dull red, then gray or milky-white color, followed by flattening and softening. The change is usually apparent by 1 year of age.[17] Smaller hemangiomas typically involute sooner than very large ones.[17] More than 90% of IHs have completed involution by 3.5 to 4 years of age.[20,21] It is important to recognize that complete involution does not equate with complete resolution of the IH. More than half of children with hemangiomas will be left with residual telangiectasias, fibrofatty tissue, or anetodermic skin. Superficial IHs are more likely to develop residual skin changes following involution compared with deep IHs (odds ratio: 8.4).[22] Combined IH and those with a steep border or a cobblestoned surface have a significantly higher risk of permanent scarring.[21]

Classification[8]: Cutaneous IH morphology can be classified based on tumor depth (superficial, deep, combined/mixed) and distribution (localized, segmental, indeterminate, multifocal).[23,24] This morphologic distinction can guide expectations as natural history, prognosis, and possible complications vary based on these classification features.

Superficial IHs are the most common of the morphologic subtypes, presenting as bright fuchsia pink to "strawberry" red vascular plaques or nodules; they involve the papillary dermis. In contrast, deep IHs present as a partially compressible, localized subcutaneous tumors with variable prominence depending upon depth in the skin, and either appear with a slight blue hue or the same color as the surrounding skin; they may be noted, on average, 1 month later than superficial IHs. Less frequently, deep IHs are not appreciated until the infant is a few months of age. Deep IHs are more likely to have a longer proliferative phase, rarely growing for months to years beyond the growth phase of other IHs, and later onset of involution compared with their superficial counterparts.[17,18] Combined (also called *mixed*) IHs have clinical features of both deep and superficial IHs. A less-common subtype of IH is distinguished by its minimal-to-absent proliferation and telangiectatic surface, referred to as IH with minimal or abortive growth,[25] has been described (Fig. 118-3). Found most commonly on the lower body, especially at acral sites, these IHs express the same histologic markers (eg, GLUT1) as typical proliferative IHs, but for unclear reasons fail to undergo the usual IH trajectory of growth.[25,26]

In addition to their individual morphology, IHs can be classified based on their distribution on the body as localized (focal), segmental, indeterminate, or multifocal, which provides valuable prognostic information.[23,24] Approximately two-thirds of IHs are localized (focal) and exhibit clear spatial containment as if arising from one central focus (Fig. 118-4).[27] On the face, localized IHs tend to present near lines of mesenchymal and ectodermal embryonic fusion.[23] Segmental hemangiomas—similar to other segmental dermatologic disease such as vitiligo and neurofibromatosis—are often plaque-like and correspond to a portion of a developmental segment or broad geographic anatomic territory (Fig. 118-5).[28] In a large study, 13.1% of IHs were segmental.[29] The patterns of facial segmental IH have been suggested to correspond to neural crest–derived facial prominences and their presence is associated with risk of PHACE (posterior fossa brain malformations, hemangiomas of the face, arterial anomalies, cardiac anomalies, and eye abnormalities).[29] Segmental IHs on the lower body confer risk of myelopathy and genitourinary anomalies in LUMBAR (lower body hemangioma and other cutaneous defects, urogenital anomalies, ulceration, myelopathy, bony deformities, anorectal malformations, arterial anomalies, and renal anomalies) syndrome (see section "Lumbar Syndrome"). Indeterminate IHs are those that are not clearly identifiable as localized or segmental; some authors consider them to be "subsegmental" (Fig. 118-6). Multifocal (multiple localized) IHs are less common, with fewer than 3% of infants presenting with 6 or more IHs.[27]

Classification of hemangiomas by subtype not only facilitates communication, but also helps predict risk of complications and need for treatment. A prospective study of more than 1000 children with IHs showed that segmental hemangiomas are 11 times more likely to experience complications and 8 times more likely to receive treatment than localized hemangiomas, even when controlled for size.[27]

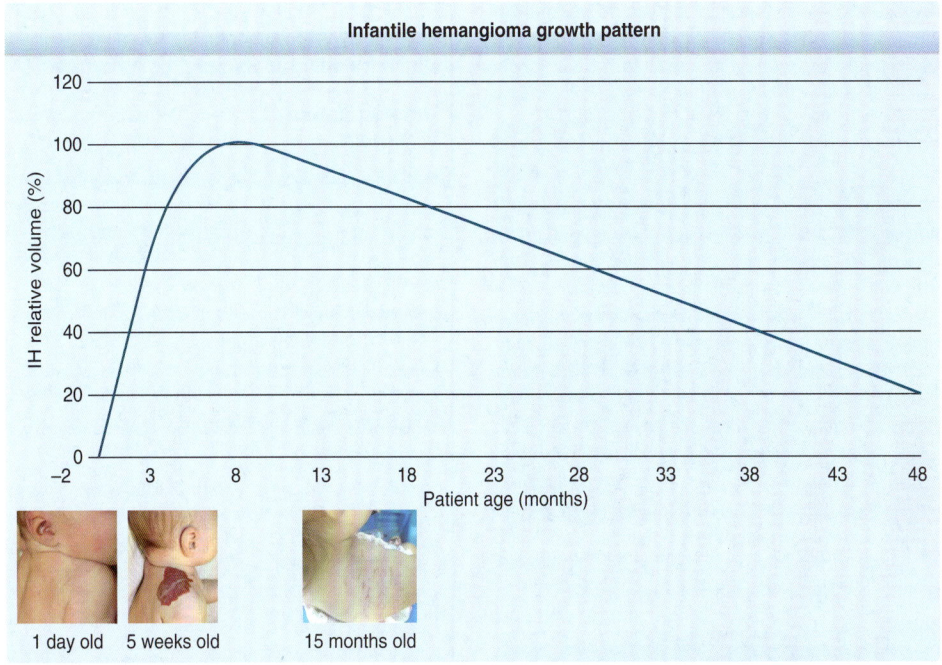

Figure 118-1 Growth characteristics of infantile hemangioma.

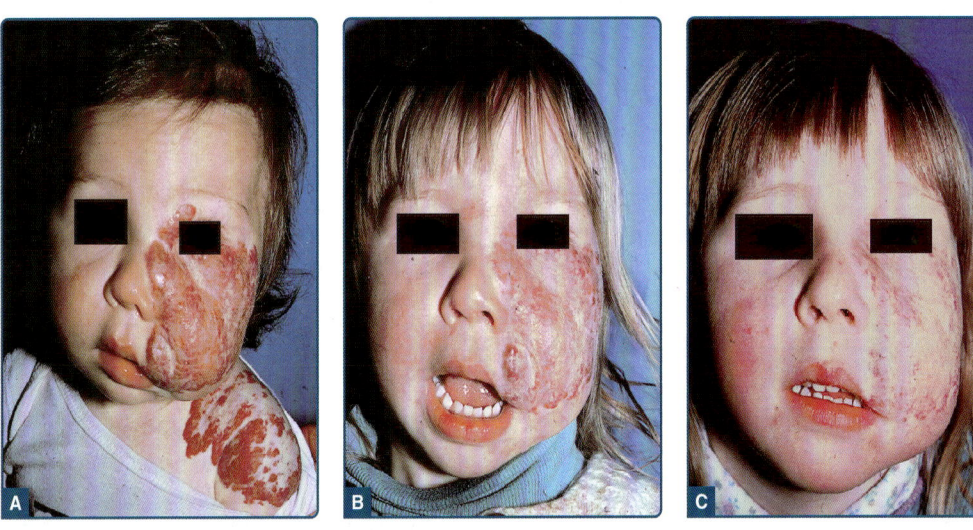

Figure 118-2 Natural history of segmental infantile hemangioma. Note the plaque-like, geographic configuration. **A,** Age 11 months, peak of proliferative phase. **B,** Age 2 years, involuting phase. **C,** Age 4 years, majority of natural involution has occurred.

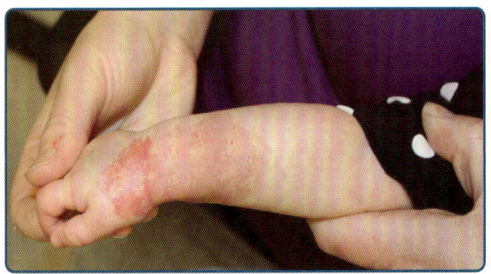

Figure 118-3 An infantile hemangioma with minimal or abortive growth on the right arm and hand of an infant.

NONCUTANEOUS FINDINGS AND COMPLICATIONS

Certain IHs have a known risk of associated complications and congenital anomalies (Table 118-3). The presence of multifocal or segmental IH is associated with a greater risk of extracutaneous disease.[15] Anatomic location is one of the most important factors affecting risk. Involvement of the central face (especially the nose and perioral skin), periocular area, neck, mandibular region, and perineum

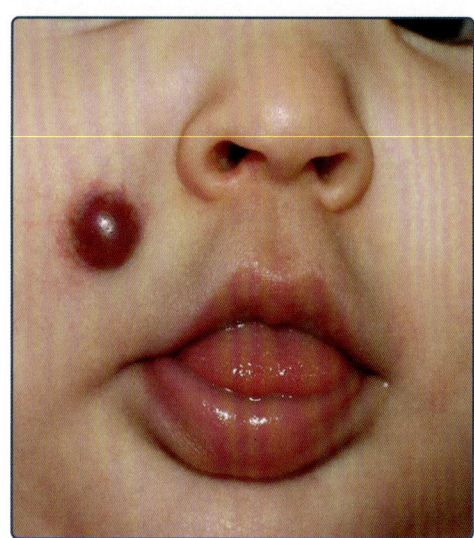

Figure 118-4 Localized infantile hemangioma on the cheek of an infant.

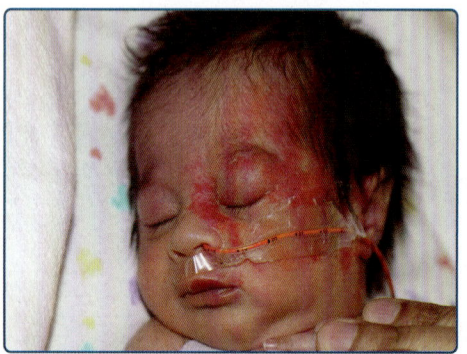

Figure 118-5 Segmental infantile hemangioma on the face, scalp, and neck of a newborn with PHACE.

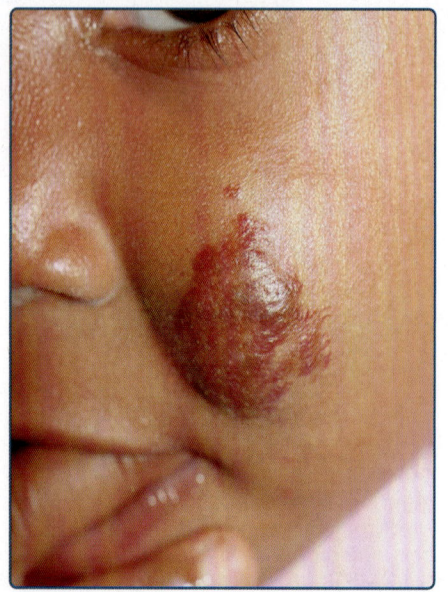

Figure 118-6 Indeterminate infantile hemangioma on the cheek of an infant 14 months of age.

TABLE 118-3
High-risk Infantile Hemangioma Features

ANATOMIC LOCATION/ MORPHOLOGY	ASSOCIATED RISK
Facial, large segmental	PHACE (posterior fossa malformations, hemangiomas, arterial anomalies, cardiac defects, eye abnormalities, sternal clefting) syndrome
Nasal tip, ear, large facial (especially with prominent deep component)	Permanent scarring, cartilage destruction, disfigurement
Periorbital and retrobulbar	Ocular axis occlusion, astigmatism, amblyopia, tear-duct obstruction
Segmental (S3)/"beard area," central neck	Airway infantile hemangioma
Perioral	Ulceration, disfigurement, feeding difficulties
Segmental overlying lumbosacral spine	Myelopathy, genitourinary anomalies
Perineal, axilla, neck, perioral	Ulceration
Multifocal	Visceral involvement (especially liver, GI tract)

should alert clinicians to possible increased risk of complications. Even though the vast majority of IHs remain asymptomatic and uncomplicated with no intervention required, complications can include ulceration, severe bleeding (less than 1% of cases), scarring, pain, and infection, with additional complications found in certain sites of involvement (eg, airway obstruction, congestive heart failure, and visual compromise). Approximately 12% of all IHs are complex, requiring specialist referral. Outcomes are greatly dependent upon timing of referral and intervention.

SYNDROMES AND ASSOCIATIONS WITH SEGMENTAL INFANTILE HEMANGIOMAS

As described above, facial segmental IH patterns correspond to developmental units and have been labeled as 4 segments (S1 to S4): frontotemporal (S1), maxillary (S2), mandibular (S3), and frontonasal (S4).[27] The frontotemporal segment (S1) is associated with cerebral, cerebrovascular, and ocular anomalies; the maxillary segment (S2) is less-frequently associated with extracutaneous involvement; the mandibular segment (S3) is correlated with airway IH, ventral developmental defects, and cardiovascular abnormalities; and the frontonasal segment (S4) encompasses the high-risk territory of the nose, including the nasal tip,[30] and confers risk of cerebral and cerebrovascular involvement (Fig. 118-7).

PHACE

Facial segmental IHs confer a risk of PHACE,[31] which is a neurocutaneous association. It is sometimes referred to as PHACES to denote the additional association of *Sternal* defects (ie, sternal clefting or supraumbilical raphe).[32] For unclear reasons, up to 90% of PHACE cases are in girls.—In addition, up to one-third of patients with facial segmental IHs with a surface area equal to or greater than 22 cm² have been reported to meet criteria for PHACE syndrome.[33-35] The frontotemporal (S1) and mandibular (S3) segments are the segments most highly associated with PHACE. There are infants with extracutaneous features of PHACE who have segmental IHs on the back of the head, upper trunk, or arm, as well as infants who have small IHs or who lack cutaneous IHs entirely.[36-39] Diagnostic criteria have been revised (Table 118-4).[40]

Congenital vascular anomalies of are the most common extracutaneous features in PHACE. Cerebral vascular anomalies occur in greater than 90% of cases, and cardiac abnormalities occur in up to 67% of cases.[30,32,33,35,41] Dysplasia, stenosis, hypoplasia, and agenesis of major cerebral and cervical vessels can occur. Coarctation of the aorta has been reported in 19% to 30% of PHACE cases, and aortic arch anomalies are uniquely complex when associated with PHACE, frequently involving long segment of the transversa and/or descending aorta.[40,42] Notably, aortic coarctation in PHACE is frequently associated with aberrant origin of both subclavian arteries arising distal to the coarctation, rendering the blood pressures of the 4 extremities incapable of demonstrating a gradient reflective of the coarctation on physical examination. Structural brain anomalies occur in approximately 40% of PHACE patients,[43] with estimates ranging widely from 30% to greater than 80%.[40] Arterial ischemic stroke is known to occur in PHACE, and often presents with seizure or hemiparesis.[44] Although the degree of risk for most infants with PHACE is unclear, risk appears highest in the setting of occlusion or significant narrowing of a major cerebral artery within or above the circle of Willis, especially with concomitant aortic coarctation.[40] Ocular anomalies are less common and typically manifest as posterior segment anomalies (eg, morning glory disc anomaly, optic nerve hypoplasia, persistent fetal vasculature, or retinal vascular anomalies) or microphthalmia. Endocrine abnormalities, including hypothy-

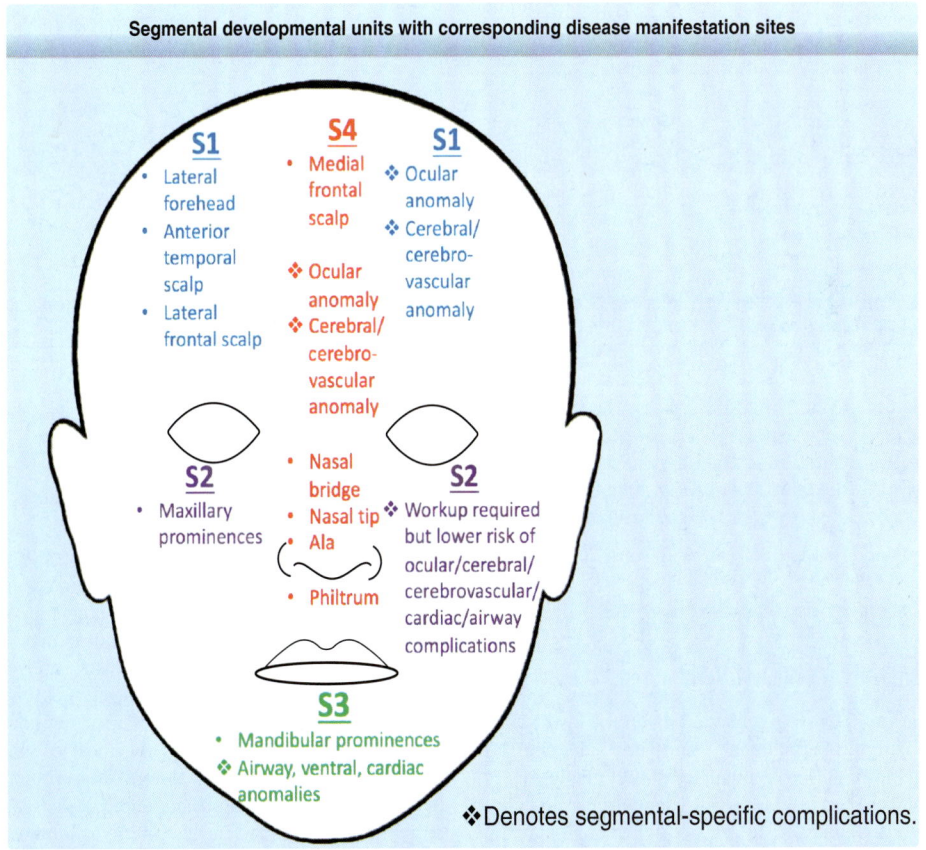

Figure 118-7 Segmental developmental units with corresponding disease manifestation sites. (Data from Haggstrom AN, Lammer EJ, Schneider RA, et al. Patterns of infantile hemangiomas: new clues to hemangioma pathogenesis and embryonic facial development. *Pediatrics.* 2006;117(3):698-703.)

TABLE 118-4
PHACE Diagnostic Criteria

ORGAN SYSTEM	MAJOR CRITERIA	MINOR CRITERIA
Arterial anomalies	Anomaly of major cerebral or cervical arteries[a] Dysplasia[b] of the large cerebral arteries Arterial stenosis or occlusion with or without moyamoya collaterals Absence or moderate-severe hypoplasia of the large cerebral and cervical arteries Aberrant origin or course of the large cerebral or cervical arteries except common arch variants such as bovine arch Persistent carotid-vertebrobasilar anastomosis (proatlantal segmental, hypoglossal, otic, and/or trigeminal arteries)	Aneurysm of any of the cerebral arteries
Structural brain	Posterior fossa brain anomalies Dandy-Walker complex Other hypoplasia/dysplasia of the mid and/or hind brain	Midline brain anomalies Malformation of cortical development
Cardiovascular	Aortic arch anomalies Coarctation of the aorta Dysplasia[a] Aneurysm Aberrant origin of the subclavian artery with or without a vascular ring	Ventricular septal defect Right aortic arch/double aortic arch Systemic venous anomalies
Ocular	Posterior segment abnormalities Persistent hyperplastic primary vitreous Persistent fetal vasculature Retinal vascular anomalies Morning glory disc anomaly Optic nerve hypoplasia Peripapillary staphyloma	Anterior segment abnormalities Microphthalmia Sclerocornea Coloboma Cataracts
Ventral/midline	Anomaly of the midline chest and abdomen Sternal defect Sternal pit Sternal cleft Supraumbilical raphe	Ectopic thyroid hypopituitarism Midline sternal papule/hamartoma
Definite PHACE		
IH >5 cm diameter of the head (including scalp) *plus* 1 major criterion or 2 minor criteria	IH of the neck, upper trunk, or trunk, and proximal upper extremity *plus* 2 major criteria	
Possible PHACE		
IH >5 cm diameter of the head (including scalp) *plus* 1 minor criterion	IH of the neck, upper trunk, or trunk, and proximal upper extremity *plus* 1 major criterion or 2 minor criteria	No IH *plus* 2 major criteria

[a]Internal carotid artery, middle cerebral artery, anterior cerebral artery, posterior cerebral artery, or vertebrobasilar system.
[b]Includes kinking, looping, tortuosity, and/or dolichoectasia.
From Garzon MC, Epstein LG, Heyer GL, et al. PHACE syndrome: consensus-derived diagnosis and care recommendations. *J Pediatr*. 2016;178:24-33.e2. With permission. Copyright © Elsevier.

roidism and hypopituitarism, with subsequent growth hormone deficiency, as well as headaches, and speech and language delays can also occur.[40,45]

LUMBAR SYNDROME

Similar to PHACE, segmental IHs on the lower body involving the perineum or lumbosacral area are risk factors for associated spinal, bony, and genitourinary anomalies (Fig. 118-8). LUMBAR syndrome describes the constellation of lower body hemangioma and other cutaneous defects, urogenital anomalies, ulceration, myelopathy, bony deformities, anorectal malformations, arterial anomalies, and renal anomalies.[46]

Similar groups of patients have been described with the acronyms PELVIS (perineal hemangioma, external genitalia malformations, lipomyelomeningocele, vesicorenal abnormalities, imperforate anus, skin tag) and SACRAL (spinal dysraphism, anogenital anomalies, cutaneous anomalies, renal and urologic anomalies, associated with angioma of lumbosacral localization).[47,48] Myelopathy is the most commonly associated extracutaneous abnormality, presenting as tethered cord or lipomyelo(meningo)cele.[46] MRI is strongly recommended in this setting as lumbosacral ultrasound is reported to result in false-negative findings given its poor sensitivity.[49,50] IHs in the setting of LUMBAR are more likely to be IHs with minimal or

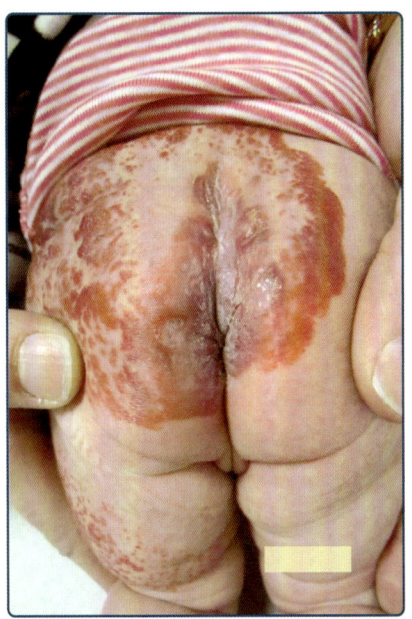

Figure 118-8 A segmental infantile hemangioma of the lower body in an infant with LUMBAR syndrome complicated by painful ulceration.

abortive growth morphology and carry a notable risk of ulceration. Underlying arterial anomalies and limb hypotrophy can occur.[46]

PERIOCULAR HEMANGIOMAS

Infants with periocular hemangiomas are at risk for anisometropia and amblyopia, which, if untreated, can lead to permanent visual loss (Fig. 118-9).[51,52] Amblyopia is the most common ocular complication, occurring in 40% to 60% of infants with untreated periocular IH.[53,54] IHs larger than 1 cm in diameter confer greater risk of amblyopia, significantly lowering the threshold to initiate treatment.[52] Direct pressure on the cornea can produce astigmatism or myopia, and the mass effect of the tumor itself can cause ptosis, proptosis, visual axis occlusion, or strabismus. Any patient with a hemangioma in the periocular area should have a prompt formal ophthalmologic evaluation with repeat visits during the rapid and late proliferative phases. In the setting of ophthalmologic complications, treatment should be initiated urgently to prevent long-term effects, including permanent blindness. Standard evaluation with an ophthalmologist trained in the care of infants should include refraction via retinoscopy following cycloplegia. Serial examinations are especially important with involvement of upper eyelid or supraorbital region. Long-term morbidity can include optic atrophy, blepharoptosis, and ocular proptosis.[55] Between 40% and 80% of periorbital IHs have permanent residual changes following involution.[56] The most favorable prognostic sign to herald normal vision following involution is the absence of asymmetrical refractive error.[54] In certain cases, MRI may be necessary to determine the presence of retrobulbar involvement.

"BEARD AREA" HEMANGIOMAS

Segment 3 IHs involving the preauricular, mandibular, chin, and neck skin (or so-called *beard area*) carry a 60% risk of causing symptomatic airway disease.[57] Airway hemangiomas often present with the insidious onset of biphasic stridor between weeks 4 and 12 of life and are often mistakenly diagnosed as tracheomalacia, upper respiratory tract infection, or croup. Without intervention, respiratory distress can ensue and become life-threatening. Prompt evaluation by a pediatric otolaryngologist and treatment is essential.[58] Parotid gland IH may have an unusually prolonged growth phase and may require treatment because of massive growth of the IH and deformity of adjacent structures. High-output congestive heart failure has been reported, although rarely.[59,60]

MULTIFOCAL HEMANGIOMAS

Approximately 15% of infants will have more than 1 hemangioma. Infants with multifocal IH have an increased risk of noncutaneous IH. Screening hepatic and abdominal ultrasound is recommended for infants presenting with 5 or more cutaneous IHs (Fig. 118-10).[61,62] In rare cases, infants can have hundreds of lesions. The term *multifocal IH with or without extracutaneous disease* has been suggested to replace the older term *diffuse neonatal hemangiomatosis*, given that it is now understood that cases reported in the older literature confused IH with multifocal lymphangioendotheliomatosis with thrombocytopenia (MLT) and other non-IH multifocal tumors. Other sites of visceral involvement are very rare in true IH. Visceral hemangiomas, including those affecting the liver, GI tract, and brain, also have been reported with solitary segmental hemangiomas.[63]

HEPATIC HEMANGIOMAS

The liver is the most common extracutaneous site for IH. Even when present, hepatic IHs are frequently asymptomatic. A minority of hepatic IHs cause morbidity, and, in rare cases, can be life threatening, causing high-output congestive heart failure, hypothyroidism, or hepatic failure. Hepatic hemangiomas can be focal, multifocal, or diffuse.[64] Focal hepatic hemangiomas are not true IHs, but are analogous to rapidly involuting congenital hemangioma (RICH) occurring in the liver. They are fully formed at birth, present without cutaneous IHs, and can cause moderately severe thrombocytopenia and coagulopathy, although not as severe as the consumptive coagulopathy of Kasabach-Merritt phenomenon. Multifocal and diffuse hepatic hemangiomas are true IHs. Multifocal infantile hepatic hemangiomas are often asymptomatic but can cause high-output congestive heart failure

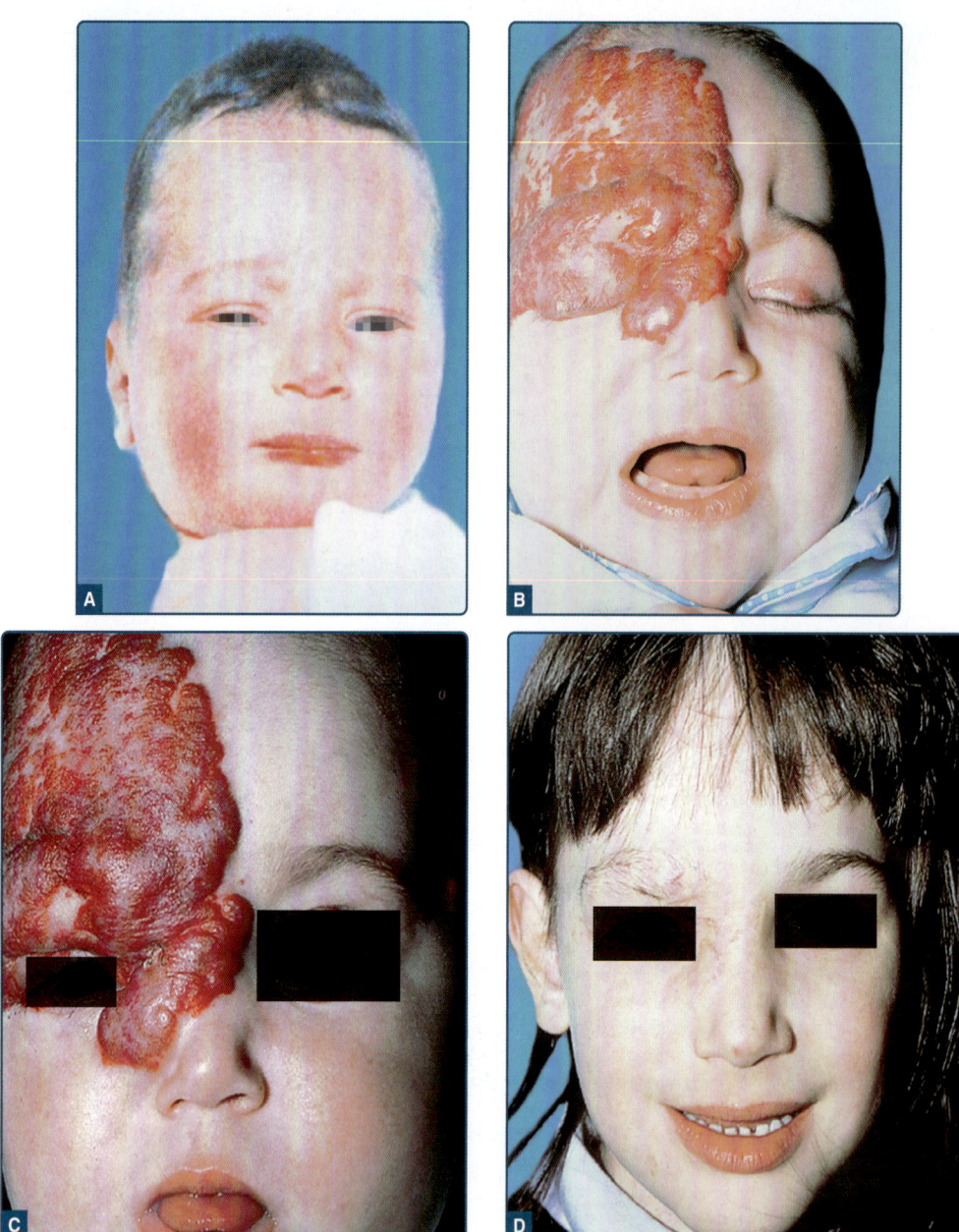

Figure 118-9 Vision-endangering segmental infantile hemangioma treated with systemic glucocorticoids. **A,** No premonitory signs of tumor seen on infant's photograph. **B,** By age 3 months, extensive infantile hemangioma infiltrating the upper lid and surrounding tissue, causing blocked vision. **C,** Eyelid opened within 2 weeks of glucocorticoid therapy. **D,** Involuted tumor at age 6 years with residual scarring.

if arteriovenous or portovenous shunting occurs. Diffuse infantile hepatic hemangiomas are less common and associated with high morbidity and mortality. In this setting, the majority of the liver parenchyma is replaced by tumor and can cause abdominal compartment syndrome and severe hypothyroidism as a consequence of tumor-related overproduction of Type III iodothyronine deiodinase. Systemic β-blocker therapy and, in severe cases, concomitant systemic corticosteroids or embolization may be required.[65,66] Aggressive thyroid hormone replacement is needed in cases with hypothyroidism.[67] In life-threatening cases, liver transplantation may be considered.

ULCERATION

Ulceration is the most common complication of IH, occurring in greater than 20% of infants in a referral

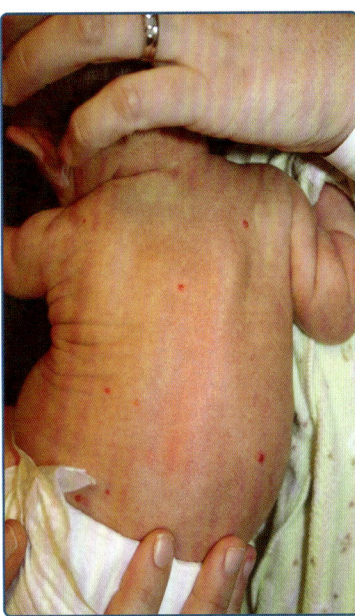

Figure 118-10 Multifocal infantile hemangiomas in an infant. There are multiple, small, superficial, pink papules on the trunk and extremities.

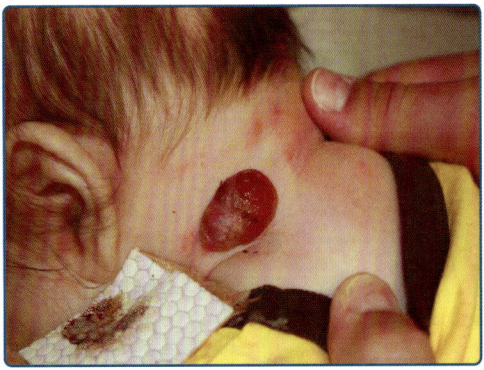

Figure 118-11 A painful ulcerated infantile hemangioma on the neck that required treatment with wound care, pulsed-dye laser, and propranolol.

ETIOLOGY AND PATHOGENESIS

IHs occur exclusively in humans and are primarily composed of endothelial cells. IHs also contain fibroblasts, pericytes, interstitial cells, and mast cells. The patterns found in segmental IHs suggest at least some IHs occur as the result of a developmental error as early as 4 to 6 weeks of gestation.[29] The pathogenesis of their development and evolution remains elusive, in part hampered by the lack of a strong in vitro system or in vivo animal model (Fig. 118-12). Research continues to highlight the complex pathophysiology[56,76-79] by which these tumors proliferate and involute. Current understanding suggests that both angiogenesis, the

setting, typically during the proliferative phase, with a median age of onset of 4 months.[27,68] It occurs most commonly in large or segmental IHs and at sites that are exposed to moisture and friction, such as the perioral, perianal, and intertriginous areas (Fig. 118-11).[68,69] Early gray-white discoloration in patients younger than 3 months is a sensitive marker of impending ulceration.[70] Secondary infection can occur, but polymicrobial colonization is more typical.[71] Treatment of the ulceration (Table 118-5) is often successful in the absence of antibiotic therapy, although localized colonization versus infection can improve with the topical mupirocin or metronidazole. If deep or persistent infection is suspected, systemic antibiotics should be prescribed.

Local wound care, barrier protection, and pain control are essential for treatment. Bio-occlusive dressings may be helpful but their usefulness is often limited by location because they do not adhere well near the mouth or in diaper area.[72,73] In these areas, thick applications of petrolatum-based ointments can be helpful. Pain can be a major issue in management. It can be minimized with an occlusive dressing, oral acetaminophen with or without codeine, and the use of very small amounts of topical lidocaine ointment no more than a few times a day.[69] Severe ulcers or those that remain unhealed after 2 to 3 weeks of appropriate wound care warrant more aggressive therapy. Options include systemic β-blocker therapy, topical β-blocker (eg, topical timolol maleate), and pulsed-dye laser (PDL). Other options less frequently employed in the β-blocker era include becaplermin 0.01% gel,[74,75] intralesional and systemic corticosteroids, and early excision.

TABLE 118-5

Management of Ulcerations

- Local wound care and barrier protection
- Compresses (wet to dry saline compresses, Burow solution) for exudative ulcers
- Occlusive dressings
- Absorbent nonstick dressings, foam dressings
- Alginate dressings (exudative ulcers)
- Petrolatum-based ointments; petroleum jelly-impregnated gauze
- Zinc oxide paste, hydrophilic petrolatum
- Pain control
- Topical lidocaine (very small amount)
- Acetaminophen with or without codeine
- Topical antibiotics (if secondary infection is suspected)
- Mupirocin ointment
- Metronidazole gel
- Aggressive therapy in ulcers that are unhealed after 2 to 3 weeks of wound care
- Systemic β-blocker therapy
- Topical β-blocker (timolol maleate)
- Pulsed-dye laser
- Becaplermin 0.01% gel
- Intralesional and systemic corticosteroids
- Early excision

development of new blood vessels from existing blood vessels, and vasculogenesis, the de novo development of blood vessels, are important in IH development. Studies show IHs to be of fetal, rather than maternal, origin,[80] and demonstrate immature mesenchymal features with similarities to the cardinal vein, an early embryologic vascular structure.[81]

The recognition that GLUT1, a red blood cell glucose transporter protein and the most reliable histologic marker of IH, which is expressed in all stages of IH, prompted new hypotheses on the pathogenesis of IH.[82,83] GLUT1 expression is absent in the normal cutaneous vasculature but is found in placental blood vessels as well as in other so-called barrier tissues, such as the blood–brain barrier. This, together with other immunohistochemical markers shared by IH and human placenta (Lewis Y antigen, merosin, Fc-γ receptor-IIb, indoleamine 2,3-deoxygenase, and Type III iodothyronine deiodinase), and the similar gene expression profiles found on DNA-based microarrays led to speculation that these tumors are of placental origin from invading angioblasts that have differentiated toward a placental phenotype.[83,84] Earlier theories of embolic placental tissue as the trigger for IH have been discredited given that both placental trophoblastic marker expression and villous architecture are absent in IH.[85]

Proliferation is differentiated by the expression of the primitive cell marker, CD133+,[86,87] found in pluripotent stem cells known as HemSCs, with demonstration of the presence of endothelial progenitor cells (CD31+, CD34+, CD133+ stem cells) (HemEPCs) in proliferative IH but absent in the involution phase.[88,89] Translational studies involving implantation of HemSCs isolated from human IH into immunodeficient mice resulted in mimicry of the IH life cycle, with development of GLUT1+ vessels and subsequent adipocyte replacement.[88] HemSCs are precursors for adipocytes, and the presence of adipocytes in involuted IH is well known. Vasculogenesis in IH is theorized to occur from the clonal expansion of circulating endothelial progenitor cells and circulating endothelial progenitor cells may be the progenitor of the endothelial cells lining IH vessels.[35] Other studies demonstrate increased amounts of angiogenic factors in proliferating IH, including basic fibroblast growth factor, vascular endothelial growth factor A, insulin-like growth factor, and matrix metalloprotease 9.[90] These angiogenic factors are downregulated during involution.

Increasing evidence supports the role of hypoxia in IH development and hypoxia is postulated to trigger neovasculogenesis in infants. Low birth weight, the most significant risk factor for IH, is known to be associated with hypoxia.[8,12] GLUT1 is upregulated in the setting of hypoxia.[35,91] Translational studies performed on proliferating IH have identified presence of multiple markers of hypoxia in addition to GLUT1, including insulin-like growth factor-2 and vascular endothelial growth factor A.[92] Histologic features differentiate between the proliferative and involuting phases of IH and shed light on the pathogenesis as well. During proliferation, the clonal nature and histologic features of endothelial cell proliferation[93,94] suggest the process to be secondary to vasculogenesis,[95] whereas involution is marked by apoptosis and capillary lumina fibrosis.[96] However, the definitive pathogenesis to explain trajectory of IH initiation, proliferation, and involution remain con-

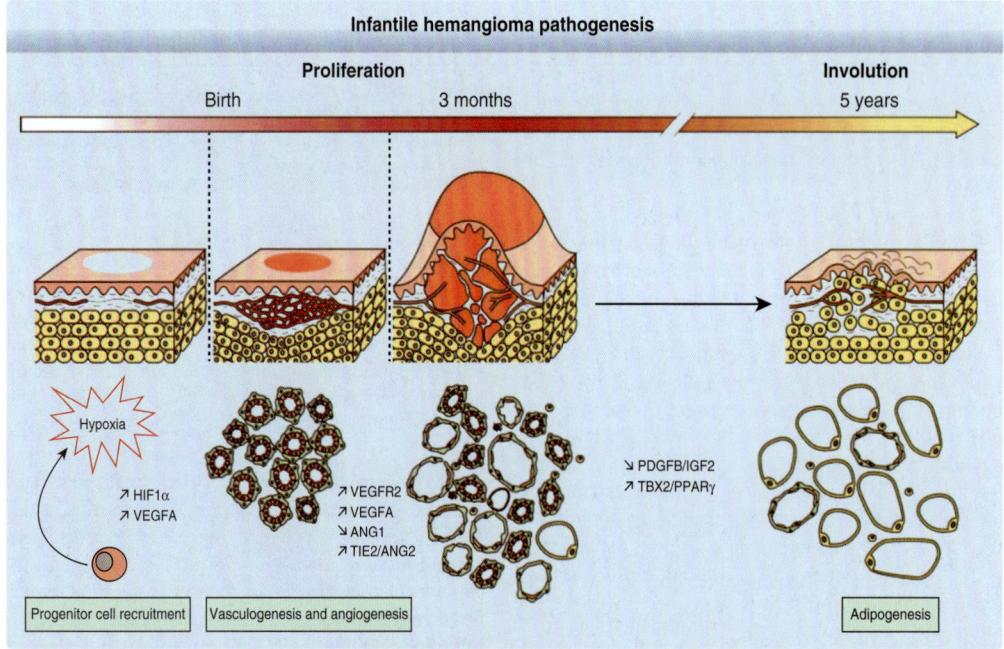

Figure 118-12 Infantile hemangioma pathogenesis. (Figure reprinted from Léauté-Labrèze C, Harper JI, Hoeger PH. Infantile haemangioma. *The Lancet*. 2017;390(10089):85-94, with permission. Copyright © Elsevier.)

troversial. At present, the most supported explanation suggests that hypoxia (in utero or in local tissue) is key[97] to stimulation of circulating endothelial progenitor cells (CD34+, CD133+ stem cells), subsequent vasculogenesis[98] with ensuing proliferation to maintain tissue oxygenation homeostasis,[97] and eventual increased apoptosis (beginning by end of first year of life) to initiate involution.[96]

DIAGNOSIS

With the exception of unusually challenging cases, the diagnosis of IH is almost exclusively clinical, based on the physical examination and clinical history.

SUPPORTIVE STUDIES

Supportive studies may be warranted in certain clinical contexts (Fig. 118-13). When necessary, ultrasound imaging offers the advantages of lack of need for sedation, lack of ionizing radiation and relatively low cost. On Doppler ultrasound, IH is a high-flow lesion and appears as a well-defined solid mass with increased vascular flow within the mass. Arterial feeder and venous drainage can be visualized. The use of MRI offers the benefit of additional anatomic detail, but its use must be weighed against both the risk of exposure to inhaled anesthesia in young infants and increased cost. The current weight of evidence does support the use of MRI and magnetic resonance angiography (MRA) in the workup of PHACE syndrome in early life.[40] Some centers experienced in the imaging of infants may be able to successfully complete an MRI in the neonatal period after feeding and swaddling ("feed-and-wrap" technique); the likelihood of compromising image quality by motion artifact increases with the age of the infant and the duration of the study. On MRI, IH appears as a T2 bright, T1 isointense mass with homogeneous, avid contrast enhancement. Internal serpiginous flow voids, indicative of arterial feeding vessels, are visible on T2-weighted imaging. MRA demonstrates early arterial enhancement.[99]

LABORATORY TESTS

Thyroid Function Tests: Hypothyroidism is a rare complication in infants with diffuse infantile hepatic hemangiomas.[100,101] The liver tumor demonstrates high levels of Type III iodothyronine deiodinase activity, which accelerates the degradation of thyroid hormone.[67,102] Infants with significant hepatic hemangiomas should have thyroid function evaluated, including triiodothyronine (T3) (the hormone consumed) and thyroid-stimulating hormone, because thyroxine (T4) levels may initially remain normal. Conversely, screening hepatic ultrasound should be performed in infants with hypothyroidism of unknown etiology even in the absence of cutaneous hemangiomas. Hypothyroidism and other endocrine abnormalities also have been reported with PHACE syndrome.

PATHOLOGY

The histopathologic appearance of IH varies markedly over the course of its life cycle. In all but the earliest phase of growth and the very end of involution, features of proliferation and involution are

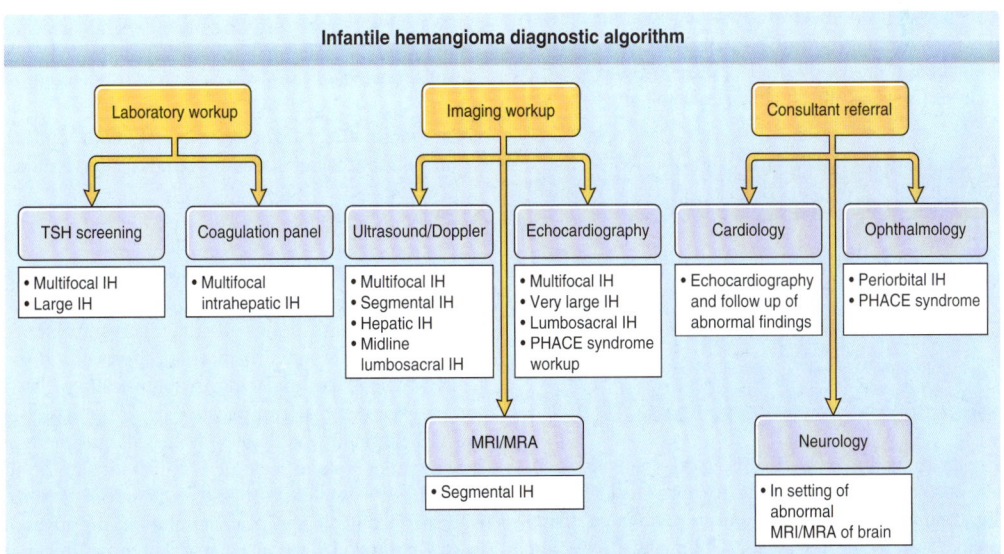

Figure 118-13 Infantile hemangioma (IH) diagnostic algorithm. PHACE, posterior fossa brain malformations, hemangiomas of the face, arterial anomalies, cardiac anomalies, and eye abnormalities; TSH, thyroid-stimulating hormone. (Adapted from Léauté-Labrèze C, Harper JI, Hoeger PH. Infantile haemangioma. *Lancet*. 2017;390(10089):85-94.)

comingled. As a complement to radiologic imaging, IH in the rapid proliferative phase are made up of unencapsulated but well-defined mass of capillaries arranged in lobules divided by fine septae or normal surrounding soft tissue, comprised of endothelial cells, pericytes, mast cells and interstitial dendritic cells. The vessels are lined with plump endothelial cells with enlarged nuclei and abundant cytoplasm with a surrounding rim of similarly plump pericytes in the absence of smooth muscle cells.[35] The appearance is somewhat similar to young pyogenic granulomas (lobular capillary hemangiomas). In early IH, markers of cellular proliferation such as Ki-67 denotes proliferation of endothelium and pericytes and normal appearing mitotic figures appear abundant. Thick-walled draining veins may be visible. In involuting IH specimens, capillaries begin to be regress and are replaced with adipocytes; mast cells are increased and apoptosis is notable. The basement membranes vessels within the IH thicken and hyalinize. At the end of involution, fibrofatty stroma is prominent and apoptotic debris in the remaining "ghost" capillaries remains.[60,64] When necessary to confirm the diagnosis on histopathologic specimen, GLUT1 immunostaining is positive in the endothelial cells lining IH capillaries at all stages of IH growth, distinguishing IH from other vascular tumors and all vascular malformations.[65,66,76,82] IHs are also CD31+ and CD34+, as noted above.

IMAGING

Presence of a segmental IH of the head, neck, and/or scalp warrants evaluation for possible PHACE to include MRI and MRA of the head/neck/chest,[40] formal ophthalmologic evaluation, and echocardiogram. Likewise, workup of possible LUMBAR syndrome includes MRI/MRA of the lumbosacral spine, pelvis, and/or lower extremity. Initial evaluation for potential hepatic IHs in the setting of multifocal IHs requires hepatic/abdominal ultrasound with Doppler flow and spectral analysis (baseline ultrasound ± serial imaging.)

DIFFERENTIAL DIAGNOSIS

Table 118-6 discusses the differential diagnosis of IH.[103]

CLINICAL COURSE AND PROGNOSIS

The prognosis of most IHs is excellent, with spontaneous involution and little to no sequelae, but a significant minority of IH result in permanent disfigurement or medical sequelae. Following involution, approximately half of all treated patients will attain normal skin, while the other half can have residual atrophy, scarring, telangiectasias, or fibrofatty soft-tissue remnant. One study of 97 untreated patients demonstrated residual skin changes in more than 68 (70%) of patients.[22] Specific IH characteristics (as previously outlined by each subclassification) are associated with increased rates of complications.[17,104] The most important factor to affect prognosis in complicated IH is timing of specialist referral for management, including initiation of therapy and workup as necessary. Certain characteristics are associated with an increased risk of complications and need for treatment (see Table 118-3).[17,104] Consideration of early treatment should be given to IH with these characteristics, depending on the specific clinical setting.

MANAGEMENT

INTERVENTIONS

The decision to initiate treatment is based on many factors, including size and location, psychosocial implications, and risks and benefits of the proposed therapy (Fig. 118-14). For the majority of small IH, active nonintervention with close observation and followup is the most appropriate approach. Especially during the first few months of life and during the rapid proliferative phase, visits should be more frequent, as often as every 1 to 2 weeks in the youngest infants.[105] Visits with parents and caregivers should emphasize education about the natural course and prognosis of IH, addressing both parental anxiety[106] and psychosocial impact on the patient and family.[107-109] Photographs of the likely outcome for a similar lesion are often helpful. Many parents experience anxiety and may find themselves subject to comments from complete strangers about their child's hemangioma.[106] Most parents of young children do not think their child is deeply affected by these reactions, but facial IHs, in particular, can cause psychological suffering once the child reaches school-age.[107,108] Potential treatment options should be discussed well ahead of entrance to elementary school.

For those IHs warranting intervention, options include pharmacologic, laser, and surgical interventions.

MEDICATIONS

Beta Blockers: With widely established efficacy in IH treatment and a more favorable risk profile compared with prior systemic treatment options, propranolol is the only medication approved by the United States Food and Drug Administration (FDA) for the treatment of complicated IH. Propranolol is the clear first-line systemic pharmacologic therapy for most moderate to severe IHs at risk for significant morbidity.[110-112] Unlike corticosteroids, which stabilize IH growth but do not cause involution, propranolol causes regression in the vast majority of cases. Rebound growth after cessation of therapy can occur, but usually responds well to retreatment.[111,112] Key criteria to warrant consideration of beta-blocker treatment initiation

TABLE 118-6
Differential Diagnosis of Infantile Hemangioma

DISORDER	AGE OF ONSET	CLINICAL EXAMINATION	DISTINGUISHING FEATURES
Vascular Anomalies			
Kaposiform hemangioendothelioma (KHE)	Congenital to infancy or later	Firm, reddish-brown to violaceous, plaque or nodule	May be associated with Kasabach-Merritt phenomenon: increased D-dimer, low fibrinogen, severe thrombocytopenia
Tufted angioma	As for KHE	Similar to KHE ± associated hair	Similar to KHE, although considered less severe on spectrum
Rapidly involuting congenital hemangiomas	Congenital; full size at birth	Often symmetric blue nodule with coarse telangiectasia; rim of pallor	High flow
Noninvoluting congenital hemangiomas	Congenital; full size at birth or minimal postnatal growth	Similar to rapidly involuting congenital hemangioma (RICH)	High flow
Pyogenic granuloma	Infancy or childhood (more commonly)	Friable vascular papule with brisk intermittent bleeding	Rarely may be multiple and congenital
Multifocal lymphangioendotheliomatosis	Congenital	Varied appearance of papules, plaques, or nodules	Thrombocytopenia (waxing and waning), potentially severe GI bleeding
Blue rubber bleb nevus syndrome	Congenital, infancy or later	Small, compressible, blue to purple papulonodules	May be confused for multifocal infantile hemangioma (IH); associated with GI bleeding ± larger venous malformation, often in thigh or pelvis
Capillary malformation (port-wine stain)	Congenital	Confluent pink to dusky pink; possibly reticulated	Reticulated may appear similar to minimal growth IH
Venous malformation	Congenital; may not be noted until later	Blue-purple compressible; growth gradual and progressive	Low flow; may be confused with deep IH
Glomuvenous malformation	Congenital in segmental plaque presentation; multifocal present later	Segmental thin plaque pink to violaceous; papules/nodules firm ± tender	Autosomal dominant; limited to skin and soft tissue
Lymphatic malformation	Macrocystic cervicofacial present at birth; microcystic often noted later	Deep, skin-colored nodule ± vascular appearing pink to purple blebs	Low flow; may be confused with deep IH
Verrucous hemangioma	Congenital	Plaque, papule, or nodule with keratotic change over time	A subtype of lymphatic malformation
Cutis marmorata telangiectatica congenita	Congenital	Reticulated, marbled pink to dusky purple ± ulceration ± limb undergrowth	May be confused with minimal growth IH or reticulated port-wine stain
Nonvascular Lesions			
Myofibroma	Congenital to infancy	Small to large plaques and nodules	May ulcerate and mimick ulcerated IH
Spitz nevus	Infancy rarely; childhood commonly	Pink to red-brown papule	Typically solitary although may have agminated presentation
Juvenile xanthogranuloma	Congenital to infancy	Pink to red-brown papules or nodules	Become yellow with time; central ulceration possible in larger lesions
Dermoid cyst	Congenital	Skin colored to slightly bluish; firm; typically mobile nodule face and scalp at sites of suture closure/embryonic fusion	May be confused with deep IH
Encephalocele	Congenital	Bluish nodule, may transilluminate in midline frontal or occipital scalp	Consider with midline deep blue nodule
Rhabdomyosarcoma	Congenital to first year in most	Firm tumoral nodule with overlying telangiectasias; embryonal rhabdomyosarcoma is multifocal and congenital	May be confused with deep or mixed IH

(Continued)

TABLE 118-6
Differential Diagnosis of Infantile Hemangioma (Continued)

DISORDER	AGE OF ONSET	CLINICAL EXAMINATION	DISTINGUISHING FEATURES
Infantile fibrosarcoma	Congenital to first 2 years	Red to blue; firm and fixed to underlying tissue	May be confused with mixed IH, but more often KHE/tufted angioma or RICH/ noninvoluting congenital hemangioma
Langerhans cell histiocytosis	Congenital, infancy or later	Seborrheic distribution in scalp and diaper area especially; red to brown papules, nodules, petechial papules	Congenital presentation has a more-favorable prognosis than presentation in infancy or later; presentation with larger nodule, often on scalp, possible
Neuroblastoma	Congenital to early infancy	Blue to violaceous nodule	Increased urine homovanillic ± vanillylmandelic acid
Congenital leukemia cutis	Congenital to neonatal	Pink, blue, or violaceous firm plaques and nodules	May be confused with multifocal IH

Adapted from Püttgen KB. Diagnosis and management of infantile hemangiomas. *Pediatr Clin North Am.* 2014;61(2):383-402.

for IH include facial deformity, active or impending functional impairment, early prevention of anticipated permanent sequelae, and mitigation of the need for surgery.[113] Positive results also have been reported in other settings, including fully proliferated IHs and airway, liver, and orbital hemangiomas.[111,114-116] Despite early controversy, most patients with PHACE can safely tolerate propranolol, although it is recommended to use the lowest effective dose, consider a slower dose titration, and to give the medication in 3 divided doses, rather than the standard twice-daily dosing, to avoid significant alterations in peak blood levels.[40] Molecular mechanisms of propranolol in effectively treating IH include lesional capillary vasoconstriction (visible IH color change within first 48 hours of use), angiogenesis inhibition (arresting growth), and induction of apoptosis (bringing about IH regression).[117] Common side effects of propranolol include sleep disturbance, acrocyanosis, and asymptomatic transient decrease in blood pressure or heart rate. Rarely observed potential important adverse effects include hypoglycemia, symptomatic hypotension or bradycardia, wheezing, bronchospasm, and diarrhea. Propranolol's efficacy has been documented in a large, international, placebo-controlled, randomized trial and numerous smaller prospective and retrospective case series and case reports, including a small multicenter randomized trial comparing oral corticosteroids to propranolol and several comparative retrospective studies.[111,112,118] A multicenter, randomized, double-blind, Phase II-III trial comprised of 456 patients investigating the efficacy of oral propranolol in IH involved 5 treatment

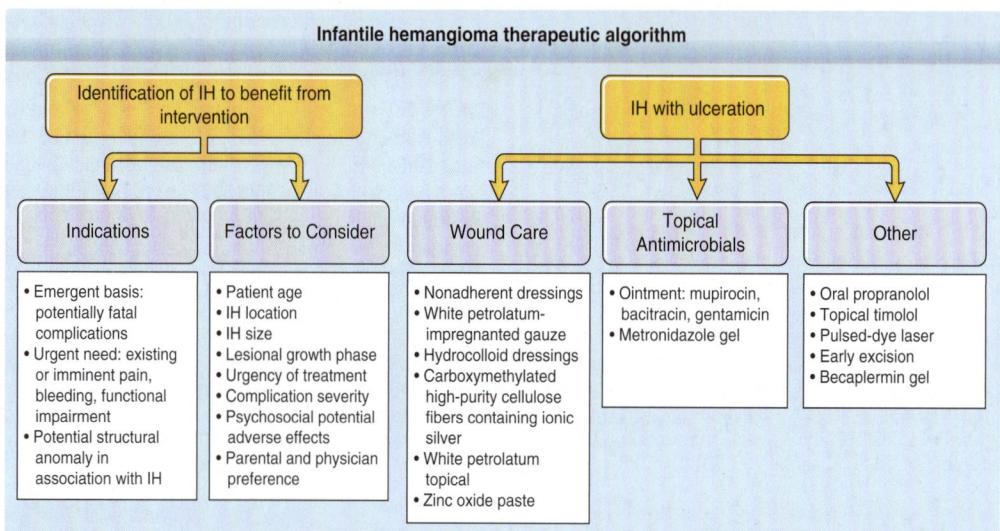

Figure 118-14 Infantile hemangioma (IH) therapeutic algorithm. (Data from Darrow DH, Greene AK, Mancini AJ, et al. Diagnosis and management of infantile hemangioma. *Pediatrics.* 2015;136(4):e1060-e1104.)

arms (1 mg/kg/day for 3 months vs 6 months' duration, 3 mg/kg/day for 3 months vs 6 months' duration, and placebo). Dosing of 3 mg/kg/day for 6 months was found to have the highest benefit-to-risk ratio with 88% of patients on this daily dose demonstrating improvement by the fifth week of treatment. In this study, side effects included a decrease in heart rate (by a mean of 7 beats per minute with observed change of heart rate within 1 hour of dose with minimal change thereafter) and a decrease in mean systolic blood pressure (by 3 mm Hg). Serious adverse events ($n = 33$) included: bronchospasm, diarrhea (3 mg/kg/day > 1 mg/kg/day), and sleep disorder (73 propranolol vs 7 placebo).[119] A study cohort involving 39 European centers with nearly 1100 total patients, reported the use patterns of propranolol in IH, with 91.4% of patients demonstrating clinically significant improvement regardless of daily maintenance dose (less than 2 mg/kg/day, 2 mg/kg/day, greater than 2 mg/kg/day) with risk of adverse events to be based upon daily maintenance dosing.[120] With report of overall IH response rate of 98% and 0.9% resistance rate in IH, propranolol has reduced the need for surgery in nasal-site-specific IH.[121-123] Given propranolol's lipophilic nature with ease of crossing the blood–brain barrier, sleep disorder can manifest in several ways (fatigue, restlessness, nightmares, insomnia), affecting 11.4% of patients, with a reported 3.7% of patients experiencing nightmares. Theoretical risks of propranolol extrapolated from adult volunteer studies in the psychology literature include impaired short-term and long-term memory, sleep quality, mood, and psychomotor function. Fatigue associated with pediatric hypertension improves over time.[124,125]

Propranolol initiation can take place in the inpatient or outpatient setting (Fig. 118-15). In determining a patient's candidacy for propranolol, family history must be obtained to ensure absence of congenital heart disease, arrhythmia, and maternal connective tissue disease. Uniformly accepted standard monitoring procedures for patients on propranolol for IH have not yet been established. However, current proposed factors favoring inpatient initiation include young age (the study on which FDA approval of propranolol was granted included infants as young as 5 weeks of age with outpatient initiation), comorbid medical conditions (eg, respiratory or cardiovascular), inadequate social support, or any preexisting concerns for blood glucose. In the outpatient setting, hypoglycemia can be prevented with anticipatory guidance, dosing propranolol with feedings, frequent feedings, and either decreasing or holding the dose in the setting of decreased oral intake.[126,127] Outpatient initiation is suitable for most otherwise healthy children beyond the neonatal period. Current published guidelines and many, but not all, physicians advocate 2-hour monitoring in the ambulatory setting for heart rate and blood pressure with first dose administered. Dosing is typically started at 1 mg/kg/day in 2 divided doses and increased by 0.5 mg/kg/day increments every 3 to 7 days to a target dose between 2 and 3 mg/kg/day. Most practitioners use 2 mg/kg/day. Slower dose escalation or lower target dose may be warranted in the setting of PHACE syndrome, ulceration or other comorbid conditions. Atenolol, a β_1-selective antagonist, and nadolol, a nonselective β-antagonist, have been used in infants for IH treatment but neither is available in liquid formulation in the United States. The main benefit of atenolol is the lack of bronchial reactivity; nadolol's advantage is its inability to cross the blood–brain barrier, thereby decreasing concerns for any potential neurocognitive side effects compared with propranolol. Only few international publications reporting the use of atenolol and nadolol in IH are available as of this writing; further studies are warranted. Likewise, further studies investigating any neurocognitive effects of propranolol are ongoing. Early evidence does not demonstrate adverse effects on neurodevelopment with use of propranolol, but comprehensive neurocognitive testing in this population has not been reported.[128]

In light of the proved efficacy of systemic beta blockers, the efficacy of topical beta blockers in IH treatment were evaluated in an effort to even further decrease side effects. Topical timolol is a nonselective beta blocker available in an ophthalmic preparation approved for the treatment of pediatric glaucoma.[129] Eight to 10 times more potent than propranolol, topical timolol was first reported as an effective option for IH treatment in 2010,[130] and continues to gain increasing acceptance and application. The systemic bioavailability of 1 intraocular drop of timolol 0.5% solution ranged from 39% to 98%, with a mean value of 78.3±24.5%.[131] Additional research on topical timolol demonstrated differences in systemic absorption based upon vehicle preparation. Compared to aqueous timolol solution (0.25% to 0.5%) with average plasma concentration of 0.46 to 1.72 ng/mL, timolol gel-forming solution (0.1% to 0.5%) was developed to decrease systemic absorption with average plasma concentration rage of 0.13 to 0.71 ng/mL. Little is known about the absorption across IH-affected skin. Several contributing factors can impact systemic absorption independent of vehicle, including application site (mucosa, ulceration, and areas under occlusion increase absorption), application size, and size of patients (neonates and especially premature infants with greater absorption as a result of increased surface-area-to-volume ratios). Timolol is metabolized by cytochrome P450 CYP2D6; poor metabolizers are likely at greater risk for adverse effects. Changes in heart rate correlate with plasma levels in timolol, thus less-significant heart rate changes were found in hydrogel formulation. Topical timolol in either vehicle had negligible pulmonary or blood pressure effects.[132] The largest powered multicenter retrospective topical (0.05%) timolol (85% gel foaming solution) study (n = 731) with a 9.5-month mean duration of treatment (83.5% of participants dosed at 1 drop twice daily) reported 3.4% adverse events (half of these noted to be local irritation at application site with 3 cases of bronchospasm and 4 cases of ulceration development). The retrospective endeavor concluded timolol was most effective in

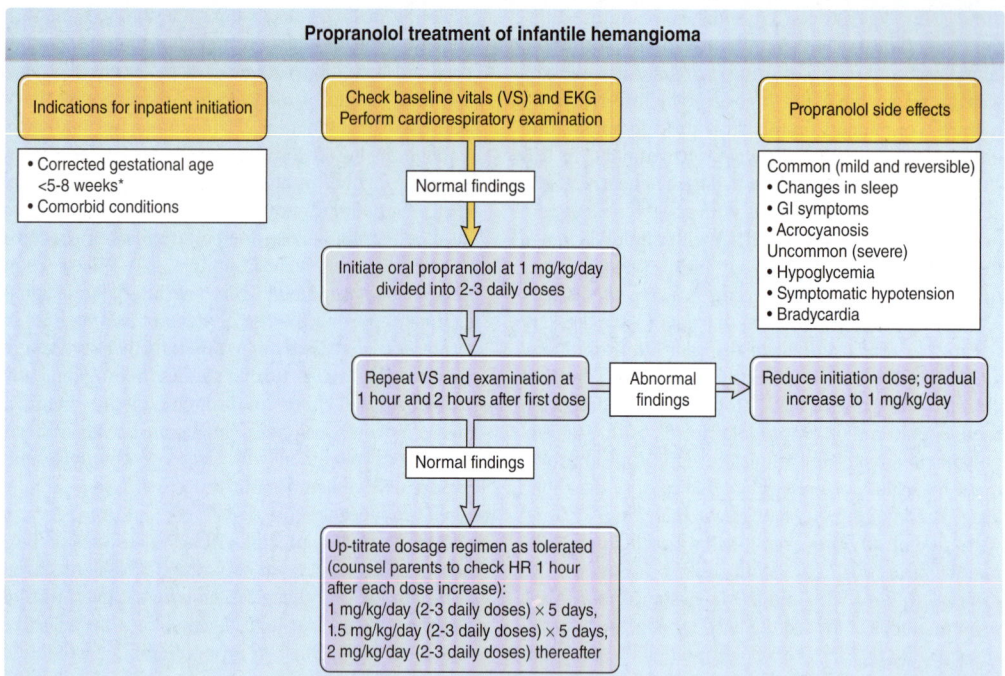

Figure 118-15 Propranolol treatment of infantile hemangioma. *Drolet BA, Frommelt PC, Chamlin SL, et al. Initiation and use of propranolol for infantile hemangioma: report of a consensus conference. *Pediatrics*. 2013;131(1):128-140; Léauté-Labrèze C, Hoeger P, Mazereeuw-Hautier J, et al. A randomized controlled trial of oral propranolol in infantile hemangioma. *N Engl J Med*. 2015;372:735-746. (Data from Drolet BA, Frommelt PC, Chamlin SL, et al. Initiation and use of propranolol for infantile hemangioma: report of a consensus conference. *Pediatrics*. 2013;131(1):128-140.)

thinner IH and with longer duration of treatment. Color improved more than overall volume, extent, and size with topical timolol use.[133]

Corticosteroids: Systemic corticosteroids, previously considered first-line treatment of deforming, endangering, or life-threatening IH, are now used rarely given the efficacy, safety and improved tolerability of beta blockers.[134] Corticosteroids are most effective during the proliferative phase, causing slowing or cessation of growth in up to 90% of cases, with actual shrinkage in approximately one-third. Although the mechanism of action is not well understood, prior studies suggest the upregulation of mitochondrial cytochrome b, clusterin/ApoJ (possible apoptotic markers), and/or interleukin-6 as markers of corticosteroid-induced cessation of IH growth.[135-137] When used, prednisone or prednisolone is given at a dose of 2 to 3 mg/kg/day, typically for 4-8 weeks followed by a tapering of varying length, depending on the age of the child and indication for treatment. A metaanalysis showed an 84% response rate with an average dose of 2.9 mg/kg for a mean of 1.8 months before tapering. Although 3 mg/kg/day is more effective (94% response) than 2 mg/kg/day (75% response), greater adverse events occur at higher doses.[138]

Short-term complications of systemic corticosteroids include cushingoid faces (71%), personality changes (irritability/fussiness) (29%), gastric irritation (21%), fungal infection (oral or perineal, 6%), and diminished gain of height (35%) and weight (42%) during treatment. More than 90% of children with diminished gain of height return to their pretreatment growth curve by 24 months of age.[139,140] Other complications include hypertension, steroid-induced myopathy, immunosuppression, and transient adrenal insufficiency.[140,141] Blood pressure should be closely monitored by the treating physician.[142] Children taking more than 2 mg/kg/day of prednisone for longer than 14 days are considered to have a deficit in cell-mediated immunity. Live viral vaccinations should be deferred in infants receiving high-dose corticosteroids. Rare cases of *Pneumocystis carinii* pneumonia has been reported in this setting, leading some physicians to use trimethoprim-sulfamethoxazole prophylaxis during treatment.[143,144]

Intralesional corticosteroids can be an effective treatment for select, relatively small, localized IHs located in high-risk sites such as the lip, nasal tip, cheek, and ear. Current use of this modality for IH is maintained by a minority of physicians with expertise in its use. Injections for periocular hemangiomas are not recommended. If used, it should only be performed by experienced ophthalmologists, given reports of retinal artery embolization and blindness.[145,146] The largest published case series of intralesional steroids found that the majority showed a greater than 50% reduction in volume, with the best results occurring in relatively superficial IHs. Adverse events occurred in 6.4% of patients and included cushingoid appearance, cutaneous atrophy and anaphylactic shock.[147]

Only few case series have reported on the efficacy of Class 1 topical corticosteroids, namely for small, superficial hemangiomas.[110,148,149]

Medications of Historical Importance (Interferon-α, Vincristine, Imiquimod):

Interferon-α, vincristine, and imiquimod were previously regarded as second-line or third-line therapeutic options for IH. Their use is no longer advocated in light of the established efficacy and more favorable side-effect profile of beta blockers. Interferon-α carries the notable risk of potential neurotoxicity, specifically spastic diplegia. A metaanalysis of 441 patients showed 11 developed irreversible spastic diplegia and 16 developed motor disturbances that were reversible on discontinuation of the drug.[150] All affected patients were younger than 1 year of age at initiation of therapy. Vincristine's use in the treatment of vascular tumors is now reserved for complicated kaposiform hemangioendothelioma (KHE) and tufted angioma (TA); its use for this indication may be eclipsed by sirolimus in future years, but further study is warranted.[151-153]

PROCEDURES

Laser Therapy: PDL, originally designed to treat port-wine stains (ie, capillary malformations), has been used to treat IH with varying results.[154] PDL was used more frequently in the treatment of IH before the discovery of propranolol. Its usefulness is primarily limited by its minimal depth of penetration (less than 2 mm).[35] Several reports have shown improvement in treating associated ulceration[155,156]; its use in diminishing residual telangiectasias and erythema after involution is well accepted. Its use in the treatment of proliferating IHs is controversial.[157] In a prospective, randomized, controlled study, 22 infants treated with either observation or PDL with epidermal cooling demonstrated significant color improvement in the PDL group, but unchanged total surface area and echo depth by 12 months' followup.[158] Another prospective study randomized children to PDL without epidermal cooling (n = 60) and observation (n = 61) groups with comparable results of (near-) complete resolution between groups at age 1 year, with a trend toward increased hypopigmentation and textural change in the PDL group. Outcomes between groups were similar at the 5-year followup of 117 children.[155] Other studies have shown good results with either the 585-nm PDL or 595-nm PDL, with varying fluencies (total energy per unit area), but several have emphasized that treatments work best for more superficial hemangiomas and are unable to halt growth of deeper components.[159-162] Severe ulceration and scarring, particularly in treating segmental hemangiomas during the proliferative phase, have been reported.[163] Although comparative studies are lacking, the same IHs that are reasonable candidates in the proliferative phase for PDL are similarly good candidates for topical timolol treatment. Expert opinion and rudimentary cost analysis support the use of medical therapy with timolol in superficial IHs over the use of PDL in most cases.[133] A conservative approach is to reserve PDL primarily for treating ulceration and for hastening resolution of erythema in IH after the proliferative phase is completed.[164]

Surgical Therapy: Surgical excision may be indicated at any time during the life cycle of an IH, but elective excision in infancy is typically neither necessary nor advocated. Proposed indications for surgical intervention of IH during infancy include an anatomically favorable site amenable to resection, a contraindication or failure of pharmacotherapy, or a high risk of ultimately necessary resection with similar scar regardless of timing of surgery. Timing of surgical intervention depends upon evolution of tumor (whether it continues to regress), anatomic location, degree of deformity, and the age of the child. Certain anatomic locations, such as the nasal tip and lip, often require surgery.[165-170] Even earlier excision may be indicated in cases where clinical characteristics, such as pedunculated IH, severe, recalcitrant ulceration, or extremely thick dermal involvement dictate that scarring will inevitably occur. In most instances, it is best to wait until regression is well under way and a more accurate assessment can be made regarding whether scarring and textural changes have occurred. Surgery during and after involution can allow reconstruction of affected adjacent structures, resection of residual excess skin or fibrofatty tissue, or scar revision. Decisions regarding this can often be made between 3 and 5 years of age, even if involution is not complete.[171] Four years serves an appropriate threshold age as most IHs have completed involution and children develop self-awareness, long-term memory, and self-esteem.[35] A standard elliptical excision is often performed; however, circular excision followed by a purse-string closure may leave a smaller scar.[172] A second stage following purse-string closure may or may not be necessary.

SCREENING

Screening for PHACE is recommended in the setting of segmental IH on the head, in infants without classic segmental IH or with a small IH who have a major anomaly seen in PHACE (eg, coarctation of the aorta or supraumbilical raphe) and in infants with 2 major criteria for PHACE as outlined in consensus guidelines from 2016.[40]

OTHER VASCULAR TUMORS

AT-A-GLANCE

- Vascular tumors in the current International Society for the Study of Vascular Anomalies classification are subdivided into (a) benign, (b) locally aggressive or borderline, or (c) malignant.
- Congenital hemangiomas are fully formed at birth. Rapidly involuting, noninvoluting, and partially involuting congenital hemangiomas are recognized subtypes.
- Tufted angiomas represent subtle pink or dusky-red patches and may evolve into plaques or nodules and have a characteristic histology.
- Kaposiform hemangioendothelioma is a locally aggressive vascular tumor, morphologically similar to but etiologically distinct from Kaposi sarcoma and can be associated with Kasabach-Merritt phenomenon. Kaposiform hemangioendothelioma exists on a spectrum with tufted angioma.
- Multifocal lymphangiomatosis with thrombocytopenia consists of cutaneous vascular papules and plaques associated with intermittent thrombocytopenia, often with GI bleeding.
- Spindle-cell hemangioma usually occurs in the extremities most often associated with Maffucci syndrome.
- Pyogenic granuloma, a rapidly growing papule or nodule with a collarette of scale or eroded surface, is very common. Treatment is excision or electrocautery.
- Congenital eccrine angiomatous hamartoma is a rare ill-defined plaque associated with increased lanugo hair and sweating.

Many other benign vascular neoplasms occur in both children and adults.[173] This section highlights selected important vascular tumors according to the 2014 ISSVA classification, which classifies vascular tumors as (a) benign, (b) locally aggressive or borderline, or (c) malignant. More comprehensive reviews of this subject can be found elsewhere.[2,173,174]

CONGENITAL HEMANGIOMAS

Hemangiomas that are fully formed tumors at the time of birth and do not proliferate in postnatal life are referred to as *congenital hemangiomas*. They are benign and much less common than IH. There are now 3 major subtypes recognized on the basis of their natural history: the rapidly involuting (RICH), noninvoluting (NICH), and partially involuting congenital hemangioma.[175,176] Recognition of the partially involuting congenital hemangioma subtype in recent years highlights that these tumors exist on a spectrum. Definitive categorization is often challenging in the immediate newborn period and can often only be made with confidence in retrospect after observation of the clinical behavior. Congenital hemangiomas have similar anatomic sites of predilection, including the head, neck, and extremities, but can occur elsewhere. They are equally common in boys and girls.[176]

RICH often appears as a raised, violaceous tumor with large, radiating veins or with overlying telangiectasia and a halo of pallor (Fig. 118-16). Central ulceration may be present. Most RICHs involute spontaneously by or before 14 months of age and usually leave residual atrophic anetodermic scar tissue.[177] A presumed RICH noted on prenatal ultrasound that involuted before birth has been reported, leaving a scar tissue at the site of the lesion.[178]

RICHs can be associated with mild to moderate thrombocytopenia and a coagulopathy characterized by elevated fibrin degradation products and low fibrinogen in the neonatal period. In contrast to Kasabach-Merritt phenomenon (discussed in section "Kaposiform Hemangioendothelioma"), the laboratory findings of cutaneous RICHs are often self-limited and uncomplicated with only supportive care generally required.[179]

Hepatic RICHs, which are the focal subtype of hepatic hemangioma, are rare, but at greater risk of complications, with associations with marked thrombocytopenia as well as severe progressive hepatic dysfunction and resultant heart failure.

NICHs are less common than RICHs and also present at birth. They are usually flatter than RICHs, presenting as a well-circumscribed round to oval, somewhat indurated or raised soft-tissue mass with overlying telangiectasias and a rim of pallor (Fig. 118-17).

Partially involuting congenital hemangioma was introduced into the vascular anomalies lexicon in 2014 and fewer than 20 cases have been reported. Partial involution occurs over the first 12 to 30 months of life (mean: 18 months) before stabilization occurs (Fig. 118-18).[176]

Somatic activating missense mutations in the genes *GNAQ* and *GNA11* are reported to cause RICH and NICH. The mutational change, alteration of glutamine at amino acid 209 (Gln209), was the same in both tumors, so does not explain their varied clinical courses.[180] The same Gln209 missense mutation is common in uveal melanoma, and postzygotic mosaic mutations in *GNAQ* and *GNA11* codons 183 or 209 have been reported in association with phakomatosis pigmentovascularis and extensive dermal melanocytosis.[181]

Indications for treatment of congenital hemangiomas are similar to those for IH, including ulceration, impairment of vital function and congestive heart failure. Excision, with or without preoperative embolization, should definitely be considered for ulceration,

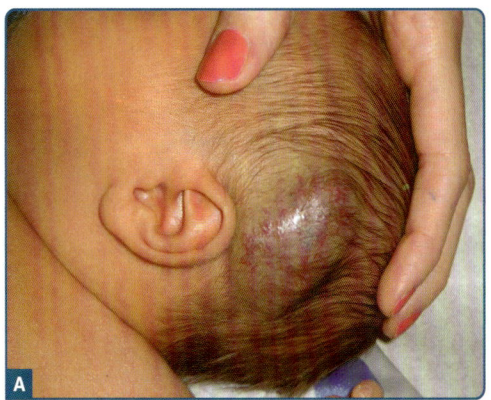

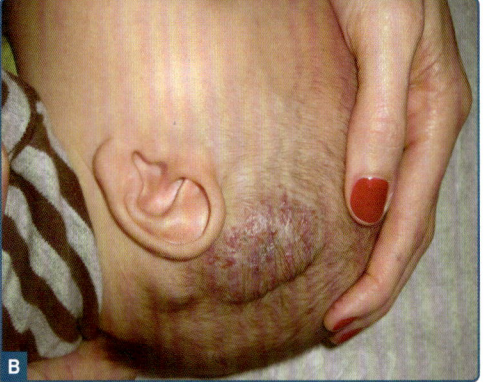

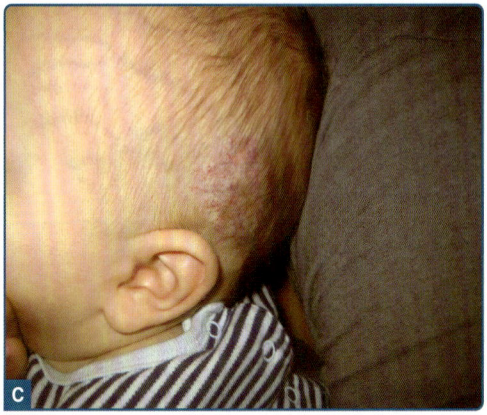

Figure 118-16 Rapidly involuting congenital hemangioma on left scalp. **A,** Infant with overlying coarse telangiectasias at 1 month of age. **B,** Early regression at age 5 months. **C,** Continued rapid involution at age 8 months.

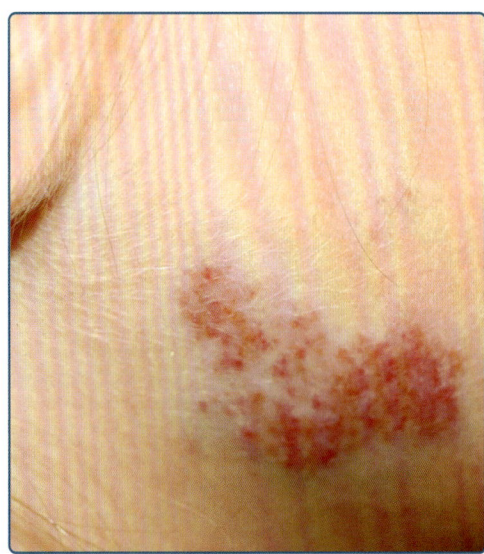

Figure 118-17 Noninvoluting congenital hemangioma on right mandible. Note the overlying telangiectasias and rim of pallor.

which can lead to severe hemorrhage, and for postinvolutional skin changes if disfiguring.[175] NICH do not go away, but are often asymptomatic; decisions regarding their removal must weigh risks and benefits of the proposed treatment.

The distinguishing pathologic features of congenital hemangiomas are lobules of capillaries with plump endothelial cells and pericytes set within densely fibrotic stroma containing hemosiderin deposits, focal lobular thrombosis, and sclerosis.[182] They are GLUT1 negative, unlike IH.[183] On ultrasound, congenital hemangiomas heterogenous with scattered calcifications possible and are generally confined to the subcutaneous fat. They are high-flow vascular tumors, often showing arteriovenous microfistulas, more common seen in NICH, on Doppler interrogation.[184]

TUFTED ANGIOMA

EPIDEMIOLOGY

TA is a rare benign vascular tumor that also has been called *angioblastoma of Nakagawa*. Although adult cases have been reported, most cases occur early in childhood and may have a protracted course. Approximately 25% of TA are congenital and 50% appear in the first year of life. There is no sex predilection.

CLINICAL FEATURES

TA display various clinical patterns and are most commonly seen on the neck, trunk, and extremities. They may present as a subtle stain-like area that later thickens, as a large, plaque-like, infiltrated, red or dusky blue-purple lesion, or as an exophytic, firm, rubbery, violaceous, cutaneous nodule (Fig. 118-19). Tenderness and overlying hyperhidrosis may occur.[185] TA are usually solitary, but multifocal cases have been reported.[186]

COMPLICATIONS

Kasabach-Merritt phenomenon (KMP) may develop in TA but this is more common with KHE (see section "Kaposiform Hemangioendothelioma").

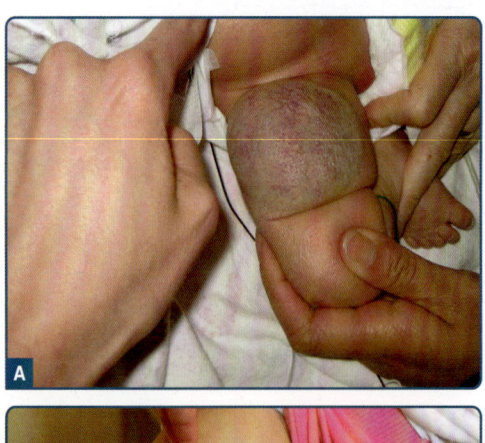
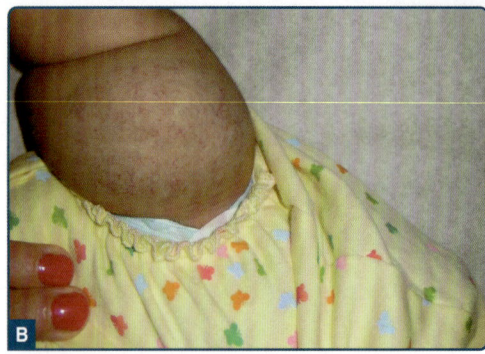
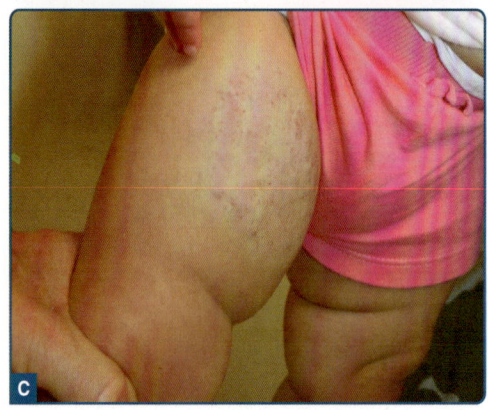
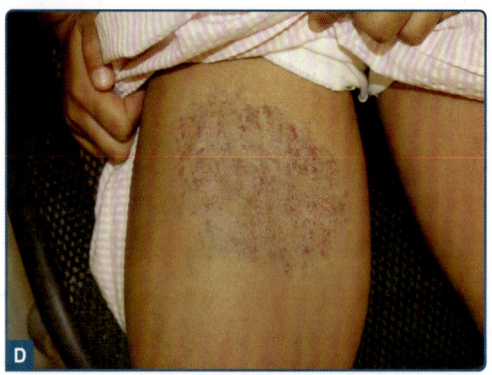

Figure 118-18 Partially involuting congenital hemangioma on the right thigh. Note the overlying telangiectasias and rim of pallor. **A,** First day of life. **B,** Early decrease in size at 6 weeks of age. **C,** At 13 months of age it is broad but flat. **D,** At 5 years of age no further involution has occurred and there is renewed prominence of superficial vessels.

ETIOLOGY AND PATHOGENESIS

Its etiology and pathogenesis are uncertain, although based on its immunostaining pattern, a lymphatic origin is likely. Unlike IH, there are no known gender or gestational age correlates.

DIAGNOSIS

Histologically, both acquired and congenital TAs demonstrate vascular tufts of tightly packed capillaries, randomly dispersed throughout the dermis in a typical "cannonball distribution" with crescentic spaces surrounding the vascular tufts, and lymphatic-like spaces within the tumor stroma.[187,188] Unlike IH, TA does not stain with GLUT1.[82] It is CD31+; D2-40, LYVE1, and PROX1 lymphatic markers, are only partially positive in surrounding vessels, helping distinguish TA from KHE.[189]

CLINICAL COURSE AND PROGNOSIS

TAs may persist unchanged or regress completely within a few years.[190] TAs that are present at birth or in the first year of life have a greater tendency to spontaneously regress than do those that appear later in life.[191] Of those TAs that regress, 95% are reported to do so within 2 years.[187]

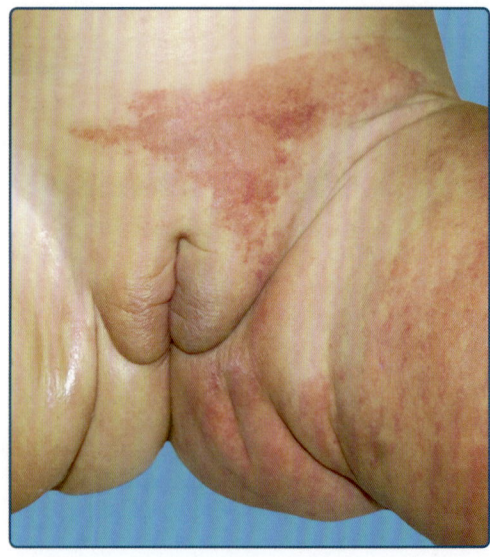

Figure 118-19 Tufted angioma (confirmed by biopsy) of the left leg, buttocks, lower abdomen in an 18-month-old child. Laboratory evaluation revealed elevated D-dimers.

MANAGEMENT

No widely accepted treatment guidelines exist for management of TA. Recommended therapies for TA, with and without KMP, include excision, compression, laser, topical or systemic corticosteroids, propranolol and chemotherapy. See "Kaposiform Hemangioendothelioma" below for a fuller discussion of therapy.

KAPOSIFORM HEMANGIOENDOTHELIOMA

EPIDEMIOLOGY

KHE is a rare vascular tumor with an estimated prevalence of 0.91 cases per 100,000 children.[192] It may be present at birth or develop in early childhood. A series of more than 100 patients reported that 60% present as neonates and 93% in infancy. Rare adult cases have been reported. Three-quarters involve the skin. It is usually reported in association with KMP, which occurs in more than 70% of cases.[192]

CLINICAL FEATURES

KHE is an infiltrative, aggressive tumor classified as locally aggressive or borderline in the ISSVA classification. It may present as a brown-red stain at birth which begins to thicken and become purpuric, or as plaques or deep-seated nodules and bulky tumors. Most cases involve the skin and musculature. KHE can occur on the extremities, especially overlying joints, trunk, head, neck. Deeper viscera including cervicothoracic, abdominal, and the retroperitoneum can be affected. Notably, KHE does not occur in the liver. Locoregional lymph node involvement may occur and likely represents multifocal disease. Distant metastases do not occur. Mediastinal or retroperitoneal disease may present with hemothorax and ascites.[141] Spontaneous involution is rare. Most reported cases have had associated KMP, but KHE can occur in the absence of a coagulopathy.[192-195] KHE may resolve with atrophic or stain-like areas, infiltrated plaques and papules, or nodules. Residual fibrosis is not rare and can result in considerable morbidity.[196]

COMPLICATIONS

Kasabach-Merritt Phenomenon: KMP refers to the presence of platelet trapping within a vascular tumor resulting in profoundly severe thrombocytopenia (typically less than 30000/μL) and associated microangiopathic hemolytic anemia and consumption of clotting factors resulting in low fibrinogen, elevated D-dimers, and varying degrees of decreased coagulation factors (Fig. 118-20). It was long considered to be a complication of "hemangioma," but it is now recognized to be a complication almost exclusively of TA and KHE, not IH.[14,197] KMP must be differentiated

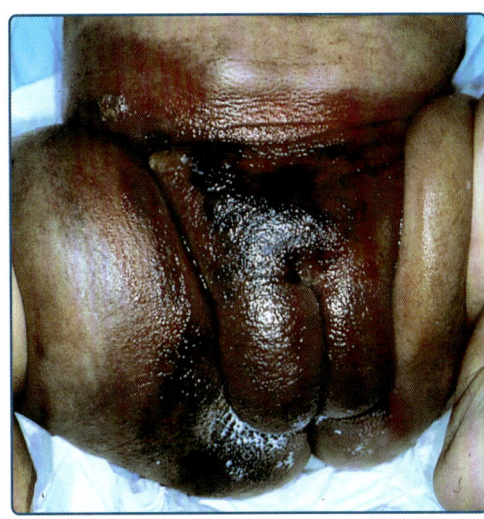

Figure 118-20 Kasabach-Merritt phenomenon secondary to kaposiform hemangioendothelioma (KHE). An indurated, purpuric tumor appeared at age 3 months and is seen here at age 8 months. KHE confirmed by MRI and biopsy. Platelet count <5000/mm³.

from the coagulopathy that can arise in association with venous and mixed venous-lymphatic malformations (sometimes erroneously called KMP) as a result of chronic clotting and consumption of clotting factors, but not primarily by platelet trapping,[198] which is more likely to be either localized or disseminated intravascular coagulopathy.

ETIOLOGY AND PATHOGENESIS

The pathogenesis of KHE and KMP is unknown. KHE and TA are thought to exist on a spectrum of severity.[192]

RISK FACTORS

Involvement across more than 1 anatomic region increases the risk of developing KMP, while KHE presenting at a later age, with superficial tumors or tumors involving only bone, appears to have a lower risk of KMP.[192]

DIAGNOSIS

Diagnosis is based upon clinical and histologic features and laboratory abnormalities, including severe thrombocytopenia, consumption of fibrinogen, elevated D-dimers, decreased coagulation factors to varying degrees, and microangiopathic hemolytic anemia.

The histology of KHE is characterized by infiltrative nodules and sheets of spindled endothelial cells with minimal atypia and infrequent mitoses lining slit-like or crescentic vessels containing hemosiderin. Edema, microthrombi, fibrosis and atypical appearing lymphatic vessels can be seen. The tumor is GLUT1 negative. Similar to TA, increased lymphatic spaces reactive with the lymphatic markers including vascular endothelial growth factor receptor-3 and D2-40 suggest a lymphatic origin, similar to that of Kaposi sarcoma.[199,200]

CLINICAL COURSE AND PROGNOSIS

The prognosis and management of KHE varies with extent and location of the tumor, in addition to the presence of KMP. Although the KHE and TA may persist, the coagulopathy of KMP usually abates by 1 year of age or sooner with treatment.

MANAGEMENT

No one treatment is uniformly effective nor are there widely accepted treatment guidelines for KHE management. KHE complicated by KMP requires more aggressive intervention than KHE in the absence of coagulopathy. Complete surgical excision, when possible, is curative, but is often not feasible given the infiltrative nature of the tumor. Systemic corticosteroids are considered first-line treatment and are often used in combination with vincristine, especially in the setting of KMP. Ticlopidine and aspirin are reported as adjunctive therapies with variable benefit. Arterial embolization may be adjunctive before planned surgery to decrease bleeding risk and may result in temporary improvement of coagulopathy and lesion size but is rarely effective as monotherapy.[201] Reports on the use of oral sirolimus, a mammalian target of rapamycin inhibitor, in this condition are promising[202,203] showing rapid reversal of the coagulopathy; results from prospective clinical trials are pending. Older literature reports use of radiation therapy, cyclophosphamide, interferon-α, actinomycin-D, and methotrexate, but these are all considered third-line therapies to be used only in the setting of failure of other agents. Platelet transfusions should be avoided unless active bleeding occurs or before surgical procedures.[204-208] The use of other blood transfusion products has proved ineffective in correction of the coagulopathy.

SPINDLE-CELL HEMANGIOMA

Spindle-cell hemangioma, also called *spindle-cell hemangioendothelioma*, is a rare benign vascular tumor most often seen with Maffucci syndrome. While the genetic mutation associated with this syndrome has been identified (IDH1 and IDH2, which produce isocitrate dehydrogenases to convert isocitrate to 2-ketoglutarate) and detected in associated cutaneous findings of this condition, the relationship of the mutations and the manifestations of this disorder remains unclear. It can occur at any age and site but the extremities are the most commonly affected. The histology is of a nodular, dense, spindle cell proliferation associated with dilated dysplastic veins. Lesions can be locally aggressive and may recur even after excision.[209]

PYOGENIC GRANULOMA (LOBULAR CAPILLARY HEMANGIOMA)

Pyogenic granuloma (PG) is also known by its correct histopathologic description *lobular capillary hemangioma*. It is one of the most common vascular tumors of infants and children and can also occur in adults, particularly in pregnant women. PG usually presents as a solitary, red, rapidly growing papule or nodule, often with a subtle collarette of scale (Fig. 118-21). Typical locations include the cheek or forehead, but virtually any body site including the mucous membranes may be affected. The rapid growth of PGs usually presents at a later age than that associated with the proliferative phase of IH, but in very young infants can cause confusion.[210] They often develop an eroded surface, with subsequent bleeding which can be profuse, resulting in the moniker *the Band-Aid disease*. Solitary and agminated PG-like lesions have rarely been reported in association with vascular anomalies including arteriovenous malformations and congenital hemangioma.[211,212]

PG does not typically involute spontaneously. Even after definitive treatment, recurrence and even satellite lesions surrounding the original PG have been reported.[213,214] Simple curettage with electrocautery is usually curative. Other options include excision, laser surgery (carbon dioxide or pulsed-dye laser), and cryotherapy. Imiquimod and timolol have been suggested as effective topical treatment options.[215,216]

MULTIFOCAL LYMPHANGIOENDO-THELIOMATOSIS WITH THROMBOCYTOPENIA

MLT—also known as *cutaneovisceral angiomatosis with thrombocytopenia*—is a rare condition that was initially

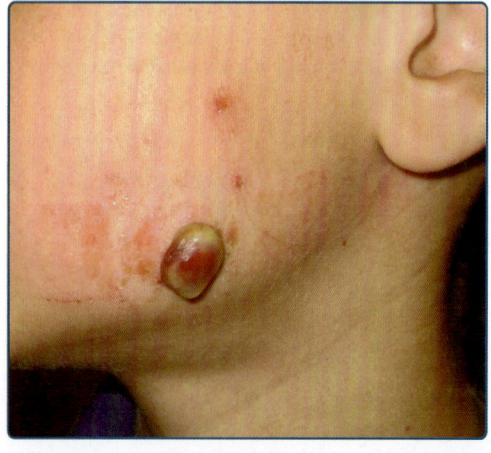

Figure 118-21 Large pyogenic granuloma on left cheek.

described in 2004, and is characterized by multiple cutaneous vascular papules and plaques that are usually congenital with development of new lesions over time.[217] It is currently unclear whether it is a vascular tumor or a vascular malformation. Some patients have prominent exophytic cutaneous vascular tumors, whereas others have subtle blueberry muffin-like papules.[218] Most affected infants have intermittent thrombocytopenia and lesions in the GI tract, leading to GI bleeding. Other reported sites of involvement include bones, synovium, lungs, liver, spleen, and brain. It is now understood that many patients previously diagnosed with "diffuse neonatal hemangiomatosis" actually had MLT.[219] Skin biopsy specimens demonstrate thin-walled vessels, some hobnailed endothelial cells, and intraluminal papillary projections similar to Dabska tumor.[217,220] Endothelial cells stain positively for CD31, CD34, and LYVE1, variably for D2-40, and are negative for GLUT1.[186,218] Prognosis varies based on extent of disease and bleeding complications. A metaanalysis reported a 65% mortality rate.[219] Effective therapy has been challenging but early experience with sirolimus has been positive, with some authors recommending it as first-line treatment.[221,222] A variety of other systemic medications have been reported with variable benefit including corticosteroids, vincristine, thalidomide, interferon-α2a, propranolol, and bevacizumab.[218,223]

PAPILLARY INTRALYMPHATIC ANGIOENDOTHELIOMA

Papillary intralymphatic angioendothelioma (PILA), also known as Dabska tumor, is a dermal nodule or a diffuse violaceous swelling on the head, neck, or extremities that is seen almost exclusively in the pediatric-age group. PILA/Dabska tumor is a low-grade vascular tumor whose rarity has made study of its long-term prognosis and optimal treatment difficult. Histopathology shows enlarged vessels with thick walls surrounded with lymphoid aggregates and smaller lymphatic vessels. The presence of "hobnail" endothelial cells inside tumoral vessels is the sine qua non of PILA/Dabska tumor.[185]

RETIFORM HEMANGIOENDOTHELIOMA

Retiform hemangioendothelioma occurs primarily in adults and has significant overlap with PILA/Dabska tumor. There is no noted sex predilection and development occurs in the second to fourth decades of life (mean age: 36 years). Histopathology demonstrates presence of retiform pattern of long, arborizing blood vessels lined by monomorphic hobnail endothelial cells. Most cases noted to have prominent lymphocytic infiltrate with focal presence of hyaline collagenous core comprising papillae, similar to PILA/Dabska tumor. Recurrence is frequent but metastatic rate is low.[224]

COMPOSITE HEMANGIOENDOTHELIOMA

Composite hemangioendothelioma is a low- to intermediate-grade malignant vascular tumor comprised of a variable combination of benign and malignant vascular components. Identification of at least 2 hemangioendothelioma variants is necessary to render this diagnosis. Epithelioid and retiform variants are most commonly observed, although foci of spindle-cell hemangioma and/or angiosarcoma-like foci can also be present.[225]

TARGETOID HEMOSIDEROTIC HEMANGIOMA

Targetoid hemosiderotic hemangioma is a benign lesion presenting as a violaceous papule, often surrounded by a pale rim and peripheral ecchymotic halo, which fades with time. Lesions usually present on the trunk or extremities and histologically consist of dilated vascular channels within intraluminal papillary projections dissecting into collagen bundles in the subcutis. Extravasated erythrocytes and hemosiderin are present, hence the designation.

CONGENITAL ECCRINE ANGIOMATOUS HAMARTOMA (SUDORIPAROUS ANGIOMA)

Congenital eccrine angiomatous hamartoma is a rare condition characterized by ill-defined plaques with increased lanugo hair and sweating at the site of the lesion. They are usually located on the extremities or abdomen. Diagnosis is established on the basis of characteristic histologic findings: closely packed eccrine sweat glands associated with dilated capillaries, a few dysplastic venous channels, and a dense collagenous matrix.[226]

REFERENCES

1. Wassef M, Blei F, Adams D, et al. Vascular anomalies classification: recommendations from the International Society for the Study of Vascular Anomalies. *Pediatrics*. 2015;136(1):e203-e214.
2. ISSVA classification of vascular anomalies. 2014. International Society for the Study of Vascular Anomalies. Available at http://www.issva.org/classification. Accessed December 2016.
3. Enjolras O, Mulliken JB. Vascular tumors and vascular malformations (new issues). *Adv Dermatol*. 1997;13:375-423.
4. Hand JL, Frieden IJ. Vascular birthmarks of infancy: resolving nosologic confusion. *Am J Med Genet A*. 2002;108(4):257-264.
5. Frieden IJ, Haggstrom AN, Drolet BA, et al. Infantile hemangiomas: current knowledge, future directions. Proceedings of a research workshop on infantile hemangiomas, April 7-9, 2005, Bethesda, Maryland, USA. *Pediatr Dermatol*. 2005;22(5):383-406.
6. Jacobs AH, Walton RG. The incidence of birthmarks in the neonate. *Pediatrics*. 1976;58(2):218-222.
7. Alper JC, Holmes LB. The incidence and significance of birthmarks in a cohort of 4,641 newborns. *Pediatr Dermatol*. 1983;1(1):58-68.
8. Hemangioma Investigator Group, Haggstrom AN, Drolet BA, et al. Prospective study of infantile hemangiomas: demographic, prenatal, and perinatal characteristics. *J Pediatr*. 2007;150(3):291-294.
9. Finn MC, Glowacki J, Mulliken JB. Congenital vascular lesions: clinical application of a new classification. *J Pediatr Surg*. 1983;18(6):894-900.
10. Kilcline C, Frieden IJ. Infantile hemangiomas: how common are they? A systematic review of the medical literature. *Pediatr Dermatol*. 2008;25(2):168-173.
11. Drolet BA, Swanson EA, Frieden IJ; Hemangioma Investigator Group. Infantile hemangiomas: an emerging health issue linked to an increased rate of low birth weight infants. *J Pediatr*. 2008;153(5):712-715, 715e1.
12. Munden A, Butschek R, Tom WL, et al. Prospective study of infantile haemangiomas: incidence, clinical characteristics and association with placental anomalies. *Br J Dermatol*. 2014;170(4):907-913.
13. Garzon MC, Drolet BA, Baselga E, et al. Comparison of infantile hemangiomas in preterm and term infants: a prospective study. *Arch Dermatol*. 2008;144(9):1231-1232.
14. Enjolras O, Gelbert F. Superficial hemangiomas: associations and management. *Pediatr Dermatol*. 1997;14(3):173-179.
15. Bruckner AL, Frieden IJ. Hemangiomas of infancy. *J Am Acad Dermatol*. 2003;48(4):477-493; quiz 494-496.
16. Tollefson MM, Frieden IJ. Early growth of infantile hemangiomas: what parents' photographs tell us. *Pediatrics*. 2012;130(2):e314-e320.
17. Chang LC, Haggstrom AN, Drolet BA, et al. Growth characteristics of infantile hemangiomas: implications for management. *Pediatrics*. 2008;122(2):360-367.
18. Ritter MR, Reinisch J, Friedlander SF, et al. Myeloid cells in infantile hemangioma. *Am J Pathol*. 2006;168(2):621-628.
19. Brandling-Bennett HA, Metry DW, Baselga E, et al. Infantile hemangiomas with unusually prolonged growth phase: a case series. *Arch Dermatol*. 2008;144(12):1632-1637.
20. Couto RA, Maclellan RA, Zurakowski D, et al. Infantile hemangioma: clinical assessment of the involuting phase and implications for management. *Plast Reconstr Surg*, 2012;130(3):619-624.
21. Baselga E, Roe E, Coulie J, et al. Risk factors for degree and type of sequelae after involution of untreated hemangiomas of infancy. *JAMA Dermatol*. 2016;152(11):1239-1243.
22. Bauland CG, Luning TH, Smit JM, et al. Untreated hemangiomas: growth pattern and residual lesions. *Plast Reconstr Surg*. 2011;127(4):1643-1648.
23. Waner M, North PE, Scherer KA, et al. The nonrandom distribution of facial hemangiomas. *Arch Dermatol*. 2003;139(7):869-875.
24. Chiller KG, Passaro D, Frieden IJ. Hemangiomas of infancy: clinical characteristics, morphologic subtypes, and their relationship to race, ethnicity, and sex. *Arch Dermatol*. 2002;138(12):1567-1576.
25. Suh KY, Frieden IJ. Infantile hemangiomas with minimal or arrested growth: a retrospective case series. *Arch Dermatol*. 2010;146(9):971-976.
26. Corella F, Garcia-Navarro X, Ribe A, et al. Abortive or minimal-growth hemangiomas: Immunohistochemical evidence that they represent true infantile hemangiomas. *J Am Acad Dermatol*. 2008;58(4):685-690.
27. Haggstrom AN, Drolet BA, Baselga E, et al. Prospective study of infantile hemangiomas: clinical characteristics predicting complications and treatment. *Pediatrics*. 2006;118(3):882-887.
28. Happle R. Superimposed segmental hemangioma of infancy. *Dermatology*. 2010;220(2):180-182.
29. Haggstrom AN, Lammer EJ, Schneider RA, et al. Patterns of infantile hemangiomas: new clues to hemangioma pathogenesis and embryonic facial development. *Pediatrics*. 2006;117(3):698-703.
30. Metry D, Heyer G, Hess C, et al. Consensus statement on diagnostic criteria for PHACE syndrome. *Pediatrics*. 2009;124(5):1447-1456.
31. PHACE Association.
32. Frieden IJ, Reese V, Cohen D. PHACE syndrome. The association of posterior fossa brain malformations, hemangiomas, arterial anomalies, coarctation of the aorta and cardiac defects, and eye abnormalities. *Arch Dermatol*. 1996;132(3):307-311.
33. Metry DW, Garzon MC, Drolet BA, et al. PHACE syndrome: current knowledge, future directions. *Pediatr Dermatol*. 2009;26(4):381-398.
34. Haggstrom AN, Garzon MC, Baselga E, et al. Risk for PHACE syndrome in infants with large facial hemangiomas. *Pediatrics*. 2010;126(2):e418-e426.
35. Darrow DH, Greene AK, Mancini AJ, et al. Diagnosis and management of infantile hemangioma. *Pediatrics*. 2015;136(4):e1060-e1104.
36. Brandon K, Burrows P, Hess C, et al. Arteriovenous malformation: a rare manifestation of PHACE syndrome. *Pediatr Dermatol*. 2011;28(2):180-184.
37. Chan YC, Eichenfield LF, Malchiodi J, et al. Small facial haemangioma and supraumbilical raphe—a forme fruste of PHACES syndrome? *Br J Dermatol*. 2005;153(5):1053-1057.
38. Nabatian AS, Milgraum SS, Hess CP, et al. PHACE without face? Infantile hemangiomas of the upper body region with minimal or absent facial hemangiomas and associated structural malformations. *Pediatr Dermatol*. 2011;28(3):235-241.
39. Antonov NK, Spence-Shishido A, Marathe KS, et al. Orbital hemangioma with intracranial vascular anomalies and hemangiomas: a new presentation of PHACE syndrome? *Pediatr Dermatol*. 2015;32(6):e267-e272.

40. Garzon MC, Epstein LG, Heyer GL, et al. PHACE syndrome: consensus-derived diagnosis and care recommendations. *J Pediatr*. 2016;178:24-33,e2.
41. Metry DW, Dowd CF, Barkovich AJ, et al. The many faces of PHACE syndrome. *J Pediatr*. 2001;139(1):117-123.
42. Bayer ML, Frommelt PC, Blei F, et al. Congenital cardiac, aortic arch, and vascular bed anomalies in PHACE syndrome (from the International PHACE Syndrome Registry). *Am J Cardiol*. 2013;112(12):1948-1952.
43. Hess CP, Fullerton HJ, Metry DW, et al. Cervical and intracranial arterial anomalies in 70 patients with PHACE syndrome. *AJNR Am J Neuroradiol*. 2010;31(10):1980-1986.
44. Siegel DH, Tefft KA, Kelly T, et al. Stroke in children with posterior fossa brain malformations, hemangiomas, arterial anomalies, coarctation of the aorta and cardiac defects, and eye abnormalities (PHACE) syndrome: a systematic review of the literature. *Stroke*. 2012;43(6):1672-1674.
45. Goddard DS, Liang MG, Chamlin SL, et al. Hypopituitarism in PHACES association. *Pediatr Dermatol*. 2006;23(5):476-480.
46. Iacobas I, Burrows PE, Frieden IJ, et al. LUMBAR: association between cutaneous infantile hemangiomas of the lower body and regional congenital anomalies. *J Pediatr*. 2010;157(5):795-801.e1-7.
47. Girard C, Bigorre M, Guillot B, et al. PELVIS syndrome. *Arch Dermatol*. 2006;142(7):884-888.
48. Stockman A, Boralevi F, Taieb A, et al. SACRAL syndrome: spinal dysraphism, anogenital, cutaneous, renal and urologic anomalies, associated with an angioma of lumbosacral localization. *Dermatology*. 2007;214(1):40-45.
49. Drolet BA, Chamlin SL, Garzon MC, et al. Prospective study of spinal anomalies in children with infantile hemangiomas of the lumbosacral skin. *J Pediatr*. 2010;157(5):789-794.
50. Tubbs RS, Wellons JC 3rd, Iskandar BJ, et al. Isolated flat capillary midline lumbosacral hemangiomas as indicators of occult spinal dysraphism. *J Neurosurg* 2004;100(2, suppl pediatrics):86-89.
51. Ceisler EJ, Santos L, Blei F. Periocular hemangiomas: what every physician should know. *Pediatr Dermatol*. 2004;21(1):1-9.
52. Schwartz SR, Blei F, Ceisler E, et al. Risk factors for amblyopia in children with capillary hemangiomas of the eyelids and orbit. *J AAPOS*. 2006;10(3):262-268.
53. Haik BG, Jakobiec FA, Ellsworth RM, et al. Capillary hemangioma of the lids and orbit: an analysis of the clinical features and therapeutic results in 101 cases. *Ophthalmology*. 1979;86(5):760-792.
54. Robb RM. Refractive errors associated with hemangiomas of the eyelids and orbit in infancy. *Am J Ophthalmol*. 1977;83(1):52-58.
55. Stigmar G, Crawford JS, Ward CM, et al. Ophthalmic sequelae of infantile hemangiomas of the eyelids and orbit. *Am J Ophthalmol*. 1978;85(6):806-813.
56. Boscolo E, Bischoff J. Vasculogenesis in infantile hemangioma. *Angiogenesis*. 2009;12(2):197-207.
57. Orlow SJ, Isakoff MS, Blei F. Increased risk of symptomatic hemangiomas of the airway in association with cutaneous hemangiomas in a "beard" distribution. *J Pediatr*. 1997;131(4):643-646.
58. Rahbar R, Nicollas R, Roger G, et al. The biology and management of subglottic hemangioma: past, present, future. *Laryngoscope*. 2004;114(11):1880-1891.
59. Reinisch JF, Kim RY, Harshbarger RJ, et al. Surgical management of parotid hemangioma. *Plast Reconstr Surg*. 2004;113(7):1940-1948.
60. Greene AK, Rogers GF, Mulliken JB. Management of parotid hemangioma in 100 children. *Plast Reconstr Surg*. 2004;113(1):53-60.
61. Hughes JA, Hill V, Patel K, et al. Cutaneous haemangioma: prevalence and sonographic characteristics of associated hepatic haemangioma. *Clin Radiol*. 2004;59(3):273-280.
62. Horii KA, Drolet BA, Frieden IJ, et al. Prospective study of the frequency of hepatic hemangiomas in infants with multiple cutaneous infantile hemangiomas. *Pediatr Dermatol*. 2011;28(3):245-253.
63. Metry DW, Hawrot A, Altman C, et al. Association of solitary, segmental hemangiomas of the skin with visceral hemangiomatosis. *Arch Dermatol*. 2004;140(5):591-596.
64. Christison-Lagay ER, Burrows PE, Alomari A, et al. Hepatic hemangiomas: subtype classification and development of a clinical practice algorithm and registry. *J Pediatr Surg*. 2007;42(1):62-67; discussion 67-68.
65. Kassarjian A, Dubois J, Burrows PE. Angiographic classification of hepatic hemangiomas in infants. *Radiology*. 2002;222(3):693-698.
66. Kassarjian A, Zurakowski D, Dubois J, et al. Infantile hepatic hemangiomas: clinical and imaging findings and their correlation with therapy. *AJR Am J Roentgenol*. 2004;182(3):785-795.
67. Ho J, Kendrick V, Dewey D, et al. New insight into the pathophysiology of severe hypothyroidism in an infant with multiple hepatic hemangiomas. *J Pediatr Endocrinol Metab*. 2005;18(5):511-514.
68. Chamlin SL, Haggstrom AN, Drolet BA, et al. Multicenter prospective study of ulcerated hemangiomas. *J Pediatr*. 2007;151(6):684-689, 689.e1.
69. Kim HJ, Colombo M, Frieden IJ. Ulcerated hemangiomas: clinical characteristics and response to therapy. *J Am Acad Dermatol*. 2001;44(6):962-972.
70. Maguiness SM, Hoffman WY, McCalmont TH, et al. Early white discoloration of infantile hemangioma: a sign of impending ulceration. *Arch Dermatol*. 2010;146(11):1235-1239.
71. Brook I. Microbiology of infected hemangiomas in children. *Pediatr Dermatol*. 2004;21(2):113-116.
72. Yan AC. Pain management for ulcerated hemangiomas. *Pediatr Dermatol*. 2008;25(6):586-589.
73. Oranje AP, de Waard-van der Spek FB, Devillers AC, et al. Treatment and pain relief of ulcerative hemangiomas with a polyurethane film. *Dermatology*. 2000;200(1):31-34.
74. Metz BJ, Rubenstein MC, Levy ML, et al. Response of ulcerated perineal hemangiomas of infancy to becaplermin gel, a recombinant human platelet-derived growth factor. *Arch Dermatol*. 2004;140(7):867-870.
75. Sugarman JL, Mauro TM, Frieden IJ. Treatment of an ulcerated hemangioma with recombinant platelet-derived growth factor. *Arch Dermatol*. 2002;138(3):314-316.
76. Boye E, Jinnin M, Olsen BR. Infantile hemangioma: challenges, new insights, and therapeutic promise. *J Craniofac Surg*. 2009;20(suppl 1):678-684.
77. Bischoff J. Progenitor cells in infantile hemangioma. *J Craniofac Surg*. 2009;20(suppl 1):695-697.
78. Chang EI, Chang EI, Thangarajah H, et al. Hypoxia, hormones, and endothelial progenitor cells in hemangioma. *Lymphat Res Biol*. 2007;5(4):237-243.

79. Barnes CM, Christison-Lagay EA, Folkman J. The placenta theory and the origin of infantile hemangioma. *Lymphat Res Biol*. 2007;5(4):245-255.
80. Pittman KM, Losken HW, Kleinman ME, et al. No evidence for maternal-fetal microchimerism in infantile hemangioma: a molecular genetic investigation. *J Invest Dermatol*. 2006;126(11):2533-2538.
81. Dadras SS, North PE, Bertoncini J, et al. Infantile hemangiomas are arrested in an early developmental vascular differentiation state. *Mod Pathol*. 2004;17(9):1068-1079.
82. North PE, Waner M, Mizeracki A, et al. GLUT1: a newly discovered immunohistochemical marker for juvenile hemangiomas. *Hum Pathol*. 2000;31(1):11-22.
83. North PE, Waner M, Mizeracki A, et al. A unique microvascular phenotype shared by juvenile hemangiomas and human placenta. *Arch Dermatol*. 2001;137(5):559-570.
84. Barnes CM, Huang S, Kaipainen A, et al. Evidence by molecular profiling for a placental origin of infantile hemangioma. *Proc Natl Acad Sci U S A*. 2005;102(52):19097-19102.
85. Bree AF, Siegfried E, Sotelo-Avila C, et al. Infantile hemangiomas: speculation on placental trophoblastic origin. *Arch Dermatol*. 2001;137(5):573-577.
86. Kleinman ME, Greives MR, Churgin SS, et al. Hypoxia-induced mediators of stem/progenitor cell trafficking are increased in children with hemangioma. *Arterioscler Thromb Vasc Biol*. 2007;27(12):2664-2670.
87. Yu Y, Flint AF, Mulliken JB, et al. Endothelial progenitor cells in infantile hemangioma. *Blood*. 2004;103(4):1373-1375.
88. Khan ZA, Boscolo E, Picard A, et al. Multipotential stem cells recapitulate human infantile hemangioma in immunodeficient mice. *J Clin Invest*. 2008;118(7):2592-2599.
89. Chen TS, Eichenfield LF, Friedlander SF. Infantile hemangiomas: an update on pathogenesis and therapy. *Pediatrics*. 2013;131(1):99-108.
90. Mihm MC Jr, Nelson JS. Hypothesis: the metastatic niche theory can elucidate infantile hemangioma development. *J Cutan Pathol*. 2010;37(suppl 1):83-87.
91. Ahrens WA, Ridenour RV 3rd, Caron BL, et al. GLUT-1 expression in mesenchymal tumors: an immunohistochemical study of 247 soft tissue and bone neoplasms. *Hum Pathol*. 2008;39(10):1519-1526.
92. Ritter MR, Dorrell MI, Edmonds J, et al. Insulin-like growth factor 2 and potential regulators of hemangioma growth and involution identified by large-scale expression analysis. *Proc Natl Acad Sci U S A*. 2002;99(11):7455-7460.
93. Boye E, Yu Y, Paranya G, et al. Clonality and altered behavior of endothelial cells from hemangiomas. *J Clin Invest*. 2001;107(6):745-752.
94. Walter JW, North PE, Waner M, et al. Somatic mutation of vascular endothelial growth factor receptors in juvenile hemangioma. *Genes Chromosomes Cancer*. 2002;33(3):295-303.
95. Nguyen VA, Furhapter C, Romani N, et al. Infantile hemangioma is a proliferation of beta 4-negative endothelial cells adjacent to HLA-DR-positive cells with dendritic cell morphology. *Hum Pathol*. 2004;35(6):739-744.
96. Razon MJ, Kraling BM, Mulliken JB, et al. Increased apoptosis coincides with onset of involution in infantile hemangioma. *Microcirculation*. 1998;5(2-3):189-195.
97. Drolet BA, Frieden IJ. Characteristics of infantile hemangiomas as clues to pathogenesis: does hypoxia connect the dots? *Arch Dermatol*. 2010;146(11):1295-1299.
98. Bielenberg DR, Bucana CD, Sanchez R, et al. Progressive growth of infantile cutaneous hemangiomas is directly correlated with hyperplasia and angiogenesis of adjacent epidermis and inversely correlated with expression of the endogenous angiogenesis inhibitor, IFN-beta. *Int J Oncol*. 1999;14(3):401-408.
99. Tekes A, Koshy J, Kalayci TO, et al. S.E. Mitchell Vascular Anomalies Flow Chart (SEMVAFC): a visual pathway combining clinical and imaging findings for classification of soft-tissue vascular anomalies. *Clin Radiol*. 2014;69(5):443-457.
100. Konrad D, Ellis G, Perlman K. Spontaneous regression of severe acquired infantile hypothyroidism associated with multiple liver hemangiomas. *Pediatrics*. 2003;112(6, pt 1):1424-1426.
101. Ayling RM, Davenport M, Hadzic N, et al. Hepatic hemangioendothelioma associated with production of humoral thyrotropin-like factor. *J Pediatr*. 2001;138(6):932-935.
102. Huang SA, Tu HM, Harney JW, et al. Severe hypothyroidism caused by type 3 iodothyronine deiodinase in infantile hemangiomas. *N Engl J Med*. 2000;343(3):185-189.
103. Puttgen KB. Diagnosis and management of infantile hemangiomas. *Pediatr Clin North Am*. 2014;61(2):383-402.
104. Metry DW. Potential complications of segmental hemangiomas of infancy. *Semin Cutan Med Surg*. 2004;23(2):107-115.
105. Hoeger PH, Harper JI, Baselga E, et al. Treatment of infantile haemangiomas: recommendations of a European expert group. *Eur J Pediatr*. 2015;174(7):855-865.
106. Williams EF 3rd, Hochman M, Rodgers BJ, et al. A psychological profile of children with hemangiomas and their families. *Arch Facial Plast Surg*. 2003;5(3):229-234.
107. Gleason T. Summer's strawberry. *J Am Acad Dermatol*. 2004;51(1)(suppl):S53-S54.
108. Greig AV, Harris DL. A study of perceptions of facial hemangiomas in professionals involved in child abuse surveillance. *Pediatr Dermatol*. 2003;20(1):1-4.
109. Tanner JL, Dechert MP, Frieden IJ. Growing up with a facial hemangioma: parent and child coping and adaptation. *Pediatrics*. 1998;101(3, pt 1):446-452.
110. Leaute-Labreze C, Dumas de la Roque E, Hubiche T, et al. Propranolol for severe hemangiomas of infancy. *N Engl J Med*. 2008;358(24):2649-2651.
111. Hogeling M, Adams S, Wargon O. A randomized controlled trial of propranolol for infantile hemangiomas. *Pediatrics*. 2011;128(2):e259-e266.
112. Price CJ, Lattouf C, Baum B, et al. Propranolol vs corticosteroids for infantile hemangiomas: a multicenter retrospective analysis. *Arch Dermatol*. 2011;147(12):1371-1376.
113. Hermans DJ, Bauland CG, Zweegers J, et al. Propranolol in a case series of 174 patients with complicated infantile haemangioma: indications, safety and future directions. *Br J Dermatol*. 2013;168(4):837-843.
114. Marsciani A, Pericoli R, Alaggio R, et al. Massive response of severe infantile hepatic hemangioma to propranolol. *Pediatr Blood Cancer*. 2010;54(1):176.
115. Fay A, Nguyen J, Jakobiec FA, et al. Propranolol for isolated orbital infantile hemangioma. *Arch Ophthalmol*. 2010;128(2):256-258.

116. Buckmiller L, Dyamenahalli U, Richter GT. Propranolol for airway hemangiomas: case report of novel treatment. *Laryngoscope*. 2009;119(10):2051-2054.
117. Storch CH, Hoeger PH. Propranolol for infantile haemangiomas: insights into the molecular mechanisms of action. *Br J Dermatol*. 2010;163(2):269-274.
118. Bauman NM, McCarter RJ, Guzzetta PC, et al. Propranolol vs prednisolone for symptomatic proliferating infantile hemangiomas: a randomized clinical trial. *JAMA Otolaryngol Head Neck Surg*. 2014;140(4):323-330.
119. Leaute-Labreze C, Hoeger P, Mazereeuw-Hautier J, et al. A randomized, controlled trial of oral propranolol in infantile hemangioma. *N Engl J Med*. 2015;372(8):735-746.
120. Wedgeworth E, Glover M, Irvine AD, et al. Propranolol in the treatment of infantile haemangiomas: lessons from the European Propranolol In the Treatment of Complicated Haemangiomas (PITCH) Taskforce survey. *Br J Dermatol*. 2016;174(3):594-601.
121. Marqueling AL, Oza V, Frieden IJ, et al. Propranolol and infantile hemangiomas four years later: a systematic review. *Pediatr Dermatol*. 2013;30(2):182-191.
122. Causse S, Aubert H, Saint-Jean M, et al. Propranolol-resistant infantile haemangiomas. *Br J Dermatol*. 2013;169(1):125-129.
123. Perkins JA, Chen BS, Saltzman B, et al. Propranolol therapy for reducing the number of nasal infantile hemangioma invasive procedures. *JAMA Otolaryngol Head Neck Surg*. 2014;140(3):220-227.
124. Langley A, Pope E. Propranolol and central nervous system function: potential implications for paediatric patients with infantile haemangiomas. *Br J Dermatol*. 2015;172(1):13-23.
125. Drolet BA, Frommelt PC, Chamlin SL, et al. Initiation and use of propranolol for infantile hemangioma: report of a consensus conference. *Pediatrics*. 2013;131(1):128-140.
126. Lawley LP, Siegfried E, Todd JL. Propranolol treatment for hemangioma of infancy: risks and recommendations. *Pediatr Dermatol*. 2009;26(5):610-614.
127. Frieden IJ, Drolet BA. Propranolol for infantile hemangiomas: promise, peril, pathogenesis. *Pediatr Dermatol*. 2009;26(5):642-644.
128. Moyakine AV, Kerstjens JM, Spillekom-van Koulil S, et al. Propranolol treatment of infantile hemangioma (IH) is not associated with developmental risk or growth impairment at age 4 years. *J Am Acad Dermatol*. 2016;75(1):59-63 e1.
129. Singh BN, Williams FM, Whitlock RM, et al. Plasma timolol levels and systolic time intervals. *Clin Pharmacol Ther*. 1980;28(2):159-166.
130. Guo S, Ni N. Topical treatment for capillary hemangioma of the eyelid using beta-blocker solution. *Arch Ophthalmol*. 2010;128(2):255-256.
131. Korte JM, Kaila T, Saari KM. Systemic bioavailability and cardiopulmonary effects of 0.5% timolol eyedrops. *Graefes Arch Clin Exp Ophthalmol*. 2002;240(6):430-435.
132. Nieminen T, Lehtimaki T, Maenpaa J, et al. Ophthalmic timolol: plasma concentration and systemic cardiopulmonary effects. *Scand J Clin Lab Invest*. 2007;67(2):237-245.
133. Puttgen K, Lucky A, Adams D, et al. Topical timolol maleate treatment of infantile hemangiomas. *Pediatrics*. 2016;138(3).
134. Al-Sebeih K, Manoukian J. Systemic steroids for the management of obstructive subglottic hemangioma. *J Otolaryngol*. 2000;29(6):361-366.
135. Hasan Q, Tan ST, Gush J, et al. Steroid therapy of a proliferating hemangioma: histochemical and molecular changes. *Pediatrics*. 2000;105(1, pt 1):117-120.
136. Hasan Q, Tan ST, Gush J, et al. Altered mitochondrial cytochrome b gene expression during the regression of hemangioma. *Plast Reconstr Surg*. 2001;108(6):1471-1476; discussion 1477-1478.
137. Hasan Q, Tan ST, Xu B, et al. Effects of five commonly used glucocorticoids on haemangioma in vitro. *Clin Exp Pharmacol Physiol*. 2003;30(3):140-144.
138. Bennett ML, Fleischer AB Jr, Chamlin SL, et al. Oral corticosteroid use is effective for cutaneous hemangiomas: an evidence-based evaluation. *Arch Dermatol*. 2001;137(9):1208-1213.
139. Boon LM, MacDonald DM, Mulliken JB. Complications of systemic corticosteroid therapy for problematic hemangioma. *Plast Reconstr Surg*. 1999;104(6):1616-1623.
140. Lomenick JP, Backeljauw PF, Lucky AW. Growth, bone mineral accretion, and adrenal function in glucocorticoid-treated infants with hemangiomas—a retrospective study. *Pediatr Dermatol*. 2006;23(2):169-174.
141. Lomenick JP, Reifschneider KL, Lucky AW, et al. Prevalence of adrenal insufficiency following systemic glucocorticoid therapy in infants with hemangiomas. *Arch Dermatol*. 2009;145(3):262-266.
142. George ME, Sharma V, Jacobson J, et al. Adverse effects of systemic glucocorticosteroid therapy in infants with hemangiomas. *Arch Dermatol*. 2004;140(8):963-969.
143. Aviles R, Boyce TG, Thompson DM. Pneumocystis carinii pneumonia in a 3-month-old infant receiving high-dose corticosteroid therapy for airway hemangiomas. *Mayo Clin Proc*. 2004;79(2):243-245.
144. Maronn ML, Corden T, Drolet BA. Pneumocystis carinii pneumonia in infant treated with oral steroids for hemangioma. *Arch Dermatol*. 2007;143(9):1224-1225.
145. O'Keefe M, Lanigan B, Byrne SA. Capillary haemangioma of the eyelids and orbit: a clinical review of the safety and efficacy of intralesional steroid. *Acta Ophthalmol Scand*. 2003;81(3):294-298.
146. Egbert JE, Paul S, Engel WK, et al. High injection pressure during intralesional injection of corticosteroids into capillary hemangiomas. *Arch Ophthalmol*. 2001;119(5):677-683.
147. Chen MT, Yeong EK, Horng SY. Intralesional corticosteroid therapy in proliferating head and neck hemangiomas: a review of 155 cases. *J Pediatr Surg*. 2000;35(3):420-423.
148. Cruz OA, Zarnegar SR, Myers SE. Treatment of periocular capillary hemangioma with topical clobetasol propionate. *Ophthalmology*. 1995;102(12):2012-2015.
149. Garzon MC, Lucky AW, Hawrot A, et al. Ultrapotent topical corticosteroid treatment of hemangiomas of infancy. *J Am Acad Dermatol*. 2005;52(2):281-286.
150. Michaud AP, Bauman NM, Burke DK, et al. Spastic diplegia and other motor disturbances in infants receiving interferon-alpha. *Laryngoscope*. 2004;114(7):1231-1236.
151. Perez J, Pardo J, Gomez C. Vincristine—an effective treatment of corticoid-resistant life-threatening infantile hemangiomas. *Acta Oncol*. 2002;41(2):197-199.
152. Fawcett SL, Grant I, Hall PN, et al. Vincristine as a treatment for a large haemangioma threatening vital functions. *Br J Plast Surg*. 2004;57(2):168-171.

153. Moore J, Lee M, Garzon M, et al. Effective therapy of a vascular tumor of infancy with vincristine. *J Pediatr Surg.* 2001;36(8):1273-1276.
154. Morelli JG, Tan OT, Yohn JJ, et al. Treatment of ulcerated hemangiomas infancy. *Arch Pediatr Adolesc Med.* 1994;148(10):1104-1105.
155. Batta K, Goodyear HM, Moss C, et al. Randomised controlled study of early pulsed dye laser treatment of uncomplicated childhood haemangiomas: results of a 1-year analysis. *Lancet.* 2002;360(9332):521-527.
156. David LR, Malek MM, Argenta LC. Efficacy of pulse dye laser therapy for the treatment of ulcerated haemangiomas: a review of 78 patients. *Br J Plast Surg.* 2003;56(4):317-327.
157. Michel JL. Treatment of hemangiomas with 595 nm pulsed dye laser dermobeam. *Eur J Dermatol.* 2003;13(2):136-141.
158. Kessels JP, Hamers ET, Ostertag JU. Superficial hemangioma: pulsed dye laser versus wait-and-see. *Dermatol Surg.* 2013;39(3, pt 1):414-421.
159. Hohenleutner U, Landthaler M. Laser treatment of childhood haemangioma: progress or not? *Lancet.* 2002;360(9332):502-503.
160. Kolde G. Early pulsed-dye laser treatment of childhood haemangiomas. *Lancet.* 2003;361(9354):348-349; author reply 349.
161. Kono T, Sakurai H, Groff WF, et al. Comparison study of a traditional pulsed dye laser versus a long-pulsed dye laser in the treatment of early childhood hemangiomas. *Lasers Surg Med.* 2006;38(2):112-115.
162. Rizzo C, Brightman L, Chapas AM, et al. Outcomes of childhood hemangiomas treated with the pulsed-dye laser with dynamic cooling: a retrospective chart analysis. *Dermatol Surg.* 2009;35(12):1947-1954.
163. Witman PM, Wagner AM, Scherer K, et al. Complications following pulsed dye laser treatment of superficial hemangiomas. *Lasers Surg Med.* 2006;38(2):116-123.
164. Anderson RR. Infant hemangiomas: a controversy worth solving. *Lasers Surg Med.* 2006;38(2):92-93.
165. Demiri EC, Pelissier P, Genin-Etcheberry T, et al. Treatment of facial haemangiomas: the present status of surgery. *Br J Plast Surg.* 2001;54(8):665-674.
166. Denk MJ, Ajkay N, Yuan X, et al. Surgical treatment of nasal hemangiomas. *Ann Plast Surg.* 2002;48(5):489-494; discussion 494-495.
167. Hochman M, Mascareno A. Management of nasal hemangiomas. *Arch Facial Plast Surg.* 2005;7(5):295-300.
168. Faguer K, Dompmartin A, Labbe D, et al. Early surgical treatment of Cyrano-nose haemangiomas with Rethi incision. *Br J Plast Surg.* 2002;55(6):498-503.
169. McCarthy JG, Borud LJ, Schreiber JS. Hemangiomas of the nasal tip. *Plast Reconstr Surg.* 2002;109(1):31-40.
170. Warren SM, Longaker MT, Zide BM. The subunit approach to nasal tip hemangiomas. *Plast Reconstr Surg.* 2002;109(1):25-30.
171. McHeik JN, Renauld V, Duport G, et al. Surgical treatment of haemangioma in infants. *Br J Plast Surg.* 2005;58(8):1067-1072.
172. Mulliken JB, Rogers GF, Marler JJ. Circular excision of hemangioma and purse-string closure: the smallest possible scar. *Plast Reconstr Surg.* 2002;109(5):1544-1554; discussion 1555.
173. Requena L, Sangueza OP. Cutaneous vascular proliferation. Part II. Hyperplasias and benign neoplasms. *J Am Acad Dermatol.* 1997;37(6):887-919; quiz 920-922.
174. Weiss SW, Goldblum JR. *Enzinger and Weiss's Soft Tissue Tumors.* 4th ed. St Louis, MO: Mosby; 2001.
175. Krol A, MacArthur CJ. Congenital hemangiomas: rapidly involuting and noninvoluting congenital hemangiomas. *Arch Facial Plast Surg.* 2005;7(5):307-311.
176. Nasseri E, Piram M, McCuaig CC, et al. Partially involuting congenital hemangiomas: a report of 8 cases and review of the literature. *J Am Acad Dermatol.* 2014;70(1):75-79.
177. Boon LM, Enjolras O, Mulliken JB. Congenital hemangioma: evidence of accelerated involution. *J Pediatr.* 1996;128(3):329-335.
178. Ozcan UA. Rapidly involuting congenital hemangioma: a case of complete prenatal involution. *J Clin Ultrasound.* 2010;38(2):85-88.
179. Baselga E, Cordisco MR, Garzon M, et al. Rapidly involuting congenital haemangioma associated with transient thrombocytopenia and coagulopathy: a case series. *Br J Dermatol.* 2008;158(6):1363-1370.
180. Ayturk UM, Couto JA, Hann S, et al. Somatic activating mutations in GNAQ and GNA11 are associated with congenital hemangioma. *Am J Hum Genet.* 2016;98(6):1271.
181. Thomas AC, Zeng Z, Riviere JB, et al. Mosaic activating mutations in GNA11 and GNAQ are associated with phakomatosis pigmentovascularis and extensive dermal melanocytosis. *J Invest Dermatol.* 2016;136(4):770-778.
182. Berenguer B, Mulliken JB, Enjolras O, et al. Rapidly involuting congenital hemangioma: clinical and histopathologic features. *Pediatr Dev Pathol.* 2003;6(6):495-510.
183. North PE, Waner M, James CA, et al. Congenital nonprogressive hemangioma: a distinct clinicopathologic entity unlike infantile hemangioma. *Arch Dermatol.* 2001;137(12):1607-1620.
184. Gorincour G, Kokta V, Rypens F, et al. Imaging characteristics of two subtypes of congenital hemangiomas: rapidly involuting congenital hemangiomas and non-involuting congenital hemangiomas. *Pediatr Radiol.* 2005;35(12):1178-1185.
185. Colmenero I, Hoeger PH. Vascular tumours in infants. Part II: vascular tumours of intermediate malignancy [corrected] and malignant tumours. *Br J Dermatol.* 2014;171(3):474-484.
186. Maronn M, Chamlin S, Metry D. Multifocal tufted angiomas in 2 infants. *Arch Dermatol.* 2009;145(7):847-848.
187. Ishikawa K, Hatano Y, Ichikawa H, et al. The spontaneous regression of tufted angioma. A case of regression after two recurrences and a review of 27 cases reported in the literature. *Dermatology.* 2005;210(4):346-348.
188. Jones EW, Orkin M. Tufted angioma (angioblastoma). A benign progressive angioma, not to be confused with Kaposi's sarcoma or low-grade angiosarcoma. *J Am Acad Dermatol.* 1989;20(2, pt 1):214-225.
189. Arai E, Kuramochi A, Tsuchida T, et al. Usefulness of D2-40 immunohistochemistry for differentiation between kaposiform hemangioendothelioma and tufted angioma. *J Cutan Pathol.* 2006;33(7):492-497.
190. Browning J, Frieden I, Baselga E, et al. Congenital, self-regressing tufted angioma. *Arch Dermatol.* 2006;142(6):749-751.
191. Okada E, Tamura A, Ishikawa O, et al. Tufted angioma (angioblastoma): case report and review of 41 cases in the Japanese literature. *Clin Exp Dermatol.* 2000;25(8):627-630.
192. Croteau SE, Liang MG, Kozakewich HP, et al. Kaposiform hemangioendothelioma: atypical features and risks of Kasabach-Merritt phenomenon in 107 refer-

rals. *J Pediatr*. 2013;162(1):142-147.
193. Lyons LL, North PE, Mac-Moune Lai F, et al. Kaposiform hemangioendothelioma: a study of 33 cases emphasizing its pathologic, immunophenotypic, and biologic uniqueness from juvenile hemangioma. *Am J Surg Pathol*. 2004;28(5):559-568.
194. Gruman A, Liang MG, Mulliken JB, et al. Kaposiform hemangioendothelioma without Kasabach-Merritt phenomenon. *J Am Acad Dermatol*. 2005;52(4):616-622.
195. Adams DM, Trenor CC 3rd, Hammill AM, et al. Efficacy and safety of sirolimus in the treatment of complicated vascular anomalies. *Pediatrics*. 2016;137(2): e20153257.
196. Enjolras O, Mulliken JB, Wassef M, et al. Residual lesions after Kasabach-Merritt phenomenon in 41 patients. *J Am Acad Dermatol*. 2000;42(2, pt 1):225-235.
197. Sarkar M, Mulliken JB, Kozakewich HP, et al. Thrombocytopenic coagulopathy (Kasabach-Merritt phenomenon) is associated with Kaposiform hemangioendothelioma and not with common infantile hemangioma. *Plast Reconstr Surg*. 1997;100(6):1377-1386.
198. Mazoyer E, Enjolras O, Laurian C, et al. Coagulation abnormalities associated with extensive venous malformations of the limbs: differentiation from Kasabach-Merritt syndrome. *Clin Lab Haematol*. 2002;24(4):243-251.
199. Debelenko LV, Perez-Atayde AR, Mulliken JB, et al. D2-40 immunohistochemical analysis of pediatric vascular tumors reveals positivity in kaposiform hemangioendothelioma. *Mod Pathol*. 2005;18(11): 1454-1460.
200. Folpe AL, Veikkola T, Valtola R, et al. Vascular endothelial growth factor receptor-3 (VEGFR-3): a marker of vascular tumors with presumed lymphatic differentiation, including Kaposi's sarcoma, kaposiform and Dabska-type hemangioendotheliomas, and a subset of angiosarcomas. *Mod Pathol*. 2000;13(2):180-185.
201. Drolet BA, Trenor CC 3rd, Brandao LR, et al. Consensus-derived practice standards plan for complicated Kaposiform hemangioendothelioma. *J Pediatr*. 2013;163(1): 285-291.
202. Blatt J, Stavas J, Moats-Staats B, et al. Treatment of childhood kaposiform hemangioendothelioma with sirolimus. *Pediatr Blood Cancer*. 2010;55(7):1396-1398.
203. Wang Z, Li K, Dong K, et al. Successful treatment of Kasabach-Merritt phenomenon arising from Kaposiform hemangioendothelioma by sirolimus. *J Pediatr Hematol Oncol*. 2015;37(1):72-73.
204. Hauer J, Graubner U, Konstantopoulos N, et al. Effective treatment of kaposiform hemangioendotheliomas associated with Kasabach-Merritt phenomenon using four-drug regimen. *Pediatr Blood Cancer*. 2007;49(6):852-854.
205. Haisley-Royster C, Enjolras O, Frieden IJ, et al. Kasabach-Merritt phenomenon: a retrospective study of treatment with vincristine. *J Pediatr Hematol Oncol*. 2002;24(6):459-462.
206. Drucker AM, Pope E, Mahant S, et al. Vincristine and corticosteroids as first-line treatment of Kasabach-Merritt syndrome in kaposiform hemangioendothelioma. *J Cutan Med Surg*. 2009;13(3):155-159.
207. Lopez V, Marti N, Pereda C, et al. Successful management of Kaposiform hemangioendothelioma with Kasabach-Merritt phenomenon using vincristine and ticlopidine. *Pediatr Dermatol*. 2009;26(3):365-366.
208. Rodriguez V, Lee A, Witman PM, et al. Kasabach-Merritt phenomenon: case series and retrospective review of the Mayo Clinic experience. *J Pediatr Hematol Oncol*. 2009;31(7):522-526.
209. Perkins P, Weiss SW. Spindle cell hemangioendothelioma. An analysis of 78 cases with reassessment of its pathogenesis and biologic behavior. *Am J Surg Pathol*. 1996;20(10):1196-1204.
210. Frieden IJ, Esterly NB. Pyogenic granulomas of infancy masquerading as strawberry hemangiomas. *Pediatrics*. 1992;90(6):989-991.
211. Barrick B, Lehman J, Tollefson M. Agminated pyogenic granuloma-like growth arising in a congenital hemangioma. *JAMA Dermatol*. 2014;150(7):781-783.
212. Baselga E, Wassef M, Lopez S, et al. Agminated, eruptive pyogenic granuloma-like lesions developing over congenital vascular stains. *Pediatr Dermatol*. 2012;29(2):186-190.
213. Patrice SJ, Wiss K, Mulliken JB. Pyogenic granuloma (lobular capillary hemangioma): a clinicopathologic study of 178 cases. *Pediatr Dermatol*. 1991;8(4):267-276.
214. Pagliai KA, Cohen BA. Pyogenic granuloma in children. *Pediatr Dermatol*. 2004;21(1):10-13.
215. Tritton SM, Smith S, Wong LC, et al. Pyogenic granuloma in ten children treated with topical imiquimod. *Pediatr Dermatol*. 2009;26(3):269-272.
216. Malik M, Murphy R. A pyogenic granuloma treated with topical timolol. *Br J Dermatol*. 2014;171(6):1537-1538.
217. North PE, Kahn T, Cordisco MR, et al. Multifocal lymphangioendotheliomatosis with thrombocytopenia: a newly recognized clinicopathological entity. *Arch Dermatol*. 2004;140(5):599-606.
218. Maronn M, Catrine K, North P, et al. Expanding the phenotype of multifocal lymphangioendotheliomatosis with thrombocytopenia. *Pediatr Blood Cancer*. 2009;52(4):531-534.
219. Glick ZR, Frieden IJ, Garzon MC, et al. Diffuse neonatal hemangiomatosis: an evidence-based review of case reports in the literature. *J Am Acad Dermatol*. 2012;67(5):898-903.
220. Prasad V, Fishman SJ, Mulliken JB, et al. Cutaneovisceral angiomatosis with thrombocytopenia. *Pediatr Dev Pathol*. 2005;8(4):407-419.
221. Droitcourt C, Boccara O, Fraitag S, et al. Multifocal lymphangioendotheliomatosis with thrombocytopenia: clinical features and response to sirolimus. *Pediatrics*. 2015;136(2):e517-e522.
222. Lanoel A, Torres Huamani AN, Feliu A, et al. Multifocal lymphangioendotheliomatosis with thrombocytopenia: presentation of two cases treated with sirolimus. *Pediatr Dermatol*. 2016;33(4):e235-e239.
223. Kline RM, Buck LM. Bevacizumab treatment in multifocal lymphangioendotheliomatosis with thrombocytopenia. *Pediatr Blood Cancer*. 2009;52(4):534-536.
224. Calonje E, Fletcher CD, Wilson-Jones E, et al. Retiform hemangioendothelioma. A distinctive form of low-grade angiosarcoma delineated in a series of 15 cases. *Am J Surg Pathol*. 1994;18(2):115-125.
225. Nayler SJ, Rubin BP, Calonje E, et al. Composite hemangioendothelioma: a complex, low-grade vascular lesion mimicking angiosarcoma. *Am J Surg Pathol*. 2000;24(3):352-361.
226. Nakatsui TC, Schloss E, Krol A, et al. Eccrine angiomatous hamartoma: report of a case and literature review. *J Am Acad Dermatol*. 1999;41(1):109-111.

Chapter 119 :: Cutaneous Lymphoma
:: Martine Bagot & Rudolf Stadler

第一百一十九章

皮肤淋巴瘤

中文导读

原发性皮肤淋巴瘤是一组异质性结外非霍奇金淋巴瘤，起源于皮肤归巢或/和皮肤驻留T细胞或B淋巴细胞的恶性克隆性转化和血液皮源性前体肿瘤。皮肤淋巴瘤被定义为在临床表现、组织病理学、免疫表型和预后方面有明显差异的异质性组。欧洲癌症研究和治疗组织(EORTC)和世界卫生组织(WHO)在2005年发布了皮肤淋巴瘤的共识分类。本章介绍了最常见的原发皮肤T细胞淋巴瘤中的蕈样肉芽肿、Sézary综合征、原发性皮肤间变性大细胞淋巴瘤和淋巴瘤样丘疹病，以及最常见的皮肤B细胞淋巴瘤中的原发性皮肤毛囊中心淋巴瘤、原发性皮肤边缘区淋巴瘤和原发性皮肤弥漫性大B细胞淋巴瘤（腿型）。这7种皮肤淋巴瘤占所有皮肤淋巴瘤的近90%。

〔粟　娟〕

Primary cutaneous lymphomas are a heterogeneous group of extranodal non-Hodgkin lymphomas arising from malignant clonal transformation of skin homing or/and skin resident T cells or B lymphocytes and hematodermic precursor neoplasias (plasmacytoid dendritic cell neoplasias). Cutaneous lymphomas (Fig. 119-1) are defined as a heterogeneous group with distinct variability in clinical presentation, histopathology, immunophenotyping, and prognosis.

Primary cutaneous lymphomas are defined entities with a completely different clinical behavior and prognosis as nodal non-Hodgkin lymphomas and require different treatment approaches.

For this reason the European Organization for Research and Treatment of Cancer (EORTC) and World Health Organization (WHO) published a consensus classification for cutaneous lymphomas in 2005.[1] This first common classification (WHO-EORTC) categorizes the entities according to lineage and then according to a combination of morphology, immunophenotype, genetic features, and clinical syndromes, and constitutes the basis for the classification of cutaneous lymphomas in the WHO classification 2008 and the revised classification of lymphoid neoplasias in 2016.[2,3] This chapter discusses the most frequent cutaneous T-cell lymphomas (CTCLs)—mycosis fungoides (MF), Sézary syndrome, primary cutaneous anaplastic large-cell lymphoma, and lymphomatoid papulosis—and the most frequent cutaneous B-cell lymphomas (CBCLs)—primary cutaneous follicle center lymphoma (PCFCL), primary cutaneous marginal zone lymphoma (PCMZL), and primary cutaneous diffuse large B-cell lymphoma (PCLBCL), leg. type. These 7 types of cutaneous lymphoma represent nearly 90% of all cutaneous lymphomas. Rare entities occurring primary in the skin are also described.

EPIDEMIOLOGY

CTCLs represent the second most common group of extranodal lymphomas after the primary GI lymphomas. The incidence of CTCLs has been increasing and is currently, in the United States, estimated to be 6.4 cases/million people between 1993 and 2002 or 7.7 cases/million people between 2001 and 2005. The incidence of CTCL increases significantly with age, with a median age at diagnosis in the mid-50s and a fourfold increase in incidence appreciated in patients older than age 70 years.[4-6]

PRIMARY CUTANEOUS T-CELL LYMPHOMAS

CTCLs are non-Hodgkin lymphomas characterized by clonal expansion of activated T-cells expressing the E-selectin ligand cutaneous lymphocyte antigen and chemokine receptors (eg, CCR4, CCR8, CCR10) that are required for their subsequent trafficking to the skin.[7-9] Clonal expansion is followed by differentiation into multiple subsets of effector and memory cells. Human skin is protected by 4 functionally-distinct populations of T cells, 2 resident and 2 recirculating, with differing territories of migration and distinct functional activities. Central memory cells (T_{CM}) retain the ability to access the peripheral blood and lymph nodes. Effector memory cells (T_{EM}), in contrast, migrate into extranodal sites, including the skin, where a subset will remain as tissue-resident memory cells (T_{RM}). The majority of T cells in the skin are T_{RM}, express a high affinity antigen receptor, and have a distinct gene expression profile. Clonal T cells in MF are commonly T_{RM}-derived, which explains their tendency to be confined to the skin. In contrast, in patients with leukemic CTCL variants (Sézary syndrome and MF with secondary leukemic involvement), tumor cells express CCR7 and L-selectin, resembling T_{CM}. This fundamental difference in the putative cell origin between Sézary syndrome (T_{CM}-derived) and MF (T_{RM}-derived) is consistent with the distinct clinical behavior. Among the recirculating cells 2 distinct populations were observed, CCR7+/L-selectin+ T_{CM} and CCR7+/L-selectin− T cells termed *migratory memory T cells* (T_{MM}). A subset of MF patients with secondary leukemic involvement, poorly demarcated patches/plaques, dermal involvement, and lymphadenopathy most probably harbor a T_{MM} clone.[10,11]

The most common forms, representing approximately 65% of CTCL, are MF and Sézary syndrome, with an annual incidence of 7.7 cases/million people. CTCL encompasses skin-limited variants such as MF and leukemic forms of the disease, including Sézary syndrome.

After MF and Sézary syndrome, the primary cutaneous CD30+ lymphoproliferative disorders, comprising lymphomatoid papulosis and cutaneous anaplastic large-cell lymphoma, represent the second most common group of CTCLs (approximately 27%).[12] Table 119-1 outlines the WHO classification of primary cutaneous lymphomas.

ETIOLOGY

The skin of a human adult contains approximately 20 billion memory T cells. Despite major advances in cellular and molecular biology revealing many details about lymphocytes, including the incredible diversity of T-cell antigen receptors, their characterization as T_{CM} or T_{EM} or T_{RM}, and the role of environmental and host genetic factors for the pathogenesis in CTCL remains unclear. In general, long-term antigen stimulation is thought to induce an inflammatory response with T-cell proliferation leading to clonal malignant T cells with continuous expansion. However, recent advances in the understanding of the molecular pathogenesis, signal transduction pathways, and disease-associated immune dysregulation helped to understand the complex pathogenesis to advance the treatment in CTCL.[10-19]

ENDOGENOUS FACTORS

As a result of the above-mentioned hypothesis of antigen stimulation, several studies have analyzed the human leukocyte antigen (HLA) background of

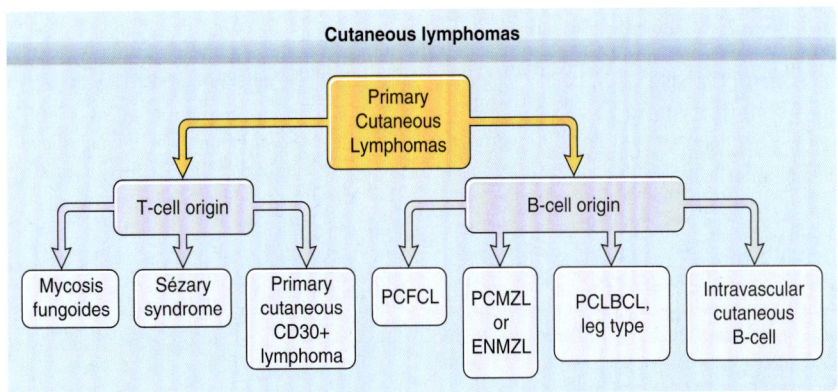

Figure 119-1 Cutaneous lymphomas. ENMZL, extranodal marginal zone lymphoma; PCFCL, primary cutaneous follicle center lymphoma; PCLBCL, primary cutaneous diffuse large B-cell lymphoma; PCMZL, primary cutaneous marginal zone lymphoma.

affected individuals. Two independent studies showed an association of distinct HLA class II molecules and MF or Sézary syndrome; that is, the alleles HLA-DRB1*11 and DQB1*03 are significantly overrepresented in these patients (Fig. 119-2).

EXOGENOUS FACTORS

Viruses have been identified as etiologic factors in at least 2 cutaneous lymphomas (human T-cell lymphotropic virus-1 [HTLV-1]-associated adult T-cell lymphoma/leukemia, and Epstein-Barr virus [EBV]-associated natural killer [NK]/T-cell lymphoma), whereas no such relation has been confirmed for MF or Sézary syndrome. All these data suggest that HTLV does not play an important role in the etiology of CTCLs, outside of HTLV-1 endemic regions, and that the only reason to screen patients for antibodies is the suspicion that the diagnosis is adult T-cell lymphoma/leukemia rather than MF. EBV as well as cytomegalovirus have been discussed as causative pathogens. EBV is associated with CD30 lymphoproliferation and with immunosuppression. Several studies show that EBV is detectable only in a minor percentage of CTCL lesions. In these studies, EBV detection was related to a poor prognosis and its presence is more likely related to immunosuppression caused by either the disease or the therapy, rather than to the etiology of CTCL. However, a strong association of EBV in a rare cutaneous lymphoproliferative disease with a hydroa vacciniforme–like appearance, which occurs mostly in people of Asian origin, has been observed.

Bacterial infections also have been implicated in the etiology of CTCLs. Of special interest has been the hypothesis that superantigens from *Staphylococcus aureus* may be responsible for chronic antigenic stimulation. In several studies, *S. aureus* has been detected in a high percentage on the skin of CTCL patients with a high tumor burden, while patients in early stage disease did not show significant differences to control groups. Although these studies conclusively demonstrate the involvement of *S. aureus* in disease exacerbation and clinical improvement following antibiotic treatment, the missing difference in *S. aureus* colonization in early stages of CTCL and control groups questions the involvement of *S. aureus* or superantigens produced by these bacteria in initiation of CTCLs.

However, *S. aureus* enterotoxin A stimulates signal transducer and activator of transcription (STAT) 3 activation, and interleukin (IL)-17 expression in cutaneous T-cell lymphoma and may play a direct role in the progression of the disease.

Besides infectious pathogens, it also has been suggested that environmental and occupational risk factors play a causative role in CTCL (see Fig. 119-2), because an indolent dermatitis often precedes the diagnosis. Exposure to carcinogens in the work environment could provide the suspected long-term antigenic stimulation for the initiation of the clonal expansion. In epidemiologic studies, several occupations, such as glass formers, potters, and paper and wood industry workers, have been associated with a higher risk for development of MF. However, the results of the different studies were not consistent, and a common denominator, like exposure to known carcinogens, could not be identified. With regard to chronic antigenic stimulation by occupational contact allergens, it has to be considered that MF arises typically on body areas like the lateral

TABLE 119-1
World Health Organization Classification of Primary Cutaneous Lymphomas

Cutaneous T-Cell and Natural Killer (NK)-Cell Lymphomas
- Mycosis fungoides
- Mycosis fungoides variants and subtypes
  - Folliculotropic mycosis fungoides
  - Pagetoid reticulosis
  - Granulomatous slack skin
- Sézary syndrome
- Adult T-cell leukemia/lymphoma
- Primary cutaneous CD30+ T-cell lymphoproliferative disorders
  - Primary cutaneous anaplastic large-cell lymphoma
  - Lymphomatoid papulosis
- Subcutaneous panniculitis-like T-cell lymphoma
- Extranodal NK/T-cell lymphoma, nasal type
- Primary cutaneous peripheral T-cell lymphoma, not otherwise specified
  - Primary cutaneous γ/δ T-cell lymphoma
  - Primary cutaneous CD8+ aggressive epidermotropic cytotoxic T-cell lymphoma
  - Primary cutaneous acral CD8+ T-cell lymphoma
  - Primary cutaneous CD4+ small–medium T-cell lymphoproliferative disorder

Cutaneous B-Cell Lymphomas
- Primary cutaneous marginal zone B-cell lymphoma
- Primary cutaneous follicle center lymphoma
- Primary cutaneous diffuse large B-cell lymphoma, leg type
- Primary cutaneous diffuse large B-cell lymphoma, other
  - Intravascular large B-cell lymphoma
- Epstein-Barr virus–positive, mucocutaneous ulcer
- Precursor hematologic neoplasm
- CD4+/CD56+ hematodermic neoplasm (plasmacytoid dendritic cell neoplasia)

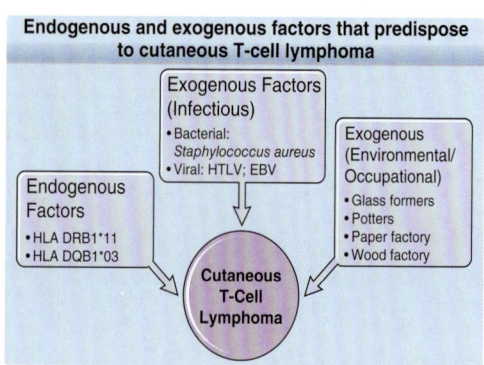

Figure 119-2 Endogenous and exogenous factors that predispose to cutaneous T-cell lymphoma. EBV, Epstein-Barr virus; HTLV, human T-cell lymphotropic virus.

trunk that are protected by clothes during working time. Also, other environmental risk factors, like consumption of alcohol, smoking, or exposure to ultraviolet (UV) radiation, were not consistently observed in association with an increased risk for CTCLs.[20-31]

PATHOGENESIS

Cutaneous T-cell lymphoma is a malignancy of skin-homing T-cells. Patients typically present with localized patches and plaques in sun-protected skin. Lymphoma cells extend from these lesions to uninvolved skin and accumulate in the superficial dermis, leading to patches/plaques and tumors. In advanced disease, malignant T cells disseminate to blood, lymph nodes and viscera. In leukemic CTCL (Sézary syndrome), malignant T-cells can comprise greater than 99% of the circulating T lymphocytes. Loss of the normal T-cell receptor (TCR) and the disappearance of normal lymphocytes lead to immunosuppression and opportunistic infections, which are the most common disease-related causes of death.

The clinical entities encompassed by the term *cutaneous T-cell lymphoma* share several components: the epidermal and/or dermal microenvironment, a clonal T-cell population, and a modulated antitumor response. A spectral karyotyping and comparative genomic hybridization studies combined with TCRγ polymerase chain reaction have demonstrated that genetically-damaged malignant T cells are present in even the earliest stages of MF, confirming that MF is a lymphoma of genetically-damaged malignant T cells even in its earliest manifestation. There is emerging evidence that the distinct clinical presentation of CTCLs may represent their derivation from different subsets of skin-homing T cells. Malignant T cells in MF have the surface phenotype of nonrecirculating T_{RM} and classic erythrodermic Sézary syndrome has malignant T cells with a surface phenotype of T_{CM}, consistent with their tendency to form stable inflammatory skin lesions versus transitory erythroderma, respectively. However, the phenotype of Sézary cells is more heterogeneous than initially reported, and Sézary cells can also present phenotypic plasticity.[10,32-37]

T_{MM} are novel skin-homing T cells. These cells express CCR7 but lack L-selectin, are present in the blood and skin of healthy individuals, and recirculate more slowly out of skin than do T_{CM}. In CTCL patients, malignant T_{MM} give rise to discrete skin lesions with ill-defined borders and peripheral blood disease, which, in the current classification, is referred to as MF with peripheral blood disease.

The fundamental difference in the putative cell of origin between Sézary syndrome (T_{CM} derived) and MF (T_{RM} derived) is consistent with their distinct clinical behaviors, as T_{CM} may be found in both, in the peripheral blood, lymph node, and skin, and are resistant to apoptosis, whereas resident T_{RM} cells remain fixed within the skin. In addition, a population of recirculating CCR7+ L-selectin– T_{MM} has been described in the skin. The contention that MF subtypes and Sézary syndrome originate from different T-cell subsets is consistent with comparative genomic hybridization (CGH), a gene expression profiling data demonstrating that these CTCL subtypes are genetically distinct. Detection of these malignant T-cell clones is critical in making the diagnosis of CTCL.[10,11]

Emerging with new molecular technology using high-throughput TCR sequencing, it has been demonstrated that the malignant T-cell clones in MF and leukemic CTCL localized to different anatomic compartments in the skin could be discriminated from benign inflammatory skin diseases.

Regulatory T cells expressing the transcription factor FOX-P3 are important in the maintenance of self-tolerance and form a minor subset of skin-resident T cells. It is discussed that a subset of Sézary patients harbor a clone that is derived from resident regulatory T cells. However, regulatory T cells represent only a minority of skin-resident T cells; the majority of T cells in the skin produce cytokines characteristic of distinct effector T-cell subsets, including T-helper (Th) 1, Th2, and Th17 cells. MF and Sézary syndrome are associated with the expression of Th2-associated genes (eg, GATA-3) and the production of Th2-associated cytokines (eg, IL-4, IL-5, IL-13), raising the possibility that a significant subset of patients may harbor Th2-derived clones.[38-44]

Alternatively, recurrence mutations activating specific signaling pathways (nuclear factor of activated T cells [NFAT], nuclear factor κB [NFκB], Janus kinase [JAK]/STAT) may provoke the acquisition of a particular phenotype independent of the cell of origin.[37]

Recent molecular studies have advanced our understanding of the molecular pathogenesis of CTCL. Recurrent deletions of 10q and 17p and amplification of 8q and 17q have been identified with robust evidence implicating deletions of TP53 und CDKN2a and amplifications of 8q containing MYC. In a recent study of the genomic landscape of cutaneous lymphomas, somatic mutations in 17 genes in CTCL were described. Frequent deletion and damaging somatic copy number variants in chromatin-modifying genes (*ARID1A* [62.5%], *CTCF* [12.5%], and *DNNT3A* [42.5%]) were found. Many genes mutated in CTCL contribute to other T-cell neoplasms, including peripheral T-cell lymphoma (*CD28*, *DNMT3A*, and *RHOA*), underscoring the importance of these genes for the malignant transformation of T cells. Consistent with this notion, mutations were found in multiple components of the TCR signaling pathway, including CD28 and the genes for TCR-associated enzymes (*PLCG1*, *PRKCQ*, and *TNFAIP3*) and transcription factors (*NFκB2*, *STAT5B*, and *ZEB1*). These genes drive the Th2 differentiation (*ZEB1*) that facilitates escape from transforming growth factor-β–mediated growth suppression (*ZEB1*) and facilitates resistance to tumor necrosis factor receptor superfamily–mediated apoptosis (*FAS* and *ARID1A*).[45,46]

In CTCL, several cytokines play a role in disease manifestation as well as in the progression of this disease. In early stages of CTCL, signaling of IL-2,

IL-7, and IL-15, which all are γc-chain cytokines using JAK1/JAK3, drives the activation of STAT5 and STAT3. As a result of downstream processes of STAT3 and STAT5, a shift from Th1 toward a Th2 phenotype of the malignant T cells can be observed. This is achieved by the transcriptional activation of the micro-RNA (miRNA)-155 by STAT5. In turn, miRNA-155 targets STAT4, leading to the downregulation of Th1 genes. In addition, STAT5 activates IL-4 expression, fostering the Th2 phenotype. This shift is associated with the progression of CTCL as Th2 responses (IL-4, IL-10) are well known mechanisms of tumor-induced immunosuppression.

Furthermore, the activation of JAK3, STAT3, and STAT5 leads to a transcriptional repression of miRNA-22, a known tumor suppressor. For CTCL, malignant T cells—CTCL cell lines as well as peripheral blood Sézary CD4+ T cells—demonstrate a reduced expression of miRNA-22. The miRNA-22 normally inhibits tumor growth and metastasis because it targets the transcription of a number of putative oncogenic genes (eg, *MYCB*, *HDAC4*, *HDAC6*, *CDK6*, and *NcoA1*). But in CTCL, a loss of these tumor-suppressive activities by miRNA-22 is observed, as the expression of miRNA-22 is directly downregulated by STAT5, leading to a faster progression of the malignant state of the T cells. These findings suggest that JAK/STAT signaling plays another key role in the pathogenesis and progression of CTCL and that JAK-inhibition could mediate a direct suppressive effect on tumor growth and metastasis (Fig. 119-3).

In addition to this, the activation of STAT3 is a critical mediator of the transformation of malignant CTCL T cells, as well as an important mediator of plasticity.[1,7] STAT3 activation leads to IL-17 production of CTCL T cells as demonstrated in vitro with CTCL cell lines, as well as by expression of IL-17 in neoplastic lymphocytes in CTCL skin lesions ex vivo. Receptors for IL-17 are expressed by various cells in the skin microenvironment of CTCL lesions, such as fibroblast, keratinocytes, and epithelial cells. Upon stimulation with IL-17 these cells produce other proinflammatory cytokines, chemokines, and angiogenic factors. It was shown that CTCL lesions exhibit increased angiogenesis, providing the suggestion that IL-17 of neoplastic T cells in CTCL influences tumorigenesis by modulating inflammation and angiogenesis in CTCL skin lesions.

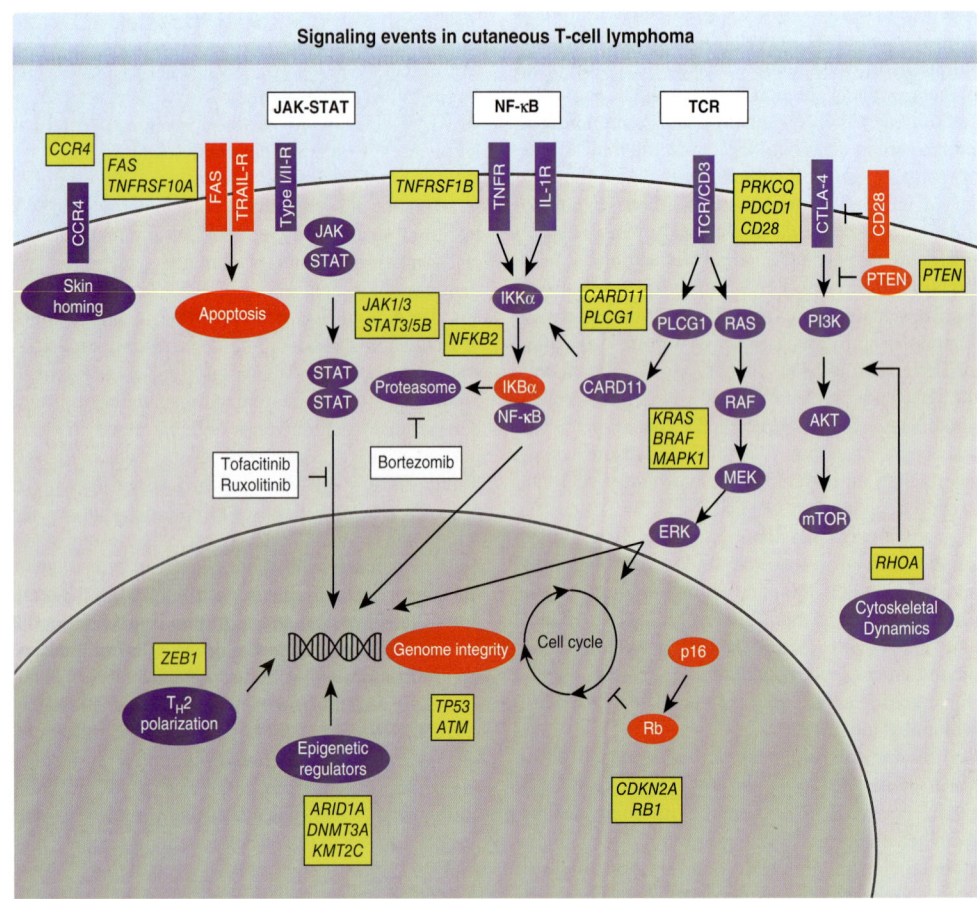

Figure 119-3 Signaling events in cutaneous T-cell lymphoma. (From Damsky WE, Choi J. Genetics of cutaneous T cell lymphoma: from bench to bedside. *Curr Treat Options Oncol.* 2016;17(7):33, with permission from Springer. Copyright © 2016.)

Therefore, targeting the initial STAT3 activation by JAK inhibition would also have beneficial effects on these indirect effects of aberrant T cells of the Th17 phenotype.

STAT3 transcriptional activity also leads to the expression of IL-21 in the aberrant T cells, which drives an autocrine signaling loop, leading to constitutive signaling via JAK1/JAK3 and the activation of STAT3. This constitutive activation of STAT3 driven by IL-21 is essential for the progression of CTCL by several mechanisms: (a) it promotes the expression of antiapoptotic proteins like bcl-2, leading to survival of malignant T cells[1]; (b) STAT3 is involved in the upregulation of the transcription of the angiogenic factor vascular endothelial growth factor; (c) it induces the expression of IL-5 and other cytokines involved in erythroderma and eosinophilia; (d) STAT3 transcriptional activities are involved in driving the plasticity of the T cells (Th2 and Th17 phenotypes) observed in advanced stages of CTCL; and (e) it induces the expression of an oncogenic miRNA, miRNA-21. The miRNA-21 is involved in the survival of malignant T cells due to antiapoptotic activities. All these reasons provide a strong rationale for targeting JAK/STAT pathways in CTCL.

Other cytokines in the microenvironment of CTCL are also involved, like IL-13, a cytokine related to the γc-chain cytokines sharing the IL-4 receptor α subunit (IL-4Rα). IL-13 belongs, therefore, to the IL-4 family and is secreted by the transformed malignant Th2 cells in CTCL, as IL-13 is highly expressed in clinically involved skin of CTCL patients. IL-13 acts as an autocrine growth factor of CTCL cells, especially in the Sézary syndrome variant of CTCL. Blockade of JAK1/JAK3 would also block IL-13 cytokine signaling, leading to the inhibition of tumor cell proliferation.[47-60]

In recent years, it has become evident that cytokine signaling plays a critical role in the pathogenesis of CTCL.

In addition to multiple defects in apoptosis, aberrant cell-cycle regulation, including inactivation of the CDKN2A-CDKN2B locus, is frequently observed in CTCL. Cyclin upregulation, including cyclin D_1, and loss of RB1 also have been described. As gene expression profiling and next-generation sequencing technologies are employed, additional pathogenic pathways, including those involved in transcription factors regulating T-cell differentiation and C-MYC, RAS, BRAF, and MEK signaling, are being identified in subsets of CTCL.[13,34]

In summary, recent research into CTCL has significantly advanced our knowledge of molecular pathogenesis, cellular origin, migratory behavior, and death signaling. As for other malignancies, the major challenge now will be to define meaningful molecular and/or phenotypic subgroups that relate to clinical behavior and/or treatment response to drugs that specifically interfere with disease-promoting signaling cascades or cellular interactions. As a result, promising treatment approaches will be based on our increasing knowledge about the molecular pathogenesis of CTCL.

MYCOSIS FUNGOIDES

DEFINITION

MF is the most common form of primary cutaneous lymphoma, accounting for approximately 40% of all cutaneous lymphomas, usually arising in mid to late adulthood (median age at diagnosis: 55-60 years) with a male predominance of 2:1. According to the WHO classification, MF is defined by its classic form, that is, by patches and plaques or variants.

CLINICAL FINDINGS

Skin Signs: Clinically, MF is categorized as patch, plaque, or tumor stage, but patients may simultaneously have more than 1 type of lesion. In early patch stage MF (Figs. 119-4 and 119-5), there are single or multiple erythematous, scaly macules and patches that vary in size and are usually well defined. The color of the lesions may vary from orange to a dusky violet-red. The distribution classically favors non–sun-exposed sites, with the "bathing trunk" and intertriginous areas predominant early in the course of the disease. The eruption may be intensely pruritic or asymptomatic, and occasionally may be transitory, disappearing spontaneously without scarring. Diagnosis at this stage may be difficult. Often a patient will recall a preceding "chronic dermatitis" for 10 to 20 years that may have been considered to be therapeutically-resistant contact dermatitis, atopic dermatitis, psoriasis, or eczema. In any patient with a dermatosis that is refractory to the

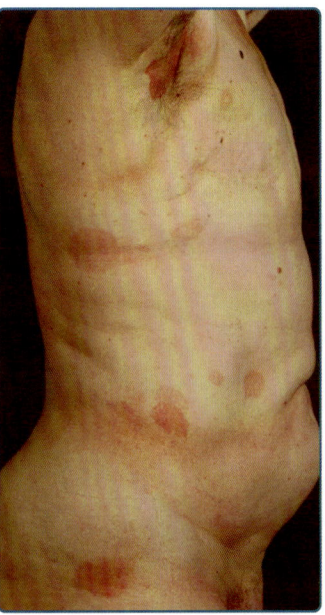

Figure 119-4 Patch lesions of mycosis fungoides in typical locations on the lateral trunk.

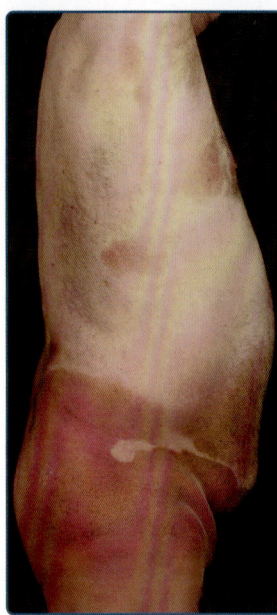

Figure 119-5 Large patch lesions of mycosis fungoides surrounding areas of uninvolved skin.

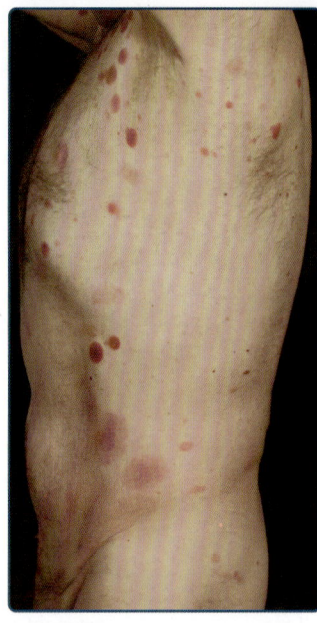

Figure 119-7 Multiple patches and plaques of mycosis fungoides on the lateral trunk. In this patient, the plaques developed rapidly and show partial central necrosis.

usual modalities of treatment, multiple biopsy specimens should be taken to pursue a diagnosis.

Patches may last for months or years before progressing to plaque stage (Fig. 119-6), or plaques may arise de novo. Plaques appear as sharply demarcated, scaly, elevated lesions that are dusky red to violaceous and variably indurated (Figs. 119-6 and 119-7). Lesions in this stage may regress spontaneously or may coalesce to form large plaques with annular, arcuate, or serpiginous borders, and may clear centrally with disease activity remaining at the periphery of the lesion. There may be purpuric hyperpigmentation or hypopigmentation and poikiloderma.

Tumors may occur anywhere on the body, but have a predilection for the face (Figs. 119-8 and 119-9) and body folds: axillae, groin, antecubital fossae, and, in women, the inframammary area. These usually occur in preexisting plaques or patches of MF; this coincides with an extension of these lesions in the vertical dimension (see Fig. 119-6). At this point, the neoplastic cells behave in a biologically-more aggressive manner, with pronounced tumor cell accumulation that leads to the clinical appearance of an expanding dermal nodule (see Fig. 119-9). De novo occurrence

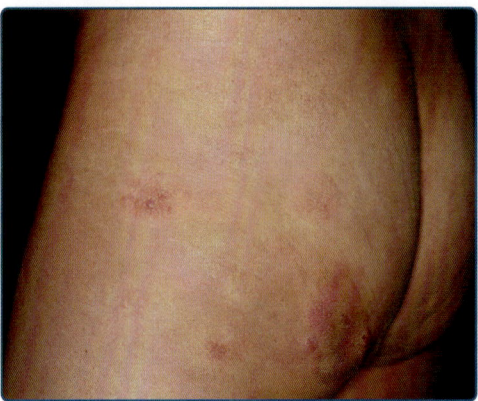

Figure 119-6 Polymorphic nature of mycosis fungoides. Patches and a plaque with a developing nodule on the left buttock.

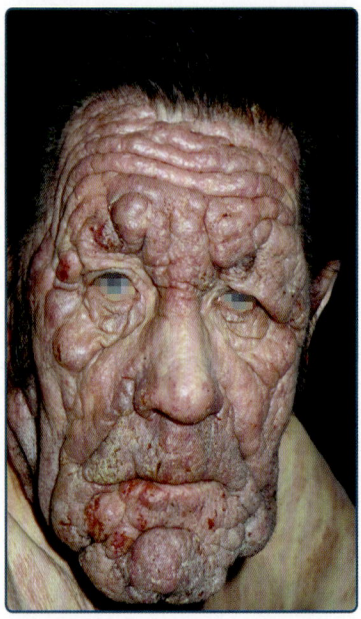

Figure 119-8 Leonine facies characterized by infiltrated plaques and tumors of cutaneous T-cell lymphoma.

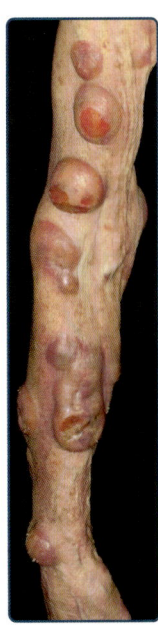

Figure 119-9 Tumor lesions of mycosis fungoides on the right arm, which are partially eroded and ulcerated.

Erythroderma (Fig. 119-10A) may start de novo or develop in MF. The nomenclature for erythrodermic phases of CTCL varies. It has been proposed that erythroderma be defined as the involvement of 80% of body surface area with lesions of ill-defined borders and that patients with a history of preexisting MF be defined as having a separate syndrome of "erythrodermic MF."

The skin is diffusely bright red with readily apparent scaling, but there may be characteristic islands of uninvolved skin. There may be sparing of the areas of skin that are frequently folded, such as the abdomen and antecubital and axillary areas. This sparing produces a finding often called the *deck chair* or *folded luggage* sign. Some patients with the erythrodermic form of CTCL develop tumors.

Other Symptoms: Patients may complain of fever, chills, weight loss, malaise, insomnia secondary to the overwhelming pruritus, and poor body temperature homeostasis. There may be hyperkeratosis, scaling and fissuring of the palms and soles, alopecia, ectropion, nail dystrophy, and ankle edema, with the integument being shiny and hidebound. These changes result in pain on walking and extreme difficulty with tasks requiring manual dexterity. Such patients experience severe restrictions by the extent and localization of their skin manifestations. Pruritus is often intense, which results in excoriation, exudation, and secondary infection that may dominate the clinical picture.

Hypopigmentated Mycosis Fungoides: Patients with dark skin develop hypopigmented MF, a variant (Table 119-2) of patch MF. This form of MF must be differentiated from vitiligo. In darker-skinned individuals, this may be the most common presentation of the disease. Patients respond to therapy with

suggests metastatic spread by cells of a malignant T-cell clone. The nodules are reddish brown or purplish red and smooth surfaced, but they often ulcerate and may become secondarily infected. Growth rate is variable. Patients with tumors tend to have a more aggressive form of the disease than patients with patch and plaque disease.

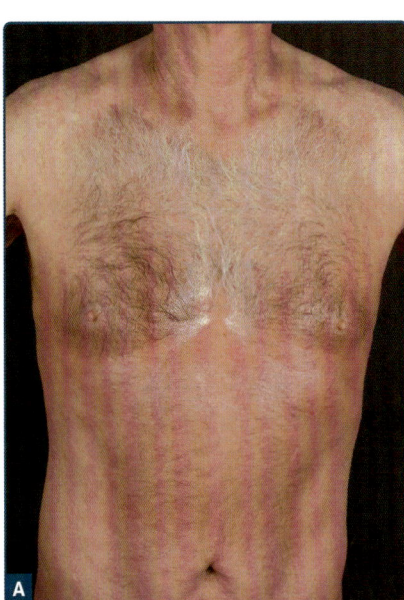
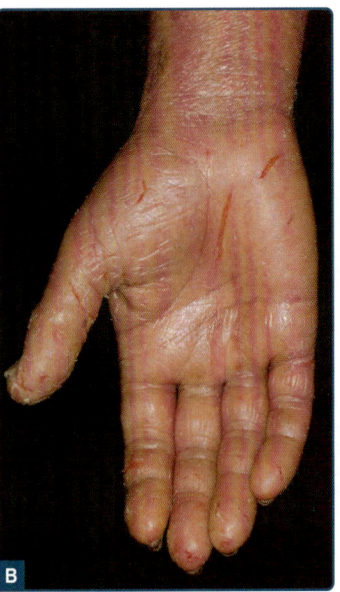
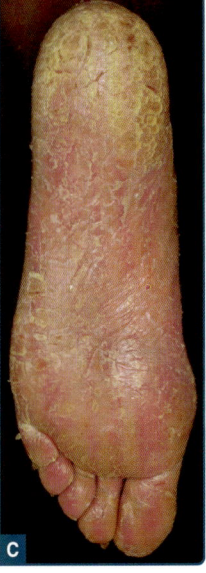

Figure 119-10 Sézary syndrome patient with erythroderma (**A**), palmar fissuring (**B**), and plantar hyperkeratosis (**C**).

TABLE 119-2
Subtypes and Variants of Mycosis Fungoides

SUBTYPES	
Erythrodermic mycosis fungoides (MF)	Develops de novo or as a progression of MF; > 80% involvement of skin surface
Hypopigmented mycosis fungoides	Common in darkly pigmented individuals; response to therapy characterized by repigmentation. Vitiligo is a differential diagnosis

repigmentation, and the reappearance of hypopigmented lesions often indicates a relapse.

HISTOPATHOLOGY

Figure 119-11 shows the characteristic histology of MF. In the patch, plaque, and also in the erythrodermic stage, there is a band-like infiltrate in the upper dermis composed of reactive T cells and neoplastic T lymphocytes, which are characterized by hyperconvoluted cerebriform nuclei. The neoplastic T cells show an epidermotropism with formation of intraepidermal Pautrier microabscesses (Figs. 119-12 and 119-13). In the tumor stage, a nodular infiltrate in the dermis is found, and the epidermal component is much less pronounced (Fig. 119-14). Immunohistologically, the malignant cells express a mature peripheral T-cell (CD4+) phenotype. Partial loss of pan–T-cell antigens such as CD7 and CD3 may be a feature of MF, but is not pathognomonic of the disease. Analysis of TCR genes typically shows a clonal rearrangement as demonstrated by polymerase chain reaction or Southern blot techniques. However, a T-cell clone is only found in half the biopsies in early stages of disease.

Thus, neither molecular tests for T-cell clonality nor phenotypic marker are of significant diagnostic value in early MF. Maybe in the near future modern molecular diagnostics, such as high-throughput technology, will be capable of detecting T-cell clones even in early MF.

Table 119-3 presents an algorithm for diagnosis of early MF.

TOX (thymocyte selection-associated high-mobility group box factor) is associated with development of CD4+, CD8– T cells in the thymus, but is suppressed in mature CD4+ T cells. It is aberrantly expressed in MF and Sézary syndrome. It was thought to help in discriminating between early MF lesions and biopsy from inflammatory skin disorders. According to recent data it could contribute the diagnosis of CTCL; however, TOX expression is not restricted to CD4+, CD8– neoplastic T cells.[61]

Table 119-4 summarizes the recommended evaluation/initial staging of the patient with MF/Sézary syndrome.

DIFFERENTIAL DIAGNOSIS

Table 119-5 summarizes the differential diagnosis of MF.

TREATMENT AND PROGNOSIS

Treatment should be stage adapted. In early disease stages, treatment should be based on skin-directed therapies alone or combined with systemic biologic response modifiers (eg, interferon α or γ, retinoids). Targeted therapies and small molecules are gaining favor as ways to debulk tumors and blood compartments as an alternative for chemotherapy approaches (see sec-

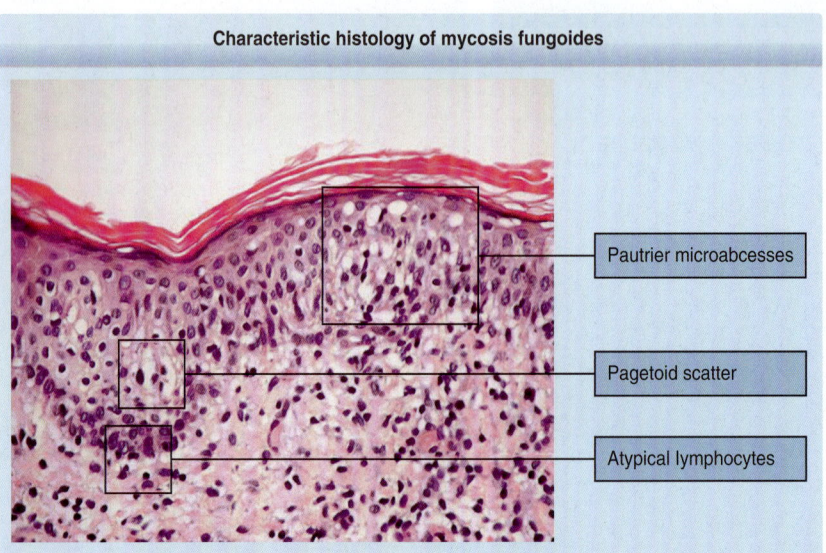

Figure 119-11 Characteristic histology of mycosis fungoides.

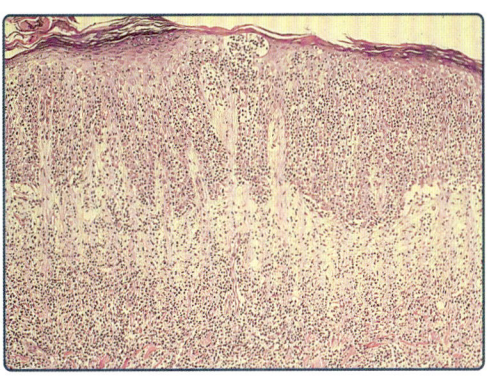

Figure 119-12 Dense mononuclear cell infiltrate extending from the papillary dermis into the epidermis. The epidermis is completely permeated by these cells, which form a Pautrier abscess.

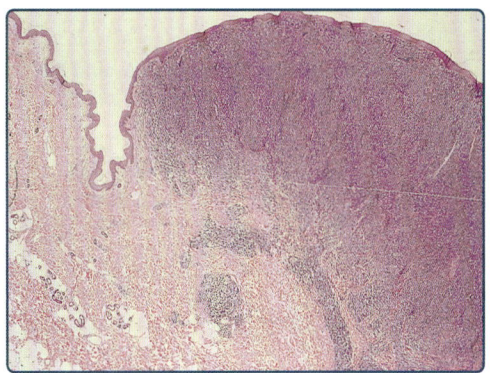

Figure 119-14 Low-power view of a mycosis fungoides tumor. The dense infiltrate extends deep into the dermis.

tions "Staging of Cutaneous T-Cell Lymphoma" and "Principles of Treatment of Cutaneous T-Cell Lymphoma"). Prognosis depends on the type and extent of skin involvement (plaque, tumor, or erythroderma), the presence of lymph node involvement, and the presence of visceral disease. Among early stage patients, 25% will progress to advanced stage. Overall, patients with MF limited to the skin have a 5-year survival rate of 80% to 100%. In contrast, patients with lymph node involvement show a 5-year survival rate of 40%.[62]

The Cutaneous Lymphoma International Consortium study published survival data and analysis based on 1275 patients with advanced MF and Sézary syndrome. The median overall survival was 63 months with 2-year and 5-year survival rates of 77% and 52%, respectively. The median overall survival for patients with Stage IIB disease was 86 months, but patients diagnosed with Stage III disease have slightly improved survival compared with patients with Stage IIB disease. Patients diagnosed with Stage IV disease had a significantly

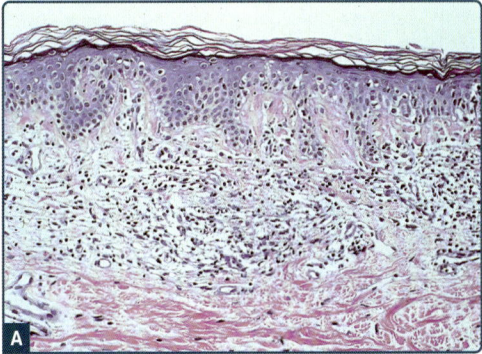

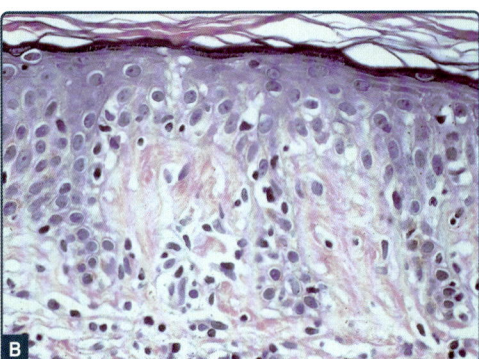

Figure 119-13 Patch stage of mycosis fungoides. **A,** Single atypical mononuclear cells in epidermis with sparse superficial perivascular infiltrate in the papillary dermis. (Hematoxylin and eosin-stained section.) **B,** High-power view of atypical cells in epidermis of same section.

TABLE 119-3
Algorithm for Diagnosis of Early Mycosis Fungoides

CRITERIA SCORING SYSTEM

- Clinical
  - Basic 2 points for basic criteria and 2 additional criteria
  - Persistent and/or progressive patches/thin plaques 1 point for basic criteria and 1 additional criterion
  - Additional
    - Non–sun-exposed location
    - Size/shape variation
    - Poikiloderma
- Histopathologic
  - Basic 2 points for basic criteria and 2 additional criteria
  - Superficial lymphoid infiltrate 1 point for basic criteria and 1 additional criterion
  - Additional
    - Epidermotropism without spongiosis
    - Lymphoid atypia
- Molecular biological
  - Clonal TCR gene rearrangement 1 point for clonality
- Immunopathologic
  - <50% CD2+, CD3+, and/or CD5+ T cells 1 point for 1 or more criteria
  - <10% CD7+ T cells
  - Epidermal/dermal discordance of CD2, CD3, CD5, or CD7

A total of 4 points is required for the diagnosis of MF based on any combination of points from the clinical, histopathologic, molecular biologic, and immunopathologic criteria

From Pimpinelli N, Olsen EA, Santucci M, et al. Defining early mycosis fungoides. *J Am Acad Dermatol.* 2005;53:1053-1063, with permission. Copyright © American Academy of Dermatology.

TABLE 119-4
Recommended Evaluation/Initial Staging of the Patient with Mycosis Fungoides/Sézary Syndrome

- Evaluation of skin lesions; measure of the percentages of body surface area of patches, plaques, and tumors
- Evaluation of localization and measures of lymph nodes
- Clinical identification of visceral disease
- Histology and immunohistology of skin lesions, and evaluation for T-cell clonality
- Histology and immunohistology of enlarged lymph nodes, and evaluation for T-cell clonality
- Blood cell count, lactate dehydrogenase, liver function tests
- Blood T-cell clonality
- Sézary cell count by cytomorphology and/or flow cytometric analysis of T-cell blood subpopulations (CD4+/CD7– and CD4+CD26–)
- Early-stage patients: chest radiograph and ultrasound of abdomen
- Late-stage patients: CT scan of chest, abdomen, and pelvis

worse survival (48 months for Stage IVA and 33 months for Stage IVB). Of 10 variables tested, 4 (Stage IV, age >60 years, large-cell transformation, and increased lactate dehydrogenase) were independent prognostic markers for worse survival. Combining these 4 factors for a prognostic index model led to the identification of 3 risk groups across stages, with significantly different 5-year survival rates: low risk (0-1) 68%, intermediate risk (2) 44%, and high risk (3-4) 28%.[63]

MYCOSIS FUNGOIDES VARIANTS

Table 119-6 outlines the clinical findings and prognosis for MF and variants.

TABLE 119-5
Differential Diagnosis of Mycosis Fungoides

Patch/Plaque Stage
- "Chronic dermatitis"
- Psoriasis
- Contact dermatitis
- Eczema
- Tinea corporis
- Vitiligo

Tumor Stage
- B-cell lymphoma
- Carcinoma cutis
- Sarcoidosis
- Deep fungal infection
- Atypical mycobacterial infection
- Leprosy
- Leishmaniasis
- Erythroderma
- Pityriasis rubra pilaris
- Psoriasis
- Atopic dermatitis
- Drug eruption
- Seborrheic dermatitis

FOLLICULOTROPIC MYCOSIS FUNGOIDES

Compared to classic MF, follicular or folliculotropic MF has classically been considered to carry a worse prognosis with 5-year survival rates of approximately 60% (follicular MF) and 41% (folliculotropic MF) by 15 years.

Clinically, folliculotropic MF presents with patches, plaques, and unusual hair loss within the lesions; occasionally, the disease may manifest with predominantly papular lesions. Folliculotropic MF preferentially involves the head and neck region and is characterized by folliculotropic T-cell infiltrates, with or without mucinous degeneration of the hair follicles. Previously, this variant was called *follicular mucinosis* or *alopecia mucinosa*. Folliculotropic MF affects mostly adults and is rarely observed in children and adolescents. Patients may have grouped follicular papules (Fig. 119-15A), acneiform lesions, indurated plaques, and, sometimes, tumors, which usually involve the head and neck region. The occurrence of hair loss within the lesions, most conspicuous on the eyebrows, an intense pruritus, and secondary bacterial infection are common.

It is important to mention that 2 newer studies show that it is possible to distinguish 2 different types of folliculotropic MF, including a subtype with a favorable prognosis.[64,65]

Distinction of folliculotropic MF-associated follicular mucinosis from benign (idiopathic follicular mucinosis) remains challenging. Although folliculotropic MF more probably displays a dense lymphocytic infiltrate with slight nuclear atypia, increased CD4-to-CD8 ratio, and a clonal rearrangement of TCR genes, the histologic or phenotypic features do not allow separating the 2 entities with certainty.

PAGETOID RETICULOSIS

Patients with pagetoid reticulosis present with a solitary psoriasiform or hyperkeratotic patch or plaque, which is usually localized on the extremities (Fig. 119-16) and is slowly progressive. Unlike in classic MF, extracutaneous dissemination has not been observed.

Pagetoid reticulosis, listed as an MF subtype in the WHO classification, shows more prominent epidermotropism and nuclear pleomorphism compared with unilesional MF, and more commonly shows a CD8+ phenotype. Furthermore, pagetoid reticulosis manifests more often as a hyperkeratotic lesion.

GRANULOMATOUS SLACK SKIN

Granulomatous slack skin is a rare subtype of MF characterized by localized areas of bulky folding of skin, with a predilection for the axillae and groin (Fig. 119-17). Light microscopy reveals a dense granulomatous infiltrate in the entire dermis. In addition to small, atypical cells with cerebriform nuclei, one

TABLE 119-6
Clinical Findings and Prognosis for Mycosis Fungoides and Variants

	CLINICAL FINDINGS	PROGNOSIS (5-YEAR SURVIVAL RATE)
Mycosis fungoides (skin limited)	Single-to-multiple erythematous scaly macules and patches on non–sun-exposed sites; plaques appear sharply demarcated, scaly, violaceous, and indurated; tumors have a predilection for the face and body folds	80%-100%
Mycosis fungoides (lymph node involvement)		40%
Folliculotropic mycosis fungoides	Characterized by patches, plaques, and hair loss within lesions; preferential involvement of head and neck	More aggressive than early mycosis fungoides; 60%
Pagetoid reticulosis	A solitary, hyperkeratotic plaque, usually on an extremity	Generally indolent behavior, recurrences and relapses may occur[a,b]
Granulomatous slack skin	Localized areas of bulky folding of the skin, on axillae and groins	Indolent course, slowly progressive with rare nodal involvement[a]
Sézary syndrome	Diffuse erythroderma, generalized lymphadenopathy, presence of circulating Sézary cells	24%-43%

[a]Martinez-Escala ME, Gonzales BR, Guitart J. Mycosis fungoides variants. *Surg Pathol Clin.* 2014;7(2):169-89.
[b]Haghighi B, Smoller B, LeBoit P, et al. Pagetoid reticulosis (Woringer-Kolopp disease): an immunophenotypic, molecular and clinicopathologic study. *Mod Pathol.* 2000;13(5):502-10.

finds macrophages and multinucleated giant cells and loss of elastic fibres. The neoplastic cells express a CD3+CD4+CD8– phenotype.

SÉZARY SYNDROME

DEFINITION

Sézary syndrome is characterized by the triad of diffuse erythroderma, generalized lymphadenopathy, and circulating malignant T cells with cerebriform nuclei, so-called Sézary cells.

Sézary syndrome is a rare form of CTCL, accounting for 3% of all cutaneous lymphomas. In contrast to MF, Sézary syndrome carries an unfavorable prognosis, with a 5-year overall survival varying from 24% to 43%.[1,63]

CLINICAL FINDINGS

The erythroderma is often accompanied by severe scaling or fissuring of the palms and soles (see Fig. 119-10), alopecia, and onychodystrophy, and may be associated with marked exfoliation, edema, lichenification, and intense pruritus. In rare cases, hyperpigmentation occurs.

LABORATORY FINDINGS

Sézary syndrome demonstrates histologic features similar to those of MF, but repeated biopsies may be necessary as specimens often show nondiagnostic findings. The clonal T cells are generally CD3+, CD4+, and CD8– by multicolor flow cytometry. As in MF, the aberrant loss of T-cell antigens, including CD2, CD3, CD4, CD5, and CD7, is frequently observed. Of these, loss

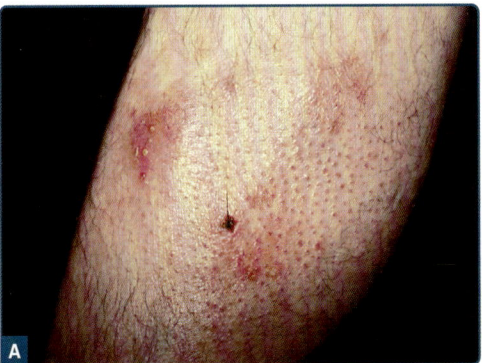 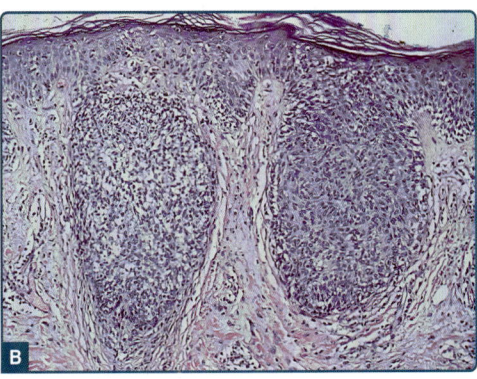

Figure 119-15 **A,** Folliculotropic mycosis fungoides. Note follicular localization and resulting hair loss. **B,** Outer root sheath of hair follicle is disrupted by T cells and mucin deposition, which leads to small cystic spaces.

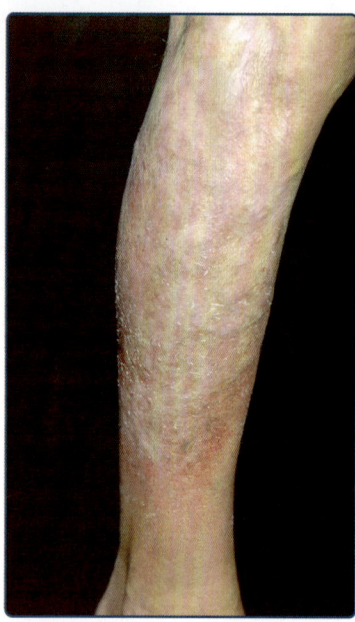

Figure 119-16 Pagetoid reticulosis. Hyperkeratotic plaque localized on the leg of a male patient.

phomas (ISCL)/EORTC TNMB staging classification, the diagnosis of Sézary syndrome requires an erythroderma with a positive T-cell clone in the peripheral blood associated with at least one B2 criterion, such as identification of more than 1000 Sézary cells/mm^3 in the blood. Sézary cells were first described in 1938 by Sézary as large, atypical, mononuclear cells with lobulated, cerebriform nuclei. However, detection of Sézary cells by cytomorphology lacks specificity for the diagnosis of Sézary syndrome as they can be found in other inflammatory erythrodermas. Other diagnosis criteria include an expanded CD4+ T-cell population resulting in a CD4-to-CD8 ratio of more than 10; loss of any or all of the T-cell antigens CD2, CD3, CD4, or CD5; and lack of CD7 and CD26.[66,67]

TREATMENT AND PROGNOSIS

Compared with patients with patch/plaque-stage MF, patients with Sézary syndrome have a markedly decreased 5-year survival rate. By the time the Sézary syndrome appears, there is very little normal immunity left. Indeed, Sézary syndrome patients often die because of infectious complications.

of CD7 expression is observed in approximately two-thirds of cases. Loss of CD26 expression, observed in the majority of cases, is also useful in the identification of Sézary cells. The aberrant expression of the major histocompatibility complex class I-binding, immunoglobulin-like receptor (KIR) CD158k/KIR3DL2, normally expressed by NK cells, was described in the majority of patients with Sézary syndrome. In the current International Society for Cutaneous Lym-

PRIMARY CUTANEOUS CD30+ LYMPHOPROLIFERATIVE DISORDERS

Primary cutaneous CD30+ lymphoproliferative disorders are the second most common form (20%-25%) of cutaneous lymphomas (CTCL). Primary cutaneous CD30+ lymphoproliferative disorders represent a spectrum of diseases, including lymphomatoid papulosis and primary cutaneous anaplastic large-cell lymphoma (ALCL).

LYMPHOMATOID PAPULOSIS

Definition: Lymphomatoid papulosis was first described by Macaulay in 1968. It is an uncommon chronic disorder (prevalence of 1.2-1.9 cases per 1,000,000 persons) characterized by recurrent, self-healing crops of papules and nodules.

Clinical Findings: Lymphomatoid papulosis is a chronic, recurrent, and self-healing papulonecrotic or papulonodular skin eruption (Fig. 119-18). The lesions typically involve the trunk and extremities, and lesions in various stages of evolution may be present concurrently.

Histopathology: Lymphomatoid papulosis is a clinically diverse disorder; in recent years a number of new pathologic and clinical variants have been described. The atypical cells express one or more T-cell

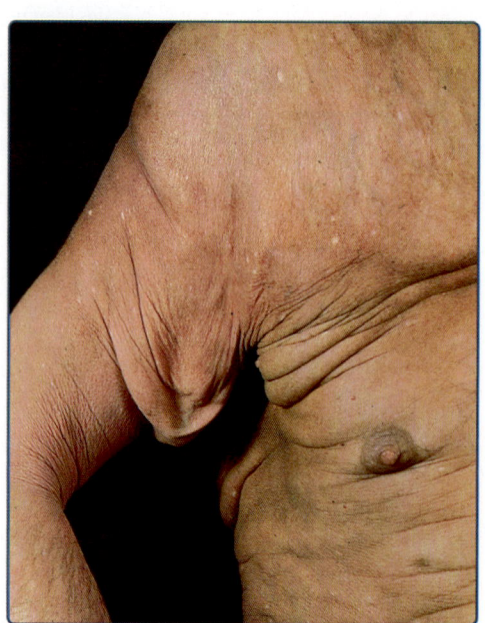

Figure 119-17 Granulomatous slack skin. Note skinfolds caused by secondary elastolysis.

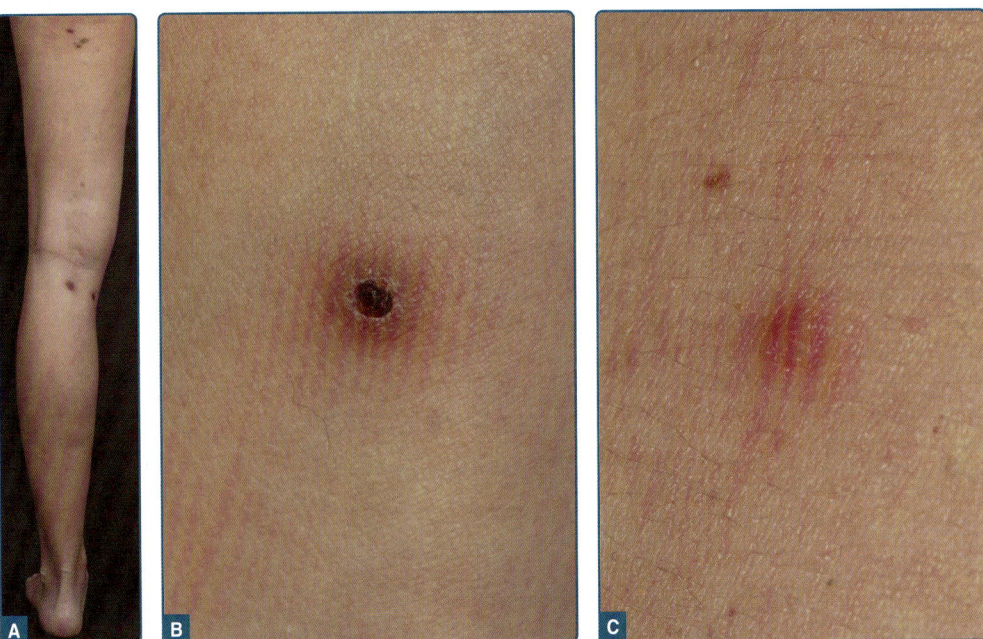

Figure 119-18 Lymphomatoid papulosis. **A,** Papular skin lesions on the right leg. The lesions may appear disseminated and grouped. **B,** Lymphomatoid papulosis papulonecrotic lesion. **C,** Lymphomatoid papulosis erythematous papulonodule.

antigens as well as the lymphoid activation antigen CD30 (Fig. 119-19).

The WHO 2016 classification recognizes the original variants Types A, B, and C, as well as the more recently described Type D (mimics primary cutaneous aggressive epidermotropic CD8+ cytotoxic T-cell lymphoma) and the angioinvasive, angiocentric Type E.

Lymphomatoid papulosis with chromosome 6p25 rearrangement (IRF4/DUSPP locus) was described by Karai et al, clinically characterized by localized papules and nodules, and histologically characterized by epidermotropic and nodular CD30+ cells. Appreciation of these variants is important, as histologically they can mimic very aggressive T-cell lymphomas, but they are clinically similar to other forms of lymphomatoid papulosis.[68,69]

Treatment and Prognosis: Because a curative therapy is not available and none of the available treatment modalities affects the natural course of the disease, the short-term benefits of active treatment should be balanced carefully against the potential side effects. Low-dose methotrexate (5-10 mg/week) is the most effective therapy to suppress development of new skin lesions. Treatment with PUVA has been reported to yield beneficial effects, but duration of response is often short-lived after discontinuation of treatment. Therefore, in patients with few, nonscarring lesions, long-term followup without active treatment should be considered.[70]

In general, lymphomatoid papulosis shows a benign clinical course and a favorable 10-year survival rate of nearly 100%. However, in a proportion of patients,

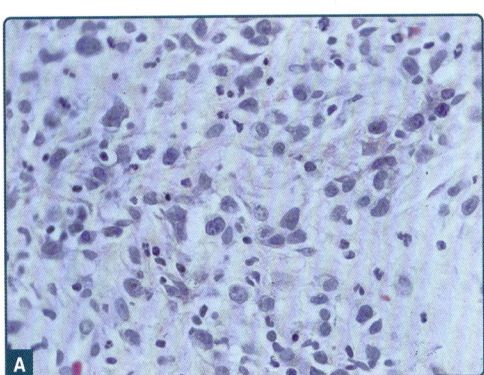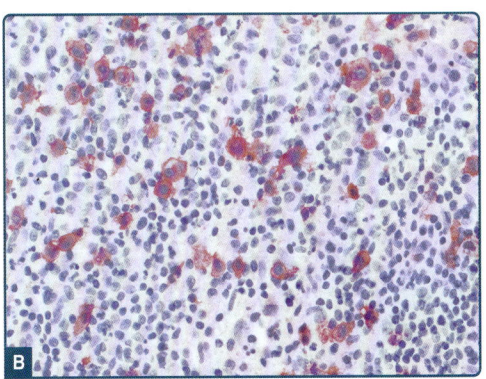

Figure 119-19 **A,** Lymphomatoid papulosis. Dermal infiltrate contains several large lymphoid cells with nuclei showing evenly dispersed chromatin and variably prominent nucleoli (so-called Type A cells). **B,** Type A with large CD30+ T cells (*red*) among admixed inflammatory cells.

estimated at 10% to 20% of cases, lymphomatoid papulosis can precede, coexist with, or follow malignant lymphoma, especially MF, Hodgkin lymphoma, and nodal ALCL. In many of these cases, the same clonal TCR rearrangements have been found in the lymphomatoid papulosis, as well as in the associated lymphoma. In the majority of lymphomatoid papulosis cases, despite the sometimes extremely long course of the disease, there is no evolution of a secondary lymphoma. Nevertheless, patients suffering from lymphomatoid papulosis should be monitored lifelong. In patients with lymphomatoid papulosis, monoclonal TCR rearrangement or histologic mixed-type may be prognostic for disease more likely to develop lymphomatoid papulosis–associated lymphomas.

CUTANEOUS ANAPLASTIC LARGE-CELL LYMPHOMA

Definition: Cutaneous ALCL is characterized by large tumor cells, of which the majority express the CD30 antigen, with no evidence or history of MF or other type of primary CTCL. Regardless of the morphology of the tumor cells (eg. anaplastic, immunoblastic, or pleomorphic large cells), the clinical presentation and behavior are identical.

Clinical Findings: CD30+ cutaneous large-cell lymphomas occur in adults and rarely in children and adolescents, with a male-to-female ratio of 1.5:1. The clinical picture is characterized by the solitary or locoregional occurrence of reddish-to-brownish nodules and tumors, which frequently ulcerate (Fig. 119-20A). Cutaneous lesions may regress spontaneously. Although secondary involvement of regional lymph nodes is observed in roughly 10% of patients, it is not necessarily associated with an unfavorable prognosis.

Histopathology: A nodular or diffuse nonepidermotropic infiltrate of large cells is seen in the dermis (see Fig. 119-20B). In the majority of cases, the neoplastic cells show an anaplastic morphology with oval or irregularly-shaped nuclei, prominent nucleoli, and an abundant cytoplasm. Less commonly, a pleomorphic or immunoblastic appearance is observed. Atypical mitotic figures are frequent. In the periphery of the lesions, inflammatory cells (eg. lymphocytes, eosinophils, and neutrophils) are present, sometimes mimicking the histologic picture seen in lymphomatoid papulosis.

The most common phenotype in primary cutaneous ALCL is that of a CD4+ T-helper phenotype. In rare cases, tumor cells express CD8+, which does not seem to be associated with an impaired prognosis. By definition, more than 75% of the tumor cells express CD30 in cohesive sheets. In contrast to nodal ALCL, which expresses anaplastic lymphoma kinase (ALK) in approximately 60% of cases, primary cutaneous ALCLs are usually negative for this marker and lack the translocation t(2;5). Unusual cases of ALK+ primary cutaneous ALCL that are associated with a translocation variant and cytoplasmic staining for ALK have been reported.

Improved criteria now exist for the recognition of ALK– ALCL in daily practice, and the actual WHO 2016 classification no longer considers this type provisional. Gene expression profiling studies show that ALK– ALCL has a signature quite close to that of ALK+ ALCL and distinct from NK/T-cell lymphomas. Newer studies illuminating the genetic landscape of ALK– ALCL have shown convergent mutations and kinase fusions that lead to constitutive

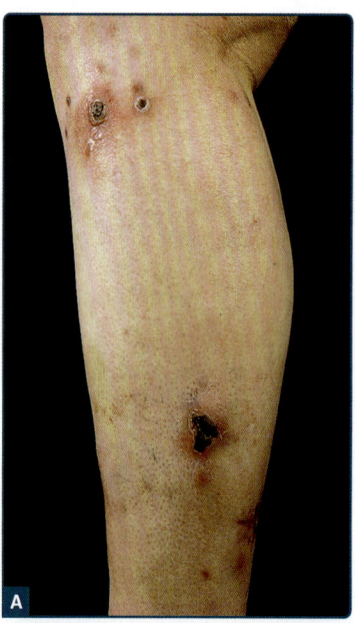

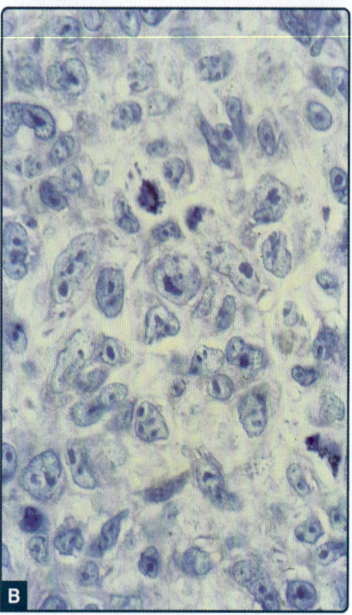

Figure 119-20 Primary cutaneous anaplastic large-cell lymphoma. **A,** Localized nodules, some with ulcerations. **B,** Pleomorphic large-cell lymphoma T-cell infiltrate.

activation of the JAK/STAT3 pathways. These studies provide a genetic rationale for the morphologic and phenotypic similarities between ALK+ and ALK– ALCL. However, not all cases of ALK– ALCL are created equal. A subset with rearrangements at the locus containing DUSP22-IRF4 in chromosome 6p25 tends to be relatively monomorphic, usually lacks cytotoxic granules, and is reported to have a better prognosis, whereas a small subset with TP63 rearrangement is very aggressive. Interestingly, the same locus in 6p25 is also implicated in lymphomatoid papulosis and primary cutaneous ALCL.[3,69,71,72]

Treatment and Prognosis: In cases of solitary or localized skin lesions, excision or radiotherapy is the treatment of choice. A successful treatment with PUVA in combination with interferon-α has been reported. If skin lesions are generalized, systemic therapy with methotrexate (20 mg/week) is preferred; vinblastine is an alternative option.

In the case of extracutaneous dissemination, treatment with cyclophosphamide, doxorubicin, vincristine, and prednisone (CHOP) is the most frequently chosen option. Brentuximab vedotin can also be regarded as a therapy of choice. This immunoconjugate is an anti-CD30 monoclonal antibody linked to monomethyl auristatin, a spindle-cell toxin that induces cell-cycle arrest. A 100% response of primary cutaneous ALCL was observed with this treatment.

In contrast to nodal ALCL, cutaneous CD30+ large-cell lymphomas have a favorable prognosis, with a disease-related 5-year survival rate of 90%.

SUBCUTANEOUS PANNICULITIS-LIKE T-CELL LYMPHOMA

Definition: Subcutaneous panniculitis-like T-cell lymphoma is defined as a cytotoxic T-cell lymphoma characterized by the presence of primarily subcutaneous infiltrates of small, medium, or large pleomorphic αβ T cells and many macrophages that predominantly affect the legs and are occasionally complicated by a hemophagocytic syndrome. Subcutaneous lymphomas with a γδ phenotype of the TCR show a more aggressive course and are classified within the cutaneous γδ T-cell lymphomas.

Clinical Findings: This lymphoma accounts for 1% of all cutaneous lymphoma and for 75% of all subcutaneous forms of T-cell lymphoma. In the revised WHO 2016 classification, this term is, by definition, restricted to cases expressing a TCR α/β phenotype.

Subcutaneous panniculitis-like T-cell lymphoma is characterized by subcutaneous nodules and plaques, which usually involve the extremities, the trunk, and, less commonly, the face. Patients may present with "B" symptoms, that is, weight loss, fever, and fatigue.

Histopathology: Histologic examination shows subcutaneous infiltrates simulating a lobular panniculitis. Infiltrates contain a mixture of neoplastic pleomorphic cells of various sizes and macrophages. Rimming of individual fat cells by neoplastic T cells is a helpful diagnostic feature.

Immunophenotyping shows that the neoplastic cells express CD3+, CD4–, CD8+, CD56–, TIA-1+, granzyme-β+, and βF1+. The expression of βF1 (TCR α/β) by immunohistochemistry is a pivotal diagnostic marker for this entity.

Treatment and Prognosis: The α/β type of the subcutaneous panniculitis-like T-cell lymphoma responds well to systemic corticosteroids with an excellent prognosis (a 5-year survival rate of 85%), which justifies an initial treatment approach with corticosteroids alone.[73-75]

EXTRANODAL NATURAL KILLER/ T-CELL LYMPHOMA, NASAL TYPE

Definition: Extranodal NK/T-cell lymphoma, nasal type, is a rare, aggressive form of primary cutaneous lymphoma that shares immunophenotypical characteristics with normal NK cells and characteristically displays a strong expression of CD56 and cytotoxic proteins, such as perforin, granzyme B, and TIA-1. This lymphoma is nearly always EBV+. The tumor cells are small, medium, or large, and usually have an NK cell or, more rarely, a cytotoxic T-cell phenotype.

The skin is the second most common site of presentation after the nasal cavity.

Clinical Findings: Extranodal NK/T-cell lymphoma either affects the nasopharynx, which leads to destruction of the nasal region (formerly described as lethal midline granuloma), or manifests in skin, subcutis, lungs, viscera, and testes. Skin lesions comprise subcutaneous tumors, erythematous plaques, ulcers, or an exanthematous eruption with macules and papules (Fig. 119-21). The clinical course is often worsened by a hemophagocytic syndrome with pancytopenia.

Histopathology: This type of lymphoma shows dense infiltrates involving the dermis and often the subcutis. Epidermotropism may be present. Prominent angiocentricity and angiodestruction are often accompanied by extensive necrosis (Fig. 119-22). Immunophenotypically, the neoplastic cells express CD56 and cytotoxic proteins (TIA-1, granzyme B, perforin), and are characteristically positive for EBV. The TCR–CD3 complex is not expressed on the surface. Clonal episome presence of EBV is typically found. TCR genes are usually in germline configuration.[3,76]

Treatment and Prognosis: Even with aggressive polychemotherapy, the disease is often lethal within months. A study of the EORTC cutaneous lymphoma group suggested that bone marrow transplantation may be the treatment of choice.

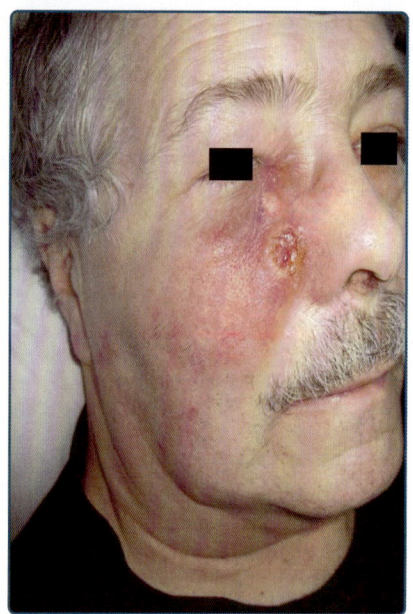

Figure 119-21 Extranodal natural killer/T-cell lymphoma, nasal type. Infiltrated and ulcerated plaque.

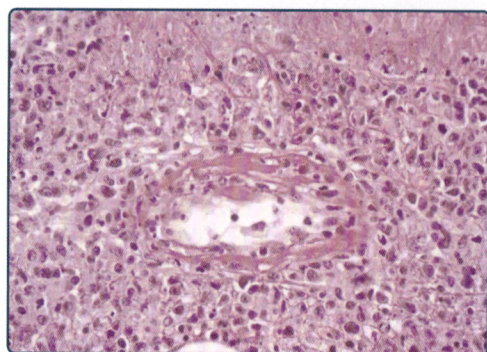

Figure 119-22 Extranodal natural killer/T-cell lymphoma, nasal type. Dense angiocentric infiltrate.

sized pleomorphic cells is observed within the dermis and, sometimes, the subcutis. Epidermotropism may be present. The neoplastic cells express a T-helper cell phenotype with frequent loss of pan–T-cell markers. Demonstration of an aberrant phenotype and of T-cell clonality, as well as predominance of pleomorphic T cells in the infiltrate, serve as useful criteria for the exclusion of pseudolymphomas, which often show an identical histologic pattern. MF is excluded by the absence of a dominant cerebriform tumor cell population.

Treatment and Prognosis: Solitary lesions are often excised for diagnostic purposes. If excision is not possible or lesions are localized, radiotherapy is the preferred mode of treatment. PUVA therapy, possibly in combination with interferon (IFN)-α, is useful in cases with disseminated lesions.

A 5-year survival rate between 60% and 90% is reported for this type of lymphoma.[77-79]

PROVISIONAL ENTITIES OF CUTANEOUS T-CELL LYMPHOMA

DEFINITION

In addition to the diseases discussed in preceding sections, a number of provisional entities are included in the revised WHO classification system. These primary CTCLs display characteristic clinical and histologic features, but the series reported remain limited and do not allow definition of a precise outcome.

PRIMARY CUTANEOUS CD4+ SMALL AND MEDIUM T-CELL LYMPHOPROLIFERATIVE DISORDER

Definition: This entity is defined clinically by papules and nodules, and histologically by a skin infiltrate composed of pleomorphic, small- and medium-sized T cells. The outcome is usually favorable but limited series have been reported.

Clinical Findings: Patients have one or several red-purplish papules or nodules with a predilection for the head and neck area. Because histologic differentiation from MF and MF-associated follicular mucinosis can raise problems, the absence of patches and plaques in pleomorphic small- and medium-sized CTCL is an important criterion.

Histopathology: Histologically, a dense, diffuse or nodular infiltrate containing small- to medium-

PRIMARY CUTANEOUS AGGRESSIVE EPIDERMOTROPIC CD8+ CYTOTOXIC T-CELL LYMPHOMA

Definition: Primary cutaneous aggressive epidermotropic CD8+ cytotoxic T-cell lymphoma is a CTCL characterized by a proliferation of CD8+ cytotoxic T cells that exhibit a strong epidermotropism and aggressive clinical behavior. Differentiation from other types of CTCL expressing a CD8+ cytotoxic T-cell phenotype, as observed in pagetoid reticulosis and rare cases of MF, lymphomatoid papulosis, and cutaneous ALCL, is based on clinical presentation, histopathology, and clinical behavior.

Clinical Findings: Primary cutaneous aggressive epidermotropic CD8+ T-cell lymphoma presents with hyperkeratotic patches and plaques, well-demarcated papules and tumors, or ulcerations. A metastatic spread to unusual sites, such as the lung, testis, CNS, and oral cavity, but not to the lymph nodes, is often observed.

Histopathology: Histologically, band-like infiltrates consisting of pleomorphic lymphocytes or immunoblasts are observed, displaying diffuse infiltration of the epidermis with variable degrees of spongiosis, intraepidermal blistering, and necrosis. The neoplastic cells express the Ki67 antigen at high frequency and are positive for CD3, CD8, CD45RA, and TIA, whereas CD2 and CD5 are frequently lost. Expression of TIA identifies these lymphomas derived from a cytotoxic T-cell subset.

Treatment and Prognosis: Even with multiagent chemotherapy, the disease shows an aggressive course and median survival is 32 months.[76,79,80]

CUTANEOUS γ/δ T-CELL LYMPHOMA

Definition: Cutaneous γ/δ T-cell lymphoma comprises the peripheral T-cell lymphomas with a clonal proliferation of mature, activated γ/δ T cells with a cytotoxic phenotype. This group includes cases previously termed *subcutaneous panniculitis-like T-cell lymphoma with a γ/δ phenotype*.[3]

Clinical Findings: Patients have disseminated ulceronecrotic nodules or tumors, particularly on the extremities, but other sites also may be affected. Involvement of mucosal and other extranodal sites is frequent, but involvement of lymph nodes, spleen, or bone marrow is uncommon. A hemophagocytic syndrome may occur.

Histopathology: Histologically, 3 major patterns of involvement can be present in the skin: epidermotropic, dermal, and subcutaneous. The neoplastic cells are generally medium to large with coarsely clumped chromatin. Large blastic cells with vesicular nuclei and prominent nucleoli are infrequent. Apoptosis and necrosis are common, often with vessel invasion. Immunohistologically, the tumor cells have a βF1−, CD3+, CD2+, CD5−, CD7+/−, CD56+ phenotype with strong expression of cytotoxic proteins. Most cases are CD4 or lack both CD4 and CD8, although CD8 may be expressed in some cases. In frozen sections, the cells are strongly positive for TCRδ (antibody testing is not available for paraffin sections). If only paraffin sections are available, the absence of βF1 may be used to conclude a γ/δ origin.[74,75]

Treatment and Prognosis: Most patients have aggressive disease resistant to multiagent chemotherapy and/or radiation therapy. Median survival is 15 months.

PRIMARY CUTANEOUS ACRAL CD8+ T-CELL LYMPHOPROLIFERATION

Definition: This entity is characterized by indolent cutaneous, CD8+ lymphoid proliferation originating predominately in the ear, with a favorable prognosis.

Clinical Features: Indolent cutaneous, CD8+ lymphoid proliferation, typically presents with solitary skin lesions on the face or at acral sites. Solitary papules or, in some cases, bilateral plaques, have been described on the feet.

Histopathology: Histologically, indolent CD8+ lymphoid proliferations are characterized by a dense dermal infiltrate of nonepidermotropic, medium-sized pleomorphic clonal CD8+ T cells, mostly of the nonactivated cytotoxic phenotype, showing, in the majority of cases, a clear cut grenz zone and a low proliferation index.

Differentiation from otherwise aggressive T-cell lymphomas bearing a cytotoxic CD8+ phenotype is fundamental to avoid unnecessary anxiety for the patient and unwarranted aggressive treatment that would be considered as part of the therapeutic algorithm for the CD8+ phenotype.

It has recently been suggested that CD68 could be a new discriminative marker, helpful in distinguishing indolent CD8+ lymphoid proliferation from other CD8+ cutaneous lymphomas in ambiguous cases.

Treatment and Prognosis: Treatment is based on local excision or radiation therapy. Complete remission lasts for years and the prognosis is excellent.[81]

STAGING OF CUTANEOUS T-CELL LYMPHOMA

After establishing the diagnosis of a CTCL, appropriate staging investigations are mandatory to exclude secondary involvement of the skin by an extracutaneous lymphoma and to determine the extent of disease. The first classification and staging system of CTCLs was published in 1979 by the MF Cooperative Group. It is recognized that this staging system does not apply to all CTCL types listed in the current WHO classification. Furthermore, the Ann Arbor system, commonly used for staging of nodal non-Hodgkin lymphomas, is not suitable for all CTCL types. Because of these facts and new data on prognostic factors, both revisions of the staging and classification for MF and Sézary syndrome and a TNM (tumor, node, metastasis) classification system for cutaneous lymphomas other than MF and Sézary syndrome have been proposed by the EORTC and the ISCL. It has to be mentioned that staging according to the TNM system has been proven to be useful for choosing an appropriate therapy for patients with MF and Sézary syndrome, but data correlating results of the TNM staging and prognosis are missing for some types of CTCLs. Staging examination for all types of CTCLs includes examination of the entire skin, chest radiography, and ultrasonography of abdominal organs and peripheral lymph nodes (cervical, axillary, and inguinal). Blood investigations should include complete blood cell count, clinical chemistry with liver enzymes, kidney function tests, and lactate dehydrogenase level, as well as T-cell clonality. Staging may be completed by CT scan and/or histologic and molecular (TCR rearrangement) investigations of suspicious lymph nodes and/or visceral organs. Staging examination should be repeated at relapse or progression of disease. A bone marrow examination is only recommended at a B2 blood rating (Table 119-7) or where there are unexplained hematologic abnormalities. However, this procedure is not of direct clinical relevance, as detection of atypical cells in the bone marrow is not an independent prognostic factor.

The aforementioned investigations allow for classification according to the TNM system (see Tables 119-4 and 119-7). Although the prognostic value and applicability of TNM staging for different CTCLs is controversial, the TNM scheme directs the decision-making process toward an appropriate therapeutic regimen for most CTCLs.

TABLE 119-7
Staging System for Mycosis Fungoides and Sézary Syndrome

STAGE	T (TUMOR)	N (LYMPH NODE)	M (METASTASES)	B (BLOOD)
IA	T1	N0	M0	B0 or B1
IB	T2	N0	M0	B0 or B1
IIA	T1 or T2	N1 or N2	M0	B0 or B1
IIB	T3	N0-N2	M0	B0 or B1
III	T4	N0-N2	M0	B0 or B1
IIIA	T4	N0-N2	M0	B0
IIIB	T4	N0-N2	M0	B1
IVA1	T1-T4	N0-N2	M0	B2
IVA2	T1-T4	N3	M0	B0-B2
IVB	T1-T4	N0-N3	M1	B0-B2

T1, patch/plaque on ≤10% of body surface; T2, patch/plaque on ≥10% of body surface; T3, skin tumor(s); T4, erythroderma; N0, normal nodes; N1, palpable nodes without clear histologic evidence of lymphoma (for N1 and N2, "a" or "b" may be added for either no [a] or detection [b] of a T-cell clone by Southern blot or polymerase chain reaction [PCR] analysis); N2, palpable nodes, histologic evidence of lymphoma, node architecture preserved; N3, palpable nodes with histologic evidence of lymphoma, effacement of node architecture; M0, no visceral involvement; M1, histologically confirmed visceral involvement. B0, ≤5% Sézary cells (for B0 and B1, "a" or "b" may be added for either no [a] or detection [b] of a T-cell clone by Southern blot or PCR analysis); B1, >5% Sézary cells but either less than 1.0 K/μL absolute Sézary cells or absence of a clonal rearrangement of the TCR or both; clonal rearrangement of the TCR in the blood and either 1.0 K/μL or more Sézary cells or one of the following 2: (a) increased CD4+ or CD3+ cells with CD4/CD8 of 10 or more or (b) increase in CD4+ cells with an abnormal phenotype (>40% CD4+/CD7− or >30% CD4+/CD26−).

PRINCIPLES OF TREATMENT OF CUTANEOUS T-CELL LYMPHOMA

Every successful strategy in managing CTCL begins with the correct diagnosis and staging. The prognosis and survival of patients does not only vary based on the type of cutaneous lymphoma but also on the stage; each lymphoma has its own best treatment to date, which is primarily stage based. Current staging is based on the proposal of the ISCL and the Cutaneous Lymphoma Task Force of the EORTC as published in the journal *Blood* in 2007.[66]

Table 119-8 outlines the international staging system for cutaneous lymphomas other than MF and Sézary syndrome.

Once the individual classification of TNMB (tumor, node, metastasis, blood) has been determined, then these cases can be rolled into the staging system for MF and Sézary syndrome.

To assess the response to a given treatment, a consensus statement of criteria was established by the International Society of Cutaneous T-cell Lymphomas, the United States Cutaneous Lymphoma Consortium, and the Cutaneous Lymphoma Task Force of the EORTC, and published in 2011.[82] A global response score for MF and Sézary syndrome was established that addresses the entire TNMB spectrum, not only the response in the skin. However, as of this writing, there are still some problems regarding staging and prediction of survival. Indeed, survival does not always correlate with conventional staging: there is an overlap between Stages IIB versus III, and IB with folliculotropic MF.

Many prognostic factors are still outside the staging system and have to be evaluated in prognostic trials.

As of this writing, the most valid prognostic factors are age older than 60 years, tumor burden, and large-cell transformation. A prognostic index model was published by Scarisbrick et al.[63]

The chronic disease course of the most frequently occurring CTCL subtypes, MF and Sézary syndrome, makes surrogate markers necessary and tumor burden is still the best surrogate marker for survival. Additional measures of symptoms, like pruritus or quality-of-life assessments, are commonly used; skin scores provide a measure of objective responses to therapy; and questionnaires guide the assessment of subjective responses to therapy. It has not been shown that reducing disease in a patient from T3 to T1 is accompanied by any survival benefit, yet it is also recognized that a cure is unattainable unless the patient is first in remission with a skin score of 0 by whatever skin scoring system is used. Thus, remission is the first step toward cure.

Treatment of CTCL ideally requires a multidisciplinary team that includes dermatologists, radiation oncologists, and hematological-medical oncologists. The National Comprehensive Cancer Network, the EORTC, and the European Medical Society of Oncology have developed treatment guidelines that might be helpful in guiding therapeutic strategies. With a chronic disease like CTCL, supportive care, addressing quality of life, and reducing symptoms like pruritus and skin infections are mandatory for improving the quality of life of patients with CTCL.[83,84]

TABLE 119-8
Staging System for Cutaneous Lymphomas Other Than Mycosis Fungoides and Sézary Syndrome

T (Tumor)
- T1: solitary skin involvement
  - T1a: a solitary lesion with a diameter <5 cm
  - T1b: a solitary lesion with a diameter >5 cm
- T2: regional skin involvement: multiple lesions limited to 1 body region or 2 contiguous body regions[a]
  - T2a: all-disease-encompassing in a circular area with a diameter <15 cm
  - T2b: all-disease-encompassing in a circular area with a diameter >15 but <30 cm
  - T2c: all-disease-encompassing in a circular area with a diameter >30 cm
- T3: generalized skin involvement
  - T3a: multiple lesions involving 2 noncontiguous body regions
  - T3b: multiple lesions involving ≥3 body regions

N (Lymph Node)
- N0: No clinical or pathologic lymph node involvement
- N1: Involvement of 1 peripheral lymph node region[b] that drains an area of current or prior skin involvement
- N2: Involvement of 2 or more peripheral lymph node regions[b] or involvement of any lymph node region that does not drain an area of current or prior skin involvement
- N3: Involvement of central lymph nodes

M (Metastases)
- M0: No evidence of extracutaneous non–lymph node disease
- M1: Extracutaneous non–lymph node disease present

[a]Definition of body regions.[61]
[b]Definition of lymph node regions is consistent with the Ann Arbor system: Peripheral sites: antecubital, cervical, supraclavicular, axillary, inguinal-femoral, and popliteal. Central sites: mediastinal, pulmonary hilar, paraaortic, iliac.

Table 119-9 outlines treatment algorithms for MF and Sézary syndrome.

TREATMENT OF EARLY STAGE MYCOSIS FUNGOIDES

Treatment of early stage MF usually involves skin-directed therapy, with or without systemic therapy. Established skin-directed therapy approaches consist of UVB phototherapy, PUVA phototherapy, topical corticosteroids, topical chlormethine, topical retinoids (eg, bexarotene), and radiation (eg, external beam radiotherapy and total skin electron beam therapy).

IMIQUIMOD AND RESIQUIMOD

Imiquimod and resiquimod are novel topical immune response modifiers belonging to the imidazoquinoline family of drugs. They are Toll-like receptor agonists that, when used topically or injected into lesions or tumors, may cause systemic effects. Both imiquimod and resiquimod induce synthesis and release of the cytokines IFN-α, tumor necrosis factor-α, IL-6, and IL-12 that all activate the adaptive immune response toward Th1 or the cell-mediated pathway, while inhibiting the Th2 pathway. Promising results have been reported with resiquimod.[85,86]

LOCAL AND TOTAL SKIN ELECTRON BEAM THERAPY

Total skin electron beam is perhaps the most effective of all skin-directed therapies. It is often used locally in patients with skin-limited disease, especially resistant plaques and tumors. Combined initial data of 11,065 patients with total skin electron beam therapy showed complete response rates close to 70%. Complete response rates are higher in patients with T1-limited disease where use of early, low-dose radiation toward solitary lesions may lead to a cure. However, total skin electron beam is usually reserved for patients with greater skin involvement than IA, especially for extensive plaques or for palliation of Sézary syndrome or prior to nonablative allogeneic stem cell transplantation.

In solitary nodules in Stage IIB disease, control may be achieved using a lower dose of 4 to 8 Gy administered for single refractory lesions or using low-dose 12 Gy total-body administration. Lower doses are effective and provide an opportunity for multiple treatments to be given without undue toxicity.[87-89]

MAINTENANCE THERAPY AND TOPICAL STEROID THERAPY

The concept of treating normal skin evolved from the clinical experiences with skin-directed therapies. There are 2 components to this approach: the treatment of normal skin during remission-induction skin-directed therapy and the treatment of normal skin during the remission-maintenance phase. Topical chemotherapy, PUVA, and total skin electron beam radiation all involve the exposure of normal skin as an integral component of their success in achieving remission. This success reflects the ability of the therapy to interrupt the critical skin-based phase of the lifecycle of a recirculating CTCL cell. Once remission has been achieved, normal skin can be maintained with lower doses and frequencies of the therapies used to clear it. Maintenance therapies have been described with PUVA, total skin application of nitrogen mustard, extracorporeal photochemotherapy (ECP), and IFN. The most commonly used maintenance therapy is PUVA or UVB irradiation. As a maintenance therapy, PUVA is initially administered at once-weekly intervals for 1 year. Beginning with the second year of treatment, the schedule is changed to every other week for another year, to every third week for the following year, and, finally, to every fourth week for 2 years. At this point, the patient should have been in remission for 5 years. Consideration should be given to stopping

TABLE 119-9
Treatment Algorithms for Mycosis Fungoides and Sézary Syndrome

		LEVEL OF EVIDENCE
Recommendations for First-Line Treatment of Mycosis Fungoides (MF) Stages IA, IB, and IIA		
Expectant policy (mainly T1a)		Level 4
SDT[a]	Topical corticosteroids (mainly T1a and T2a)	Level 3
	UVB (ultraviolet B) (mainly T1a and T2a)	Level 2
	PUVA (psoralen and ultraviolet A)	Level 2
	Localized radiotherapy (RT) (for localized MF including pagetoid reticulosis)	Level 4
Recommendations for Second-Line Treatment of MF Stages IA, IB, and IIA		
Systemic therapies[b]		
	Retinoids[c]	Level 2
	Interferon (IFN)-α	Level 2
Total skin electron beam (TSEB) (mainly T2b)		Level 2
Low-dose methotrexate (MTX)		Level 4
Recommendations for First-Line Treatment of MF Stage IIB		
Systemic therapies[b]		
	Retinoids[c]	Level 2
	IFN-α	Level 2
TSEB		Level 2
Monochemotherapy (gemcitabine, pegylated liposomal doxorubicin)		Level 4
Low-dose MTX		Level 4
Localized RT[d]		Level 4
Recommendations for Second-Line Treatment of MF Stage IIB		
Polychemotherapy[e]		Level 3
Allogeneic stem cell transplantation[f]		Level 3
Recommendations for First-Line Treatment of MF Stages IIIA and IIIB		
Systemic therapies[b]		
	Retinoids[c]	Level 2
	IFN-α	Level 2
Extracorporeal photochemotherapy (ECP)[g]		Level 3
Low-dose MTX		Level 4
TSEB		Level 2
Recommendations for Second-Line Treatment of MF Stages IIIA and IIIB		
Monochemotherapy (gemcitabine, pegylated liposomal doxorubicin)		Level 3
Allogeneic stem cell transplantation[h]		Level 3
Recommendations for Treatment of MF Stages IVA and IVB[i]		
Chemotherapy (gemcitabine, pegylated liposomal doxorubicin, CHOP, and CHOP-like polychemotherapy)[j]		Level 3
Radiotherapy (TSEB and localized)[k]		Level 4
Alemtuzumab (mainly in B2)		Level 4
Allogeneic stem cell transplantation		Level 3
Recommendations for First-Line Treatment of Sézary Syndrome		
ECP[p]		Level 3
Chlorambucil + prednisone		Level 3
Systemic therapies in combination with ECP or PUVA		
	Retinoids[c]	Level 3
	IFN-α	Level 3
Low-dose MTX		Level 4

(Continued)

TABLE 119-9
Treatment Algorithms for Mycosis Fungoides and Sézary Syndrome (*Continued*)

	LEVEL OF EVIDENCE
Recommendations for Second-Line Treatment of Sézary Syndrome	
Chemotherapy (gemcitabine, pegylated liposomal doxorubicin, CHOP, and CHOP-like polychemotherapy)	Level 3
Alemtuzumab	Level 4
Allogeneic stem cell transplantation[h]	Level 3
Agents That Can Be Used for Maintenance After Remission Has Been Achieved in MF and Sézary Syndrome[i]	
ECP	
IFN-α	
Low-dose MTX	
Mechlorethamine	
PUVA	
Retinoids	
Topical corticosteroids	
UVB	

[a]Skin-directed therapy.
[b]The following agents are most commonly combined with PUVA; combinations with other modalities and with each other are also widely used.
[c]Including retinoic acid receptor (RAR) and retinoid X receptor (RXR) agonists.
[d]Used as add-on treatment in combination with systemic and other SDTs.
[e]CHOP (cyclophosphamide, doxorubicin, vincristine, and prednisone) is the most widely used regimen with a number of variants and other combinations available.
[f]Should be restricted to exceptional patients, see text for details.
[g]ECP can be used alone or in combination with skin-directed and other systemic therapies.
[h]Should be restricted to exceptional patients.
[i]For treatment of MF Stage IVA1, recommendations for Sézary syndrome might apply.
[j]Monochemotherapy should be preferentially used.
[k]Used alone or in combination with systemic therapies.
[l]Options are listed alphabetically and should be chosen to be effective, tolerable, easy to use, and efficient. Oxford Center for Evidence-Based Medicine levels are generally 5.
Adapted from Trautinger F, Eder J, Assaf C, et al. EORTC consensus recommendations for the treatment of mycosis fungoides/Sézary syndrome—update 2017. *Eur J Cancer.* 2017;77:57-74.

therapy at this point. A cure is defined as freedom from disease for 8 years off all therapy. This definition arose from the experience with nitrogen mustard treatment and total skin electron beam radiotherapy showing that after a patient achieves a remission off therapy for 5 to 8 years, late relapse is extremely rare. This would imply that malignant cutaneous T cells recirculate without causing lesions for up to 5 years. With 5 years of intermittent PUVA, it is less likely that one of these cells will survive, but it is still possible. After therapy has been discontinued, patients should not be considered cured unless they remain clear of disease for 8 years.[88,89]

The management of suspected relapse often includes the use of topical glucocorticoids and reflects the critical role this modality can play in the treatment of suspicious lesions. Early in the course of CTCL and in a relapse of the disease in a patient in remission, the T-cell activation process can be blunted by the aggressive use of topical glucocorticoids. Indeed, most patients have a history of using these agents before a firm diagnosis is made. A regimen for treating early lesions of MF is twice-daily applications of a class I topical glucocorticoid for 8 weeks. This regimen is one of the first-line modalities for suspected relapse, and it can help to identify those patients who need to undergo a 4-week "washout" before repeated biopsies are performed.

ERYTHRODERMA

In erythrodermic CTCLs, immune dysfunction and inflammatory processes initiated by the malignant cells result in total skin redness, scaling, and discomfort. It is not surprising that immune-based therapies take the forefront in the management of these disorders. The 3 major biologic response modifiers (BRMs) used in the treatment of erythrodermic CTCLs are (a) oral retinoids, (b) ECP via an intravenous route, and (c) subcutaneous injections of IFN-α (Table 119-10). In the clinical trials of these agents, patients have undergone monotherapy for what has usually been heavily pretreated refractory disease. In practice, these treatments are often used as first-line monotherapy in erythroderma, and other agents are incorporated for combination therapies if the response is incomplete. With these agents, partial responses are more common than complete responses. Thus, if the goal is remission, combination therapy is used more commonly than monotherapy. If the goal is palliation, monotherapy with a BRM is often sufficient. The BRMs differ in terms of their administration, side effects, interactions with other therapy modalities, and availability.[83]

RETINOID THERAPY

First-generation retinoids, such as isotretinoin, have limited effect on CTCL. The synthetic retinoid bexarotene binds the retinoid X receptor with high selectivity, whereas the other available retinoids have less-specific binding patterns. In monotherapy trials, bexarotene was used at 300 mg/m². Responses were seen in patients in all stages of the disease: plaques, erythroderma, and tumors. Responses paralleled the secondary end points: decreases in overall body surface area involved and in overall tumor aggregate area, and improvement in pruritus. Erythrodermic patients may experience increased desquamation during the first few weeks of oral bexarotene therapy. Improvement typically starts by week 12 of therapy.

Although there appeared to be a dose–response relationship with respect to efficacy, the higher dosages were also associated with a higher rate of adverse events and dose-limiting toxicities. Of these, hypertriglyceridemia, hypercholesterolemia, neutropenia, and central hypothyroidism were most common. Elevations in lipid levels occurred rapidly, within 2 to 4 weeks, and were associated with serious, but reversible, pancreatitis. Monitoring of lipids and the use of lipid-lowering drugs were helpful in controlling the lipid levels. Dosage reduction of bexarotene capsules was also required in some patients. Drug interactions of oral bexarotene with gemfibrozil and warfarin have been observed.

Patients started on bexarotene therapy develop central hypothyroidism with low levels of thyroid-stimulating hormone and free thyroxine within weeks of starting the medication. Symptoms of hypothyroidism may be subtle and include feeling fatigued and feeling cold, which may wrongly be attributed to the disease itself. Supplementation with levothyroxine while taking bexarotene alleviates the symptoms and improves tolerance of treatment. The condition is reversible within weeks of stopping therapy. There is no immunosuppression with bexarotene therapy. Patients taking bexarotene typically have monthly monitoring visits to follow lipid, liver, and thyroid parameters.[90-94]

EXTRACORPOREAL PHOTOCHEMOTHERAPY

Refer to Chap. 199, "Photochemotherapy and Photodynamic Therapy" for an in-depth discussion of ECP.

ECP involves the treatment of a portion of a patient's lymphocyte compartment with 8-methoxypsoralen in the presence of UVA light, followed by reinfusion of these cells. The treatment is performed via an intravenous line that feeds into an UVA-radiation device, and the procedure typically requires the patient to remain recumbent for 3 hours. Treatments are conducted on 2 consecutive days every 4 weeks. Erythrodermic CTCLs can be managed with ECP monotherapy, but treatment of other disease stages with monotherapy has not been rigorously studied. In a multicenter study involving

TABLE 119-10
Biologic Response Modifiers for the Treatment of Erythrodermic Cutaneous T-cell Lymphomas

		DOSE OPTIONS	TIME TO EXPECTED CLINICAL RESPONSE	SIDE EFFECTS AND ADVERSE REACTIONS
Retinoid therapy		Bexarotene, 300 mg/m²	12 weeks	Hypertriglyceridemia, hypercholesterolemia, neutropenia, central hypothyroidism, pancreatitis (reversible)
Extracorporeal photochemotherapy		Photopheresis, with 8-methoxypsoralen and ultraviolet A, on 2 consecutive days every 4 weeks	4-6 months	See Chap. 198 ("Phototherapy")
Interferon-α therapy		3 million units, 3×/week, increasing to a maximally tolerated dose (~9 million units/day)	3-6 months	Flu-like symptoms, chronic fatigue; risk for long-term neurologic toxicity (depression, neuropathy, dementia, and myelopathy); thyroiditis, liver, bone marrow toxicity
Targeted monoclonal antibodies	Alemtuzumab	Varies, according to protocol (see text)		Cytomegalovirus reactivation, opportunistic infections at higher doses
	Brentuximab vedotin	1.2-1.8 mg/kg every 3 weeks	12 weeks	Peripheral neuropathy (reversible in most)

erythrodermic CTCL patients, approximately one-fourth had a complete response, one-fourth had no response, and the remainder had partial responses. However, it is clear that even a partial response can improve the quality of life of these patients. Improvement sometimes began as early as 6 weeks into therapy, but some patients did not show complete lesion clearance until 12 months after starting therapy. There were occasional temporary responses immediately after a 2-day cycle of therapy. On average, after 4 to 6 months there was typically a gradual and permanent decrease in erythema, scaling, and pruritus. Patients often notice more subtle changes, such as the return of body hair, loss of rigors, and a return of the ability to sweat. Partial responses may also decrease the morbidity these patients experience in terms of infectious complications. More heavily involved and inflamed skin is more readily colonized, providing both a reservoir and access point for microbes to invade the host. Thus, cutaneous improvement can also minimize complications of CTCLs.

The clinical experiences with ECP for erythrodermic MF and Sézary syndrome suggest that the therapeutic response may well be based in the immune system. One feature is that when less than 5% of the malignant lymphocyte pool is photoinactivated with 8-methoxypsoralen and UVA light, clinical responses can be seen, with more than 95% of the malignant lymphocytes disappearing over time. It also appears that most immunocompetent patients respond. Patients, who were heavily pretreated, with longer disease durations, were less responsive. Also, patients with normal or only slightly decreased CD8+ lymphocyte levels were responsive to ECP. In one study, total skin electron beam radiotherapy was combined with ECP in patients with Stage T3 and Stage T4 disease. Comparison of patients receiving skin-directed radiotherapy plus BRM with historic controls who underwent electron beam radiotherapy at the same institution demonstrated the impact of ECP, because patients in the skin-directed therapy plus BRM group showed significantly longer survival.[95,96]

INTERFERON-α THERAPY

In the treatment of CTCLs, the most-studied IFN is IFN-α; however, clinical studies regarding the use of IFN-β and IFN-γ in the treatment of CTCLs have also been conducted. The initial studies using IFN-α as monotherapy showed rates of complete responses that varied from 10% to 27% with treatment durations of less than 6 months. Again, the heterogeneity of the disease and the pretreatments patients underwent before may affect outcomes and make comparisons with other modalities impossible. IFN-α is typically started at 3 million units, 3 times a week, and can be increased to a maximally tolerated dose, typically in the range of 9 million units/day. As with the other BRMs, the response to IFN is gradual, and 3 to 6 months are needed to determine the maximal response. After patients achieve a maximal response, IFN dosage can be lowered to a maintenance level.

All IFNs have similar toxicities. Initially IFN therapy is complicated by a flu-like illness that is characterized by fever, headache, myalgia, and fatigue. As this wears off, patients are often left with a slight feeling of chronic fatigue. The long-term toxicity that causes most concern is neurologic: depression, neuropathy, dementia, and myelopathy. Autoimmune phenomena, such as thyroiditis, may occur. Furthermore, toxic effects of the liver and bone marrow may occur. Monitoring of IFN therapy includes blood counts along with questionnaires assessing the impact on the patient's quality of life.[97]

TARGETED MONOCLONAL ANTIBODIES

Alemtuzumab: Alemtuzumab is a humanized monoclonal antibody that targets CD52, expressed on most T and B lymphocytes and NK cells. Lundin et al[97A] reported a response rate of 50% to 70% in patients with CTCL. Because of prolonged depression of T, B, and NK cells in the original dosage schedule and immunosuppression, this treatment led to reactivation of cytomegalovirus and other opportunistic infections.

Alternative dosage schedules with lower doses and subcutaneous administration have been investigated. Querfeld et al[97B] reported a favorable response when intravenous alemtuzumab was followed with lower-dose subcutaneous antibody. A different schedule was proposed by Bernengo et al[99]; 4 patients received 3 mg alemtuzumab on day 1, 10 mg on day 3, and then 15 mg on alternate days. Bernengo et al reported 86% response rates in 12 of 14 refractory Sézary syndrome patients, including 3 complete remissions.

However, Rei Watanabe[98] showed that low-dose alemtuzumab is a highly effective and generally well tolerated therapy for refractory CTCL (ie, CTCL patients with peripheral blood disease).

Low-dose alemtuzumab is effective in patients with blood involvement (leukemic disease) but ineffective in MF, reflecting the fact that MF derives from distinct T-cell subsets. Patients with malignant T cells with blood disease have the phenotype of CCR7+ L-selectin+ T_{CM} that are migratory and recirculate between skin, blood, and lymph nodes, whereas MF T cells are derived from nonmigratory skin-resident T_{RM}. Low-dose alemtuzumab depletes all circulating T cells and depletes skin in recirculating malignant T cells, leading to complete, and often durable, remissions in 50% of patients while sparing benign T cells in skin. Based on the clinical experience of Rachael Clark,[98A] alemtuzumab should be used in patients with or without adjuvant skin-directed therapy and in patients with diffuse cutaneous erythema, but some investigators caution against its use in patients with preexisting plaques and/or tumors.[98,99]

Brentuximab Vedotin: The antibody drug conjugate brentuximab vedotin is an anti-CD30 monoclonal antibody conjugated via a highly stable protease cleavable linker with monomethyl auristatin E, an antitubulin agent. It is U.S. Food and Drug Administration approved for the treatment of relapsed-refractory Hodgkin lymphoma and ALCL.

In the past, CD30 has been identified as an excellent therapeutic target in lymphomas that express CD30. Histologically it is uniquely expressed in Hodgkin lymphoma, ALCL, and normal activated T, B, and NK cells, but is not expressed in normal tissues. Monoclonal antibodies that interact with CD30 are thought to induce apoptosis by initiating CD30 signaling.

CD30 is highly expressed on the surface of primary cutaneous ALCL and subtypes of lymphomatoid papulosis and variably expressed in MF morphologic subtypes, including large-cell transformed MF. The first results of Phase II clinical trials in CTCL were published recently. In the Phase II trial of brentuximab vedotin in MF or Sézary syndrome by Kim et al,[101] the overall global response was 70% among the 30 evaluable patients. CD30 expression assessed by immunohistochemistry was highly variable with a median CD30 maximum expression of 13% (range: 0%-100%); those with less than 5% CD30 expression had a lower likelihood of global response than those with greater than or equal to 5% CD30 expression. The detection of abundant macrophages CD163+ M2 type in the tumor milieu suggested that brentuximab may target these macrophages in addition to the malignant T cells and disrupt their tumor-promoting function. The detection also suggested that these CD30-bearing macrophages may offer an additional source of monomethyl auristatin E to the nearby malignant T cells.

The other Phase II study was published by Duvic et al[100] in patients with CD30 lymphoproliferative disorder or CD30 MF/Sézary syndrome. The evaluable 48 patients showed an overall response rate of 73% and a complete response rate of 35%. The median time to response was 12 weeks, and duration of response was 32 weeks (range: 3-93 weeks). All patients with lymphomatoid papulosis or primary cutaneous ALCL responded.

The most common side effect is the induction of peripheral neuropathy. Although reversible in most of the cases, some experienced irreversible neuropathy. The recommended dose of brentuximab vedotin is 1.8 mg/kg every 3 weeks; to overcome its side effects, a lower dosage of 1.2 mg/kg is recommended or prolongation of the interval between doses.

Currently, brentuximab vedotin in the treatment of CTCL is being studied in an open-label Phase III ALCANZA Study Group trial,[100A] which is comparing brentuximab vedotin with physicians' choices, either bexarotene or methotrexate, in patients with relapsed CD30+ MF or primary cutaneous ALCL.[100,101]

Mogamulizumab: Mogamulizumab is a defucosylated anti-CCR4 monoclonal antibody. It targets CCR4, a chemokine receptor that is preferentially expressed by Th2 and regulatory T cells in MF and Sézary syndrome patients. In response to its ligands, CCL17 (TARC) and CCL22 (MDC), CCR4 promotes T-cell migration to the skin. These CCR4 ligands are produced by keratinocytes, dendritic cells, and macrophages, and are abundant within MF/Sézary syndrome–involved skin. A recently described subset of peripheral T-cell lymphoma expresses CCR4 as part of the transcriptional repertoire of GATA-3, the master transcriptional regulator driving Th2 differentiation. GATA-3 is not only expressed by regulatory T cells, residing within various sites such as the skin, but also by MF/Sézary syndrome cells, and may drive CCR4 expression in these cells.

In addition to its role in regulating cell homing and trafficking, CCR4 engagement may also promote cell growth and survival. However, cells can become desensitized to CCR4 through receptor internalization, a homeostatic regulatory mechanism. Clearly, CCR4 has a pathogenic role in MF/Sézary syndrome and other T-cell lymphoproliferative disorders and is an attractive therapeutic target.

Mogamulizumab depletes CCR4-expressing cells by antibody-dependent cell-mediated cytotoxicity. Targeting the chemokine receptor CCR4, Duvic et al demonstrated that mogamulizumab is well tolerated and has significant clinical activity, with an overall response rate of 36% and a median duration of time to response of 1.4 months in heavily pretreated patients with MF and Sézary syndrome. The same group showed that in addition to antibody-dependent cell-mediated cytotoxicity, mogamulizumab depletes regulatory T cells, an important therapeutic target in many human cancers because of the role of regulatory T cells in suppressing host antitumor immunity.

Mogamulizumab is currently being evaluated worldwide in a Phase III trial comparing mogamulizumab with the histone deacetylase inhibitor vorinostat.[102,102A]

SINGLE-AGENT CHEMOTHERAPY

More than 20 years ago, Bunn et al[103] at the National Institutes of Health concluded that multiagent chemotherapy was not superior to sequential conservative therapies with respect to overall survival in advanced CTCL. Therefore, the therapeutic approach was more concentrated to reduce systemic side effects to a single-agent chemotherapy shown to be as effective. Choice of therapy is based on stage, concomitant medical condition, and prior treatment, as each agent has unique side effects and efficacy profile.

Methotrexate, pegylated liposomal doxorubicin, gemcitabine, and pentostatin have all been studied in Phase II trials of CTCL patients.[84]

Gemcitabine: Gemcitabine hydrochloride, a nucleoside analog of deoxycytidine that inhibits DNA synthesis has shown activity against solid tumors as well as hematologic malignancies. In a number of small studies, gemcitabine, given as a dosage of 1200 mg/m^2 administered for 3 or 4 weeks for 3 courses, has shown overall response rates of 70.5% with a median duration of 15 months. Duvic et al demonstrated that a lower dose of gemcitabine (1000 mg/m^2 once per week for 3 weekly cycles) produced an overall response rate of 68% in 25 patients with advanced stage and refractory MF. It was especially active in MF patients with cutaneous tumors. Gemcitabine can be used in combination with bexarotene maintenance therapy to manage the plaques and patches of MF. It can also be alternated with liposomal doxorubicin infusion to prolong the duration of chemotherapy. The adverse effects of gemcitabine have most frequently involved bone marrow suppression (leukopenia), anemia, and, especially, thrombocytopenia.[104,105]

Pegylated Liposomal Doxorubicin: Pegylated liposomal doxorubicin is a new formulation of doxorubicin in which the drug is encapsulated in liposomes and stabilized by the attachment of polyethylene glycol (ie, pegylation) to the liposomal surface, resulting in increased half-life and improved accumulation in tumor tissues. Toxicity profile is characterized by dose-limiting mucosal and cutaneous adverse effects, in particular palmar-plantar erythrodysesthesia syndrome reporting up to 20% of treated patients.

In a prospective multicenter controlled trial by the EORTC, patients with Stage IIB, IIIB, or IVA MF, refractory or recurrent after at least 2 previous systemic therapies, were treated with 6 cycles of pegylated liposomal doxorubicin 20 mg/m^2 on days 1 and 15 over a single 28-day cycle. The primary end point was response rate. Among the 49 patients, the overall response rate was 48% with 6.1% complete remission. The median progression-free survival was 6.2 months. Toxicity (grades III to IV) was observed in 20% of the treated patients.[106]

The trial has produced benchmark data in a defined population of patients with MF in need of cytotoxic therapy. The efficacy is reasonable, and patients are allowed to use liposomal encapsulated doxorubicin as a debulking agent.

Pralatrexate: Pralatrexate, a novel antifolate with a high affinity for the reduced folate carrier (RFC-1), a novel mechanism of resistance when compared with methotrexate, was associated with an overall response rate of 29% in patients with relapsed or refractory peripheral T-cell lymphoma. A total of 12 patients with transformed MF were included in the study. Many of these patients had received more than 5 prior systemic therapies, including CHOP or CHOP-like regimens. However, results of a dose-finding study were reported in a larger cohort of CTCL patients. In this study, published by Horwitz et al,[106A] the optimal dose was identified as 15 mg/m^2, given weekly 3 weeks out of 4, and was associated with an overall response rate of 43%. In an effort to reduce the incidence of mucositis, folic acid and vitamin B_{12} supplementation was routinely provided to these patients. However, pralatrexate has not been studied in a randomized trial against established compounds in CTCL.[107]

ALLOGENEIC STEM CELL TRANSPLANTATION

Younger patients with advanced stage CTCL (Stage IIB or greater) who fail to respond to first-line therapy are now being considered for nonablative allogeneic hematopoietic stem cell transplantation.

Patients need to have a related or unrelated matched donor and be physically and emotionally able to undergo the procedure. The therapeutic concept is based on the existence of a graft-versus-T-cell-lymphoma effect particularly using nonmyeloablative conditions. Selected patients have achieved long-term remission and curative responses.

Duarte et al reported on the long-term outcome of allogeneic hematopoietic stem cell transplantation for patients with MF and Sézary syndrome. These data show that patients with advanced stage MF and Sézary syndrome continue to benefit from allogenic hematopoietic cell transplantation over time, with an overall survival of 46% at 5 years and 44% at 7 years, and progression-free survival of 32% at 5 years and 30% at 7 years. Disease-relapse progression is a main cause of posttransplantation failure; a total of 45% of patients experience relapse progression at a medium of 3.8 months after hematopoietic stem cell transplantation. In a multivariable analysis, a number of disease and transplantation factors showed an independent impact on patient outcomes. The analysis focused on nonrelapse mortality, which was borderline associated with transplants from unrelated donors. Relapse was highly significantly associated with myeloablative conditioning versus nonmyeloablative and with a poor performance score at hematopoietic cell transplantation (Karnofsky score <70). Patients must be treated with allogeneic transplantation after having achieved complete or nearly complete remission.[108,109]

PRIMARY CUTANEOUS B-CELL LYMPHOMAS

Primary CBCLs (Table 119-11) are B-lymphocyte–derived malignancies that develop in the skin without extracutaneous involvement at the time of diagnosis and account for 20% to 25% of primary cutaneous lymphomas. The incidence of CBCL is estimated at 3 cases per 1,000,000 persons per year based on surveillance epidemiology and end results registry data.[110]

The PCMZL/extranodal marginal zone lymphoma and the PCFCL are indolent subtypes, whereas the PCLBCL, leg type has an intermediate to aggressive clinical behavior.

These 3 entities (ie, PCMZL, PCFCL, and PCLBCL) together comprise 97% of the CBCL.[111-113]

ETIOLOGY

As for CTCL, an infectious trigger has been hypothesized to be involved in the etiology of CBCL. A strong association of gastric extranodal marginal zone lymphomas and *Helicobacter pylori* infection is well known. In a minority of PCMZLs from European patients, but not in American or Asian patients, *Borrelia burgdorferi* has been detected. A newer study suggests that, based on immunoglobulin expression, 2 types of PCMZLs can be distinguished. In the most frequent PCMZL subtype, B cells expressing class-switched immunoglobulin (Ig) heavy chains, including IgG and to a lesser extend IgA or IgE, are observed. In a majority of cases, diffuse proliferation of IgM+ MCXCR3-expressing B cells is observed, which is associated with fewer infiltrating T cells and a skewed CD4-to-CD8 ratio toward an increased number of CD4+ T cells. In IgM+ cases, extracutaneous localization of disease is frequently observed, suggesting that cutaneous localizations of extranodal mucosal-associated lymphoid tissue from class-switched and non–class-switched immunoglobulin heavy chains result from distinct pathologic processes.

Detailed studies on immunoglobulin heavy-chain expression showed that PCMZL showed IgG_4 expression in 39% of cases. There was no evidence of IgG_4-related disease in any of these patients pointing to a localized immunologic IgG_4-driven process. In clinical management, these observations are helpful, as the marginal zone lymphomas presenting skin that expresses IgG_4 will invariably be PCMZL.

A viral agent, in particular hepatitis C virus, also is suspected to be relevant in the etiology of CBCL, but the results of the studies are contradictory.[110-116]

PATHOGENESIS

Because of the rarity of the CBCL subtypes, studies investigating pathogenetic events in CBCL have been mainly conducted on a small number of cases. However, in recent years, considerable progress in understanding the pathogenesis of CBCL has been made.

A phenomenon called *aberrant somatic hypermutation*, which has been reported in nodal B-cell lymphomas, has been detected in the 3 main types of CBCL. This term describes the activity of the enzyme activation–induced deaminase, which contributes to the process of affinity maturation of immunoglobulins by somatic hypermutation, in regions of the genome that do not encode immunoglobulin genes. If this process occurs in oncogene-containing gene loci, in association with the loss of the physiologically high-fidelity DNA repair mechanisms, tumorigenic mutations may occur and contribute to lymphomagenesis.[79]

Furthermore, genetic investigations demonstrated distinct differences of CBCL subtypes. A genetic basis for differentiation of histologic skin PCFCL with a diffuse growth pattern of large cells and PCLBCL, leg type, was shown. The gene expression profiles of these entities were consistent with either germinal center B cells for PCFCL or activated B cells for PCLBCL, leg type. Similar results were found in a study focusing on proapoptotic and antiapoptotic genes. While PCLBCL, leg type with a poor prognosis had a genetic profile called *activate apoptosis cascade*, PCFCL and cases of PCLBCL, leg type with a favorable prognosis had a high expression level for genes that are associated with an antitumoral cytotoxic immune response. These findings also explain why PCFCL has a more favorable prognosis than PCLBCL, leg type.

TABLE 119-11
Summary of Cutaneous B-Cell Lymphomas

	AGE AT DIAGNOSIS	NATURE OF DISEASE	CLINICAL FINDINGS	CELL OF ORIGIN	IMMUNOHISTOCHEMICAL CHARACTERISTICS	TREATMENT
Primary cutaneous follicle center lymphoma (PCFCL)	Median age at diagnosis is 58 years	Indolent	Solitary or grouped firm, painless erythematous plaques and tumors, head and trunk commonly affected	Clonal centrocytes and centroblasts	CD19+, CD20+, CD79a, CD10, Bcl6+[a]	Radiotherapy; immune therapy for disseminated lesions
Extranodal marginal zone lymphoma (EMZL)/primary cutaneous marginal zone lymphoma (PCMZL)	Median age at diagnosis is 55 years; female predominant	Indolent	Violaceous papules, plaques, or nodules; occur on multiple locations	Small B lymphocytes, marginal zone cells, lymphoplasmacytoid cells, plasma cells	CD20, CD79a, Bcl2+; plasma cells may express CD138, CD79a	Radiotherapy; systemic antibiotics if *Borrelia burgdorferi* associated; chlorambucil, rituximab, intralesional interferon
Primary cutaneous diffuse large B-cell lymphoma, leg type	Median age at diagnosis is 65 years; female predominant	Intermediate to aggressive	Solitary or clustered bluish erythematous plaques and tumors located on 1 or both legs	Large B cells	CD20+, CD79a, IRF4-MUM-1+, FOXP1+, cytoplasmic immunoglobulin M ± D, Bcl2+, Bcl6+	Rituximab, cyclophosphamide, hydroxydaunorubicin, Oncovin, prednisolone, bendamustine + rituximab regimen

[a]May be Bcl2+ with nodal disease.

Furthermore, PCMZLs were found to arise in a different pathogenetic background than extranodal marginal zone lymphomas. The main differences were the high percentage of CXCR3− PCMZLs, which also, in contrast to other extranodal marginal zone lymphoma, exhibited an immunoglobulin class switch and a Th2 cytokine milieu. It remains to be investigated how this relates to the presence of plasmacytoid dendritic cells in PCMZL, which were also found in cutaneous pseudolymphomas, but not in diffuse large B-cell lymphomas and only rarely in PCFCL.[113,117-124]

PRIMARY CUTANEOUS FOLLICULAR CENTER LYMPHOMA

DEFINITION

PCFCL can be defined as a neoplasm of clonal centrocytes (small and large cleaved follicle center cells) and centroblasts (large follicle center cells with prominent nucleoli) with or without formation of follicles.

CLINICAL FINDINGS

PCFCL usually presents with solitary or grouped firm, painless, erythematous plaques and tumors that are preferentially located on the head and trunk, and rarely present on the leg. Patients with PCFCL have a median age of 58 years at diagnosis, and adult males are affected nearly twice as often as adult females. Occasionally, an annular erythema can be observed in the surrounding area (Fig. 119-23A). A typical finding is the occurrence of lesions in a circumscribed area of the head and neck region or the trunk, but rarely on the legs.

HISTOPATHOLOGY

These tumors are composed of medium to large follicle center cells containing a mixture of centrocytes and centroblasts arranged in a follicular or diffuse growth pattern (see Fig. 119-23B). The neoplastic cells express the pan–B-cell markers CD19, CD20, and CD79a, and express the germinal center marker Bcl6. Expression of CD10 is particularly observed in cases with a follicular growth pattern. Unlike primary cutaneous B-cell lymphoma, leg type, expression of IRF4-MUM-1, FOXP1, and cytoplasmic immunoglobulin is generally not observed. In contrast to nodal follicular center lymphomas, in most studies PCFCLs uncommonly express Bcl2 and generally do not contain the translocation t(14;18). Gene expression studies demonstrate that PCFCLs have a gene expression profile resembling germinal center B-cell–like diffuse large B-cell lymphomas. Genomic studies found c-REL amplification in 63% of cases and deletions of 14q32.33 in 68% of cases.

TREATMENT AND PROGNOSIS

PCFCLs are indolent lymphomas that rarely metastasize to extracutaneous localizations and their prognosis is excellent with a 5-year survival of greater than 95%. Approximately 5% of PCFCLs develop on the legs and these cases have a more aggressive behavior. Radiotherapy (30 Gy) is the preferred treatment for PCFCL (Table 119-12). Relapses are observed in 30% of cases, but these do not herald an adverse prognosis and can be retreated with radiotherapy. For relapses a palliative dose of 4 Gy can be used, which will result in effective local control in 90% of cases. Immune therapy, such as administration of IFN-α or monoclonal antibodies against CD20, may be beneficial in cases with disseminated lesions.[124,125]

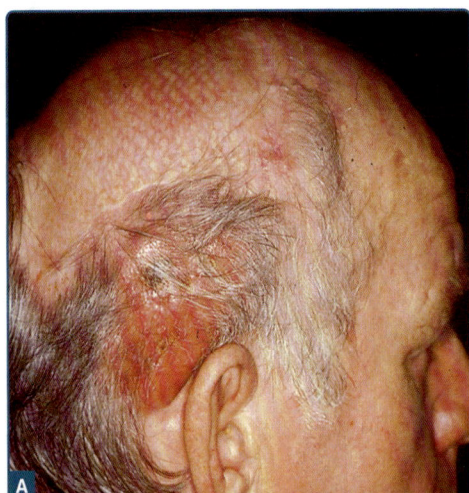 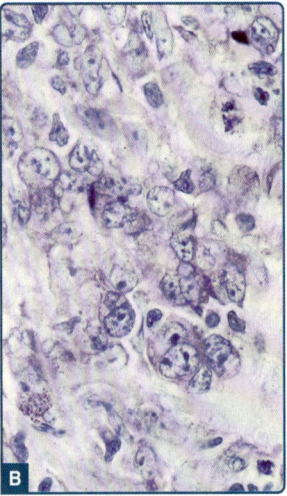

Figure 119-23 Primary cutaneous follicle center lymphoma. **A,** Tumor in the head area surrounded by erythema. **B,** The cellular infiltrate consists of a mixture of centrocytes, a number of centroblasts, and reactive T cells.

EXTRANODAL MARGINAL ZONE B-CELL LYMPHOMA

DEFINITION

PCMZL or extranodal marginal zone lymphoma is an indolent B-cell lymphoma composed of small B lymphocytes, marginal zone cells, lymphoplasmacytoid cells, and plasma cells, which are initially localized in the marginal zone of a follicular center. In the current WHO classification, it is classified within the extranodal marginal zone lymphoma of mucosa-associated lymphatic tissue. In a subgroup of PCMZL, *B. burgdorferi* is thought to have an etiologic role.

CLINICAL FINDINGS

PCMZLs are seen most commonly on the upper extremities or the trunk and occur at a median age of 55 years; they predominate in females. Patients have small red-to-violaceous papules, plaques, or nodules that, in contrast to the lesions of PCFCL, frequently occur in multiple locations. PCMZL accounts for 25% of primary CBCLs.

HISTOPATHOLOGY

The histologic infiltrate includes marginal zone (centrocyte-like) cells, plasmacytoid cells, and plasma cells. Typically, the marginal zone cells express CD20, CD79a, and Bcl2, but are negative for CD5, CD10, and Bcl6. Plasma cells express CD138 and CD79a, and show monotypic cytoplasmic immunoglobulin light-chain expression on paraffin sections.[118,119,126,127]

TREATMENT AND PROGNOSIS

PCMZLs have been described in relation to tick bites and antigen injection, which suggests that chronic antigenic stimulation may play a role in the pathogenesis of these lymphomas. PCMZLs are indolent lymphomas and scattered lesions can be treated with radiotherapy (see Table 119-12). In case of detection of *B. burgdorferi*, a systemic antibiotic treatment should be given first. For widespread lesions a wait-and-see approach can be adopted and symptomatic lesions can be treated with surgery, topical or intralesional steroids, or low-dose radiotherapy. In addition, systemic therapy with chlorambucil or rituximab and intralesional treatment with IFN-α or rituximab are reported to lead to complete responses in a majority of patients.[117]

TABLE 119-12
Treatment Algorithms for Cutaneous B-Cell Lymphomas

DISEASE TYPE AND EXTENT	FIRST-LINE THERAPY	ALTERNATIVE THERAPIES
Primary Cutaneous Marginal Zone Lymphoma		
Solitary/localized	Local radiotherapy	Interferon (IFN)-α intralesional
	Excision	Rituximab intralesional
	Antibiotics[a]	Intralesional steroids
Multifocal	Wait-and-see	IFN-α intralesional
	Local radiotherapy	Rituximab intralesional
	Chlorambucil[b]	Topical or intralesional steroids
	Rituximab IV	
	Antibiotics[a]	
Primary Cutaneous Follicle Center Lymphoma		
Solitary/localized	Local radiotherapy	IFN-α intralesional
	Excision	Rituximab intralesional
Multifocal	Wait-and-see	R-CVP/CHOP[c]
	Local radiotherapy	
	Rituximab IV	
Primary Cutaneous Diffuse Large B-Cell Lymphoma, Leg Type		
Solitary/localized	R-CHOP ± IFRT	Local radiotherapy
		Rituximab IV
Multifocal	R-CHOP	Rituximab IV

Abbreviations: CHOP, cyclophosphamide, doxorubicin, vincristine, and prednisone; IFRT, involved-field radiotherapy; R-CHOP, rituximab, cyclophosphamide, doxorubicin, vincristine, and prednisone; R-CVP, rituximab, cyclophosphamide, vincristine, and prednisone.

[a]In case of evidence for *Borrelia burgdorferi* infection.
[b]Or other single or combination regimens appropriate for low-grade B-cell lymphomas.
[c]In exceptional cases or for patients developing extracutaneous disease.
Adapted from Senff NJ, Noordijk EM, Kim YH, et al. European Organization for Research and Treatment of Cancer and International Society for Cutaneous Lymphoma consensus recommendations for the management of cutaneous B-cell lymphomas. *Blood*. 2008;112(5):1600-09, with permission.

PRIMARY CUTANEOUS DIFFUSE LARGE B-CELL LYMPHOMA, LEG TYPE

DEFINITION

PCLBCL, leg type, has been identified as a distinct clinical entity because of its perceived poor outcome compared with the indolent subtypes described above. This entity shows an intermediate, and in some patients aggressive, clinical course. It is defined by tumors composed of large B cells that present in the overwhelming majority of cases on the legs, but can also arise at other locations. The majority of patients with PCLBCL, leg type, have aberrations on chromosome 9p21, and loss of this region, which contains the *CDKN2A* gene, is associated with a worse prognosis.[128,129]

CLINICAL FINDINGS

PCLBCL, leg type affects elderly patients (older than age 65 years), with a predominance in females. Typically, patients have solitary or clustered bluish erythematous plaques and tumors located on one or, sometimes, both legs (Fig. 119-24A); approximately 10% of patients present with lesions at other sites than the legs. Ulceration is common and sometimes leads to the misdiagnosis of an ulcer from chronic venous insufficiency.

HISTOPATHOLOGY

The diffuse infiltrate shows sheets of immunoblasts and centroblasts with few mixed reactive cells (see Fig. 119-24B). The neoplastic cells express CD20 and CD79a, and, unlike PCFCL, are strongly positive for Bcl2, IRF4-MUM1, and FOXP1, and have cytoplasmic expression of IgM ± IgD. Bcl6 is expressed in most cases, whereas CD10 is generally absent. In line with the immunophenotypic profile, PCLBCL, leg type has a gene expression profile resembling activated B cells diffuse large B-cell lymphoma. In addition, PCLBCL, leg type expresses activation-induced cytidine desaminase, solves thermotic hypermutation of the immunoglobulin genes, and harbors mutations in the *Bcl6*, *Myc*, *Rho-TTF*, and *PAX5* genes, which are indicative of ectopic somatic hypermutation. Translocations have been observed for Myc in up to 43% of PCLBCL, leg type cases, and Bcl6 in up to 46% of PCLBCL, leg type cases. Studies on copy number alterations describe high-level amplifications for the *Bcl2* gene in 67% of cases and loss of CDKN2a in 23% to 42% of patients. Loss of CDKN2a expression either by gene deletion or promoter methylation correlates with an adverse prognosis.

TREATMENT AND PROGNOSIS

PCLBCL, leg type, belongs to the intermediate-aggressive group of CBCLs and should preferentially be treated with rituximab, cyclophosphamide, hydroxydaunorubicin, Oncovin (vincristine), and prednisolone (R-CHOP) (see Table 119-12). In general, age-adapted polychemotherapy combined with rituximab showed a better outcome than polychemotherapy regimens alone.[125] Because PCLBCL, leg type, occurs in elderly women (older than age 80 years), less-toxic regimens like bendamustine combined with rituximab could also be recommended. Despite this treatment, recurrences are observed in the majority of patients, and disease-related 5-year survival is approximately 50%.

PRIMARY CUTANEOUS DIFFUSE LARGE B-CELL LYMPHOMA, OTHER

PCLBCL, other, covers diffuse large B-cell lymphomas that do not belong to either PCLBCL, leg type, or PCFCL. These cases may represent a skin manifestation of systemic lymphomas. T-cell/histocyte-rich B-cell lymphomas with skin lesions only are also included; these cases show, in contrast to their nodal counterparts, an excellent prognosis.

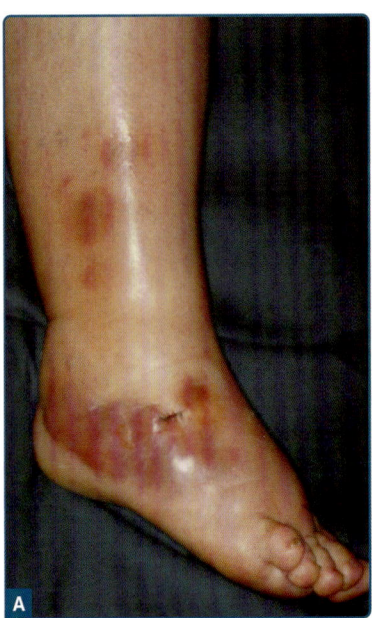 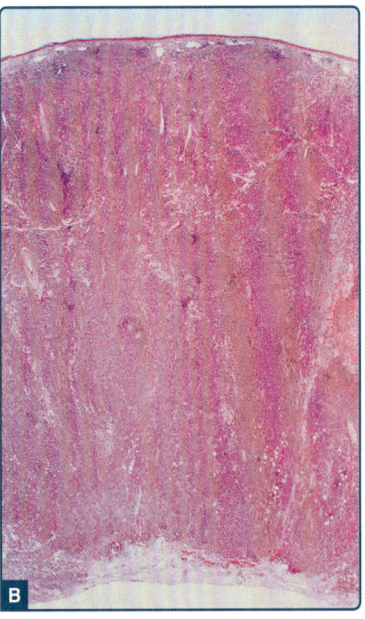

Figure 119-24 Primary cutaneous diffuse large B-cell lymphoma, leg type. **A,** Nodules and tumors on the right leg. **B,** Histology shows a diffuse infiltrate of large B cells with centroblasts, large centrocytes, and numerous immunoblasts.

INTRAVASCULAR CUTANEOUS B-CELL LYMPHOMA

Intravascular CBCL is characterized by clusters of large neoplastic B cells within dermal and subcutaneous blood vessels. Occasionally, slight extravascular infiltrates of atypical cells are observed. Clinically, red to bluish, indurated plaques occur on the legs or trunk. Sometimes, a panniculitis-like pattern can be seen. Multiagent chemotherapy is the preferred mode of treatment.[130,131]

STAGING OF CUTANEOUS B-CELL LYMPHOMA

The International Society for Cutaneous Lymphoma and the Cutaneous Lymphoma Task Force of the EORTC developed a proposal for a tumor-node-metastases (TNM) classification for cutaneous lymphomas, other than MF and Sézary syndrome (see Table 119-4). Recommended staging procedures for primary cutaneous B-cell lymphomas (PCBL) included thorough physical examination, laboratory studies, including a complete blood cell count, blood chemistry, including lactate dehydrogenase level, and, if indicated, a serum electrophoresis to exclude monoclonal gammopathy and/or flow cytometry on peripheral blood.

In endemic regions, *Borrelia* serologic testing and polymerase chain reaction of skin biopsy specimens should be performed.

Imaging studies include a contrast-enhanced CT scan with or without positron emission tomography, for chest, abdomen, and pelvis, and if lesions arose on the head and neck area, of the neck. Bone marrow biopsy and aspirate are required in PCFCL and PCLBCL, leg type, but are not required in patients presenting with a B-cell lymphoma in the skin with histologic features suggesting a follicular center lymphoma or marginal zone lymphoma, unless indicated by other staging assessments. However, a study by Senff et al[131A] demonstrated bone marrow involvement at diagnosis in 22 (11%) of 193 PCFCLs in 9 patients. Bone marrow involvement was the only extracutaneous localization. Because these patients with skin and bone marrow localization had significantly worse prognoses than patients with only skin lesions, it was suggested that bone marrow examination should be considered in these patients.

The proposed staging system for CBCL has been investigated in retrospective studies, demonstrating that the TNM system is a useful tool when documenting the extent of disease in CBCLs and for providing prognostic information in PCLBCL, leg type.

PRINCIPLES OF TREATMENT OF CUTANEOUS B-CELL LYMPHOMA

Treatment of primary CBCLs (see Table 119-12) should be adapted to the favorable prognosis of these lymphomas, in particular of PCFCL and PCMZL. Because no curative regimen has been defined as of this writing, therapy depends on the lymphoma and the dissemination of cutaneous lesions. In the case of solitary lesions, complete excision of the tumor may be proposed. Alternatively, or in the case of few localized lesions, local irradiation (a single dose of 3-4 Gy; total dose of 30-40 Gy) by X-ray or electron beam is effective. When this regimen is used, long-lasting remissions can be achieved.[125,132]

Systemic treatment is recommended for disseminated PCMZL or PCFCL with anti-CD20 antibodies. For relapse of indolent CBCLs with disseminated lesions a wait-and-see strategy combined with treatment of symptomatic lesions may be followed.

Systemic treatment regimens are recommended in cases of PCLBCL, leg type, and in PCFCL with localization on the legs, as these PCFCLs have a worse prognosis, as well as when secondary extracutaneous manifestations are present. Polychemotherapy (6 cycles of CHOP or COP [cyclophosphamide, vincristine, and prednisone]) in combination with an anti-CD20 antibody is recommended. In patients who would not tolerate such an aggressive treatment, local radiotherapy or rituximab monotherapy may be considered.

PRECURSOR NEOPLASMS

BLASTIC PLASMACYTOID DENDRITIC CELL NEOPLASM

DEFINITION

According to the current WHO classification, blastic plasmacytoid dendritic cell neoplasm (BPDCN) is classified as an acute myeloid leukemia–related precursor neoplasm that derives from precursors of plasmacytoid dendritic cells. BPDCN is an orphan disease with a very aggressive clinical course that results in median survival times of 12 to 14 months.

CLINICAL FINDINGS

BPDCN usually occurs in elderly patients with a median age between 60 and 70 years. However, BPDCN can present at any age, even in children. More often BPDCN occurs in men (male-to-female ratio: 3:1) but has no known racial or ethnic predilection. Patients typically present with asymptomatic solitary or multiple skin lesions, such as nodules, plaques, or bruise-like lesions that can range in size from a few millimeters to 10 cm (Fig. 119-25). The skin lesions can be associated with erythema, hyperpigmentation, purpura, or ulceration. Extracutaneous disease is present in most patients at diagnosis, often involving the regional lymph nodes. As the disease continues to progress, the peripheral blood and bone marrow become involved.

In 10% to 20% of patients with BPDCN, coincident myelodysplasia that can subsequently lead to the development of acute myelomonocytic leukemia is identified.

HISTOPATHOLOGY

In cutaneous lesions, BPDCN typically infiltrates the dermis but spares the epidermis. As the disease progresses, it frequently extends into the subcutaneous fat. The neoplastic cells tend to aggregate in the superficial to mid dermis in a perivascular and/or periadnexal distribution, although, less frequently, they may be seen as a lichenoid infiltrate in the superficial dermis. At high magnification, BPDCN is characterized by a monotonous population of small to medium cells with irregular nuclear contours, fine to evenly dispersed chromatin, 1 to 3 small nucleoli, and scant to moderate amounts of cytoplasm.

By immunohistochemistry, the BPDCN cells typically express CD56, CD4, CD123, and T-cell leukemia/lymphoma 1 (TCL1). They can also express other plasmacytoid dendritic cell–associated antigens, such as blood dendritic cell antigen 2 (BDCA-2)/CD303 and the IFN-α–dependent molecule MxA.

PATHOGENESIS

BPDCN cells demonstrate a recurrent recombination of deletions in several tumor-suppressor genes, including *RB1*, *CDKN1B*, *CDKN2A*, and tumor protein P53 (*TP53*). The *TET2* gene (ten-eleven translocation-2) located on band 4q24 is mutated in BPDCN, myelodysplastic syndromes, chronic myelomonocytic leukemia, and acute myelomonocytic leukemia, which provides addition evidence that BPDCN is a myeloid-related neoplasm.

Targeted ultradeep sequencing revealed recurrent and mutually exclusive mutation of cancer genes in BPDCN. In 33 BPDCN samples, point mutations in *NRAS* (27.3%), *ATM* (21.2%), *MET*, *KRAS*, *IDH2*, and *KIT* (9.1% each) occurred. Moreover, *NRAS*, *KRAS*, and *ATM* mutations were found to be mutually exclusive. *CDKN2A* deletions were detected in 27.3% of the cases, followed by deletion of *RB1* (9.1%). The mutual exclusive distribution of some mutations may point to different subgroups of BPDCN, the biologic significance of which remains to be explored.[131,133,134]

TREATMENT AND PROGNOSIS

BPDCN is associated with a highly aggressive clinical course and thus a poor prognosis (median survival of 14 months). Although systemic chemotherapy is the first choice for treatment of this disease, gemcitabine may be useful to control the initial disease so that the patient can be referred as fast as possible for bone marrow transplantation.[135,136]

Another possibly promising approach is to address the IL-3 receptor CD123 by an immunoconjugate.[137]

REFERENCES

1. Willemze R, Jaffe ES, Burg G, et al. WHO-EORTC classification for cutaneous lymphomas. *Blood*. 2005;105:3768-3785.
2. Swerdlow SH, Campo E, Harris NL, et al. *WHO Classification of Tumours of Hematopoetic and Lymphoid Tissues*. 4th ed. Lyon, France: IARC Press; 2008.
3. Swerdlow SH, Campo E, Harris NL, et al. The 2016 revision of the World Health Organization classification of lymphoid neoplasms. *Blood*. 2016;127:2375-2390.
4. Weinstock MA, Gardstein B. Twenty-year trends in the reported incidence of mycosis fungoides and associated mortality. *Am J Public Health*. 1999;89:1240-1244.
5. Bradford PT, Devesa SS, Anderson WF, et al. Cutaneous lymphoma incidence pattern in the United States: a population-based study of 3884 cases. *Blood*. 2009;113:5064-5073.
6. Korgavkar K, Xiong M, Weinstock MA. Changing incidence trends in cutaneous lymphoma. *JAMA Dermatol*. 2013;149:1295-1299.
7. Clark RA, Chong B, Mirchandani N, et al. The vast majority of CLA+ T cells are resident in normal skin. *J Immunol*. 2006;176:4431-4439.
8. Reiss Y, Proudfoot AE, Power CA, et al. CC chemokine receptor (CCR)4 and the CCR 10 ligand cutaneous T cell-attracting chemokine (CTACK) in lymphocyte trafficking in inflamed skin. *J Exp Med*. 2001;194:1541-1547.

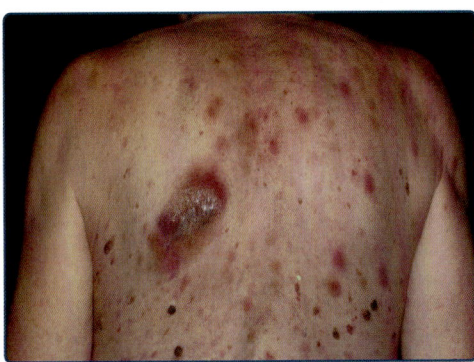

Figure 119-25 Blastic plasmacytoid dendritic cell neoplasm. Multiple lesions on the back. The large tumor was the initial site of manifestation (centrally located is the scar of a biopsy). The multiple small lesions developed in a short period of time.

9. Homey B, Alenius H, Muller A, et al. CCL27-CCR10 interactions regulate T cell-mediated skin inflammation. *Nat Med*. 2002;8:157-165.
10. Kirsch IR, Watanabe R, O'Malley JT, et al. TCR sequencing facilitates diagnoses and identifies mature T cells as the cell of origin in CTCL. *Sci Transl Med*. 2015;7:308ra158.
11. Watanabe R, Gehad A, Yang C, et al. Human skin is protected by four functionally and phenotypically discrete populations of resident and recirculating memory T cells. *Sci Transl Med*. 2015;7:279ra39.
12. Assaf CGS, Steinhoff M, Nashan D, et al. Cutaneous lymphomas in Germany: an analysis of the central cutaneous lymphoma registry of the German Society of Dermatology (DDG). *J Dtsch Dermatol Ges*. 2007;5:662-668.
13. Wilcox RA. Cutaneous T-cell lymphoma: 2016 Update on diagnosis, risk-stratification, and management. *Am J Hematol*. 2016;91:152-165.
14. Tan RS, Butterworth CM, McLaughlin H, et al. Mycosis fungoides—a disease of antigen persistence. *Br J Dermatol*. 1974;91:607-616.
15. Jackow CM, McHam JB, Friss A, et al. HLA-DR5 and DQB1*03 class II alleles are associated with cutaneous T-cell lymphoma. *J Invest Dermatol*. 1996;107:373-376.
16. Hodak E, Lapidoth M, Kohn K, et al. Mycosis fungoides: HLA class II associations among Ashkenazi and non-Ashkenazi Jewish patients. *Br J Dermatol*. 2001;145:974-980.
17. Pancake BA, Zucker-Franklin D, Coutavas EE. The cutaneous T cell lymphoma, mycosis fungoides, is a human T cell lymphotropic virus-associated disease. A study of 50 patients. *J Clin Invest*. 1995;95:547-550.
18. Zendri E, Pilotti E, Perez M, et al. The HTLV tax-like sequences in cutaneous T-cell lymphoma patients. *J Invest Dermatol*. 2008;128:489-492.
19. Courgnaud V, Duthanh A, Guillot B, et al. Absence of HTLV-related sequences in skin lesions and peripheral blood of cutaneous T-cell lymphomas. *J Invest Dermatol*. 2009;129:2520-2522.
20. Pawlaczyk M, Filas V, Sobieska M, et al. No evidence of HTLV-I infection in patients with mycosis fungoides and Sezary syndrome. *Neoplasma*. 2005;52:52-55.
21. Bazarbachi A, Soriano V, Pawson R, et al. Mycosis fungoides and Sezary syndrome are not associated with HTLV-I infection: an international study. *Br J Haematol*. 1997;98:927-933.
22. De Francesco MA, Gargiulo F, Esteban P, et al. Polymorphism analysis of Epstein-Barr virus isolates of lymphoblastoid cell lines from patients with mycosis fungoides. *J Med Microbiol*. 2004;53:381-387.
23. Novelli M, Merlino C, Ponti R, et al. Epstein-Barr virus in cutaneous T- cell lymphomas: evaluation of the viral presence and significance in skin and peripheral blood. *J Invest Dermatol*. 2009;129:1556-1561.
24. Quintanilla-Martinez L, Kimura H, Jaffe ES. EBV-positive T-cell lymphoproliferative disorders of childhood. In: Swerdlow SH, Campo E, Harris NL, et al, eds. *WHO Classification of Tumours of Haematopoetic and Lymphoid Tissues*. 4th ed. Lyon, France: IARC Press; 2008:278.
25. Vonderheid EC, Bigler RD, Hou JS. On the possible relationship between staphylococcal superantigens and increased Vbeta5.1 usage in cutaneous T-cell lymphoma. *Br J Dermatol*. 2005;152:825-826.
26. Jackow CM, Cather JC, Hearne V, et al. Association of erythrodermic cutaneous T-cell lymphoma, superantigen-positive *Staphylococcus aureus*, and oligoclonal T-cell receptor V beta gene expansion. *Blood*. 1997;89:32-40.
27. Tokura Y, Yagi H, Ohshima A, et al. Cutaneous colonization with staphylococci influences the disease activity of Sézary syndrome: a potential role for bacterial superantigens. *Br J Dermatol*. 1995;133:6-12.
28. Talpur R, Bassett R, Duvic M. Prevalence and treatment of *Staphylococcus aureus* colonization in patients with mycosis fungoides and Sézary syndrome. *Br J Dermatol*. 2008;159:105-112.
29. Willerslev-Olsen A, Krejsgaard T, Lindahl LM, et al. *Staphylococcus aureus* enterotoxin A (SEA) stimulates STAT3 activation and IL-17 expression in cutaneous T-cell lymphoma. *Blood*. 2016;127:1287-1296.
30. Whittemore AS, Holly EA, Lee IM, et al. Mycosis fungoides in relation to environmental exposures and immune response: a case-control study. *J Natl Cancer Inst*. 1989;81:1560-1567.
31. Morales-Suárez-Varela MM, Olsen J, Johansen P, et al. Occupational risk factors for mycosis fungoides: a European multicenter case-control study. *J Occup Environ Med*. 2004;46:205-211.
32. Girardi M, Heald PW, Wilson LD. The pathogenesis of mycosis fungoides. *N Engl J Med*. 2004;350:1978-1988.
33. Dummer R, Willers J, Kamarashev J, et al. Pathogenesis of cutaneous lymphomas. *Semin Cutan Med Surg*. 2000;19:78-86.
34. Chung GC, Poligone B. Cutaneous T cell lymphoma: an update on pathogenesis and systemic therapy. *Curr Hematol Malig Rep*. 2015;10:468-476.
35. Moins-Teisserenc H, Daubord M, Clave E, et al. CD158k is a reliable marker for diagnosis of Sézary syndrome and reveals an unprecedented heterogeneity of circulating malignant cells. *J Invest Dermatol*. 2015;135:247-257.
36. van Doorn R, van Kester MS, Dijkman R, et al. Oncogenomic analysis of mycosis fungoides reveals major differences with Sezary syndrome. *Blood*. 2009;113:127-136.
37. Vaque JP, Gomez-Lopez G, Monsalvez V, et al. PLCG1 mutations in cutaneous T-cell lymphomas. *Blood*. 2014;123:2034-2043.
38. Heid JB, Schmidt A, Oberle N, et al. FOXP31CD25- tumor cells with regulator function in Sezary syndrome. *J Invest Dermatol*. 2009;129:2875-2885.
39. Krejsgaard T, Odum N, Geisler C, et al. Regulator T cells and immunodeficiency in mycosis fungoides and Sezary syndrome. *Leukemia*. 2012;26:424-432.
40. Wilcox RA, Wada DA, Ziesmer SC, et al. Monocytes promote tumor cell survival in T cell lymphoproliferative disorders and are impaired in their ability to differentiate into mature dendritic cells. *Blood*. 2009;114:2936-2944.
41. Berger CL, Tigelaar R, Cohen J, et al. Cutaneous T-cell lymphoma: malignant proliferation of T-regulatory cells. *Blood*. 2005;105:1640-1647.
42. Clark RA. Skin-resident T cells: the ups and downs of on-site immunity. *J Invest Dermatol*. 2010;130:362-370.

43. Wang T, Feldman AL, Wada DA, et al. GATA-3 expression identifies a high-risk subset of PTCL, NOS with distinct molecular and clinical features. *Blood*. 2014;123:3007-3015.
44. Vowels BR, Lessin SR, Cassin M, et al. Th2 cytokine mRNA expression in skin in cutaneous T-cell lymphoma. *J Invest Dermatol*. 1994;103:669-673.
45. Choi J, Goh G, Walradt T, et al. Genomic landscape of cutaneous T cell lymphoma. *Nat Genet*. 2015;47:1011-1011.
46. McGirt LY, Jia P, Baerenwald DA, et al. Whole-genome sequencing reveals oncogenic mutations in mycosis fungoides. *Blood*. 2015;126:508-519.
47. Netchiporouk E, Litvinov IV, Moreau L, et al. Deregulation in STAT signaling is important for cutaneous T-cell lymphoma (CTCL) pathogenesis and cancer progression. *Cell Cycle*. 2014;13:3331-3335.
48. Kim YH, Liu HL, Mraz-Gernhard S, et al. Long-term outcome of 525 patients with mycosis fungoides and Sezary syndrome: clinical prognostic factors and risk for disease progression. *Arch Dermatol*. 2003;139:857-866.
49. Wasik MA. IL-13 as a novel growth factor in CTCL. *Blood*. 2015;125:2737-2738.
50. Rubio Gonzalez B, Zain J, Rosen ST, et al. Tumor microenvironment in mycosis fungoides and Sézary syndrome. *Curr Opin Oncol*. 2016;28:88-96.
51. Sibbesen NA, Kopp KL, Litvinov IV, et al. JAK3, STAT3, and STAT5 inhibit expression of MiR-22, a novel tumor suppressor microRNA, in cutaneous T-cell lymphoma. *Oncotarget*. 2015;6:20555-20569.
52. Ballabio E, Mitchell T, van Kester MS, et al. MicroRNA expression in Sezary syndrome: identification, function, and diagnostic. *Blood*. 2010;116:1105-1113.
53. Abraham RM, Zhang Q, Odum N, et al. The role of cytokine signaling in the pathogenesis of cutaneous T-cell lymphoma. *Cancer Biol Ther*. 2011;12:1019-1022.
54. Krejsgaard T, Ralfkiaer U, Clasen-Linde E, et al. Malignant cutaneous T-cell lymphoma cells express IL-17 utilizing the JAK3/Stat3 signaling pathway. *J Invest Dermatol*. 2011;131:1331-1338.
55. van der Fits L, Out-Luiting JJ, van Leeuwen MA, et al. Autocrine IL-12 stimulation is involved in the maintenance of constitutive STAT3 activation in Sézary syndrome. *J Invest Dermatol*. 2012;132:440-447.
56. Krejsgaard T, Vetter-Kauczok CS, Woetmann A, et al. JAK3- and JNK-dependent vascular endothelial growth factor expression in cutaneous T-cell lymphoma. *Leukemia*. 2006;20:1759-1766.
57. van der Fits L, van Kester MS, Qin Y, et al. MicroRNA-21 expression in CD4+ T cells is regulated by STAT 3 and is pathologically involved in Sézary syndrome. *J Invest Dermatol*. 2011;131:762-768.
58. Geskin LJ, Viragova S, Stolz DB, et al. Interleukin-13 is overexpressed in cutaneous T-cell lymphoma cells and regulates their proliferation. *Blood*. 2015;125:2798-2805.
59. Schwartz DM, Bonelli M, Gadina M, et al. Type I/II cytokines, JAKs, and new strategies for treating autoimmune diseases. *Nat Rev Rheumatol*. 2016;12:25-36.
60. Chung GC, Poligone B. Cutaneous T cell lymphoma: an update on pathogenesis and systemic treatment. *Curr Hematol Malig Rep*. 2015;10:468-476.
61. Schrader AM, Jansen PM, Willemze R. TOX expression in cutaneous T-cell lymphomas: an adjunctive diagnostic marker that is not tumor specific and not restricted to the CD4(+) CD8(-) phenotype. *Br J Dermatol*. 2016;175:382-386.
62. Scarisbrick JJ, Kim YH, Whittaker SJ, et al. Prognostic factors, prognostic indices and staging in mycosis fungoides and Sézary syndrome: where are we now? *Br J Dermatol*. 2014;170:1226-1236.
63. Scarisbrick JJ, Prince HM, Vermeer MH, et al. Cutaneous Lymphoma International Consortium study of outcome in advanced stages of mycosis fungoides and Sézary syndrome: effect of specific prognostic markers on survival and development of a prognostic model. *J Clin Oncol*. 2015;33:3766-3773.
64. van Santen S, Roach RE, van Doorn R, et al. Clinical staging and prognostic factors in folliculotropic mycosis fungoides. *JAMA Dermatol*. 2016;1;152(9):992-1000.
65. Hodak E, Amitay-Laish I, Atzmony L, et al. New insights into folliculotropic mycosis fungoides (FMF): a single-center experience. *J Am Acad Dermatol*. 2016;75:347-355.
66. Olsen, E., Vonderheid E, Pimpinelli N, et al. Revisions to the staging and classification of mycosis fungoides and Sezary syndrome: a proposal of International Society for Cutaneous Lymphomas (ISCL) and the Cutaneous Lymphoma Task Force of the European Organization of Research and Treatment of Cancer (EORTC). *Blood*. 2007;110: 1713-1722.
67. Kim YH, Willemze R, Pimpinelli N, et al. TNM classification system for primary cutaneous lymphomas other than mycosis fungoides and Sezary syndrome: a proposal of the International Society for Cutaneous Lymphomas (ISCL) and the Cutaneous Lymphoma Task Force of the European Organization of Research and Treatment of Cancer (EORTC). *Blood*. 2007;110:479-484.
68. Burg G, Kempf W, Cozzio A, et al. WHO/EORTC classification of cutaneous lymphomas 2005: histological and molecular aspects. *J Cutan Pathol*. 2005;32:647-674.
69. Kempf W. Cutaneous CD30-positive lymphoproliferative disorders. *Surg Pathol Clin*. 2014;7:203-228.
70. Kempf W, Pfaltz K, Vermeer MH, et al. European Organization for Research and Treatment of Cancer (EORTC), International Society of Cutaneous Lymphoma (ISCL) and United States Cutaneous Lymphoma Consortium (USCLC) consensus recommendations for the treatment of primary cutaneous CD30-positive lymphoproliferative disorders: lymphomatoid papulosis and primary cutaneous anaplastic large-cell lymphoma. *Blood*. 2011;118:4024-4035.
71. Kadin ME, Carpenter C. Systemic and primary cutaneous anaplastic large cell lymphomas. *Semin Hematol*. 2003;40:244-256.
72. Massone C, El-Shabrawi-Caelen L, Kerl H, et al. The morphologic spectrum of primary cutaneous anaplastic large T-cell lymphoma: a histopathologic study on 66 biopsy specimens from 47 patients with report of rare variants. *J Cutan Pathol*. 2008;35:46-53.
73. Kempf W, Mitteldorf C. Pathologic diagnosis of cutaneous lymphomas. *Dermatol Clin*. 2015;33:655-681.
74. Willemze R, Jansen PM, Cerroni L, et al. Subcutaneous panniculitis-like T-cell lymphoma: definition, classification, and prognostic factors: an EORTC Cutaneous Lymphoma Group Study of 83 cases. *Blood*. 2008;111:838-845.

75. Guitart J, Weisenburger DD, Subtil A, et al. Cutaneous gamma delta T-cell lymphomas: a spectrum of presentations with overlap with other cytotoxic lymphomas. *Am J Surg Pathol*. 2012;36:1656-1665.
76. Kempf W, Kazakov D, Kerl K. Cutaneous lymphomas an update part 1: T-cell and natural killer/T-cell lymphomas and related conditions. *Am J Dermatopathol*. 2014;36:105-123.
77. Garcia-Herrera A, Colomo L, Camos M, et al. Primary cutaneous small/medium CD4+ T-cell lymphomas: a heterogeneous group of tumors with different clinicopathologic features and outcome. *J Clin Oncol*. 2008;26:3364-3371.
78. James E, Sokhn JK, Gibson JF, et al. CD4+ primary cutaneous small/medium-sized pleomorphic T-cell lymphoma: a retrospective case series and review of the literature. *Leuk Lymphoma*. 2015;56:951-957.
79. Beltraminelli H, Leinweber B, Kerl H, et al. Primary cutaneous CD4+ small-/medium-sized pleomorphic T-cell lymphoma: a cutaneous nodular proliferation of pleomorphic T lymphocytes of undetermined significance? A study of 136 cases. *Am J Dermatopathol*. 2009;31:317-322.
80. Berti E, Tomasini D, Vermeer MH, et al. Primary cutaneous CD8-positive epidermotropic cytotoxic T cell lymphomas. A distinct clinicopathological entity with an aggressive clinical behavior. *Am J Pathol*. 1999;155:483-492.
81. Kluk J, Kai A, Koch D, et al. Indolent CD8-positive lymphoid proliferation of acral sites: three further cases of a rare entity and an update on a unique patient. *J Cutan Pathol*. 2016;43:125-136.
82. Olsen EA, Whittaker S, Kim YH, et al. Clinical end points and response criteria in mycosis fungoides and Sézary syndrome: a consensus statement of the International Society for Cutaneous Lymphomas, the United States Cutaneous Lymphoma Consortium, and the Cutaneous Lymphoma Task Force of the European Organisation for Research and Treatment of Cancer. *J Clin Oncol*. 2011;29:2598-2607.
83. Trautinger F, Knobler R, Willemze R, et al. EORTC consensus recommendations for the treatment of mycosis fungoides/Sézary syndrome. *Eur J Cancer*. 2006;42:1014-1030.
84. Duvic M. Choosing a systemic treatment for advanced stage cutaneous T-cell lymphoma: mycosis fungoides and Sézary syndrome. *Hematology Am Soc Hematol Educ Program*. 2015;2015:529-544.
85. Martinez-Gonzalez MC, Verea-Hernando MM, Yebra-Pimental MT, et al. Imiquimod in mycosis fungoides. *Eur J Dermatol*. 2008;18:148-152.
86. Rook AH, Gelfand JC, Wysocka M, et al. Topical resiquimod can induce disease regression and enhance T-cell effector functions in cutaneous T-cell lymphoma. *Blood*. 2015;126:1452-1461.
87. Kamstrup, MR, Lindahl LM, Gniadecki R, et al. Low-dose total skin electron beam therapy as a debulking agent for cutaneous T-cell lymphoma: an open-label prospective phase II study. *Br J Dermatol*. 2012;166:399-404.
88. Hoppe, RT, Harrison C, Travallaee M, et al. Low-dose total skin electron beam therapy as an effective modality to reduce disease burden in patients with mycosis fungoides: results of a pooled analysis from 3 phase-II clinical trials. *J Am Acad Dermatol*. 2015;72:286-292.
89. Stadler R. Optimal combination with PUVA: rationale and clinical trial update. *Oncology (Williston Park)*. 2007;21(2)(suppl 1):29-32.
90. Duvic M, Hymes K, Heald P, et al. Bexarotene is effective and safe for treatment of refractory advanced-stage cutaneous T-cell lymphoma: multinational phase II-III trial results. *J Clin Oncol*. 2001;19:2456-2471.
91. Duvic M, Martin AG, Kim Y, et al. Phase 2 and 3 clinical trial of oral bexarotene (Targretin capsules) for the treatment of refractory or persistent early-stage cutaneous T-cell lymphoma. *Arch Dermatol*. 2001;137:581-593.
92. Whittaker S, Ortiz P, Dummer R, et al. Efficacy and safety of bexarotene combined with psoralen-ultraviolet A (PUVA) compared with PUVA treatment alone in stage IB-IIA mycosis fungoides: final results from the EORTC Cutaneous Lymphoma Task Force phase III randomized clinical trial (NCT00056056). *Br J Dermatol*. 2012;167:678-687.
93. Assaf C, Bagot M, Dummer R, et al. Minimizing adverse side-effects of oral bexarotene in cutaneous T-cell lymphoma: an expert opinion. *Br J Dermatol*. 2006;155:261-266.
94. Gniadecki R, Assaf C, Bagot M, et al. The optimal use of bexarotene in cutaneous T-cell lymphoma. *Br J Dermatol*. 2007;157:433-440.
95. Knobler R, Berlin G, Calzavara-Pinton P, et al. Guidelines on the use of extracorporeal photopheresis. *J Eur Acad Dermatol Venereol*. 2014;28(suppl 1):1-37.
96. Dippel E, Schrag H, Goerdt S, et al. Extracorporeal photopheresis and interferon-alpha in advanced cutaneous T-cell lymphoma. *Lancet*. 1997;350:32-33.
97. Stadler R, Otte HG, Luger T, et al. Prospective randomized multicenter clinical trial on the use of interferon-2a plus acitretin versus interferon-2a plus PUVA in patients with cutaneous T-cell lymphoma stages I and II. *Blood*. 1998;92:3578-3581.
97A. Lundin J, Hagberg H, Repp R, et al. Phase 2 study of alemtuzumab (anti-CD52 monoclonal antibody) in patients with advanced mycosis fungoides/Sezary syndrome. *Blood*. 2003;101(11):4267-4272.
97B. Querfeld C, Mehta N, Rosen ST, et al. Alemtuzumab for relapsed and refractory erythrodermic cutaneous T-cell lymphoma: a single institution experience from the Robert H. Lurie Comprehensive Cancer Center. *Leuk Lymphoma*. 2009;50(12):1969-1976.
98. Watanabe R, Teague JE, Fisher DC, et al. Alemtuzumab therapy for leukemic cutaneous T-cell lymphoma: diffuse erythema as a positive predictor of complete remission. *JAMA Dermatol*. 2014;150:776-779.
98A. Clark RA, Watanabe R, Teague JE, et al. Skin effector memory T cells do not recirculate and provide immune protection in alemtuzumab-treated CTCL patients. *Sci Transl Med*. 2012 Jan 18;4(117):117ra7.
99. Bernengo MG, Quaglino P, Comessatti A, et al. Low-dose intermittent alemtuzumab in the treatment of Sézary syndrome: clinical and immunological findings in 14 patients. *Haematologica*. 2007;92:784-794.
100. Duvic M, Tetzlaff MT, Gangar P, et al. Results of a phase II trial of brentuximab vedotin for CD30+ cutaneous T-cell lymphoma and lymphomatoid papulosis. *J Clin Oncol*. 2015;33:3759-3765.
100A. Prince HM, Kim YH, Horwitz SM, et al; ALCANZA Study Group. Brentuximab vedotin or physician's choice in CD30-positive cutaneous T-cell lymphoma (ALCANZA): an international, open-label, randomised, phase 3, multicentre trial. *Lancet*. 2017 Aug 5;390(10094):555-566.

101. Kim YH, Tavallaee M, Sundram U, et al. Phase II investigator-initiated study of brentuximab vedotin in mycosis fungoides and Sézary syndrome with variable CD30 expression level: a multi-institution collaborative project. *J Clin Oncol.* 2015;33:2750-2758.
102. Duvic M, Pinter-Brown LC, Foss FM, et al. Phase 1/2 study of mogamulizumab, a defucosylated anti-CCR4 antibody, in previously treated patients with cutaneous T-cell lymphoma. *Blood.* 2015;125:1883-1889.
102A. Kim YH, Bagot M, Pinter-Brown L, et al. Anti-CCR4 monoclonal antibody mogamulizumab versus vorinostat in previously treated cutaneous T-cell lymphoma (MAVORIC): an international, randomized, phase 3 trial. *Lancet Oncol,* in press.
103. Bunn PA, Hoffmann SJ, Norris D, et al. Systemic therapy of cutaneous T-cell lymphomas (mycosis fungoides and the Sézary syndrome). *Ann Intern Med.* 1994;121:592-602.
104. Marchi E, Alinari L, Tani M, et al. Gemcitabine as frontline treatment for cutaneous T-cell lymphoma: phase II study of 32 patients. *Cancer.* 2005;104:2437-2441.
105. Duvic M, Talpur R, Wen S, et al. Phase II evaluation of gemcitabine monotherapy for cutaneous T-cell lymphoma. *Clin Lymphoma Myeloma.* 2006;7:51-58.
106. Dummer R, Quaglino P, Becker JC, et al. Prospective international multicenter phase II trial of intravenous pegylated liposomal doxorubicin monochemotherapy in patients with stage IIB, IVA, or IVB advanced mycosis fungoides: final results from EORTC 21012. *J Clin Oncol.* 2012;30:4891-4897.
106A. Horwitz SM, Kim YH, Foss F, et al. Identification of an active, well-tolerated dose of pralatrexate in patients with relapsed or refractory cutaneous T-cell lymphoma. *Blood.* 2012;119(18):4115-4122.
107. O'Connor OA, Pro B, Pinter-Brown L, et al. Pralatrexate in patients with relapsed or refractory peripheral T-cell lymphoma: results from the pivotal PROPEL study. *J Clin Oncol.* 2011;29:1182-1189.
108. Lechowicz MJ, Lazarus HM, Carreras J, et al. Allogeneic hematopoietic cell transplantation for mycosis fungoides and Sezary syndrome. *Bone Marrow Transplant.* 2014;49:1360-1365.
109. Duarte RF, Boumendil A, Gabriel I, et al. Long-term outcome of allogeneic hematopoietic cell transplantation for patients with mycosis fungoides and Sézary syndrome: a European Society for Blood and Marrow Transplantation Lymphoma Working Party extended analysis. *J Clin Oncol.* 2014;32:3347-3348.
110. Smith BD, Smith GL, Cooper DL, et al. The cutaneous B-cell lymphoma prognostic index: a novel prognostic index derived from a population-based registry. *J Clin Oncol.* 2005;23:3390-3395.
111. Zinzani PL, Quaglino P, Pimpinelli N, et al.; Italian Study Group for Cutaneous Lymphomas. Prognostic factors in primary cutaneous B-cell lymphoma: the Italian Study Group for Cutaneous Lymphomas. *J Clin Oncol.* 2006;24:1376-1382.
112. Senff NJ, Hoefnagel JJ, Jansen PM, et al. Reclassification of 300 primary cutaneous B-cell lymphomas according to the new WHO-EORTC classification for cutaneous lymphomas: comparison with previous classifications and identification of prognostic markers. *J Clin Oncol.* 2007;25:1381-1387.
113. Kerl H, Kodama K, Cerroni L. Diagnostic principles and new developments in primary cutaneous B-cell lymphomas. *J Dermatol Sci.* 2004;34:167-175.
114. Hallermann C, Kaune KM, Gesk S, et al. Molecular cytogenetic analysis of chromosomal breakpoints in the IGH, MYC, BCL6, and MALT1 gene loci in primary cutaneous B-cell lymphomas. *J Invest Dermatol.* 2004;123:213-219.
115. Vermeer MH, Willemze R. Recent advances in primary cutaneous B-cell Lymphoma. *Curr Opin Oncol.* 2014;26:230-236.
116. Kodama K, Massone C, Chott A, et al. Primary cutaneous large B-cell lymphomas: clinicopathologic features, classification, and prognostic factors in a large series of patients. *Blood.* 2005;106:2491-2497.
117. Golling P, Cozzio A, Dummer R, et al. Primary cutaneous B-cell lymphomas—clinicopathological, prognostic and therapeutic characterisation of 54 cases according to the WHO-EORTC classification and the ISCL/EORTC TNM classification system for primary cutaneous lymphomas other than mycosis fungoides and Sézary syndrome. *Leuk Lymphoma.* 2008;49:1094-1103.
118. Servitje O, Estrach T, Pujol RM, et al. Primary cutaneous marginal zone B-cell lymphoma: a clinical, histopathological, immunophenotypic and molecular genetic study of 22 cases. *Br J Dermatol.* 2002;147:1147-1158.
119. Hoefnagel JJ, Vermeer MH, Jansen PM, et al. Primary cutaneous marginal zone B-cell lymphoma: clinical and therapeutic features in 50 cases. *Arch Dermatol.* 2005;141:1139-1145.
120. Dijkman R, Tensen CP, Buettner M, et al. Primary cutaneous follicle center lymphoma and primary cutaneous large B-cell lymphoma, leg type, are both targeted by aberrant somatic hypermutation but demonstrate differential expression of AID. *Blood.* 2006;107:4926-4929.
121. Deutsch AJ, Frühwirth M, Aigelsreiter A, et al. Primary cutaneous marginal zone B-cell lymphomas are targeted by aberrant somatic hypermutation. *J Invest Dermatol.* 2009;129:476-479.
122. Liu M, Schatz DG. Balancing AID and DNA repair during somatic hypermutation. *Trends Immunol.* 2009;30:173-181.
123. Hoefnagel JJ, Dijkman R, Basso K, et al. Distinct types of primary cutaneous large B-cell lymphoma identified by gene expression profiling. *Blood.* 2005;105:3671-3678.
124. Senff NJ, Zoutman WH, Vermeer MH, et al. Fine-mapping chromosomal loss at 9p21: correlation with prognosis in primary cutaneous diffuse large B-cell lymphoma, leg type. *J Invest Dermatol.* 2009;129:1149-1155.
125. Grange F, Joly P, Barbe C, et al. Improvement of survival in patients with primary cutaneous diffuse large B-cell lymphoma, leg type, in France. *JAMA Dermatol.* 2014;150:535-541.
126. van Maldegem F, van Dijk R, Wormhoudt TA, et al. The majority of cutaneous marginal zone B-cell lymphomas expresses class-switched immunoglobulins and develops in a T-helper type 2 inflammatory environment. *Blood.* 2008;112:3355-3361.
127. Kutzner H, Kerl H, Pfaltz MC, et al. CD123-positive plasmacytoid dendritic cells in primary cutaneous marginal zone B-cell lymphoma: diagnostic and pathogenetic implications. *Am J Surg Pathol.* 2009;33:1307-1313.
128. van Galen JC, Hoefnagel JJ, Vermeer MH, et al. Profiling of apoptosis genes identifies distinct types of

primary cutaneous large B cell lymphoma. *J Pathol.* 2008;215:340-346.
129. Senff NJ, Hoefnagel JJ, Jansen PM, et al. Reclassification of 300 primary cutaneous B-cell lymphomas according to the new WHO-EORTC classification for cutaneous lymphomas: comparison with previous classifications and identification of prognostic markers. *J Clin Oncol.* 2007;25:1581-1587.
130. Brandenburg A, Humme D, Terhorst D, et al. Long-term outcome of intravenous therapy with rituximab in patients with primary cutaneous B-cell lymphomas. *Br J Dermatol.* 2013;169:1126-1132.
131. Stenzinger A, Endris V, Pfarr N, et al. Targeted ultra-deep sequencing reveals recurrent and mutually exclusive mutations of cancer genes in blastic plasmacytoid dendritic cell neoplasm. *Oncotarget.* 2014;5:6404-6412.
131A. Senff NJ, Kluin-Nelemans HC, Willemze R. Results of bone marrow examination in 275 patients with histological features that suggest an indolent type of cutaneous B-cell lymphoma. *Br J Haematol.* 2008 Jul;142(1):52-56.
132. Neelis KJ, Schimmel EV. Vermeer MH, et al. Low-dose palliative radiotherapy for cutaneous B- and T-cell lymphomas. *Int J Radiat Oncol Biol Phys.* 2009;74:154-158.
133. Shi Y, Wang E. Blastic plasmacytoid dendritic cell neoplasm. A clinicopathologic review. *Arch Pathol Lab Med.* 2014;138:564-569.
134. Julia F, Dalle S, Duru G, et al. Blastic plasmacytoid dendritic cell neoplasms. Clinico-immunohistochemical correlations in a series of 91 patients. *Am J Surg Pathol.* 2014;38:673-680.
135. Aoki T, Suzuki R, Kuwatsuka Y, et al. Long-term survival following autologous and allogeneic stem cell transplantation for blastic plasmacytoid dendritic cell neoplasm. *Blood.* 2015;125:3559-3562.
136. Julia F, Petrella T, Beylot-Barry M, et al. Blastic plasmacytoid dendritic cell neoplasm: clinical features in 90 patients. *Br J Dermatol.* 2013;169:579-586.
137. Frankel AE, Woo JH, Ahn C, et al. Activity of SL401, a targeted therapy directed to interleukin-3 receptor in blastic plasmacytoid dendritic cell neoplasm patients. *Blood.* 2014;124:385-392.

Chapter 120 :: Cutaneous Pseudolymphoma
Werner Kempf, Rudolf Stadler, & Martine Bagot

第一百二十章
皮肤假性淋巴瘤

中文导读

皮肤假性淋巴瘤是指一组皮肤疾病，可定义为在临床和/或组织学上模拟皮肤淋巴瘤的良性淋巴增生过程。这些疾病在临床、组织学和免疫表型表现上不同，病因也不同。本章分为10节：①定义；②历史；③分类；④诊断；⑤病程；⑥结节性假性淋巴瘤；⑦假性蕈样肉芽肿；⑧其他富淋巴细胞浸润的疾病；⑨良性淋巴细胞血管内增生；⑩总结。

第一节介绍了皮肤假性淋巴瘤的定义及诱发因素，包括感染性因素、注射疫苗、异物以及药物等。

第二节介绍了皮肤假性淋巴瘤的命名历程。

第三节介绍了皮肤假性淋巴瘤的不同分类方法，可根据病因有主要的淋巴细胞成分或表型分类。

第四节介绍了诊断包括组织学检查、诊断检查（包括病史和体查）以及外周血淋巴细胞、嗜酸性粒细胞、感染性病原体的血清学检查，必要时行放射检查。

第五节介绍了皮肤假性淋巴瘤的病程是高度多变的，活检后可能会消退，但有些持续几个月甚至几年。由药物或过敏原引起的可复发。

第六节结节性假淋巴瘤，介绍了皮肤B细胞假性淋巴组织瘤、皮肤T细胞和混合性假性淋巴瘤、CD30+T细胞假性淋巴瘤、假性淋巴瘤性毛囊炎及其他形式的结节性假性淋巴管瘤的临床表现、组织病理学、鉴别诊断、病因、流行病学、实验室检查、临床病程与预后。

第七节假性蕈样肉芽肿，重点介绍了淋巴瘤样接触性皮炎、淋巴瘤样药物反应、光化性类网状细胞增多症、免疫缺陷CD8+T细胞假性淋巴瘤等的临床表现、实验室检查、诊断与鉴别诊断、临床病程、预后和治疗。

第八节其他富淋巴细胞浸润的疾病，概述了肢端假淋巴母细胞瘤、淋巴浆细胞性斑块、皮肤浆细胞增多症、皮肤炎性假瘤、CASTLEMAN病的基本特征及治疗方法，详细介绍了血管淋巴样增生伴嗜酸性粒细胞增多症的临床特点、组织病理学、免疫表型和分子检测、临床病程、治疗和预后。

第九节良性淋巴细胞血管内增生，介绍了其可表达或不表达CD30，常发生在有炎症性皮肤病或皮肤创伤的区域，如硬化性苔癣可出现。

第十节总结了临床与病理的对照是皮肤假性淋巴瘤与皮肤淋巴瘤鉴别诊断最重要的环节，消除感染性因素或避免暴露于病原体是治疗的第一步。

〔粟 娟〕

AT-A-GLANCE

- Cutaneous pseudolymphomas are benign lymphoproliferations that clinically and/or histologically simulate cutaneous lymphomas.
- They exhibit a wide range of clinical, histological, and immunophenotypic features and can be triggered by different infectious and non-infectious agents.
- Clinicopathological correlation plays an important role in the differentiation from cutaneous lymphomas.
- Therapy includes avoidance of exposure to the causative agent, immunomodulating agents or ablative approaches.

DEFINITION

The term *cutaneous pseudolymphoma* refers to a group of skin diseases that can be defined as benign lymphoproliferative processes that clinically and/or histologically simulate cutaneous lymphomas. These diseases differ in their clinical, histologic, and immunophenotypic presentation, and are of different etiologies (Table 120-1).

A broad spectrum of causative factors known to induce cutaneous pseudolymphomas (PSLs) have been identified. Infectious agents, such as spirochetal bacteria (*Borrelia burgdorferi* sp., *Treponema pallidum*), viruses (eg, parapoxviruses), infestations (eg, scabies), insect bites, injection of vaccines or antigens for hyposensitization, foreign bodies such as tattoos and metals, and drugs have been identified as causative factors for PSL. All cases without identifiable cause are referred to as an idiopathic form of PSL.

HISTORICAL ASPECTS

Various synonyms have been introduced and several terms are still nowadays used to describe PSLs of the skin. For the first time the concept of PSL (pseudomalignancy) had been introduced by M. Kaposi in 1891 (Table 120-2).[1] In 1923, Biberstein coined the term *lymphocytoma cutis*.[2] Subsequently, in 1943, Bäfverstedt used the designation *lymphadenosis benigna cutis*.[3] Lever introduced the term *pseudolymphoma of Spiegler and Fendt* in 1967, and in 1969, Caro and Helwig employed the term *cutaneous lymphoid hyperplasia*.[4] Many other terms were proposed and referred mostly to B-cell PSLs. Among T-cell PSLs, actinic reticuloid was first described in 1969.[5] In the 1980s the designation cutaneous PSL for B-cell–dominated and T-cell–dominated processes became more widely used and accepted.[6] Synonymously, the term *atypical lymphoid proliferation* is often employed by pathologists and dermatopathologists.

CLASSIFICATION

Various approaches have been proposed to categorize cutaneous PSL. For example, according to the etiology, the predominant lymphocytic component (T, B, or mixed cells) or distinct clinical features (eg, acral papular angiokeratoma of childhood).[7-9]

Categorization of PSL according to etiology or histology and phenotype into T-cell and B-cell PSL is widely used in textbooks. In daily work, clinicians or pathologists encountering infiltrates suspicious of being a PSL cannot recognize the etiology and the phenotype at first glance; further diagnostic workup is needed. Moreover, it has to be emphasized that the composition of the infiltrate is determined mostly by genetic and immunologic factors of the host rather than the causative agent per se, as the same agents can, in many instances, induce B-cell PSL and T-cell PSL as well.

From a practical point of view, cutaneous PSL presenting as a solitary or multiple nodule(s), which clinically and histologically simulate lymphoma, can be distinguished from other forms of PSL, which mimic cutaneous T-cell lymphoma on histologic grounds alone, and are summarized under the term *pseudo–mycosis fungoides* (pseudo-MF). In addition, there are numerous infectious and noninfectious conditions that are characterized by a lymphocyte-rich infiltrate and are prone to be misinterpreted as cutaneous lymphoma primarily on histologic grounds.

Thus, this chapter is divided into the following sections: (a) nodular PSL simulating clinically and histologically T-cell or B-cell lymphoma; (b) PSLs mimicking histologically mycosis fungoides (so called pseudo-MF); (c) other skin disorders with lymphocyte-rich infiltrates; and (d) benign intravascular proliferation of lymphocytes (simulating intravascular lymphoma) (see Table 120-1).

DIAGNOSTIC APPROACH

The clinical presentation of cutaneous PSL ranges from a solitary nodule to clustered or disseminated papules to erythroderma.[8,10] The histologic analysis plays a crucial role in the diagnostic approach to cutaneous PSLs. Different infiltrate patterns (nodular infiltrate vs epidermotropic infiltrates), the size of the lymphocytes (mostly small cells; occasionally medium and large cells), immunophenotype (T-cell vs B-cell; CD4 vs CD8; CD30) can be distinguished. Molecular studies for clonality and infectious agents, especially *Borrelia burgdorferi*, are adjunctive diagnostic tools. It is important to emphasize that the detection of a clonal T-cell or B-cell population per se does not indicate the presence of malignant lymphoma. Moreover some PSL cases have been reported to harbor clonal T or B cells.[11-14] Thus, both the histologic and the molecular findings always need to be interpreted in synopsis with the clinical context; that is, the clinicopathologic correlation is essential to achieve the final diagnosis.

The diagnostic workup includes the medical history (particularly exposure to arthropods, allergens, and drugs) and physical examination including palpatory evaluation of lymph nodes, examination of peripheral blood (lymphocytosis, eosinophilia, serology for infectious agents, especially *B. burgdorferi*, syphilis, HIV). Because PSLs represent benign lymphocytic prolifera-

TABLE 120-1
Spectrum of Cutaneous Pseudolymphoma

1. Nodular pseudolymphoma
B-cell pseudolymphoma (PSL)
T-cell PSL
    CD30+ T-cell PSL
Mixed PSL
Pseudolymphomatous folliculitis
Causes:
Infections: Borrelia burgdorferi
             Treponema pallidum
             α-Herpesviruses
             Parapoxviruses
             Molluscum contagiosum virus
Drugs: Anticonvulsants, vaccines
Arthropod bites, infestations, leeches (*Hirudo medicinalis*)
Lymphomatoid reaction to tattoo and metals

2. PSLs—histologic simulators of mycosis fungoides ("pseudo-MF")
Lymphomatoid contact dermatitis
Lymphomatoid drug reaction
Actinic reticuloid
Immunodeficiency-associated cutaneous CD8+ infiltrates
B. burgdorferi–associated T-cell infiltrates
Papuloerythroderma Ofuji
Clonal dermatitis

3. Other disorders with lymphocyte-rich infiltrates
Acral persistent angiokeratoma
Lymphoplasmacytic plaque
Cutaneous plasmacytosis
Cutaneous inflammatory pseudotumor
Angiolymphoid hyperplasia with eosinophilia
T-cell–rich angiomatoid polypoid pseudolymphoma of the skin
Castleman disease
             Lymphocytic infiltration of the skin
             Palpable arciforme migratory erythema
             Lichen sclerosus, pityriasis lichenoides, vitiligo
             Pigmented purpuric dermatoses
             Morphea (inflammatory stage)
             Lupus tumidus, lupus panniculitis

4. Benign intravascular proliferation of lymphocytes
Benign intravascular proliferation of lymphoid blasts
Benign atypical intravascular CD30+ T-cell proliferation

TABLE 120-2
Terminology of Cutaneous Pseudolymphoma—Historical Aspect

Year	Term
1891	Sarcomatosis cutis (M. Kaposi)[1]
1910	Sarcoid Spiegler-Fendt (Darier)[114]
1923	Lymphocytoma cutis (Biberstein)[2]
1943	Lymphadenosis benigna cutis (Bäfverstedt)[3]
1969	Cutaneous lymphoid hyperplasia (Caro and Helwig)[4]
1982	Cutaneous pseudolymphoma (Burg et al)[6]

ular lesions, monotypic expression of immunoglobulin light chains, detection of T-cell or B-cell clonality, or other inconsistent or unexpected histologic or phenotypic findings, radiologic staging (computed tomography or positron emission tomography-computed tomography) should be considered to exclude primary or secondary cutaneous lymphoma mimicking PSL.

COURSE

The course of cutaneous PSLs is highly variable. Resolution may occur after biopsy, but some lesions may persist over several months or even years. Recurrences can be observed particularly after reexposure to the inducing agent in cases that are caused by drugs or allergens. Progression of PSL has been reported, but is a very rare event, if it exists at all.[15] It remains unclear whether PSL in fact progressed to overt lymphoma (eg, by acquisition of chromosomal aberrations or persisting antigenic stimulus resulting in permanent proliferation of lymphocytes) or whether those cases represent cutaneous lymphomas from the very beginning, but could not be recognized as such by histologic, phenotypic, or molecular findings in their very early disease stages.

NODULAR PSEUDOLYMPHOMA

PSLs that present with a solitary nodule or with multiple nodules simulate cutaneous T-cell and B-cell lymphomas on clinical and histologic grounds. They represent one of the most common forms of PSL, but no detailed data on the overall prevalence of B-cell PSLs have been reported. Histologically they can be classified according to the predominant lymphocytic subset into B-cell, T-cell, and mixed (T-cell/B-cell) PSL.[8,10] This classification is rather artificial as B-cell PSL always contains T cells and vice versa. T-cell PSL often harbors a variable number of B cells. Nevertheless, the distinction into the 3 histologic and phenotypic subtypes of nodular PSL remains useful for the differential diagnosis, which also has to be considered for the potential cause of the pseudolymphomatous reaction.

Avoidance of reexposure to the inducing agent (eg, vaccines, allergen injection, other drugs, *Hirudo medicinalis* treatment, acupuncture, and tattoo) is the most important step to prevent persistence and recurrence of nodular PSL. Solitary lesions can be treated by complete surgical excision, topical or intralesional corticosteroids, cryotherapy, or laser therapy (Table 120-3). If those therapeutic approaches are not successful, radiation therapy may be considered. In patients with multiple PSL lesions, particularly those with idiopathic multifocal PSL, systemic corticosteroids, intralesional interferon-α, or hydroxychloroquine may be therapeutic options. Hydroxychloroquine inhibits the activity of plasmacytoid dendritic cells, which are found in the majority of B-cell PSLs as clusters in close vicinity to

TABLE 120-3
Treatment of Nodular Pseudolymphoma

1. Avoidance or elimination of the causative agent (eg, contact allergen)
2. Antibiotic treatment for infection-associated pseudolymphoma (eg, *Borrelia*-associated-cell pseudolymphoma)
3. Surgical excision, cryotherapy, laser treatment
4. Topical/intralesional steroids or interferon-α
5. Systemic steroids, hydroxychloroquine

T cells and plasma cells, and may represent the driving force in induction and maintenance of the PSLs.[16,17]

CUTANEOUS B-CELL PSEUDOLYMPHOMA

B-cell PSL is often also referred as lymphocytoma cutis or cutaneous lymphoid hyperplasia.

CLINICAL FEATURES

B-cell PSL most commonly presents with a nodule or plaque. The face, especially the nose and the cheeks, the upper trunk, and the arms are the most commonly involved sites. A male-to-female ratio of 2:1 has been described.[18] Approximately 67% of the patients with B-cell PSLs are younger than age 40 years and less than 10% are children and adolescents.[4]

The localized form of B-cell PSL that presents with a solitary nodule measuring up to 4 cm, is the most common presentation. One-third of patients develop multiple nodules or a miliarial form in which the lesions are papules measuring only a few millimeters in diameter.[19]

HISTOLOGY

All nodular B-cell PSLs essentially share the same growth pattern and composition of the infiltrate. There is a dense nodular infiltrate, predominantly located in the reticular dermis and occasionally extending into the superficial parts of the subcutis. The infiltrate is mostly composed of small lymphocytes with chromatin dense nuclei and reactive germinal centers containing tingible body macrophages. The lymphocytes do not show nuclear atypia. There is an admixture of plasma cells, which usually do not form aggregates but are rather diffusely scattered throughout the infiltrate. Eosinophils and a granulomatous component can be observed in some cases. There is an admixture of a variable number of T cells, which usually account for less than 30% of the infiltrate. Immunophenotyping reveals that the majority of the infiltrate is represented by CD19+, CD20+, and CD79a+ B cells. The cells in the reactive follicles express bcl-6, but are negative for bcl-2, whereas the small B cells in the interfollicular area express bcl-2, but are negative for bcl-6. The networks of CD21+ follicular dendritic cells are sharply demarcated and regularly structured. Polytypic expression of immunoglobulin (Ig) light chains κ and λ by plasma cells is found by immunohistochemistry or in situ hybridization. Molecular studies demonstrate lack of monoclonal rearrangement of Ig heavy-chain genes by polymerase chain reaction (PCR) or Southern blot analysis.

DIFFERENTIAL DIAGNOSES

The differential diagnosis of B-cell PSLs primarily includes other B-cell infiltrates with a follicular pattern; that is, primary cutaneous marginal zone lymphoma (PCMZL) and primary cutaneous follicle center lymphoma (PCFCL) or their nodal or other extranodal counterparts presenting with secondary cutaneous infiltrates (Table 120-4). The architecture and composition of the infiltrate in PCMZL is very similar to that of B-cell PSL as both present with nodular infiltrates in the reticular dermis and superficial subcutis.[20] In comparison with B-cell PSL, the plasma cells in PCMZL are usually more prominent and found in sheets, particularly at the periphery of the infiltrates. The most important histopathologic diagnostic finding is the monotypic expression of Ig light chains in PCMZL with a ratio of at least 5:1 and ranging up to 10:1 for the expression of 1 of the 2 Ig light chains. The presence and number of eosinophils are not a useful finding for discrimination between B-cell PSL and PCMZL. Detection of a clonal B-cell population can be used as an additional diagnostic hint for PCMZL, but such deletion is only found in 50% to 70% of PCMZL cases, thereby limiting its diagnostic value for distinguishing between B-cell PSL and PCMZL. The other important differential diagnosis to be considered is PCFCL, which is characterized by the predominance of centrocyte-like differentiated tumor cells arranged in large neoplastic follicles. In addition, tingible body macrophages are only found in a small minority of PCFCLs compared to those found in B-cell PSLs with readily identifiable tingible body macrophages as part of the reactive follicles.[21] Furthermore, a low proliferative activity in the neoplastic follicles of PCFCL is a characteristic finding, which contrasts with the high proliferative activity in the reactive germinal centers of B-cell PSLs. The networks of CD21+ follicular dendritic cells in PCFCL are irregular and disrupted in contrast to the sharply demarcated and regularly structured networks in B-cell PSLs. A clonal B-cell population can be detected in the majority of PCFCL detected by PCR or Southern blot analysis. It should be mentioned that the vast majority of PCFCL do not express bcl-2 by the neoplastic centrocyte-like differentiated cells. Consequently, the expression of bcl-2 is not of diagnostic value for distinguishing PCFCL from B-cell PSL. In cases with expression of bcl-2 by

TABLE 120-4
Comparison of B-Cell Pseudolymphoma and Cutaneous B-Cell Lymphomas

	B-CELL PSEUDOLYMPHOMA	PRIMARY CUTANEOUS MARGINAL ZONE LYMPHOMA	PRIMARY CUTANEOUS FOLLICLE CENTER LYMPHOMA
Gender (male-to-female ratio)	3:1	1:2	1:1.5
Age	<40 years	30-50 years	>50 years
Localization	Face > upper trunk > arms	Upper trunk > arms > face/head	Head/neck > upper trunk
Clinical features	Solitary nodule	Solitary or multiple nodules	Solitary or multiple nodules and plaques
Histology	Nodular infiltrate	Nodular infiltrate	Nodular infiltrate
	Reactive germinal centers with tingible body macrophages	Reactive germinal centers with tingible body macrophages	Neoplastic germinal centers; lack of polarization
	Small lymphocytes	Tumor cells with lymphoplasmacytoid (or, rarely, with monocytoid) differentiation	Tumor cells with centrocyte-like differentiation
	Plasma cells scattered	Plasma cells in small sheets	Few plasma cells
Phenotype	Small lymphocytes: CD20+ B cells > CD3+ T cells	Tumor cells: CD20+, bcl-2+, bcl-6–	Tumor cells: CD20+, bcl-2–, bcl-6+
	Germinal centers: bcl-2–, bcl-6+; high proliferative activity; sharply demarcated networks of follicular dendritic cells	Germinal centers: bcl-2–, bcl-6+; high proliferative activity; sharply demarcated networks of follicular dendritic cells	Germinal centers: bcl-2–, bcl-6+; low proliferative activity; irregular networks of follicular dendritic cells
	Polytypic expression of immunoglobulin light chains	Monotypic expression of immunoglobulin light chains	Usually no significant expression of immunoglobulin light chains
Molecular findings	Polyclonal	Monoclonal (70% to 80%)	Monoclonal (80% to 90%)

the centrocyte-like tumor cells, secondary cutaneous infiltration by a nodal follicle center lymphoma has to be considered because nodal follicle center lymphoma exhibits expression of bcl-2 by the neoplastic cells as the result of an underlying t(14;18) translocation in the majority of the cases. Other differential diagnoses include cutaneous infiltrates of B-cell chronic lymphocytic leukemia or small cell lymphocytic lymphoma, although the cutaneous infiltrates of small cell lymphocytic lymphoma usually do not show reactive germinal centers.

Clonality studies in B-cell PSLs are of limited value in distinguishing B-cell PSLs from cutaneous B-cell lymphomas as approximately 10% to 20% of PSLs harbor a clonal B-cell population.[12,22] In some studies, an even higher percentage of cases with clonal B cells were detected in nodular PSL.[23] In lesions with rather subtle infiltrates, pseudoclonality should always be ruled out as it represents a diagnostic pitfall.[24]

ETIOLOGY

A broad range of causes for B-cell PSLs has been identified. In addition to B-cell PSLs being caused by *Borrelia burgdorferi* sp. infection, insect bites, or injection of vaccines or antigens for hyposensitization, B-cell PSLs can be caused by acupuncture treatment, tattoos, metals in piercing rings and earrings, and drugs.

BORRELIA-ASSOCIATED B-CELL PSEUDOLYMPHOMA

EPIDEMIOLOGY

The terms *lymphocytoma cutis* and *lymphadenosis cutis benigna* are used synonymously for cases caused by *B. burgdorferi* infection. Approximately 1% of clinically apparent *Borrelia burgdorferi* sp. infections manifest as B-cell PSLs. A female preponderance (male-to-female ratio: 2:1) is observed in some, but not all, studies. This form of B-cell PSLs has more often been reported in whites than in African Americans. *Borrelia*-associated B-cell PSLs affects typically children and occurs in early adulthood, but may be seen in all age groups, with most patients being younger than age 40 years.

CLINICAL FINDINGS

A solitary red to violaceous dome-shaped nodule usually develops in *Borrelia*-induced B-cell PSLs, but in approximately 10% to 15% of patients, multifocal skin lesions can be observed. The face and scalp, and especially the earlobes, nipples, and scrotum, are the preferred sites for *Borrelia*-induced B-cell PSLs, but the trunk and extremities also may be involved (Fig. 120-1). Regional lymphadenopathy can be present.

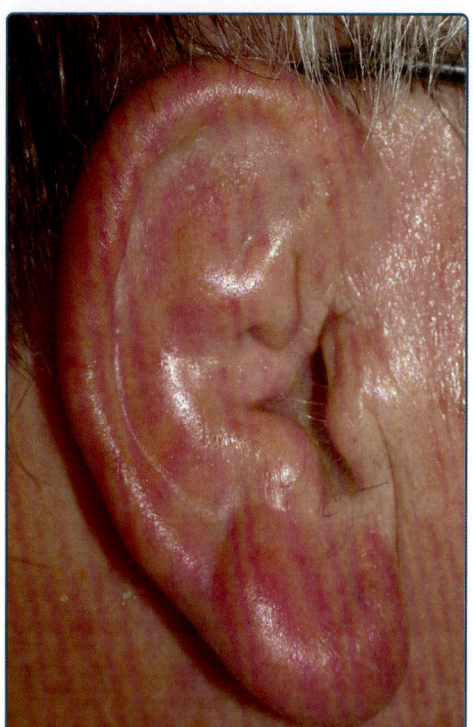

Figure 120-1 *Borrelia*-associated nodular B-cell lymphoma (lymphocytoma cutis, lymphadenosis cutis benigna): violaceous nodule on the earlobe.

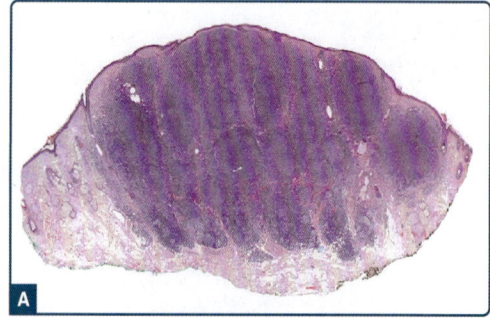
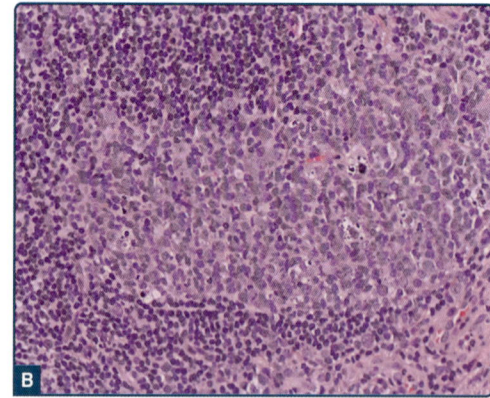

Figure 120-2 *Borrelia*-associated B-cell pseudolymphoma, histology: nodular lymphocytic infiltrate (**A**) with reactive germinal centers containing tingible body macrophages (**B**).

LABORATORY TESTS

Histologically, the archetypic pattern of a dense dermal nodular infiltrate of small B cells and reactive germinal centers is found (Fig. 120-2).[14] In *Borrelia*-associated B-cell PSL, the germinal centers tend to be larger and confluent with only a small mantle zone, and in some cases there is a lack of polarization.[14,22] Because of the confluence of the large germinal centers, the lesions resemble the neoplastic follicles in PCFCL (follicular growth pattern).[22] Plasma cells are almost always present and are found particularly at the periphery of the infiltrates.

In rare cases of so-called large cell lymphocytoma associated with *Borrelia* infection, a predominance of blasts, resembling centroblasts and immunoblasts, are found simulating the findings in large B-cell lymphoma.[25] Those cases are prone to be misdiagnosed as diffuse large B-cell lymphoma.

In the vast majority of the cases of *Borrelia*-associated B-cell PSLs, molecular studies show a polyclonal rearrangement of IgH genes, but detection of monoclonal B cells has been observed and thus does not exclude the diagnosis of *Borrelia*-induced B-cell PSL.[14]

Serology shows antibodies against *B. burgdorferi* with variable pattern; that is, IgG and IgM or only 1 class of antibodies may be detectable and elevated. Nevertheless, cases with negative serologic findings can be seen[14]; consequently, negative serology does not exclude *Borrelia*-induced B-cell PSL. Molecular studies for the detection of *B. burgdorferi* DNA by PCR are a helpful adjunctive diagnostic tool with a sensitivity of approximately 70%.[26]

Diagnosis is based on histology, the clinical context (history of tick bite, localization at predilection site), serologic findings and/or detection of *B. burgdorferi* DNA in the tissue by PCR.

CLINICAL COURSE, PROGNOSIS, AND TREATMENT

In *Borrelia*-associated B-cell PSLs, antibiotics (see Table 120-3) are the first-line therapy and prevent other complications from *Borrelia* infection, such as arthritis and carditis.

CUTANEOUS T-CELL AND MIXED PSEUDOLYMPHOMA

Nodular T-cell PSL is characterized by a dense dermal T-cell–rich nodular infiltrate, which is accompanied by variable number of B cells, which can reach up to 30% of the entire infiltrate.[27] Mixed forms of PSL contain an equal number of T-cells and B-cells.

EPIDEMIOLOGY

There are no detailed epidemiologic data on the prevalence of T-cell or mixed PSL. They affect patients of both genders and all age and ethnic groups.

ETIOLOGY AND PATHOGENESIS

All causes identified in B-cell PSLs also can be found as underlying stimuli in T-cell and mixed PSLs. In approximately 5% of cases, drugs are identified as the causative stimulus in T-cell PSL. Most cases, however, are without known cause and therefore referred to as idiopathic T-cell PSL or mixed PSL.

CLINICAL FEATURES

T-cell and mixed PSL usually presents with a solitary or multiple red to violaceous nodules similar to B-cell PSL (Fig. 120-3).

LABORATORY TESTS

Histologically, T-cell and mixed PSL present in most cases with a dense nodular infiltrate extending throughout the entire dermis and into the superficial parts of the subcutis (Fig. 120-4). The infiltrates are predominantly composed of small lymphocytes with chromatin-dense nuclei, but a variable number of slightly enlarged (up to medium-sized) lymphocytes with chromatin-dense nuclei can be found. There is an admixture of a variable number of eosin-

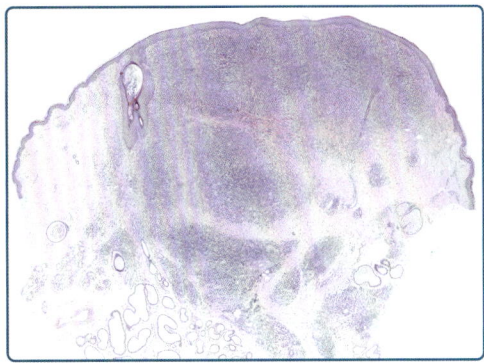

Figure 120-4 Nodular T-cell pseudolymphoma, histology: nodular infiltrate composed mostly of small lymphocytes. No follicles are present.

ophils, histiocytes, plasma cells (ranging from a few up to small clusters). The B cells can be arranged in small aggregates, but, rarely, germinal centers are found. Granuloma formation can be observed. There may be exocytosis of T lymphocytes into the epithelia of the hair follicles, but usually there is no significant exocytosis of lymphocytes into the overlying interfollicular epidermis (lack of epidermotropism).

Immunohistochemistry shows that, in most cases, the majority of the small lymphocytes are CD4+ CD30– T cells. There may be an admixture of a few CD30+ blasts representing activated lymphocytes.

Clonality studies reveal a polyclonal infiltrate in the majority of T-cell PSLs, but PSLs with clonal T cells have been reported and are referred to as *clonal PSLs*. Some of those cases may progress to overt lymphoma and may rather represent very early stages of lymphomagenesis than real PSLs.

DIFFERENTIAL DIAGNOSIS

Differential diagnosis of nodular T-cell and mixed PSLs includes cutaneous CD4+ small-/medium-sized T-cell lymphoma/lymphoproliferative disorder (CD4+ SMT-LPD) according to the World Health Organization (WHO) 2008 classification and the revised WHO 2016 classification, which show overlapping histologic and immunophenotypic features.[28,29] The CD4+ SMT-LPD also presents usually with a solitary lesion located mostly on the head and neck area and shows an indolent course (Fig. 120-5). Because nodular T-cell PSL and cutaneous CD4+ SMT-LPD cannot be distinguished with certainty based on clinical or histopathologic or phenotypic features, some authors consider them to represent the same process. Therefore, the encompassing term *cutaneous CD4+ small/medium T-cell lymphoproliferative disorder* has been introduced in the updated WHO 2016 classification to emphasize the indolent nature of this process. The expression of programmed cell death protein 1 (PD-1), originally thought to be a discriminative marker, is not of diagnostic value.

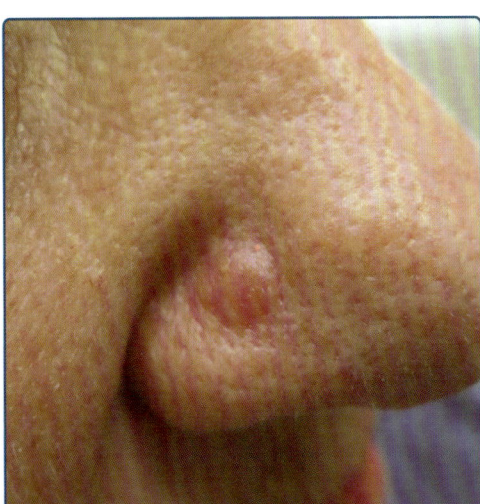

Figure 120-3 Nodular T-cell pseudolymphoma: erythematous nodule on the nose.

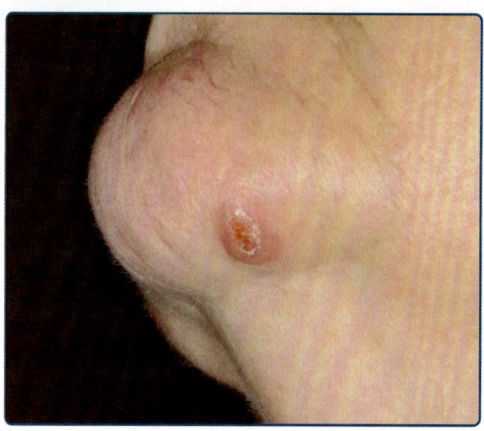

Figure 120-5 Cutaneous CD4+ small-/medium-sized T-cell lymphoproliferative disorder: nodular lesion on the chin.

Nodular T-cell PSLs should be differentiated from mycosis fungoides (MF) in tumor stage because MF tumor stage may rarely present with small to medium-sized T cells without a significant number of large cells. In MF, however, the small and medium-sized cells show a higher degree of nuclear atypia than in CD4+ SMT-LPD. The distinction between MF, CD4+ SMT-LPD, and T-cell PSL has to be based on the clinical presentation with patches and plaques preceding the tumors in MF in contrast to the mostly solitary nodule without preceding patch(es) and plaque(s) in T-cell PSL. The differential diagnosis further includes secondary cutaneous infiltrates of angioimmunoblastic T-cell lymphoma (AITL), in which the small CD4+ and PD-1+ T cells are accompanied by a significant number of B cells. The clinical context with B symptoms, serologic findings, the nodal involvement shown by radiologic staging examinations, a high proliferation rate in AITL infiltrates, and the association with Epstein-Barr virus in some of the cases of AITL, are useful findings for distinguishing AITL from nodular T-cell PSL.

Among inflammatory skin disorders, lupus erythematosus (particularly the tumidus type) has to be considered, which also can present with dense dermal lymphocytic infiltrates. In those cases, however, vacuolization at the interface of the hair follicle epithelium and interstitial mucin deposits are present. In addition, the clinical presentation allows differentiation from nodular T-cell PSLs.

CLINICAL COURSE, PROGNOSIS, AND TREATMENT

T-cell and mixed PSL can resolve spontaneously after withdrawal of the underlying cause, but may persist for longer periods (months or years). If no spontaneous regression is observed after biopsy, surgical excision, cryotherapy, laser treatment, topical/intralesional steroids, or interferon represent therapeutic options.[30] T-cell PSL usually does not recur unless the underlying stimulus persists (eg, a drug). As in B-cell PSL, avoidance of the underlying stimulus is the effective preventive measure to avoid recurrence.

CD30+ T-CELL PSEUDOLYMPHOMA

CD30+ PSL represents a histologic subtype of T-cell PSL of the skin that is characterized by the presence of medium-sized to large atypical CD30+ T cells.[31,32] T-cell–rich pseudolymphomatous infiltrates with admixture of CD30+ cells have been reported in the context of lymphomatoid drug eruptions, nodular scabies, and arthropod bite reactions, as well as viral infections, particularly parapoxvirus-associated disorders such as Orf disease[33] and milker nodule, as well as molluscum contagiosum and herpes virus infections (for a review see reference 31). Among noninfectious disorders, CD30+ pseudolymphomatous infiltrates have been described in drug eruptions, hidradenitis, and injuries by corals.[34]

In CD30+ PSL, immunohistochemistry shows enlarged, that is, medium-sized to even large, CD30+ blast-like cells that are usually found as single units scattered throughout the infiltrate, which is otherwise dominated by small T cells (Fig. 120-6). In contrast to CD30+ lymphomas, CD30+ PSLs do not, in most of the cases, harbor a clonal T-cell population. Because of the presence of enlarged CD30+ cells, lymphomatoid papulosis (particularly histologic Type A) and cutaneous anaplastic large cell lymphoma (ALCL) have to be considered as differential diagnoses. In contrast to lymphomatoid papulosis and ALCL, the CD30+ cells in CD30+ PSL are usually not arranged in aggregates. Moreover, the significant number of B cells and plasma cells argues for a reactive process, that is, PSL, as they are usually absent or only present in a small number in lymphomatoid papulosis and ALCL. In addition, in contrast to lymphomatoid papulosis, expression of 5hmC in the CD30+ cells in CD30+ PSL is preserved and can serve as an additional diagnostic marker.[35]

Treatment of CD30+ PSL is directed against the underlying cause of the disease.

PSEUDOLYMPHOMATOUS FOLLICULITIS

This PSL variant was first described in 1988 by Kibbi and coworkers.[36] It presents with a solitary nodule located on the face that measures less than 1.5 cm and is similar or identical identical to the clinical manifestation found in cutaneous CD4+ SMT-LPD.[37] A miliarial form of B-cell pseudolymphomatous folliculitis has been described.[19] Histologically, half of the cases carry the features of nodular B-cell PSLs and the remaining

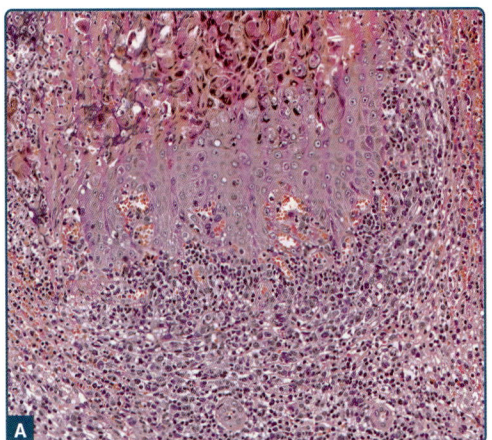

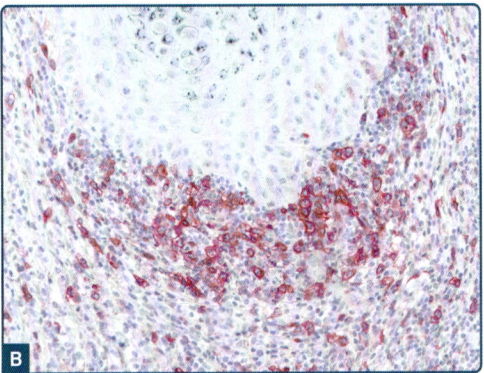

Figure 120-6 CD30+ pseudolymphoma. **A,** Infiltrates of atypical lymphocytes in molluscum contagiosum. **B,** Expression of CD30 by the medium-sized to large atypical lymphocytes.

all cases.[37] The course and treatment is similar to other forms of nodular PSL and CD4+ SMT-LPD.

OTHER FORMS OF NODULAR PSEUDOLYMPHOMA

On clinical grounds alone T-cell, B-cell, or mixed PSL cannot be discerned. In addition, some agents may induce T-cell and B-cell PSL so that an unequivocal correlation between the causative factor and the composition of the PSL is not possible. Nevertheless, the clinical context may provide essential information regarding the etiology of PSL, especially for those cases resulting from tattoos or metals (piercing, earrings), or PSL caused by exposure to leaches and acupuncture.

PERSISTENT NODULAR ARTHROPOD BITE REACTIONS AND NODULAR SCABIES

In both conditions longstanding pruritic papules and nodules are found with a predilection for the elbows, trunk, genitalia, and axillary, as well as inguinal folds. The lesions tend to be red-brown and may be excoriated. Mites or scybala are rarely found in the epidermis overlying the dense dermal lymphocytic infiltrates. A delayed-type hypersensitivity reaction is considered to be the underlying trigger factor for the formation of the T-cell–rich infiltrates.

Histologically the epidermis often shows features of pruriginous reaction with acanthosis and hyperparakeratosis. There is a wedge-shaped dermal infiltrate predominantly composed of small lymphocytes with admixture of eosinophils and occasional plasma cells (Fig. 120-8). Formation of flame figures can be seen particularly in cases with numerous eosinophils. In the center of the infiltrates, hypereosinophilic collagen bundles are found. The vessels show plump endothelia. In the majority of nodular arthropod bite

cases carry the features of nodular T-cell PSLs. The lymphocytic infiltrates are located throughout the entire dermis and may extend into the subcutis and are arranged around the hair follicles (Fig. 120-7). A Grenz zone may be present. There is exocytosis of lymphocytes into the hair follicles often showing broadened epithelia.[38] In half of the cases, atypical lymphocytes are found. Half of the cases harbor aggregates of histiocytes. An admixture of numerous dendritic cells with expression of CD1a and S-100 was identified in

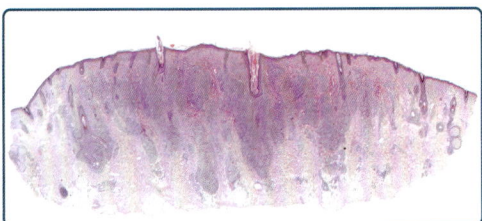

Figure 120-7 Pseudolymphomatous folliculitis, histology: dense dermal lymphocytic infiltrates with perifollicular accentuation.

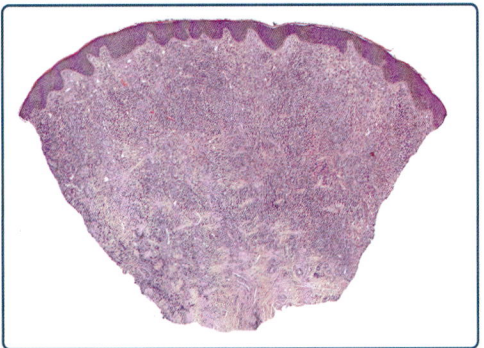

Figure 120-8 Nodular arthropod bite reaction, histology: wedge-shaped dermal infiltrate composed of lymphocytes and numerous eosinophils.

reactions, the infiltrate is dominated by T cells. Rarely, B-cell–rich forms with germinal centers may be seen. There can be an admixture of medium to even large atypical-appearing CD30+ lymphocytes (see section "CD30+ pseudolymphomas").[31,32,39] In those cases, distinguishing CD30+ pseudolymphomas from lymphomatoid papulosis can be challenging. There is no clonal rearrangement of T cells in nodular arthropod bite reactions and nodular scabies.

Persistent arthropod bite reactions have to be differentiated from exaggerated bite reactions, which can occur in patients with B-cell chronic lymphocytic leukemia and other leukemias.[40] In those patients, hematologic examination may be considered. Moreover, lymphomatoid papulosis (Type A), Hodgkin lymphoma, and nodular secondary syphilis are histologically differential diagnoses.

The lesions in nodular arthropod bite reactions and nodular scabies may be longstanding and persist for several months. Antiscabietic treatment is ineffective. Excision, intralesional corticosteroids, or topical immunomodulators may be considered if spontaneous regression does not occur or topical steroids are ineffective.[41]

PSEUDOLYMPHOMA CAUSED BY LEECHES (*HIRUDO MEDICINALIS*) THERAPY

The distribution of the lesions corresponds to the exposure to leeches (*H. medicinalis*) which are commonly found on the lower back or over areas that have been treated for hematoma after trauma or surgery (Fig. 120-9).[42] A diffuse form has been described.[43] Both T-cell and B-cell predominant forms were observed. Hypothetically bacteria residing in the leeches are transferred to the host during the blood meal and induce the pseudolymphomatous reaction.

NODULAR PSEUDOLYMPHOMA CAUSED BY DRUGS

PSL caused by drugs show a variety of clinical, histologic, and phenotypic manifestations. Some of the

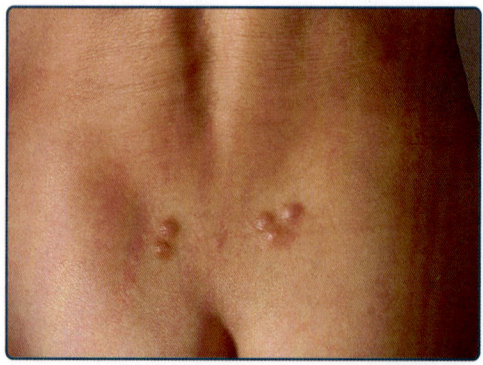

Figure 120-9 Pseudolymphoma caused by leeches (*Hirudo medicinalis*): characteristic localization of the pseudolymphoma.

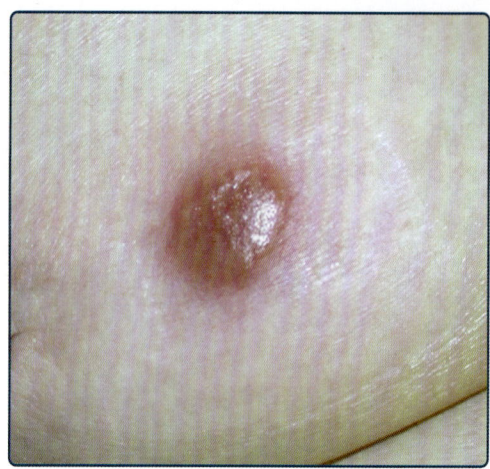

Figure 120-10 Nodular T-cell pseudolymphoma caused by anticonvulsant (phenytoin): erythematous nodule on the right breast.

drugs, like anticonvulsants, may induce nodular PSL (Fig. 120-10), as well as other histologic manifestations (see below).[27,44,45] Clinically, drug-related nodular PSL may present with a solitary or multiple nodules.[44]

Histologically, nodular drug-related PSL presents with the typical histologic features of nodular T-cell or B-cell PSL.[46,47] The lymphocytes in nodular T-cell PSLs may show subtle nuclear atypia. Proliferation rate is low, approximately 10%. In B-cell PSLs, the typical immunophenotypic features as outlined above are found. In T-cell PSLs, immunohistochemistry reveals a predominance of CD4 lymphocytes and admixture of a variable number of CD30+ lymphocytes.[48] Loss of pan–T-cell markers is not observed. In most cases, there is no monoclonal rearrangement of T-cell receptor γ genes or IgH genes.

Diagnosis of lymphomatoid drug eruption is challenging, particularly as the latency between onset of medication and development of drug eruption can be very long (several months up to years).

Differential diagnosis depends on the phenotype. In B-cell nodular PSL, differential diagnosis includes cutaneous marginal zone lymphoma and follicle center lymphoma. In CD4+ T-cell rich forms of drug-related nodular PSL, the differential diagnoses include cutaneous CD4+ SMT-LPD, MF, and Sézary syndrome.

Withdrawal of the drug is the first step in the management of drug-related PSL. Surgical excision or intralesional injection of corticosteroids may be considered, if spontaneous regression is delayed. One has to be aware that drug-related nodular PSL may persist for several months even after withdrawal of the causative drug. Reexposure to the drug may elicit a relapse of the PSL.

PSEUDOLYMPHOMA AT DRUG AND VACCINE INJECTION SITES

Solitary or multiple PSL may also develop after injection of vaccines to prevent infectious diseases

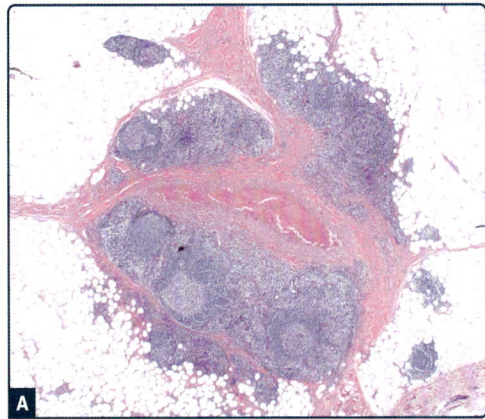

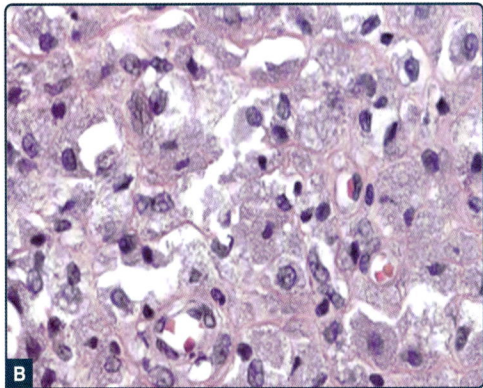

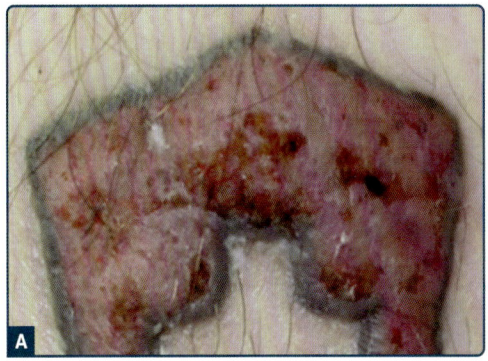

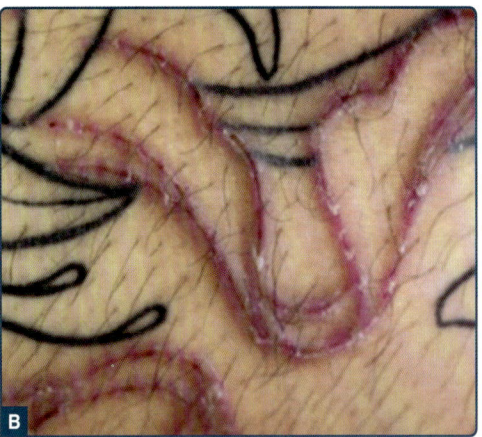

Figure 120-11 Pseudolymphoma caused by allergen injection: **A,** Subcutaneous B-cell–rich infiltrate with formation of follicles. Note the central area with the histiocyte-rich infiltrate. **B,** The histiocytes show a grayish granular cytoplasm containing aluminum hydroxide–bound vaccine.

Figure 120-12 A and **B,** Pseudolymphoma in association with tattoo: Infiltration within the area of red tattoo component.

or after injection of allergens for hyposensitization. They are typically found in the subcutaneous tissue at the injection site.[49] The histologic features show B-cell–rich infiltrates with reactive germinal centers. In the center of the infiltrates, an accumulation of histiocytes can be seen (Fig. 120-11).[50,51] The histiocytes show a cytoplasm with a granular gray-blue aspect, which seems to represent aluminium hydroxide–bound vaccines.[52]

PSEUDOLYMPHOMA IN ASSOCIATION WITH TATTOOS OR METALS

Pseudolymphomatous infiltrates arising in tattoos and caused by metals in earrings or piercings share similar features.[53,54] In tattoos, the lymphocytic infiltrates mostly arise and remain limited to areas with red tattoo dye (Fig. 120-12). Cinnabar, a mercuric sulfide, is the most commonly used dye for red tattoos. In addition, PSLs also have been observed in blue or green tattoos, for which cobalt and chrome salts are employed. The PSL to the tattoo dye can be regarded as a delayed-type hypersensitivity reaction. Clinically, mostly papules, nodules, or plaque-like infiltrates develop within 1 compartment of the tattoo. They are usually asymptomatic. The latency between application of the tattoo dye and occurrence of the PSL is highly variable, ranging from months to years.[55] Histologically, a lichenoid component with a band-like superficial infiltrate, interface changes, and exocytosis of lymphocytes, as well as a deeper lymphocytic infiltrate in the mid and deep dermis with admixture of eosinophils, is present leading to a pseudolymphomatous appearance.[56] The lymphocytes are small and do not display significant nuclear atypia. Patch test to mercury or other substances in the tattoo dyes may reveal delayed type hypersensitivity, but the test also may be negative.[55] Therapy is challenging and includes intralesional injections of corticosteroids, laser therapy, or excision if small papulonodular lesions are present.

INFECTIONS WITH LYMPHOCYTE-RICH INFILTRATES SIMULATING LYMPHOMA

Various infections, particularly those caused by viruses and parasites, may show dense lymphocyte-rich infiltrates, thereby simulating a lymphoma. Among infections with parasites, cutaneous leishmaniasis histologically simulates lymphoma by its nodular infiltrate composed of numerous lymphocytes, including plasma cells and histiocytes. The lack of nuclear atypia and detection of the parasite either by special stains, immunohistochemistry or by molecular techniques enables cutaneous leishmaniasis to be differentiated from cutaneous lymphoma. Not only histologic can findings in cutaneous leishmaniasis simulate lymphoma, but the clinical aspects occasionally can resemble B-cell PSL.[57,58]

In infections with herpes simplex virus and varicella zoster virus, occasionally lymphocyte-rich infiltrates without the pathognomonic epithelial changes can be observed and have been referred to as *herpes incognito*. Both lymphocytes with slightly enlarged and atypical-appearing chromatin-dense nuclei and enlarged CD30+ lymphocytes may be found in herpes incognito, making those infiltrates subject to being mistaken for lymphoma infiltrates. Detection of viral antigens by immunohistochemistry and/or detection of viral DNA by PCR enable identification of those infiltrates as herpes virus–related T-cell reactions.

Parapoxvirus infection may induce cytomorphologic changes and expression of CD30 by the infiltrating T cells, which makes distinguishing them from pleomorphic lymphocytes in the context of anaplastic large-cell lymphoma challenging (see Fig. 120-6).[31,32] The presence of epithelial changes with inclusion bodies typical for parapoxvirus infection, the absence of loss of T-cell markers, and the lack of monoclonal rearrangement of T-cell receptor–γ genes help to distinguish those infiltrates from cutaneous T-cell lymphoma. However, the diagnosis is based on the detection of the virus by immunohistochemistry, electron microscopy, or PCR.

PSEUDOLYMPHOMAS-HISTOLOGIC MYCOSIS FUNGOIDES SIMULATORS

The term *pseudo-MF* describes a group of disorders of different etiologies that histologically mimic MF. Because the histologic evaluation suggests MF or another form of epidermotropic cutaneous T-cell lymphoma, the clinicopathologic correlation is crucial to avoid misinterpreting the histologic findings as a lymphoma and for assigning the findings to a distinct reactive skin disease, such as PSL.

Histologically, the diseases described in this section have in common a dermal, either band-like or perivascular, infiltrate of mostly small lymphocytes, which show exocytosis into the epidermis and may exhibit subtle nuclear atypia, thereby simulating epidermotropic cutaneous T-cell lymphoma (CTCL). Phenotyping reveals either a predominance of CD4+ or CD8+ cells. In addition, a variable expression of CD30 can be seen in some cases of pseudo-MF. As in other forms of PSL, the lymphocytes are polyclonal in the majority of cases. In some diseases, such as pityriasis lichenoides et varioliformis acuta, a significant percentage of clonal T cells is found, but does not indicate malignancy or a risk of progression to lymphoma.

Differential diagnoses include primarily MF or Sézary syndrome. In cases with a predominantly CD8+ infiltrate, differential diagnosie include CD8+ MF, Sézary syndrome, cutaneous CD8+ aggressive epidermotropic cytotoxic T-cell lymphoma, and lymphomatoid papulosis (Types D and E). Profound nuclear atypia, predominance of medium-sized to large cells, loss of pan T-cell markers, and monoclonal rearrangement of T-cell receptor genes, are findings in favor of CTCL.

As in other forms of PSL, the treatment focuses on avoiding exposure to the causative agents, such as allergens in lymphomatoid contact dermatitis and drugs in lymphomatoid drug eruption. In addition, topical corticosteroids or immunomodulators and ultraviolet (UV) light therapy are used. Systemic steroids and immunosuppressive drugs, such as cyclosporine, may be indicated in severe forms of PSL.

LYMPHOMATOID CONTACT DERMATITIS

Lymphomatoid contact dermatitis (LCD) is a chronic contact dermatitis that histologically simulates MF.[59] Various antigens, including nickel sulfate, gold, zinc, paraphenylenediamine, textile dye, and several other antigens, have been identified as culprits.[60] LCD occurs mostly in adults and affects both genders.

Clinically, LCD manifests with eczematous erythematous and scaly papules, patches, plaques, and, in rare cases, erythroderma (Fig. 120-13). The lesions are pruritic.

Histopathologically there is a superficial band-like infiltrate with variable exocytosis of lymphocytes into the epidermis, which may show spongiosis or spongiotic vesicles. Intraepidermal accumulations of Langerhans cells (so-called pseudo Pautrier collections) can be found. Some of the lymphocytes can show slightly convoluted nuclei, but nuclear atypia is not prominent.

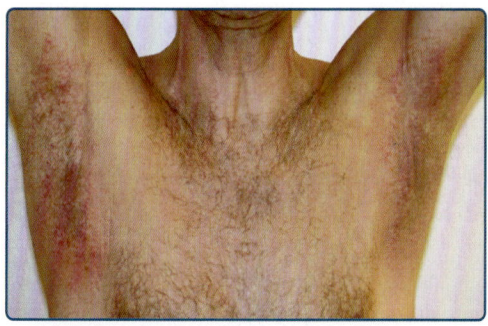

Figure 120-13 Lymphomatoid contact dermatitis: eczematous lesions in both axillae caused by contact allergy to fragrance components.

There is an admixture of eosinophils. The ratio of CD4+ to CD8+ lymphocytes is inconspicuous, but there can be an admixture of slightly enlarged CD30+ cells representing activated lymphocytes.

Differentiation of LCD from MF is based on the presence of variable degree of spongiosis, the lack of significant atypia of lymphocytes, an inconspicuous CD4-to-CD8 ratio, and the absence of loss of T-cell markers in LCD. Monoclonal T cells have been reported in LCD and do not indicate lymphoma. Sensitization against the allergen(s) is documented by patch test and is an essential diagnostic criterion for proving a diagnosis of LCD.[61]

The course of LCD is chronic, particularly if exposure to the allergen cannot be avoided. The treatment follows the general recommendation for the treatment of other forms of contact dermatitis with avoidance of exposure to the allergen and suppression of the immunologic reaction against the allergen mostly by topical corticosteroids or topical immunomodulators. In addition, UV light–based strategies or systemic immunosuppression may be effective.

LYMPHOMATOID DRUG REACTION

Apart from its nodular form, drug-related PSL commonly presents with maculopapular or papular eruptions. A large number of drug classes that induce various forms of lymphomatoid drug eruptions have been described.[8,62]

In this form of lymphomatoid drug reaction, a band-like infiltrate in the upper dermis, with variable degrees of exocytosis of lymphocytes, is found.[63] Vacuolar alteration at the dermoepidermal junction and apoptotic keratinocytes may be present. The lymphocytes may show an irregular nuclear contour (ie, nuclear atypia) (Fig. 120-14 A, B). Eosinophils are commonly found, but also may be absent. Immunohistochemistry reveals either a predominance of CD4+ or CD8+ lymphocytes and an admixture of a variable number of CD30+ lymphocytes (Fig. 120-14C).[48] Loss of pan T-cell markers is not observed.

Differential diagnosis includes epidermotropic CTCL, particularly MF and Sézary syndrome. Lining up of lymphocytes along the junctional zone, nuclear atypia of the lymphocytes, loss of pan T-cell markers, and monoclonal rearrangement of T-cell receptor-γ genes favor MF or Sézary syndrome. Moreover, expression of PD-1 and TOX (thymocyte selection-associated high-mobility group box factor) by the majority of the lymphocytes was found in Sézary syndrome, but not in inflammatory erythrodermas.[64] Cases with CD8+ infiltrates showing exocytosis of lymphocytes have to be distinguished from CD8+ MF (patches and plaques), CD8+ lymphomatoid papulosis (especially Type D or Type E), and pityriasis lichenoides et varioliformis acuta (PLEVA). Drug-related CD30+ PSL simulates lymphomatoid papulosis (Type A or Type B).[65] Occasionally,

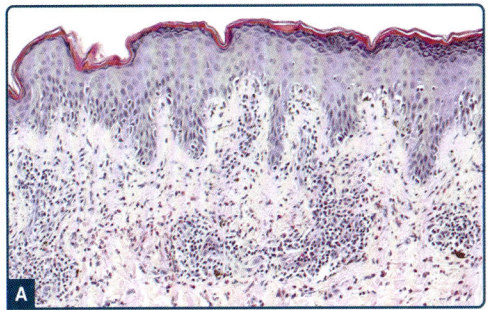

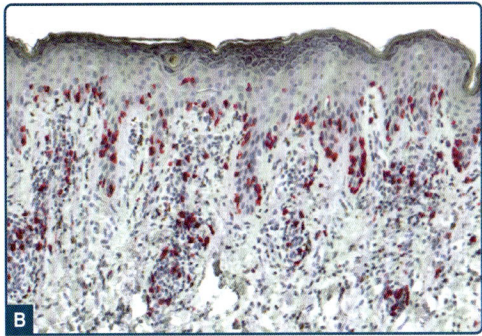

Figure 120-14 Lymphomatoid drug reaction, histology: lymphocytic infiltrate with exocytosis of lymphocytes into the epidermis and nuclear atypia of the lymphocytes (**A**) with expression of CD8 (**B**).

the lymphocytes in lymphomatoid drug eruptions exhibit remarkable nuclear atypia so that distinction from lymphoma is very challenging or even impossible by histology alone. Clinicopathologic correlation and history are mandatory to reach the final diagnosis in drug-related PSL.

As in the nodular form of drug-related PSL, withdrawal of the drug is the essential step in the management. Lymphomatoid drug eruption can persist for several months and reexposure to the drug may elicit a relapse of the PSL. Systemic, intralesional, or topical steroids are used for treatment.

ACTINIC RETICULOID

Actinic reticuloid represents a chronic multifactorial dermatitis with severe photosensitivity to a broad spectrum of wavelengths, which histologically mimics epidermotropic CTCL.[5]

CLINICAL FINDINGS

It affects mostly middle-aged and older men.[66] It presents with persistent erythematous lichenoid papules and plaques on light-exposed skin areas, particularly on the face and neck. In some patients infiltration on the face leads to a facies leonina-like aspect (Fig. 120-15). Progression into erythroderma can be observed. Lichenification and erosions usually occur

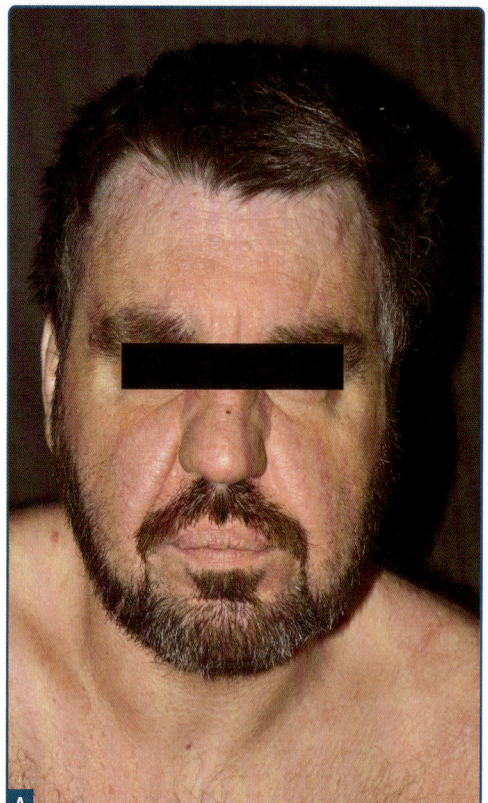

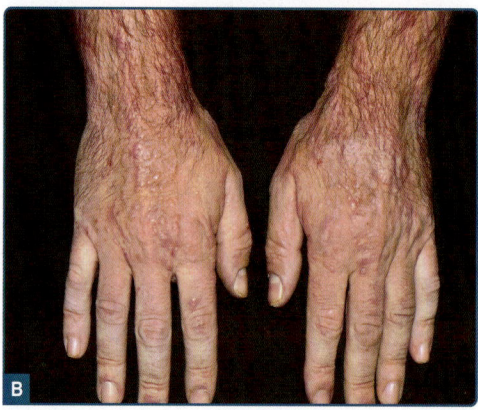

Figure 120-15 Actinic reticuloid: diffuse infiltration and erythema and papules on the face (**A**) and papules on the back of the hands (**B**).

over time. The skin lesions are accompanied by intense pruritus.

LABORATORY TESTS

Histologically, there is psoriasiform hyperplasia of the epidermis, slight spongiosis, and compact orthokeratosis with focal parakeratosis. In the upper dermis there is an infiltrate arranged in a perivascular, but also interstitial, distribution and composed of small lymphocytes, eosinophils, and plasma cells. Coarse bundles of collagen arranged in vertical streaks are found in the papillary dermis. Multinucleated fibroblasts may be present. The lymphocytes may show slightly atypical nuclei and exocytosis into the overlying epidermis. Immunohistochemistry reveals a predominance of CD8+ T cells.[67]

In the peripheral blood, an increased number of CD8+ T cells (reversed CD4-to-CD8 ratio) is characteristic for actinic reticuloid, particularly in erythrodermic patients.[66] The atypical circulating lymphocytes show indented nuclei. Phototesting, including positive photo patch tests, reveals sensitization to 1 or multiple allergens.

DIAGNOSIS AND DIFFERENTIAL DIAGNOSIS

The diagnosis of actinic reticuloid is based on the presence of persistent infiltrated plaques and papules on light-exposed skin areas, photo sensitivity to a broad spectrum of wavelengths, and histologic findings with a predominance of CD8+ slightly atypical lymphocytes and variable degree of exocytosis, as well as the presence of circulating CD8+ lymphocytes in the peripheral blood.[67]

Based on clinical and/or histologic grounds, MF and/or Sézary syndrome have to be considered. CD8+ MF shows a more pronounced epidermotropism and nuclear atypia of the lymphocytes. Moreover, CD8+ MF is usually located on UV-protected body regions in contrast to actinic reticuloid displaying a distribution in light-exposed areas. Particularly in patients with actinic reticuloid presenting with erythroderma, Sézary syndrome represents an important differential diagnosis. In contrast to actinic reticuloid with a predominance of CD8+ lymphocytes, Sézary syndrome is characterized by clonal CD4+ atypical lymphocytes in the skin and the peripheral blood, lymphadenopathy, alopecia, and palmoplantar hyperkeratosis.

CLINICAL COURSE, PROGNOSIS, AND TREATMENT

Actinic reticuloid shows a longstanding highly chronic course. In addition to UV light protection with sunscreens, topical steroids and topical immunomodulators can be used, but show variable efficacy. Among systemic drugs, cyclosporine may be effective. Photo hardening with UV-B irradiation to induce photo tolerance was reported to produce a good response in one series.[67]

CD8+ T-CELL PSEUDOLYMPHOMA IN IMMUNODEFICIENCY

In patients with immunodeficiency, in particular HIV infection, infiltrates of CD8+ lymphocytes mimicking MF may develop. Fewer than 50 cases of CD8+

infiltrates in HIV-infected patients have been reported as of this writing. The etiology and pathogenesis of these infiltrates is largely unknown, but may be related to severe immunodeficiency as the cutaneous CD8+ infiltrates occur in advanced HIV infection with low numbers of CD4+ cells. A variety of clinical presentations have been described, including disseminated, often pruritic papules, or a diffuse, mildly pruritic papular eruption.[68,69] In addition, palmoplantar hyperkeratosis and erythroderma were observed. The dermal infiltrates of CD8+ lymphocytes are accompanied by exocytosis of CD8+ lymphocytes into the epidermis. The lymphocytes may show subtle nuclear atypia. Molecular studies revealed a polyclonal nature.

The course of the cutaneous CD8+ infiltrates per se is indolent in most patients, but is considered as a sign for bad overall prognosis, which is mostly determined by the severe lymphopenia of CD4+ T cells. In most patients remission was achieved when receiving highly active antiretroviral therapy, and in moderately immunosuppressed patients methotrexate was shown to be effective.[70,71]

This condition seems not to be exclusively limited to patients with HIV infection, as similar features were recently described in a renal transplant recipient.[72]

BORRELIA-ASSOCIATED T-CELL PSEUDOLYMPHOMA

With the exception of erythema migrans, *Borrelia* infection of the skin most commonly manifests with B-cell–predominant infiltrates, including plasma cells, such as lymphocytoma cutis. Recently *B. burgdorferi* infections with T-cell–rich infiltrates have been reported.[73,74] The dermal T-cell infiltrate was either band-like or diffuse and displayed focal epidermotropism with lining-up of lymphocytes along the junctional zone. The lymphocytes show slight nuclear atypia. In addition, a minor interstitial histiocytic component of the infiltrate can be observed. Both the histologic features that mimic MF and the clinical aspect with patches resembling MF represent a diagnostic pitfall in some of the affected individuals. Other clinical presentations included the typical findings of erythema migrans or acrodermatitis chronica atrophicans. Treatment with antibiotics results in remission.

PAPULOERYTHRODERMA OFUJI

Papuloerythroderma Ofuji is a rare pruritic erythrodermic dermatosis that clinically can simulate CTCL.[75] Association with drugs, Hodgkin lymphoma, visceral malignancies, and immunodeficiency syndromes have been reported. In some patients,[76,77] papuloerythroderma Ofuji was described as a manifestation of MF, in others as a disease accompanying MF.[78]

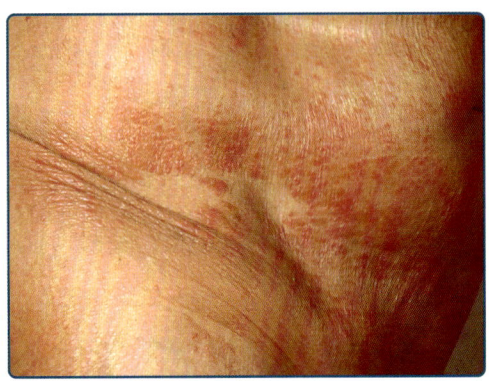

Figure 120-16 Papuloerythroderma Ofuji: papules with confluence to plaques and spared areas.

Papuloerythroderma Ofuji was originally described in Japanese patients, but similar cases have been reported from other geographic regions. The median age is 70 years. It occurs more frequently in males than in females. Clinically, papuloerythroderma Ofuji manifests with disseminated solid papules. The coalescing brownish papules are flat-topped and observed mainly on the flexor surfaces of the extremities. The axillae, inguinal regions, antecubital and popliteal fossae, and big furrows on the abdomen are spared ("deckchair" sign; Fig. 120-16).[79]

Histology shows eczematous features with acanthosis, spongiosis and hyperparakeratosis, and a dermal lymphocytic infiltrate with admixture of plasma cells, eosinophils, and neutrophils is found. Exocytosis of neutrophils and eosinophils may be observed.[80] Immunohistochemistry shows numerous dendritic cells and mature T cells in the dermis. The most common abnormal laboratory findings were eosinophilia and an elevated serum IgE level. There should be a search for immunodeficiency, especially HIV infection.

The clinical differential diagnoses include Sézary syndrome. Papuloerythroderma Ofuji can be distinguished from Sézary syndrome because, unlike Sézary syndrome, papuloerythroderma Ofuji lacks nuclear atypia of the lymphocytes and circulating atypical lymphocytes.

The prognosis of papuloerythroderma Ofuji is good, if there is no underlying malignancy. UV light treatment including psoralen and ultraviolet A (PUVA), bath PUVA, UV-B in combination with topical steroids, etretinate, Re-PUVA, oral steroids, and cyclosporine have been described as effective therapeutic approaches.[11-14]

INFLAMMATORY DISORDERS AS CTCL AND CLONAL DERMATITIS

Various disorders, which are discussed in other chapters, are characterized by a T-cell–rich infiltrate and exocytosis of lymphocytes into the epidermis, making the disorders prone to be misinterpreted as epidermotropic CTCL. These disorders include lichen planus, lichen sclerosus et atrophicans, pigmented purpuric dermatitis, and pityriasis lichenoides.[65,81-83] Furthermore, inflammatory diseases with lymphocyte-rich dermal and/or subcutaneous infiltrates, such as lupus erythematosus (particularly the tumid type) and lupus panniculitis, have to be differentiated from other forms of CTCL including subcutaneous panniculitis-like T-cell lymphoma.

DETECTION OF T-CELL CLONES IN INFLAMMATORY SKIN DISEASES

Highly sensitive methods to assess clonality, such as PCR combined with temperature gradient gel electrophoresis or denaturing gradient gel electrophoresis and automated high-resolution fragment analysis, allow detection of clonal T cells, which may comprise as little as 1% of all infiltrating cells. Clonal T-cell populations have been found in some cases in the above mentioned inflammatory skin conditions, for example, in lichen planus and lichen sclerosus et atrophicans, in which clonal T cells were found in 6% (lichen planus) and 13% (lichen sclerosus et atrophicans) of the cases. Remarkably, a monoclonal rearrangement of *TCR* genes is commonly found in pityriasis lichenoides harboring clonal T cells in up to 60% of cases.[82,84] The significance of these T-cell clones is unclear. As a consequence for the diagnostic workup of lymphocyte-rich infiltrates, detection of a clonal T-cell population cannot be used as a sufficient finding to diagnose CTCL.[13] The presence of clonal T cells within an infiltrate may merely represent a predominance of 1 or more T-cell clones in the context of an immunologic reaction that may be induced and maintained by certain antigens. In contrast to cutaneous lymphomas with persistence of a single T-cell clone during disease evolution, the T-cell clones in inflammatory skin disorders are transient and change over time. As a consequence the detection of clonal T-cells in inflammatory disorders underlines the necessity to correlate the results of clonality assays with the clinical, histologic, and immunophenotypic findings to achieve the final diagnosis.[85]

CLONAL DERMATITIS

Apart from the above-mentioned well-characterized and distinct inflammatory skin diseases that may harbor clonal T cells in some cases, clonality studies employing PCR techniques led to the identification of cases with chronic, nonspecific dermatitis harboring T-cell clones. Those cases have been referred to as "clonal dermatitis."[86] Approximately 25% of clonal dermatitis cases progress to overt CTCL within 5 years.[86] These observations indicate that at least some cases of "clonal dermatitis" may represent CTCL precursor lesions. Clonal dermatitis would thus be one of the earliest manifestations of CTCL, harboring a dominant T-cell clone but lacking histologic features diagnostic for CTCL.

LYMPHOCYTIC INFILTRATION OF THE SKIN AND PALPABLE ARCIFORME MIGRATORY ERYTHEMA

Lymphocytic infiltration of the skin Jessner-Kanof (LIS) and palpable arciform migratory erythema of Clark (PAME) have been regarded by some authors as T-cell PSLs, and by others as lupus-like eruptions.

The clinical presentation in PAME led to its designation with infiltrated annular erythema developing into large migrating lesions.[87] The trunk is the predilection site. Histology shows dense perivascular and periadnexal predominantly lymphocytic infiltrate. There is no admixture of plasma cells and interstitial mucin deposits such as in lupus erythematosus are absent. Immunohistochemistry reveals an infiltrate dominated by T cells with admixture of B cells and histiocytes. The lymphocytes are polyclonal. The histology is very similar to the findings in LIS.[88] Phenotypically, the infiltrate in LIS is mostly composed of CD8+ lymphocytes.[89] We consider PAME and LIS to represent the same process because of the similarities in clinical presentation, histology, and course. Both processes may respond to topical steroids, oral antibiotics, and UV-A1.[88] There is a tendency for relapses.

OTHER DISORDERS WITH LYMPHOCYTE-RICH INFILTRATES

ACRAL PSEUDOLYMPHOMATOUS ANGIOKERATOMA

Acral pseudolymphomatous angiokeratoma (APA) was originally described as occurring in children (hence the original name *acral pseudolymphomatous angiokeratoma of childhood* [APACHE]), but it has been shown that it also affects adults.[90-92] Some authors consider the lesions to represent persistent arthropod bite reactions, whereas others categorize APA as a benign vascular process with a prominent lymphocytic infiltrate, that is, a form of cutaneous PSL.[90,92] Consequently, the term *papular pseudolymphoma* has been proposed.[92]

Clinically, APA manifests as a unilateral eruption of clustered red to violaceous angiomatous papules (diameter: 1 to 5 mm) on acral sites, that is, hands and

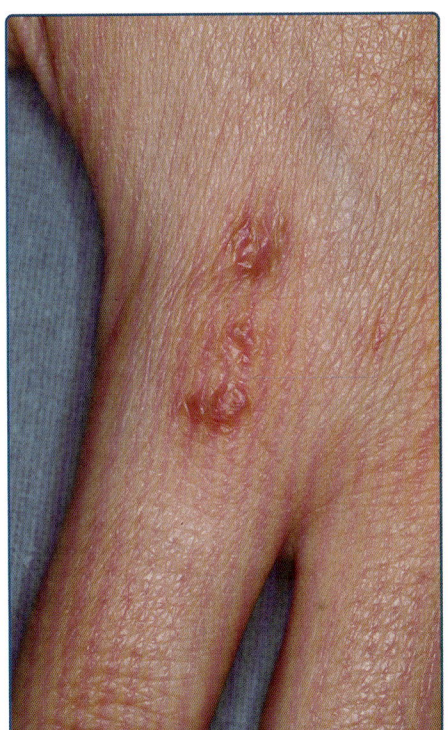

Figure 120-17 Acral pseudolymphomatous angiokeratoma of childhood (APACHE): grouped papules on the hand of an 8-year old girl. (Used with permission from Prof. Dr. S. Lautenschlager, Zurich, Switzerland.)

feet (Fig. 120-17).[90] Coalescence of the lesions can be seen. Longitudinal splitting of the nails, onycholysis, and nail deformities may occur.

The histology of APA shows a dense infiltrate of small lymphocytes, eosinophils, plasma cells, and histiocytes. Within the infiltrate there are thick-walled vessels lined by plump endothelia. Diagnosis is based on clinicopathologic correlation. The accompanying infiltrate is composed of small, well-differentiated lymphocytes admixed with a few plasma cells and histiocytes, including histiocytic giant cells. In some instances, a few eosinophils may be present. Immunohistochemistry demonstrates that the lymphocytes are polyclonal T cells and B cells, with B cells occasionally forming small aggregates. The histologic differential diagnoses of APACHE include lymphomatoid drug eruptions and arthropod bite reaction.

Similar histologic findings, but clinically manifesting as a solitary, polypoid, erythematous papule, was described under the term T-cell–rich angiomatoid polypoid PSL of the skin.[93] Its nosologic relationship to APACHE remains to be determined.

APACHE is a benign process. No reoccurrences have been reported following treatment. When left untreated, the lesions can regress, show a waning-and-waxing course, or remain unchanged for months or years.

Destruction of the lesions by curettage, intralesional corticosteroids, or high-potency topical corticosteroids under occlusion has been used for treatment and resulted in complete remission.[91]

LYMPHOPLASMACYTIC PLAQUE

Lymphoplasmacytic plaque (LPP) is a recently described rare skin disease that is considered to be a form of PSL of unknown etiology. Originally it was reported in children with the pretibial region as predilection site, and referred to as isolated primary cutaneous plasmacytosis in children and pretibial LPP.[94,95] A recent study indicates that LPP can also affect adults and involve the trunk and arms. Consequently, we prefer the term *lymphoplasmacytic plaque*.[96] There is a female preponderance.

Clinically, LPP shows a distinct presentation characterized by a longstanding plaque or circumscribed, often linear arranged, reddish and brownish papules and plaques (Fig. 120-18).[96,97] Histology reveals a dense dermal lymphohistiocytic infiltrate with numerous polyclonal plasma cells accounting for up to 25% of the entire infiltrate. The infiltrate is superficial, band-like, or deep nodular and interstitial, often accentuated around adnexal structures or blood vessels (Fig. 120-19). Interstitial histiocytic granulomas around sclerotic collagen bundles (so-called pseudorosettes) with histiocytic giant cells and an increased number of vessels can be seen.[96]

LPP have to be differentiated from other conditions containing plasma cells and histiocytes, such

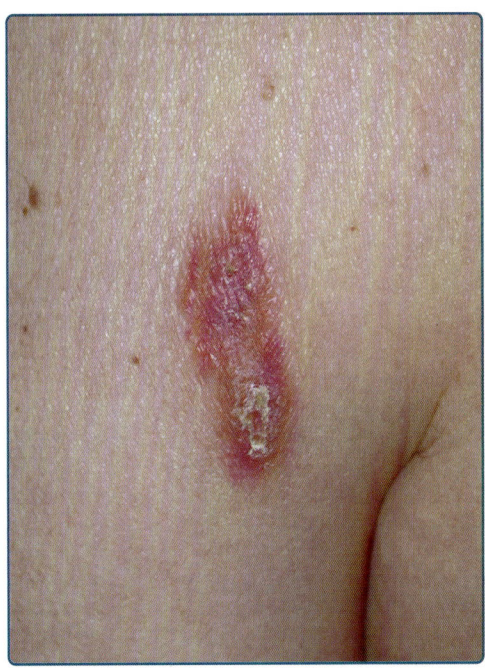

Figure 120-18 Lymphoplasmacytoid plaque: longstanding erythematous plaque on the lateral aspect of the left upper arm.

as primary cutaneous plasmocytosis, lymphocytoma cutis, cutaneous marginal zone lymphoma, primary and secondary cutaneous plasmocytoma, and infections (eg, fungal, mycobacterial, treponemal). An infectious process should always be ruled out by serology, special stains, and molecular pathologic techniques. The diagnosis of LPP is based on clinicopathologic correlation.

LPP and APA show overlapping clinical and histologic features, such as female predominance and a predilection for the extremities, especially the legs, as well as a lymphohistiocytic infiltrate and polyclonal plasma cells. It has been postulated that both entities (APACHE and LPP) belong to the same spectrum of diseases and represent a plasma cell–rich PSL with a prominent vascular component.

The course of LPP is longstanding up to several years. Surgical excision is the first-line treatment, especially as other therapies are not effective.[96]

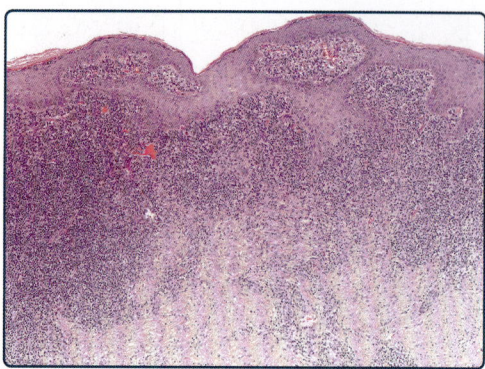

Figure 120-19 Lymphoplasmacytoid plaque, histology: epidermal hyperplasia and dense dermal infiltrate of lymphocytes and histiocytes.

CUTANEOUS PLASMOCYTOSIS

Cutaneous plasmocytosis is a rare disease that has been reported in Asian countries, especially Japan. It mostly affects adults.[98,99] It is characterized by multiple, brownish, small plaques and nodules occurring all over the body. Histology shows dermal infiltrates composed predominantly of mature polyclonal plasma cells.[98,99] In some patients, signs of a systemic involvement (eg, lymphadenopathy, hepatosplenomegaly, hypergammaglobulinemia, increased levels of interleukin-6 in the serum, and elevated erythrocyte sedimentation rate) can be found. Treatment includes PUVA, steroids, and chemotherapeutic approaches.

CUTANEOUS INFLAMMATORY PSEUDOTUMOR

The term *inflammatory pseudotumor* has been used to describe 2 conditions that today are considered to be distinct entities, namely, plasma cell granuloma and inflammatory myofibroblastic tumor.[100] Inflammatory pseudotumor is a benign process of unknown etiology. Clinically, it manifests as longstanding dermal or subcutaneous nodules of firm consistency. Histologically, a circumscribed nodular infiltrate of small lymphocytes, numerous plasma cells arranged in sheets, and histiocytes is found in plasma cell granuloma. Reactive germinal centers may be found. In inflammatory myofibroblastic tumor, a prominent spindle-cell component of myofibroblasts with expression of ALK (anaplastic lymphoma kinase) and a lymphocytic infiltrate with plasma cells are the characteristic findings. Surgical excision results in complete remission.

ANGIOLYMPHOID HYPERPLASIA WITH EOSINOPHILIA

Angiolymphoid hyperplasia with eosinophilia (ALHE) represents a proliferation of blood vessels with prominent endothelia accompanied by a dense infiltrate of T-cells and B-cells in conjunction with eosinophils. It was first described in 1969 by Wells and Whimster.[101] Nowadays ALHE is commonly regarded to be an angioproliferative process resulting from the presence of prominent, bizarrely shaped blood vessels and epithelioid endothelia leading to its alternative synonymous designation as epithelioid hemangioma.[102,103] Most authors consider ALHE as a hyperplastic process in response to tissue damage and formation of vascular shunts.

The relationship of ALHE to Kimura disease is a matter of debate, but most experts consider them as distinct clinicopathologic entities. The lesions in Kimura disease tend to be larger and deeper and are accompanied by peripheral blood eosinophilia as well as enlarged lymph nodes.

EPIDEMIOLOGY AND PATHOGENESIS

ALHE and Kimura disease affect both genders without sex predominance.[103] Most patients are in the third or fourth decade of life. Arteriovenous shunts may underlie the formation of blood vessels seen in ALHE and Kimura disease.

CLINICAL FEATURES

ALHE presents as angiomatous pink to red-brown papules or nodule(s) most commonly found on the head and neck, especially on the face and ears, but also occurring at the extremities and genital area (Fig. 120-20). The lesions may be asymptomatic or be associated with pruritus, pain, or bleeding.

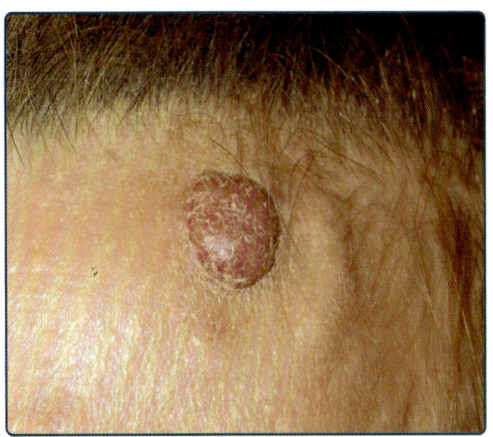

Figure 120-20 Angiolymphoid hyperplasia with eosinophilia: nodular infiltrate on the left forehead.

HISTOPATHOLOGY, IMMUNOPHENOTYPING, AND MOLECULAR TESTS

The dermal and/or subcutaneous nodules are composed of a proliferation of postcapillary vessels and a dense lymphocytic infiltrate (Fig. 120-21). The vessels are lined by prominent endothelial cells with a round or oval nucleus, an abundant eosinophilic cytoplasm, and an epithelioid or hobnail appearance. The infiltrate contains small lymphocytes, reactive germinal centers, and eosinophils.[104] Immunohistochemistry shows expression of CD31 and ERG by the endothelia, but no reactivity for podoplanin/D2-40. Immunohistochemical studies demonstrate that the majority of lymphocytes are of T-cell lineage. Admixed B cells may form lymphoid follicles. In Kimura disease the lymphoid component with germinal centers predominates over the proliferation of vessels. Clonal T cells have been detected in both ALHE and in Kimura disease.[105,106] In ALHE, the majority of those cases showed a protracted and therapy-resistant course with recurrences.

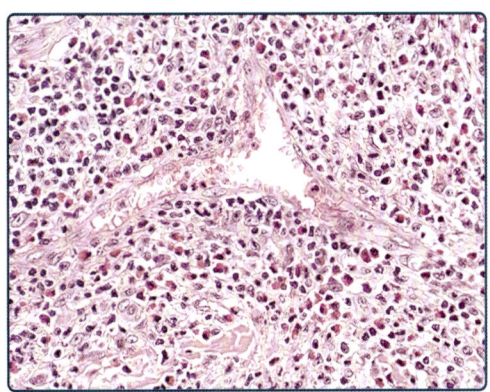

Figure 120-21 Angiolymphoid hyperplasia with eosinophilia, histology: vessels with prominent endothelia embedded in a dense infiltrate of lymphocytes and eosinophils.

DIFFERENTIAL DIAGNOSIS

Differential diagnosis includes pyogenic granuloma, which shows lobularly proliferation of vessels accompanied by a mixed-cellular infiltrate. Among lymphomas, specific infiltrates of adult T-cell lymphoma/leukemia (AITL) should be considered as they also show an increased number of vessels as well as an infiltrate composed of T cells and B cells with slight nuclear atypia. The T cells in AITL, however, are atypical, proliferatively active, and express markers of follicular helper T cells such as PD-1, ICOS, bcl-6, CD10, and CXCL-13.

CLINICAL COURSE, PROGNOSIS, AND TREATMENT

There is no spontaneous regression of ALHE lesions. Recurrences are common, particularly after surgical resection.[103,107] Surgery, cryotherapy, and laser ablation, as well as methotrexate and interferon-α, have been used to treat ALHE.[108] If an arteriovenous shunt can be identified as an underlying triggering factor, the shunt should be removed by, for example, embolization.

CASTLEMAN DISEASE

Castleman disease is a benign lymphoproliferative disorder with 2 variants: the hyaline vascular type and the plasma cell variant. The plasma cell variant can be associated with POEMS syndrome (*p*olyneuropathy, *o*rganomegaly, *e*ndocrinopathy, *m* protein, and *s*kin changes).[109] Castleman disease most commonly is located in the lymph nodes (mediastinal or generalized) and rarely affects the skin.[110] Histologically, the hyaline vascular type is more common with small lymphocytes that surround the germinal centers in a concentrically whorled pattern. This type is more common in younger patients. The plasma cell type shows large follicles and an interfollicular zone rich in blood vessels and plasma cells. The prognosis of Castleman disease with localized extranodal lesions is favorable. Therapy depends on the extent of the disease and includes surgical excision, radiation, and chemotherapy.

BENIGN INTRAVASCULAR PROLIFERATION OF LYMPHOCYTES

Recently, benign intravascular proliferation of lymphoid blasts with or without expression of CD30 has been reported. This condition arises in areas with inflammatory skin diseases or trauma of the skin.[111-113] Pathogenetically, obstruction of lymphatics by lichen sclerosus with disrupted immune cell trafficking may result in the accumulation of activated CD30+ lymphocytes. The lymphocytes are large and have

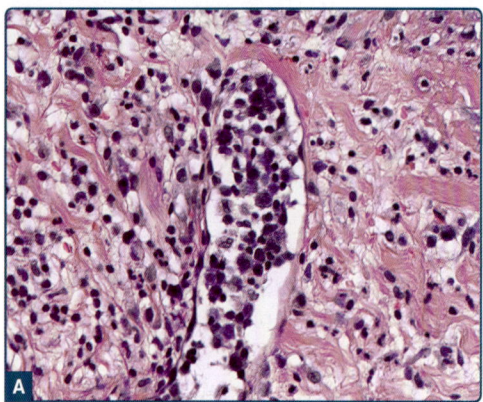

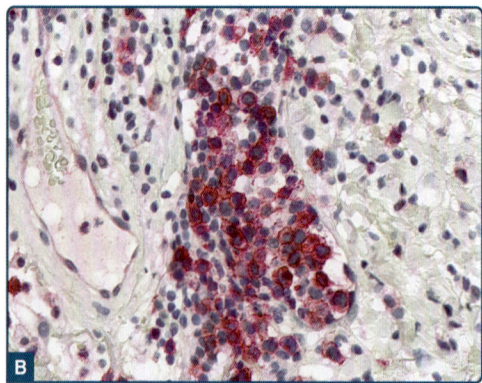

Figure 120-22 Intravascular lymphoid proliferation, histology: Intralymphatic accumulation of blast-like lymphoid cells (**A**) with expression of CD30 (**B**).

a blast-like morphology (Fig. 120-22). They express T-cell markers (CD3, CD4) and, in some cases, CD30. There is no association with Epstein-Barr virus infection. Clonality studies reveal the polyclonal nature of the process. Intravascular lymphoma is the most important differential diagnosis as it is an aggressive lymphoma with various phenotypic forms (B cell, T cell, or natural killer/T cell). In addition, benign intravascular proliferation of lymphoid cells needs to be distinguished from intralymphatic histiocytosis representing a reactive proliferation of histiocytes in the lumina of lymphatics in patients with rheumatoid arthritis or orthopedic metal implants.

SUMMARY

Cutaneous PSL refers to a group of lymphocyte-rich infiltrates that clinically and/or histologically simulate cutaneous lymphomas.[115] Clinicopathologic correlation is essential to achieve the final diagnosis in cutaneous PSL and to differentiate it from cutaneous lymphomas. Elimination of infectious agents (eg, by antibiotics or antiviral drugs) or avoidance of exposure to the causative agent (eg, LCD and drug reactions) are the first step in the management in addition to immunomodulating agents (eg, corticosteroids, UV light treatment) or ablative approaches (eg, surgical excision, cryotherapy).

REFERENCES

1. Kaposi M. *Pathologie und Therapie der Hautkrankheiten*. 4th ed. Vienna, Austria: Urban und Schwartzenberg; 1893.
2. Biberstein H. Lymphozytom. *Z Haut Geschlechtskr*. 1923;6:70-71.
3. Bäfverstedt B. Ueber lymphadenosis benigna cutis. Eine klinische pathologisch-anatomische Studie. *Acta Derm Venereol Suppl (Stockh)*. 1944;24(suppl XI):1-102.
4. Caro WA, Helwig HB. Cutaneous lymphoid hyperplasia. *Cancer*. 1969;24:487-502.
5. Ive FA, Magnus IA, Warin RP, et al. "Actinic reticuloid"; a chronic dermatosis associated with severe photosensitivity and the histological resemblance to lymphoma. *Br J Dermatol*. 1969;81(7):469-485.
6. Burg G, Braun-Falco O. *Cutaneous Lymphomas, Pseudolymphomas and Related Disorders*. Berlin, Germany: Springer-Verlag; 1983.
7. Rijlaarsdam JU, Willemze R. Cutaneous pseudolymphomas: classification and differential diagnosis. *Semin Dermatol*. 1994;13(3):187-196.
8. Ploysangam T, Breneman DL, Mutasim DF. Cutaneous pseudolymphomas. *J Am Acad Dermatol*. 1998;38(6, pt 1):877-895.
9. Gilliam AC, Wood GS. Cutaneous lymphoid hyperplasias. *Semin Cutan Med Surg*. 2000;19(2):133-141.
10. van Vloten WA, Willemze R. The many faces of lymphocytoma cutis. *J Eur Acad Dermatol Venereol*. 2003;17(1):3-6.
11. Hammer E, Sangueza O, Suwanjindar P, et al. Immunophenotypic and genotypic analysis in cutaneous lymphoid hyperplasias. *J Am Acad Dermatol*. 1993;28(3):426-433.
12. Bouloc A, Delfau-Larue MH, Lenormand B, et al. Polymerase chain reaction analysis of immunoglobulin gene rearrangement in cutaneous lymphoid hyperplasias. French Study Group for Cutaneous Lymphomas. *Arch Dermatol*. 1999;135(2):168-172.
13. Holm N, Flaig MJ, Yazdi AS, et al. The value of molecular analysis by PCR in the diagnosis of cutaneous lymphocytic infiltrates. *J Cutan Pathol*. 2002;29(8):447-452.
14. Colli C, Leinweber B, Mullegger R, et al. Borrelia burgdorferi-associated lymphocytoma cutis: clinicopathologic, immunophenotypic, and molecular study of 106 cases. *J Cutan Pathol*. 2004;31(3):232-240.
15. Goodlad JR, Davidson MM, Hollowood K, et al. *Borrelia burgdorferi*-associated cutaneous marginal zone lymphoma: a clinicopathological study of two cases illustrating the temporal progression of *B. burgdorferi*-associated B-cell proliferation in the skin. *Histopathology*. 2000;37(6):501-508.
16. Kempf W, Kerl H, Kutzner H. CD123-positive plasmacytoid dendritic cells in primary cutaneous marginal zone B-cell lymphoma: a crucial role and a new lymphoma paradigm. *Am J Dermatopathol*. 2009;32(2):194-196.
17. Kutzner H, Kerl H, Pfaltz MC, et al. CD123-positive plasmacytoid dendritic cells in primary cutaneous marginal zone B-cell lymphoma: diagnostic and pathogenetic implications. *Am J Surg Pathol*. 2009;33(9):1307-1313.
18. Brodell RT, Santa Cruz DJ. Cutaneous pseudolymphomas. *Dermatol Clin*. 1985;3(4):719-734.
19. Moulonguet I, Ghnassia M, Molina T, et al. Miliarial-type perifollicular B-cell pseudolymphoma (lymphocytoma cutis): a misleading eruption in two women. *J Cutan Pathol*. 2012;39(11):1016-1021.
20. Baldassano MF, Bailey EM, Ferry JA, et al. Cutaneous lymphoid hyperplasia and cutaneous marginal

20. zone lymphoma: comparison of morphologic and immunophenotypic features. *Am J Surg Pathol*. 1999;23(1):88-96.
21. Leinweber B, Colli C, Chott A, et al. Differential diagnosis of cutaneous infiltrates of B lymphocytes with follicular growth pattern. *Am J Dermatopathol*. 2004;26(1):4-13.
22. Boudova L, Kazakov DV, Sima R, et al. Cutaneous lymphoid hyperplasia and other lymphoid infiltrates of the breast nipple: a retrospective clinicopathologic study of fifty-six patients. *Am J Dermatopathol*. 2005;27(5):375-386.
23. Nihal M, Mikkola D, Horvath N, et al. Cutaneous lymphoid hyperplasia: a lymphoproliferative continuum with lymphomatous potential. *Hum Pathol*. 2003;34(6):617-622.
24. Boer A, Tirumalae R, Bresch M, et al. Pseudoclonality in cutaneous pseudolymphomas: a pitfall in interpretation of rearrangement studies. *Br J Dermatol*. 2008;159(2):394-402.
25. Grange F, Wechsler J, Guillaume JC, et al. *Borrelia burgdorferi*-associated lymphocytoma cutis simulating a primary cutaneous large B-cell lymphoma. *J Am Acad Dermatol*. 2002;47(4):530-534.
26. Kempf W, Flaig MJ, Kutzner H. Molecular diagnostics in infectious skin diseases. *J Dtsch Dermatol Ges*. 2013;11(suppl 4):50-58.
27. Rijlaarsdam JU, Scheffer E, Meijer CJ, et al. Cutaneous pseudo-T-cell lymphomas. A clinicopathologic study of 20 patients. *Cancer*. 1992;69(3):717-724.
28. Bergman R, Khamaysi Z, Sahar D, et al. Cutaneous lymphoid hyperplasia presenting as a solitary facial nodule: clinical, histopathological, immunophenotypical, and molecular studies. *Arch Dermatol*. 2006;142(12):1561-1566.
29. Leinweber B, Beltraminelli H, Kerl H, et al. Solitary small- to medium-sized pleomorphic T-cell nodules of undetermined significance: clinical, histopathological, immunohistochemical and molecular analysis of 26 cases. *Dermatology*. 2009;219(1):42-47.
30. Tomar S, Stoll HL, Grassi MA, et al. Treatment of cutaneous pseudolymphoma with interferon alfa-2b. *J Am Acad Dermatol*. 2009;60(1):172-174.
31. Kempf W. CD30+ lymphoproliferative disorders: histopathology, differential diagnosis, new variants, and simulators. *J Cutan Pathol*. 2006;33(suppl 1):58-70.
32. Werner B, Massone C, Kerl H, et al. Large CD30-positive cells in benign, atypical lymphoid infiltrates of the skin. *J Cutan Pathol*. 2008;35(12):1100-1107.
33. Gonzalez LC, Murua MA, Perez RG, et al. CD30+ lymphoma simulating Orf. *Int J Dermatol*. 2010;49(6):690-692.
34. Fukamachi S, Sugita K, Sawada Y, et al. Drug-induced CD30+ T cell pseudolymphoma. *Eur J Dermatol*. 2009;19(3):292-294.
35. De Souza A, Tinguely M, Pfaltz M, et al. Loss of expression of 5-hydroxymethylcytosine in CD30-positive cutaneous lymphoproliferative disorders. *J Cutan Pathol*. 2014;41(12):901-906.
36. Kibbi AG, Scrimenti RJ, Koenig RR, et al. A solitary nodule of the left cheek. Pseudolymphomatous folliculitis. *Arch Dermatol*. 1988;124(8):1272-1273, 1276.
37. Arai E, Okubo H, Tsuchida T, et al. Pseudolymphomatous folliculitis: a clinicopathologic study of 15 cases of cutaneous pseudolymphoma with follicular invasion. *Am J Surg Pathol*. 1999;23(11):1313-1319.
38. Petersson F. Pseudolymphomatous folliculitis with marked lymphocytic folliculo- and focal epidermotropism—expanding the morphologic spectrum. *Am J Dermatopathol*. 2011;33(3):323-325.
39. Gallardo F, Barranco C, Toll A, et al. CD30 antigen expression in cutaneous inflammatory infiltrates of scabies: a dynamic immunophenotypic pattern that should be distinguished from lymphomatoid papulosis. *J Cutan Pathol*. 2002;29(6):368-373.
40. Liu KC, Hsu CK, Lee JY. Insect bite-like reaction in association with chronic lymphocytic leukemia. *Int J Dermatol*. 2015;54(10):1191-1193.
41. Almeida HL Jr. Treatment of steroid-resistant nodular scabies with topical pimecrolimus. *J Am Acad Dermatol*. 2005;53(2):357-358.
42. Smolle J, Cerroni L, Kerl H. Multiple pseudolymphomas caused by *Hirudo medicinalis* therapy. *J Am Acad Dermatol*. 2000;43(5, pt 1):867-869.
43. Altamura D, Calonje E, Liau J, et al. Diffuse cutaneous pseudolymphoma due to therapy with medicinal leeches. *JAMA Dermatol*. 2014;150(7):783-784.
44. Braddock SW, Harrington D, Vose J. Generalized nodular cutaneous pseudolymphoma associated with phenytoin therapy. Use of T-cell receptor gene rearrangement in diagnosis and clinical review of cutaneous reactions to phenytoin. *J Am Acad Dermatol*. 1992;27(2, pt 2):337-340.
45. Albrecht J, Fine LA, Piette W. Drug-associated lymphoma and pseudolymphoma: recognition and management. *Dermatol Clin*. 2007;25(2):233-244, vii.
46. Kardaun SH, Scheffer E, Vermeer BJ. Drug-induced pseudolymphomatous skin reactions. *Br J Dermatol*. 1988;118(4):545-552.
47. Magro CM, Crowson AN. Drugs with antihistaminic properties as a cause of atypical cutaneous lymphoid hyperplasia. *J Am Acad Dermatol*. 1995;32(3):419-428.
48. Pulitzer MP, Nolan KA, Oshman RG, et al. CD30+ lymphomatoid drug reactions. *Am J Dermatopathol*. 2013;35(3):343-350.
49. Goerdt S, Spieker T, Wolffer LU. Multiple cutaneous B-cell pseudolymphomas after allergen injections. *J Am Acad Dermatol*. 1996;34(6):1072-1074.
50. Maubec E, Pinquier L, Viguier M, et al. Vaccination-induced cutaneous pseudolymphoma. *J Am Acad Dermatol*. 2005;52(4):623-629.
51. Chong H, Brady K, Metze D, et al. Persistent nodules at injection sites (aluminium granuloma)—clinicopathological study of 14 cases with a diverse range of histological reaction patterns. *Histopathology*. 2006;48(2):182-188.
52. Cerroni L, Borroni RG, Massone C, et al. Cutaneous B-cell pseudolymphoma at the site of vaccination. *Am J Dermatopathol*. 2007;29(6):538-542.
53. Blumental G, Okun MR, Ponitch JA. Pseudolymphomatous reaction to tattoos. Report of three cases. *J Am Acad Dermatol*. 1982;6(4, pt 1):485-488.
54. Iwatsuki K, Yamada M, Takigawa M, et al. Benign lymphoplasia of the earlobes induced by gold earrings: immunohistologic study on the cellular infiltrates. *J Am Acad Dermatol*. 1987;16(1, pt 1):83-88.
55. Lubach D, Hinz E. A pseudolymphomatous reaction in tattooing [in German]. *Hautarzt*. 1986;37(10):573-575.
56. Amann U, Luger TA, Metze D. Lichenoid pseudolymphomatous tattooing reaction [in German]. *Hautarzt*. 1997;48(6):410-413.
57. Yavuzer R, Akyurek N, Ozmen S, et al. Leishmania cutis with B-cell cutaneous hyperplasia. *Plast Reconstr Surg*. 2001;108(7):2177-2178.
58. Flaig MJ, Rupec RA. Cutaneous pseudolymphoma in association with *Leishmania donovani*. *Br J Dermatol*. 2007;157(5):1042-1043.
59. Gomez-Orbaneja J, Diez LI, Lozano JL, et al. Lymphomatoid contact dermatitis: a syndrome produced by

epicutaneous hypersensitivity with clinical features and a histopathologic picture similar to that of mycosis fungoides. *Contact Dermatitis*. 1976;2(3):139-143.
60. Uzuncakmak TK, Akdeniz N, Ozkanli S, et al. Lymphomatoid contact dermatitis associated with textile dye at an unusual location. *Indian Dermatol Online J*. 2015;6(suppl 1):S24-S26.
61. Martinez-Moran C, Sanz-Munoz C, Morales-Callaghan AM, et al. Lymphomatoid contact dermatitis. *Contact Dermatitis*. 2009;60(1):53-55.
62. Wolf IH, Cerroni L, Fink-Puches R, et al. The morphologic spectrum of cutaneous pseudolymphomas [in German]. *J Dtsch Dermatol Ges*. 2005;3(9):710-720; quiz 721.
63. Souteyrand P, d'Incan M. Drug-induced mycosis fungoides-like lesions. *Curr Probl Dermatol*. 1990;19:176-182.
64. Klemke CD, Booken N, Weiss C, et al. Histopathological and immunophenotypical criteria for the diagnosis of Sezary syndrome in differentiation from other erythrodermic skin diseases: a European Organisation for Research and Treatment of Cancer (EORTC) Cutaneous Lymphoma Task Force Study of 97 cases. *Br J Dermatol*. 2015;173(1):93-105.
65. Kempf W, Kazakov DV, Palmedo G, et al. Pityriasis lichenoides et varioliformis acuta with numerous CD30+ cells: A variant mimicking lymphomatoid papulosis and other cutaneous lymphomas. A clinicopathologic, immunohistochemical, and molecular biological study of 13 cases. *Am J Surg Pathol*. 2012;36(7):1021-1029.
66. Toonstra J, Henquet CJ, van Weelden H, et al. Actinic reticuloid. A clinical photobiologic, histopathologic, and follow-up study of 16 patients. *J Am Acad Dermatol*. 1989;21(2, pt 1):205-214.
67. Toonstra J. Actinic reticuloid. *Semin Diagn Pathol*. 1991;8(2):109-116.
68. Longacre TA, Foucar K, Koster F, et al. Atypical cutaneous lymphoproliferative disorder resembling mycosis fungoides in AIDS. Report of a case with concurrent Kaposi's sarcoma. *Am J Dermatopathol*. 1989;11(5):451-456.
69. Egbers RG, Do TT, Su L, et al. Rapid clinical change in lesions of atypical cutaneous lymphoproliferative disorder in an HIV patient: a case report and review of the literature. *Dermatol Online J*. 2011;17(9):4.
70. Sbidian E, Battistella M, Rivet J, et al. Remission of severe CD8(+) cytotoxic T cell skin infiltrative disease in human immunodeficiency virus-infected patients receiving highly active antiretroviral therapy. *Clin Infect Dis*. 2010;51(6):741-748.
71. Ingen-Housz-Oro S, Sbidian E, Ortonne N, et al. HIV-related CD8+ cutaneous pseudolymphoma: efficacy of methotrexate. *Dermatology*. 2013;226(1):15-18.
72. Bayal C, Büyükbani N, Seckin D, et al. Cutaneous atypical papular CD8+ lymphoproliferative disorder at acral sites in a renal transplant patient. *Clin Exp Dermatol*. 2017;42(8):902-905.
73. Tee SI, Martinez-Escaname M, Zuriel D, et al. Acrodermatitis chronica atrophicans with pseudolymphomatous infiltrates. *Am J Dermatopathol*. 2013;35(3):338-342.
74. Kempf W, Kazakov DV, Hubscher E, et al. Cutaneous borreliosis associated with T cell-predominant infiltrates: a diagnostic challenge. *J Am Acad Dermatol*. 2015;72(4):683-689.
75. Ofuji S, Furukawa F, Miyachi Y, et al. Papuloerythroderma. *Dermatologica*. 1984;169(3):125-130.
76. Sugita K, Kabashima K, Nakamura M, et al. Drug-induced papuloerythroderma: analysis of T-cell populations and a literature review. *Acta Derm Venereol*. 2009;89(6):618-622.
77. Torchia D, Miteva M, Hu S, et al. Papuloerythroderma 2009: two new cases and systematic review of the worldwide literature 25 years after its identification by Ofuji et al. *Dermatology*. 2010;220(4):311-320.
78. Shah M, Reid WA, Layton AM. Cutaneous T-cell lymphoma presenting as papuloerythroderma—a case and review of the literature. *Clin Exp Dermatol*. 1995;20(2):161-163.
79. Aste N, Fumo G, Conti B, et al. Ofuji papuloerythroderma. *J Eur Acad Dermatol Venereol*. 2000;14(1):55-57.
80. Bech-Thomsen N, Thomsen K. Ofuji's papuloerythroderma: a study of 17 cases. *Clin Exp Dermatol*. 1998;23(2):79-83.
81. Toro JR, Sander CA, LeBoit PE. Persistent pigmented purpuric dermatitis and mycosis fungoides: simulant, precursor, or both? A study by light microscopy and molecular methods. *Am J Dermatopathol*. 1997;19(2):108-118.
82. Magro C, Crowson AN, Kovatich A, et al. Pityriasis lichenoides: a clonal T-cell lymphoproliferative disorder. *Hum Pathol*. 2002;33(8):788-795.
83. Citarella L, Massone C, Kerl H, et al. Lichen sclerosus with histopathologic features simulating early mycosis fungoides. *Am J Dermatopathol*. 2003;25(6):463-465.
84. Dereure O, Levi E, Kadin ME. T-Cell clonality in pityriasis lichenoides et varioliformis acuta: a heteroduplex analysis of 20 cases. *Arch Dermatol*. 2000;136(12):1483-1486.
85. Lor P, Krueger U, Kempf W, et al. Monoclonal rearrangement of the T cell receptor gamma-chain in lichenoid pigmented purpuric dermatitis of Gougerot-Blum responding to topical corticosteroid therapy. *Dermatology*. 2002;205(2):191-193.
86. Wood GS. Analysis of clonality in cutaneous T cell lymphoma and associated diseases. *Ann N Y Acad Sci*. 2001;941:26-30.
87. Abeck D, Ollert MW, Eckert F, et al. Palpable migratory arciform erythema. Clinical morphology, histopathology, immunohistochemistry, and response to treatment. *Arch Dermatol*. 1997;133(6):763-766.
88. Wagner G, Bartsch S, Rose C, et al. Palpable arciforme migratory erythema [in German]. *Hautarzt*. 2012;63(12):965-968.
89. Poenitz N, Dippel E, Klemke CD, et al. Jessner's lymphocytic infiltration of the skin: a CD8+ polyclonal reactive skin condition. *Dermatology*. 2003;207(3):276-284.
90. Kaddu S, Cerroni L, Pilatti A, et al. Acral pseudolymphomatous angiokeratoma. A variant of the cutaneous pseudolymphomas. *Am J Dermatopathol*. 1994;16(2):130-133.
91. Okada M, Funayama M, Tanita M, et al. Acral angiokeratoma-like pseudolymphoma: one adolescent and two adults. *J Am Acad Dermatol*. 2001;45(6)(suppl):S209-S211.
92. Wagner G, Rose C, Sachse MM. Papular pseudolymphoma of adults as a variant of acral pseudolymphomatous angiokeratoma of children (APACHE). *J Dtsch Dermatol Ges*. 2014;12(5):423-424.
93. Dayrit JF, Wang WL, Goh SG, et al. T-cell-rich angiomatoid polypoid pseudolymphoma of the skin: a clinicopathologic study of 17 cases and a proposed nomenclature. *J Cutan Pathol*. 2011;38(6):475-482.
94. Gilliam AC, Mullen RH, Oviedo G, et al. Isolated benign primary cutaneous plasmacytosis in children: two illustrative cases. *Arch Dermatol*. 2009;145(3):299-302.
95. Fried I, Wiesner T, Cerroni L. Pretibial lymphoplasmacytic plaque in children. *Arch Dermatol*. 2010;146(1):95-96.

96. Mitteldorf C, Palmedo G, Kutzner H, et al. Diagnostic approach in lymphoplasmacytic plaque. *J Eur Acad Dermatol Venereol*. 2015;29(11):2206-2215.
97. Moulonguet I, Hadj-Rabia S, Gounod N, et al. Tibial lymphoplasmacytic plaque: a new, illustrative case of a recently and poorly recognized benign lesion in children. *Dermatology*. 2012;225(1):27-30.
98. Uhara H, Saida T, Ikegawa S, et al. Primary cutaneous plasmacytosis: report of three cases and review of the literature. *Dermatology*. 1994;189(3):251-255.
99. Honda R, Cerroni L, Tanikawa A, et al. Cutaneous plasmacytosis: report of 6 cases with or without systemic involvement. *J Am Acad Dermatol*. 2013;68(6):978-985.
100. El Shabrawi-Caelen L, Kerl K, Cerroni L, et al. Cutaneous inflammatory pseudotumor—a spectrum of various diseases? *J Cutan Pathol*. 2004;31(9):605-611.
101. Wells GC, Whimster IW. Subcutaneous angiolymphoid hyperplasia with eosinophilia. *Br J Dermatol*. 1969;81(1):1-14.
102. Requena L, Sangueza OP. Cutaneous vascular proliferation. Part II. Hyperplasias and benign neoplasms. *J Am Acad Dermatol*. 1997;37(6):887-919; quiz 920-922.
103. Adler BL, Krausz AE, Minuti A, et al. Epidemiology and treatment of angiolymphoid hyperplasia with eosinophilia (ALHE): a systematic review. *J Am Acad Dermatol*. 2016;74(3):506-512.e11.
104. Olsen TG, Helwig EB. Angiolymphoid hyperplasia with eosinophilia. A clinicopathologic study of 116 patients. *J Am Acad Dermatol*. 1985;12(5, pt 1):781-796.
105. Chim CS, Fung A, Shek TW, et al. Analysis of clonality in Kimura's disease. *Am J Surg Pathol*. 2002;26(8):1083-1086.
106. Kempf W, Haeffner AC, Zepter K, et al. Angiolymphoid hyperplasia with eosinophilia: evidence for a T-cell lymphoproliferative origin. *Hum Pathol*. 2002;33(10):1023-1029.
107. Al-Jitawi S, Oumeish OY. Angiolymphoid hyperplasia with tissue eosinophilia. *Int J Dermatol*. 1989;28(2):114-118.
108. Sagi L, Halachmi S, Levi A, et al. Combined pulsed dye and CO_2 lasers in the treatment of angiolymphoid hyperplasia with eosinophilia. *Lasers Med Sci*. 2016;31(6):1093-1096..
109. Dispenzieri A. POEMS syndrome: 2014 update on diagnosis, risk-stratification, and management. *Am J Hematol*. 2014;89(2):214-223.
110. Skelton HG, Smith KJ. Extranodal multicentric Castleman's disease with cutaneous involvement. *Mod Pathol*. 1998;11(1):93-98.
111. Riveiro-Falkenbach E, Fernandez-Figueras MT, Rodriguez-Peralto JL. Benign atypical intravascular CD30(+) T-cell proliferation: a reactive condition mimicking intravascular lymphoma. *Am J Dermatopathol*. 2013;35(2):143-150.
112. Kempf W, Keller K, John H, et al. Benign atypical intravascular CD30+ T-cell proliferation: a recently described reactive lymphoproliferative process and simulator of intravascular lymphoma: report of a case associated with lichen sclerosus and review of the literature. *Am J Clin Pathol*. 2014;142(5):694-699.
113. Calamaro P, Cerroni L. Intralymphatic proliferation of T-cell lymphoid blasts in the setting of hidradenitis suppurativa. *Am J Dermatopathol*. 2016;38(7):536-540.
114. Darier J. Die cutanen und subcutanen Sarkoide. Ihre Beziehungen zum Sarkom, zum Lymphodermie, zur Tuberkulose usw. *Monatschr Prakt Dermatol*. 1910; 50:419-451.
115. Mitteldorf C, Kempf W. Cutaneous pseudolymphoma. *Surg Pathol Clin*. 2017;10:455-476.

Chapter 121 :: Neoplasias and Hyperplasias of Muscular and Neural Origin
:: Hansgeorg Müller & Heinz Kutzner

第一百二十一章
肌肉和神经源性肿瘤与增生

中文导读

本章分为6节，包括肌肉来源和神经来源的良性肿瘤、恶性肿瘤及错构瘤等，介绍了各种平滑肌肿瘤、横纹肌肿瘤、周围神经鞘瘤、良性神经鞘瘤（神经瘤）、良性神经鞘肿瘤及其他肌肉和神经源性肿瘤与增生的流行病学、临床表现、组织病理学、临床病程、预后及管理。

〔粟 娟〕

TUMORS OF SMOOTH MUSCLE

Cutaneous tumors with smooth muscle differentiation Table 121-1) can be categorized according to their microanatomical origin: (a) arrector pili muscles, (b) smooth muscle of genital skin, including scrotum (dartos muscle), vulva, nipple and areolar region, and (c) walls of blood vessels. Each of these sources of smooth muscle can give rise to benign superficial smooth muscle tumors (leiomyomas) as well as their malignant counterparts (leiomyosarcomas).[1] Anecdotally, smooth muscle also has been reported in organoid and blue nevi.[2] Of note, smooth muscle tumors arising in deep soft tissues (eg, abdominal cavity, pelvis, retroperitoneum), and visceral organs (including uterine tumors) often show overlapping morphologic and immunohistochemical features with cutaneous tumors, but form different clinicopathologic categories because biologic potential, clinical prognosis, and criteria for malignancy depend primarily on location.[3,4] Histologically, the constituent cells of smooth muscle lesions are spindled and contain abundant brightly eosinophilic cytoplasm as well as blunt-ended (cigar-shaped) nuclei. Smooth muscle antigens, including α-smooth muscle actin (α-SMA), muscle-specific actin, desmin, and h-caldesmon are readily identified by immunohistochemistry. Atypical intradermal smooth muscle neoplasms and leiomyosarcomas often at least focally express epithelial markers, and sporadic cases may express S-100 protein.[5,6] Figure 121-1 provides an overview of the diagnosis of cutaneous tumors with smooth muscle differentiation. The spectrum of cutaneous smooth muscle lesions includes leiomyomas, leiomyosarcomas, and smooth muscle hamartomas.

LEIOMYOMA

AT-A-GLANCE

- Synonyms: superficial leiomyoma; leiomyoma cutis; superficial benign smooth muscle tumor.

- Benign neoplasm of the skin with smooth muscle differentiation occurring in 3 categories: piloleiomyoma (synonym: pilar leiomyoma), solitary genital (including dartoic, vulvar, nipple and areolar) leiomyoma, and angioleiomyoma.

- Commonly presents as solitary or multiple, firm, reddish-brown papulonodule with a predilection

- for the face, back, and extensor surfaces of the extremities.
- Multiple piloleiomyomas usually develop during adolescence in the setting of a multiple cutaneous and uterine leiomyomatosis syndrome resulting from a germline mutation in the fumarate hydratase (*FH*) gene.

EPIDEMIOLOGY

Cutaneous leiomyomas are reported to be relatively uncommon. In the experience of Orellana-Diaz and associates, based on surgical material, the incidence was 34 out of 85,349 pathology specimens (0.04%).[7] This study probably underestimates the large number of asymptomatic, usually unrecognized lesions. The relative incidence of the various leiomyoma subtypes is unknown. Although formerly considered to represent the more common subgroup, pilar leiomyomas are probably less frequent than previously thought and are potentially outnumbered by those originating from genital sites.[8]

ETIOLOGY AND PATHOGENESIS

Superficial benign smooth muscle tumors segregate into (a) piloleiomyomas (Fig. 121-2) deriving from the arrector pili muscles, (b) leiomyomas of genital sites (Fig. 121-3) and the nipple and the areola (Fig. 121-4), deriving from specialized smooth muscle of genital skin (dartoic, vulvar, mammillary, areolar), and (c) angioleiomyomas (Fig. 121-2), deriving from smooth muscle tissue of vessel walls. Pilar leiomyoma usually afflicts adolescents, although rare cases are present at birth or appear during early childhood.[9] Lesions are more often multiple than solitary. Up to several hundred lesions may develop. A positive family history with an autosomal dominant inheritance pattern can be detected in a minority of patients.[10] Recent evidence implies that most patients presenting with multiple cutaneous leiomyomas have a germline loss-of-function mutation in the fumarate hydratase gene (*FH*), mapped to chromosome 1q42.3-43 and encoding an enzyme that functions as part of the Krebs cycle by converting fumarate to malate.[11-13] The gene may also act as tumor suppressor gene. The vast majority of women with multiple cutaneous leiomyomas develop early-onset uterine leiomyomas with the cutaneous tumors typically occurring in the late second or third decade of life prior to the diagnosis of uterine lesions.[14] This syndrome, known as multiple cutaneous and uterine leiomyomatosis (Reed syndrome, multiple leiomyomatosis, familial leiomyomatosis cutis et uteri),[15] also can be associated with early-onset renal cell carcinoma of the papillary Type II, the tubule-papillary type, and the collecting duct type, a condition referred to as hereditary leiomyomatosis and renal cell cancer

Table 121-2.[16] Renal tumors present at relatively advanced stages in approximately 10% to 16% of individuals with hereditary leiomyomatosis and renal cell cancer and tend to occur more commonly in adult females than in adult males with this syndrome.[17,18] The specific risk to women with hereditary leiomyomatosis and renal cell cancer of developing uterine leiomyosarcoma is unknown.

CLINICAL FINDINGS

Piloleiomyomas typically appear as multiple, firm, brown-red to pearly discrete papulonodules that in the nascent stage are more easily palpable than visible. Sites of predilection include the face and back, and the extensor sites of the extremities. Solitary piloleiomyomas are commonly slightly larger than the tumors in individuals presenting with multiple lesions, reaching 2 cm or greater in diameter.[19] Lesions on the trunk are typically multiple ("cutaneous leiomyomatosis"; Fig. 121-5) and can be arranged in a diffuse (disseminated), blaschkoid, segmental (zosteriform), or, rarely, symmetrical distribution.[9,20] They may coalesce to form plaques or display an agminated, clustered, or linear pattern.[21] Anecdotal cases of Type 2 segmental manifestations of hereditary cutaneous leiomyomatosis have been reported.[22] The tumors are frequently associated with spontaneous or secondary pain, particularly by exposure to cold. It is unclear whether the produced pain results from a contraction of the muscle fibers, local compression of nearby located nerves, or an increased number of nerve bundles.[1] Genital leiomyomas of the nipple–areolar region are rare and usually small, seldom exceeding 2 cm in diameter. Scrotal leiomyomas present as firm nodules. Vulval tumors, typically arising in the labia majora, and scrotal tumors tend to be larger, measuring 1 to 5 cm and 1 to 14 cm in diameter, respectively.[23] Angioleiomyomas occur preferentially as slowly enlarging nodules of several years' duration on the extremities, particularly the lower leg. They are more frequent in females, except for those tumors in the oral cavity where the opposite holds true.[24]

HISTOPATHOLOGY

Pilar leiomyoma is a dermal-based tumor, but focal involvement of the superficial subcutis may occasionally be present. The cellular neoplasms are ill defined and composed of bland-appearing spindle cells containing blunt-ended, cigar-shaped nuclei with eosinophilic cytoplasm arranged in interweaving fascicles (Fig. 121-6). In contrast to angioleiomyomas, the lesions blend in an irregular fashion with the surrounding dermal collagen and adjacent pilar muscle. The central tumor parts are usually devoid of connective tissue and consist of densely packed bundles of smooth muscle fibers. A nodular and well-circumscribed growth pattern is infrequently encountered. Neither atypia nor mitotic activity is seen in piloleiomyomas. In contrast to leiomyomas of the uterus and deep soft tissue,

TABLE 121-1
Tumors of Muscular Differentiation Involving the Skin Comprise 2 Large Subgroups

	TUMORS OF SMOOTH MUSCLE					TUMORS OF STRIATED MUSCLE			
	PILAR LEIOMYOMA	GENITAL LEIOMYOMA	ANGIOLEIOMYOMA	LEIOMYSARCOMA	SMOOTH MUSCLE HAMARTOMA	RHABDOMYOMA	RHABDOMYOSARCOMA	RHABDOMYOMATOUS MESENCHYMAL HAMARTOMA	NEUROMUSCULAR HAMARTOMA
Incidence	Uncommon	Uncommon	Uncommon	Rare	Very rare	Very rare	Very rare	Extremely rare	Extremely rare
Age & gender	Adolescence M:F = 1:1	Adolescence M:F = 1:1	Adults (30 to 50 years of age) M:F = 1:2	Adults (40 to 60 years of age) M>F	Birth M:F = 1:1	Children to adults M>F	Neonates to adults M>F	Neonate M>F	Children <2 years of age and adults
Location	Back, extensor sites of upper extremities, face, etc	Tunica dartos, labium majus, nipple, areola	Strong predilection for extremities, particularly lower leg	Hair-bearing areas of lower extremities, scalp, trunk	Trunk or extremities	Head and neck region, vulva	Most commonly on the head and neck region or the extremities	Midline region of the skin in the head and neck region, most frequently on the chin	Large nerve trunks (brachial and sciatic), cranial nerves
Size	0.5 to 2 cm	0.5 to 14 cm	0.5 to 2 cm	1 to 4 cm	1 to 10 cm	0.5 to 10 cm	1 to 15 cm	0.5 to 2 cm	
Clinical presentation	Brown-red to pearly, firm papulonodule, solitary or multiple lesions	Firm nodule	Firm, slowly growing, subcutaneous mass	Firm nodule with hyperpigmentation and erythema of the involved skin	Skin-colored or lightly pigmented patch or plaque, may show hyperpigmentation and/or hypertrichosis	Round or polypoid mass (adult rhabdomyoma), subcutaneous mass (fetal rhabdomyoma)	Rapidly growing, subcutaneous or ulcerated mass; "blueberry muffin baby"	Small dome-shaped papule or polypoid pedunculated lesion	Solitary mass
Symptoms	Episodic pain	Usually painless	Pain or tenderness in 50% of cases	Pain or tenderness occasionally present	Pseudo-Darier sign	Usually painless	May limit range of motion	Usually painless	Neurologic symptoms
Genetics	Hereditary variant (multiple lesions): loss-of-function germline mutation in the fumarate hydratase gene (*FH*), chromosome 1q42.3-43			May develop as secondary malignancy in the setting of hereditary retinoblastoma, alterations of the retinoblastoma 1 (Rb1) locus		*PTCH* (patched hedgehog gene) mutations for fetal rhabdomyomas in the setting of nevoid basal cell carcinoma syndrome	80% of adult-type rhabdomyosarcomas have the *PAX3-FOXO1A* or *PAX7-FOXO1A* fusion gene		

(Continued)

TABLE 121-1
Tumors of Muscular Differentiation Involving the Skin Comprise 2 Large Subgroups (Continued)

	TUMORS OF SMOOTH MUSCLE					TUMORS OF STRIATED MUSCLE			
	PILAR LEIOMYOMA	GENITAL LEIOMYOMA	ANGIOLEIOMYOMA	LEIOMYOSARCOMA	SMOOTH MUSCLE HAMARTOMA	RHABDOMYOMA	RHABDOMYOSARCOMA	RHABDOMYOMATOUS MESENCHYMAL HAMARTOMA	NEUROMUSCULAR HAMARTOMA
Histopathologic features	Dermal tumor, interweaving fascicles of spindle cells containing blunt-ended, cigar-shaped nuclei with brightly eosinophilic cytoplasm	Ill-defined fascicles of spindle cells containing blunt-ended, cigar-shaped nuclei with brightly eosinophilic cytoplasm	Well-demarcated nodule of smooth muscle tissue punctuated with thick-walled vessels with partially open lumina	Intersecting fascicles of large, atypical spindle cells, nuclear atypia, mitosis, necrosis	Well-defined and thickened smooth muscle fibers haphazardly oriented in reticular dermis; some fibers are attached to hair follicles	Adult rhabdomyoma: eosinophilic polygonal cells with small, peripherally placed nuclei and intracellular vacuoles	Rhabdomyoblasts, multinucleated giant cells, areas of necrosis, high mitotic index	Mixture of mature-appearing adipose and skeletal muscle tissue, adnexal structures, blood vessels, and nerves	Bundles of perpendicularly oriented skeletal muscles intermingled with small nerve fascicles
Immunohistochemical features	h-Caldesmon, desmin, α-smooth muscle actin (SMA), muscle-specific actin (MSA)	h-Caldesmon, desmin, α-SMA, MSA	h-Caldesmon, desmin, α-SMA, MSA	h-Caldesmon, desmin, α-SMA, MSA	h-Caldesmon, desmin, α-SMA, MSA	Desmin, MSA	Myogenin (myogenic factor 4) and MyoD1 (myogenic differentiation 1)	Myogenin and MyoD1	Myogenin and MyoD1
Management	Surgical excision	Surgical excision	Surgical excision	Wide surgical excision with >3 cm margins	Surgical excision	Surgical excision	Multidisciplinary approach	Surgical excision	Surgical excision
Associated syndromes	HLRCC (hereditary leiomyomatosis and renal cell cancer)				Michelin tire baby syndrome	Nevoid basal cell carcinoma syndrome			
Other	Early-onset uterine leiomyomas, 15% lifetime risk for renal cell cancer (!) HLRCC (early-onset uterine leiomyomas, 10%-16% lifetime risk for renal cell cancer)		Symptoms may be paroxysmal with worsening by light touch, temperature, or hormonal change		Dermal leiomyomas ("intradermal smooth muscle neoplasms") have an excellent prognosis	Overlapping features with Becker melanosis	Cardiac rhabdomyomas are associated with tuberous sclerosis		Multiple lesions occur in the setting of associated congenital abnormalities

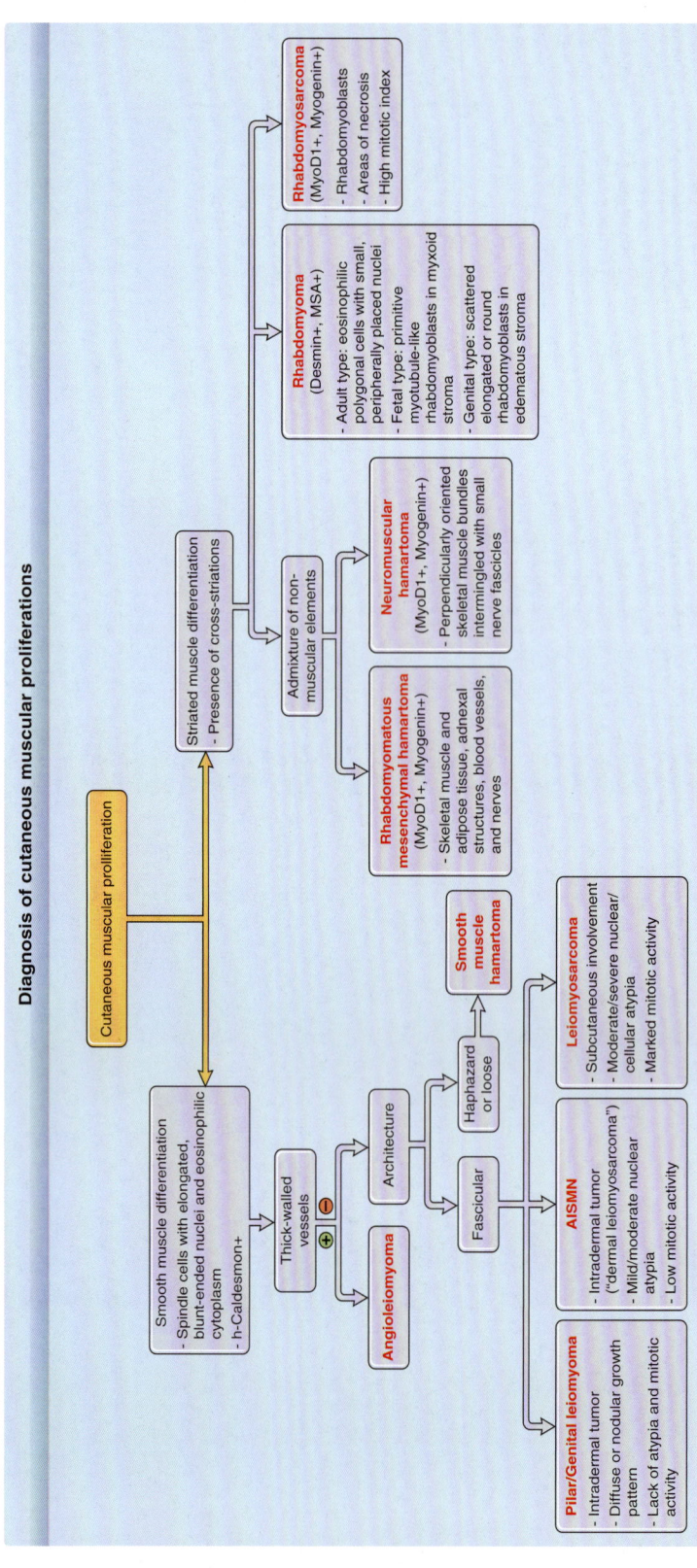

Figure 121-1 Diagnosis of cutaneous muscular proliferations. AISMN, atypical intradermal smooth muscle neoplasm; MSA, muscle-specific actin; MyoD1, myogenic differentiation 1.

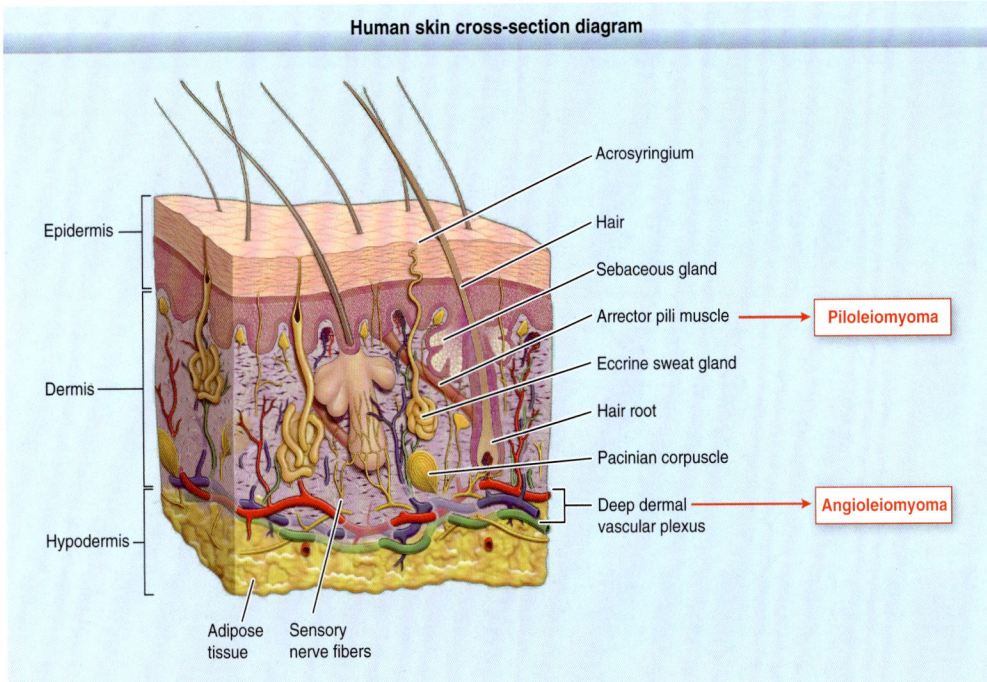

Figure 121-2 Piloleiomyomas, deriving from the arrector pili muscles, and angioleiomyomas, deriving from smooth muscle tissue of vessel walls.

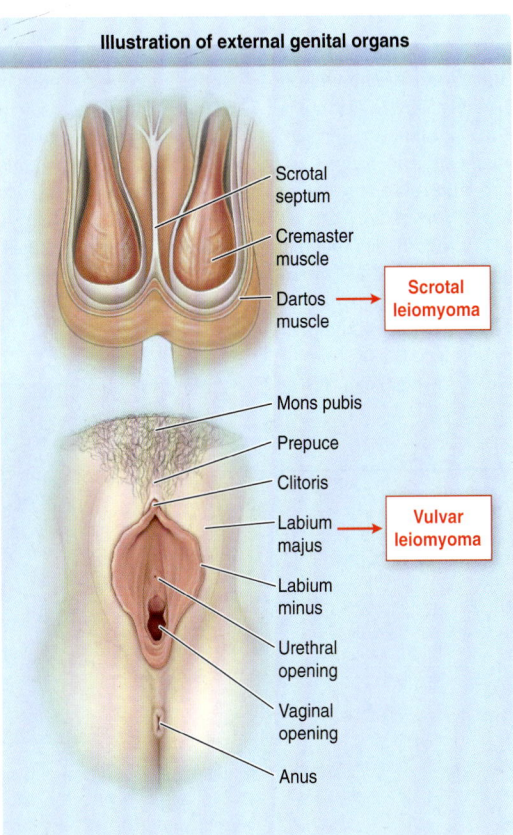

Figure 121-3 Leiomyomas of genital sites, deriving from specialized smooth muscle of genital skin (dartoic, vulvar). **Top**, Scrotal leiomyomas. **Bottom**, Vulvar leiomyomas.

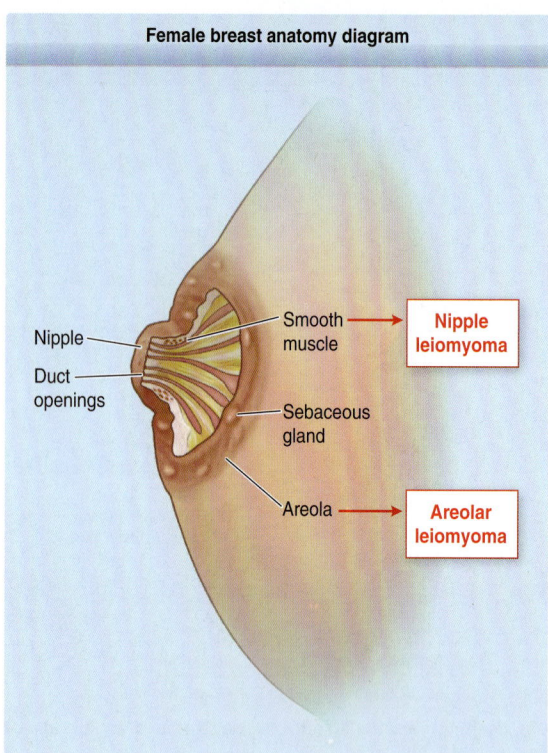

Figure 121-4 Leiomyomas of the nipple and the areola, deriving from specialized smooth muscle of skin (mammillary, areolar).

cutaneous tumors with cellular atypia but without mitotic activity can be comfortably labeled "symplastic leiomyomas." α-Smooth muscle actin (Fig. 121-7B), desmin (Fig. 121-7C), muscle-specific actin, and h-caldesmon are strongly and diffusely expressed in virtually all piloleiomyomas. *FH* mutation carriers have FH-deficient cutaneous and uterine leiomyomas defined as negative FH staining by immunohistochemistry (Fig. 121-7D), but loss of FH protein expression also may be observed in sporadic cases.[25,26] The presence of multiple FH-deficient cutaneous piloleiomyomas in adolescents should raise the suspicion for an underlying Reed syndrome and prompt for a detailed family history assessment. Genital leiomyomas display a greater range of histologic appearance (eg, spindle-cell or epithelioid cell type, myxoid variants), tend to be more cellular, and often have ill-defined or focally infiltrative margins.[27] Angioleiomyomas are well-demarcated nodules of smooth muscle tissue punctuated with thick-walled vessels with partially open lumina (Fig. 121-8A). The inner layers of smooth

TABLE 121-2
Diagnostic Criteria for Hereditary Leiomyomatosis and Renal Cell Carcinoma

Major Criteria (High Likelihood of HLRCC)
- Multiple cutaneous leiomyomata with at least 1 biopsy proven/ histologically confirmed

Minor Criteria (Suspicious for HLRCC)
- Solitary cutaneous leiomyoma and family history of HLRCC
- Early-onset renal tumors of Type 2 papillary histology
- Multiple early-onset (<40 years of age) symptomatic uterine fibroids

Definitive Diagnosis
- Positive germline *FH*-mutation test

HLRCC, hereditary leiomyomatosis and renal cell cancer.

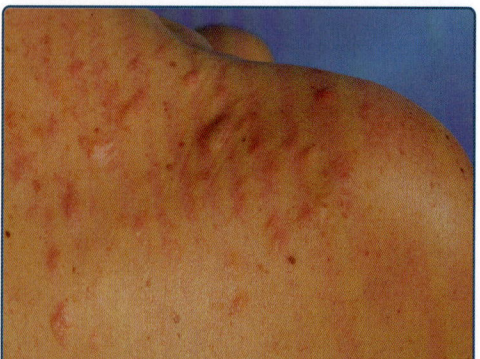

Figure 121-5 Clinical photograph showing multiple leiomyomas involving the shoulder area. (Image from the collection of Sonja Radakovic, MD, and Teresa Valero, MD, Department of Dermatology, Medical University of Vienna, Austria. Used with permission.)

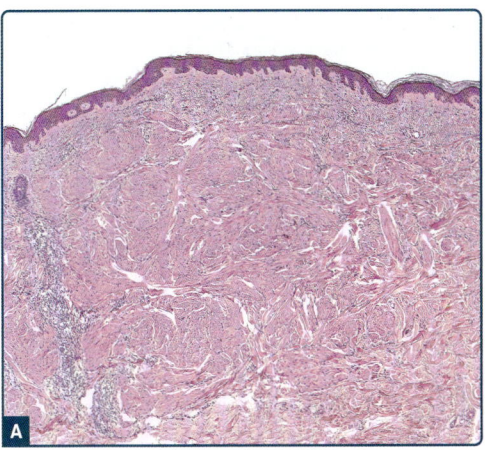

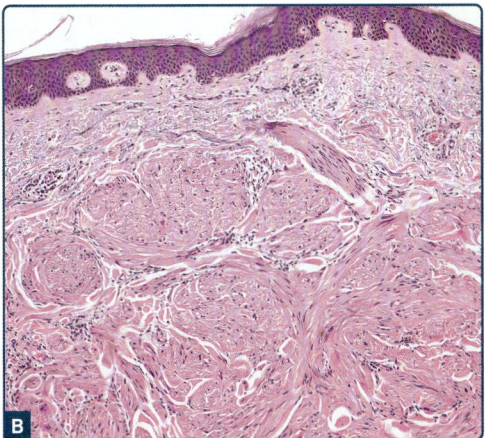

Figure 121-6 A, Photomicrograph of a pilar leiomyoma showing an ill-defined dermal-based tumor composed of interweaving fascicles of spindle cells (hematoxylin-and-eosin [H&E], ×20 magnification). **B,** Well-differentiated elongated spindle cells with blunt-ended, cigar-shaped nuclei and abundant fibrillary eosinophilic cytoplasm (H&E, ×100 magnification).

muscle of the vessel are arranged circumferentially, and the outer layers blend with the less-well-ordered peripheral smooth fibers (Fig. 121-8B).

DIFFERENTIAL DIAGNOSIS

The clinical differential diagnosis of cutaneous leiomyomas comprises a broad spectrum of solitary, agminated, and widespread dermal-centered papulonodular lesions, including dermatofibromas (fibrous histiocytomas), dermal melanocytic nevi, neurofibromas, schwannomas, (angio)lipomas, adnexal tumors, and metastases. Cellular and atypical dermatofibroma variants are in the main histopathologic differential diagnosis with the constituent cells being slenderer and less-well-ordered, and lacking myofibrils. The differential diagnosis with leiomyosarcoma and smooth muscle hamartoma is discussed in sections "Etiology and Pathogenesis (for leiomyosarcoma)" and "Etiology and Pathogenesis (for smooth muscle hamartoma)".

CLINICAL COURSE AND PROGNOSIS

At present, cutaneous leiomyomas are generally considered not to undergo malignant transformation. Recurrence after complete excision is unusual. The genetic predisposition of females with hereditary leiomyomatosis and renal cell cancer to early-onset uterine leiomyomas and of affected individuals of both sexes to early-onset renal cell cancer requires adequate screening. The lifetime renal cancer risk for *FH* mutation carriers is estimated to be 15%.[28]

MANAGEMENT

Simple excision is curative and the appropriate treatment for those tumors that are symptomatic or of cosmetic concern and amenable to surgical treatment. CO_2 laser ablation, cryotherapy, and electrosurgery are alternative treatment modalities that have been used for cutaneous leiomyomatosis, where surgical excision is not feasible.[29] Symptomatic treatment options include nitroglycerin, nifedipine, phenoxybenzamine, gabapentin, intralesional botulinum toxin, and topical analgesics.[30-34]

LEIOMYOSARCOMA

AT-A-GLANCE

- Malignant smooth muscle tumor comprising 2 subtypes with respect to location and prognosis: *dermal* leiomyosarcomas arising from the arrector pili or genital smooth muscle and *subcutaneous* leiomyosarcomas (synonym: superficial leiomyosarcomas) probably arising from vascular smooth muscle.

- Most commonly presents in males between the fifth and seventh decades as solitary tumors on the scalp or hair-bearing areas of the lower extremities.

- Leiomyosarcomas confined to the dermis are considered to have no metastatic potential and are referred to as *atypical intradermal smooth muscle neoplasms*.

- Tumors involving the subcutaneous adipose tissue warrant the designation leiomyosarcoma and metastasize in approximately 30% to 40% of cases. Wide local excision is required.

EPIDEMIOLOGY

Leiomyosarcomas account for 5% to 10% of soft-tissue sarcomas. They are principally tumors of adults,

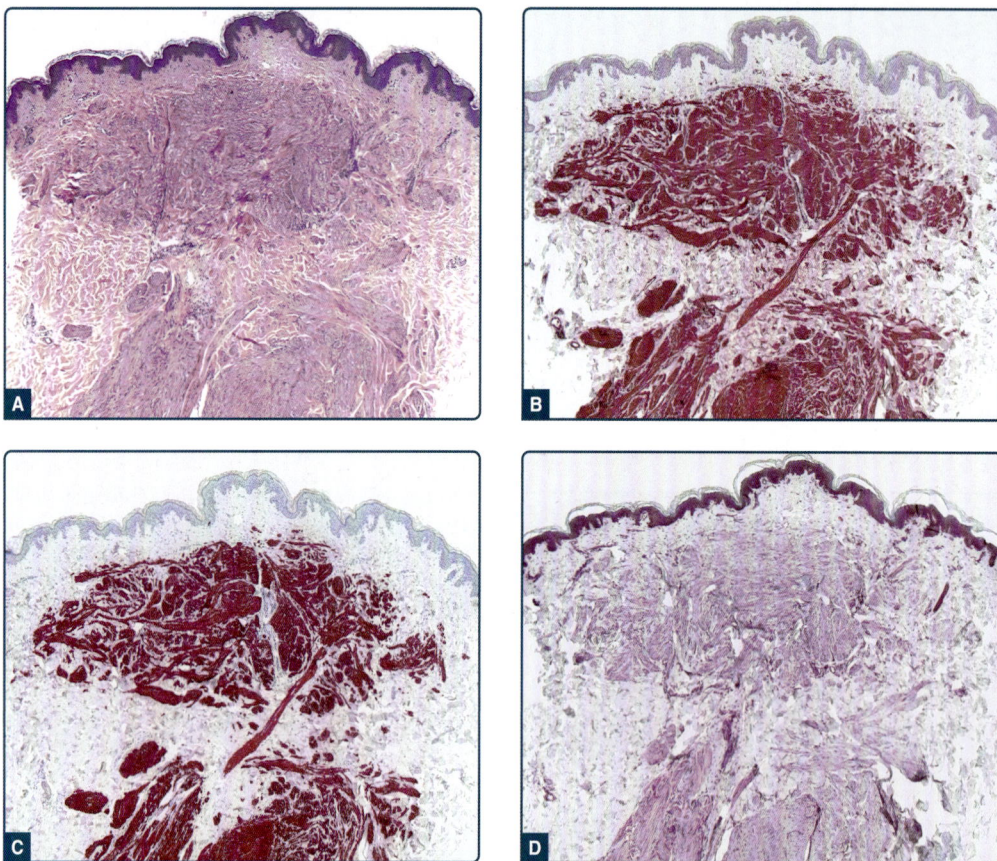

Figure 121-7 **A**, Photomicrograph of a pilar leiomyoma from a *FH*-mutation carrier (hematoxylin-and-eosin [H&E], ×40 magnification). Diffuse and strong expression of α-smooth muscle actin (**B**; anti–α-smooth muscle actin, ×40 magnification) and desmin (**C**; anti-desmin, ×40 magnification) accompanied by an almost complete loss of FH expression (**D**; anti-FH, ×40 magnification).

but occur in all age groups, and no gender predilection is known. Atypical intradermal smooth muscle neoplasms (see section "Etiology and Pathogenesis") affect middle-aged to elderly adults, with a male-to-female ratio of nearly 5:1.[35,36]

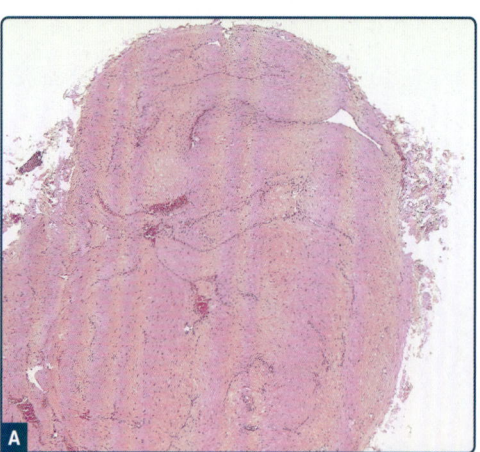
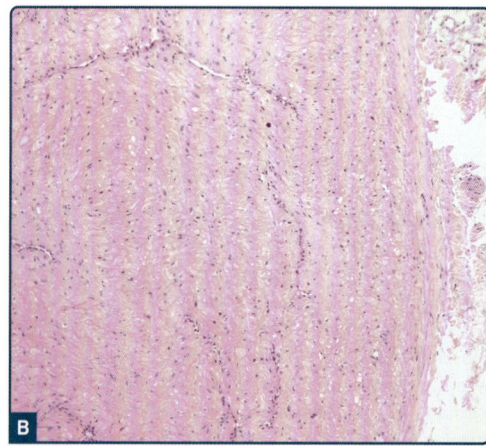

Figure 121-8 Histologic appearance of an angioleiomyoma. **A,** Sharply circumscribed nodular smooth muscle cell proliferation within which multiple vascular channels are present (hematoxylin-and-eosin [H&E], ×20 magnification). **B,** Densely packed fascicles of bland smooth muscle cells surrounding vascular channels (H&E, ×100 magnification).

ETIOLOGY AND PATHOGENESIS

It is useful to divide superficial leiomyosarcomas into 2 site-related subgroups because of their significant clinical and biologic differences: (a) dermal leiomyosarcomas deriving from arrector pili muscles or smooth muscle at genital sites, and (b) subcutaneous leiomyosarcomas probably deriving from vascular smooth muscle. Although the designation *cutaneous leiomyosarcoma* in the past referred to neoplasms originating in the dermis or subcutis, this term should be restricted to tumors that arise from the dermis and only secondarily involve the subcutis. When limited to the dermis, the tumors may recur locally but, to the best of our knowledge, have no metastatic potential; as a result, the "leiomyosarcoma" designation has been recently challenged. Consequently, it has been proposed that dermal tumors with smooth muscle differentiation displaying atypia and mitotic activity (1 to 2 mitosis/10 high-power field [HPF]) be termed *atypical intradermal smooth muscle neoplasms (AISMN)*, although this designation has not been universally accepted.[35] At present, these tumors are continued to be diagnosed as leiomyosarcoma. Tumors arising from the dermis and displaying invasion into the subcutaneous tissue warrant the designation *cutaneous leiomyosarcoma* and rarely metastasize. The vast majority of leiomyosarcomas that are centered in the subcutis arise from vessels and thus resemble leiomyosarcomas of soft tissue with respect to biologic and clinical behavior, and ultimate prognosis. Those tumors are termed *subcutaneous leiomyosarcomas* (synonym: superficial leiomyosarcomas) and carry a substantial risk of metastasis. Leiomyosarcomas rarely occur in radiation fields or following trauma but may develop as a second malignancy in the setting of hereditary retinoblastoma.[37,38] Alterations of the retinoblastoma 1 locus can be identified in a minority of sporadic leiomyosarcomas as well.[39] Even though well-differentiated areas mimicking leiomyoma are frequently present in a leiomyosarcoma, this is not regarded as evidence of malignant transformation. Moreover, the predilection of leiomyosarcomas to the subcutis, in contrast to the predominantly intradermal location of leiomyomas, is indicative of the contrary. Cutaneous leiomyosarcomas arise de novo, whereas cutaneous leiomyomas, to the best of our knowledge, are not thought to undergo malignant transformation.

CLINICAL FINDINGS

Cutaneous leiomyosarcomas typically present as solitary lesions and have a predilection for hair-bearing areas of lower extremities, and to a lesser extent, to the scalp and trunk, but can occur ubiquitously. There is a male predominance, and most tumors appear between the fifth and seventh decades of life.[40] The tumors usually present as deep-seated, firm nodules with occasional ulceration and hyperplasia of the epidermis. Dermal tumors are typically fixed to the epidermis and rarely exceed 3 cm in diameter, whereas subcutaneous lesions may rapidly develop into larger, well-circumscribed tumor nodules. Hyperpigmentation and erythema of the involved skin is common (Fig. 121-9). Leiomyosarcomas arising from uterine and retroperitoneal uterine primary tumors rarely present as "secondary leiomyosarcomas" with multiple dermal or subcutaneous nodules in the skin.

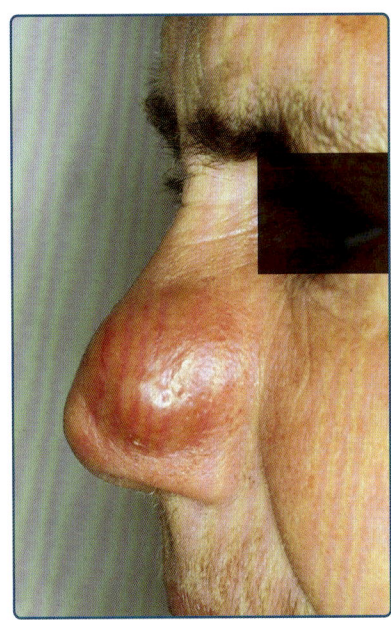

Figure 121-9 Cutaneous leiomyosarcoma on the nose. A firm nodule with erythema and hyperpigmentation of the involved skin is seen. (Image from the collection of Arno Rütten, MD, Dermatopathology Friedrichshafen. Used with permission.)

HISTOPATHOLOGY

Leiomyosarcomas are composed of intersecting fascicles of atypical spindle cells (Fig. 121-10). Dermal-based tumors appear ill-defined, with tumor fascicles ramifying through the surrounding collagen and pilar arrector muscle. Tumors with involvement of the subcutis appear more circumscribed because of the pseudocapsule that is generated by compression of the adjacent collagenous tissue. Most tumors are well-differentiated (low-grade) or moderately differentiated (intermediate grade) tumors and the tumor cells demonstrate the characteristic cytomorphology indicative of smooth muscle differentiation; that is, large, elongated fusiform cells with abundant brightly eosinophilic cytoplasm, variably blunt-ended nuclei, and well-defined cell borders. Intratumoral hemorrhage, necrosis, and hyalinization are rarely observed. Tumor giant cells may be detected. Poorly differentiated (high-grade) tumors exhibit marked nuclear pleomorphism and a high mitotic rate (>10 mitosis/10 HPF). Identification of cells with pathognomonic nuclear features is essential for correct diagnosis. Myxoid, epithelioid cell, granular cell, and sclerosing/desmoplastic variants

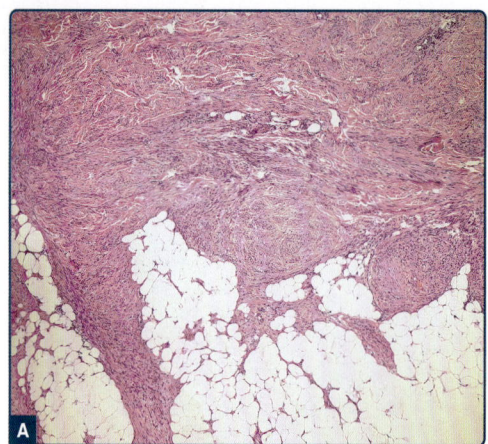

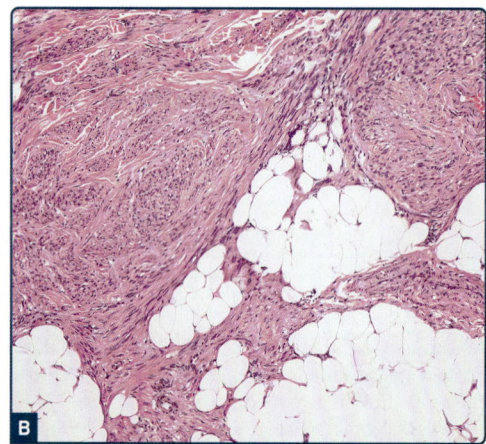

Figure 121-10 Histologic examination of a cutaneous leiomyosarcoma. **A,** Ill-defined atypical dermal spindle-cell tumor displaying a diffusely infiltrative growth pattern (hematoxylin-and-eosin [H&E], ×20 magnification). **B,** Fascicles of atypical spindle cells with hyperchromatic, pleomorphic nuclei infiltrate the surrounding collagen and the subcutaneous fatty tissue (H&E, ×100 magnification).

have been reported.[41] Tumors that are predominantly composed of pleomorphic cells are known as pleomorphic leiomyosarcoma. AISMN (see "Etiology and Pathogenesis" above) are limited to the dermis and typically display a mixed nodular and infiltrative growth pattern (Fig. 121-11A). Only minimal involvement of the superficial subcutaneous fat with a pushing border is allowed for the designation AISMN. The constituent cells display a typical smooth muscle cell morphology and, in contrast to pilar leiomyoma, mild to moderate atypia and mitotic activity (1 to 2 mitoses/10 HPF; Fig. 121-11B). Recurrent tumors often present with a nodular growth pattern, marked nuclear atypia, and a higher mitotic rate. AISMN are usually positive for α-SMA, muscle-specific actin, desmin, and h-caldesmon. Approximately 50% of cases show focal cytokeratin expression. Detection of smooth muscle antigens is particularly important for the diagnosis of poorly differentiated (high-grade) leiomyosarcomas. α-SMA and muscle-specific actin are present in most leiomyosarcomas. h-Caldesmon is a specific, but less-sensitive (approximately 40%) smooth muscle antigen.[42] Desmin expression is variable, and if present, only focally, or even absent in high-grade tumors. Expression of epithelial membrane antigen (EMA) and cytokeratin is seen in 30% to 40% of leiomyosarcomas.[43]

DIFFERENTIAL DIAGNOSIS

The clinical differential diagnosis comprises all lesions appearing as solitary, growing, dermal or subcutaneous nodule: dermatofibroma, dermatofibrosarcoma, neurofibroma, squamous cell carcinoma (SCC), atypical fibroxanthoma, pleomorphic dermal sarcoma, melanoma, adnexal tumors, and cysts. Definitive diagnosis requires histopathologic confirmation. On histology, the differential diagnosis for leiomyosarcoma includes both nonpleomorphic spindle-cell tumors, such as cellular dermatofibroma, cellular schwannoma, malignant peripheral nerve sheath

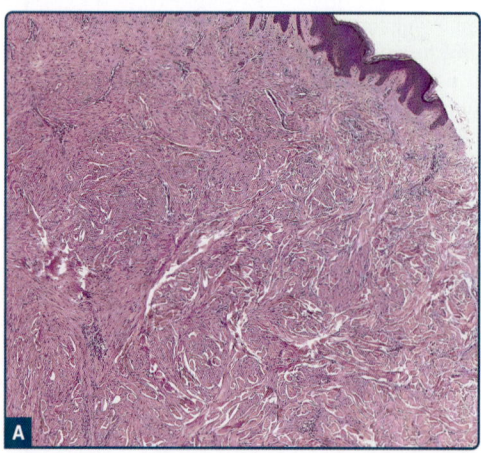

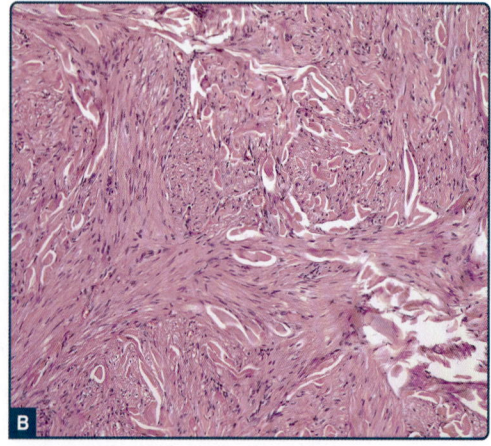

Figure 121-11 Photomicrograph of an atypical intradermal smooth muscle neoplasm. **A,** The tumor is confined to the dermis and fascicles of tumor cells ramify through dermal collagen bundles (hematoxylin-and-eosin [H&E], ×20 magnification). **B,** The tumor cells show mild nuclear atypia and mitotic activity (H&E, ×100 magnification).

tumor (MPNST), myopericytoma, myofibroma, as well as various pleomorphic spindle-cell tumors. In addition, well-differentiated leiomyosarcoma must be delineated from cutaneous leiomyoma. The differential diagnosis versus non–smooth muscle tumors requires immunophenotyping. It must be noted, however, that the distribution and intensity of muscle markers in dedifferentiated tumor areas are strikingly diminished compared to well-differentiated and moderately differentiated areas. Moreover, focal expression of actin or desmin is not necessarily indicative of myoid differentiation, because myofibroblasts also display these phenotypes. Tumors arising from vascular smooth muscle, such as subcutaneous leiomyosarcoma, often show a desmin-negative/h-caldesmon–positive phenotype.[44] In contrast to AISMN, cellular dermatofibroma lacks the well-defined tumor bundles, blunt-ended nuclei, nuclear atypia, and bright eosinophilic appearance. α-SMA and desmin (myofibroblasts) can be focally positive, but h-caldesmon is consistently negative. Atypical dermatofibroma is composed of pleomorphic, plump and spindled fibrohistiocytic cells displaying marked nuclear atypia including bizarre multinucleated giant cells. α-SMA, desmin, and CD34 are sometimes focally positive. It can be distinguished from AISMN by its mixed fascicular and storiform architecture, the heterogeneous tumor cells, and absence of h-caldesmon expression. Cellular schwannoma is an encapsulated neoplasm composed of spindle cells that form a compact fascicular growth pattern and show diffuse expression of S-100 protein. MPNST shows loss of SOX10, neurofibromin, and p16 expression. Myopericytoma/myofibroma typically display a whorled perivascular arrangement of tumor cells with less-abundant eosinophilic cytoplasm and areas with dilated blood vessels. Immunohistochemical staining for α-SMA and h-caldesmon is positive in almost all cases, but desmin expression is restricted to approximately 10% of cases. Leiomyosarcomas that arise on the head and neck must be distinguished from pleomorphic spindle-cell neoplasms arising in sun-damaged skin such as spindle-cell (sarcomatoid) SCC, melanoma, spindle-cell angiosarcoma, atypical fibroxanthoma, and pleomorphic dermal sarcoma. Similar to spindle-cell SCC cell carcinoma, AISMN and leiomyosarcomas are often focally positive for keratin, but desmin and h-caldesmon are not expressed in SCC. The presence of an overlying atypical lentiginous melanocytic hyperplasia and/or a junctional tumor component as well as expression of S-100 protein, HMB-45, MART-1, MITF, SOX10, and NGFR/p75(NTR) should be excluded to distinguish high-grade leiomyosarcoma occurring in severely sun-damaged skin from malignant melanoma. Spindle-cell angiosarcoma can be delineated by search for classical morphologic features (multilayering, papillary structures, irregular anastomosing blood vessels) and immunophenotyping for ERG, a marker expressed in benign and malignant vascular endothelial cells. Spindle-cell variants of atypical fibroxanthoma and pleomorphic dermal sarcoma may pose a significant diagnostic challenge and both are diagnoses of exclusion. The tumors arise almost exclusively in actinically damaged skin of the head and neck area of older adults. Focal areas with scattered epithelioid and histiocytic tumor cells, multinucleated giant cells, and brisk mitotic activity are usually present. Weak positivity for α-SMA may be present and atypical fibroxanthoma is frequently positive for CD10, while tumor cells stain negative for S-100 protein, melanocytic differentiation antigens, cytokeratins, desmin, h-caldesmon, and ERG. The presence of epithelial-like areas or an in situ component facilitates the diagnosis of spindle-cell SCC (sarcomatoid SCC), but both components may be completely absent. By immunohistochemistry, spindled tumor cells in sarcomatoid SCC often at least focally express broad-spectrum keratins (eg, clone MNF116 and/or AE1/AE3), as well as nuclear p63.

CLINICAL COURSE AND PROGNOSIS

The prognosis of cutaneous leiomyosarcomas is almost always favorable, with the majority of tumors cured with a timely wide surgical excision. This is, in part, contributable to the fact that most tumors are small (<2 cm) and highly-differentiated (low-grade). AISMN have an a particularly excellent prognosis but incompletely excised tumors bear a recurrence rate of 20% to 30% with margin status representing the only predictor of local recurrence.[35] Although quantification of risk of metastatic spread in cutaneous leiomyosarcoma is difficult, tumor size, degree of subcutaneous involvement, high histologic grade, and previous local reoccurrence are considered as risk factors. In general, leiomyosarcomas confined to the dermis do not metastasize, whereas those with subcutaneous involvement metastasize in approximately 30% to 40% of cases.[45-47] Metastatic dissemination occurs commonly hematogenously to the lung, and regional lymph may be occasionally involved.

MANAGEMENT

As the overwhelming majority of cutaneous leiomyosarcomas are potentially curable, initial eradication of the tumors by wide surgical excision with at least 3-cm margins and careful histologic examination of surgical margins is the treatment of choice. Given its substantial risk for local recurrence, complete excision with negative margins is also the appropriate therapy for AISMN. Recurrent leiomyosarcomas confer an increased risk of eventual metastasis because of their distinct propensity for a larger tumor size at diagnosis and infiltration of deeper structures. Mohs micrographic surgery has been used as an alternative treatment modality with a reported recurrence rate of 14%.[48]

SMOOTH MUSCLE HAMARTOMA

AT-A-GLANCE

- Hyperplasia of dermal smooth muscles fibers giving rise to a rare hamartoma.
- Solitary flesh-colored patch or plaque typically occurring in the lumbar region during childhood or early adolescence.
- Follicular prominence, hypertrichosis, and variable pigmentation are frequent.
- Clinical and histopathologic association with the nevus of Becker.

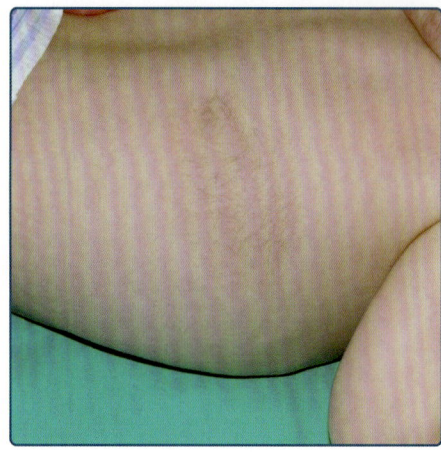

Figure 121-12 Congenital smooth muscle hamartoma on the lower back of an infant. The tumor presents as a skin-colored patch with hypertrichosis. (Image from the collection of Antonio Torrelo, MD, Department of Pediatric Dermatology, Hospital del Niño Jesús, Madrid, Spain. Used with permission.)

EPIDEMIOLOGY

Smooth muscle hamartoma was initially described by Stokes in 1923.[49] The lesions are usually present from birth, but exceptional cases of an acquired variant have been reported. The estimated prevalence is approximately 1 in 2600 live births.[50]

ETIOLOGY AND PATHOGENESIS

Smooth muscle hamartoma of the skin is a benign hamartomatous proliferation consisting of well-defined smooth muscle located in the dermis. The etiology is unknown. Familial occurrence has been reported. Some of the acquired cases appear to represent acquired smooth muscle secondary to chronic lymphedema.

CLINICAL FINDINGS

Smooth muscle hamartoma typically presents as skin-colored or lightly pigmented patch or plaque measuring up to 10 cm in diameter with a predilection for the lumbar region of the trunk, the buttocks, and the proximal extremities (Fig. 121-12). The spectrum of clinical presentations comprises solitary lesions, agminated lesions, and a generalized variant with excess symmetrical skin folds (known as *Michelin tire baby syndrome*), as well as occasional hypertrichosis and follicular dimpling.[51,52] All forms can display variable hyperpigmentation and hypertrichosis. Small papules may be detectable within the lesions and sensitive to transient piloerection following rubbing (pseudo-Darier sign). Smooth muscle bundles may also occur in the nevus of Becker, a pigmentary hamartoma with its onset in adolescence, characterized by invariable hyperpigmentation and hypertrichosis. Given their overlapping histologic and clinical features, smooth muscle hamartoma and Becker melanosis can be regarded as varying morphologic expressions of the same hamartomatous process involving the pilar unit and the arrector pili muscles.[53]

HISTOPATHOLOGY

There are well-defined and thickened smooth muscle fibers haphazardly oriented in reticular dermis (Fig. 121-13). Some surround or are attached to hair follicles. Commonly, there are thin retractions spaces separating the muscle bundles from the adjacent collagen. The overlying epidermis may show mild hyperpigmentation of the basal layer, acanthosis and papillomatosis. The constituent cells express α-SMA and desmin. The surrounding stroma may contain a high number of cells positive for CD34.

DIFFERENTIAL DIAGNOSIS

Differential diagnosis of cutaneous smooth muscle hamartoma includes leiomyoma, Becker nevus, congenital melanocytic nevus, neurofibroma, connective tissue nevus, and solitary mastocytoma. Leiomyomas usually appear as papulonodules rather than as plaques. Histologic distinction of cutaneous leiomyomas from smooth muscle hamartomas of the skin is not always clearcut and may substantially relate more to differences in clinical presentation than histologic features. The smooth muscle fibers in leiomyomas are arranged in interweaving fascicles that blend with the adjacent dermal collagen fibers whereas smooth muscle hamartomas are composed of discrete smooth muscle fibers set in dermal collagen.

CLINICAL COURSE AND PROGNOSIS

To the best of our knowledge, smooth muscle hamartomas do not undergo malignant transformation. A

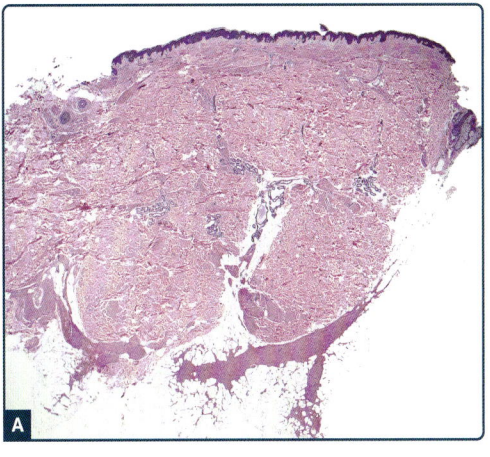 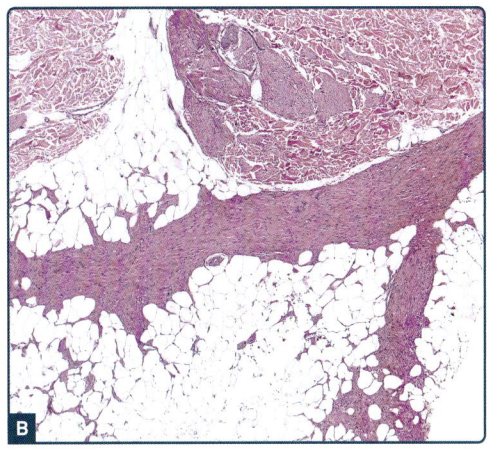
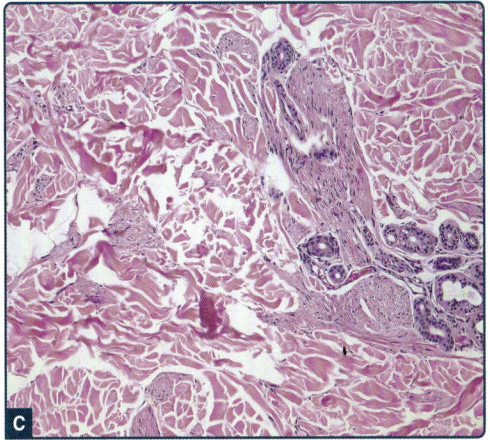 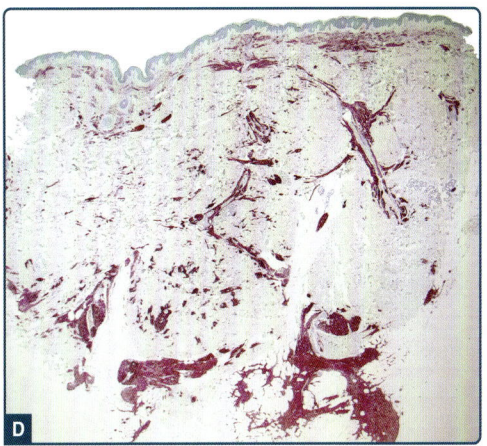

Figure 121-13 Photomicrograph of a congenital smooth muscle hamartoma. Proliferation of scattered, well-demarcated, haphazardly arranged bundles of smooth muscle throughout the dermis (**A**; hematoxylin-and-eosin [H&E], ×4 magnification) and the superficial subcutaneous fatty tissue (**B**; H&E, ×10 magnification). **C,** Short fascicles of smooth muscle cells with characteristic elongated, spindle-shaped to blunt-ended nuclei (H&E, ×100 magnification). **D,** The constituent cells are immunoreactive for desmin (anti-desmin, ×4 magnification).

melanocytic nevus has been reported in association with a smooth muscle hamartoma. A naevus flammeus also was present in 1 case. Individuals presenting with the generalized form may have variety of congenital anomalies that have been reported in babies with multiple symmetric circumferential rings of folded skin ("Michelin tire baby syndrome").[54]

MANAGEMENT

Treatment may be indicated for cosmetic purposes. Lesions may be amenable for surgical excision.

TUMORS OF STRIATED MUSCLE

Tumors of striated muscle (see Table 121-1) segregate into genuine neoplasms with striated muscle differentiation (rhabdomyoma and rhabdomyosarcoma) and nonneoplastic hamartomas (rhabdomyomatous mesenchymal hamartoma and neuromuscular hamartoma). Figure 121-1 provides an overview of the diagnosis of cutaneous tumors with striated muscle differentiation.

RHABDOMYOMA

AT-A-GLANCE

- Benign neoplasm of striated muscle presenting as adult, fetal, or genital type.
- Most commonly located on the head and neck of males.
- Fetal rhabdomyoma may be associated with nevoid basal cell carcinoma syndrome.
- Surgical removal is the treatment of choice.

EPIDEMIOLOGY

Rhabdomyomas are much less common than rhabdomyosarcomas and account for no more than 2% all of striated muscle neoplasms.[55] There are 2 main categories of rhabdomyomas: cardiac and extracardiac. For practical reasons extracardiac rhabdomyomas are further subcategorized into 3 clinical and morphologic subtypes: adult-type, fetal-type, and genital-type rhabdomyomas. Fetal-type and adult-type rhabdomyomas affect mostly men (male-to-female ratio is 3:1). In 20% to 30% cases of adult-type rhabdomyomas, multiple lesions develop in the same patient.

ETIOLOGY AND PATHOGENESIS

Rhabdomyomas are benign neoplasms of striated muscle differentiation. Cardiac tumors are associated with tuberous sclerosis. The prevalence rates of cardiac rhabdomyomas in patients with tuberous sclerosis range from 47% to 67%, as assessed by repeated echocardiography, whereas extracardiac rhabdomyomas do not occur in the setting of tuberous sclerosis.[56,57] There are repeated reports in the literature documenting an association of fetal rhabdomyoma with the nevoid basal cell carcinoma syndrome.[58] Mutations in the *PTCH1* tumor-suppressor gene have been identified in this syndrome.

CLINICAL FINDINGS

Among the group of extracardiac rhabdomyomas, 3 clinically and morphologically different subtypes can be defined: (a) the *adult type*, a slowly enlarging mass that is almost always arising in the head and neck area of middle-aged and elderly adults (mean age: 60 years) that causes neither tenderness nor pain; (b) the *fetal type*, an exceptionally rare tumor that also principally occurs in the head and neck region in both children and adults; and (c) the *genital type*, a small polypoid lesion detected nearly always in the vagina or vulva of middle-aged women. The designation as *adult* or *fetal* refers to the tumor's resemblance to adult or fetal skeletal muscle, not to the age of the patient.

HISTOPATHOLOGY

Microscopically, adult rhabdomyoma is composed of variously sized, deeply eosinophilic polygonal cells with small, peripherally placed nuclei and occasional intracellular vacuoles (Fig. 121-14). The histologic spectrum of fetal rhabdomyoma recapitulates fetal skeletal muscle: "Classic" or "myxoid" fetal rhabdomyoma is chiefly composed of primitive oval or spindle-shaped cells and a richly myxoid stroma. "Intermediate" or "cellular" fetal rhabdomyoma consists of intersecting bundles of differentiated eosinophilic myofibrils containing cross-striations, fewer or absent spindle-shaped mesenchymal cells, and sparse or no myxoid stroma. Irrespective of cellularity, the nuclei are bland and lack atypia, pleomorphism, and anaplasia; in addition, most cases lack mitosis.

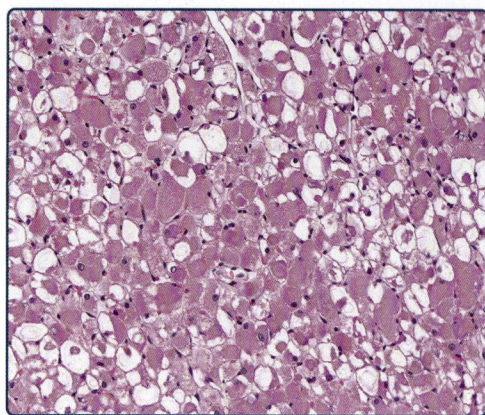

Figure 121-14 Histologic appearance of an adult rhabdomyoma. There are round and polygonal cells with small, peripherally placed nuclei and deeply eosinophilic, finely granular cytoplasm arranged in solid sheets (hematoxylin-and-eosin [H&E] ×100 magnification).

DIFFERENTIAL DIAGNOSIS

Differential diagnosis of rhabdomyomas includes granular cell tumor, hibernoma, paraganglioma, and embryonal rhabdomyosarcoma.

CLINICAL COURSE AND PROGNOSIS

Cardiac rhabdomyomas often regress spontaneously by age, but this has not been observed for extracardiac rhabdomyomas. Adult-type rhabdomyoma carries an estimated 42% risk of local recurrence following incomplete excision, while only rare reports of local recurrences of fetal rhabdomyomas exist.[59,60] As of this writing, there is no valid evidence for the concept that fetal rhabdomyoma represents an early stage in the development of adult rhabdomyoma.

MANAGEMENT

Extracardiac rhabdomyomas are readily curable by surgical excision.

RHABDOMYOSARCOMA

AT-A-GLANCE

- Malignant soft-tissue neoplasm with primitive skeletal muscle differentiation.
- Most common soft-tissue sarcoma in children and adolescents.
- Presents as subcutaneous or ulcerated mass on the head and neck or the extremities; rare cause of "blueberry muffin baby."

- Highly variable prognosis, with 5-year survival rates ranging from 30% to 95%.
- Multidisciplinary therapeutic approach of surgery and chemotherapy ± radiotherapy is needed.

EPIDEMIOLOGY

Rhabdomyosarcoma (RMS) is the most frequent soft-tissue sarcoma in children and adolescents and one of the most common soft-tissue sarcomas in young adults. The estimated annual incidence in children is approximately 4.3 cases per million children per year, accounting for approximately 5% of all pediatric cancers and approximately 50% of soft-tissue sarcomas in children younger than age 15 years.[61] The tumor rarely occurs in individuals older than 45 years of age and has been estimated to account for 3% of all sarcomas in adults.[62] There is a slight male predominance.

ETIOLOGY AND PATHOGENESIS

RMS is a primitive malignant soft-tissue sarcoma that shows some differentiation toward skeletal muscle. Because the tumor often arises in at sites in which skeletal muscle tissue is normally absent or scant, it is not suggested to arise from skeletal muscle cells. Embryonal RMS appears to arise from the undifferentiated mesoderm. Genetic factors are implicated by the rare occurrence in siblings, the association of the tumor with other neoplasms, and the infrequent presentation at birth. In one study, approximately 30% of children with RMS had a congenital anomaly.[63] Based on histologic criteria, RMS can be generally divided into 3 broad subsets: *embryonal* rhabdomyosarcoma (ERMS), *alveolar* rhabdomyosarcoma (ARMS), and *anaplastic* (*undifferentiated*) RMS (also known as *pleomorphic* RMS). Within the ERMS subtype, there are 2 histopathologic variants with superior outcome, botryoid and spindle cell. Sclerosing RMS and epithelioid RMS represent other proposed variants. ERMS is the most common (60%) followed by ARMS (20%). ERMS is associated with an 11p15.5 loss of heterozygosity.[64] Approximately 60% of tumors diagnosed histologically as ARMS have a $t^{2;13}$(q35;q14) translocation and approximately 20% carry a $t^{1;13}$(p36;q14) translocation, resulting in a *PAX3-FOXO1A* and a *PAX7-FOXO1A* fusion, respectively.[65,66]

CLINICAL FINDINGS

RMS can occur at various anatomic sites throughout the body. The most common primary tumor sites include the head and neck region, followed by the genitourinary tract, the retroperitoneum, and the extremities. primaries. Cutaneous manifestation is rare and usually recognizable as a rapidly growing mass of several months' duration that results from expansion of an underlying soft-tissue lesion and may eventually become ulcerated (Fig. 121-15). RMS is often palpable and limits motion. The tumor also may be encountered in areas where the expanding neoplasm reaches the body surface (eg, eyelid, anal region). Primary cutaneous origin is very rare. Neonatal ARMS presenting with cutaneous and subcutaneous metastases is a very rare cause of "blueberry muffin baby."

HISTOPATHOLOGY

The presence of rhabdomyoblasts is essential for the diagnosis of RMS. Rhabdomyoblasts are large round, spindle-shaped, or elongated ("strap"-shaped) cells with deeply eosinophilic granular cytoplasm rich in thick and thin filaments that may show cross-striations, reflecting sarcomere formation and advancement of differentiation. The cells in RMS may exhibit a marked primitive ovoid or primitive spindle-shaped, small, round, pleomorphic, clear, or even elongated-fusiform cytomorphology with cigar-shaped nuclei and prominent nucleoli resembling smooth muscle cells. Multinucleated giant cells and areas of necrosis may be present. In rare cases of ARMS, viable cells are virtually absent. Mitotic index is high. ERMS typically consists of small, round or spindle-shaped cells with alternating cellular and myxoid zones. ARMS displays a characteristic alveolar growth pattern with central loss of cellular cohesion in cellular nests and adherence of the peripheral cell layer to fibrovascular septa. Various immunohistochemical markers have been applied to the diagnosis of RMS. However, diagnostic accuracy is variable in routine practice and of limited utility. Given their high sensitivity and specificity for RMS, the myogenic markers myogenin (myogenic factor 4) and myogenic differentiation 1 (MyoD1) have the highest diagnostic value in the setting of pediatric "small, blue, round-cell tumor"(see section "Epidemiology, Etiology,

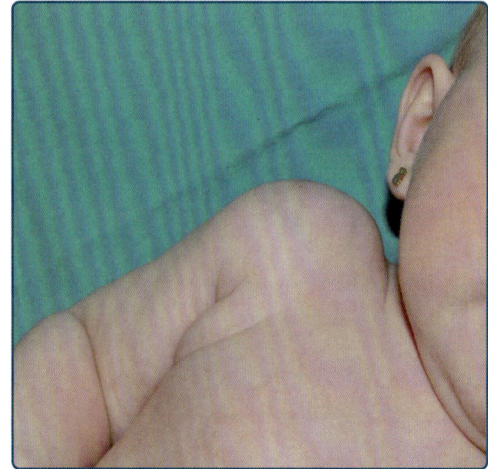

Figure 121-15 Rhabdomyosarcoma presenting as a subcutaneous mass on the shoulder of an infant. (Image from the collection of Antonio Torrelo, MD, Department of Pediatric Dermatology, Hospital del Niño Jesús, Madrid, Spain. Used with permission.)

and Pathogenesis").[67] Approximately 80% of ARMS have the *PAX3-FOXO1A* or *PAX7-FOXO1A* fusion.

DIFFERENTIAL DIAGNOSIS

Differential diagnosis of RMS includes other malignant neoplasms composed of primitive cells with minimal or no differentiation ("small, blue, round-cell tumors of childhood") and poorly differentiated spindle-cell sarcomas in children and young adults. Immunohistochemical analysis using a panel of stains is basically indispensable to delineate RMS from its histologic mimickers, including neuroblastoma, Ewing sarcoma, lymphoma, melanoma, poorly differentiated angiosarcoma, granulocytic sarcoma, synovial sarcoma, pleomorphic leiomyosarcoma, and undifferentiated pleomorphic sarcoma. Pleomorphic RMS and pleomorphic leiomyosarcoma may exhibit a quite similar cytomorphology. As desmin is positive in both tumors, specific skeletal muscle markers, including monoclonal myoglobin and MyoD1 and/or myogenin, must be included in the antibody panel. Of note, CD99, a highly sensitive marker of Ewing sarcoma, is sometimes detectable in ERMS and ARMS.[68]

CLINICAL COURSE AND PROGNOSIS

Although generally considered as poor, the prognosis of RMS is highly variable among affected individuals and has improved dramatically in the recent decades. The International Classification of RMS distinguishes 4 main categories with respect to prognosis: (a) superior prognosis (botryoid RMS, spindle-cell RMS), (b) intermediate prognosis (ERMS), (c) poor prognosis (ARMS, undifferentiated sarcoma), and (d) subtypes whose prognosis is not presently evaluable (RMS with rhabdoid features).[69] Notably, the prognosis of RMS has improved substantially since 1970 with 5-year-survival rates ranging from approximately 20% to 30% for undifferentiated sarcoma to 90% to 95% for botryoid RMS.

MANAGEMENT

Treatment of RMS requires a multidisciplinary approach including a biopsy or surgical removal of the tumor and chemotherapy with or without radiotherapy.

RHABDOMYOMATOUS MESENCHYMAL HAMARTOMA

First described in 1986 by Hendrick and associates as *striated muscle hamartoma* and renamed in 1989 by Mills as *rhabdomyomatous mesenchymal hamartoma*, this extremely rare cutaneous entity usually presents in the midline of newborns (synonym: *congenital midline hamartoma*).[70,71] It may arise as a solitary lesion in an otherwise healthy neonates or occur as multiple lesions in the setting of uncommon ectodermal/mesodermal abnormalities. Anecdotal cases have been diagnosed in adults. Rhabdomyomatous mesenchymal hamartoma clinically presents as a small dome-shaped papule or polypoid pedunculated lesion in the midline region of the skin in the head and neck region, most frequently on the chin. Unusual sites include the oral cavity, nasal vestibule, vagina, and the anal region. Histologically, the lesion is composed of disordered mixture of mature-appearing adipose and skeletal muscle tissue, adnexal structures and sometimes blood vessels and nerves (synonym: *hamartoma of cutaneous adnexa and mesenchyma*). The differential diagnosis includes nevus lipomatosus superficialis and fibrous hamartoma of infancy, both of which lack skeletal muscle fibers. Moreover, rhabdomyomatous mesenchymal hamartoma must also be distinguished from cutaneous ERMS and neuromuscular hamartoma (see "Neuromuscular Hamartoma" below). Rare cases of rhabdomyomatous mesenchymal hamartoma may undergo spontaneous regression. Local excision is an adequate treatment option.

NEUROMUSCULAR HAMARTOMA

Neuromuscular hamartoma, also called *benign Triton tumor* or *neuromuscular choristoma*, is a rare developmental lesion composed of skeletal muscle and nerve muscle elements. Of the fewer than 50 cases reported in the literature, the majority presented in children younger than 2 years of age as solitary masses involving large nerve trunks, principally the brachial plexus and the sciatic nerve.[72] Tumors arising from intracranial nerves are typically detected during adult life (Fig. 121-16). Owing to their locations, neuromuscular hamartomas commonly cause neurologic symptoms. Cutaneous manifestation without major nerve involvement is exceedingly rare, with only a few reported cases in the literature. The histogenesis of this entity remains controversial. Histologic appearance is characterized by bundles of perpendicularly oriented skeletal muscles intermingled with multiple small nerve fascicles. Total excision of neuromuscular hamartoma is often challenging because of its association with a major nerve. Given its benignity, treatment should thus be aimed at amelioration of symptoms and maintaining the integrity of the nerve.

PERIPHERAL NERVE SHEATH TUMORS

Peripheral nerve sheath tumors constitute the vast majority of neural proliferations presenting in the skin and the subcutis Table 121-3). These tumors arise from, or differentiate toward, one or more elements of the peripheral nervous system. The entire spectrum can be

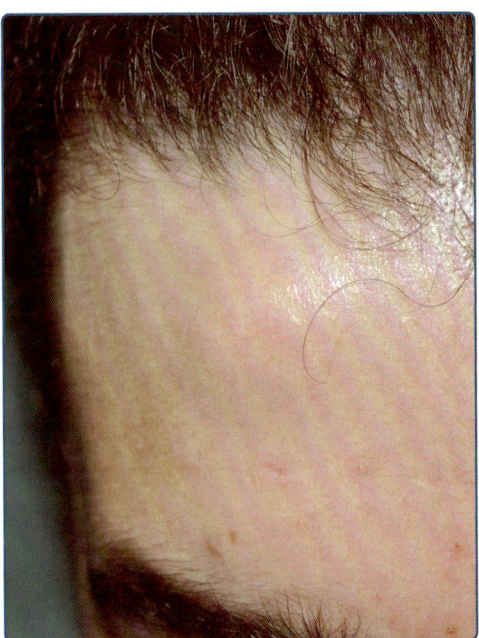

Figure 121-16 Neuromuscular hamartoma on the forehead of a teenager. (Image from the collection of Antonio Torrelo, MD, Department of Pediatric Dermatology, Hospital del Niño Jesús, Madrid, Spain. Used with permission.)

protein.[74] Axons contain the specific intermediate filament type designated neurofilament, and myelinated axons contain myelin basic protein. Figure 121-17 provides an overview of the diagnosis of cutaneous neural proliferations.

BENIGN NERVE SHEATH TUMORS (NEUROMAS)

AT-A-GLANCE

- Nonneoplastic nerve sheath proliferations occurring in distinct clinicopathologic settings.
- Consist of both axons and Schwann cells at a ratio of approximately 1:1.
- Presents as flesh-colored papules or nodules; occasionally painful.
- Treatment is excision.

TRAUMATIC (AMPUTATION) NEUROMA

EPIDEMIOLOGY

The incidence of traumatic neuromas varies widely in the literature, with a reported range of 10% to 30% for symptomatic traumatic neuromas.[75,76] They can present at any age.

ETIOLOGY AND PATHOGENESIS

Traumatic neuromas are regenerative proliferations that result after sectioning or traumatization of a nerve in any way so that its continuity cannot be reestablished. As a result, a guided growth of axons in a proximal–distal axis through tubes of proliferating Schwann cells is not possible and the disorganized proliferation of the proximal nerve gives rise to a *traumatic neuroma*.[77] They may be painful as a result of abnormal synapse formation and signaling within the tangle of nerve fascicles.

CLINICAL FINDINGS

Traumatic neuromas present as firm, oval, flesh-colored, occasionally painful papules or nodules in the subcutis or deeper soft tissues. They occur at sites of previous trauma, in amputation stumps, and in scars.[78]

HISTOPATHOLOGY

Histologically, traumatic neuromas are composed of a haphazard proliferation of nerve fascicles, includ-

broadly subdivided for practical purposes into genuine nerve sheath neoplasms and nonneoplastic proliferations, including hamartomatous tumors.[73] From a clinical perspective, peripheral nerve sheath tumors often resemble each other and most tumors are benign. However, some neoplasms may occur in the setting of an underlying clinical syndrome, and their correct diagnosis can therefore facilitate the recognition of an important genetic disorder and, ultimately, better patient management. In addition, malignant transformation of neurofibromas is an acknowledged phenomenon in a subset of patients with neurofibromatosis 1 (NF-1). The sheath of peripheral nerves is composed by 3 different cell types: (a) Schwann cells, which give rise to the 3 main entities of cutaneous peripheral nerve sheath tumors: neuromas, schwannomas (neurilemomas), neurofibromas, and their variants; (b) perineurial cells, which are considered specific fibroblasts that give rise to perineuriomas and differ from Schwann cells by lacking a basement membrane; and (c) nonspecific mesenchymal cells (eg, fibroblasts, mast cells), which are predominantly located in the endoneurium, that is, the space between the individual nerve fibers. The various types of peripheral nerve sheath tumors contain the same principal constituents of a peripheral nerve—Schwann cells, axons, fibroblasts, and stroma tissue. However, the proportion and architectural arrangement of these basic units varies according to the tumor type. Schwann cells are considered as neural crest–derived cells and express S-100 protein but not EMA, whereas perineurial cells are generally viewed as mesodermal derived cells and express EMA, GLUT1 (glucose transporter 1), and claudin-1, but not S-100

TABLE 121-3
Cutaneous Proliferations with Neural Differentiation

	TRAUMATIC NEUROMA	PALISADED ENCAPSULATED NEUROMA	SCHWANNOMA	NEUROFIBROMA	NERVE SHEATH MYXOMA	PERINEURIOMA	GRANULAR CELL TUMOR	MPNST
Incidence	Uncommon	Rare	Uncommon	Very common	Rare	Rare	Rare	Very rare
Age & gender	Any M:F = 1:1	Adults (20 to 50 years of age) M:F = 1:1	Adults (20 to 60 years of age) M:F = 1:1	Adults (20 to 80 years of age) M:F = 1:1	Any (mean age: 36 years) Males > Females	Any (mean age: 46 years) M:F = 1:2	Adults (20 to 80 years of age) M:F = 1:3	Adults (20 to 50 years of age) Males > Females
Location	Trauma sites, amputation stumps, scars	90% Face (nose, lip, cheek), 10% extrafacial	Head and neck area, flexural aspects of extremities	Localized type: trunk, head Diffuse type: head, neck Plexiform type: anywhere	Extremities (hand/fingers, knee/pretibial region, ankle/foot)	Sclerosing type: digits and palms Deep soft-tissue type: trunk, legs	65% Head and neck area (mainly tongue, oral mucosa, hard palate), 35% elsewhere	Proximal extremities and trunk
Size	0.5 to 2 cm	0.2 to 0.6 cm	1 to 4 cm	0.2 to 2 cm (localized type)	0.5 to 2.5 cm	0.5 to 1.5 cm	0.2 to 3 cm	>5 cm
Clinical presentation	Oval, firm, flesh-colored papule or nodule	Small, immobile, firm, rubbery, skin-colored or pink, dome-shaped papule or nodule	Soft, slowly growing, skin-colored to yellowish, dermal or subcutaneous nodule	Soft, skin-colored, dome-shaped or pedunculated papule or nodule	Soft, skin-colored, multinodular mass	Firm, flesh-colored, superficial papule or nodule	Flesh-colored or brownish-red, firm nodule with a smooth, rough, or verrucous surface	Enlarging palpable mass
Symptoms	Itching, prickling, pain in 10% to 30% of cases	Asymptomatic	Asymptomatic; pain, tenderness, neurologic symptoms may occur	Asymptomatic; positive "button-hole" sign	Asymptomatic	Usually asymptomatic	Asymptomatic; pruritus or tenderness may occur	Radicular pain, paresthesia, motor weakness
Genetics		MEN2B: gain-of-function germline mutations in RET (10q11.21)	Sporadic and NF-2–associated tumors: inactivation of NF2 (22q12.2); Schwannomatosis: inactivation of SMARCB1/INI1, (22q11.23)	Sporadic and NF-1–associated tumors: inactivation of NF1 (17q11.2); genetic heterogeneity (eg, loss-of-function variants, gene deletions)		Often mutations or deletions of the NF2 gene	LEOPARD syndrome: germline missense mutations in PTPN11 (12q24.13)	Sporadic, radiotherapy- and NF-1–associated tumors: inactivation of NF1 (17q11.2), CDKN2A (9p21.3), PRC2 (EED or SUZ12)

(Continued)

TABLE 121-3
Cutaneous Proliferations with Neural Differentiation (Continued)

	TRAUMATIC NEUROMA	PALISADED ENCAPSULATED NEUROMA	SCHWANNOMA	NEUROFIBROMA	NERVE SHEATH MYXOMA	PERINEURIOMA	GRANULAR CELL TUMOR	MPNST
Histopathologic features	Haphazard proliferation of nerve fascicles including myelinated axons, Schwann cells, fibroblasts, and perineural cells; collagenous stroma	Well-circumscribed tumor with partial encapsulation; multiple closely packed Schwann cell fascicles and abundant axons; interfascicular clefting	Well-circumscribed encapsulated tumor; parenchyma composed of Schwann cells; hypercellular areas with nuclear palisades alternate with hypocellular areas	Poorly circumscribed to well-circumscribed, usually nonencapsulated, haphazard proliferation of Schwann cells with slender, wavy nuclei, fibroblasts, perineurial cells, mast cells	Nonencapsulated multilobulated or multinodular tumor with abundant myxoid matrix; epithelioid, stellate-shaped, multipolar, spindled Schwann cells	Well-circumscribed nonencapsulated tumor with whorled, storiform, or lamellar growth pattern; spindle cells with elongated, bipolar cytoplasmic processes; usually collagenous stroma	Poorly circumscribed nodule; polygonal cells with abundant, fine to coarsely granular cytoplasm and round, dark nuclei; pseudoepitheliomatous hyperplasia	Poorly circumscribed unencapsulated tumor with fibrosarcoma-like appearance; cells arranged in sweeping fascicles; cellular and myxoid areas alternate ("marbleized" pattern), mitotic activity
Immunohistochemical features	NF+, EMA+/–, S-100+	NF+, EMA+, S-100+	NF–, EMA+, S-100+	NF+/–, S-100+, EMA–	S-100+, GFAP+, NSE+	EMA+, GLUT1+, claudin-1+	S-100+, NSE+, CD68+	S-100+/–, H3K27me3+/–
Management	Reapposition, surgical excision	Surgical excision	Surgical excision	Surgical excision	Surgical excision	Surgical excision	Surgical excision	Surgical excision, radiotherapy and/or chemotherapy
Associated syndromes		Multiple mucosal neuromas occur in the setting of MEN2B	5% with multiple meningiomas; 3% with NF-2; 2% with multiple schwannomas	Plexiform type almost unique to NF-1; diffuse type usually associated with NF-1			Multiple granular cell tumors are an associated feature of LEOPARD syndrome	Approximately 50% of MPNSTs occur in the setting of NF-1; 8% to 13% lifetime risk of MPNST in NF-1
Other	"Rudimentary polydactyly" is regarded as a variant		Multiple schwannomas ("schwannomatosis"): multiple cranial, spinal and peripheral schwannomas without vestibular tumors	Malignant transformation of plexiform type into MPNST occurs in approximately 4% of cases		Malignant transformation of soft-tissue perineurioma into malignant perineurioma is very uncommon	Malignant granular cell tumors are very rare	1-Year local reoccurrence rate of 40%; 1-year distant metastasis rate of 50%

EMA, epithelial membrane antigen; GFAP, glial fibrillary acidic protein; GLUT1, glucose transporter 1; LEOPARD, lentigines, electrocardiographic abnormalities, ocular hypertelorism, pulmonary stenosis, abnormalities of genitalia, retardation of growth, and deafness; M:F, male-to-female ratio; MEN, multiple endocrine neoplasia; MPNST, malignant peripheral nerve sheath tumor; NF, neurofibromatosis; NSE, neuron-specific enolase.

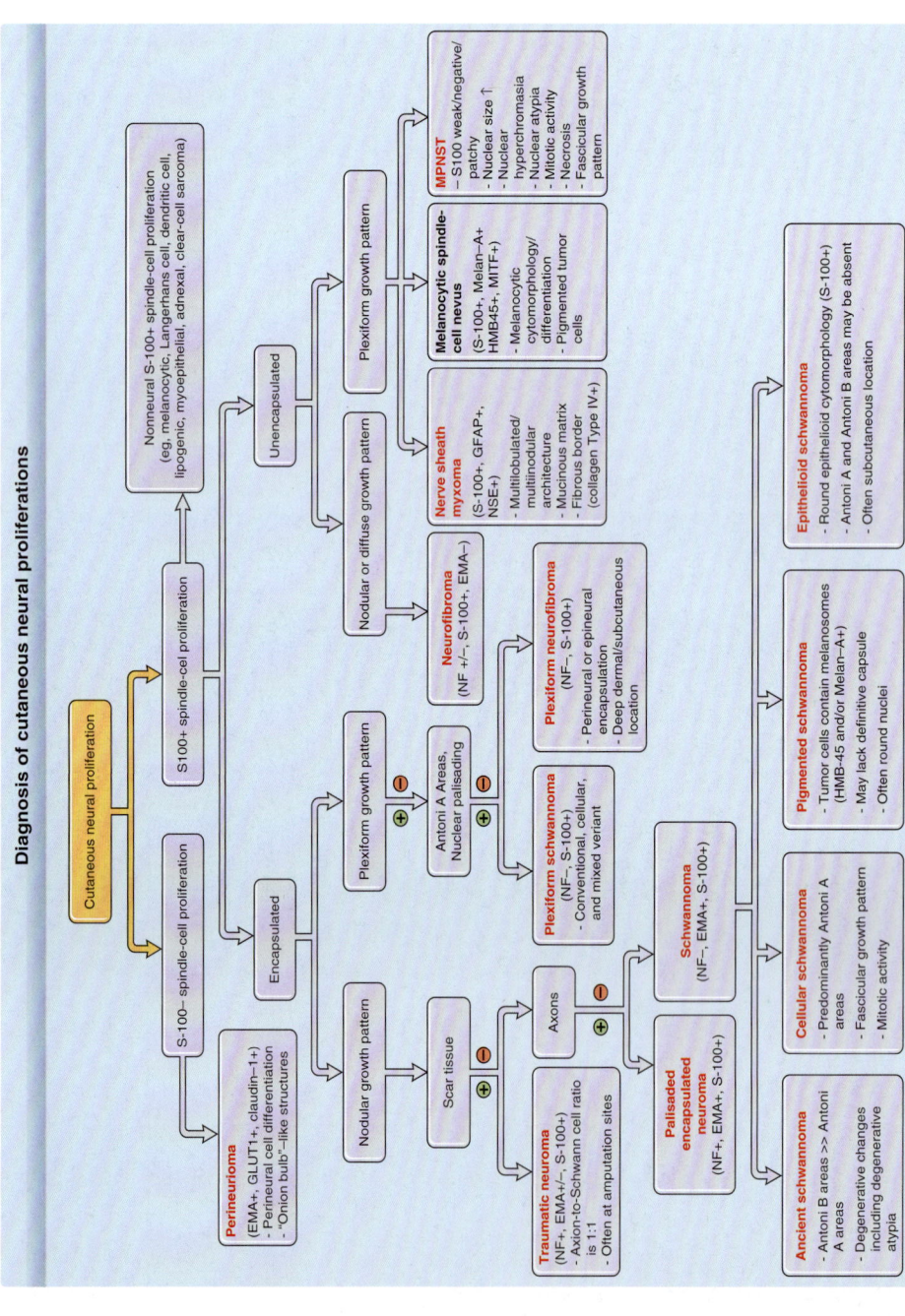

Figure 121-17 Diagnosis of cutaneous neural proliferations. −, Negative; +, positive; EMA, epithelial membrane antigen; GLUT1, glucose transporter 1; HMB45, melanocytic differentiation antigen; Melan-A, melanocytic differentiation antigen; MITF, microphthalmia-associated transcription factor; NF, neurofilament; NSE, neuron-specific enolase; S-100, S-100 protein.

ing axons with their myelin sheaths, Schwann cells, and fibroblasts embedded in a collagenous stroma. Concentric condensations of fibrous tissue around individual fascicles may be present. Perineurial cells, expressing EMA, surround each fascicle Table 121-4).

DIFFERENTIAL DIAGNOSIS

Differential diagnosis of traumatic neuromas includes granuloma, dermatofibroma, neurofibroma, schwannoma, and hypertrophic scar.

MANAGEMENT

Effective treatment of painful traumatic neuroma remains a challenge. Following nerve injury, an attempt should thus be made to reappose the disconnected nerve ends to enable regeneration in an orderly fashion. Once a neuroma has developed, a nerve block provides temporary pain relief. Surgical excision of the lesion and reposition of the proximal nerve stump into a scar-free area is the conventional therapy.[79]

RUDIMENTARY POLYDACTYLY

EPIDEMIOLOGY

The vast majority of cases presents in newborns or in early childhood. Recognition in adult life is rare.[80]

ETIOLOGY AND PATHOGENESIS

The designation "rudimentary polydactyly" is applied to a nodular tumor that rarely appears on the ulnar surface of the proximal fifth finger and contains a disordered proliferation of nerve fascicles analogous to a classical conventional neuroma. The lesion has been traditionally viewed as a variant of amputation neuroma at the site of a supernumerary sixth digit that has undergone autoamputation in utero. This concept has been challenged and it has been suggested that such proliferations are neural malformations unrelated to a supernumerary digit.[81]

CLINICAL FINDINGS

Raised nodule on the ulnar border of the proximal fifth finger (Fig. 121-18).

HISTOPATHOLOGY

Multiple bundles of nerve fibers embedded in connective tissue in the upper dermis, and in dermal papillae. Numerous Meissner corpuscles are present.

DIFFERENTIAL DIAGNOSIS

The diagnosis is usually suspected by the history of a solitary nodular lesion at the ulnar site of the fifth finger since birth or early childhood.

MANAGEMENT

Primary suture ligation of accessory digits in infancy may lead to the subsequent development of a genuine traumatic neuroma. Primary surgical excision with

TABLE 121-4
Immunohistochemical Staining of Neural Hyperplasias and Neoplasms

NEURAL PROLIFERATION	S-100 PROTEIN	NEUROFILAMENT	EPITHELIAL MEMBRANE ANTIGEN	OTHER
Traumatic neuroma	+	+	+	Neuron-specific enolase positive
Palisaded encapsulated neuroma	+	+	+ for the capsule	
Schwannoma	+	−	+ for the capsule only	Vimentin positive
Neurofibroma	+	Variable	−	CD34 positive
Plexiform neurofibroma	+	−	−	
Nerve sheath myxoma	+	−	+ in adjacent dense collagen	GFAP positive; CD57 positive; collagen Type IV pericellular positive
Perineurioma	−	−	+	Claudin-1 positive; GLUT1 positive
Malignant peripheral nerve sheath tumor	+	+	Variable	Vimentin variable; cytokeratin negative; neuron-specific enolase positive
Primitive neuroectodermal tumor	+ if differentiated	−	−	Neuron-specific enolase positive; CD99 positive
Granular cell tumor	+	−	−	Neuron-specific enolase positive

−, Negative; +, positive; GFAP, glial fibrillary acidic protein; GLUT1, glucose transporter 1.

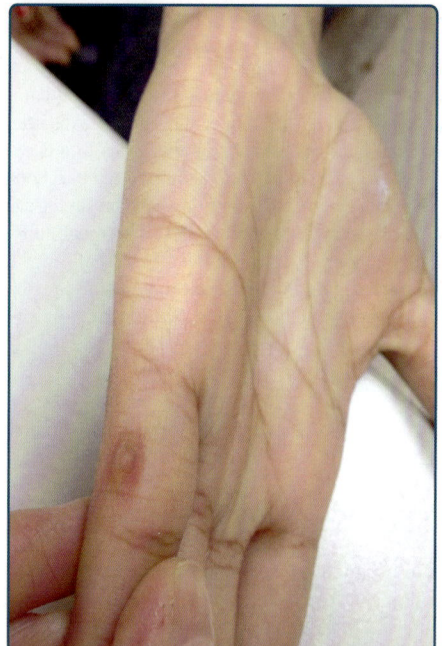

Figure 121-18 Rudimentary polydactyly on the left hand. The lesion was excised because of paresthesia. (Image from the collection of Mar Llamas-Velasco, MD, Hospital Universitario de La Princesa, Madrid, Spain. Used with permission.)

high transection and retraction of the accessory digital nerve prevents postoperative neuroma formation.[82]

PALISADED ENCAPSULATED NEUROMA

EPIDEMIOLOGY

Palisaded encapsulated neuromas (PENs), also described as "solitary circumscribed neuromas," appear during adulthood, mostly in the third to fifth decade. Males and females are equally affected.[83] PENs account for approximately 25% of all cutaneous nerve sheath tumors.[84]

ETIOLOGY AND PATHOGENESIS

PEN can be conceptualized as a morphologically distinctive hamartomatous overgrowth of Schwann cells and axons of a cutaneous peripheral nerve.[83] It is not associated with trauma, multiple endocrine neoplasia syndrome Type 2B (MEN2B), or neurofibromatosis. The etiology is unknown.

CLINICAL FINDINGS

PENs commonly appear as small, asymptomatic, flesh-colored, firm papules or nodules (Fig. 121-19). They may arise at any location, but approximately 90%

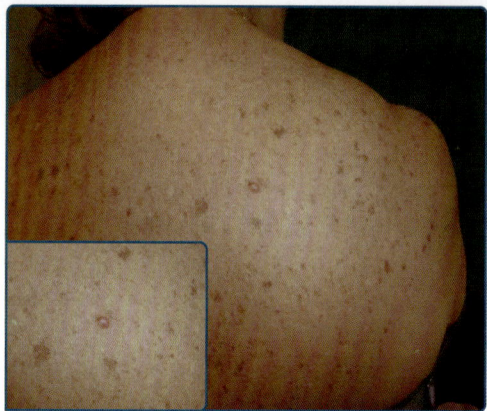

Figure 121-19 Palisaded encapsulated neuroma on the upper back. (Image from the collection of Mar Llamas-Velasco, MD, Hospital Universitario de La Princesa, Madrid, Spain. Used with permission.)

of cases are diagnosed in the area of the face, primarily around the nose and lips.[84] Rare cases on the distal extremities have been described.[85]

HISTOPATHOLOGY

PENs usually present as nodular or polypoid, well-circumscribed, dermal-based tumors that are surrounded by a thin perineurial connective tissue capsule (Fig. 121-20A). Multinodular and plexiform growth patterns are described.[86] The solid proliferations are composed of multiple closely packed fascicles of Schwann cells and abundant axons. The variably oriented fascicles are commonly separated by clefts (Fig. 121-20B). Parallel arrangement of nuclei ("nuclear palisading") may occasionally be found, but distinct Verocay body formation is rare. The perineurial cell-rich capsule stains for EMA (Fig. 121-20C). The spindle-shaped tumor cells stain for S-100 protein (Fig. 121-20D), and numerous axons can be readily identified by staining for neurofilament protein (Fig. 121-20E) (see Table 121-4).[87,88]

DIFFERENTIAL DIAGNOSIS

Differential diagnosis of PEN includes dermal melanocytic nevus, basal cell carcinoma, adnexal tumor, and neurofibroma. Schwannoma and neurofibroma are in the main histopathologic differential diagnosis. PENs typically lack the variety of stromal changes that are frequently encountered in these tumors. Focal hypercellularity and minor degrees of nuclear palisading reminiscent of schwannoma may be found in PENs, but they differ by the absence of Verocay bodies and the presence of axons. Occasionally, the spindle cells in PEN lack a fascicular pattern, as seen in neurofibroma. In contrast to PEN, neurofibroma is not encapsulated in the dermis.

MANAGEMENT

Complete surgical excision of the tumor is curative.

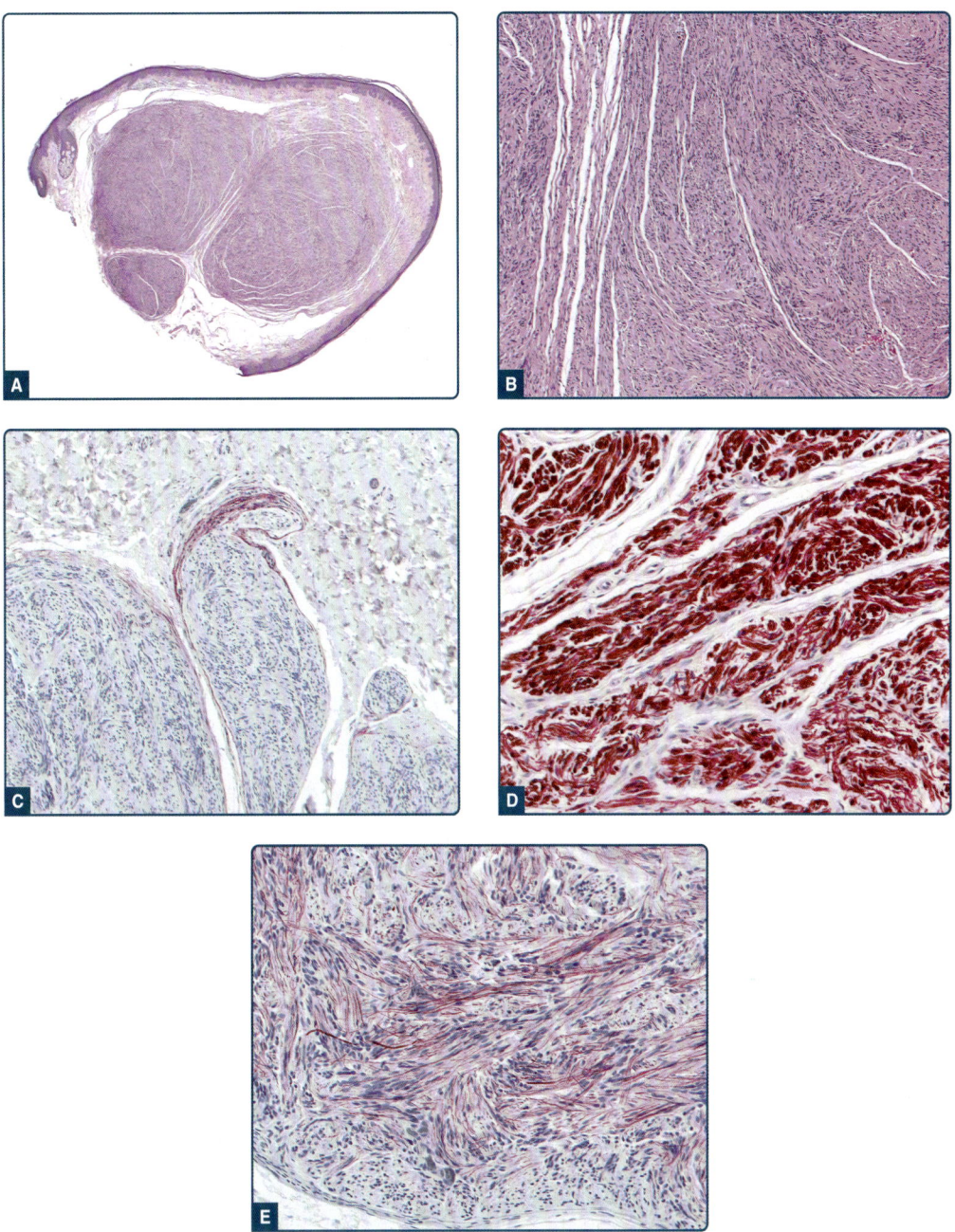

Figure 121-20 Photomicrograph of a palisaded encapsulated neuroma. **A,** Presentation as a dermal-based tumor that is partially surrounded by a thin connective tissue capsule is typical (hematoxylin-and-eosin [H&E], ×20 magnification). **B,** Short fascicles of closely packed Schwann cells that are separated by clefts (H&E, ×100 magnification). The capsule stains for epithelial membrane antigen (EMA) (**C**; anti-EMA, ×100 magnification), the tumor cells stain diffusely positive for S-100 protein (**D**; anti–S-100 protein, ×100 magnification), and numerous intratumoral axons can be identified with staining for neurofilament protein (**E**; anti-neurofilament protein, ×100 magnification).

MUCOSAL NEUROMAS AND MULTIPLE ENDOCRINE NEOPLASIA SYNDROME TYPE 2B

EPIDEMIOLOGY

The exact incidence of mucosal neuromas is not clear. Lesions occurring in the setting of MEN2B manifest during the first few decades in life. The prevalence of MEN2B has been derived from epidemiologic studies as 1 in 600,000 patients[89] to 1 in 4,000,000 patients.[90]

ETIOLOGY AND PATHOGENESIS

MEN2B is an autosomal dominant condition caused by gain-of-function germline mutations of the RET protooncogene, which encodes a receptor tyrosine kinase and maps to chromosome 10q11.2. At least 95% of MEN2B cases are the result of a point mutation in exon 16 (M918/T).[90]

CLINICAL FINDINGS

MEN2B is characterized by the early development of medullary thyroid carcinoma in all affected individuals and the occurrence of pheochromocytomas in approximately 50% of individuals. In contrast to MEN2A, clinically significant parathyroid disease is absent, but patients with MEN2B have additional malformations (Marfanoid habitus, facial dysmorphism), as well as mucosal neuromas and diffuse ganglioneuromatosis of the GI tract.

Multiple mucosal neuromas are the most consistent and distinctive clinical manifestation of MEN2B, occurring in 100% of patients.[91] As they may represent the initial manifestation of this life-threatening syndrome, early recognition of these marker lesions is essential for establishing a timely diagnosis. Neuromas appear by the age of 2 years as pink, pedunculated, painless papules on the mucosal surfaces of the eyelids, lips, tongue, and intestines. The lips become diffusely hypertrophied and bulging (or "blubbery") over time, and submucosal nodules may be present on the vermilion border of the lips. Neuromas of the eyelids may cause thickening and eversion of the upper eyelid margins. Other cutaneous signs of MEN2B include café-au-lait spots, facial lentigines, and hyperpigmentation of the hands and feet. Mucocutaneous neuromas also have been reported in association with the spectrum of genetic disorders caused by PTEN (phosphatase and tensin homolog) mutations, that is, the PTEN hamartoma–tumor syndrome.[92]

HISTOPATHOLOGY

Histologically, lesions are composed of irregular, tortuous, hyperplastic nerves with a prominent perineurium lying in the submucosal tissue.

DIFFERENTIAL DIAGNOSIS

Differential diagnosis of mucosal neuromas and MEN2B includes mucosal neuromas occurring in PTEN hamartoma–tumor syndrome, mucocele, and PEN.

MANAGEMENT

In MEN2B, management should be aimed at (a) identification of individuals with germline gain-of-function mutations of the RET gene associated with MEN2B and (b) reduction of morbidity and mortality in high-risk individuals via either prophylactic thyroidectomy or screening for medullary thyroid cancer (catecholamine urine testing, serum calcium and parathyroid hormone levels). Patients with clinical evidence of MEN2B as well as all at-risk members of kindreds in which a germline RET pathogenic variant has been identified should undergo genetic analysis of the RET gene. Relatives who do not carry the genetic mutation are not at risk for developing the disease. Prophylactic thyroidectomy during the first 6 to 12 months of life is advised for individuals with an identified germline RET pathogenic variant, because medullary thyroid cancer develops at an early age in affects individuals.[92]

BENIGN NERVE SHEATH NEOPLASMS

AT-A-GLANCE

- Schwannomas are benign encapsulated nerve sheaths neoplasms derived from the proliferation of Schwann cells and lack axons.
- Neurofibromas are benign nonencapsulated nerve sheath tumors composed of all elements of a peripheral nerve. Plexiform neurofibroma is linked to NF-1 and has a potential for malignant transformation.
- Usually presents as isolated lesions, but multiple neurofibromas are found in neurofibromatosis Type 1 and multiple schwannomas found in neurofibromatosis Type 2, in schwannomatosis, or in association with multiple meningiomas.
- Treatment is simple excision of schwannomas and localized neurofibromas is curative. Resection of diffuse and plexiform neurofibromas is performed when tumors are severely disfiguring or severely compromise functionality.

SCHWANNOMA

EPIDEMIOLOGY

Schwannomas occur at all ages but mostly between the ages of 20 and 60 years. Women are slightly more affected than men.[73] According to a population-based study by Antinheimo and associates approximately 90% of schwannomas arise sporadically, 5% in individuals with multiple meningiomas (with or without NF-2), 3% in those with NF-2 (detailed in Chap. 135), and 2% in individuals with multiple schwannomas.[93] In contrast to plexiform neurofibromas, which are considered a clinical hallmark of NF-1, the association of plexiform schwannomas with neurofibromatosis Type 2 and with schwannomatosis is approximately 5% each.[94]

ETIOLOGY AND PATHOGENESIS

Schwannomas are genuine true nerve sheath neoplasms that are derived the proliferation of Schwann cells within nerve sheaths and are thus surrounded by a true capsule consisting of epineurium. Historically, they have been termed *neurinomas*, *neurolem(m)omas*, or *neurilem(m)omas*. Approximately 60% of sporadic and NF-2–associated schwannomas harbor inactivating mutations of the *NF2* gene located at 22q12.2, and in approximately one-third of schwannomas there is chromosomal loss of 22q. All schwannomas, including sporadic and syndromic tumors, lack merlin, the protein product of *NF2*, suggesting the presence of either undetectable mutations or epigenetic modification in the remaining tumors.[95,96] The tumors grow within a capsule and are almost entirely composed of Schwann cells. They remain attached to the parent nerve, which, on pathologic examination, may occasionally be detected at the periphery. Sites of predilection include the peripheral nerves at the flexor sites of the upper and lower extremities, followed by the cranial and cervical nerves, particularly the division of the eighth cranial nerve, which gives rise to vestibular schwannomas (formerly known as *acoustic neuromas*).[97] They also occur in spinal roots and on the tongue. Deeply seated schwannomas are mostly found in the retroperitoneum and in the posterior mediastinum.

CLINICAL FINDINGS

Cutaneous schwannomas (Fig. 121-21) present as soft, slowly growing, skin-colored to yellowish dermal or subcutaneous nodules. They are usually solitary and measure 1 to 4 cm in diameter.[78] When attached to a small nerve, the tumors are highly movable in several axes. Small tumors are usually asymptomatic, but pain, tenderness, and neurologic symptoms may occur in larger lesions and as a consequence of forceful displacement of tumors.[97] Plexiform schwannomas, which represent approximately 15% of all cutaneous schwannomas, may be clinically recognizable as intradermal multinodular masses.

Multiple Schwannomas: Schwannomatosis, also known as neurilemmomatosis, is a genetic disorder characterized by multiple cranial, spinal and peripheral schwannomas, without vestibular schwannomas or other signs of NF-1 or NF-2. The reported incidence of this recently recognized entity ranges from 1.40,000 to 1.7 million, with most studies suggesting an incidence analogous to that of NF-2.[93] The genetics of schwannomatosis is complex. Schwannomatosis occurs mostly sporadically, likely representing new mutations, but cases of autosomal dominant transmission have been reported. Sporadic cases may occasionally show mosaicism for the *NF2* mutation, reflecting the phenotype overlap between patients with NF-2 and patients with sporadic schwannomatosis. Somatic mutations of the *NF2* gene are frequently detected in schwannomas of schwannomatosis patients, but germline transmission of schwannomatosis occurs by involvement of the tumor-suppressor gene *SMARCB1*, also known as *INI1*.[98] The vast majority of schwannomatosis patients harbor somatic *SMARCB1* and *NF2* mutations in affected tissues. Notably, SMARCB1 has been reported not to play a role in solitary sporadic schwannomas.[99]

HISTOPATHOLOGY

Schwannomas are well-circumscribed, encapsulated, nodular true nerve sheath proliferations, usually limited to the subcutis. The tumor parenchyma is exclusively composed of Schwann cells. Neither axons nor perineurial cells are detectable. The surrounding fibrous capsule consists of epineurium and residual nerve fibers. Schwannomas commonly grow as uninodular eccentric masses, resulting in displacement of the nerve of origin. Apart from plexiform schwannomas, intradermal occurrence is rare and has been mostly reported in the setting of schwannomatosis or NF-2. The constituent tumor cells show a typical Schwann cell appearance with elongated slender nuclei and elongated eosinophilic cytoplasmic processes. The hallmark of schwannomas is the pattern of 2 alternating tissue areas (Fig. 121-22A). In the areas of high cellularity (called *Antoni A*), compact spindle-shaped Schwann cells are arranged in short bundles or interlacing fascicles. The tumor cells have

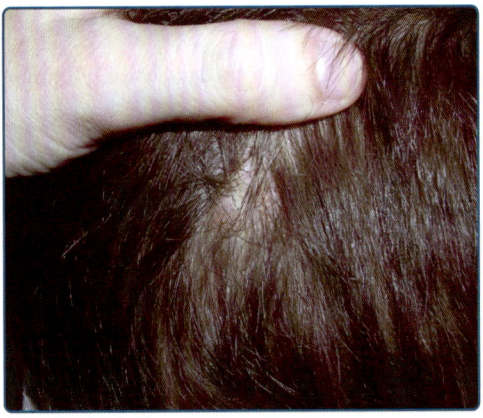

Figure 121-21 Schwannoma on the scalp of a child with neurofibromatosis Type II. (Image from the collection of Marta Feito-Rodríguez, MD, Department of Dermatology, Hospital Universitario La Paz, Spain. Used with permission.)

indistinct cytoplasmic borders and their nuclei are frequently twisted. The nuclei of adjacent cells may be tightly aligned, creating stacks of nuclear *palisades*. A *Verocay body* is formed by a horizontal arrangement of 2 rows of elongated palisading nuclei that are separated by acellular zones made up of stacked cytoplasmic processes of the tumor cells (Fig. 121-22B).[100] The areas of low cellularity (called *Antoni B*) consist of widely separated and haphazardly arranged spindle or oval tumor cells in a loosely textured myxoid matrix with delicate collagen fibers and large, irregularly spaced, partially thrombosed blood wells with thickened walls caused by dense fibrosis. Antoni B tissue may represent degenerated Antoni A tissue and typically shows varying changes indicative of degeneration, such as hyalinization, cyst formation, hemorrhage, fibrosis, and, occasionally, calcification. The relative proportions of Antoni A and Antoni B areas vary considerably, and they may blend indiscernibly or change abruptly. Tumors of long duration may develop substantial degenerative changes in association with marked nuclear atypia. The nuclei are large and hyperchromatic, but lack mitotic figures. Numerous inflammatory cells are commonly present. These tumors behave as classic schwannomas and are thus comfortably termed *ancient schwannomas*.[101] *Cellular schwannomas* are defined as tumors composed exclusively or predominantly of Antoni A areas (ie, Antoni B areas not exceeding 10%) that lack Verocay bodies. Low mitotic activity and focal areas of necrosis may be present. *Plexiform schwannomas* are characterized by a plexiform pattern (Fig. 121-23) that is often associated with multinodularity. They have a propensity for the skin and may present in the dermis and or in the subcutis, and infrequently in deep soft tissues. Similar to classic schwannomas, they are encapsulated and often cellular, thus frequently qualifying as cellular schwannomas. Schwannomas composed predominantly or exclusively of small rounded Schwann cells arranged singly, in cohesive nests, or in cords within a collagenous or partially myxoid stroma have been referred to as *epithelioid schwannomas*. In *melanotic (pigmented) schwannomas*, Schwann cells contain melanosomes and are immunoreactive with melanocytic markers (eg, HMB-45). The highly cellular tumors are composed of spindled and epithelioid cells and carry a 10% risk of malignant transformation. The psammomatous subvariant (*psammomatous melanotic schwannomas*) is associated with the Carney complex in half of the cases.[102] Additional rare variants include the (pseudo) glandular, neuroblastoma-like, and the microcystic-reticular variant. Schwannomas stain strongly and diffusely positive for S-100 protein (see Table 121-4).

DIFFERENTIAL DIAGNOSIS

Clinical differential diagnosis of schwannomas includes lipoma, cyst, leiomyoma, adnexal tumors, and MPNST. Histologically, schwannomas must be distinguished from PEN (see "Palisaded Encapsulated Neuroma" before) and neurofibromas by their growth

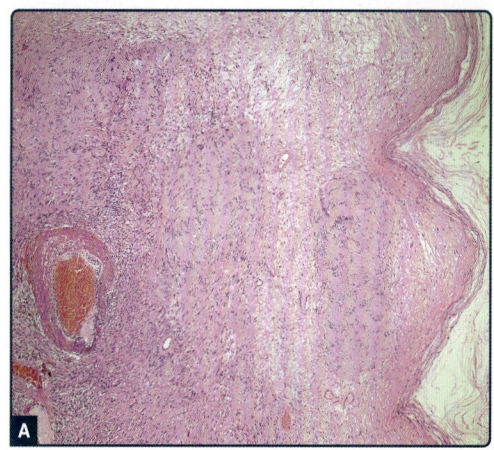

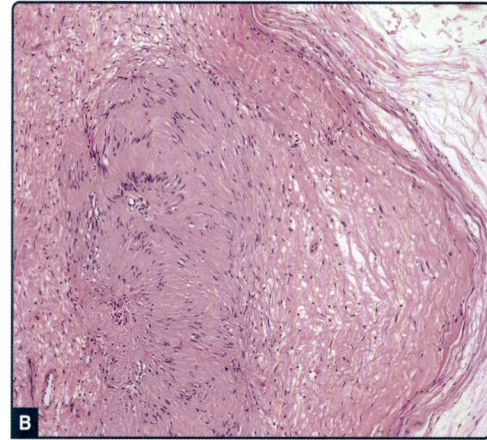

Figure 121-22 Photomicrograph of a schwannoma. **A,** Nodular, well-circumsribed, encapsulated tumor composed of fascicles of plump spindle cells. Characteristic zonation of alternating hypercellular areas (Antoni A) and hypocellular areas (Antoni B), and hyalinized, thick-walled blood vessels are seen. **B,** Foci of nuclear palisades surrounding aggregates of cytoplasmic processes (Verocay bodies) are present.

pattern and cellular composition. In contrast to PEN, most schwannomas are composed of both hypercellular and hypocellular areas, and are without intervening clefts. Verocay bodies are usually present, but are rare in PEN. Neurofibromas are noncapsulated and differ from schwannomas with respect to cellular composition (see "Neurofibroma" below). Cellular schwannomas may occasionally exhibit Antoni A areas with broad, long, sweeping tumor fascicles arranged in a herringbone pattern and may thus partially mimic leiomyosarcoma, fibrosarcomatous dermatofibrosarcoma protuberans or fibrosarcoma. Plexiform schwannoma must be critically distinguished from plexiform neurofibroma (see section "Epidemiology"), which is pathognomonic for NF-1 and has a propensity for malignant transformation, as well as from plexiform MPNST, plexiform fibrohistiocytic tumor, plexiform granular cell tumor, and traumatic neuroma.

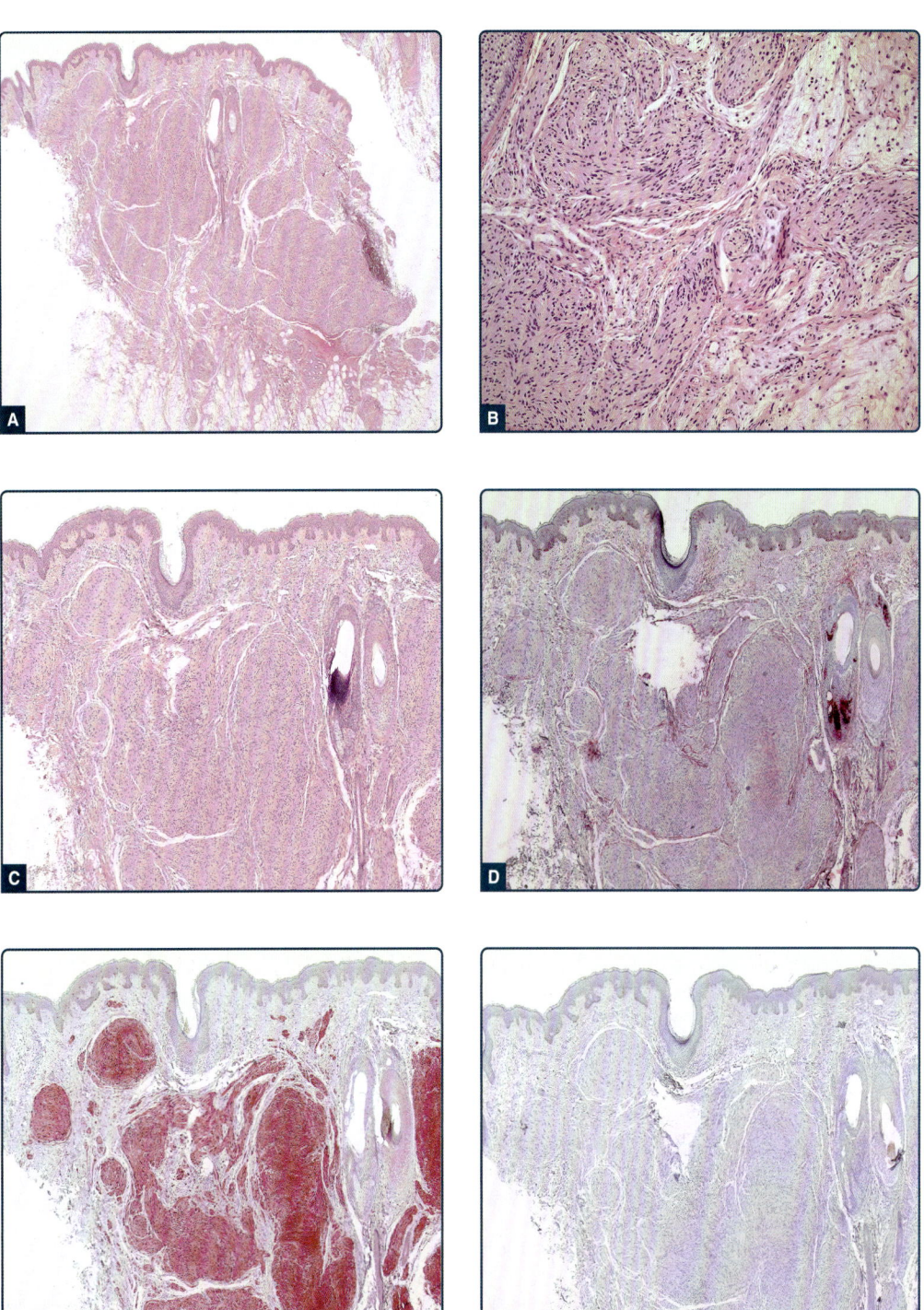

Figure 121-23 Photomicrograph of a plexiform schwannoma in a child with neurofibromatosis-2. **A,** Multinodular, well-circumscribed, encapsulated tumor composed of uniform spindle cells in a plexiform pattern (hematoxylin-and-eosin [H&E], ×4 magnification). **B,** Characteristic cellular Antoni A areas with vague nuclear palisades are present (H&E, ×100 magnification). Tumor masses (**C**; H&E, ×10 magnification) are surrounded by an epithelial membrane antigen (EMA)-positive perineurial capsule (**D**; anti-EMA, ×10 magnification), the tumor cells stain diffusely positive for S-100 protein (**E**; anti–S-100 protein, ×10 magnification). **F,** Neurofilament protein expression is negative because of an absence of axons (anti-neurofilament protein, ×10 magnification). (Image from the collection of Elena Ruíz Bravo-Burguillos, MD, Department of Pathology, Hospital Universitario La Paz, Madrid, Spain. Used with permission.)

CLINICAL COURSE AND PROGNOSIS

Malignant transformation of classic schwannomas is exceedingly rare but has been observed. The biologic behavior of melanotic schwannomas is difficult to predict and slightly more than 10% of melanotic schwannomas undergo malignant transformation[73]; 50% of the psammomatous variant are associated with the Carney syndrome.[102]

MANAGEMENT

Simple excision is the treatment of choice. Plexiform schwannomas have been associated with an increased risk of local recurrence following incomplete excision.

NEUROFIBROMA

EPIDEMIOLOGY

Localized sporadic neurofibromas are common benign tumors that, like their inherited counterparts, have no gender predilection. Most lesions arise in individuals between the ages of 20 and 30 years. Multiple neurofibromas that arise in a segmental or widespread distribution should raise suspicion for one of several types of NF.[103] Plexiform neurofibromas are pathognomonic of NF-1.

ETIOLOGY AND PATHOGENESIS

Neurofibromas are benign nerve sheath proliferations that are composed of all elements of a peripheral nerve.[73] In contrast to neuromas, the relative ratio of axons to Schwann cells is less than 1:1. Neurofibromas can occur sporadically or in the context of NF-1, which is covered in detail in Chap. 135. NF-1 is inherited as an autosomal dominant trait with a high rate of penetrance. Only half of the patients with this trait have affected family members, with the remainder of affected individuals representing de novo mutations.[104] The *NF-1* gene maps to the long arm of chromosome 17 (17q11.2). More than 1000 pathogenic allelic variants have been identified. The *NF1* gene product is a cytoplasmic protein called *neurofibromin 1*, which is considered to have diverse functions in many different tissues. Although not all functional aspects of neurofibromin 1 are understood, it regulates activation of the Ras intracellular signaling pathway in Schwann cells.[105,106]

CLINICAL FINDINGS

There are 3 main subtypes of neurofibromas based on architectural growth patterns: (a) localized neurofibromas, (b) diffuse neurofibromas, and (c) plexiform neurofibromas. The localized form is by far the most

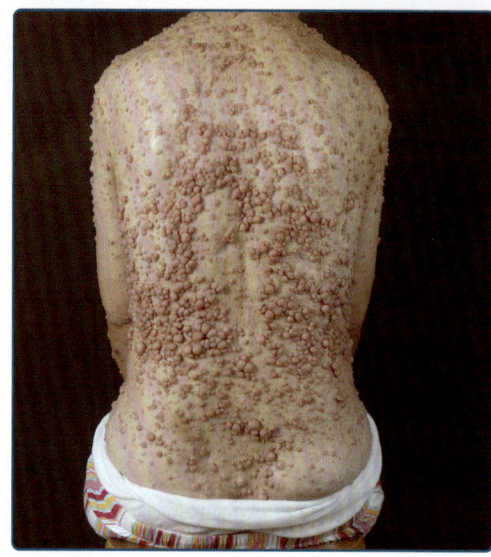

Figure 121-24 Clinical photograph showing multiple neurofibromas on the back of a patient with neurofibromatosis Type I ("NF1 microdeletion syndrome"). (Image from the collection of Robert Gruber, MD, Dermatology, Venereology and Allergology, Medical University of Innsbruck, Innsbruck, Austria. Used with permission.)

common type, representing 90% of all tumors.[107] The majority are solitary lesions that are not associated with NF-1. Multiple tumors arise in patients with NF-1 (Fig. 121-24). *Localized neurofibromas* present as slowly growing, skin-colored, soft or rubbery, papules or nodules. They may enlarge to protuberant or pedunculated tumors, but rarely exceed 5 cm in diameter. The tumors tend to invaginate on pressure (the *buttonhole sign*). They are usually asymptomatic, but may be pruritic. *Diffuse neurofibromas* mainly affect children and young adults and are most frequently located within the subcutaneous tissues of the head and neck; 90% are solitary lesions and not associated with NF-1. Clinically, the diffuse variant typically causes a plaque-like elevation of the skin with thickening of the entire subcutis. *Plexiform neurofibromas* are characterized by diffuse involvement of a long nerve segment and its branches, forming bag-like or pedunculated rope-like masses that feel similar to a "bag of worms" on palpation. These tumors can be associated with massive soft-tissue overgrowth, resulting in functional impairment. They usually occur in early childhood and are pathognomonic of NF-1. A subset of plexiform neurofibromas presents with hyperpigmentation and hypertrichosis of the overlying skin and has been termed *pigmented neurofibroma* (Fig. 121-25).[108]

HISTOPATHOLOGY

Localized solitary neurofibromas are dermal-centered, nonencapsulated, loosely textured proliferations composed of Schwann cells, perineurial cells, mast cells, and plump fibroblasts arranged haphazardly in a variably collagenous and myxoid matrix (Fig. 121-26A). The delicate tumor cell fascicles are usually only a single-layer thick and the cells contain oval or "wavy," spindle-shaped nuclei and a scant, indefinite cytoplasm (Fig. 121-26B). The matrix can be variably mucinous, sclerosing or hyalinized. Occasionally nuclear palisades can occur, but true Verocay formation is exceedingly rare. Nuclear pleomorphism may be present, but mitoses are rare. Diffuse neurofibromas demonstrate a similar cytomorphology but display a diffusely infiltrative growth pattern with involvement of adjacent structures such as the skin appendages and considerable subcutaneous extension along connective tissue septa. The correct diagnosis of plexiform neurofibromas is crucial for establishing the diagnosis of NF-1. The tumors rarely arise in the dermis and consist of a tortuous mass of numerous large nerve fascicles embedded in a matrix composed of collagen, mucin, fibroblasts, and Schwann cells (Fig. 121-27). Initially, the tumor is confined to the epineurium. Upon continued growth, tumor cells spill out into soft tissue. These areas may mimic areas of diffuse neurofibroma, and tumors in NF-1 patients can show both plexiform and diffuse areas. Plexiform neurofibromas may display nuclear atypia. Because this neurofibroma type carries the highest risk of malignant transformation, careful evaluation of areas with high cellularity and severe atypia is crucial. In pigmented plexiform neurofibroma, there is melanocytic hyperplasia at the dermoepidermal junction and a proliferation of single pigmented melanocytes with occasional small nests in the papillary dermis, and scattered within underlying neurofibromatous tissue.[109] A variant characterized by 2 distinct cell types and pseudorosette formation has been described as *dendritic cell neurofibroma with pseudorosettes* (Fig. 121-28).[110]

DIFFERENTIAL DIAGNOSIS

Clinical differential diagnosis of neurofibroma includes dermal melanocytic nevus, soft fibroma, neuroma, lipoma, dermatofibroma, and MPNST. Histopathologic differential diagnosis includes dermatofibroma, neural nevus, neuroma, plexiform schwannoma, MPNST, desmoplastic melanoma, and dermatofibrosarcoma protuberans. Plexiform schwannomas, in contrast to plexiform neurofibromas, are encapsulated tumors that consist exclusively of Schwann cells presenting a

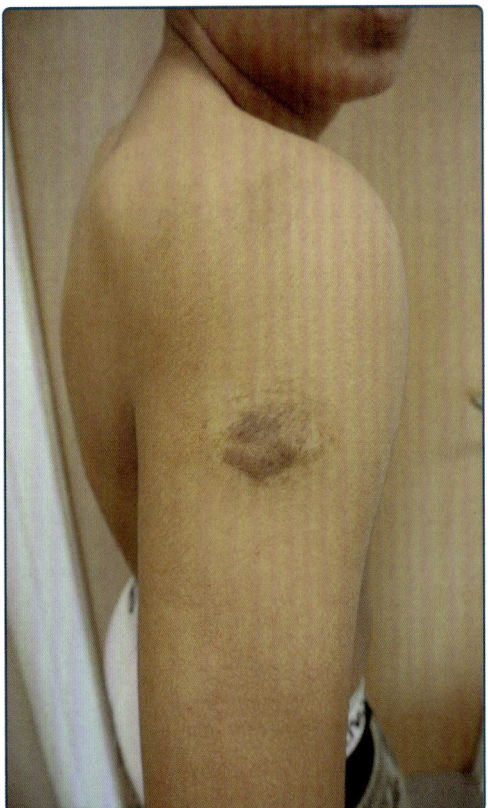

Figure 121-25 Pigmented neurofibroma, a variant of plexiform neurofibroma with hyperpigmentation and hypertrichosis of the overlying skin, on the upper arm. (Image from the collection of Robert Gruber, MD, Dermatology, Venereology and Allergology, Medical University of Innsbruck, Innsbruck, Austria. Used with permission.)

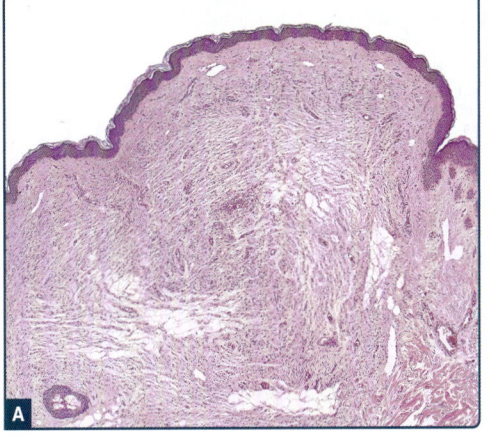

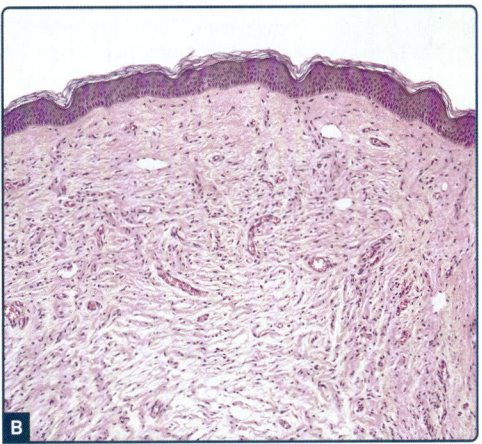

Figure 121-26 Histologic appearance of localized neurofibroma. **A,** Nonencapsulated, loosely textured, dermal proliferation of spindle cells in a variably collagenous and myxoid matrix (hematoxylin-and-eosin [H&E], ×20 magnification). **B,** Delicate tumor cell fascicles composed of short to more elongated spindle cells elongated, "wavy" nuclei and scant indefinite cytoplasm (H&E, ×100 magnification).

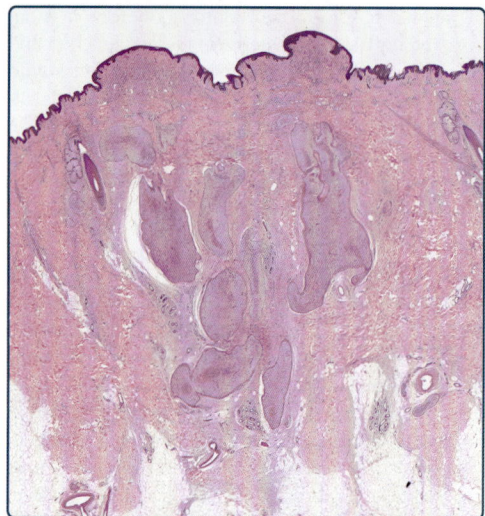

Figure 121-27 Photomicrograph of a plexiform neurofibroma. The tumor consists of multiple tortuous nodules and cords that result from irregular replacement and expansion of peripheral nerve fascicles. In contrast to localized neurofibroma, this neurofibroma variant is more circumscribed (hematoxylin-and-eosin [H&E], ×40 magnification).

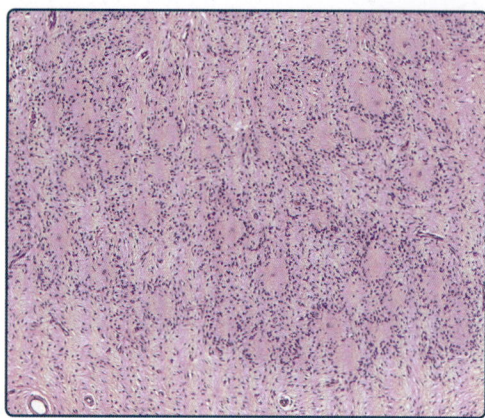

Figure 121-28 Histologic appearance of a dendritic cell neurofibroma with pseudorosettes (hematoxylin-and-eosin [H&E], ×100 magnification). Small, dark, lymphocyte-like cells are grouped concentrically around cells with larger pale-staining nuclei and clear eosinophilic cytoplasm.

plexiform arrangement. The histopathologic delineation of a neurofibroma with atypical histologic features from a low-grade MPNST is challenging because these lesions represent a histologic continuum (see section "Histopathology"). Desmoplastic malignant melanoma may be composed of deceptively bland cells with wavy nuclei, virtually mimicking neurofibroma. Important clues to the diagnosis of melanoma include the presence of significant solar elastosis, atypical junctional melanocytic hyperplasia and/or an in situ component, the presence of very long, hyperchromatic cells, a "packeted" growth pattern, dense fibrosis, and deep nodular lymphoid aggregates. Immunohistochemistry is of limited value in this situation, as both tumors express S-100 protein, and more specific melanocytic differentiation antigens (eg, Melan-A, HMB-45, MITF [microphthalmia-associated transcription factor]) are essentially never positive in desmoplastic melanoma. CD34 immunoreactivity in a "fingerprint" pattern has been reported to be more typical of neurofibroma than desmoplastic melanoma.[111] Pigmented neurofibromas can be distinguished from pigmented forms of dermatofibrosarcoma protuberans (Bednar tumor), formerly known as *storiform pigmented neurofibroma*. The Bednar tumor is characterized by a repetitive storiform pattern and uniform fibroblastic tumor cells that express CD34 and lack expression of S-100 protein.

CLINICAL COURSE AND PROGNOSIS

Plexiform neurofibroma has a potential for malignant transformation, and is a recognized precursor for MPNST in NF-1 patients.[112] The clinical course, prognosis, and management of patients NF-1 are discussed in Chap. 135.

MANAGEMENT

Simple excision of sporadic neurofibromas is curative. Surgical intervention is currently the best treatment option for plexiform neurofibromas, but complete tumor resection is not always possible. Treatment with arterial embolization and surgical resection has been reported in a patient with a giant plexiform neurofibroma.[113] Treatment of large tumors should be aimed at resection of rapidly enlarging masses, symptomatic and functional improvement, and enhancement of cosmesis in disfiguring disease.[114] Recurrence of plexiform neurofibromas is common.

NERVE SHEATH MYXOMA

EPIDEMIOLOGY

Nerve sheath myxoma is an uncommon benign nerve sheath tumor. It occurs at all ages, but the peak incidence is in the fourth decade. Both sexes are roughly equally affected. Almost 90% of cases arise on the extremity, particularly the fingers and the knee/pretibial region.[115]

ETIOLOGY AND PATHOGENESIS

Nerve sheath myxoma, first described in 1969 by Harkin and Reed, has been a controversial entity for decades. In 1980, Gallagher and Helwig used the term *neurothekeoma* to describe the same tumor.[115] Because some neurothekeomas have a myxoid stroma, both entities were for many years regarded as neural tumors at either end of a histopathologic spectrum. In

2005, Fetsch and associates characterized nerve sheath myxomas as distinct true nerve sheath tumors perhaps related to schwannoma and unrelated to cellular and mixed-type neurothekeomas.[116] This concept was further substantiated by differential gene expression profiling of nerve sheath myxomas and neurothekeomas that confirm a peripheral nerve sheath origin for dermal nerve sheath myxomas and suggest a fibrohistiocytic origin for neurothekeomas.[117]

CLINICAL FINDINGS

The tumors are solitary, superficial, slow growing, and usually painless. The size ranges from 0.5 cm to 2.5 cm in diameter.

HISTOPATHOLOGY

Histologically, the nonencapsulated tumors form distinct multilobulated or multinodular masses with abundant myxoid matrix and a peripheral fibrous border (Fig. 121-29A). They are dermal centered but frequently extend into the superficial subcutaneous tissue.[118] The tumors are composed of small epithelioid Schwann cells arranged in cords, nests or syncytial-like aggregates (Fig. 121-29B). In addition, a variable amount of multipolar Schwann cells with a ring-like appearance, and scattered spindled and stellate-shaped Schwann cells are present. Nuclear hyperchromatism and nuclear atypia are occasionally present. Mitotic figures are rare. The tumor cells strongly express S-100 protein (Fig. 121-29C), glial fibrillary acidic protein, neuron specific enolase, and CD57 (see Table 121-4). They are bordered by collagen IV. EMA-positive perineurial cells are typically present in small numbers, primarily in the fibrous tissue directly adjacent to the myxoid nodules.

DIFFERENTIAL DIAGNOSIS

Clinical differential diagnosis includes myxoid or ganglion cyst, adnexal tumor, dermal melanocytic nevus, and neurothekeoma. Histopathologic differential diagnosis of nerve sheath myxoma includes schwannoma, neuroma, and myxoid neurofibroma, as well as cellular and mixed-type neurothekeoma. *Cellular neurothekeoma*, first described by Rosati and associates in 1986,[119] is a dermal neoplasm of presumed fibrohistiocytic lineage.[120] It commonly occurs on the head, neck, and upper body of young adults, with a slight female predominance. On histology, these tumors are poorly circumscribed, typically being composed of nests and fascicles of epithelioid and spindle-shaped cells. The tumor cells do not express S-100 protein, but are essentially always positive for NK1-C3 antibody. The marker PGP9.5 (protein gene product 9.5) is frequently expressed. Immunoreactivity for CD10, MITF (microphthalmia-associated transcription factor), α-SMA, vimentin, and CD86 has been reported. The *mixed type* of neurothekeomas shows overlapping features of nerve sheath myxoma and cellular neurothekeoma.

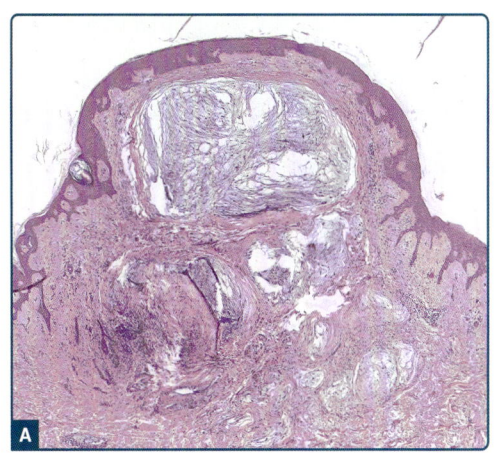

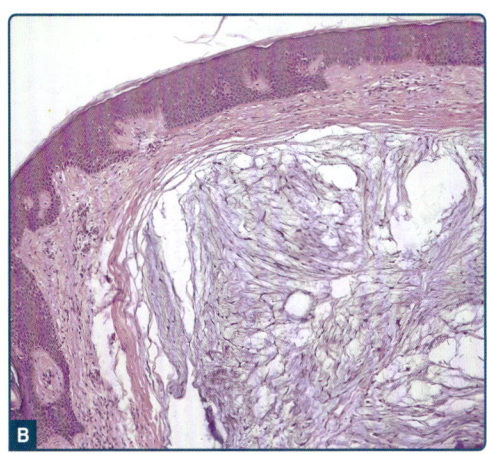

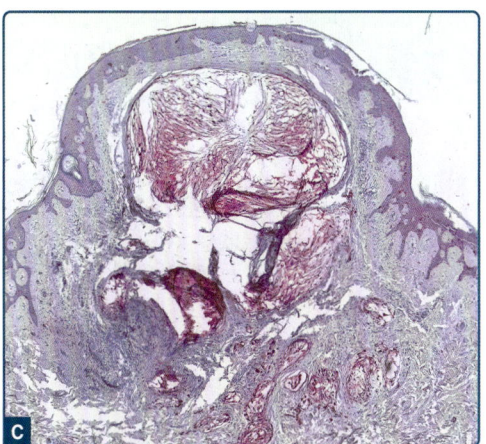

Figure 121-29 Photomicrograph of a nerve sheath myxoma. **A,** Well-circumscribed, nonencapsulated, multinodular, dermal tumor with a myxoid stroma and a peripheral fibrous border (hematoxylin-and-eosin [H&E], ×20 magnification). **B,** Spindled, stellate-shaped, multipolar, and epithelioid Schwann cells arranged in syncytial-like aggregates are seen (H&E, ×100 magnification). **C,** The tumor cells strongly express S-100 protein (anti–S-100 protein, ×100 magnification).

CLINICAL COURSE AND PROGNOSIS

Nerve sheath myxomas are benign but recur in almost 50% of cases, often after incomplete excisions.[116]

MANAGEMENT

Nerve sheath myxomas are managed by simple excision.

PERINEURIOMA

EPIDEMIOLOGY

Perineuriomas are uncommon benign tumors that comprise less than 1% of nerve sheath tumors. Epidemiologic data are scarce. Cutaneous and soft-tissue perineuriomas have a male-to-female ratio of 1:2.

ETIOLOGY AND PATHOGENESIS

Perineurial cells are of mesenchymal origin and form a sheath for peripheral nerves. A perineurioma is a benign peripheral nerve sheath tumor composed exclusively of perineurial cells that occurs in the dermis, subcutis, or soft tissue. Neither intraneural nor extraneural perineuriomas appear to be associated with NF-1 or NF-2, but chromosome 22 deletions have been seen.[121,122]

CLINICAL FINDINGS

There are 2 forms of perineurioma: One form is intraneural and presents as a fusiform swelling of a major nerve, often with signs of mononeuropathy.

The other form of perineurioma is extraneural. It usually arises in soft tissue, but cutaneous examples are increasingly being reported. Cutaneous perineuriomas present as firm, flesh-colored, superficial nodules, usually ranging from 0.5 to 1.5 cm in diameter. Larger variants have been reported, usually in soft tissues.[121] Perineuriomas are most commonly reported on the leg or trunk. The sclerosing perineurioma is a distinctive variant that most commonly presents on fingers and palms of young adults.

HISTOPATHOLOGY

Histologically, intraneural perineuriomas are circumscribed nonencapsulated proliferations of delicate spindle cells with elongated, bipolar cytoplasmic processes (Fig. 121-30A). There are small aggregates and bundles with individual cells oriented either parallel to each other or forming small whorls composed of multiple concentric layers ensheathing a central axon and Schwann cell ("onion bulbs") (Fig. 121-30B).[123] The stroma can vary from densely collagenous (principally in the sclerosing variant) to myxoid in character. The "onion bulb"-like structures of concentric circles are an important clue to the diagnosis but are also a characteristic finding in *localized hypertrophic neuropathy*, with which it has no relationship at all.[124,125] The cells in perineurioma clearly differentiate along perineurial lines, as shown by ultrastructure and immunohistochemistry, whereas the "onion bulbs" of hypertrophic neuropathy are composed of Schwann cells. The *sclerosing perineurioma* shows a heavily collagenous background, whereas the *reticular (retiform) perineurioma* is composed of anastomosing cords of fusiform cells that wrap around islands of fibromyxoid stroma. The *epithelioid perineurioma* is composed of epithelioid cells with eosinophilic cytoplasm. Perineuriomas stain positive for EMA (Fig. 121-30C) and negative for S-100 and neurofilament. Most cases also express GLUT1 (Fig. 121-30D) and claudin-1 (Fig. 121-30E) (see Table 121-4).

DIFFERENTIAL DIAGNOSIS

Differential diagnosis of perineurioma includes dermal nevus, dermatofibroma, and infundibular cyst.

TREATMENT

Excision is curative.

MALIGNANT TUMORS OF NERVE

MALIGNANT NERVE SHEATH TUMORS

AT-A-GLANCE

- Malignant nerve sheath tumors are also known as neurofibrosarcoma, neurogenic sarcoma, neurosarcoma or malignant schwannoma.
- Two percent of nerve sheath tumors are malignant peripheral nerve sheath tumors (MPNSTs).
- Approximately 50% of MPNSTs occur in neurofibromatosis Type 1.
- Clinical presentation: enlarging masses in the deep soft tissues.
- Treatment is a multimodality approach.
- Outcome is poor, with 5-year survival rates of 10% to 50%.

EPIDEMIOLOGY

MPNSTs account for approximately 2% of all nerve sheath tumors. In most large studies, approximately 50% of MPNSTs occur in the context of NF-1.[126] The estimated lifetime risk of MPNST in patients with NF-1 is 8% to 13%.[127] Individuals with microdeletions of the

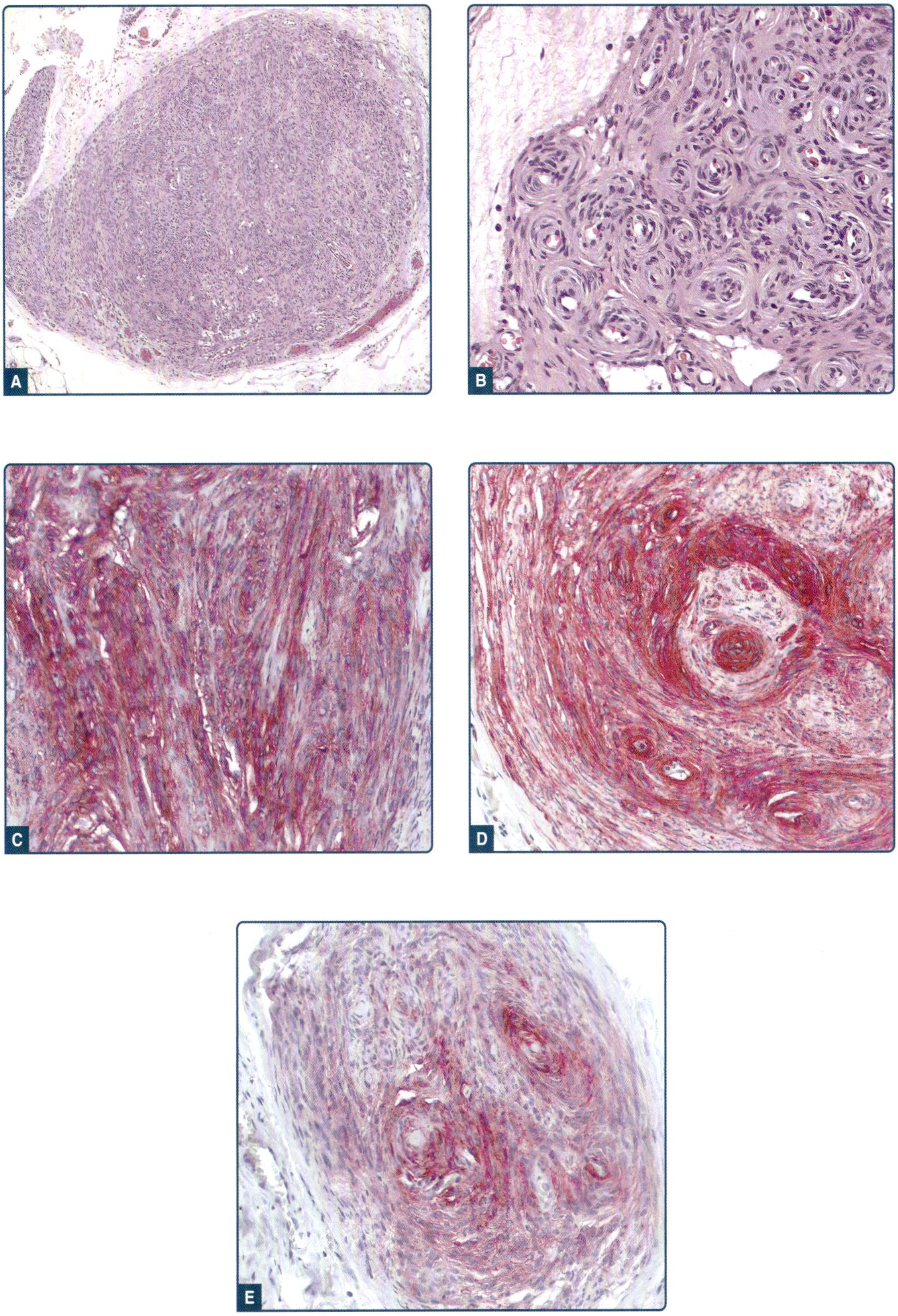

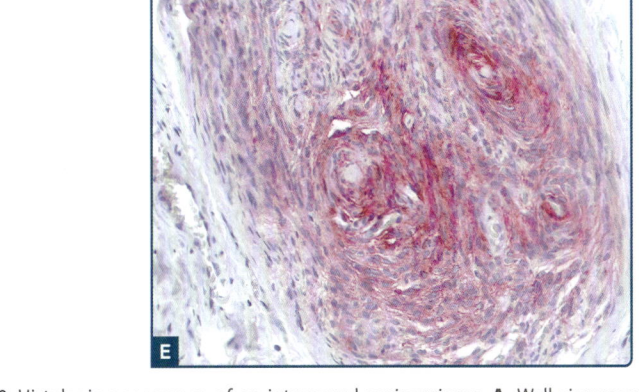

Figure 121-30 Histologic appearance of an intraneural perineurioma. **A,** Well-circumscribed, unencapsulated, dermal centered, nodular tumor composed of bland spindled perineurial cells forming characteristic "onion bulb"-like structures (hematoxylin-and-eosin [H&E], ×20 magnification). **B,** Onion-bulb formations consist of perineurial cells wrapping around individual axons and residual Schwann cells (H&E, ×100 magnification). The tumor cells stain positive for EMA (anti–epithelial membrane antigen, ×100 magnification) **(C)**, GLUT1 (anti–glucose transporter-1, ×100 magnification) **(D)**, and claudin-1 (anti–claudin-1, ×100 magnification) **(E)**.

NF1 gene have a lifetime risk of 16% to 26%.[128] Young and middle-aged adults are most commonly affected.

ETIOLOGY AND PATHOGENESIS

MPNST is the preferred designation for a tumor arising from or showing differentiation toward the various elements of the nerve sheath. Historically, MPNST also has been called *neurofibrosarcoma, neurogenic sarcoma, neurosarcoma,* and *malignant schwannoma.* MPNST may arise (a) from a peripheral nerve, (b) from a preexisting benign nerve sheath tumor, or, rarely, (c) de novo. The main benign precursors to MPNST are plexiform neurofibroma and massive soft-tissue neurofibroma in the setting of NF-1. Approximately 10% to 20% of sporadic cases occur as postirradiation tumors after a latent period of 15 years.[126] Malignant transformation of schwannoma into MPNST is rare.[129]

CLINICAL FINDINGS

MPNSTs arise predominantly in deep soft tissues of the proximal extremities and present as enlarging masses (Fig. 121-31). Pain is more prevalent in patients with NF-1, and pain or sudden enlargement of a longstanding tumor in the setting of NF-1 should raise should raise the suspicion of malignant transformation.

HISTOPATHOLOGY

MPNST is a cellular tumor composed of tight wavy or interlacing fascicles of spindle cells (Fig. 121-32A). The tumor typically presents typically with fibrosarcoma-like appearance: densely cellular areas alternate with less cellular areas, creating a marble-like effect. The constituent cells exhibit a malignant Schwann cell morphology, that is, asymmetrically tapered spindle cells with hyperchromatic, wavy, buckled, or comma-shaped nuclei and a pale cytoplasm (Fig. 121-32B). However, in the majority of cases there is a mixed proliferation of Schwann cells, perineurial cells, fibroblastic cells, and primitive cells. Nuclear palisading is uncommon. A plexiform and an epithelioid variant (malignant epithelioid schwannoma) have been described. Heterologous elements occur in 10% to 15% of cases in the form of cartilage and bone, or, less commonly, skeletal muscle (so called malignant triton tumor), smooth muscle, angiosarcoma, or well-differentiated glands (MPNST with glands). A rare subset of MPNSTs with perineurial differentiation has been termed *perineurial MPNST*. This variant stains positive for EMA and negative for S-100 protein. Immunohistochemistry is of limited value in the diagnosis of MPNST. At most, 50% of tumors show a focal or patchy expression of S-100 protein. The partial or even complete loss of S-100 expression in MPNST is one of the most useful distinctions from benign Schwann cell tumors. CD34 is frequently expressed and glial fibrillary acidic protein is positive in 30% to 40% of cases (see Table 121-4).

DIFFERENTIAL DIAGNOSIS

Clinical differential diagnosis of MPNSTs includes neurofibroma, schwannoma, lipoma, and cyst. Desmo-

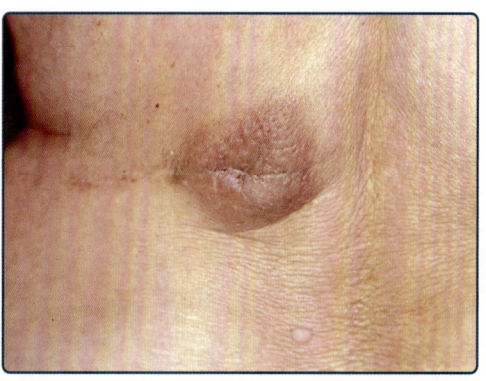

Figure 121-31 Malignant peripheral nerve sheath tumor on the lower back. (Image from the collection of Arno Rütten, MD, Dermatopathology Friedrichshafen. Used with permission.)

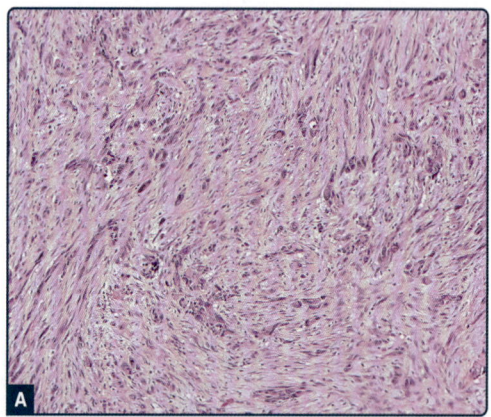

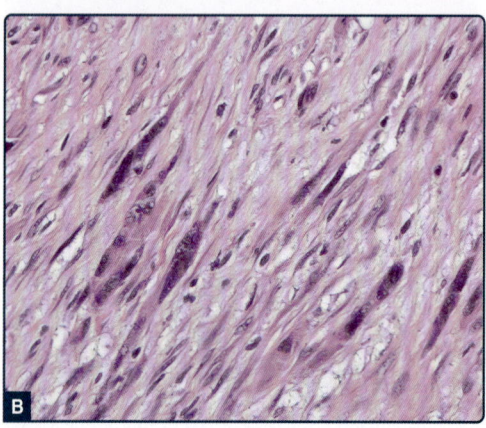

Figure 121-32 Histologic examination of a MPNST. **A,** The tumor is composed of highly cellular fascicles of atypical spindle cells (hematoxylin-and-eosin [H&E], ×20 magnification). **B,** Asymmetrically tapered spindle cells with hyperchromatic buckled nuclei and indistinct cytoplasm are seen (H&E, ×100 magnification).

plastic melanoma, cellular schwannoma and a variety of sarcomas, primarily synovial sarcoma, leiomyosarcoma, RMS, adult-type fibrosarcoma, dedifferentiated liposarcoma, and clear-cell sarcoma, are in the main histopathologic differential diagnosis. Moreover, low-grade MPNST may demonstrate very scarce mitotic activity and thus mimic neurofibroma with atypical features (see section "Histopathology"). The minimal criteria for the delineation of a MPNST from a benign nerve sheath tumor are: (a) marked cell crowding, (b) generalized nuclear enlargement (3 times normal neurofibroma cells), (c) nuclear hyperchromasia, and (d) a mitotic rate greater than 5 per 10 HPF. In the setting of NF-1, the presence of any mitotic activity in a neurofibroma warrants the diagnosis of low-grade MPNST. Desmoplastic melanomas present as fibrosing spindle-cell melanomas in chronically sun-damaged skin, typically the head and neck area. In addition to the superficial location, there is often a junctional component of atypical melanocytes and a strong expression of S-100 protein. Complete loss of SOX10, neurofibromin, or p16 expression, or the presence of epidermal growth factor receptor immunoreactivity are helpful in differential diagnosis with cellular schwannoma.[130] Synovial sarcoma is characterized by a t(X;18) balanced translocation and shows strong nuclear staining for TLE1 as well as consistently negative staining for glial fibrillary acidic protein.

CLINICAL COURSE AND PROGNOSIS

MPNSTs are high-grade sarcomas with a high tendency of local recurrence and distant metastasis. Prognosis is poor, with local recurrences developing in approximately 40% of patients and metastases developing in 40% to 60% of patients within 12 months of surgery on average.[126] Overall 5-year survival rates range from approximately 50% in sporadic patients to 10% to 35% in NF-1 patients.

MANAGEMENT

The management of patients with MPNST involves a multimodality approach. Complete surgical resection and adjuvant radiation therapy are required for good local tumor control. The response rates to cytotoxic chemotherapy in metastatic disease are low.

PRIMITIVE NEUROECTODERMAL TUMOR

EPIDEMIOLOGY, ETIOLOGY, AND PATHOGENESIS

Primitive neuroectodermal tumors (PNETs) are a group of highly malignant tumors composed of small round cells of neuroectodermal origin. Peripheral PNET and Ewing sarcoma represent ends of a morphologic spectrum known as the Ewing family of tumors. They both express the cell surface product of the *MIC2* gene, CD99, and both carry a consistent chromosomal translocation (t11;22) (q24;q12). PNETs are primarily a disease of childhood with a median age at diagnosis of 9 years of age. PNETs represent 2.8% of all primary cerebral tumors of childhood and adolescence.

CLINICAL FINDINGS

PNETs can metastasize to the skin.[131] Most peripheral PNETs/Ewing sarcomas are located in deep soft tissue.[132] With neuroblastoma, cutaneous metastases can be very numerous and involve multiple sites. In approximately 50% of patients with such metastases, they were the initial clinical presentation. Extremely rare cases of peripheral PNETs arising as primary cutaneous or subcutaneous tumors also have been reported.

HISTOPATHOLOGY

PNETs consist of small, round, basophilic ("blue") cells. Homer Wright rosettes can be present. If the tumor is differentiated, S-100 protein, neuron-specific enolase, and CD99 are positive.

DIFFERENTIAL DIAGNOSIS

Differential diagnosis of PNET includes neurofibroma, lipoma, and cyst.

MANAGEMENT

Treatment is surgical. A wide margin of excision and a young age correlated with improved survival in a series of patients with extraskeletal Ewing sarcoma.

MISCELLANEOUS TUMORS

GRANULAR CELL TUMOR

AT-A-GLANCE

- Neural tumor composed of large granular-appearing eosinophilic cells.
- Most common single anatomic site is the tongue.
- Malignant transformation is exceedingly rare.
- Treatment is excision.

EPIDEMIOLOGY

Granular cell tumors (GCTs) are relatively rare. The major majority arise in adults with a male-to-female ratio of 1:3. Approximately 10% to 15% have multiple lesions.

ETIOLOGY AND PATHOGENESIS

Although originally considered by Abrikossoff to be a muscle tumor, the expression of S-100 protein, myelin proteins, and myelin-associated glycoprotein has resulted in the reclassification of GCT as a tumor of Schwann cell origin.

CLINICAL FINDINGS

GCTs are small, asymptomatic or occasionally tender or pruritic, skin-colored, firm nodules usually located in the dermis or subcutis. They are slow growing and rarely exceed 3 cm in diameter. GCTs may present in various anatomical sites but have a strong predilection for the tongue and the dermis of the head and neck region, and the breast. GCTs also have been reported in the genitalia, esophagus, and larynx.[133]

HISTOPATHOLOGY

GCTs are ill-defined, dermal-based, nodular proliferations composed of sheets of large polyhedral cells. The cells have distinct cell borders, small, round, central nuclei, and abundant fine to coarsely granular cytoplasm (Fig. 121-33). The cytoplasmic granules stain strongly with the periodic acid-Schiff stain and retain this characteristic after diastase digestion. The overlying epithelium often shows prominent pseudoepitheliomatous hyperplasia, a feature that can lead to a mistaken diagnosis of SCC on superficial biopsies. Dermal tumors often extent into the subcutaneous tissue. Cells infiltrate between collagen bundles and tend to grow along small nerves and muscle fibers. Rarely, a plexiform or dermatofibroma-like growth pattern is present.[134] GCTs usually express S-100 protein, CD68, NGFR-5, MITF, NK1-C3, neuron specific enolase, and PGP9.5 (see Table 121-4). Rare cases of GCT show focal Melan-A positivity.[135] Malignant GCTs are extremely rare, accounting for only 1-2% of all GTCs.[136] *Atypical GCTs* are histologically defined by the presence of 1 or 2 of the following criteria: spindling of the tumor cells, necrosis, diffuse pleomorphism, prominent nucleoli, a high nuclear-to-cytoplasmic ratio, and a mitotic activity of greater than 2 per 10 HPF. Neoplasms that meet 3 or more of these criteria are classified as *malignant GCTs*, and GCTs with focal pleomorphism but none of the other criteria are classified as benign.[137]

DIFFERENTIAL DIAGNOSIS

Differential diagnosis of GCTs includes adnexal tumors, melanocytic nevi, dermatofibroma, and SCC of the tongue. On histology, various other tumor entities may present with a granular cell variant, such as dermatofibroma, leiomyosarcoma, melanoma, and angiosarcoma. Congenital granular cell tumor is a

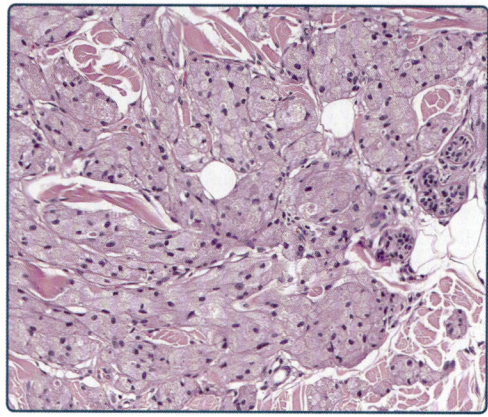

Figure 121-33 Photomicrograph of a granular cell tumor composed of sheets of polygonal cells with abundant granular eosinophilic cytoplasm, small, round, mostly central nuclei, and distinct cell borders. The present case shows a markedly collagenized stroma (hematoxylin-and-eosin [H&E], ×100 magnification).

rare benign neoplastic growth affecting the gingival mucosa of neonates.

CLINICAL COURSE AND PROGNOSIS

Benign and atypical GCTs have an excellent outcome with no metastasis. Local recurrence and metastasis are relatively common in malignant GCTs. Poor prognostic factors associated with malignant GCT include large tumor size, older patient age, increased mitotic activity, and Ki-67 greater than 10%.[137]

MANAGEMENT

Local surgical excision is the treatment of choice.

CENTRAL NERVOUS SYSTEM HETEROTOPIA

CNS heterotopias are composed of ectopic neural tissue and are divided into neuroglial heterotopia (nasal glioma) and meningeal heterotopia (MH).

NEUROGLIAL HETEROTOPIA

AT-A-GLANCE

- Rare congenital lesion commonly referred to as *nasal glioma*.
- Developmental anomaly consists of mature displaced neuroglial tissue; not a true neoplasm.
- Most often presents as a round, firm papule on the nose.
- Rarely connected to intracranial cavity.

Epidemiology: Heterotopic neuroglial tissue or nasal gliomas are rare congenital lesions.[138]

Etiology and Pathogenesis: Neuroglial heterotopias represent displaced mature neuroglial tissue that is entrapped in dural diverticula. This occurs during craniofacial development and sometimes does not regress. These lesions are now considered malformations[139] rather than neoplasms, as the designation *nasal glioma* implies.

Clinical Findings: Heterotopic neuroglial tissue occurs as a solitary, firm, papule, often vascular appearing, most commonly in or on the nose but also can be present on the face, scalp, lip, tongue, oropharynx, nasopharynx, or orbit.

Histopathology: There are various admixtures of neurons, astrocytes, oligodendrocytes, ependyma, and choroid plexus. There may be significant fibrosis, which can obscure the neuroglial component[139,140]

Differential Diagnosis: Differential diagnosis of neuroglial heterotopia includes encephalocele, dermoid cyst, hemangioma, intracranial astrocytoma or meningioma with nasal extension, lymphatic malformation, lymphoma/plasmacytoma, and carcinoid tumor.

Clinical Course and Prognosis: Neuroglial heterotopias can be connected to the intracranial cavity, and therefore CT and/or MRI of the head is imperative before biopsy or excision. In one small series, 3 of 10 patients had lesions that extended into the intracranial cavity.[141]

Management: Surgical excision is the treatment of choice.

MENINGEAL HETEROTOPIA

AT-A-GLANCE

- Rare lesion characterized by meningothelial elements in skin.
- Occurs in children secondary to developmental defect; occurs in adults secondary to extension of intracranial meningioma.
- Can be connected to intracranial cavity.

Epidemiology: Heterotopic meningeal tissue is a rare condition that presents most commonly in the neonatal period but also can be seen in adults. Rare familial cases have been reported.[142,143]

Etiology and Pathogenesis: Meningeal heterotopia is characterized by meningothelial elements

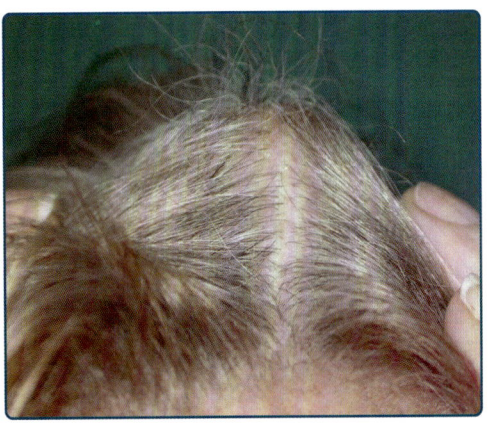

Figure 121-34 Meningeal heterotopia in adulthood: Slowly enlarging nodule on the scalp of a 67-year-old woman with an evolution period of 10 years. (Image from the collection of Mar Llamas-Velasco, MD, Hospital Universitario de La Princesa, Madrid, Spain. Used with permission.)

present in the skin.[142] This condition is also known as *cutaneous meningioma, rudimentary meningocele, acroleic meningocele,* and *meningeal hamartoma.* In adults, these lesions usually represent cutaneous or subcutaneous extension of an aggressive intracranial meningioma and are commonly referred to as cutaneous meningiomas. In children, they are often referred to as rudimentary meningoceles and most likely represent a developmental defect related to abnormal attachment and closure of the neural tube during embryogenesis. There is evidence to suggest that rudimentary meningoceles represent an atretic form of a meningocele.[142] Some lesions may contain a central lumen and be connected to the dura by a fibrous band running through a skull or vertebral defect.

Clinical Findings: Meningeal heterotopia typically presents as a skin-colored nodule on the scalp over the midline or along the spine (Fig. 121-34). In children, they can be associated with the "hair collar" sign, in which a ring of long, dark, coarse hair surrounds a midline scalp nodule (Fig. 121-35). In adults with cutaneous meningiomas, the intracranial component itself surprisingly may cause few neurologic symptoms, and patients may actually present because of an enlarging nodule on their scalp.

Histopathology: Microscopic examination reveals a mass composed of meningothelial elements in the superficial and deep dermis surrounded by dense collagen bundles.[142] The meningothelial cells contain round nuclei with stippled chromatin and clear cytoplasm.[143] Occasionally, a whorled pattern can be observed. Psammoma bodies, collagen bodies, and calcification are variably present.[142,143]

Differential Diagnosis: Differential diagnosis of meningeal heterotopia includes meningocele, encephalocele, aplasia cutis, and epidermal/pilar cyst.

Clinical Course and Prognosis: These lesions can be connected to the intracranial cavity, and, therefore, radiographic imaging is necessary before any invasive procedure such as biopsy or excision.

Management: The treatment of choice is surgical excision.

CUTANEOUS GANGLIONEUROMA AND GANGLION CELL TUMOR

Ganglioneuromas are neoplasms composed of mature ganglion cells, that are usually intermingled with fascicles of spindle cells of Schwann cell origin. Pure ganglion cell tumors do not contain the Schwann cell component. They are usually seen as deep-seated tumors of the autonomic nervous system. Primary cutaneous ganglioneuromas are exceedingly rare. The majority develops after birth. Clinically, they present as nondescript small papules or nodules. Of the half dozen or so reported cases,[144,145] only 1 case was congenital. These lesions have to be distinguished from cutaneous metastases from a neuroblastoma, which can mature into ganglioneuroma. Furthermore, some plexiform neurofibromas in patients with neurofibromatosis arise in autonomic ganglia and can therefore contain residual, entrapped ganglion cells.[146]

MYXOPAPILLARY EPENDYMOMA

Myxopapillary ependymoma is a peculiar variant of ependymoma that typically arises intradurally from the filum terminale of the spinal cord. However, histologically identical lesions also rarely occur as primary extradural tumors of the sacrococcygeal soft tissue, where they present as subcutaneous masses. They are thought to arise from subcutaneous ependymal rests, which are quite common in this region.[147] These tumors generally present in young patients as a sacrococcygeal or, more rarely, a gluteal mass that is asymptomatic in most cases and can reach a size of several centimeters. Histologically, they are composed of papillae covered by ependymal cells. The cores of the papillae contain abundant myxoid ground substance, hence the name. Although intradural myxopapillary ependymomas are usually benign, the subcutaneous type is more aggressive with a significant risk of local recurrence and even metastasis.[147]

REFERENCES

1. Holst VA, Junkins-Hopkins JM, Elenitsas R. Cutaneous smooth muscle neoplasms: clinical features, histologic findings, and treatment options. *J Am Acad Dermatol*. 2002;46:477-490; quiz, 491-494.
2. Burden PA, Gentry RH, Fitzpatrick JE. Piloleiomyoma arising in an organoid nevus: a case report and review of the literature. *J Dermatol Surg Oncol*. 1987;13:1213-1218.
3. Hornick JL, Fletcher CD. Criteria for malignancy in nonvisceral smooth muscle tumors. *Ann Diagn Pathol*. 2003;7:60-66.
4. Miettinen M. Smooth muscle tumors of soft tissue and non-uterine viscera: biology and prognosis. *Mod Pathol*. 2014;27(suppl 1):S17-S29.
5. Iwata J, Fletcher CD. Immunohistochemical detection of cytokeratin and epithelial membrane antigen in leiomyosarcoma: a systematic study of 100 cases. *Pathol Int*. 2000;50:7-14.
6. Swanson PE, Stanley MW, Scheithauer BW, et al. Primary cutaneous leiomyosarcoma. A histological and immunohistochemical study of 9 cases, with ultrastructural correlation. *J Cutan Pathol*. 1988;15:129-141.
7. Orellana-Diaz O, Hernandez-Perez E. Leiomyoma cutis and leiomyosarcoma: a 10-year study and a short review. *J Dermatol Surg Oncol*. 1983;9:283-287.
8. Yokoyama R, Hashimoto H, Daimaru Y, et al. Superficial leiomyomas. A clinicopathologic study of 34 cases. *Acta Pathol Jpn*. 1987;37:1415-1422.
9. Henderson CA, Ruban E, Porter DI. Multiple leiomyomata presenting in a child. *Pediatr Dermatol*. 1997;14:287-289.
10. Thyresson HN, Su WP. Familial cutaneous leiomyomatosis. *J Am Acad Dermatol*. 1981;4:430-434.
11. Tomlinson IP, Alam NA, Rowan AJ, et al. Germline mutations in FH predispose to dominantly inherited uterine fibroids, skin leiomyomata and papillary renal cell cancer. *Nat Genet*. 2002;30:406-410.
12. Martinez-Mir A, Gordon D, Horev L, et al. Multiple cutaneous and uterine leiomyomas: refinement of the genetic locus for multiple cutaneous and uterine leiomyomas on chromosome 1q42.3-43. *J Invest Dermatol*. 2002;118:876-880.
13. Chuang GS, Martinez-Mir A, Engler DE, et al. Multiple cutaneous and uterine leiomyomata resulting from

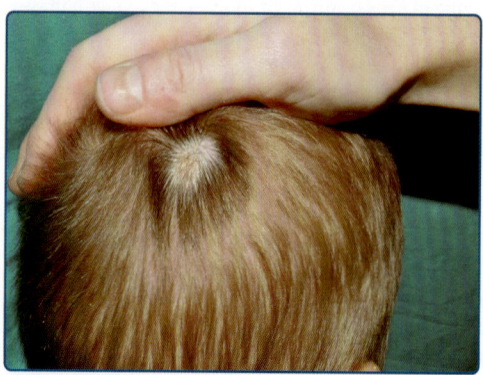

Figure 121-35 Meningeal heterotopia in childhood: A hairless patch on the scalp of an infant with the "hair collar" sign, present since birth. (Image from the collection of Antonio Torrelo, MD, Department of Pediatric Dermatology, Hospital del Niño Jesús, Madrid, Spain. Used with permission.)

missense mutations in the fumarate hydratase gene. *Clin Exp Dermatol.* 2006;31:118-121.
14. Varol A, Stapleton K, Roscioli T. The syndrome of hereditary leiomyomatosis and renal cell cancer (HLRCC): the clinical features of an individual with a fumarate hydratase gene mutation. *Australas J Dermatol.* 2006;47:274-276.
15. Reed WB, Walker R, Horowitz R. Cutaneous leiomyomata with uterine leiomyomata. *Acta Derm Venereol.* 1973;53:409-416.
16. Launonen V, Vierimaa O, Kiuru M, et al. Inherited susceptibility to uterine leiomyomas and renal cell cancer. *Proc Natl Acad Sci U S A.* 2001;98:3387-3392.
17. Toro JR, Nickerson ML, Wei MH, et al. Mutations in the fumarate hydratase gene cause hereditary leiomyomatosis and renal cell cancer in families in North America. *Am J Hum Genet.* 2003;73:95-106.
18. Alam NA, Barclay E, Rowan AJ, et al. Clinical features of multiple cutaneous and uterine leiomyomatosis: an underdiagnosed tumor syndrome. *Arch Dermatol.* 2005;141:199-206.
19. Stout AP. Solitary cutaneous and subcutaneous leiomyoma. *Am J Cancer.* 1937:435-469.
20. Agarwalla A, Thakur A, Jacob M, et al. Zosteriform and disseminated lesions in cutaneous leiomyoma. *Acta Derm Venereol.* 2000;80:446.
21. Fisher WC, Helwig EB. Leiomyomas of the skin. *Arch Dermatol.* 1963;88:510.
22. Konig A, Happle R. Type 2 segmental cutaneous leiomyomatosis. *Acta Derm Venereol.* 2001;81:383.
23. Newman PL, Fletcher CD. Smooth muscle tumours of the external genitalia: clinicopathological analysis of a series. *Histopathology.* 1991;18:523-529.
24. Gutmann J, Cifuentes C, Balzarini MA, et al. Angiomyoma of the oral cavity. *Oral Surg Oral Med Oral Pathol.* 1974;38:269-273.
25. Llamas-Velasco M, Requena L, Kutzner H, et al. Fumarate hydratase immunohistochemical staining may help to identify patients with multiple cutaneous and uterine leiomyomatosis (MCUL) and hereditary leiomyomatosis and renal cell cancer (HLRCC) syndrome. *J Cutan Pathol.* 2014;41:859-865.
26. Harrison WJ, Andrici J, Maclean F, et al. Fumarate hydratase-deficient uterine leiomyomas occur in both the syndromic and sporadic settings. *Am J Surg Pathol.* 2016;40:599-607.
27. Tavassoli FA, Norris HJ. Smooth muscle tumors of the vulva. *Obstet Gynecol.* 1979;53:213-217.
28. Menko FH, Maher ER, Schmidt LS, et al. Hereditary leiomyomatosis and renal cell cancer (HLRCC): renal cancer risk, surveillance and treatment. *Fam Cancer.* 2014;13:637-644.
29. Christenson LJ, Smith K, Arpey CJ. Treatment of multiple cutaneous leiomyomas with CO2 laser ablation. *Dermatol Surg.* 2000;26:319-322.
30. Fernandez-Pugnaire MA, Delgado-Florencio V. Familial multiple cutaneous leiomyomas. *Dermatology.* 1995;191:295-298.
31. Tiffee JC, Budnick SD. Multiple cutaneous leiomyomas. Report of a case. *Oral Surg Oral Med Oral Pathol.* 1993;76:716-717.
32. Batchelor RJ, Lyon CC, Highet AS. Successful treatment of pain in two patients with cutaneous leiomyomata with the oral alpha-1 adrenoceptor antagonist, doxazosin. *Br J Dermatol.* 2004;150:775-776.
33. Alam M, Rabinowitz AD, Engler DE. Gabapentin treatment of multiple piloleiomyoma-related pain. *J Am Acad Dermatol.* 2002;46(2)(suppl case reports):S27-S29.
34. Onder M, Adisen E. A new indication of botulinum toxin: leiomyoma-related pain. *J Am Acad Dermatol.* 2009;60:325-328.
35. Kraft S, Fletcher CD. Atypical intradermal smooth muscle neoplasms: clinicopathologic analysis of 84 cases and a reappraisal of cutaneous "leiomyosarcoma." *Am J Surg Pathol.* 2011;35:599-607.
36. Massi D, Franchi A, Alos L, et al. Primary cutaneous leiomyosarcoma: clinicopathological analysis of 36 cases. *Histopathology.* 2010;56:251-262.
37. Laskin WB, Silverman TA, Enzinger FM. Postradiation soft tissue sarcomas. An analysis of 53 cases. *Cancer.* 1988;62:2330-2340.
38. Francis JH, Kleinerman RA, Seddon JM, Abramson DH. Increased risk of secondary uterine leiomyosarcoma in hereditary retinoblastoma. *Gynecol Oncol.* 2012;124:254-259.
39. Panelos J, Beltrami G, Scoccianti G, et al. Prognostic significance of the alterations of the G1-S checkpoint in localized leiomyosarcoma of the peripheral soft tissue. *Ann Surg Oncol.* 2011;18:566-571.
40. Kaddu S, Beham A, Cerroni L, et al. Cutaneous leiomyosarcoma. *Am J Surg Pathol.* 1997;21:979-987.
41. Diaz-Cascajo C, Borghi S, Weyers W. Desmoplastic leiomyosarcoma of the skin. *Am J Dermatopathol.* 2000;22:251-255.
42. Watanabe K, Kusakabe T, Hoshi N, et al. h-Caldesmon in leiomyosarcoma and tumors with smooth muscle cell-like differentiation: its specific expression in the smooth muscle cell tumor. *Hum Pathol.* 1999; 30:392-396.
43. Miettinen M. Immunoreactivity for cytokeratin and epithelial membrane antigen in leiomyosarcoma. *Arch Pathol Lab Med.* 1988;112:637-640.
44. Matsuyama A, Hisaoka M, Hashimoto H. Vascular leiomyosarcoma: clinicopathology and immunohistochemistry with special reference to a unique smooth muscle phenotype. *Pathol Int.* 2010;60:212-216.
45. Fields JP, Helwig EB. Leiomyosarcoma of the skin and subcutaneous tissue. *Cancer.* 1981;47:156-169.
46. Jensen ML, Jensen OM, Michalski W, et al. Intradermal and subcutaneous leiomyosarcoma: a clinicopathological and immunohistochemical study of 41 cases. *J Cutan Pathol.* 1996;23:458-463.
47. Dahl I, Angervall L. Cutaneous and subcutaneous leiomyosarcoma. A clinicopathologic study of 47 patients. *Pathol Eur.* 1974;9:307-315.
48. Auroy S, Contesso G, Spatz A, et al. Primary cutaneous leiomyosarcoma: 32 cases [in French]. *Ann Dermatol Venereol.* 1999;126:235-242.
49. Stokes JH. Nevus pilaris with hyperplasia of nonstriated muscle. *Arch Dermatol Syph.* 1923;7:479.
50. Zvulunov A, Rotem A, Merlob P, et al. Congenital smooth muscle hamartoma. Prevalence, clinical findings, and follow-up in 15 patients. *Am J Dis Child.* 1990;144:782-784.
51. Gerdsen R, Lagarde C, Steen A, et al. Congenital smooth muscle hamartoma of the skin: clinical classification. *Acta Derm Venereol.* 1999;79:408-409.
52. Jang HS, Kim MB, Oh CK, et al. Linear congenital smooth muscle hamartoma with follicular spotted appearance. *Br J Dermatol.* 2000;142:138-142.
53. de la Espriella J, Grossin M, Marinho E, et al. Smooth muscle hamartoma: anatomoclinical charac-

54. Schnur RE, Herzberg AJ, Spinner N, et al. Variability in the Michelin tire syndrome. A child with multiple anomalies, smooth muscle hamartoma, and familial paracentric inversion of chromosome 7q. *J Am Acad Dermatol*. 1993;28:364-370.
55. Kawada H, Kawada J, Iwahara K, et al. Multiple cutaneous rhabdomyomas in a child. *Eur J Dermatol*. 2004;14:418-420.
56. Harding CO, Pagon RA. Incidence of tuberous sclerosis in patients with cardiac rhabdomyoma. *Am J Med Genet*. 1990;37:443-446.
57. Nir A, Tajik AJ, Freeman WK, et al. Tuberous sclerosis and cardiac rhabdomyoma. *Am J Cardiol*. 1995; 76:419-421.
58. Yang S, Zhao C, Zhang Y, et al. Mediastinal fetal rhabdomyoma in nevoid basal cell carcinoma syndrome: a case report and review of the literature. *Virchows Arch*. 2011;459:235-238.
59. Kapadia SB, Meis JM, Frisman DM, et al. Adult rhabdomyoma of the head and neck: a clinicopathologic and immunophenotypic study. *Hum Pathol*. 1993;24:608-617.
60. Kapadia SB, Meis JM, Frisman DM, et al. Fetal rhabdomyoma of the head and neck: a clinicopathologic and immunophenotypic study of 24 cases. *Hum Pathol*. 1993;24:754-765.
61. Dasgupta R, Rodeberg DA. Update on rhabdomyosarcoma. *Semin Pediatr Surg*. 2012;21:68-78.
62. Hawkins WG, Hoos A, Antonescu CR, et al. Clinicopathologic analysis of patients with adult rhabdomyosarcoma. *Cancer*. 2001;91:794-803.
63. Ruymann FB, Maddux HR, Ragab A, et al. Congenital anomalies associated with rhabdomyosarcoma: an autopsy study of 115 cases. A report from the Intergroup Rhabdomyosarcoma Study Committee (representing the Children's Cancer Study Group, the Pediatric Oncology Group, the United Kingdom Children's Cancer Study Group, and the Pediatric Intergroup Statistical Center). *Med Pediatr Oncol*. 1988;16:33-39.
64. Anderson J, Gordon A, McManus A, et al. Disruption of imprinted genes at chromosome region 11p15.5 in paediatric rhabdomyosarcoma. *Neoplasia*. 1999;1:340-348.
65. Mercado GE, Barr FG. Fusions involving PAX and FOX genes in the molecular pathogenesis of alveolar rhabdomyosarcoma: recent advances. *Curr Mol Med*. 2007;7:47-61.
66. Parham DM, Qualman SJ, Teot L, et al. Correlation between histology and PAX/FKHR fusion status in alveolar rhabdomyosarcoma: a report from the Children's Oncology Group. *Am J Surg Pathol*. 2007;31:895-901.
67. Wang NP, Marx J, McNutt MA, et al. Expression of myogenic regulatory proteins (myogenin and MyoD1) in small blue round cell tumors of childhood. *Am J Pathol*. 1995;147:1799-1810.
68. Folpe AL, Hill CE, Parham DM, et al. Immunohistochemical detection of FLI-1 protein expression: a study of 132 round cell tumors with emphasis on CD99-positive mimics of Ewing's sarcoma/primitive neuroectodermal tumor. *Am J Surg Pathol*. 2000;24:1657-1662.
69. Newton WA Jr, Gehan EA, Webber BL, et al. Classification of rhabdomyosarcomas and related sarcomas. Pathologic aspects and proposal for a new classification—an Intergroup Rhabdomyosarcoma Study. *Cancer*. 1995;76:1073-1085.
70. Hendrick SJ, Sanchez RL, Blackwell SJ, et al. Striated muscle hamartoma: description of two cases. *Pediatr Dermatol*. 1986;3:153-157.
71. Mills AE. Rhabdomyomatous mesenchymal hamartoma of skin. *Am J Dermatopathol*. 1989;11:58-63.
72. Maher CO, Spinner RJ, Giannini C, et al. Neuromuscular choristoma of the sciatic nerve. Case report. *J Neurosurg*. 2002;96:1123-1126.
73. Antonescu C, Scheithauer BW, Woodruff JM. *Tumors of the Peripheral Nervous System Atlas of Tumor Pathology, 4th series, Fascicle 19*. Washington, DC: Armed Forces Institute of Pathology, 2013:1-553.
74. Pina-Oviedo S, Ortiz-Hidalgo C. The normal and neoplastic perineurium: a review. *Adv Anat Pathol*. 2008;15:147-164.
75. Schley MT, Wilms P, Toepfner S, et al. Painful and nonpainful phantom and stump sensations in acute traumatic amputees. *J Trauma*. 2008;65:858-864.
76. van der Avoort DJ, Hovius SE, Selles RW, et al. The incidence of symptomatic neuroma in amputation and neurorrhaphy patients. *J Plast Reconstr Aesthet Surg*. 2013;66:1330-1334.
77. Mathews GJ, Osterholm JL. Painful traumatic neuromas. *Surg Clin North Am*. 1972;52:1313-1324.
78. Reed ML, Jacoby RA. Cutaneous neuroanatomy and neuropathology. Normal nerves, neural-crest derivatives, and benign neural neoplasms in the skin. *Am J Dermatopathol*. 1983;5:335-362.
79. Vernadakis AJ, Koch H, Mackinnon SE. Management of neuromas. *Clin Plast Surg*. 2003;30:247-268, vii.
80. Upjohn E, Barlow R, Robson A. Rudimentary polydactyly in an adult: an unusual presentation to a dermatological surgery unit. *Australas J Dermatol*. 2006;47:206-208.
81. Brehmer-Andersson EE. Penile neuromas with multiple Meissner's corpuscles. *Histopathology*. 1999; 34:555-556.
82. Leber GE, Gosain AK. Surgical excision of pedunculated supernumerary digits prevents traumatic amputation neuromas. *Pediatr Dermatol*. 2003;20:108-112.
83. Reed RJ, Fine RM, Meltzer HD. Palisaded, encapsulated neuromas of the skin. *Arch Dermatol*. 1972; 106:865-870.
84. Dakin MC, Leppard B, Theaker JM. The palisaded, encapsulated neuroma (solitary circumscribed neuroma). *Histopathology*. 1992;20:405-410.
85. Jokinen CH, Ragsdale BD, Argenyi ZB. Expanding the clinicopathologic spectrum of palisaded encapsulated neuroma. *J Cutan Pathol*. 2010;37:43-48.
86. Argenyi ZB, Cooper PH, Santa Cruz D. Plexiform and other unusual variants of palisaded encapsulated neuroma. *J Cutan Pathol*. 1993;20:34-39.
87. Albrecht S, Kahn HJ, From L. Palisaded encapsulated neuroma: an immunohistochemical study. *Mod Pathol*. 1989;2:403-406.
88. Fletcher CD. Solitary circumscribed neuroma of the skin (so-called palisaded, encapsulated neuroma). A clinicopathologic and immunohistochemical study. *Am J Surg Pathol*. 1989;13:574-580.
89. Marx SJ. Multiple endocrine neoplasia. In Melmed S, Polonsky KS, Larson PR, Kronenberg HM, eds. *Williams Textbook of Endocrinology*. 12th ed. Philadelphia, PA: Elsevier Saunders; 2011:1728-1767.

90. Moline J, Eng C. Multiple endocrine neoplasia type 2: an overview. *Genet Med.* 2011;13:755-764.
91. Pujol RM, Matias-Guiu X, Miralles J, et al. Multiple idiopathic mucosal neuromas: a minor form of multiple endocrine neoplasia type 2B or a new entity? *J Am Acad Dermatol.* 1997;37:349-352.
92. Schaffer JV, Kamino H, Witkiewicz A, et al. Mucocutaneous neuromas: an underrecognized manifestation of PTEN hamartoma-tumor syndrome. *Arch Dermatol.* 2006;142:625-632.
93. Antinheimo J, Sankila R, Carpen O, et al. Population-based analysis of sporadic and type 2 neurofibromatosis-associated meningiomas and schwannomas. *Neurology.* 2000;54:71-76.
94. Berg JC, Scheithauer BW, Spinner RJ, et al. Plexiform schwannoma: a clinicopathologic overview with emphasis on the head and neck region. *Hum Pathol.* 2008;39:633-640.
95. Roche PH, Bouvier C, Chinot O, et al. Genesis and biology of vestibular schwannomas. *Prog Neurol Surg.* 2008;21:24-31.
96. Stemmer-Rachamimov AO, Xu L, Gonzalez-Agosti C, et al. Universal absence of merlin, but not other ERM family members, in schwannomas. *Am J Pathol.* 1997;151:1649-1654.
97. Whitaker WG, Droulias C. Benign encapsulated neurilemoma: a report of 76 cases. *Am Surg.* 1976;42:675-678.
98. Hulsebos TJ, Plomp AS, Wolterman RA, et al. Germline mutation of INI1/SMARCB1 in familial schwannomatosis. *Am J Hum Genet.* 2007;80:805-810.
99. Patil S, Perry A, Maccollin M, et al. Immunohistochemical analysis supports a role for INI1/SMARCB1 in hereditary forms of schwannomas, but not in solitary, sporadic schwannomas. *Brain Pathol.* 2008;18:517-519.
100. Joshi R. Learning from eponyms: Jose Verocay and Verocay bodies, Antoni A and B areas, Nils Antoni and schwannomas. *Indian Dermatol Online J.* 2012;3:215-219.
101. Argenyi ZB, Balogh K, Abraham AA. Degenerative ("ancient") changes in benign cutaneous-schwannoma. A light microscopic, histochemical and immunohistochemical study. *J Cutan Pathol.* 1993;20:148-153.
102. Carney JA. Psammomatous melanotic schwannoma. A distinctive, heritable tumor with special associations, including cardiac myxoma and the Cushing syndrome. *Am J Surg Pathol.* 1990;14:206-222.
103. Huson SM, Compston DA, Clark P, et al. A genetic study of von Recklinghausen neurofibromatosis in south east Wales. I. Prevalence, fitness, mutation rate, and effect of parental transmission on severity. *J Med Genet.* 1989;26:704-711.
104. Friedman JM. Epidemiology of neurofibromatosis type 1. *Am J Med Genet.* 1999;89:1-6.
105. Xu GF, Lin B, Tanaka K, et al. The catalytic domain of the neurofibromatosis type 1 gene product stimulates ras GTPase and complements ira mutants of *S. cerevisiae*. *Cell.* 1990;63:835-841.
106. Marchuk DA, Saulino AM, Tavakkol R, et al. cDNA cloning of the type 1 neurofibromatosis gene: complete sequence of the NF1 gene product. *Genomics.* 1991;11:931-940.
107. Murphey MD, Smith WS, Smith SE, et al. From the archives of the AFIP. Imaging of musculoskeletal neurogenic tumors: radiologic-pathologic correlation. *Radiographics.* 1999;19:1253-1280.
108. Williamson DM, Suggit RI. Pigmented neurofibroma. *Br J Dermatol.* 1977;97:685-688.
109. Schaffer JV, Chang MW, Kovich OI, et al. Pigmented plexiform neurofibroma: distinction from a large congenital melanocytic nevus. *J Am Acad Dermatol.* 2007;56:862-868.
110. Michal M, Fanburg-Smith JC, Mentzel T, et al. Dendritic cell neurofibroma with pseudorosettes: a report of 18 cases of a distinct and hitherto unrecognized neurofibroma variant. *Am J Surg Pathol.* 2001;25:587-594.
111. Yeh I, McCalmont TH. Distinguishing neurofibroma from desmoplastic melanoma: the value of the CD34 fingerprint. *J Cutan Pathol.* 2011;38:625-630.
112. McCarron KF, Goldblum JR. Plexiform neurofibroma with and without associated malignant peripheral nerve sheath tumor: a clinicopathologic and immunohistochemical analysis of 54 cases. *Mod Pathol.* 1998;11:612-617.
113. Velez R, Barrera-Ochoa S, Barastegui D, et al. Multidisciplinary management of a giant plexiform neurofibroma by double sequential preoperative embolization and surgical resection. *Case Rep Neurol Med.* 2013;2013:987623.
114. Wise JB, Cryer JE, Belasco JB, et al. Management of head and neck plexiform neurofibromas in pediatric patients with neurofibromatosis type 1. *Arch Otolaryngol Head Neck Surg.* 2005;131:712-718.
115. Gallager RL, Helwig EB. Neurothekeoma—a benign cutaneous tumor of neural origin. *Am J Clin Pathol.* 1980;74:759-764.
116. Fetsch JF, Laskin WB, Miettinen M. Nerve sheath myxoma: a clinicopathologic and immunohistochemical analysis of 57 morphologically distinctive, S-100 protein- and GFAP-positive, myxoid peripheral nerve sheath tumors with a predilection for the extremities and a high local recurrence rate. *Am J Surg Pathol.* 2005;29:1615-1624.
117. Sheth S, Li X, Binder S, et al. Differential gene expression profiles of neurothekeomas and nerve sheath myxomas by microarray analysis. *Mod Pathol.* 2011;24:343-354.
118. Goldstein J, Lifshitz T. Myxoma of the nerve sheath. Report of three cases, observations by light and electron microscopy and histochemical analysis. *Am J Dermatopathol.* 1985;7:423-429.
119. Rosati LA, Fratamico FC, Eusebi V. Cellular neurothekeoma. *Appl Pathol.* 1986;4:186-191.
120. Hornick JL, Fletcher CD. Cellular neurothekeoma: detailed characterization in a series of 133 cases. *Am J Surg Pathol.* 2007;31:329-340.
121. Robson AM, Calonje E. Cutaneous perineurioma: a poorly recognized tumour often misdiagnosed as epithelioid histiocytoma. *Histopathology.* 2000;37:332-339.
122. Sciot R, Dal Cin P, Hagemeijer A, et al. Cutaneous sclerosing perineurioma with cryptic NF2 gene deletion. *Am J Surg Pathol.* 1999;23:849-853.
123. Emory TS, Scheithauer BW, Hirose T, et al. Intraneural perineurioma. A clonal neoplasm associated with abnormalities of chromosome 22. *Am J Clin Pathol.* 1995;103:696-704.
124. Mentzel T, Dei Tos AP, Fletcher CD. Perineurioma (storiform perineurial fibroma): clinico-pathological analysis of four cases. *Histopathology.* 1994;25:261-267.

125. Tsang WY, Chan JK, Chow LT, et al. Perineurioma: an uncommon soft tissue neoplasm distinct from localized hypertrophic neuropathy and neurofibroma. *Am J Surg Pathol.* 1992;16:756-763.
126. Goldblum JR, Folpe AL, Weiss SW, eds. *Enzinger and Weiss's Soft Tissue Tumors.* 6th ed. Philadelphia, PA: Saunders/Elsevier; 2014.
127. Evans DG, Baser ME, McGaughran J, et al. Malignant peripheral nerve sheath tumours in neurofibromatosis 1. *J Med Genet.* 2002;39:311-314.
128. De Raedt T, Brems H, Wolkenstein P, et al. Elevated risk for MPNST in NF1 microdeletion patients. *Am J Hum Genet.* 2003;72:1288-1292.
129. Woodruff JM, Selig AM, Crowley K, et al. Schwannoma (neurilemoma) with malignant transformation. A rare, distinctive peripheral nerve tumor. *Am J Surg Pathol.* 1994;18:882-895.
130. Pekmezci M, Reuss DE, Hirbe AC, et al. Morphologic and immunohistochemical features of malignant peripheral nerve sheath tumors and cellular schwannomas. *Mod Pathol.* 2015;28:187-200.
131. Wesche WA, Khare VK, Chesney TM, et al. Nonhematopoietic cutaneous metastases in children and adolescents: thirty years experience at St. Jude Children's Research Hospital. *J Cutan Pathol.* 2000;27:485-492.
132. Hashimoto H, Enjoji M, Nakajima T, et al. Malignant neuroepithelioma (peripheral neuroblastoma). A clinicopathologic study of 15 cases. *Am J Surg Pathol.* 1983;7:309-318.
133. Lack EE, Worsham GF, Callihan MD, et al. Granular cell tumor: a clinicopathologic study of 110 patients. *J Surg Oncol.* 1980;13:301-316.
134. Lee J, Bhawan J, Wax F, et al. Plexiform granular cell tumor. A report of two cases. *Am J Dermatopathol.* 1994;16:537-541.
135. Gleason BC, Nascimento AF. HMB-45 and Melan-A are useful in the differential diagnosis between granular cell tumor and malignant melanoma. *Am J Dermatopathol.* 2007;29:22-27.
136. Ordonez NG. Granular cell tumor: a review and update. *Adv Anat Pathol.* 1999;6:186-203.
137. Fanburg-Smith JC, Meis-Kindblom JM, Fante R, et al. Malignant granular cell tumor of soft tissue: diagnostic criteria and clinicopathologic correlation. *Am J Surg Pathol.* 1998;22:779-794.
138. Marina MB, Zurin AR, Muhaizan WM, et al. Heterotopic neuroglial tissue presenting as oral cavity mass with intracranial extension. *Int J Pediatr Otorhinolaryngol.* 2005;69:1587-1590.
139. Argenyi ZB. Cutaneous neural heterotopias and related tumors relevant for the dermatopathologist. *Semin Diagn Pathol.* 1996;13:60-71.
140. Amin A, Monabati A, Kumar PV, et al. Nasal glioma (neuroglial heterotopia) mimicking an astrocytoma: case report. *Ear Nose Throat J.* 2005;84:657-658.
141. Pensler JM, Ivescu AS, Ciletti SJ, et al. Craniofacial gliomas. *Plast Reconstr Surg.* 1996;98:27-30.
142. El Shabrawi-Caelen L, White WL, Soyer HP, et al. Rudimentary meningocele: remnant of a neural tube defect? *Arch Dermatol.* 2001;137:45-50.
143. Miyamoto T, Mihara M, Hagari Y, et al. Primary cutaneous meningioma on the scalp: report of two siblings. *J Dermatol.* 1995;22:611-619.
144. Gambini C, Rongioletti F. Primary congenital cutaneous ganglioneuroma. *J Am Acad Dermatol.* 1996;35:353-354.
145. Hammond RR, Walton JC. Cutaneous ganglioneuromas: a case report and review of the literature. *Hum Pathol.* 1996;27:735-738.
146. Rios JJ, Diaz-Cano SJ, Rivera-Hueto F, et al. Cutaneous ganglion cell choristoma. Report of a case. *J Cutan Pathol.* 1991;18:469-473.
147. Kline MJ, Kays DW, Rojiani AM. Extradural myxopapillary ependymoma: report of two cases and review of the literature. *Pediatr Pathol Lab Med.* 1996;16:813-822.

Chapter 122 :: Lipogenic Neoplasms
:: Thomas Mentzel & Thomas Brenn

第一百二十二章

脂肪源性肿瘤

中文导读

脂肪源性肿瘤是皮肤和软组织中最大的间叶性肿瘤，其中浅层和深层脂肪源性肿瘤在发病率、形态学特征和预后方面存在显著差异，了解这些差异对于避免误诊和治疗失误非常重要。本章分14节：介绍了脂肪瘤、脂肪瘤病、神经脂肪瘤病、浅表脂肪瘤样痣、脂肪母细胞瘤/脂肪母细胞瘤病、血管脂肪瘤、梭形细胞脂肪瘤和多形性脂肪瘤、软骨样脂肪瘤、肌脂瘤、冬眠瘤、不典型脂肪瘤样肿瘤与分化型脂肪肉瘤、去分化脂肪肉瘤、黏液样脂肪肉瘤、多形性脂肪肉瘤的流行病学、临床表现、病因和发病机制、组织学表现、鉴别诊断、临床病程、预后和治疗。

〔粟　娟〕

AT-A-GLANCE

- Lipogenic neoplasms represent the most frequent mesenchymal neoplasms.
- Lipogenic neoplasms include benign neoplasms (eg, lipoma, angiolipoma), intermediate, locally aggressive, nonmetastasizing neoplasms (eg, atypical lipomatous tumor), and clearly malignant lesions (eg, pleomorphic liposarcoma).
- Anatomic site, depth, and size are responsible for striking differences in regard to incidence, morphology, and prognosis.
- The clinical presentation of lipogenic neoplasms is usually nonspecific.
- The majority of lipogenic neoplasms is characterized by distinct cytogenetic abnormalities that may have diagnostic and therapeutic value.
- Surgical excision is the treatment of choice; in cases of malignant neoplasms not amenable for complete excision radiation therapy, however, chemotherapy or target-like therapy may be used.

Although lipogenic neoplasms represent the largest single group of mesenchymal tumors in the skin and in soft tissues, there are significant differences in regard to incidence, morphologic features, and prognosis between superficial and deep-seated lipogenic neoplasms that are important to know to avoid misdiagnosis and therapeutic errors. Whereas liposarcomas in deep soft tissues represent the most common sarcomas in adults, they are exceedingly rare in purely dermal location. Cases of spindle-cell/pleomorphic lipoma arising in the subcutis are encapsulated and occur predominantly in the neck and shoulder region of elderly male patients. In contrast, purely dermal spindle-cell/pleomorphic lipomas are ill-defined, infiltrative lesions that occur equally in both genders and show a broad anatomic distribution. The prognosis of atypical lipomatous tumor ("well-differentiated liposarcoma") is strongly related to site and size of the neoplasms. Cases of atypical lipomatous tumor, arising in the retroperitoneum, intraabdominal, in the mediastinum and in the spermatic cord are associated with a poor clinical prognosis. These neoplasms often achieve a large size, recur repeatedly, and may cause death in a high number of cases as a result of uncontrolled local effects. In striking contrast, cases of atypical lipomatous tumor arising in surgically amenable soft tissue of the extremities usually do not recur after complete excision, and in general superficially located liposarcomas have a relatively good prognosis.

LIPOMA

> **AT-A-GLANCE**
>
> - Lipoma is one of the most common benign mesenchymal neoplasms in adults.
> - Lipomas are composed of mature white adipocytes.
> - Lipomas show varying cytogenetic abnormalities.
> - Although surgical excision is curative, cases of intramuscular lipoma show a higher recurrence rate.

EPIDEMIOLOGY

Lipoma is the most common benign mesenchymal neoplasm and tends to occur in adults without gender predilection. Cases in childhood and multiple lesions are rare.

CLINICAL FEATURES

Lipomas usually present as a painless, slowly growing mass involving the subcutaneous tissue of the trunk, neck, or extremities; involvement of the hands and feet is uncommon. Superficial lipomas are typically small, measuring less than 5 cm. In contrast, deep-seated intramuscular and intermuscular lipomas may reach a considerable size. Parosteal lipoma arises on the surface of bone, and so-called lipoma arborescens represents a villous lipomatous proliferation of the synovial membrane.[1] Lipomas may be seen as a manifestation of Gardner syndrome, and multiple lipomas together with macrocephaly, lymphangiomas, and hemangiomas are noted in Bannayan syndrome (Table 122-1).[2]

ETIOLOGY AND PATHOGENESIS

Lipomas are cytogenetically heterogeneous and the most common abnormalities include aberrations involving 12q13-15, rearrangements involving 6p21-23, and deletions involving 13q.[3] The *HMGA2* gene, localized at 12q14.3, plays an important role in the pathogenesis of some lipomas, and a recombination of *HMGA2* with several genes has been reported.[4]

HISTOLOGIC FEATURES

Classical subcutaneously located lipomas are well-circumscribed, encapsulated and lobulated lesions composed of mature adipocytes with thin and hypocellular fibrous septa containing thin-walled capillaries (Fig. 122-1). There is only slight variation in size and shape of adipocytes and no nuclear atypia is present. Immunohistochemically, tumor cells are negative for p16, MDM2, and CDK4. Cases of lipoma may show posttraumatic changes with fat necrosis and inflammation, and the presence of numerous histiocytes containing enlarged nuclei that show a cytoplasmic staining for p16, MDM2, and CDK4 may mimic features of more aggressive atypical lipomatous tumor. Cases of lipoma may contain abundant fibrous tissue (fibrolipoma), cartilage (chondrolipoma) or bone (osteolipoma) (Fig. 122-2). Purely dermal lipomas are unencapsulated and rather ill-defined lesions (Fig. 122-3), and if sweat ducts and sweat glands are present within the lesion, the term *adenolipoma* has been used. Intramuscular and intermuscular lipomas are ill-defined, infiltrating neoplasms (Fig. 122-4) and preexisting skeletal muscle fibers often show features of atrophy.

DIFFERENTIAL DIAGNOSIS

Angiolipoma is characterized by a variable increased number of blood vessels containing fibrin thrombi,

TABLE 122-1
Syndromes Where Lipogenic Tumors Are Found

SYNDROME	ASSOCIATED TUMORS
Gardner syndrome	Familial adenomatous polyposis, desmoid-fibromatosis, lipomas, osteomas, cysts
Bannayan-Riley-Ruvalcaba syndrome	Macrocephaly, lipomas, lymphangiomas, hamartomas, intestinal polyposis, lentigines
Cowden syndrome	Hamartomas, trichilemmomas, lipomas, oral papillomas, palmoplantar keratoses
Goldenhar-Gorlin syndrome	Intracranial lipomas, hydrocephalus, oculoauriculovertebral dysplasia
Myoclonus epilepsy and ragged-red fibers syndrome	Symmetric lipomas
CLOVE syndrome	Congenital lipomatous overgrowth, vascular malformations, epidermal nevi
Ekbom syndrome	Cervical lipomas, cerebellar ataxia, photomyoclonus, skeletal deformities

and often present as painful multiple lesions. Cases of atypical lipomatous tumor are characterized by striking variations in size and shape of lipogenic cells, and the presence of enlarged and hyperchromatic nuclei. The fibrous septa in atypical lipomatous tumor often contain atypical cells and lipoblasts may be present. Immunohistochemically, a focal expression of p16 is seen in atypical lipomatous tumor, and in a number of cases a focal nuclear staining for MDM2 and CDK4 is present. Fluorescence in situ hybridization (FISH) analysis reveals amplification of *MDM2* and *CDK4* in cases of atypical lipomatous tumor.

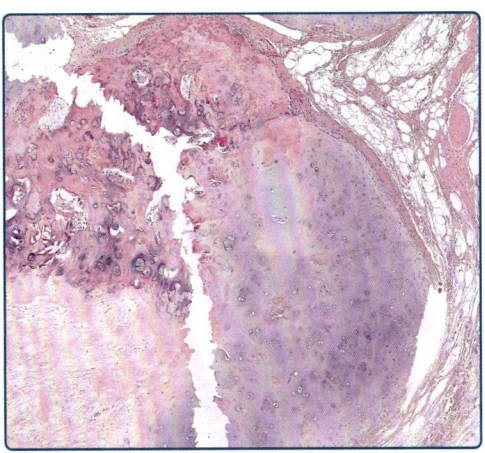

Figure 122-2 Chondrolipoma. An example of lipoma with prominent chondrous metaplasia.

CLINICAL COURSE, PROGNOSIS, AND TREATMENT

Classical lipomas are entirely benign and recur only rarely; in contrast, intramuscular and intermuscular lipoma shows a higher rate of local recurrences (up to 20%).[5] The transition of a preexisting lipoma to an atypical lipomatous tumor represents an exceedingly rare phenomenon.[6] Surgical excision is curative.

LIPOMATOSIS

AT-A-GLANCE

- Lipomatosis is characterized by a diffuse overgrowth of mature adipose tissue infiltrating through preexisting structures.
- Different clinical presentations are known.

EPIDEMIOLOGY AND CLINICAL FINDINGS

Diffuse lipomatosis occurs predominantly in children and rarely in adults. It is characterized by a diffuse overgrowth of mature lipogenic tissue involving subcutaneous tissue and skeletal muscle of the trunk and the extremities; in addition, osseous involvement may be seen. Pelvic lipomatosis is seen more frequently in black males, whereas symmetric lipomatosis (Madelung disease) develops in middle-aged men of Mediterranean origin and has a predilection for the neck, shoulder, and proximal upper limbs. In addition, peripheral neuropathy is a common finding in these patients. HIV-positive patients treated with protease inhibitors may develop lipodystrophy with increased fat tissue at the neck, the breast, and visceral organs, and steroid lipomatosis is seen in patients on hormonal therapy or suffering

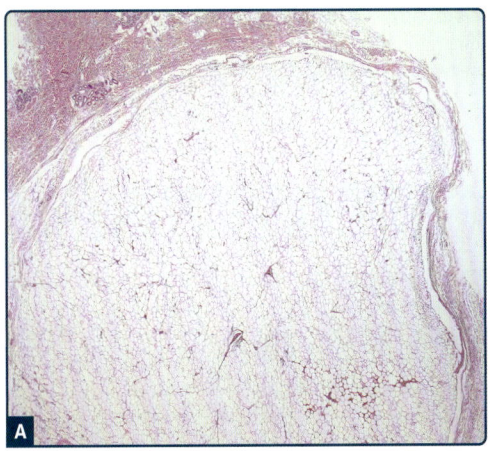
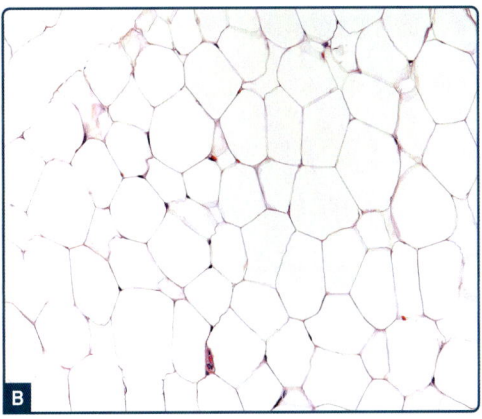

Figure 122-1 Lipoma. Subcutaneously located lipomas are well-circumscribed, often encapsulated lipogenic lesions (**A**), composed of mature univacuolated adipocytes showing only mild variation in size and shape (**B**).

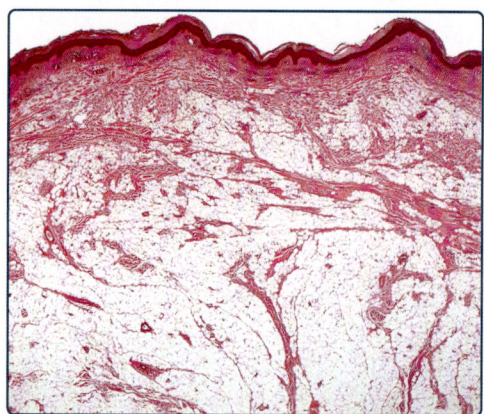

Figure 122-3 Intradermal lipoma. Mature lipogenic cells diffusely infiltrate preexisting dermal collagen bundles.

from increased endogenous production of adrenocortical steroids.

ETIOLOGY AND PATHOGENESIS

Generally, the basic mechanisms in lipomatosis are not well understood; however, an association with mitochondrial dysfunction has been reported, and multiple deletions of mitochondrial DNA, as well as point mutations in mitochondrial genes, have been found.[7]

HISTOLOGIC FEATURES

The gross appearance and the histologic features are the same for all of the different subtypes of lipomatosis. Poorly circumscribed, infiltrating, soft, yellow, fat tissue that is identical to normal fat is seen.

CLINICAL COURSE, PROGNOSIS, AND TREATMENT

Palliative surgical excision of the fat tissue is the treatment of choice; however, all forms of lipomatosis tend to recur, and massive accumulation of fat tissue may cause considerable clinical problems.

LIPOMATOSIS OF NERVE

AT-A-GLANCE

- Lipomatosis of nerve is a rare lesion seen in infants and children.
- Lipomatosis of nerve is a growing mass with a predilection for the hand.
- Lipomatosis of nerve shows a proliferation of adipose and fibrous tissue within the epineurium and perineurium, mainly of the median nerve.

EPIDEMIOLOGY

Lipomatosis of nerve, also known as fibrolipomatous hamartoma of nerve, arises most frequently at birth or in early childhood, and may be associated with macrodactyly of the digits innervated by the affected nerve.[8]

CLINICAL FEATURES

Clinically, the patients present with a slowly growing mass that is often associated with pain, paresthesia, and sensor or motor deficits. The median nerve and its branches, followed by the ulnar nerve, are most commonly affected, whereas an involvement of cranial nerves and the brachial plexus is seen only rarely.[9,10]

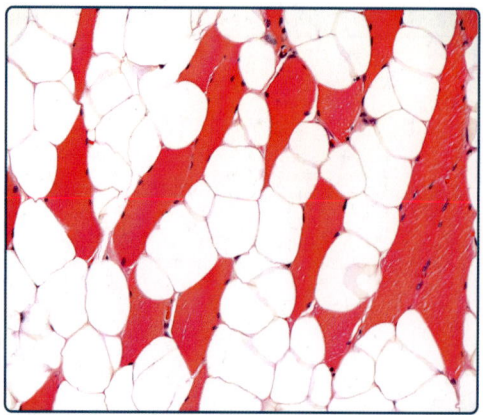

Figure 122-4 Intramuscular lipoma. Mature lipogenic cells show an infiltrative growth pattern within skeletal muscle fibers.

HISTOLOGIC FEATURES

Grossly, a fusiform enlargement of the affected nerve is seen, and histologically, the epineurial and perineurial compartments of the affected nerve are infiltrated by mature adipose tissue and collagenous fibrous tissue (Fig. 122-5). Concentric perineurial fibrosis is present, and, rarely, metaplastic bone formation has been reported.[11]

CLINICAL COURSE, PROGNOSIS, AND TREATMENT

Lipomatosis of nerve is an entirely benign lesion; surgical excision may cause severe damage of the affected nerve.

NEVUS LIPOMATOSIS SUPERFICIALIS

AT-A-GLANCE

- Nevus lipomatosis superficialis (Hoffmann-Zurhelle) represents a rare type of connective tissue nevus that affects children and young adults.
- Nevus lipomatosis superficialis is usually found as a plaque-like, solitary lesion, which arises predominantly at the buttock, lumbar back, and posterior thigh.
- The lesions are composed of mature adipose tissue and connective tissue components.

EPIDEMIOLOGY

Nevus lipomatosus superficialis is a rare form of connective tissue nevus that usually affects children and young adults in the first decades of life with an equal gender distribution.

CLINICAL FEATURES

Cases of nevus lipomatosus superficialis present as plaques, papules, or solitary lesions with a predilection for the buttocks, upper posterior thighs, and lumbar back. A generalized form is extremely rare. The lesions are unilateral, and sometimes a linear or zosteriform arrangement is noted.

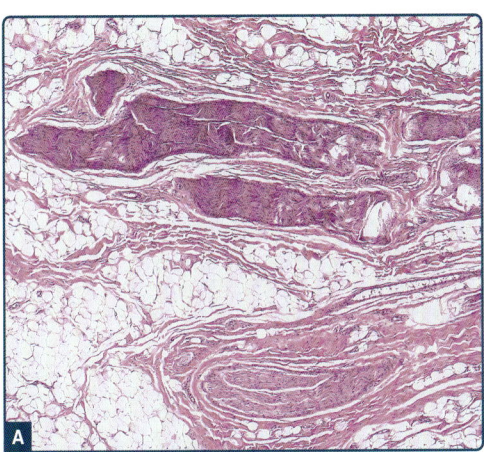
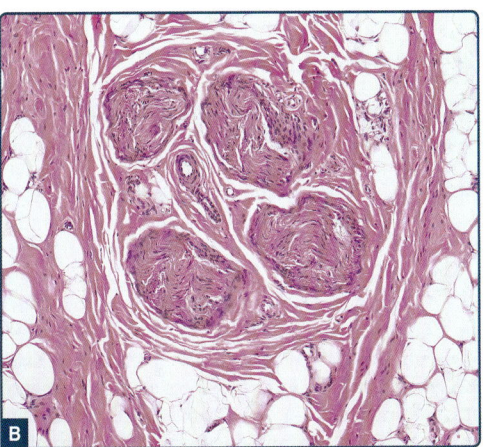

Figure 122-5 Lipomatosis of nerve. **A,** Epineural infiltration of lipogenic cells and collagenous fibrous tissue separating nerve bundles. **B,** Note the perineural fibrosis.

HISTOLOGIC FEATURES

Histologically, the ill-defined lesions are composed of mature adipose tissue that replaces the dermis. In addition, thickening of collagen bundles, as well as an increase of elastic fibers in deeper parts of the dermis and an increase of fibroblasts, may be seen. The overlying epidermis may show slight acanthosis and hyperpigmentation (Fig. 122-6).

DIFFERENTIAL DIAGNOSIS

Rare dermal spindle-cell lipoma is composed of mature adipose tissue associated with bland spindled tumor cells that stain positively for CD34, show loss of Rb-1 expression, and the often myxoid

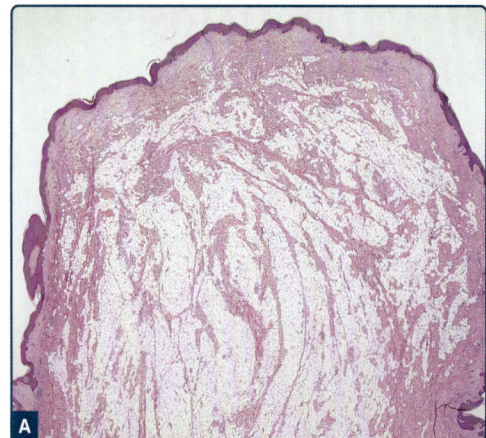

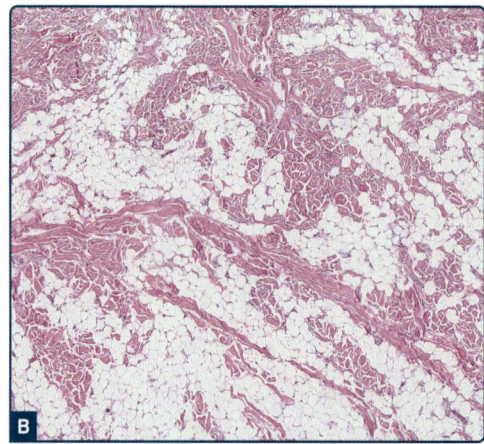

Figure 122-6 Nevus lipomatosus superficialis. Polypoid lesion with diffuse infiltration of the dermis by mature lipogenic cells (**A**), with typically hyalinized collagen bundles (**B**).

stroma contains hyalinized collagen fibers and mast cells.

LIPOBLASTOMA/ LIPOBLASTOMATOSIS

AT-A-GLANCE

- Lipoblastomas/lipoblastomatosis are benign lipogenic neoplasms arising predominantly in infancy and early childhood.
- Lipoblastomas/lipoblastomatosis are well-circumscribed, lobulated lesions composed of lipogenic cells showing a spectrum of maturation from primitive mesenchymal cells and lipoblasts to mature adipocytes.
- Lipoblastomas/lipoblastomatosis show characteristic genetic changes.

EPIDEMIOLOGY

Lipoblastomas/lipoblastomatosis are rare, benign neoplasms of embryonal white fat arising predominantly in infants and young children, with a male predominance.[12-14] Infrequently, tumors are congenital or occur in young adults.[15]

CLINICAL FEATURES

Cases of lipoblastoma/lipoblastomatosis tend to occur on the trunk, at the extremities, and in the head and neck region, whereas visceral involvement and involvement of the retroperitoneum, pelvis, mediastinum, and the abdominal cavity is rarely seen. Most cases present as painless, slowly growing lesions. Lipoblastoma is a rather well-circumscribed neoplasm whereas lipoblastomatosis is characterized by an infiltrative growth that often extends into deeper structures. A significant number of patients have disorders of the CNS, such as seizures, autism, developmental delay, congenital anomalies, and/or Sturge-Weber syndrome.[14]

ETIOLOGY AND PATHOGENESIS

Cytogenetically, the majority of analyzed cases of lipoblastoma/lipoblastomatosis show aberrations involving chromosome 8, and a recurrent translocation involving chromosome band 8q11-13 with rearrangements of the *PLAG1* gene.[16]

HISTOLOGIC FEATURES

Lipoblastoma represents a well-circumscribed, lobulated tumor composed of an admixture of mature and immature lipogenic cells separated by fibrovascular septa (Fig. 122-7). Lobulation is less prominent in cases of lipoblastomatosis that show an infiltrative growth pattern. Lipoblasts are seen in different stages of development, and varying amounts of myxoid stroma with primitive spindled cells and a plexiform vascular pattern (reminiscent of the vascular pattern in myxoid liposarcoma) may be present (Figs. 122-8 and 122-9). Even though some tumors are predominantly composed of mature adipocytes as a manifestation of maturation, the characteristic lobular growth and the presence of fibrous septa are helpful clues for the diagnosis. A fibroblastic proliferation, chondroid metaplasia, or extramedullary hematopoiesis is seen occasionally. The lipogenic cells demonstrate an expression of S-100 protein, PLAG1, and CD34,[14] the spindled cells stain often positively for desmin.[17] Interestingly, cases of

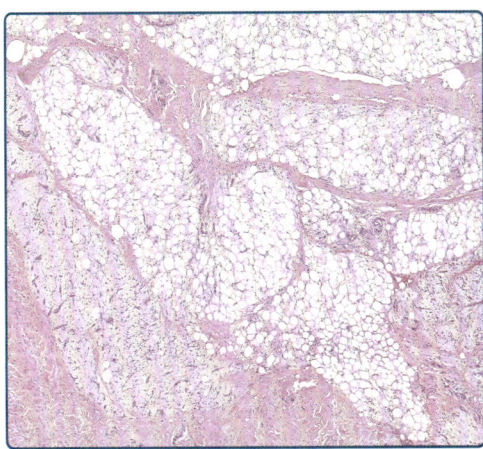

Figure 122-7 Lipoblastoma: lipoblastoma represents a well-circumscribed lipogenic neoplasm showing multi-lobulation and collagenous fibrous septa.

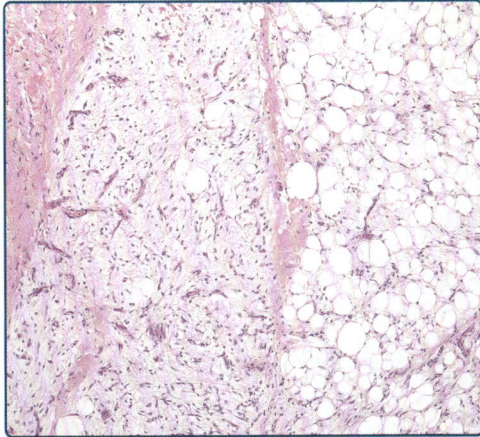

Figure 122-8 Lipoblastoma. Areas of lipogenic cells are admixed with myxoid areas showing a plexiform vascular pattern.

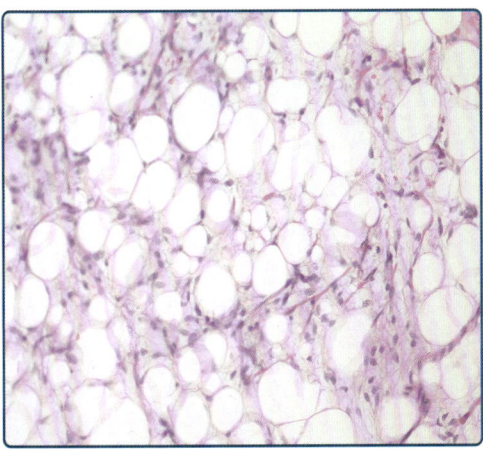

Figure 122-9 Lipoblastoma. Lipogenic cells in different stages of development are present.

lipoblastoma may stain positively for p16, which represents a diagnostic pitfall in the distinction to atypical lipomatous tumor.[18]

DIFFERENTIAL DIAGNOSIS

Myxoid liposarcoma represents one of the most important differential diagnoses of lipoblastoma/lipoblastomatosis; however, this diagnosis in patients younger than 10 years of age is exceedingly rare. In older children, adolescents, and young adults, the differentiation can be quite problematic. A striking lobulation and lack of hyperchromatic nuclei support the diagnosis of lipoblastoma/lipoblastomatosis; in addition, different molecular changes are helpful for the correct diagnosis. Further differential diagnoses include lipoma, lipofibromatosis, hibernoma, and atypical lipomatous tumor. Rare lipoblastoma-like tumor of the vulva arises in adults; the tumor lacks PLAG1 expression and shows loss of Rb-1.[19]

CLINICAL COURSE, PROGNOSIS, AND TREATMENT

Lipoblastoma/lipoblastomatosis has an excellent prognosis despite their potential to invade locally and their considerable size as seen in a number of cases. The reported rate of local recurrences is up to 46%,[14] which is caused by incomplete excision or confined to diffuse-type lesions (lipoblastomatosis). There is no risk of tumor progression, metastasis, or malignant transformation.

ANGIOLIPOMA

AT-A-GLANCE

- Angiolipoma is a common, often painful, entirely benign lipogenic lesion.
- Angiolipoma affects young adults; multiple lesions often are seen.
- Angiolipoma contains a variable number of thin-walled vessels that may contain fibrin thrombi.

EPIDEMIOLOGY

Subcutaneous angiolipomas are frequent mesenchymal tumors that occur predominantly in young males; a familial incidence has been described.[20]

CLINICAL FEATURES

Angiolipomas tend to be multifocal and often present as painful and tender subcutaneous lesions that occur predominantly on the forearm followed by the trunk, upper arm, and legs.

ETIOLOGY AND PATHOGENESIS

In contrast to lipomas, all investigated angiolipomas have had a normal karyotype, and because cases of cellular angiolipoma can be almost exclusively composed of blood vessels, it has been speculated, that these lesions represent hemangiomas instead of lipomas.[21]

HISTOLOGIC FEATURES

Histologically, angiolipomas are well-circumscribed, encapsulated nodular lesions composed of mature adipocytes, a variable number of thin-walled capillaries, which may contain fibrin thrombi, and stromal spindled cells (Figs. 122-10 and 122-11). In cases of cellular angiolipoma the vessels predominate and lipogenic cells may be absent (Fig. 122-12).

DIFFERENTIAL DIAGNOSIS

The presence of fibrin thrombi and clinical features are helpful in the distinction of angiolipoma from cases of lipoma with an increased number of vessels. Cellular angiolipoma has to be distinguished from vascular neoplasms such as Kaposi sarcoma, kaposiform hemangioendothelioma, spindle-cell hemangioma, and angiosarcoma.

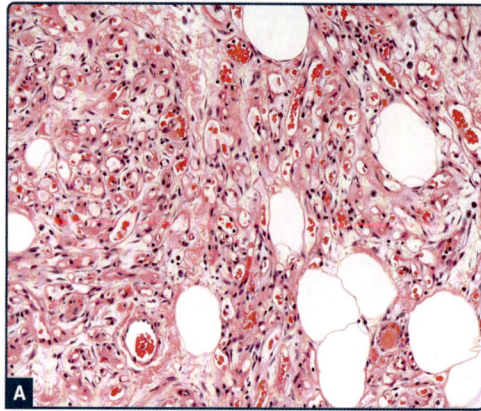
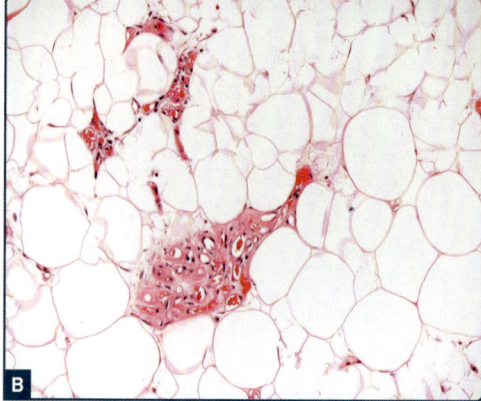

Figure 122-11 Angiolipoma. **A,** Narrow and dilated, thin-walled capillaries are admixed with mature adipocytic tissue. **B,** The adipocytic component can predominate.

CLINICAL COURSE, PROGNOSIS, AND TREATMENT

The clinical behavior of angiolipomas is entirely benign and simple resection is curative.

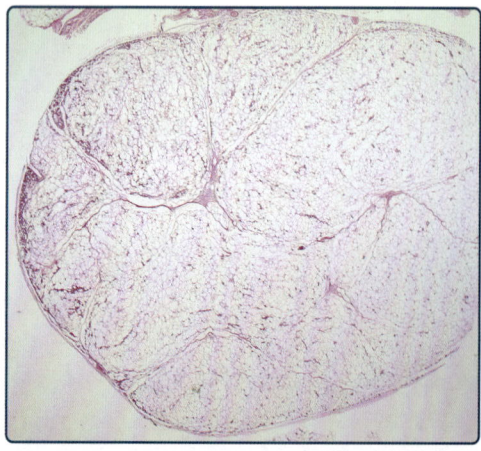

Figure 122-10 Angiolipoma. Low-power view shows an encapsulated, subcutaneously located lipogenic neoplasm with an increased number of vessels in the periphery.

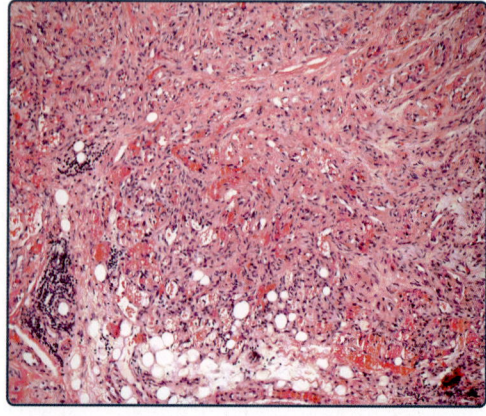

Figure 122-12 Cellular angiolipoma. Predominant vascular component mimicking a vascular neoplasm.

SPINDLE-CELL LIPOMA AND PLEOMORPHIC LIPOMA

AT-A-GLANCE

- Spindle-cell lipoma and pleomorphic lipoma represent a morphologic continuum of a single clinicopathologic entity.
- Spindle-cell lipoma and pleomorphic lipoma are related to mammary myofibroblastoma and cellular angiofibroma.
- Classical cases of spindle-cell lipoma and pleomorphic lipoma occur as encapsulated subcutaneous lesions arising predominantly on the posterior neck, shoulder, and upper back of elderly males.
- Purely dermal spindle cell lipoma and pleomorphic lipoma represent ill-defined, infiltrative lesions, show a broad anatomic distribution, and no gender preference.
- Spindle-cell lipoma is composed of mature adipocytes and CD34+, bland spindled cells; multinucleated, CD34+ giant cells are present in pleomorphic lipoma.
- Atypical spindle cell lipomatous tumor and atypical pleomorphic lipomatous tumor represent intermediate, locally aggressive, nonmetastasizing neoplasms.

EPIDEMIOLOGY

Spindle-cell lipoma and pleomorphic lipoma form a morphologic spectrum of a single clinicopathologic entity with significant clinical, morphologic, and cytogenetic overlap. The majority of these rare neoplasms are seen in elderly males; very rarely have familial spindle-cell lipomas with multiple lesions in the affected patients have been reported.[22] In contrast, purely dermal lipomas show no gender preference.[23]

CLINICAL FEATURES

Spindle-cell lipoma and pleomorphic lipoma usually present as an asymptomatic, often longstanding, mobile tumor in the subcutaneous tissue. The majority of these lesions are seen on the posterior neck, shoulder, and upper back. Infrequently, the face, oral cavity, and extremities are affected.[24,25] Purely dermal spindle-cell lipoma and pleomorphic lipoma show a broad anatomic distribution.[23]

ETIOLOGY AND PATHOGENESIS

The karyotype of spindle-cell and pleomorphic lipomas is complex and frequently hypodiploid with frequent partial losses and few balanced rearrangements. Many cases show monosomy and partial losses involving chromosomes 13 and 16.[3] Given the overlapping clinical, histologic, and molecular features between spindle-cell lipoma, cellular angiofibroma, and mammary-type myofibroblastoma, these tumors probably represent points along a spectrum of a single clinicopathologic entity.[26,27]

HISTOLOGIC FEATURES

Subcutaneous spindle-cell lipoma represents an encapsulated lesion composed of mature adipocytes and a variable number of cytologically bland spindled tumor cells set in a collagenous and myxoid stroma containing blood vessels, hyalinized rope-like collagen fibers and, often, mast cells (Fig. 122-13). Mitotic activity is virtually absent. The spindled cells can predominate, and

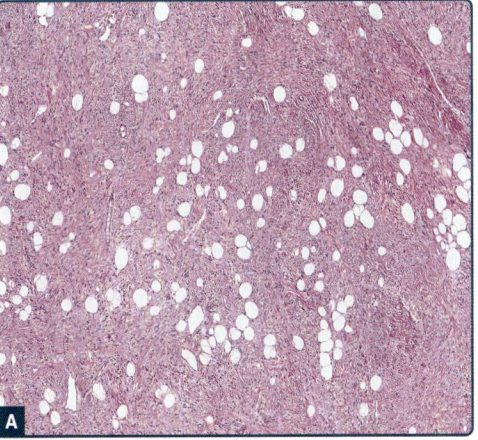

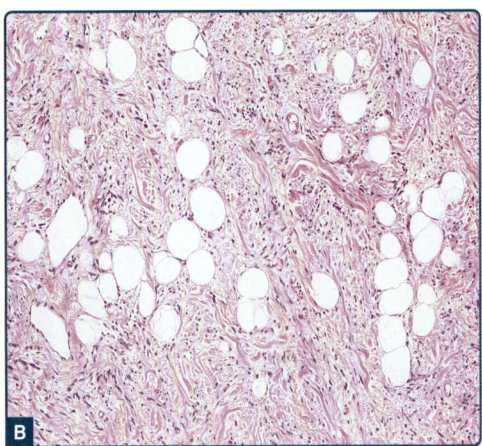

Figure 122-13 Spindle-cell lipoma. **A,** Mature adipocytes are admixed with short, loosely arranged spindled tumor cells. **B,** Hyalinized, rope-like collagen fibers are present.

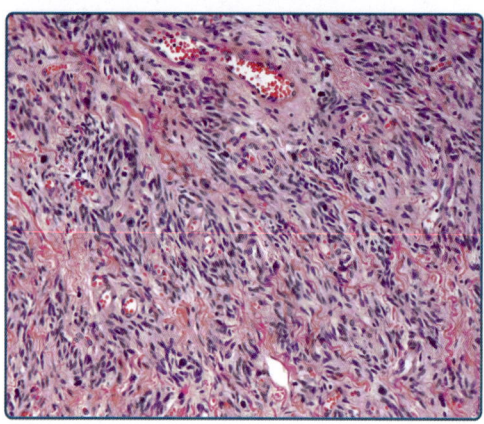

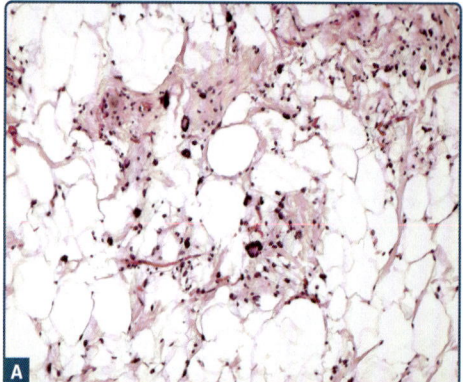

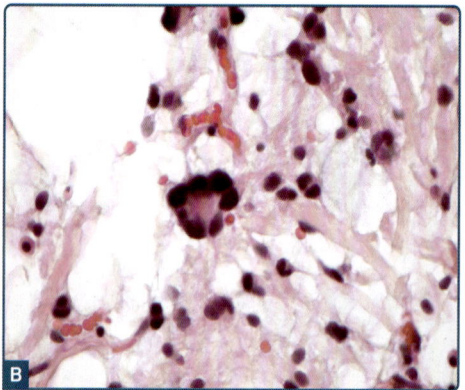

Figure 122-14 Spindle-cell lipoma. The spindled cells can predominate. Note scattered mast cells.

even cases without lipogenic cells have been reported that may cause significant diagnostic problems (Fig. 122-14).[28] Occasionally, prominent myxoid stromal changes are seen, and numerous slit-like spaces resembling vascular channels are present in the so-called pseudoangiomatous variant (Fig. 122-15).[29]

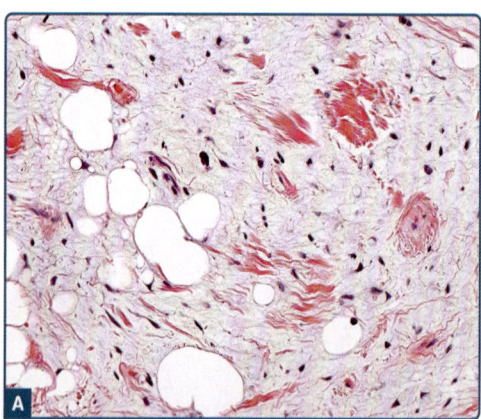

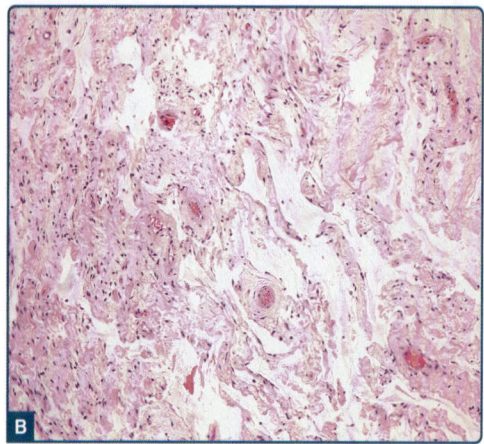

Figure 122-15 Spindle-cell lipoma. **A,** Prominent myxoid stromal changes; note that the tumor cell nuclei are slightly enlarged and hyperchromatic. **B,** Slit-like spaces are seen in the pseudoangiomatous variant.

Figure 122-16 Pleomorphic lipoma. **A,** The characteristic floret-like multinucleated giant cells contain overlapping hyperchromatic nuclei in a circular or semicircular arrangement. **B,** Higher-power view of a floret-like tumor giant cell set in a myxoid stroma with scattered mast cells.

Scattered lipoblasts may be present in otherwise typical cases of spindle-cell lipoma. The characteristic feature of pleomorphic lipoma is the additional presence of multinucleated giant cells with radially arranged nuclei (floret-like giant cells; Fig. 122-16); both low-fat and fat-free pleomorphic lipomas also have been reported.[30] Purely dermal cases of spindle-cell lipoma

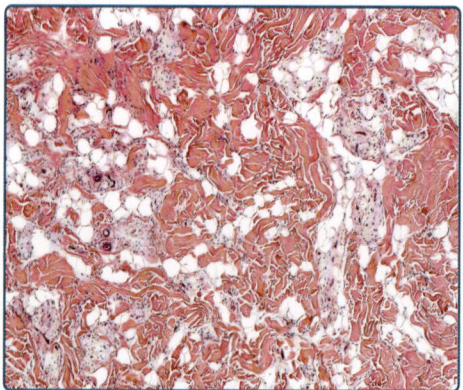

Figure 122-17 Dermal spindle-cell lipoma. Intradermal lesions are less circumscribed and show a diffuse infiltration of preexisting dermal collagen bundles.

and pleomorphic lipoma are in contrast unencapsulated and infiltrative mimicking a more aggressive neoplasm (Fig. 122-17). Infrequently, cases of spindle-cell lipoma and pleomorphic lipoma arise at unusual anatomic sites and show an infiltrative pattern and significant atypia of lipogenic cells, as well as of spindled and pleomorphic giant cells (Fig. 122-18). These cases are designated as atypical spindle cell lipomatous

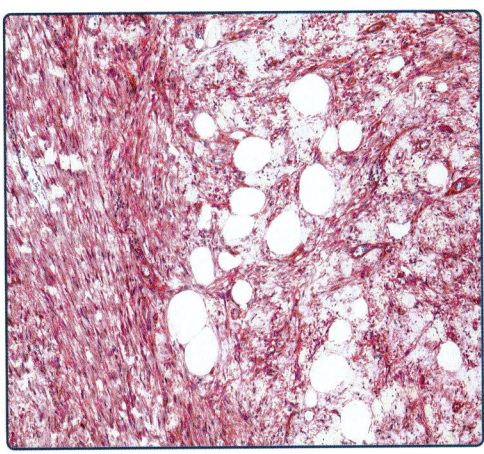

Figure 122-19 Spindle-cell lipoma Tumor cells stain positively for CD34.

tumor and atypical pleomorphic lipomatous tumor, and show a clinical behavior comparable to atypical lipomatous tumor.[31,32,32A,32B] Immunohistochemically, spindled cells and pleomorphic tumor giant cells stain positively for CD34 (Fig. 122-19), and show loss of the expression of Rb-1 (Fig. 122-20).[33] Very rarely an expression of desmin and S-100 protein by spindled cells has been reported.[34,35]

DIFFERENTIAL DIAGNOSIS

Atypical lipomatous tumor shows striking variation of size and shape of the lipogenic cells and significant atypia with the presence of enlarged and hyperchromatic nuclei. In addition, a focal nuclear expression of MDM2 and CDK4 may be seen; FISH analysis reveals *MDM2* and *CDK4* amplification. Cases of solitary fibrous tumor may contain fat cells and tumor cells stain positively for CD34 as well. However, solitary fibrous tumor is characterized by a varying cellularity,

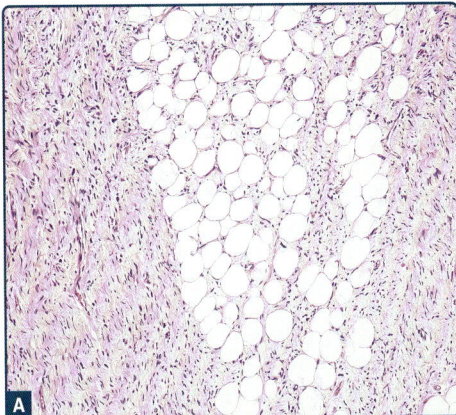

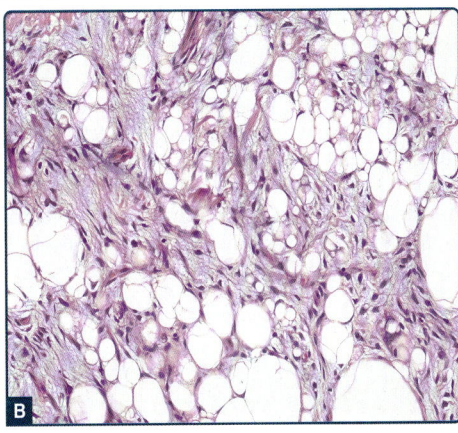

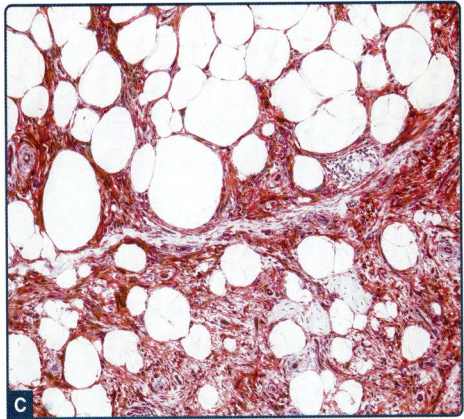

Figure 122-18 Atypical spindle cell lipoma. **A,** An irregular admixture of lipogenic cells with spindle-shaped tumor cells. **B,** Both components show at least sight nuclear atypia with enlarged and hyperchromatic nuclei; in addition lipoblastic cells are noted. **C,** Immunohistochemically, spindled cells stain positively for CD34.

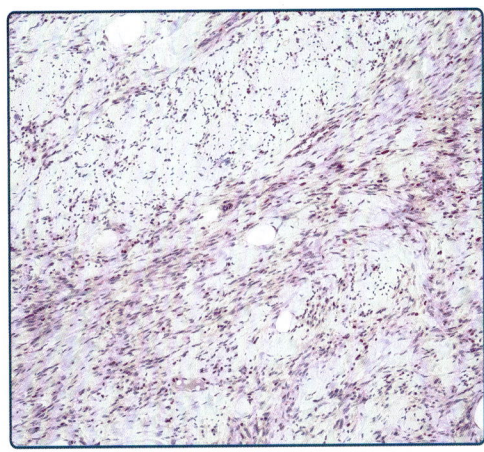

Figure 122-20 Spindle-cell lipoma. Tumor cells show loss of the expression of Rb1.

the presence of hemangiopericytoma-like blood vessels, and tumor cells that show nuclear expression of STAT6. Dermatofibrosarcoma protuberans is composed of CD34+ spindled cells, however, these neoplasms show a diffuse, honey-comb infiltration of the subcutaneous tissue and different genetic changes.

CLINICAL COURSE, PROGNOSIS, AND TREATMENT

Spindle-cell and pleomorphic lipomas are entirely benign, although local recurrences occur rarely. Cases of atypical spindle cell lipomatous tumor and pleomorphic lipomatous tumor are locally aggressive neoplasms and show an increased rate of local recurrences.[31,32]

CHONDROID LIPOMA

AT-A-GLANCE

- Chondroid lipoma represents a rare benign lipogenic neoplasm.
- Chondroid lipoma is seen more frequently in female patients.
- Chondroid lipoma arises predominantly in deep soft tissues of the extremities.
- Chondroid lipoma is composed of adipocytes, lipoblasts, and small vacuolated cells.
- Tumor cells in chondroid lipoma are set in a myxoid–chondroid matrix.
- A recurrent t(11;16)(q13;p13) is seen in cases of chondroid lipoma.

EPIDEMIOLOGY

Chondroid lipoma, first described in 1993,[36] is a very rare lipogenic neoplasm and arises predominantly in adults, with a predilection for females.

CLINICAL FEATURES

The majority of cases of chondroid lipoma presents as a painless, deep-seated mass, and may show a history of recent growth. The proximal extremities and limb girdles are the most frequently affected anatomic sites,[36,37] but the trunk and the head and neck region, including the oral cavity,[38] also may be affected. The neoplasms arise usually in deep subcutaneous tissue, fascia, and skeletal muscle.

ETIOLOGY AND PATHOGENESIS

Ultrastructural studies confirmed the lipogenic differentiation in cases of chondroid lipoma, and a spectrum of differentiation ranging from primitive mesenchymal cells, with features of prelipoblasts, to lipoblasts, preadipocytes, and mature adipocytes, has been reported.[36,39] Cytogenetically, a balanced translocation involving chromosomes 11 and 16, t(11;16)(q13;p12-13) with a *C11orf95-MKL2* fusion gene product has been found,[40] and cyclin D1 (*CCND1*) expression without abnormalities of the *CCND1* locus has been reported.[41]

HISTOLOGIC FEATURES

Chondroid lipomas are usually deep-seated, well-circumscribed, encapsulated, nodular, and lobulated neoplasms. The neoplasms are composed of a variable admixture of mature adipocytes, multivacuolated lipoblasts with enlarged and hyperchromatic nuclei, and small, round cells containing an eosinophilic and vacuolated cytoplasm displaying a range of lipoblastic differentiation and containing small lipid droplets and periodic acid–Schiff–positive glycogen (Figs. 122-21, 122-22, and 122-23). The tumor cells are set in a myxoid–chondroid stroma and positive Alcian blue stainings at low pH indicate the presence of sulfated chondroitin. The lesions contain many vessels, and areas of hemorrhage, fibrosis, and calcification may be present. Mature lipogenic cells stain positively for S-100 protein, and, occasionally, a focal expression of pancytokeratin by lipogenic cells can be seen.

DIFFERENTIAL DIAGNOSIS

Given the depth and size of the lesion associated with the presence of nuclear atypia and lipoblasts,

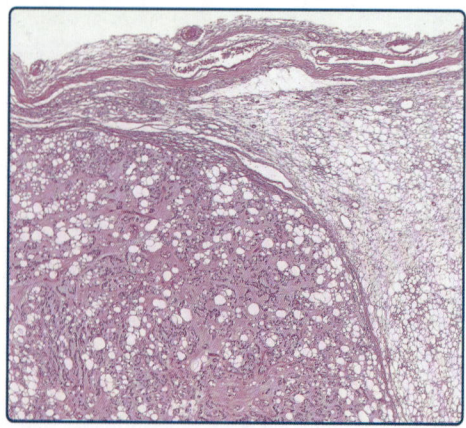

Figure 122-21 Chondroid lipoma. Encapsulated lipogenic neoplasm with a lobular growth.

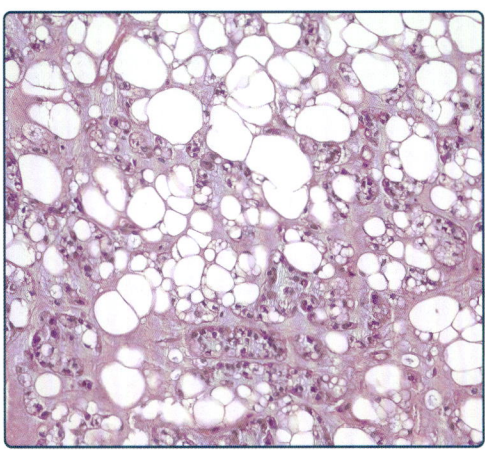

Figure 122-22 Chondroid lipoma. Univacuolated and multivacuolated lipoblasts are admixed with mature adipocytes.

benign chondroid lipoma has to be distinguished from more aggressive neoplasms, including atypical lipomatous tumor, myxoid liposarcoma, extraskeletal myxoid chondrosarcoma, and myoepithelioma of soft tissues.

CLINICAL COURSE, PROGNOSIS, AND TREATMENT

Chondroid lipoma represents an entirely benign lipogenic neoplasm and simple surgical excision is curative. Local recurrences are rare and neither malignant transformation nor metastases have been reported as of this writing.

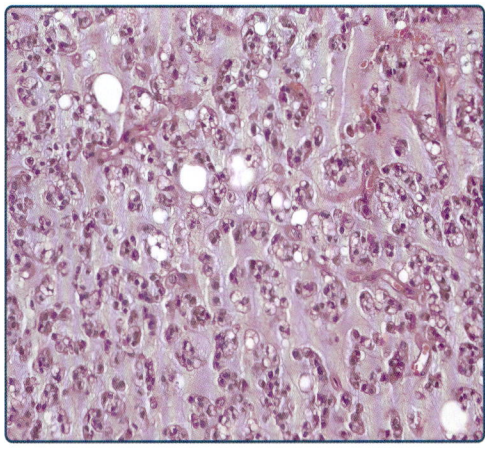

Figure 122-23 Chondroid lipoma. In addition, small, round tumor cells containing an eosinophilic and vacuolated cytoplasm are seen.

MYOLIPOMA

AT-A-GLANCE

- Myolipoma is a very rare benign mesenchymal neoplasm of deep soft tissue.
- Myolipoma occurs predominantly in females.
- Myolipoma is composed of an irregular mixture of mature adipocytes and smooth muscle cells.

EPIDEMIOLOGY

Myolipoma represents a very rare neoplasm of soft tissues occurring in adult patients with a female predominance.[42]

CLINICAL FEATURES

Cases of myolipoma tend to occur in deep soft tissue of the retroperitoneum, abdominal cavity, and inguinal region, whereas an involvement of subcutaneous tissue of the extremities and the trunk is only rarely seen.[42] Although these lesions may reach a considerable size, they are often found incidentally.

ETIOLOGY AND PATHOGENESIS

HMGA2 alterations have been reported in cases of myolipoma, and most recently a fusion of the *HMGA2* and *C9orf92* genes with t(9;12)(p22;q14) has been detected.[43]

HISTOLOGIC FEATURES

Myolipoma of soft tissues is a well-circumscribed or encapsulated lesion composed of fascicles of cytologically bland smooth muscle cells associated with a variable amount of mature fat (Fig. 122-24). No cytologic atypia, mitoses, or thick-walled vessels are present. Immunohistochemically, smooth muscle cells stain positively for alpha-smooth muscle actin, desmin, and h-caldesmon (Fig. 122-25), and an expression of estrogen and progesterone receptors has been reported.[44] No expression of HMB-45 by smooth muscle cells and no expression of MDM2 and CDK4 by lipogenic cells are noted.

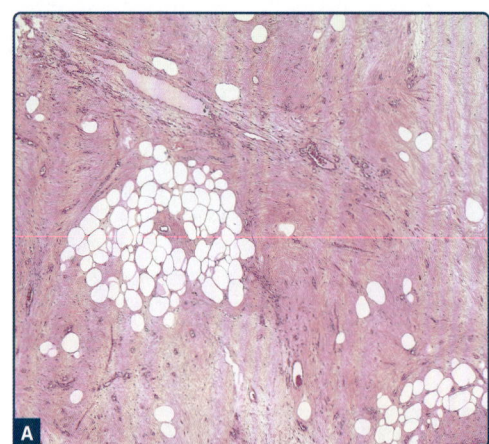

DIFFERENTIAL DIAGNOSIS

The differential diagnosis for myolipoma of soft tissues includes atypical lipomatous tumor, dedifferentiated liposarcoma, well-differentiated leiomyosarcoma, and angiomyolipoma.

CLINICAL COURSE, PROGNOSIS, AND TREATMENT

Despite the large size, myolipoma of soft tissues represents an entirely benign mesenchymal neoplasm, and complete excision is curative.

HIBERNOMA

AT-A-GLANCE

- Hibernoma represents a benign neoplasm of brown fat.
- Hibernoma usually arises in adults and the most common anatomic site is the thigh.
- Cases of atypical lipomatous tumor and myxoid liposarcoma may contain hibernoma-like areas.

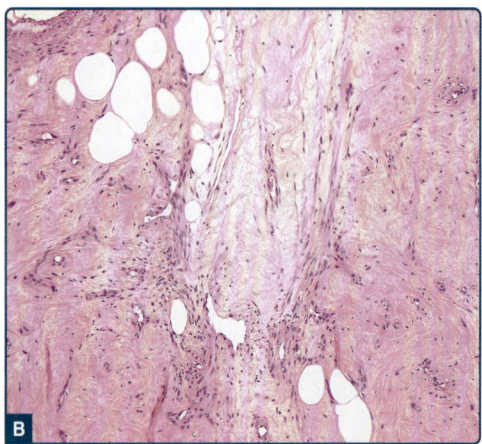

Figure 122-24 Myolipoma. **A,** Mature adipocytic cells are admixed with bland spindled cells. **B,** The myogenic spindled cells contain an eosinophilic cytoplasm and bland spindled nuclei.

EPIDEMIOLOGY

Hibernoma is a rare neoplasm, and occurs predominantly in young adults, whereas it is only rarely seen in children and the elderly. Males are slightly more frequently affected than females.

CLINICAL FEATURES

Hibernoma represents a painless, slowly growing, mobile tumor arising in the subcutis or in deep soft tissues. The most common anatomic site for hibernoma is the thigh followed by the trunk, the chest wall, the shoulder area, the upper extremity, and the head and neck area.[45] Rarely, hibernoma arises intraabdominally, in the retroperitoneum, in the mediastinum, or intraosseous.[46,47]

ETIOLOGY AND PATHOGENESIS

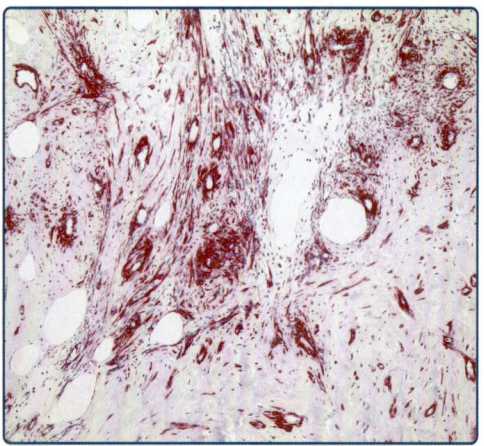

Figure 122-25 Myolipoma. Eosinophilic spindled tumor cells stain positively for h-caldesmon, confirming their smooth muscle differentiation.

The reported karyotypes of hibernoma appear to be more complex than those in other benign lipogenic neoplasms, and structural rearrangements involving chromosome band 11q13-21 have been detected.[48]

HISTOLOGIC FEATURES

Hibernomas are well-circumscribed, lobular neoplasms containing a capillary network and are composed of a variable number of brown fat cells admixed with white fat cells and stromal cells. Typical hibernomas are composed of large, polygonal, brown fat cells with multivacuolation, granular cytoplasm, and a small, centrally located nucleus admixed with mature white fat cells (Fig. 122-26). The eosinophilic variant is composed of predominantly brown fat cells with a deeply eosinophilic and granular cytoplasm, the pale cell variant contains mostly large brown fat cells with palely staining vacuolated cytoplasm, and the mixed subtype is intermediate between the two. In addition, myxoid, spindle-cell, and lipoma-like variants are known.[45] Prominent cytologic atypia and increased proliferative activity are not present. Immunohistochemically, tumor cells stain positively for S-100 protein and for uncoupling protein, a protein unique to brown adipocyte mitochondria.[49] The spindled cells may express CD34.

DIFFERENTIAL DIAGNOSIS

Scattered brown fat cells as well as hibernoma-like areas may be present in cases of myxoid liposarcoma and atypical lipomatous tumor that have to be distinguished from hibernoma. Further differential diagnoses include granular cell tumor and spindle-cell lipoma.

CLINICAL COURSE, PROGNOSIS, AND TREATMENT

Hibernoma is an entirely benign lipogenic neoplasm, and complete excision is curative.

ATYPICAL LIPOMATOUS TUMOR AND WELL-DIFFERENTIATED LIPOSARCOMA

AT-A-GLANCE

- Atypical lipomatous tumor and well-differentiated liposarcoma are synonyms and describe lipogenic neoplasms with identical morphologic and cytogenetic features.
- Atypical lipomatous tumor represents a locally aggressive, nonmetastasizing neoplasm.
- Anatomic location, size, and depth of the lesions are important prognostic predictors.
- Neoplasms arising at sites amenable to surgical excision (ie, extremities) show a low rate of local recurrence, risk of dedifferentiation, and mortality.
- In striking contrast, neoplasms arising in the retroperitoneum, intraabdominal cavity, or in paratesticular location, where complete excision is difficult or not achievable, are characterized by a high rate of local recurrence, a high risk of dedifferentiation, and a poor clinical outcome.
- The known morphologic variants have no prognostic value.

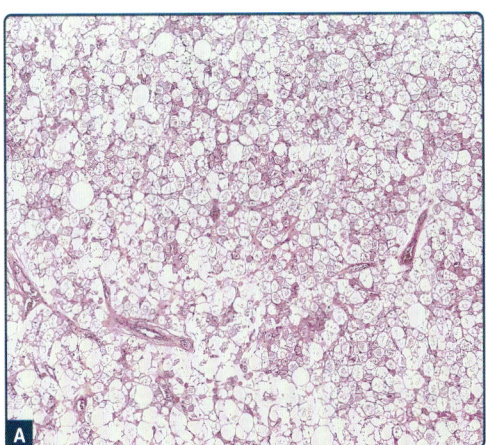
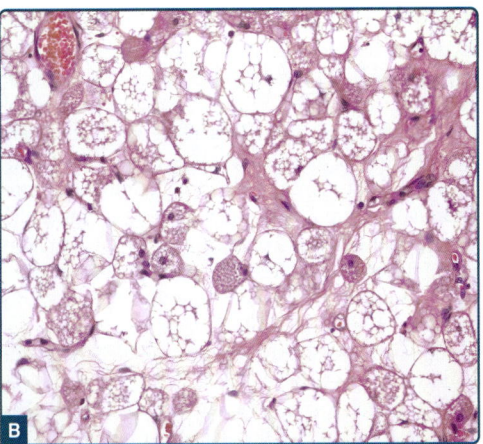

Figure 122-26 Hibernoma. **A,** Mature adipocytes are admixed with large multivacuolated cells and smaller eosinophilic cells. **B,** Vacuolated tumor cells with centrally placed nuclei and a clear or eosinophilic granular cytoplasm.

EPIDEMIOLOGY

Atypical lipomatous tumor represents the largest single group of clinically aggressive lipogenic neoplasms, and liposarcomas in general are the most frequent sarcomas in adults. The majority of neoplasms occurs in middle-age adults, with a peak incidence in the sixth decade.[50-54] Cases in children are extremely rare, but have been described.[55,56]

CLINICAL FEATURES

Cases of atypical lipomatous tumor occur usually in deep soft tissues. The subcutaneous tissue may be occasionally involved, but purely dermal lesions that may present as a skin tag are extremely rare (Fig. 122-27).[57] The predominantly affected site is the musculature of the extremities, especially the thigh, followed by the retroperitoneum, the abdominal cavity, the groin, the paratesticular region, and the mediastinum. However, also other anatomic locations are rarely involved, as it is the oral cavity, the orbit, the larynx, and the vulva.[58-61] An enlarging painless mass is the typical presenting sign and tumors may grow to a very large size before becoming symptomatic, especially in retroperitoneal and intraabdominal locations.

ETIOLOGY AND PATHOGENESIS

Cases of atypical lipomatous tumor are characterized cytogenetically by supernumerary ring and giant marker chromosomes derived from the 12q13-15 region and resulting in consistent amplification of the *MDM2* and *CDK4* genes.[62,63]

HISTOLOGIC FEATURES

Atypical lipomatous tumors are typically large, well-circumscribed and lobulated lesions, and in retroperitoneal and intraabdominal locations, multiple discontinuous neoplasms may be present. Morphologically, atypical lipomatous tumor can be divided into 3 main subtypes; however, especially in large neoplasms of the retroperitoneum, more than 1 variant may be present. The most frequent adipocytic (lipoma-like) variant is composed of relatively mature adipocytic cells with marked variations in size and shape showing scattered enlarged and hyperchromatic nuclei. In addition, atypical stromal cells with enlarged nuclei located in fibrous septa, as well as multivacuolated lipoblasts, may be present; however, lipoblasts may be entirely absent (Fig. 122-28). The second most frequent sclerosing variant that is frequently seen in the retroperitoneal and paratesticular locations is characterized by the presence of enlarged stromal cells with large and hyperchromatic nuclei set in a paucicellular, fibrillary, collagenous stroma, and scattered atypical lipogenic cells and lipoblasts (Fig. 122-29). Rare, inflammatory atypical lipomatous tumors are mainly seen in retroperitoneal and intraabdominal locations, and show a prominent inflammatory infiltrate that mimics features of a lymphoma or an inflammatory pseudotumor.[64] So-called well-differentiated spindle-cell liposarcoma[65] shows a predilection for the subcutaneous tissue of the shoulder girdle and the limbs and is composed of slightly atypical spindled cells with enlarged, hyperchromatic nuclei arranged in fascicles and whorls set in a fibrous and/or myxoid stroma associated with atypical adipocytic cells. Genetic studies emphasize that these neoplasms most likely represent atypical spindle cell lipomatous tumor with a clinical behavior almost identical to atypical lipomatous tumor.[31,32,66] Very rarely, a heterologous differentiation with osseous or myogenic elements is seen. The term

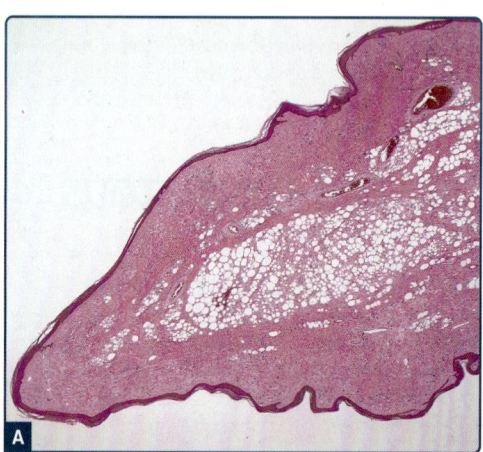

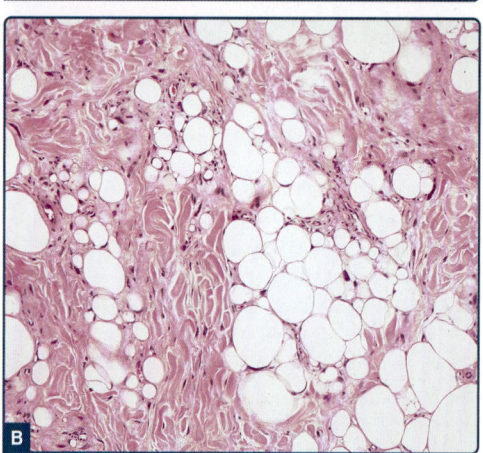

Figure 122-27 Dermal atypical lipomatous tumor. **A,** A polypoid lesion, clinically diagnosed as a skin tag, has been excised. **B,** Histologically, an atypical lipomatous tumor composed of atypical stromal cells and atypical lipogenic cells with enlarged hyperchromatic nuclei and scattered lipoblasts is seen.

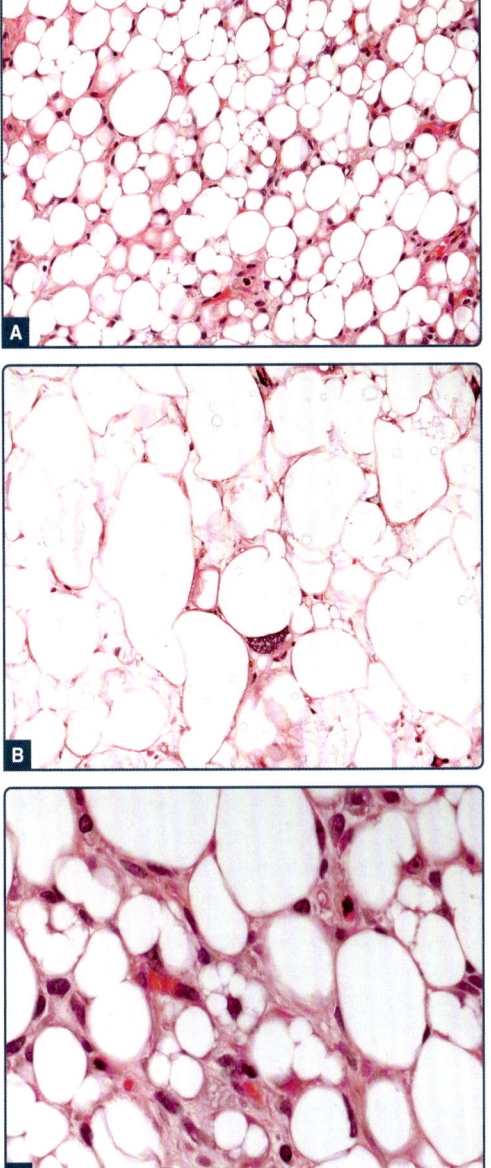

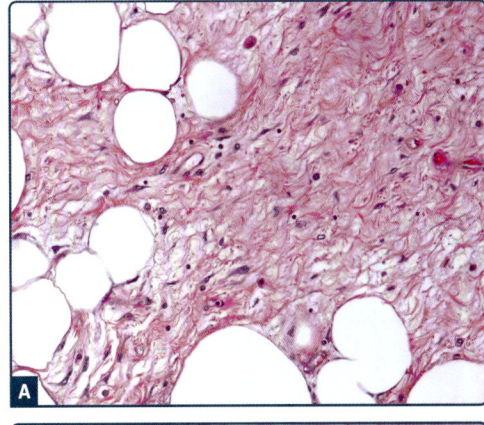

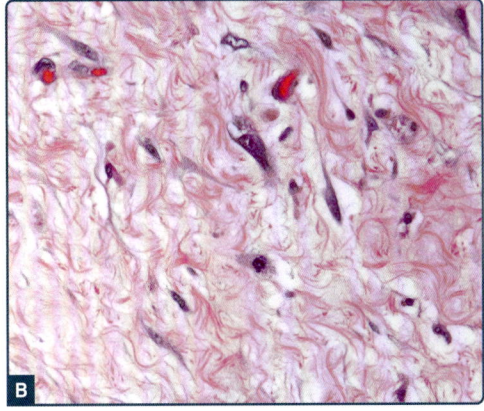

Figure 122-29 Atypical lipomatous tumor. **A,** The presence of a paucicellular stroma with admixed adipocytes characterizes the sclerosing variant. **B,** Note the presence of bizarre-appearing stromal cells set in a fibrillary stroma.

Figure 122-28 Atypical lipomatous tumor. **A,** The lipoma-like variant is composed of lipogenic cells showing marked variation in size and shape. Scattered, enlarged, hyperchromatic nuclei and vacuolated lipogenic cells are noted. Higher-power view reveals enlarged and hyperchromatic nuclei (**B**), as well as multivacuolated lipoblasts (**C**).

lipoleiomyosarcoma has been applied to lesions showing morphologic features of atypical lipomatous tumor and well-differentiated leiomyosarcoma.[67] Immunohistochemically, focal expression of p16, as well as nuclear staining for MDM2 and/or CDK4, is helpful in the differential diagnoses to other lipogenic and nonlipogenic lesions. However, especially, very well-differentiated examples of atypical lipomatous tumor may not show MDM2 and/or CDK4 expression by immunohistochemistry. In these cases, FISH analysis may be very helpful.[68,69]

DIFFERENTIAL DIAGNOSIS

In contrast to atypical lipomatous tumor, typical cases of lipoma are composed of mature adipocytes without nuclear atypia and lipoblasts, and do not stain positively for p16, MDM2, and CDK4. However, traumatized lipomas may contain numerous histiocytes with enlarged nuclei that show a cytoplasmic staining for p16, MDM2, and CDK4, and may mimic a more aggressive neoplasm. Lipoblastoma is composed of a varying number of lipoblasts and may stain positively for p16,[18] but the presence of a lobular lesion with characteristic septa, and the lack of MDM2/CDK4 expression are of help in the differential diagnosis. Spindle-cell lipoma and pleomorphic lipoma may contain scattered lipoblasts, but lack atypia, and neoplastic cells are negative for MDM2 and/or CDK4. Dedifferentiated liposarcoma contains a nonlipogenic component with strong expression of p16, MDM2, and CDK4. Angiomyolipoma is characterized by the presence of thick-walled blood vessels and a perivascular myogenic component staining positively for myogenic marker and HMB-45. Rare cases of massive localized lymphedema simulate clinically and histologically atypical lipomatous tumor,[70] but no significant atypia and no expression of p16, MDM2, and CDK4 are noted in these lesions.

CLINICAL COURSE, PROGNOSIS, AND TREATMENT

The clinical behavior and the prognosis of atypical lipomatous tumor is strongly dependent on the anatomic site, the depth, and the size of the neoplasms. Surgical treatment is curative for lesions arising superficially, and at surgically amenable anatomic sites such as the extremities. The estimated rate of progressing to dedifferentiated liposarcoma is less than 2% with a mortality rate of virtually zero for cases arising at these anatomic locations. In striking contrast, cases of atypical lipomatous tumor arising in deep soft tissues of the retroperitoneum, the mediastinum, intraabdominal cavity, and paratesticular location, where complete surgical excision is problematic and not possible, tend to recur locally, may cause death as a result of uncontrolled local effects, and have a risk of dedifferentiation of more than 20%. The overall mortality of atypical lipomatous tumor in the retroperitoneum is more than 80%.[53,71] Surgical excision is the primary therapeutic approach in cases of atypical lipomatous tumor; adjuvant chemotherapy and radiotherapy may be used in advanced cases.

DEDIFFERENTIATED LIPOSARCOMA

AT-A-GLANCE

- Dedifferentiated liposarcoma represents the morphologic form of progression of atypical lipomatous tumor.
- Dedifferentiated liposarcoma most frequently occurs in the retroperitoneum and intraabdominal cavity as a large tumor mass.
- An abrupt or gradual transition from an atypical lipomatous tumor to a nonlipogenic sarcomatous component is seen in dedifferentiated liposarcoma.
- The nonlipogenic component shows a variable morphology, and a heterologous differentiation is seen in a significant number of cases.
- Dedifferentiated liposarcoma shows the same karyotypic changes as atypical lipomatous tumor.
- Dedifferentiated liposarcoma is best regarded as an intermediate-grade sarcoma (grade 2 of malignancy).

EPIDEMIOLOGY

Dedifferentiated liposarcoma represents the most common pleomorphic sarcoma in the retroperitoneum, and typically affects adult patients in the sixth decade.[72] Dedifferentiation as a morphologic form of tumor progression represents a time-dependent phenomenon, and occurs in approximately 90% of cases as a de novo presentation, whereas 10% develop it in a local recurrence.

CLINICAL FEATURES

The majority of dedifferentiated liposarcomas occur in the retroperitoneum, intraabdominal, and paratesticular locations, whereas an involvement of deep soft tissues of the extremities is seen more rarely. Other rare locations include the trunk, and the head and neck region, presentation in subcutaneous tissue is very rare.[73] Typically, cases of dedifferentiated liposarcoma present as a large painless mass, and are found in the retroperitoneum and intraabdominal locations by chance. A recent increase in size of a longstanding deep-seated mass in the extremities may indicate dedifferentiation in an atypical lipomatous tumor.

ETIOLOGY AND PATHOGENESIS

The karyotypic findings in dedifferentiated liposarcoma are similar to those seen in atypical lipomatous tumor; however, coamplification involving 1p32 and 6q23 with activation of the *JUN* and *ASK2* genes has been reported.[74]

HISTOLOGIC FEATURES

Histologically, an abrupt or gradual transition from areas showing features of atypical lipomatous tumor to nonlipogenic sarcoma areas is characteristic for dedifferentiated liposarcoma (Fig. 122-30). The extent and the morphology of the nonlipogenic component are variable, but in most cases, the dedifferentiated component shows features of a high-grade, undifferentiated, pleomorphic sarcoma (Fig. 122-31). Especially in the retroperitoneum and intraabdominal locations, intermediate-grade or high-grade myxofibrosarcoma areas are present. Occasionally, a low-grade dedifferentiation is noted that mimics features of low-grade fibrosarcoma or desmoid fibromatosis (Fig. 122-32). Heterologous differentiation is seen in approximately 10% of cases, and most often a myogenic or osteosarcomatous/chondrosarcomatous differentiation is detected (Fig. 122-33). More rarely angiosarcomatous

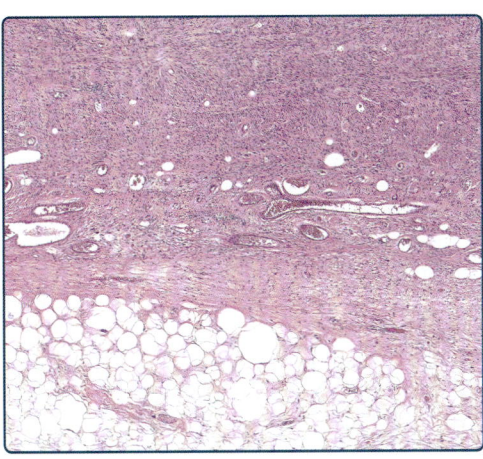

Figure 122-30 Dedifferentiated liposarcoma. A rather abrupt transition from areas showing features of an atypical lipomatous tumor (button) to a nonlipogenic sarcoma is seen.

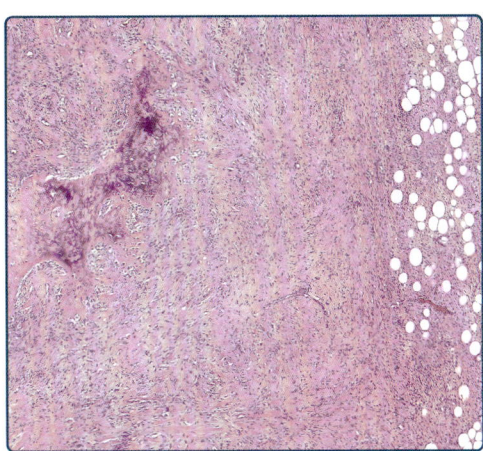

Figure 122-33 Dedifferentiated liposarcoma. A heterologous, osteosarcomatous differentiation with focal calcification is noted in this case.

and meningothelial-like whorls have been reported.[75] Interestingly, the dedifferentiated component may show a lipoblastic differentiation that resembles pleomorphic liposarcoma, but molecular changes are identical to classical dedifferentiated liposarcoma.[76] Immunohistochemically, a strong expression of p16, MDM2, and CDK4 is seen, especially in the nonlipogenic component (Fig. 122-34). Heterologous myogenic differentiation is reflected by positive staining for myogenic (actin, desmin, h-caldesmon, myogenin), osteosarcomatous (SATB2), chondrosarcomatous (S-100 protein), or angiosarcomatous (CD31, ERG) immunohistochemical markers (Fig. 122-35).

DIFFERENTIAL DIAGNOSIS

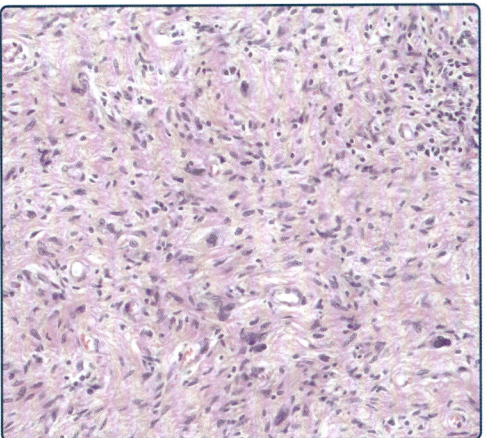

Figure 122-31 Dedifferentiated liposarcoma. The nonlipogenic component often shows features of a rather undifferentiated, pleomorphic sarcoma.

Given the variable morphology of the nonlipogenic component, the differential diagnosis of dedifferentiated liposarcoma is broad and includes pleomorphic liposarcoma, myxofibrosarcoma, GI stromal tumor, leiomyosarcoma, rhabdomyosarcoma, malignant solitary fibrous tumor, rare fibrosarcoma, and desmoid fibromatosis. In addition, large lipomas with cytologic atypia and atypical spindle cell lipomatous tumor and atypical pleomorphic lipomatous tumor have to be considered, especially when dealing with a small biopsy.

CLINICAL COURSE, PROGNOSIS, AND TREATMENT

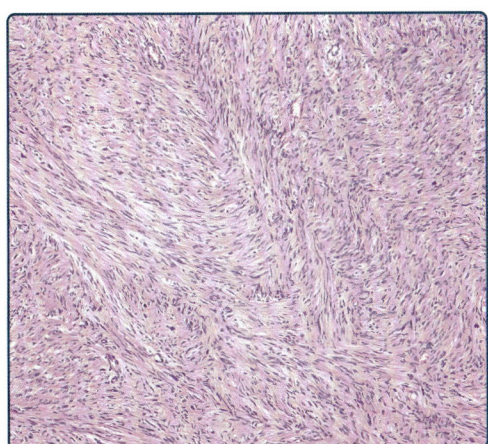

Figure 122-32 Dedifferentiated liposarcoma. Infrequently, a low-grade dedifferentiation with features of a low-grade fibroblastic sarcoma is noted.

Dedifferentiated liposarcoma is characterized by a protracted clinical course with a high risk for local recurrences and a locally aggressive growth. Almost all cases arising in the retroperitoneum and intraabdominal locations recur if followed long enough. However, in contrast to many other high-grade sarcomas, the

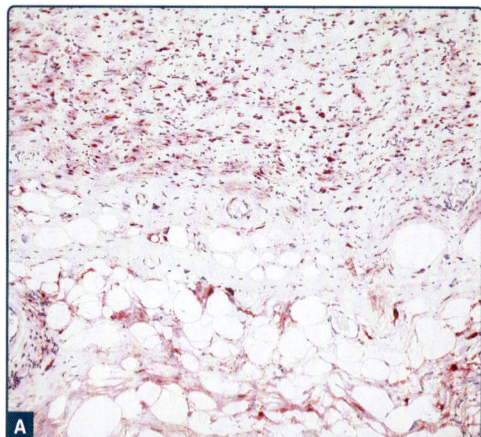

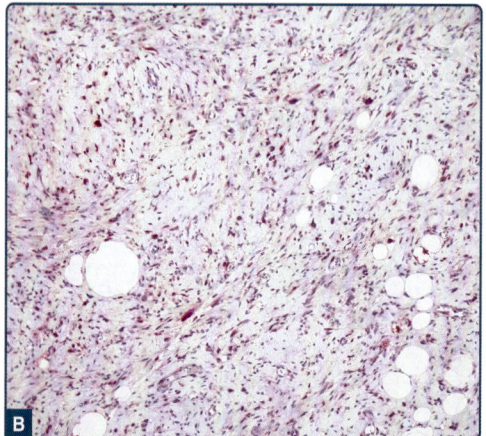

Figure 122-34 Dedifferentiated liposarcoma. Immunohistochemically, an expression of p16 (**A**) and MDM2 (**B**) is seen in the lipogenic and in the nonlipogenic component.

overall risk of distant metastatic spread is estimated at approximately 15% to 20%.[72,77] It can be speculated that the absence of complex karyotypic aberrations and the rarity of p53 mutations in cases of dedifferentiated liposarcoma[78] may explain the better outcome. As in cases of atypical lipomatous tumor, the anatomic location is the most important prognostic factor in dedifferentiated liposarcoma, and cases arising in retroperitoneum and intraabdominal locations are associated with a poor prognosis. It has been shown that myogenic differentiation and the histologic grade of the nonlipogenic tumor component are important prognostic parameters.[79] The extent of dedifferentiation is prognostically not predictive. Complete surgical removal represents the treatment of choice; however, especially in the retroperitoneum and in intraabdominal locations, this is often impossible. New therapeutic options targeting the gene products of chromosome 12 or inhibitors of the Akt-mTOR and MAPK (mitogen-activated protein kinase) pathways are under discussion for use in nonresectable cases.[80,81]

MYXOID LIPOSARCOMA

AT-A-GLANCE

- Myxoid liposarcoma usually occurs in deep soft tissues of the extremities, particularly the thigh, of middle-aged adults.
- Myxoid liposarcoma is composed of small, primitive, mesenchymal cells and lipoblasts in varying stages of differentiation with a characteristic vascular pattern.
- The presence of a round cell component is of adverse significant prognostic importance.
- Myxoid liposarcoma is characterized by *FUS-DDIT3* or *EWSR1-DDIT3* rearrangements.

EPIDEMIOLOGY

Myxoid liposarcoma represents the second most frequent variant of liposarcoma and approximately 5% of all soft-tissue sarcomas in adults. Most cases of myxoid liposarcoma arise in young to middle-aged adults; however, a significant number of cases are seen in children and adolescents, representing the most frequent variant of liposarcoma in this age group, and these cases may show unusual morphologic features.[82] In addition an expression of cancer testis antigens, ie, PRAME is seen.[82A]

CLINICAL FEATURES

Cases of myxoid liposarcoma present as a large, painless mass in deep soft tissues of the extremities, and the majority of neoplasms arise on the thigh. Only rarely, myxoid liposarcoma is seen in the subcutis and in the retroperitoneum or intraabdominal locations. The monoclonal origin of cases multifocal myxoid liposarcoma confirms an unusual metastatic pattern in these cases.[83]

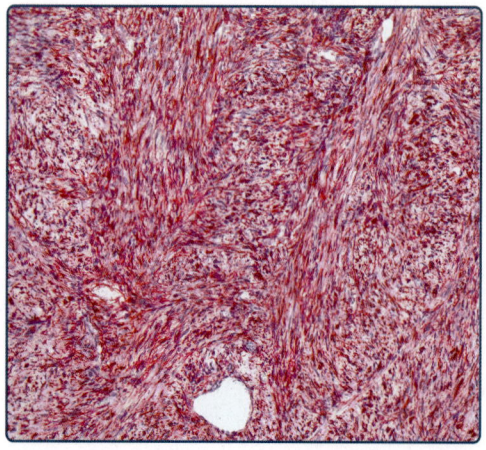

Figure 122-35 Dedifferentiated liposarcoma. Heterologous myogenic differentiation with strong expression of desmin by nonlipogenic spindled tumor cells.

ETIOLOGY AND PATHOGENESIS

Cytogenetically, myxoid liposarcoma is characterized by a recurrent translocation t(12;16)(q13;p11) with *FUS-DDIT3* fusion in the majority of cases; more rarely, a t(12;22)(q13:q12) with *EWSR1-DDIT3* fusion is present.[84,85]

HISTOLOGIC FEATURES

The nodular neoplasms are composed of an admixture of uniform, cytologically bland, small, oval, mesenchymal tumor cells, and small, univacuolated or bivacuolated lipoblasts set in a prominent myxoid stroma with microcystic spaces and characteristic branching, thin-walled blood vessels (Fig. 122-36). These well-differentiated neoplasms lack significant cytologic atypia, mitoses, and tumor necrosis. Myxoid/round-cell liposarcoma, and predominantly round-cell liposarcoma, is characterized by progression to more cellular areas containing enlarged round tumor cells with enlarged and overlapping round nuclei (Fig. 122-37). Rarely, myxoid liposarcoma may show prominent adipocytic differentiation mimicking morphologic features of atypical lipomatous tumor (Fig. 122-38),[86] which also has been reported in cases treated with neoadjuvant therapy.[87] In addition, cases of myxoid liposarcoma may show a prominent spindle-cell component (spindle-cell myxoid liposarcoma) or a pleomorphic component (pleomorphic myxoid liposarcoma), and these features are mainly seen in young patients.[82] Immunohistochemically, S-100 protein is variably positive in the high-grade, round-cell component.

DIFFERENTIAL DIAGNOSIS

The differential diagnosis includes benign lesions as lipoblastoma and chondroid lipoma, as well as malignant neoplasms of different lines of differentiation (myxofibrosarcoma, low-grade fibromyxoid sarcoma, extraskeletal myxoid chondrosarcoma, myxoid malignant melanoma).

CLINICAL COURSE, PROGNOSIS, AND TREATMENT

Myxoid liposarcoma tends to recur and may develop distant metastases in up to 40% of patients, and metastases at unusual locations in soft tissues or bone often are observed. Patients with "multifocal" disease at presentation have a poor prognosis, and adverse histologic features include the presence of a round-cell differentiation (>5%), tumor necrosis, p53 overexpression, and *CDKN2A* aberrations.[88,89] It has been shown that advanced cases of myxoid liposarcoma can be treated successfully with trabectedin.[90-92]

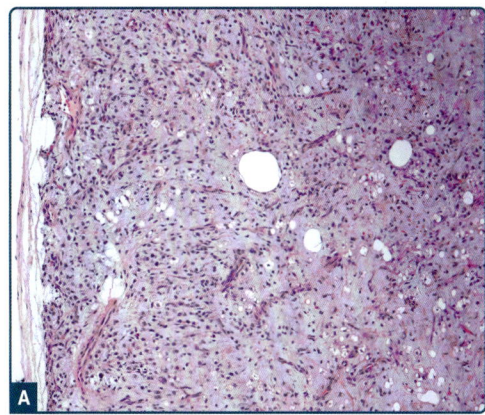
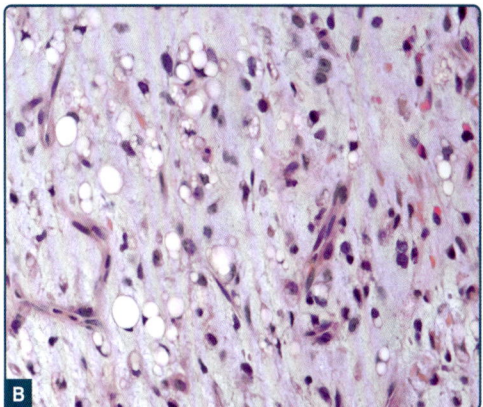
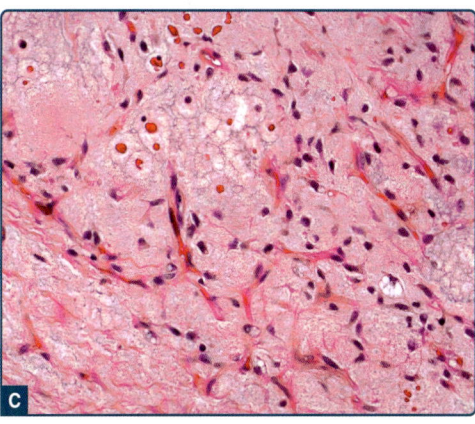

Figure 122-36 Myxoid liposarcoma. **A,** The myxoid neoplasms are lobulated and composed of immature mesenchymal cells and atypical lipogenic cells. Note the increased cellularity in the periphery. **B,** The presence of univacuolated, bivacuolated, and multivacuolated lipoblasts and cytologically bland oval-shaped cells set in a myxoid stroma is a characteristic feature. **C,** Note the delicate branching, capillary sized vessels.

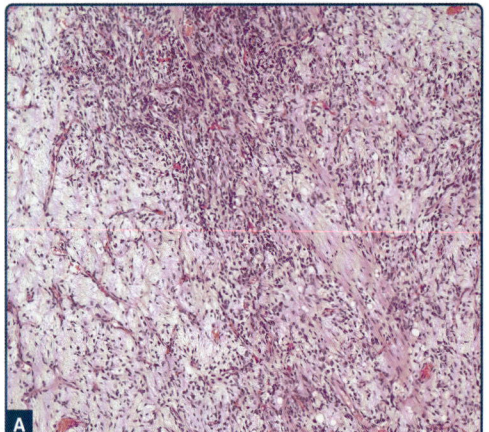

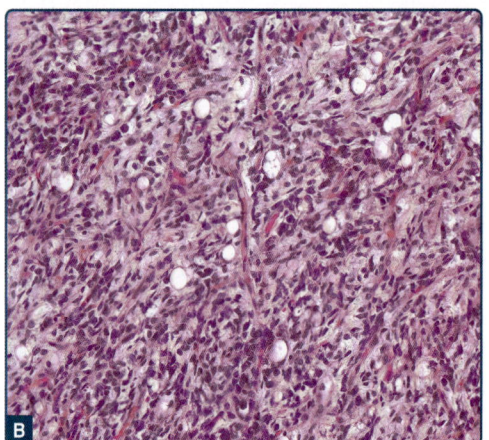

Figure 122-37 Myxoid/round cell liposarcoma. **A,** Areas of increased cellularity with slightly enlarged round tumor cells containing round nuclei are seen. **B,** High-grade round-cell liposarcoma is composed predominantly of enlarged round tumor cells without prominent pleomorphism. Note the characteristic vascular pattern and the presence of lipoblasts.

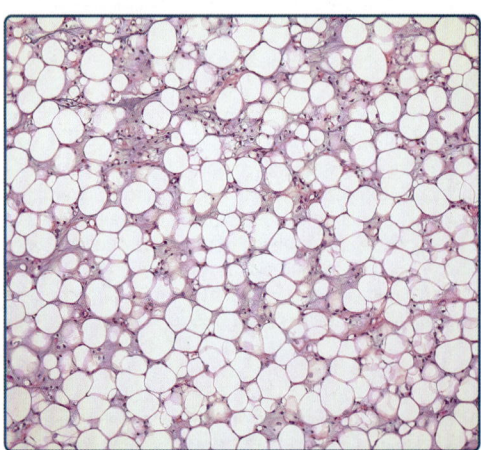

Figure 122-38 Lipogenic myxoid liposarcoma. In some cases of myxoid liposarcoma, a predominant lipogenic differentiation is seen mimicking an atypical lipomatous tumor.

PLEOMORPHIC LIPOSARCOMA

AT-A-GLANCE

- Pleomorphic liposarcoma represents a high-grade sarcoma containing a variable number of pleomorphic lipoblasts.
- Pleomorphic liposarcoma shows a predilection for the extremities of adults.
- Pleomorphic liposarcoma arises either de novo or represents the morphologic form of progression of atypical lipomatous tumor/dedifferentiated liposarcoma.

EPIDEMIOLOGY

Pleomorphic liposarcoma represents the rarest subtype of liposarcoma (5%) and arises predominantly in the elderly with a slight male predominance.[93,94]

CLINICAL FEATURES

Clinically, pleomorphic liposarcoma usually presents as a fast growing neoplasm in deep soft tissues of the extremities (lower > upper extremities), while the trunk, the retroperitoneum, the abdominal cavity, the head and neck region, and the pelvis are only rarely involved. A small but significant number of cases of pleomorphic liposarcoma arise in subcutaneous tissues, whereas purely dermal neoplasms are exceedingly rare (Fig. 122-39).[94-96]

ETIOLOGY AND PATHOGENESIS

Cytogenetically, many cases of pleomorphic liposarcoma closely resemble other pleomorphic sarcomas and show complex structural rearrangements. However, it has been shown that a small, but significant, number of cases reveal *MDM2* and *CDK4* amplifications, which suggests that these neoplasms represent a tumor progression from atypical lipomatous tumor/dedifferentiated liposarcoma.[76,97]

HISTOLOGIC FEATURES

The well-circumscribed or infiltrative neoplasms show features of a high-grade pleomorphic sarcoma

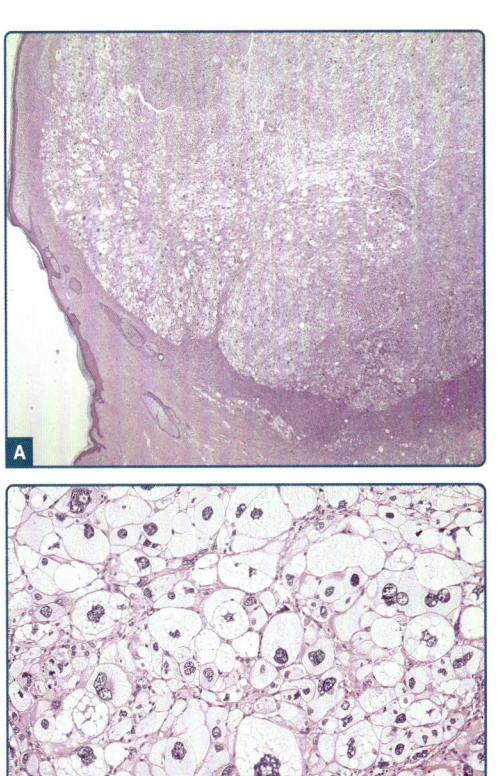

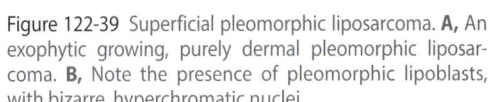

Figure 122-39 Superficial pleomorphic liposarcoma. **A,** An exophytic growing, purely dermal pleomorphic liposarcoma. **B,** Note the presence of pleomorphic lipoblasts, with bizarre, hyperchromatic nuclei.

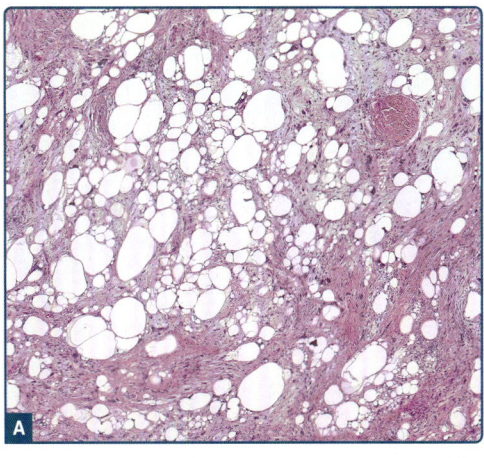

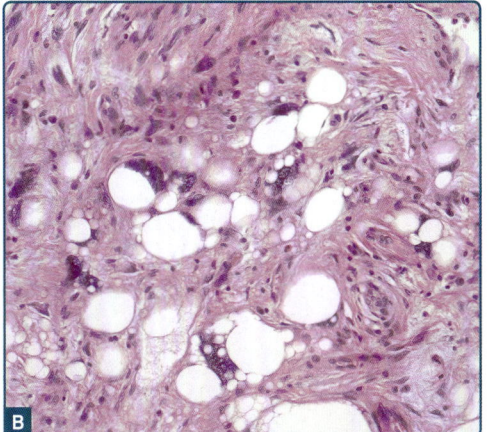

Figure 122-40 Pleomorphic liposarcoma. **A** and **B,** Pleomorphic lipoblasts and atypical lipogenic cells are irregularly admixed with sarcoma cells.

(high-grade fibrosarcoma or "malignant fibrous histiocytoma") containing pleomorphic spindled cells and multinucleated tumor giant cells admixed with a variable number of pleomorphic lipoblasts. These pleomorphic lipoblasts contain enlarged and bizarre, hyperchromatic nuclei scalloped by cytoplasmic lipid droplets, and are scattered throughout the pleomorphic sarcoma or are arranged in larger sheets (Fig. 122-40). Often intracellular and extracellular eosinophilic droplets are noted. Many cases show morphologic features similar to intermediate-grade or high-grade myxofibrosarcoma with scattered pleomorphic lipoblasts (Fig. 122-41). The epithelioid variant of pleomorphic liposarcoma is characterized by large, densely packed, epithelioid tumor cells with abundant eosinophilic cytoplasm and vesicular nuclei resembling renal clear cell carcinoma or adrenal cortical carcinoma.[98] Immunohistochemically, tumor cells in pleomorphic liposarcoma may stain positively for actins, cytokeratins, CD34, and, rarely, desmin.

DIFFERENTIAL DIAGNOSIS

Dedifferentiated liposarcoma contains an atypical lipomatous tumor component and no pleomorphic lipoblasts. The presence of at least scattered pleomorphic lipoblasts in pleomorphic liposarcoma is important in the differential diagnosis to other pleomorphic, high-grade sarcomas (myxofibrosarcoma, leiomyosarcoma, rhabdomyosarcoma), as well as poorly differentiated, sarcomatoid melanoma and carcinoma.

CLINICAL COURSE, PROGNOSIS, AND TREATMENT

Pleomorphic liposarcoma represents a high-grade sarcoma with a local recurrence and metastatic rate of 30-50%, and an estimated overall 5-year survival rate

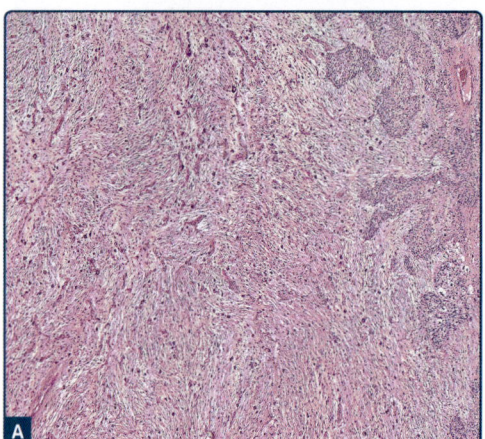

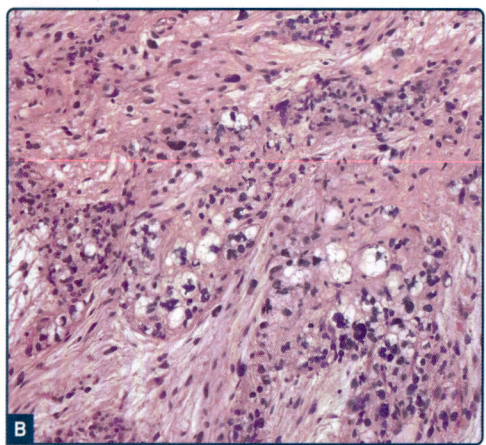

Figure 122-41 Pleomorphic liposarcoma. **A,** The neoplasm shows features of a higher grade myxofibrosarcoma. **B,** Pleomorphic lipoblasts are present at the right side.

of 50% to 60%. The lung is the preferred metastatic site. The treatment is surgical excision with radiation and chemotherapy for advanced cases.

REFERENCES

1. Nielsen GP, Mandahl N. Lipoma. In: Fletcher CDM, Bridge JA, Hogendoorn PCW, et al. *World Health Organization Classification of Tumours of Soft Tissue and Bone*. Lyon, France: IARC; 2013.
2. Bannayan GA. Lipomatosis, angiomatosis, and macrocephalia. A previously undescribed congenital syndrome. *Arch Pathol*. 1971;92(1):1.
3. Sandberg AA. Updates on the cytogenetics and molecular genetics of bone and soft tissue tumors: lipoma. *Cancer Genet Cytogenet*. 2004;150(2):93.
4. Petit MM, Mols R, Schoenmakers ET, et al. LPP, the preferred fusion partner gene of HMGIC in lipomas, is a novel member of the LIM protein gene family. *Genomics*. 1996;36(1):118.
5. Fletcher CDM, Martin-Bates E: Intramuscular and intermuscular lipoma: neglected diagnoses. *Histopathology*. 1988;12(3):275.
6. Kuhnen C, Mentzel T, Lehnhardt M, et al. Lipoma and atypical lipomatous tumor within the same neoplasia: evidence for a continuous transition [in German]. *Pathologe*. 2010;31(2):129.
7. Klopstock T, Naumann M, Seibel P, et al. Mitochondrial DNA mutations in multiple symmetric lipomatosis. *Mol Cell Biochem*. 1997;174(1-2):271.
8. Ruppert V, Friedel R, Mentzel T, et al. Fibrolipomatous hamartoma of nerve—a rare etiology of macrodactyly. A case report [in German]. *Handchir Mikrochir Plast Chir*. 1999;31(1):53.
9. Silverman TA, Enzinger FM. Fibrolipomatous hamartoma of nerve. A clinicopathologic analysis of 26 cases. *Am J Surg Pathol*. 1985;9(1):7.
10. Price AJ, Compson JP, Calonje E. Fibrolipomatous hamartoma of nerve arising in the brachial plexus. *J Hand Surg Br*. 1995;20(1):16.
11. Drut R. Ossifying fibrolipomatous hamartoma of the ulnar nerve. *Pediatr Pathol*. 1988;8(2):179.
12. Collins MH, Chatten J. Lipoblastoma/lipoblastomatosis: a clinicopathologic study of 25 tumors. *Am J Surg Pathol*. 1997;21(1):1131.
13. Mentzel T, Calonje E, Fletcher CDM. Lipoblastoma and lipoblastomatosis: a clinicopathological study of 14 cases. *Histopathology*. 1993;23(6):527.
14. Coffin CM, Lowichik A, Putman A. Lipoblastoma (LPB): a clinicopathologic and immunohistochemical study of 59 cases. *Am J Surg Pathol*. 2009;33(11):1705.
15. de Saint Aubain Somerhausen N, Coindre JM, Debiec-Rychter M, et al. Lipoblastoma in adolescents and young adults: report of six cases with FISH analysis. *Histopathology*. 2008;52(3):294.
16. Hibbard MK, Kozakewich HP, Dal Cin P, et al. PLAG1 fusion oncogenes in lipoblastoma. *Cancer Res*. 2000;60(17):4869.
17. Kubota F, Matsuyama A, Shibuya R, et al. Desmin positivity in spindle cells: under-recognized immunophenotype in lipoblastoma. *Pathol Int*. 2013;63(7):353.
18. Cappellesso R, d'Amore ES, Dall'Igna P, et al. Immunohistochemical expression of p16 in lipoblastomas. *Hum Pathol*. 2016;47(1):64.
19. Mirkovic J, Fletcher CDM. Lipoblastoma-like tumor of the vulva. Further characterization in 8 new cases. *Am J Surg Pathol*. 2015;39(9):1290.
20. Abbasi NR, Brownell I, Fangman W. Familial multiple angiolipomatosis. *Dermatol Online J*. 2007;13(1):3.
21. Sciot R, Akerman M, Dal Cin P, et al. Cytogenetic analysis of subcutaneous angiolipoma: further evidence supporting its difference from ordinary pure lipomas: a report of the CHAMP study group. *Am J Surg Pathol*. 1997;21(4):441.
22. Fanburg-Smith JC, Devaney KO, Miettinen M, et al. Multiple spindle cell lipomas: a report of 7 familial and 11 nonfamilial cases. *Am J Surg Pathol*. 1998;22(1):40.
23. French CA, Mentzel T, Kutzner H, et al. Intradermal spindle cell/pleomorphic lipoma. A distinct subset. *Am J Dermatopathol*. 2000;22(6):496.
24. Billings SD, Henley JD, Summerlin DJ, et al. Spindle cell lipoma of the oral cavity. *Am J Dermatopathol*. 2006;28(1):28.
25. Akaike K, Suehara Y, Takagi T, et al. Spindle cell lipoma of the wrist, occurring in a distinctly rare location. A case report with review of the literature. *Int J Clin Exp Pathol*. 2015;8(3):3299.
26. Flucke U, van Krieken JH, Mentzel T. Cellular angiofibroma: analysis of 25 cases emphasizing its relationship to spindle cell lipoma and mammary-type myofibroblastoma. *Mod Pathol*. 2011;24(1):82.

27. Howitt BE, Fletcher CDM. Mammary-type myofibroblastoma: clinicopathologic characterization in a series of 143 cases. *Am J Surg Pathol*. 2016;40(3):361.
28. Billings SD, Folpe AL. Diagnostically challenging spindle cell lipoma: a report of 34 "low-fat" and "fat-free" variants. *Am J Dermatopathol*. 2007;29(5):437.
29. Hawley IC, Krausz T, Evans DJ, et al. Spindle cell lipoma–a pseudoangiomatous variant. *Histopathology*. 1994;24(6):565.
30. Sachdeva MP, Goldblum JR, Rubin BP, et al. Low-fat and fat-free pleomorphic lipoma: a diagnostic challenge. *Am J Dermatopathol*. 2009;31(5):423.
31. Mentzel T, Palmedo G, Kuhnen C. Well-differentiated spindle cell liposarcoma ("atypical spindle cell lipomatous tumor") does not belong to the spectrum of atypical lipomatous tumor but has a close relationship to spindle cell lipoma: clinicopathologic, immunohistochemical, and molecular analysis of six cases. *Mod Pathol*. 2010;23(5):729.
32. Creytens D, van Gorp J, Savola S, et al. Atypical spindle cell lipoma: a clinicopathological, immunohistochemical, and molecular study emphasizing its relationship to classical spindle cell lipoma. *Virchows Arch*. 2014;465(1):97.
32A. Marino-Enriquez A, Nascimento AF, Logon AH, et al. Atypical spindle cell lipomatous tumor: clinicopathologic characterization of 232 cases demonstrating a morphologic spectrum. *Am J Surg Pathol*. 2017;41(2):234.
32B. Creytens D, Mentzel T, Ferdinande L, et al. "Atypical" pleomorphic lipomatous tumor: a clinicopathologic, immunohistochemical and molecular study of 21 cases, ephasizing its relationship to atypical spindle cell lipomatous tumor and suggesting a morphologic spectrum (atypical spindle cell/pleomorphic lipomatous tumor). *Am J Surg Pathol*. 2017;41(11):1443.
33. Chen BJ, Marino-Enriquez A, Fletcher CDM, et al. Loss of retinoblastoma protein expression in spindle cell/pleomorphic lipomas and cytogenetically related tumors: an immunohistochemically study with diagnostic implications. *Am J Surg Pathol*. 2012;36(8):1119.
34. Tardio JC, Aramburu JA, Santonja C. Desmin expression in spindle cell lipomas: a potential diagnostic pitfall. *Virchows Arch*. 2004;445(4):354.
35. Mentzel T, Rütten A, Hantschke M, et al. S-100 protein expression of spindle cells in spindle cell lipoma: a diagnostic pitfall. *Virchows Arch*. 2016;469(4):435.
36. Meis JM, Enzinger FM. Chondroid lipoma. A unique tumor simulating liposarcoma and myxoid chondrosarcoma. *Am J Surg Pathol*. 1993;17(11):1103.
37. Mentzel T, Remmler K, Katenkamp D. Chondroid lipoma. Clinicopathological, immunohistochemical, and ultrastructural analysis of six cases of a distinct entity in the spectrum of lipomas. *Pathologe*. 1999;20(6):330.
38. Villarroel Dorrego M, Papp Y, Shelley MJ, et al. Chondroid lipoma of the tongue: a report of two cases. *Oral Maxillofac Surg*. 2014;18(2):219.
39. Nielsen GP, O'Connell JX, Dickersin GR, et al. Chondroid lipoma, a tumor of white fat cells. A brief report of two cases with ultrastructural analysis. *Am J Surg Pathol*. 1995;19(11):1272.
40. Flucke U, Tops BB, de Saint Aubain Somerhausen N, et al. Presence of C11orf95-MKL2 fusion is a consistent finding in chondroid lipomas: a study of eight cases. *Histopathology*. 2013;62(6):925.
41. de Vreeze RS, van Coevorden F, Boerrigter L, et al. Delineation of chondroid lipoma: an immunohistochemical and molecular biological analysis. *Sarcoma*. 2011;2011:638403.
42. Meis JM, Enzinger FM. Myolipoma of soft tissue. *Am J Surg Pathol*. 1991;15(12):121.
43. Panagopoulos I, Gorunova L, Agostini A, et al. Fusion of the HMGA2 and C9orf92 genes in myolipoma with t(9;12)(p22;q14). *Diagn Pathol*. 2016;11(1):22.
44. Fernandez-Aguilar S, de Saint Aubain Somerhausen N, Dargent JL, et al. Myolipoma of soft tissue: an unusual tumor with expression of estrogen and progesterone receptors. Report of two cases and review of the literature. *Acta Obstet Gynecol Scand*. 2002;81(11):1088.
45. Furlong MA, Fanburg-Smith JC, Miettinen M. The morphologic spectrum of hibernoma: a clinicopathologic study of 170 cases. *Am J Surg Pathol*. 2001;25(6):809.
46. Baldi A, Santini N, Mellone P, et al. Mediastinal hibernoma: a case report. *J Clin Pathol*. 2004;57(9):993.
47. Kumar R, Deaver MT, Czerniak BA, et al. Intraosseous hibernoma. *Skeletal Radiol*. 2011;40(5):641.
48. Mertens F, Rydholm A, Brosjö O, et al. Hibernomas are characterized by rearrangements of chromosome bands 11q13-21. *Int J Cancer*. 1994;58(4):503.
49. Zancanaro C, Pelosi G, Accordini C, et al. Immunohistochemical identification of the uncoupling protein in human hibernoma. *Biol Cell*. 1994;80(1):75.
50. Enzinger FM, Winslow DJ. Liposarcoma. A study of 103 cases. *Virchows Arch Pathol Anat Physiol Klin Med*. 1962;335:367.
51. Kindblom LG, Angervall L, Svendsen P. Liposarcoma a clinicopathologic, radiographic and prognostic study. *Acta Pathol Microbiol Scand*. 1975;253:1.
52. Evans HL. Liposarcoma: a study of 55 cases with a reassessment of its classification. *Am J Surg Pathol*. 1979;3(6):507.
53. Weiss SW, Rao VK. Well-differentiated liposarcoma (atypical lipoma) of deep soft tissue of the extremities, retroperitoneum, and miscellaneous sites. A follow-up study of 92 cases with analysis of the incidence of "dedifferentiation." *Am J Surg Pathol*. 1992;16(11):1051.
54. Evans HL. Atypical lipomatous tumor, its variants, and its combined forms: a study of 61 cases, with a minimum follow-up of 10 years. *Am J Surg Pathol*. 2007;31(1):1.
55. Shmookler BM, Enzinger FM. Liposarcoma occurring in children. An analysis of 17 cases and review of the literature. *Cancer*. 1983;52(3):567.
56. Kuhnen C, Mentzel T, Fisseler-Eckhoff A, et al. Atypical lipomatous tumor in a 14-year-old patient. Distinction from lipoblastoma using FISH-analysis. *Virchows Arch*. 2002;441(3):299.
57. Paredes BE, Mentzel T. Atypical lipomatous tumor/"well-differentiated liposarcoma" of the skin clinically presenting as a skin tag: clinicopathologic, immunohistochemical, and molecular analysis of 2 cases. *Am J Dermatopathol*. 2011;33(6):603.
58. Nascimento AF, McMenamin ME, Fletcher CDM. Liposarcomas/atypical lipomatous tumors of the oral cavity: a clinicopathologic study of 23 cases. *Ann Diagn Pathol*. 2002;6(2):83.
59. Cai YC, McMenamin ME, Rose G, et al. Primary liposarcoma of the orbit: a clinicopathologic study of seven cases. *Ann Diagn Pathol*. 2001;5(5):255.
60. Wenig BM, Weiss SW, Gnepp DR. Laryngeal and hypolaryngeal liposarcoma. A clinicopathologic study of 10 cases with a comparison to soft-tissue counterparts. *Am J Surg Pathol*. 1990;14(2):134.

61. Nucci MR, Fletcher CDM. Liposarcoma (atypical lipomatous tumors) of the vulva: a clinicopathologic study of six cases. *Int J Gynecol Pathol*. 1998:17(1):17.
62. Rosai J, Akerman M, Dal Cin P, et al. Combined morphological and karyotypic study of 59 atypical lipomatous tumors. Evaluation of their relationship and differential diagnosis with other adipose tissue tumors (a report of the CHAMP study group). *Am J Surg Pathol*. 1996;20(10):1182.
63. Sandberg AA. Updates on the cytogenetics and molecular genetics of bone and soft tissue tumors: liposarcoma. *Cancer Genet Cytogenet*. 2004;155(1):1.
64. Kraus MD, Guillou L, Fletcher CDM. Well-differentiated inflammatory liposarcoma: an uncommon and easily overlooked variant of a common sarcoma. *Am J Surg Pathol*. 1997;21(5):518.
65. Dei Tos AP, Mentzel T, Newman PL, et al. Spindle cell liposarcoma, a hitherto unrecognized variant of liposarcoma. Analysis of six cases. *Am J Surg Pathol*. 1994;18(9):913.
66. Italiano A, Chambonniere ML, Attias R, et al. Monosomy 7 and absence of 12q amplification in two cases of spindle cell liposarcoma. *Cancer Genet Cytogenet*. 2008;184(2):99.
67. Folpe AL, Weiss SW. Lipoleiomyosarcoma (well-differentiated liposarcoma with leiomyosarcomatous differentiation): a clinicopathologic study of nine cases including one with dedifferentiation. *Am J Surg Pathol*. 2002;26(6):742.
68. Binh MB, Sastre-Garau X, Guillou L, et al. MDM2 and CDK4 immunostainings are useful adjuncts in diagnosing well-differentiated and dedifferentiated liposarcoma subtypes: a comparative analysis of 559 soft tissue neoplasms with genetic data. *Am J Surg Pathol*. 2005;29(10):1340.
69. Thway K, Flora R, Shah C, et al. Diagnostic utility of p16, CDK4, and MDM2 as an immunohistochemical panel in distinguishing well-differentiated and dedifferentiated liposarcomas from other adipocytic tumors. *Am J Surg Pathol*. 2012;36(3):462.
70. Farshid G, Weiss SW. Massive localized lymphedema in the morbidly obese: a histologically distinct reactive lesion simulating liposarcoma. *Am J Surg Pathol*. 1998;22(10):1277.
71. Lucas DR, Nascimento AG, Sanjay BK, et al. Well-differentiated liposarcoma. The Mayo Clinic experience with 58 cases. *Am J Clin Pathol*. 1994;102(5):677.
72. Henricks WH, Chu YC, Goldblum JR, et al. Dedifferentiated liposarcoma: a clinicopathological of 155 cases with a proposal for an expanded definition of dedifferentiation. *Am J Surg Pathol*. 1997;21(3):271.
73. Yoshikawa H, Ueda T, Mori S, et al. Dedifferentiated liposarcoma of the subcutis. *Am J Surg Pathol*. 1996;20(12):1525.
74. Chibon F, Mariani O, Derre J, et al. ASK1 (MAP3K5) as a potential therapeutic target in malignant fibrous histiocytomas with 12q14-q15 and 6q23 amplifications. *Genes Chromosomes Cancer*. 2004;40(1):32.
75. Nascimento AG, Kurtin PJ, Guillou L, et al. Dedifferentiated liposarcoma: a report of nine cases with a peculiar neurallike whorling pattern associated with metaplastic bone formation. *Am J Surg Pathol*. 1998;22(8):945.
76. Marino-Enriquez A, Fletcher CDM, Dal Cin P, et al. Dedifferentiated liposarcoma with "homologous" lipoblastic (pleomorphic liposarcoma-like) differentiation: clinicopathologic and molecular analysis of a series suggesting revised diagnostic criteria. *Am J Surg Pathol*. 2010;34(8):1122.
77. McCormick D, Mentzel T, Beham A, et al. Dedifferentiated liposarcoma. Clinicopathological analysis of 32 cases suggesting a better prognosis subgroup among pleomorphic sarcomas. *Am J Surg Pathol*. 1994;18(12):1213.
78. Dei Tos AP, Doglioni C, Piccinin S, et al. Molecular abnormalities of the p53 pathway in dedifferentiated liposarcoma. *J Pathol*. 1997;181(1):8.
79. Gronchi A, Collini P, Miceli R, et al. Myogenic differentiation and histologic grading are major prognostic determinants in retroperitoneal liposarcoma. *Am J Surg Pathol*. 2015;39(5):383.
80. Thway K, Jones RL, Noujaim J, et al. Dedifferentiated liposarcoma: updates on morphology, genetics, and therapeutic strategies. *Adv Anat Pathol*. 2016;23(1):30.
81. Ishii T, Kohashi K, Iura K, et al. Activation of the Akt-mTOR and MAPK pathways in dedifferentiated liposarcoma. *Tumour Biol*. 2016;37(4):4767.
82. Alaggio R, Coffin CM, Weiss SW, et al. Liposarcomas in young patients: a study of 82 cases occurring in patients younger than 22 years of age. *Am J Surg Pathol*. 2009;33(5):645.
82A. Hemminger JA, Toland AE, Scharschmidt TJ, et al. Expression of cancer testis antigens MAGEA1, MAGEA3, ACRBP, PRAME, SSX2, and CTAG2 in myxoid and round cell liposarcoma. *Mod Pathol*. 2014;27(9):1238.
83. Antonescu CR, Elahi A, Healey JH, et al. Monoclonality of multifocal myxoid liposarcoma: confirmation by analysis of TLS-CHOP or EWS-CHOP rearrangements. *Clin Cancer Res*. 2000;6(7):2877.
84. Knight JC, Renwick PJ, Dal Cin P, et al. Translocation t(12;16)(q13;p11) in myxoid liposarcoma and round cell liposarcoma: molecular and genetic analysis. *Cancer Res*. 1995;55(1):24.
85. Dal Cin P, Sciot R, Panagopoulos I, et al. Additional evidence of a variant translocation t(12;22) with EWS/CHOP fusion in myxoid liposarcoma: clinicopathological features. *J Pathol*. 1997;182(4):437.
86. Iwasaki H, Ishiguro M, Nishio J, et al. Extensive lipoma-like changes of myxoid liposarcoma: morphologic, immunohistochemical, and molecular cytogenetic analyses. *Virchows Arch*. 2015;466(4):453.
87. Wang WL, Katz D, Araujo DM, et al. Extensive adipocytic maturation can be seen in myxoid liposarcomas treated with neoadjuvant doxorubicin and ifosfamide and pre-operative radiation therapy. *Clin Sarcoma Res*. 2012;2(1):25.
88. Antonescu CR, Tschernyavsky SJ, Decuseara R, et al. Prognostic impact pf p53 status, TLS-CHOP fusion transcript structure, and histological grade in myxoid liposarcoma: a molecular and clinicopathologic study of 82 cases. *Clin Cancer Res*. 2001;7(12):3977.
89. Haniball J, Sumathi VP, Kindblom LG, et al. Prognostic factors and metastatic patterns in primary myxoid/round cell liposarcoma. *Sarcoma*. 2011;2011:538085.
90. Gronchi A, Bui BN, Bonvalot S, et al. Phase II clinical trial of neoadjuvant trabectedin in patients with advanced localized myxoid liposarcoma. *Ann Oncol*. 2012;23(3):771.
91. Grosso F, Jones RL, Demetri GD, et al. Efficacy of trabectedin (ecteinascidin-743) in advanced pretreated myxoid liposarcoma: a retrospective study. *Lancet Oncol*. 2007;8(7):595.
92. Grosso F, Sanfilippo R, Virdis E, et al. Trabectedin in myxoid liposarcomas (MLS): a long-term analysis of a single-institution series. *Ann Oncol*. 2009;20(8):1439.
93. Gebhard S, Coindre JM, Michels JJ, et al. Pleomorphic liposarcoma: clinicopathologic, immunohistochemical,

and follow-up analysis of 63 cases: a study from the French Federation of Cancer Centers Sarcoma Group. *Am J Surg Pathol*. 2002;26(5):601.
94. Hornick JL, Bosenberg MW, Mentzel T, et al. Pleomorphic liposarcoma: clinicopathologic study of 57 cases. *Am J Surg Pathol*. 2004;28(10):1257.
95. Dei Tos AP, Mentzel T, Fletcher CDM. Primary liposarcoma of the skin: a rare neoplasm with unusual high grade features. *Am J Dermatopathol*. 1998;20(4):332.
96. Gardner JM, Dandekar M, Thomas D, et al. Cutaneous and subcutaneous pleomorphic liposarcoma: a clinicopathologic study of 29 cases with evaluation of MDM2 gene amplification in 26. *Am J Surg Pathol*. 2012;36(7):1047.
97. Boland JM, Weiss SW, Oliveira AM, et al. Liposarcomas with mixed well-differentiated and pleomorphic features: a clinicopathologic study of 12 cases. *Am J Surg Pathol*. 2010;34(6):837.
98. Miettinen M, Enzinger FM. Epithelioid variant of pleomorphic liposarcoma: a study of 12 cases of a distinctive variant of high-grade liposarcoma. *Mod Pathol*. 1999;12(7):722.

Metabolic, Genetic, and Systemic Diseases

PART 21

第二十一篇 代谢性、遗传性和全身性疾病

Chapter 123 :: Cutaneous Changes in Nutritional Disease
:: Albert C. Yan

第一百二十三章
营养性疾病的皮肤改变

中文导读

营养是生物体消耗和吸收食物营养以生存、生长和维持内稳态的一系列复杂事件。适当的营养包括平衡摄入关键的宏量营养素和必需的微量营养素。宏量营养素由碳水化合物、蛋白质和脂质组成，微量营养素是维生素和矿物质。人体无法合成这些分子，当这种平衡出现紊乱时，就会导致临床疾病——营养不足或营养过剩。

本章回顾了营养性疾病状态下观察到的重要临床特征，主要分为4个部分，首先介绍了与宏量营养素相关的疾病，包括蛋白质-能量营养不良（PEM）、必需脂肪酸缺乏等的流行病学、病因与发病机制、皮肤改变的临床特征、实验室检查、鉴别诊断及治疗；随后介绍了与微量元素相关的疾病，包括脂溶性维生素中维生素A缺乏症与维生素A中毒、胡萝卜素血症与胡萝卜素黄皮病、维生素D、维生素E及维生素K相关疾病，水溶性维生素相关疾病介绍了维生素B_1、维生素B_2、维生素B_3（烟酸）、维生素B_6（吡哆醇）、维生素B_9（叶酸）、维生素B_{12}（钴胺）、维生素C（抗坏血酸）、生物素（维生素H）相关疾病；然后介绍了矿物质相关疾病，包括门克斯病，以及硒、锰、铁、锌缺乏与中毒的相关疾病特征；最后特别介绍了坏疽性口炎的流行病学、病因与发病机制、临床表现与治疗。

本章最后总结了诊断的关键是熟悉与这些疾病相关的临床表现的范围，并在评估有皮肤表现或可能提示营养病因的皮肤病患者时，对这些疾病保持适当的怀疑。对疑似营养性疾病患者的适当评估应从详细的饮食和用药史开始，询问既往史和家族史，并仔细检查皮肤，特别注意头发、指甲和黏膜的状况。

〔粟　娟〕

PROTEIN ENERGY MALNUTRITION

AT-A-GLANCE

- *Marasmus* is caused by chronic global nutrient deficiency and characterized by dry, loose, and wrinkled skin with a loss of subcutaneous fat.
- *Kwashiorkor* is caused by inadequate protein or fat in the context of ongoing carbohydrate intake and characterized by generalized edema with a "flaky paint" dermatosis.
- In modern industrialized settings, kwashiorkor may result from excessive intake of rice beverages (young children), anorexia and associated eating disorders (adolescents and young adults), and GI surgery, especially bariatric surgical procedures (adults).
- Particular attention should be given to preventing refeeding syndrome, which is characterized by electrolyte abnormalities.

Nutrition is the complex series of events by which living organisms consume and assimilate foods and other nutrients to live, grow, and maintain homeostasis. Proper nutrition involves the consumption of key macronutrients in balanced tandem with essential micronutrients. Consisting of carbohydrates, proteins, and lipids, macronutrients are those nutrients that are needed in large quantities by an organism to both fuel metabolic processes and provide the substrate for building and maintaining cellular structure. By contrast, micronutrients are vitamins and minerals, which, although necessary to good health, are required in relatively minute quantities. Because humans are unable to synthesize these molecules, clinical disease results when disturbances occur in that equilibrium—most commonly from nutrient deficiencies, but also from an unbalanced ratio of consumed nutrients, or, less commonly, from nutrient excesses.

With an improved understanding of the role of diet in health and the advent of nutritional supplements, longstanding named scourges, such as scurvy, beriberi, and pellagra, have largely become diseases of historical interest. Even so, nutritional diseases remain problematic in developing countries and in settings of war, famine, and poverty. In industrialized countries, nutritional diseases may still arise among the disenfranchised—the homeless and those suffering from alcoholism or other forms of substance abuse. Individuals at risk also include those with derangements in their normal diets, such as might be encountered with eating disorders or unusual dietary habits, as well as with parenteral nutrition. Hypercatabolic states, exemplified by those with cancer, AIDS, hepatic or renal disease, and certain disease states such as carcinoid syndrome, may develop nutrient deficiencies even in the face of normal intake as a consequence of increased metabolic requirements. Excessive nutrient losses may occur as a result of decreased absorption arising from GI diseases such as cystic fibrosis, inflammatory bowel disease, celiac disease, or following GI surgery, especially bariatric procedures. Those receiving chronic medications, such as anticonvulsants or antibiotics, may experience impaired utilization of their nutrients when their medications interfere with GI absorption and normal metabolism. Impaired utilization may derive from underlying genetic metabolic defects, enzyme deficiencies, hepatic disease, or drug–nutrient interactions. In contrast, syndromes of nutrient excess generally stem from dietary surplus or iatrogenic therapeutic intake.

Because macronutrients and micronutrients are intrinsically involved in multiple biochemical pathways, disorders of nutrition may produce extracutaneous consequences. Moreover, those at risk for one nutrient deficiency may be suffering from other concomitant deficiencies as well. Appropriate evaluation of the patient with suspected nutritional disease should commence with a detailed history of dietary and medication intake, a review of past medical and family history, and careful inspection of the skin with special attention to the status of hair, nails, and mucous membranes. Even though some skin findings may be pathognomonic for certain nutritional disorders, physical findings are more often nondiagnostic. Laboratory analysis of blood and urine nutrient levels may be useful, but poor correlation with tissue levels limits their utility. Radiologic imaging studies may also offer corroboration for diseases such as scurvy, rickets, or beriberi. Clinical improvement following replacement therapy may represent the best or only means to confirm the clinical diagnosis of some nutritional deficiencies. This chapter reviews the important clinical features observed in nutritional disease states.

MACRONUTRIENTS

PROTEIN-ENERGY MALNUTRITION

EPIDEMIOLOGY

Malnutrition is a medical concern of global significance. The United Nations estimates that more than 2 billion individuals worldwide are malnourished.[1] As of 2017, estimates are that 150 million children younger than 5 or a quarter of children in this age group, suffered from malnutrition. Approximately 5 million children younger than age 5 years die from malnutrition each year.[2] The global response to malnutrition in financial terms exceeds $3.5 billion.[1]

In developing countries, malnutrition most commonly arises as a result of inadequate dietary intake, often compounded by disease. War, famine, and poverty states often aggravate the inadequate access to food, which may arise from political unrest, natural disasters, infectious diseases, seasonal and climactic factors, insufficient food production, lack of education, poor sanitation, regional and religious practices, and the limited availability of health care.[3] The availability of food in these settings may be limited to diets of corn, rice, and sometimes beans, which provide inadequate amounts of macronutrients and micronutrients. In industrialized countries such as the United States, less than 1% of children nationally suffer from protein-energy malnutrition (PEM). When it is encountered, chronic illness, malabsorption, presumed food allergies, food aversion, nutritional ignorance, and fad diets are more typical etiologies.

ETIOLOGY AND PATHOGENESIS

PEM refers to a spectrum of disorders describing varying degrees of protein and calorie deficiency. Several subtypes of PEM have been defined on the basis of relative deficiencies in protein and total calorie intake.

Children with marasmus are defined as those with severe wasting and stunting and are at less than 60% of expected body weight for age. The term *marasmus* derives from the Greek *marasmos*, meaning wasting. These changes are the result of chronic and global nutrient deficiencies, often because of a lack of available food. Children with kwashiorkor have body weights less than 60% to 80% of that expected for age, generally as a result of being fed grain-derived foods without adequate accompanying protein or fat. This might occur in geographic areas where grains are more plentiful, but more expensive proteins and fats are not. In fact, the term *kwashiorkor* derives from the Ghanaian term for "the one who is deposed," referring to the child who is weaned off of breastmilk onto a carbohydrate-rich but often protein-poor diet when the next child is born. The exclusive use of rice beverages, so-called rice milk products, as a substitute for baby formulas—either because of their lower cost or because of their perceived hypoallergenicity—has been linked to the development of kwashiorkor among infants in the United States as well as other countries.[4-8] A hybrid form of malnutrition in which stunting is associated with edema has been termed *marasmic kwashiorkor*.

The pathophysiology of these disorders can also be conceptualized as adapted and nonadapted forms of starvation. In adapted starvation (marasmus), decreased intake of all macronutrients, particularly carbohydrates, results in suppressed insulin production. As a result, catabolic hormones act unopposed and allow the appropriate conversion of glycogen into glucose. In the early stages of adapted starvation, muscle breakdown occurs within the first 24 hours, which permits gluconeogenesis to release glucose into the systemic circulation. Later, fat breakdown creates ketone bodies, which can also be utilized by the brain and CNS. This reduces the need for further muscle breakdown and, therefore, ammonia synthesis, so that lean body mass and some protein synthesis can be spared. In prolonged states of adapted starvation, wasting occurs and lean body mass is eventually used when all other sources are expended; in the absence of additional nutrient intake, the organism dies. In nonadapted starvation states (kwashiorkor), an imbalance results when intake of carbohydrate is increased relative to decreased intake of protein and fat. In this setting, insulin production is not appropriately suppressed. Without concomitant fat and protein intake, insulin inhibits protein synthesis. Hypoproteinemia, edema, and diarrhea develop, and without protein synthesis, affected individuals are unable to manufacture lipoproteins so fats accumulate, resulting in a fatty liver; more importantly, necessary immune proteins are not produced so patients become susceptible to opportunistic infection and septicemia, which represent major causes of mortality in these patients.

Although the concepts of adapted and nonadapted starvation provide convenient explanations for why some children develop marasmus and others develop kwashiorkor, some controversy exists. For instance, aflatoxins have been detected with greater frequency in patients with kwashiorkor than in those with marasmus.[9] Also, the role of oxidative and nitrosative stress in kwashiorkor is supported by data showing that patients with edematous PEM have lower levels of erythrocyte glutathione and total plasma antioxidants than healthy controls.[10]

CLINICAL FINDINGS

Childhood is marked by periods of significant and rapid growth and development, and nutritional deprivation often manifests as alterations in these patterns of normal growth and development. Failure to thrive, a key finding in patients with PEM, may appear first as wasting in which patients have poor weight gain, and eventually, as decreased rates of linear growth (stunting). Various measurements have been recommended as markers for malnutrition, and include body weight and length/height ratio relative to age, body mass index, triceps, or middle upper arm circumference, as well as skin and hair characteristics.[11,12] Suboptimal neurodevelopmental outcomes, heightened susceptibility to infection, and increased mortality also may be observed in chronically malnourished children.

Marasmus typically affects infants younger than 1 year of age. The physical findings of marasmus include dry, thin, loose, wrinkled skin resulting from loss of subcutaneous fat with an emaciated appearance (Table 123-1 and Fig. 123-1).[13] Hair growth slows and examination may reveal easy hair loss leading to thin, fine, brittle hair and alopecia. Increased lanugo hair also may be present. Nails may also show signs of fissuring with impaired growth.[14] As the body mobilizes all endogenous energy stores to survive, both subcutaneous fat and muscle mass are lost. The loss of buccal fat pads creates the aged or wizened appearance attributed to children with marasmus that has been referred to disparagingly as "monkey facies" (Fig. 123-2). Perianal fat loss can lead to rectal prolapse and abdominal muscle hypotonia may result in abdominal distension.[15] Constipation may alternate with periods of diarrhea that may or may not be associated with concomitant GI tract infection. Angular cheilitis and mucous membrane changes also have been observed in patients with marasmus.[16] Patients often show both decreased resting body temperature and bradycardia.

The hallmark features of kwashiorkor—also known as edematous or "wet" PEM—include failure to thrive in association with edema and is primarily noted in children between 6 months and 5 years of age (Table 123-2). Children are often irritable, but may become lethargic and apathetic. In contrast to marasmus, skin findings are common in kwashiorkor. The generalized dermatitis in edematous PEM has been likened to flaking enamel paint, with the pattern of skin fissuring suggesting cracked or "crazy" pavement (Fig. 123-3). Increased pigmentation of skin may be observed on extensor surfaces of the arms and legs. Hair often changes from its natural color, typically developing a red tint before further pigment dilution results in light, gray-white hair (Fig. 123-4B). If a child experiences intermittent periods of kwashiorkor and improved nutrition, alternate bands of light and dark color within the hair shaft may be observed and has been referred to as the "flag sign" (Fig. 123-4A).

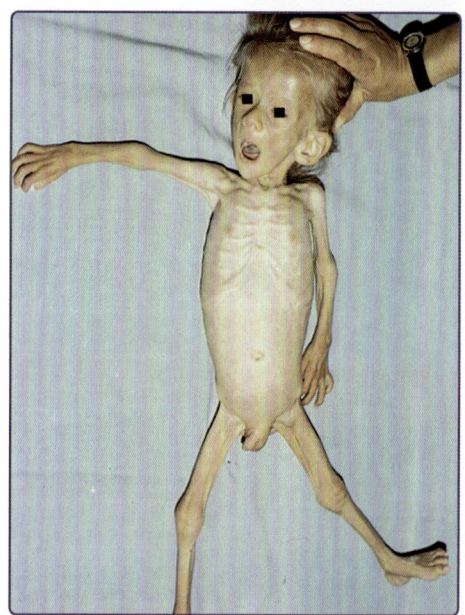

Figure 123-1 Marasmus. General appearance with advanced disease.

Increased lanugo hair can also be noted in kwashiorkor. In addition to the peripheral edema, a direct consequence of hypoproteinemia, distension of the abdomen is noted as a result of fatty infiltration of the liver.

Adults also may be at risk for PEM, particularly those suffering from chronic illnesses, eating disorders such as anorexia nervosa, and the elderly. The prevalence of PEM in adult dialysis patients has been estimated at

TABLE 123-1
Clinical Features of Marasmus

- Affects infants younger than age 1 year
- Failure to thrive
- Dry, thin, loose, wrinkled skin
- Hair loss; fine, brittle hair; alopecia
- Fissuring and impaired growth of nails
- Loss of subcutaneous fat and muscle mass
- Loss of buccal fat (monkey facies)
- Rectal prolapse, abdominal distension
- Diarrhea, constipation
- Angular cheilitis

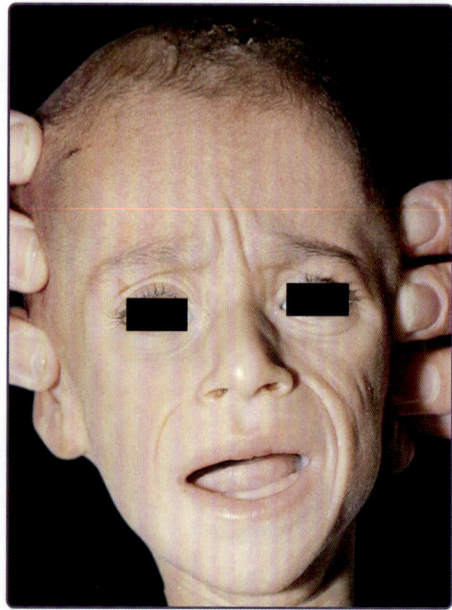

Figure 123-2 Marasmus. "Monkey facies" in an Arab infant, with wrinkled skin and loss of subcutaneous fat.

TABLE 123-2
Clinical Features of Kwashiorkor

- Affects children between 6 months and 5 years of age
- Failure to thrive, edema
- Irritability, lethargy, apathy
- Generalized dermatitis likened to "flaking enamel paint," "cracked pavement"
- Increased pigmentation on arms and legs
- Hair color changes (red tint → gray-white; "flag sign")
- Distension of abdomen

25% to 50% and is posited to occur as a result of semi-starvation with inadequate caloric and protein intake, possibly complicated by the presence of a chronic systemic inflammatory response to dialysis.[17,18] Cases of macronutrient PEM have been reported as a complication of bariatric surgery.[19-21] The manifestations of PEM in adults may be less prominent, manifesting more as xerosis or acquired ichthyosis, and may be the result of decreased sebaceous gland secretions or concurrent micronutrient deficiency.[22] Hyperpigmentation at characteristic sites also may be present, including the perioral, periocular, and malar areas. Diffuse telogen effluvium, lanugo, and thin, dry, dull hair also has been reported in adult PEM.[23]

LABORATORY TESTING

Initial laboratory testing in PEM as recommended by the World Health Organization[24] includes screening for hypoglycemia and anemia, and an investigation into potential comorbid infectious diseases. Because patients with PEM are at a significantly increased risk of serious infection, urinalysis for bacterial infection, blood smear for malaria parasites, and examination of feces for blood, ova, and parasites are essential. Skin testing for tuberculosis should be performed. Chest radiography may demonstrate concomitant signs of bacterial pneumonia, tuberculosis, heart failure, rickets, and fractures. Patients with kwashiorkor

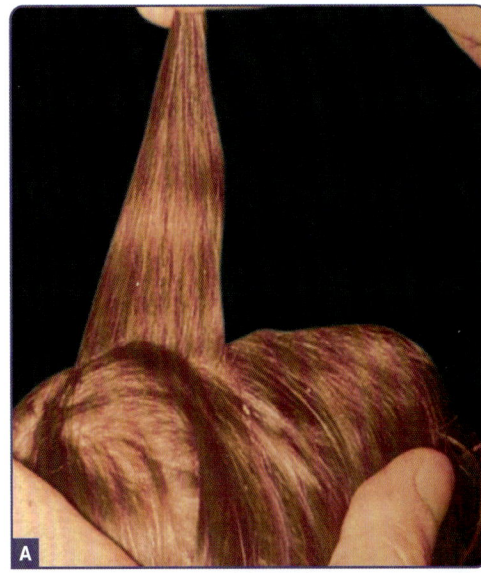

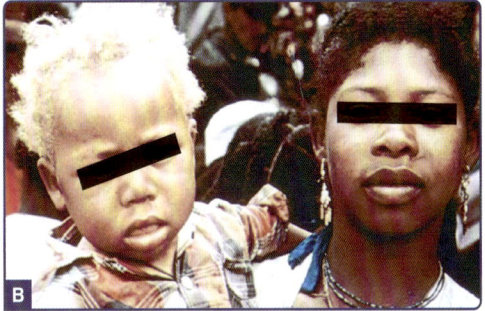

Figure 123-4 A, Flag sign in a Salvadoran child. **B,** Hypomelanization of the hair and skin.

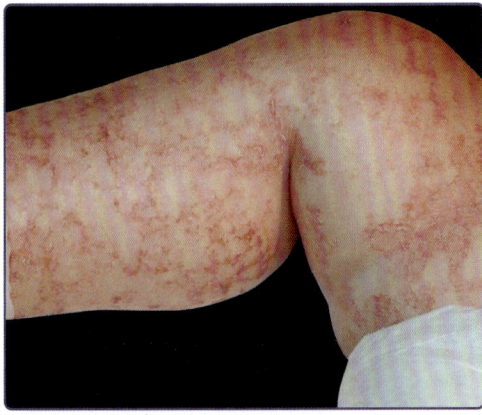

Figure 123-3 The "flaky paint" or "crazy pavement" dermatitis of kwashiorkor.

will also demonstrate hypoproteinemia, which may help guide treatment and prognosis. Evaluation of electrolyte levels before treatment should be interpreted with caution, as refeeding will likely alter mineral balances.

Elevated soluble CD14 levels are associated with indicators of protein-energy wasting, such as low body mass index and muscle atrophy, and increased mortality in hemodialysis patients. CD14 is a coreceptor that triggers immune activation in response to various ligands, including endotoxins and bacterial products. In patients with chronic renal failure on hemodialysis, increased soluble CD14 is associated with elevated markers of systemic inflammation, such as C-reactive protein, interleukin 6, fibrinogen, and plasma pentraxin 3. This suggests a possible link between chronic inflammation, PEM, and mortality in hemodialysis patients.[25] In one recent study, C-reactive protein elevation of greater than 15 mg/L and low phosphate in the context of PEM were documented as risk factors for greater mortality.[26]

Histologic evaluation is generally unnecessary because the clinical features in association with an appropriate history are diagnostic. However, histologic evaluation of the skin reveals increased thickness of the stratum corneum, atrophy of the granular layer, increased basal layer pigmentation, reduction of collagen fibers, and crowding of elastic fibers. Atrophy of the hair appendages with sparing of the sweat gland apparatus can also be noted.[27]

DIFFERENTIAL DIAGNOSIS

Table 123-3 outlines the differential diagnosis of PEM.

TREATMENT

Patients with severe PEM often require hospitalization because of the concurrent risks of hypoglycemia, hypothermia, dehydration, and sepsis. Individuals who are not awake and responsive may require intravenous hyperalimentation during the initial stages of therapy; care must be taken to avoid excessively rapid rehydration because of the risks of congestive heart failure. Oral refeeding using oral rehydration salts containing a mixture of essential electrolytes, at least until diarrhea subsides, or fortified formulas as soon as these can be tolerated, is generally preferred. Because severely malnourished children are relatively immunocompromised, empiric antibiotic therapy may be considered on admission for suspected sepsis, and any identified infections should appropriately addressed.[24]

ESSENTIAL FATTY ACIDS

AT-A-GLANCE

- *Function:* cell membrane fluidity, inflammatory mediators, and lamellar granule formation in the stratum corneum.
- *Sources:* fish oil and vegetable oil.

EPIDEMIOLOGY

Naturally occurring essential fatty acids (EFAs) deficiency states are uncommon in humans. Cases of deficiency arise, instead, from inadequate intake, malabsorption, or excessive loss. In the past, parenteral nutrition was a common cause of EFA deficiency, but with the introduction of lipid supplementation during parenteral nutrition in 1975, the incidence of EFA deficiency has decreased substantially. However, acquired EFA deficiency may arise as a result of recent attempts at lipid minimization. Neonates receiving lipid emulsions as an adjunct to parenteral nutrition for more than 21 days are at increased risk of parenteral nutrition-associated liver disease. There has been some interest in substituting soybean oil emulsions in lieu of fish oil emulsions to reduce the risk of hepatopathy, but their use has been linked to an increased incidence of EFA deficiency.[28]

Patients at risk for EFA deficiency include those with poor dietary intake, including alcoholics and patients with anorexia nervosa, and those with malabsorptive conditions such as biliary disease, inflammatory bowel disease, postgastrointestinal surgery (eg, bariatric surgery), and may represent one of the primary etiologies for the rash observed in cystic fibrosis patients.[29] Premature low-birthweight infants are born with inadequate EFA stores and are also at risk.

ETIOLOGY AND PATHOGENESIS

EFAs represent a group of 18-carbon, 20-carbon, or 22-carbon polyunsaturated fatty acids that cannot be synthesized de novo by the human body. The ω-3 series of fatty acids is found in fish oils, and is derived from α-linoleic acid. The ω-6 series is found in vegetable oils, and is derived from linoleic acid.[13] Linoleic acid and α-linoleic acid are the 2 EFAs that serve as precursors for other EFAs and thus must be obtained from dietary intake. In cell membranes, EFAs increase lipoprotein unsaturation to modulate cell membrane fluidity. Arachidonic acid, a derivative of linoleic acid, is converted into prostaglandins, eicosanoids, and leukotrienes. In the epidermis, linoleic acid contributes to lamellar granule formation in the stratum corneum. Therefore, EFAs play a number of key roles in maintaining homeostasis.

CLINICAL FINDINGS

Skin manifestations of EFA deficiency include: xerosis and scaly, diffuse erythema, and associated intertriginous erosions. Poor wound healing, traumatic purpura secondary to capillary fragility, brittle nails, and alopecia may be observed. Affected individuals may also demonstrate hyperpigmentation or hypopigmentation of the hair (Table 123-4). Extracutaneous findings include fatty liver infiltration, increased susceptibility to infection, a blunted immune response, anemia, thrombocytopenia, and growth retardation.

LABORATORY TESTING

In EFA deficiency states, linoleic acid levels are low and the enzymes that normally convert linoleic acid to arachidonic acid use oleic acid to create an abnormal byproduct. Consequently, laboratory evaluation

TABLE 123-3
Differential Diagnosis of Protein-Energy Malnutrition

- Acrodermatitis enteropathica
- Atopic dermatitis
- Seborrheic dermatitis
- Langerhans cell histiocytosis

TABLE 123-4
Skin Manifestations of Essential Fatty Acid Deficiency

- Xerosis
- Scaly erythema, intertriginous erosions
- Traumatic purpura, poor wound healing
- Brittle nails, alopecia
- Hyperpigmentation and hypopigmentation of hair

---

would demonstrate decreased levels of linoleic and arachidonic acids, and elevated plasma levels of an abnormal intermediary, 5,8,11-eicosatrienoic acid. Measurements documenting an increased ratio (≥0.2) of this abnormal intermediary relative to arachidonic acid are diagnostic for EFA deficiency.

TREATMENT

Although topical application of sunflower seed and safflower oils that contain linoleic acid may improve the clinical cutaneous findings of EFA deficiency,[30] topical absorption is unpredictable[31] and optimal treatment typically consists of oral or intravenous supplementation of EFA. To prevent EFA deficiency, EFA should represent 1% to 2% of total daily calories.[32]

MICRONUTRIENTS

FAT-SOLUBLE VITAMINS

AT-A-GLANCE

- Vitamins A, D, E, and K.
- Vitamin A deficiency is the most common cause of preventable childhood blindness in the world.
- Carotenemia results from excess carotene not converted to vitamin A in the intestinal mucosa deposits in stratum corneum.
- Understanding of the full function of vitamin D is still evolving.
- Vitamin D supplementation is recommended for exclusively breastfed infants, and others who have inadequate oral intake or sun exposure.
- Hemorrhagic disease of the newborn results from vitamin K deficiency and can present with a spectrum of bleeding, from ecchymoses to intracranial hemorrhage.

VITAMIN A (RETINOL)

Etiology and Pathogenesis: Vitamin A is a fat-soluble vitamin important in retinal photoreceptor function, epithelial proliferation, and keratinization. The two most clinically important metabolites of vitamin A are retinal, which is a key component of rhodopsin generation, and retinoic acid, which regulates cell differentiation.[33] Dietary intake of vitamin A derives from both plant and animal sources. Plant sources include dark, green, leafy vegetables, red palm oil, and brightly colored fruits such as papaya, mango, carrots, tomatoes, apricots, and cantaloupe. In plants, the vitamin A precursor beta-carotene can be found as a 2-molecule complex of the carotenoid known as retinal. The retinal can be later reduced to retinol in the intestinal villous cells. Animal sources of vitamin A include egg yolk, liver, fish, fortified milk, and other dairy products. In animal sources, vitamin A exists as retinyl esters, which are hydrolyzed to retinol in the intestinal lumen and absorbed into intestinal mucosal cells. All retinol vitamin A alcohol is esterified to retinyl esters within the intestinal mucosa, released into the bloodstream bound to chylomicrons, and then transported to the liver for storage. Here, retinol can be stored as retinyl esters in the liver; when needed, this storage form may be converted to retinol and bound to retinol binding protein and transthyretin and circulated throughout the body.

VITAMIN A DEFICIENCY

Epidemiology: Vitamin A deficiency (VAD) can result in both cutaneous and ocular complications. It is, in fact, the most common cause of preventable blindness in children, according to the World Health Organization. VAD also is associated with defects in immune regulation.

Etiology and Pathogenesis: The primary causes of VAD continue to be inadequate intake, fat malabsorption states, and liver disease. In the United States, inadequate intake can be seen in individuals with eating disorders, restrictive diets, and chronic illness. Because vitamin A is fat-soluble, conditions associated with malabsorption of fat, such as pancreatic or biliary tract disease, celiac disease, Crohn disease, Shwachman-Diamond syndrome, cystic fibrosis, cholestatic liver disease, chronic intestinal parasitic infection, and gastric bypass surgery, can predispose a person to VAD.

Clinical Findings: Table 123-5 outlines the manifestations of VAD. The earliest manifestations are ocular changes. Impaired dark adaptation (nyctalopia), is followed by xerophthalmia, and as corneal keratin desquamates and overgrowth of *Corynebacterium xerosis* on the sclera occurs, white patches known as *Bitot spots* develop. Severe deficiency may lead to corneal xerosis, ulceration, and keratomalacia, which may result in corneal perforation, prolapse of the iris, and blindness (Fig. 123-5).

The cutaneous findings of VAD are the result of abnormal keratinization. Mild deficiency may manifest as xerosis and scaling, whereas more-severe deficiency may result in deep skin fissuring referred to as *dermomalacia*. Squamous metaplasia of the salivary glands, as well as of the nasal and oral mucosa, may occur, leading

TABLE 123-5
Manifestations of Vitamin A Deficiency

- **Ocular**
  - Impaired dark adaption
  - Xerophthalmia
  - Corneal xerosis, ulceration, keratomalacia
  - Corneal perforation, blindness
- **Cutaneous, Mucocutaneous**
  - Xerosis
  - Skin fissuring (dermatomalacia)
  - Phrynoderma
  - Mucosa
  - Xerostomia
  - Hypotonia
  - Hypogeusia

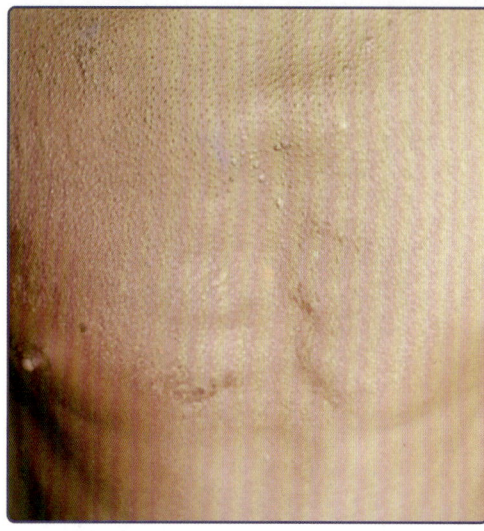

Figure 123-6 Vitamin A deficiency. Typical perifollicular hyperkeratosis of the chest in a Tanzanian adult male.

to xerostomia, hyposmia, and hypogeusia. Laryngeal, bronchial, and vaginal mucosa can also become involved.

Phrynoderma, "toad skin" (Greek for toad + skin), is typically associated with VAD. These keratotic follicular papules often first develop on the anterolateral thighs and posterolateral upper arms, which then spread to extensory surfaces of the extremities, shoulders, abdomen, back, buttocks, face, and posterior neck (Fig. 123-6). Lucius Nicholas noted the association between this hyperkeratotic folliculitis or phrynoderma with VAD in 1933, when he observed these cutaneous findings among East African workers who developed night blindness and xerophthalmia.[34] Although originally reported in association with VAD, phrynoderma is a nonspecific finding that can be observed with deficiencies in B-complex vitamins, vitamin C, vitamin E, EFA deficiency, PEM, and general malnutrition states.[35]

Laboratory Testing: Vitamin A levels can be measured from serum. Normal serum levels are between 20 and 50 mcg/dL (Table 123-6). Recently, assessment for the hydrolysis of retinoyl glucuronide to retinoic acid has shown promise as an adjunctive test for VAD. Retinoyl glucuronide is a water-soluble form of vitamin A that is not absorbed or hydrolyzed to retinoic acid in vitamin A–replete humans. The presence of serum retinoic acid for 4 hours after oral administration of retinoyl glucuronide is correlated with low serum retinol.[36]

Treatment: An international unit is equivalent to 0.3 mcg of retinol or 0.6 mcg of beta-carotene.[37] The recommended daily allowance (RDA) of vitamin A is between 700 mcg (adult females) to 900 mcg (adult males) (Table 123-7), with younger individuals requiring a lower intake of vitamin A. Lower levels are recommended during pregnancy and higher levels are recommended during lactation. Recommended treatment of VAD is 600 to 3000 mcg of oral vitamin A daily until symptoms resolve and serum levels normalize. Repletion dosages depend on the age of the patient, and require conversion to the appropriate food-related equivalent.[38]

VITAMIN A TOXICITY

Additional information is found in Chap. 213.

Epidemiology: In 1856, Elisha Kent Kane published his 2-volume *Arctic Explorations*, which included accounts of vitamin A toxicity that resulted after his team ingested polar bear liver during his expedition. The toxic substance in polar bear liver was later identified as vitamin A. Since that time, studies have shown

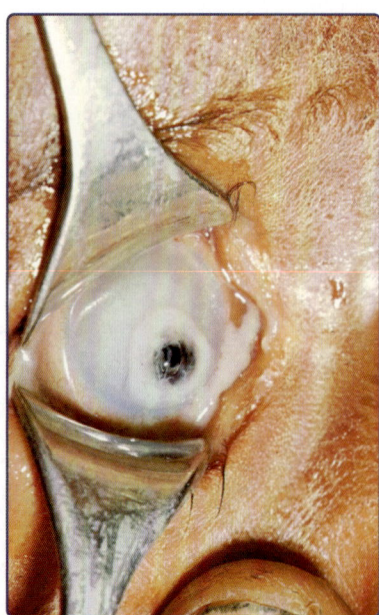

Figure 123-5 Vitamin A deficiency, advanced keratomalacia, in a 5-month-old Arab child. Note hyperkeratosis of facial skin. Serum vitamin A level was 2 mcg/dL (normal: 20-50 mcg/dL).

TABLE 123-6
Diagnostic Tests for Vitamin Deficiency

CONDITION	LABORATORY TESTS	NORMAL VALUES[a]	DEFICIENCY[a]
Vitamin A	Serum vitamin A levels/plasma retinol	20-50 mcg/dL	<20 mcg/dL (<0.70 μmol/L)–deficiency[c]
	Relative dose–response test: serum retinoic acid in serum after oral retinoyl administration glucuronide	In normal states, oral retinoyl administration leads to a *decrease* in serum retinoic acid	Serum retinoic acid *increase* of at least 20% indicates low liver vitamin A reserves
Vitamin D (calcitriol)	Serum 25-hydroxyvitamin D levels	≥50 nmol/L (≥20 ng/mL)[d]	<30 nmol/L (<12 ng/mL)–deficiency[d] 30-50 nmol/L (12-20 ng/mL)–inadequate for bone health[d]
Vitamin K (phytonadione)	Prothrombin time (PT) Activated partial thromboplastin time (PTT) Serum vitamin K des-γ-carboxy prothrombin (DCP)	11-13 seconds[e]	>13 seconds[e]
Vitamin B_1 (thiamine)	Erythrocyte thiamine transketolase	0-15%[f]	15%-25%–marginal deficiency[f] >25%–deficiency[f]
Vitamin B_2 (riboflavin)	Erythrocyte glutathione reductase activity coefficient Total riboflavin excretion	≤1.2 120 mcg/day[g]	1.2-1.4–marginal deficiency[e] >1.4–deficiency[g] <40 mcg/day–deficiency[g]
Vitamin B_3 (niacin)	Urinary *N*-methylnicotinamide and pyridone[b]	1	≤1–deficiency
Vitamin B_6 (pyridoxine)	Plasma pyridoxal-5-phosphate	>30 nmol/L[f]	20-30 nmol/L–marginal deficiency[h] <20 nmol/L–deficiency[h]
Vitamin B_9 (folate)	Serum folic acid levels Erythrocyte folate concentration	>3 ng/mL[i] >140 ng/mL[i]	<3 ng/mL[i] <140 ng/mL[i]
Vitamin B_{12} (cobalamin)	Serum cobalamin levels	350 ng/mL or higher[j]	<350 ng/mL[j] 1000 nmol/L–deficiency[j]
	Methylmalonic acid levels	<280 nmol/L[k]	>400 nmol/L[k]
Vitamin C (ascorbic acid)	Leukocyte ascorbate levels	>11.4 μM (0.2 mg/dL)[k]	<75 mg/L; <11.4 μM or 0.2 mg/dL–deficiency[l]

[a]There may be a wide range of normal values between laboratories. Values also differ between age groups.
[b]Urinary excretion of *N*-methyl-2-pyridone-5-carboxamide decreases to a greater extent than *N*-methylnicotinamide.
[c]Data from the National Institutes of Health (NIH), Office of Dietary Supplements. Vitamin A fact sheet for health professionals. https://ods.od.nih.gov/factsheets/VitaminA-HealthProfessional/ and Ross A. Vitamin A and carotenoids. In: Shils M, Shike M, Ross A, et al, eds. *Modern Nutrition in Health and Disease*. 10th ed. Baltimore, MD: Lippincott Williams & Wilkins; 2014.
[d]Data from the NIH, Office of Dietary Supplements. Vitamin D fact sheet for health professionals. t https://ods.od.nih.gov/factsheets/VitaminD-HealthProfessional/.
[e]Data from the NIH, Office of Dietary Supplements. Vitamin K fact sheet for health professionals. https://ods.od.nih.gov/factsheets/list-all/VitaminK/.
[f]Data from the NIH, Office of Dietary Supplements. Thiamin fact sheet for health professionals. https://ods.od.nih.gov/factsheets/Thiamin-HealthProfessional/.
[g]Data from the NIH, Office of Dietary Supplements. Riboflavin fact sheet for health professionals. https://ods.od.nih.gov/factsheets/Riboflavin-HealthProfessional/.
[h]Data from the NIH, Office of Dietary Supplements. Vitamin B_6 fact sheet for health professionals. https://ods.od.nih.gov/factsheets/VitaminB6-HealthProfessional/.
[i]Data from the NIH, Office of Dietary Supplements. Folate fact sheet for health professionals. https://ods.od.nih.gov/factsheets/Folate-HealthProfessional/.
[j]Data from the NIH, Office of Dietary Supplements. Vitamin B_{12} fact sheet for health professionals. https://ods.od.nih.gov/factsheets/VitaminB12-HealthProfessional/.
[k]Data from the NIH, Office of Dietary Supplements. Vitamin C fact sheet for health professionals. https://ods.od.nih.gov/factsheets/list-all/VitaminC/.

that animal livers contain exceptionally high amounts of vitamin A.

Vitamin A toxicity is the result of excess intake of vitamin A and can occur on an acute or chronic basis. Acute toxicity occurs when excessive amounts of vitamin A are ingested over a period of several hours or days. Toxicity typically results when intake exceeds 20 times the RDA in a child or 100 times the RDA in an adult. Chronic toxicity results from daily ingestion of greater than 25,000 IU (international units) for more than 6 years or greater than 100,000 IU for more than 6 months of preformed vitamin A. Children appear to be more sensitive to vitamin A intake than adults. Individuals most at risk for toxicity include patients taking systemic vitamin A derivatives for the treatment of dermatologic conditions such as acne, psoriasis, and ichthyosis. The other population at risk includes vitamin food faddists who consume large quantities of nonprescription vitamin A supplements.[39] Two notable episodes of vitamin A toxicity occurred in the 1950s when very high levels of vitamin A supplementation were added to infant formulas and the 1970s when high doses of vitamin A were used to treat a variety of dermatologic diseases.[40]

Vitamin A derivatives have been studied in chemoprevention of keratinocytic carcinomas, such as

TABLE 123-7
Summary of Recommended Daily Allowances in Vitamin Deficiency

DEFICIENCY	RDA	TREATMENT DOSE
Vitamin A	Adult (males): 900 mcg[a] Adult (females): 700 mcg[a]	600-3000 mcg/day until symptoms resolve
Vitamin D (calcitriol)	RDA: 15 mcg[b]	200-400 mcg/day × 2-3 months
Vitamin E (tocopherol)	RDA: 15 mg/day[c]	Deficiency states rare
Vitamin K (phytonadione)	Adult (males): 120 mcg[d] Adult (females): 90 mcg[d]	Acute: Fresh-frozen plasma Parenteral or intramuscular (IM) 5-10 mg vitamin K per day
Vitamin B_1 (thiamine)	Adult (males): 1.2 mg[e,f] Adult (females): 1.1 mg[f]	Beriberi: 50-100 mg/day for 1-2 weeks, IV or IM, then oral supplementation until recovered
Vitamin B_2 (riboflavin)	Adult (males): 1.3 mg[g,h] Adult (females): 1.1 mg[h]	Infants, children: 1-3 mg/day Adults: 10-20 mg/day
Vitamin B_3 (niacin)	15-20 mg of niacin or 60 mg of exogenous tryptophan	500 mg/day of nicotinamide or nicotinic acid
Vitamin B_6 (pyridoxine)	Adult (males): 2 mg/day Adult (females): 1.6 mg/day Infants: 0.3 mg/day	Replacement therapy of 100 mg of pyridoxine per day
Vitamin B_9 (folate)	400 mcg/day[i]	1-5 mg of folic acid per day; rule out concurrent vitamin B_{12} deficiency
Vitamin B_{12} (cobalamin)	RDA: 2.4 mcg[j]	Cyanocobalamin 1 mg/week per month
Vitamin C (ascorbic acid)	Adult (males): 90 mg[k] Adult (females): 75 mg[k]	100-300 mg
Biotin	Neonate: 30 mcg Adults: 100-200 mcg	Acquired deficiency: 150 mcg/day until resolution of symptoms Holocarboxylase synthetase

[a]Data from the National Institutes of Health (NIH), Office of Dietary Supplements. Vitamin A fact sheet for health professionals. https://ods.od.nih.gov/factsheets/VitaminA-HealthProfessional/.
[b]Data from the NIH, Office of Dietary Supplements. Vitamin D fact sheet for health professionals. https://ods.od.nih.gov/factsheets/VitaminD-HealthProfessional/.
[c]Data from the NIH, Office of Dietary Supplements. Vitamin E fact sheet for health professionals. https://ods.od.nih.gov/factsheets/VitaminE-HealthProfessional/.
[d]Data from the NIH, Office of Dietary Supplements. Vitamin K fact sheet for health professionals. https://ods.od.nih.gov/factsheets/list-all/VitaminK/.
[e]Approximately 0.5 mg/1000 kcal.
[f]Data from the NIH, Office of Dietary Supplements. Thiamin fact sheet for health professionals. https://ods.od.nih.gov/factsheets/Thiamin-HealthProfessional/.
[g]Approximately 0.6 mg/1000 kcal.
[h]Data from the NIH, Office of Dietary Supplements. Riboflavin fact sheet for health professionals. https://ods.od.nih.gov/factsheets/Riboflavin-HealthProfessional/.
[i]Data from the NIH, Office of Dietary Supplements. Folate fact sheet for health professionals. https://ods.od.nih.gov/factsheets/Folate-HealthProfessional/.
[j]Data from the NIH, Office of Dietary Supplements. Vitamin B_{12} fact sheet for health professionals. https://ods.od.nih.gov/factsheets/VitaminB12-HealthProfessional/.
[k]Data from the NIH, Office of Dietary Supplements. Vitamin C fact sheet for health professionals. https://ods.od.nih.gov/factsheets/list-all/VitaminC/.

squamous cell and basal cell carcinomas. A large, blinded, randomized, controlled study of elderly men with a history of 2 keratinocytic carcinomas in the 5 years prior to initiation of the study compared topical tretinoin 0.1% cream to placebo. Surprisingly, the study was terminated 6 months early because of a statistically significant increase in all-cause mortality in the tretinoin group compared to the placebo group.[41] Analysis of this increased risk was limited by its post hoc nature and suggests that further studies are needed to clarify this association. Rare cases of iatrogenic intoxication have been reported in association with excessive use of vitamin A as a nutritional supplement.[42]

TABLE 123-8
Manifestations of Vitamin A Toxicity

- Dry, scaly skin with desquamation
- Peeling of palms and soles, follicular hyperkeratosis
- Cheilitis, fissuring of lips and angles of mouth
- Alopecia
- Anorexia, nausea, vomiting
- Myalgias, arthralgias
- Blurred vision, pseudotumor cerebri
- Skeletal changes: premature closure of the epiphyses, spontaneous bone fractures

Clinical Findings: Table 123-8 outlines manifestations of vitamin A toxicity. Individuals with acute vitamin A toxicity have dry, scaly skin, with large areas of desquamation and fissuring of the lips and angles of the mouth. Other signs and symptoms include headache, fatigue, anorexia, nausea, vomiting, blurred vision, pseudotumor cerebri, myalgias, arthralgias, and bone pain and swelling. An early cutaneous sign of chronic vitamin A toxicity in adults is dryness of the lips, which may progress to diffuse, dry, pruritic, scaly skin with peeling of palms and soles, alopecia, follicular hyperkeratosis, and hyperpigmentation of the face and neck. Anorexia, fatigue, and weight loss may also occur. It is interesting to note that follicular hyperkeratosis may occur in the settings of both VAD and toxicity.

In children, chronic toxicity presents as coarse hair with diffuse alopecia, coarse skin with generalized exfoliation, hyperpigmentation, and exfoliative cheilitis. Associated pseudotumor cerebri with headaches and papilledema, and in infants may a bulging fontanelle may be present. Skeletal changes are common with vitamin A toxicity, and may present with growth retardation secondary to premature closure of the epiphyses and spontaneous bone fractures. Proposed mechanisms for the pathologic bone findings seen in vitamin A toxicity involves antagonism between vitamin A-mediated and vitamin D-mediated intracellular signaling pathways and interactions with calcium-regulating hormones.[23,39]

Laboratory Testing: Laboratory findings in patients with hypervitaminosis A include elevated levels of calcium and alkaline phosphatase. This alteration in calcium homeostasis can lead to calcification of tendons, ligaments, and soft tissues. Deposition of excess vitamin A in adipose tissue and perisinusoidal fibrosis of the liver, which can lead to cirrhosis, are the most significant effect of long-term vitamin A toxicity.

Treatment: Almost all of the symptoms of vitamin A toxicity subside after the excess vitamin intake is discontinued, with the exception of liver cirrhosis and consequences of pseudotumor cerebri.

CAROTENEMIA AND CAROTENODERMA

Epidemiology: While hypervitaminosis A is a disease that causes a broad spectrum of clinical findings, excessive intake of carotene results in a benign disorder characterized by yellow-orange skin pigmentation. The condition was described as "carotenemia" in 1919 by Hess and Meyers who reported a connection between yellow skin pigmentation and increased serum carotene levels.[43] During World War I and World War II, carotenemia was more commonly seen because of the dietary shift from a meat-based diet to a more plant-based diet as a result of food shortages.

As antioxidants, carotenoids also have been studied in cancer prevention. A recent metaanalysis and systematic review was concordant with other past studies showing no significant benefit in reducing the incidence of cancer or cardiovascular disease.[44]

Interestingly, beta-carotene supplementation of 20 to 30 mg per day was associated with an increased risk of lung and gastric cancers.[45,46] Beta-carotene supplementation is also associated with an increased risk of aggressive prostate cancer.[47] Animal studies suggest that excessive carotenoids may increase cyclic adenosine monophosphate signaling and cause deleterious effects on oxidative stress pathways, leading to the increased risk of malignancy.[48,49]

Etiology and Pathogenesis: Carotenes are not synthesized endogenously and are obtained through intake of carotene-rich foods. Plant carotenes are converted to vitamin A in the GI tract, but approximately one-third of carotene is directly absorbed. Several factors can affect carotene absorption, including thyroid hormone, pancreatic lipase and bile acid concentrations, processing of foods, and dietary fat and fiber content. Hypothyroid patients notice an elevation of carotene levels as a result of decreased conversion to retinol. Pancreatic lipase and bile acids digest carotene so that a deficiency of these enzymes from pancreatic or biliary or hepatic dysfunction could result in elevated carotene levels. Mashing, cooking, and pureeing fruits and vegetables increase the availability of carotene because cell membranes are ruptured in the process. Dietary fiber decreases absorption. Because carotene is fat-soluble, a high-fat meal increases absorption. Patients with conditions that lead to hyperlipidemia, like diabetes mellitus, nephrotic syndrome, and hypothyroidism, also predispose patients to carotenemia because of a linear relationship between the amount of β-lipoprotein and carotene. Impaired conversion of carotene to vitamin A in patients with hypothyroidism and liver disease further contributes to carotenemia. Some patients with anorexia nervosa can present with carotenemia because of increased intake of vegetables. Other groups at risk for carotenemia are food faddists, those with excessive intake of nutritional supplements, dried seaweed (nori), carrots, and papayas, and infants ingesting a large amount of pureed vegetables.[50-52]

Clinical Findings: Excessive ingestion of carotenes does not result in hypervitaminosis A because the slow conversion of carotene to vitamin A in the intestinal mucosa is not rapid enough to produce toxic amounts of vitamin A.

Carotene deposits in the stratum corneum because of its high lipid content. The yellow discoloration of skin secondary to carotenemia is called carotenoderma. The carotene is excreted by sebaceous glands and in sweat, so the yellow pigmentation appears first on the face, predominantly in the nasolabial folds and forehead, and then progresses to manifest diffusely, especially on the palms and soles. The pigmentation is particularly noticeable in artificial light. Of note, carotenoderma, in contrast to jaundice, spares mucous membranes, like the sclera.

Laboratory Testing: Carotenemia does not occur until serum levels reach 3 to 4 times normal levels, greater than 250 mcg/dL, and is detectable approximately 4 to 7 weeks following initiation of a carotenoid-rich diet.

Treatment: Treatment involves discontinuation of excessive carotene intake, and carotenoderma typically fades as the intake of carotene decreases.

VITAMIN D (CALCITRIOL)

Etiology and Pathogenesis: Vitamin D is essential for regulation of calcium and phosphorus metabolism. Vitamin D acts on the GI tract to increase dietary calcium and phosphate absorption, stimulates increased bone resorption of calcium and phosphate, and stimulates the renal tubules to increase reabsorption of calcium and phosphate.

Humans obtain vitamin D from 2 sources: dietary intake and synthesis in the skin from exposure to ultraviolet light. Common dietary sources of vitamin D include fortified milk, fish oil, and fish such as salmon, sardines, herring, tuna, cod, and shrimp. Vitamin D can also be synthesized in the epidermis from the precursor molecule 7-dehydrocholesterol (provitamin D_3) by ultraviolet light in the 290 to 320 nm range. Previtamin D_3 then undergoes a spontaneous, temperature-dependent isomerization to vitamin D_3 (cholecalciferol), which enters the dermal capillaries. At this point, endogenous vitamin D_3 joins with exogenous D_2 (ergocalciferol) for hydroxylation in the liver to 25-hydroxyvitamin D. This molecule travels to the kidney where it is again hydroxylated to make mature vitamin D (1,25-hydroxyvitamin D, also known as calcitriol).

The most common disorder seen with vitamin D is vitamin D-deficient rickets related to decreased dietary intake of vitamin D. Several genetic causes of rickets also deserve mention. Two types of vitamin D-dependent rickets have been described. Type I represents an autosomal recessive defect in renal vitamin D–1α-hydroxylase, and is therefore treated with supplements of 1,25-hydroxyvitamin D. Type II, also referred to as hereditary vitamin D–resistant rickets, is associated with a rare autosomal recessive end-organ resistance to physiologic levels of 1,25-hydroxyvitamin D. Supplementation with high doses of 1,25-hydroxyvitamin D and calcium may overcome this resistance.

A surge in interest regarding the multisystem effect of vitamin D has spurred numerous studies. Evidence suggests that vitamin D deficiency is associated with increased systolic blood pressures,[53] fasting plasma glucose and insulin concentrations,[54] risk of cardiovascular disease,[55-57] risk of hip fractures in postmenopausal women,[58] and colon cancer mortality.[59] Vitamin D deficient individuals have an increased rate of all-cause mortality when compared to those who are vitamin D replete.[57,60] Studies into the function of vitamin D in the immune system have indicated that vitamin D is involved in the innate immune response. Toll-like receptor activation triggers expression of vitamin D receptor and vitamin D–1α-hydroxylase, which promotes macrophage activation.[61] A low vitamin D level is associated with an increased risk of active *Mycobacterium tuberculosis* infection.[62]

Vitamin D–deficient rickets continues to occur in modern times. Groups at risk for vitamin D deficiency include those with inadequate diet, malabsorption, and decreased exposure to sunlight. This includes the elderly or debilitated who have decreased sun exposure or decreased vitamin intake; patients on anticonvulsant therapy; those with malabsorption from GI surgery, celiac disease, or pancreatic or biliary disease; those with chronic renal failure; dark-skinned individuals living in areas with poor sun exposure; and breastfed babies who are exclusively breastfed without vitamin supplementation.

A recent resurgence in vitamin D–deficient rickets has prompted further evaluation of those at risk. A review of 166 cases of rickets in the United States between 1986 and 2003 showed that most cases presented between 4 and 54 months of age. Eighty-three percent were African American or black and 96% were breastfed.[63]

These results emphasized that exclusively breastfed infants, especially those with dark skin tones, may require vitamin supplementation. In response to the continued increase in cases of vitamin D–deficient rickets, the American Academy of Pediatrics in 2003 identified 3 populations who should be given supplemental vitamin D (200 IU): (a) all breastfed infants unless they take in 500 mL/day of fortified formula or milk; (b) all non-breastfed infants taking in less than 500 mL/day of fortified formula or milk; and (c) children and adolescents who do not obtain regular sun exposure, do not ingest at least 500 mL of fortified milk a day, or do not take a multivitamin with at least 200 IU vitamin D.[64]

Vitamin D–deficient rickets is associated with congenital ichthyoses, such as lamellar ichthyosis,[65-67] nonbullous ichthyosiform erythroderma,[68] X-linked ichthyosis,[66] and epidermolytic hyperkeratosis,[69] as well as photosensitive disorders such as xeroderma pigmentosum.[70] Factors contributing to vitamin D deficiency include avoidance of sun exposure, excessive transepidermal calcium loss, defective vitamin D synthesis in affected skin, and decreased intestinal calcium absorption secondary to systemic retinoid therapy.

There is increasing interest in the role of vitamin D and its deficiency in skin cancer risk. Vitamin D is thought to have antiproliferative properties that may influence the development of skin cancer.[71] Some emerging evidence indicates that vitamin D deficiency is associated with increased Breslow thickness of melanoma[72,73] and may correlate to some degree with nevus count. However, the exact relationship between vitamin D levels and skin cancer development remain uncertain as to whether increasing vitamin levels will have a causal influence on reducing skin cancer at this time.

Given the movement to encourage sunscreen use, there is concern regarding secondary vitamin D deficiency. Theoretically, regular use of the recommended amount of sunscreen can decrease 25-hydroxyvitamin D levels, but with real-life application of inadequate amounts of sunscreen and the tendency for increased sun exposure in individuals wearing sunscreen, there seems to be no significant impact on the incidence of vitamin D deficiency.[74]

At the same time, it appears that only limited sunlight exposure is necessary to produce adequate amounts of vitamin D_3. For patients with Fitzpatrick skin Type II, it has been calculated that only 5 minutes of summertime noon sun 2 to 3 times a week provides adequate vitamin D production to satisfy physiologic requirements (see also Chap. 17).[75,76]

Clinical Findings: The classic manifestations of vitamin D–deficient rickets are skeletal (Table 123-9). Calcium and phosphorus deficiency leads to poor calcification of new bones, resulting in fraying and widening of the metaphysis. This can be seen at costochondral junctions of the anterior ribs, creating the well-known "rachitic rosary." Poor calcification of the skull bones results in craniotabes, a softening of the skull bones giving them a ping-pong ball feel. As the bones become weaker, they cannot support the weight of the child and progressive lateral bowing of the lower extremities occurs. Other findings can include frontal bossing, widening of the wrists, scoliosis, hypotonia, fractures, dental defects, and, rarely, hypocalcemic seizures or tetany. Early radiographic signs of rickets include widening of the epiphyseal plate and blurring of the epiphyseal and metaphyseal junction. If the disease progresses, deformities at the growth plate develop, including cupping, splaying, formation of cortical spurs, and stippling. The bone cortices appear thinner and generalized osteopenia is noted.

A potentially fatal manifestation of vitamin D deficiency is a dilated cardiomyopathy. In a report of 16 British cases, 3 infants died and 6 additional infants were successfully resuscitated from cardiopulmonary arrest.[77] Importantly, the cardiomyopathy is responsive to vitamin D supplementation and can result in complete resolution.[77-79]

Vitamin D–dependent rickets Type II also is associated with cutaneous features that are clinically indistinguishable from the syndrome of generalized atrichia associated with mutations in the hairless gene.[80,81] Affected patients in both conditions are born with hair. However, within a few months after birth, scalp and body hair are lost with the exception of eyebrows and eyelashes. Small papules and cysts representing abnormal, rudimentary hair structures characteristically develop on the face and scalp. These cysts typically show disintegration of the lower two-thirds of the follicular unit. While the cutaneous features—notably the alopecia and cysts—are phenotypically and histologically identical, these are distinct clinical entities (Table 123-10).

TABLE 123-9
Clinical Manifestations of Rickets

- Rachitic rosary
- Craniotabes, frontal bossing
- Lateral bowing of lower extremities
- Widening of wrists, scoliosis, fractures
- Dental defects
- Rarely hypocalcemic seizures

TABLE 123-10
Comparison of Vitamin D–Resistant Rickets and Generalized Atrichia

VITAMIN D–RESISTANT RICKETS TYPE I	GENERALIZED ATRICHIA
Chromosome 12q14	Chromosome 8p12
Mutations in vitamin D receptor (Zn finger)	Mutations in human hairless gene (Zn finger)
End-organ unresponsiveness to vitamin D	Defect in catagen remodeling
Atrichia with papules and milia; + eyebrows/eyelashes	Atrichia with papules and milia; + eyebrows/eyelashes
Alopecia by 1-3 months of age	Alopecia by 40 days to 4 months

Laboratory Testing: In addition to the clinical and radiologic signs of rickets, laboratory examination may be helpful. Elevated alkaline phosphatase levels and low serum 25-hydroxyvitamin D levels are often useful laboratory indicators of vitamin D deficiency (see Table 123-6). In the early stages of rickets, parathyroid hormone levels increase to compensate, but this compensatory mechanism becomes inadequate if the deficiency continues.

Treatment: The recommended daily value of vitamin D is 5 to 10 mcg (see Table 123-7). Treatment includes oral vitamin D repletion with dihydroxyvitamin D in addition to a calcium-rich diet. Supplementation with 200 to 400 mcg vitamin D per day until resolution of symptoms, approximately 2 to 3 months, is usually adequate.[82] Additional therapy can include judicious sun exposure.

Two additional therapies can be used in cases of hepatic rickets, which is unresponsive to oral vitamin D supplementation because of decreased intraluminal bile salts. D-α-Tocopheryl polyethylene glycol-1000 succinate (TPGS), a water-soluble vitamin E that forms micelles at low concentrations, enhances vitamin D absorption and successfully treated 8 pediatric cases of hepatic rickets. These patients maintained adequate levels of vitamin D while on continued TPGS and vitamin D supplementation, without elevation of vitamin E levels.[83] Promoting cutaneous synthesis of vitamin D through ultraviolet radiation successfully treated 2 cases of hepatic rickets secondary to chronic cytomegalovirus hepatitis and to Alagille syndrome.[84] Ultraviolet light therapy also has treated an Asian male with poor dietary intake of vitamin D.[85]

VITAMIN E (TOCOPHEROL)

Vitamin E is rarely associated with deficiency or excess states of disease. Found in oils and shortenings, as well as various fortified grains, dark-green leafy vegetables, legumes, nuts, avocado, and small fishes such as herring and sardines.[86] Because it is a fat-soluble vitamin, excessive intake may augment the effects of anticoagulant medications leading to purpura and propensity for hemorrhage.[87] Deficiency states are rare. However, ataxia with isolated vitamin E deficiency is a rare and severe spinocerebellar neurodegenerative disorder with autosomal recessive inheritance. Patients with mutations in the α-tocopherol transfer protein are unable to properly transfer α-tocopherol from lysosomes into lipoproteins that results in a predisposition to oxidative stress in affected cells.[88-90]

VITAMIN K (PHYTONADIONE)

Etiology and Pathogenesis: Vitamin K is a necessary cofactor in the carboxylation of glutamate residues on coagulation factors II, VII, IX, and X, and proteins C and S. Dietary vitamin K, phylloquinone, is found in green, leafy vegetables, certain legumes, soybeans, cereals, and beef liver. Phylloquinone is actively transported in the distal small bowel. Approximately half of the body's vitamin K is obtained though these dietary sources, and the other half is synthesized by GI flora as menaquinones, which are passively absorbed in the distal small bowel and colon.

Vitamin K is derived from the German word *Koagulationsvitamin*, which literally translates to mean "clotting vitamin." In the early 1900s, Henrik Dam of Denmark discovered an "antihemorrhagic factor" that reversed diet-induced bleeding disorders in chicks. In 1943, Edward Doisy and Henrik Dam were awarded the Nobel Prize in Physiology and Medicine for their separate work on isolating vitamin K.

Clinical Findings: Vitamin K deficiency leads to impaired coagulation and hemorrhage, which in neonates is referred to as hemorrhagic disease of the newborn (HDN). Neonates are particularly prone to vitamin K deficiency because of poor transplacental transfer, low dietary intake, and a sterile bowel. HDN is divided into early presentation and late presentation. The incidence of early HDN is 0.25% to 1.7% and causes unexpected bleeding in the first week of life in an otherwise healthy neonate. It can present as ecchymoses, cephalohematomas or nasal, subgaleal, umbilical, intestinal, or intracranial hemorrhages. Late HDN is defined by the American Academy of Pediatrics as unexpected bleeding from severe vitamin K deficiency in 2- to 12-week-old infants who are primarily breastfed and who received no or inadequate neonatal vitamin K prophylaxis.[91] Vitamin K deficiency beyond the newborn period is rare, but may result from malabsorption, liver disease, inadequate dietary intake, or medications. Fat malabsorption occurs in conditions such as regional ileitis, topical sprue, celiac disease, cystic fibrosis, pancreatic insufficiency, and biliary obstruction. Antibiotic use can result in vitamin K deficiency by altering the populations of normal bowel flora. Coumarin interferes with vitamin K epoxide reductase, an enzyme important in the recycling of inactive vitamin K into its active form. Other medications that can interfere with vitamin K metabolism include anticonvulsants (phenytoin), rifampin, isoniazid, high-dose salicylates, cholestyramine, and cephalosporins.[13,92] Vitamin K deficiency in older children and adults can present as purpura, ecchymoses, gingival bleeding, and GI, genitourinary, and retroperitoneal hemorrhage.

Laboratory Testing: Because vitamin K is a key cofactor in the coagulation pathway, deficiency of vitamin K typically manifests as elevations in both prothrombin time and activated partial thromboplastin time. Serum levels of vitamin K can also be measured (see Table 123-6).

Although des-γ-carboxy prothrombin, also known as the abnormal "protein induced by vitamin K absence," can be a sensitive indicator for vitamin K deficiency, its presence also has been strongly linked to certain malignancies, in particular, hepatocellular carcinoma. It appears that hepatocellular carcinoma cells produce des-γ-carboxy prothrombin directly rather than as a byproduct of low vitamin K levels, which may be normal in patients with hepatocellular carcinoma.[93]

Treatment: Neonatal prophylaxis is traditionally with a single intramuscular dose of 0.5 to 1.0 mg vitamin K. There have been some studies regarding the use of oral vitamin K prophylaxis, but there is no definitive data on efficacy, safety, or bioavailability.[91]

Acute treatment is with fresh-frozen plasma to replace deficient coagulation factors. Vitamin deficiency can also be treated with parenteral or intramuscular 5 to 10 mg vitamin K per day to correct severe deficiency (see Table 123-7).

WATER-SOLUBLE VITAMINS

VITAMIN B$_1$ (THIAMINE)

Etiology and Pathogenesis: Disorders of thiamine may have broad-ranging implications because thiamine is an essential coenzyme for 3 separate enzymes involved in nicotinamide adenine dinucleotide phosphate synthesis, carbohydrate metabolism, and deoxyribose and ribose synthesis. Thiamine is used as a coenzyme for transketolase in the pentose phosphate pathway to produce nicotinamide adenine

AT-A-GLANCE

- B complex vitamins, vitamin C, biotin.
- Niacin supplementation should be given with isoniazid therapy to prevent pellagra, characterized by a photosensitive dermatitis, diarrhea, dementia, and death.
- Vitamin C is an essential cofactor in multiple biologic reactions, including collagen synthesis. Deficiency causes scurvy, which presents with follicular hyperkeratosis, curled corkscrew hairs, and a bleeding diathesis.

dinucleotide phosphate. Thiamine pyrophosphate acts as a coenzyme in pyruvate dehydrogenase and α-ketoglutarate dehydrogenase, which are involved in oxidative decarboxylation reactions in the metabolism of carbohydrates and branched-chain amino acids.

Epidemiology: Thiamine is obtained from whole grains, enriched bread products, dried peas and beans, potatoes, and fish. Polished rice eliminates the thiamine-containing husk and predisposes to thiamine deficiency.

Disorders of thiamine excess are extremely rare. Most arise as a result of intravenous administration for suspected thiamine deficiency in the context of chronic alcoholism. Local irritation at the site of intravenous administration, generalized pruritus, and anaphylactic or anaphylactoid reactions have been described.[94] Neurotoxicity can occur in experimental settings when thiamine is administered directly into the CNS.[95] In general, thiamine excess states are extremely rare in humans.

Beriberi refers to a thiamine deficiency state. The word is derived from Sinhalese meaning "extreme weakness." The symptoms of beriberi have been recognized in East Asian countries for thousands of years because polished white rice is a dietary staple. The Japanese navy observed in the 1890s that beriberi could be eradicated by adding meat, fish, and vegetables to the diet.[96] Beriberi became an epidemic in the Dutch East Indies in the late 1800s. Christiaan Eijkman was part of the medical team stationed in the Dutch East Indies to study beriberi. In 1929, Eijkman was awarded the Nobel Prize in Physiology and Medicine for his work, starting in 1886, studying the effect of polished rice and unpolished rice on the incidence of beriberi in chickens. Through a series of detailed experiments on populations of chickens fed various diets and injected with various bacteria, he concluded that there was a direct correlation between diet and beriberi, but like many, had initially misattributed the cause to a nonexistent infectious agent in polished rice. In 1926, Barend Coenraad Petrus Jansen and William Frederick Donath successfully isolated thiamine from rice polishings, and Robert Williams was able to synthesize thiamine in the 1930s.[97]

Predisposing factors for pediatric thiamine deficiency include unsupplemented parenteral nutrition, breastfed infants of thiamine-deficient mothers, congestive heart failure,[98] certain metabolic disorders,[99] and severe malnutrition. In adults, aside from chronic alcoholism, cases of thiamine deficiency are associated with bariatric surgery,[100] food refusal in severe depression,[101] renal disease,[102,103] congestive heart failure (most likely related to furosemide administration which inhibits thiamine absorption),[104,105] lymphoma,[106] bezoar,[107] and complicated obesity.[108]

Clinical Findings: Thiamine deficiency in the United States is now rare. Early signs include irritability, apathy, restlessness, and vomiting. As the disease progresses, neurologic signs of Wernicke encephalopathy may develop, such as ophthalmoplegia, ataxia, nystagmus, and characteristic laryngeal nerve paralysis resulting in aphonia, which is a classic manifestation of infantile beriberi. Other symptoms include congestive heart failure, tachycardia, dyspnea, and cyanosis. In 2003, a series of infants presenting with ophthalmoplegia as a manifestation of Wernicke encephalopathy was reported in Israel as a result of a thiamine-deficient infant soy formula. In all these cases, a prodromal illness was observed. Early symptoms included vomiting, anorexia, diarrhea, lethargy, irritability, and developmental delay. Upbeat nystagmus and ophthalmoplegia were the primary neurologic signs. Following treatment, those with early disease had complete recovery, but those with severe disease had residual neurologic complications.[109]

Adult beriberi has been categorized into dry and wet forms. Dry beriberi describes a symmetric distal peripheral neuropathy involving both sensory and motor systems. Wet beriberi includes neuropathy and signs of cardiac involvement, including cardiomegaly, cardiomyopathy, congestive heart failure, peripheral edema, and tachycardia. Rarely, wet beriberi can be associated with pulmonary hypertension that is reversible after thiamine supplementation.[110] A red, burning tongue and peripheral edema also have been observed with wet beriberi.

Laboratory Testing: Diagnosis of thiamine deficiency is made by measurement of erythrocyte thiamine transketolase or blood thiamine concentration (see Table 123-6). The more reliable measure is erythrocyte thiamine transketolase before and after thiamine pyrophosphate stimulation, represented as a percentage of thiamine pyrophosphate effect. Normal values are up to 15%.

Treatment: Because thiamine is a cofactor in a variety of metabolic pathways, daily thiamine requirements are calculated from an individual's ideal total caloric intake, with current recommendations indicating 0.5 mg per 1000 kcal.

Treatment of thiamine deficiency can be via intravenous, intramuscular, or oral routes of administration. Usually, treatment of beriberi is initiated with IV or intramuscular thiamine of 50 to 100 mg per day for 7 to 14 days; oral supplementation is then provided until full recovery is documented (see Table 123-7).

VITAMIN B_2 (RIBOFLAVIN)

Etiology and Pathogenesis: Riboflavin was discovered in 1879 as a fluorescent yellow-green substance found in milk. Its chemical structure was later determined in 1933. Riboflavin is used in 2 coenzymes, flavin mononucleotide (FMN) and flavin-adenine dinucleotide, both of which are involved in oxidation-reduction reactions in cellular respiration and oxidative phosphorylation. These 2 enzymes are also involved in pyridoxine (vitamin B_6) metabolism. Newer studies suggest that riboflavin deficiency may contribute to increased plasma homocysteine levels, impaired handling of iron, and night blindness.[111]

Riboflavin is typically obtained through dairy products, nuts, meat, eggs, whole grain and enriched bread products, fatty fish, and green leafy vegetables. A small amount of dietary riboflavin is present as free riboflavin; most are found as flavin-adenine dinucleotide or flavin mononucleotide. Dietary flavin-adenine dinucleotide and flavin mononucleotide are hydrolyzed to riboflavin by brush-border membranes or enterocytes. Free riboflavin in the intestinal lumen is then taken up by active transport in the proximal small bowel.

Deficiency states can be caused by decreased intake, inadequate absorption, phototherapy, and underlying metabolic disorder. Alcoholics, elderly, and adolescents are groups at risk for riboflavin deficiency secondary to poor nutritional intake. Malabsorption after gastric bypass surgery can also predispose individuals to riboflavin deficiency.[112] In areas of India, China, and Iran, riboflavin deficiency is endemic because of their dependence on an unenriched cereal diet. Infants of riboflavin-deficient mothers are also at risk of deficiency because breastmilk concentrations of the vitamin are proportional to maternal concentrations. Once weaned from the breast, these infants are at additional risk if they are not transitioned to milk. When confounded by PEM, riboflavin deficiency may be worsened because the usual renal compensatory mechanism of increased riboflavin absorption is impaired in this setting. Visible light phototherapy for jaundiced neonates causes photodecomposition of riboflavin.[113] Certain drugs also affect riboflavin levels through effects on absorption or metabolic inhibition. Chlorpromazine and other tricyclic drugs inhibit transport of riboflavin in the GI tract predisposing to deficiency states.[114] Borate displaces riboflavin from binding sites, increases urinary riboflavin excretion, and inhibits riboflavin-dependent enzymes, thereby contributing to riboflavin deficiency.[115] The neurodegenerative disorder, Brown-Vialetto-Van Laere syndrome is characterized by hearing loss and pontobulbar palsy, and has been linked to mutations in RFVT2 and RFVT3, riboflavin transporter genes that result in riboflavin deficiency.[116]

Clinical Findings: Signs of acute riboflavin deficiency include a deep-red erythema, epidermal necrolysis, and mucositis. The severity of symptoms depends on the severity of deficiency (Table 123-11).[117]

Clinical signs of chronic riboflavin deficiency or ariboflavinosis begin 3 to 5 months after initiation of an inadequate diet. Skin and mucous membrane findings predominate. Initially, angular stomatitis manifests as small papules at the corners of the mouth that enlarge and ulcerate before developing into macerated fissures that extend laterally and often bleed (Fig. 123-7). Pronounced cheilosis with erythema, xerosis, and vertical fissuring of lips can occur. Early glossitis appears as prominent lingual papillae, but after these papillae are lost, the tongue becomes smooth, swollen, and magenta in color. The dermatitis of riboflavin deficiency resembles seborrheic dermatitis in that it involves the nasolabial folds, nostrils, nasal bridge, forehead, cheeks, and posterior auricular regions. Flexural areas of the limbs also may be affected. Plugging of the sebaceous glands (dyssebacia) may be observed around the nose. The dermatitis can affect the genitalia, more often to a greater extent in males than in females. A red, confluent, crusty, or lichenified dermatitis of the scrotum often spreads to involve the inner thighs. In general, the dermatitis is worse in areas of chafing or trauma. Infants frequently manifest the dermatitis in the inguinal areas. In older individuals, the dermatitis is often more pronounced in facial creases and wrinkles, and if incontinent, can involve the perianal and buttock areas. Cutaneous findings are not aggravated by light exposure, but are exacerbated by heavy physical activity. Ocular findings are also a prominent feature of this disorder with photophobia and conjunctivitis being most notable. *Oculo-orogenital syndrome* is the term used to describe this constellation of symptoms.

Laboratory Testing: A normochromic, normocytic anemia may be observed. Erythrocyte glutathione reductase activity can be used as a screening test (see Table 123-6), but a trial of riboflavin supplementation

TABLE 123-11
Clinical Signs of Riboflavin Deficiency
Acute
▪ Erythema
▪ Epidermal necrolysis
▪ Mucositis
Chronic
▪ Angular stomatitis
▪ Cheilosis with erythema, xerosis, and fissuring
▪ Glossitis
▪ Seborrheic dermatitis-like dermatitis affecting typical sites and flexural areas of limbs and genitalia
▪ Photophobia and conjunctivitis

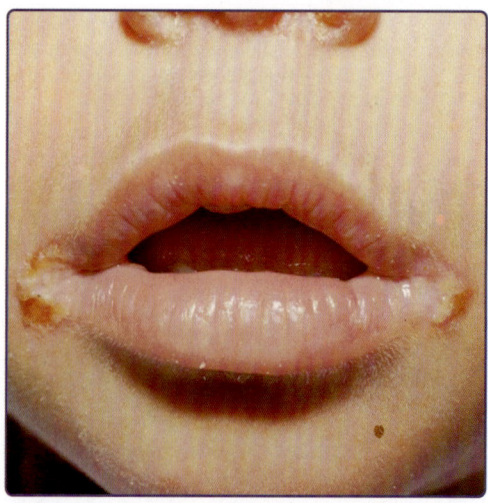

Figure 123-7 Riboflavin deficiency. Angular stomatitis with maceration in an Arab child. Riboflavin excretion in the urine was diminished.

is often the most optimal method to confirm a riboflavin deficiency.

Treatment: The recommended daily value of riboflavin is 0.6 mg per 1000 kcal. Treatment of deficient infants and children is 1 to 3 mg per day, and for deficient adults, 10 to 20 mg per day (see Table 123-7).

VITAMIN B$_3$ (NIACIN)

Etiology and Pathogenesis: Niacin is a vitamin cofactor that can be obtained for the diet or synthesized endogenously from the essential amino acid tryptophan. Niacin is found in whole grains and enriched bread products, nuts, dairy products, liver, animal meat, mushrooms, and dried beans. Dietary niacin exists primarily in the form of nicotinamide-adenine dinucleotide (NAD) and nicotinamide-adenine dinucleotide phosphate (NADP). NAD and NADP are hydrolyzed in the intestinal lumen to form nicotinamide. Nicotinamide can be converted to nicotinic acid by intestinal bacteria or be absorbed into plasma. Nicotinamide and nicotinic acid then travel to the liver, kidney, enterocytes, where they are converted back to NAD and NADP. These 2 agents act as hydrogen donors and acceptors in oxidation-reduction reactions involved in the synthesis and metabolism of carbohydrates, fatty acids, and proteins.

Deficiency of niacin or vitamin B$_3$ results in pellagra.

Historical Background: In 1735, Gasper Casal noted poor peasants in northern Spain were particularly affected by a skin disorder referred to then as "mal de la rose," so named because of the reddish, glossy rash on the dorsum of the hands and feet. He noted that these peasants were all poor, ate mainly maize, and rarely ate fresh meat. Francois Thierty published the first description of pellagra in 1755, but it was Francesco Frapoli who coined the name *pellagra* after the Italian words "pelle," meaning skin, and "agra," meaning rough.

During the 19th century, the cause of many diseases was attributed to infectious agents, and pellagra had been thought to be related to some infectious microorganism. While working as for the United States Public Health Service, Joseph Goldberger first suggested that pellagra might be caused by an amino acid deficiency in 1922, and that a dietary "pellagra-preventive factor" existed. Pellagra was endemic in the southern United States in the early 1900s because of a ubiquitous diet consisting principally of corn bread, molasses, and pork fat. Beginning in 1914, Goldberger worked with 2 orphanages and 1 sanitarium in the South. By increasing the amount of fresh animal meat and vegetables available at the 3 institutions, Goldberger was able to significantly decrease the incidence of pellagra. He went on to investigate pellagra among male prisoners. Using 12 prisoners from the Mississippi State Penitentiary and offering prisoners pardons as an incentive to participate, he successfully demonstrated that pellagra could be induced by a monotonous cereal-based, low calorie, and protein diet. To disprove the allegation that pellagra was caused by an infectious agent, he subjected 16 volunteers to the blood, urine, feces, and epidermal scales of pellagrous patients and showed that they were not predisposed to develop pellagra.[118] Goldberger died before he identified the pellagra-preventive factor, but in 1937, Conrad Elvanhjem identified niacin as the antipellagra factor.[119]

Pellagra remains endemic in parts of the world, including South Africa, China, and India, where corn and maize continue to be a dietary mainstay. Corn and maize contain bound niacin, so without alkaline hydrolysis to release the niacin, it is unavailable for absorption. Jowar, a type of millet found in parts of India, contains adequate levels of niacin, but large quantities of leucine interfere with the conversion of tryptophan to niacin.[120] Although Mexicans have a predominantly maize-based diet, pellagra is relatively uncommon because preparation of the maize includes washing it in lime water, which releases the complexed niacin.

Because niacin is absorbed from the GI tract, GI disorders can predispose to pellagra. Impaired absorption of tryptophan and niacin occurs in patients with jejunoileitis, gastroenterostomy, prolonged diarrhea, chronic colitis, ulcerative colitis, cirrhosis, Crohn disease, and subtotal gastrectomy.[121] Patients with Hartnup disease, a rare autosomal recessive disorder, develop pellagra-like symptoms in childhood. This is caused by a defect in the neutral brush-border system, resulting in malabsorption of amino acids, including tryptophan. Alcoholics develop pellagra from a combination of poor diet and malabsorption. Overly restrictive diets from eating disorders, such as anorexia nervosa, presumed food allergies, and food faddism can also cause pellagra.

Patients with increased metabolic needs as seen in carcinoid syndrome can develop pellagra. Normally, approximately 1% of tryptophan is metabolized to serotonin, but in carcinoid syndrome, an excessive amount, approximately 60%, of tryptophan is converted to serotonin. Because of this diversion of tryptophan to serotonin production, less tryptophan is available to make niacin.

Medications can also induce pellagra symptoms. Isoniazid is a competitive inhibitor of NAD because of their similar structures, and also impairs pyridoxine functioning, which is essential for niacin synthesis from tryptophan. 5-Fluorouracil inhibits conversion of tryptophan to niacin, and 6-mercaptopurine inhibits NAD phosphorylase, which inhibits NAD production. Other implicated medications include phenytoin, chloramphenicol, azathioprine, sulfonamides, and antidepressants.[122]

Clinical Findings: Pellagra is classically described with the four Ds of (a) dermatitis, (b) diarrhea, (c) dementia, and (d) death. The characteristic dermatitis begins as painful, erythematous, pruritic patches in photodistributed areas. The skin becomes progressively more edematous, and several days later may develop vesicles and bullae, which can rupture, leaving crusted erosions, or develop into brown scales. Over time, the skin thickens into sharply demarcated, keratotic, hyperpigmented plaques. Painful fissures can develop in the palms and soles, resembling goose skin. The dorsum of the hands is the most commonly affected site, and when the rash extends proximally, more on the radial than ulnar side, it forms the "gauntlet" of pellagra (Fig. 123-8A). A butterfly distribution may be apparent on the face when it extends from the nose to the cheeks, chins, and lips. When the dermatitis affects the upper central portion of the chest and neck, it is referred to as "Casal's necklace" (Fig. 123-8B). It can sometimes extend down over the sternum to create a "cravat." Mucous membrane involvement may manifest as cheilitis, angular stomatitis, a red tongue, and ulceration of the buccal mucosa and vulva. Half and half nails also may be present (Table 123-12).[123]

TABLE 123-12
Clinical Manifestations of Pellagra

- Painful pruritic dermatitis in photoexposed areas
- May be vesicular, crusted, and develops into scaly, keratotic plaques
- Dorsum of hands ("gauntlet"), neck ("Casal's necklace"), dorsa of feet ("gaiter" of pellagra); butterfly distribution in face
- Angular stomatitis, cheilitis, glossitis
- Diarrhea, nausea, vomiting, abdominal pain, anorexia
- Insomnia, fatigue, nervousness, apathy, impaired memory, depression, psychosis, dementia

GI symptoms may represent the earliest signs of pellagra. Diarrhea, nausea, vomiting, abdominal pain, and anorexia have been reported. Neurologic symptoms, such as insomnia, fatigue, nervousness, apathy, impaired memory, and depression, can progress to psychosis and dementia in later stages. Without treatment, pellagra leads to death from multiorgan failure.

Laboratory Testing: Diagnosis is primarily made on clinical grounds and through a rapid response to vitamin supplementation. However, measurement of urinary metabolites of niacin—*N*-methylnicotinamide and pyridone—may be used to aid in the diagnosis (see Table 123-6). Histologic examination of skin biopsies from affected skin areas may demonstrate depletion of Langerhans cells whose absence are thought to allow for more prolonged inflammation at these sites.[124]

Treatment: The recommended daily value of niacin is 15 to 20 mg of niacin (see Table 123-6), or approximately 60 mg of exogenous tryptophan. Treatment with 500 mg per day of nicotinamide or nicotinic acid is given over several weeks. Nicotinamide is preferred over nicotinic acid because nicotinic acid is frequently associated with headache and flushing. Neuropsychiatric symptoms may remit after 24 to 48 hours of treatment, but skin lesions often take 3 to 4 weeks to clear.[125]

VITAMIN B_6 (PYRIDOXINE)

Etiology and Pathogenesis: Pyridoxine deficiency was elucidated by Albert Szent-Gyorgi in 1934 while studying pellagra in rats. Esmond Snell identified the 2 other forms of vitamin B_6 and worked extensively to clarify the biochemical properties of these molecules in the mid-1900s.

Vitamin B_6 describes 3 interchangeable molecules: pyridoxine, pyridoxamine, and pyridoxal. Humans are unable to synthesize any of these molecules, but, fortunately, they are widely available in both plant and animal products. Meats, whole grains, vegetables, and nuts are the best sources for vitamin B_6. Processing of these foods can decrease the amount of vitamin available. They are absorbed through passive diffusion in the jejunum and undergo phosphorylation to become components of active coenzymes. The most common form existing is pyridoxal-5-phosphate. Vitamin B_6 is employed in multiple pathways, including the

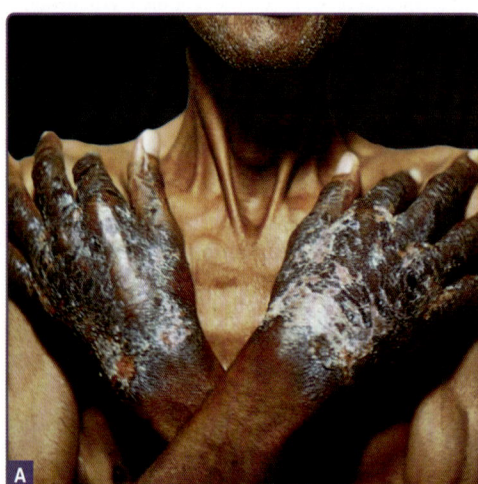

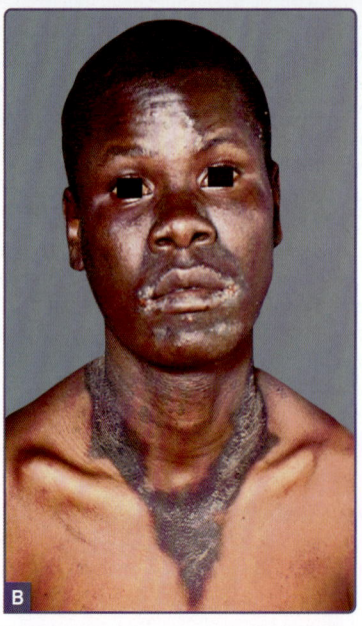

Figure 123-8 Pellagra. Acute dermatosis. **A,** "Glove" or "gauntlet" exudative and crusted lesions on the hands. **B,** "Casal's necklace" on the neck with facial involvement.

decarboxylation and transamination of amino acids, gluconeogenesis, and conversion of tryptophan to niacin, sphingolipid synthesis, prostaglandin synthesis, and neurotransmitter synthesis. As such, clinical features of pyridoxine deficiency may overlap with those of niacin deficiency.

As a consequence of the availability of dietary vitamin B_6, deficiency is seldom caused by inadequate intake, but can occur in alcoholics as the result of poor diet. More commonly, malabsorption and medication-induced deficiency is etiologic. Small-bowel disorders, such as Crohn disease and celiac disease, can interfere with absorption and produce deficiency. Medications that are implicated in causing deficiency include isoniazid, hydralazine, penicillamine, and oral contraceptives. Isoniazid, hydralazine, and penicillamine bind to pyridoxal-5-phosphate to increase excretion or decrease activity of the coenzyme. Bariatric surgery has been reported as an infrequent cause of pyridoxine deficiency.

Clinical Findings: Vitamin B_6 toxicity from excessive intake does not typically produce skin findings, although it can be associated with peripheral neuropathy.

Vitamin B_6 deficiency classically presents as a seborrheic-like dermatitis of the face, scalp, neck, shoulders, buttocks, and perineum. Clinical features overlap those of niacin deficiency including features of photodermatitis, glossitis, and cheilitis. Glossitis appears as redness, burning, and ulceration of the tongue, leading to flattening of the filiform papillae. Other areas of oral mucosa also become red and ulcerated, resulting in angular stomatitis, cheilosis, and conjunctivitis. This condition produces an oculo-orogenital syndrome quite similar to that seen with riboflavin deficiency.[126] Neurologic signs include somnolence, peripheral neuropathy, paresthesias, weakness, and confusion. Other signs and symptoms are nonspecific, and include nausea, vomiting, depression, anorexia, and anemia. The clinical manifestations of vitamin B_6 deficiency often resemble pellagra because vitamin B_6 is needed for the conversion of tryptophan to niacin.

Laboratory Testing: Vitamin B_6 can be evaluated by mean measurement of plasma pyridoxal-5-phosphate. Low levels of plasma pyridoxal-5-phosphate indicate deficiency (see Table 123-6).

Treatment: Recommended daily values of pyridoxine depend on age and gender. Adult males require at least 2 mg per day; adult females require at least 1.6 mg per day; and infants require approximately 0.3 mg per day (see Table 123-7). Treatment involves discontinuation of inciting medication and initiating replacement therapy of 100 mg of pyridoxine per day. Oral lesions resolve in days, skin, and hematologic changes resolve in weeks and neurologic symptoms over several months.[13]

VITAMIN B_9 (FOLATE)

Etiology and Pathogenesis: Folate can be found in almost all foods, particularly in liver, wheat bran and other grains, leafy green vegetables, and dried beans. Tetrahydrofolate, the coenzyme form of folate, is used for single-carbon transfers in amino acid, purine, and pyrimidine metabolism. The poor diets of alcoholics, malabsorption, and medications can produce folate deficiency. Malabsorptive states (such as celiac disease, chronic diarrhea, following total gastrectomy) and antifolate medications (such as methotrexate, trimethoprim, oral contraceptives, and pyrimethamine) can produce folate deficiency. The antiepileptics phenobarbital and phenytoin can also lead to folate deficiency states through induction of microsomal hepatic enzymes by antiepileptics, which deplete folate stores.[127] In children, folate deficiency also can be associated with excessive boiling of milk or a goat's milk diet. Human milk has greater bioavailability of folate when compared with goat's milk.[128,129]

Clinical Findings: As with vitamin B_{12} deficiency, the primary manifestation is hematologic: hypersegmented neutrophils, followed by macrocytosis and megaloblastic anemia. Neutropenia, thrombocytopenia, diarrhea, and irritability also may be observed. In contradistinction to vitamin B_{12} deficiency, folate deficiency is not associated with neurologic symptoms.

Mucocutaneous findings include glossitis with atrophy of the filiform papillae, angular cheilitis, mucosal ulceration, perirectal ulcerations, perineal seborrheic dermatitis, and diffuse brown hyperpigmentation concentrated in the palmar creases and flexures.[130,131]

Laboratory Testing: Macrocytic and megaloblastic anemia with hypersegmentation of neutrophils is suggestive. Diagnostic confirmation can be accomplished through measurement of serum folic acid levels (see Table 123-6).

Treatment: Folic acid supplementation is typically curative. Discontinuation of antifolate agents is recommended if involved. Ruling out concurrent vitamin B_{12} deficiency is crucial before initiating treatment of folate deficiency. If vitamin B_{12} deficiency is present but not treated, the hematologic symptoms may be respond to folate, but the neurologic symptoms will progress. Treatment involves 1 to 5 mg of folic acid per day (see Table 123-7).

VITAMIN B_{12} (COBALAMIN)

Historical Background: Some controversy exists as to who documented the earliest report of pernicious anemia. Thomas Addison is often credited with the first published description in 1855, but others, like

James Combe and Antoine Biemer, also deserve some measure of credit. Pernicious anemia was a recognized entity in the late 1800s, and strides were made in the early 20th century toward a better understanding of pernicious anemia. As understanding of other diseases, such as pellagra and beriberi, began to emerge, researchers began to wonder if pernicious anemia was also caused by a dietary deficiency. In 1920, George Whipple published results from studies he had done on anemic dogs. Whipple induced anemia in dogs by bleeding them. After trials of different foods to recover the hemoglobin level, Whipple observed the greatest improvement with liver. George Minot and William Murphy won the 1934 Nobel Prize in Physiology and Medicine along with Whipple for their work in documenting that meat and liver could be employed to treat anemic patients.[132,133]

Around the same time, William Castle used controls and patients with pernicious anemia to prove that an essential interaction between meat (extrinsic factor) and a component of normal human gastric secretions (intrinsic factor) were required for resolution of anemia. Finally, in 1948, Karl Folkers and colleagues successfully crystallized vitamin B_{12} and in 1964 Philippus Hoedenmaeker showed that Castle's intrinsic factor was produced by the gastric parietal cell. The well-known Schilling test to assess intrinsic factor deficiency was described by Robert Schilling in 1953.[134]

Etiology and Pathogenesis: Vitamin B_{12} is an important coenzyme for 2 biochemical pathways in humans. The first enzyme uses methylcobalamin as a coenzyme for methyltransferase to methylate homocysteine to methionine, which is used in DNA, protein, and lipid metabolism. The second requires 5'-adenosylcobalamin to catalyze the reaction by methylmalonyl coenzyme A (CoA) mutase to convert methylmalonic acid to succinyl-CoA, which is used in fat and carbohydrate metabolism.

Vitamin B_{12} is found primarily in animal products, with liver, eggs, milk, beef, and organ meats being excellent sources. Gastric acid separates vitamin B_{12} from food proteins so it can bind to intrinsic factor in the duodenum. This complex is taken up by specific ileal receptors in the terminal ileum. In the enterocyte, vitamin B_{12} dissociates from intrinsic factor and enters the portal circulation bound to transcobalamin II for transport to tissues. Between 1% and 5% of free cobalamin is absorbed along the intestinal wall by passive diffusion. The body is able to store large amounts of vitamin B_{12}, so symptoms of deficiency often take 3 to 6 years to develop.

Epidemiology: Causes of vitamin B_{12} deficiency can be divided into 3 groups: inadequate intake, malabsorption, and other. Elderly individuals and psychiatric patients with poor diets (including those with anorexia nervosa), and strict vegetarians and their breastfed infants are most likely to become deficient from inadequate intake. Cases related to malabsorption can be further divided into 4 groups: (a) decreased gastric acid states leaving more B_{12} food-bound (chronic proton pump inhibitors and histamine H_2 receptor blockers); (b) decreased intrinsic factor (pernicious anemia, atrophic gastritis, postgastrectomy); (c) microbial competition in the gut (bacterial overgrowth, *Diphyllobothrium latum* infection); and (d) impaired absorption (Crohn disease, Whipple disease, Zollinger-Ellison syndrome, celiac disease, short-bowel syndrome). The other causes of cobalamin deficiency relate to inborn errors of transport or metabolism.[135]

Clinical Findings: Vitamin B_{12} deficiency manifests primarily in 4 systems. As with cases of folate deficiency, mucocutaneous manifestations include glossitis, angular cheilitis, hair depigmentation, and cutaneous hyperpigmentation. Glossitis is characterized by an atrophic, red, and painful tongue with atrophy of the filiform papillae, which is referred to as *Hunter glossitis*. Early vitamin B_{12} deficiency can manifest as a linear glossitis.[136] Hair depigmentation may be localized or diffuse. Hyperpigmentation can be diffuse and symmetric or few scattered macules. The greatest concentration is usually observed on the hands, nails, and face, with the most commonly affected areas being the palmar creases, flexural regions, and pressure points. This hyperpigmentation often resembles Addison disease, but patients show no evidence of adrenal insufficiency.[137-140]

Three proposed hypotheses exist regarding the pathophysiology of the hyperpigmentation. Vitamin B_{12} maintains glutathione in reduced form, which is used to regulate tyrosinase, an enzyme necessary in melanogenesis. In B_{12} deficiency, increased tyrosinase activity results in hypermelanosis. Another proposed hypothesis involves defective melanin transport between melanocytes and keratinocytes. Finally, megaloblastic changes in keratinocytes from B_{12} deficiency may affect melanin distribution.[13,23,139,140]

The importance of cobalamin deficiency lies in its association with the classically described neurologic manifestations of subacute combined degeneration of the dorsal and lateral spinal column. Generalized weakness with paresthesias progresses to ataxia and symmetric loss of vibration and proprioception, worse in the lower extremities, eventuating in severe weakness, spasticity, paraplegia, and incontinence. Other neurologic findings include apathy, somnolence irritability, memory loss, dementia, and psychosis. Early neurologic findings may present before hematologic signs.

Laboratory Testing: The hematologic findings are similar to those found in folate deficiency, namely macrocytic anemia and hypersegmented neutrophils. Bone marrow biopsy reveals a hypercellular marrow secondary to disordered maturation.

Deficiency is diagnosed by measuring serum cobalamin levels, with levels less than 200 pg/mL indicating definite B_{12} deficiency and 200 to 300 pg/mL being borderline low (see Table 123-6).

Treatment: Treatment depends on treating the cause of deficiency and supplementing with vitamin B_{12}. Oral and parenteral supplementations have both been used. Oral supplementation can even be used in patients with pernicious anemia, but require much larger doses of enteral B$_{12}$ than when parental as absorption has to be through the intrinsic-factor-independent mechanism. Supplementation with cyanocobalamin of some form is 1 mg per week for 1 month (see Table 123-7). If symptoms persist, or if deficiency is to be a long-term problem, as in pernicious anemia, then additional supplementation is with 1 mg of cyanocobalamin every month.

VITAMIN C (ASCORBIC ACID)

Etiology and Pathogenesis: Vitamin C is an antioxidant and essential cofactor in several biologic reactions, including collagen biosynthesis, prostaglandin metabolism, fatty acid transport, and norepinephrine synthesis. Humans are unable to synthesize ascorbic acid because they lack gulonolactone oxidase, an enzyme most other animals possess and use to convert glucose to ascorbic acid. Other organisms that require ascorbic acid include the guinea pig, the fruit bat, and certain fish and bird species.

The majority of Western dietary vitamin C is obtained from fruits and vegetables, like potatoes, tomatoes, berries, citrus fruits, and green vegetables. Vitamin C is absorbed in the distal small bowel. Most dietary vitamin C is completely absorbed, but there is a decrease in absorption as dietary intake increases. Vitamin C is found in greatest concentration in the pituitary, adrenal glands, liver, leukocytes, and eyes. Depletion of body stores occurs after 1 to 3 months of a deficient diet.

As a water-soluble vitamin, ascorbic acid excess states are not typically associated with significant clinical disease. However, vitamin C deficiency is a disease of both great clinical importance and of great historical significance. Vitamin C deficiency results in scurvy.

Historical Background: Scurvy, the disease of vitamin C deficiency, has been documented since antiquity. Ancient Greek, Roman, and Egyptian texts describe cases of scurvy. The *Ebers Papyrus*, which dates to approximately 1552 BCE, documents cases of scurvy that were successfully treated with onions. Scurvy plagued sailors for hundreds of years before its cause was fully understood. One of the earliest reports dates to the 1497 expedition of India by Vasco da Gama. On this journey, many of the crew members developed scurvy, but da Gama noted that their symptoms improved after they traded for fresh oranges with locals in East Africa. After their supply of fresh oranges were depleted, da Gama observed the symptoms returned, so at their next landfall, they again sought locals with oranges to cure their disease. Other ships were not as fortunate as da Gama's crew. George Anson's pursuit of Spanish ships in 1740-1744 began with more than 1400 crew members. By the end of the 4-year journey, he returned with only 145 of his original crew members with only four killed in enemy action and more than 1300 having died from scurvy.[141]

In 1747, James Lind devised one of the earliest clinical trials to investigate crew members from the HMS *Salisbury* who were afflicted with scurvy. Lind selected 12 seamen with severe scurvy and divided them into 6 groups of 2, and each group was assigned to receive a different dietary therapy: hard apple cider, elixir of vitriol, vinegar, sea water, two oranges and one lemon daily for 6 days, and a medicinal paste. Lind published his findings in his *Treatise of the Scurvy* in 1753 where he concluded that oranges and lemons were the most effective treatment for scurvy.[142] Although Lind's findings were published in 1753, it was not until 1793 that lemon juice became a required daily provision on long sea voyages under the advice of Gilbert Blaine.[143]

As the incidence of scurvy decreased at sea, several epidemics on land occurred. The Great Potato Famine of 1845-1848, World War I, and World War II were times of nutritional impoverishment. The armies of the Crimean War and American Civil War, Arctic explorers, and California gold rush communities suffered from scurvy in large numbers. In the late 19th and early 20th centuries, an explosion in cases of infantile scurvy occurred in the United States because of the trend toward heated milk and proprietary foods. As shown by James Lind, heating of vitamin C decreased its biologic activity. Alfred Hess reported that pasteurization of milk likewise decreases its vitamin C concentration.[144] Proprietary food at that time was of poor nutritional quality. Interestingly, most of the affected infants were from affluent families who thought they were providing superior nutrition for their children.[145] Vitamin C was isolated by Albert Szent-Gyorgyi in 1927 when he isolated a compound found in high concentrations in the adrenal cortex, oranges, cabbages, and paprika.

Etiology and Pathogenesis: Causes of scurvy include insufficient vitamin C intake, increased vitamin requirement, and increased loss. Inadequate intake is the most common cause. Elderly individuals living alone may have limited diets as a result of poverty, immobility, poor dentition, poor access to groceries, or dementia.[146,147] Alcoholics, food faddists, individuals with presumed food allergies, and cancer patients may have decreased overall dietary intake or may simply avoid fruit and vegetables.[148] Iatrogenic scurvy occurs when physicians recommend dietary restrictions for certain conditions, such as ulcerative colitis, Whipple disease, peptic ulcers, and gastroesophageal reflux, or with inadequate vitamin supplementation with parenteral nutrition. Increased vitamin C requirements are encountered with certain drugs, including aspirin, indomethacin, tetracycline, oral contraceptives, corticosteroids, and tobacco smoking. Scurvy has been reported as a complication of interleukin-2 treatment of metastatic renal cell carcinoma.[149] Peritoneal dialysis and hemodialysis can induce scurvy because the water-soluble vitamin is removed during the dialyzing process.[150] Scurvy also has been reported among patients receiving liver transplantations.[151] One series highlighted associations between scurvy and patients suffering from thalassemia, neurologic disease, and those receiving chemotherapy or bone marrow transplantations.[152]

TABLE 123-13
Clinical Manifestations of Scurvy

Skin	• Follicular keratotic plugging • Corkscrew hairs • Perifollicular purpura • Lower-extremity edema with ecchymosis • Poor wound healing and dehiscence
Mucosa	• Swelling, ecchymoses, and bleeding of gingiva • Hemorrhagic gingivitis, necrosis, loss of teeth
Other organs	• Hemorrhagic intraarticular, subperiosteal, intramuscular, disruption of growth plates, bowing of bones, depressed sternum • Epistaxis, hematuria, GI, and cerebral hemorrhage

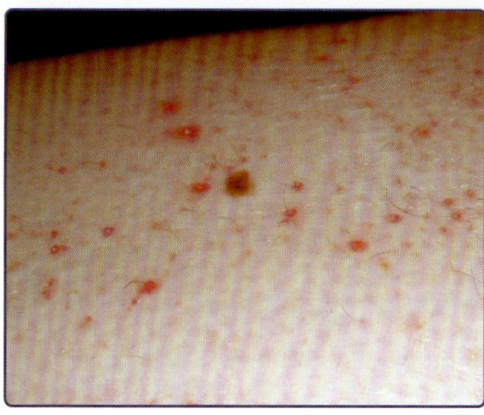

Figure 123-9 Vitamin C deficiency in an 18-year-old girl after GI surgery. Note the "corkscrew" or "swan-neck" hairs associated with perifollicular purpura.

Impaired collagen synthesis is the basis for many cutaneous manifestation of scurvy. Ascorbic acid is required for the hydroxylation of proline residues on procollagen, allowing the formation of hydrogen–hydrogen bonding in the triple helix of mature collagen. Without ascorbic acid, the polypeptides are unstable and unable to form stable triple helices. This results in decreased collagen secretion from fibroblasts, increased collagen solubility, and unstable collage fibrils. This abnormal collagen creates pathology in skin, mucous membranes, blood vessels, and bone, leading to the 4 Hs of scurvy: hemorrhagic signs, hyperkeratosis of hair follicles, hypochondriasis, and hematologic abnormalities (Table 123-13).

Clinical Manifestations: Table 123-13 outlines the clinical manifestations of scurvy. The earliest cutaneous sign of scurvy is phrynoderma, which is the enlargement and keratosis of hair follicles, especially on the posterolateral aspect of the arms, resembling keratosis pilaris. The keratotic plugging generalizes, extending to the back, buttocks, posterior thighs, calves, and shins. The hairs within these plugged follicles become curled, resulting in corkscrew hairs. The corkscrew hair results from impaired keratin crosslinks by disulfide bonds. As the disease progresses, the follicles turn red from congestion and proliferation of surrounding blood vessels, then turn purple, and finally red and hemorrhagic (Fig. 123-9). This palpable perifollicular purpura is characteristically found on the legs. Lower-extremity edema is often referred to as "woody edema," which is associated with pain and ecchymosis. Other nonspecific cutaneous findings include xerosis and acne. Poor wound healing, and even dehiscence of old wounds, involving skin and bone, can occur because vitamin C is necessary for wound healing and maintenance of healed wounds. Hemorrhage in the nail bed is noted as subungual linear (splinter) hemorrhages.

Oral manifestations are common. Gingival disease manifests as swelling, ecchymoses, bleeding, and loosening of teeth. Interdental and marginal gingivae become red, smooth, swollen, and shiny before becoming purple, black, and necrotic. This hemorrhagic gingivitis is secondary to poor osteodentin formation, which produces softer teeth that are prone to infection. Existing gingivitis and poor dentition predispose to more severe disease, but those without teeth do not develop hemorrhagic gingivitis.

Hemorrhage can occur in areas other than the skin, mouth, and nails. Bone disease is a frequent manifestation in children. Hemorrhage can be intraarticular, intramuscular, and subperiosteal. All of the above can lead to pain and disruption of the growth plates. Bowing of the long bones and a depressed sternum with and outward projection of the end of the ribs are noted on musculoskeletal examination. Metaphyseal spurs with marginal fractures (Pelkan sign), a ring of increased density surrounding the epiphysis (Wimberger sign), widening of the zone of provisional calcification (white line of Frankl), and a transverse band of radiolucency in the metaphysis (scurvy line or Trümmerfeld zone) are seen on radiographs of extremities. Periosteal bleeding may occur. Epistaxis, hematuria, intracerebral hemorrhage, subconjunctival hemorrhage, and GI hemorrhage have been reported. Weakness, fatigue, emotional lability, hypochondriasis, weight loss, arthralgias, hypotension, anorexia, and diarrhea are nonspecific findings associated with vitamin C deficiency.

The causes of a normochromic, normocytic anemia are multifactorial, including blood loss from hemorrhage, intravascular hemolysis, intracellular iron depletion, and decreased folate levels.

Laboratory Testing: Scurvy is a clinical diagnosis, but when unsure of the diagnosis, measurement of leukocyte ascorbate level can be helpful. Levels less than 75 mg/L indicate a deficient state (see Table 123-6).

Treatment: Recommended daily intake of vitamin C is 40 to 60 mg of ascorbic acid. With vitamin C supplementation, clinical symptoms rapidly improve within several days following initiation of supplementation. Therapeutic doses of 100 to 300 mg of ascorbic acid are administered daily until symptoms completely resolve (see Table 123-7).

BIOTIN

Etiology and Pathogenesis: Biotin is an essential cofactor for 4 carboxylating enzymes: (a) acetyl-CoA carboxylase in fatty acid synthesis and lipogenesis; (b) pyruvate carboxylase in gluconeogenesis; and (c) propionyl-CoA carboxylase and (d) 3-methylcrotonyl-CoA carboxylase, both of which are involved in amino acid catabolism.

Eggs, liver, milk, peanuts, mushrooms, chocolates, and hazelnuts are common sources of biotin. Release of protein-bound dietary biotin depends on pancreatic biotinidase. Free biotin diffuses across the gut to bind to plasma proteins. Because biotin is found in many dietary sources and can be synthesized by enteric bacteria, deficiency is uncommon. In 1941, Paul Gyorgy found that avidin in egg white bound and inactivated biotin. Virgil Sydenstricker took this observation and induced biotin deficiency by feeding normal volunteers raw-egg-white-rich diets. Avidin, a protein found in egg whites, binds free biotin in the bowel, thereby preventing absorption of both dietary and synthesized biotin. Although an uncommon cause of biotin deficiency, individuals following fad diets high in raw egg whites can be at risk for deficiency.[153] Biotin deficiency may arise from long-term parenteral nutrition without biotin supplementation.[154] Individuals on unsupplemented parenteral nutrition and on long-term antibiotics are particularly at risk because the antibiotics eradicate biotin-producing enteric flora.[155] Anticonvulsants, such as valproic acid, carbamazepine, and phenytoin, can increase biotin catabolism or impair liver function, leading to biotin deficiency.[156-158] A series of biotin deficiency cases were reported in Japan secondary to an elemental infant formula without supplemental biotin.[159,160]

Clinical Findings: Symptoms can develop 3 to 6 months after initiation of unsupplemented parenteral nutrition or a raw-egg-white-rich diet, but appear earlier in infants because of the greater biotin requirement for growth. The cutaneous manifestations are similar to those of acrodermatitis enteropathica (AE) and EFA deficiency (see section "Essential Fatty Acids") (Table 123-14). An erythematous, scaling, and crusting dermatitis usually begins around the eyes, nose, and mouth, and continues to involve multiple periorificial areas, including the perianal region. Alopecia, conjunctivitis, and glossitis also are associated. Neurologic findings include irritability, lethargy, paresthesias, hypotonia, developmental delay, and myalgias. Nausea and anorexia also have been described.

Two inborn errors of metabolism, both autosomal-recessive multiple-carboxylase deficiencies, also alter normal biotin metabolism. The neonatal (early onset) form is associated with a defect in holocarboxylase synthetase. This enzyme is used to catalyze the formation of the amide bond that links biotin to several carboxylase enzymes. Symptoms develop during the first 6 weeks of life and the condition is typically fatal. Patients present with a bright red scaling dermatosis that starts on the scalp, eyebrows, and eyelashes, which can spread to involve the perioral, perinasal, and intertriginous regions. Hair thinning can progress to patchy or total alopecia. Holocarboxylase synthetase deficiency can also present as a collodion membrane and subsequent ichthyosis.[161] Neurologic findings are common and manifest as difficulty feeding and breathing, hypotonia, ataxia, seizures, lethargy, and global developmental delay. Associated metabolic derangements are metabolic acidosis, mild-to-moderate hyperammonemia, lactic acidosis, ketoacidosis, and organic aciduria, all of which can be exacerbated by intercurrent illness.[162]

The juvenile (infantile or late-onset) form presents after 3 months of age and is caused by biotinidase deficiency. Biotinidase is found in pancreatic secretions to recycle endogenous biotin and release protein-bound dietary biotin. Because symptoms derive from a relative biotin deficiency, large supplemental doses of biotin are used to treat this disorder. In biotinidase deficiency, children present with a scaly, erythematous periorificial dermatitis. Severe cases develop lichenification, crusting, and eroded lesions, which can become infected by *Candida*. Keratoconjunctivitis, total alopecia, including eyebrows and eyelashes, and glossitis are associated mucocutaneous findings. Ataxia, developmental delay, hypotonia, seizures, optic nerve atrophy, hearing loss, and myoclonic spasms are common neurologic findings. Hypertonia does not rule out this deficiency.[163] Sensorineural hearing loss is preventable with early diagnosis of biotinidase deficiency, but once present, is irreversible.[164] In contrast, the metabolic encephalopathy is reversible once appropriate therapy is initiated.[165] Like holocarboxylase synthetase deficiency, metabolic acidosis, lactic acidosis, and organic aciduria are found. Humoral and cellular immunodeficiencies can predispose to cutaneous and systemic infections.

Laboratory Testing: If dietary history is not explanatory, consultation to evaluate for inborn errors of metabolism is recommended in children who present with findings suggestive of a biotin deficiency. Biotinidase levels, serum amino acids, urine organic acids, carnitine studies, and ammonia may be helpful in differentiating this disorder from other metabolic diseases.

Treatment: The recommended daily value increases from 30 mcg in neonates to 100 to 200 mcg in adults (see Table 123-7). Acquired deficiency is treated with 150 mcg of biotin per day until resolution of symptoms. Although holocarboxylase synthetase deficiency can be treated with 10 to 40 mg of biotin per

---

TABLE 123-14

Clinical Manifestations of Biotin Deficiency and Multiple Carboxylase Deficiency

- Erythematous, crusting, scaly dermatitis around eyes, nose, mouth, and other periorificial areas
- Alopecia, glossitis, conjunctivitis
- Irritability, lethargy, paresthesias, hypotonia, developmental delay

day to reverse cutaneous symptoms, neurologic deficits may persist. Patients with biotinidase deficiency are treated with 5 to 10 mg of biotin and have better clinical outcomes than that seen with holocarboxylase synthetase deficiency.

MINERALS

AT-A-GLANCE

- Cutaneous changes associated with iron deficiency include koilonychia, spoon-shaped nails; brittle, lusterless hair; aphthous stomatitis; and angular stomatitis.
- Acrodermatitis enteropathica is an inherited defect in the intestinal zinc transporter ZIP4.
- Zinc deficiency presents with a periorificial and acral eczematous and erosive dermatitis.
- Zinc status can be measured by serum zinc or alkaline phosphatase, a zinc-dependent enzyme.
- Menkes disease is an X-linked disorder of intestinal copper transport, and results in characteristic kinking of the hair and neurologic deficits.

COPPER

Etiology and Pathogenesis: Copper is an essential component of several metalloenzymes, including tyrosinase and lysyl oxidase. Tyrosinase is involved in melanin biosynthesis, and lysyl oxidase deaminates lysine and hydroxylysine in the first step in collagen crosslinking. Other copper enzymes are involved in catecholamine production, free radical detoxification, and oxidation-reduction reactions.

Epidemiology: Copper is found in fish, oysters, whole grains, beef and pork liver, chocolate, eggs, and raisins. Copper deficiency is uncommon, but can result from malnutrition, malabsorptive states, chronic unsupplemented parenteral nutrition, infants with a strictly cow's-milk diet, and excessive intake of antacids, zinc, iron, or vitamin C, that can interfere with absorption. Celiac disease, cystic fibrosis, gastric bypass surgery, and short-bowel syndrome lead to malabsorption of dietary copper.

Clinical Findings: Clinical manifestations in these cases include hypopigmentation of hair and skin and bony abnormalities (osteoporosis, fractures, periosteal reaction, and flaring of anterior ribs). Copper deficiency myeloneuropathy presents as a progressive and symmetric sensory loss and motor weakness of both upper and lower extremities.[166-168] All sensory modalities are affected. If untreated, optic nerve involvement may occur, with permanent vision loss.[168] Copper supplementation prevents further neurologic deterioration, but recovery of function is not guaranteed.

Laboratory Testing: Microcytic anemia, neutropenia, hypocupremia, and hypoceruloplasminemia can be observed. Neutropenia is the earliest and most common sign of copper deficiency and is a sensitive measure of treatment adequacy.

Treatment: Treatment is with supplemental copper in the diet.

COPPER AND MENKES DISEASE

Epidemiology: Menkes disease, also known as kinky hair disease, was described by John Menkes in 1962 as a multifocal degenerative disease of gray matter. The connection between copper deficiency and demyelinating disease was first suggested in the 1930s by Australian veterinarians after observing ataxia in lambs born to mothers grazing in copper-deficient pastures. Menkes described 5 male infants born into an English-Irish family who showed an X-linked syndrome of neurologic degeneration, particular hair, and failure to thrive. The incidence of Menkes disease ranges from 1 in 100,000 to 1 in 250,000 live births.

Etiology and Pathogenesis: The Menkes gene, *MNK*, was identified on chromosome Xq13 in 1993. The protein product is a copper-transporting *P*-type adenosine triphosphatase, which is expressed in almost all tissues, except the liver. Mutations in *MNK* lead to decreased concentrations of copper because of impaired intestinal absorption and consequent decreased activity of cuproenzymes.

Clinical Findings: Classically, signs of Menkes disease begin at 2 to 3 months of age, although neonatal indicators include preterm labor, large cephalohematomas, hypothermia, hypoglycemia, and jaundice. The characteristic facies of Menkes disease is a cherubic appearance with a depressed nasal bridge, ptosis, and reduced facial movements. At 2 to 3 months of age, there is loss of developmental milestones, hypotonia, seizures, and failure to thrive. Structural changes in the hair are seen, with the general appearance of short, sparse, lusterless, tangled, and depigmented hair. The eyebrows have the same steel wool appearance as scalp hair. On light microscopy, pili torti is classically seen. Monilethrix, segmental shaft narrowing, and trichorrhexis nodosa, small beaded swelling of the hair shaft with fractures at regular intervals, also may be observed. Other cutaneous findings include follicular hyperkeratosis and soft, inelastic, depigmented skin, especially at the nape of the neck, axillae, and trunk. A high-arched palate and delayed tooth eruption may be noted on oral examination (Table 123-15).

Neurologic deficits represent the major morbidity in this disorder. Profound truncal hypotonia with poor head control is typical, while appendicular tone may be increased. Deep tendon reflexes are hyperactive. Suck and cry remain strong. Optic disks are pale with impaired visual fixation and tracking. Hearing

> **TABLE 123-15**
> **Clinical Features of Menkes Disease**
>
> - Depressed nasal bridge, ptosis, and reduced facial movements
> - Loss of developmental milestones, hypotonia, seizures, hypothermia, and failure of thrive
> - Steel wool appearance of hair: short, sparse lusterless, tangled, and depigmented. Microscopically: pili torti, trichorrhexis nodosa
> - Follicular hyperkeratosis, inelastic depigmented skin at nape of neck, axillae, and trunk
> - Arched palate, delayed tooth eruption
> - Severe neurologic deficits
> - Bony and renal changes, including bone fractures and subdural hematoma

remains normal. Developmental arrest occurs at occasional smiling and babbling. Bony changes most often involve the extremities and the skull, and less often the thorax, vertebrae, and pelvis. They include osteoporosis, metaphyseal widening and lateral spur formation, ossification of sutures, a diaphyseal periosteal reaction, and scalloping of the posterior aspects of the vertebral bodies, and subperiosteal new bone formation. Patients are at increased risk of bone fractures and subdural hematomas which may resemble those seen with nonaccidental trauma (child abuse).[169] Renal involvement as hydronephrosis, hydroureter, and diverticula of the bladder can occur. Elongation and tortuosity of many large vessels lead to severe arterial disease, a frequent cause of death by 3 to 4 years of age.

Laboratory Testing: Diagnosis is through the clinical history, physical examination, and reduced levels of serum ceruloplasmin and copper.

Treatment: Early treatment with copper histidinate has resulted in good outcomes, including normal neurodevelopmental milestones, in some patients. Initiation of therapy in older patients may be helpful in alleviation of symptoms like irritability and insomnia.[170,171]

SELENIUM

Etiology and Pathogenesis: Selenium is an essential component of glutathione peroxidase, an antioxidant. Selenium is found in seafood, red meat, egg yolks, grain products, and chicken. The amount of selenium available in cereal grains depends on the selenium content of the soil where it was grown. An area with low soil selenium is Keshan, China, where selenium deficiency in humans is endemic. Selenium-deficient soil is seen in the context of heavy erosion of the surface soil, resulting in trace mineral depletion.[172,173]

SELENIUM DEFICIENCY

Epidemiology: Selenium deficiency is primarily seen in geographic areas where low soil selenium exists, but can also occur in the context of restricted protein diets, unsupplemented parenteral nutrition, malabsorption states, and increased losses.[174,175]

Clinical Findings: Two disorders are attributed to selenium deficiency: Keshan disease and Keshin-Beck (or Kashin-Bek) disease. These diseases have only been reported in endemic areas of Asia.

Keshan disease is a multifocal myocarditis leading to fatal cardiomyopathy that is seen primarily in women and young children in endemic areas. Acute or chronic insufficiency of cardiac function, cardiomegaly, arrhythmias, and electrocardiographic abnormalities have been noted. Muscle pain and weakness with hepatic congestion, mesenteric lymphadenosis, erythrocyte macrocytosis without anemia, and pancreatic exocrine dysfunction also have been seen. Cutaneous findings in these patients have included white nail beds, similar to those of Terry's nails in hepatic cirrhosis, and hypopigmentation of skin and hair (pseudoalbinism). These findings resolve with selenium supplementation.

Keshin-Beck disease is an osteoarthropathy that affects the epiphyseal and articular cartilage and the epiphyseal growth plates, resulting in enlarged joints, and shortened fingers and toes.

Laboratory Testing: Diagnosis of selenium deficiency is through measurement of plasma selenium levels and glutathione peroxidase activity.

Treatment: Selenium supplementation is used for both acute correction and long-term maintenance.

SELENIUM EXCESS

Epidemiology: Selenium toxicity can be acutely fatal. Cases of toxicity have been associated with increased soil selenium. Marco Polo described findings consistent with selenium poisoning in Western China during his explorations in 1295. In the 1960s, reports of selenium toxicity came out of Enshi County in Hubei, China. The cause of this endemic toxicity arose from coal contaminated with selenium that was then used to fertilize the soil.[176] Sporadic cases of selenium intoxication secondary to excess supplement ingestion have been reported.[177] Additional cases of acute selenium toxicity have been documented after ingestion of glass blue (used in stained glass manufacturing),[178] selenite broth (enriched culture media used to isolate *Salmonella* bacilli), and gun bluing agent (a finishing product for firearms).[179]

Clinical Findings: Hair becomes dry and brittle in association with an exfoliative dermatitis on the scalp, often resulting in broken hairs and alopecia. Nails also become brittle with white horizontal streaking on the surface. Breaks in the wall of then nail eventually leads to nail loss. The new nail is fragile and thickened with a rough surface. Nails, hair, and teeth can all develop a reddish hue. Skin on the extremities and neck can become red, swollen, blistered, and occasionally ulcerate that heal slowly. Neurologic complaints of peripheral anesthesia, hyperreflexia, numbness, convulsions, and paralysis have been reported. Nausea, vomiting, diarrhea, garlic or sour-milk breath odor, and hypersalivation can occur. Severe corrosive hemorrhagic gastritis can progress into a deep gastric ulcer after acute intoxication. Acute tubular necrosis of the kidneys with the potential for acute renal failure requiring dialysis may also complicate selenium toxicity.[180]

Laboratory Testing: Screening of plasma can be used to document elevation selenium levels.

Treatment: Treatment involves removal of the source of excess selenium and supportive care for complications.

TABLE 123-16
Cutaneous Features of Iron Deficiency

Nails	• Fragile, longitudinally ridged • Lamellated brittle nails → thinning, flattening of nail plate, koilonychia
Hair	• Lusterless, dry, focally narrow and split hair shafts, heterochromia of black hair; hair loss
Mucous membranes	• Aphthous stomatitis, angular stomatitis, glossodynia, atrophied tongue papillae
Blue sclerae	
Pruritus	

MANGANESE

Etiology and Pathogenesis: Manganese activates glycosyltransferases used in the synthesis of glycosaminoglycans and glycoproteins and is used in 2 metalloenzymes (pyruvate carboxylase and superoxide dismutase). Manganese is also found in high concentrations in melanocytes. Reported cases of manganese deficiency are rare. Manganese deficiency was reported during a study of vitamin K requirements, when a study participant was accidentally placed on a manganese-deficient diet. He developed a mild dermatitis, reddening of his black hair, slowed hair and nail growth, and occasional nausea and vomiting with moderate weight loss. A subsequent study of manganese-deficient states showed no hair changes, but miliaria crystallina developed in half the subjects, and disappeared after repletion. Long-term parenteral nutrition without adequate supplementation can induce manganese-deficient states.[181] Likewise, in cases where manganese is supplemented in parenteral nutrition, hypermagnesemia can occur, which is associated with neurologic sequelae.[182] More recently, loss-of-function mutations in the manganese-zinc dication transporter gene, *SLC39A8*, are associated with glycosylation and mitochondrial disorders.[183] Affected patients demonstrated hypotonia, intellectual disability, variable short stature, strabismus, and cerebellar atrophy.[184] An exome-wide association study identified a mutation in the this transporter that is associated with dilated cardiomyopathy.[185]

IRON

Iron is used in several biologic pathways, including heme synthesis, oxidation-reduction reactions, collagen synthesis, and as a cofactor for enzymes such as succinic dehydrogenase, monoamine oxidase, and glycerophosphate oxidase. Iron is found in red meats, egg yolks, dried beans, nuts, dried fruits, green leafy vegetables, and enriched grain products.

IRON DEFICIENCY

Iron deficiency continues to be an international problem that crosses socioeconomic and ethnic divides. Deficiency states result from inadequate intake or chronic blood loss. Groups at high risk include infants, menstruating females, and individuals with chronic GI bleeding. Infants on an iron-fortified formula are at risk for deficiency 3 to 6 months after transitioning to cow's-milk formula because of the lower iron content of cow's milk.[186]

Skin changes seen in iron deficiency involve the skin, mucous membranes, hair, and nails (Table 123-16). Moderate iron deficiency causes fragile, longitudinally ridged, lamellated, or brittle nails. As deficiency progresses, the nail plate shows thinning, flattening, and a spoon-shaped convexity known as *koilonychia*. The index and third fingernails are usually the most severely involved. Even after iron replacement therapy begins, koilonychia resolves slowly.

Hair changes include a lusterless, brittle, dry, and focally narrow or split hair shafts, likely caused by impaired keratin production. Heterochromia of black scalp hair with alternating segments of dark brown, white, and liver bands have been described. Cunningham noted, in 1932, that hair loss occurred in iron deficiency, but Hard was the first to show an etiologic connection between iron-deficiency anemia and diffuse scalp hair loss.[187,188] However, the role of iron deficiency in hair loss continues to be a controversial topic.[189,190]

Mucous membrane manifestations include aphthous stomatitis, angular stomatitis, glossodynia, and absent or atrophied tongue papillae. Blue sclerae that persists after iron replacement is likely secondary to impaired collagen synthesis. Generalized pruritus of variable severity has been reported in some individuals with iron deficiency, and sometimes associated with dermatitis herpetiformis. Plummer-Vinson syndrome is an iron-deficiency-associated syndrome encountered predominantly in middle-aged women with microcytic anemia, dysphagia, glossitis, koilonychia, and angular stomatitis. This is considered to be a precancerous phenomenon, associated with carcinoma of the mouth or upper respiratory tract.

Iron deficiency in a microcytic anemia is diagnosed by measurement of serum iron levels, ferritin, total iron binding capacity, transferrin saturation, as well as free or zinc protoporphyrin levels. Treatment involves appropriate iron supplementation. Low zinc levels may aggravate iron-deficiency anemia, and if present, may require correction as well.

IRON EXCESS

Chronic iron overload, hemosiderosis, can be associated with tissue injury, which is called *hemochromatosis*. Hyperpigmentation and ichthyosis-like changes of the skin are seen. Associated findings are cirrhosis of the liver, diabetes mellitus, and cardiomyopathy.

ZINC

Zinc is an important micronutrient that is an essential component of many metalloenzymes involved in a variety of metabolic pathways and cellular functions, and is particularly important in protein and nucleic acid synthesis. Adequate zinc levels are also important for wound healing and for T-cell, neutrophil, and natural killer cell function. Zinc homeostasis depends on adequate zinc absorption and maintenance of appropriate intracellular and extracellular zinc levels, as well as its regulated transport across luminal surfaces. Dietary sources of zinc include meat, fish, shellfish, eggs, dairy products, and legumes, with the highest and most bioavailable forms of zinc found in meats, fish, and shellfish. Other vegetables, fruits, and refined carbohydrates contain very little zinc. Phytates (found in cereal grains, legumes, and nuts) and fiber interfere with intestinal zinc absorption. Human breastmilk contains very high levels of zinc during the first 1 to 2 months of lactation, averaging 3 mg/L; subsequently, zinc levels decrease. Human breastmilk also contains a zinc-binding ligand that increases the bioavailability of breastmilk zinc. Although cow's-milk formula contains higher levels of zinc, the bioavailability is significantly less than that in human breastmilk.

Enteral zinc absorption occurs in the small intestine. Zinc excretion occurs primarily via the GI tract via pancreatic and intestinal secretions, with lesser amounts excreted in the urine complexed to free amino acids. There are more than 27 genes encoding transporter proteins for zinc. Two important families of zinc transporter proteins, including *ZnT* (zinc transporter) genes and Zip (Zrt-like and Irt-like proteins) transporters, have been identified in humans.

Although total-body zinc is stored primarily in the bones, muscles, prostate, and skin, there is no free exchange of stored zinc, and metabolic needs must be met by a continual supply of dietary zinc. In plasma, approximately 50% of the total zinc is complexed with albumin, while the remainder is bound to other serum proteins, including transferrin and α_2-macroglobulin, or to free amino acids. Plasma levels may decrease transiently in response to intercurrent illness, surgery, or other stressors. Excess plasma zinc levels inhibit copper absorption, possibly through competitive inhibition of a common divalent cationic transporter. Zinc deficiency also results in impaired mobilization of hepatic retinol stores and is associated with impaired night vision (nyctalopia). Conversely, excessive calcium intake can interfere with normal zinc absorption, likely also a result of competitive inhibition.

ZINC DEFICIENCY

Epidemiology: Zinc deficiency occurs worldwide. Populations at special risk include patients with intestinal malabsorption syndromes liver disease, anorexia nervosa or food faddism, extensive cutaneous burns, and nephritic syndrome. Iatrogenic zinc deficiency may result from prolonged parenteral or enteral nutrition that contains inadequate zinc levels to meet the metabolic demands. Certain rural populations with diets high in phytates, as have been reported in certain parts of Iran, Turkey, and the former Yugoslavia, are also at risk for acquired zinc deficiency (AZD).

Etiology and Pathogenesis: Zinc deficiency may be either inherited, a form commonly referred to as AE, or acquired, and therefore referred to as AZD.

AZD may results from states associated with inadequate intake, impaired absorption, or increased excretion, including pregnancy, lactation, extensive cutaneous burns, generalized exfoliative dermatoses, food faddism, parenteral nutrition, anorexia nervosa, and even excessive sweating. Intestinal malabsorption syndromes, such as inflammatory bowel disease and cystic fibrosis, result in impaired intestinal absorption of zinc, whereas alcoholism and nephrotic syndrome result in increased renal zinc losses. Penicillamine has been reported to cause zinc deficiency in a patient with Wilson disease. Ornithine transcarbamylase deficiency also is associated with zinc deficiency.

Acute AZD secondary to impaired absorption of zinc, inadequate intake, or excessive renal or intestinal losses may result in a clinical picture that resembles AE and occurs also in adults (Fig. 123-10). This is also seen as a complication to bariatric surgery.

A chronic or subacute form of zinc deficiency is also recognized. These patients often have zinc levels in the mildly deficient range (40 to 60 mcg/dL). Clinical manifestations include growth retardation in children and adolescents, hypogonadism in males, dysgeusia, poor appetite, poor wound healing, abnormal dark adaptation, and impaired mentation. Cutaneous manifestations, when present, are usually less striking and present predominantly as a psoriasiform dermatitis involving the hands and feet and, occasionally, the knees.

AE, the inherited form of zinc deficiency, is a rare autosomal recessive disorder of zinc absorption. These infants have a defect in an intestinal zinc transporter, the human ZIP4 protein encoded on the *SLC39A4* gene. Mutations in this gene prevents appropriate enteral zinc absorption.[191-193]

AE classically presents during infancy on weaning from breastmilk to formula or cereal, which have lower zinc bioavailability than breastmilk. There is a form of AZD that may also present during infancy but, in contrast to AE, these infants become symptomatic

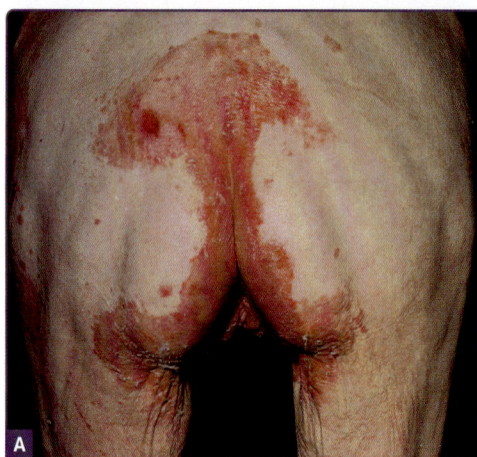

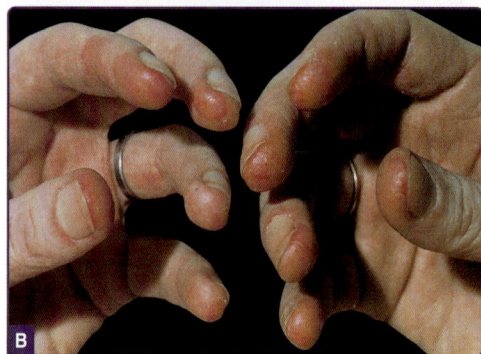

Figure 123-10 Zinc deficiency. **A,** There are plaques of dry, scaly, eczematous skin around the buttocks. The lesions often become secondarily infected with *Candida albicans*. **B,** Hands. The fingers are enlarged, and there are paronychia and bright erythema on the terminal phalanges.

TABLE 123-17
Clinical Features of Acrodermatitis Enteropathica
■ Eczematous and erosive dermatitis
■ Preferentially localized to periorificial and acral areas
■ Alopecia
■ Diarrhea
■ Lethargy, irritability
■ Whining and crying
■ Superinfection with *Candida albicans* and *Staphylococcus aureus*

nonspecific, acrally distributed, symmetric, eczematous dermatitis. Over time, bullae and erosions with a characteristic peripheral crusted border develop (Fig. 123-11). Vitiligo-like depigmented patches have been described.[196] In addition to dry and brittle hair,

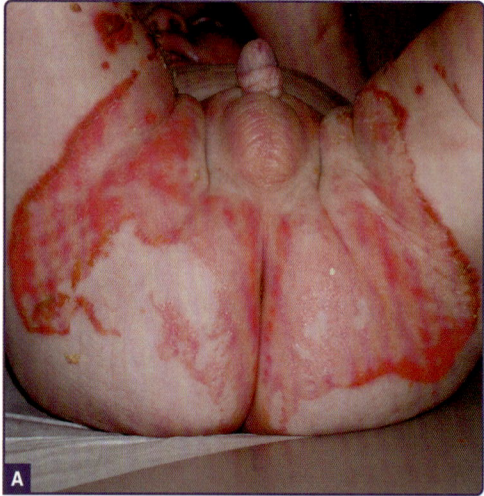

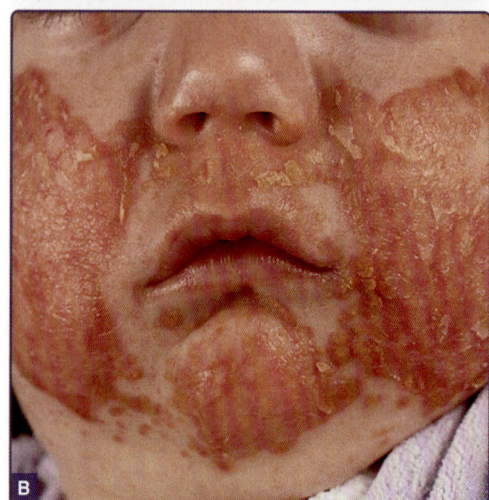

Figure 123-11 A, Patient with acrodermatitis enteropathica. These clinical findings resolved within 2 weeks of initiating zinc supplementation. **B,** This crusted and scaly, erosive, and sharply demarcated eruption appeared shortly after weaning. The child was highly irritable, whining and crying, and had diarrhea.

while breastfeeding and improve after weaning to formula or table foods. Many of these reported infants were premature, but cases also have been reported in full-term infants. The mothers of these infants have a presumed defect in mammary excretion of zinc into their breastmilk, resulting in inadequate zinc intake in their infants.[194,195] In a single case evaluated by the author of this chapter (ACY), breastmilk zinc deficiency occurred as a result of excessive maternal intake of calcium that the mother was taking in the belief that calcium supplements might mitigate postpartum depression. Measured breastmilk zinc levels were significantly decreased and rebounded to normal levels upon discontinuation of maternal calcium supplementation. Measurement of breastmilk zinc levels is a useful tool and is diagnostic when less than 70 mcg/dL.

AE presents soon after weaning in affected infants or during the fourth to tenth week of life in infants who are not breastfed. The classic features of AE include alopecia, diarrhea, lethargy, and an acute eczematous and erosive dermatitis favoring periorificial (perioral, periocular, anogenital) and acral areas (hands and feet) (Table 123-17). The cutaneous findings are highly characteristic and often present initially as a

alternating dark and light bands with polarized light can be seen.[197] Patients also appear to be predisposed to systemic infections as a result of impaired cell-mediated immunity, and superinfection with *Candida albicans* and bacteria, usually *Staphylococcus aureus*, is common. Delayed wound healing, acute paronychia, conjunctivitis, blepharitis, and photophobia also may be observed. Diarrhea may be prominent but is not seen in all cases. If untreated, the disease is fatal.

Laboratory Testing: A low plasma zinc level is the gold standard for diagnosing zinc deficiency. Use of contaminated needles, catheters, and sample tubes may lead to erroneously high measured zinc levels. Contact with collection tubes with rubber stoppers should be avoided as they may contain high levels of zinc. Normal plasma zinc levels range from 70 to 250 mcg/dL. Measurement of serum alkaline phosphatase—a zinc-dependent enzyme—is another useful and rapid indicator of zinc status, as alkaline phosphatase may be low-normal; serum alkaline phosphatase will increase with zinc supplementation, thus confirming the diagnosis.

In cases in which the plasma zinc level is equivocal and the diagnosis is uncertain, skin biopsy for routine histology may be helpful. The characteristic features are variable psoriasiform hyperplasia with confluent parakeratosis, spongiosis and pallor of the upper epidermis, focal dyskeratosis, and variable epidermal atrophy. However, these findings are not specific; and may be seen in a number of other nutritional deficiencies.

Treatment: Zinc supplementation with either an enteral or parenteral formulation is appropriate. Clinical response is usually rapid, with initial improvement noted within several days. Irritability and whining disappear first, followed by improvement of skin lesions. Although several zinc formulations are available, the most commonly used enteral formulation is zinc sulfate. Zinc chloride is recommended for parenteral supplementation.

In children, 0.5 to 1.0 mg/kg of elemental zinc given as 1 to 2 daily doses is recommended for mild-to-moderate zinc deficiency. Higher doses may be required in cases of AZD caused by intestinal malabsorption. In adults, 15 to 30 mg of elemental zinc per day is usually sufficient in cases of AZD. Serum zinc levels should be monitored during therapy. Patients with AE require lifelong treatment. Patients with AZD may need variable levels of supplementation, depending on their underlying disease. Of note, excess zinc levels may interfere with copper metabolism.

ZINC TOXICITY

Zinc toxicity has been reported with exposure to zinc-containing fumes, intravenous poisoning, and ingestion of large amounts of zinc. There are no cutaneous manifestations, but patients may present with severe vomiting, nausea, lethargy, dizziness, neuropathy, and dehydration. Hypocupremia may result.

NOMA

AT-A-GLANCE

- Devastating gangrene of the soft and hard tissue of the face found in developing countries.
- Malnutrition, vitamin deficiencies, and immune dysregulation create an environment for this rapidly progressive destructive polymicrobial infection.

EPIDEMIOLOGY

Noma (necrotizing ulcerative stomatitis, stomatitis gangrenosa, or cancrum oris) is a devastating gangrenous condition that destroys soft and hard tissue of the face; predominantly, it affects children between the ages of 1 to 7 years. The word *noma* originates from the Greek word νομη, which means to graze or devour, which reflects the rapid progression of this condition.

In 1848, Tourdes was the first to define noma as

> a gangrenous disease affecting the mouth and face of children living in poor hygiene conditions and suffering from debilitating diseases, especially eruptive fevers. Beginning with an ulcer on the oral mucosa rapidly spreading outside and destroying the soft and hard tissues of the face—and almost always fatal.[198]

As public health initiatives improved sanitation in developed countries, the global epidemiology of noma likewise improved. In general, noma has become a rare occurrence in developed countries and is predominantly encountered now only in parts of Africa, Latin America, and Asia. Intermittent epidemics of noma were noted during World War I, the malaria epidemic in 1938, and World War II in the Belsen and Auschwitz concentration camps.[199] In response to reports from humanitarian organizations, the World Health Organization declared noma a health priority in 1994. The World Health Organization estimates the worldwide incidence of noma to be 500,000 cases per year with a 79% mortality rate. An estimated 25,000 children are affected in the developing countries bordering the Sahara every year.[200] Unfortunately, the data on the incidence of noma are likely an underestimation of the true incidence as less than 10% of affected individuals actually seek medical care.[201] The high mortality rate and rapid progression of disease means that many patients die before reaching medical attention. Moreover, many cultures perceive noma as a curse on the family, so affected children are often ignored or hidden. Finally, the nomadic lifestyles of many patients make them difficult to register and follow.

An increase in noma has been observed in developed countries since 2000, mostly in association with immunosuppressive therapy, HIV/AIDS, and severe combined immunodeficiency.[202]

Noma neonatorum is thought to be a related but separate entity from noma. The original description by Ghosal, in 1978, described 35 premature and low-birthweight infants in India who developed gangrenous lesions on their noses, eyelids, oral cavities, anal regions, and genitalia. These infants had *Pseudomonas aeruginosa* isolated from their skin lesions and many of their blood cultures. This condition is almost uniformly fatal. Since Ghosal's description, clinical experience has shown that preterm and low-birthweight newborns, especially those with severe intrauterine growth retardation, are at highest risk. The causative organism is usually *Pseudomonas*, but *Escherichia coli*, *Klebsiella*, and staphylococci have occasionally been isolated. Because most cases of noma neonatorum are caused by *Pseudomonas*, some researchers have wondered if it is really ecthyma gangrenosum.[63] Almost all reported cases have been from India, China, Lebanon, or Israel, but there was 1 reported case in the United States in 2002.

ETIOLOGY AND PATHOGENESIS

The pathogenesis of noma is a complex, and yet undefined, interaction between infection, impaired host defense, and malnutrition. The one known risk factor for noma is poverty. There are no reported cases of noma in well-nourished African children. An epidemiologic study in a Nigerian hospital in 2002 revealed that 98% of affected children lived in very poor homes with an average of 7 children per family.[64]

Malnutrition and associated vitamin deficiencies contribute to the pathogenesis of noma. Deficiencies in vitamin A, B_6, C, and E, and the trace elements iron and zinc, and the amino acids cysteine, methionine, serine, and glycine have been identified as possible contributing factors to immune dysfunction in the malnourished. Adrenal hyperfunction in PEM also has been implicated in depression of cell-mediated immunity, and decrease in mucosal resilience. Early malnutrition and chronic infections resulting from early weaning from breastmilk may also represent predisposing factors.[203]

In the early 1940s, Albert Eckstein proposed that acute necrotizing gingivitis, a painful inflammation and necrosis of the interdental papillae, was the precursor to noma. He hypothesized that progression to necrotic stomatitis and noma occurred if appropriate dental hygiene and antibiotics were not initiated. Acute necrotizing gingivitis is associated with poor oral hygiene, stress, and malnutrition. However, any oral mucosal ulceration or trauma, including tooth eruption and viral ulcers, can develop into noma.[204]

Patients with noma frequently have a recent history of debilitating infections, with measles and malaria being the most frequent. Unfortunately, the causative link between these preceding infections and noma remains unclear. Studies in Nigeria show that the frequencies of malaria in northern and southern regions are equal, but the prevalence of noma in the north is higher than in the south. The link between measles and noma appears stronger, but still elusive. The ulcerative oral lesions in patients with measles are one proposed site of initiation of noma.[205]

Noma is a polymicrobial infection, with *Prevotella intermedia* and *Fusobacterium necrophorum* being the 2 most frequently isolated organisms.[206] Other frequently identified organisms are *Tannerella forsythensis*, *Peptostreptococcus micros*, *Campylobacter*, streptococci, and enteric Gram-negative rods. Although organisms are isolated from noma lesions, there is a low likelihood of transmissibility. There are no reports of outbreaks in families or villages after 1 child develops noma. Groupings of noma seem to be more associated with common risk factors rather than true transmission.

CLINICAL FINDINGS

The prodrome of noma is not well documented because of late presentation to medical care and rapid progression. Parents often describe fever and apathy. Early acute noma often presents with soreness of the mouth, halitosis, tenderness of the lip or cheek, cervical lymphadenopathy, and purulent oral discharge. The intraoral lesion is a necrotizing stomatitis generally starting on the alveolar margin and extending to the mucosal surface of the cheek. This evolution is rapid, taking 24 to 48 hours. Swelling and blue-black discoloration of the skin overlying the intraoral lesion develops and rapidly becomes necrotic with well-defined borders. As it becomes black, this necrotic zone expands and forms a classic cone shape, cone gangreneux, with internal destruction greater than external involvement (Fig. 123-12). Laboratory investigation

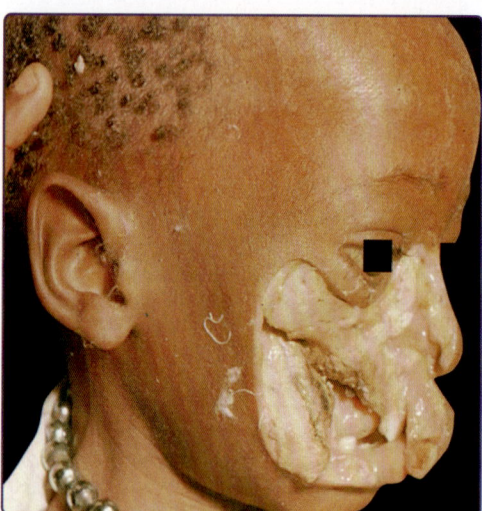

Figure 123-12 Cancrum oris (noma). Massive destruction of the face in a Tanzanian child.

TABLE 123-18
Clinical Presentation of Noma

- Rapid progression of soreness of mouth, halitosis, purulent oral discharge, tenderness of lips and cheeks
- Necrotizing stomatitis starting at alveolar margin and extending to mucosal surface of cheek
- Swelling and blue-black discoloration of cheek → cone-shaped black necrosis, tissue destruction, and ulceration

often shows severe anemia, a high white blood cell count, and hypoalbuminemia (Table 123-18).

Healing noma lesions are also difficult to manage because of the extensive fibrous scars. These scars can lead to strictures of the mouth, severe dental malposition, defective speech, and even complete closure of the mouth from contractures.

TREATMENT

Management of acute noma is geared toward minimizing damage, but invasive intraoral procedures are contraindicated. Key goals of acute management are:

- Correction of dehydration and electrolyte imbalances.
- Treatment of predisposing disease, ie, malaria, measles, HIV, tuberculosis.
- Antibiotics: Some researchers recommend broad-spectrum antibiotics, whereas others believe that metronidazole is adequate because anaerobic organisms predominate.
- Oral hygiene with chlorhexidine digluconate rinses.
- Nutritional rehabilitation—oral, enteral, or parenteral.
- Local wound care.
- Physiotherapy to reduce strictures from fibrous scarring.

Surgical intervention should not occur until the acute phase has ended, and is aimed at restoring function and improving appearance to allow patients to reintegrate into society.

CONCLUSION

Nutritional disorders arise most commonly as a result of nutrient deficiencies, but may also derive from imbalances in nutrients or at times from nutrient excess. Because macronutrients and micronutrients play roles in multiple biochemical pathways, these disorders often present with clinical features in a variety of organ systems. The key to diagnosis is in having a familiarity with the range of clinical presentations associated with these disorders and maintaining an appropriate index of suspicion for these disorders when evaluating dermatologic patients with skin findings or a history that might suggest a nutritional etiology.

ACKNOWLEDGMENTS

The author gratefully acknowledges Melinda Jen, MD, and Kara N. Shah, MD, PhD, for their contributions to this chapter in previous editions.

REFERENCES

1. World Health Organization. *Malnutrition in the Crosshairs*. http://www.who.int/nutrition/pressrelease-FAOWHO-symposium-malnutrition/en/. Accessed March 24, 2017.
2. World Health Organization. *Nutrition for Health and Development: A Global Agenda for Combating Malnutrition*. Geneva, Switzerland: World Health Organization; 2000.
3. UNICEF. *The State of the World's Children*. New York, NY: Oxford University Press; 1998.
4. Katz KA, Mahlberg MJ, Honig PJ, et al. Rice nightmare: kwashiorkor in 2 Philadelphia-area infants fed Rice Dream beverage. *J Am Acad Dermatol*. 2005;52:S69-S72.
5. Kuhl J, Davis MD, Kalaaji AN, et al. Skin signs as the presenting manifestation of severe nutritional deficiency: report of 2 cases. *Arch Dermatol*. 2004;140:521-524.
6. Liu T, Howard RM, Mancini AJ, et al. Kwashiorkor in the United States: fad diets, perceived and true milk allergy, and nutritional ignorance. *Arch Dermatol*. 2001;137:630-636.
7. Mori F, Serranti D, Barni S, et al. A kwashiorkor case due to the use of an exclusive rice milk diet to treat atopic dermatitis. *Nutr J*. 2015;14:83.
8. Fourreau D, Peretti N, Hengy B, et al. Pediatric nutrition: Severe deficiency complications by using vegetable beverages, four cases report [in French]. *Presse Med*. 2013;42(2):e37-e43.
9. Hatem NL, Hassab HM, Abd Al-Rahman EM, et al. Prevalence of aflatoxins in blood and urine of Egyptian infants with protein-energy malnutrition. *Food Nutr Bull*. 2005;26:49-56.
10. Fechner A, Böhme C, Gromer S, et al. Antioxidant status and nitric oxide in the malnutrition syndrome kwashiorkor. *Pediatr Res*. 2001;49:237-243.
11. Barness L. *Nutrition and Nutritional Disorders*. 14th ed. Philadelphia, PA: WB Saunders; 1992.
12. Mei Z, Grummer-Strawn LM, de Onis M, et al. The development of a MUAC-for-height reference, including a comparison to other nutritional status screening indicators. *Bull World Health Organ*. 1997;75:333-341.
13. Miller S. Nutritional deficiency and the skin. *J Am Acad Dermatol*. 1989;21:1-30.
14. Prendiville J, Manfredi L. Skin signs of nutritional disorders. *Semin Dermatol*. 1992;11:88-97.
15. Müller O, Krawinkel M. Malnutrition and health in developing countries. *CMAJ*. 2005;173:279-286.
16. Ruiz-Maldonado R, Orozco-Ovarrubias L. *Skin Manifestations of Nutritional Disorders*. Malden, MA: Blackwell Publishing; 2006.
17. Bistrian B, McCowen K, Chan S. Protein-energy malnutrition in dialysis patients. *Am J Kidney Dis*. 1999;33:172-175.
18. Lacquaniti A, Bolignano D, Campo S, et al. Malnutrition in the elderly patient on dialysis. *Ren Fail*. 2009;31:239-245.

19. Malinowski S. Nutritional and metabolic complications of bariatric surgery. *Am J Med Sci*. 2006;331:219-225.
20. Pitt R, Labib PL, Wolinski A, et al. Iatrogenic kwashiorkor after distal gastric bypass surgery: the consequences of receiving multinational treatment. *Eur J Clin Nutr*. 2016;70(5):635-636.
21. Boutin D, Cante V, Levillain P, et al. Adult kwashiorkor: a rare complication of bariatric surgery [in French]. *Ann Dermatol Venereol*. 2015;142(2):99-103.
22. Strumia R. Dermatologic signs in patients with eating disorders. *Am J Clin Dermatol*. 2005;6:165-173.
23. Ryan A, Goldsmith L. Nutrition and the skin. *Clin Dermatol*. 1996;14:389-406.
24. World Health Organization. *Management of Severe Malnutrition: A Manual for Physicians and Other Senior Health Workers*. Geneva, Switzerland: World Health Organization; 1999.
25. Raj DS, Carrero JJ, Shah VO, et al. Soluble CD14 levels, interleukin 6, and mortality among prevalent hemodialysis patients. *Am J Kidney Dis*. 2009;54:1072-1080.
26. Rytter MJ, Babirekere-Iriso E, Namusoke H, et al. Risk factors for death in children during inpatient treatment of severe acute malnutrition: a prospective cohort study. *Am J Clin Nutr*. 2017;105(2):494-502.
27. Thavaraj V, Sesikeran B. Histopathological changes in skin of children with clinical protein energy malnutrition before and after recovery. *J Trop Pediatr*. 1989;35:105-108.
28. Ernst KD. Essential fatty acid deficiency during parenteral soybean oil lipid minimization. *J Perinatol*. 2017;37(6):695-697.
29. Darmstadt G, McGuire J, Ziboh V. Malnutrition-associated rash of cystic fibrosis. *Pediatr Dermatol*. 2000;17:337-347.
30. Friedman Z, Shochat SJ, Maisels MJ, et al. Correction of essential fatty acid deficiency in newborn infants by cutaneous application of sunflower-seed oil. *Pediatrics*. 1976;58:650-654.
31. Hunt CE, Engel RR, Modler S, et al. Essential fatty acid deficiency in neonates: Inability to reverse deficiency by topical applications of EFA-rich oil. *J Pediatr*. 1978;92:603-607.
32. Duerksen D, McCurdy K. Essential fatty acid deficiency in a severely malnourished patient receiving parenteral nutrition. *Dig Dis Sci*. 2005;50:2386-2388.
33. Bates C. Vitamin A. *Lancet*. 1995;345:31-35.
34. Nicholls L. Phrynoderma: a condition due to vitamin deficiency. *Ind Med Gaz*. 1933;68:681.
35. Maronn M, Allen D, Esterly N. Phrynoderma: a manifestation of vitamin A deficiency?... The rest of the story. *Pediatr Dermatol*. 2005;22:60-63.
36. Sarma PC, Goswami BC, Gogoi K, et al. A new approach to the assessment of marginal vitamin A deficiency in children in suburban Guwahati, India: hydrolysis of retinoyl glucuronide to retinoic acid. *Br J Nutr*. 2009;101:794-797.
37. National Institutes of Health, Office of Dietary Supplements. Dietary Supplement Ingredient Database. https://dietarysupplementdatabase.usda.nih.gov/ingredient_calculator/help.php. Accessed March 25, 2017.
38. National Institutes of Health: Office of Dietary Supplements. Vitamin A Fact Sheet for Health Professionals. https://ods.od.nih.gov/factsheets/VitaminA-Health-Professional/. Accessed March 25, 2017.
39. Penniston K, Tanumihardjo S. The acute and chronic toxic effects of vitamin A. *Am J Clin Nutr*. 2006;83:191-201.
40. Brooke P. Diseases of nutrition and metabolism. *Adv Dermatol*. 1993;8:155-171; discussion 172.
41. Weinstock MA, Bingham SF, Lew RA, et al. Topical tretinoin therapy and all-cause mortality. *Arch Dermatol*. 2009;145:18-24.
42. Baineni R, Gulati R, Delhi CK. Vitamin A toxicity presenting as bone pain. *Arch Dis Child*. 2017;102(6):556-558.
43. Hess A, Meyers V. Carotenemia. A new clinical picture. *JAMA*. 1919;73:1743-1745.
44. Schwingshackl L, Boeing H, Stelmach-Mardas M, et al. Dietary supplements and risk of cause-specific death, cardiovascular disease, and cancer: a systematic review and meta-analysis of primary prevention trials. *Adv Nutr*. 2017;8(1):27-39.
45. Druesne-Pecollo N, Latino-Martel P, Norat T, et al. Beta-carotene supplementation and cancer risk: A systematic review and meta-analysis of randomized controlled trials. *Int J Cancer*. 2009;127(1):172-184.
46. Satia JA, Littman A, Slatore CG, et al. Long-term use of beta-carotene, retinol, lycopene, and lutein supplements and lung cancer risk: Results from the VITamins And Lifestyle (VITAL) study. *Am J Epidemiol*. 2009;169:815-828.
47. Neuhouser ML, Barnett MJ, Kristal AR, et al. Dietary supplement use and prostate cancer risk in the Carotene and Retinol Efficacy Trial. *Cancer Epidemiol Biomarkers Prev*. 2009;18:2202-2206,
48. Al-Wadei HA, Schuller HM. Non-genomic inhibitory signaling of beta-carotene in squamous cell carcinoma of the lungs. *Int J Oncol*. 2009;34:1093-1098.
49. van Helden YG, Keijer J, Heil SG, et al. Beta-carotene affects oxidative stress-related DNA damage in lung epithelial cells and in ferret lung. *Carcinogenesis*. 2009;30:2070-2076.
50. Maharshak N, Shapiro J, Trau H. Carotenoderma—a review of the current literature. *Int J Dermatol*. 2003;42:178-181.
51. Sale T, Stratman E. Carotenemia associated with green bean ingestion. *Pediatr Dermatol*. 2004;21:657-659.
52. Takita Y, Ichimiya M, Hamamoto Y, et al. A case of carotenemia associated with ingestion of nutrient supplements. *J Dermatol*. 2006;33:132-134.
53. Judd SE, Nanes MS, Ziegler TR, et al. Optimal vitamin D status attenuates the age-associated increase in systolic blood pressure in white Americans: results from the third National Health and Nutrition Examination Survey. *Am J Clin Nutr*. 2008;87:136-141.
54. Liu E, Meigs JB, Pittas AG, et al. Plasma 25-hydroxyvitamin d is associated with markers of the insulin resistant phenotype in nondiabetic adults. *J Nutr*. 2009;139:329-334.
55. Kendrick J, Targher G, Smits G, et al. 25-Hydroxyvitamin D deficiency is independently associated with cardiovascular disease in the Third National Health and Nutrition Examination Survey. *Atherosclerosis*. 2009;205:255-260.
56. Wang TJ, Pencina MJ, Booth SL, et al. Vitamin D deficiency and risk of cardiovascular disease. *Circulation*. 2008;117:503-511.
57. Dobnig H, Pilz S, Scharnagl H, et al. Independent association of low serum 25-hydroxyvitamin D and 1,25-dihydroxyvitamin D levels with all-cause and cardiovascular mortality. *Arch Intern Med*. 2008; 168:1340-1349.
58. Cauley JA, Parimi N, Ensrud KE, et al. Serum 25 hydroxyvitamin D and the risk of hip and non-spine fractures in older men. *J Bone Miner Res*. 2010;25(3):545-553.

59. Wu K, Feskanich D, Fuchs CS, et al. A nested case control study of plasma 25-hydroxyvitamin D concentrations and risk of colorectal cancer. *J Natl Cancer Inst*. 2007;99:1120-1129.
60. Melamed ML, Michos ED, Post W, et al. 25-Hydroxyvitamin D levels and the risk of mortality in the general population. *Arch Intern Med*. 2008;168:1629-1637.
61. Liu PT, Stenger S, Li H, et al. Toll-like receptor triggering of a vitamin D-mediated human antimicrobial response. *Science*. 2006;311:1770-1773.
62. Nnoaham K, Clarke A. Low serum vitamin D levels and tuberculosis: a systematic review and metaanalysis. *Int J Epidemiol*. 2008;37:113-119.
63. Freeman A, Mancini A, Yogev R. Is noma neonatorum a presentation of ecthyma gangrenosum in the newborn? *Pediatr Infect Dis J*. 2002;21:83-85.
64. Obiechina A, Arotiba J, Fasola A. Cancrum oris (noma). Level of education and occupation of parents of affected children in Nigeria. *Odontostomatol Trop*. 2000;23:11-14.
65. Sethuraman G, Khaitan BK, Dash SS, et al. Ichthyosiform erythroderma with rickets: report of five cases. *Br J Dermatol*. 2008;158:603-606.
66. Thacher TD, Fischer PR, Pettifor JM, et al. Nutritional rickets in ichthyosis and response to calcipotriene. *Pediatrics*. 2004;114:e119-e123.
67. Sathish Kumar T, Scott XJ, Simon A, et al. Vitamin D deficiency rickets with lamellar ichthyosis. *J Postgrad Med*. 2007;53:215-217.
68. Dayal D, Kumar L, Singh M. Non-bullous ichthyosiform erythroderma with rickets. *Indian Pediatr*. 2002;39:207-208.
69. Nayak S, Behera SK, Acharjya B, et al. Epidermolytic hyperkeratosis with rickets. *Indian J Dermatol Venereol Leprol*. 2006;72:139-142.
70. Kuwabara A, Tsugawa N, Tanaka K, et al. High prevalence of vitamin D deficiency in patients with xeroderma pigmetosum-A under strict sun protection. *Eur J Clin Nutr*. 2015;69(6):693-6.
71. Ombra MN, Paliogiannis P, Doneddu V, et al. Vitamin D status and risk for malignant cutaneous melanoma: recent advances. *Eur J Cancer Prev*. 2017;26(6):532-541.
72. Wyatt C, Lucas RM, Hurst C, et al. Vitamin D deficiency at melanoma diagnosis is associated with higher Breslow thickness. *PLoS One*. 2015;10(5):e0126394.
73. Caini S, Boniol M, Tosti G, et al. Vitamin D and melanoma and non-melanoma skin cancer risk and prognosis: a comprehensive review and meta-analysis. *Eur J Cancer*. 2014;50(15):2649-2658.
74. Norval M, Wulf H. Does chronic sunscreen use reduce vitamin D production to insufficient levels? *Br J Dermatol*. 2009;161:732-736.
75. Holick MF. Sunlight "D"ilemma: risk of skin cancer or bone disease and muscle weakness. *Lancet*. 2001;357:4-6.
76. Lim HW, Gilchrest BA, Cooper KD, et al. Sunlight, tanning booths, and vitamin D. *J Am Acad Dermatol*. 2005;52:868-876.
77. Maiya S, Sullivan I, Allgrove J, et al. Hypocalcaemia and vitamin D deficiency: an important, but preventable, cause of life-threatening infant heart failure. *Heart*. 2008;94:581-584.
78. Amirlak I, Al Dhaheri W, Narchi H. Dilated cardiomyopathy secondary to nutritional rickets. *Ann Trop Paediatr*. 2008;28:227-230.
79. Kosecik M, Ertas T. Dilated cardiomyopathy due to nutritional vitamin D deficiency rickets. *Pediatr Int*. 2007;49:397-399.
80. Bergman R, Schein-Goldshmid R, Hochberg Z, et al. The alopecias associated with vitamin D-dependent rickets type IIA and with hairless gene mutations: a comparative clinical, histologic, and immunohistochemical study. *Arch Dermatol*. 2005;141:343-351.
81. Miller J, Djabali K, Chen T, et al. Atrichia caused by mutations in the vitamin D receptor gene is a phenocopy of generalized atrichia caused by mutations in the hairless gene. *J Invest Dermatol*. 2001;117:612-617.
82. Wagner CL, Greer FR; American Academy of Pediatrics Section on Breastfeeding; American Academy of Pediatrics Committee on Nutrition. Prevention of rickets and vitamin D deficiency in infants, children, and adolescents. *Pediatrics*. 2008;122(5):1142-1152. Erratum in: *Pediatrics*. 2009;123(1):197.
83. Argao EA, Heubi JE, Hollis BW, et al. d-Alpha-tocopheryl polyethylene glycol-1000 succinate enhances the absorption of vitamin D in chronic cholestatic liver disease of infancy and childhood. *Pediatr Res*. 1992;31:146-150.
84. Kooh SW, Roberts EA, Fraser D, et al. Ultraviolet irradiation for hepatic rickets. *Arch Dis Child*. 1989;64:617-619.
85. Dent CE, Round JM, Rowe DJ, et al. Effect of chapattis and ultraviolet irradiation on nutritional rickets in an Indian immigrant. *Lancet*. 1973;1:1282-1284.
86. U.S. Department of Health and Human Services, Department of Agriculture. *Dietary Guidelines for Americans, 2005*. 6th ed. Washington, DC: U.S. Government Printing Office; 2005.
87. Thomson C, Sarubin-Fragakis A. Vitamin, minerals, and phytochemicals. In: Hark L, Morrison G, eds. *Medical Nutrition and Disease: A Case-based Approach*. Malden, MA: Blackwell Publishing; 2003.
88. Copp RP, Wisniewski T, Hentati F, et al. Localization of alpha-tocopherol transfer protein in the brains of patients with ataxia with vitamin E deficiency and other oxidative stress related neurodegenerative disorders. *Brain Res*. 1999;822:80-87.
89. Ouahchi K, Arita M, Kayden H, et al. Ataxia with isolated vitamin E deficiency is caused by mutations in the alpha-tocopherol transfer protein. *Nat Genet*. 1995;9:141-145.
90. Qian J, Atkinson J, Manor D. Biochemical consequences of heritable mutations in the alpha-tocopherol transfer protein. *Biochemistry*. 2006;45:8236-8242.
91. American Academy of Pediatrics Committee on Fetus and Newborn. Controversies concerning vitamin K and the newborn. *Pediatrics*. 2003;112:191-192.
92. Goskowicz M, Eichenfield L. Cutaneous findings of nutritional deficiencies in children. *Curr Opin Pediatr*. 1993;5:441-445.
93. Fujiyama S, Morishita T, Hashiguchi O, et al. Plasma abnormal prothrombin (des-gamma-carboxy prothrombin) as a marker of hepatocellular carcinoma. *Cancer*. 1988;61:1621-1628.
94. Wrenn K, Murphy F, Slovis C. A toxicity study of parenteral thiamine hydrochloride. *Ann Emerg Med*. 1989;18:867-870.
95. Snodgrass S. Vitamin neurotoxicity. *Mol Neurobiol*. 1992;6:41-73.
96. Carpenter K. *Beriberi, White Rice, and Vitamin B*. Berkeley, CA: University of California Press; 2000.
97. Hardy A. Beriberi, vitamin B1 and world food policy, 1925-1970. *Med Hist*. 1995;39:61-77.
98. Hanninen SA, Darling PB, Sole MJ, et al. The prevalence of thiamin deficiency in hospitalized patients

with congestive heart failure. *J Am Coll Cardiol.* 2006;47:354-361.
99. Kara B, Genç HM, Uyur-Yalçın E, et al. Pyruvate dehydrogenase-E1α deficiency presenting as recurrent acute proximal muscle weakness of upper and lower extremities in an 8-year-old boy. *Neuromuscul Disord.* 2017;27(1):94-97.
100. Lawton AW, Frisard NE. Visual loss, retinal hemorrhages, and optic disc edema resulting from thiamine deficiency following bariatric surgery complicated by prolonged vomiting. *Ochsner J.* 2017;17(1):112-114.
101. Dias SP, Diogo MC, Capela C, et al. Wernicke's encephalopathy due to food refusal in a patient with severe depressive disorder. *J Neurol Sci.* 2017;375:92-93.
102. Ubukata M, Amemiya N, Nitta K, et al. Serum thiamine values in end-stage renal disease patients under maintenance hemodialysis. *Int J Vitam Nutr Res.* 2016 [Epub ahead of print].
103. Zhang F, Masania J, Anwar A, et al. The uremic toxin oxythiamine causes functional thiamine deficiency in end-stage renal disease by inhibiting transketolase activity. *Kidney Int.* 2016;90(2):396-403.
104. Teigen LM, Twernbold DD, Miller WL. Prevalence of thiamine deficiency in a stable heart failure outpatient cohort on standard loop diuretic therapy. *Clin Nutr.* 2016;35(6):1323-1327.
105. Katta N, Balla S, Alpert MA. Does long-term furosemide therapy cause thiamine deficiency in patients with heart failure? A focused review. *Am J Med.* 2016;129(7):753.e7-753.e11.
106. Masood U, Sharma A, Nijjar S, et al. B-cell lymphoma, thiamine deficiency, and lactic acidosis. *Proc (Bayl Univ Med Cent).* 2017;30(1):69-70.
107. Huertas-González N, Hernando-Requejo V, Luciano-García Z, et al. Wernicke's encephalopathy, wet beriberi, and polyneuropathy in a patient with folate and thiamine deficiency related to gastric phytobezoar. *Case Rep Neurol Med.* 2015;2015:624807.
108. Nath A, Tran T, Shope TR, et al. Prevalence of clinical thiamine deficiency in individuals with medically complicated obesity. *Nutr Res.* 2017;37:29-36.
109. Fattal-Valevski A, Kesler A, Sela BA, et al. Outbreak of life-threatening thiamine deficiency in infants in Israel caused by a defective soy-based formula. *Pediatrics.* 2005;115:e233-e238.
110. Park JH, Lee JH, Jeong JO, et al. Thiamine deficiency as a rare cause of reversible severe pulmonary hypertension. *Int J Cardiol.* 2007;121:e1-e3.
111. Powers H. Riboflavin (vitamin B-2) and health. *Am J Clin Nutr.* 2003;77:1352-1360.
112. Clements R, Katasani VG, Palepu R, et al. Incidence of vitamin deficiency after laparoscopic Roux-en-Y gastric bypass in a university hospital setting. *Am Surg.* 2006;72:1196-1202; discussion 203-204.
113. Gromisch DS, Lopez R, Cole HS, et al. Light (phototherapy)-induced riboflavin deficiency in the neonate. *J Pediatr.* 1977;90:118-122.
114. Tomei S, Yuasa H, Inoue K, et al. Transport functions of riboflavin carriers in the rat small intestine and colon: Site difference and effects of tricyclic-type drugs. *Drug Deliv.* 2001;8:119-124.
115. Pinto J, Rivlin R. Drugs that promote renal excretion of riboflavin. *Drug Nutr Interact.* 1987;5:143-151.
116. Menezes MP, O'Brien K, Hill M, et al. Auditory neuropathy in Brown-Vialetto-Van Laere syndrome due to riboflavin transporter RFVT2 deficiency. *Dev Med Child Neurol.* 2016;58(8):848-854.
117. Roe D. Riboflavin deficiency: mucocutaneous signs of acute and chronic deficiency. *Semin Dermatol.* 1991;10:293-295.
118. Kraut A. *Goldberger's War: The Life and Work of a Public Health Crusader.* New York, NY: Hill and Wang; 2003.
119. Rajakumar K. Pellagra in the United States: a historical perspective. *South Med J.* 2000;93:272-277.
120. Karthikeyan K, Thappa D. Pellagra and skin. *Int J Dermatol.* 2002;41:476-481.
121. MacDonald A, Forsyth A. Nutritional deficiencies and the skin. *Clin Exp Dermatol.* 2005;30:388-390.
122. Kaur S, Goraya JS, Thami GP, et al. Pellagrous dermatitis induced by phenytoin. *Pediatr Dermatol.* 2002;19:93.
123. Cakmak SK, Gönül M, Aslan E, et al. Half-and-half nail in a case of pellagra. *Eur J Dermatol.* 2006;16(6):695-696.
124. Yamaguchi S, Miyagi T, Sogabe Y, et al. Depletion of epidermal Langerhans cells in the skin lesions of pellagra patients. *Am J Dermatopathol.* 2017;39(6):428-432.
125. Isaac S. The "gauntlet" of pellagra. *Int J Dermatol.* 1998;37:599.
126. Friedli A, Saurat J. Images in clinical medicine. Oculo-orogenital syndrome—a deficiency of vitamins B2 and B6. *N Engl J Med.* 2004;350:1130.
127. Kishi T, Fujita N, Eguchi T, et al. Mechanism for reduction of serum folate by antiepileptic drugs during prolonged therapy. *J Neurol Sci.* 1997;145:109-112.
128. Swiatlo N, O'Connor DL, Andrews J, et al. Relative folate bioavailability from diets containing human, bovine and goat milk. *J Nutr.* 1990;120:172-177.
129. Semchuk G, Allen O, O'Connor D. Folate bioavailability from milk-containing diets is affected by altered intestinal biosynthesis of folate in rats. *J Nutr.* 1994;124:1118-1125.
130. Downham T, Rehbein H, Taylor K. Letter: hyperpigmentation and folate deficiency. *Arch Dermatol.* 1976;112:562.
131. Jucgla A, Sais G, Berlanga J, et al. Hyperpigmentation of the flexures and pancytopenia during treatment with folate antagonists. *Acta Derm Venereol.* 1997;77:165-166.
132. Okuda K. Discovery of vitamin B12 in the liver and its absorption factor in the stomach: a historical review. *J Gastroenterol Hepatol.* 1999;14:301-308.
133. Rasmussen S, Fernhoff P, Scanlon K. Vitamin B12 deficiency in children and adolescents. *J Pediatr.* 2001;138:10-17.
134. Chanarin I. Historical review: a history of pernicious anaemia. *Br J Haematol.* 2000;111:407-415.
135. Oh R, Brown D. Vitamin B12 deficiency. *Am Fam Physician.* 2003;67:979-986.
136. Graells J, Ojeda RM, Muniesa C, et al. Glossitis with linear lesions: an early sign of vitamin B12 deficiency. *J Am Acad Dermatol.* 2009;60:498-500.
137. Ahuja S, Sharma R. Reversible cutaneous hyperpigmentation in vitamin B12 deficiency. *Indian Pediatr.* 2003;40:170-171.
138. Hoffman C, Palmer D, Papadopoulos D. Vitamin B12 deficiency: a case report of ongoing cutaneous hyperpigmentation. *Cutis.* 2003;71:127-130; quiz 138-140.
139. Mori K, Ando I, Kukita A. Generalized hyperpigmentation of the skin due to vitamin B12 deficiency. *J Dermatol.* 2001;28:282-285.
140. Simşek OP, Gönç N, Gümrük F, et al. A child with vitamin B12 deficiency presenting with pancytopenia

140. and hyperpigmentation. *J Pediatr Hematol Oncol.* 2004;26:834-836.
141. Hirschmann J, Raugi G. Adult scurvy. *J Am Acad Dermatol.* 1999;41:895-906; quiz 907-910.
142. Lind J. *A Treatise on the Scurvy in Three Parts.* 3rd ed. London, UK: S. Crowder, D. Wilson, G. Nicholls, T. Cadell, T. Becket, and Co; 1772.
143. Brown S. *Scurvy.* New York, NY: Thomas Dunne Books; 2003.
144. Hess A. *Scurvy, Past and Present.* Philadelphia, PA: JB Lippincott; 1920.
145. Rajakumar K. Infantile scurvy: a historical perspective. *Pediatrics.* 2001;108:E76.
146. Francescone M, Levitt J. Scurvy masquerading as leukocytoclastic vasculitis: a case report and review of the literature. *Cutis.* 2005;76:261-266.
147. Pimentel L. Scurvy: historical review and current diagnostic approach. *Am J Emerg Med.* 2003;21:328-332.
148. Weinstein M, Babyn P, Zlotkin S. An orange a day keeps the doctor away: scurvy in the year 2000. *Pediatrics.* 2001;108:E55.
149. Alexandrescu DT, Dasanu CA, Kauffman CL. Acute scurvy during treatment with interleukin-2. *Clin Exp Dermatol.* 2008;34(7):811-814.
150. Blumberg A, Hanck A, Sander G. Vitamin nutrition in patients on continuous ambulatory peritoneal dialysis (CAPD). *Clin Nephrol.* 1983;20:244-250.
151. Hatuel H, Buffet M, Mateus C, et al. Scurvy in liver transplant patients. *J Am Acad Dermatol.* 2006;55:154-156.
152. Golriz F, Donnelly LF, Devaraj S, et al. Modern American scurvy-experience with vitamin C deficiency at a large children's hospital. *Pediatr Radiol.* 2017;47(2):214-220.
153. Baugh C, Malone J, Butterworth CJ. Human biotin deficiency. A case history of biotin deficiency induced by raw egg consumption in a cirrhotic patient. *Am J Clin Nutr.* 1968;21:173-182.
154. Carlson GL, Williams N, Barber D, et al. Biotin deficiency complicating long-term total parenteral nutrition in an adult patient. *Clin Nutr.* 1995;14:186-190.
155. Mock DM, Baswell DL, Baker H, et al. Biotin deficiency complicating parenteral alimentation: diagnosis, metabolic repercussions, and treatment. *J Pediatr.* 1985; 106:762-769.
156. Mock D, Dyken M. Biotin catabolism is accelerated in adults receiving long-term therapy with anticonvulsants. *Neurology.* 1997;49:1444-1447.
157. Mock DM, Mock NI, Nelson RP, et al. Disturbances in biotin metabolism in children undergoing long-term anticonvulsant therapy. *J Pediatr Gastroenterol Nutr.* 1998;26:245-250.
158. Schulpis KH, Karikas GA, Tjamouranis J, et al. Low serum biotinidase activity in children with valproic acid monotherapy. *Epilepsia.* 2001;42:1359-1362.
159. Fujimoto W, Inaoki M, Fukui T, et al. Biotin deficiency in an infant fed with amino acid formula. *J Dermatol.* 2005;32:256-261.
160. Higuchi R, Noda E, Koyama Y, et al. Biotin deficiency in an infant fed with amino acid formula and hypoallergenic rice. *Acta Paediatr.* 1996;85:872-874.
161. Arbuckle H, Morelli J. Holocarboxylase synthetase deficiency presenting as ichthyosis. *Pediatr Dermatol.* 2006;23(2):142-144.
162. Seymons K, De Moor A, De Raeve H, et al. Dermatologic signs of biotin deficiency leading to the diagnosis of multiple carboxylase deficiency. *Pediatr Dermatol.* 2004;21:231-235.
163. Rathi N, Rathi M. Biotinidase deficiency with hypertonia as unusual feature. *Indian Pediatr.* 2009;46:65-67.
164. Genc GA, Sivri-Kalkanoğlu HS, Dursun A, et al. Audiologic findings in children with biotinidase deficiency in Turkey. *Int J Pediatr Otorhinolaryngol.* 2007;71:333-339.
165. Desai S, Ganesan K, Hegde A. Biotinidase deficiency: A reversible metabolic encephalopathy. Neuroimaging and MR spectroscopic findings in a series of four patients. *Pediatr Radiol.* 2008;38:848-856.
166. Goodman BP, Mistry DH, Pasha SF, et al. Copper deficiency myeloneuropathy due to occult celiac disease. *Neurologist.* 2009;15:355-356.
167. Kumar N, Low P. Myeloneuropathy and anemia due to copper malabsorption. *J Neurol.* 2004;251:747-749.
168. Naismith RT, Shepherd JB, Weihl CC, et al. Acute and bilateral blindness due to optic neuropathy associated with copper deficiency. *Arch Neurol.* 2009;66:1025-1027.
169. Droms RJ, Rork JF, McLean R, et al. Menkes disease mimicking child abuse. *Pediatr Dermatol.* 2017;34(3):e132-e134.
170. Kaler S. Diagnosis and therapy of Menkes syndrome, a genetic form of copper deficiency. *Am J Clin Nutr.* 1998;67:1029S-1034S.
171. Menkes J. Menkes disease and Wilson disease: two sides of the same copper coin. Part II: Wilson disease. *Eur J Paediatr Neurol.* 1999;3:245-253.
172. Ge K, Yang G. The epidemiology of selenium deficiency in the etiological study of endemic diseases in China. *Am J Clin Nutr.* 1993;57:259S-263S.
173. Litov R, Combs GJ. Selenium in pediatric nutrition. *Pediatrics.* 1991;87:339-351.
174. de Berranger E, Colinet S, Michaud L, et al. Severe selenium deficiency secondary to chylous loss. *JPEN J Parenter Enteral Nutr.* 2006;30:173-174.
175. Kanekura T, Yotsumoto S, Maeno N, et al. Selenium deficiency: report of a case. *Clin Exp Dermatol.* 2005;30:346-348.
176. Yang GQ, Wang SZ, Zhou RH, et al. Endemic selenium intoxication of humans in China. *Am J Clin Nutr.* 1983;37:872-881.
177. Centers for Disease Control (CDC). Selenium intoxication–New York. *MMWR Morb Mortal Wkly Rep.* 1984;33:157-158.
178. Kise Y, Yoshimura S, Akieda K, et al. Acute oral selenium intoxication with ten times the lethal dose resulting in deep gastric ulcer. *J Emerg Med.* 2004;26:183-187.
179. Hunsaker D, Spiller H, Williams D. Acute selenium poisoning: suicide by ingestion. *J Forensic Sci.* 2005;50:942-946.
180. Kamble P, Mohsin N, Jha A, et al. Selenium intoxication with selenite broth resulting in acute renal failure and severe gastritis. *Saudi J Kidney Dis Transpl.* 2009;20:106-111.
181. Dickerson R. Manganese intoxication and parenteral nutrition. *Nutrition.* 2001;17:689-693.
182. Fitzgerald K, Mikalunas V, Rubin H, et al. Hypermanganesemia in patients receiving total parenteral nutrition. *JPEN J Parenter Enteral Nutr.* 1999;23:333-336.
183. Park JH, Hogrebe M, Grüneberg M, et al. SLC39A8 deficiency: a disorder of manganese transport and glycosylation. *Am J Hum Genet.* 2015;97(6):894-903.
184. Boycott KM, Beaulieu CL, Kernohan KD, et al. Autosomal-recessive intellectual disability with cerebellar atrophy syndrome caused by mutation of the manganese and zinc transporter gene SLC39A8. *Am J Hum Genet.* 2015;97(6):886-893.
185. Esslinger U, Garnier S, Korniat A, et al. Exome-wide association study reveals novel susceptibility genes

to sporadic dilated cardiomyopathy. *PLoS One.* 2017;12(3):e0172995.
186. Balint J. Physical findings in nutritional deficiencies. *Pediatr Clin North Am.* 1998;45:245-260.
187. Rushton D. Nutritional factors and hair loss. *Clin Exp Dermatol.* 2002;27:396-404.
188. Sato S. Iron deficiency: structural and microchemical changes in hair, nails, and skin. *Semin Dermatol.* 1991;10:313-319.
189. Sinclair R. There is no clear association between low serum ferritin and chronic diffuse telogen hair loss. *Br J Dermatol.* 2002;147:982-984.
190. Trost L, Bergfeld W, Calogeras E. The diagnosis and treatment of iron deficiency and its potential relationship to hair loss. *J Am Acad Dermatol.* 2006;54:824-844.
191. Küry S, Dréno B, Bézieau S, et al. Identification of SLC39A4, a gene involved in acrodermatitis enteropathica. *Nat Genet.* 2002;31:239-240.
192. Wang K, Zhou B, Kuo YM, et al. A novel member of a zinc transporter family is defective in acrodermatitis enteropathica. *Am J Hum Genet.* 2002;71:66-73.
193. Wang K, Pugh EW, Griffen S, et al. Homozygosity mapping places the acrodermatitis enteropathica gene on chromosomal region 8q24.3. *Am J Hum Genet.* 2001;68:1055-1060.
194. Chew AL, Chan I, McGrath JA, et al. Infantile acquired zinc deficiency resembling acrodermatitis enteropathica. *Clin Exp Dermatol.* 2005;30:594-595.
195. Leverkus M, Kütt S, Bröcker EB, et al. Nutritional zinc deficiency mimicking acrodermatitis enteropathica in a fully breast-fed infant. *J Eur Acad Dermatol Venereol.* 2006;20:1380-1381.
196. Inamadar A, Palit A. Acrodermatitis enteropathica with depigmented skin lesions simulating vitiligo. *Pediatr Dermatol.* 2007;24(6):668-669.
197. Traupe H, Happle R, Gröbe H, et al. Polarization microscopy of hair in acrodermatitis enteropathica. *Pediatr Dermatol.* 1986;3:300-303.
198. Tourdes J. *Du noma ou du sphacèle de la bouche chez les enfants.* Strasbourg, France: Faculté de Médecine de Strasbourg; 1848.
199. Baratti-Mayer D, Pittet B, Montandon D, et al. Noma: an "infectious" disease of unknown aetiology. *Lancet Infect Dis.* 2003;3:419-431.
200. Fieger A, Marck KW, Busch R, et al. An estimation of the incidence of noma in north-west Nigeria. *Trop Med Int Health.* 2003;8:402-407.
201. Enwonwu C. Noma—the ulcer of extreme poverty. *N Engl J Med.* 2006;354:221-224.
202. Enwonwu C, Falkler WJ, Phillips R. Noma (cancrum oris). *Lancet.* 2006;368:147-156.
203. Enwonwu C, Phillips R, Ferrell C. Temporal relationship between the occurrence of fresh noma and the timing of linear growth retardation in Nigerian children. *Trop Med Int Health.* 2005;10:65-73.
204. Enwonwu C. Noma. A neglected scourge of children in sub-Saharan Africa. *Bull World Health Organ.* 1995;73:541-545.
205. Koźmińska-Kubarska A, Talleyrand D, Bakatubia M. Cutaneous complications during measles in Zairian children: noma-like postmeasles ulcerations. *Int J Dermatol.* 1982;21:465-469.
206. Falkler WJ, Enwonwu C, Idigbe E. Isolation of *Fusobacterium necrophorum* from cancrum oris (noma). *Am J Trop Med Hyg.* 1999;60:150-156.

Chapter 124 :: The Porphyrias
:: Eric W. Gou & Karl E. Anderson

第一百二十四章

卟啉病

中文导读

卟啉病是由血红素生物合成途径中8种酶的异常引起的代谢性疾病。除皮肤迟发性卟啉病（PCT）是由于途径中第五种酶的获得性缺陷而引起，其余均源于途径酶的突变。卟啉病被分为肝性或红细胞生成性疾病，根据其临床特征分为皮肤型或急性型。由卟啉病引起的症状、体征和组织学结果是非特异性的，而卟啉和卟啉前体的模式使特定的诊断和治疗成为可能。本章分为7节：①历史视角；②血红素的合成及其功能；③迟发性皮肤卟啉病（PCT）；④肝红细胞生成性卟啉病（HEP）；⑤先天性红细胞生成性卟啉病（CEP）；⑥红细胞生成性卟啉病（EPP）；⑦急性肝卟啉病。

第一节介绍了卟啉病的第一次描述是在1874年由舒尔茨提出的。在接下来的几十年里，对途径酶及其基因进行了研究，发现了多个突变。在这些进展的基础上，已经引入并正在开发更多的治疗方法。

第二节介绍了血红素的合成分为8步，每一步都由不同的酶催化。这些酶中的前3个和最后3个在线粒体中，其余4个是胞质的。大约85%的血红素合成发生在骨髓中，以支持血红蛋白的形成，其余的主要发生在肝脏，主要是内质网中的细胞色素P450酶（CYPS）。

第三节介绍了PCT的临床特征、易感因素、病因及发病机制、诊断、易感基因的鉴定及治疗，其中提到了PCT是最常见的卟啉病，其特征是皮肤脆性增加和手背及其他暴露部位在阳光下慢性起疱。其根本原因是肝细胞中的尿卟啉原脱氨酶活性不足，尿卟啉原和其他高度羧化的卟啉原在肝细胞中积聚并被氧化成相应的卟啉。PCT对静脉切开术或小剂量羟氯喹反应良好。

第四节介绍了HEP是非常罕见的卟啉病，为家族性（2型）PCT的纯合子（或复合杂合子）形式，其特征是慢性严重光敏引起的水疱性皮肤病变，本节主要从临床特征、病因及发病机制、诊断及治疗对该病进行了介绍。

第五节介绍了CEP是由于大量缺乏尿卟啉原III合成酶，导致血红蛋白合成过程中异构体I卟啉原特别是尿卟啉原I和辅卟啉原I在骨髓中积累所致。卟啉通常在红细胞、血浆和尿液中显著升高，并导致慢性严重的光敏反应。本节介绍了其病因及发病机制、临床特征、诊断及治疗。

第六节介绍了EPP是儿童最常见的卟啉病类型，它是由血红素生物合成途径的最后一种酶——铁螯合酶（FECH）功能丧失突变所致。本节主要从病因及发病机制、临床特征、诊断及治疗对该病进行了介绍。

第七节急性肝卟啉病，介绍了其流行病学、病因与发病机制、临床表现、诱因、诊断与治疗。

〔粟 娟〕

INTRODUCTION

Porphyrias are metabolic diseases caused by abnormalities of the 8 enzymes in the heme biosynthetic pathway. All but one arise from mutation of a pathway enzyme; the exception is porphyria cutanea tarda (PCT), which develops as an acquired deficiency of the fifth enzyme in the pathway with or without a mutation. Porphyrias are classified as hepatic or erythropoietic based on whether heme precursors first accumulate in liver or bone marrow, the tissues that most actively synthesize heme. Porphyrias are categorized clinically based on their clinical features as either *cutaneous* or *acute* (Table 124-1). Cutaneous porphyrias are due to overproduction and accumulation of photosensitizing porphyrins. Most, as exemplified by PCT, cause chronic blistering and scarring on sun-exposed areas of skin, whereas protoporphyrias produce an acute, severe, and mostly nonblistering reaction to light, often leaving few if any chronic skin changes. Acute porphyrias are characterized by neurologic symptoms and elevated levels of the porphyrin precursors, δ-aminolevulinic acid (ALA) and porphobilinogen (PBG). Porphyrins also accumulate in acute porphyrias, and sometimes achieve levels in plasma sufficient to cause cutaneous blistering, as exemplified especially by variegate porphyria (VP). In some porphyrias, damage to other organs, such as liver and kidney, may also occur. Symptoms, signs, and histologic findings caused by porphyrias are nonspecific, whereas patterns of porphyrins and porphyrin precursors enable specific diagnoses and treatments (Table 124-2).

HISTORICAL PERSPECTIVE

The first known description of porphyria was in 1874 by Schultz. He described a 33-year-old man with photosensitivity since 3 months of age with associated anemia, splenomegaly, and red urine.[1,2] T. McCall Anderson in 1898 described 2 brothers with blistering of sun-exposed skin, extensive scarring of facial features, and red urine.[3] These patients are thought to have had congenital erythropoietic porphyria (CEP), a very rare and severe cutaneous porphyria. Acute porphyria was first described by Stokvis in 1888 in an elderly woman with symptoms after taking sulphonal, a sedative related to barbiturates; she developed dark red urine and later died.[4] In 1923, Archibald Garrod proposed the term *inborn errors of metabolism* to describe a number of inherited metabolic disorders, including the porphyrias.[5] Porphyrias were first classified as hepatic or erythropoietic in 1954.[6] Treatment of porphyria cutanea tarda by phlebotomy was introduced by Ippen in 1961.[7] In 1970, an inherited enzyme deficiency was first described in acute intermittent porphyria,[8] and hemin therapy was first introduced for this condition in 1971.[9] In the decades that followed, the enzymes of the pathway and their genes were characterized and multiple mutations found in each of the porphyrias. Also, regulation of heme synthesis especially in liver and bone marrow has become better understood. Based on these advances, additional treatments have been introduced and are being developed.

HEME SYNTHESIS AND FUNCTIONS

Heme, or iron protoporphyrin IX, is synthesized in eukaryotic cells in 8 steps, each catalyzed by a different enzyme (Fig. 124-1). The first and last 3 of these enzymes are in the mitochondria and the other 4 are cytosolic. The first enzyme, δ-aminolevulinic acid synthase (ALAS), combines glycine and succinyl-coenzyme A to produce the amino acid δ-aminolevulinic acid (ALA), also known as 5-aminolevulinic acid. Two molecules of ALA are then combined to form a pyrrole, porphobilinogen (PBG). Four molecules of PBG are joined to form a linear tetrapyrrole, hydroxymethylbilane (HMB). HMB is a substrate for the fourth enzyme, which inverts one of the pyrrole rings of HMB and cyclizes the molecule to create uroporphyrinogen III, the first porphyrin in the pathway. This asymmetric molecule undergoes a series of decarboxylations and an oxidation to form protoporphyrin IX. Iron is then inserted to form heme. With the exception of protoporphyrin IX, the porphyrin intermediates in this pathway are in their reduced forms (ie, porphyrinogens).[10] The end product heme consists of an iron atom in the ferrous (reduced) state (Fe^{2+}) bound to the 4 pyrrolic nitrogens of the porphyrin macrocycle (Fig. 124-1), leaving 2 unoccupied electron pairs. Heme is the prosthetic group for many essential hemoproteins. In hemoglobin, for example, one unoccupied electron pair is coordinated with a histidine residue of the globin chain while the other is available to bind molecular oxygen.

Hemin is the chemical term for the oxidized form of heme, ferric protoporphyrin IX, which has only one residual positive charge, and can be isolated

TABLE 124-1
Human Porphyrias: Specific Enzymes Affected by Mutations, Modes of Inheritance, Classification, and Major Types of Clinical Features

PORPHYRIA[a]	AFFECTED ENZYME	KNOWN MUTATIONS	INHERITANCE	CLASSIFICATION	PRINCIPAL CLINICAL FEATURES
X-linked protoporphyria (XLP)	δ-Aminolevulinic acid (ALA) synthase–erythroid specific form (ALAS2)	4 (gain of function)	Sex linked	Erythropoietic	Nonblistering photosensitivity
δ-Aminolevulinic acid dehydratase porphyria (ADP)	ALA dehydratase (ALAD)	10	Autosomal recessive	Hepatic[b]	Neurovisceral
Acute intermittent porphyria (AIP)	Hydroxymethylbilane synthase (HMBS)	>400	Autosomal dominant	Hepatic	Neurovisceral
Congenital erythropoietic porphyria (CEP)	Uroporphyrinogen III synthase (UROS)	48	Autosomal recessive	Erythropoietic	Neurovisceral
Porphyria cutanea tarda (PCT)	Uroporphyrinogen decarboxylase (UROD)	121 (includes HEP)	Autosomal dominant[c]	Hepatic	Blistering photosensitivity
Hepatoerythropoietic porphyria (HEP)	UROD	—	Autosomal recessive	Hepatic[b]	Blistering photosensitivity
Hereditary coproporphyria (HCP)	Coproporphyrinogen oxidase (CPOX)	64	Autosomal dominant	Hepatic	Neurovisceral; blistering photosensitivity (uncommon)
Variegate porphyria (VP)	Protoporphyrinogen oxidase (PPOX)	174	Autosomal dominant	Hepatic	Neurovisceral; blistering photosensitivity (common)
Erythropoietic protoporphyria (EPP)	Ferrochelatase (FECH)	189	Autosomal recessive	Erythropoietic	Nonblistering photosensitivity

[a]Porphyrias are listed in the order of the affected enzyme in the heme biosynthetic pathway.
[b]These porphyrias also have erythropoietic features, including increases in erythrocyte zinc protoporphyrin.
[c]UROD inhibition in PCT is mostly acquired, but an inherited deficiency of the enzyme predisposes in familial (type 2) disease.

from blood and other tissues in the chloride form. *Hemin* also refers generically to biologics, namely, lyophilized *hematin* (heme hydroxide) and heme arginate, which are available for treatment of acute porphyrias.

Approximately 85% of heme synthesis occurs in the bone marrow to support hemoglobin formation, with the remainder mostly in the liver, primarily for cytochrome P450 enzymes (CYPs) found in the endoplasmic reticulum.[11] All other tissues synthesize heme in smaller amounts. Examples of the numerous other vital hemoproteins include myoglobin, mitochondrial respiratory cytochromes, nitric oxide synthase, and catalase.

Heme synthesis in the liver is regulated primarily by the activity of δ-aminolevulinic acid synthase 1 (ALAS1, the housekeeping form of ALAS, the first enzyme in the pathway), with repression of synthesis of this enzyme and its import into mitochondria by heme, the end product of the pathway. In the marrow, heme and globin synthesis are closely coordinated during erythropoietin signaling. Expression of ALAS2, the erythroid-specific form of ALAS, and a number of other pathway enzymes, are stimulated by heme or iron and by erythroid-specific *cis*-acting elements including GATA-1 and NF-E2, culminating with phosphorylation of ferrochelatase (FECH), the final enzyme in heme synthesis.[12]

PORPHYRIA CUTANEA TARDA

AT-A-GLANCE

- Characterized by skin friability and blistering lesions on sun-exposed areas of skin
- Caused by inhibition of hepatic uroporphyrinogen decarboxylase (UROD) activity
- This leads to excess amounts of highly carboxylated porphyrins in liver, plasma, urine, and feces in diagnostic patterns
- Genetic factors that predispose may include mutations of UROD (heterozygous, only in ~20% of cases) and hemochromatosis (HFE)
- Acquired susceptibility factors (alcohol, smoking, secondary iron overload, chronic hepatitis C, HIV, and estrogen) are often multiple
- Responds readily to repeated phlebotomy while following serum ferritin, or low-dose hydroxychloroquine

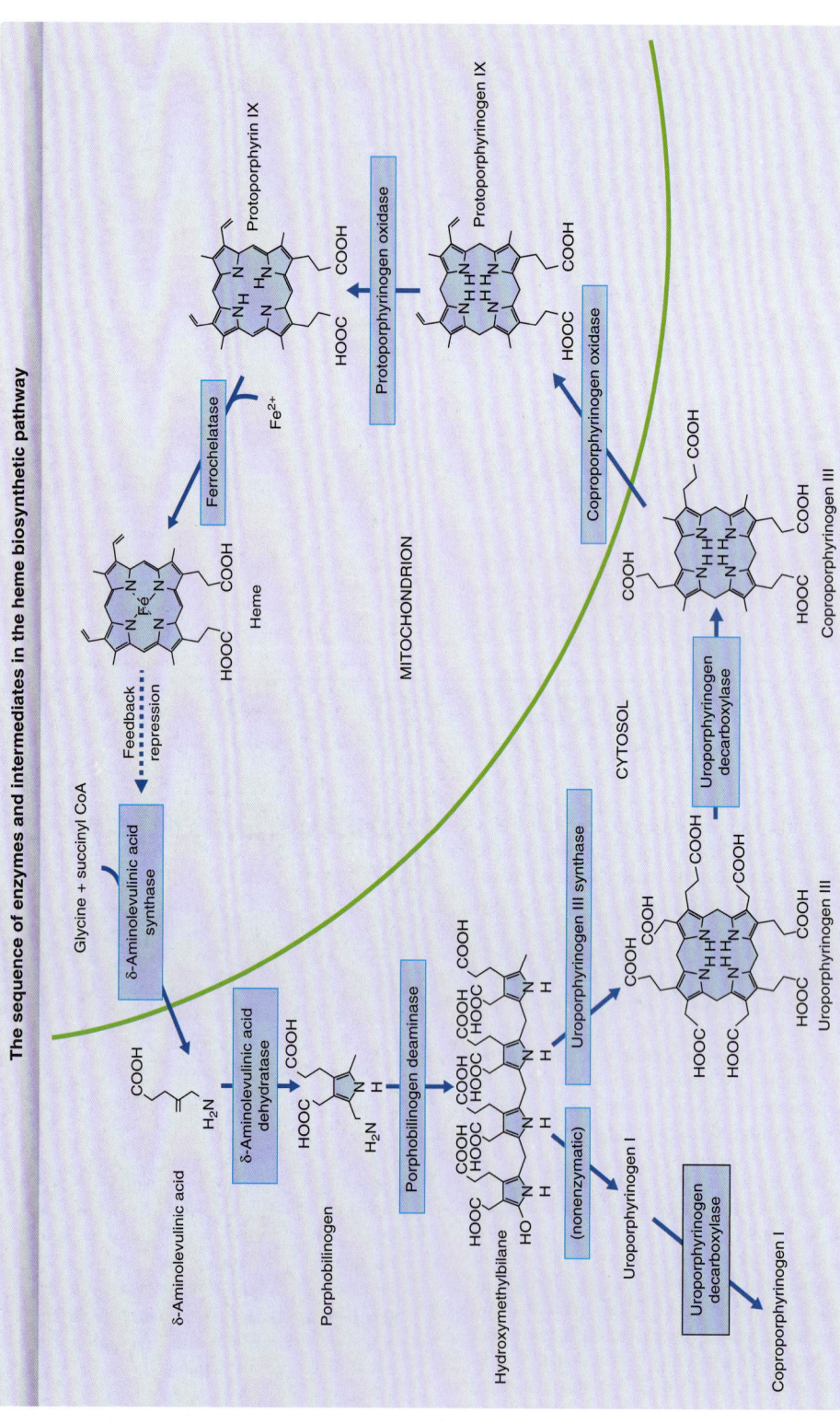

Figure 124-1 The sequence and chemical structures of intermediates in the heme biosynthetic pathway and localization of the 8 pathway enzymes in mitochondria or the cytosol. δ-Aminolevulinic acid synthase exists as a house-keeping form (ALAS1), found in all tissues, and an erythroid-specific form (ALAS2) found only in marrow erythroid cells. As shown here, the synthesis of ALAS1 in liver is under sensitive feedback control by the end product heme.

TABLE 124-2
Major Biochemical Abnormalities (in Bold) and Other Differentiating Measurements in the Human Porphyrias[a]

PORPHYRIA	ERYTHROCYTES	PLASMA	URINE	STOOL
ADP*	• **Increased zinc protoporphyrin**	• **Increased ALA** • PBG and porphyrin levels normal or slightly increased	• **Increased ALA** • **Increased coproporphyrin III** • PBG and other porphyrin levels normal or slightly increased	• Porphyrin levels normal or slightly increased
AIP	• **PBGD usually decreased**[§]	• **Increased ALA and PBG** • Porphyrin levels normal or slightly increased • Peak fluorescence ~620 nm[b]	• **Increased ALA, PBG, and porphyrins (often mostly uroporphyrin)**	• Porphyrin levels normal or slightly increased
CEP	• **Uroporphyrin I; coproporphyrin I**	• **Uroporphyrin I; coproporphyrin I** • Peak fluorescence ~620 nm[b]	• **Uroporphyrin I; coproporphyrin I**	• **Coproporphyrin I**
PCT	• Porphyrin levels normal or slightly increased	• **Uroporphyrin, heptacarboxyl porphyrin** • Peak fluorescence ~620 nm[b]	• **Uroporphyrin, heptacarboxyl porphyrin**	• **Uroporphyrin, heptacarboxyl porphyrin, coproporphyrin III, isocoproporphyrins**
HEP	• **Zinc protoporphyrin**			
HCP	• Porphyrin levels normal or slightly increased	• Porphyrins normal or increased[c] • Peak fluorescence ~620 nm[b]	• **ALA, PBG,** coproporphyrin III	• **Coproporphyrin III**
VP	• Porphyrin levels normal or slightly increased	• Protoporphyrins usually increased • **Peak fluorescence ~626 nm**[b]	• **ALA, PBG,** coproporphyrin III	• **Coproporphyrin III, protoporphyrin**
EPP and XLP	• **Metal-free protoporphyrin**[d]	• **Protoporphyrin** • **Peak fluorescence ~634 nm**[b]	• ALA, PBG, porphyrins normal	• Protoporphyrin normal or modestly increased

[a]Abbreviations as in Table 124-1.
[b]Fluorescence emission peak of diluted plasma at neutral Ph.
[c]Increased in the presence of skin lesions.
[d]Metal-free protoporphyrin approximately 85%-100% of the total in EPP, and 50%-85% in XLP.

PCT is the most common porphyria, and is characterized by the development of skin friability and chronic, blistering lesions on the dorsal aspects of the hands and other sun-exposed areas of skin usually in mid- or late life.[13] The underlying cause is deficient uroporphyrinogen deaminase (UROD) activity in hepatocytes, where uroporphyrinogen and other highly carboxylated porphyrinogens accumulate and are oxidized to the corresponding porphyrins. In active cases, hepatic UROD activity is reduced to less than ~20% of normal. PCT is an iron-related disorder and develops only in the presence of normal or increased amounts of hepatic iron. Multiple susceptibility factors contribute to iron accumulation, oxidative stress, and generation of a UROD inhibitor in hepatocytes, and are important to identify in individual patients. This is the only porphyria that can develop in absence of the mutation of the affected enzyme.[14] Heterozygous *UROD* mutations are found in ~20% of patients, but these do not cause PCT in the absence of other susceptibility factors.

PCT is the most readily treated porphyria, responding well to either phlebotomy or low-dose hydroxychloroquine. But the disease must first be differentiated from other less common porphyrias that cause identical skin lesions but are unresponsive to these treatments.

CLINICAL FEATURES

PCT usually develops in the fourth or fifth decade of life, most commonly in males. Fluid-filled blisters and bullae are found especially on the dorsal hands (Fig. 124-2), the most sun-exposed areas of the body, and often arise after minor or inapparent trauma as a result of increased skin friability. Blisters may also occur on the forearms, face, ears, neck, legs, and feet. These rupture easily, leaving erosions that may become dry and crusted and heal slowly (Fig. 124-2). Eroded areas of skin are prone to bacterial infection. Residual scarring and hyper- and hypopigmentation are prominent with prolonged disease. Milia may precede or follow vesicle formation. Facial hypertrichosis and hyperpigmentation (Fig. 124-3) are common, may even occur in the absence of blistering, and are cosmetically problematic, especially in women.[16] Severe thickening of affected areas of skin, sometimes with associated calcification, can resemble systemic sclerosis and is termed *pseudoscleroderma*. Neurologic symptoms characteristic of the acute porphyrias are not seen in PCT.

Rare childhood cases have often been associated with UROD mutations and cancer chemotherapy[15] (Fig. 124-3). The disease may develop during

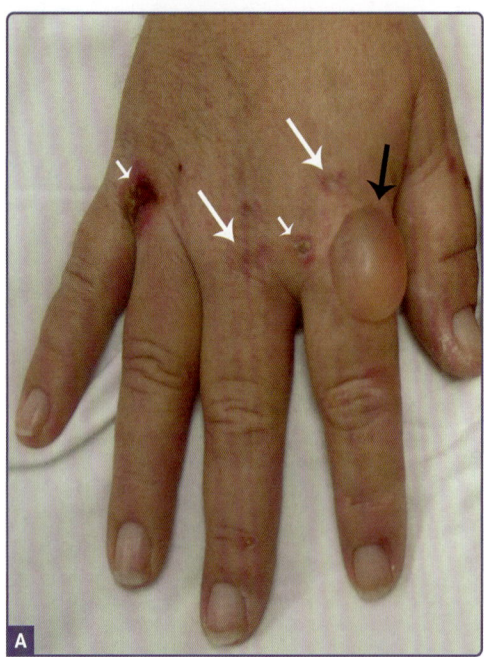

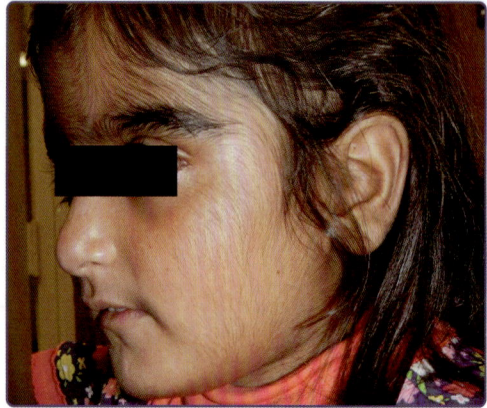

Figure 124-3 Marked hypertrichosis and hyperpigmentation due to porphyria cutanea tarda that developed in a child with an inherited *UROD* mutation after chemotherapy for leukemia, as previously reported.[15]

Mild abnormalities in liver function tests are found in almost all cases. Fresh hepatic tissue exhibits strong red fluorescence on exposure to long-wave ultraviolet light (Fig. 124-4), reflecting massive accumulation of porphyrins. Liver histopathology is nonspecific and usually includes increased iron, increased fat, hepatocyte necrosis and inflammation, which in many cases reflects the effects of alcohol or hepatitis C infection. Cirrhosis is unusual at the onset of PCT. The risk of HCC is increased, especially with more prolonged disease, perhaps due partly to concomitant susceptibility factors that themselves can cause chronic liver damage and fibrosis.[18-20]

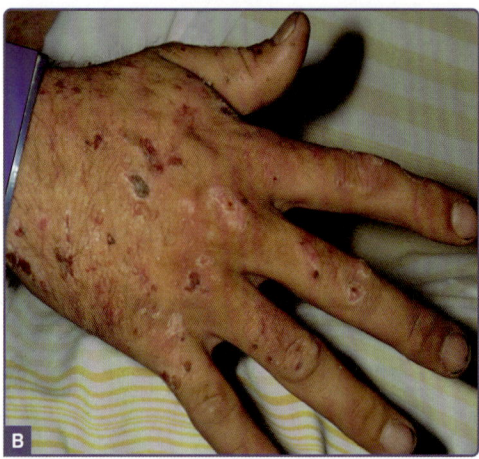

Figure 124-2 Characteristic skin lesions in PCT occur most commonly on the dorsal hands and are indistinguishable from those seen in other blistering cutaneous porphyrias (especially variegate porphyria) and pseudoporphyria. **A,** Blisters (short black arrow) often form after minor trauma, rupture to leave superficial ulcerations that may crust over (short white arrows) and leave atropic areas (long arrows) that heal slowly. **B,** Blisters are fragile, so often the only lesions present are chronic, such as erosions, crusts and scarring.

SUSCEPTIBILITY FACTORS

PCT is a multifactorial disorder, with many common susceptibility factors contributing to the disease, none of which is present in every patient. These include genetic factors, viral infections, and chemical exposures. Patients almost always possess multiple such factors, which have other health implications.[21] For example, in a large series of 143 patients with PCT in the United States, the most common susceptibility factors were ethanol use (87%), smoking (81%), chronic hepatitis C (69%), and *HFE* (hemochromatosis) mutations (53%).[22] These factors are common in the general population but do not by themselves cause PCT to develop. Additional susceptibility factors are likely to be identified in the future.

UROD MUTATIONS

Most PCT patients do not have a *UROD* mutation and are said to have sporadic (type 1) disease. Approximately 20% of patients have a heterozygous predisposing *UROD* mutation and are labeled as familial (type 2) PCT. Such mutations are inherited as autosomal

pregnancy, possibly related to effects of increased estrogen. Reported associations with cutaneous and systemic lupus erythematosus are unexplained. PCT associated with end-stage renal disease is usually more severe, because urinary excretion of porphyrins is impaired, and porphyrins are poorly dialyzed. The resulting plasma porphyrin levels can equal those seen in congenital erythropoietic porphyria (CEP) and be associated with severe bacterial infections and mutilation.[17]

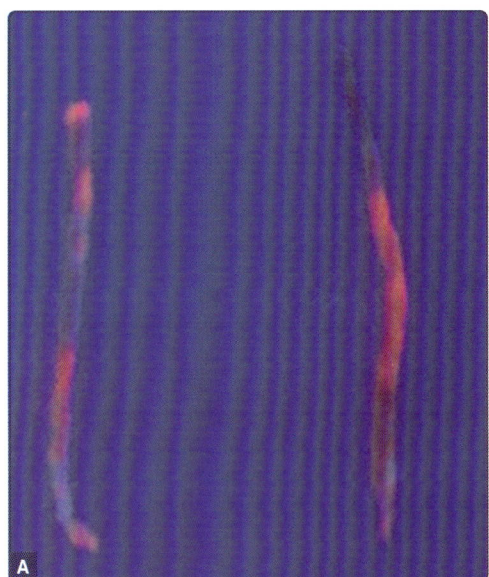

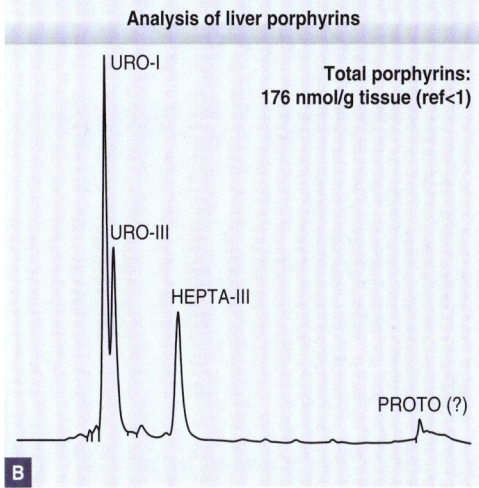

Figure 124-4 **A,** Fresh liver biopsy tissue showing bright red fluorescence under longwave ultraviolet light (Wood lamp) reflecting marked accumulation of highly carboxylated porphyrins in hepatocytes. **B,** Analysis of liver porphyrins from the same biopsy (total porphyrins 176 nmol/g tissue, ref <1) with a predominance of uroporphyrins I and III and heptacarboxyl porphyrin III on separation of porphyrins by high-performance liquid chromatography (HPLC); this pattern resembles that found in plasma and urine. (Image used with permission from Heather Stevenson-Lerner, MD, PhD; HPLC used with permission from V.M.S. Ramanujam, PhD).

dominant traits, but with low penetrance, so most type 2 patients present sporadically, having no known relatives with PCT. Having such a mutation is a susceptibility factor that does not cause PCT in the absence of other acquired or inherited susceptibility factors. HEP is the homozygous form of type 2 PCT, and resembles CEP clinically. At least 100 different mutations of the *UROD* gene, mostly missense mutations occurring in 1 or a few families, have been identified in type 2 PCT and HEP (Table 124-1). Type 3 refers to rare families with more than 1 affected individuals but no *UROD* mutation. All 3 PCT types are clinically identical, although disease onset is sometimes earlier in type 2.[23]

IRON AND HEMOCHROMATOSIS GENE (*HFE*) MUTATIONS

Iron stores are always normal or increased in PCT, whereas iron deficiency is protective. Iron provides an oxidative environment in hepatocytes and facilitates generation of a UROD inhibitor, but does not itself directly inhibit UROD. The *C282Y* mutation of the *HFE* gene, the major mutation causing hemochromatosis in whites, is more prevalent in both sporadic and familial PCT than in unaffected individuals. Up to 10% to 20% of patients may be *C282Y* homozygotes, and these may experience earlier onset of disease.[23,24] In southern Europe, where the *C282Y* is less prevalent, the *H63D* mutation is more commonly associated with PCT.[25] *HFE* mutations impair sensing of serum iron, thereby reducing hepatic hepcidin production. Because circulating levels of hepcidin are inappropriately low, downregulation of enterocyte ferroportin by hepcidin is impaired, leading to inappropriately high intestinal iron absorption. Hepatic hepcidin expression is also reduced in PCT patients without *HFE* mutations, because some other susceptibility factors reduce expression of this hormone, as noted below.[26]

ALCOHOL

PCT has long been associated with alcohol abuse. Alcohol and its metabolites may predispose to onset of PCT by inducing hepatic ALAS1 and CYPs, generating reactive oxygen species, and causing mitochondrial injury, lipid deposition, depletion of reduced glutathione and other antioxidant defenses, increasing production of endotoxin and activating Küpffer cells. Alcohol intake can also reduce hepcidin expression.[26]

SMOKING AND CYTOCHROME P450 ENZYMES

Smoking is frequently associated with alcohol use but is regarded as an independent risk factor in PCT.[21] Smoking may increase oxidative stress in hepatocytes and induces hepatic CYPs, including CYP1A2 which is important for development of uroporphyria in rodent models of PCT.[27,28] Hepatic CYPs are often increased in human PCT,[29] but it is unclear which CYPs contribute to the disease. However, a more inducible *CYP1A2* variant was found to be more common in PCT than in normal subjects.[30,31]

ESTROGENS

Estrogen use is common in women with PCT.[21,32,33] The disease has also occurred in some men treated with estrogen for prostate cancer.[32] Female rats or males receiving estrogens are more susceptible to development of chemically-induced uroporphyria than untreated males.[34] The mechanism for this predisposition is not certain, but may be secondary to generation of reactive oxygen species.[14,35]

HEPATITIS C

Hepatitis C promotes hepatocyte steatosis, iron accumulation, mitochondrial dysfunction, oxidative stress and dysregulation of hepcidin expression.[36,37] The prevalence of chronic hepatitis C in PCT ranges from 21% to 92% in various countries, and always exceeds the prevalence of this viral infection in the general population. Only an estimated 0.05% of individuals with chronic hepatitis C develop PCT.[38] Large differences in the prevalence of this viral infection in PCT in different countries reflects the considerable geographic variation in prevalence of this infection in at-risk populations.

HIV

PCT is less commonly associated with HIV infection, which may be present with or without HCV coinfection.[39] PCT can be the initial manifestation of HIV infection. The mechanism for the association with HIV infection and possible relationships to specific antiretroviral therapies are not established.

ANTIOXIDANTS

Reduced plasma levels of ascorbate and carotenoids have been noted in some patients with PCT.[40-42] Rodents with ascorbate deficiency are more susceptible to development of uroporphyria.[43]

CHEMICAL EXPOSURE AND DRUGS

A large outbreak of PCT occurred in eastern Turkey in the 1950s during a period of food shortage when the population consumed seed wheat treated with the fungicide hexachlorobenzene.[44] Smaller outbreaks and individual cases of the disease have occurred after exposures to other chemicals such as 2,3,7,8-tetrachlorodibenzo-*p*-dioxin (TCDD, dioxin).[45] These and related chemicals cause biochemical features of PCT in laboratory animals and cultured hepatocytes.[10,14]

ETIOLOGY AND PATHOGENESIS

PCT develops when hepatic UROD activity is reduced to ~20% of normal.[14] With enzyme inhibition, the amount of UROD protein remains at its genetically determined level in the liver.[46,47] As previously discussed, about 20% of patients are heterozygous for UROD mutations and are more susceptible to developing PCT, because their UROD activity in the liver (as well as other tissues) is half-normal from birth. PCT does not manifest in these individuals unless further reduction of UROD activity occurs in the liver. A UROD inhibitor, characterized as a *uroporphomethene*, was identified in a mouse model that spontaneously develops biochemical features of PCT. This inhibitor is a product of partial oxidation of uroporphyrinogen, possibly generated by 1 or more CYPs (Fig. 124-5).[49]

UROD sequentially decarboxylates uroporphyrinogen I and III (each with 8 carboxyl side groups) to coproporphyrinogen I and III (each with 4 carboxyl

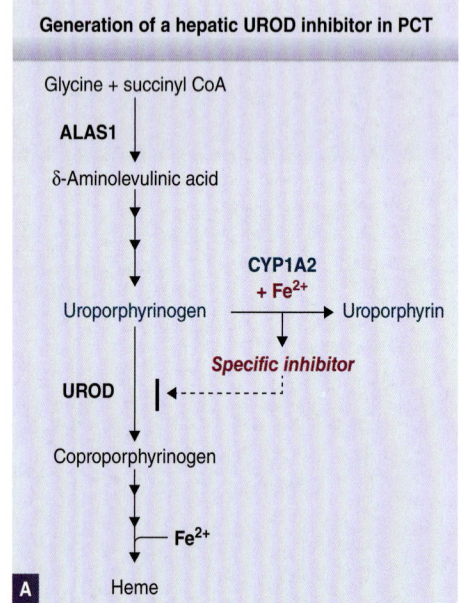

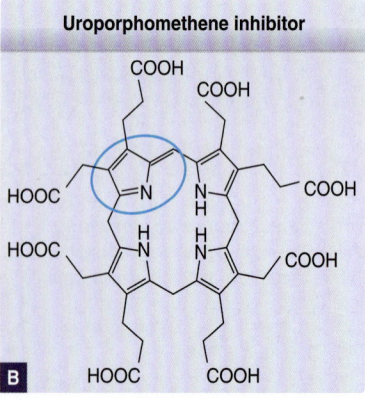

Figure 124-5 **A,** Schema for generation of a specific inhibitor of uroporphyrinogen decarboxylase in the liver in the presence of iron, cytochrome P450 enzymes (especially CYP1A2) and oxidative stress in PCT. (Modified from Anderson KE. Porphyria cutanea tarda: A possible role for ascorbic acid. *Hepatology.* 2007;45(1):6-8; with permission. Copyright © 2007, John Wiley & Sons.[48]) **B,** A UROD inhibitor has been isolated as a uroporphomethene, a uroporphyrinogen molecule that is partially oxidized at one ring (circled in blue) and its adjacent methyl bridge.

groups), respectively. Both isomers are substrates for UROD, but uroporphyrinogen III is preferred. (The next enzyme in the pathway is specific for coproporphyrinogen III as a substrate, so uroporphyrinogen I and coproporphyrin I are not heme precursors.) When hepatic UROD is inhibited, uroporphyrinogen I and III and the intermediates in the reaction (ie, I and III isomers of hepta-, hexa-, and pentacarboxyl porphyrinogen) accumulate as the corresponding oxidized porphyrins, and are eventually transported in plasma to the skin, causing photosensitivity, and to the kidneys for excretion. Biliary and fecal porphyrins are also increased. Porphyrins in their oxidized state are reddish, fluorescent, and photosensitizing, whereas porphyrinogens do not have these properties. The polycyclic aromatic structure of oxidized porphyrins contains delocalized electrons, which increase in energy level on exposure to violet light (at a wavelength of ~410 nm). This energy may be released at a higher wavelength as red fluorescent light or transferred to molecular oxygen, forming reactive singlet state oxygen and other reactive oxygen species. These may damage cutaneous cellular constituents or cause mast cell degranulation and complement activation.[50,51] Damage to the subepidermal layers of skin makes the skin friable and prone to blistering.[50,51]

DIAGNOSIS

PCT develops most commonly in adult males in association with factors such as excess alcohol use, smoking and chronic hepatitis C, and in females, particularly with estrogen use. The presentation is usually characteristic, but it must be remembered that adults with variegate porphyria (VP), hereditary coproporphyria (HCP) or pseudoporphyria, and children or adults with congenital erythropoietic porphyria (CEP) or hepatoerythropoietic porphyria (HEP) can present with identical skin lesions. Therefore, it is essential to establish a laboratory diagnosis of PCT before initiating treatment.

First-line testing (ie, screening) for PCT is measurement of total plasma or urine porphyrins. Normal results may indicate a diagnosis of pseudoporphyria. Because elevated porphyrins, especially in urine, is common in liver disease and other medical conditions, a finding of increased porphyrins and does not itself support a diagnosis of porphyria. Therefore, if first-line testing is positive, the following are suggested to establish a diagnosis and exclude other less common porphyrias that can cause similar skin manifestations and often be misdiagnosed as PCT:

- Fluorescence scanning of diluted plasma at neutral pH.[52] The porphyria most commonly misdiagnosed as PCT is VP,[53] and is rapidly and reliably recognized by plasma scanning and finding an emission peak at ~626 nm, in contrast to ~620 nm for PCT and other blistering cutaneous porphyrias.
- Fractionation of urine or plasma porphyrins, which will show a predominance of uroporphyrin, and hepta-, hexa-, and pentacarboxyl, porphyrins in PCT. This pattern of predominance of highly carboxylated porphyrins is not fully diagnostic, as it can occur in other much less common porphyrias that can be misdiagnosed as PCT especially when they present in adults.
- Total erythrocyte porphyrins, which are normal or modestly elevated in PCT, but markedly elevated in rare cases of CEP, HEP, or homozygous HCP or VP. These usually present in infancy, but can first become manifest in adults, sometimes in associated with a clonal myeloproliferative or myelodysplastic disorder.
- Fecal porphyrins may be normal or modestly increased in PCT, with a complex pattern that includes isocoproporphyrins. These atypical tetracarboxylporphyrins are formed when pentacarboxylporphyrinogen accumulates in liver as a result of UROD inhibition and undergoes premature decarboxylation by CPOX, the next enzyme in the pathway, forming dehydroisocoproporphyrinogen. The latter is excreted in bile and undergoes oxidation by intestinal bacteria to isocoproporphyrins.[54] In contrast to PCT, fecal porphyrins are markedly elevated in CEP, HCP, and VP, with a predominance of coproporphyrin I in CEP, coproporphyrin III in HCP, and both coproporphyrin III and protoporphyrin in VP.
- Urine ALA is normal or modestly increased in PCT, and PBG is always normal. Levels of these porphyrin precursors may be elevated in the acute hepatic porphyrias, AIP, HCP and VP.

An increase of plasma porphyrins and demonstration of a predominance of highly carboxylated porphyrins is essential for diagnosis of PCT in patients with advanced renal disease, although the reference range is higher in this population.[55] Advanced renal disease is commonly associated with altered erythropoiesis and resulting increases in erythrocyte zinc protoporphyrin, which should not be attributed to PCT or other porphyria. Patients with AIP and end-stage renal disease sometimes present with blistering skin lesions that resemble PCT.[56]

Although not required for diagnosis of PCT, skin biopsy reveals characteristic but nonspecific findings such as subepidermal blistering and deposition of periodic acid–Schiff-positive material around blood vessels and fine fibrillar material in the upper dermis and at the dermoepithelial junction. Deposits of immunoglobulins and complement are also found.[57] These histologic changes are also seen in other cutaneous porphyrias as well as pseudoporphyria, a poorly understood condition that presents with lesions that closely resemble PCT, but with plasma porphyrins that are not significantly increased.[58]

IDENTIFICATION OF SUSCEPTIBILITY FACTORS

All PCT patients should be questioned or examined for the following susceptibility factors, some of which are modifiable: alcohol and estrogen use, smoking, hepatitis C and HIV infection, and *HFE* and *UROD* mutations. Use of drugs that exacerbate acute porphyrias are seldom implicated in PCT. Although familial (type 2) cases of PCT can be identified by half-normal erythrocyte UROD activity, *UROD* mutation analysis is more dependable. This full analysis of susceptibility factors helps explain the disease in individual cases and may affect management. Moreover, some of these factors also have medical implications of their own. Serum ferritin should be measured and may influence choice of treatment.

THERAPY

Treatment with phlebotomy or low-dose hydroxychloroquine is highly effective in both sporadic and familial forms of PCT. These should be initiated only after the diagnosis is certain, because they are not effective in other porphyrias. It may be reasonable to start treatment after plasma porphyrin results, including fluorescence scanning,[52] are consistent with PCT and have excluded VP and pseudoporphyria. Patients should be advised to stop smoking and alcohol consumption. Use of estrogen and drugs known to induce hepatic heme synthesis should be discontinued if possible. Estrogen replacement therapy, preferably transdermal, can be considered, if needed, after PCT is in remission.[59] Adequate intake of ascorbic acid and other nutrients should be established. Removal of 1 or more susceptibility factors can lead to improvement, but the response is slow or unpredictable.[60]

Repeated phlebotomy to reduce hepatic iron is the preferred treatment at most institutions. Removal of 450 mL blood at 2-week intervals is guided by the serum ferritin level, with a target of 15 to 20 ng/mL (ie, near the lower limit of normal). Measurement of hematocrit and ferritin at each session allows monitoring to prevent symptomatic anemia and assess progress toward the target ferritin level. Phlebotomies are stopped when the ferritin from the previous visit is 25 to 30 ng/L, and ferritin is measured to confirm that the target level was reached. At that point, porphyrin levels may not have become completely normal and skin lesions are not completely resolved. Additional iron depletion is not beneficial and leads to anemia. Most patients require 6 to 8 phlebotomies for biochemical and clinical remission, but additional sessions may be necessary, especially if the baseline serum ferritin level is markedly elevated. Decreases in plasma (or serum) porphyrin levels tend to lag behind serum ferritin, but will normalize within weeks after phlebotomies are completed.[61,62] Friability of skin may persist for some time after porphyrin levels are normal, until healing and repair of the subepidermal layer of the skin is complete. Subsequent phlebotomies are generally not needed, with the exception of patients homozygous or compound heterozygous for the *C282Y HFE* mutation, as current guidelines for hemochromatosis recommend maintaining a ferritin level between 50 and 100 ng/mL.[63] Relapse of PCT may occur, often related to resumption of alcohol use, but usually responds to retreatment. Following porphyrin levels after remission can detect recurrences early so that retreatment can be reinstituted promptly.

A low-dose regimen of hydroxychloroquine (or chloroquine) is an effective alternative to phlebotomies, and is the preferred approach at some institutions.[14,64-70] These 4-aminoquinoline antimalarials do not appear to deplete hepatic iron, but mobilize porphyrins that have accumulated in lysosomes and other intracellular organelles in hepatocytes. Full therapeutic doses of these drugs rapidly mobilize porphyrins and induce an acute hepatitis, characterized by fever, malaise, nausea, and marked increases in urinary and plasma porphyrins and photosensitivity, but followed by remission.[71] Unmasking of previously unrecognized PCT with use of chloroquine for malaria prophylaxis has been described.[72] A low-dose regimen (hydroxychloroquine 100 mg or chloroquine 125 mg [one half of a standard tablet] twice weekly) is recommended to achieve remission and avoid the side effects of full doses of these drugs.[64,67,68] Treatment is continued until plasma or urine porphyrins are normalized for at least a month. Patients who respond poorly may require alternate therapy with phlebotomy.[71] These medications are associated with a small risk of retinopathy,[73] which may be lower with hydroxychloroquine. Therefore, patients should be screened by an ophthalmologist before treatment.[74] Comparison of treatment with phlebotomy or hydroxychloroquine (100 mg twice weekly), showed that time to remission (normal plasma porphyrin levels) was comparable with these treatments.[70] Treatment with an iron chelator such as desferrioxamine is much less efficient for removal of iron than phlebotomy, but can be considered if both phlebotomy and low-dose hydroxychloroquine are contraindicated.[75]

Treatment of hepatitis C with interferon-based regimens is lengthy and often not successful. Therefore we have first treated PCT, which is usually more symptomatic, and after achieving remission, then treated coexisting hepatitis C. Interferon-based treatment regimens commonly cause anemia, which usually precludes phlebotomy for PCT, and are sometimes associated with relapse of previously treated PCT.[76] Experience with low-dose hydroxychloroquine during concurrent treatment of hepatitis C is limited. The new direct-acting antivirals can treat this infection rapidly and dependably, and studies are under way to collect evidence whether they should be used instead of phlebotomy or low-dose hydroxychloroquine as initial treatment of PCT associated with hepatitis C.[76]

PCT associated with end-stage renal disease is often difficult to treat. Phlebotomy is effective if supported, as needed, by starting or increasing the dose of erythropoietin.[17,77,78] High-flux hemodialysis may provide some benefit.[79] Renal transplantation can lead to remission presumably because of resumption of endogenous erythropoietin production and reduced hepcidin levels.[80]

Periodic screening for hepatocellular carcinoma should include liver imaging by abdominal ultrasonography or computed tomography. As in other liver diseases, this should be guided by evidence of cirrhosis or hepatic fibrosis, which may be assessed by liver biopsy or indirectly by elastography, and the presence of other causes of liver disease.

HEPATOERYTHROPOIETIC PORPHYRIA

AT-A-GLANCE

- HEP is the homozygous form of familial (type 2) PCT, with mutation of both *UROD* alleles resulting in severely deficient UROD activity
- HEP resembles CEP, with blistering lesions on sun-exposed areas of skin, usually starting in childhood
- Biochemical findings resemble PCT, but with substantial elevation of erythrocyte zinc protoporphyrin
- Patients should avoid sunlight. Treatment with phlebotomy or low-dose hydroxychloroquine is not effective.

This very rare form of porphyria is the homozygous (or compound heterozygous) form of familial (type 2) PCT and is characterized by blistering skin lesions from chronic, severe photosensitivity.

CLINICAL FEATURES

HEP presents with onset of blistering skin lesions, hypertrichosis, scarring, hemolytic anemia, and red urine typically in early childhood. Sclerodermoid skin changes are sometimes prominent. The cutaneous manifestations resemble those found in PCT, but are usually much more severe. Unusually mild cases and onset during adult life have been reported.[81]

ETIOLOGY AND PATHOGENESIS

Patients with HEP have inherited a *UROD* mutation from each parent. Numerous *UROD* mutations associated with PCT or UROD have been identified. Erythrocyte UROD activity is 5% to 30% of normal in HEP. As homozygosity for a *UROD* null allele is lethal, at least one of the mutant *UROD* alleles must produce some enzyme protein with catalytic activity. Expression studies in eukaryotic cells suggest that some mutations may destabilize the enzyme protein in a tissue-specific manner.[82] Excess porphyrins are primarily generated in the liver. Zinc protoporphyrin accumulates in the marrow and is markedly elevated in erythrocytes.

DIAGNOSIS

Biochemical findings in HEP resemble PCT, with predominant accumulation and excretion of uroporphyrin, heptacarboxyl porphyrin, and isocoproporphyrins. In contrast to PCT, erythrocyte zinc protoporphyrin is substantially increased. Erythrocyte UROD activity is markedly diminished, and molecular studies should demonstrate mutations affecting both *UROD* alleles.

THERAPY

Patients with HEP should be advised to avoid sunlight. Phlebotomy and hydroxychloroquine have shown little or no benefit.[83] Patients should avoid susceptibility factors known to be important in PCT. Oral charcoal was helpful in a severe case associated with dyserythropoiesis, likely due to trapping of porphyrins in the intestinal lumen and preventing their enterohepatic circulation.[84] Retrovirus-mediated gene transfer studies suggest that correction of the HEP defect through gene replacement therapy may be applicable in the future.[85]

CONGENITAL ERYTHROPOIETIC PORPHYRIA

AT-A-GLANCE

- As a result of mutation of both uroporphyrinogen III synthase (UROS) alleles resulting in severe loss of activity of UROS and elevations of uroporphyrin I and coproporphyrin I
- Characterized by subepidermal scarring and bullous lesions affecting light-exposed areas
- Diagnosis is established by markedly elevated uroporphyrin I and coproporphyrin I in erythrocytes, urine, plasma, and feces and identification of causative mutations
- Hematopoietic stem cell transplantation at a young age is potentially curative
- Strict light avoidance can prevent chronic, disfiguring skin disease

Cases of CEP, also known as Günther disease, were first described in 1874 and 1898.[3] CEP is due to substantial deficiency of uroporphyrinogen III synthase (UROS), which results in accumulation of isomer I porphyrinogens, especially uroporphyrinogen I and coproporphyrinogen I, in the marrow during hemoglobin synthesis. Porphyrins are usually markedly elevated in erythrocytes, plasma and urine and cause chronic, severe photosensitivity

ETIOLOGY AND PATHOGENESIS

UROS catalyzes the formation of uroporphyrinogen III from hydroxymethylbilane (HMB) in the cytosol (Fig. 124-1). This reaction involves inverting one of the 4 pyrroles (ring D) of the linear tetrapyrrole and formation of a porphyrin macrocycle with an asymmetric arrangement of side chains. In the absence of this enzyme, HMB spontaneously cyclizes to form uroporphyrinogen I, which is symmetrical. UROD, the next enzyme in the pathway, will metabolize both uroporphyrinogen I and III to coproporphyrinogen I and III, respectively. However, coproporphyrinogen I is a dead-end product because the next enzyme in the heme biosynthetic pathway accepts only coproporphyrinogen III as a substrate.

More than 48 mutations of the *UROS* gene have been identified, and more severe mutations are associated with more severe clinical manifestations.[86] A GATA-1 mutation described in one case associated with beta-thalassemia indicates that a genetic defect outside the heme biosynthetic pathway can cause CEP.[87]

Marrow normoblasts in CEP display marked microscopic fluorescence due to porphyrin accumulation.[88] Increased porphyrin concentrations in circulating erythrocytes cause cell damage due to exposure to light in the dermal capillaries. Hemolysis and increased uptake of damaged cells by the spleen leads to splenomegaly as a common finding in CEP. Ineffective erythropoiesis in the marrow contributes to anemia. Excess porphyrins are transported in erythrocytes and plasma to the skin and lead to chronic and usually severe photosensitivity.

CLINICAL FEATURES

CEP is characterized by subepidermal bullous lesions affecting light-exposed areas such as the dorsal hands, fingers and face (Fig. 124-6), which often leads to scarring and areas of hyper- and hypopigmentation. Cutaneous lesions resemble those found in PCT, but with much higher porphyrin levels causing more prominent hyperpigmentation, scarring, contraction, and loss of fingers and facial features. Milder disease is often misdiagnosed as PCT, and rare onset in adults may be associated with myelodysplastic or myeloproliferative disorders with expansion of a clone of erythrocyte precursors carrying a *UROS* mutation.[90] The disease may be recognized in utero as a cause of fetal hydrops.[91] In most cases, photosensitivity is noted soon after birth. Erythrodontia (brown staining of the teeth) is caused by porphyrin deposition in developing teeth in utero. Porphyrins are also deposited in bone.[92] Pathologic fractures and other bony abnormalities may result from bone marrow expansion and vitamin D deficiency resulting from avoidance of sunlight.

Anemia resulting from intravascular hemolysis and ineffective erythropoiesis can be severe and require repeated red blood cell transfusions. Uncorrected anemia can further stimulate erythropoiesis and contribute to increased porphyrin production. Peripheral blood smears reveal polychromasia, poikilocytosis, anisocytosis, and basophilic stippling of erythrocytes and increases in reticulocytes and nucleated red blood cells. The liver and nervous system are not affected in CEP. A mother with CEP successfully delivered a healthy, unaffected infant with erythrodontia as a result of porphyrins crossing placenta.[93]

DIAGNOSIS

CEP can be recognized in utero by large amounts of porphyrins measured in amniotic fluid or fetal blood. CEP is often diagnosed shortly after birth when pink to brownish staining of the diapers is noted, with red fluorescence under long-wave ultraviolet light. Urinary, erythrocyte, and plasma porphyrins are markedly increased, with a predominance of uroporphyrin I and coproporphyrin I. Fecal porphyrins are markedly increased and are predominantly coproporphyrin I. Protoporphyrin IX is sometimes the predominant porphyrin in erythrocytes, especially in milder cases. DNA studies to identify causative mutations are important for confirming the diagnosis, genetic counseling, and prenatal diagnosis in subsequent pregnancies.

THERAPY

An individualized, multidisciplinary approach is required.[99] Patients should be advised to avoid sunlight, skin trauma, and infections to avoid severe scarring and loss of facial features and digits. Topical sunscreens that absorb ultraviolet A and B light are marginally beneficial because the harmful light is mostly visible; oral beta-carotene is also not effective.[94] Patients may require erythrocyte transfusions for severe anemia[95] and an iron chelator to avoid the sequelae of iron overload.[96] Hydroxyurea to reduce erythropoiesis and porphyrin production also may be considered.[97] Splenectomy may be beneficial if hypersplenism is contributing to significant anemia, leucopenia or thrombocytopenia. Ascorbic acid and α-tocopherol improved anemia in one patient.[98] Oral charcoal was reportedly beneficial in another.[84] Use of oral charcoal, splenectomy, and chronic hypertransfusion were associated with complications, without appreciable clinical benefit and negative impact on health-related quality of life in a large case series.[99]

Hematopoietic stem cell transplantation is curative and is the treatment of choice for young patients with severe disease.[100] Successful transplantation results in marked clinical improvement and reduction in porphyrin levels. Gene therapy is being explored using retroviral and lentiviral vectors and hematopoietic stem cells in patients with CEP.[101,102]

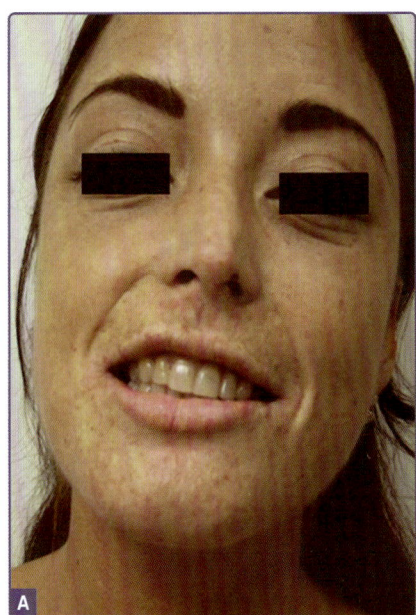
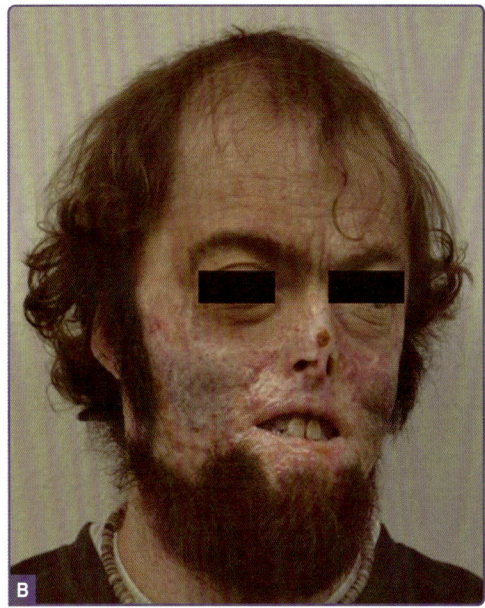
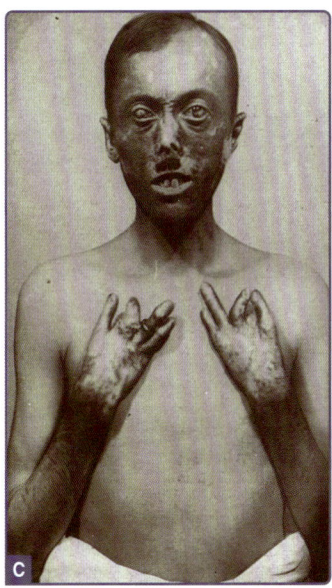

Figure 124-6 Three cases of congenital erythropoietic porphyria of different severity. Patient A had mild disease, strictly avoided sunlight, and manifested only mild skin contraction of the skin on the face, perioral scarring, and mild scarring of the dorsal hands and fingers with developmentally small, shortened fingers (not shown). Patient B also had mild disease with progressive scarring of the face, hands, and fingers from not avoiding sunlight. (Reprinted from Gou E, Phillips JD, Anderson KE. The porphyrias. In: Gilbert-Barness E, Barness L, Farrell PM, eds. *Metabolic Diseases*. Amsterdam: IOS Press BV; 2017:543-575,[10] Copyright 2017, with permission from IOS Press. The publication is available at IOS Press through https://www.iospress.nl/book/metabolic-diseases/. Patient C is Mr. Petry, who was historically important having worked in the laboratory of the porphyrin chemist Hans Fischer, where he provided samples for early studies of porphyrin chemistry; he had severe disease and survived to age 34. From Günther H. In: Schittenhelm A, ed. *Handbuch der Krankheiten der Blutes und der Blutbildenden Organe*. Vol 2. Berlin: Springer; 1925; with permission. Copyright © 1925.[89])

PROTOPORPHYRIAS

AT-A-GLANCE

- EPP is the third most common porphyria and the most common in children
- It results from mutation of both ferrochelatase (FECH) alleles; one with a severe mutation and in most families the other with a predisposing alteration that is common in the population
- XLP is less common and results from gain-of-function mutations of ALAS2
- Both are characterized by an acute, mostly nonblistering type of cutaneous photosensitivity and risk of liver damage.
- Diagnosis is established by marked elevation of erythrocyte protoporphyrin, which is predominantly metal-free protoporphyrin (not zinc protoporphyrin)
- Management emphasizes light avoidance and photoprotection

Erythropoietic protoporphyria (EPP) is the most common type of porphyria in children and the third most common in adults, with reported prevalence ranging between 0.5 and 1.5 cases per 100,000 individuals.[103-105] It results from loss-of-function mutation of ferrochelatase (FECH), the last enzyme of the heme biosynthetic pathway. But the protoporphyria phenotype can result from mutation of other genes. X-linked protoporphyria (XLP) results from gain-of-function mutation of ALAS2, the erythroid-specific form of the first enzyme in the pathway, and comprises ~5% of protoporphyria cases.[106] Protoporphyria with increased ALAS2 activity can also result from mutation of mitochondrial CLPX.[107] With rare exceptions, symptoms in all protoporphyrias begin in early childhood with an acute and nonblistering type of cutaneous photosensitivity. Protoporphyric hepatopathy is a potentially fatal complication occurring in less than 5% of patients.

ETIOLOGY AND PATHOGENESIS

EPP is caused by mutation of ferrochelatase (FECH, which catalyzes insertion of iron into protoporphyrin IX, the last step of the heme biosynthetic pathway; Fig. 124-1). FECH deficiency results in the accumulation of the substrate protoporphyrin particularly in marrow reticulocytes. Inheritance of EPP has been described as autosomal dominant with variable penetrance. But since the discovery that mutation of both FECH alleles is required, it is now best described as autosomal recessive. In most families, a severe *FECH* mutation, of which at least 189 have been described, is *trans* to a low-expression (hypomorphic) variant allele (IVS3-48C/T).[108-110] The change in DNA sequence in the low-expression allele results in increased use of an aberrant splice site that produces an mRNA more prone to degradation and a decreased steady-state level of wildtype FECH mRNA.[110] This *FECH* allele occurs in 10% of whites, and by itself has no phenotype. Its frequency varies widely in other populations; its prevalence is higher in east Asians but very low in Africa, accounting for geographic differences in the prevalence of EPP.[103-110]

Cases with 2 severe *FECH* mutations, 1 inherited from each parent, but without the low-expression allele, have been described. At least 1 allele must allow enough FECH enzyme to be synthesized for adequate synthesis of heme. These cases are sometimes associated with seasonal palmar keratoderma, neurologic symptoms, less-than-expected increases in erythrocyte protoporphyrin, and absence of liver dysfunction.[111]

Adult-onset cases of EPP have been described in patients with a myeloproliferative or myelodysplastic syndrome, in which there is expansion of a clone of hematopoietic cells carrying a *FECH* mutation.[112,113] For example, a patient with a myeloproliferative disorder developed severe EPP due to clonal expansion of erythroid precursor cells with a *FECH* deletion *trans* to a hypomorphic *FECH* allele, and died of EPP-induced liver disease.[114]

An X-linked pattern of inheritance in some patients with protoporphyria who lacked *FECH* mutations led to discovery of gain-of-function mutations of *ALAS2* (the only gene encoding an enzyme in the heme biosynthetic pathway found on the X chromosome).[106] These mutations lead to an approximately 3-fold increase in enzymatic activity of the ALAS protein and accumulation of protoporphyrin IX, which indicates that FECH activity is the next rate-limiting step in erythroid heme synthesis.[106] Two members of a family in France were recently found to have protoporphyria without mutation of *FECH* or *ALAS2*, but with a loss-of-function mutation of *CLPX* inherited as an autosomal dominant trait, resulting in decreased degradation of ALAS2 and overproduction of ALA and protoporphyrin.[107]

In EPP, the excess protoporphyrin found in circulating erythrocytes is primarily metal-free rather complexed with zinc, in contrast to many other conditions that increase erythrocyte protoporphyrin that is mostly zinc protoporphyrin (eg, lead intoxication, iron deficiency, anemia of chronic disease, hemolytic states). Excess metal-free protoporphyrin in plasma, which originates from the marrow, where hemoglobin synthesis is active, as well as from circulating erythrocytes, is taken up by hepatocytes, excreted in bile and feces, and may undergo enterohepatic recirculation. Protoporphyrin is hydrophobic as it only possesses 2 hydroxyl groups and is not excreted in urine. Erythrocytes in XLP and protoporphyria due to a CLPX mutation contain increased amounts of both metal-free and zinc-complexed protoporphyrin.

Excitation of porphyrins by ultraviolet light generates free radicals and singlet oxygen,[115] which in EPP can lead to complement activation, peroxidation of lipids,[116] crosslinking of membrane proteins,[117] and polymorphonuclear chemotaxis, resulting in skin pathology.[118] Nonspecific findings on skin histopathology include thickened capillary walls in the papillary dermis surrounded by deposition of amorphous hyalinelike and periodic acid–Schiff (PAS)-positive mucopolysaccharides, complement, and immunoglobulins.[119] Basement membrane abnormalities are less marked than in other forms of cutaneous porphyria.[120]

Protoporphyric hepatopathy occurs in less than 5% of patients. It may cause chronic abnormalities in liver function tests with progression to cirrhosis, or present acutely with rapid progression and require urgent liver transplantation. Other causes of liver damage, such as alcoholic or nonalcoholic steatohepatitis or viral hepatitis, can predispose patients to this condition by impairing protoporphyrin excretion and thereby increasing circulating protoporphyrin to levels that accelerate damage to the liver. Excess protoporphyrin is cholestatic, forms crystalline structures in hepatocytes, and impairs mitochondrial function.[121,122] Accumulated protoporphyrin may appear as brown pigment in hepatocytes, Küpffer cells, and biliary canaliculi and as doubly refractive inclusions with a "Maltese cross" appearance under polarizing microscopy.[123]

TABLE 124-3
Clinical Manifestations in a Series of 32 Cases of Erythropoietic Protoporphyria

SYMPTOMS AND FINDINGS	INCIDENCE (% OF TOTAL)
Burning	97
Edema	94
Itching	88
Erythema	69
Scarring	19
Vesicles	3
Anemia	27
Cholelithiasis	12
Abnormal liver function results	4

Data from Bloomer J, Wang Y, Singhal A, et al. Molecular studies of liver disease in erythropoietic protoporphyria. *J Clin Gastroenterol.* 2005;39(4 suppl 2):S167-S175.[124]

CLINICAL FEATURES

Disease manifestations in a series of 32 patients with EPP are summarized in Table 124-3. Acute cutaneous photosensitivity, which is seldom seen by physicians, is the most prominent symptom described as stinging, burning, or tingling pain that may develop within minutes of sunlight exposure, followed by erythema and edema (described as solar urticaria) (Fig. 124-7), and systemic manifestations that may last for several days. Petechiae or purpura may occur with prolonged exposure. Children are unable to describe these symptoms, but parents may observe crying, skin swelling, and erythema after exposure to sunlight. Hands and face are most often affected, and symptoms are worse during spring and summer. Patients are sensitive to sunlight, either direct or passing through window glass, and also to artificial light, including operating room lights.[125] Among 226 patients in North America, the mean age at symptom onset was 4.4 years, and higher protoporphyrin levels were associated with earlier age of onset, less sun tolerance, and more frequent reports of liver function abnormalities. On average, male patients with XLP had higher erythrocyte protoporphyrin levels than patients with EPP (3574 vs 1669 μg/dL; P <.001). Symptom severity and protoporphyrin levels varied markedly among female XLP patients owing to random X-chromosomal inactivation.[126]

Because patients are prompted by pain and learn to avoid sunlight, chronic skin changes are uncommon and usually subtle. These may include leathery hyperkeratotic skin on the dorsae of the hands and finger joints, mild scarring, labial grooving, and separation of the nail plate (onycholysis), developing with frequent sun exposure (Fig. 124-8). Bullae, skin fragility, hypertrichosis, hyperpigmentation, severe scarring, and mutilation, as seen in other cutaneous porphyrias, are rare. Pregnancy is reported to lower erythrocyte

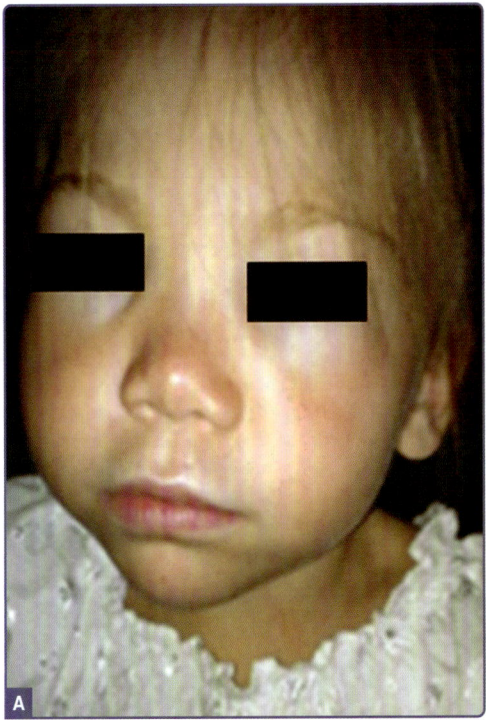
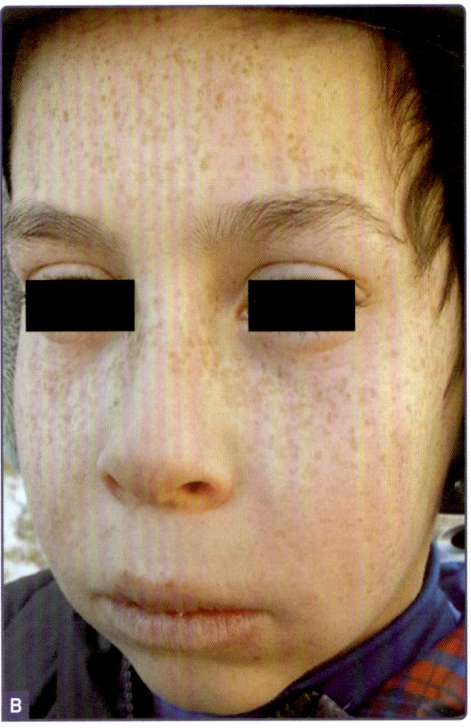

Figure 124-7 Acute swelling and erythema of the face in 2 children with EPP after exposure to sunlight. In the second child, only the lower face, which was not shielded by a ski mask, was affected.

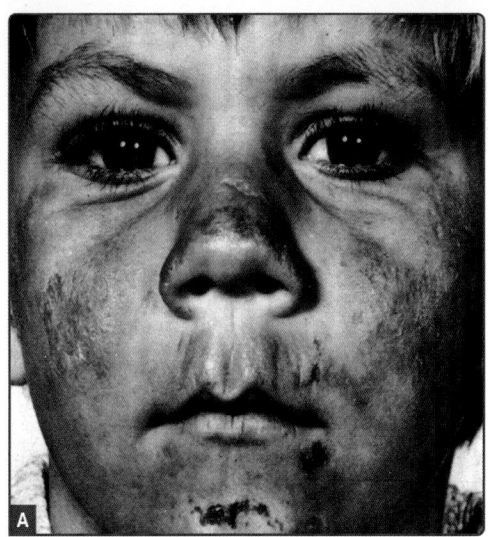

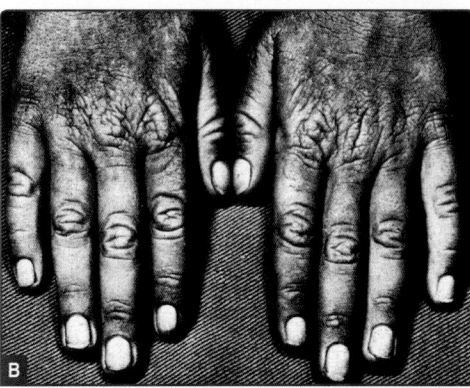

Figure 124-8 Chronic skin manifestations in a 6-year-old child with EPP resulting from repeated light reactions, including facial ulcerations and scarring, labial grooving, and thickened skin on the dorsal hands and loss of lanulae of the fingernails. (Reproduced from Schmidt H, Snitker G, Thomsen K, Lintrup J. Erythropoietic protoporphyria. A clinical study based on 29 cases in 14 families. *Arch Dermatol.* 1974;110(1):58-64; with permission. Copyright © 1974 American Medical Association. All rights reserved.[127])

protoporphyrin levels somewhat and increase tolerance to sunlight.[128]

Mild iron-deficiency anemia with microcytosis, decreased transferrin saturation, in the low part of the normal range of serum ferritin is seen in 20% to 50% of cases of EPP.[129,130] There is little evidence for impaired erythropoiesis or abnormal iron absorption or metabolism,[131-133] and hemolysis is absent or mild.

Neurovisceral manifestations are absent in uncomplicated EPP, but protoporphyric hepatopathy may be complicated by severe motor neuropathy similar to that seen in the acute porphyrias.[134] Autosomal recessive EPP associated with palmar keratoderma also has been associated with unexplained neurologic symptoms.[111]

Gallstones containing large amounts of protoporphyrin are common, and form from excretion of large amounts of water-insoluble protoporphyrin in bile. Such stones may be symptomatic and require cholecystectomy at an early age.[135] Liver function and liver protoporphyrin content are usually normal in EPP. Protoporphyric hepatopathy results from the cholestatic effects of protoporphyrin presented in excess amounts to the liver. Rarely, this is the major presenting feature of EPP.[136] Circulating protoporphyrin levels increase markedly as impairment of biliary excretion progresses. Operating room lights during liver transplantation or other prolonged surgery, especially in patients with hepatopathy, can cause marked photosensitivity with extensive burns of the skin and peritoneum, and can be avoided by use of special filters.[137,138]

DIAGNOSIS

Painful, nonblistering photosensitivity occurring at any age with few chronic skin changes should suggest a diagnosis of protoporphyria. Measurement of total erythrocyte protoporphyrin and, if elevated, measurement of the proportions of metal-free and zinc protoporphyrin will establish or exclude this diagnosis. Elevation of total erythrocyte protoporphyrin is not specific for EPP, because it is increased, with a predominance of erythrocyte zinc protoporphyrin, in many conditions such as homozygous porphyrias (other than most cases of CEP), iron deficiency, lead poisoning, anemia of chronic disease,[139] hemolytic conditions,[140] and many other erythrocyte disorders. But an increase in erythrocyte protoporphyrin comprised predominantly of metal-free protoporphyrin is a finding unique to protoporphyrias. FECH catalyzes the formation of both zinc protoporphyrin and heme (iron protoporphyrin), and when this enzyme is deficient, formation of both is impaired and the accumulating protoporphyrin remains mostly metal free. In XLP, FECH activity is normal but its capacity is exceeded by an excess amount of substrate, so the protoporphyrin that accumulates is usually mostly metal free.

Clinicians who wish to screen for EPP and XLP should be aware of major pitfalls in measuring erythrocyte protoporphyrin for this purpose and should use a laboratory that report results correctly as "total erythrocyte protoporphyrin" and "metal-free protoporphyrin." The now obsolete term "free erythrocyte protoporphyrin," abbreviated "FEP," was widely used to describe iron-free protoporphyrin before the 1970s. This was before it was discovered that this increase is due to zinc protoporphyrin in lead poisoning, iron deficiency, and the many other conditions, but to metal-free protoporphyrin in EPP. Some laboratories (Quest and LabCorp) measure erythrocyte protoporphyrin by hematofluorometry, which only measures zinc protoporphyrin and was developed for screening for lead poisoning and not protoporphyrias; their use of the misleading and obsolete terms "free protoporphyrin" and "FEP" falsely indicate that metal-free protoporphyrin was measured. ARUP measures the total amount correctly but if that is elevated does not fractionate metal-free and zinc protoporphyrin, which is essential to show that the increase is due to protoporphyrias. Testing for protoporphyrias is carried out correctly in the United States by the Porphyria Laboratory at the University of Texas Medical Branch and Mayo Medical Laboratories.[141]

Plasma porphyrins are increased in most but not all cases of EPP and are particularly susceptible to photodegradation during sample processing.[142] A plasma fluorescence peak of diluted plasma at neutral pH near 634 nm can help confirm a diagnosis of EPP.[53] Fecal porphyrin levels are normal or somewhat increased and consist mostly of protoporphyrin. Urine porphyrins are normal, except in patients with protoporphyric hepatopathy, which causes increases in urinary coproporphyrin, as is typical for hepatic dysfunction of any cause.

THERAPY

Photoprotection, especially avoidance of sunlight exposure, is the primary therapeutic intervention in EPP. This necessitates changes in lifestyle and the working environment and other avoidance behaviors that greatly impair quality of life. Protective clothing and hats are essential for most patients when outdoors. Topical sunblocks containing zinc oxide or titanium dioxide can provide some benefit. Sunscreens that absorb UV wavelengths are not beneficial. Orally administered beta-carotene, thought to quench activated oxygen radicals,[143] can increase sunlight tolerance.[144] A daily dose of 120 to 180 mg or higher is recommended to achieve serum beta-carotene levels of 600 to 800 µg/dL, which can be assessed 3 to 4 weeks after a dose change.[125] However, skin discoloration from carotenemia may be difficult cosmetically especially for children. Oral cysteine at doses of 500 mg twice daily may also quench excited oxygen species and increase tolerance to sunlight in EPP.[145] Afamelanotide, a synthetic analog of α-melanocyte–stimulating hormone mimics the naturally occurring hormone and increases melanin production in melanocytes, resulting in increased skin pigmentation and better sunlight tolerance in patients with EPP or XLP.[146,147] Afamelanotide is currently approved for restricted use in the European Union and Switzerland and is under review by the US Food and Drug Administration for use in patients with EPP and XLP. Cimetidine, which inhibits hepatic CYPs, was reported to decrease photosensitivity in 3 children with EPP.[148] This is not recommended because the proposed inhibition of ALAS2 and lowering of protoporphyrin levels have not been documented.[149]

Mild iron deficiency in protoporphyrias is unexplained and is thought by some to be beneficial (by limiting up-regulation of ALAS2 by iron), but is also potentially detrimental (by further limiting iron incorporation into protoporphyrin). Some patients have noted that iron supplementation increases photosensitivity, but increases in erythrocyte or plasma protoporphyrin levels have not been documented, to our knowledge. On the other hand, clinical and biochemical improvement have been noted in some individual cases of EPP and XLP with iron supplementation.[150,151] The effects of iron supplementation in patients with protoporphyrias and low serum ferritin levels is currently under study by the Porphyrias Consortium in the United States.

Exposure to alcohol, hepatotoxic drugs, or drugs and hormones that increase hepatic porphyrin and heme synthesis or impair hepatic excretory function should be avoided as a precaution.[152,153] Erythrocyte and plasma porphyrin levels, liver function tests, serum ferritin, and serum vitamin D levels should be monitored yearly. Daily intake of 800 international units of vitamin D and 1000 mg of calcium is recommended because EPP patients must avoid sunlight exposure.

Protoporphyric hepatopathy may resolve spontaneously or with treatment, especially if it was triggered by a reversible cause of liver dysfunction, such as viral infection or alcohol.[120,154] This life-threatening complication is usually treated with a combination of interventions including cholestyramine,[122,155,156] ursodeoxycholic acid,[157] vitamin E, red blood cell transfusions,[158] plasma exchange, and intravenous hemin with the aim to reduce plasma and erythrocyte protoporphyrin levels and the amount of protoporphyrin delivered to the liver. This may bridge patients to liver transplantation or even spontaneous improvement.[159] Liver transplantation is as successful as in other liver diseases, although a recurrence rate in the new liver of 69% at 5 years has been reported.[160,161] Acute motor neuropathy has developed in some patients with protoporphyric liver disease after transfusion[162] or liver transplantation,[134,163] and is sometimes reversible with administration of hemin and plasmapheresis prior to transplantation.[164] Bone marrow transplantation is effective in EPP,[165] and sequential bone marrow transplantation after liver transplantation can prevent recurrence of liver disease.[166]

ACUTE HEPATIC PORPHYRIAS

AT-A-GLANCE

- The acute porphyrias are characterized by intermittent acute neurologic symptoms, but can develop chronic blistering lesions in 3 of these conditions, VP, HCP, and AIP (in advanced renal disease).
- Neurovisceral manifestations include abdominal pain, vomiting, extremity pain, seizures, and muscle weakness due to motor neuropathy.
- Urine porphobilinogen is elevated especially during acute attacks. Fluorometric scanning of plasma porphyrin and patterns of fecal porphyrins are most useful for distinguishing the specific acute porphyria.
- Cutaneous manifestations are prevented by avoidance of sunlight.
- Acute neurovisceral attacks are prevented by avoiding exacerbating factors and best treated with hemin infusion

The 4 acute porphyrias, δ-aminolevulinate dehydratase deficiency porphyria (ADP), acute intermittent porphyria (AIP), hereditary coproporphyria (HCP), and variegate porphyria (VP) result from loss-of-function mutation of the second, third, sixth, and seventh enzymes in the heme biosynthetic pathway, respectively, and are characterized by neurologic symptoms occurring mostly as intermittent acute exacerbations. However, chronic blistering skin lesions resembling PCT can occur in 3 of these conditions. They are common in VP, uncommon in HCP, in AIP occur only with advanced renal disease, and are not described in ADP.[167]

ADP is extremely rare, with only 6 cases reported; unlike the other acute porphyrias, its inheritance is autosomal recessive.[168] (It will not be discussed further in this chapter.) The enzyme deficiencies in the other acute porphyrias are inherited as autosomal dominant traits with low penetrance (see Table 124-1). AIP is the most common acute hepatic porphyria worldwide. The prevalence of AIP has been estimated to be 1 to 2 per 100,000 in Europe,[169] that of HCP was estimated to be 0.2 per 100,000 in Denmark,[170] and that of VP in Finland reported at 1.3 per 100,000.[171] VP is especially common in South Africa among whites of Dutch descent due a founder effect, with an estimated prevalence of 300 per 100,000[172], and almost all cases share the same *PPOX* mutation (R59W).

ETIOLOGY AND PATHOGENESIS

At least 400 *PBGD/HMBS* mutations have been identified in AIP, 64 *CPOX* mutations in HCP[173] and 174 *PPOX* mutations in VP[86] (Table 124-1). Mutation types include missense, nonsense, splicing, deletion, and insertion mutations. PBGD catalyzes the assembly of HMBS, a linear tetrapyrrole, from 4 molecules of PBG. CPOX catalyzes the 2-step oxidative decarboxylation at a single active site of coproporphyrinogen III to yield protoporphyrinogen IX, with intermediate formation of harderoporphyrinogen, a tricarboxyl porphyrinogen. PPOX catalyzes the dehydrogenation of protoporphyrinogen IX to form protoporphyrin IX. Neurovisceral symptoms in the acute hepatic porphyrias are associated with accumulation of the porphyrin precursors delta-aminolevulinic acid (ALA) and porphobilinogen (PBG). Symptoms may result from neurotoxic effects of ALA and/or from heme deficiency in neuronal or vascular tissue.[174] Porphyrins accumulate in all of these disorders and most commonly in sufficient amounts to cause chronic blistering skin manifestations in VP.

CLINICAL FEATURES

Typical neurovisceral manifestations of the acute porphyrias include abdominal pain, vomiting, extremity pain, seizures, and muscle weakness due to motor neuropathy. Several factors are recognized to contribute to attacks in AIP, HCP, and VP, including drugs, hormones, and dietary factors. Risk of chronic hypertension, renal disease, and hepatocellular carcinoma are increased. Very rare cases of homozygous AIP, HCP, and VP have presented with severe photosensitivity and neurologic impairment early in life but without acute attacks.[174] A variant form of homozygous HCP termed harderoporphyria is due to *CPOX* mutations that prematurely release harderoporphyrinogen from the enzyme before the second decarboxylation occurs.[175]

PRECIPITATING FACTORS

Known endogenous and exogenous factors can precipitate acute attacks in heterozygotes and are additive in individual patients. Many known factors cause induction of hepatic ALAS1, and this leads to accumulation of pathway intermediates. Some individuals remain susceptible to repeated attacks despite avoidance of known precipitants. Additional unknown factors, including undiscovered modifying genes, are likely to contribute.

DRUGS AND OTHER EXOGENOUS CHEMICALS

Most drugs that are harmful in acute porphyrias are known to induce hepatic CYPs and ALAS1. Induction of CYPs (the most abundant hemoproteins in liver) increases demand for newly synthesized heme.[176] Examples of drugs known to be harmful and safe are shown in Table 124-4. Updated drug safety databases are found at the websites of the American Porphyria Foundation (www.porphyriafoundation.com) and the European Porphyria Network (www.porphyria-europe.com). Smoking is known to increase hepatic CYPs in humans, probably from effects of inhaled polycyclic aromatic hydrocarbons, and is associated with more frequent symptoms.[177] Ethanol and other alcohols also induce ALAS1 and some CYPs, and have been implicated in causing attacks.[178,179]

ENDOCRINE FACTORS

Symptoms often develop after puberty and occur more commonly in women, suggesting that endogenous female hormones contribute to the onset of symptoms. Progesterone, synthetic progestins, and certain metabolites of testosterone are potent inducers of ALAS1 and CYPs and have been associated with acute attacks of porphyria. Increases in progesterone in the luteal phase of the menstrual cycle are most likely responsible for cyclic attacks in AIP, HCP, and VP. Estrogens have been considered harmful, but do not have the inducing effects of progestins on ALAS1 and CYPs, and reports of attacks when they are administered without a progestin are few. But as discussed

TABLE 124-4
A Partial List of Drugs Known to Be Unsafe or Safe in the Acute Porphyrias

UNSAFE		SAFE
Alcohol	Meprobamate[a] (also mebutamate,[a] tybutamate[a])	Acetaminophen
Barbiturates[a]		Aspirin
Carbamazepine[a]		Atropine
Carisoprodol[a]	Methyprylon	Bromides
Clonazepam (high doses)	Metoclopramide[a]	Cimetidine
	Phenytoin[a]	Erythropoietin[a,b]
Danazol[a]	Primidone[a]	Gabapentin
Diclofenac[a] and possibly other NSAIDs	Progesterone and synthetic progestins[a]	Glucocorticoids
		Insulin
	Pyrazinamide[a]	Levetiracetam
Ergots	Pyrazolones (aminopyrine, antipyrine)	Narcotic analgesics
Estrogens[a,c]		
Ethchlorvynol[a]	Rifampin[a]	Penicillin and derivatives
Glutethimide[a]	Succinimides (ethosuximide, methsuximide)	
Griseofulvin[a]		Phenothiazines
Mephenytoin	Sulfonamide antibiotics[a]	Ranitidine[a,b]
	Valproic acid[a]	Streptomycin
		Vigabatrin

[a]Porphyria is listed as a contraindication, warning, precaution, or adverse effect in US labeling for these drugs.

[b]Although porphyria is listed as a precaution in US labeling; these drugs are regarded as safe by other sources.

[c]Estrogens–unsafe for porphyria cutanea tarda but can be used with caution in the acute porphyrias.

Note: More complete and frequently updates sources, such as the websites of the American Porphyria Foundation (www.porphyriafoundation.com/) and the European Porphyria Initiative (www.porphyria-europe.com/), should be consulted before using drugs not listed here.

Modified from Anderson KE, Bloomer JR, Bonkovsky HL, et al. Recommendations for the diagnosis and treatment of the acute porphyrias. *Ann Intern Med.* 2005;142(6):439-450; with permission.[167]

earlier, estrogen use is a common susceptibility factor in women with PCT. Diabetes mellitus may decrease the frequency of attacks and lower porphyrin precursor levels, likely because of high glucose levels.[180]

PREGNANCY

Most women with AIP report that pregnancy is well tolerated.[181] However, attacks sometimes become more frequent during pregnancy, which may be due to harmful drugs (eg, metoclopramide)[182,183] or reduced caloric intake with hyperemesis gravidarum. Attacks during pregnancy should be treated with hemin, unless they are mild. Termination of pregnancy is rarely indicated for an acute attack of porphyria.

NUTRITION

Reduced intake of calories and carbohydrate to lose weight or during an illness or surgery can precipitate attacks. In these circumstances, peroxisomal proliferator-activated cofactor 1α (PGC-1α) is up-regulated in the liver, which induces ALAS1 and increases ALA and PBG. These effects can be prevented or reversed by administration of carbohydrate.[184,185] Starvation may also induce hepatic heme oxygenase,[186] which may deplete hepatic heme and contribute to ALAS1 induction.

DIAGNOSIS

Urinary PBG is elevated during acute attacks of AIP, HCP and VP, but often less so, and more transiently, in HCP and VP than in AIP; further testing readily differentiates these 3 conditions. Skin lesions resembling PCT are rare in AIP and occur only in the presence of advanced renal disease with increases in plasma levels of both PBG and porphyrins. In HCP and VP, urine porphyrins (especially uroporphyrin and coproporphyrin) are also elevated, but this finding by itself is nonspecific and does not readily differentiate these porphyrias from each other. Fecal porphyrin levels are markedly increased in both HCP and VP and are predominantly coproporphyrin III in HCP, and both coproporphyrin III and protoporphyrin in VP. The fecal coproporphyrin III/I ratio is sensitive for diagnosis of HCP, even in asymptomatic stages of the disease.[187]

Plasma porphyrin concentration is commonly elevated in VP and seldom increased in AIP and HCP, unless there are cutaneous manifestations. A specific feature of VP is a plasma porphyrin fluorescence maximum at neutral pH of ~626 nm, which represents protoporphyrin bound covalently to plasma proteins.[188] This fluorometric scanning method is more effective than examination of fecal porphyrins for detecting asymptomatic VP,[189] and is especially useful for rapidly differentiating VP from PCT, which displays a fluorescence peak at ~620 nm. Erythrocyte PBGD activity is decreased in most AIP patients and normal in HCP and VP. Assays for CPOX and PPOX require cells containing mitochondria and are not widely available. DNA studies are most reliable for identifying asymptomatic carriers, once the familial mutation is identified.

Homozygous cases of AIP, HCP, and VP demonstrate more severe increases in porphyrin precursors and porphyrins, including erythrocyte zinc protoporphyrin. Harderoporphyria is identified by elevations in both coproporphyrin III and harderoporphyrin III in feces and erythrocytes.[190]

THERAPY

Cutaneous manifestations of VP and HCP, though identical to the blistering skin lesions seen in PCT, do not respond to phlebotomies or low-dose hydroxychloroquine. Therefore, avoidance of sunlight and use of protective clothing is most important. Long-term avoidance of precipitating factors may lower chronically elevated porphyrin levels, but to our knowledge this has not been documented. Patients with AIP, renal failure, and associated cutaneous manifestations should be considered for renal or combined hepatic and renal transplantation.[191]

For acute attacks, hospitalization is usually advisable for treatment of severe symptoms, intravenous therapies and monitoring of respiration, electrolytes, and nutritional status. Milder recurring attacks that respond rapidly to treatment are sometimes managed as outpatients. Precipitating factors, such as harmful drugs are removed. Pain, nausea, and vomiting usually require narcotic analgesics, chlorpromazine or another phenothiazine, or ondansetron. Short-acting benzodiazepines are given for anxiety and insomnia.[167] β-Adrenergic-blocking agents can be used to control tachycardia and hypertension, unless contraindicated by hypovolemia or heart failure.[192] Treatment for seizures should focus on correcting hyponatremia, if present. Most anticonvulsant drugs are potentially harmful in acute porphyrias. Clonazepam may be less harmful than phenytoin, barbiturates, or valproic acid.[193,194]

The identification and long-term avoidance of factors precipitating acute neurovisceral attacks is essential. Yearly screening for hepatocellular carcinoma is recommended after 50 years of age, especially in those with persistent increases in porphyrin precursors or porphyrins.

Hemin is the most effective treatment for acute attacks, and is available in the United States as lyophilized hematin (Panhematin, Recordati Rare Diseases), and as heme arginate (Normosang, Orphan Europe) in Europe and South Africa.[195,196] Intravenously infused hemin is taken up primarily by hepatocytes where it reconstitutes the regulatory heme pool and represses the synthesis of ALAS1, leading to dramatic reduction in ALA, PBG, and porphyrins, and more rapid resolution of symptoms.[197]

Hemin therapy should be initiated for moderate to severe attacks, and for mild attacks unresponsive to carbohydrate loading.[167,195,198] Infusion of 3 to 4 mg/kg daily for 4 days is standard therapy and may be extended if a response is incomplete within this time. Hemin has been administered safely during pregnancy.[167,195,196] Reconstitution of hematin with 25% human albumin is recommended, as degradation products that form when using sterile water may cause infusion site phlebitis and limit future venous access.[167,199] A transient coagulopathy with thrombocytopenia and prolongation of prothrombin and partial thromboplastin times is also prevented with use of albumin.[200,201] Side effects of hemin may include fever, aching, malaise, and rarely hemolysis, anaphylaxis, and circulatory collapse.[202,203] Hemin administered once or twice weekly is an option for preventing frequent, noncyclic attacks.[204,205]

CARBOHYDRATE LOADING

Administration of carbohydrates downregulates PGC-1α and the induction of hepatic ALAS1, thereby decreasing production of porphyrin precursors. However, this is less effective than hemin and should be used only for mild attacks (without severe pain requiring opioids, paresis, seizures or hyponatremia),[167] or until hemin becomes available. Intravenous treatment with 300 to 500 g of IV glucose is usually administered as a 10% solution, with careful monitoring to avoid hyponatremia due to administration of large volumes of free water.[167] Oral glucose polymer solutions may be given if tolerated.

REFERENCES

1. Moore M, McColl K. *Disorders of Porphyrin Metabolism*. New York, NY: Plenum; 1987.
2. Schultz J. *Ein fall von pemphigus, kompliziert durch lepra visceralis*. Greifswald: Greifswald University; 1874.
3. Anderson TM. Hydroa aestivale in two brothers, complicated with the presence of haematoporphyrin in the urine. *Br J Dermatol.* 1898;10:1.
4. Stokvis BJ. Over Twee Zeldsame Kleuerstoffen in Urine van Zicken. *Ned Tijdschr Geneeskd.* 1889;13:409.
5. Garrod AE. *Inborn Errors of Metabolism*. London: Hodder & Stoughton; 1923.
6. Schmid R, Schwartz S, Watson CJ. Porphyrin content of bone marrow and liver in the various forms of porphyria. *Arch Intern Med.* 1954;93:167-190.
7. Ippen H. Treatment of porphyria cutanea tarda by phlebotomy. *Semin Hematol.* 1977;14:253-259.
8. Strand LJ, Felsher BF, Redeker AG, et al. Heme biosynthesis in intermittent acute porphyria: decreased hepatic conversion of porphobilinogen to porphyrins and increased delta-aminolevulinic acid synthetase activity. *Proc Natl Acad Sci U S A.* 1970;67:1315-1320.
9. Bonkowsky HL, Tschudy DP, Collins A, et al. Repression of the overproduction of porphyrin precursors in acute intermittent porphyria by intravenous infusions of hematin. *Proc Natl Acad Sci U S A.* 1971;68(11):2725-2729.
10. Gou EW, Phillips JD, Anderson KE. The porphyrias. In: Gilbert-Barness E, Barness L, Farrell P, eds. *Metabolic Diseases*. Amsterdam: IOS Press BV; 2017:543-575.
11. Granick S, Sassa S. δ-Aminolevulinic acid synthase and the control of heme and chlorophyll synthesis. In: Vogel HJ, ed. *Metabolic Regulation*. New York, NY: Academic Press; 1971:77.
12. Chung J, Wittig JG, Ghamari A, et al. Erythropoietin signaling regulates heme biosynthesis. *Elife.* 2017;6.
13. Bissell DM, Anderson KE, Bonkovsky HL. Porphyria. *N Engl J Med.* 2017;377(9):862-872.
14. Elder GH. Porphyria cutanea tarda and related disorders (Chap. 88). In: Kadish KM, Smith K, Guilard R, eds. *Porphyrin Handbook, Part II*. Vol 14. San Diego, CA: Academic Press; 2003:67-92.
15. Thawani R, Moghe A, Idhate T, et al. Porphyria cutanea tarda in a child with acute lymphoblastic leukemia. *Q J Med.* 2016;109(3):191-192.
16. Boffa MJ, Reed P, Weinkove C, et al. Hypertrichosis as the presenting feature of porphyria cutanea tarda. *Clin Exp Dermatol.* 1995;20(1):62-64.
17. Anderson KE, Goeger DE, Carson RW, et al. Erythropoietin for the treatment of porphyria cutanea tarda in a patient on long-term hemodialysis. *N Engl J Med.* 1990;322:315-317.
18. Cassiman D, Vannoote J, Roelandts R, et al. Porphyria cutanea tarda and liver disease. A retrospective analysis of 17 cases from a single centre and review of the literature. *Acta Gastroenterol Belg.* 2008;71(2):237-242.

19. Gisbert JP, Garcia-Buey L, Alonso A, et al. Hepatocellular carcinoma risk in patients with porphyria cutanea tarda. *Eur J Gastroenterol Hepatol.* 2004;16(7):689-692.
20. Rossmann-Ringdahl I, Olsson R. Porphyria cutanea tarda in a Swedish population: risk factors and complications. *Acta Derm Venereol.* 2005;85(4):337-341.
21. Egger NG, Goeger DE, Payne DA, et al. Porphyria cutanea tarda: multiplicity of risk factors including HFE mutations, hepatitis C, and inherited uroporphyrinogen decarboxylase deficiency. *Dig Dis Sci.* 2002;47(2):419-426.
22. Jalil S, Grady JJ, Lee C, et al. Associations among behavior-related susceptibility factors in porphyria cutanea tarda. *Clin Gastroenterol Hepatol.* 2010; 8(3):297-302, 302.e1.
23. Brady JJ, Jackson HA, Roberts AG, et al. Co-inheritance of mutations in the uroporphyrinogen decarboxylase and hemochromatosis genes accelerates the onset of porphyria cutanea tarda. *J Invest Dermatol.* 2000;115(5):868-874.
24. Roberts AG, Whatley SD, Nicklin S, et al. The frequency of hemochromatosis-associated alleles is increased in British patients with sporadic porphyria cutanea tarda. *Hepatology.* 1997;25(1):159-161.
25. Dereure O, Aguilar-Martinez P, Bessis D, et al. HFE mutations and transferrin receptor polymorphism analysis in porphyria cutanea tarda: a prospective study of 36 cases from southern France. *Br J Dermatol.* 2001;144(3):533-539.
26. Ajioka RS, Phillips JD, Weiss RB, et al. Down-regulation of hepcidin in porphyria cutanea tarda. *Blood.* 2008; 112(12):4723-4728.
27. Sinclair PR, Gorman N, Walton HS, et al. CYP1A2 is essential in murine uroporphyria caused by hexachlorobenzene and iron. *Toxicol Appl Pharmacol.* 2000; 162(1):60-67.
28. Smith AG, Clothier B, Carthew P, et al. Protection of the Cyp1A2(–/–) null mouse against uroporphyria and hepatic injury following exposure to 2,3,7,8-tetrachlorodibenzo-p-dioxin. *Toxicol Appl Pharmacol.* 2001;173(2):89-98.
29. Blekkenhorst GH, Eales L, Pimstone NR. Activation of uroporphyrinogen decarboxylase by ferrous iron in porphyria cutanea tarda. *S Afr Med J.* 1979;56(22):918-920.
30. Christiansen L, Bygum A, Jensen A, et al. Association between CYP1A2 polymorphism and susceptibility to porphyria cutanea tarda. *Hum Genet.* 2000; 107(6):612-614.
31. Wickliffe JK, Abdel-Rahman SZ, Lee C, et al. CYP1A2*1F and GSTM1 alleles are associated with susceptibility to porphyria cutanea tarda. *Mol Med.* 2011;17(3-4):241-247.
32. Grossman ME, Bickers DR, Poh-Fitzpatrick MB, et al. Porphyria cutanea tarda. Clinical features and laboratory findings in 40 patients. *Am J Med.* 1979;67(2):277-286.
33. Sixel-Dietrich F, Doss M. Hereditary uroporphyrinogen-decarboxylase deficiency predisposing porphyria cutanea tarda (chronic hepatic porphyria) in females after oral contraceptive medication. *Arch Dermatol Res.* 1985;278(1):13-16.
34. Legault N, Sabik H, Cooper SF, et al. Effect of estradiol on the induction of porphyria by hexachlorobenzene in the rat. *Biochem Pharmacol.* 1997;54(1):19-25.
35. Liehr JG. Vitamin C reduces the incidence and severity of renal tumors induced by estradiol or diethylstilbestrol. *Am J Clin Nutr.* 1991;54(6)(suppl):S1256-S1260.
36. Fujita N, Sugimoto R, Motonishi S, et al. Patients with chronic hepatitis C achieving a sustained virological response to peginterferon and ribavirin therapy recover from impaired hepcidin secretion. *J Hepatol.* 2008;49(5):702-710.
37. Nishina S, Hino K, Korenaga M, et al. Hepatitis C virus-induced reactive oxygen species raise hepatic iron level in mice by reducing hepcidin transcription. *Gastroenterology.* 2008;134(1):226-238.
38. Younossi Z, Park H, Henry L, et al. Extrahepatic manifestations of hepatitis C: a meta-analysis of prevalence, quality of life, and economic burden. *Gastroenterology.* 2016;150(7):1599-1608.
39. Wissel PS, Sordillo P, Anderson KE, et al. Porphyria cutanea tarda associated with the acquired immune deficiency syndrome. *Am J Hematol.* 1987;25(1):107-113.
40. Percy VA, Naidoo D, Joubert SM, et al. Ascorbate status of patients with porphyria cutanea tarda symptomatica and its effect on porphyrin metabolism. *S Afr J Med Sci.* 1975;40(4):185-196.
41. Rocchi E, Casalgrandi G, Masini A, et al. Circulating pro- and antioxidant factors in iron and porphyrin metabolism disorders. *Ital J Gastroenterol Hepatol.* 1999;31(9):861-867.
42. Sinclair PR, Gorman G, Shedlofsky SI, et al. Ascorbic acid deficiency in porphyria cutanea tarda. *J Lab Clin Med.* 1997;130:197-201.
43. Gorman N, Zaharia A, Trask HS, et al. Effect of iron and ascorbate on uroporphyria in ascorbate-requiring mice as a model for porphyria cutanea tarda. *Hepatology.* 2007;45(1):187-194.
44. Schmid R. Cutaneous porphyria in Turkey. *N Engl J Med.* 1960;263:397-398.
45. Calvert GM, Sweeney MH, Fingerhut MA, et al. Evaluation of porphyria cutanea tarda in U.S. workers exposed to 2,3,7,8-tetrachlorodibenzo-p-dioxin. *Am J Ind Med.* 1994;25(4):559-571.
46. Elder GH, Urquhart AJ, de Salamanca RE, et al. Immunoreactive uroporphyrinogen decarboxylase in the liver in porphyria cutanea tarda. *Lancet.* 1985;2(8449):229-233.
47. Moran MJ, Fontanellas A, Brudieux E, et al. Hepatic uroporphyrinogen decarboxylase activity in porphyria cutanea tarda patients: the influence of virus C infection. *Hepatology.* 1998;27(2):584-589.
48. Anderson KE. Porphyria cutanea tarda: a possible role for ascorbic acid. *Hepatology.* 2007;45(1):6-8.
49. Phillips JD, Bergonia HA, Reilly CA, et al. A porphomethene inhibitor of uroporphyrinogen decarboxylase causes porphyria cutanea tarda. *Proc Natl Acad Sci U S A.* 2007;104(12):5079-5084.
50. Sarkany RP. Making sense of the porphyrias. *Photodermatol Photoimmunol Photomed.* 2008;24(2):102-108.
51. Pigatto PD, Polenghi MM, Altomare GF, et al. Complement cleavage products in the phototoxic reaction of porphyria cutanea tarda. *Br J Dermatol.* 1986;114(5):567-573.
52. Poh-Fitzpatrick MB. A plasma porphyrin fluorescence marker for variegate porphyria. *Arch Dermatol.* 1980;116(5):543-547.
53. Poh-Fitzpatrick MB, Lamola AA. Direct spectrophotometry of diluted erythrocytes and plasma: a rapid diagnostic method in primary and secondary porphyrinemias. *J Lab Clin Med.* 1976;87:362-370.
54. Elder GH. The metabolism of porphyrins of the isocoproporphyrin series. *Enzyme.* 1974;17(1):61-68.
55. Poh-Fitzpatrick MB, Sosin AE, Bemis J. Porphyrin levels in plasma and erythrocytes of chronic hemodialysis patients. *J Am Acad Dermatol.* 1982;7(1):100-104.
56. Sardh E, Andersson DE, Henrichson A, et al. Porphyrin precursors and porphyrins in three patients with

acute intermittent porphyria and end-stage renal disease under different therapy regimes. *Cell Mol Biol (Noisy-le-grand)*. 2009;55(1):66-71.
57. Dabski C, Beutner EH. Studies of laminin and type IV collagen in blisters of porphyria cutanea tarda and drug-induced pseudoporphyria. *J Am Acad Dermatol*. 1991;25(1, pt 1):28-32.
58. Bajaj D, Pachyala A, Singal A. Porphyria cutanea tarda is a biochemical and not histological diagnosis. *Gastroenterol Hepatol Open Access*. 2016;5(8).
59. Bulaj ZJ, Franklin MR, Phillips JD, et al. Transdermal estrogen replacement therapy in postmenopausal women previously treated for porphyria cutanea tarda. *J Lab Clin Med*. 2000;136(6):482-488.
60. Topi GC, Amantea A, Griso D. Recovery from porphyria cutanea tarda with no specific therapy other than avoidance of hepatic toxins. *Br J Dermatol*. 1984;111(1):75-82.
61. Ratnaike S, Blake D, Campbell D, et al. Plasma ferritin levels as a guide to the treatment of porphyria cutanea tarda by venesection. *Australas J Dermatol*. 1988;29(1):3-7.
62. Rocchi E, Gibertini P, Cassanelli M, et al. Serum ferritin in the assessment of liver iron overload and iron removal therapy in porphyria cutanea tarda. *J Lab Clin Med*. 1986;107:36-42.
63. Bacon BR, Adams PC, Kowdley KV, et al. Diagnosis and management of hemochromatosis: 2011 practice guideline by the American Association for the Study of Liver Diseases. *Hepatology*. 2011;54(1):328-343.
64. Ashton RE, Hawk JLM, Magnus IA. Low-dose oral chloroquine in the treatment of porphyria cutanea tarda. *Br J Dermatol*. 1984;3:609-613.
65. Bruce AJ, Ahmed I. Childhood-onset porphyria cutanea tarda: successful therapy with low-dose hydroxychloroquine (Plaquenil). *J Am Acad Dermatol*. 1998;38(5, pt 2):810-814.
66. Freesemann A, Frank M, Sieg I, et al. Treatment of porphyria cutanea tarda by the effect of chloroquine on the liver. *Skin Pharmacol*. 1995;8(3):156-161.
67. Kordac V, Semradova M. Treatment of porphyria cutanea tarda with chloroquine. *Br J Dermatol*. 1974;90:95-100.
68. Taljaard JJF, Shanley BC, Stewart-Wynne EG, et al. Studies on low dose chloroquine therapy and the action of chloroquine in symptomatic porphyria. *Br J Dermatol*. 1972;87(3):261-269.
69. Timonen K, Niemi KM, Mustajoki P. Skin morphology in porphyria cutanea tarda does not improve despite clinical remission. *Clin Exp Dermatol*. 1991;16(5):355-358.
70. Singal AK, Kormos-Hallberg C, Lee C, et al. Low-dose hydroxychloroquine is as effective as phlebotomy in treatment of patients with porphyria cutanea tarda. *Clin Gastroenterol Hepatol*. 2012;10(12):1402-1409.
71. Sweeney GD, Jones KG. Porphyria cutanea tarda: clinical and laboratory features. *Can Med Assoc J*. 1979;120(7):803-807.
72. Thornsvard MAJCT, Guider BA, Kimball DB. An unusual reaction to chloroquine-primaquine. *JAMA*. 1976;235(16):1719-1720.
73. Malkinson FD, Levitt L. Hydroxychloroquine treatment of porphyria cutanea tarda. *Arch Dermatol*. 1980;116(10):1147-1150.
74. Marmor MF, Kellner U, Lai TY, et al. Revised recommendations on screening for chloroquine and hydroxychloroquine retinopathy. *Ophthalmology*. 2011;118(2):415-422.
75. Rocchi E, Cassanelli M, Ventura E. High weekly intravenous doses of desferrioxamine in porphyria cutanea tarda. *Br J Dermatol*. 1987;117(3):393-396.
76. Singal AK, Venkata KVR, Jampana S, et al. Hepatitis C treatment in patients with porphyria cutanea tarda. *Am J Med Sci*. 2017;353(6):523-528.
77. Shieh S, Cohen JL, Lim HW. Management of porphyria cutanea tarda in the setting of chronic renal failure: a case report and review. *J Am Acad Dermatol*. 2000;42(4):645-652.
78. Yaqoob M, Smyth J, Ahmad R, et al. Haemodialysis-related porphyria cutanea tarda and treatment by recombinant human erythropoietin. *Nephron*. 1992;60(4):428-431.
79. Carson RW, Dunnigan EJ, DuBose TDJ, et al. Removal of plasma porphyrins with high-flux hemodialysis in porphyria cutanea tarda associated with end-stage renal disease. *J Am Soc Nephrol*. 1992;2(9):1445-1450.
80. Stevens BR, Fleischer AB, Piering F, et al. Porphyria cutanea tarda in the setting of renal failure: response to renal transplantation. *Arch Dermatol*. 1993;129(3):337-339.
81. Armstrong DK, Sharpe PC, Chambers CR, et al. Hepatoerythropoietic porphyria: a missense mutation in the UROD gene is associated with mild disease and an unusual porphyrin excretion pattern. *Br J Dermatol*. 2004;151(4):920-923.
82. Phillips JD, Parker TL, Schubert HL, et al. Functional consequences of naturally occurring mutations in human uroporphyrinogen decarboxylase. *Blood*. 2001;98(12):3179-3185.
83. Bundino S, Topi GC, Zina AM, et al. Hepatoerythropoietic porphyria. *Pediatr Dermatol*. 1987;4(3):229-233.
84. Pimstone NR, Gandhi SN, Mukerji SK. Therapeutic efficacy of oral charcoal in congenital erythropoietic porphyria. *N Engl J Med*. 1987;316(7):390-393.
85. Fontanellas A, Mazurier F, Moreau-Gaudry F, et al. Correction of uroporphyrinogen decarboxylase deficiency (hepatoerythropoietic porphyria) in Epstein-Barr virus-transformed B-cell lines by retrovirus-mediated gene transfer: fluorescence-based selection of transduced cells. *Blood*. 1999;94(2):465-474.
86. Balwani M, Desnick RJ. The porphyrias: advances in diagnosis and treatment. *Blood*. 2012;120(23):4496-504. [Erratum In: *Blood*. 2013;122(17):3090.]
87. Phillips JD, Steensma DP, Pulsipher MA, et al. Congenital erythropoietic porphyria due to a mutation in GATA1: the first trans-acting mutation causative for a human porphyria. *Blood*. 2007;109(6):2618-2621.
88. Watson CJ, Perman V, Spurrell FA, et al. Some studies of the comparative biology of human and bovine porphyria erythropoietica. *Trans Assoc Am Physicians*. 1958;71:196-209.
89. Günther H. In: Schittenhelm A, ed. *Handbuch der Krankheiten der Blutes und der Blutbildenden Organe*. Vol 2. Berlin: Springer; 1925.
90. Sassa S, Akagi R, Nishitani C, et al. Late-onset porphyrias: what are they? *Cell Mol Biol (Noisy-le-grand)*. 2002;48(1):97-101.
91. Verstraeten L, Van Regemorter N, Pardou A, et al. Biochemical diagnosis of a fatal case of Gunther's disease in a newborn with hydrops foetalis. *Eur J Clin Chem Clin Biochem*. 1993;31(3):121-124.
92. Desnick RJ, Astrin KH. Congenital erythropoietic porphyria: advances in pathogenesis and treatment. *Br J Haematol*. 2002;117(4):779-795.

93. Hallai N, Anstey A, Mendelsohn S, et al. Pregnancy in a patient with congenital erythropoietic porphyria. *N Engl J Med.* 2007;357(6):622-623.
94. Seip M, Thune PO, Eriksen L. Treatment of photosensitivity in congenital erythropoietic porphyria (CEP) with beta-carotene. *Acta Derm Venereol.* 1974;54(3):239-240.
95. Haining RG, Cowger ML, Labbe RF, et al. Congenital erythropoietic porphyria. II. The effects of induced polycythemia. *Blood.* 1970;36(3):297-309.
96. Piomelli S, Poh-Fitzpatrick MB, Seaman C, et al. Complete suppression of the symptoms of congenital erythropoietic porphyria by long-term treatment with high-level transfusions. *N Engl J Med.* 1986;314(16):1029-1031.
97. Guarini L, Piomelli S, Poh-Fitzpatrick MB. Hydroxyurea in congenital erythropoietic porphyria [letter]. *N Engl J Med.* 1994;330(15):1091-1092.
98. Fritsch C, Bolsen K, Ruzicka T, et al. Congenital erythropoietic porphyria. *J Am Acad Dermatol.* 1997;36(4):594-610.
99. Katugampola RP, Anstey AV, Finlay AY, et al. A management algorithm for congenital erythropoietic porphyria derived from a study of 29 cases. *Br J Dermatol.* 2012;167(4):888-900.
100. Dupuis-Girod S, Akkari V, Ged C, et al. Successful match-unrelated donor bone marrow transplantation for congenital erythropoietic porphyria (Gunther disease). *Eur J Pediatr.* 2005;164(2):104-107.
101. Geronimi F, Richard E, Lamrissi-Garcia I, et al. Lentivirus-mediated gene transfer of uroporphyrinogen III synthase fully corrects the porphyric phenotype in human cells. *J Mol Med (Berl).* 2003;81(5):310-320.
102. Kauppinen R, Glass IA, Aizencang G, et al. Congenital erythropoietic porphyria: prolonged high-level expression and correction of the heme biosynthetic defect by retroviral-mediated gene transfer into porphyric and erythroid cells. *Mol Genet Metab.* 1998;65(1):10-17.
103. Marko PB, Miljkovic J, Gorenjak M, et al. Erythropoietic protoporphyria patients in Slovenia. *Acta Dermatovenerol Alp Pannonica Adriat.* 2007;16(3):99-102, 104.
104. Parker M, Corrigall AV, Hift RJ, et al. Molecular characterization of erythropoietic protoporphyria in South Africa. *Br J Dermatol.* 2008;159(1):182-191.
105. Holme SA, Anstey AV, Finlay AY, et al. Erythropoietic protoporphyria in the U.K.: clinical features and effect on quality of life. *Br J Dermatol.* 2006;155(3):574-581.
106. Whatley SD, Ducamp S, Gouya L, et al. C-terminal deletions in the *ALAS2* gene lead to gain of function and cause X-linked dominant protoporphyria without anemia or iron overload. *Am J Hum Genet.* 2008;83(3):408-414.
107. Yien YY, Ducamp S, van der Vorm LN, et al. Mutation in human *CLPX* elevates levels of δ-aminolevulinate synthase and protoporphyrin IX to promote erythropoietic protoporphyria. *Proc Natl Acad Sci U S A.* 2017;114(38):E8045-E8052.
108. Gouya L, Deybach JC, Lamoril J, et al. Modulation of the phenotype in dominant erythropoietic protoporphyria by a low expression of the normal ferrochelatase allele. *Am J Hum Genet.* 1996;58(2):292-299.
109. Gouya L, Puy H, Lamoril J, et al. Inheritance in erythropoietic protoporphyria: a common wild-type ferrochelatase allelic variant with low expression accounts for clinical manifestation. *Blood.* 1999;93(6):2105-2110.
110. Gouya L, Puy H, Robreau AM, et al. The penetrance of dominant erythropoietic protoporphyria is modulated by expression of wildtype FECH. *Nat Genet.* 2002;30(1):27-28.
111. Holme SA, Whatley SD, Roberts AG, et al. Seasonal palmar keratoderma in erythropoietic protoporphyria indicates autosomal recessive inheritance. *J Invest Dermatol.* 2009;129(3):599-605.
112. Aplin C, Whatley SD, Thompson P, et al. Late-onset erythropoietic porphyria caused by a chromosome 18q deletion in erythroid cells. *J Invest Dermatol.* 2001;117(6):1647-1649.
113. Shirota T, Yamamoto H, Hayashi S, et al. Myelodysplastic syndrome terminating in erythropoietic protoporphyria after 15 years of aplastic anemia. *Int J Hematol.* 2000;72(1):44-47.
114. Goodwin RG, Kell WJ, Laidler P, et al. Photosensitivity and acute liver injury in myeloproliferative disorder secondary to late-onset protoporphyria caused by deletion of a ferrochelatase gene in hematopoietic cells. *Blood.* 2006;107(1):60-62.
115. Spikes JD. Porphyrins and related compounds as photodynamic sensitizers. *Ann N Y Acad Sci.* 1975;244:496-508.
116. Goldstein BD, Harber LC. Erythropoietic protoporphyria: lipid peroxidation and red cell membrane damage associated with photohemolysis. *J Clin Invest.* 1972;51(4):892-902.
117. Schothorst AA, van Steveninck J, Went LN, et al. Photodynamic damage of the erythrocyte membrane caused by protoporphyrin in protoporphyria and in normal red blood cells. *Clin Chim Acta.* 1972;39(1):161-170.
118. Lim HW, Poh-Fitzpatrick MB, Gigli I. Activation of the complement system in patients with porphyrias after irradiation in vivo. *J Clin Invest.* 1984;74(6):1961-1965.
119. Ryan EA. Histochemistry of the skin in erythropoietic protoporphyria. *Br J Dermatol.* 1966;78(10):501-518.
120. Poh-Fitzpatrick MB. The erythropoietic porphyrias. *Dermatol Clin.* 1986;4(2):291-296.
121. Berenson MM, Kimura R, Samowitz W, et al. Protoporphyrin overload in unrestrained rats: biochemical and histopathologic characterization of a new model of protoporphyric hepatopathy. *Int J Exp Pathol.* 1992;73(5):665-673.
122. Bloomer JR. The liver in protoporphyria. *Hepatol.* 1988;8(2):402-407.
123. Bloomer JR, Enriquez R. Evidence that hepatic crystalline deposits in a patient with protoporphyria are composed of protoporphyrin. *Gastroenterology.* 1982;82(3):569-573.
124. Bloomer J, Wang Y, Singhal A, et al. Molecular studies of liver disease in erythropoietic protoporphyria. *J Clin Gastroenterol.* 2005;39(4)(suppl 2):S167-S175.
125. Mathews-Roth MM. Systemic photoprotection. *Dermatol Clin.* 1986;4(2):335-339.
126. Balwani M, Naik H, Anderson KE, et al. Clinical, biochemical, and genetic characterization of North American patients with erythropoietic protoporphyria and X-linked protoporphyria. *JAMA Dermatol.* 2017;153(8):789-796.
127. Schmidt H, Snitker G, Thomsen K, et al. Erythropoietic protoporphyria. A clinical study based on 29 cases in 14 families. *Arch Dermatol.* 1974;110(1):58-64.
128. Poh-Fitzpatrick MB. Human protoporphyria: reduced cutaneous photosensitivity and lower erythrocyte porphyrin levels during pregnancy. *J Am Acad Dermatol.* 1997;36(1):40-43.
129. Balwani M, Doheny D, Bishop DF, et al. Loss-of-function ferrochelatase and gain-of-function erythroid

5-aminolevulinate synthase mutations causing erythropoietic protoporphyria and X-linked protoporphyria in North American patients reveal novel mutations and a high prevalence of X-linked protoporphyria. *Mol Med.* 2013;19:26-35.
130. Holme SA, Worwood M, Anstey AV, et al. Erythropoiesis and iron metabolism in dominant erythropoietic protoporphyria. *Blood.* 2007;110(12):4108-4110.
131. Bossi K, Lee J, Schmeltzer P, et al. Homeostasis of iron and hepcidin in erythropoietic protoporphyria. *Eur J Clin Invest.* 2015;45(10):1032-1041.
132. Risheg H, Chen FP, Bloomer JR. Genotypic determinants of phenotype in North American patients with erythropoietic protoporphyria. *Mol Genet Metab.* 2003;80(1-2):196-206.
133. Turnbull A, Baker H, Vernon-Roberts B, et al. Iron metabolism in porphyria cutanea tarda and in erythropoietic protoporphyria. *Q J Med.* 1973;42:341-355.
134. Rank JM, Carithers R, Bloomer J. Evidence for neurological dysfunction in end-stage protoporphyric liver disease. *Hepatology.* 1993;18(6):1404-1409.
135. Doss MO, Frank M. Hepatobiliary implications and complications in protoporphyria, a 20-year study. *Clin Biochem.* 1989;22(3):223-229.
136. Singer JA, Plaut AG, Kaplan MM. Hepatic failure and death from erythropoietic protoporphyria. *Gastroenterology.* 1978;74(3):588-591.
137. Key NS, Rank JM, Freese D, et al. Hemolytic anemia in protoporphyria: possible precipitating role of liver failure and photic stress. *Am J Hematol.* 1992;39(3):202-207.
138. Wahlin S, Srikanthan N, Hamre B, et al. Protection from phototoxic injury during surgery and endoscopy in erythropoietic protoporphyria. *Liver Transpl.* 2008;14(9):1340-1346.
139. Hastka J, Lasserre JJ, Schwarzbeck A, et al. Zinc protoporphyrin in anemia of chronic disorders. *Blood.* 1993;81(5):1200-1204.
140. Anderson KE, Sassa S, Peterson CM, et al. Increased erythrocyte uroporphyrinogen-I-synthetase, δ-aminolevulinic acid dehydratase and protoporphyrin in hemolytic anemias. *Am J Med.* 1977;63(3):359-364.
141. Gou EW, Balwani M, Bissell DM, et al. Pitfalls in erythrocyte protoporphyrin measurement for diagnosis and monitoring of protoporphyrias. *Clin Chem.* 2015;61(12):1453-1456.
142. Poh-Fitzpatrick MB, DeLeo VA. Rates of plasma porphyrin disappearance in fluorescent vs. red incandescent light exposure. *J Invest Dermatol.* 1977;69(6):510-512.
143. Mathews-Roth MM, Pathak MA, Fitzpatrick TB, et al. Beta carotene therapy for erythropoietic protoporphyria and other photosensitivity diseases. *Arch Dermatol.* 1977;113(9):1229-1232.
144. Minder EI, Schneider-Yin X, Steurer J, et al. A systematic review of treatment options for dermal photosensitivity in erythropoietic protoporphyria. *Cell Mol Biol (Noisy-le-grand).* 2009;55(1):84-97.
145. Mathews-Roth MM, Rosner B. Long-term treatment of erythropoietic protoporphyria with cysteine. *Photodermatol Photoimmunol Photomed.* 2002;18(6):307-309.
146. Langendonk JG, Balwani M, Anderson KE, et al. Afamelanotide for erythropoietic protoporphyria. *N Engl J Med.* 2015;373(1):48-59.
147. Lane AM, McKay JT, Bonkovsky HL. Advances in the management of erythropoietic protoporphyria-role of afamelanotide. *Appl Clin Genet.* 2016;9:179-189.
148. Tu JH, Sheu SL, Teng JM. Novel treatment using cimetidine for erythropoietic protoporphyria in children. *JAMA Dermatol.* 2016;152(11):1258-1261.
149. Langendonk JG, Wilson J. Insufficient evidence of cimetidine benefit in protoporphyria. *JAMA Dermatol.* 2017;153(2):237-237.
150. Bentley DP, Meek EM. Clinical and biochemical improvement following low-dose intravenous iron therapy in a patient with erythropoietic protoporphyria. *Br J Haematol.* 2013;163(2):289-291.
151. Landefeld C, Kentouche K, Gruhn B, et al. X-linked protoporphyria: iron supplementation improves protoporphyrin overload, liver damage and anaemia. *Br J Haematol.* 2016;173(3):482-484.
152. Gordeuk VR, Brittenham GM, Hawkins CW, et al. Iron therapy for hepatic dysfunction in erythropoietic protoporphyria. *Ann Intern Med.* 1986;105(1):27-31.
153. Mercurio MG, Prince G, Weber FL, et al. Terminal hepatic failure in erythropoietic protoporphyria. *J Am Acad Dermatol.* 1993;29(5, pt 2):829-833.
154. Bonkovsky HL, Schned AR. Fatal liver failure in protoporphyria: synergism between ethanol excess and the genetic defect. *Gastroenterology.* 1986;90(1):191-201.
155. Bloomer JR. Pathogenesis and therapy of liver disease in protoporphyria. *Yale J Biol Med.* 1979;52(1):39-48.
156. Kniffen JC. Protoporphyrin removal in intrahepatic porphyrastasis. *Gastroenterology.* 1970;58:1027.
157. Gross U, Frank M, Doss MO. Hepatic complications of erythropoietic protoporphyria. *Photodermatol Photoimmunol Photomed.* 1998;14(2):52-57.
158. Bechtel MA, Bertolone SJ, Hodge SJ. Transfusion therapy in a patient with erythropoietic protoporphyria. *Arch Dermatol.* 1981;117(2):99-101.
159. Van Wijk HJ, Van Hattum J, Delafaille HB, et al. Blood exchange and transfusion therapy for acute cholestasis in protoporphyria. *Dig Dis Sci.* 1988;33(12):1621-1625.
160. McGuire BM, Bonkovsky HL, Carithers RL Jr, et al. Liver transplantation for erythropoietic protoporphyria liver disease. *Liver Transpl.* 2005;11(12):1590-1596.
161. Wahlin S, Stal P, Adam R, et al. Liver transplantation for erythropoietic protoporphyria in Europe. *Liver Transpl.* 2011;17(9):1021-1026.
162. Todd DJ, Callender ME, Mayne EE, et al. Erythropoietic protoporphyria, transfusion therapy and liver disease. *Br J Dermatol.* 1992;127(5):534-537.
163. Nordmann Y. Erythropoietic protoporphyria and hepatic complications. *J Hepatol.* 1992;16(1-2):4-6.
164. Muley SA, Midani HA, Rank JM, et al. Neuropathy in erythropoietic protoporphyrias. *Neurology.* 1998;51(1):262-265.
165. Poh-Fitzpatrick MB, Wang X, Anderson KE, et al. Erythropoietic protoporphyria: Altered phenotype after bone marrow transplantation for myelogenous leukemia in a patient heteroallelic for ferrochelatase gene mutations. *J Am Acad Dermatol.* 2002;46(6):861-866.
166. Rand EB, Bunin N, Cochran W, et al. Sequential liver and bone marrow transplantation for treatment of erythropoietic protoporphyria. *Pediatrics.* 2006;118(6):e1896-e1899.
167. Anderson KE, Bloomer JR, Bonkovsky HL, et al. Recommendations for the diagnosis and treatment of the acute porphyrias. *Ann Intern Med.* 2005;142(6):439-450.
168. Akagi R, Kato N, Inoue R, et al. delta-Aminolevulinate dehydratase (ALAD) porphyria: the first case in

North America with two novel ALAD mutations. *Mol Genet Metab.* 2006;87(4):329-336.
169. Goldberg A, Moore MR, McColl KEL, et al. Porphyrin metabolism and the porphyrias. In: Ledingham DA, Warrell DA, Wetherall DJ, eds. *Oxford Textbook of Medicine.* Oxford: Oxford University Press; 1987:9136.
170. With TK. Hereditary coproporphyria and variegate porphyria in Denmark. *Dan Med Bull.* 1983;30(2):106-112.
171. Mustajoki P. Variegate porphyria. Twelve years' experience in Finland. *Q J Med.* 1980;49(194):191-203.
172. Eales L, Day RS, Blekkenhorst GH. The clinical and biochemical features of variegate porphyria: an analysis of 300 cases studied at Groote Schuur Hospital, Cape Town. *Int J Biochem.* 1980;12(5-6):837-853.
173. Meyer UA, Schuurmans MM, Lindberg RLP. Acute porphyrias: pathogenesis of neurological manifestations. *Semin Liver Dis.* 1998;18(1):43-52.
174. Grandchamp B, Phung N, Nordmann Y. Homozygous case of hereditary coproporphyria. *Lancet.* 1977;2(8052-8053):1348-1349.
175. Schmitt C, Gouya L, Malonova E, et al. Mutations in human CPO gene predict clinical expression of either hepatic hereditary coproporphyria or erythropoietic harderoporphyria. *Hum Mol Genet.* 2005;14(20):3089-3098.
176. Podvinec M, Handschin C, Looser R, et al. Identification of the xenosensors regulating human 5-aminolevulinate synthase. *Proc Natl Acad Sci U S A.* 2004;101(24):9127-9132.
177. Lip GYH, McColl KEL, Goldberg A, et al. Smoking and recurrent attacks of acute intermittent porphyria. *Br Med J.* 1991;302(6775):507.
178. Louis CA, Sinclair JF, Wood SG, et al. Synergistic induction of cytochrome-P450 by ethanol and isopentanol in cultures of chick embryo and rat hepatocytes. *Toxicol Appl Pharmacol.* 1993;118(2):169-176.
179. Thunell S, Floderus Y, Henrichson A, et al. Alcoholic beverages in acute porphyria. *J Stud Alcohol.* 1992;53(3):272-276.
180. Andersson C, Bylesjo I, Lithner F. Effects of diabetes mellitus on patients with acute intermittent porphyria. *J Intern Med.* 1999;245(2):193-197.
181. Kauppinen R. Prognosis of acute porphyrias and molecular genetics of acute intermittent porphyria in Finland. Thesis, University of Helskinki; 1992.
182. Milo R, Neuman M, Klein C, et al. Acute intermittent porphyria in pregnancy. *Obstet Gynecol.* 1989;73(3, pt 2):450-452.
183. Shenhav S, Gemer O, Sassoon E, et al. Acute intermittent porphyria precipitated by hyperemesis and metoclopramide treatment in pregnancy. *Acta Obstet Gynecol Scand.* 1997;76(5):484-485.
184. Handschin C, Lin J, Rhee J, et al. Nutritional regulation of hepatic heme biosynthesis and porphyria through PGC-1alpha. *Cell.* 2005;122(4):505-515.
185. Welland FH, Hellman ES, Gaddis EM, et al. Factors affecting the excretion of porphyrin precursors by patients with acute intermittent porphyria. I. The effect of diet. *Metabolism.* 1964;13:232-250.
186. Thaler MM, Dawber NH. Stimulation of bilirubin formation in liver of newborn rats by fasting and glucagon. *Gastroenterology.* 1977;72(2):312-315.
187. Blake D, McManus J, Cronin V, et al. Fecal coproporphyrin isomers in hereditary coproporphyria. *Clin Chem.* 1992;38(1):96-100.
188. Longas MO, Poh-Fitzpatrick MB. A tightly bound protein-porphyrin complex isolated from the plasma of a patient with variegate porphyria. *Clin Chim Acta.* 1982;118(2-3):219-228.
189. Hift RJ, Davidson BP, van der Hooft C, et al. Plasma fluorescence scanning and fecal porphyrin analysis for the diagnosis of variegate porphyria: precise determination of sensitivity and specificity with detection of protoporphyrinogen oxidase mutations as a reference standard. *Clin Chem.* 2004;50(5):915-923.
190. Nordmann Y, Grandchamp B, De Verneuil H, et al. Harderoporphyria: a variant hereditary coproporphyria. *J Clin Invest.* 1983;72(3):1139-1149.
191. Wahlin S, Harper P, Sardh E, et al. Combined liver and kidney transplantation in acute intermittent porphyria. *Transpl Int.* 2010;23(6):e18-e21.
192. Bonkowsky HL, Tschudy DP. Hazard of propranolol in treatment of acute porphyria (letter). *Br Med J.* 1974;4(5935):47-48.
193. Bonkowsky HL, Sinclair PR, Emery S, et al. Seizure management in acute hepatic porphyria: risks of valproate and clonazepam. *Neurology.* 1980;30(6):588-592.
194. Larson AW, Wasserstrom WR, Felsher BF, et al. Posttraumatic epilepsy and acute intermittent porphyria: effects of phenytoin, carbamazepine, and clonazepam. *Neurology.* 1978;28(8):824-828.
195. Mustajoki P, Nordmann Y. Early administration of heme arginate for acute porphyric attacks. *Arch Intern Med.* 1993;153(17):2004-2008.
196. Tenhunen R, Mustajoki P. Acute porphyria: treatment with heme. *Semin Liver Dis.* 1998;18(1):53-55.
197. Bonkovsky HL, Healey JF, Lourie AN, et al. Intravenous heme-albumin in acute intermittent porphyria: evidence for repletion of hepatic hemoproteins and regulatory heme pools. *Am J Gastroenterol.* 1991;86(8):1050-1056.
198. Harper P, Wahlin S. Treatment options in acute porphyria, porphyria cutanea tarda, and erythropoietic protoporphyria. *Curr Treat Options Gastroenterol.* 2007;10(6):444-455.
199. Anderson KE, Bonkovsky HL, Bloomer JR, et al. Reconstitution of hematin for intravenous infusion. *Ann Intern Med.* 2006;144(7):537-538.
200. Green D, Reynolds N, Klein J, et al. The inactivation of hemostatic factors by hematin. *J Lab Clin Med.* 1983;102(3):361-369.
201. Jones RL. Hematin-derived anticoagulant. Generation in vitro and in vivo. *J Exp Med.* 1986;163(3):724-439.
202. Daimon M, Susa S, Igarashi M, et al. Administration of heme arginate, but not hematin, caused anaphylactic shock. *Am J Med.* 2001;110(3):240.
203. Khanderia U. Circulatory collapse associated with hemin therapy for acute intermittent porphyria. *Clin Pharm.* 1986;5(8):690-692.
204. Marsden JT, Guppy S, Stein P, et al. Audit of the use of regular haem arginate infusions in patients with acute porphyria to prevent recurrent symptoms. *JIMD Rep.* 2015;22:57-65.
205. Anderson KE, Collins S. Open-label study of hemin for acute porphyria: clinical practice implications. *Am J Med.* 2006;119(9):801.e19-801.e24.

Chapter 125 :: Amyloidosis
:: Peter D. Gorevic & Robert G. Phelps

第一百二十五章

淀粉样变性

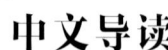

中文导读

　　淀粉样蛋白是一种病理实体，其特征是存在细胞外的均一的透明物质，通过特殊染色可呈现为细胞外深紫色或红色物质，其另一特征是淀粉样物质存在戊聚糖。淀粉样疾病的不同形式是由构成纤维的亚单位蛋白质来区分的，其中11种涉及皮肤和/或有皮肤表现。

　　本章首先介绍了系统性淀粉样变性的所有表现形式，都可能与隐匿性或显性皮肤受累有关，包括眶周紫癜、巨舌症、舌结节。同时概述了其流行病学特征。

　　接下来介绍了局限性淀粉样变性，包括鼻咽（喉）、眼部、泌尿生殖道和肺淀粉样变性，以及可能发生在不同部位的淀粉样瘤，表125-3列出了常见的皮肤淀粉样变性及其特征，主要类型有黄斑型、丘疹/苔藓型和混合型/双相型皮肤淀粉样变性，分别概述了常见及罕见类型的临床特点、流行病学特点、诊断探讨。

　　最后还介绍了淀粉样变性疾病的治疗策略，对于系统性淀粉样变，首先采用的策略是降低前体蛋白水平与使用抗细胞因子治疗、大剂量地塞米松等，另一策略是抑制导致纤维形成的聚集现象，第三种方法是利用免疫疗法中和低聚物，促进组织淀粉样蛋白的清除。对于皮肤淀粉样变性，若由系统性引起，治疗策略与系统性淀粉样变的策略相同，同时可采用局部治疗手段，包括刮除、切除、局部外用和病灶内类固醇、局部外用钙调神经磷酸酶抑制药、小剂量口服环磷酰胺和环孢素等。

〔梁　娟〕

AT-A-GLANCE

- There are 36 types of amyloid disease, defined by the subunit proteins that constitute the fibrils in these disorders, 11 of which involve the skin.
- Cutaneous amyloidosis may reflect a systemic form of amyloid, or be localized to the skin and/or mucous membranes.
- Precursors of fibril subunit proteins may circulate in blood and/or be synthesized locally; they may be wildtype or mutant molecules that can be typed by DNA sequencing.
- Amyloid in skin may be sampled by lesional biopsy or abdominal fat pad aspiration or biopsy; it is characterized by metachromasia and apple-green birefringence after staining with Congo red, or yellow-green fluorescence after staining with thioflavin T.
- Deposits may localize to the papillary dermis (macular and lichen amyloidosis) or be characterized by congophilic angiopathy and involvement of adnexal structures (nodular amyloidosis).
- Amyloid can be typed by immunohistochemistry, immunoelectron microscopy, and/or laser capture mass spectroscopy followed by protein sequencing.
- Treatment of amyloid diseases is determined by the fibril subunit protein, associated clinical manifestations, and whether disease is systemic or localized.
- Treatment strategies include suppression of precursor protein, disruption of oligomers and/or fibrils, and/or enhanced clearance of deposits.
- Localized cutaneous amyloidoses present specific challenges and opportunities for diagnosis and therapy because of the accessibility of skin lesions, association in some cases with defined genetic abnormalities, and multifactorial etiologies for itch in pathogenesis.

DEFINITION

Amyloid is a pathologic entity characterized by the presence of mostly extracellular homogenous hyaline material that is typically metachromatic, as seen by color changes of dyes such as Congo red (actually orange in solution), crystal violet (which yields a deep red-purple color on a blue background), or sodium sulfate Alcian blue (reacts with proteoglycan in amyloid deposits to yield a green color). Other stains that can be used include cotton dyes such as Sirius red (a polyazo dye) and Pagoda red. Amyloid is further defined in tissue section as yielding apple-green birefringence by polarizing microscopy after staining with Congo red, and as having typical yellow-green fluorescence after staining with thioflavin T. Ultrastructurally, the main constituents of deposits are fibrils which are 10 to 15 nm in diameter, and variable in length, that accumulate in the extracellular space, and can be visualized by electron microscopy.

A second feature of all amyloid deposits is the presence of a pentraxin, serum amyloid P-component (SAP). In addition to the fibril and SAP, deposits are enriched in heparan sulfate proteoglycan, as well as a number of proteins that have been identified by extraction of amyloid from tissue. These other substances include several apolipoproteins, notably apoE, apoJ, and apoA4.[1] Thus the diagnosis of amyloidosis is rigorously defined by the appearance, tinctorial properties and ultrastructural features of biopsied material (Table 125-1).

AMYLOID DISEASES RELEVANT TO DERMATOLOGY

Different forms of amyloid disease are distinguished by the subunit proteins that constitute the fibril, 36 of which have been described, each associated with distinct clinical entities,[2] 11 known to involve the skin and/or have cutaneous manifestations (Table 125-2). The current list of 36 subunit proteins includes 6 different apolipoproteins, notably the high-density lipoprotein-associated serum amyloid A (apoSAA), an acute-phase reactant that forms the amyloid in reactive or secondary (AA) amyloidosis, and 2 members of the immunoglobulin gene superfamily, immunoglobulin light chain (AL), the major constituent of primary or myeloma-associated amyloidosis, and β_2-microglobulin (Aβ_2m), the subunit protein in patients on longstanding hemodialysis or chronic peritoneal dialysis (dialysis amyloidosis). Fibril subunit proteins arise from soluble precursors, most of which can be found in blood, but which also may be synthesized by cells contiguous to the amyloid deposits. They may be wildtype (WT) (ie, have the same amino acid sequence as the physiologic precursor), but in several forms of amyloidosis they have been found to have single nucleotide and amino acid substitutions, corresponding to point mutations in the DNA sequence. These mutations characterize familial forms of amyloidosis, in which multiple members of a kindred are affected by distinct organ-specific clinical syndromes, but may also occur in apparently sporadic cases of amyloidosis. More than 500 different mutations in subunit proteins, or in proteins strongly associated with several forms of amyloidosis, have been identified, providing diagnostic genetic markers for several important forms of amyloid disease.[3]

PATHOGENESIS

Following synthesis in the cell of origin, precursor proteins may adopt a number of configurations, some of which may be normal folding intermediates important for intracellular processing and secretion. Cellular

TABLE 125-1
Histologic Criteria for the Definition of Amyloid

- Homogenous-hyaline
- Mostly extracellular
- Typical 10 to 15 nm fibrils by electron microscopy
- Metachromasia
- Congo red birefringence
- Thioflavin T yellow-green fluorescence
- Multiple chemical types

SYSTEMIC FORMS OF AMYLOIDOSIS

The majority of patients seen in tertiary care centers have systemic forms of amyloidosis, most commonly AL, AA, and amyloidosis caused by transthyretin (ATTR), a thyroid transport protein also known as prealbumin. In a 2013 series from the United Kingdom, 65% of patients with systemic amyloid were AL, 18% AA, 7% WT ATTR, and 10% mutant ATTR.[5] In AL, high levels of a monoclonal immunoglobulin (Ig) light chain are produced by an aberrant plasma cell population, associated with frank or smoldering multiple myeloma in 10% to 20%. Sustained elevated levels of SAA are triggered by proinflammatory cytokines, notably interleukin (IL)-6, which may be a result of chronic infections or rheumatic or autoinflammatory diseases. In ATTR, the conversion of circulating WT or mutant TTR may be reflected in relatively low levels of precursor protein as a result of a "sink" effect in which precursor may deposit onto existing amyloid. Organ system involvement for AL is clinically diverse, with cardiac, renal and neurologic disease being particularly important; in AA amyloidosis, approximately 80% renal involvement occurs, and is the cause of morbidity and mortality, with lesser involvement of the GI tract (20%) and heart; ATTR may present as overlapping syndromes of neuropathy, cardiomyopathy, GI, vitreous, and occasional leptomeningeal amyloidosis.[6]

factors that contribute to protein misfolding include membrane interactions, altered cell chemistry, post-translational modifications, crowding, and pathogenic mutations; in both the intracellular and extracellular milieu, acidification, temperature, protein concentration, and oxidative stress may be important.[4]

Prior to the formation of amyloid fibrils, precursor proteins may adopt the configuration of amorphous aggregates, oligomers, and other intermediates, which may be demonstrable in vitro, and in several cases in vivo. Aggregates have not yet accumulated cofactors, such as SAP and heparan sulfate proteoglans, but appear to be important in mediating distinct functional abnormalities that are demonstrable in association with, or preceding, amyloid deposition, as well as inducing apoptosis and cell death. In addition, several precursor proteins undergo proteolysis as part of the conversion to insoluble fibrils, with specific cleavage products being the main form of subunit protein retrieved from deposits. However, the precursor–product relationships of amorphous aggregates, oligomers, and alternative fibrillar states have yet to be fully defined (Fig. 125-1).[1,4]

Less-common forms of systemic amyloidosis include several heredofamilial syndromes that have been prominently associated with nephropathic amyloidosis (apoA2, apoCII and apoCIII, fibrinogen, lysozyme), and lattice dystrophy, cutis laxa, and cranial

TABLE 125-2
Nomenclature for Amyloid Fibril Proteins with Known Cutaneous Involvement, Including Precursor Proteins, Major Organ System Disease, and Skin Manifestations

FIBRIL PROTEIN	PRECURSOR PROTEIN	TARGET ORGANS	CUTANEOUS INVOLVEMENT
AL	Immunoglobulin light chain	All except CNS	Pinch/postproctoscopic purpura; nodules; waxy plaques; congophilic angiography; macroglossia
Aβ$_2$M	β$_2$-Microglobulin	Musculoskeletal	Subcutaneous and lingual nodules
AA	Serum amyloid A	All except CNS	Fat pad aspiration/biopsy
ATTR	Transthyretin	Nervous system; heart; vitreous	Periorbital purpura; nodules; fat pad aspiration/biopsy
AApoAI	Apolipoprotein AI	Heart; liver; kidney; nervous system	C-terminal variants affect larynx and skin; yellow and maculopapular squamous lesions
ALys	Lysozyme	Kidney	Variants may present with sicca, have adenopathy, petechial rash/bruising
AGel	Gelsolin	Cornea; peripheral nervous system	Cutis laxa; pruritus; ecchymoses; alopecia
ACys	Cystatin C	Cerebral hemorrhages	Asymptomatic
AGal7	Galectin 7	Localized cutaneous	Lichen/macular amyloidosis
AIns	Insulin	Iatrogenic	Injection site (insulin pump)
AEnf	Enfuvirtide	Iatrogenic (HIV medicine)	Local injection site

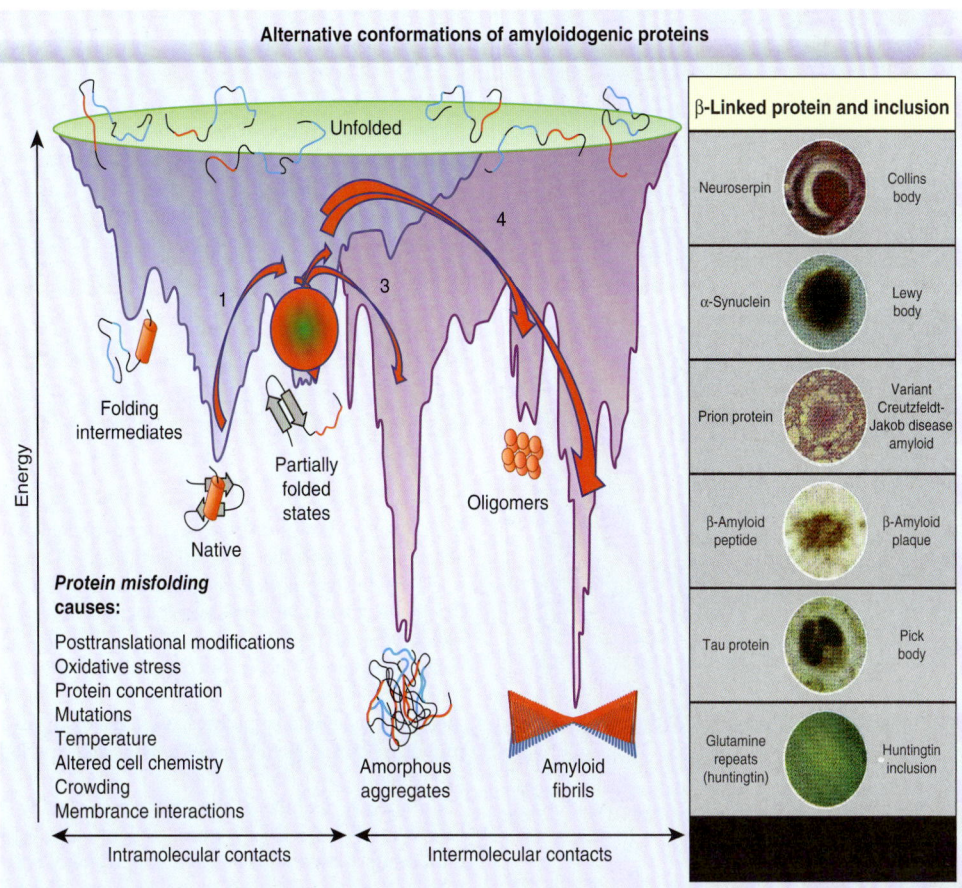

Figure 125-1 Alternative conformations of amyloidogenic proteins, including amorphous aggregates, oligomers and fibrils, and factors implicated in fibrillogenesis. Amyloidosis within the spectrum of aggregation disorders, several of which are implicated in neurodegeneration. (Adapted by permission from Springer Nature: Hartl FU, Hayer-Hartl M. Converging concepts of protein folding in vitro and in vivo. *Nat Struct Mol Biol.* 2009;16(6):574-81. Copyright © 2009.)

neuropathy (gelsolin).[3]

Although dominant organ involvement may define clinical presentation in each of the systemic amyloidoses, there is often diffuse involvement that may become more apparent as disease progresses, or is apparent at postmortem. Organ-dominant disease may significantly influence the prognosis of patients with AL, with cardiac involvement accounting for a 1-year mortality of approximately 45% and a median survival time of 6 to 14 months compared to a subset of patients with soft-tissue (eg, macroglossia, submandibular swelling), bone, and joint disease, among whom 2- to 3-year survivals are not uncommon. In AA, most patients have glomerular disease, presenting as proteinuria/nephrotic syndrome; however, there also may be interstitial and vascular amyloid, which may present as an elevation in creatinine, or renal insufficiency, without significant proteinuria. WT and mutant ATTR may present as carpal tunnel syndrome with amyloid retrievable from the flexor retinaculum in cases that have been available for study. Although most mutant ATTR are associated with neuropathy, approximately 50% also have cardiomyopathy, which may dominate the clinical presentation in patients with specific mutations associated with late-onset disease.

SKIN DISEASE IN SYSTEMIC AMYLOIDS

All forms of systemic amyloid may be associated with occult or overt cutaneous involvement, again with variable clinical presentations. Overt presentations include pinch and periorbital purpura in approximately 10% of patients with AL (Fig. 125-2) and a smaller number with ATTR. Macroglossia, lingual nodules, or lateral ridging, are unique to AL (Fig. 125-3) and $A\beta_2m$. Dermatologic signs may be found in as many as one-third of patients with AL amyloid. Almost any site has been described, including face, neck and fingers. Sclerodermoid and bullous lesions may be found rarely[7]; hair and nail changes can also occur. In AL, fissured masses may be present focally or diffusely in the papillary or reticular dermis. A common and often diagnostic feature is the presence of amyloid in the walls of small or

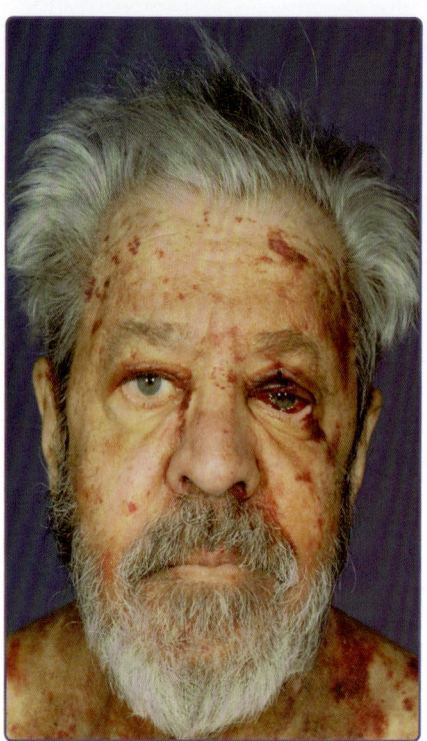

Figure 125-2 Pinch, periorbital and facial purpura in a patient with known systemic AL amyloidosis. Patient grew a beard to avoid the trauma/purpura associated with shaving.

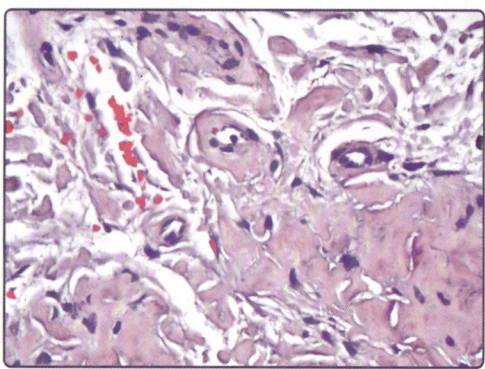

Figure 125-4 AL amyloidosis showing deposits in the dermis and walls of capillaries (hematoxylin and eosin, ×10 magnification).

medium-sized blood vessels (Fig. 125-4), causing vascular wall weakening and hemorrhage.

Overt cutaneous involvement is rare in AA amyloidosis; however this form of amyloid may complicate inflammatory cutaneous disorders, most notably in patients with severe inflammation complicating Hidradenitis suppurativa, pyoderma gangrenosum/ inflammatory bowel disease, and some patients with severe and uncontrolled psoriatic arthritis. AA amyloidosis may also complicate autoinflammatory diseases that have distinctive skin lesions such as erysipelas-like erythema (familial Mediterranean fever), cold urticaria (some of the cryopyrinopathies), erythematous macules and papules (hyper-IgD syndrome), and migratory edematous patches or periorbital edema (tumor necrosis factor receptor-associated periodic syndrome).

Cutaneous manifestations may occasionally be found in the hereditary forms of amyloid. ATTR may be associated with eyelid and peripheral ecchymoses, atrophic scars, bullous lesions, thickened skin, and xerosis[8]; cutis laxa is a major manifestation of AGel[9]; yellow and maculopapular squamous rashes may complicate carboxyterminal variants of AApoAI[10]; and petechial rashes/easy bruising have been described in some variants of ALys[11]; asymptomatic skin deposition has been found for ALys and ACys[12] (see Table 125-2).

EPIDEMIOLOGY OF THE SYSTEMIC AMYLOIDS

The overall incidence of systemic amyloid is 5 to 12 cases per million-person years in large series reported from the Mayo Clinic, the United Kingdom amyloidosis referral center, and Scandinavia.[5,13] During the 20th century, the percent contribution of AA amyloid resulting from chronic infection decreased, correlating with an increased representation of associated rheumatologic, inflammatory bowel and autoinflammatory diseases such as familial Mediterranean fever. There are an estimated 5000 to 10,000 cases of AA amyloid in Europe and North America. Approximately 100,000 persons are affected by familial Mediterranean fever worldwide; in Turkey, Syria, Egypt, and Israel, it is a common cause of AA, and is responsible for a significant percent of renal disease caused by amyloidosis. Each year, 1275 to 3200 new cases of AL amyloid are reported, giving an estimate

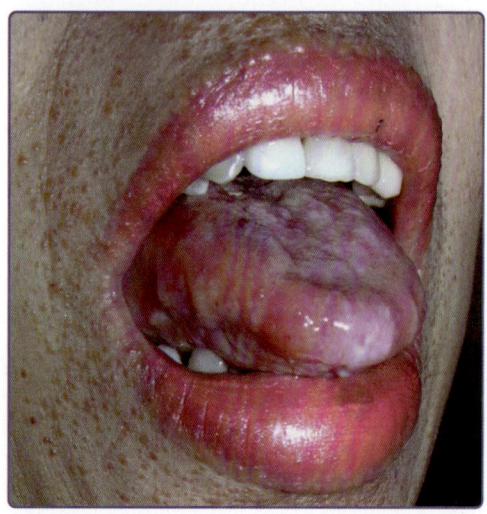

Figure 125-3 Macroglossia with lateral ridging caused by the impression of adjacent teeth in a patient with known systemic AL amyloidosis. Note the perioral macules with a waxy appearance also caused by cutaneous amyloid.

of 15,000 patients in the United States and Europe. The overall incidence of familial amyloid polyneuropathy caused by ATTR is 0.3 cases per year per million persons, or 5000 to 10,000 cases worldwide. However, there are wide variations in incidence for the most common Met30 ATTR mutation, which is endemic in northern Portugal and the north of Sweden. The Ile122 ATTR mutation is carried by 4% of the African American and African Caribbean populations, and in parts of west Africa.[3,13,14]

LOCALIZED AMYLOIDOSIS

Excluding CNS amyloid associated with neurodegenerative diseases, localized forms of amyloid account for approximately 10% of patients seen in referral centers. They include nasopharyngeal (laryngeal), ocular, genitourinary, and pulmonary amyloidoses, as well as amyloidomas that may occur in a variety of locations. Symptoms reflect the specific organ system (eg, hoarseness in laryngeal amyloid, gross hematuria in genitourinary amyloid, and subconjunctival masses, often mistaken for lymphomas). The large majority of cases of localized amyloid that have been characterized biochemically appear to be AL, with evidence in some cases that the aggregates are being synthesized by clonal contiguous plasma cells. Even though patients are routinely evaluated for systemic involvement, disease may remain stable or only extend locally even with prolonged periods of observation, with cures reported if full resection is feasible.[15]

CUTANEOUS AMYLOIDOSES[16]

Table 125-3 lists common cutaneous amyloidoses and their characteristics.

Cutaneous amyloid diseases may have heterogenous manifestations, depending on the location of amyloid deposition within the dermis or epidermis. Localized cutaneous amyloidoses are often restricted to the papillary dermis, whereas in systemic disorders, the subpapillary layers, dermal appendages and blood vessels are frequently involved.[17] Vascular involvement may be apparent as congophilic angiopathy, causing petechiae, purpura, or ecchymoses, which typically occur over the upper chest wall, or in a periorbital distribution distinct from that seen in purpura from other causes (eg, vasculitis) (see Fig. 125-2). Involvement of the upper dermis may cause thickening, apparent as waxy papules and plaques, or nodules (see Fig. 125-3). Nodules may be single or multiple in systemic or localized AL amyloid, sometimes growing to a large size[18] if untreated (Fig. 125-5), and can also involve the face. Three major types of primary cutaneous amyloidosis have been described: macular (~35%), papular/lichen (~35%), and mixed/biphasic (~15%),[19] in addition to rarer disease entities.

MACULAR AMYLOIDOSIS

Macular amyloidosis commonly presents in the interscapular region as a pigmented patch of varying size. It can occur in other sites, such as the extensor surface of the arms, thighs, and shins. Typical is a rippled salt-and-pepper appearance with alternating hyperpigmentation and hypopigmentation (Fig. 125-6). It is more common in women and patients with a darker complexion. The pathology of macular amyloidosis is subtle and easily missed without clinical correlation. Within the papillary dermis are small collections of amyloid globules, or "corpuscles." These can be irregularly scattered and not found in every rete. A useful clue (as in lichen amyloidosis) is the presence of rare melanin-containing histiocytes encircling these deposits. Often, special stains are necessary to demonstrate

TABLE 125-3
Common Cutaneous Amyloidoses

	EPIDEMIOLOGY	COMMONLY AFFECTED SITES	CLINICAL APPEARANCE	PATHOLOGIC FEATURES
Macular amyloidosis	~35% of cutaneous amyloidosis cases; women of darker complexion more commonly affected	Interscapular region, extensor surfaces of arms, thighs, and shins	"Salt-and-pepper" appearance with alternating hyper- and hypopigmentation	Mild epidermal hyperkeratosis; collections of amyloid "corpuscles" within papillary dermis; melanin-containing histiocytes encircle the deposits
Lichen amyloidosis	~35% of cutaneous amyloidosis; most common subtype; men in their fifth to sixth decades are more commonly affected	Shins and forearms, occasionally upper back	Linear rows of firm, pigmented, grouped, hyperkeratotic papules that can evolve into plaques	Epidermis is acanthotic and papillomatous with basal layer hyperpigmentation and elongated rete ridges; small collections of amphophilic material in papillary dermis surrounded by melanophages
Biphasic cutaneous amyloidosis	~15% of cases	Characteristics of both macular and lichen amyloidosis	Overlapping clinical features	Overlapping pathologic features

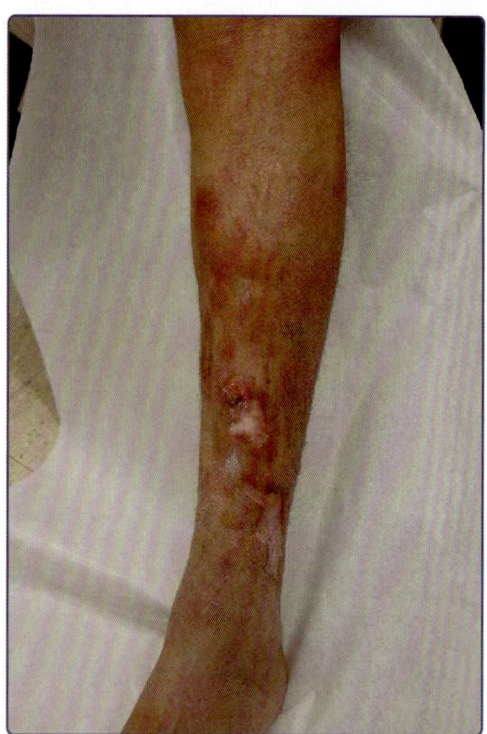

Figure 125-5 Multiple large and confluent nodules developed on the shin of a patient with nodular amyloidosis, noting the site of biopsy shown in **Fig. 125-4**. Followed over several years, the patient had no indication of systemic AL amyloid or plasma cell dyscrasia on repeated evaluations.

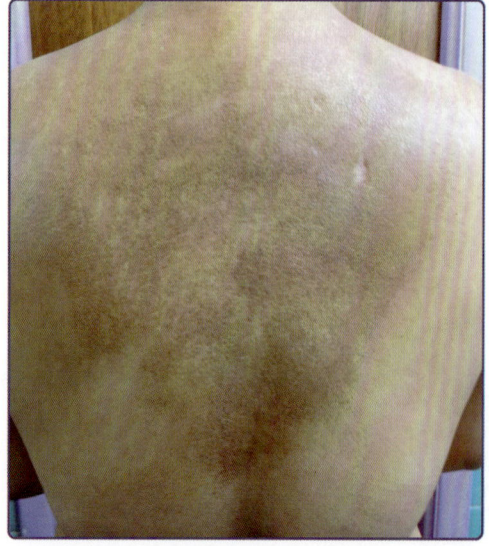

Figure 125-6 Interscapular area of a patient showing edge-shaped rippled hypopigmentation and hyperpigmentation consistent with macular amyloidosis.

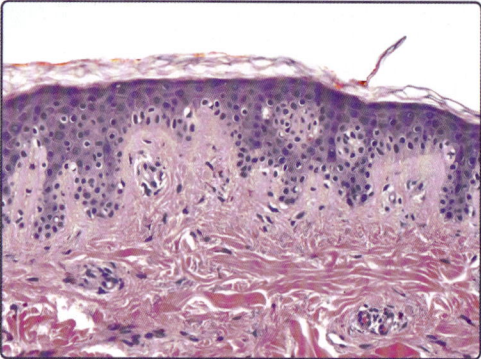

Figure 125-7 Dermis of a patient with macular amyloidosis showing scattered melanin and rare foci of amyloid (hematoxylin and eosin, ×20 magnification).

the amyloid. The extent of epidermal changes is minimal with only mild hyperkeratosis (Fig. 125-7).

LICHEN AMYLOIDOSIS

Lichen amyloidosis is the most common type of cutaneous amyloidosis. It usually presents later in life, predominantly in the fifth and sixth decades, and is more common in men and patients with a higher Fitzpatrick skin type. The initial symptom of this disorder is intense pruritus that may improve with sun exposure and worsen during periods of stress. Hyperpigmented lesions are presumed to be secondary to scratching. Clinically, lesions often occur on the shins and forearms as linear rows of firm pigmented grouped hyperkeratotic papules that can evolve into large plaques (Fig. 125-8); the upper back also can be involved. As a result of the intense pruritus, the epidermis is often acanthotic and papillomatous with a compact horn; hyperkeratosis, hyperpigmentation of basal keratinocytes and elongation of rete ridges is typical. Basal cell vacuolar changes may occur with intraepidermal cytoid bodies. Within or adjacent to the lesion, changes of lichen simplex chronicus may occur. Within the broadened papillary dermis, there are small collections of amphophilic material often surrounded by melanophages (macrophages with engulfed melanin) (Figs. 125-9 and 125-10).

BIPHASIC CUTANEOUS AMYLOIDOSIS

Biphasic cutaneous amyloidosis refers to the concurrent presence of macular amyloidosis and lichen amyloidosis. This entity may also exist as a form in combination with blisters and poikilodermic skin lesions.[19]

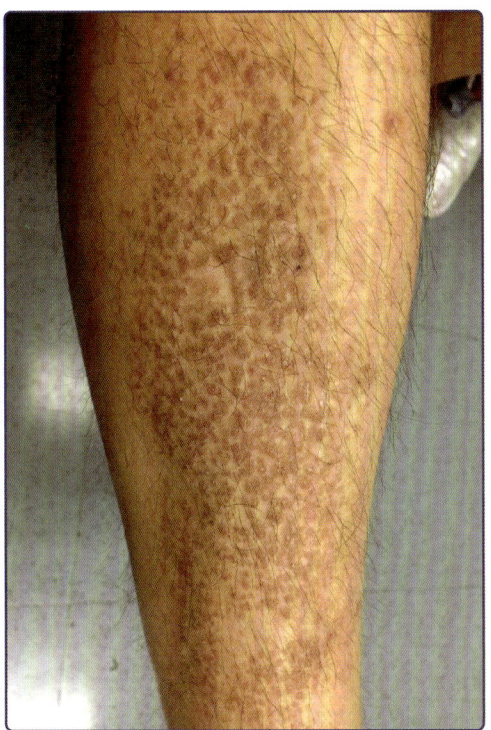

Figure 125-8 Linear keratotic papules on the shin characteristic for lichen amyloidosis.

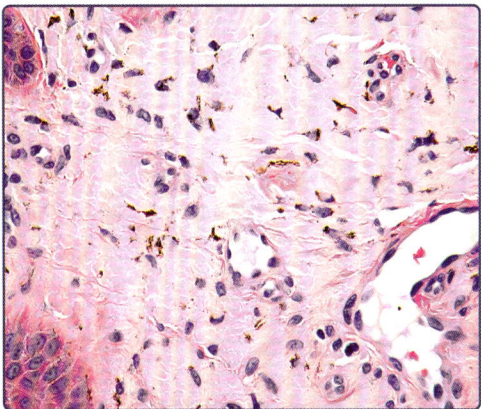

Figure 125-10 Characteristic appearance of amyloid: fissured small globules in the dermis, surrounded by melanophages, in lichen amyloidosis (hematoxylin and eosin, ×20 magnification).

VARIANT FORMS OF LOCALIZED CUTANEOUS AMYLOIDOSIS

- Towel-associated amyloidosis induced by prolonged contact with nylon towels.[20]
- Anosacral amyloidosis has been described mainly in Chinese and Japanese patients presenting with brownish patches of plaques in the anosacral region. It is often associated with lichenification, and most patients report pruritus. Amyloid deposits are found in the papillary dermis with pigment incontinence.[21]
- Notalgia paresthetica amyloidosis isolated sensory neuropathy that typically occurs on the back may be associated with amyloid, likely resulting from prolonged pruritus and scratching.[22]
- Friction melanosis or amyloidosis prolonged contact with sponges, towels, plant sticks and leaves. In the opinion of the authors and others, these most likely represent variants of macular or lichen amyloidosis, with a similar pathology[23,24]
- Lichen amyloidosis of the auricular concha hyperpigmentation of the bowl of the ear; likely a variant of lichen amyloidosis.[25]

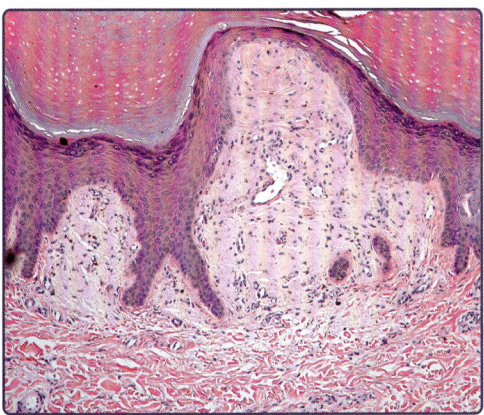

Figure 125-9 Beneath an acanthotic and papillomatous epidermis, a widened dermal papillae contains amyloid globules (hematoxylin and eosin, ×4 magnification).

NODULAR AMYLOIDOSIS

Patients present with 1 or more deep-seated lesions that have a waxy or nodular appearance. They can appear as papules, nodules, or plaques (see Fig. 125-5). Common sites include the feet and trunk.[26] Deposition may occur as discrete amorphous areas between collagen bundles. Nodular amyloidosis may be unique to the skin, although vascular involvement is common (Fig. 125-11). AL is the amyloid type of the large majority of cases that have been characterized biochemically, and the presence of monotypic plasma cells contiguous to nodules has suggested local synthesis (Fig. 125-12); nevertheless, followup for the development of a plasma cell dyscrasia or lymphoproliferative disease is indicated for these patients. In addition, up to 25% of nodular amyloidosis may be associated with primary Sjögren syndrome, a disease in which there may be an increased incidence of non-Hodgkin lymphoma of mucosa-associated lymphoid tissue.[27]

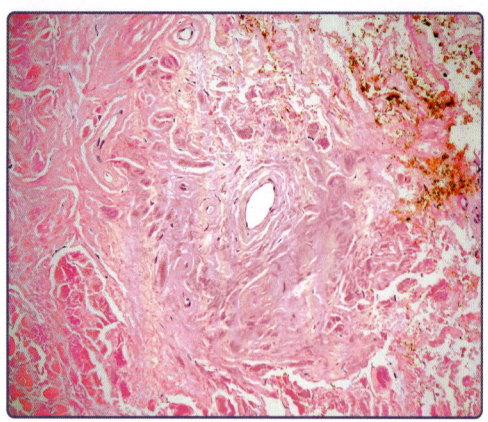

Figure 125-11 Diffuse deposits of amyloid completely replacing the dermis and surrounding blood vessels in nodular amyloidosis (hematoxylin and eosin, ×4 magnification).

Cutaneous amyloidomas of β_2-microglobulin have also rarely been described in patients with dialysis amyloidosis.[28]

AMYLOID ADJACENT TO TUMORS

Although not evident clinically, it is not uncommon to find collections of amyloid adjacent to keratocytic tumors such as basal cell carcinoma, Bowen disease, squamous cell carcinoma, or associated with more benign lesions such as seborrheic or actinic keratoses. Between 66% and 77% of basal cell carcinomas, particularly the nodular type, have been reported to have amyloid deposits within the tumor stroma.[29,30]

CUTIS LAXA IN FAMILIAL AMYLOID CAUSED BY MUTANT GELSOLIN

Originally described in Finland as Meretoja syndrome, the gelsolin mutation has a worldwide distribution and manifests as lattice corneal dystrophy, Type 4, cranial and peripheral neuropathies, and, in some families, prominent renal involvement. Cutis laxa starts on the face, usually in the fifth decade of life, and is apparent as premature aging, but then becomes more generalized. The consequences of skin atrophy may be xerosis, easy bruising with minor trauma, loss of body and scalp hair and occasional lichen amyloidosis. Gelsolin amyloid tends to deposit adjacent to basement structures, including the subdermis and eccrine sweat glands, in dermal blood vessels, and between collagen and elastic fibers.[9]

TRANSTHYRETIN AMYLOIDOSIS

Amyloid can be found in the walls of small blood vessels, freely in the dermis as small fissured collections, and diffusely in adipose tissue between adipocytes (Fig. 125-13).[8]

INJECTION-SITE AMYLOIDOSES

Localized forms of amyloid that result from therapeutics with amyloidogenic propensity have been found in association with insulin pumps and with the use of

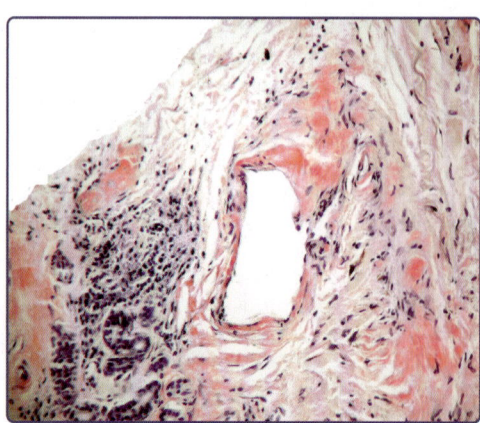

Figure 125-12 Small collection of plasma cells adjacent to nodular amyloid (Congo red, ×10 magnification). Immunohistology may reveal the same light chain in the amyloid as is produced by the adjacent plasma cells.

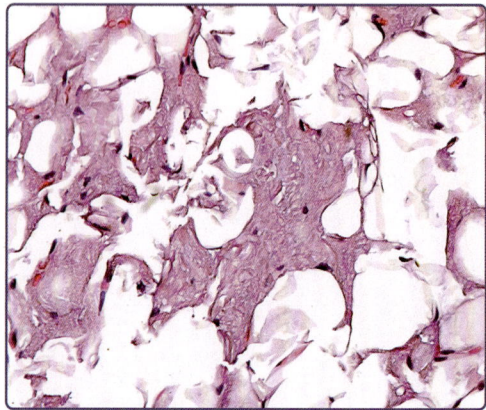

Figure 125-13 Transthyretin amyloid, late stage, apparent on abdominal fat pad biopsy, with fissured masses of amyloid replacing and surrounding adipocytes (hematoxylin and eosin, ×4 magnification).

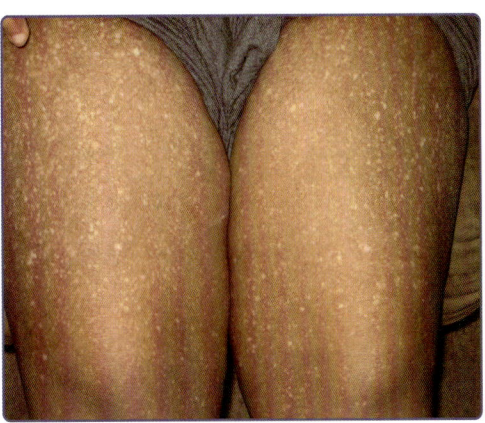

Figure 125-14 Spotted hypopigmentation on a hyperpigmented background in a patient with amyloidosis cutis dyschromica.

enfuvirtide (Fuzeon). Enfuvirtide is a second-line antiretroviral agent used in patients with multidrug resistance to HIV. It comes in a form that is reconstituted for subcutaneous injection, which may result in large, red-yellow, subcutaneous nodules at the sites of injection. Biochemical characterization of these amyloids has been carried out by mass spectroscopy and sequence analysis, and fibrillogenesis demonstrated in vitro.[31]

AMYLOIDOSIS CUTIS DYSCHROMICA

Amyloidosis cutis dyschromica is a rare condition in which patients develop progressive diffuse hyperpigmentation and hypopigmentation and atrophy (Fig. 125-14). It usually has no other associations, though occasional patients have neurologic changes, or signs and symptoms consistent with connective tissue disease. Pathogenesis is unknown, although photosensitivity has been implicated. Amyloid is usually localized within the papillary dermis, and stains with antikeratin antibodies.[32,33]

EPIDEMIOLOGY OF CUTANEOUS AMYLOIDOSES

Macular amyloidosis has a high incidence in Asia, the Middle East, and South America, but is rarely seen in Europe and North America. Macular lesions predominate in studies from Indonesia, Turkey, and India, although papular lesions were more common in one study from Kuala Lumpur. The highest incidence has been reported from southern China and Taiwan, and in most series, the female predominance is overwhelming. Familial cases are estimated to account for up to 10% overall, and have been associated with specific gene defects, including mutations in the oncostatin M receptor (OSMR), interleukin-31 receptor A (IL31RA), and the RET protooncogene.[17]

Cutaneous lichen amyloidosis defines a variant of the multiple endocrine neoplasia 2A syndrome, which is primarily (~95%) associated with medullary thyroid cancer (MTC), and less commonly with pheochromocytoma (30% to 50%) or primary hyperparathyroidism (20% to 30%) and mutations in the RET (rearranged during transfection) protooncogene, which causes constitutive activation of the transmembrane tyrosine kinase receptor. In this syndrome, lichen amyloidosis may occur in childhood before MTC, with most reported cases being the codon 634 mutations, which is estimated to give a 30% likelihood of developing lichen amyloidosis, with 77% affected individuals being women.[34] In one Chinese family with MTC associated with cutaneous amyloidosis, disease was associated with a RET S891A mutation coexisting with a novel OSMR variant, G513D, in 3 family members, with clinical data suggesting a synergism between the 2 mutations that may be driving the clinical phenotype.[35]

GENETICS AND PRURITUS IN CUTANEOUS AMYLOIDOSIS

Recent studies have identified receptors in skin additional to those responsible for histamine effects, including the Mas-related G-protein–coupled receptors, and the transient receptor potential vanilloid Type 1, some of which have been identified in sensory neurons and may respond to histamine, heat, or capsaicin.[36] Particular interest has been directed to OSMR, which encodes OSMRb, a component of both the OSM Type II receptor and the IL-31 receptor. IL-31 has been implicated in pruritus associated with atopic dermatitis, prurigo nodularis and cutaneous T-cell lymphoma (Sézary syndrome).[37] Thirteen heterozygous mutations in OSMRb have been described in association with familial primary cutaneous amyloidosis, most in the extracellular fibronectin III repeat domains central to receptor dimerization with gp-130 (IL-6) or IL-31RA. One heterozygous missense mutation in IL-31RA also has been reported in association with familial lichen amyloidosis.[38] Lesional skin was found to have increased apoptosis of keratinocytes, epidermal hyperinnervation, cytokeratin-5 specific antibody reactivity, increased epidermal expression of IL-31 receptors, and elevated tissue/serum IL-31 levels.[39,40]

Although keratinocyte apoptosis appears to be a central event in the pathogenesis of lichen amyloidosis, and cytokeratin immunohistology a valuable adjunct to diagnosis, recent studies provide evidence that the amyloid fibrils in this disorder may be attributed to subsequences of galectin 7 (Gal7). Early extraction studies yielded codepositing keratin epitopes, as well as P-component, actin, and apoE (enriched in apoE4 in 2 studies), and Gal7, results which could be confirmed by immunohistology[17,41]; however, only Gal7 was found to bind thioflavin T. This protein is one of a family of β-galactoside–binding proteins, only expressed in stratified epithelia, particularly abundant in the stratum spinosum, through which postmitotic keratinocytes move from the basal layer of the epithelium and transform into flattened, enucleated cells connected by tight junctions that secrete keratins to the extracellular matrix; it is markedly induced during keratinocyte apoptosis. Subsequences of Gal7 were found to be fibrillogenic in vitro, corresponding to fragments generated by enzymes known to be active during apoptosis, and modulated by coassociated actin.[42] The exact relationship of these findings to keratinocyte apoptosis and the clinical symptoms of itch are active areas of investigation.

TABLE 125-5
Differential Diagnosis of Cutaneous Amyloidoses

- *Interscapular:* lichen simplex chronicus; lichen sclerosis and atrophicus; postinflammatory hyperpigmentation; dorsal macular pigmentary incontinence; fixed drug eruption; notalgia paresthetica; poikiloderma; scleroderma/morphea
- *Shins:* prurigo nodularis; atopic eczema; pretibial myxedema; hypertrophic lichen planus
- *Nodules:* cutaneous lymphomas; nevus lipomatosis; nodular cutaneous neoplasms; nodular pseudolymphomas
- *Waxy deposits:* sebaceous keratosis; xanthomas
- *Periorbital purpura:* dermatomyositis/heliotrope; posttraumatic raccoon eyes
- *Pinch purpura:* vasculitic purpura; pigmented purpuric dermatoses; thrombocytopenic purpura; trichinosis

AN APPROACH TO THE DIAGNOSIS OF CUTANEOUS AMYLOIDOSIS

Table 125-4 outlines the diagnosis of patients with known or suspected cutaneous amyloidosis.

INITIAL EVALUATION

Patients with cutaneous amyloidosis may present to dermatologists for evaluation, or as referrals from specialists who suspect amyloid involving the skin. The specialist referral might be an individual in whom the diagnosis of systemic amyloid is suspected or known, and in whom skin lesions are to be examined and possibly studied pathologically; patients presenting to a dermatologist might include patients with cutaneous findings that include macular, lichen, or nodular amyloid in the differential diagnosis (Table 125-5).

Initial evaluation should include a cataloging of comorbid medical conditions, such as carpal tunnel syndrome or other forms of neuropathy, enquiry regarding easy bruising, petechial rash, or ecchymoses, localized areas of pruritus on the upper back or shins, a search for multiple lesions, pinch or periorbital purpura, and an evaluation for macroglossia or lateral ridging of the tongue. Macular or papular lesions should be examined for a waxy appearance suggestive of amyloidosis. Some patients may be able to volunteer a family history of amyloid diseases; others may be aware of multiple relatives known to have neuropathy, renal or cardiac disease, or affected by periodic fever syndromes. A family history of cutaneous disease may be relevant in considering a patient with suspected macular or lichen amyloidosis from Southeast Asia or South America.

TABLE 125-4
Diagnosis of Patients with Known or Suspected Cutaneous Amyloidosis

- *History:* evidence of systemic disease, and which organ systems may be involved; onset of disease in general and cutaneous lesions/pruritus in particular
- *Family history:* include ethnicity, and familial clustering of conditions known to be associated with amyloid
- *Laboratory:* immunoglobulin clonality for AL, elevated acute-phase reactants for AA, low TTR levels for ATTR
- *Genetic testing:* TTR, MEFV, RET, others in specialty laboratory test results
- *Skin lesions:* waxy deposits, macroglossia or lingual nodules; nodules, macules, lichen, and variants; single or multiple lesions; evidence of increased vascular fragility; hyperkeratosis/hyperpigmentation; cutis laxa
- *Biopsy:* lesional skin or abdominal fat pad; Congo red or thioflavin T; subpapillary amyloid or congophilic angiography/involvement of adnexa
- *Immunohistochemistry:* generic (eg, P-component), fibril subunit specific (L-chain, TTR, GAL7), or coassociating (keratin, actin)-specific antibodies; immunoelectron microscopy
- *Mass spectroscopy:* protein (AL variable; mutations) sequences and coassociating molecules

LABORATORY

In addition to routine studies, specific laboratory testing may be suggestive for certain forms of systemic amyloidosis. For both systemic and localized AL amyloidosis, this includes a measurement of quantitative immunoglobulins (IgG, IgA, and IgM isotypes), serum and urine immunofixation, and a measurement of serum κ and λ free light chains, which will identify a clonal population of immunoglobulin light chains in more than 95% of patients with systemic AL disease, and a much lower number of patients with localized AL disease. For AA, an elevated erythrocyte sedimentation rate, as well as specific acute-phase reactants, such as C-reactive protein and fibrinogen, serve as surrogates for elevated levels of SAA protein, which can directly be measured in panels of acute-phase reactants available for profiling rheumatoid arthritis or inflammatory bowel disease. For suspected ATTR, an assay for serum TTR levels and TTR gene-sequence analysis may serve to identify a specific mutations, although it should be noted that up to 25% of patients also are found to have monoclonal immunoglobulins as an incidental finding.

PATHOLOGY

Congo red binding to several forms of cutaneous amyloid may be weak and inferior to the use of thioflavin T or Pagoda red as diagnostic reagents; in addition, the interpretation of apple-green birefringence may be obscured by the small amount of amyloid in early lesions, and because of background white birefringence attributable to collagen in the dermis.[30] To this end, a modified Congo Red immunohistochemical overlay has been suggested to improve diagnosis,[43] and a luminescent conjugated oligothiophene, h-FTAA (heptamer formyl thiophene acetic acid), was developed to improve selectivity and sensitivity.[44] The immunohistochemistry of amyloid in tissue has proven to be a valuable adjunct to confirming proper diagnosis and guiding treatment, although its applicability to cutaneous amyloid presents certain caveats not found in other organ systems. A panel of polyclonal or monoclonal antibodies for the identification and typing of amyloid in tissue includes anti–P-component, anti-apoE, anti–κ Ig light chain, and anti–λ Ig light chain, anti-TTR, anti-AA, anti-β_2m, and generic or specific anti-keratin antibodies. In particular, the utility of antibodies to P-component as an immunohistologic surrogate marker for amyloid in tissue may be limited by the fact that this protein is an elastic fiber microfibrillar sheath-associated protein in normal skin,[45] as well as in cutis laxa associated with Meretoja syndrome,[9] and other dermal elastolytic conditions. Anti-TTR antibodies have been used to uncover amyloid in skin of patients with advanced ATTR (Fig. 125-15), and anti–keratin antibodies to type and define the distribution of localized cutaneous amyloidosis (Fig. 125-16). Among the organ-limited cutaneous amyloidoses, association with basal keratinocytes has been reflected in the identification of cytokeratin (CK)-5 as a major constituent of amyloid deposits and suggested a role of keratinocyte apoptosis in pathogenesis. In addition, other cytokeratins are positive immunochemically to varying degrees in lichen amyloidosis (CK5 > 1 > 14 > 10) and cutaneous amyloidosis associated with tumors and keratoses (CKL5 > 1 > 10 > 14).[17] For all forms of localized cutaneous amyloid, diagnosis may be improved by immunohistochemistry using pan CK antibodies, or monoclonal reagents, such as 34βE12 (anti–keratin 903), which is reactive with CK5, CK1, CK10, and CK14.[46] The identification of deposits as fibrils distinct from collagen or elastic fibers can be established by electron microscopy (Fig. 125-17). The utility of anti-κ or anti-λ antisera is limited by their specificity for determinants in the constant region of the Ig light chain, which may be lost during the proteolysis that is a concomitant of fibril

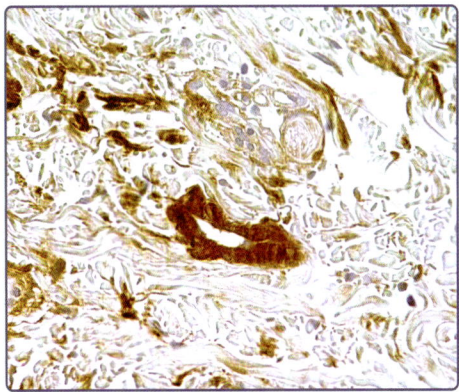

Figure 125-15 Anti-transthyretin (TTR) (prealbumin) antibodies highlighting a blood vessel in a patient with amyloidosis transthyretin (ATTR) amyloid attributable to familial amyloid polyneuropathy (hematoxylin and eosin (H&E), diaminobenzidine, ×10 magnification).

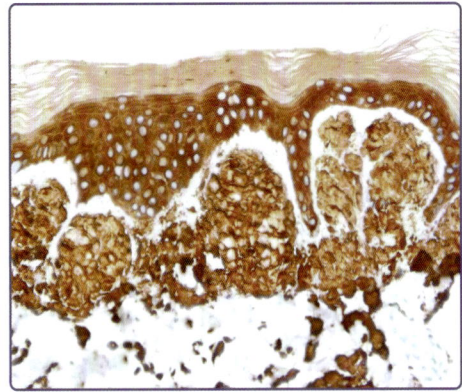

Figure 125-16 Anti–keratin 903 antibodies highlighting amyloid in expanded dermal papillae (hematoxylin and eosin (H&E), diaminobenzidine, ×4 magnification).

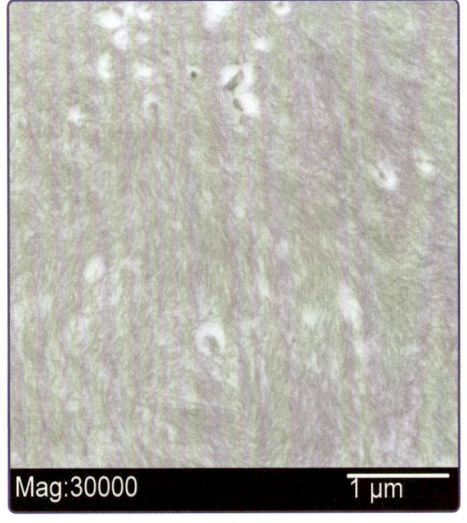

Figure 125-17 Electron micrograph showing thin filaments of amyloid in the dermis measuring 7 to 10 nm in thickness (uranyl acetate, lead citrate, ×30,000 magnification).

formation; improved specificity has been reported by immunofluorescence, using specific imaging dyes, and by immunoelectron microscopy. Treatment of tissue by autoclaving with potassium permanganate causes loss of Congo red affinity for AA and Aβ_2m; prolonged autoclaving affects binding of AL but not ATTR.[47] Although immunohistochemistry has been validated as a technique of typing amyloids in tissue section, antibodies specific for some forms are not yet commercially available, and the importance of in-house quality controls has been emphasized.[43]

BIOCHEMISTRY

The diagnostic value of skin biopsy as a noninvasive way to diagnose systemic amyloids was first reported in the 1970s, and has been perfected as the abdominal fat pad aspiration or fat pad biopsy, both of which are office procedures with minimal morbidity.[48] Aspiration has been used to screen for Congo red–positive material among fat globules (so-called fat rings), and can be modified for proteomic studies, quantitation of specific precursor proteins, and immunoelectron microscopy[49]; biopsy can be used to assess the morphology of amyloid in subcutaneous fat, for immunohistochemistry, and to isolate and sequence amyloid proteins by mass spectroscopy.[50] Using this technique, the diagnosis of AL can be established in 80% to 90% of cases, and AA in 75% to 80%, with a lower (~40%) yield for ATTR.[49] Laser capture microdissection of amyloid from formalin-fixed amyloidotic tissue, followed by trypsin digestion, mass spectroscopy, and direct sequence analysis of peptides, has been validated for the typing of amyloid in various tissues, including cutaneous lesions and abdominal fat pad biopsies. This methodology also has been adapted for the identification of pathogenic mutations in cases of hereditary amyloid and for the identification of Ig light chain subgroups in systemic and localized AL amyloidosis.[51] It also provides a profile of colocalizing proteins, such as P-component, keratins, and apoE, which may be important in pathogenesis.

TREATMENT STRATEGIES FOR AMYLOID DISEASES

SYSTEMIC AMYLOIDS

The onset of amyloid deposition may be preceded over many years by the presence of a mutant precursor protein, excess Ig light chain, or elevated SAA levels in blood; functional abnormalities, such as pruritus, may also anticipate the appearance of characteristic skin lesions or MTC in familial cases of lichen amyloidosis. Identification of genetic abnormalities, either reflecting fibril subunit proteins, proteolysis, or coassociating conditions, allows for the potential to identify persons at risk and initiate prophylactic therapies early in the course of disease. For the systemic amyloidoses, lowering the level of precursor protein correlates with clinical improvement and even regression of amyloid for SAA (with anticytokine therapy) and AL (with chemotherapies largely adapted from evolving myeloma protocols); in particular, the use of anti–IL-6 for AA amyloidosis, and high-dose dexamethasone, melphalan, thalidomide analogs, proteasome inhibitors, and anti-CD38 monoclonal antibodies have proven effective in reducing Ig light chain production by aberrant plasmablasts in AL amyloid.[13,52] Ongoing trials have demonstrated the ability of silencing RNAs and antisense oligonucleotides to knock down the levels of mutant and wildtype TTR in blood, and are assessing efficacy for the clinical manifestations of polyneuropathy and/or cardiomyopathy. An alternative approach that has reached licensing is to use TTR tetramer stabilizers (diflunisal/tafamidis) to prevent dissociation to the monomer stage, which is the direct precursor of oligomers, amorphous aggregates, and fibrils in ATTR.[53]

An alternative strategy is to focus on inhibiting the aggregation phenomena responsible for oligomerization or fibril formation. This may occur at the deposition phase of amyloid formation, or to interfere with formed fibrils by intercalating at the sites of intermolecular contact critical for β-pleated sheet formation. Agents that may be active as fibril disrupters that have progressed to clinical testing include (a) doxycycline (ATTR, AL, Aβ_2m), which disrupts fibril formation and mature fibrils, as well as inhibiting matrix metalloproteinase (MMP)-9; and the nutraceuticals[54]; (b) epigallocatechin-3-gallate (green tea) (ATTR, Aβ-Alzheimer disease; AApoA2, transforming growth factor (TGF) β$_1$-lattice corneal dystrophy, Type 1), which disrupts mature fibrils and suppresses markers of oxidative stress; and (c) curcumin (ATTR; Aβ), which induces oligomerization to a nontoxic "off pathway."[55] Low-molecular-weight aggregation inhibitors include β-sheet breaker peptides, Fab, scFv or single chain camelid nanobodies, and peptide inhibitors of adhesive segments.[56]

A third approach is to use immunotherapy to neutralize oligomers and facilitate the clearance of tissue amyloid. Critical to this approach is to design antibodies that are specific for shared conformational epitopes rather than the native precursor protein, accessibility to the target conformers, and the safe elicitation of macrophage-dependent clearance mechanisms. Currently, an anti-AL antibody with specificity for amyloid and oligomers is undergoing Phase III clinical trials, and antibodies to P-component are being tested as generic agents for systemic amyloids following depletion of serum, but not tissue amyloid–associated, SAP with a proline-derived small molecule that binds the pentamers together and facilitates their clearance from blood.[57,58]

THERAPY FOR CUTANEOUS AMYLOIDOSES

Currently, treatment of cutaneous manifestations associated with systemic amyloids has followed the general strategies outlined above.[17] However, accessibility of skin amyloid allows for direct delivery to the sites of pathology. Early studies used dimethylsulfoxide (DMSO), based on a suggestion that it might be able to disaggregate AL fibrils, possible antiinflammatory effects, and deep permeability at the sites of application; general applicability, however was limited by the acrid smell and difficulty in obtaining preparations that were free of contaminants. Newer studies in patients with macular and lichen amyloidosis have reported rapid and significant improvement in pruritus and hyperpigmentation, although not resolution of amyloid on followup biopsies.[59]

The main concern for nodular amyloid is the potential for progression to systemic AL, which has been reported as up to 50%; therefore, the main therapeutic challenge is to assess for monoclonal gammopathy and for other organ involvement. More rarely, evaluation of nodular amyloidosis may reveal that a patient has primary Sjögrens disease, a syndrome characterized by dry eyes and dry mouth (sicca syndrome) sometimes associated with major hematologic, pulmonary, GI or renal involvement. This may in turn suggest the use of systemic treatments for sicca (eg, sialogogues) or Disease Modifying Agents (DMARDs) such as hydroxychloroquine or methotrexate for systemic disease. Absent any indication of systemic AL, treatment is determined by the size, location, and multiplicity of the cutaneous nodules. Lesions in locations such as the foot or temple have been effectively treated with curettage, excision, and, rarely, intralesional methotrexate or ablative laser therapy; a 9% risk of local reoccurrence has been reported, and long-term followup recommended if localized AL is documented by special studies.[17,26]

Treatment of localized cutaneous amyloidoses overlaps the spectrum of macular and papular (lichen) variants, with a specific target of interrupting the cycle of pruritus, scratching, and lichenification. Common treatments that have been used in small series include topical and intralesional steroids, topical calcineurin inhibitors, low-dose oral cyclophosphamide, dermabrasion, and cyclosporine. Small series have reported successes with carbon dioxide resurfacing surgical laser, yttrium-aluminum-garnet laser, tocoretinate (a synthetic esterified compound of tocopherol and retinoic acid), narrowband ultraviolet B light therapy, and a combination of psoralen and ultraviolet A with acitretin. Resurfacing, neodymium-doped yttrium-aluminum-garnet, and pulsed-dye laser treatments have been recommended because of the lack of scarring or pigmentary changes; in some instances, improvement in histology and resolution of amyloid have been reported.[60]

In general, antihistamines are ineffective for the treatment of pruritus in this disorder, likely reflecting the lack of generation of histamine or involvement of histamine receptors in observed pathology. An alternative focus has been on the common occurrence of dysesthesias correlating with lichenoid skin lesions, and changes in epidermal nerve fiber density that have been demonstrated on biopsies. Topical capsaicin 0.025%, which releases neuropeptides from C-fibers, and prevents their deposition, may be tried, and there may be role for inhibitors of nonhistamine pruritogens and receptors currently being considered.[36] Lastly, antagonists of IL-31 receptors or its receptor have been under development for the treatment of atopic dermatitis, and might also have relevance to ameliorating the itch of lichen amyloidosis.[37]

ACKNOWLEDGMENTS

Research support from the Seaver Foundation is gratefully acknowledged.

REFERENCES

1. Kisilevsky R, Raimondi S, Bellotti V. Historical and current concepts of fibrillogenesis and in vivo amyloidogenesis: implications of amyloid tissue targeting. *Front Mol Biosci*. 2016;3:17.
2. Sipe JD, Benson MD, Buxbaum JN, et al. Amyloid fibril proteins and amyloidosis: chemical identification and clinical classification International Society of Amyloidosis 2016 Nomenclature Guidelines. *Amyloid*. 2016;23(4):209-213.
3. Gorevic PD. Genetic factors in the amyloid diseases. *Up-To-Date*. 2016.
4. Merlini G, Bellotti V. Molecular mechanisms of amyloidosis. *N Engl J Med*. 2003;349(6):583-596.
5. Pinney JH, Smith CJ, Taube JB, et al. Systemic amyloidosis in England: an epidemiological study. *Br J Haematol*. 2013;161:525-532.
6. Wechalekar AD, Gillmore JD, Hawkins PN. Systemic amyloidosis. *Lancet*. 2016;387(10038):2641-2654.
7. Brownstein MH, Helwig EB. The cutaneous amyloidoses. II. Systemic forms. *Arch Dermatol*. 1970;102(1):20-28.
8. Lanoue J, Wei N, Gorevic P, et al. Cutaneous manifestations of familial transthyretin amyloid polyneuropathy. *Am J Dermatopathol*. 2016;38(10):719-725.
9. Kiuru-Enari S, Keski-Oja J, Haltia M. Cutis laxa in hereditary gelsolin amyloidosis. *Br J Dermatol*. 2005;152(2):250-257.
10. Muscardin L, Cota C, Donati P, et al. Hereditary apolipoprotein A1 amyloidosis with cutaneous and cardiac involvement: a long familial history. *Eur J Dermatol*. 2014;24(2):261-263.
11. Sattianayagam PT, Gibbs SD, Rowczenio D, et al. Hereditary lysozyme amyloidosis—phenotypic heterogeneity and the role of solid organ transplantation. *J Intern Med*. 2012;272(1):36-44.
12. Benedikz E, Blöndal H, Gudmundsson G. Skin deposits in hereditary cystatin C amyloidosis. *Virchows Arch A Pathol Anat Histopathol*. 1990;417(4):325-331.
13. Nienhuis HL, Bijzet J, Hazenberg BP. The prevalence and management of systemic amyloidosis in western countries. *Kidney Dis (Basel)*. 2016;2(1):10-19.
14. Jacobson DR, Alexander AA, Tagoe C, et al. The prevalence and distribution of the amyloidogenic transthyretin (TTR) V122I allele in Africa. *Mol Genet Genomic Med*. 2016;4(5):548-556.
15. Mahmood S, Bridoux F, Venner CP, et al. Natural history and outcomes in localised immunoglobulin light-chain amyloidosis: a long-term observational study. *Lancet Haematol*. 2015;2(6):e241-e250.

16. Brownstein MH, Helwig EB. The cutaneous amyloidoses. I. Localized forms. *Arch Dermatol*. 1970;102(1):8-19.
17. Schreml S, Szeimies RM, Vogt T, et al. Cutaneous amyloidoses and systemic amyloidoses with cutaneous involvement. *Eur J Dermatol*. 2010;20(2):152-160.
18. Haverkampf S, Evert K, Schröder J, et al. Nodular cutaneous amyloidosis resembling a giant tumor. *Case Rep Dermatol*. 2016;8(1):22-25.
19. Brownstein MH, Hashimoto K, Greenwald G. Biphasic amyloidosis: link between macular and lichenoid forms. *Br J Dermatol*. 1973;88(1):25-29.
20. Yoshida A, Takahashi K, Tagami H, et al. Lichen amyloidosis induced on the upper back by long-term friction with a nylon towel. *J Dermatol*. 2009;36(1):56-59.
21. Wang WJ, Huang CY, Chang YT, et al. Anosacral cutaneous amyloidosis: a study of 10 Chinese cases. *Br J Dermatol*. 2000;143(6):1266-1269.
22. Bernhard JD. Macular amyloidosis, notalgia paresthetica and pruritus: three sides of the same coin? *Dermatologica*. 1991;183(1):53-54.
23. Mysore V, Bhushnurmath SR, Muirhead DE, et al. Frictional amyloidosis in Oman—a study of ten cases. *Indian J Dermatol Venereol Leprol*. 2002;68(1):28-32.
24. Siragusa M, Ferri R, Cavallari V, et al. Friction melanosis, friction amyloidosis, macular amyloidosis, towel melanosis: many names for the same clinical entity. *Eur J Dermatol*. 2001;11(6):545-548.
25. Kandhari R, Ramesh V, Singh A. Asymptomatic conchal papules. Lichen amyloidosis of the auricular concha. *Indian J Dermatol Venereol Leprol*. 2013;79(3):445-447.
26. Konopinski JC, Seyfer SJ, Robbins KL, et al. A case of nodular cutaneous amyloidosis and review of the literature. *Dermatol Online J*. 2013;19(4):10.
27. Wey SJ, Chen YM, Lai PJ, et al. Primary Sjögren syndrome manifested as localized cutaneous nodular amyloidosis. *J Clin Rheumatol*. 2011;17(7):368-370.
28. Gargallo V, Angulo L, Hernández E, et al. Massive subcutaneous masses on the back related to β2-microglobulin amyloidosis. *JAMA Dermatol*. 2015;151(5):564-565.
29. Apaydin R, Gürbüz Y, Bayramgürler D, et al. Cytokeratin contents of basal cell carcinoma, epidermis overlying tumour, and associated stromal amyloidosis: an immunohistochemical study. *Amyloid*. 2005;12(1):41-47.
30. Westermark P. Localized amyloidoses and amyloidoses associated with aging outside the central nervous system. In: Pickens MM, Dogan A, Herrera GA, eds. *Amyloid and Related Disorders: Surgical Pathology and Clinical Correlations*. New York, NY: Humana Press; 2012:81-103.
31. D'Souza A, Theis JD, Vrana JA, et al. Pharmaceutical amyloidosis associated with subcutaneous insulin and enfuvirtide administration. *Amyloid*. 2014;21(2):71-75.
32. Fernandes, NF, Mercer SE, Kleinerman R, et al. Amyloidosis cutis dyschromica associated with atypical Parkinsonism, spasticity and motor weakness in a Pakistani female. *J Cutan Pathol*. 2011;38(10):827-831.
33. Mahon C, Oliver F, Purvis D, et al. Amyloidosis cutis dyschromica in two siblings and review of the epidemiology, clinical features and management in 48 cases. *Australas J Dermatol*. 2015. [Epub ahead of print]
34. Scapineli JO, Ceolin L, Puñales MK, et al. MEN 2A-related cutaneous lichen amyloidosis: report of three kindred and systematic literature review of clinical, biochemical and molecular characteristics. *Fam Cancer*. 2016;15(4):625-633.
35. Qi XP, Zhao JQ, Chen ZG, et al. RET mutation p.S891A in a Chinese family with familial medullary thyroid carcinoma and associated cutaneous amyloidosis binding OSMR variant p.G513D. *Oncotarget*. 2015;6(32):33993-34003.
36. Sanders KM, Nattkemper LA, Yosipovitch G. Advances in understanding itching and scratching: a new era of targeted treatments. *F1000Res*. 2016;5.
37. Cevikbas F, Kempkes C, Buhl T, et al. Role of interleukin-31 and oncostatin M in itch and neuroimmune communication. In: Carstens E, Akiyama T, eds. *Itch: Mechanisms and Treatment*. Boca Raton, FL: CRC Press; 2014.
38. Wali A, Liu L, Takeichi T, et al. Familial primary localized cutaneous amyloidosis results from either dominant or recessive mutations in OSMR. *Acta Derm Venereol*. 2015;95(8):1005-1007.
39. Tanaka A, Arita K, Lai-Cheong JE, et al. New insight into mechanisms of pruritus from molecular studies on familial primary localized cutaneous amyloidosis. *Br J Dermatol*. 2009;161(6):1217-1224.
40. Dousset L, Seneschal J, Boniface K, et al. A Th2 cytokine interleukin-31 signature in a case of sporadic lichen amyloidosis. *Acta Derm Venereol*. 2015;95(2):223-224.
41. Miura Y, Harumiya S, Ono K, et al. Galectin-7 and actin are components of amyloid deposit of localized cutaneous amyloidosis. *Exp Dermatol*. 2013;22(1):36-40.
42. Ono K, Fujimoto E, Fujimoto N, et al. In vitro amyloidogenic peptides of galectin-7: possible mechanism of amyloidogenesis of primary localized cutaneous amyloidosis. *J Biol Chem*. 2014;289(42):29195-29207.
43. Linke RP. On typing amyloidosis using immunohistochemistry. Detailed illustrations, review and a note on mass spectrometry. *Prog Histochem Cytochem*. 2012;47(2):61-132.
44. Sjölander D, Röcken C, Westermark P, et al. Establishing the fluorescent amyloid ligand h-FTAA for studying human tissues with systemic and localized amyloid. *Amyloid*. 2016;23(2):98-108.
45. Breathnach SM, Hintner H. Amyloid P-component and the skin. *Clin Dermatol*. 1990;8(2):46-54.
46. Yoneda, K. Watanabe H, Yanagihara M, et al. Immunohistochemical staining properties of amyloids with anti-keratin antibodies using formalin-fixed, paraffin-embedded sections. *J Cutan Pathol*. 1989;16(3):133-136.
47. Fernandez-Flores A. Cutaneous amyloidosis: a concept review. *Am J Dermatopathol*. 2012;34(1):1-14.
48. Westermark P. Amyloid diagnosis, subcutaneous adipose tissue, immunohistochemistry and mass spectrometry. *Amyloid*. 2011;18:175-176.
49. Brambilla F, Lavatelli F, Di Silvestre D, et al. Reliable typing of systemic amyloidoses through proteomic analysis of subcutaneous adipose tissue. *Blood*. 2012;119(8):1844-1847.
50. Vrana JA, Theis JD, Dasari S, et al. Clinical diagnosis and typing of systemic amyloidosis in subcutaneous fat aspirates by mass spectrometry-based proteomics. *Haematologica*. 2014;99(7):1239-1247.
51. Kourelis TV, Dasari S, Theis JD, et al. Clarifying immunoglobulin gene usage in systemic and localized immunoglobulin light chain amyloidosis by mass spectrometry. *Blood*. 2017;129(3):299-306.
52. Muchtar E, Buadi FK, Dispenzieri A, et al. Immunoglobulin light-chain amyloidosis: from basics to new developments in diagnosis, prognosis and therapy. *Acta Haematol*. 2016;135(3):172-190.
53. Gertz MA, Benson MD, Dyck PJ, et al. Diagnosis, prognosis, and therapy of transthyretin amyloidosis. *J Am Coll Cardiol*. 2015;66(21):2451-2466.

54. Stoilova T, Colombo L, Forloni G, et al. A new face for old antibiotics: tetracyclines in treatment of amyloidoses. *J Med Chem*. 2013;56(15):5987-6006.
55. Stefani M, Rigacci S. Beneficial properties of natural phenols: highlight on protection against pathological conditions associated with amyloid aggregation. *Biofactors*. 2014;40(5):482-493.
56. De Genst E, Messer A, Dobson CM. Antibodies and protein misfolding: from structural research tools to therapeutic strategies. *Biochim Biophys Acta*. 2014;1844(11):1907-1919.
57. Gertz MA, Landau H, Comenzo RL, et al. First-in-human phase I/II study of NEOD001 in patients with light chain amyloidosis and persistent organ dysfunction. *J Clin Oncol*. 2016;34(10):1097-1103.
58. Richards DB, Cookson LM, Berges AC, et al. Therapeutic clearance of amyloid by antibodies to serum amyloid P component. *N Engl J Med*. 2015;373(12):1106-1114.
59. Krishna A, Nath B, Dhir GG, et al. Study on epidemiology of cutaneous amyloidosis in northern India and effectiveness of dimethylsulphoxide in cutaneous amyloidosis. *Indian Dermatol Online J*. 2012;3(3):182-186.
60. Al Yahya RS. Treatment of primary cutaneous amyloidosis with laser: a review of the literature. *Lasers Med Sci*. 2016;31(5):1027-1035.

Chapter 126 :: Xanthomas and Lipoprotein Disorders
:: Vasanth Sathiyakumar, Steven R. Jones, & Seth S. Martin

第一百二十六章
黄色瘤和脂蛋白紊乱

中文导读

黄色瘤主要是指由皮肤或肌腱中多余的脂质堆积而成的斑块或结节，其本身并不是一种疾病，是各种脂蛋白紊乱的征兆，可能源于原发性血脂异常，也可能是系统性疾病导致继发性血脂异常所引起的皮肤改变。本章分7节：①历史视角；②流行病学；③临床特点；④病因和发病机制；⑤诊断；⑥鉴别诊断；⑦临床管理。

第一节历史视角，介绍了对临床黄色瘤的认识早于现代血脂异常几十年，黄色瘤的分类随着对血脂异常病因的发现而不断完善，介绍了各大指南指出的监测血脂的重要性。

第二节介绍了不同种族间血脂异常患病率无明显差异。血脂异常继发性病因的流行更为明显，包括糖尿病、甲状腺功能障碍、慢性肾脏疾病等，但在这些患者中黄色瘤的直接患病率尚不清楚。

第三节介绍了黄色瘤的皮肤表现、其他表现及并发症。临床上分为发疹型、结节型、腱状型或平面型，分布部位不一。部分特殊黄色瘤可累及黏膜，也可累及内脏器官、眼部结构、中枢神经系统和骨骼系统。其并发症包括美容和功能缺陷或局部疼痛，眼部受累可引起失明等，若由严重的全身性疾病引起还可导致死亡。

第四节介绍了黄色瘤形成的主要原因是血清乳糜微粒和脂蛋白的积累，最终沉积在皮肤内。其病因分为：原发性血脂异常，可能带有遗传或家族成分；继发性血脂异常，通常是后天性的，但可能暴露出潜在的遗传易感性；或正常血脂状态，其中没有潜在的血脂异常。

第五节介绍了黄色瘤的准确诊断可发现潜在的全身性疾病或高脂血症，有助于确定早期生活方式和治疗方案，减缓临床动脉粥样硬化性心血管疾病的进展。目前诊断手段包括支持性研究和实验室检测手段、组织病理学和影像学检查。

第六节表126-1概述了黄色瘤、平面黄色瘤、发疹性黄瘤、腱性和结节性黄瘤、疣状黄瘤和播散性黄瘤的鉴别诊断。

第七节介绍了黄色瘤治疗的基石包括解决潜在的高脂血症，通常是通过改变生活方式和药物治疗，此外手术、冷冻或激光等用于美容目的，同时提到了咨询和筛查的重要性。

〔粟　娟〕

AT-A-GLANCE

- Xanthomas are plaques or nodules consisting of an abnormal excess of lipid primarily in the skin or tendons.

- Clinically, xanthomas may be divided into eruptive, tuber-eruptive or tuberous, tendinous, or planar forms. Two traditionally noninherited variations include verruciform and disseminated xanthomas, both of which have a propensity for largely noncutaneous manifestations.

- Xanthomas are not disease entities themselves but are signs of various lipoprotein disorders, which may be primary lipid disorders or secondary disorders from a variety of causes including hepatic, hematologic, and endocrine sources.

- The key pathogenesis of xanthoma formation consists of the downstream formation of foam cells, which involves an interplay of various lipoproteins including chylomicrons, very-low-density lipoproteins (VLDLs), chylomicron and VLDL remnant lipoproteins, low-density lipoproteins, and high-density lipoproteins.

- Primary dyslipidemias, designated as Types I to V, have been historically categorized into various phenotypes described by Fredrickson, Levy, and Lees, based on the elevated lipoprotein fractions found in serum.

- Diagnosis of xanthoma is based on clinical and morphologic characteristics of the lesions and identifying the underlying lipid disorder.

- Treatment of xanthoma is aimed at the underlying lipid disorder, and typically involves lifestyle changes (diet, weight loss, smoking cessation) and medications (statins, adjuvant agents, PCSK9 inhibitors).

- Young patients with xanthomas and those with suspected familial dyslipidemias should be referred for genetic testing and counseling.

DEFINITIONS

Xanthomas are plaques or nodules consisting of an accumulation of excess of lipid primarily in the skin or tendons, resulting in the formation of foam cells. Not a disease entity in themselves, xanthomas are signs of various lipoprotein disorders and are occasionally seen without underlying metabolic effects. Xanthomas may arise from primary dyslipidemias or may be the cutaneous manifestations of systemic disorders resulting in secondary dyslipidemia.

HISTORICAL PERSPECTIVE

Primary dyslipidemias have been traditionally grouped into 6 major phenotypes (Types I, IIa, IIb, III, IV, and V) classified by Fredrickson, Levy, and Lees in a series of seminal papers from the 1960s.[1] By visually assessing samples of patient serum and directly measuring cholesterol content through ultracentrifugation, precipitation, and electrophoresis techniques, Fredrickson, Levy, and Lees quantified the size, composition, and density of various lipoproteins, including chylomicrons, low-density lipoprotein (LDL), and very-low-density lipoprotein (VLDL). At the time of publication, 5 phenotypes were proposed based on the predominant lipoprotein present in serum with a sixth phenotype later added to this scheme in the 1970s by Goldstein and colleagues.[2]

The World Health Organization formally adopted the Fredrickson-Levy-Lees classification in 1972 using a biochemical phenotypic classification and incorporated clinical dyslipidemias associated with the various combinations of elevated apolipoprotein B (apoB) containing lipoproteins. Interestingly, the adoption of the Fredrickson-Levy-Lees classification occurred prior to the recognition of HDL as an important contributor to dyslipidemia. Although the basis of these definitions is rooted in which serum lipoprotein is elevated; as of this writing there is no consensus on absolute values used to define an excess state. However, after the discovery of apolipoprotein E (apoE) as a significant factor in dyslipidemia development in the 1970s, increasing use of genetic testing involving quantification and identifying mutations in apolipoproteins has helped confirm the diagnosis for many patients with primary dyslipidemias.

Since the adaptation of the World Health Organization classification, various systemic diseases have been linked to secondary dyslipidemias and xanthoma formation, including nephrotic syndrome, hepatic abnormalities, and thyroid dysfunction. These disease entities are increasingly recognized as important causes of dyslipidemia.

Yet, the recognition of clinical xanthomas predated the modern-day characterization of dyslipidemias by decades. Planar xanthomas were first reported in the medical literature in the early 1900s. Xanthoma disseminatum was described in 1938, and diffuse normolipemic plane xanthoma was first reported in 1962.[3]

Regardless of the etiology of dyslipidemia—primary or secondary—worldwide clinical lipid guidelines emphasize the importance of monitoring dyslipidemia to initiate and intensify therapy directed at non-HDL, apoB-containing lipoproteins. The 2002 National Cholesterol Education Program guidelines focused on low-density lipoprotein cholesterol (LDL-C) as the main target for disease management.[4] The 2013 American College of Cardiology/American Heart Association joint *Guideline on the Treatment of Blood Cholesterol* recognized dyslipidemia as a modifiable risk factor in patients with known atherosclerotic cardiovascular disease, and recommended primary prevention statin-therapy for high-risk patients.[5] In 2016, the American College of Cardiology released an Expert Consensus Statement highlighting the role of nonstatin therapies for further LDL-C lowering in patients with dyslipidemia.[6]

EPIDEMIOLOGY

Because xanthomas are signs of underlying dyslipidemia, little data is available regarding the prevalence of xanthomas themselves. Xanthelasmas, a specific type of xanthoma involving the eyelids, constitute 6% of eyelid tumors according to one study.[7] There is no specific age or gender bias toward xanthoma formation, except in the rare xanthoma disseminatum variation that tends to affect younger males in a 2:1 predilection compared to younger females, and in patients with homozygous familial hypercholesterolemia in which xanthomas may be seen as early as the first decade of life.[3]

However, identifying the prevalence of underlying dyslipidemia—either primary or secondary—may serve as a surrogate predictor for possible xanthoma formation. Based on the National Health and Nutrition Examination Survey, a cross-population sample of children and adults living in the United States, an estimated 53% of all U.S. adults have some form of lipid abnormalities, with 27% of adults manifesting high LDL-C and 30% with high triglyceride levels. Nearly 21% of U.S. adults have multiple lipid abnormalities.[8] Even among children and adolescents, almost 20% were reported to have some form of dyslipidemia.[9] When assessing hyperlipidemias within the Multi-Ethnic Study of Atherosclerosis, nearly 30% were characterized with dyslipidemias. The Multi-Ethnic Study of Atherosclerosis study includes participants from 4 major race groups, namely, whites, African Americans, Hispanic Americans, and Chinese Americans. There were no significant differences in the prevalence of dyslipidemia among the races.[10]

Excluding familial hypercholesterolemia (Type IIa), which has a prevalence in the United States and in Europe in the range of 1 in 200 to 250 individuals with upwards of 34 million patients diagnosed worldwide, relatively few studies have directly assessed the prevalence of the Fredrickson-Levy-Lees phenotypes in large, modern, crosspopulation cohorts.[11,12] In a cross-population cohort from the Very Large Database of Lipids study, the prevalence of the various phenotypes were as follows: Type I <0.01%; Type IIa 4.5%; Type IIb 1.7%; Type III 0.1%; Type IV 7.5%; and Type V 0.04%. These frequencies changed depending on concomitant HDL levels, such that at lower HDL levels the frequencies of Types IIb, IV, and V increased. The opposite trend was seen with the Type IIa phenotype. Smaller studies have suggested Types IIa (7%), IV (41%), and IIb (51%) are relatively common among primary dyslipidemias, with Types I, III, and V much more uncommon.[13]

Lipoprotein lipase and apolipoprotein CII deficiencies are identified causes of the Type I phenotype yet only range from less than 1 to 1-2 per 1 million in the general population. Genetic studies suggest founder populations in Canada and the Netherlands, where prevalence is still rare but slightly increased to 20 per million in the general population. Familial combined dyslipidemia (Type IIb) is found in 0.5% to 2% of the general population and in upwards of 10% in those with known cardiovascular disease. Dysbetalipoproteinemia, or the Type III phenotype, is reported in 1 in 10,000 adults and familial hypertriglyceridemia has been reported to have a population prevalence of 0.5 to 1.0 in 10,000 adults.[14,15]

The prevalence of secondary causes of dyslipidemias is more readily apparent. Nearly 10% of Americans have diabetes; upwards of 12% of the U.S. population will develop some form of thyroid dysfunction; and nearly 14% of Americans have a form of chronic kidney disease.[16,17] However, of those who have a form of dyslipidemia or are at risk of developing dyslipidemia from a secondary cause, the direct prevalence of xanthomas is unknown.

CLINICAL FEATURES

CUTANEOUS FINDINGS

Xanthomas are clinically divided into eruptive, tuberoeruptive or tuberous, tendinous, or planar forms.[18] Two traditionally noninherited variations are verruciform and disseminated xanthomas, both of which have a propensity for largely noncutaneous manifestations.

Eruptive xanthomas are multiple, small, red-yellow papules, usually less than 5 mm in size, that may appear suddenly and are arranged in crops on the extensor surface of the extremities and the buttocks, often forming a confluent rash (Fig. 126-1).[19] They are associated with severe hypertriglyceridemia, usually resulting from accumulation of chylomicrons as in Types I and V dyslipidemia, and may be aggravated by underlying diabetes, obesity, excessive ethanol intake, and drugs such as retinoids, estrogen therapy, and protease inhibitors (Fig. 126-2). Eruptive xanthomas also follow the Koebner phenomenon; that is, lesions may appear secondary to direct skin trauma.

Tuberous xanthomas are nodules that are localized to pressure areas including the extensor surfaces of the elbows, knees, knuckles, and buttocks (Figs. 126-3 and 126-4).[20] Rarely, they can be found on the face.

Tendinous xanthomas are firm, subcutaneous nodules found in fascia, ligaments, Achilles tendons, or extensor tendons of the hands, knees, and elbows (Fig. 126-5 and 126-6).[21] They may occasionally appear as tophus-like lesions over the great toe and be mistaken for gout, and may be uncovered by direct trauma.

Planar xanthomas are yellow macules, soft papules, or plaques found commonly on the upper eyelids near the inner canthus (xanthelasma palpebrarum or xanthelasma), the wrists and palms (xanthoma striatum palmare), and in intertriginous areas (Fig. 126-7 and 126-8).[22] Xanthelasmas may be found in patients with elevated LDL-C levels, but most often occur in patients with relatively normal lipid levels and the occurrence of these lesions on the eyelids is usually not associated

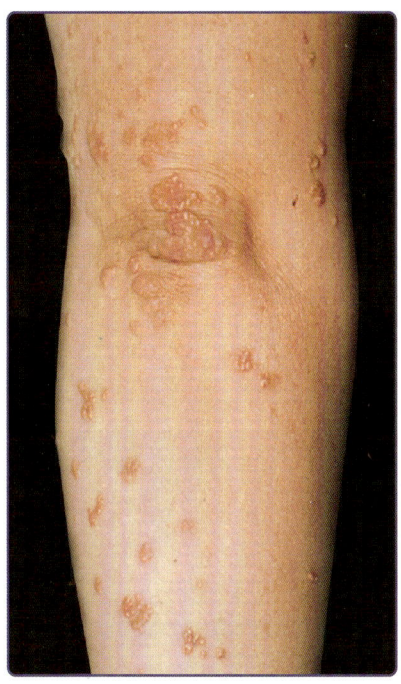

Figure 126-1 Example of eruptive xanthoma.

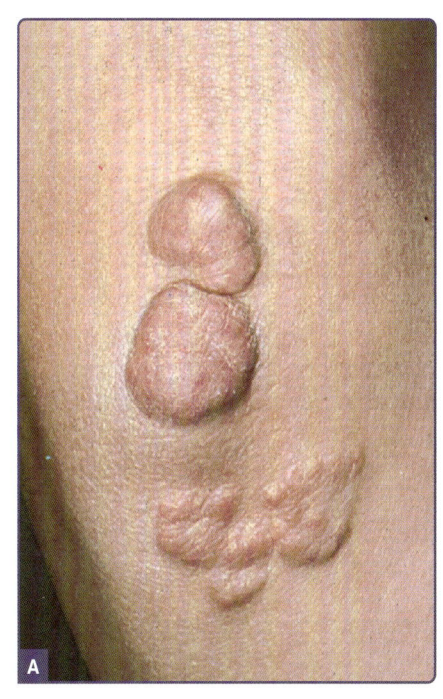

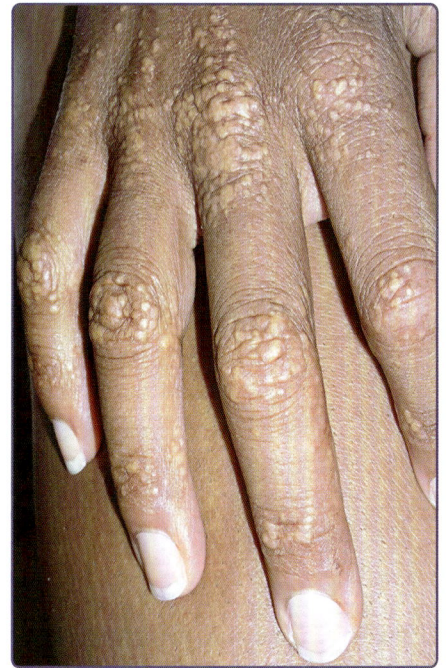

Figure 126-2 Example of eruptive xanthoma in a patient with severe chylomicronemia.

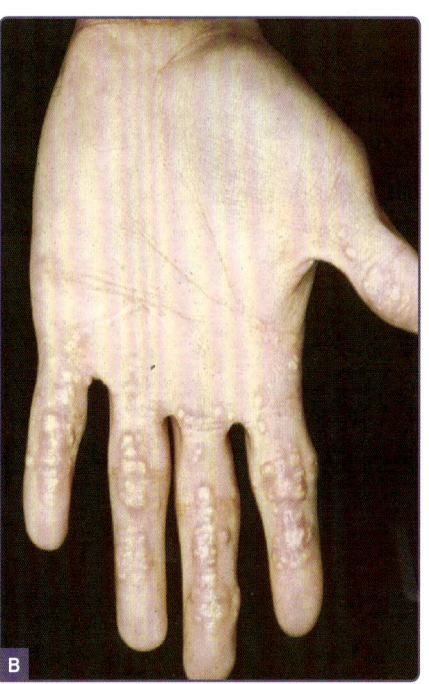

Figure 126-3 Examples of tuberoeruptive and tuberous xanthomas. **A,** Knee. **B,** Palm.

with coronary heart disease.[23] A variation of this disorder, known as giant xanthelasma palpebrarum, may involve all 4 eyelids.

Patients with Type III dyslipidemia and accumulation of chylomicron and VLDL remnant lipoproteins may develop a characteristic variant xanthoma characterized by yellow-orange discoloration of the cutaneous creases of the palmar skin.[24-26]

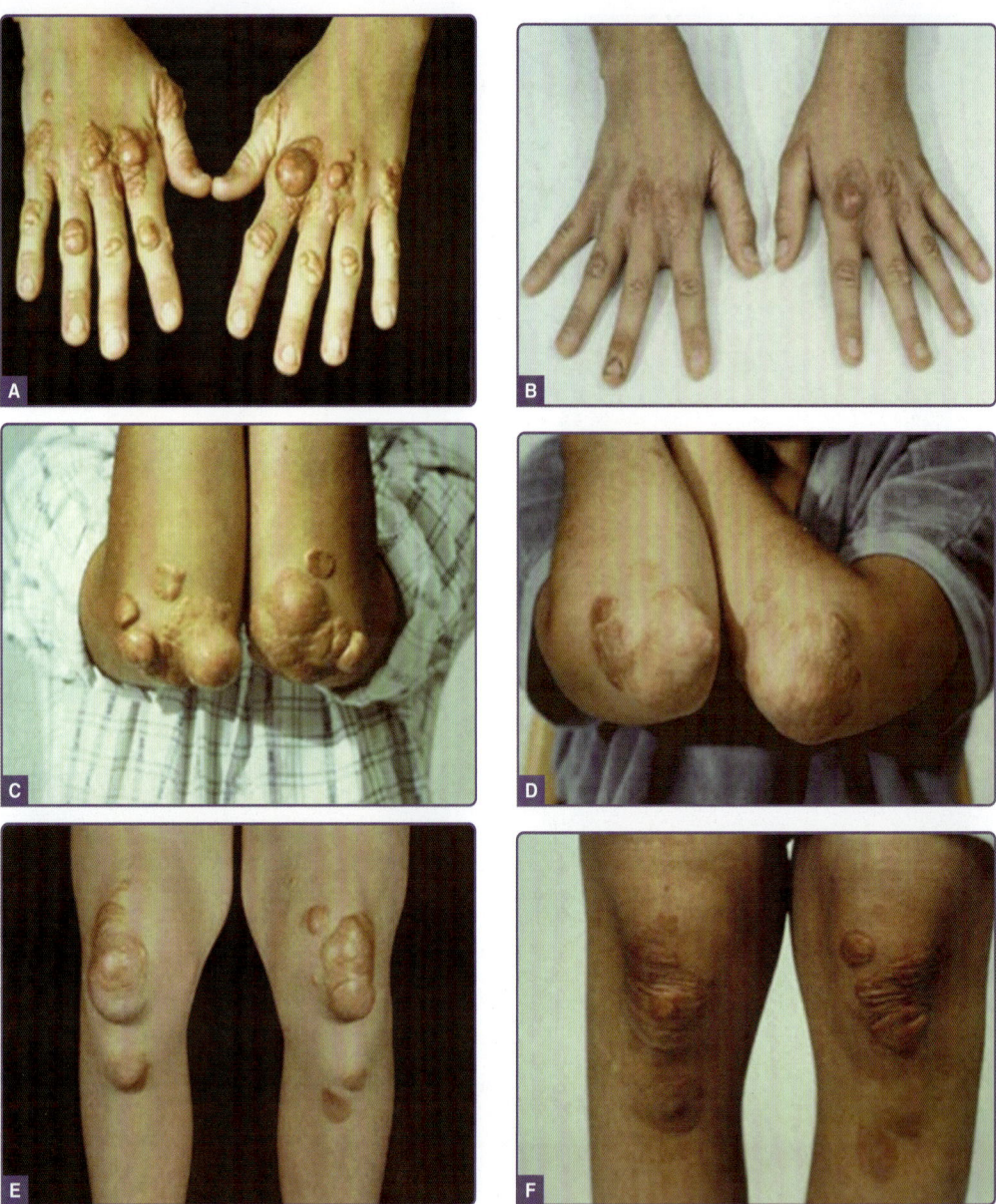

Figure 126-4 Examples of tuberoeruptive xanthomas. **A, B,** Hands. **C, D,** Elbows. **E, F,** Knees. Panels **D, E,** and **F** demonstrate regression of these lesions after lipid-lowering therapy.

NONCUTANEOUS FINDINGS

Patients with verruciform xanthoma mainly have oral mucosal involvement with lesions appearing in polypoid or sessile forms.[27] Cutaneous lesions are largely limited to the perineum and scrotum in males, and are associated with the CHILD (congenital hemidysplasia with ichthyosiform erythroderma and limb defects) syndrome or epidermolysis bullosa.

Xanthoma disseminatum involves xanthoma formation and histiocyte proliferation within common mucocutaneous sites, but also can involve visceral organs, ocular structures, the CNS, and the skeletal system.[28-30] Without any known familial inheritance, the disease is thought to evolve as a reactive phenomenon with only a handful of cases reported in medical literature over the past century. Variations of the disease include a persistent form, a progressive form with systemic involvement, and an uncommon self-limited disease state. Because all types of xanthoma are associated with underlying dyslipidemia, noncutaneous findings may also include atherosclerotic disease in any vascular bed. However, most clinically important lesions include coronary atherosclerosis, carotid stenosis, peripheral vascular disease, and intracranial lesions.

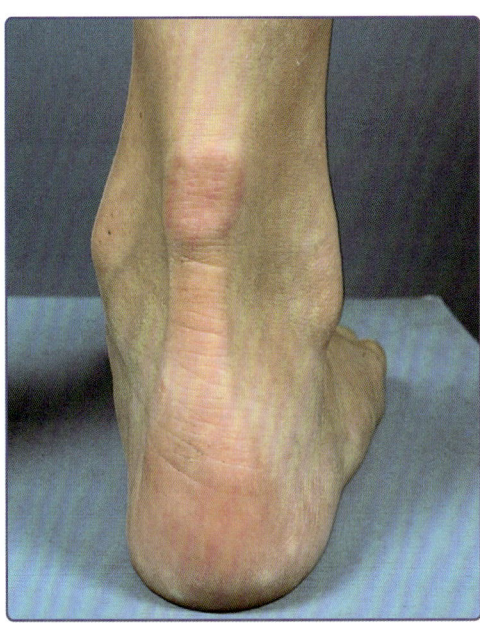

Figure 126-5 Example of tendon xanthoma.

A subset of patients with tendinous xanthomas develop cerebrotendinous xanthomas, which manifest as intracranial lesions causing neurologic dysfunction, including dementia and cerebellar ataxia.[31] These patients have only modest elevations in plasma cholesterol levels, and are unable to convert cholesterol to chenodeoxycholate, a major bile acid, because of defects in the sterol 27-hydroxylase gene. The result of this defect is accumulation of cholestanol, which can be noted by gas chromatography.[32] The condition is inherited in an autosomal recessive pattern. Typical treatment consists of chenodeoxycholic acid in concert with statin therapy.[33,34]

Some patients may develop sitosterolemia, or a retention and elevation of plant-based sterols in the serum. This condition is caused by a mutation of the ABCG5/G8 transporter (discussed in "Pathogenesis" section), which is important for intestinal absorption of sterols. These patients may develop tendinous xanthomas with the overall clinical picture imitating familial hypercholesterolemia (also discussed in "Primary (Genetic) Dyslipidemias" section). Distinguishing this entity from familial hypercholesterolemia is important, as first-line therapy consists of ezetimibe, usually in combination with statin-based therapy, and sometimes bile acid sequestrants.

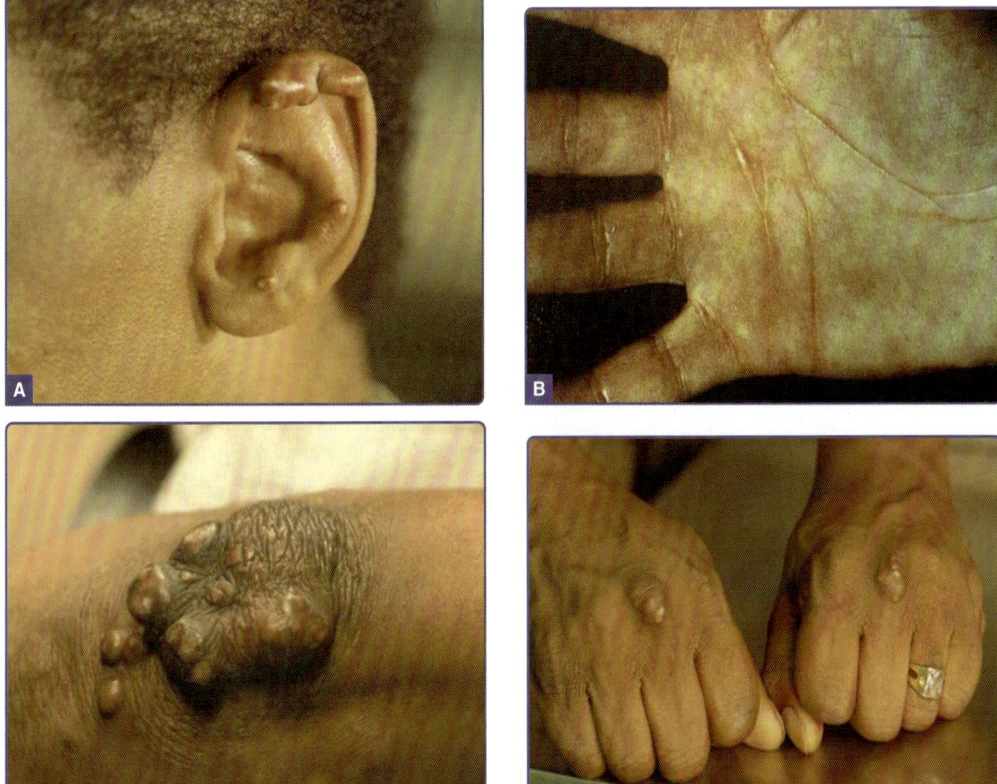

Figure 126-6 Examples of tuberoeruptive xanthomas. **A,** Ears. **C,** Elbows. **D,** Hands. **B,** An example of a palmar xanthoma is seen in the hand creases.

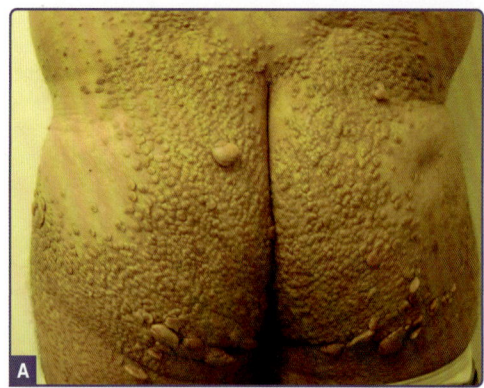

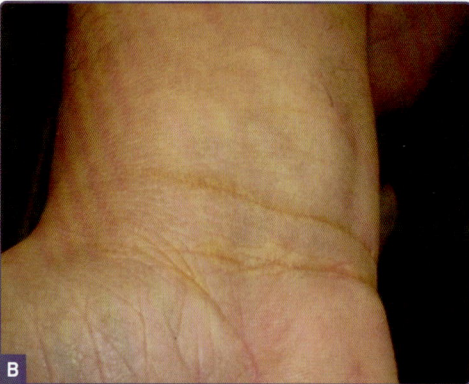

Figure 126-7 Examples of tuberoeruptive and palmar xanthomas in a patient with apoAI deficiency. **A,** Located in the lower back and buttocks. **B,** Palmar xanthomas.

COMPLICATIONS

Morbidity from cutaneous xanthomas is largely limited to cosmetic and functional defects or localized pain depending on the site of involvement. Patients with flexural surface lesions may have restricted range of motion, whereas those with xanthelasmas may develop obstructive blindness. However, any further morbidity or mortality from isolated cutaneous lesions is rare.

Nonetheless, various case reports have linked the presence of cutaneous xanthomas to underlying systemic diseases other than primary disorders of lipid metabolism, which carry significant mortality. For example, planar xanthomas may be the first sign of underlying hematologic abnormalities and may be associated with chronic microcytic anemia or hematologic malignancies.[22,35,36]

Patients with xanthoma disseminatum are at further increased risk for morbidity. Involvement of the GI tract may result in dysphagia, whereas airway involvement may cause dyspnea. Ocular involvement may involve the cornea or conjunctiva and lead to blindness.[37] Intracranial lesions may present similarly as cerebrotendinous xanthoma and can cause a number of motor or sensory deficits secondary to hydrocephalus or epileptic episodes. Involvement of the skeletal system may result in subclinical osteolytic lesions, overt fractures, or the development of rheumatoid arthritis.[28] Rarer forms are associated with Budd-Chiari syndrome and may result in marked hepatic dysfunction.

Mortality in patients with xanthomas stems from the underlying dyslipidemia, which places patients at increased risk for clinical atherosclerotic cardiovascular disease, including obstructive atherosclerosis, myocardial infarction, and stroke. Patients with severely elevated triglycerides resulting from accumulation of chylomicrons are prone to significant morbidity from repeated episodes of acute pancreatitis.

ETIOLOGY AND PATHOGENESIS

PATHOGENESIS

The key pathogenesis of xanthoma formation results from accumulations of serum chylomicrons and lipoproteins, which eventually deposit within the skin. After diffusion of serum lipoproteins through capillary walls and deposition in skin and tendons, monocytes incorporate LDL and other lipid subtypes through scavenger receptors. This results in the formation of foam cells, which clinically manifest as xanthomas. Foam cells may also develop secondary to in situ lipid synthesis by the macrophage itself, and lipid that has been extravasated by the capillaries may also recruit additional foam cells into an already established xanthoma by inducing vascular cellular adhesion.[38,39] Local factors, such as heat, movement, and friction, may increase lipid capillary leakage and lead to underlying inflammation and recruitment of macrophages, resulting in downstream formation of xanthomas. Because of the central role of lipids in the formation of

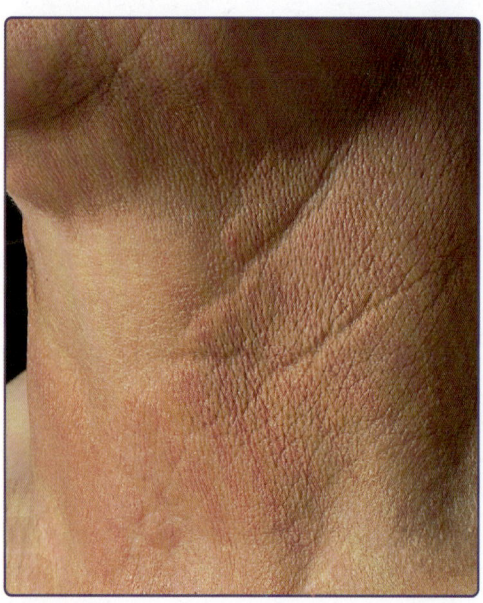

Figure 126-8 Example of plane xanthoma in a patient with lymphoma.

xanthomas, an understanding of cholesterol and lipoprotein pathophysiology is essential (Fig. 126-9).

Cholesterol, the most abundant sterol in plasma, is primarily produced from an endogenous pathway (ie, synthesized in cells in the body, especially the liver) or, to a lesser extent, absorbed via an exogenous pathway through intestinal uptake.[40] Cholesterol, primarily in its esterified form, linking a fatty acid moiety at the 3-hydroxy position, is a core component of lipoprotein. Cholesterol serves as a precursor for bile acids; helps form steroid hormones, including estrogen, testosterone, and cortisol; and maintains the integrity and structure of cell membranes.[39,41-43]

Dietary cholesterol through the exogenous pathway is transported from the intestine via the Niemann-Pick C-like protein 1 transporter. Cholesterol in the

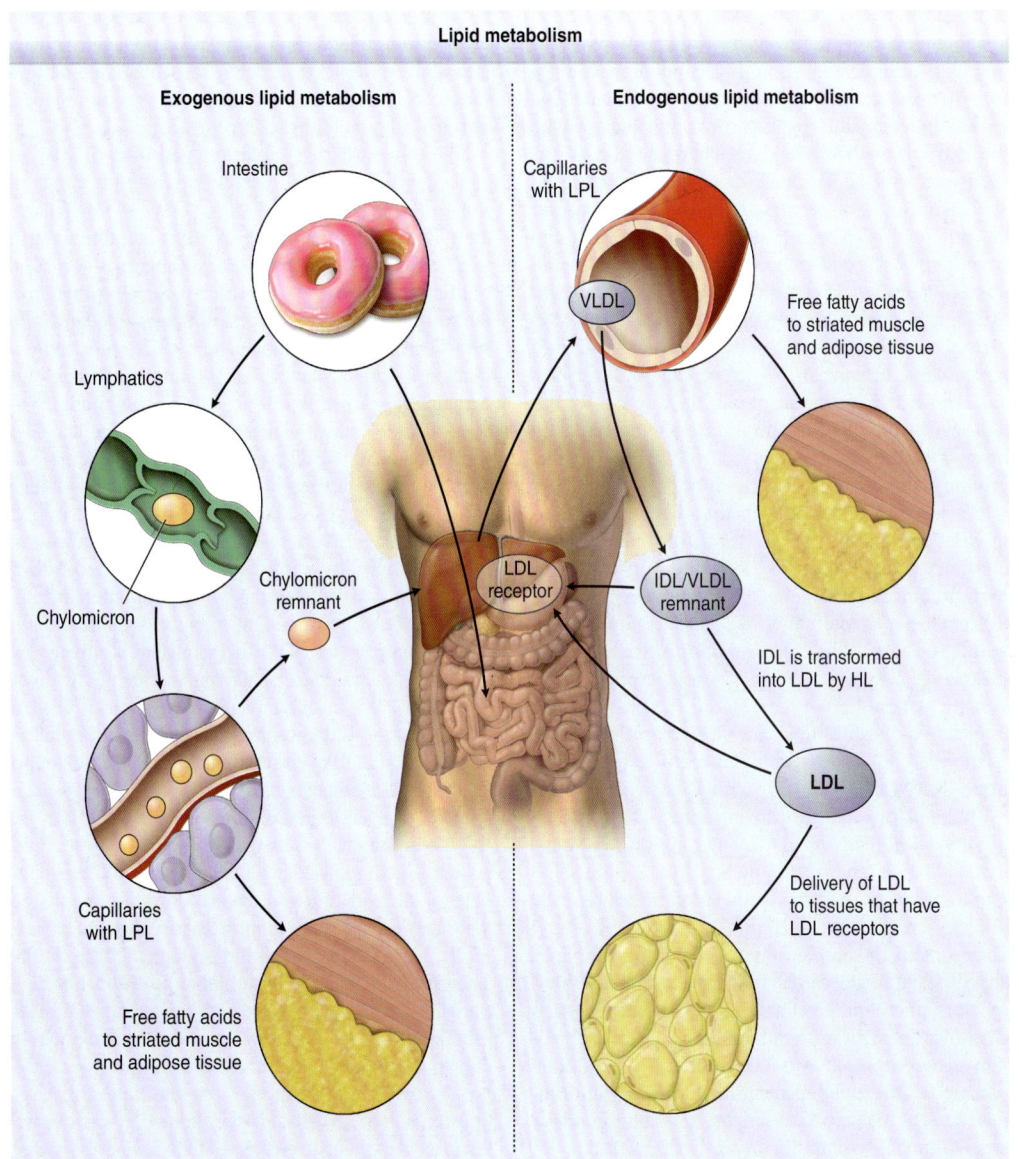

Figure 126-9 Overview of lipid metabolism with an emphasis on exogenous and endogenous pathways. The exogenous pathway consists of triglycerides in the intestines packaged into chylomicrons in the intestinal enterocytes. Capillary lipoprotein lipase (LPL), which requires apoCII as a cofactor, hydrolyzes the triglycerides and releases fatty acids for uptake by various tissues. The remaining chylomicron particle, called a *chylomicron remnant*, is recycled by the liver in a process that requires apoE as a ligand for the low-density lipoprotein (LDL) receptors in the liver. The endogenous pathway involves the hepatic production of very-low-density lipoprotein (VLDL) and the delivery of free fatty acids to peripheral tissues. Similar to chylomicron metabolism, LPL hydrolyzes triglycerides and releases fatty acids for peripheral tissue uptake. VLDL remnants are called intermediate-density lipoproteins (IDLs). IDLs may be removed from circulation via the LDL receptor or be transformed into LDL by hepatic lipase (HL) in the liver. LDL may bind to the LDL receptor for clearance or deposit within luminal walls.

intestinal cell is largely packaged into chylomicrons for entry into the bloodstream, stored in the intestine as either free cholesterol or cholesteryl ester, or transported back into the intestinal lumen via the action of the 2 adenosine triphosphate–binding cassette transporters (ABCG5 and ABCG8).[44] Nearly 50% of the intestinal cholesterol and more than 95% of the intestinal β-sitosterol and campesterol are transported into the intestinal lumen and are not absorbed. Of note, patients who have defects in ABCG5 and ABCG8 have elevated plasma levels of β-sitosterol.

The endogenous pathway of cholesterol synthesis involves multiple reduction and condensation steps to form mevalonate, a key intermediate molecule. The terminal step in this pathway involves the enzyme β-hydroxy-β-methylglutaryl-coenzyme A (HMG-CoA) reductase, which is the rate limiting step in cholesterol synthesis and the target of statin-based therapies. After an additional 19 steps, mevalonate is transformed into cholesterol.[40] The endogenous pathway is regulated in a negative feedback mechanism based on the amount of exogenous cholesterol absorbed.

In plasma, lipoproteins are the transporters of lipid molecules and consist of cholesterol, triglycerides, and a surface layer of phospholipids functioning as a detergent, allowing these hydrophobic molecules to be mobilized in the aqueous environment of plasma. Lipoproteins contain specific apolipoproteins that interact with specific enzymes and receptors, and in combination with the specific lipid composition of the particle, define its class and function. The hydrophobic components of lipoproteins, including cholesteryl ester and triglyceride, are carried within the core of the spherical lipoprotein particles. Plasma lipoproteins are classified based on size and density, ranging from very large triglyceride-rich lipoproteins with a density of less than 0.94 g/mL (chylomicrons) to small HDL molecules of density up to 1.21 g/mL.[1,39,41]

Chylomicrons made in the intestine have a plasma density of less than 0.93 g/mL, and range in weight (50 to 1000×10^6 Da) and size (diameter: 75 to 1200 nm).[41,42,45] These particles predominantly contain triglyceride (85% by weight) and include 3% cholesteryl ester.[39] They contain fat-soluble vitamins, including vitamin A as retinyl palmitate, carotenoids, vitamin D, vitamin E as α-tocopherol or γ-tocopherol, and vitamin K. Each chylomicron particle has an apoB48, and after chylomicrons are released into the lymphatic system, they pick up additional lipoproteins including apolipoprotein AI (apoAI), apoAIV, and the C apolipoproteins (apoCI, apoCII, and apoCIII).

After chylomicrons are transported to the serum, lipoprotein lipase (LPL) on the surfaces of adipocytes and myocytes cleave free fatty acids off the glycerol backbones of trygiclerides.[46] ApoCII acts as a cofactor for LPL in this reaction, whereas apoAV promotes LPL-mediated triglyceride lipolysis. The free fatty acids are taken up by adjacent cells, or bind to albumin for transport to other tissues including the liver. In adipocytes, the free fatty acids are converted back into triglyceride as a form of energy storage. ApoCIII inhibits the process of lipolysis.

After the majority of chylomicron triglyceride has been removed, chylomicrons obtain cholesteryl ester from HDL in exchange for triglyceride via the action of HDL-specific cholesteryl ester transfer protein (CETP). The remainder of the chylomicron, now called a chylomicron remnant, is taken up by the liver through the binding of surface apoE to the hepatic LDL or lipoprotein receptor-related protein (LRP) receptor. In the process of metabolizing into remnant particles, chylomicrons transfer apoAI, apoAIV, apoAV, and the C apolipoproteins to HDL, but still retain their apoB48 and apoE. Of note, the plasma residence time of chylomicron triglyceride is roughly 5 to 10 minutes compared to 5 hours for apoB48.[39,41,45]

VLDLs, which have plasma densities of 0.93 to 1.006 g/mL, are synthesized in the liver and range in molecular weight (10 to 80×10^6 Da) and size (diameter: 30 to 80 nm).[1,39] These particles are abundant in triglyceride (60% by weight) and contain 10% cholesteryl ester. These lipoproteins are proteomically similar to chylomicrons but approximately one-tenth the typical chylomicron diameter at the time of secretion, contain a higher proportion of cholesterol ester, and contain the larger apoB100. Additional apolipoproteins include CI, CII, CIII, and E. In the prandial state, the average daily production of apoB100 in humans is approximately 20 mg/kg/day.[39] When VLDLs enter plasma, the particles obtain apoE from HDL. VLDL triglyceride is removed similarly to chylomicrons via LPL, with free fatty acids converted into triglyceride in adipocytes for energy storage. After the action of LPL, remnant VLDL particles are known as intermediate-density lipoproteins (IDLs), which have roughly equal amounts of cholesterol and triglyceride.[47] The liver internalizes IDL through the binding surface IDL apoE to the LDL and LRP receptors. Remaining serum IDL is converted to LDL by the enzyme hepatic lipase, found on the surface of liver cells.[39]

LDLs, the end product of VLDL catabolism, are the predominant plasma lipoproteins. These lipoproteins have molecular weights of 2×10^6 Da, diameters of 18 to 25 nm, and plasma densities of 1.019 to 1.063 g/mL.[1,39,41,48] These particles are rich in cholesteryl ester (40% by weight) and contain 5% triglyceride. The predominant protein in LDL is apoB100, but LDL particles may contain trace amounts of CI, CII, CIII, and apoE. In adults, LDL contains approximately 60% to 70% of total cholesterol and roughly 80% to 90% of the total apoB. LDL apoB has a plasma residence of approximately 3.5 days, and is taken up by various tissues through the LDL receptor.[39] LDL has been divided into large LDL (density 1.019 to 1.044 g/mL) and small dense LDL (density 1.044 to 1.063 g/mL). Small dense LDL is considered more atherogenic than large LDL, yet specifically measuring small dense LDL does not clearly improve risk prediction over and above total LDL particle or apoB concentrations.[49]

HDLs (density 1.063 to 1.21 g/mL) contain variable proportions of triglyceride, cholesterol, and cholesterol ester, dependent on particle size.[1,39,41,50] The major proteins of HDL are apoAI and apoAII. HDL-specific apoAI has a residence time of approximately 4.5 days. HDLs are key participants in reverse cholesterol transport, in which HDL particles obtain cholesterol from cells in peripheral tissues, and then deliver cholesterol to the liver for excretion or transfer it to triglyceride-rich lipoproteins in exchange for triglyceride via the action of CETP.[39] In HDL, the enzyme lecithin–cholesterol acyltransferase catalyzes the formation of the cholesteryl esters, which are later transferred to lipoproteins via CETP. Decreased HDL-C of less than 40 mg/dL is often considered a significant cardiovascular risk factor.

ETIOLOGIES AND RISK FACTORS

Etiologies of xanthomas may be categorized into (a) primary dyslipidemias, which may carry a heritable or familial component; (b) secondary dyslipidemias, which are typically acquired but may unmask an underlying genetic predisposition; or (c) normolipemic states in which there is no underlying dyslipidemia. The normolipemic state is much rarer compared to primary and secondary dyslipidemias.

PRIMARY (GENETIC) DYSLIPIDEMIAS

Type I hyperlipidemias are characterized by an increase in serum chylomicrons. Deficiencies or functional defects in LPL or apoCII, both of which have autosomal recessive inheritance, are common genetic mutations underlying this disorder.[51] Without the ability to cleave triglycerides in peripheral tissues, chylomicrons accumulate with triglyceride levels 10 to 100 times above normal serum triglyceride limits. Serum triglyceride levels are commonly above 1000 mg/dL, but morbidity may be seen at much lower levels. Severe hypertriglyceridemia can lead to episodic eruptive xanthomas that may quickly subside without intervention. Other clinical manifestations include frequent episodes of acute pancreatitis, neuropathy, arthralgias, hepatosplenomegaly, and lipemia retinalis, which may herald the development of eruptive xanthomas.[52] Repeated episodes of acute pancreatitis may lead to chronic pancreatitis and eventual diabetes, which itself is a risk factor for further dyslipidemia.

Type IIa hyperlipidemias are commonly caused by familial hypercholesterolemia and result in abnormally high circulating levels of LDL-C. Mutations either in the LDL receptor, which clears circulating LDL, or in apoB, which serves as a cofactor in the binding between LDL and its receptor, are common genetic defects.[11,12,53] Rarer causes of familial hypercholesterolemia include (a) the autosomal recessive form resulting from defects in LDL receptor adaptor protein 1 (LDLRAP1), which helps traffic LDL bound to LDL receptors intracellularly for degradation, and (b) mutations in proprotein convertase subtilisin/kexin type 9 (PCSK9). PCSK9 also promotes degradation of LDL receptors and therefore results in less availability of LDL receptors on the surface of hepatocytes and other cells.[54]

Familial hypercholesterolemia is typically classified into heterozygous or homozygous forms. The homozygous form manifests with cardiovascular disease and xanthoma formation at a much younger age. Familial hypercholesterolemia is further categorized into 1 of 5 classes.[55] Class I involves a complete absence of LDL receptor synthesis; Class II involves a defect in transportation of the LDL receptor from the endoplasmic reticulum to the Golgi apparatus within cells; Class III involves abnormal binding between the LDL receptor and LDL as a result of mutations in the receptor itself or in apoB; Class IV involves correct binding between the LDL receptor and LDL, with a defect in endocytosis of LDL; and Class V results from dysregulation in recycling of the LDL receptor. Patients with familial hypercholesterolemia or Type IIa hyperlipidemia in general are prone to developing tendinous xanthomas, especially over the Achilles tendon. Such xanthomas can also be seen in patients who synthesize excess cholestanol or overabsorb plant sterols. Both cholestanol and plant sterols (β-sitosterol and campesterol) are then carried in excess on LDL particles.

Type IIb hyperlipidemia is commonly caused by familial combined hyperlipidemia, resulting in elevated LDL and VLDL concentrations. Although the condition is inherited, other factors, including excessive alcohol intake, obesity, hypothyroidism, and diabetes, may exacerbate the expression of this disorder. The pathogenesis stems from an increase in hepatic VLDL production, although the exact mechanisms contributing to VLDL overproduction are still not clear. Postulated mechanisms include increased free fatty acid delivery to the liver; decreased LPL activity either from mutations, insulin resistance, or increased apoCIII concentrations; an increase in dense LDL particles from CETP overactivity or an increase in VLDL precursors; insulin resistance from the aforementioned factors (ie, obesity, alcohol intake); and defects in adipose tissue metabolism.[56,57] Elevated LDL may be a result of heterozygous mutations in LPL and possible mutations in *APOA5* and *APOC3*. Xanthomas are rarely seen with Type IIb hyperlipidemia.

The Type III phenotype, referred to as dysbetalipoproteinemia, results in elevated concentrations of remnant lipoprotein particles, either chylomicron remnants or VLDL remnants including IDL. A defect in apoE 2/2 is a major causative factor and has implications in the development of hyperlipidemia and eventual atherosclerosis.[58] As discussed in "Pathogenesis" section, apoE plays a central role in the clearance of triglyceride-rich particles by facilitating the binding of remnant particles to the LDL and LRP receptors. Defects in this protein therefore result in elevated remnant particle concentration, which is highly atherogenic and leads to the development of characteristic palmar xanthomas. Most causes of hyperlipidemia and subsequent xanthoma formation occur with homozygous defects; those with a heterozygous defect may, paradoxically, have decreased cholesterol because of a compensatory upregulation in LDL receptor concentration, increased binding of apoB100 to the LDL-receptor instead, and decreased conversion of VLDL to LDL resulting in lower serum concentrations of LDL.[14,15] As with the aforementioned dyslipidemias, concomitant secondary causes, such as nephrosis, obesity, and diabetes, may be required for phenotypic expression in heterozygous patients. Ongoing work evaluating polymorphisms in other interacting cofactors, such as mutations in apoCIII and apoAV, continues to mold the pathophysiology underlying this genetic disorder.[59] Aside from palmar xanthomas, tuberoeruptive xanthomas are the most common xanthoma seen with Type III disorders.

The Type IV disorder, known as familial hypertriglyceridemia, results in an isolated elevation of VLDL. This phenotype is relatively common and, as a result of increased triglyceride synthesis, results in increased VLDL synthesis and secretion.[60,61] There is no concomitant increase in LDL, which distinguishes this disorder from the Type IIb hyperlipidemia; triglycerides are carried in plasma primarily by VLDL, distinguishing this disorder from the Type I hyperlipidemia where elevated triglyceride levels are a result of the accumulation of chylomicrons. Although VLDL carries apoB and is considered atherogenic, the increase in risk of cardiovascular disease with familial hypertriglyceridemia is modest in isolation given normal or even low levels of LDL and apoB.[60,61] However, the dyslipidemia is associated with obesity, diabetes, and development of insulin resistance, and these patients are at substantially elevated cardiovascular risk. The exact molecular basis underlying excess VLDL secretion is not known. As with other conditions associated with hypertriglyceridemia, eruptive xanthomas may be seen, but are rare in comparison with hyperchylomicronemic dyslipidemias. Most patients are without cutaneous manifestations of the dyslipidemia.

The Type V dyslipidemia consists of elevated VLDL and chylomicrons; consequently, patients are at increased risk of eruptive xanthomas secondary to hypertriglyceridemia. The genetic mechanisms underlying this disorder result from a combination of the aforementioned mutations, resulting in Types I and IV dyslipidemia. It is commonly seen in the setting of diabetes with underlying Type IV dyslipidemia, progressing to increasing extent of impairment in LPL activity or high dietary fat intake and chylomicron accumulation, and hyperchylomicronemia in combination with underlying excess VLDL concentration typical of common diabetic dyslipidemia.

It is important to note that the Fredrickson-Levy-Lees categories do not factor HDL-C levels or lipoprotein(A) levels into its schema. This was a limitation noted by the authors in their original papers. They specifically recognized that further genetic dyslipidemias would be discovered with more advanced genotyping and fractionation techniques. To this point, tuberoeruptive xanthomas may be observed in marked HDL deficiency. Other known genetic lipoprotein disorders not formerly classified by Fredrickson, Levy, and Lees that are associated with premature coronary heart disease include heritable lipoprotein(A) levels in excess of the 80th population percentile and seen in approximately 20% of families with premature coronary heart disease, and familial hypoalphalipoproteinemia (isolated low HDL-C <40 mg/dL), which may be seen in 5% of families.[39,62,63] Patients with disorders impairing HDL reverse cholesterol transport function occasionally develop tendinous or tuberoeruptive xanthomas, although cutaneous xanthomas are rarely attributable to elevations in lipoprotein(A).

SECONDARY (ACQUIRED) HYPERLIPIDEMIA

Many of the aforementioned genetic dyslipidemias require secondary, acquired causes of hyperlipidemia for phenotypic expressions, including xanthomas. Several categories of secondary hyperlipidemia have been identified, including hematologic, hepatic, nephrotic, endocrinologic/metabolic, and drug-induced.

Various types of xanthomas, including tuberoeruptive and planar xanthomas, have been observed in patients with hematologic and oncologic abnormalities, including monoclonal gammopathies, multiple myeloma, lymphoma, and various forms of leukemia.[64,65] Immunoglobulins may bind to plasma lipoprotein particles and, in some cases, markedly delay the clearance of chylomicron remnants or VLDL remnants, resulting in combined hyperlipidemia or dysbetalipoproteinemia. Solid tumors also have been linked to elevated LDL and triglyceride concentrations, possibly the result of a shared pathway in cellular proliferation and endogenous cholesterol formation through the mevalonate pathway, which increases the guanosine triphosphatases Ras and Rho.[66] An alternative explanation linking malignancy and dyslipidemia may be the existence of an underlying metabolic syndrome, which has been demonstrated to be a risk factor for cancer development.[67]

Hepatic causes of dyslipidemia include prolonged biliary tree obstruction leading to the accumulation of serum cholesterol,[68] which may take the form of a novel lipoprotein-like particle Lp-X.[69] Common causes of chronic biliary obstruction include primary biliary cirrhosis and secondary biliary obstruction, leading to hypercholesterolemia. Long-term hypercholesterolemia may lead to plane xanthomas (beige-orange plaques on hands, feet, and trunk), xanthelasma, and, occasionally, tuberous xanthomas. Patients with prolonged biliary obstruction may also manifest jaundice, pruritus, and hyperpigmentation of the skin. Treatment involves relieving the underlying cause of obstruction.

Metabolic and endocrinologic causes of dyslipidemia include pregnancy, thyroid disorders, and the metabolic syndrome spectrum, which includes obesity and diabetes. Expected changes during normal pregnancy include hypertrophy of maternal adipocytes and a subsequent increase in insulin and hormonal (ie, estrogen and progesterone) secretion, which leads to a disproportionate increase in lipogenesis (especially triglyceride formation) compared to lipolysis.[70]

Patients with predisposed hypertriglyceridemia are nevertheless at increased risk for eruptive xanthoma formation in pregnancy with the added stimulus of pregnancy-induced triglyceridemia.

Thyroid dysfunction is well established as a modifiable factor in dyslipidemia, with a direct, linear relationship observed between increasing thyroid-stimulating hormone levels and total cholesterol, LDL-C, and triglycerides.[71] Thyroid hormones, particularly triiodothyronine (T_3), upregulate LDL receptors by increasing LDL receptor gene expression, increasing the activity of LPL, and increasing the affinity of remnant particles to the LDL receptor. As a result, hypothyroidism may promote increased concentrations of serum lipid subfractions through the reversal of these mechanisms, but also by increasing insulin resistance, increasing overall obesity, and decreasing the function of CETP.[71] Because of the mixed effects of decreased thyroid levels on lipid metabolism, clinical hypothyroidism may mimic the Type IIa or Type III phenotypes. Patients are therefore at increased risks for tendon xanthoma formation or eruptive xanthomas.

Diabetes is perhaps the most important factor on the metabolic syndrome/obesity spectrum. Because of decreased peripheral insulin resistance and resultant lipolysis with free fatty acid delivery to hepatic cells, patients with diabetes have increased rates of production and secretion of VLDL.[72] Peripheral LPL, which is stimulated by insulin, may be decreased in patients with diabetes. Finally, postprandial chylomicrons may have defective clearance in diabetes. The combination of these mechanisms may lead to a number of lipid disorders, including chylomicronemia, hypertriglyceridemia, increased LDL, and increased VLDL.[72] Consequently, all types of xanthomas may be seen in patients prone to dyslipidemia with underlying diabetes.

Several drugs and toxins may result in dyslipidemia. Because of the extensive list of known therapeutics that affect lipid metabolism, general trends in lipid metabolism based on therapeutic category are discussed here. Drugs that increase LDL concentration include protease antineoplastic agents (ie, danazol with a 10% to 40% increase), antiretroviral therapy (ie, protease inhibitors with a 15% to 30% increase), anabolic steroids (20% increase), immunosuppressant agents (0% to 50% increase), and thiazide diuretics (5% to 10% increase).[73] Several drugs that increase serum triglyceride levels include estrogen (40% increase), antiretrovirals (15% to 200% increase), immunosuppressant agents (0 to 70% increase), thiazide diuretics (5% to 15% increase), beta-blockers (10% to 40% increase), and antipsychotics (20% to 50% increase).[73]

NORMOLIPEMIC XANTHOMAS

Interestingly, the 2 nonheritable types of xanthomas without a predilection for cutaneous manifestations are often seen in normolipemic patients. Because of the rarity of xanthoma disseminatum, few risk factors have been found. Verruciform xanthomas may be uncovered by chronic inflammatory states and local oromucosal trauma, given the propensity for mucosal lesions. Prior studies have failed to find a link to human papillomavirus or other preceding viral infections.[27,74] However, poor oral hygiene, prior dental abscesses, mechanical stimuli, tobacco abuse, alcohol exposure, dental implants, and overall immunocompromise are postulated as risk factors.

The even rarer diffuse normolipemic plane xanthoma is characterized by symmetric plaques found diffusely in the neck, flexural areas, and upper trunk.[22,23,75] This entity is associated with hematologic disorders, including multiple myeloma and monoclonal gammopathies.[75] Disorders in the reticuloendothelial system also are linked to diffuse xanthoma formation.

DIAGNOSIS

Accurate diagnosis of xanthoma is important as it can point to underlying systemic disease or hyperlipidemia. Even though the morbidity from cutaneous xanthomas is limited, pinpointing hyperlipidemia may help identify early lifestyle and treatment options that would help slow the progression of clinical atherosclerotic cardiovascular disease.

SUPPORTIVE STUDIES AND LABORATORY TESTING

For primary hyperlipidemias, the traditional methodologies used by Fredrickson, Levy, and Lees included direct lipid fractionation through electrophoresis and ultracentrifugation.[1] In modern-day medicine, the initial standard approach is to order a plasma lipid profile. This test provides a measurement of the concentration of total cholesterol, triglyceride, HDL-C, and calculated LDL-C. A total cholesterol of greater than 240 mg/dL and associated LDL-C value of greater than 160 mg/dL are classified as elevated and are associated with an increased cardiovascular risk, with cholesterol less than 200 mg/dL and LDL-C less than 100 mg/dL being classified as optimal for the majority of patients. A triglyceride level of greater than 1000 mg/dL is classified as markedly elevated and is associated with an increased risk of pancreatitis, as well as eruptive xanthomas.

Occasionally, patients will have elevated total cholesterol levels as a result of elevated levels of β-sitosterol (>225 μmol/mmol of total cholesterol) and campesterol (>270 μmol/mmol of total cholesterol) as seen in phytosterolemia, or elevated cholestanol as seen in cerebrotendinous xanthomatosis. These abnormalities may only be detected by measuring plasma sterols using gas chromatography.

Although the definition of the primary hyperlipidemia is based on which lipoprotein subfraction(s) is (are) present and elevated in concentration, as of this writing there is no formal consensus on what cutoffs should be used for these definitions. Furthermore, while total cholesterol and HDL-C are provided in the lipid panel, obtaining direct measurement of lipoprotein subfractions, including VLDL, IDL, LDL, and chylomicrons, is only possible through more complex assays such as ultracentrifugation.[76] Other methodologies are now clinically available, such as ion mobility and nuclear magnetic resonance spectroscopy, to measure lipoprotein particle concentrations.[77,78]

Recently, an algorithm proposed by Sniderman and colleagues classifies patients into one of the Fredrickson-Levy-Lees phenotypes based on 3 lipid parameters: total cholesterol, apoB concentration, and triglyceride levels.[79] This algorithm has not yet been validated in large-scale studies. Definitive classification relies on genotyping, including apoE status.

Depending on the underlying clinical suspicion, further tests may be warranted to assess secondary causes of dyslipidemia. Fasting glucose tolerance testing and hemoglobin A_{1c} values help with diagnosing diabetes. In patients with proteinuria noted on standard urinalysis, a 24-hour urine protein collection may be warranted to assess for nephrotic syndrome. Both diabetes and renal disorders are associated with elevated triglycerides and decreased HDL-C. Both hypothyroidism and obstructive liver disease (with elevated levels of alkaline phosphatase and total bilirubin) are often associated with elevated LDL-C. Hypothyroidism is associated, typically, with elevated thyroid-stimulating hormone levels, but decreased free thyroxine (T_4) levels. Hepatocellular disease or fatty liver with elevated transaminases is often observed in patients with hypertriglyceridemia. For hematologic conditions, serum and urine protein electrophoresis, serum free light chains, and immunofixation assays may help identify conditions such as multiple myeloma and monoclonal gammopathy if the clinical suspicion is high. Certain tumor markers, such as carcinoembryonic antigen, cancer antigen 19-9, and prostate-specific antigen may help identify solid malignancies if history points to one.

Serum genetic testing is described in the "Counseling and Screening" section.

PATHOLOGY

Foam cells are macrophages that contain lipid and are histopathologically characteristic of xanthomas (Fig. 126-10). Slight variations in associated cells and surrounding material (eg, amount of fibrosis and inflammatory cells) may be seen, depending on the type of xanthoma.[31,37,80-82] For example, eruptive xanthomas often consist of lymphoid cells, histiocytes, neutrophils, and, frequently, free lipid in the dermis.[19,81] Tuberous xanthomas contain foam cells and cholesterol clefts.[20] Cholesterol is doubly refractile, whereas other types of lipid are not. Tendon xanthomas are histopathologically similar to tuberous xanthomas; however, xanthelasmas can be differentiated by their superficial location.[31,32] Along with the foam cells, xanthelasmas may reveal striated muscle, vellus hair, and/or a thinned epidermis,

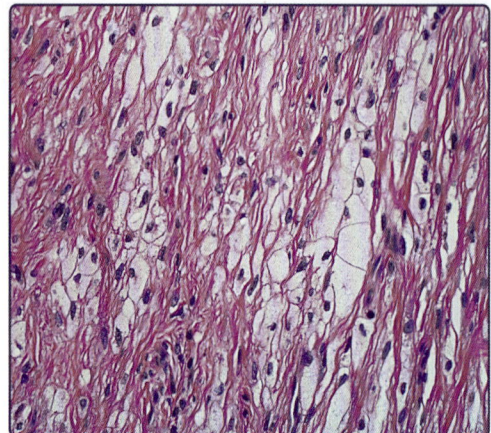

Figure 126-10 Example of foam cells seen histologically from a tuberous xanthoma.

indicative of the superficial location.[7] Both tuberous and tendinous xanthomas may have associated fibrosis, with greater degrees of fibrosis indicating older lesions.

Although the diagnosis of xanthomas is made clinically, certain histopathologic considerations may help differentiate similar appearing lesions. Necrobiotic xanthogranuloma, a primarily granulomatous disease that may be mistaken for planar xanthoma, largely involves degenerated collagen, granulomatous inflammation, multinucleate giant cells, cholesterol clefts, and lymphoid follicles on pathology specimens.[83] Basal cell carcinoma, which may be mistaken for xanthelasmas with a similar "waxy" appearance, involves proliferation of the basal epithelial layer, whereas sebaceous hyperplasia results in an increase in the number of sebaceous glands.[7] Eruptive xanthomas may be mistaken for granuloma annulare, which may involve histiocytes, necrobiosis, multinucleated giant cells, fibrin deposition, and perivascular and interstitial lymphocytes. Tendinous xanthomas sometimes clinically appear as rheumatoid nodules, gouty tophi, or erythema elevatum diutinum. Rheumatoid nodules appear as granulomatous tissue with multinucleated giant cells, histiocytes, plasma cells, and eosinophils, whereas gouty tophi may appear as edematous synovium with characteristic uric acid crystals under polarized light.[84] Finally, verrucous xanthomas may be confused for condylomata, which appear as vacuolated keratinocytes and stain positive for human papillomavirus, or squamous cell carcinoma, which consists of a proliferation in the squamous epithelial layer.[74]

IMAGING

Imaging is usually unnecessary for the diagnosis of xanthomas, as clinical appearance and laboratory tests typically suffice. In cases where diagnosis is unclear, ultrasonography or MRI may be considered. In ultrasonography, xanthomas typically appear as hypoechoic nodules with an overall heterogeneous pattern. Under MRI, xanthomas appear as hyperintense lesions on T1-weighted and T2-weighted images with possible diffuse reticulate patterns.[85] The use of positron emission tomography has been reported in cases of xanthoma disseminatum to aid in prognosticating the extent of disease.[86]

Imaging may be necessary, however, to further diagnose secondary causes of dyslipidemia. For thyroid abnormalities, diagnostic algorithms involve the use of both thyroid ultrasonography and sestamibi scans. Abnormal liver function tests may involve the use of ultrasonography, triple-phase CT scans, or MRI for further characterization of possible lesions. Renal disorders typically involve the use of renal ultrasonography to assess parenchymal changes and urinary system abnormalities, including obstruction and dilation. Underlying hematologic or oncologic disorders require imaging-based staging, which is beyond the scope of this chapter.

For patients with diagnosed primary dyslipidemias, evaluating for coronary artery disease, especially with a history of chest pain, may involve noninvasive or invasive imaging. Noninvasive stress tests involve transthoracic echocardiograms, nuclear imaging, positron emission tomography, or MRI. For a global assessment of coronary artery disease without a stress test, specialized CT scans to assess for coronary artery calcium or coronary CT angiograms may be appropriate. In patients who are thought to have hemodynamically significant coronary lesions, invasive coronary arteriograms may be indicated. Intravascular ultrasonography has been used to assess for plaque burden in clinical trials, but is not considered a clinical tool aside from its use in percutaneous coronary interventional procedures.

DIFFERENTIAL DIAGNOSIS

Table 126-1 outlines the differential diagnoses of xanthelasma, planar xanthomas, eruptive xanthomas, tendinous and tuberous xanthomas, verrucous xanthomas, and xanthoma disseminatum.

TABLE 126-1
Differential Diagnoses

- For xanthelasma: sebaceous hyperplasia, juvenile xanthogranuloma, syringoma, nodular basal cell carcinoma
- For planar xanthomas: necrobiotic xanthogranuloma, syringeal palmar keratoderma, digital fibromatosis
- For eruptive xanthomas: generalized granuloma annulare, molluscum contagiosum, subepidermal calcified nodules, xanthoma disseminatum, sarcoidosis
- For tendinous and tuberous xanthomas: rheumatoid nodules, gouty tophi, subcutaneous granuloma annulare, erythema elevatum diutinum
- For verrucous xanthomas: condylomata, oral papilloma, verrucous carcinoma, squamous cell carcinoma
- For xanthoma disseminatum: benign cephalic histiocytosis, reticulohistiocytoma, juvenile xanthogranuloma, generalized eruptive histiocytoma, progressive nodular histiocytosis

MANAGEMENT

The cornerstone of xanthoma therapy involves addressing the underlying hyperlipidemia, typically through lifestyle changes and medication management. Even though xanthomas themselves have relatively benign courses and are usually treated for cosmetic purposes, the underlying dyslipidemia may progress to atherosclerotic cardiovascular disease and warrants further treatment consideration. This is especially important given the morbidity and mortality stemming from any untreated, underlying dyslipidemia.

INTERVENTIONS

LIFESTYLE–EXERCISE

Lifestyle changes represent the initial intervention for all lipid disorders, as reflected in clinical guidelines, including those from the National Cholesterol Education Program, American College of Cardiology, American Heart Association, and National Lipid Association.[87] Increased aerobic physical activity (at least 30 min/day of walking, riding on a bicycle, or some other weekly activity totaling 900 kcal of energy expenditure) as well as weight control are important for preventing diabetes, lowering total cholesterol and LDL-C by up to 3.9 mg/dL, lowering triglycerides by approximately 7.1 mg/dL, and raising HDL-C levels by 1.9 to 2.5 mg/dL.[87] Greater benefits are seen in patients with established cardiovascular disease. Physical inactivity may result in the opposite trends in lipid values.

LIFESTYLE–SMOKING

Tobacco abuse has a similar effect to physical inactivity, and may lower HDL-C levels while concomitantly increasing total cholesterol, LDL-C, and triglyceride levels.[88] Smoking cessation aids include nicotine patches and nicotine gum, while prescription medications include bupropion and varenicline. Tobacco use reduces activity of LPL and will tend to exacerbate hypertriglyceridemic dyslipidemias.

LIFESTYLE–DIET

In patients with elevated LDL-C and other high-risk patients with known atherosclerotic cardiovascular disease, referral to a nutritionist for dietary restriction is appropriate. Prior systematic reviews have shown patients referred for counseling have reductions in total cholesterol and LDL-C. Dietary management involves goals set forth by therapeutic diets such as the Mediterranean diet, which is high in monounsaturated fats and limits consumption of red meat and dairy products, and the Portfolio Diet, which is plant based and consists of soluble fiber, soy, plant sterols, and almonds. These diets may further reduce total cholesterol and LDL-C levels.[87]

Diets specifically targeted toward lowering chylomicron concentrations and triglycerides include a fat-restricted diet, typically less than 15% of total calories in hyperchylomicronemia syndromes. Furthermore, a low glycemic, carbohydrate-restricted diet is recommended in insulin-resistance states and hypertriglyceridemic disorders (eg, Types IIb and IV) where the problem is mainly excess VLDL secretion.

LIFESTYLE–WEIGHT MANAGEMENT

Excess weight or obesity is the most common "second hit" in secondary dyslipidemias and will exacerbate insulin resistance in a variety of tissues and organs, result in hypersecretion of VLDL, contribute to the formation of the metabolic syndrome and its related disorders, and reduce LPL activity. Pathogenic effects from excess adipocytes, termed *adiposopathy* or *sick fat*, may result in excess hyperlipidemia through impaired fatty acid storage and subsequent increases in circulating free fatty acids.[89] Based on recommendations from the American College of Cardiology, American Heart Association, and The Obesity Society, even sustained weight losses of 3% to 5% will result in beneficial effects on triglyceride and blood glucose levels. Overweight adults should aim for a 500 to 750 kcal/day energy deficit, which typically amounts to 1200 to 1500 kcal/day for women and 1500 to 1800 kcal/day for men.[90]

MEDICATIONS

STATIN THERAPY

Statins are the first-line pharmacotherapy for lowering LDL-C. The rate-limiting enzyme in endogenous cholesterol synthesis is HMG-CoA reductase. Statins competitively inhibit this enzyme, decreasing cellular cholesterol synthesis by up to 80%. The cells in the body respond by increasing the level and activity of surface LDL receptors, enhancing the clearance of LDL particles from the bloodstream.[91] Statins may also improve endothelial function, increase plaque stability, and prevent thrombus formation. Statins are typically categorized based on their potency, the lipid-lowering effect per unit dose of the particular statin, and intensity, which represents the overall lipid-lowering effect of the therapy. High-potency, high-intensity statin therapies include rosuvastatin 20 mg or 40 mg and atorvastatin 40 mg or 80 mg daily. Common reported side effects include an increased propensity for diabetes (particularly in those predisposed) and, rarely, hemorrhagic stroke and rhabdomyolysis.

Several trials have evaluated the efficacy and potency of statin therapy in both primary and secondary prevention. Within the context of dyslipidemia, the American College of Cardiology and American Heart Association combined guidelines strongly recommend the use of statin therapy in individuals with established atherosclerotic cardiovascular disease and 3 other "statin benefit groups" in which statins may be considered based on clinician–patient risk discussions. These groups include those with LDL-C levels equal to or greater than 190 mg/dL, those with diabetes within an age range of 40 to 75 years with LDL-C values ranging between 70 and 189 mg/dL, and those with 10-year estimated risks of 7.5% or greater of developing a clinical atherosclerotic event, including myocardial infarctions or strokes.[5] The group with LDL-C levels equal to or greater than 190 mg/dL includes patients for whom there is a high clinical suspicion of familial hypercholesterolemia.

ADJUVANT THERAPY

Second-line medication therapy often includes ezetimibe, a specific inhibitor of the Niemann-Pick C-like protein 1 transporter, which is responsible for dietary cholesterol and plant sterol absorption within intestinal cells.[92] The use of ezetimibe is supported by multiple international guidelines, including the European Society of Cardiology and the National Institute for Health and Clinical Excellence. Recently, the 2016 Consensus Statement from the American College of Cardiology suggested the use of ezetimibe in patients with LDL-C equal to or greater than 190 mg/dL who are on statin therapy for secondary prevention and who have failed to achieve at least a 50% reduction in LDL-C levels on maximally tolerated statins.[6] Side effects are few, it is usually well tolerated with rare side effects include headaches and diarrhea.

Fibrates are common agents used to help lower triglyceride levels by 40% to 60%, and are especially useful in patients with elevated VLDL and chylomicrons.[93] Through activation of nuclear peroxisome-proliferator-activated receptors (PPARs), fibrates directly induce genes responsible for triglyceride catabolism, including PPAR-mediated synthesis of apoAI and apoAII needed for HDL formation, as well as PPAR-mediated increase in LPL activity. Fibrates may consequently raise HDL-C levels by 15% to 25% dependent on triglyceride levels, and are often used as adjuvant therapy to statins to further reduce rates of cardiovascular events or as therapy to manage hyperchylomicronemia for prevention of pancreatitis. Side effects include dyspepsia and myopathy.

Other agents that may help further reduce triglycerides include niacin, which may cause triglyceride reductions of 30% to 50% and also raise HDL-C levels by 20% to 30%. The exact mechanism of niacin is not precisely known, although it may lower the release of adipose free fatty acids and increase the activity of LPL. Common side effects include flushing, pruritus, and, occasionally, GI symptoms, including nausea and vomiting.

Omega-3 fatty acids may also help reduce triglycerides by 25% to 50%, but may increase LDL-C levels by 5% to 10%.[93,94] The increase in LDL-C is usually without increase in LDL particle concentration. Omega-3 fatty acids in fish oil are thought to be anti-inflammatory mediators and direct inhibitors of hepatic VLDL secretion through decreased triglyceride synthesis among other mechanisms, including inhibition of diacylglycerol acyltransferase, which catalyzes the final step in triacylglycerol synthesis.[95]

Lomitapide was approved by the U.S. Food and Drug Administration (FDA) in 2012 for use in patients with homozygous familial hypercholesterolemia.[96] The agent inhibits microsomal triglyceride transfer protein, which is responsible for loading triglycerides onto apoB in hepatic VLDL particles. LDL-C reductions in small studies ranged from 30% to 50%. Adverse events included diarrhea, hepatic toxicity, and embryotoxicity in pregnant patients. As a result of these toxicities, the use of the drug is restricted to a subset of certified physicians. Mipomersen subsequently was approved by the FDA in 2013 in patients with homozygous familial hypercholesterolemia. The mechanism of action involves direct binding of apoB messenger RNA, leading to decreased production of apoB, a key protein in VLDL, IDL, and LDL particle constitution.[97] Small trials have demonstrated LDL-C decreases of 25% to 47%, with side effects including injection-site reactions, flu-like symptoms, and increase in transaminases.

PCSK9 INHIBITORS

The FDA has approved a new class of injectable medications, PCSK9 inhibitors, for the treatment of dyslipidemias in patients refractory to standard medical therapy. PCSK9 normally binds to LDL receptors on the surface of cells, mainly hepatocytes, and induces their clearance via phagocytosis and subsequent degradation. By blocking the action of PCSK9, these inhibitors increase the availability of surface LDL receptors, thereby helping to clear circulating LDL.[54] Currently, 2 formulations are clinically available: evolocumab and alirocumab. FDA indications currently are limited to patients with familial hypercholesterolemia or those with established atherosclerotic cardiovascular disease who are on diet therapy and maximally tolerated statin therapy, and in need of additional LDL-C lowering. Early randomized controlled trials showed robust LDL-C lowering in a variety of patient populations and that clinically approved PCSK9 inhibitor regimens reduce LDL-C by approximately 60% on average. Subsequent studies with evolocumab have shown plaque regression and the large clinical outcomes trial FOURIER (Further Cardiovascular Outcomes Research With PCSK9 Inhibition in Patients With Elevated Risk) met its primary end point for cardiovascular event reduction. Adverse effects may include myalgia, ophthalmologic complaints, headaches and neurologic dysfunction, and injection-site reactions.

FUTURE OPTIONS

Several novel medications are in clinical development, most notably CETP inhibition, which has failed to improve clinical outcomes in the first 3 large outcomes trials.[98] Other targets include adenosine triphosphate-citrate lyase and adenosine monophosphate-activated protein kinase (ETC-1002), as well as thyromimetics.

TREATMENT OF SECONDARY DYSLIPIDEMIAS

Specific medical management of secondary dyslipidemias, including, for example, hepatic, endocrinologic, and renal causes, are beyond the scope of this chapter. However, recognition of secondary causes and their associated treatments should be initiated in any patient with overt dyslipidemia.

PROCEDURES

BIOPSY

Although the diagnosis of xanthomas is made on a clinical basis, biopsies may help in the diagnosis depending on the suspicion for alternate etiologies (Table 126-2). Specific histopathologic patterns expected with xanthomas and other diseases were previously discussed in the Pathology section.

SURGERY AND RELATED OPTIONS

Definitive management and removal of xanthomas involve surgical resection, especially if they cause functional impairment, and treatment of the underlying dyslipidemia. Surgery also may be pursued for mainly cosmetic reasons, especially with xanthelasmas. Other treatment options for xanthelasmas include ablative laser therapy or cryotherapy. Lesions may improve with lipid-lowering therapy. However, lesions will usually recur if the underlying dyslipidemia is not treated. In patients with homozygous familial hypercholesterolemia, a variety of surgical options have been tried without sustained clinical response. These include ileal bypass, portacaval shunt, and, in severe cases, liver transplantation to replenish functional LDL receptors. However, with the advent of apoB lipoprotein apheresis and PCSK9 inhibitors, surgical options are considered only in refractory cases.

ApoB LIPOPROTEIN PHERESIS AND PLASMAPHERESIS

ApoB lipoprotein apheresis has been approved by the FDA for patients who are not at LDL-C goals despite standard medical therapy. It is typically used in patients with homozygous familial hypercholesterolemia and, occasionally, in those with severe elevation in elevations in lipoprotein(A) and recurrent atherosclerotic cardiovascular events. The process involves extracorporeal removal of apoB particles, including VLDL and LDL on a weekly or biweekly basis through

TABLE 126-2
Characteristics of the Fredrickson-Levy-Lees Dyslipidemias

FREDRICKSON-LEVY-LEES PHENOTYPE	DEFECT	LIPOPROTEIN EXCESS	XANTHOMA TYPE
Type I (familial lipoprotein lipase [LPL] deficiency or familial hyperchylomicronemia)	Decreased LPL or apolipoprotein CII deficiencies	Chylomicrons	Eruptive
Type IIa (familial hypercholesterolemia or familial defective apolipoprotein B100)	Low-density lipoprotein (LDL) receptor defect	LDL	Tendinous Tuberous Xanthelasma intertriginous
Type IIb (familial combined dyslipidemia)	LDL receptor defect	LDL + very-low-density lipoprotein (VLDL)	Rarely seen
Type III (dysbetalipoproteinemia)	Apoprotein E 2/2 defect	Remnant particles	Palmar Tuberous Tuberoeruptive
Type IV (familial hypertriglyceridemia)	Increased VLDL production	VLDL	Rarely eruptive
Type V	Apolipoprotein CII deficiency and increased VLDL	VLDL + chylomicrons	Eruptive Rarely palmar

an apoB-avid adsorbent column.[99] Expected LDL-C reduction is 50% to 75% per session, with 30% reduction over a several-month time averaged interval. Similar to dialysis, patients often have venous access through port or through an arteriovenous fistula, and side effects include hypotension, anemia, and headaches. Small studies suggest a reduction in the progression of atherosclerosis and incidence of myocardial infarctions in patients undergoing apoB lipoprotein apheresis.

Plasmapheresis is a related procedure and is used for severe chylomicronemia to remove chylomicrons and replenish functional LPL and apoCII in the setting of severe episodes of recurrent pancreatitis.

COUNSELING AND SCREENING

In addition to nutritional and smoking cessation counseling, two other forms of counseling include individual genetic screening and family screening. The most commonly tested primary dyslipidemia is familial hypercholesterolemia, but even this may be underdiagnosed in the United States, as less than 10% of cases are recognized. More than 1500 genetic defects in the LDL receptor, as well as mutations in apoB100 and PCSK9, have been identified. If patients meet clinical criteria for familial hypercholesterolemia, it is reasonable to consider pedigree analysis of first-degree and second-degree relatives, and perform genetic testing both for the patient and first-degree family members. Cascade genetic testing involves testing second-degree family members only if first-degree members test positive.[53] Even if patients do not meet overt criteria for familial hypercholesterolemia but clinical suspicion is still high, genetic testing may still be performed as these individuals (a) still have a chance for passing mutations to offspring, (b) may have elevated cholesterol levels at a later testing period, placing them at high risk for cardiovascular disease, and (c) may not have phenotypic expression of the disease. Furthermore, knowing the specific type of mutation (eg, if there are mutations in PCSK9) may further help tailor therapy for maximum lipid-lowering effect. However, it is important to note that upward of 40% of patients meeting clinical criteria may not test positive for any known genetic mutations.[11]

Hypertriglyceridemic states are only being genetically verified in very specialized centers. The Type III phenotype is most commonly investigated with apoE genotyping[100] in patients with suspected Type III dyslipidemia.

Xanthomas in children are uncommon and must always be investigated. The differential diagnosis for xanthomas in children includes homozygous familial hypercholesterolemia, phytosterolemia/sitosterolemia, cerebrotendinous xanthomatosis, and Alagille syndrome.

Alagille syndrome is an inherited syndrome of biliary hypoplasia leading to elevated serum cholesterol.[101] Children with Alagille syndrome have a characteristic facies with a prominent forehead, hypertelorism, pointed chin, and nasal dystrophy. Serum cholesterol is elevated when patients are young, but can decrease over time. Cirrhosis develops in approximately 12% of patients. Treatment includes medical management or, if cirrhosis develops, liver transplantation. Xanthomas have been found to resolve after liver transplantation.

ACKNOWLEDGMENTS

The authors acknowledge Dr. Ernst J. Schaefer and Dr. Raul D. Santos for their authorship in the previous edition of this chapter.

REFERENCES

1. Fredrickson DS, Levy RI, Lees RS. Fat transport in lipoproteins—an integrated approach to mechanisms and disorders. *N Engl J Med*. 1967;276(1):34-44.
2. Goldstein JL, Schrott HG, Hazzard WR, et al. Hyperlipidemia in coronary heart disease II. Genetic analysis of lipid levels in 176 families and delineation of a new inherited disorder, combined hyperlipidemia. *J Clin Invest*. 1973;52(7):1544-1568.
3. Khezri F, Gibson LE, Tefferi A. Xanthoma disseminatum: effective therapy with 2-chlorodeoxyadenosine in a case series. *Arch Dermatol*. 2011;147(4):459-464.
4. National Cholesterol Education Program (NCEP) Expert Panel on Detection, Evaluation, and Treatment of High Blood Cholesterol in Adults (Adult Treatment Panel III). Third report of the National Cholesterol Education Program (NCEP) Expert Panel on Detection, Evaluation, and Treatment of High Blood Cholesterol in Adults (Adult Treatment Panel III) final report. *Circulation*. 2002;106(25):3143-3421.
5. Stone NJ, Robinson JG, Lichtenstein AH, et al. 2013 ACC/AHA guideline on the treatment of blood cholesterol to reduce atherosclerotic cardiovascular risk in adults: a report of the American College of Cardiology/American Heart Association Task Force on Practice Guidelines. *J Am Coll Cardiol*. 2014;63(25, pt B):2889-2934.
6. Lloyd-Jones DM, Morris PB, Ballantyne CM, et al. 2016 ACC expert consensus decision pathway on the role of non-statin therapies for LDL-cholesterol lowering in the management of atherosclerotic cardiovascular disease risk: a report of the American College of Cardiology Task Force on Clinical Expert Consensus Documents. *J Am Coll Cardiol*. 2016;68(1):92-125.
7. Deprez M, Uffer S. Clinicopathological features of eyelid skin tumors. A retrospective study of 5504 cases and review of literature. *Am J Dermatopathol*. 2009;31(3):256-262.
8. Tóth PP, Potter D, Ming EE. Prevalence of lipid abnormalities in the United States: the National Health and Nutrition Examination Survey 2003-2006. *J Clin Lipidol*. 2012;6(4):325-330.
9. Kit BK, Kuklina E, Carroll MD, et al. Prevalence of and trends in dyslipidemia and blood pressure among US children and adolescents, 1999-2012. *JAMA Pediatr*. 2015;169(3):272.
10. Goff DC, Bertoni AG, Kramer H, et al. Dyslipidemia prevalence, treatment, and control in the multi-ethnic study of atherosclerosis (MESA): gender, ethnicity, and coronary artery calcium. *Circulation*. 2006;113(5):647-656.
11. Santos RD, Maranhao RC. What is new in familial hypercholesterolemia? *Curr Opin Lipidol*. 2014;25(3):183-188.
12. Nordestgaard BG, Chapman MJ, Humphries SE, et al. Familial hypercholesterolaemia is underdiagnosed and undertreated in the general population: guidance for clinicians to prevent coronary heart disease: consensus statement of the European Atherosclerosis Society. *Eur Heart J*. 2013;34(45):3478-3490a.
13. Albuquerque EM, de Faria EC, Oliveira HC, et al. High frequency of Fredrickson's phenotypes IV and IIb in Brazilians infected by human immunodeficiency virus. *BMC Infect Dis*. 2005;5(1):47.
14. Mahley RW, Huang Y, Rall SC. Pathogenesis of type III hyperlipoproteinemia (dysbetalipoproteinemia). Questions, quandaries, and paradoxes. *J Lipid Res*. 1999;40(11):1933-1949.
15. Schaefer JR. Unraveling hyperlipidemia type III (dysbetalipoproteinemia), slowly. *Eur J Hum Genet*. 2009;17(5):541-542.
16. Menke A, Casagrande S, Geiss L, et al. Prevalence of and trends in diabetes among adults in the United States, 1988-2012. *JAMA*. 2015;314(10):1021.
17. Centers for Disease Control and Prevention, National Center for Chronic Disease Prevention and Health Promotion. *National Chronic Kidney Disease Fact Sheet*, 2017. https://www.cdc.gov/diabetes/pubs/pdf/kidney_factsheet.pdf. Accessed May 29th, 2018.
18. Sprecher DL, Schaefer EJ, Kent KM, et al. Cardiovascular features of homozygous familial hypercholesterolemia: analysis of 16 patients. *Am J Cardiol*. 1984;54(1):20-30.
19. Kashif M, Kumar H, Khaja M. An unusual presentation of eruptive xanthoma. *Medicine (Baltimore)*. 2016;95(37):e4866.
20. Fujiwara S, Oka M, Kunisada M, et al. Severe xanthomatosis with prominent tuberous xanthomas on the cheeks and the nasal dorsum in a patient with type IIa hyperlipoproteinemia. *Eur J Dermatol*. 2013;23(4):517-518.
21. Terasaki F, Morita H, Harada-Shiba M, et al. Familial hypercholesterolemia with multiple large tendinous xanthomas and advanced coronary artery atherosclerosis. *Intern Med*. 2013;52(5):577-581.
22. Groszek E, Abrams JJ, Grundy SM. Normolipidemic planar xanthomatosis associated with benign monoclonal gammopathy. *Metabolism*. 1981;30(9):927-935.
23. Esmat S, Abdel-Halim MRE, Fawzy MM, et al. Are normolipidaemic patients with xanthelasma prone to atherosclerosis? *Clin Exp Dermatol*. 2015;40(4):373-378.
24. Brewer HB, Zech LA, Gregg RE, et al. NIH conference. Type III hyperlipoproteinemia: diagnosis, molecular defects, pathology, and treatment. *Ann Intern Med*. 1983;98(5, pt 1):623-640.
25. Burnside NJ, Alberta L, Robinson-Bostom L, et al. Type III hyperlipoproteinemia with xanthomas and multiple myeloma. *J Am Acad Dermatol*. 2005;53(5):S281-S284.
26. Sharma D, Thirkannad S. Palmar xanthoma—an indicator of a more sinister problem. *Hand (N Y)*. 2010;5(2):210-212.
27. Beutler BD, Cohen PR. Verruciform genital-associated (vegas) xanthoma: report of a patient with verruciform xanthoma of the scrotum and literature review. *Dermatol Online J*. 2015;21(8).
28. Gupta P, Khandpur S, Vedi K, et al. Xanthoma disseminatum associated with inflammatory arthritis and synovitis—a rare association. *Pediatr Dermatol*. 2015;32(1):e1-e4.
29. Zak IT, Altinok D, Neilsen SSF, et al. Xanthoma disseminatum of the central nervous system and cranium. *AJNR Am J Neuroradiol*. 2006;27(4):919-921.
30. Büyükavci M, Selimoglu A, Yildirim U, et al. Xanthoma disseminatum with hepatic involvement in a child. *Pediatr Dermatol*. 2005;22(6):550-553.
31. Razi SM, Gupta AK, Gupta DC, et al. Cerebrotendinous xanthomatosis (a rare lipid storage disorder): a case report. *J Med Case Rep*. 2016;10(1):103.
32. Parente F, Vesnaver M, Massie R, et al. An unusual cause of Achilles tendon xanthoma. *J Clin Lipidol*. 2016;10(4):1040-1044.
33. Bhattacharyya AK, Connor WE. β-Sitosterolemia and

xanthomatosis. *J Clin Invest*. 1974;53(4):1033-1043.

34. Salen G, Starc T, Sisk CM, et al. Intestinal cholesterol absorption inhibitor ezetimibe added to cholestyramine for sitosterolemia and xanthomatosis. *Gastroenterology*. 2006;130(6):1853-1857.

35. Horne MK, Merryman P, Cullinane A, et al. In vitro characterization of a monoclonal IgG(kappa) from a patient with planar xanthomatosis. *Eur J Haematol*. 2008;80(6):495-502.

36. Guidry J, Thompson W, Sonabend M. Chronic myelomonocytic leukemia can present with diffuse planar xanthoma. *Dermatol Online J*. 2014;20(7).

37. Kim JY, Jung HD, Choe YS, et al. A case of xanthoma disseminatum accentuating over the eyelids. *Ann Dermatol*. 2010;22(3):353-357.

38. Yu X-H, Fu Y-C, Zhang D-W, et al. Foam cells in atherosclerosis. *Clin Chim Acta*. 2013;424:245-252.

39. Schaefer EJ. Lipoproteins, nutrition, and heart disease. *Am J Clin Nutr*. 2002;75(2):191-212.

40. Mazein A, Watterson S, Hsieh W-Y, et al. A comprehensive machine-readable view of the mammalian cholesterol biosynthesis pathway. *Biochem Pharmacol*. 2013;86(1):56-66.

41. Feingold KR, Grunfeld C. *Introduction to Lipids and Lipoproteins*. 2000. http://www.ncbi.nlm.nih.gov/pubmed/26247089. Accessed February 20, 2017.

42. Ramasamy I. Recent advances in physiological lipoprotein metabolism. *Clin Chem Lab Med*. 2014;52(12):1695-1727.

43. Jun KR, Park H-I, Chun S, et al. Effects of total cholesterol and triglyceride on the percentage difference between the low-density lipoprotein cholesterol concentration measured directly and calculated using the Friedewald formula. *Clin Chem Lab Med*. 2008;46(3):371-375.

44. Yu X-H, Qian K, Jiang N, et al. ABCG5/ABCG8 in cholesterol excretion and atherosclerosis. *Clin Chim Acta*. 2014;428:82-88.

45. Julve J, Martín-Campos JM, Escolà-Gil JC, et al. Chylomicrons: advances in biology, pathology, laboratory testing, and therapeutics. *Clin Chim Acta*. 2016;455:134-148.

46. Kobayashi J, Mabuchi H. Lipoprotein lipase and atherosclerosis. *Ann Clin Biochem*. 2015;52(6):632-637.

47. Ooi EM, Russell BS, Olson E, et al. Apolipoprotein B-100-containing lipoprotein metabolism in subjects with lipoprotein lipase gene mutations. *Arterioscler Thromb Vasc Biol*. 2012;32(2):459-466.

48. Gibbons GF, Wiggins D, Brown A-M, et al. Synthesis and function of hepatic very-low-density lipoprotein. *Biochem Soc Trans*. 2004;32(pt 1):59-64.

49. Jungner I, Sniderman AD, Furberg C, et al. Does low-density lipoprotein size add to atherogenic particle number in predicting the risk of fatal myocardial infarction? *Am J Cardiol*. 2006;97(7):943-946.

50. Zhou L, Li C, Gao L, et al. High-density lipoprotein synthesis and metabolism (review). *Mol Med Rep*. 2015;12(3):4015-4021.

51. Brahm AJ, Hegele RA. Chylomicronaemia—current diagnosis and future therapies. *Nat Rev Endocrinol*. 2015;11(6):352-362.

52. Gaudet D, Brisson D, Tremblay K, et al. Targeting APOC3 in the familial chylomicronemia syndrome. *N Engl J Med*. 2014;371(23):2200-2206.

53. Santos RD, Frauches TS, Chacra AP. Cascade screening in familial hypercholesterolemia: advancing forward. *J Atheroscler Thromb*. 2015;22(9):869-880.

54. Sattar N, Preiss D, Robinson JG, et al. Lipid-lowering efficacy of the PCSK9 inhibitor evolocumab (AMG 145) in patients with type 2 diabetes: a meta-analysis of individual patient data. *Lancet Diabetes Endocrinol*. 2016;4(5):403-410.

55. Marais AD. Familial hypercholesterolaemia. *Clin Biochem Rev*. 2004;25(1):49-68.

56. Gaddi A, Cicero AF, Odoo FO, et al; Atherosclerosis and Metabolic Diseases Study Group. Practical guidelines for familial combined hyperlipidemia diagnosis: an up-date. *Vasc Health Risk Manag*. 2007;3(6):877-886.

57. van Greevenbroek MM, Stalenhoef AF, de Graaf J, et al. Familial combined hyperlipidemia. *Curr Opin Lipidol*. 2014;25(3):176-182.

58. Yu J-T, Tan L, Hardy J. Apolipoprotein E in Alzheimer's disease: an update. *Annu Rev Neurosci*. 2014;37(1):79-100.

59. Evans D, Aberle J, Beil FU. Resequencing the apolipoprotein A5 (APOA5) gene in patients with various forms of hypertriglyceridemia. *Atherosclerosis*. 2011;219(2):715-720.

60. Berglund L, Brunzell JD, Goldberg AC, et al. Evaluation and treatment of hypertriglyceridemia: an Endocrine Society clinical practice guideline. *J Clin Endocrinol Metab*. 2012;97(9):2969-2989.

61. Yuan G, Al-Shali KZ, Hegele RA. Hypertriglyceridemia: its etiology, effects and treatment. *CMAJ*. 2007;176(8):1113-1120.

62. Loscalzo J. Lipoprotein(a). A unique risk factor for atherothrombotic disease. *Arteriosclerosis*. 10(5):672-679.

63. Jacobson TA. Lipoprotein(a), cardiovascular disease, and contemporary management. *Mayo Clin Proc*. 2013;88(11):1294-1311.

64. Segner S, Theate I, Poiré X, et al. Diffuse xanthomatosis as a presenting feature of multiple myeloma. *Eur J Haematol*. 2010;84(5):460-461.

65. Buezo GF, Porras JI, Fraga J, et al. Coexistence of diffuse plane normolipaemic xanthoma and amyloidosis in a patient with monoclonal gammopathy. *Br J Dermatol*. 1996;135(3):460-462.

66. Bielecka-Dąbrowa A, Hannam S, Rysz J, et al. Malignancy-associated dyslipidemia. *Open Cardiovasc Med J*. 2011;5:35-40.

67. Mozessohn L, Earle C, Spaner D, et al. The association of dyslipidemia with chronic lymphocytic leukemia: a population-based study. *J Natl Cancer Inst*. 2016;109(3).

68. Yazgan Y, Oncu K, Kaplan M, et al. Malignant biliary obstruction increases significantly serum lipid levels: a novel biochemical tumor marker? *Hepatogastroenterology*. 2012;59(119):2079-2082.

69. Seidel D, Alaupovic P, Furman RH. A lipoprotein characterizing obstructive jaundice. I. Method for quantitative separation and identification of lipoproteins in jaundiced subjects. *J Clin Invest*. 1969;48(7):1211-1223.

70. Mukherjee M; American College of Cardiology. *Dyslipidemia in Pregnancy*. 2014. http://www.acc.org/latest-in-cardiology/articles/2014/07/18/16/08/dyslipidemia-in-pregnancy. Accessed February 19, 2017.

71. Rizos CV, Elisaf MS, Liberopoulos EN. Effects of thyroid dysfunction on lipid profile. *Open Cardiovasc Med J*. 2011;5:76-84.

72. Goldberg IJ. Diabetic dyslipidemia: causes and consequences. *J Clin Endocrinol Metab*. 2001;86(3):965-971.

73. Herink M, Ito MK. *Medication Induced Changes in Lipid and Lipoproteins*. 2015. http://www.ncbi.nlm.nih.gov/pubmed/26561699. Accessed February 19, 2017.

74. Hegde U, Doddawad VG, Sreeshyla H, et al.

Verruciform xanthoma: a view on the concepts of its etiopathogenesis. *J Oral Maxillofac Pathol*. 2013;17(3): 392-396.
75. Cohen YK, Elpern DJ. Diffuse normolipemic plane xanthoma associated with monoclonal gammopathy. *Dermatol Pract Concept*. 2015;5(4):65-67.
76. Martin SS, Blaha MJ, Elshazly MB, et al. Comparison of a novel method vs the Friedewald equation for estimating low-density lipoprotein cholesterol levels from the standard lipid profile. *JAMA*. 2013;310(19):2061-2068.
77. Quest Diagnostics. *Your Cardio IQ Report. An in-Depth Assessment of CVD Risk to Help Individualize Treatment*. http://www.questdiagnostics.com/home/physicians/testing-services/condition/cardiovascular/cardio-iq-report.html. Accessed March 5, 2017.
78. LabCorp. *Lipid Cascade With Reflex to Lipoprotein Particle Assessment by NMR (With Graph)*. https://www.labcorp.com/test-menu/30431/lipid-cascade-with-reflex-to-lipoprotein-particle-assessment-by-nmr-with-graph. Accessed March 5, 2017.
79. Sniderman A, Couture P, de Graaf J. Diagnosis and treatment of apolipoprotein B dyslipoproteinemias. *Nat Rev Endocrinol*. 2010;6(6):335-346.
80. Yang G-Z, Li J, Wang L-P. Disseminated intracranial xanthoma disseminatum: a rare case report and review of literature. *Diagn Pathol*. 2016;11(1):78.
81. Digby M, Belli R, McGraw T, et al. Eruptive xanthomas as a cutaneous manifestation of hypertriglyceridemia: a case report. *J Clin Aesthet Dermatol*. 2011;4(1):44-46.
82. Dabski K, Winkelmann RK. Generalized granuloma annulare: histopathology and immunopathology. Systematic review of 100 cases and comparison with localized granuloma annulare. *J Am Acad Dermatol*. 1989;20(1):28-39.
83. Fernández-Herrera J, Pedraz J. Necrobiotic xanthogranuloma. *Semin Cutan Med Surg*. 2007; 26(2):108-113.
84. Veys EM, De Keyser F. Rheumatoid nodules: differential diagnosis and immunohistological findings. *Ann Rheum Dis*. 1993;52(9):625-626.
85. Fernandes Ede Á, Santos EH, Tucunduva TC, et al. Achilles tendon xanthoma imaging on ultrasound and magnetic resonance imaging [in Portuguese]. *Rev Bras Reumatol*. 2015;55(3):313-316.
86. Jin S, Chae SY, Chang SE, et al. A case of xanthoma disseminatum: evaluation and monitoring by 18F-fluorodeoxyglucose positron emission tomography/computed tomography. *Br J Dermatol*. 2014;170(5): 1177-1181.
87. Kelly RB. Diet and exercise in the management of hyperlipidemia. *Am Fam Physician*. 2010;81(9): 1097-1102.
88. Rao Ch S, Subash YE. The effect of chronic tobacco smoking and chewing on the lipid profile. *J Clin Diagn Res*. 2013;7(1):31-34.
89. Bays HE, Toth PP, Kris-Etherton PM, et al. Obesity, adiposity, and dyslipidemia: A consensus statement from the National Lipid Association. *J Clin Lipidol*. 2013;7(4):304-383.
90. Jensen MD, Ryan DH, Apovian CM, et al. 2013 AHA/ACC/TOS guideline for the management of overweight and obesity in adults. *Circulation*. 2014;129(25) (suppl 2):S102-S138.
91. Collins R, Reith C, Emberson J, et al. Interpretation of the evidence for the efficacy and safety of statin therapy. *Lancet*. 2016;388(10059):2532-2561.
92. Battaggia A, Donzelli A, Font M, et al. Clinical efficacy and safety of ezetimibe on major cardiovascular endpoints: systematic review and meta-analysis of randomized controlled trials. *PLoS One*. 2015;10(4):e0124587.
93. Ito MK. Long-chain omega-3 fatty acids, fibrates and niacin as therapeutic options in the treatment of hypertriglyceridemia: a review of the literature. *Atherosclerosis*. 2015;242(2):647-656.
94. Weitz D, Weintraub H, Fisher E, et al. Fish oil for the treatment of cardiovascular disease. *Cardiol Rev*. 2010;18(5):258-263.
95. Barter P, Ginsberg HN. Effectiveness of combined statin plus omega-3 fatty acid therapy for mixed dyslipidemia. *Am J Cardiol*. 2008;102(8):1040-1045.
96. Blom DJ, Fayad ZA, Kastelein JJ, et al; LOWER Investigators. LOWER, a registry of lomitapide-treated patients with homozygous familial hypercholesterolemia: rationale and design. *J Clin Lipidol*. 2016;10(2): 273-282.
97. Panta R, Dahal K, Kunwar S. Efficacy and safety of mipomersen in treatment of dyslipidemia: a meta-analysis of randomized controlled trials. *J Clin Lipidol*. 2015;9(2):217-225.
98. Eyvazian VA, Frishman WH. Evacetrapib. *Cardiol Rev*. 2017;25(2):1.
99. McGowan MP. Emerging low-density lipoprotein (LDL) therapies: management of severely elevated LDL cholesterol—the role of LDL-apheresis. *J Clin Lipidol*. 2013;7(3):S21-S26.
100. Evans D, Beil FU, Aberle J. Resequencing the APOE gene reveals that rare mutations are not significant contributory factors in the development of type III hyperlipidemia. *J Clin Lipidol*. 2013;7(6):671-674.
101. Turnpenny PD, Ellard S. Alagille syndrome: pathogenesis, diagnosis and management. *Eur J Hum Genet*. 2012;20(3):251-257.

Chapter 127 :: Fabry Disease
:: Atul B. Mehta & Catherine H. Orteu

第一百二十七章

Fabry病

中文导读

Fabry病（法布里病）又称为α-半乳糖苷酶A缺乏症。本章分为8节：①流行病学；②病因和发病机制；③皮肤表现；④其他表现；⑤诊断；⑥鉴别诊断；⑦预后与临床病程；⑧治疗。

第一节介绍了Fabry病是第二大最常见的溶酶体储存障碍，估计发病率在1∶40,000到1∶170,000之间。

第二节介绍了Fabry病是一种罕见的X连锁代谢疾病，由溶酶体酶α-半乳糖苷酶A部分或完全缺乏引起。由于这种酶的缺乏，带有末端α-半乳糖残基的中性鞘磷脂积累在不同组织和液体的溶酶体中。

第三节介绍了其皮肤表现，包括血管角皮瘤为主的皮肤血管病变、"假性肢端肥大症"面部特征、下肢水肿和淋巴水肿、出汗减少、雷诺现象。

第四节介绍了Fabry病的非皮肤性表现，儿童期通常与嗜睡、疲倦、疼痛、皮肤异常、感觉器官改变，以及胃肠功能障碍有关。成年期的早期，出现淋巴水肿、蛋白尿和肾脏心脏或中枢/脑血管病的首发体征。在成年期的后期，症状包括上述情况的恶化和更严重的器官功能障碍。

第五节介绍了Fabry病的确诊通常会延迟，从症状出现到诊断的平均时间为15年，必须通过血浆、血清或白细胞中的α-半乳糖苷酶A活性缺陷并鉴定致病突变来确诊。

第六节介绍了不同的临床表现鉴别诊断不一。血管角化瘤的临床诊断可能比较困难，可能需要仔细检查皮肤诊断。广泛性的血管角化瘤可见于其他溶酶体储存障碍，在鉴别诊断中应予以考虑。

第七节预后与临床病程，提到了男性的预期寿命为58.2岁，女性的预期寿命为75.4岁。肾功能衰竭以前是最常见的死亡原因，但现在心脑血管疾病越来越常见。

第八节中表127-5概述了Fabry病的治疗。法布里病是一种多系统疾病，应该在多学科环境中对患者进行评估，治疗包括对症处理、特异性酶替代疗法以及一些基因治疗和造血细胞移植等新疗法。

〔粟 娟〕

AT-A-GLANCE

- Incidence estimated at 1:3200 to 1:170,000 population in all ethnicities.
- X-linked lysosomal storage disorder.
- Highly penetrant in males; female heterozygotes have variable expressivity.
- Partial or complete deficiency of α-galactosidase A with deposition of glycosphingolipids (mostly globotriaosylceramide).
- Classical variants affect predominantly skin, kidneys, heart, eyes, and brain.
- Life expectancy shortened by 20 years in males and 15 years in females.
- Later onset variants are milder and predominantly involve a single organ (eg, renal or cardiac).
- Dermatologic manifestations include angiokeratoma, telangiectases, "pseudoacromegalic" facies, hypohidrosis and hyperhidrosis, lymphoedema, and Raynaud phenomenon.
- Light microscopy shows ectatic upper dermal vessels, peripheral epidermal acanthosis, and variable hyperkeratosis.
- Electron microscopy shows intracytoplasmic, electron-dense, vacuolar "Zebra bodies."
- Treatment is symptomatic, enzyme replacement; chaperone therapy (for amenable mutations).

EPIDEMIOLOGY

Fabry disease (α-galactosidase A deficiency) is generally considered the second most prevalent lysosomal storage disorder, after Gaucher disease,[1,2] with an estimated incidence ranging between 1:40,000 and 1:170,000 persons. All ethnic groups are affected. Neonatal screening studies reveal a higher incidence of mutations in the *GLA* gene and some of the affected individuals suffer from milder variants of the disease, which are associated with significant residual enzyme activity. These may occur with much higher frequency (eg, 1:3200) as suggested by a recent survey of neonates in Northern Italy.[3] A study of more than 7000 neonates in Japan suggests an incidence of pathogenic mutations of approximately 1:7000[4] and a similar incidence has been reported from Europe.[5] These variants often have predominant involvement of a single organ (eg, heart or kidney) and have onset in adult life. A study of the Taiwan Chinese population revealed an unexpectedly high prevalence of the cardiac-variant Fabry-causing mutation IVS4+919G>A among newborns (approximately 1:1600 males), as well as patients with idiopathic hypertrophic cardiomyopathy.[6]

ETIOLOGY AND PATHOGENESIS

Fabry disease (Online Mendelian Inheritance in Man #301500) is a rare X-linked metabolic disorder caused by the partial or complete deficiency of a lysosomal enzyme, α-galactosidase A (Fig. 127-1). As a result of this enzyme deficiency, neutral sphingolipids with terminal α-galactosyl residues (predominantly globotriaosylceramide [Gb3]) accumulate in the lysosomes of different tissues and fluids (epithelial cells of glomeruli and tubules of the kidneys; cardiac myocytes; ganglion cells of the autonomic system; cornea; endothelial, perithelial, and smooth muscle cells of blood vessels; and histiocytic and reticular cells of connective tissue). Elevated levels of globotriaosylsphingosine, which is the deacylated derivative of Gb3, correlate with disease severity in males and females. Globotriaosylsphingosine inhibits the activity of α-galactosidase A and it has been suggested that elevated levels in females could be of pathogenic significance.[7] Clinical onset is variable (Fig. 127-2). Although the condition is X linked, heterozygous females are frequently affected and may be as severely affected as hemizygous males.[8] Clinical symptoms typically occur a decade or so later in females than in males and organ damage in females is usually less severe than in males. Variable expression in females is attributed to the Lyon hypothesis whereby 1 X chromosome is inactivated on a random basis in the female, while the other provides the genetic information. The mutant X chromosome is more likely to be expressed in a range of tissues in symptomatic females with Fabry disease.[9]

The gene *GLA* for α-galactosidase A is located at the Xq22.1 region. More than 600 mutations have been identified in the *GLA* gene,[10-12] including missense, nonsense mutations, and single amino acid deletions and insertions. Most of these mutations are "private," having been identified only in individual families. Some (eg, the p.N215S mutation) are associated with single-organ or late-onset variants and patients have normal levels of urinary Gb_3, despite having clinical evidence of Fabry disease.

CUTANEOUS MANIFESTATIONS

CUTANEOUS VASCULAR LESIONS

ANGIOKERATOMA

Angiokeratomas, are the cutaneous hallmark of Fabry disease.[11-13] Present in 70% of males and 39% of females,[13,14] angiokeratomas are pinpoint to 4 mm

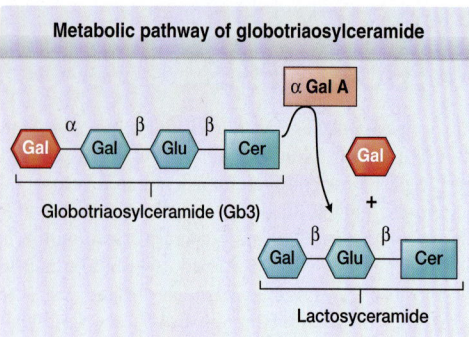

Figure 127-1 Metabolic pathway of globotriaosylceramide. α-Galactosidase A (α Gal A) metabolizes globotriaosylceramide to galactose (Gal) and lactosylceramide. Cer, ceramide; Glu, glucose.

diameter, dark-red to blue-black, macular and papular lesions that do not blanch on pressure (Fig. 127-3). Overlying hyperkeratosis is variable and frequently absent at sites other than the genitalia and umbilicus. Angiokeratomas appear between the ages of 5 and 15 years in males and the ages of 8 and 25 years in females.[15-17] They were a presenting feature in 50 (14.2%) of 352 pediatric patients,[18] in 114 (31.7%) of 359 adult males (n = 359), and in 13 (11.2%) of 118 adult females (n = 118).[19] They may be widespread or grouped. In males, lesions are typically within the "bathing trunk" area (genitals, buttocks, lower abdomen, umbilicus, groins, inner thighs and sacrum). Angiokeratomas are also seen on the proximal limbs, particularly their medial aspects, the elbows and knees, the palms and soles, and over the distal phalanges of the digits (Fig. 127-4). Lesions may occur on the lips, particularly along the vermilion

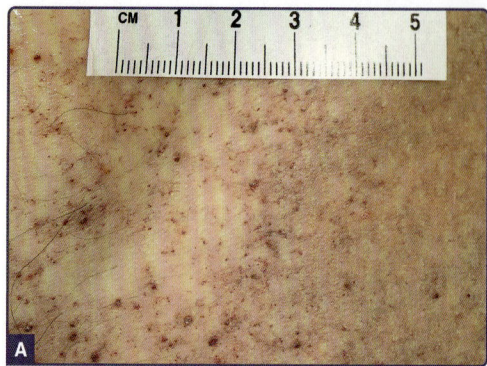

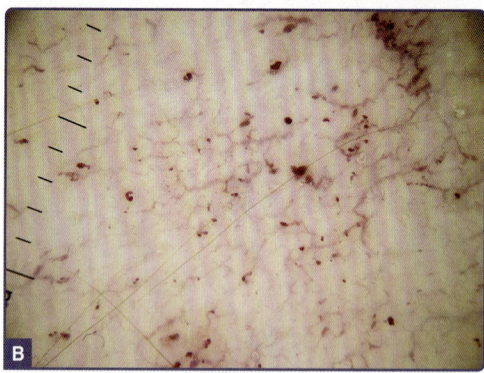

Figure 127-3 A, Angiokeratomas and telangiectatic vessels on the flank of a patient with angiokeratoma corporis diffusum. **B,** Dermatoscopic view showing angiokeratomas and upper dermal vessel tortuosity.

border, and occasionally on the mucosal surfaces (Fig. 127-5). They rarely occur elsewhere on the face. In females, angiokeratomas are usually sparsely distributed (Fig. 127-6), and may occasionally occur in a dermatomal distribution.[13] The most common sites are the trunk and proximal limbs.[13] Female genital lesions are relatively infrequent.

HISTOPATHOLOGY

Histology typically shows dilated, ectatic capillaries in the papillary dermis, a variably thinned epidermis centrally, with epidermal acanthosis at the edges of the lesion, and variable degrees of overlying focal compact orthohyperkeratosis (Fig. 127-7A). Endothelial, perithelial, perineural, eccrine, smooth muscle cells, and fibroblasts are filled with cytoplasmic vacuoles containing glycosphingolipid that can be visualized with toluidine blue stains.[20] Characteristic, electron-dense, lamellated, intracytoplasmic vacuolar inclusions (Zebra bodies) are typically seen on electron microscopy (Fig. 127-7B-D).[21] They exhibit a pattern of alternating light and dark 4- to 6-nm bands. These inclusions may be present in biopsies of angiokeratoma or from normal skin. They may be absent in the skin of heterozygous females. Electron microscopy and immunoelectron microscopy using

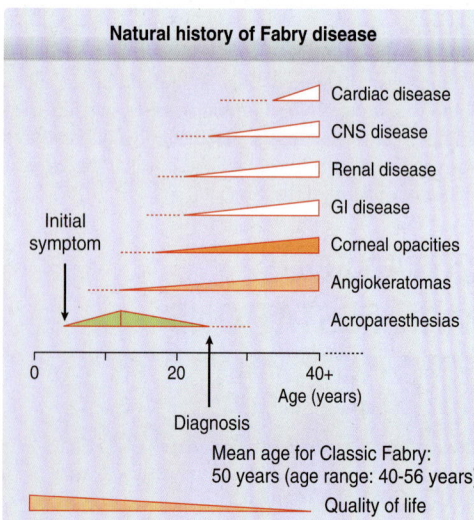

Figure 127-2 Natural history of Fabry disease. Acroparesthesias, angiokeratomas, corneal opacities, and GI symptoms are often the first manifestations. Diagnosis is usually delayed and occurs around the second decade.

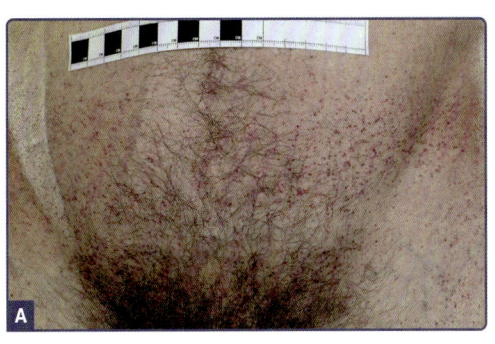
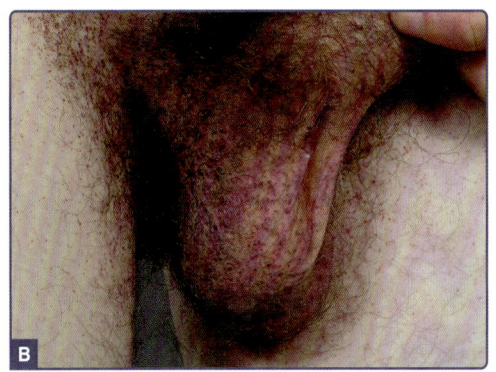
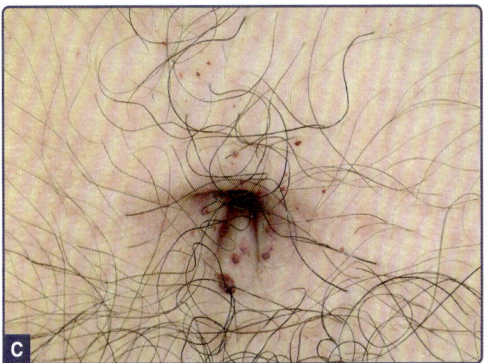
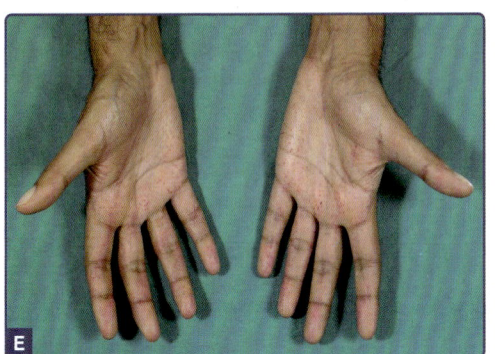
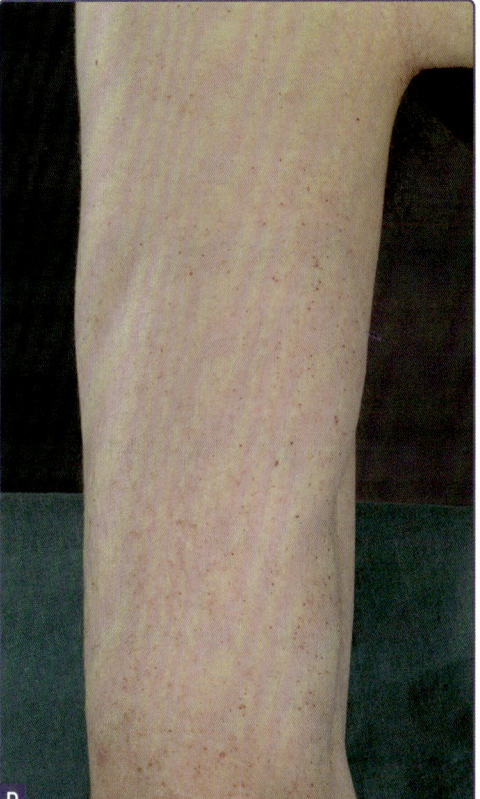
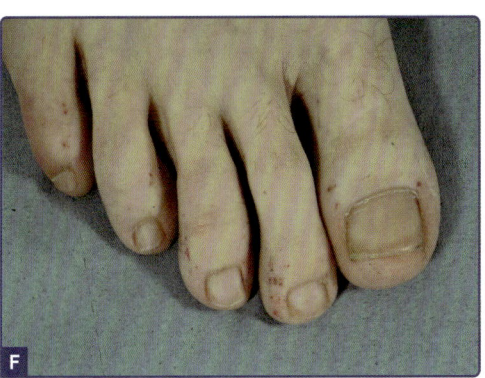

Figure 127-4 Distribution of angiokeratomas in Fabry males with complete phenotypic expression of disease. **A,** Lower abdomen; **B,** scrotum and medial thighs; **C,** umbilicus; **D,** upper limb; **E,** palms; **F,** toes.

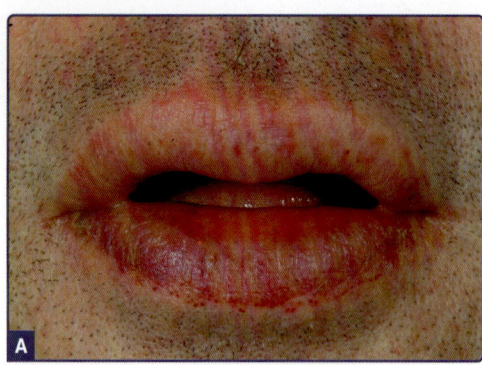 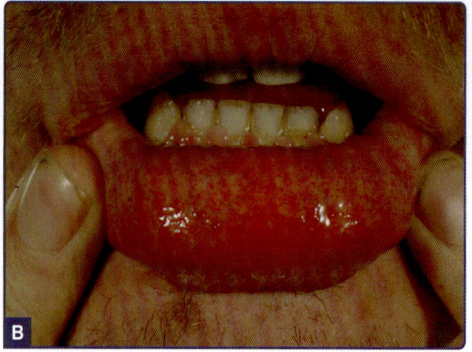

Figure 127-5 Angiomatous lesions on the lips. **A**, Concentrated along the vermilion border; **B**, on the mucosal surface of the lower lip.

anti-Gb3 antibodies are useful tools when other diagnostic tests are inconclusive.[22]

ANGIOMAS AND TELANGIECTASES

Up to a third of Fabry males and two-thirds of Fabry females do not have angiokeratomas.[16,17] A proportion have no cutaneous vascular lesions,[1] others have 1- to 2-mm diameter bright red macular angiomatous lesions, which could represent early angiokeratomas or macular hemangiomas clinically.[11] Patients with widespread papular angiomas, clinically and histologically in keeping with cherry angiomas, are also recognized. In one series, patients with a predominantly cardiac phenotype (N215S mutation) rarely had classical angiokeratoma, but a third of males in this group had widespread (>100) cherry angiomas.[23] Because the prevalence of cherry angiomas in the general population may be as high as 50%,[18] their significance in patients with Fabry disease is not clear. Telangiectases are also common,[13] and may be distinguished from angiokeratomas and macular and cherry angiomas by the presence of blanching on diascopic pressure. Registry data show that they are more common in males (23%) than females (9%).[13,14] Although based on patient recall, data suggest that telangiectases appear later than angiokeratomas, with a mean age at onset of 26 years in males (SD 17, range: 3-70 years) and 42 years in females (SD 22, range: 5-73 years).[13] In a majority of cases, telangiectases occur at sun-exposed sites such as the face and V of the neck, often in patients with skin Type I or Type II. Occasionally, telangiectases may be seen at unusual sites, such as the flanks, groin, and elbow and knee flexures. Dermoscopy of these areas reveals dilated, tortuous upper dermal vessels (see Fig. 127-3). This tends to occur in patients with widespread angiokeratoma and full phenotypic expression of disease.

RELATIONSHIP TO DISEASE SEVERITY

In both sexes, the presence of cutaneous vascular lesions, namely telangiectases and/or angiokeratomas, is associated with higher disease severity scores and a higher prevalence of major organ involvement.[13,14] Thus, cerebrovascular involvement (stroke and transient ischemic attack) was present in 38% of females and 32% of males with cutaneous vascular lesions, but in only 12% of females and 9% of males without. Cardiac involvement occurred in 80% of females and 73% of males with cutaneous vascular lesions versus 38% of females and 49% of males without; renal involvement occurred in 62% of females and 72% of males with cutaneous vascular lesions versus 29% of females and 42% of males without. Similar differences are observed for hypertension, eye, ear, GI, and other neurologic involvement.[14] These findings demonstrate the importance of dermatologic assessment and its possible predictive value in terms of systemic morbidity.

Figure 127-6 Sparsely distributed pinpoint dark-red macular and papular lesions on the trunk of a Fabry female.

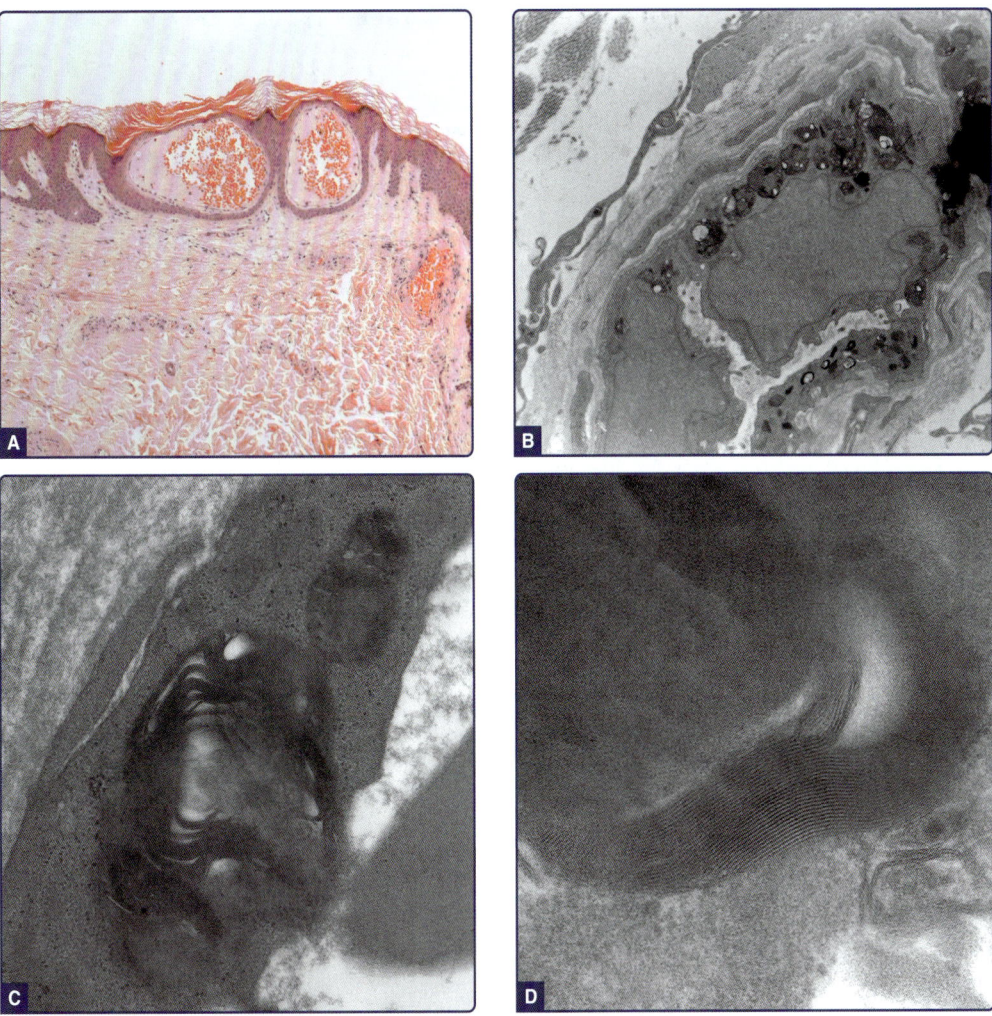

Figure 127-7 Histopathologic features of angiokeratoma. **A,** Light microscopy. Dilated capillaries in the papillary dermis with overlying epidermal thinning and mild orthohyperkeratosis. Acanthotic epidermis at the periphery. Hematoxylin and eosin (H&E) stain ×40 magnification. **B-D,** Electron microscopy. **B,** Multiple electron-dense inclusions in a cutaneous vascular endothelial cell (×9000 magnification). **C,** At higher power a lamellar or "zebra" body is seen (×63,000 magnification). **D,** At highest power (×223,000 magnification) light and dark bands with a periodicity of 4 to 6 nm are identified.

FACIAL FEATURES

A "pseudoacromegalic" facial appearance has been described in some families with Fabry disease (Fig. 127-8). This feature is documented in 2 larger studies. An assessment of 38 patients by a panel of 3 clinical geneticists was based on standardized medical photography[24] and identified (in order of decreasing frequency) periorbital fullness, prominent ear lobes, bushy eyebrows, recessed forehead, pronounced nasal angle, generous nose/bulbous nasal tip, prominent supraorbital ridges, shallow midface, full lips, prominent nasal bridge, broad alar base, coarse features, posteriorly rotated ears, and prognathism. A second study, in which facial dysmorphism was objectively assessed by three-dimensional dense surface modeling and anthropometric analysis using a three-dimensional photogrammetric camera, facial features in 20 males and 22 females with Fabry disease were compared to controls.[25] This study confirmed, in males, and less prominently in females, the presence of the facial features noted above. The presence of these facial features should prompt appropriate investigations for Fabry disease.

The Fabry face appears more common in patients with widespread angiokeratomas and classical disease at the more-severe end of the spectrum. Moderate or marked facial changes were present in 26 (63%) of 41 males with a classical disease phenotype; 16 (61%) of the 26 males had angiokeratoma corporis diffusum. In contrast, facial features were present to a very mild degree (periorbital puffiness only) in 2 (10.5%) of 19 males with a predominantly cardiac phenotype of disease.[14]

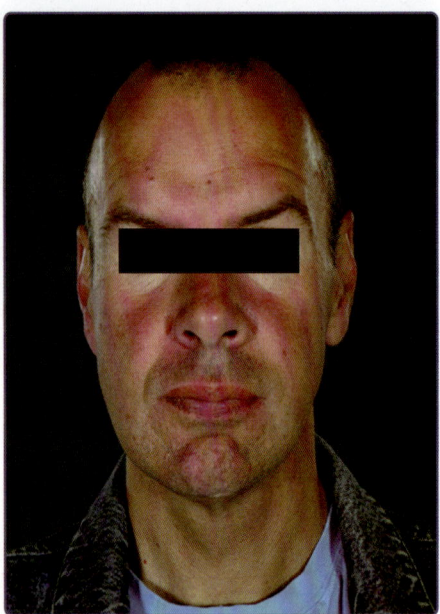

Figure 127-8 Typical facial features: prominent supraorbital ridges, periorbital fullness, large bitemporal width, bushy eyebrows, broad nasal base, full lips, and prominent chin.

LOWER-LIMB EDEMA AND LYMPHEDEMA

Edema and lymphedema, particularly affecting the limbs, is frequently observed in Fabry patients (Fig. 127-9). Lymphedema was cited in the original description of Fabry disease and is recognized in other lysosomal storage diseases such as α-N-acetylgalactosaminidase deficiency.[26] Case reports document it as an unusual presenting feature of the condition,[27] and some suggest that familial lymphedema and Fabry disease might be linked.[28] Registry data from the Fabry Outcome Survey on more than 700 patients confirm that reversible peripheral edema of the lower limbs was present in 25% of Fabry males and 17% of Fabry females; lymphedema was present in 16% of Fabry males and 7% of Fabry females. The mean age of onset was 37 years for males (range: 13-70 years) and a decade or so later for females.[13] This is significantly more than the documented UK community prevalence of 1.33 per 1000 population.[29] In the community it is 5 times more common in women. The mechanism underlying the changes is unclear, and the presence of the changes does not correlate with renal or cardiac involvement. Contributory factors may include glycosphingolipid accumulation,[30] recurrent edema, and primary abnormality of the lymphatics.[31,32] Using the technique of fluorescence microlymphography and measurement of lymph capillary pressure, Amann-Vesti et al demonstrated fragmentation of the microlymphatic network in 5 of 5 hemizygous males and 5 of 5 heterozygous females but in none of 12 healthy controls. Severe structural and functional changes in the initial lymphatics of the skin were present, even when lymphedema was not manifest.[32] Significantly higher serum levels of vascular endothelial growth factor (VEGF)-A, a glycoprotein known to stimulate endothelial cell migration and proliferation, and to increase microvascular permeability and vasodilation, have been identified in Fabry patients.[33]

The possibility that abnormalities in expression or function of recently identified mediators of lymphangiogenesis (VEGF-C/-D and VEGF-Rs)[34] may be involved in the development of lymphedema in Fabry disease remains to be investigated.

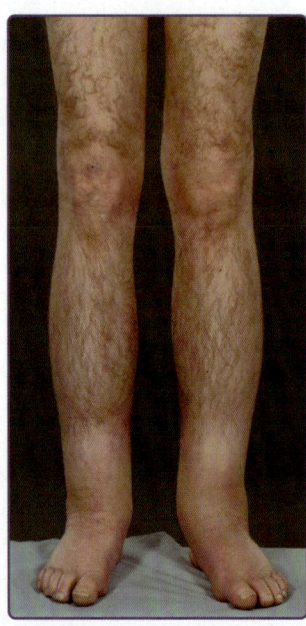

Figure 127-9 Bilateral lower-limb lymphedema in a 43-year-old Fabry male.

ABNORMALITIES OF SWEATING

Reduced sweating is a classical feature of Fabry disease and thought largely to be a consequence of autonomic neuropathy, although substrate accumulation within sweat glands may play a role.[35,36] Hypohidrosis was reported by 53% of males and 28% of females, with earlier onset in males (mean age: 23 vs 26 years). Anhidrosis was described by 25% of males, but only 4% of females.[8] Heat intolerance is a commonly associated and disabling symptom, resulting in reduced exercise tolerance, nausea, dyspnea, light-headedness, and headache, or complete collapse with loss of consciousness. Previous studies[36,37] demonstrated an improvement in sweating in Fabry patients undergoing enzyme replacement therapy (ERT). Hyperhidrosis may also occur, more often in females than males: 44 (11.9%) of 369 females versus 22 (6.4%) of 345 males.[38] This is higher than the estimated prevalence of 1.0% to 2.8% of the general population in the United States.[39] In a majority of Fabry patients, hyperhidrosis affects palms and soles and is not generalized.[38]

RAYNAUD PHENOMENON

"Cold intolerance" and the development of pain in the extremities in cold environments is a frequent complaint among Fabry patients. Registry data has documented Raynaud phenomenon in 57 (8%) of 710 females and 71 (11%) of 644 males (data from Fabry Outcome Survey).[14] Two newer studies identified Raynaud phenomenon in 15.3% to 38% of Fabry patients.[40,41] This is significantly higher than the prevalence of 3% to 22% reported in the general population, in which males are less commonly affected (0.5% to 16%) than females (2.5% to 22%).[41] The reversal of the sex ratio and high prevalence in males suggest a possible causal link to the underlying Fabry disease. In a fluoroscopic nailfold capillaroscopy study[42] that examined 25 Fabry patients (17 males), significantly more bushy capillaries and clusters were identified in cases (72%) than controls (10%). Morphologic and functional abnormalities of nailfold capillaries were present. In a further capillaroscopic study of 32 Fabry patients, 25 (78%) of whom were on ERT, the only significant difference identified was an increase in ramification of capillaries.[41] Although the abnormal vasoreactivity of digital vessels could be related to autonomic dysfunction, abnormalities of nitric oxide synthetase, and increased oxidative stress in vascular endothelium and smooth muscle, might also be important triggers.[43]

NONCUTANEOUS FINDINGS

The noncutaneous findings in Fabry disease are illustrated in Figure 127-2 and listed in Table 127-1 in relation to their typical age of onset. Fabry disease is a progressive, multisystem disorder that typically results in a global reduction in quality of life for affected individuals. Symptoms in childhood typically relate to lethargy, tiredness, pain, cutaneous abnormalities, changes to sensory organs, and, often, GI disturbances. In early adulthood, patients may suffer extension of any of the above symptoms and often develop lymphedema, proteinuria and the first signs of renal, cardiac, or CNS/cerebrovascular disease. In late adulthood (age >30 years), symptoms include worsening of the above and more-severe organ dysfunction (cardiac disease, renal disease, and cerebrovascular disease).

NEUROLOGIC FINDINGS

Acroparesthesias occur in 80% to 90% of affected individuals and typically occur in the first decade.[16]

TABLE 127-1
Noncutaneous Findings

- Renal
  - Chronic renal failure
- Cardiovascular
  - Hypertension
  - Coronary vascular disease
  - Left ventricle hypertrophy
  - Valve disease
  - Arrhythmias
  - Elevated high-density lipoprotein
- Neurologic/psychiatric
  - Acroparesthesias
  - Cerebrovascular disease
  - Dementia
  - Depression
  - Increased suicide ideation
- Ocular
  - Cornea verticillata
  - Conjunctival vessel aneurysms
  - Increased tortuosity of retinal vessels
  - Fabry cataract
- GI
  - Diarrhea
  - Nausea
  - Vomiting
  - Postprandial flank pain
  - Malabsorption
- Others
  - Hearing loss and tinnitus
  - Hypothyroidism
  - Obstructive airway disease
  - Osteopenia and osteoporosis
  - Anemia

Patients describe the sensation as pain, feeling like pins and needles in hands and feet often radiating proximally. Triggers include increased body temperature, exercise, and stress. Pain typically declines over time, which may be the result of damage to nerve fibers as a result of inflammation and substrate accumulation.

SENSORY ORGAN ABNORMALITIES

The most common ocular finding is cornea verticillata (opacities in the cornea characterized by 1 or more lines radiating from near the center of the cornea), which occurs in more than 90% of Fabry males and 70% of Fabry males. Other changes include increased tortuosity of retinal vessels, optic atrophy, cataracts, and lenticular changes. The extent of ocular abnormalities correlates with the overall extent of the disease.[44] Ocular changes also correlate with the genotype, and are more severe in subjects with nonsense mutations.[45] Tinnitus and high-frequency sensorineural hearing loss are also common manifestations, occurring in more than 50% of patients.[16]

Sudden deafness and dizziness resulting from vestibular pathology can also occur.[16]

GASTROINTESTINAL CHANGES

Cramping abdominal pain, nausea, diarrhea and, occasionally, constipation are frequent, and are often the presenting symptom.[46] The pathogenesis is probably related to neurologic abnormalities.

ORGAN DAMAGE IN FABRY DISEASE

RENAL MANIFESTATIONS

Renal manifestations are seen in more than 90% of males.[16] Microalbuminuria and hyperfiltration are early features; proteinuria is typically seen in the third and fourth decades; and progressive decline in renal filtering capacity occurs. Females frequently show proteinuria, although progression to end-stage renal failure is less common. A renal variant of Fabry disease has been described in patients with decreased,[1] but not absent, α-galactosidase A activity; these patients lack other characteristic manifestations.

CARDIAC MANIFESTATIONS

Cardiac manifestations are a constant feature and increasingly recognized as the major cause of death in both male and female patients.[47] Substrate deposition can be demonstrated throughout the myocardium, valves, and conduction system, and is often accompanied by an inflammatory cell infiltrate. A common presentation is with left ventricular hypertrophy, but mitral valve prolapse, arrhythmia, and coronary artery disease can all be present. A cardiac variant[1] has been described in patients with reduced, but not absent, α-galactosidase A activity, and presents later in life (often when patient is older than age 40 years) with predominant cardiac symptoms. MRI scanning has a valuable role in detecting early involvement and in demonstrating scarring, which is a feature of advanced disease.[48]

CEREBROVASCULAR MANIFESTATIONS

Cerebrovascular manifestations include ischemic or hemorrhagic strokes occurring early in life, and transient ischemic attack and strokes affecting the posterior circulation. Stroke is often reported as the presenting feature of Fabry disease and Fabry disease should be considered in the differential diagnosis of young patients with cryptogenic stroke.[49] There is an increased prevalence of factor V Leiden among Fabry patients who have suffered stroke.[50] Cognitive impairment can be demonstrated among older males and females with Fabry disease.[51]

OTHER MANIFESTATIONS

Global manifestations of Fabry disease include lethargy, tiredness, failure to thrive in children, and anemia. Depression is frequent and often underdiagnosed, affecting up to 50% of Fabry males and females.[52] Sexual activity is often affected by the presence of angiokeratomas in the genital region and can lead to decreased self-esteem and libido. Autonomic dysfunction is underrecognized and can lead to hyperhidrosis, abnormal tear and saliva formation, abnormal cardiac reactivity, GI dysmobility, altered pain and temperature perception, and peripheral edema. Endocrine abnormalities are uncommon but osteopenia and hypothyroidism[53] are well described. Pulmonary abnormalities are underrecognized; Fabry disease can lead to an obstructive airways pattern[54] in some patients, but asthma is the presenting feature in other patients. In contrast to other lysosomal storage disorders, cognitive impairment is not generally seen; however, older patients (older than age 50 years) are increasingly seen with memory loss, global intellectual deterioration, and personality change.[51]

DIAGNOSIS

The definitive diagnosis of Fabry disease is usually delayed, with a mean time between the onset of symptoms and diagnosis of 15 years.[55] The diagnosis must be confirmed by the demonstration of deficient α-galactosidase A activity in plasma, serum, or leukocytes and the identification of the pathogenic mutation. Female patients have variable, and, occasionally, even normal levels of enzyme activity, making DNA confirmation of the diagnosis essential.

Biopsy of tissues, such as skin and kidney, demonstrates the presence of lipid deposition and multilamellated myelin bodies in electron micrographs (see Fig. 127-7). As Gb3 deposition starts in utero, prenatal diagnosis can be performed from chorionic villi or culture of amniotic cells, where low α-galactosidase A activity can be demonstrated.[1] There is an increasing recognition of the importance of late-onset mutations; and it is very important that the pathogenicity of the mutation should be confirmed. Measurement of globotriaosylsphingosine can add valuable information.[56]

DIFFERENTIAL DIAGNOSIS

The pain associated with acroparesthesia is often misdiagnosed as rheumatoid arthritis, rheumatic fever, erythromelalgia, Raynaud disease, or simply as "growing pains."[16]

TABLE 127-2
Differential Diagnosis of Angiokeratomas

LOCALIZED FORMS	ANGIOKERATOMA CORPORIS DIFFUSUM
Angiokeratoma of Fordyce	Fucosidosis
Angiokeratoma of the vulva	Aspartylglycosaminuria
Angiokeratoma of Mibelli	Galactosialidosis
Solitary papular angiokeratoma	Schindler/Kanzaki disease
Angiokeratoma circumscriptum	β-Mannosidosis
	GM_1-gangliosidosis/β-galactosidase
	Sialidosis
	Idiopathic

The clinical diagnosis of angiokeratomas in Fabry disease may be difficult. Careful inspection of the skin may be required to distinguish them from purpura, petechiae, and angioma serpiginosum. They should also be distinguished from the solitary and localized forms of angiokeratoma that occur in the absence of underlying systemic disease (Tables 127-2 and 127-3).[57]

Widespread angiokeratomas occur in other lysosomal storage disorders which should be considered in the differential diagnosis. They include fucosidosis,[58] where more than 50% of patients have the changes, α-N-galactosaminidase deficiency and galactosialidosis (47% to 50%) (see Tables 127-2 and 127-4). In addition to the distinct enzyme deficiency in each of these storage diseases and other clinical features, angiokeratomas from Fabry disease can be differentiated by electron microscopic examination by the characteristic electron-dense, lamellar (zebra-like) inclusions within endothelial and other cell types.[59-62] Chloroquine therapy may result in storage of biochemically and ultrastructurally similar inclusions in many of the same cells as Fabry disease and may result in similar clinical manifestations, including the development of angiokeratoma.[63] Widespread angiokeratomas have also been described in association with tuberous sclerosis,[64] juvenile dermatomyositis,[65] and without an associated metabolic disorder.[66]

PROGNOSIS AND CLINICAL COURSE

Earlier studies suggested that males with Fabry disease typically die in the fourth or fifth decade, and females live perhaps 15 years longer. More recently, the life expectancy for males has been estimated as 58.2 years (compared to 74.7 in the general U.S. population) and 75.4 years for females (compared to 80 years in the general U.S. population).[67] There is also evidence that, whereas renal failure was previously the most common cause of death, cardiac disease and cerebrovascular disease are increasingly common. Some of these changes may be a result of the impact of ERT.[67,68]

TREATMENT

Table 127-5 outlines Fabry disease treatment. Fabry disease is a multisystem disorder and patients should be assessed within a multidisciplinary setting.

TABLE 127-3
Clinical Features of Different Types of Angiokeratoma

TYPE	AGE AT ONSET (YR)	SEX	CLINICAL ASPECT	BODY SITE	INHERITED	ASSOCIATION
Fabry	5-12	Both, males > females	Multiple, clustered dark-red to blue-black macules and papules; larger lesions warty (1-4 mm)	Any part of the body, especially bathing trunk area, umbilicus, lips	Yes, X-linked	Acroparesthesias, heart and renal failure, stroke, cornea verticillata, deafness, etc.
Mibelli	10-15	Both, female > males	Grouped, warty, dark-red papules (1-5 mm)	Lateral aspect and dorsa of fingers and toes, hands, and feet	Yes, autosomal dominant	Acrocyanosis and chilblains
Fordyce	>60	Male	Multiple warty, blue-black papules (1-4 mm)	Genitals, mainly scrotum	No	Local venous hypertension
Vulva	>60	Female	Grouped, warty, blue-black papules (1-4 mm)	Vulva	No	Local venous hypertension
Solitary papular	10-40	Both	Single dark-red to black keratotic papules (2-10 mm) often bleed/thrombose	Any part of the body, especially in lower extremities	No	—
Circumscriptum	Usually early onset or at birth	Both	Unilateral plaque keratotic dark-red papules, may bleed	Lower legs or foot may be zosteriform[53]	No	Cobb syndrome; vascular malformations

TABLE 127-4
Differential Diagnosis of Angiokeratoma Corporis Diffusum

GROUP	NAME	ENZYME DEFICIENCY	GENE	ELECTRON MICROSCOPY FINDINGS[55]	CLINICAL FINDINGS	DERMATOLOGIC FINDINGS
Sphingolipidoses	Fabry (OMIM #301500)	α-Galactosidase A	Xq22	Electron-dense lysosomal deposits	Acroparesthesias, heart and renal failure, stroke, cornea verticillata	Angiokeratoma corporis diffusum, telangiectasias, hypohidrosis/anhidrosis, lymphedema
	GM_1-gangliosidosis (OMIM #230500)	β-Galactosidase	3p21-3pter	Electron-lucent lysosomal dilation	Facial dysmorphism, hematologic signs, mental retardation, organomegaly	Angiokeratoma corporis diffusum
Glycoproteinoses	Aspartylglucosaminuria (OMIM #208400)	Aspartylglycosaminidase	4q32-33	Electron-lucent lysosomal dilation	Coarse facies, macroglossia, organomegaly, ocular findings, cardiac valve involvement	Angiokeratoma corporis diffusum, facial angiofibromas, oral fibromatosis, and leukokeratosis
	Fucosidosis (OMIM #230000)	α-Fucosidase	1p34	Electron-lucent lysosomal dilation	Mental retardation, coarse facies, growth retardation, recurrent respiratory tract infections, dysostosis multiplex, visceromegaly	Angiokeratoma corporis diffusum, widespread telangiectasias, acrocyanosis, purple transverse distal nail bands, increased vasculature in hands and feet, sweating abnormalities
	β-Mannosidosis (OMIM #248510)	β-Mannosidase	4q22-q25	Electron-lucent lysosomal dilation	Mental retardation, neuropathy, hearing loss, recurrent infections	Angiokeratoma corporis diffusum in bathing trunk area
	Sialidosis II (OMIM #256550)	Neuraminidase	6p21.3	Electron-lucent lysosomal dilation	Mental retardation, dysostosis multiplex, vacuolated lymphocytes, subtle coarse facial features	Angiokeratoma corporis diffusum
Multiple enzyme deficiency	Galactosialidosis (OMIM #256540)	β-Galactosidase and neuraminidase	20q13.1	Electron-lucent lysosomal dilation	Dwarfism, gargoyle facies, mental retardation, seizures, corneal clouding, dysostosis multiplex, and hearing loss	Angiokeratoma corporis diffusum scattered along entire body, especially knees, elbows, and bathing trunk area
	Kanzaki (OMIM #104170)	α-N-acetylgalactosaminidase	22q11	Electron-lucent lysosomal dilation	Mental retardation, coarse facial features, ocular signs, hearing loss, neuropathy	Angiokeratoma corporis diffusum of entire body, more dense on the bathing trunk area, axillae, and breasts Telangiectasias on lips and oral mucosa

OMIM, Online Mendelian Inheritance in Man.

TABLE 127-5
Treatment: A Multidisciplinary Approach Is Always Advisable
Symptomatic
Angiokeratomas
▪ Liquid nitrogen
▪ Electrocoagulation
▪ Surgical excision
▪ Laser (pulsed-dye 585 nm, neodynium YAG [Nd:YAG] 1064 nm, combined pulsed-dye and Nd:YAG) and intense pulsed light
Lymphedema
▪ Manual lymphatic drainage massage and compression
Hyperhidrosis
▪ Aluminium chloride hexahydrate
▪ Electrophoresis
▪ Botulinum toxin
▪ Glycopyrrolate sodium
Raynaud phenomenon
▪ Avoid smoking, cold and vasoconstrictor therapies
▪ Losartan
▪ Diltiazem
▪ Fluoxetine
▪ Sildenafil
Pain
▪ Avoid triggers
▪ Diphenylhydantoin
▪ Carbamazepine
▪ Gabapentin
Stroke
▪ Antiplatelet
▪ Anticoagulant
Hearing
▪ Hearing aid devices
▪ Avoid noise trauma
Lungs
▪ Avoid smoking
▪ Bronchodilators
GI
▪ Pancrelipase
▪ Metoclopramide
Cardiovascular
▪ Antihypertensive drugs
▪ Antiarrhythmia drugs
▪ Artificial pacemakers
▪ Implantable defibrillators
▪ Coronary bypass
Chronic renal failure
▪ Angiotensin converting enzyme inhibitors
▪ Hemodialysis
▪ Allograft transplant
Specific
Enzyme replacement
▪ α-Galactosidase B (Fabrazyme)
▪ α-Galactosidase A (Replagal)
▪ Migalastat (for patients with amenable mutations)

The advent of ERT has meant that patients and families are increasingly assessed in a specialist center, where they will have access to a physician or pediatrician, dermatologist, and possibly cardiologist/nephrologist/neurologist. Access to audiologists, ophthalmologists, gastroenterologists, and psychiatrists/counselors, as well as to genetic counselors and nurses is desirable and available at larger centers.

SYMPTOMATIC THERAPIES

Individual end-organ manifestations of disease are treated symptomatically (see Table 127-5).

SKIN-DIRECTED THERAPIES

Although clearance of Gb3 from the skin following ERT is reported,[69,70] this does not necessarily translate to clearance of angiokeratomas. The variety of vascular lesions seen in Fabry disease can, however, be treated effectively with quasicontinuous wave and pulsed lasers, and intense pulsed light systems.[71,72] Newer lasers, which combine a high-powered pulsed-dye laser and a 1064-nm long-pulse Nd:YAG laser penetrate deeper and seem to work particularly well for the larger genital angiokeratomas.[73,74]

Prophylactic therapy with grade II graduated below-knee compression hosiery can prevent the development of lymphedema in patients whose edema is still fully reversible. Once lymphedema is established, control can be maintained in up to 80% of patients by regular skin care, exercise, manual lymphatic draining and/or self-massage, and the use of appropriate specialist bandaging and hosiery for lymphedema.[75]

There is some evidence that hypohidrosis improves with ERT.

For those patients with hyperhidrosis, treatment options include the use of topical aluminium chloride hexahydrate, tap water iontophoresis and local botulinum toxin injections, oral glycopyrrolate sodium up to 2 mg three times daily (a well-tolerated anticholinergic with minimal side effects, provided there are no cardiac contraindications) and chemical or endoscopic sympathectomy.[76,77]

For patients with cold extremities, standard measures, such as stopping smoking, avoiding vasoconstricting medications such as beta-blockers, and maintaining warm hands and feet with suitable clothing during winter months are generally recommended. Drug therapies with proven efficacy for Raynaud phenomenon in other patient groups include angiotensin II receptor antagonists, calcium channel blockers, fluoxetine, and sildenafil.[78,79] Possible cardiac and renal contraindications should be taken into account before prescribing these drugs in Fabry patients.

THERAPIES DIRECTED AT OTHER ORGAN SYSTEMS

Pain is the most disturbing and early symptom, and can sometimes be partially managed with diphenylhydantoin, carbamazepine, or gabapentin. Patients should be encouraged to identify, and try to avoid, their personal precipitating factors.

For the primary or secondary prevention of stroke and other vascular pathologies, such as retinal artery occlusion, antiplatelet and anticoagulant therapy might be needed.

Metoclopramide and pancrelipase are used to reduce GI symptoms. Hypertension must be controlled, as it significantly affects 3 of the most affected organs: the kidney, brain, and heart. Angiotensin-receptor blockade should be undertaken at the first sign of proteinuria and is an important adjunct to ERT in slowing the decline in renal function. Fabry patients are good candidates for kidney transplant in the event of end-stage renal failure and the role of ERT in this situation is to preserve the function of other organs. Ancillary care from a cardiac perspective includes consideration of antiarrhythmics, artificial pacemakers, and surgery, including septal ablation and cardiac transplantation.

SPECIFIC THERAPEUTICS: ENZYME REPLACEMENT THERAPY

Two formulations of ERT have been developed: agalsidase beta (Genzyme) and agalsidase alpha (Replagal). Only agalsidase beta is licensed in the United States, whereas both formulations are available in most other parts of the world. Agalsidase beta is administered at a dose of 1 mg/kg biweekly and is manufactured using a recombinant technology in a Chinese hamster ovary cell line. Agalsidase alpha is given at a dose of 0.2 mg/kg biweekly and is manufactured using a gene activation methodology in a human fibroblast cell line. The efficacy of both ERT formulations has been demonstrated in randomized controlled trials,[80-82] and both improve biochemical (eg, levels of Gb3 in plasma, urine, and tissue biopsy) and clinical parameters. The main clinical parameters chosen for study are renal function, pain, cardiac size and function, and quality of life.[83] Long-term effectiveness (with data over 10 years) has been demonstrated in Registry studies of both preparations.[84,85] Both preparations are considered safe and well tolerated. The main side effects are infusion related (fever, temperature) and both preparations can induce antibody formation. However, the impact of antibodies on clinical effectiveness has not been demonstrated. The 2 ERT formulations are generally considered to be of equivalent effectiveness when used at their licensed doses.[86] The optimum time for commencement of treatment has not been established. ERT is recommended for all symptomatic males and at the first sign of organ dysfunction in females. Patients receiving ERT should be regularly monitored with serial measurements of pain, quality of life, and renal and cardiac function. Their data should be entered onto Registries wherever possible.[87] ERT improves hearing and GI symptoms. Direct beneficial effects of ERT on CNS abnormalities have not been demonstrated and enzymes cannot cross the blood–brain barrier.

NEW TREATMENTS

Chaperone-based enzyme enhancement therapy consists of small molecules that rescue misfolded/mistrafficked enzymes from the lysosomes and transport them to the endoplasmic reticulum. Chaperone-based therapy can be administered orally and has demonstrated activity in subjects with amenable mutations and residual activity.[88] Migalastat has been approved by the regulatory authorities in both the United States and Europe.

Substrate deprivation (inhibition of an early step in the synthesis of glycosphingolipids) and the infusion of galactose are other therapeutic options that are still in the research stage.

Gene therapy and hematopoietic cell transplantation are still being developed.

GENETIC COUNSELING

All families that have a member with Fabry disease should have an opportunity to receive genetic counseling. Given the X-linked nature of Fabry disease, female patients have a 50% chance of transmitting the gene to both their sons and daughters, whereas male patients will have no affected sons and 100% of daughters affected. The genotype–phenotype variability should also be stressed, especially among patients with subtle manifestations.

REFERENCES

1. Mehta A, Hughes DA. Fabry disease. In: Adam, MP, Ardinger HH, Pagon RA, et al, eds. *GeneReviews*. Seattle, WA: University of Washington; 2017. https://www.ncbi.nlm.nih.gov/books/NBK1292/. Accessed January 5, 2017.
2. Meikle PJ, Hopwood JJ, Clague AE, et al. Prevalence of lysosomal storage disorders. *JAMA*. 1999;281(3):249-254.
3. Spada M, Pagliardini S, Yasuda M, et al. High incidence of later-onset Fabry disease revealed by newborn screening. *Am J Hum Genet*. 2006;79(1):31-40.
4. Inoue T, Hattori K, Ihara K, et al. Newborn screening for Fabry disease in Japan: prevalence and genotypes of Fabry disease in a pilot study. *J Hum Genet*. 2013;58(8):548-552.
5. Mechtler TP, Stary S, Mez TF, et al. Neonatal screening for lysosomal storage disorders; feasibility and incidence from a nationwide study in Austria. *Lancet*. 2012;379(9813):335-341.
6. Hsu TR, Sung SH, Change FP, et al. Endomyocardial biopsies in patients with left ventricular hypertrophy and a common later-onset Fabry mutation (IV54+919G>A). *Orphanet J Rare Dis*. 2014;9:96.

7. Aerts JM, Groener JE, Kuiper S, et al. Elevated globotriaosylsphingosine is a hallmark of Fabry disease. *Proc Natl Acad Sci U S A*. 2008;105:2812-2817.
8. Wilcox WR, Oliveira JP, Hopkin RJ, et al. Females with Fabry disease frequently have major organ involvement: lessons from the Fabry Registry. *Mol Genet Metab*. 2008;93(2):112-128.
9. Echevarria L, Benistan K, Toussaint A, et al. X chromosome inactivation in female patients with Fabry disease. *Clin Genet*. 2016;89::44-54.
10. Desnick RJ, Ioannou YA, Eng CM, et al. Alpha-galactosidase A deficiency: Fabry disease. In: Valle D, Beaudet AL, Vogelstein B, et al, eds. *The Online Metabolic and Molecular Bases of Inherited Disease*. New York, NY: McGraw-Hill; 2014.
11. Anderson W. A case of angiokeratoma. *Br J Dermatol*. 1898;10:113-117.
12. Fabry J. Ein Beitrag zur Kenntnis der Purpura haemorrhagica nodularis (Purpura papulosa haemorrhagica Hebrae). *Arch Dermatol Syph*. 1898;43:187-200.
13. Orteu CH, Jansen T, Lidove O, et al. Fabry disease and the skin: data from FOS the Fabry outcome survey. *Br J Dermatol*. 2007;157(2):331-337.
14. Dhoat S, Orteu CH, Navarro C, et al. Patients with Fabry disease with cutaneous vascular lesions have higher disease severity scores and more multisystem involvement: data from 1354 patients registered on FOS, the Fabry outcome survey. *Br J Dermatol*. 2009;161(suppl 1):45.
15. Ramaswami U, Whybra C, Parini R, et al. Clinical manifestations of Fabry disease in children: data from FOS—the Fabry Outcome Survey. *Acta Paediatr*. 2006;95:86-92.
16. MacDermott KD, Holmes A, Miners AH. Anderson-Fabry disease: clinical manifestations and impact of disease in a cohort of 98 hemizygous males. *J Med Genet*. 2001;38:750-760.
17. MacDermott KD, Holmes A, Miners AH. Anderson-Fabry disease: clinical manifestations and impact of disease in a cohort of 60 obligate carrier females. *J Med Genet*. 2001;38:769-775.
18. Hopkin RJ, Bissler J, Banikazemi M, et al. Characterization of Fabry disease in 352 pediatric patients in the Fabry Registry. *Pediatr Res*. 2008;64:550.
19. Mehta A, Ricci R, Widmer U, et al. Fabry disease defined: baseline clinical manifestations of 366 patients in the Fabry Outcome Survey. *Eur J Clin Invest*. 2004;34:236-242.
20. Larralde M, Boggio P, Amartino H, et al. Fabry disease: a study of 6 hemizygous men and 5 heterozygous women with emphasis on dermatologic manifestations. *Arch Dermatol*. 2004;140 (12):1440-1446.
21. Navarro C, Teijeira S, Dominguez C, et al. Fabry disease: an ultrastructural comparative study of skin in hemizygous and heterozygous patients. *Acta Neuropathol*. 2006;7:1-8.
22. Kanekura T, Fukushige T, Kanda A, et al. Immunoelectron-microscopic detection of globotriaosylceramide accumulated in the skin of patients with Fabry disease. *Br J Dermatol*. 2005;153(3):544-548.
23. Orteu CH, Mehta AB, Dhoat S, et al. Fabry disease and angiokeratoma corporis diffusum are not synonymous: cutaneous vascular lesions and facial features in 100 patients with Fabry disease. *Br J Dermatol*. 2009;161(suppl 1):46.
24. Ries M, Moore DF, Robinson CJ, et al. Quantitative dysmorphology assessment in Fabry disease. *Genet Med*. 2006;8(2):96-101.
25. Cox-Brinkman J, Vedder A, Hollak C, et al. Three-dimensional face shape in Fabry disease. *Eur J Hum Genet*. 2007;15(5):535-542.
26. Chabas A, Coll MJ, Aparicio M, et al. Mild phenotypic expression of alpha-N-acetylgalactosaminidase deficiency in two adult siblings. *J Inherit Metab Dis*. 1994;17(6):724-731.
27. Lozano F, Garcia-Talavera R, Gomez-Alonso A. An unusual cause of lymphoedema—confirmed by isotopic lymphangiography. *Eur J Vasc Surg*. 1988;2(2):129-131.
28. Gemignani F, Pietrini V, Tagliavini F, et al. Fabry's disease with familial lymphedema of the lower limbs. Case report and family study. *Eur Neurol*. 1979;18(2):84-90.
29. Moffatt CJ, Franks PJ, Doherty DC, et al. Lymphoedema: an underestimated health problem. *Q J Med*. 2003;96(10):731-738.
30. Jansen T, Bechara FG, Orteu CH, et al. The significance of lymphoedema in Fabry Disease. *Acta Paediatr Suppl*. 2005;447:117.
31. Gitzelmann G, Widmer U, Bosshard NU, et al. Lymphoedema in Fabry disease: pathology and therapeutic perspectives. *Acta Paediatr Suppl*. 2006;451:122.
32. Amann-Vesti BR, Gitzelmann G, Widmer U, et al. Severe lymphatic micrangiopathy in Fabry disease. *Lymphat Res Biol*. 2003;1(3):185-189.
33. Zampetti A, Gnarra M, Borsini W, et al. Vascular endothelial growth factor (VEGF-a) in Fabry disease: association with cutaneous and systemic manifestations with vascular involvement. *Cytokine*. 2013;61(3):933-939.
34. Lohela M, Bry M, Tammela T, et al. VEGFs and receptors involved in angiogenesis versus lymphangiogenesis. *Curr Opin Cell Biol*. 2009;21(2):154-165.
35. Cable WJ, Kolodny EH, Adams RD. Fabry disease, impaired autonomic function. *Neurology*. 1982;32:498-450.
36. Hilz MJ, Brys M, Marthol H, et al. Enzyme replacement therapy improves function of C-, Adelta-, and Abeta-nerve fibers in Fabry neuropathy. *Neurology*. 2004;62(7):1066-1072.
37. Schiffman R, Floeter MK, Dambrosia JM, et al. Enzyme replacement therapy improves peripheral nerve and sweat function in Fabry disease. *Muscle Nerve*. 2003;28(6):703-710.
38. Lidove O, Ramaswami U, Jaussaud R, et al. Hyperhidrosis: a new and often early symptom in Fabry disease. International experience and data from the Fabry Outcome Survey. *Int J Clin Pract*. 2006;60(9):1053-1059.
39. Strutton DR, Kowalski JW, Glaser DA, et al. US prevalence of hyperhidrosis and impact on individuals with axillary hyperhidrosis: results from a national survey. *J Am Acad Dermatol*. 2004;51(2):241-248.
40. Germain DP, Atanasiu OI, Akrout-Marouene J, et al. Raynaud's phenomenon associated with Fabry disease. *J Inherit Metab Dis*. 2015;38(2):367-368.
41. Deshayes S, Auboire L, Jaussaud R, et al Prevalence of Raynaud phenomenon and nailfold capillaroscopic abnormalities in Fabry disease: a cross-sectional study. *Medicine (Baltimore)*. 2015;94(20):e780.
42. Wasik JS, Simon RW, Meier T, et al. Nailfold capillaroscopy: specific features in Fabry disease. *Clin Hemorheol Microcirc*. 2009;42(2):99-106.
43. Cooke JP, Marshall JM. Mechanisms of Raynaud's disease. *Vasc Med*. 2005;10(4):293-307.
44. Sodi A, Ioannidis AS. Mehta A, et al. Ocular manifestations of Fabry disease: data from the Fabry Outcome Survey. *Br J Ophthalmol*. 2007;91(2):210-214.

45. Pitz S, Kalkum G, Arash L, et al. Ocular signs correlate well with disease severity and genotype in Fabry disease. Data from FOS. *PLoS One*. 2015;10(3): e0120814.
46. Hoffman B, Schwarz M, Mehta A, et al. Gastrointestinal symptoms in 342 patients with Fabry disease: prevalence and response to enzyme replacement therapy. *Clin Gastroenterol Hepatol*. 2007;5(12):1447-1453.
47. Linhart A, Kampmann C, Zamorano JL, et al. Cardiac manifestations of Anderson Fabry disease: results from the International Fabry Outcome Survey. *Eur Heart J*. 2007;28(10):1228-1235.
48. Sado DM, White SK, Piechnik SK, et al. Identification and assessment of Anderson-Fabry disease by cardiovascular magnetic resonance noncontrast myocardial T1 mapping. *Circ Cardiovasc Imaging*. 2013;6(3):392-398.
49. Rolfs A, Bottcher T, Zschiesche M, et al. Prevalence of Fabry disease in patients with cryptogenic stroke: a prospective study. *Lancet*. 2005;366:1794-1796.
50. Lenders M, Karabul N, Dunting T, et al. Thromboembolic events in Fabry disease and the impact of factor V Leiden. *Neurology*. 2015;84(10):1009-1016.
51. Löhle M, Hughes D, Milligan A, et al. Clinical prodromes of neurodegeneration in Anderson Fabry disease. *Neurology*. 2015;84(14):1454-1464.
52. Cole AL, Lee PJ, Hughes DA, et al. Depression in adults with Fabry disease: a common and under-diagnosed problem. *J Inherit Metab Dis*. 2007;30:943-951.
53. Hauser AC, Gessl A, Lorenz M, et al. High prevalence of subclinical hypothyroidism in patients with Anderson-Fabry disease. *J Inherit Metab Dis*. 2005;28:715-722.
54. Magage S, Lubanda JC, Susa Z, et al. Natural history of the respiratory involvement in Anderson-Fabry disease. *J Inherit Metab Dis*. 2007;30:790-799.
55. Mehta AB, Lewis S, Laverey C. Treatment of lysosomal storage disorders. *BMJ*. 2003;327(7413):462-463.
56. Niemann M, Rolfs A, Störk S, et al. Gene mutations versus clinically relevant phenotypes: lyso-Gb3 defines Fabry disease. *Circ Cardiovasc Genet*. 2014;7:8-16.
57. Schiller PI, Itin PH. Angiokeratomas: an update. *Dermatology*. 1996;193(4):275-282.
58. Fleming C, Rennie A, Fallowfield M, et al. Cutaneous manifestations of fucosidosis. *Br J Dermatol*. 1997; 136(4):594-597.
59. Kanzaki T, Yokota M, Irie F, et al. Angiokeratoma corporis diffusum with glycopeptiduria due to deficient lysosomal alpha-N-acetylgalactosaminidase activity. Clinical, morphologic and biochemical studies. *Arch Dermatol*. 1993;129:460-465.
60. Rodriguez-Serna M, Botella-Estrada R, Chabas A, et al. Angiokeratoma corporis diffusum associated with beta-mannosidase deficiency. *Arch Dermatol*. 1996;132(10):1219-1222.
61. Paller SA. Metabolic disorders characterized by angiokeratomas and neurologic dysfunction. *Neurol Clin*. 1987;5(3):441-446.
62. Kanitakis J, Allombert C, Doebelin B, et al. Fucosidosis with angiokeratoma. Immunohistochemical & electron microscopic study of a new case and literature review. *J Cutan Pathol*. 2005;32(7):506-511.
63. Albay D, Adler SG, Philipose J, et al. Chloroquine-induced lipidosis mimicking Fabry disease. *Mod Pathol*. 2005;18(5):733-738.
64. Gil-Mateo MP, Miquel FJ, Velasco AM, et al. Widespread angiokeratomas and tuberous sclerosis. *Br J Dermatol*. 1996;135:280.
65. Shannon PL, Ford M. Angiokeratomas in juvenile dermatomyositis. *Pediatr Dermatol*. 1999;16:448.
66. Marsden J, Allen R. Widespread angiokeratomas without evidence of metabolic disease [Letter]. *Arch Dermatol*. 1987;123:1125.
67. Waldek S, Patel MR, Banikazemi M, et al. Life expectancy and cause of death in males and females with Fabry disease: findings from the Fabry Registry. *Genet Med*. 2009;11(11):1-7.
68. Mehta A, Clarke JT, Giugliani R, et al. Natural course of Fabry disease: changing pattern of causes of death in FOS–Fabry Outcome Survey. *J Med Genet*. 2009;46(8):548-552.
69. Eng CM, Banikazemi M, Gordon RE, et al. A phase 1/2 clinical trial of enzyme replacement in Fabry disease: pharmacokinetic, substrate clearance, and safety studies. *Am J Hum Genet*. 2001;68(3):711-722.
70. Thurberg BL, Randolph Byers H, Granter SR, et al. Monitoring the 3-year efficacy of enzyme replacement therapy in Fabry disease by repeated skin biopsies. *J Invest Dermatol*. 2004;122(4):900-908.
71. Ross BS, Levine VJ, Ashinoff R. Laser treatment of acquired vascular lesions. *Dermatol Clin*. 1997;15(3): 385-396.
72. Morais P, Santos AL, Baudrier T, et al. Angiokeratomas of Fabry successfully treated with intense pulsed light. *J Cosmet Laser Ther*. 2008;10(4):218-222.
73. Pfirrmann G, Raulin C, Karsai S. Angiokeratoma of the lower extremities: successful treatment with a dual-wavelength laser system (595 and 1064 nm). *J Eur Acad Dermatol Venereol*. 2009;23(2):186-187.
74. Ozdemir M, Baysal I, Engin B, et al. Treatment of angiokeratoma of Fordyce with long-pulse neodymium-doped yttrium aluminium garnet laser. *Dermatol Surg*. 2009;35(1):92-97.
75. Rockson SG. Diagnosis and management of lymphatic vascular disease. *J Am Coll Cardiol*. 2008;52(10): 799-806.
76. Ram R, Lowe NJ, Yamauchi PS. Current and emerging therapeutic modalities for hyperhidrosis, part 1: conservative and non-invasive treatments. *Cutis*. 2007;79(3):211-217.
77. Ram R, Lowe NJ, Yamauchi PS. Current and emerging therapeutic modalities for hyperhidrosis, part 2: moderately invasive and invasive procedures. *Cutis*. 2007;79(4):281-288.
78. Pope JE. The diagnosis and treatment of Raynaud's phenomenon. *Drugs*. 2007;67(4):517-525.
79. Coleiro B, Marshall SE, Denton CP, et al. Treatment of Raynaud's phenomenon with the selective serotonin reuptake inhibitor fluoxetine. *Rheumatology (Oxford)*. 2001;40(9):1038-1043.
80. Schiffmann R, Kopp JB, Austin HA 3rd, et al. Enzyme replacement therapy in Fabry disease: a randomized controlled trial. *JAMA*. 2001;285:2743-2749.
81. Eng CM, Guffon N, Wilcox WR, et al. Safety and efficacy of recombinant human alpha-galactosidase A replacement therapy in Fabry's disease. *N Engl J Med*. 2001;345:9-16.
82. Hughes DA, Elliott PM, Shah J, et al. Effects of enzyme replacement therapy on the cardiomyopathy of Anderson-Fabry disease: a randomised, double-blind, placebo-controlled clinical trial of agalsidase alfa. *Heart*. 2008;94(2):153-158.
83. Mehta AB, Beck M, Elliott P, et al. Evidence of benefit of 5 years of enzyme replacement therapy with agalsidase alfa in patients with Fabry disease—a report from the Fabry Outcome Survey (FOS) *Lancet*. 2009;374:1986-1996.
84. Germain DP, Charrow J, Desnick RJ, et al. Ten-year outcome of enzyme replacement therapy with agalsidase

beta in patients with Fabry disease. *J Med Genet.* 2015;52(5):353-358.
85. Beck M, Hughes D, Kampmann C, et al. Long term effectiveness of agalsidase alfa enzyme replacement therapy in Fabry disease: a Fabry Outcome Survey analysis. *Mol Genet Metab Rep.* 2015;3:21-27.
86. Sirrs SM, Bichet DG, Casey R, et al. Outcomes of patients treated through the Canadian Fabry Disease Initiative. *Mol Genet Metab.* 2014;11(4):499-506.
87. Biegstraaten M, Arngrímsson R, Barbey F, et al. Recommendations for initiation and cessation of enzyme replacement therapy in patients with Fabry disease: the European Fabry Working Group consensus document. *Orphanet J Rare Dis.* 2015;10:36.
88. Germain DP, Hughes DA, Nicholls K, et al. Treatment of Fabry's disease with pharmacologic chaperone migalastat. *N Engl J Med.* 2016;375:545-555.

Chapter 128 :: Calcium and Other Mineral Deposition Disorders
:: Janet A. Fairley & Adam B. Aronson

第一百二十八章

钙和其他矿物沉积紊乱

中文导读

本章主要介绍了钙和尿酸沉积紊乱所致的相关疾病。首先介绍了钙的生理功能主要包括骨骼肌和心肌收缩、神经传递和凝血的关键物质，骨骼中的主要矿物质；然后讲到至少有3种调节激素控制血清中的离子钙浓度：甲状旁腺激素、降钙素、1，25-二羟基维生素D3；随后介绍了营养不良性钙化的病因包括结缔组织病、脂膜炎、弹力纤维假黄瘤等遗传性疾病，基底细胞癌和化脓性肉芽肿等皮肤肿瘤，以及感染因素等；接下来介绍了转移性钙化的病因包括慢性肾功能衰竭、维生素D增多症、肿瘤性钙质沉着症；同时介绍了特发性钙化、医源性钙化、原发性骨化的特征及治疗；最后介绍了痛风的流行病学、发病机制、临床特征、实验室检查和病理学、治疗。

AT-A-GLANCE

- Results from the deposition of calcium salts in the dermis, subcutaneous tissue, or vascular endothelium when the local calcium concentration exceeds its solubility in the tissue.
- Clinically, it may be categorized as dystrophic, metastatic, idiopathic, or iatrogenic.
- Pathology shows aggregates of calcium that stain with Alizarin red S or von Kossa stains.
- Ossification may occur secondary to calcification or primarily in genetic syndromes.
- Treatment is often difficult.

CALCIUM

Calcium is involved in many physiologic processes. It is key to skeletal muscle and myocardial contraction, neurotransmission, and blood coagulation. In addition, it is the primary mineral in the bony skeleton. On the cellular level, its diverse functions include transmission of information into and between cells, regulation of plasma membrane potential, and exocytosis. Only over the last 20 years has its effect on skin been fully appreciated. Calcium regulates major functions in the epidermal keratinocytes including proliferation, differentiation, and cell–cell adhesion.[1-6]

REGULATORY HORMONES

At least 3 regulatory hormones control the ionic calcium concentration in serum: (1) parathyroid hormone (PTH), (2) calcitonin, and (3) 1,25-dihydroxyvitamin D_3 (1,25(OH)$_2$D$_3$).

PTH is an 84–amino acid, single-chain polypeptide that is synthesized in the parathyroid glands. Under normal conditions, a decrease in the serum concentration of ionized calcium results in an increase in PTH production, whereas an increase in the serum concentration of ionized calcium results in a decrease in PTH production. In the kidney, PTH increases renal tubular reabsorption of calcium and increases renal clearance of phosphate. PTH also acts directly on the bone to increase the plasma calcium concentration. It does this acutely by mobilizing calcium from bone into the extracellular fluid. Osteocytes and osteoblasts are the presumed target cells for this effect. PTH also stimulates osteoclastic bone resorption, possibly by stimulating osteoblasts to release factors that activate osteoclasts. PTH together with a decreased plasma phosphate concentration stimulates 1α-hydroxylase activity in the kidney, causing an increase in the plasma concentration of 1,25(OH)$_2$D$_3$. 1,25(OH)$_2$D$_3$ increases intestinal absorption of calcium.

Calcitonin is a 32–amino acid polypeptide that is produced by parafollicular or C cells of the thyroid gland. Calcium is the primary stimulant for calcitonin secretion. Calcitonin lowers the serum calcium concentration, primarily through osteoclast inhibition, but whether it plays a major role in serum calcium metabolism outside of the neonatal period in vivo is unclear.

Vitamin D_3, or cholecalciferol, is a secosteroid (steroid with a "broken" ring) formed by the opening of the β ring of 7-dehydrocholesterol. In humans, this formation occurs in the basal layer of the epidermis. First, there is an ultraviolet B-mediated conversion of 7-dehydrocholesterol to previtamin D_3. Previtamin D_3 then undergoes thermal isomerization to form vitamin D_3. To become biologically active, vitamin D_3 must first be hydroxylated at carbon position 25 in the liver and then at carbon position 1α by the enzyme 1α-hydroxylase in the kidney. 1α-Hydroxylase is tightly regulated. PTH and calcitonin increase its activity, whereas calcium, phosphate, and 1,25(OH)$_2$D$_3$ inhibit it.[7]

1,25(OH)$_2$D$_3$, similarly to PTH, increases the concentration of plasma calcium. Its primary action is to stimulate the active transport of calcium across the intestine. 1,25(OH)$_2$D$_3$ also increases the plasma calcium concentration by mobilizing calcium from bone.[8] The simultaneous presence of PTH appears to be necessary for this effect.

1,25(OH)$_2$D$_3$ also plays a major role in the growth and differentiation of tissues, including skin.[9] 1,25(OH)$_2$D$_3$ acts through its nuclear receptor (vitamin D receptor [VDR]), which is a member of the superfamily of steroid/thyroid/retinoid nuclear receptors. In the skin, receptors for 1,25(OH)$_2$D$_3$ are present on epidermal keratinocytes, pilosebaceous structures, and in the dermis.[10-13] In human keratinocyte cultures, 1,25(OH)$_2$D$_3$ causes a dose-dependent decrease in proliferation, an increase in morphologic differentiation, and an increase in terminal differentiation markers.[14] Cultured human keratinocytes can also convert 25(OH)D$_3$ to 1,25(OH)$_2$D$_3$, suggesting that the epidermis may regulate its own growth and differentiation by endogenously produced 1,25(OH)$_2$D$_3$.[14] The mechanism by which 1,25(OH)$_2$D$_3$ may induce differentiation of epidermal cells may be through calcium, because calcium is required for terminal differentiation of keratinocytes. 1,25(OH)$_2$D$_3$ may facilitate calcium entry into cells and, through induction of calcium-binding proteins, facilitate the ability of calcium to regulate various cellular processes.

ABERRANT CALCIFICATION AND OSSIFICATION

Despite the careful regulation of serum calcium, calcification and ossification of cutaneous and subcutaneous tissues may occur.[15] Calcification is the deposition of insoluble calcium salts; when it occurs in cutaneous tissues, it is known as *calcinosis cutis*. Ossification is the formation of true bony tissue by the deposition of calcium and phosphorus in a proteinaceous matrix as hydroxyapatite crystals. Cutaneous calcification may be divided into 4 major categories: (1) dystrophic, (2) metastatic, (3) idiopathic, and (4) iatrogenic (Table 128-1). Dystrophic calcification is the most common type of calcinosis cutis and occurs as a result of local tissue injury. Although calcium and phosphate metabolism and serum levels are normal, local tissue abnormalities, such as alterations in collagen, elastin, or subcutaneous fat may trigger calcification. The internal organs usually remain unaffected. Metastatic calcification is the precipitation of calcium salts in normal tissue secondary to an underlying defect in calcium and/or phosphate metabolism. The calcification may be widespread and, in addition to the skin, affects predominantly blood vessels, kidneys, lungs, and gastric mucosa. All patients presenting with signs of cutaneous calcification should receive a calcium and phosphate metabolic evaluation. Idiopathic calcification occurs without identifiable underlying tissue abnormalities, abnormal calcium, and/or phosphate metabolism. Cutaneous calcification also may be iatrogenic. Cutaneous ossification most commonly occurs secondary to local tissue alteration or preexisting calcification. Any calcifying disorder of the skin may ossify secondarily. Rarely, primary cutaneous ossification may occur without underlying tissue abnormalities or preexisting calcification.

TABLE 128-1
Calcinosis Cutis Subtypes

CATEGORIES OF CALCINOSIS CUTIS	SERUM CALCIUM	SERUM PHOSPHATE	CAUSE	ASSOCIATED CONDITIONS
Dystrophic	Normal	Normal	Local tissue injury	Connective tissue diseases Panniculitis Inherited disorders Cutaneous neoplasms Infections
Metastatic	Elevated or normal	Elevated or normal	Precipitation of calcium salts in normal tissue due to underlying defect in calcium and/or phosphate metabolism	Chronic renal failure Hypervitaminosis D Milk-alkali syndrome Tumoral calcinosis
Idiopathic	Normal	Normal	unknown	
Iatrogenic	Normal	Normal	Local injury	IV calcium chloride IV calcium gluconate therapy

DYSTROPHIC CALCIFICATION

CONNECTIVE TISSUE DISEASES

Dystrophic calcification frequently occurs in connective tissue diseases.[16] Scleroderma, including the limited cutaneous form previously known as CREST syndrome (*c*alcinosis cutis, *R*aynaud phenomenon, *e*sophageal dysfunction, *s*clerodactyly, *t*elangiectasia) are notable examples that are frequently associated with calcinosis cutis (Fig. 128-1; Chap. 63). In these disorders, nodules and plaques of calcium deposits may occur in the skin, subcutaneous tissue, muscle, or tendons. The calcium deposits most commonly occur on the upper extremities, especially on the fingers and wrists, but may occur in any area subject to trauma or motion. As the calcifications enlarge, they may ulcerate and exude a chalky material.

Dystrophic calcification also occurs in dermatomyositis (Chap. 62). It is more commonly associated with juvenile rather than adult-onset dermatomyositis (formerly in about 50% to 70% of children as opposed to 20% of adults); nevertheless, the more aggressive early treatment of juvenile dermatomyositis has been associated with a decrease in the occurrence of dystrophic calcification.[17] The calcification tends to occur 2 to 3 years after disease onset and most frequently appears on the elbows, knees, shoulders, and buttocks.[18] The calcium deposits may be painful and can ulcerate. They also may exude a chalky material, form sinuses, and become chronically infected. In a condition known as calcinosis universalis, calcium salt deposition may become quite extensive, progressing along fascial planes of skin and muscle, forming an "exoskeleton," and leading to significant morbidity and mortality. Calcinosis cutis in dermatomyositis is difficult to treat; however, if the patient survives long enough, the calcified nodules may improve spontaneously. Although uncommon, calcinosis cutis has been described in all clinical subsets of lupus erythematosus and scleroderma.[19-22]

There is no standard treatment for dystrophic calcification. A diet low in calcium and phosphate along with aluminum hydroxide has been reported to arrest or facilitate regression of the calcified nodules.[23] Disodium etidronate also has been used with some success.[24] Several series report long-term treatment with diltiazem improves the calcinosis in some patients.[25,26] Other reported treatments include warfarin, colchicine, probenecid, bisphosphonates, and sodium thiosulfate.[16,27] Occasionally, calcium deposits must be removed surgically to clear sinus tracts, ulcers, or chronic infections.

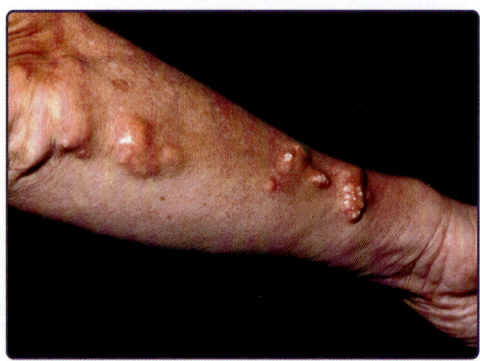

Figure 128-1 Dystrophic calcification in limited cutaneous systemic sclerosis (formerly CREST syndrome: *c*alcinosis cutis, *R*aynaud phenomenon, *e*sophageal dysfunction, *s*clerodactyly, *t*elangiectasia).

PANNICULITIS

Pancreatic enzyme panniculitis (Chap. 73) is a lobular panniculitis that commonly demonstrates dystrophic calcification. It occurs in patients with pancreatitis or pancreatic adenocarcinoma and is presumably caused by the action of liberated pancreatic enzymes on subcutaneous fat. The fatty acids formed by lipolysis may combine with calcium and form calcium soap.

In subcutaneous fat necrosis of the newborn, erythematous, well-defined nodules and plaques occur during the first few weeks of life over the cheeks, back, buttocks, and extremities.[28,29] The affected infants are generally otherwise healthy, and the nodules and plaques usually clear spontaneously. Occasionally, the lesions calcify, and in a small subset of patients symptomatic hypercalcemia may develop, sometimes several months after birth.

INHERITED DISORDERS

Dystrophic calcification occurs in patients with pseudoxanthoma elasticum (PXE; Chap. 72). PXE is a hereditary disorder of elastic tissue characterized by progressive calcification of elastin fibers, primarily within the skin, Bruch's membrane of the retina, and the cardiovascular system. Mutations in the *ABCC6* gene (ATP-binding cassette) have been found in PXE patients.[30] This gene is thought to play a critical role in transmembrane transport. These patients also have significantly reduced serum levels of fetuin-A, an antimineralization protein, which may allowed increased calcification of elastic fibers.[31] Most patients with PXE have normal calcium phosphate metabolism, but a few have been identified who have abnormal calcium, phosphate, and/or vitamin D metabolism. Patients in this subset may develop metastatic calcification in the form of calcified or ossified tumors, calcification of the falx cerebri, and arterial calcification.[32-34]

Ehlers-Danlos syndrome (EDS; Chap. 72) is a group of inherited disorders of fibrillar collagen metabolism. Mutations in the collagen genes or enzymes that regulate collagen biosynthesis have been determined to underlie a number of EDS subtypes.[35-37] The skin characteristically shows hyperelasticity and fragility with formation of pseudotumors and large gaping scars. Subcutaneous calcified nodules, termed *spheroids* or *spherules*, may appear and are thought to represent calcified ischemic fat lobules.[38,39] Calcification of healing surgical incisions also has been reported in patients with EDS.[40]

Dystrophic calcification has been observed in patients with porphyria cutanea tarda (Chap. 124).[41,42] Sclerodermoid plaques with dystrophic calcification have occurred on the preauricular area, scalp, neck, and dorsa of the hands. Ulceration with transepidermal elimination of sheets of calcium is also rarely reported. Other genetic disorders in which calcification may occur include Werner syndrome, Rothmund–Thomson syndrome, and cerebral amyloid angiopathy (Chap. 130).[43,44]

CUTANEOUS NEOPLASMS

Dystrophic calcification occurs in association with a variety of benign and malignant cutaneous neoplasms. Often the neoplasms also show ossification in the surrounding stroma.

Pilomatricomas (Chap. 109) are the most common cutaneous neoplasms that manifest calcification and ossification. Approximately 75% of pilomatricomas show calcification and 15% to 20% show ossification.[45,46] Ossification usually occurs within the connective tissue adjacent to the shadow cells, probably through metaplasia of fibroblasts into osteoblasts. High levels of the adherens junction protein β-catenin have been identified in pilomatricomas due to mutations in the APC gene or by activating mutations in b-catenin gene. B-catenin signaling is a necessary for bone morphogenic protein 2–dependent ossification.[47,48]

A large number of other neoplasms may be associated with calcification and ossification, including pilar cyst, basal cell carcinoma, intradermal nevi (probably as a result of inflammation or folliculitis), desmoplastic malignant melanoma, atypical fibroxanthoma, pyogenic granuloma, hemangioma, neurilemmoma, trichoepithelioma, and seborrheic keratoses.[49-53] Mixed tumors (chondroid syringomas) may also show calcification and ossification. However, unlike other neoplasms, the ossification occurs within the tumor via ossification of the chondroid cells, much like endochondral bone formation occurring in the epiphyses of bones.

INFECTIONS

Infectious agents may produce enough cutaneous damage to cause dystrophic calcification. Parasitic infections that may result in calcinosis cutis include onchocerciasis (*Onchocerca volvulus*) and cysticercosis (*Taenia solium*).[54,55] Calcinosis cutis in annular plaques also has been reported as a complication of intrauterine herpes simplex infection.[56]

OTHER

Dystrophic calcification has been reported in a variety of settings where local tissue injury occurs, such as in scarring caused by burns, trauma, neonatal heel sticks, surgery, and keloids.[57-61]

METASTATIC CALCIFICATION

CHRONIC RENAL FAILURE

Metastatic calcification most commonly occurs in chronic renal failure and takes the form of either benign nodular calcification or calciphylaxis. In chronic renal failure, decreased clearance of phosphate results in hyperphosphatemia. In addition, the impaired production of $1,25(OH)_2D_3$ results in a decrease in calcium absorption from the intestine and decreased serum calcium levels. The hypocalcemia results in increased PTH production and secondary hyperparathyroidism. Elevated levels of PTH cause bone resorption and mobilization of calcium and phosphate into the serum, leading to normalization of the serum calcium concentration but marked hyperphosphatemia. If the solubility product of calcium and phosphate is exceeded, metastatic calcification may occur, resulting in benign nodular calcification or calciphylaxis. In benign nodular calcification, the calcifications typically occur at periarticular sites, and their size and number tend to correlate with the degree of hyperphosphatemia. The lesions are usually asymptomatic except for mass effect and disappear with normalization of calcium and phosphate levels, though they may require surgical removal if interfering with function. Deposition of calcium in the skin also has been reported following subcutaneous administration of low-molecular-weight heparin in 2 renal transplant patients, which resolved following cessation of nadoparin.[62]

Calciphylaxis is a life-threatening disorder characterized by progressive vascular calcification, soft tissue necrosis, and ischemic necrosis of the skin (Chap. 137).[63] Clinically, it presents as firm, extremely painful, reticulated violaceous plaques associated with soft tissue necrosis and ulceration (Fig. 128-2). The lesions may occur anywhere, but the lower extremities are most frequently involved. The mortality rate is estimated to be approximately 80%, usually as a result of gangrene and sepsis.

Histopathologically, there is medial calcification of small and medium-sized arteries with intimal hyperplasia, primarily in dermal and subcutaneous tissues. Calciphylaxis occurs almost exclusively in patients with a history of chronic renal failure and prolonged secondary hyperparathyroidism. However, there exist rare reports of the occurrence of calciphylaxis in the absence of renal failure.[64] Most of the patients reported are female, and there may be an association with obesity, poor nutritional status, and diabetes.[65,66]

The pathogenesis of calciphylaxis remains controversial. Experiments in a rat model suggested that calciphylaxis may be triggered by exposure to a sensitizing agent (PTH, dihydrotachysterol, or vitamin D) followed by a challenging agent (metal salts, albumin, or corticosteroids).[67] However, the clinical description and histopathology of the animal lesions differ from the human disease. Protein C dysfunction also has been described in a subset of patients with calciphylaxis, but this more likely is a marker for a coagulation defect that predisposes this group to calciphylaxis.[68] More recently, it has been proposed that conversion of vascular smooth muscle cells into osteoblast-like cells is a critical step in the development of progressive vascular calcification as is seen in calciphylaxis. This conversion may be stimulated by phosphates, substances that stimulate inflammation in the vascular wall and bone morphogenic protein (BMP)-2. Other proteins that are currently under study as potential effectors, both positive and negative, are BMP-7, osteoprotegerin, matrix Gla protein, fetuin-A, and phosphatonins.[69]

The current therapy of calciphylaxis involves a multifaceted approach. The calcium-phosphate product should be normalized by methods including low calcium dialysis, use of phosphate binders that combine calcium acetate and magnesium carbonate, sodium thiosulfate, and parathyroidectomy in those instances where medical management fails. Other possible treatments include pamidronate, cinacalcet, hyperbaric oxygen, and low-dose tissue plasminogen activator.[70,71] There is increasing evidence for the use of sodium thiosulfate for the treatment of calciphylaxis. Sodium thiosulfate has antioxidant effect and also enhances calcium chelation; however, its exact mechanism of action in calciphylaxis remains unknown.[72] Aggressive management of wound infections and judicious use of debridement may help lower the incidence of sepsis and death in these patients.

HYPERVITAMINOSIS D

Chronic ingestion of vitamin D in supraphysiologic doses (50,000–100,000 units/d) may produce hypervitaminosis D.[73] The initial signs and symptoms of hypervitaminosis D are attributable to hypercalcemia and hypercalciuria, and include weakness, lethargy, headache, nausea, and polyuria. Metastatic calcification and nephrolithiasis may also occur.

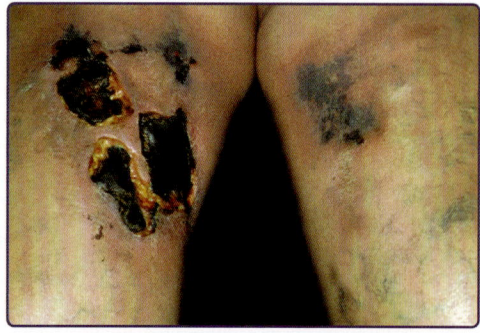

Figure 128-2 Calciphylaxis. The lesions develop as violaceous plaques that may progress to necrotic ulcers, as shown in this patient.

MILK–ALKALI SYNDROME

Milk–alkali syndrome is characterized by excessive ingestion of calcium-containing foods or antacids, leading to hypercalcemia.[74] Complications other than the acute manifestations of hypercalcemia include irreversible renal failure, nephrocalcinosis, and subcutaneous calcification, occurring predominantly in periarticular tissues.

TUMORAL CALCINOSIS

Tumoral calcinosis (TC) is a disorder characterized by the deposition of calcific masses around major joints, such as hips, shoulders, elbows, and knees. The masses are intramuscular or subcutaneous and may enlarge to sizes causing significant impairment of joint function. Usually, the overlying skin is normal, but associated ulceration and calcinosis cutis may occur. It generally occurs in otherwise healthy adolescents. Tumoral calcinosis may be either sporadic or familial. The familial type may be associated with hyperphosphatemia or normophosphatemia. Inactivating mutations in either the *GALNT3*, KLOTHO, or *FGF23* genes may lead to hyperphosphatemic TC.[75-77] *GALNT3* encodes a glycosyltransferase (*N*-acetylgalactosaminyltransferase 3 or ppGalNAc-T3) that initiates mucin-type *O*-glycosylation. It is hypothesized that FGF23, an important regulator of phosphate homeostasis, must be glycosylated by ppGalNAc-T3 to function properly. Normophosphatemic familial TC has been associated with mutations resulting in the absence of SAMD9, an anti-inflammatory protein that also has been suggested to be a tumor suppressor. Surgical excision is the treatment of choice, but phosphate deprivation via dietary restriction and antacids that impair phosphate absorption has met with some success.[78]

OTHER DISORDERS

Other systemic disorders associated with hypercalcemia and/or hyperphosphatemia are reported to cause metastatic calcification. These include neoplasms associated with bony destruction, such as lymphoma, leukemia, multiple myeloma, and metastatic carcinoma.[79-81] Sarcoidosis also may be associated with metastatic calcification.[82]

IDIOPATHIC CALCIFICATION

Calcified nodules characterize idiopathic calcification of the scrotum. The lesions usually appear in otherwise healthy males and tend to increase in size and number with time.[83] Eventually, they may break down and exude a chalky material. Controversy exists over the etiology of this disorder.[84-87] The largest series of patients as of this writing with calcified nodules of the scrotum ($n = 100$) exhibit a spectrum of histologic findings from clear-cut calcification of an epidermal cyst, to inflamed cyst with partial loss of the epithelia lining, to calcium deposits, suggesting that these nodules form from dystrophic calcification of cysts and obliteration of the cyst wall.[87] Excision of the lesions is the treatment of choice, although patients may continue to develop nodules at other sites. Idiopathic calcification of the penis, vulva, and breast also has been reported.[88,89]

Subepidermal calcified nodules appear on the exposed areas of the head and the extremities, usually in children.[90] They may be congenital or acquired and typically appear as hard, 3- to 10-mm solitary lesions, although multiple lesions may occur. Some investigators believe the lesions represent calcified sweat gland hamartomas.[91]

Reports have described the appearance of milialike idiopathic calcinosis cutis on the dorsa of hands and forearms of patients with Down syndrome.[92-94] Some of the calcifications are associated with syringomas.

IATROGENIC CALCIFICATION

Cutaneous calcification may be iatrogenic. Calcinosis cutis is a complication of IV calcium chloride and calcium gluconate therapy.[95] Calcified nodules may appear at sites of extravasation, probably as a result of an elevated tissue concentration of calcium and tissue damage. A secondary inflammatory response results, following which calcium deposits are either absorbed or transepidermally eliminated. In a rabbit model of iatrogenic calcification, intralesional triamcinolone injection decreased inflammation and ulceration. Minor trauma and prolonged contact with calcium salts can lead to calcinosis cutis in a variety of settings.[96,97] It has occurred in patients undergoing electroencephalography with saturated calcium chloride electrode paste.[98] Cutaneous calcification of skin graft donor sites after the application of calcium alginate dressings also has been reported.[99] Transient deposits of calcium in the skin and other soft tissues also have been reported after liver transplantation.[100] It is hypothesized that these transient deposits are caused by the large amounts of calcium- and citrate-containing blood products used during surgery, combined with metabolic abnormalities in the perioperative period.

PRIMARY OSSIFICATION

Primary ossification of cutaneous and subcutaneous tissues rarely occurs without underlying tissue abnormalities or preexisting calcification. However, there are 3 well-described ossifying syndromes[101]: fibrodysplasia ossificans progressiva (FOP), and 2 GNAS-associated disorders, Albright hereditary osteodystrophy (AHO), and progressive osseous heteroplasia (POH). Other primary ossification disorders reported in the literature, such as platelike osteoma cutis (also termed primary osteoma cutis, isolated osteoma, or widespread osteoma) probably are variants of the described ossifying syndromes or represent a group of poorly described primary ossification disorders.

FIBRODYSPLASIA OSSIFICANS PROGRESSIVA

FOP is an autosomal-dominant syndrome characterized by the progressive ossification of deep connective tissues leading to significant morbidity and mortality.[102] Ossification is of the endochondral type and involvement of the skin occurs as a result of direct extension from underlying tissues; thus, it is rare for it to initially present to the dermatologist. Dysmorphic great toes are a characteristic feature of FOP. Other features include abnormal phalanges of the hands, hearing loss (both conductive and sensorineural), sparse scalp hair, cognitive impairment (usually mild), cataracts, persistence of primary teeth, and severe growth retardation.

Gain-of-function point mutations in the activin (*ACVR1/ALK2*) gene have been identified as the cause of FOP. Most cases represent spontaneous mutations but in a few families parental germ-line mosaicism has been identified.[103] Activin (also known as activinlike kinase 2 [ALK2]) is a bone morphogenic protein Type I receptor and its mutation leads to overactive BMP signaling, leading to ectopic bone formation.

ALBRIGHT HEREDITARY OSTEODYSTROPHY, PROGRESSIVE OSSEOUS HETEROPLASIA, AND PLATELIKE OSTEOMA CUTIS

AHO, and POH, are closely related syndromes that are characterized by intramembranous bone formation in skin. Heterozygous, inactivating mutations in the gene encoding for the α-subunit of the stimulatory G protein of adenyl cyclase (GNAS1), a negative regulator of bone formation, have been identified in both of these disorders.[101,104,105] In addition, some patients have been described in which features of both disorders are present.[106] Several families have demonstrated an "imprinting" effect; inheritance of an inactivating mutation in GNAS1 from the mother results in pseudohypoparathyroidism Type Ia, whereas paternal inheritance leads to POH.[107,108] In addition, different splice variants are expressed solely by maternal or paternal alleles. AHO more commonly arises from maternally inherited mutations but no clear genotype–phenotype correlation has yet been established between these disorders. Those patients described as platelike osteoma cutis appear to be formes frustes of AHO or POH.

AHO is an autosomal dominantly inherited syndrome characterized by the ossification of cutaneous and subcutaneous tissues in childhood. AHO generally follows a limited course, and significant deformity and physical impairment are rare. Patients typically have brachydactyly dimpling over the metacarpophalangeal joints (Albright sign), obesity, round or moon facies, short stature, and mental retardation. Most patients have a deficient end-organ response to PTH or "pseudohypoparathyroidism" with hypocalcemia, hyperphosphatemia, and elevated levels of PTH. Other patients have "pseudopseudohypoparathyroidism" with normal serum levels of calcium and phosphorus.

POH is characterized by progressive ossification of skin and deep tissues during infancy or childhood.[109,110] Ossification usually begins in the dermis and progresses to involve deeper tissues, such as muscle, as well as overlying skin. Skin involvement has been described as a papular eruption resembling "rice grains" and having a "gritty" consistency (Fig. 128-3). When well developed, there are weblike areas of ectopic bone formation. The bone formation is most commonly intramembranous (50%), but also may be endochondral (20%) or both (30%). To meet criteria for POH, a patient must have progressive heterotopic ossification, 2 or fewer signs of AHO, and no parathyroid hormone resistance. Secondary orthopedic problems, such as limb-length discrepancy or ankylosis of the joint, may arise if cutaneous ossification is severe enough to limit motion. Other clinical features of POH include low birth weight (usually at or below the 5th percentile).[111]

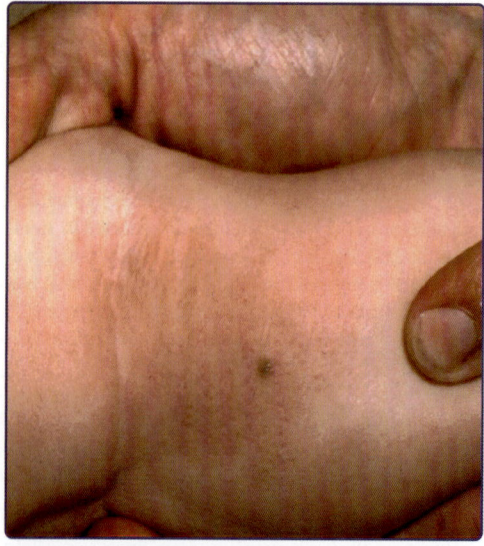

Figure 128-3 Progressive osseous heteroplasia. The appearance of the skin in progressive osseous heteroplasia can be subtle, but the lesions have a distinctive textural change that feels like rice grains in the skin.

OTHER

Miliary osteoma cutis of the face most commonly occurs as multiple small, firm nodules on the faces of young women with a history of acne vulgaris. However, there are reports of multiple miliary osteoma cutis in older patients without acne vulgaris or other underlying skin disease.[112]

GOUT

Gout is a clinical syndrome caused by a group of heterogeneous diseases characterized by deposition of monosodium urate crystals in synovial fluid and joints with or without hyperuricemia, renal disease, or nephrolithiasis.[113,114] It occurs in both acute and chronic forms. Classically, the acute presentation is that of sudden-onset lower extremity peripheral joint inflammatory synovitis. The most commonly affected sites are the first metatarsophalangeal joint and the ankle. In the chronic form, aggregates of crystals are deposited in tissue, especially in skin and around joints. Although skin disease is often asymptomatic, periarticular and osseous deposition may lead to bone destruction.

EPIDEMIOLOGY

Gout affects over 8 million Americans and has historically been described as a disease that affects men, though it also affects women.[115] Recent epidemiologic studies demonstrate that on average, women develop gout a decade later than men, and that female patients with gout are more likely to have renal insufficiency or to be taking diuretics.[116] Obesity has been linked to gout, and both diseases have increased in incidence over the last 3 decades. Recognized risk factors for gout include consumption of alcohol and purine-rich foods such as meat and seafood. Consumption of low-fat dairy products may be protective.[117] Gouty attacks in children are so uncommon that this diagnosis should prompt an evaluation for a malignant or genetic cause.

PATHOGENESIS

Hyperuricemia is a risk factor for gout, but acute gouty arthritis may also occur in patients with normal serum uric acid levels. Patients with serum uric acid levels greater than 7 mg/dL have a 22% chance of developing gout over a 5-year period; accordingly, many patients with elevated serum uric acid levels may never develop gouty arthritis.[118]

Uric acid is the end product of purine catabolism. In most fish, amphibians, and nonprimate mammals, purine-generated uric acid is degraded through uricase (a uric acid oxidase).[114] In primates, including humans, the uricase gene is silenced by 2 mutations. The absence of uricase, along with extensive reabsorption of filtered urate, results in plasma urate levels that are 10 times that of most other mammals.[114] When plasma urate levels exceed its limit of solubility, it may precipitate in tissues.

Hyperuricemia results from either overproduction or underexcretion of uric acid. Ninety percent of patients with gout are under excreters.[118] Conversely, less than 10% of patients with hyperuricemia or gout excrete excessive quantities of uric acid in a 24-hour urine collection. Table 128-2 presents a classification of hyperuricemia. It is usually in the excessive excreters that identifiable mutations in mechanisms regulating protein nucleotide synthesis can be found. The most common mutations are in hypoxanthine-guanine phosphoribosyltransferase, glucose-6-phosphatase, or fructose-1-phosphatase, and can result in either partial or complete deficiency of these enzymes. These mutations are inherited by X-linked or autosomal recessive means (in the latter two); therefore, a family history of gout or early presentation may be a clue toward the existence of one of these mutations. The Lesch–Nyhan syndrome, well described but very rare, is an extremely severe form of hypoxanthine-guanine phosphoribosyltransferase deficiency associated with mental retardation, gout, and self-mutilation.[118]

Genetic determinants of gout in the presence of hyperuricemia are still being elucidated. Genomewide association studies have identified 28 loci of associated common genetic variants. Distinct pathways of renal and gut excretion of uric acid with glycolysis are implicated in hyperuricemia, as well as a mechanism of extrarenal uric acid underexcretion with major urate loci SLC2A9 and ABCG2, respectively.[119]

TABLE 128-2
Classification of Hyperuricemia

Overproduction of uric acid
- Primary hyperuricemia
  - Idiopathic
  - Hypoxanthine-guanine phosphoribosyltransferase deficiency
  - Phosphoribosylpyrophosphate synthetase superactivity
- Secondary hyperuricemia
  - Excessive dietary purine intake
  - Increased nucleotide turnover (eg, myeloproliferative and lymphoproliferative disorders, hemolytic disease, psoriasis)

Diminished excretion of uric acid
- Primary hyperuricemia
  - Idiopathic
- Secondary hyperuricemia
  - Diminished renal function
  - Inhibition of tubular urate secretion by competitive anions (eg, keto- and lactic acidosis)
  - Enhanced tubular urate reabsorption

Dehydration, diuretics
- Miscellaneous
  - Hypertension
  - Hyperparathyroidism
  - Certain drugs (eg, cyclosporine, pyrazinamide, ethambutol, low-dose salicylates)
  - Lead nephropathy

Uric acid underexcretion is idiopathic in patients with hyperuricemia. The anatomic appearance and physiologic function of the kidney appear normal; however, drug-induced alteration of renal tubular function in these patients can precipitate gouty attacks. These pharmacologic agents include loop diuretics, low-dose cyclosporine, and salicylates.

Precipitating causes of an acute gouty attack are not well understood. Studies have shown the presence of intracellular monosodium urate crystals in synovial fluid of asymptomatic patients, suggesting that inflammation in gout is chronic. There must be an unidentified trigger in the acute attack that incites a more robust inflammatory response. Monocytes are present and secrete cytokines, including tumor necrosis factor alpha (TNF-α), interleukin 1, interleukin 6, and interleukin 8. Neutrophils are then attracted to the site as well; they ingest the crystals and release multiple inflammatory mediators, initiating further inflammation and tissue damage.[114,118]

CLINICAL MANIFESTATIONS

Gout can be divided into 4 stages: (1) asymptomatic hyperuricemia, (2) acute gouty arthritis, (3) intercritical gout (between gouty attacks), and (4) chronic tophaceous gout.[118] Patients are often asymptomatic for years, requiring no therapeutic intervention in the absence of other evidence of disease (eg, arthritis, nephrolithiasis, or renal insufficiency).

Acute gouty arthritis usually occurs in middle age and primarily affects a single joint in the lower extremities, the first metatarsophalangeal joint being the most common site of initial involvement (podagra).[113,118] Clinically, the affected joint is erythematous and exquisitely tender to palpation. This may be confused with a sprain, a septic joint, or cellulitis. Cytokine release can lead to fever and systemic symptoms, confounding the picture further. The differential diagnosis also includes other forms of arthritis (psoriatic, reactive, rheumatoid, or osteoarthritis) and pseudogout (chondrocalcinosis).[118]

Intercritical gout describes the interval that occurs between attacks of gout, an interval of between 6 months and 2 years. As attacks continue, they tend to be polyarticular, more severe, and of longer duration. Chronic tophaceous gout describes gout where patients rarely have asymptomatic periods. Urate crystals may be found in the soft tissues, cartilage, and tendons (Fig. 128-4A).[118] Lesions that occur in the skin are referred to as tophi and are a pathognomonic sign of gout. They have been reported in a variety of unusual places as well, including the nasal dorsum.[120] They may be confused with rheumatoid nodules, calcinosis cutis, or granuloma annulare, and aspiration or biopsy may prove useful in confirming the diagnosis.

LABORATORY PRESENTATION AND PATHOLOGY

Laboratory analysis may reveal elevated uric acid levels, but this finding is not necessary for the diagnosis of gout. Leukocytosis and elevated sedimentation rate are often seen during acute arthritic attacks. Accurate diagnosis rests on the demonstration of intracellular, negatively birefringent, needle-shaped crystals by polarized microscopy. Histopathologic examination of a gouty tophus reveals granulomatous inflammation surrounding yellow–brown urate crystals or needlelike spaces in a radial arrangement, representing crystals dissolved during processing (see Figs. 128-4B and 128-5).[121]

TREATMENT

The goal of therapy in acute gouty attacks is analgesia and reduction in inflammation. The main options to choose from are nonsteroidal anti-inflammatory

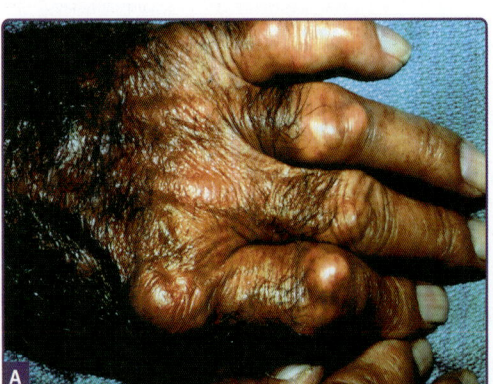 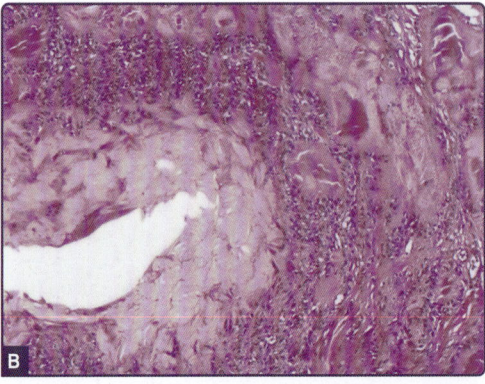

Figure 128-4 Gouty tophi. **A,** Tender nodules overlying joints and tendons, which may drain chalky white material. **B,** Histopathology shows granulomatous "fluffy" appearing infiltrate surrounding radially arranged needle-like spaces.

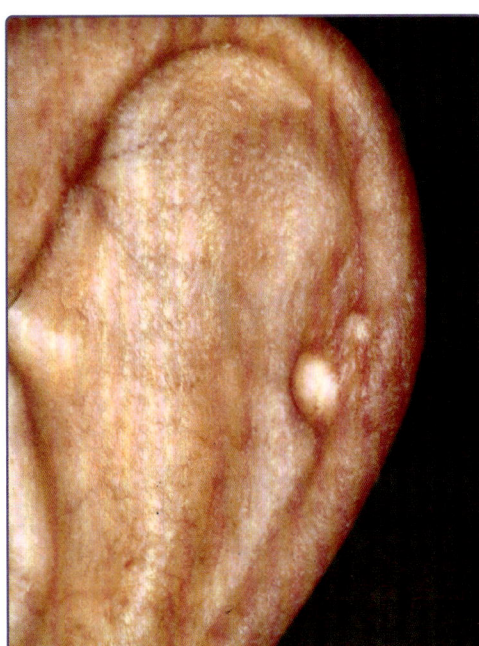

Figure 128-5 Gouty tophi on helix.

drugs, colchicine, and corticosteroids. Indomethacin has been shown in randomized controlled trials to decrease pain, as has colchicine. Colchicine may have adverse GI side effects; however, a newer dosing regimen for colchicine use in acute attacks appears to greatly reduce the incidence of GI symptoms.[121] This regimen of 1.2 mg of colchicine followed in 1 hour by 0.6 mg also reduces drug–drug interactions mediated by colchicine inhibition of P-glycoprotein and cytochrome 3A4 pathways. Severe adverse reaction and deaths have been reported when colchicine is combined with other strong inhibitors of one or both pathways (eg, clarithromycin, erythromycin, and cyclosporine).[122] Indomethacin can precipitate acute renal failure in patients with underlying renal disease. Corticosteroids, both oral and intraarticular, are also believed to be effective. Because patients with gout are typically older with many comorbidities, therapy should be individualized. Treatment should continue for 7 to 10 days after the acute attack, and prophylactic therapy may be continued for 3 to 6 months.[113,118]

In patients with history of only one gouty attack, a conservative management approach can be used. This includes avoidance of drugs that decrease the excretion of uric acid such as thiazide or loop diuretics, aspirin, pyrazinamide, or niacin. Patients should maintain adequate hydration, lose weight, control hypertension and hyperlipidemia, and make diet adjustments by decreasing purine intake. Effectiveness of limiting cholesterol, fat, meat, and alcohol has never been studied, but should be advocated to avoid the need for lifelong oral therapy.[118,123]

Uric acid–lowering therapy is likely necessary in patients with chronic tophaceous gout or those who have had more than one gouty attack. It is also indicated in patients with history of gout and renal calculi, extremely high values of serum uric acid, high serum uric acid levels in the setting of a known familial history of gout (eg, where there is a known deficiency of one of the relevant enzymes previously described), and as prophylaxis for patients receiving acute courses of chemotherapy.

The goal of urate-lowering drugs is to maintain the serum urate level consistently at less than 6 mg/dL (5 mg/dL in patients with tophi or frequent attacks). Uricosuric therapy is ideal in younger patients (age less than 60 years) with normal kidneys who are under-excreters of uric acid. Uricosurics include probenecid, sulfinpyrazone, and benzbromarone.[124,125] The major risks associated with these medicines include hypersensitivity reactions and increased risk of uric acid nephrolithiasis (avoided by alkalinizing the urine). Unfortunately, most patients with gout do not fit this "ideal" situation. Benzbromarone is not commercially available in the United States; though potent, it may cause severe hepatotoxicity.[125]

For all other patients, xanthine oxidase inhibitors are used. Allopurinol is the first-line drug for lowering serum urate.[123] It decreases production of uric acid, and is indicated for patients with nephrolithiasis, renal impairment, those who failed uricosuric agents, with myeloproliferative disorders on chemotherapy, and patients with hyperuricemia due to enzyme abnormalities. Dosages must be reduced in patients with renal failure. Twenty percent of patients taking allopurinol report side effects, and 5% discontinue medication as a result. Side effects include dyspepsia, headache, diarrhea, a pruritic papular eruption, thrombocytopenia, and hepatic function abnormalities. Allopurinol hypersensitivity syndrome is rare and includes fever, urticaria, leukocytosis, eosinophilia, interstitial nephritis, acute renal failure, granulomatous hepatitis, and toxic epidermal necrolysis. A second xanthine oxidase inhibitor is febuxostat, labeled for use at 40 mg once daily.[124,125] It appears to be roughly equivalent to allopurinol. However, it does show higher efficacy in the setting of renal impairment, when allopurinol, but not febuxostate, must be reduced.[125]

Uricases are an additional class of therapeutic agents used in treating urate disorders. The nonpegylated recombinant fungal enzyme rasburicase is FDA approved for short-course therapy to prevent tumor lysis syndrome.[124] It is highly immunogenic, and its plasma half-life is less than 24 hours. IV pegloticase, another uricase, is approved in patients with refractory chronic gout. Pegylation of uricases with production of PEG multimers has decreased the immunogenicity and increased the serum half-life to days or weeks. Infusion reactions may be seen, and include flushing, urticaria, hypotension, and anaphylaxis. All uricase therapies may induce oxidative stress, which can lead to methemoglobinemia or anemia, occurring more often but not confined to glucose-6-phosphate dehydrogenase–deficient (G6PD-deficient) individuals.[124] The role of pegylated uricases in treating urate disease remains to be determined.

Lesinurad is a recently Food and Drug Administration (FDA)–approved selective uric acid reabsorption inhibitor. It inhibits URAT1, a urate transporter that is responsible for most renal reabsorption of uric acid. It also inhibits OAT4, a transporter associated with diuretic-induced hyper uricemia. Lesinurad is administered with a xanthine oxidase inhibitor in those patients who have not achieved control with the xanthine oxidase inhibitor alone.[126]

ACKNOWLEDGMENTS

The authors thank John S. Walsh, MD, and Warren W. Piette, MD, for their work on this chapter in previous editions.

REFERENCES

1. Hennings H, Michael D, Cheng C, et al. Calcium regulation on growth and differentiation of mouse epidermal cells in culture. *Cell.* 1980;19(1):245.
2. Yuspa SH. Chapter IV. In: Skerrow D, Skerrow C, eds. *Methods of Skin Research.* Sussex, UK: John Wiley; 1985:213.
3. Yuspa SH, Kilkenny AE, Steinert PM, et al. Expression of murine epidermal differentiation markers is tightly regulated by restricted extracellular calcium concentrations in vitro. *J Cell Biol.* 1989;109(3):1207.
4. Milstone LM. Calcium modulates the growth of human keratinocytes in confluent culture. *Epithelia.* 1987;1:129.
5. Hu Z, Bonifas JM, Beech J, et al. Mutations in *ATP2C1*, encoding a calcium pump, cause Hailey-Hailey disease. *Nat Genet.* 2000;24(1):61.
6. Sakuntabhai A, Burge S, Monk S, et al. Spectrum of novel *ATP2A2* mutations in patients with Darier's disease. *Hum Mol Gen.* 1999;8:1611.
7. Holick MF, MacLaughlin JA, Clark MB, et al. Photosynthesis of previtamin D_3 in human skin and the physiological consequences. *Science.* 1980;210(4466):203.
8. Deluca HF, Schnoes HK. Vitamin D. Recent advances. *Annu Rev Biochem.* 1983;52:411-439.
9. Bikle DD. Vitamin D regulated keratinocyte differentiation. *J Cellular Biochem.* 2004;92(3):436-444.
10. Clemens TL, Adams JS, Horiuchi N, et al. Interaction of 1,25 dihydroxyvitamin D with keratinocytes and fibroblasts from skin of normal subjects and a subject with vitamin D dependent Rickets, Type II: a model for the study of the mode of action of 1,25(OH)2D3. *J Clin Endocrinol Metab.* 1983;56(4):824.
11. Eli C, Marx SJ. Nuclear uptake of 1,25 dihydroxy3H cholecalciferol in dispersed fibroblasts cultured from normal human skin. *Proc Natl Acad Sci U S A.* 1981;79:2562.
12. Feldman D, Chen T, Cone C, et al. Vitamin D resistant rickets with alopecia: cultured skin fibroblasts elicit defective cytoplasmic receptors and unresponsiveness to 1,25 dihydroxyvitamin D in rat skin. *Endocrinol Metab.* 1982;55:1020.
13. Simpson RU, DeLuca HF. Characterization of a receptor like protein for 1,25 dihydroxyvitamin D in rat skin. *Proc Natl Acad Sci U S A.* 1980;77(10):5822-5826.
14. Pillai S, Bikle DD, Elias PM, et al. Vitamin D and epidermal differentiation. Evidence for a role of endogenously produced vitamin D metabolites in keratinocyte differentiation. *Skin Pharmacol.* 1988;1(3):149-160.
15. Walsh JS, Fairley JA. Calcifying disorders of the skin. *J Am Acad Dermatol.* 1995;33(5, pt 1):693-706.
16. Boulman N, Slobodin G, Rozenbaum M, et al. Calcinosis in rheumatic diseases. *Semin Arthritis Rheum.* 2005;34(6):805-812.
17. Cook DC, Rosen FS, Banker BQ. Dermatomyositis and focal scleroderma. *Pediatr Clin North Am.* 1963;10:979.
18. Bowyer SL, Blane CE, Sullivan DB, et al. Childhood dermatomyositis. Factors predicting functional outcome and development of dystrophic calcification. *J Pediatr.* 1983;103(6):882-888.
19. Rothe MJ, Grant-Kels JM, Rothfield NF, et al. Extensive calcinosis cutis with systemic lupus erythematosus. *Arch Dermatol.* 1990;126:1060.
20. Marzano AV, Kolesnikova LV, Gasparini G, et al. Dystrophic calcinosis cutis in subacute lupus. *Dermatology.* 1999;198(1):90-92.
21. Ueki H, Takei Y, Nakagawa S. Cutaneous calcinosis in localized discoid lupus erythematosus. *Arch Dermatol.* 1980;116(2):196-197.
22. Carette S, Urowitz MB. Systemic lupus erythematosus and diffuse soft tissue calcification. *J Dermatol.* 1983;22:416.
23. Wang WJ, Lo WL, Wong CK. Calcinosis cutis in juvenile dermatomyositis. Remarkable response to aluminum hydroxide therapy. *Arch Dermatol.* 1988;124(11):1721-1722.
24. Rabens SF, Bethune JE. Disodium etidronate therapy for dystrophic cutaneous calcification. *Arch Dermatol.* 1975;11:357.
25. Palmieri GM, Sebes JI, Aelion JA, et al. Treatment of calcinosis with diltiazem. *Arthritis Rheum.* 1995;38(11):1646-1654.
26. Dolan AL, Kassimos D, Gibson T, et al. Diltiazem induces remission of calcinosis in scleroderma. *Br J Rheumatol.* 1995;34(6):576-578.
27. Fuchs D, Fruchter L, Fishel B, et al. Colchicine suppression of local inflammation due to calcinosis in dermatomyositis and progressive systemic sclerosis. *Clin Rheum.* 1986;5(4):527-530.
28. Shackelford GD, Barton LL, McAlister WH. Calcified subcutaneous fat necrosis in infancy. *J Can Assoc Radiol.* 1975;26(3):203-207.
29. Martin MM, Steven EM. Subcutaneous fat necrosis of the newborn associated with subcutaneous fat necrosis and calcification. *Am J Dis Child.* 1962;104:235.
30. Struk B, Cai L, Zäch S, et al. Mutations of the gene encoding the transmembrane transporter protein ABC-C6 cause pseudoxanthoma elasticum. *J Mol Med (Berl).* 2000;78(5):282-286.
31. Hendig D, Schulz V, Arndt M, et al. Role of serum fetuin-A, a major inhibitor of systemic calcification, in pseudoxanthoma elasticum. *Clin Chem.* 2006;52(2):227-234.
32. Choi GS, Kang DS, Chung JJ, et al. Osteoma cutis coexisting with cutis laxa-like pseudoxanthoma elasticum. *J Am Acad Dermatol.* 2000;43(2, pt 2):337-339.
33. Buka R, Wei H, Sapadin A, et al. Pseudoxanthoma elasticum and calcinosis. *J Am Acad Dermatol.* 2000;43(2, pt 1):312-315.
34. Mallette LE, Mechanick JI. Heritable syndrome of pseudoxanthoma elasticum with abnormal phosphorus and vitamin D metabolism. *Am J Med.* 1987;83(6):1157-1162.

35. Giunta C, Steinmann B. Compound heterozygosity for a disease-causing G1489D and disease-modifying G530S substitution in COL5A1 of a patient with the classical type of Ehlers-Danlos syndrome: an explanation of intrafamilial variability? *Am J Med Genet.* 2000;90(1):72-79.
36. Richards AJ, Martin S, Nicholls AC, et al. A single base mutation in *COL5A2* causes Ehlers-Danlos syndrome type II. *J Med Genet.* 1998;35(10):846-848
37. Imamura Y, Scott IC, Greenspan DS. The pro-alpha3(V) collagen chain. Complete primary structure, expression domains in adult and developing tissues, and comparison to the structures and expression domains of the other types V and XI procollagen chains. *J Biol Chem.* 2000;275(12):8749-8759.
38. Novice FM, Collison DW, Burgdorf WHC, et al. *Dysplasias and Malformations: Handbook of Genetic Skin Disorders.* Philadelphia, PA: WB Saunders; 1994:298.
39. Linnemann MP, Johnson VW. Ehlers-Danlos syndrome presenting with torsion of stomach. *Proc R Soc Med.* 1975;68:330.
40. Rees TD, Wood-Smith D, Converse J, et al. The Ehlers-Danlos syndrome. *Plast Reconstr Surg.* 1963;32:39.
41. Grossman ME, Bickers DR, Poh-Fitzpatrick MB, et al. Porphyria cutanea tarda. Clinical features and laboratory findings in 40 patients. *Am J Med.* 1979;67(2):277-286.
42. Wilson PR. Porphyria cutanea tarda with cutaneous "scleroderma" and calcification. *Australas J Dermatol.* 1989;30(2):93-96.
43. Murata K, Nakashima H. Werner's syndrome. Twenty-four cases and review of the Japanese medical literature. *J Am Geriatr Soc.* 1982;30(5):303-308.
44. Aydemir EH, Onsun N, Ozan S, et al. Rothmund-Thomson syndrome with calcinosis universalis. *J Dermatol.* 1988;27(8):591-592.
45. Peterson WC, Hult AM. Calcifying epithelioma of Malherbe. *Arch Dermatol.* 1964;90:404.
46. Forbis R, Helwig EB. Pilomatrixoma (calcifying epithelioma). *Arch Dermatol.* 1961;83:606.
47. Chan EF. Pilomatricomas contain activating mutations in beta-catenin. *J Am Acad Dermatol.* 2000;43(4):701-702.
48. Chen Y, Whetstone HC, Youn A, et al. B-Catenin signaling pathway is crucial for bone morphogenetic protein 2 to induce new bone formation. *J Biol Chem.* 2007;282(1):526-533.
49. Leppard BJ, Sanderson KB. The natural history of trichilemmal cysts. *Br J Dermatol.* 1976;94(4):379-390.
50. Walsh JS, Perniciaro C, Randle HW. Calcifying basal cell carcinomas. *Dermatol Surg.* 1999;25(1):49-51.
51. Roth SI, Stowell Re, Helwigeb. Cutaneous ossification. Report of 120 cases and review of the literature. *Arch Pathol.* 1963;76:44.
52. Moreno A, Lamarca J, Martinez R, et al. Osteoid and bone formation in desmoplastic malignant melanoma. *J Cutan Pathol.* 1986;13(2):128-134.
53. Chen KTK. Atypical fibroxanthoma of the skin with osteoid production. *Arch Dermatol.* 1980;116(1):113-114.
54. Browne SG. Calcinosis circumscripta of the scrotal wall. The etiological role of *Onchocerca volvulus. Br J Dermatol.* 1962;74:136-140.
55. Pastel A, Grupper C. Subcutaneous calcification, generalized calcinosis in nodular chains. Cysticercosis [in French]. *Bull Soc Fr Dermatol Syphligr.* 1969;76(1):28-31.
56. Beers BB, Flowers FP, Sherertz EF, et al. Dystrophic calcinosis cutis secondary to intrauterine herpes simplex. *Pediatr Dermatol.* 1986;3(3):208-211.
57. Coskey RJ, Mehregan AH. Calcinosis cutis in a burn scar. *J Am Acad Dermatol.* 1984;11:666.
58. Ellis IO, Foster MC, Womack C. Plumber's knee. Calcinosis cutis after repeated trauma in a plumber. *Br Med J.* 1984;288(6432):1723.
59. Leung A. Calcification following heel sticks. *J Pediatr.* 1985;106(1):168.
60. Katz I, LeVine M. Bone formation in laparotomy scars. Roentgen findings. *AJR Am J Roentgenol.* 1960;84:248.
61. Redmond WJ, Baker SR. Keloidal calcification. *Arch Dermatol.* 1983;119:270.
62. van Haren FM, Ruiter DJ, Hilbrands LB. Nadoparin-induced calcinosis cutis in renal transplant recipients. *Nephron.* 2001;87(3):279-282.
63. Weenig RH, Sewell LD, Davis MD, et al. Calciphylaxis: natural history, risk factor analysis and outcome. *J Am Acad Dermatol.* 2007;56(4):569-579.
64. Fader DJ, Kang S. Calciphylaxis without renal failure. *Arch Dermatol.* 1996;132:837.
65. Walsh JS, Fairley JA. Calciphylaxis. *J Am Acad Dermatol.* 1996;35:786.
66. Bleyer AJ, Choi M, Igwemezie B, et al. A case control study of proximal calciphylaxis. *Am J Kidney Dis.* 1998;32(3):376-383.
67. Selye H. *Calciphylaxis.* Chicago: University of Chicago Press; 1962.
68. Mehta RL, Scott G, Sloand JA, et al. Skin necrosis with acquired protein C deficiency in patients with renal failure and calciphylaxis. *Am J Med.* 1990;88(3):252-257.
69. Stompor T. An overview of the pathophysiology of vascular calcification in chronic kidney disease. *Perit Dial Int.* 2007;27(suppl 2):S215-S222.
70. Hafner J, Keusch G, Wahl C, et al. Uremic small-artery disease with medial calcification and intimal hyperplasia (so-called calciphylaxis): a complication of chronic renal failure and benefit from parathyroidectomy. *J Am Acad Dermatol.* 1995;33(6):954-962.
71. Robinson MR, Augustine KK, Korman NJ. Cinacalcet for the treatment of calciphylaxis. *Arch Dermatol.* 2007;143:2.
72. Peng T, Zhuo Y, Jun M, et al. A systematic review of sodium thiosulfate in treating calciphylaxis in chronic kidney disease patients [published online ahead of print June 11, 2017]. *Nephrology (Carlton).* doi:10.111/neph.13081.
73. Wilson CW, Wingfield WL, Toone EC. Vitamin D poisoning with metastatic calcification. *Am J Med.* 1953;14(1):116-123.
74. Wermer P, Kuscher M, Riley EA. Reversible metastatic calcification associated with excessive milk and alkali intake. *Am J Med.* 1953;14:108-115.
75. Topaz O, Bergman R, Mandel U, et al. Absence of intraepidermal glycosyltransferase ppGalNAc-T3 expression in familial tumoral calcinosis. *Am J Dermatopathol.* 2005;27(3):211-215.
76. Topaz O, Shurman DL, Bergman R, et al. Mutations in GALNT3, encoding a protein involved in O-linked glycosylation, cause familial tumoral calcinosis. *Nat Genet.* 2004;36(6):579-581.
77. Kato K, Jeanneau C, Tarp MA, et al. Polypeptide GalNAc-transferase T3 and familial tumoral calcinosis. Secretion of fibroblast growth factor 23 requires O-glycosylation. *J Biol Chem.* 2006;281(27):18370-18377.
78. Sprecher E. Familial tumoral calcinosis: from char-

78. acterization of a rare phenotype to the pathogenesis of ectopic calcification. *J Invest Dermatol.* 2010;130(2):652-660.
79. Panicek DM, Harty MP, Sciucetella CJ, et al. Calcification in untreated mediastinal lymphoma. *Radiology.* 1988;166(3):735-736.
80. Abe M, Segami H, Wakasa H. Hypercalcemia and metastatic calcification in adult T-cell leukemia-pathogenesis of hypercalcemia. *Fukushima J Med Sci.* 1985;31(2):85-97.
81. Raper RF, Ibels LS. Osteosclerotic myeloma complicated by diffuse arteritis, vascular calcification and extensive cutaneous necrosis. *Nephron.* 1985;39(4):389-392.
82. Kroll JJ, Shapiro L, Koplon BS, et al. Subcutaneous sarcoidosis with calcification. *Arch Dermatol.* 1972;106(6):894-895.
83. Shapiro L, Plutt N, Torres-Rodriques VM. Idiopathic calcinosis of the scrotum. *Arch Dermatol.* 1970;102(2):199-204.
84. Wright S, Navsaria H, Leigh IM. Idiopathic scrotal calcinosis is idiopathic. *J Am Acad Dermatol.* 1991;24(5, pt 1):727-730.
85. Swinehart JW, Golitz LE. Scrotal calcinosis. Dystrophic calcification of epidermoid cysts. *Arch Dermatol.* 1982;118(12):985-988.
86. Bhawan J, Nalhotra R, Frank S. The so-called idiopathic calcinosis. *Arch Dermatol.* 1983;119(9):709.
87. Dubey S, Sharma R, Maheshwari V. Scrotal calcinosis: idiopathic or dystrophic. *Dermatol Online J.* 2010;16(2):5.
88. Hutchinson IF, Abel BJ, Susskind W. Idiopathic calcinosis cutis of the penis. *Br J Dermatol.* 1980;102(3):341-343.
89. Balfour PJ, Vincenti AC. Idiopathic vulvar calcinosis. *Histopathology.* 1991;18(2):183-184.
90. Woods B, Kellaway TD. Cutaneous calculi. Subepidermal calcified nodules. *Br J Dermatol.* 1963;75:1-11.
91. Shmunes E, Wood MG. Subepidermal calcified nodules. *Arch Dermatol.* 1972;105(4):593-597.
92. Schepis C, Siragusa M, Palazzo R, et al. Perforating milia-like idiopathic calcinosis cutis and periorbital syringomas in a girl with Down syndrome. *Pediatr Dermatol.* 1994;11(3):258-260.
93. Smith ML, Golitz LE, Morelli JG, et al. Milia-like idiopathic calcinosis cutis in Down's syndrome. *Arch Dermatol.* 1989;125(11):1586-1587.
94. Maroon M, Tyler W, Marks VJ. Calcinosis cutis associated with syringomas. A transepidermal elimination disorder in a patient with Down syndrome. *J Am Acad Dermatol.* 1990;23(2, pt 2):372-375.
95. Goldminz D, Barnhill R, McGuire J, et al. Calcinosis cutis following extravasation of calcium chloride. *Arch Dermatol.* 1988;124(6):922-925.
96. Wheeland RG, Roundtree JM. Calcinosis cutis resulting from percutaneous penetration and deposition of calcium. *J Am Acad Dermatol.* 1985;12(1, pt 2):172-175.
97. Clendenning WE, Auerbach R. Traumatic calcium deposition in the skin. *Arch Dermatol.* 1964;89:360-363.
98. Schoenfeld RJ, Grekin JN, Mehregan A. Calcium deposition in the skin. A report of four cases following electroencephalography. *Neurology.* 1965;15:477-480.
99. Davey RB, Sparnon AL, Byard RW. Unusual donor site reactions to calcium alginate dressings. *Burns.* 2000;26(4):393-398.
100. Munoz SJ, Nagelberg SB, Green PJ, et al. Ectopic soft tissue calcium deposition following liver transplantation. *Hepatology.* 1988;8(3):476-483.
101. Adegbite NS, Xu M, Kaplan FS, et al. Diagnosis and mutational spectrum of progressive osseous heteroplasia (POH) and other forms of GNAS-based heterotopic ossification. *Am J Med Genet.* 2008;146A(14):1788-1796.
102. Cohen RB et al. The natural history of heterotopic ossification in patients who have fibrodysplasia ossificans progressiva. A study of forty-four patients. *J Bone Joint Surg Am.* 1993;75(2):215-219.
103. Pignolo RJ, Shore EM, Kaplan FS. Fibrodysplasia ossificans progressiva: clinical and genetic aspects. *Orphanet J Rare Dis.* 2011;6:80.
104. Eddy MC, Jan De Beur SM, Yandow SM, et al. Deficiency of the alpha-subunit of the stimulatory G protein and severe extraskeletal ossification. *J Bone Miner Res.* 2000;15(11):2074-2083.
105. Yeh GL, Mathur S, Wivel A, et al. GNAS1 mutation and Cbfa1 misexpression in a child with severe congenital platelike osteoma cutis. *J Bone Miner Res.* 2000;15(11):2063-2073.
106. Bastepe M, Juppner H. Identification and characterization of two new, highly polymorphic loci adjacent to GNAS1 on chromosome 20q13.3. *Mol Cell Probes.* 2000;14(4):261-264.
107. Urtizberea JA, Testart H, Cartault F, et al. Progressive osseous heteroplasia. Report of a family. *J Bone Joint Surg Br.* 1998;80(5):768-771.
108. Shore EM, Ahn J, Jan de Beur S, et al. Paternally inherited inactivating mutations of the GNAS1 gene in progressive osseous heteroplasia. *N Engl J Med.* 2002;346(2):99-106.
109. Kaplan FS, Craver R, MacEwen GD, et al. Progressive osseous heteroplasia: a distinct developmental disorder of heterotopic ossification. *J Bone Joint Surg Am.* 1994;76(3):425-436.
110. Miller ES, Esterly NB, Fairley JA, et al. Progressive osseous heteroplasia: report of two cases. *Arch Dermatol.* 1996;132(7):787-791.
111. Pignolo RJ, Ramaswamy G, Fong JT, et al. Progressive osseous heteroplasia: diagnosis, treatment and prognosis. *Appl Clin Genet.* 2015;8:37-48.
112. Levell NJ, Lawrence CM. Multiple papules on the face. *Arch Dermatol.* 1994;130(3):373-374.
113. Wilson JF. In the clinic. Gout. *Ann Intern Med.* 2010;152(3):ITC21.
114. Choi HK, Mount DB, Reginato AM; American College of Physicians; American Physiological Society. Pathogenesis of gout. *Ann Intern Med.* 2005;143(7):499-516.
115. Zhu Y, Pandya BJ, Choi HK. Prevalence of gout and hyperuricemia in the US general population: the National Health and Nutrition Examination Survey 2007-2008. *Arthritis Rheum.* 2011;63(10):3136-3141.
116. Harrold LR, Yood RA, Mikuls TR, et al. Sex differences in gout epidemiology, evaluation, and treatment. *Ann Rheum Dis.* 2006;65(10):1368-1372.
117. Lee SJ, Terkeltaub RA, Kavanaugh A. Recent developments in diet and gout. *Curr Opin Rheumatol.* 2006;18(2):193-198.
118. Harris ED, Ruddy S, Kelley WN. *Kelley's Textbook of Rheumatology.* Philadelphia, PA: Elsevier Saunders; 2005, Chaps 65, 68, 87, and 103.
119. Merriman TR. An update on the genetic architecture of hyperuricemia and gout. *Arthritis Res Ther.* 2015;17:98.
120. Hughes JP, Di Palma S, Rowe-Jones J. Tophaceous gout presenting as a dorsal nasal lump. *J Laryngol*

121. Ackerman AB, Boer A, Benin B, et al. *Histological Diagnosis of Inflammatory Skin Disease*. 2nd ed. Philadelphia, PA: Williams and Wilkins, 1997.
122. Terkeltaub RA, Furst DE, Bennett K, et al. High versus low dosing of oral colchicine for early acute gout flare. Twenty-four-hour outcome of the first multicenter, randomized, double-blind, placebo-controlled, parallel-group, dose-comparison colchicine study. *Arthritis Rheum*. 2000;62(2):2010.
123. Sutaria S, Katbamna R, Underwood M. Effectiveness of interventions for the treatment of acute and prevention recurrent gout: a systematic review. *Rheumatology (Oxford)*. 2006;45(11):1422-1431.
124. Terkeltaub R. The management of gout and hyperuricemia. In: Hochberg MC, Gavallese EM, Silman AJ, et al, eds. *Rheumatology*. Philadelphia, PA: Mosby; 2010.
125. Chohan S, Becker MA. Update on emerging urate lowering therapies. *Curr Opin Rheumatol*. 2009;21(2):143-149.
126. Haber SL, Fente G, Fenton SN, et al. Lesinurad: a novel agent for management of chronic gout. *Ann Pharmacother*. 2018;52(7):690-696.

Chapter 129 :: Graft-Versus-Host Disease
:: Kathryn J. Martires & Edward W. Cowen

第一百二十九章
移植物抗宿主病

中文导读

移植物抗宿主病（GVHD）根据发病时间可分为急性GVHD和慢性GVHD。本章分10节，分别从①流行病学；②病因和发病机制；③临床表现；④诊断；⑤鉴别诊断；⑥并发症；⑦预后与临床病程；⑧预防；⑨治疗；⑩慢性口腔和外阴阴道疾病的治疗，对移植物抗宿主病进行了系统介绍。

第一节介绍了急性GVHD发生在大约40%完全匹配的同胞捐献者和80%不匹配的无血缘关系的HCT受体中，近年来已将急性GVHD的发生率降低到10%，皮肤受累通常是评估急性GVHD（81%）的第一个指标。慢性GVHD的风险估计也相差很大，从37%～47%不等，其中GVHD硬化症的发生率在3.6%～22.6%之间。

第二节病因和发病机制，介绍了急性GVHD传统上被认为是由T辅助细胞Th1介导的，而Th2机制被认为在慢性GVHD中占主导地位。

第三节介绍了急性GVHD最常见的表现是掌侧和足底表面及耳部出现红斑、暗斑和丘疹，可迅速形成弥漫性麻疹样皮疹。慢性GVHD临床特征分为诊断性或特异性，诊断性皮肤特征包括扁平苔藓样病变和硬化性皮肤改变，同时提到了相关体格检查结果和组织病理学检查的重要性。

第四节介绍了急性GVHD皮肤受累的诊断是基于临床病理对照，特别需要排除药物和感染性因素。62%的慢性移植物抗宿主病患者检测到自身抗体，提到了识别疾病活动性的特定生物标志物是急性和慢性移植物抗宿主病研究的重点领域。

第五节介绍了急性GVHD的鉴别诊断是广泛的，尤其具有挑战性，往往与麻疹样药疹和植入综合征难以区分，慢性移植物抗宿主病的表现多种多样，有许多其他潜在的鉴别诊断。

第六节介绍了慢性GVHD可引起皮肤糜烂和溃疡，可能导致继发感染，硬化性改变导致关节功能受限，可能导致功能障碍和关节挛缩。此外皮肤鳞状细胞癌和黑色素瘤患者通过伏立康唑的长期治疗而风险增加。

第七节预后与临床病程，介绍了慢性GVHD是HCT患者原发病复发后死亡的第二大原因，硬化性皮肤也可能是更严重疾病的标志。许多系统危险因素预示着不良预后，包括从急性到慢性GVHD的进行性受累病史、血小板减少（低于10万个/mL）、胆红素升高、年龄增大、胃肠道症状以及6个月后对治疗无反应。

第八节介绍了慢性GVHD预防始于移植前选择HLA配型最匹配的供者，某些情况下，还包括T细胞耗尽或移植物操作。此外，皮肤癌筛查和关于光保护措施的患者教育是所有HCT患者特别是慢性GVHD患者的关键预防策略。

第九节分别介绍了急性ＧＶＨＤ和慢性GVHD的治疗方案。

第十节特别提到了慢性口腔和外阴阴道疾病的治疗，局限的口腔黏膜疾病可以通过使用高效局部糖皮质类固醇外用制剂来控制，若需要口服类固醇时，局部抗感染药应与抗真菌制剂联合使用。与慢性外阴阴道疾病相关的生殖器糜烂和裂缝可每晚使用丙酸氯倍他索软膏治疗，他克莫司软膏已被广泛用于维持治疗。继发阴道瘢痕/粘连可以用扩张器、手法松解、手术来治疗。

〔粟　娟〕

AT-A-GLANCE

- Acute graft-versus-host disease (GVHD) is a serious and potentially life-threatening sequelae of allogeneic hematopoietic stem cell transplantation. Skin manifestations range from a mild, asymptomatic morbilliform eruption to full-thickness skin loss resembling toxic epidermal necrolysis. Hepatic involvement is characterized by elevated total bilirubin. GI disease manifests as abdominal pain, nausea/vomiting, and secretory diarrhea.

- The most important risk factor for chronic GVHD is a history of acute GVHD. Other important factors include human leukocyte antigen incompatibility, older age, female donor/male recipient, and peripheral blood stem cell source (vs bone marrow).

- Chronic GVHD of the skin may resemble lichen planus, lichen sclerosus, morphea, systemic sclerosis, or eosinophilic fasciitis. The presentation can be remarkably variable, however, and may resemble folliculitis, keratosis pilaris, or psoriasis. Both epidermal and sclerotic skin manifestations may present at sites of trauma.

- Patients with chronic GVHD may manifest other autoimmune skin diseases, such as vitiligo and alopecia areata.

- The pathogenesis of chronic GVHD is poorly understood and nearly every organ system is at risk. The skin, oral mucosa, eyes, GI tract, and lungs are most frequently involved. In many cases, organ system disease resembles known autoimmune conditions.

- Topical steroids and topical calcineurin inhibitors are used to treat mild, skin-limited chronic GVHD, and systemic steroids are first line in the treatment of moderate to severe chronic GVHD.

- Optimal dermatologic management of chronic GVHD of the skin requires an understanding of other organ involvement, infection status, and cancer relapse risk. Close communication with the transplantation physician and a "team approach" to multispecialty management is needed.

EPIDEMIOLOGY

Approximately 50,000 hematopoietic stem cell transplantation (HCT) procedures are performed worldwide each year for an expanding array of hematologic malignancies and marrow failure syndromes, metabolic disorders, and immunodeficiencies. HCT may use autologous, syngeneic, or allogeneic donor hematopoietic stem cells (HCs). During autologous transplantation, the patient's own HCs are returned to the patient following preparative chemotherapy with or without radiation. Allogeneic HCT (allo-HCT) is the transfer of HCs from a related (nonidentical) or unrelated donor to a recipient. Syngeneic transplantation is the transfer of HCs between identical twins. Graft-versus-host disease (GVHD) is the primary cause of non–relapse-related morbidity and mortality in allo-HCT, and also rarely occurs following transplantation of solid organs, transfusion of blood products, and autologous transplantation.

Transplantation regimens have advanced rapidly since the first successful allo-HCT was performed in 1968.[1] Peripheral blood is now the primary source of donor HCs at many transplantation centers because of decreased risks of relapse and improved survival, although bone marrow transplantation is associated with reduced risk of GVHD.[2] Reduced intensity and nonmyeloablative conditioning permitted older patients and others who would not tolerate myeloablative chemotherapy a chance for cure with HCT.[3] Umbilical cord blood has gained prominence as a stem cell source in both pediatric and adult HCT given the low risks of GVHD and high engraftment rates.[4] Donor leukocyte infusions, the administration of additional donor HCs to the recipient weeks or even months after HCT, may be used to augment graft-versus-malignancy effect, but also may trigger GVHD activity.[5]

These evolving trends in HCT, in conjunction with other known donor/recipient risk variables (Table 129-1), contribute to a wide range of reported GVHD incidence. The degree of human leukocyte antigen (HLA) mismatch between donor and recipient remains the single most important predictor of GVHD.[6] A history of acute GVHD, in turn, confers

TABLE 129-1
Major Risk Factors for the Development of Graft-Versus-Host Disease

- Human leukocyte antigen (HLA) incompatibility
- Patient age (elderly > adult > pediatric)
- Female donor (especially multiparous)/male recipient
- Stem cell source (peripheral blood > bone marrow > cord blood)
- T-cell replete graft
- Unrelated donor
- Donor leukocyte infusion
- Interruption or rapid tapering of immunosuppression
- Total body irradiation in pretransplantation conditioning regimen[11]

the greatest risk of developing chronic disease.[7] Acute GVHD develops in approximately 40% of fully matched sibling donor HCTs and 80% of mismatched unrelated HCT recipients.[8] However, changing peritransplantation regimens, including use of cyclophosphamide and antithymocyte globulin has reduced the rate of acute GVHD in recent years to as low as 10%.[9] Risk estimates of chronic GVHD also vary widely from 37% to 47%,[2] but data from the Centers for International Bone Marrow Transplant Research demonstrate a gradual increase in chronic GVHD incidence over more than a decade.[10] Confounding factors, such as improved posttransplantation survival, may be influencing the apparent trend in increasing chronic GVHD incidence.[7]

Skin involvement is often the first indicator of acute GVHD (81%), followed by GI (54%) and liver disease (50%).[12] Similarly, the majority of patients who develop chronic GVHD manifest skin symptoms at some point in their disease course. Although sclerotic involvement is less common than "lichenoid" GVHD and tends to occur later post-HCT, sclerotic features, particularly deep-seated fascial changes, may have an insidious onset, and "lichenoid" involvement is not a prerequisite to the development of sclerotic features.

The incidence of sclerosis in chronic GVHD has been reported to be between 3.6% and 22.6%.[10,11,13,14]

ETIOLOGY AND PATHOGENESIS

Table 129-2 compares acute GVHD with chronic GVHD. The fundamental concept of GVHD is encompassed by the balance between immunosuppression, induced by the conditioning regimen and GVHD prophylaxis, and immune system (graft) activation. In 1966, Billingham proposed 3 basic requirements for GVHD: (a) immunocompetent transplanted cells, (b) host antigens recognizable by the transplanted cells and lacking in the donor, and (c) a host incapable of mounting an immune response to the transplanted cells.[15] The immunocompetent cells are T cells, targeting HLAs expressed on host tissues, as well as key minor histocompatibility antigens (eg, HY, HA-3).[16] An allogeneic response to these minor antigens is thought to partially explain the development of GVHD in 40% of recipients of HLA-identical grafts.

Host autoreactive T cells may also play a role in disease pathogenesis.[17] Tissue damage, infection, and pretransplantation conditioning modifies the inflammatory response through proinflammatory cytokine production and antigen-presenting cell activation.[18] Antigen-presenting cell activation may be mediated by damage-associated molecular patterns and pathogen-associated molecular patterns released from damaged skin, gut, and vascular tissue.[19] Demonstration of lichen planus-like and sclerotic chronic GVHD at sites of injury and viral infection has highlighted a likely role for Type I interferons, which are known to play a critical role in the innate immune response to cellular damage and viral infection.[20]

Acute GVHD has traditionally been considered T-helper cell (Th) 1–mediated, while Th2 mechanisms

TABLE 129-2
Comparison of Acute with Chronic Graft-Versus-Host Disease

	ACUTE GVHD	CHRONIC GVHD
Time to onset[a]	Usually <100 days after transplantation	Usually >100 days after transplantation
Immune pathways	T-helper (Th)-1 and Th17 mediated	Th2 and Th17 mediated
Cellular response	T cells (cytotoxic T cells) play a major role; also natural killer cells Decreased regulatory T cells	B cells play a major role; also T cells, plasma cells Tissue macrophages Decreased regulatory T cells
Inflammatory mediators	Tumor necrosis factor Interferon-γ Interleukin (IL)-1 IL-2	B-cell activating factor Platelet-derived growth factor Transforming growth factor-β IL-6 IL-21 B-cell autoantibodies (ANA, anti-dsDNA)
Histologic features *(cutaneous)*	Necrotic keratinocytes with dermal lymphocytic infiltrate Basal vacuolar interface alterations *or* subepidermal cleft formation *or* epidermal–dermal separation (depending on severity)	Vacuolar interface dermatitis with dyskeratotic keratinocytes Sclerosis of the upper dermis Epidermal atrophy, hyperkeratosis, follicular plugging

[a]Classic presentation; however, features and timing may overlap. (See revised classification in Fig. 129-1.)
ANA, anti-nuclear antibody; dsDNA, double-stranded DNA; GVHD, graft-versus-host disease.

were thought to predominate in chronic GVHD. It is now known that Th17 pathways also play a role in the pathogenesis of both disease processes.[21] Donor interleukin (IL)-17A, derived from Th17 cells, promotes skin fibrosis. There also is increased IL-17 messenger RNA in skin of chronic GVHD patients, as well as higher levels of Th17-promoting cytokines including IL-6 and IL-21, and transcription factor STAT3.[21-23]

Following activation of host antigen-presenting cells, T-cell activation and differentiation drives the response in acute GVHD. T-cell activation results in a massive release of proinflammatory cytokines, causing damage to the organs and tissues.[24] The final effector phase of acute GVHD is characterized by cell damage via cytotoxic T cells, natural killer cells, and soluble inflammatory mediators, including tumor necrosis factor (TNF), interferon-γ, and IL-1.[18]

Regulatory T cells are known to play a key role in inhibiting GVHD.[25] Acute GVHD may target secondary lymphoid organs, which may result in loss of regulatory T-cell production.[17] Decreased T-regulatory cells are associated with severity of acute GVHD and poor response to GVHD treatment.[26] Although many therapies for acute GVHD target T cells, particularly IL-2 or its receptor (CD25), these approaches may have the unintended consequence of adversely impacting the CD4+CD25+ regulatory T-cell population.[27]

The pathophysiology of chronic GVHD is less-well understood, but may share the same activating and regulatory mechanisms as acute GVHD.[19] Chronic GVHD is also associated with decreased numbers of regulatory T cells.[28] Natural killer cells and regulatory B cells may also serve roles in preventing GVHD.[29,30]

Chronic GVHD is thought to be at least partly mediated through Th2 interaction with B cells and autoantibody induction. B cells may act as antigen-presenting cells, priming T cells to respond to HLA antigens in cases of partial matching, or minor histocompatibility antigens, and high-titers of antibodies directed against minor histocompatibility antigens are associated with chronic GVHD, particularly histocompatibility Y (HY) antigen.[31] Similarly, soluble levels of B-cell activating factor (BAFF), a cytokine which inhibits apoptosis of B cells and promotes differentiation into plasma cells, correlate with chronic GVHD activity.[32] B-cell autoantibodies have been shown to associate with Th17 cells in skin, and perpetuate GVHD in mice.[33]

The role of B-cell function in chronic GVHD is supported by reports of success of use of the anti-CD20 antibody rituximab in chronic GVHD.[34] Patients who respond well to rituximab have higher circulating levels of activated B cells.[35] Administration of rituximab in preparative regimens also has been associated with lower incidence and severity of acute GVHD.[36] Autoantibody formation (eg, antinuclear antibody, anti–double-stranded DNA antibody) is a frequent finding in chronic GVHD, although the antibodies lack the specificity of typical autoimmune disease.[37]

The mechanisms responsible for chronic GVHD-induced fibrosis in the skin and elsewhere (eg, bronchiolitis obliterans) remains uncertain. Platelet-derived growth factor (PDGF) may activate transforming growth factor-β, a potent profibrotic cytokine capable of stimulating collagen production, abrogating metalloproteinase activity, and sensitizing fibroblasts to a constitutive-activated state via autocrine signaling.[38-40] Stimulatory antibodies targeting the PDGF receptor have been proposed as the etiology of fibrosis in GVHD and systemic sclerosis.[39] However, the significance of these antibodies remains unclear and other studies have failed to correlate PDGFR antibody with severity of chronic GVHD.[41] Kinase inhibition of intracellular PDGF signaling is a targeted therapeutic approach in sclerotic chronic GVHD.

Macrophages are known to play a role in the tissue-repair response contributing to fibrosis,[42] and have been shown to accumulate in fibrotic lesions in chronic GVHD.[43] Macrophages in GVHD tissue are of donor origin, and may be efficient in generating antibodies that may contribute to GVHD pathogenesis, including transforming growth factor-β.[19] Macrophages may also represent potential therapeutic targets.

In recent years, genome-wide association studies have begun to define individual genetic risk factors for GVHD.[44] Studies have revealed that single-nucleotide polymorphisms in *NOD2* (nucleotide-binding oligomerization domain-2), *TNF*, and *IL-10* are associated with GVHD. Single-nucleotide polymorphisms in *BANK1*, *CD247*, and *HLA-DPA-1* are associated with development of sclerotic GVHD.[45]

CLINICAL FINDINGS

HISTORY

Accurate diagnosis of acute GVHD is challenging, and requires a thorough assessment and clinicopathologic correlation. Because the skin eruption (and histology) may be nonspecific in the context of several potential differential diagnoses, a careful history is invaluable. Key factors include assessment of the primary disease for which the patient underwent an organ transplant procedure, stem cell source (eg, peripheral blood, bone marrow, umbilical cord blood), type of transplant (eg, allogeneic, syngeneic, autologous), degree of HLA match, use of a related versus unrelated donor, and T-cell depletion of the graft. Additional factors include agents used for GVHD prophylaxis and the pretransplantation conditioning regimen. The use of particular chemotherapeutic agents such as cytarabine may render the differential diagnosis of toxic erythema of chemotherapy more likely.[46] Reduced intensity conditioning and nonmyeloablative conditioning may be associated with increased risk of sclerotic chronic GVHD,[11] and may delay the onset of acute GVHD symptoms beyond the 100-day period.[47] The timing of engraftment, new medication exposures, virus status of both the donor and recipient (eg, cytomegalovirus), and evidence of other organ involvement (eg, elevated total bilirubin, diarrhea) provide additional data for clinicopathologic correlation. Bilirubin elevation and diarrhea, however, are nonspecific, and may be related to concomitant viral infection, drug toxicity and bile duct obstruction.

Features of acute GVHD following recent blood transfusion should raise concern for transfusion-associated GVHD (TA-GVHD). TA-GVHD is an often-fatal sequelae of administration of cellular blood products to immunocompromised HCT recipients. As a result, all blood products given to HCT recipients must be irradiated. TA-GVHD may also occur following transfusion of unirradiated blood products to children with congenital immunodeficiency. TA-GVHD may also occur in the immunocompetent setting following transfusion of an unirradiated blood product that contains donor lymphocytes that are homozygous for the HLA haplotype of the recipient, typically when transfusion occurs from a relative or genetically similar person. For example, in Japan where the genetic background of the population is more homogenous, the estimated risk of randomly receiving blood from a homozygous donor is 1 in 874.[48] In this form of TA-GVHD, the donor lymphocytes in the blood product are not recognized as foreign, leading to a GVHD reaction similar to classic acute GVHD. Beginning 10 days after transfusion, fever and skin rash (histologically consistent with GVHD) develops, followed by liver dysfunction and diarrhea. Death from pancytopenia usually occurs within several weeks.[49]

As with acute disease, a new diagnosis of chronic GVHD is best made based by history, cutaneous examination, and histology. A previous history of acute GVHD is the single greatest risk factor for chronic disease. When there is no cessation of acute GVHD prior to development of chronic GVHD, it is considered progressive, and carries the poorest prognosis. In contrast, quiescent disease is the onset of chronic disease after previous resolution of acute GVHD symptoms. Chronic GVHD is considered de novo when there is no prior history of acute GVHD. Traditionally, acute GVHD occurs within 100 days posttransplantation, while symptoms after 100 days are considered chronic GVHD. However, because acute symptoms may develop after 100 days posttransplantation and chronic symptoms may develop before then, the revised classification of acute and chronic GVHD symptoms includes additional subtypes of GVHD with overlapping features or timing of acute and chronic symptoms (Fig. 129-1).[50] Recent tapering of immunosuppressant medication or donor leukocyte infusion given to augment the graft-versus-malignancy response are potential triggers of skin activity. Donor leukocyte infusions, in particular, may present with an acute GVHD skin eruption consistent with acute GVHD rather than the eruption of chronic disease. Cutaneous or systemic infection may also induce a flare of skin GVHD, as will drug reactions, which can result in a diagnostic challenge given the clinical and histologic similarities between viral exanthem, drug eruption, and GVHD.[51] Intense ultraviolet (UV) exposure may also trigger skin GVHD. Important clues to sclerotic and fascial disease includes a new-onset edema of an extremity, muscle cramping, decreased flexibility, and complaints of skin tightness, particularly at the waistband and brassiere-line,[52] and at sites of prior injury or trauma, such as intravenous access sites or radiation fields.[53]

Although GVHD in other organ systems may not necessarily flare in synchrony with skin involvement, the presence of other organ system involvement is helpful when the cutaneous features are nondiagnostic. Therefore, a thorough review of systems should be conducted to assess for organ involvement. Common GVHD symptoms include oral and ocular sicca and oral pain, particularly with spicy foods. The presence of genital discomfort or pain also suggests GVHD. Dysphagia may indicate the presence of esophageal strictures or webbing. Bronchiolitis obliterans manifests as dry cough, wheezing, and dyspnea, but requires pulmonary function tests and CT scans to rule out infection

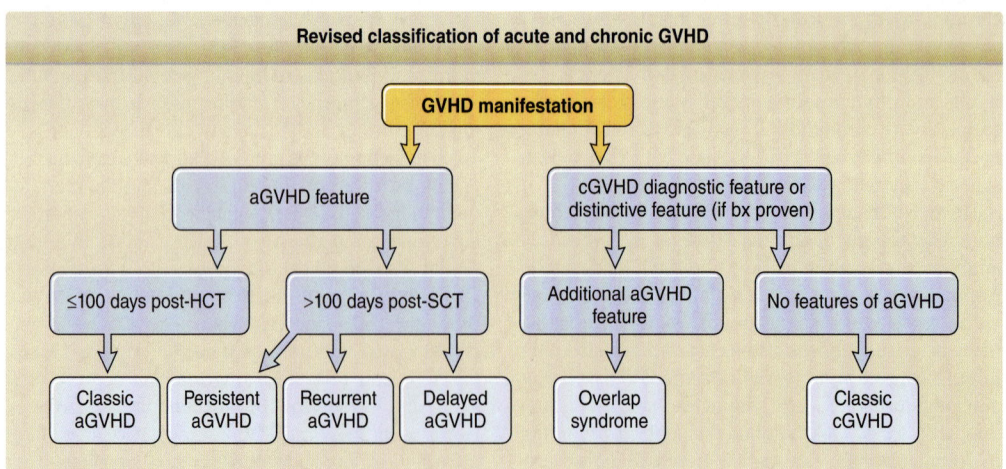

Figure 129-1 Revised classification of acute and chronic graft-versus-host disease (GVHD). aGVHD, acute graft-versus-host disease; bx, biopsy; cGVHD, chronic graft-versus-host disease; HCT, hematopoietic cell transplantation; SCT, stem cell transplantation. (Adapted from Jagasia MH, Greinix HT, Arora M, et al. National Institutes of Health consensus development project on criteria for clinical trials in chronic graft-versus-host disease: I. The 2014 Diagnosis and Staging Working Group report. *Biol Blood Marrow Transplant*. 2015;21:389-401.e1.)

and other etiologies. Also common, but less specific, are symptoms of fatigue, poor appetite, and weakness.[54,55]

Finally, it is important to remember that despite the phenotypic variability in chronic GVHD of the skin, not every skin manifestation in a patient after HCT is caused by GVHD, so a careful dermatologic history to detect other possible diagnoses is prudent.

CUTANEOUS PRESENTATION

The most common presentation of acute GVHD begins with erythematous-dusky macules and papules of the volar and plantar surfaces and ears that may rapidly become a diffuse morbilliform exanthem (Fig. 129-2A and B; Table 129-3). Very early involvement may manifest as erythema limited to hair follicles (Fig. 129-2C). A

TABLE 129-3
Acute Graft-Versus-Host Disease Organ System Manifestations

Skin
- Erythema of palms, soles, ears
- Perifollicular erythema
- Generalized exanthem
- Bullae/necrolysis

Gastrointestinal
- Abdominal pain
- Anorexia
- Ileus
- Mucositis
- Vomiting
- Secretory diarrhea

Liver
- Endothelialitis
- Pericholangitis
- Cholestatic hyperbilirubinemia

TABLE 129-4
Acute Graft-Versus-Host Disease Staging[56]

STAGE	SKIN	HISTOLOGY	DIARRHEA (500 mL/day)	BILIRUBIN (mg/dL)
0	–	–	≤500	≤2
1	<25% body surface area (BSA)	Focal or diffuse vacuolar interface	>500 or persistent anorexia, nausea, vomiting	2 to 2.9
2	25% to 50% BSA	Dyskeratotic keratinocytes	≥1000	3 to 5.9
3	>50% BSA	Subepidermal clefting	≥1500	6 to 14.9
4	Erythroderma with bullae or desquamation	Loss of epidermis	≥2000 or severe abdominal pain ± ileus	≥15

TABLE 129-5
Clinical Features of Chronic Graft-Versus-Host Disease[50]

	DIAGNOSTIC	DISTINCTIVE	OTHER	COMMON (SEEN IN BOTH ACUTE AND CHRONIC GVHD)
Skin	• Poikiloderma • Lichen sclerosus–like lesions • Lichen planus–like eruption • Morphea-like lesions • Sclerotic features	• Depigmentation (including vitiligo) • Papulosquamous lesions	• Sweat impairment • Ichthyosis • Keratosis pilaris • Hypopigmentation • Hyperpigmentation	• Erythema • Maculopapular rash • Pruritus
Nails	–	• Dystrophy • Longitudinal ridging, splitting, or brittle features • Onycholysis • Pterygium unguis • Nail loss (symmetric, most nails)	–	–
Hair	–	• New-onset scarring or nonscarring scalp alopecia • Loss of body hair • Scaling	• Thinning scalp hair, typically patchy • Coarse or dull hair • Premature gray hair	–

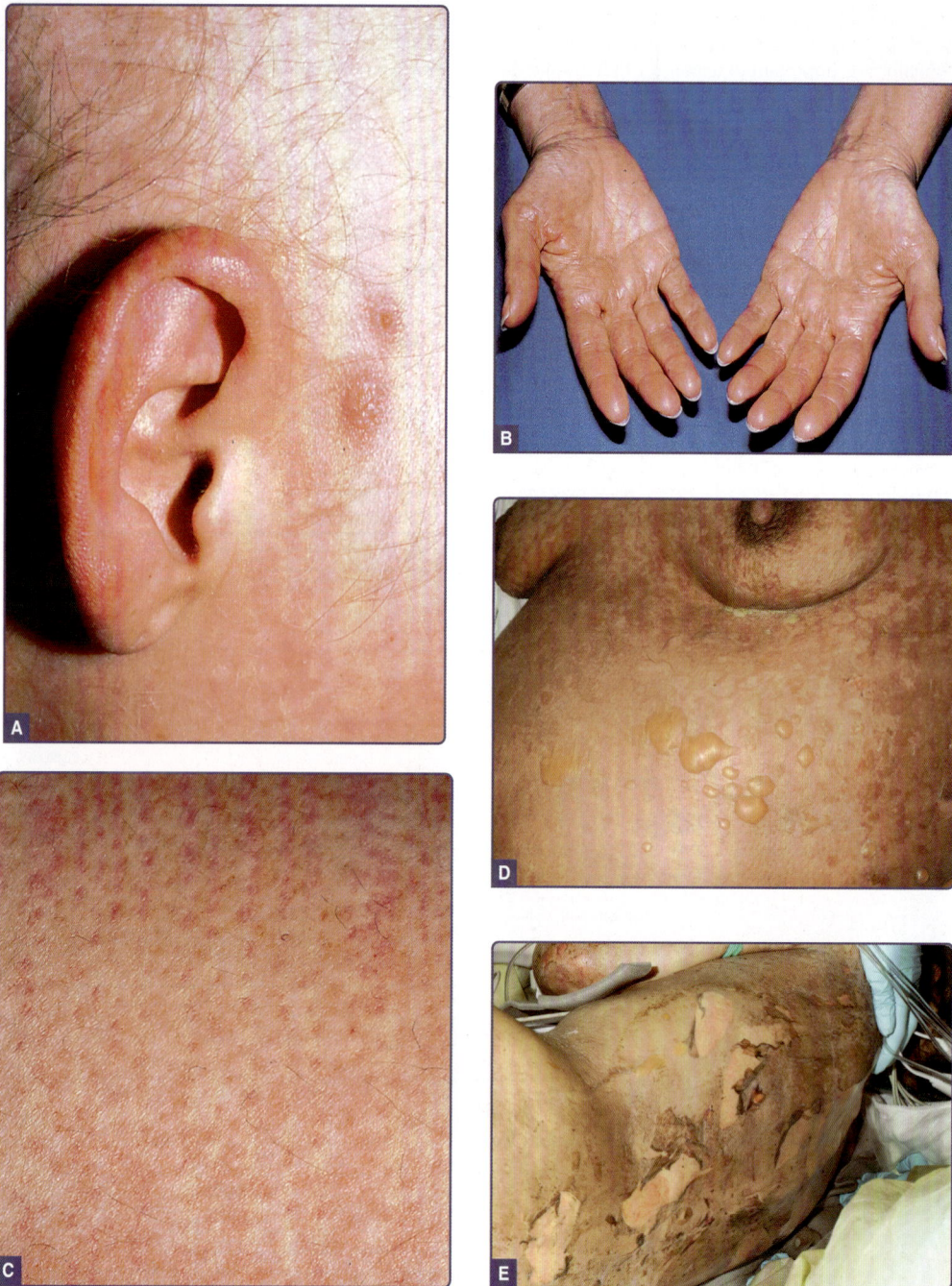

Figure 129-2 Spectrum of acute graft-versus-host skin manifestations. Acute cutaneous graft-versus-host reaction. Erythematous macules involving the ears (**A**), palms (**B**), and soles are characteristic of early cutaneous involvement. **C,** Follicular graft-versus-host disease (GVHD). Perifollicular involvement is an early manifestation of skin involvement. **D,** GVHD-associated necrolysis. Acute GVHD with bullae formation following donor leukocyte infusion for relapsed acute lymphoblastic leukemia following allogeneic hematopoietic cell transplantation. **E,** Skin sloughing in a toxic epidermal necrolysis–like presentation of acute GVHD.

predisposition for acral and perifollicular sites may help distinguish new-onset acute GVHD from other morbilliform eruptions, although these features are not always present. Pruritus is variable and is also not useful to distinguish acute GVHD from other causes.

Erythroderma and, in severe cases, spontaneous bullae (Fig. 129-2D) with skin sloughing resembling toxic epidermal necrolysis may develop (Fig. 129-2E). Widespread erythrodermic involvement, particularly skin sloughing, portends a very poor prognosis. Acute

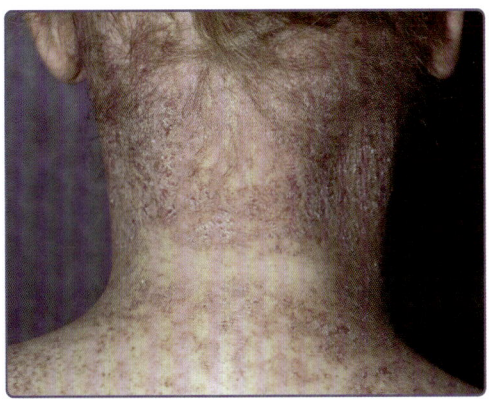

Figure 129-3 Lichen planus-like chronic graft-versus-host disease. Reticulate violaceous plaques with dry scale on the posterior neck and upper back.

GVHD is staged based on percent body surface area involvement with concordant histologic findings, as well as degree of bilirubin elevation and diarrhea (Table 129-4).[56] In contrast to chronic disease, postinflammatory pigmentary changes following acute GVHD are uncommon.

Clinical features of chronic skin GVHD are classified as *diagnostic* or *distinctive*. Diagnostic criteria establish the presence of chronic GVHD without the need for further testing or evidence of other organ involvement, while distinctive criteria warrant skin biopsy or establishment of additional organ involvement (Table 129-5). Diagnostic cutaneous features of GVHD include poikiloderma, lichen planus–like lesions, and sclerotic skin changes.[50] There is a growing appreciation of the tremendous variability in the clinical presentation of chronic skin GVHD. Previously, especially in the organ transplant community, skin findings in chronic GVHD were dichotomized as "lichenoid" or "sclerodermoid." The term *lichenoid GVHD* had been used to denote any involvement of the skin in which erythema or scaling was present; however, "lichenoid" is a histologic pattern, not a clinical one, and, therefore, usage of it is best reserved to pathologic description.

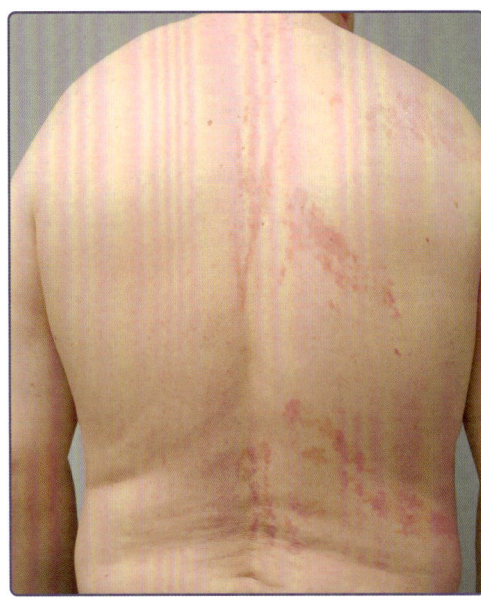

Figure 129-5 Blaschkoid chronic graft-versus-host disease (GVHD). Lichen planus–like chronic GVHD presenting unilaterally in a Blaschkoid distribution of the right-side of the back. (Used with permission from Milan J. Anadkat, MD.)

Furthermore, although chronic GVHD may resemble lichen planus (Fig. 129-3), other epidermal patterns are frequently observed, such as ichthyosis, poikiloderma (Fig. 129-4), and skin lesions resembling lupus erythematosus, keratosis pilaris, or psoriasis.[57] A linear form of chronic GVHD resembling lichen planus has been described, which may present following Blaschko lines (Fig. 129-5). Postinflammatory hyperpigmentation is common following the resolution of epidermal involvement, particularly in darkly pigmented individuals, and may persist for many months after the skin disease becomes quiescent.

The fibrosing manifestations of chronic GVHD are also remarkably variable, and the term *sclerodermoid*

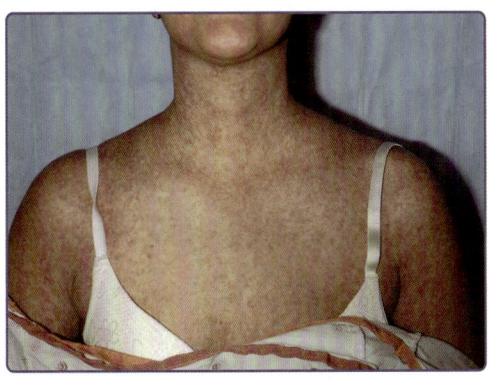

Figure 129-4 Poikilodermic chronic graft-versus-host disease. Hypopigmentation, hyperpigmentation, and erythema on the chest and proximal arms.

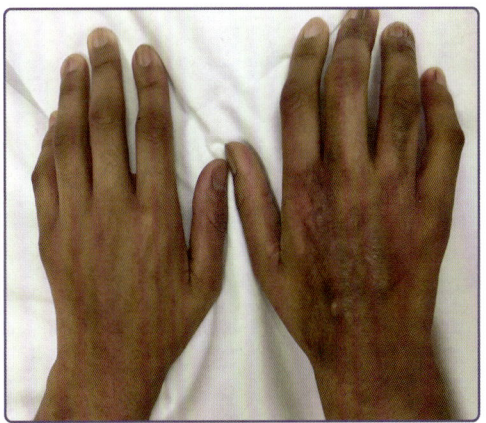

Figure 129-6 Morphea-like hyperpigmented, shiny sclerotic plaques of the dorsal hands and fingers causing functional disability.

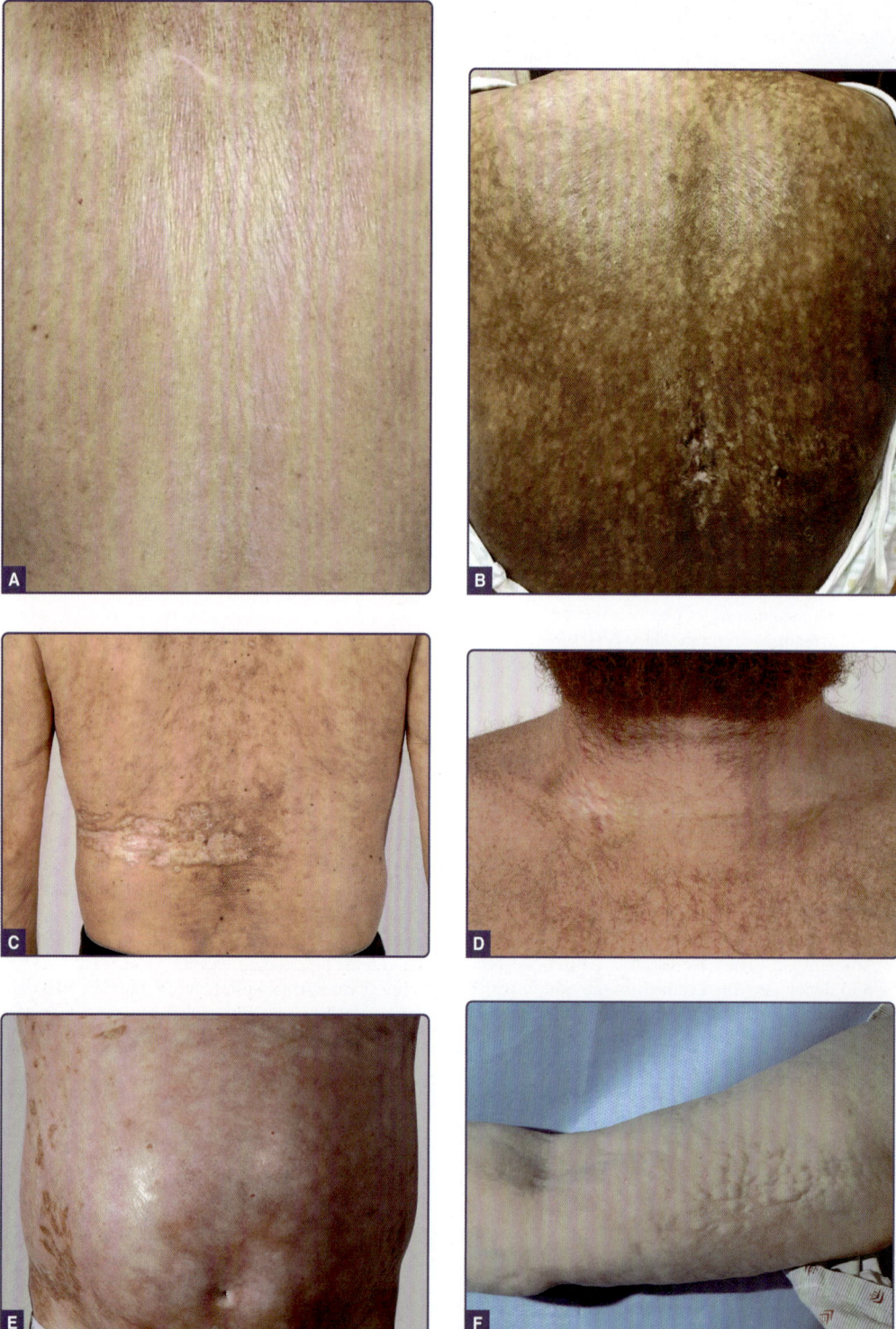

Figure 129-7 Clinical spectrum of sclerotic graft-versus-host disease (GVHD) skin manifestations. **A,** Guttate white plaques on the upper back resembling lichen sclerosus. **B,** Hypopigmentation and hyperpigmentation with extensive superficial and deep dermal sclerosis on the back. **C,** Morphea-like sclerotic plaques in the distribution of a prior zoster infection at this site of the left back and flank. **D,** Morphea-like sclerotic plaques at sites of previous indwelling line placement near the clavicle (isotopic response). **E,** Diffuse dermal sclerosis resembling scleroderma on the anterior torso with patchy hyperpigmentation. **F,** Subcutaneous fibrosis of chronic GVHD. There is prominent rippling with a firm nodular texture extending along the medial arm resembling eosinophilic fasciitis. There is associated decreased range of motion at the elbow.

is an inadequate descriptor of the varied tissue abnormalities in the dermis, subcutaneous tissue, and fascia. As in systemic sclerosis, an edematous phase may herald the onset of skin fibrosis, but in contrast to systemic sclerosis, the face, fingers, and toes are usually spared, and the typical acral-to-proximal progression characteristic of systemic sclerosis is not commonly seen in chronic GVHD. Certainly, many cases do involve the hands and fingers, but occur more proximal to the fingertips (Fig. 129-6).[58] Early superficial fibrotic involvement resembles lichen sclerosus. In contrast to traditional lichen sclerosus, which is much less common on the skin than the genital region, lichen sclerosis in GVHD patients often manifests on the skin as porcelain-white atrophic plaques on the upper back (Fig. 129-7A). A common pattern of GVHD-associated fibrosis involves patchy sclerotic plaques with hypopigmentation and hyperpigmentation mimicking morphea (Fig. 129-7B). Sclerosis of this type may exhibit an isomorphic response, localizing to the sites of minor skin trauma, particularly the waistband area,[52] or may develop at sites of previous scar formation (Fig. 129-7C) or radiation. It also has been associated with an isotopic response, developing at sites of prior zoster infection (Fig. 129-7D).[53] Diffuse dermal involvement may result in a "pipestem" appearance of the lower extremities with marked reduction in limb volume and overlying shiny hidebound skin with loss of hair resembling scleroderma (Fig. 129-7E). Deeper involvement of the subcutaneous fat results in irregular hyperpigmented sclerotic plaques with intervening areas of edematous skin closely resembling deep morphea/morphea profunda.[59] Bullae may develop at sites of fibrosis, particularly on the lower legs, as a result of dermal edema, as has been described in bullous morphea profunda.[60] Patchy hyperpigmentation ("leopard spots") may be visible prior to the diagnosis of dermal sclerotic involvement.[61] Dermal sclerosis results in decreased ability to pinch the skin.

Primary involvement of the subcutaneous fat and fascia results in a diffuse firm, rippled pattern to the skin resembling eosinophilic fasciitis (see Fig. 129-7F).[62] Features of overlying epidermal GVHD involvement and pigmentary changes may be absent. Fascial involvement is often most visible on the medial arms and thighs and be accentuated by abduction and supination of the arm. Prominent "grooving" demarcating fascial bundles and along the path of superficial vessels may be observed. Careful palpation of the skin is helpful in detecting deep-seated irregularities in skin texture and differentiation from cellulite. Examination of patients while they are lying down on the examination table may help to reveal rippling or pseudocellulite of the abdomen.[54] Dermal fibrosis or fascial involvement without overlying dermal thickening may lead to progressive loss of joint range of motion and contracture formation. Unlike in systemic sclerosis, chronic GVHD tends to affect large joints, including the shoulders, elbows, wrists, hips, and ankles.[58] Range of motion may be assessed through simple maneuvers on physical examination including flexion/extension (arms/shoulders), abduction/adduction (thighs), and prayer sign (wrists, fingers). It may be helpful to have children sit cross-legged on the examination table to determine range-of-motion abnormalities of the hips.[54] Fasciitis may be associated with cramping, polymyositis, and arthritis.

Nail involvement in chronic GVHD typically results in longitudinal ridging and thin, easily broken nails. Partial or complete anonychia and dorsal pterygium formation may occur.[50] Other findings include onycholysis, periungual erythema, and paronychia.[63]

Other skin sequelae of chronic GVHD include milia formation, porokeratosis, often on the buttock area,[64] angiomatosis,[65] nipple hyperkeratosis,[66] vitiligo, and alopecia, either diffuse or focal areas of alopecia areata.[67] A verrucous acral keratosis form of GVHD has been described, resembling common warts on the fingers, but distinguished by the presence of vacuolar interface and dyskeratotic keratinocytes on histology.[68]

Multiple manifestations of sclerotic and nonsclerotic skin disease may be present in the same individual, making accurate quantification of disease activity challenging. A number of different instruments are currently under investigation to measure skin involvement, most commonly the National Institutes of Health (NIH) Consensus organ-specific severity scoring system, in which the skin composite score in separated into body surface area and specific skin features.[50] Other tools include the Vienna Skin Score,[69] the Hopkins skin sclerosis and fasciitis scores,[70] and the Lee symptom scale and skin subscale.[55] The modified Rodnan score, which is validated for use in systemic sclerosis,[71] has not been validated for use in sclerotic GVHD, and may be of limited value for fascial disease.

RELATED PHYSICAL FINDINGS

Acute GVHD is primarily a disorder of the skin, GI tract, and liver (see Table 129-3), typically presenting with skin rash, new-onset elevation of total bilirubin, and/or voluminous diarrhea. By contrast, chronic GVHD is remarkably diverse in its breadth of organ system manifestations (Table 129-6). The most frequently affected sites are skin and nails, oral mucosa, eyes, liver, lungs, and marrow (usually thrombocytopenia).[7] Esophageal webs/strictures, vaginovulvar disease, myositis, nephrotic syndrome, and pericarditis are less-frequent sequelae of chronic disease.

Mucosal disease is second only to skin involvement in frequency in chronic GVHD. Erythema, lichen planus–like changes with Wickham striae, erosions and ulcerations, and mucoceles are the most common manifestations. The buccal mucosa is most commonly affected, followed by the lips, tongue, and soft palate. Patients often also experience sicca symptoms, and pain from erosions may limit oral intake.[54] Dryness and violaceous erythema of the lips are common. Genital involvement significantly impairs sexual

TABLE 129-6
Signs and Symptoms of Chronic Graft-Versus-Host Disease Based on National Institutes of Health Consensus Criteria

Mucosal Involvement	Ophthalmologic
Oral mucosa	- Blepharitis
- Erythema	- Cicatricial conjunctivitis
- Gingivitis	- Confluent punctuate keratopathy
- Lichen planus-like[a]	- **Dry, gritty, or painful sensation in eyes**
- **Mucocele**	- Periorbital hyperpigmentation
- Mucosal atrophy	- Photophobia
- Mucositis	*GI*
- Pain	- **Anorexia**, nausea, vomiting, **diarrhea**, weight loss, failure to thrive
- Pseudomembrane	- Esophageal web[a]
- Ulcer	- Esophageal upper third stricture/stenosis[a]
- Xerostomia	- Exocrine pancreatic insufficiency
Genital mucosa	*Hematopoietic and immune*
- Lichen planus–like[a]	- Autoantibodies (autoimmune hemolytic anemia, immune thrombocytopenic purpura)
- Lichen sclerosus–like[a]	- Eosinophilia
- Phimosis or urethral meatus scarring or stenosis[a]	- Hypogammaglobulinemia/hypergammaglobulinemia
- Vulvar erosions/fissures/ulcers	- Lymphopenia
- Vaginal scarring or clitoral/labial agglutination[a]	- **Thrombocytopenia**
Muscle, Fascia, Joint Involvement	- Raynaud phenomenon
- Arthralgia or arthritis	*Hepatic*
- Edema	- Elevated total bilirubin
- Fasciitis[a]	- Elevated alkaline phosphatase
- Joint stiffness or contractures secondary to fasciitis or sclerosis[a]	- **Elevated transaminases**
- **Muscle cramps**	*Neurologic*
- Myasthenia gravis	- Peripheral neuropathy
- Myositis or polymyositis	*Pulmonary*
Other Organ System Involvement	- Air trapping and bronchiectasis on CT
Cardiovascular	- **Bronchiolitis obliterans diagnosed by biopsy**[a] **or syndrome**
- Pericardial effusion	- Cryptogenic organizing pneumonia
- Cardiac conduction abnormality or cardiomyopathy	- Pleural effusions
	- Restrictive lung disease
	Renal
	- Nephrotic syndrome

[a]Diagnostic features of chronic graft-versus-host disease (GVHD) based on NIH Consensus Criteria. Other signs and symptoms listed are not considered sufficient to establish a diagnosis of chronic GVHD without further testing or evidence of other organ system involvement. The most common GVHD manifestations are shown in **bold**.

Adapted from Jagasia MH, Greinix HT, Arora M, et al. National Institutes of Health consensus development project on criteria for clinical trials in chronic graft-versus-host disease: I. The 2014 Diagnosis and Staging Working Group report. *Biol Blood Marrow Transplant.* 2015;21:389-401.e1.

function and quality of life and may be overlooked if a specific examination and directed questions regarding genital symptoms are not undertaken. Involvement of the penis may induce phimosis. Vulvovaginal involvement presents as erythema, erosions/fissures, vestibulitis, vaginal stenosis, labial resorption, or complete agglutination of the introitus leading to hematocolpos (Fig. 129-8).[72]

The 2014 chronic GVHD NIH Consensus Development Project provided precise terminology for organ-specific diagnostic manifestations of chronic GVHD in the setting of HCT (see Table 129-6).[50]

HISTOPATHOLOGY

Table 129-4 shows the histologic grading scale for acute GVHD. The hallmark feature of acute GVHD is the presence of necrotic keratinocytes accompanied by a dermal lymphocytic infiltrate (usually sparse) and basal vacuolar interface alteration (Fig. 129-9). Early GVHD involvement with follicular erythema correlates with involvement limited to the hair follicle. Subepidermal cleft formation (grade III) is indicative of more-severe involvement, whereas complete separation of epidermis from dermis (grade IV) correlates with clinical findings resembling toxic epidermal necrolysis. Grade IV involvement may be impossible to differentiate histologically from drug-induced toxic epidermal necrolysis and requires careful clinical correlation. The presence of eosinophils has been used to argue against a diagnosis of GVHD; however, it cannot be reliably used to distinguish between GVHD and drug hypersensitivity.[73] Engraftment syndrome is a poorly understood phenomenon at the time of neutrophil engraftment following autologous HCT or allo-HCT and is characterized by a nonspecific erythematous skin eruption, fever, and

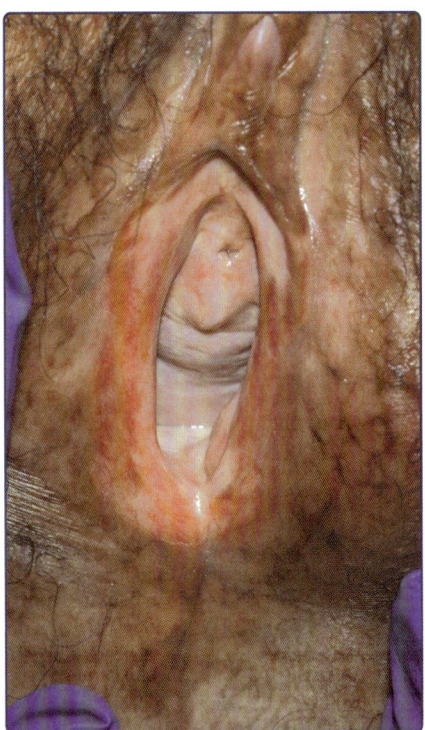

Figure 129-8 Severe chronic graft-versus-host disease (GVHD) of the vulva. The labia minora are partially resorbed with residual vulvitis and atrophic mucosa. Surrounding reticulate hyperpigmentation of the nonmucosal skin is consistent with postinflammatory changes of chronic GVHD.

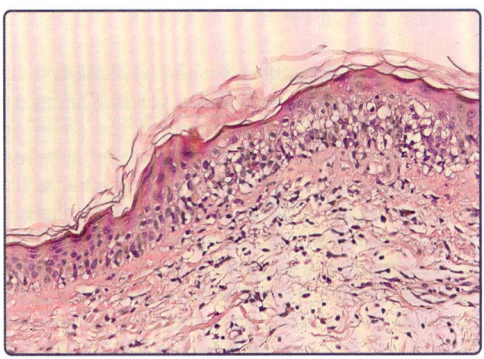

Figure 129-9 Histopathologic features of acute cutaneous graft-versus-host disease, grade II. Inflammation of the upper dermis is present, with extension of lymphocytes into the dermis and interface change.

pulmonary edema.[74] Histologically, it may not be possible to distinguish engraftment rash from early (grade I) acute GVHD.

Epidermal changes in chronic GVHD may be indistinguishable from those of acute disease and are characterized by vacuolar interface dermatitis and epidermal dyskeratotic keratinocytes (Fig. 129-10A). Adnexal structures are often affected. Sclerotic involvement of the upper dermis may resemble lichen sclerosus, with epidermal atrophy, hyperkeratosis, follicular plugging, and a pale, homogenized appearance of the upper dermis collagen (Fig. 129-10B). Sclerotic GVHD is characterized by thickened collagen bundles, increased numbers of fibroblasts, loss of periadnexal fat, and periadnexal inflammation, and may be indistinguishable from morphea and scleroderma. Subcutaneous and fascial involvement accordingly demonstrates changes in the fat septae and fascia, including thickening, edema, and fibrosis. An inflammatory infiltrate, consisting of variable numbers of lymphocytes, histiocytes, and eosinophils may be seen.[57,75]

Histology of oral mucosal GVHD reflects similar interface changes as those seen in epidermal GVHD, but without associated acanthosis. Lymphocytic infiltration of the salivary glands resembles changes seen in Sjögren syndrome.[75,76]

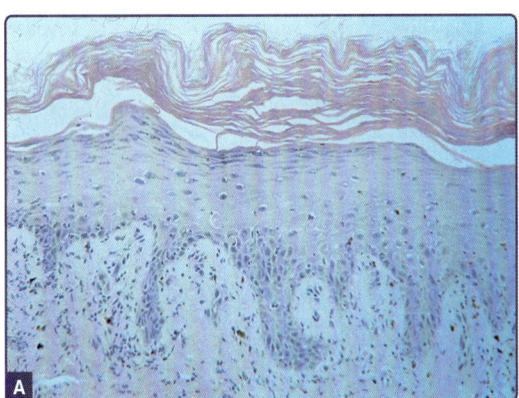
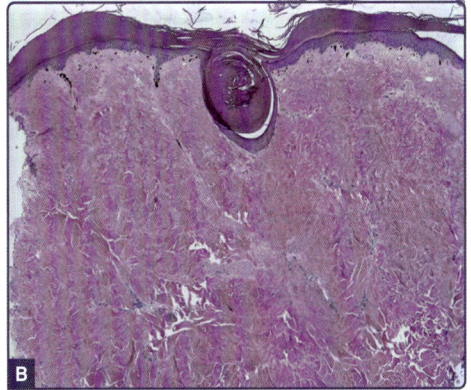

Figure 129-10 Histologic features of epidermal and sclerotic-type chronic cutaneous graft-versus-host disease. **A,** Histopathologic features of a lichen planus–like reaction. Acanthosis, hypergranulosis, hyperkeratosis, and pointed rete ridges are present. The inflammatory infiltrate is less dense than that usually seen in idiopathic lichen planus. **B,** Sclerotic-type graft-versus-host disease. There is mild, compact hyperkeratosis of the epidermis with keratin plugging. There is hyalinization of the collagen throughout the dermis with loss of appendageal structures.

DIAGNOSIS

LABORATORY TESTS

Diagnosis of acute GVHD skin involvement is based on clinicopathologic correlation, particularly exclusion of drugs and infectious causes. Total bilirubin levels and quantification of diarrhea volume are used in conjunction with skin disease to stage the disease (see Table 129-3). The presence of a neutrophil count greater than 0.5×10^9/L and a platelet count greater than 20×10^9/L indicates engraftment, and brings engraftment syndrome into the differential diagnosis of acute GVHD.[74]

In recent years, genome-wide association and proteomic studies have helped identify potential biomarkers in GVHD patients. Candidate markers found to have diagnostic and prognostic value for acute GVHD include TNF receptor-1, IL-2 receptor-α, IL-8, hepatocyte growth factor, and regenerating islet-derived 3α. Elevated levels of these markers have been associated with increased likelihood of nonresponse, as well as poorer survival.[77] Additional markers whose increased expressed may be associated with acute GVHD include BAFF, IL-33, CXCL-10, and CXCL-11.[78]

In chronic GVHD, circulating B-cell subsets and decreased T-regulatory cells are associated with disease.[28,37,69,79] BAFF, CXCL-9, elafin, aminopeptidase N, soluble-type IL-2 receptor-α, IL-4, IL-6, and TNF also are associated with diagnostic usefulness in chronic GVHD.[80-82] TNF has shown both diagnostic and prognostic value in chronic disease.[83] Although autoimmune markers may be seen in the majority of patients after allo-HCT, their presence is generally not specific for the development of chronic GVHD manifestations. In an NIH cohort, autoantibodies were identified in 62% of chronic GVHD patients, and multiple antibodies in 35% of patients. The most frequent antibodies were antinuclear antibody (29%) and rheumatoid factor (13%).[37] Other autoantibodies that have been reported in GVHD patients include anti–double-stranded DNA, anti-PDGF, and anti-HY.[31,39,84] Identifying specific biomarkers of disease activity is an area of research emphasis in acute and chronic GVHD.[82]

SPECIAL TESTS (INCLUDING IMAGING STUDIES)

Suspicion of subcutaneous sclerotic and fascial disease and myositis may be confirmed by MRI, particularly in cases in which definitive sclerotic changes are not observed or when a fascial or muscle biopsy is deferred.[85]

High-frequency ultrasound,[86] digital heat mapping, and durometry also have been used to study sclerosis of the skin in GVHD, but are not widely available in clinical practice.

TABLE 129-7
Differential Diagnosis of Graft-Versus-Host Disease

Acute Graft-Versus-Host Disease (GVHD)
- Drug eruption
- Eruption of lymphocyte recovery
- Rash of engraftment syndrome
- Transient acantholytic dermatosis
- Toxic epidermal necrolysis (for stage IV disease)
- Toxic erythema of chemotherapy
- Viral exanthem

Chronic GVHD
Epidermal involvement
- Drug eruption
- *Demodex* folliculitis
- Eczematous drug eruption
- Lichen planus
- Pityriasis lichenoides chronica
- *Pityrosporum* folliculitis
- Psoriasis

Sclerotic involvement
- Eosinophilic fasciitis
- Lichen sclerosus
- Morphea
- Nephrogenic systemic fibrosis
- Radiation dermatitis
- Systemic sclerosis

DIFFERENTIAL DIAGNOSIS

The differential diagnosis of acute GVHD is broad, and especially challenging as the clinical and histologic features are often indistinguishable from morbilliform drug eruption and engraftment syndrome, the latter of which follows neutrophil recovery and presents with a morbilliform eruption, fever, and pulmonary edema. It also may be accompanied by elevated total bilirubin and diarrhea, and appears histologically similar to acute GVHD.[74] Although engraftment syndrome is thought to occur sooner posttransplantation than GVHD, hyperacute GVHD can present within this window as well. Engraftment syndrome tends to be more steroid-responsive compared to acute GVHD. Toxic erythema of chemotherapy may occur up to 1 week after transplantation, and encompasses multiple skin reactions to chemotherapy. Chemotherapeutic agents commonly associated with toxic erythema of chemotherapy include cytarabine, anthracycline, 5-FU, capecitabine, taxanes, and methotrexate.[46,87] Another differential diagnosis to consider is eruption of lymphocyte recovery, which represents immune system recovery approximately 3 weeks after chemotherapy, and may be associated with fever. Viral reactivation is common post-HCT, including human herpesvirus-6 reactivation, cytomegalovirus, and Epstein-Barr virus, which may present as morbilliform eruptions.

As the presentation of chronic GVHD is quite varied, there are many other potential differential diagnoses. An important consideration is that not every cutaneous finding in the post-HCT setting represents

GVHD. Biopsy can be useful in helping to distinguish nondiagnostic presentations. One important differential diagnosis in these patients is *Demodex* folliculitis, which increasingly occurs in the immunosuppressed setting in HCT recipients. Table 129-7 outlines the differential diagnosis of graft-versus-host disease.

COMPLICATIONS

Skin erosions and ulceration caused by chronic GVHD may lead to secondary infection. Wound-healing in these patients is often slow and difficult in the setting of systemic corticosteroids and certain GVHD therapies (eg, sirolimus).[88] Sclerotic changes resulting in restriction in joint function may lead to functional disability and joint contractures. Restrictive lung disease may result from sclerotic involvement of the torso. HCT survivors are at increased risk for melanoma and nonmelanoma skin cancer because of previous exposure to ionizing radiation, GVHD-associated immune dysregulation, and immunosuppressive treatment of GVHD.[89-91] Both cutaneous squamous cell carcinoma and melanoma also may be increased by long-term treatment with voriconazole, a potent photosensitizer, which may be employed for antifungal treatment or prophylaxis.[92,93] Multiple squamous cell carcinomas also have been reported after psoralen and ultraviolet A (PUVA) therapy for GVHD.[94] Treatment of skin cancers in these patients is challenging because of the increased risk of infection and poor wound healing.

PROGNOSIS AND CLINICAL COURSE

Although the presence of GVHD is associated with a decreased risk of malignancy relapse, GVHD leads to significant morbidity, especially in patients with steroid-refractory disease. Chronic GVHD is the second leading cause of long-term mortality in HCT patients after recurrence of primary disease.[95] Extensive (>50%) skin involvement[96] and "lichenoid" skin histology also may be associated with poorer survival. The association between sclerotic skin and mortality is thought to relate to higher doses of immunosuppression required, and therefore increased risk of infection. Sclerotic skin is likely also a marker of more-severe disease, such as lung disease, which may directly impact mortality.

A number of systemic risk factors portend a poor prognosis, including a history of progressive involvement from acute to chronic GVHD,[97] thrombocytopenia (fewer than 100,000 cells/mL),[56] elevated bilirubin,[98] older age, GI symptoms, and lack of response to therapy at 6 months.[97]

PREVENTION

GVHD prevention begins prior to transplantation with selection of the most closely HLA-matched donor, the GVHD prophylaxis regimen, and, in some cases, T-cell depletion or manipulation of the graft. T-cell depletion is accomplished through ex vivo T-cell–negative selection or enrichment of the CD34+ stem cell population, or more commonly through in vivo treatment with anti–T-cell therapy, such as posttransplantation cyclophosphamide,[99] or alemtuzumab, an anti-CD52 monoclonal antibody.[100,101] Other strategies for T-cell modulation, including IL-2 and antibodies targeting IL-17 and IL-21. have been used to attempt to induce the expansion of T-regulatory cells.[102,103] Even though T-cell modulation may lead to higher rates of graft failure, cancer relapse, and infection, studies show that strategies aimed at reducing the incidence of GVHD may lead to improved overall mortality.[104,105] Prophylactic immunosuppressive therapy is initiated concomitantly with the administration of the hematopoietic graft, but, as with T-cell depletion, such therapy must be balanced with the potential for diminished graft-versus-leukemia/lymphoma effect and long-term infection risk. One of the most important strategies has been increasing use of antihuman T-lymphocyte immune globulin (or antithymocyte globulin) as part of the conditioning regimen,[106,107] which has shown efficacy in acute and chronic GVHD. Administration of antithymocyte globulin in this setting has been shown to significantly reduce the incidence of chronic GVHD at 2 years, and lead to discontinuation of immunosuppression with a trend toward improved survival.[108] Sirolimus is an mammalian target of rapamycin inhibitor that has been used in prophylactic regimens in combination with standard therapy or in place of calcineurin inhibitors, and which may have the advantage of improved tolerance compared to calcineurin inhibitors.[109,110]

Similar to solid-organ transplantation, skin cancer screening and patient education regarding photoprotective measures is a key preventive strategy in all HCT patients, especially those who develop chronic GVHD.[111] Patients are also at elevated risk of systemic infection; consequently, implementation of preventive infectious disease recommendations and careful monitoring for cutaneous infection, particularly in patients with chronic skin erosions/ulcerations, is prudent. Finally, patient education regarding early signs of skin sclerosis and fascial involvement, including skin tightness, edema, muscle cramping, and range-of-motion restriction, may facilitate early diagnosis and initiation of treatment.

TREATMENT

MANAGEMENT OF ACUTE GRAFT-VERSUS-HOST DISEASE

Treatment of acute GVHD is usually initiated in the hospital, given the proximity to the date of HCT and the need for close observation. Patients with mild (grade I) skin involvement without hepatic or GI symptoms may respond to high-potency topical steroids. However, more-severe skin involvement or the presence of internal organ involvement necessitates treatment with systemic corticosteroids. Patients with moderate-to-severe acute GVHD may warrant treatment with methylprednisone 1 to 2 mg/kg/day; however, lower doses may be adequate to control disease. Patients with skin sloughing require meticulous skin care, infection surveillance, and fluid management similar to toxic epidermal necrolysis. Approximately 50% of patients respond to systemic corticosteroids; however those who require additional therapy typically receive increased doses of their GVHD prophylaxis (most commonly tacrolimus, cyclosporine, or methotrexate) or additional therapy, including horse antithymocyte globulin, extracorporeal photopheresis (ECP), and mycophenolate mofetil.[112] Mycophenolate mofetil is particularly helpful in patients with acute GVHD limited to the skin, with a large case series demonstrating a 92.3% response.[113] Other agents include alemtuzumab,[100] basiliximab,[114] inolimumab,[115] daclizumab,[116] etanercept,[117] infliximab,[118] denileukin diftitox, pentostatin,[119] sirolimus,[120] and mesenchymal stem cells.[121] Levine and colleagues[117] demonstrated complete remission of skin symptoms in 81% of patients treated with steroids and etanercept, compared to steroids alone (complete remission = 47%). Similarly, infliximab has also shown success in acute treatment-refractory skin GVHD (33% to 60%).[118] Immunosuppression to treat acute GVHD must always be weighed against the risk of infection and dampening of the graft-versus-leukemia effect.

Administration of ECP is sometimes preferred prior to increased immunosuppression. ECP is thought to modulate alloreactive T-cell and dendritic cell activity. During ECP, the white cell compartment of the blood is removed from the patient via pheresis, mixed with 8-methoxypsoralen, irradiated with UVA light, and then returned to the patient. In a pooled analysis of studies examining ECP, the overall response rate was 84% for acute skin GVHD.[122] In a randomized trial, the addition of ECP to systemic steroids resulted in higher response rates, particularly for skin-only acute GVHD.[123] Limitations to ECP include the time commitment for the procedure—requiring several hours on 2 consecutive days for 1 cycle, the requirement and cost of a dedicated pheresis center, potentially prolonged vascular access, and fluid imbalance. The optimal frequency and duration of ECP treatment is unclear. Typically, 1 cycle is given weekly, followed by tapering as a response is achieved. Phototherapy (UVA1,[124] PUVA,[125] narrow band UVB[126]) also has been used for acute GVHD,[127] but is logistically challenging in the inpatient setting and should be administered cautiously to avoid inducing erythema.

In a 2008 study, 39 (71%) of 55 participants with steroid-resistant acute GVHD sustained a complete or partial response to mesenchymal stem cell infusion.[128] Responses were seen regardless of mesenchymal stem cell source (HLA-matched, haploidentical, or third-party unmatched donors), and immunogenicity was not observed. In a Phase I study, response rates of 67.5% were reported, with 27.5% experiencing a complete response.[121] The immunomodulatory mechanism of mesenchymal stem cells is unclear in GVHD, but may be through the induction of T-regulatory cells.

MANAGEMENT OF CHRONIC GRAFT-VERSUS-HOST DISEASE

The dermatologist should play a key role in the multidisciplinary approach to chronic GVHD management, beginning with careful assessment of the subtype and extent of skin involvement. Together with an understanding of other organ system activity, infection risk, relapse risk, and GVHD prognostic risk factors, a decision regarding the appropriateness of topical, physical (eg, phototherapy), and systemic therapy can then be made. If systemic therapy is prescribed by the transplant physician, periodic dermatologic monitoring is advised to differentiate adverse drug reactions or other new skin disease from GVHD, to assess cutaneous disease response, and to monitor for infection and skin malignancy.

For mild chronic skin GVHD without sclerotic features, including lichen planus–like, ichthyotic, and papulosquamous types, topical steroids may be used either alone or in conjunction with systemic steroids with close followup and screening for more significant or systemic disease.[129] Treatment typically includes mid- to high-potency topical steroids with topical calcineurin inhibitors[130] applied twice daily, potentially under occlusion for thicker or refractory lesions. Topical calcineurin inhibitors are particularly useful for treatment of areas at high risk of skin atrophy, such as the face (including the lips) and intertriginous surfaces. Extensive application of topical calcineurin inhibitors, however, can lead to systemic absorption.[131] Additional objectives of topical therapy include relief of pruritus and prevention of skin breakdown and infection. Regular moisturization to maintain skin integrity and strict photoprotection should also be employed. Pruritus without rash can be treated with low-potency topical steroids and menthol-based creams. Although systemic antihistamines at higher-than-standard dosing are often helpful, caution should be taken to avoid inducing or exacerbating oral and ocular sicca symptoms.[132]

Phototherapy may be appropriate for patients with limited epidermal or sclerotic disease in whom systemic therapy is not otherwise warranted (eg, without internal organ system involvement), or in whom systemic immunosuppressive therapy is contraindicated (eg, active infection). Data are limited to anecdotal cases and case series. Longer-wavelength UVA (340 to 400 nm; UVA-1) may be particularly beneficial for fibrosing forms of chronic GVHD.[124] UVA-1 does not require psoralen ingestion/topical, and penetrates deeper into the dermis than full-spectrum UVA. UVA-1 is thought to increase the synthesis of matrix metalloproteinases, and decrease the synthesis of procollagen though IL-1 and IL-6. It may also reduce levels of transforming growth factor-β, TNF, IL-8, and IL-10. Although UVA-1 is not yet widely available in the Unites States, it appears to be well tolerated, acceptable for pediatric use, and is not associated with persistent photosensitivity, carcinogenic risk, or potential GI issues that may occur with oral psoralen use. The largest series describes skin softening following UVA-1 treatment of sclerotic-type GVHD in 17 (70.8%) of 24 GVHD patients, with the best response rate in patients receiving high-dose UVA-1.[133] In a study of medium-dose UVA-1 phototherapy in 7 patients with lichenoid GVHD and 3 with sclerotic GVHD, all 3 patients with sclerotic GVHD demonstrated partial response or improvement.[134] Ständer and colleagues[135] described softening of skin lesions, improved joint mobility, and healing of skin erosions in 5 adult patients with medium-dose UVA-1 and 1 child treated with low-dose UVA-1. Calzavara Pinton and colleagues[136] described 5 patients with sclerotic involvement treated with UVA-1 therapy with complete resolution in 3 patients and partial response in 2 patients. Although UVA-1 may accentuate pigmentary abnormalities, the risk of skin cancer is significantly less than the risk associated with PUVA.[137] PUVA has shown limited efficacy in treating GVHD and is associated with potential phototoxicity and risk of skin cancer.[138] Narrow band UVB also has been used, with some response in patients with primarily "lichenoid" disease.[126,139] Care must be taken in administering phototherapy, as UV radiation may trigger flares of cutaneous disease. Skin cancer risk assessment and concurrent use of photosensitizing medications should also be considered. Voriconazole therapy, in particular, is an important photosensitizer in this setting and may increase the risk of squamous cell carcinoma and melanoma.[92,93]

First-line treatment of moderate to severe GVHD is high-dose systemic steroids, usually in combination with other immunosuppressive agents.[129] Long-term systemic therapy is often required for patients with moderate-to-severe disease (3 or more organs involved, moderate or severe involvement in any organ, or lung involvement).[50] Combination therapy with azathioprine, thalidomide, mycophenolate mofetil, Plaquenil, and sirolimus have suggested no significant benefit over prednisone alone for first-line therapy.[129] Calcineurin inhibitors should be used in combination with systemic steroids, and can be particularly helpful in moderating steroid dependence.[140]

Among the myriad of systemic treatments that have been used in patients with chronic GVHD who cannot be tapered from systemic corticosteroids or who are steroid-refractory, no single treatment has demonstrated proven superiority. There are no U.S. Food and Drug Administration–approved treatments for chronic GVHD. Determination of a preferred second-line or salvage agent has been complicated by poor understanding of the disease process and a lack of high-quality clinical trials. The need to spur clinical trial development in the field of chronic GVHD was acknowledged by the chronic GVHD NIH Consensus Project, which included a standardized system of organ system assessments and recommendations for clinical trial design.[50] Unfortunately, validated measures of cutaneous disease activity still have limitations, and are not routinely implemented in clinical care.[141] Ideally, dermatologic collaboration in future therapeutic trials will permit better quantification of cutaneous disease response. Response should be assessed 8 to 12 weeks after initiation of a systemic treatment. If patients progress after 4 weeks, a new treatment option should be offered.[129] Significant sclerotic disease may require substantially longer treatment periods to determine an effect.

ECP is a major salvage therapy in steroid-refractory chronic GVHD, especially in patients with evidence of skin sclerosis at high risk of adverse effects from systemic immunosuppression. ECP has an excellent safety profile, but is limiting in that it requires sustained venous access. A pooled analysis of ECP studies for chronic GVHD found an overall response rate of 71% for cutaneous disease.[122] In a large retrospective analysis of 71 patients, response was seen in 61% with best response was seen in 44 (61%) of patients, most notably in the skin. Thrombocytopenia was associated with a lower response rate.[142] Patients with classic chronic GVHD and overlap acute and chronic GVHD demonstrated superior survival after treatment with ECP.[143] ECP may be particularly useful for patients with deep-seated sclerotic involvement of the subcutaneous tissue and fascia. Although GVHD-related fasciitis resembles eosinophilic fasciitis, in contrast to eosinophilic fasciitis, GVHD-related fasciitis does not respond well to steroid therapy and may result in significant long-term functional disability. Several case reports describe successful use of ECP for GVHD-related fasciitis.[144]

Imatinib mesylate, a multikinase inhibitor with activity against bc-abl, c-kit, PDGFR, and other kinases, has been reported to have a modest benefit at doses lower than are typically administered for treatment of chronic myeloid leukemia (adult: 400 mg daily; children 260 mg/m^2 daily) as the drug in GVHD patients is poorly tolerated. In a prospective study specifically for sclerotic skin GVHD, Baird and colleagues[145] observed a partial response in 5 of 14 patients, with an average range-of-motion improvement of 26%. The drug is generally well tolerated in the setting of treatment of chronic myelogenous leukemia; however, side effects are common in the GVHD setting and include hypophosphatemia, fatigue, nausea, diarrhea, edema, and muscle cramping. The modest effect reported is in line with a large series reporting limited efficacy,[146] despite many prior case series and other studies revealing more promising results.[147-149] Ibrutinib, a small-molecule inhibitor of Bruton tyrosine kinase, has shown preclinical efficacy in mouse models of GVHD, and clinical trials are ongoing.[150-152]

TABLE 129-8
Other Potential Systemic Treatments of Chronic Skin Graft-Versus-Host Disease

Immunosuppressive Agents
- Mycophenolate mofetil[156]
- Calcineurin inhibitors (cyclosporine, tacrolimus)[157]

Chemotherapeutic Agents
- Thalidomide[158]
- Azathioprine[159]
- Methotrexate[160]
- Pentostatin[161]

Antimicrobial Agents
- Cyclophosphamide[162]
- Clofazimine[163]
- Hydroxychloroquine[132]

Small Molecule Inhibitors
- Imatinib,[145] dasatinib, nilotinib
- Sirolimus[155]
- Ruxolitinib,[153] tofacitinib[154]
- Vorinostat[164]
- Erlotinib[165]

Antibodies and Fusion Proteins
- Antithymocyte globulin[108]
- Rituximab[35]
- Infliximab, etanercept[166]
- Alefacept[167]
- Denileukin diftitox, basiliximab, daclizumab[116]

Cytokines
- Low-dose interleukin-2[168]

Cellular Therapies
- T-reg adoptive therapy[169]
- Mesenchymal stem cell therapy[170]

Radiation
- Total nodal irradiation[171]
- Thoracoabdominal irradiation[172]

Other
- Retinoids[173]
- Intravenous immunoglobulin[174]
- Extracorporeal photopheresis[122]
- Bortezomib[175]
- Vismodegib[176]

---

during treatment with ruxolitinib.[153]

Sirolimus also has been used therapeutically in chronic GVHD, with a Phase II trial demonstrating clinical response in 15 (79%) of 19 patients.[155] Table 129-8 lists systemic second-line therapies for chronic GVHD.

SUPPORTIVE CARE

Supportive care including physical and occupational therapy is especially important in patients with skin sclerosis and fasciitis leading to joint contractures. Weight-bearing exercise for 30 minutes daily 5 days per week are important for preserving range of motion and bone health. Deep-tissue massage may be helpful to preserve range of motion in patients with fasciitis.[132]

TREATMENT OF CHRONIC ORAL AND VULVOVAGINAL DISEASE

Limited oral mucosal disease can be controlled with application of a high-potency topical corticosteroid gel or paste (fluocinonide gel 0.05%, clobestasol gel 0.05%, triamcinolone 0.1% dental paste). Solutions of dexamethasone 0.5 mg/mL and prednisolone 15 mg/mL also may be used as rinses, and are beneficial for widespread involvement and should be swished in the mouth for 4 to 6 minutes 4 to 6 times daily.[177] Refractory lesions may respond to intralesional triamcinolone injection. Topical application of tacrolimus 0.1% ointment also may be used in conjunction with steroids and for maintenance; however, systemic absorption has been reported. Calcineurin inhibitors also can be constituted as oral solutions. Topical antiinflammatories should be used in combination with an anti-yeast wash (nystatin) as to avoid secondary *Candida* infection in the setting of oral steroids. Cyclosporine and azathioprine rinses also may be used for refractory disease, but require pharmacy compounding. Patients with salivary gland disease should avoid oral antihistamines as well as other xerogenic medications (selective serotonin reuptake inhibitors, tricyclic antidepressants). Dental hygiene is very important in patients with decreased salivary function and home fluoride treatment is frequently recommended. Salivary stimulants (eg, sugar-free gum) and sialogogue therapy (cevimeline, pilocarpine) are recommended for patients with severe salivary gland dysfunction.[132] Although sclerotic involvement of perioral skin involvement is uncommon, in this setting aggressive systemic therapy is indicated.

Genital erosions and fissures associated with chronic vulvovaginal disease may be treated with clobetasol propionate ointment nightly, which should be tapered

---

Rituximab has immunoregulatory effects in patients with chronic GVHD, and data suggesting elevated levels of BAFF in chronic GVHD patients supports this.[32] In a prospective, multicenter randomized trial, a significant clinical response in skin sclerosis and joint range of motion was seen in 27% of patients receiving rituximab, compared to 36% of patients receiving imatinib. Among rituximab patients, those with higher circulating activated B cells were more likely to have treatment success.[35]

Inhibitors of Janus kinase (JAK)/signal transducer and activator of transcription (STAT) signaling, ruxolitinib and tofacitinib, have also shown promising preclinical and early clinical results.[153,154] One study reported an 81.5% response rate in 54 patients with acute GVHD and 84.4% response rate for 41 patients with chronic GVHD treated with ruxolitinib. Cytopenias and cytomegalovirus reactivation were observed

to a maintenance level of 2 to 3 times weekly. Fluocinolone 0.025% ointment can be used in cases of mild disease or for maintenance in cases of treated severe disease. Additionally, tacrolimus ointment has been commonly employed for maintenance therapy in this area. If estrogen is not contraindicated, hormone replacement via topical cream, vaginal ring, or oral replacement may improve genital skin integrity. Limited vaginal scarring/synechiae can be treated with dilators or manual lysing; however, thick vaginal scarring may require surgical intervention.[178]

REFERENCES

1. Gatti R, Meuwissen H, Allen H, et al. Immunological reconstitution of sex-linked lymphopenic immunological deficiency. *Lancet*. 1968;292:1366-1369.
2. Stem Cell Trialists' Collaborative Group. Allogeneic peripheral blood stem-cell compared with bone marrow transplantation in the management of hematologic malignancies: an individual patient data meta-analysis of nine randomized trials. *J Clin Oncol*. 2005;23:5074-5087.
3. Slavin S, Nagler A, Naparstek E, et al. Nonmyeloablative stem cell transplantation and cell therapy as an alternative to conventional bone marrow transplantation with lethal cytoreduction for the treatment of malignant and nonmalignant hematologic diseases. *Blood*. 1998;91:756-763.
4. Brunstein CG, Barker JN, Weisdorf DJ, et al. Umbilical cord blood transplantation after nonmyeloablative conditioning: impact on transplantation outcomes in 110 adults with hematologic disease. *Blood*. 2007;110:3064-3070.
5. Lokhorst HM, Wu K, Verdonck LF, et al. The occurrence of graft-versus-host disease is the major predictive factor for response to donor lymphocyte infusions in multiple myeloma. *Blood*. 2004;103:4362-4364.
6. Laughlin MJ, Eapen M, Rubinstein P, et al. Outcomes after transplantation of cord blood or bone marrow from unrelated donors in adults with leukemia. *N Engl J Med*. 2004;351:2265-2275.
7. Lee SJ, Vogelsang G, Flowers ME. Chronic graft-versus-host disease. *Biol Blood Marrow Transplant*. 2003;9:215-233.
8. Shlomchik WD. Graft-versus-host disease. *Nat Rev Immunol*. 2007;7:340-352.
9. Arora M, Cutler CS, Jagasia MH, et al. Late acute and chronic graft-versus-host disease after allogeneic hematopoietic cell transplantation. *Biol Blood Marrow Transplant*. 2016;22:449-455.
10. Arai S, Arora M, Wang T, et al. Increasing incidence of chronic graft-versus-host disease in allogeneic transplantation: a report from the Center for International Blood and Marrow Transplant Research. *Biol Blood Marrow Transplant*. 2015;21:266-274.
11. Martires KJ, Baird K, Steinberg SM, et al. Sclerotic-type chronic GVHD of the skin: clinical risk factors, laboratory markers, and burden of disease. *Blood*. 2011;118:4250-4257.
12. Flowers ME, Parker PM, Johnston LJ, et al. Comparison of chronic graft-versus-host disease after transplantation of peripheral blood stem cells versus bone marrow in allogeneic recipients: long-term follow-up of a randomized trial. *Blood*. 2002;100:415-419.
13. Chosidow O, Bagot M, Vernant JP, et al. Sclerodermatous chronic graft-versus-host disease. Analysis of seven cases. *J Am Acad Dermatol*. 1992;26:49-55.
14. Uhm J, Hamad N, Shin EM, et al. Incidence, risk factors, and long-term outcomes of sclerotic graft-versus-host disease after allogeneic hematopoietic cell transplantation. *Biol Blood Marrow Transplant*. 2014;20:1751-1757.
15. Billingham RE. The biology of graft-versus-host reactions. *Harvey Lect*. 1966;62:21-78.
16. Bleakley M, Riddell SR. Molecules and mechanisms of the graft-versus-leukaemia effect. *Nat Rev Cancer*. 2004;4:371-380.
17. Wu T, Young JS, Johnston H, et al. Thymic damage, impaired negative selection, and development of chronic graft-versus-host disease caused by donor CD4+ and CD8+ T cells. *J Immunol*. 2013;191:488-499.
18. Ferrara JL, Levine JE, Reddy P, et al. Graft-versus-host disease. *Lancet*. 2009;373:1550-1561.
19. MacDonald KP, Hill GR, Blazar BR. Chronic graft-versus-host disease: biological insights from pre-clinical and clinical studies. *Blood*. 2017;129(1):13-21.
20. Hakim FT, Memon S, Jin P, et al. Upregulation of IFN-inducible and damage-response pathways in chronic graft-versus-host disease. *J Immunol*. 2016;197:3490-3503.
21. Gartlan KH, Markey KA, Varelias A, et al. Tc17 cells are a proinflammatory, plastic lineage of pathogenic CD8+ T cells that induce GVHD without antileukemic effects. *Blood*. 2015;126:1609-1620.
22. Harris T, Grosso JF, Yen HR, et al. Cutting edge: an in vivo requirement for STAT3 signaling in TH17 development and TH17-dependent autoimmunity. *J Immunol*. 2007;179:4313-4317.
23. Yi T, Chen Y, Wang L, et al. Reciprocal differentiation and tissue-specific pathogenesis of Th1, Th2, and Th17 cells in graft-versus-host disease. *Blood*. 2009;114:3101-3112.
24. Antin JH, Ferrara JL. Cytokine dysregulation and acute graft-versus-host disease. *Blood*. 1992;80:2964-2968.
25. Edinger M, Hoffmann P, Ermann J, et al. CD4+CD25+ regulatory T cells preserve graft-versus-tumor activity while inhibiting graft-versus-host disease after bone marrow transplantation. *Nat Med*. 2003;9:1144-1150.
26. Magenau JM, Qin X, Tawara I, et al. Frequency of CD4(+)CD25(hi)FOXP3(+) regulatory T cells has diagnostic and prognostic value as a biomarker for acute graft-versus-host-disease. *Biol Blood Marrow Transplant*. 2010;16:907-914.
27. Zeiser R, Nguyen VH, Beilhack A, et al. Inhibition of CD4+CD25+ regulatory T-cell function by calcineurin-dependent interleukin-2 production. *Blood*. 2006;108:390-399.
28. Zorn E, Kim HT, Lee SJ, et al. Reduced frequency of FOXP3+ CD4+CD25+ regulatory T cells in patients with chronic graft-versus-host disease. *Blood*. 2005;106:2903-2911.
29. Iwata Y, Matsushita T, Horikawa M, et al. Characterization of a rare IL-10-competent B-cell subset in humans that parallels mouse regulatory B10 cells. *Blood*. 2011;117:530-541.
30. Kheav VD, Busson M, Scieux C, et al. Favorable impact of natural killer cell reconstitution on chronic graft-versus-host disease and cytomegalovirus reactivation after allogeneic hematopoietic stem cell transplantation. *Haematologica*. 2014;99:1860-1867.
31. Miklos DB, Kim HT, Miller KH, et al. Antibody responses to H-Y minor histocompatibility antigens correlate with chronic graft-versus-host disease and disease remission. *Blood*. 2005;105:2973-2978.

32. Sarantopoulos S, Stevenson KE, Kim HT, et al. Altered B-cell homeostasis and excess BAFF in human chronic graft-versus-host disease. *Blood*. 2009;113:3865-3874.
33. Jin H, Ni X, Deng R, et al. Antibodies from donor B cells perpetuate cutaneous chronic graft-versus-host disease in mice. *Blood*. 2016;127:2249-2260.
34. Cutler C, Miklos D, Kim HT, et al. Rituximab for steroid-refractory chronic graft-versus-host disease. *Blood*. 2006;108:756-762.
35. Arai S, Pidala J, Pusic I, et al. A randomized phase II crossover study of imatinib or rituximab for cutaneous sclerosis after hematopoietic cell transplantation. *Clin Cancer Res*. 2016;22:319-327.
36. Nakasone H, Sahaf B, Miklos DB. Therapeutic benefits targeting B-cells in chronic graft-versus-host disease. *Int J Hematol*. 2015;101:438-451.
37. Kuzmina Z, Gounden V, Curtis L, et al. Clinical significance of autoantibodies in a large cohort of patients with chronic graft-versus-host disease defined by NIH criteria. *Am J Hematol*. 2015;90:114-119.
38. Ochs LA, Blazar BR, Roy J, et al. Cytokine expression in human cutaneous chronic graft-versus-host disease. *Bone Marrow Transplant*. 1996;17:1085-1092.
39. Svegliati S, Olivieri A, Campelli N, et al. Stimulatory autoantibodies to PDGF receptor in patients with extensive chronic graft-versus-host disease. *Blood*. 2007;110:237-241.
40. Zhang Y, McCormick LL, Desai SR, et al. Murine sclerodermatous graft-versus-host disease, a model for human scleroderma: cutaneous cytokines, chemokines, and immune cell activation. *J Immunol*. 2002;168:3088-3098.
41. Spies-Weisshart B, Schilling K, Böhmer F, et al. Lack of association of platelet-derived growth factor (PDGF) receptor autoantibodies and severity of chronic graft-versus-host disease (GvHD). *J Cancer Res Clin Oncol*. 2013;139:1397-1404.
42. Duffield JS, Forbes SJ, Constandinou CM, et al. Selective depletion of macrophages reveals distinct, opposing roles during liver injury and repair. *J Clin Invest*. 2005;115:56-65.
43. Alexander KA, Flynn R, Lineburg KE, et al. CSF-1-dependant donor-derived macrophages mediate chronic graft-versus-host disease. *J Clin Invest*. 2014;124:4266-4280.
44. Hansen JA, Chien JW, Warren EH, et al. Defining genetic risk for GVHD and mortality following allogeneic hematopoietic stem cell transplantation. *Curr Opin Hematol*. 2010;17:483-492.
45. Inamoto Y, Martin PJ, Flowers ME, et al. Genetic risk factors for sclerotic graft-versus-host disease. *Blood*. 2016;128:1516-1524.
46. Baack BR, Burgdorf WH. Chemotherapy-induced acral erythema. *J Am Acad Dermatol*. 1991;24:457-461.
47. Mielcarek M, Martin PJ, Leisenring W, et al. Graft-versus-host disease after nonmyeloablative versus conventional hematopoietic stem cell transplantation. *Blood*. 2003;102:756-762.
48. Ohto H, Yasuda H, Noguchi M, et al. Risk of transfusion-associated graft-versus-host disease as a result of directed donations from relatives. *Transfusion (Paris)*. 1992;32:691-693.
49. Rühl H, Bein G, Sachs UJ. Transfusion-associated graft-versus-host disease. *Transfus Med Rev*. 2009;23:62-71.
50. Jagasia MH, Greinix HT, Arora M, et al. National Institutes of Health consensus development project on criteria for clinical trials in chronic graft-versus-host disease: I. The 2014 Diagnosis and Staging Working Group report. *Biol Blood Marrow Transplant*. 2015;21:389-401.e1.
51. Paun O, Phillips T, Fu P, et al. Cutaneous complications in hematopoietic cell transplant recipients: impact of biopsy on patient management. *Biol Blood Marrow Transplant*. 2013;19:1204-1209.
52. Patel AR, Pavletic SZ, Turner ML, et al. The isomorphic response in morphea-like chronic graft-versus-host disease. *Arch Dermatol*. 2008;144:1229-1231.
53. Martires KJ, Baird K, Citrin DE, et al. Localization of sclerotic-type chronic graft-vs-host disease to sites of skin injury: potential insight into the mechanism of isomorphic and isotopic responses. *Arch Dermatol*. 2011;147:1081-1086.
54. Carpenter PA. How I conduct a comprehensive chronic graft-versus-host disease assessment. *Blood*. 2011;118:2679-2687.
55. Lee SK, Cook EF, Soiffer R, et al. Development and validation of a scale to measure symptoms of chronic graft-versus-host disease. *Biol Blood Marrow Transplant*. 2002;8:444-452.
56. Przepiorka D, Weisdorf D, Martin P, et al. 1994 Consensus Conference on Acute GVHD Grading. *Bone Marrow Transplant*. 1995;15:825-828.
57. Hymes SR, Turner ML, Champlin RE, et al. Cutaneous manifestations of chronic graft-versus-host disease. *Biol Blood Marrow Transplant*. 2006;12:1101-1113.
58. Hymes SR, Alousi AM, Cowen EW. Graft-versus-host disease: part I. Pathogenesis and clinical manifestations of graft-versus-host disease. *J Am Acad Dermatol*. 2012;66:515.e1-e18; quiz 533-534.
59. Fett N, Werth VP. Update on morphea: part I. Epidemiology, clinical presentation, and pathogenesis. *J Am Acad Dermatol*. 2011;64:217-228.
60. Su WP, Greene SL. Bullous morphea profunda. *Am J Dermatopathol*. 1986;8:144-147.
61. Peñas PF, Jones-Caballero M, Aragüés M, et al. Sclerodermatous graft-vs-host disease: clinical and pathological study of 17 patients. *Arch Dermatol*. 2002;138:924-934.
62. Schaffer JV, McNiff JM, Seropian S, et al. Lichen sclerosus and eosinophilic fasciitis as manifestations of chronic graft-versus-host disease: expanding the sclerodermoid spectrum. *J Am Acad Dermatol*. 2005;53:591-601.
63. Sanli H, Arat M, Oskay T, et al. Evaluation of nail involvement in patients with chronic cutaneous graft versus host disease: a single-center study from Turkey. *Int J Dermatol*. 2004;43:176-180.
64. Alexis AF, Busam K, Myskowski PL. Porokeratosis of Mibelli following bone marrow transplantation. *Int J Dermatol*. 2006;45:361-365.
65. Kaffenberger BH, Zuo RC, Gru A, et al. Graft-versus-host disease-associated angiomatosis: a clinicopathologically distinct entity. *J Am Acad Dermatol*. 2014;71:745-753.
66. Sanli H, Ekmekci P, Kusak F, et al. Hyperkeratosis of the nipple associated with chronic graft versus host disease after allogeneic haematopoietic cell transplantation. *Acta Derm Venereol*. 2003;83:385-386.
67. Zuo RC, Naik HB, Steinberg SM, et al. Risk factors and characterization of vitiligo and alopecia areata in patients with chronic graft-vs-host disease. *JAMA Dermatol*. 2015;151:23-32.
68. Park JH, Lester L, Kim J, et al. Acral verruca-like presentation of chronic graft-vs.-host disease. *J Cutan Pathol*. 2016;43:236-241.
69. Greinix HT, Pohlreich D, Maalouf J, et al. A single-

70. Jacobsohn DA, Rademaker A, Kaup M, et al. Skin response using NIH consensus criteria vs Hopkins scale in a phase II study for steroid-refractory chronic GVHD. *Bone Marrow Transplant*. 2009;44:813-819.

71. Furst DE, Clements PJ, Steen VD, et al. The modified Rodnan skin score is an accurate reflection of skin biopsy thickness in systemic sclerosis. *J Rheumatol*. 1998;25:84-88.

72. Spiryda LB, Laufer MR, Soiffer RJ, et al. Graft-versus-host disease of the vulva and/or vagina: diagnosis and treatment. *Biol Blood Marrow Transplant*. 2003;9:760-765.

73. Marra DE, McKee PH, Nghiem P. Tissue eosinophils and the perils of using skin biopsy specimens to distinguish between drug hypersensitivity and cutaneous graft-versus-host disease. *J Am Acad Dermatol*. 2004;51:543-546.

74. Cornell RF, Hari P, Drobyski WR. Engraftment syndrome after autologous stem cell transplantation: an update unifying the definition and management approach. *Biol Blood Marrow Transplant*. 2015;21:2061-2068.

75. Shulman HM, Kleiner D, Lee SJ, et al. Histopathologic diagnosis of chronic graft-versus-host disease: National Institutes of Health consensus development project on criteria for clinical trials in chronic graft-versus-host disease: II. Pathology Working Group Report. *Biol Blood Marrow Transplant*. 2006;12:31-47.

76. Horn TD, Rest EB, Mirenski Y, et al. The significance of oral mucosal and salivary gland pathology after allogeneic bone marrow transplantation. *Arch Dermatol*. 1995;131:964-965.

77. Levine JE, Logan BR, Wu J, et al. Acute graft-versus-host disease biomarkers measured during therapy can predict treatment outcomes: a Blood and Marrow Transplant Clinical Trials Network study. *Blood*. 2012;119:3854-3860.

78. Ahmed SS, Wang XN, Norden J, et al. Identification and validation of biomarkers associated with acute and chronic graft versus host disease. *Bone Marrow Transplant*. 2015;50:1563-1571.

79. Miura Y, Thoburn CJ, Bright EC, et al. Association of Foxp3 regulatory gene expression with graft-versus-host disease. *Blood*. 2004;104:2187-2193.

80. Kitko CL, Levine JE, Storer BE, et al. Plasma CXCL9 elevations correlate with chronic GVHD diagnosis. *Blood*. 2014;123:786-793.

81. Tanaka J, Imamura M, Kasai M, et al. Th2 cytokines (IL-4, IL-10 and IL-13) and IL-12 mRNA expression by concanavalin A-stimulated peripheral blood mononuclear cells during chronic graft-versus-host disease. *Eur J Haematol*. 1996;57:111-113.

82. Paczesny S, Hakim FT, Pidala J, et al. National Institutes of Health consensus development project on criteria for clinical trials in chronic graft-versus-host disease: III. The 2014 Biomarker Working Group Report. *Biol Blood Marrow Transplant*. 2015;21:780-792.

83. Ritchie D, Seconi J, Wood C, et al. Prospective monitoring of tumor necrosis factor alpha and interferon gamma to predict the onset of acute and chronic graft-versus-host disease after allogeneic stem cell transplantation. *Biol Blood Marrow Transplant*. 2005;11:706-712.

84. Fujii H, Cuvelier G, She K, et al. Biomarkers in newly diagnosed pediatric-extensive chronic graft-versus-host disease: a report from the Children's Oncology Group. *Blood*. 2008;111:3276-3285.

85. Clark J, Yao L, Pavletic SZ, et al. Magnetic resonance imaging in sclerotic-type chronic graft-vs-host disease. *Arch Dermatol.Dermatology*. 2009;145:918-922.

86. Tedstone JL, Richards SM, Garman RD, et al. Ultrasound imaging accurately detects skin thickening in a mouse scleroderma model. *Ultrasound Med Biol*. 2008;34:1239-1247.

87. Bolognia JL, Cooper DL, Glusac EJ. Toxic erythema of chemotherapy: a useful clinical term. *J Am Acad Dermatol*. 2008;59:524-529.

88. Dean PG, Lund WJ, Larson TS, et al. Wound-healing complications after kidney transplantation: a prospective, randomized comparison of sirolimus and tacrolimus. *Transplantation*. 2004;77:1555-1561.

89. DePry JL, Vyas R, Lazarus HM, et al. Cutaneous malignant neoplasms in hematopoietic cell transplant recipients: a systematic review. *JAMA Dermatol*. 2015;151:775-782.

90. Curtis RE, Rowlings PA, Deeg HJ, et al. Solid cancers after bone marrow transplantation. *N Engl J Med*. 1997;336:897-904.

91. Leisenring W, Friedman DL, Flowers ME, et al. Nonmelanoma skin and mucosal cancers after hematopoietic cell transplantation. *J Clin Oncol*. 2006;24:1119-1126.

92. Cowen EW, Nguyen JC, Miller DD, et al. Chronic phototoxicity and aggressive squamous cell carcinoma of the skin in children and adults during treatment with voriconazole. *J Am Acad Dermatol*. 2010;62:31-37.

93. Miller DD, Cowen EW, Nguyen JC, et al. Melanoma associated with long-term voriconazole therapy: a new manifestation of chronic photosensitivity. *Arch Dermatol*. 2010;146:300-304.

94. Altman JS, Adler SS. Development of multiple cutaneous squamous cell carcinomas during PUVA treatment for chronic graft-versus-host disease. *J Am Acad Dermatol*. 1994;31:505-507.

95. Wingard JR, Majhail NS, Brazauskas R, et al. Long-term survival and late deaths after allogeneic hematopoietic cell transplantation. *J Clin Oncol*. 2011;29:2230-2239.

96. Akpek G, Zahurak ML, Piantadosi S, et al. Development of a prognostic model for grading chronic graft-versus-host disease. *Blood*. 2001;97:1219-1226.

97. Wingard JR, Piantadosi S, Vogelsang GB, et al. Predictors of death from chronic graft-versus-host disease after bone marrow transplantation. *Blood*. 1989;74:1428-1435.

98. Pavletic SZ, Smith LM, Bishop MR, et al. Prognostic factors of chronic graft-versus-host disease after allogeneic bone marrow stem-cell transplantation. *Am J Hematol*. 2005;78:265-274.

99. Robinson TM, O'Donnell PV, Fuchs EJ, et al. Haploidentical bone marrow and stem cell transplantation: experience with post-transplantation cyclophosphamide. *Semin Hematol*. 2016;53:90-97.

100. Gibbs SD, Herbert KE, McCormack C, et al. Alemtuzumab: effective monotherapy for simultaneous B-cell chronic lymphocytic leukaemia and Sézary syndrome. *Eur J Haematol*. 2004;73:447-449.

101. Pérez-Simón JA, Kottaridis PD, Martino R, et al. Nonmyeloablative transplantation with or without alemtuzumab: comparison between 2 prospective studies in patients with lymphoproliferative disorders. *Blood*. 2002;100:3121-3127.

102. Kennedy-Nasser AA, Ku S, Castillo-Caro P, et al. Ultra low-dose IL-2 for GVHD prophylaxis after allogeneic hematopoietic stem cell transplantation mediates

expansion of regulatory T cells without diminishing antiviral and antileukemic activity. *Clin Cancer Res.* 2014;20:2215-2225.
103. Bucher C, Koch L, Vogtenhuber C, et al. IL-21 blockade reduces graft-versus-host disease mortality by supporting inducible T regulatory cell generation. *Blood.* 2009;114:5375-5384.
104. Bacigalupo A, Lamparelli T, Barisione G, et al. Thymoglobulin prevents chronic graft-versus-host disease, chronic lung dysfunction, and late transplant-related mortality: long-term follow-up of a randomized trial in patients undergoing unrelated donor transplantation. *Biol Blood Marrow Transplant.* 2006;12:560-565.
105. MacMillan ML, Weisdorf DJ, Davies SM, et al. Early antithymocyte globulin therapy improves survival in patients with steroid-resistant acute graft-versus-host disease. *Biol Blood Marrow Transplant.* 2002;8:40-46.
106. Kröger N, Zabelina T, Krüger W, et al. In vivo T cell depletion with pretransplant anti-thymocyte globulin reduces graft-versus-host disease without increasing relapse in good risk myeloid leukemia patients after stem cell transplantation from matched related donors. *Bone Marrow Transplant.* 2002;29:683-689.
107. Kumar, A. et al. Antithymocyte globulin for acute-graft-versus-host-disease prophylaxis in patients undergoing allogeneic hematopoietic cell transplantation: a systematic review. *Leukemia.* 2012;26:582-588.
108. Kröger N, Solano C, Bonifazi F. Antilymphocyte globulin for prevention of chronic graft-versus-host disease. *N Engl J Med.* 2016;374:43-53.
109. Bejanyan N, Rogosheske J, DeForTE, et al. Sirolimus and mycophenolate mofetil as calcineurin inhibitor-free graft-versus-host disease prophylaxis for reduced-intensity conditioning umbilical cord blood transplantation. *Biol Blood Marrow Transplant.* 2016;22: 2025-2030.
110. Armand P, Kim HT, Sainvil MM, et al. The addition of sirolimus to the graft-versus-host disease prophylaxis regimen in reduced intensity allogeneic stem cell transplantation for lymphoma: a multicentre randomized trial. *Br J Haematol.* 2016;173:96-104.
111. Inamoto Y, Shah NN, Savani BN, et al. Secondary solid cancer screening following hematopoietic cell transplantation. *Bone Marrow Transplant.* 2015;50: 1013-1023.
112. Martin PJ, Inamoto Y, Flowers ME, et al. Secondary treatment of acute graft-versus-host disease: a critical review. *Biol Blood Marrow Transplant.* 2012;18: 982-988.
113. Hattori K, Doki N, Kurosawa S, et al. Mycophenolate mofetil is effective only for involved skin in the treatment for steroid-refractory acute graft-versus-host disease after allogeneic hematopoietic stem cell transplantation. *Ann Hematol.* 2017;96(2):319-321.
114. Piñana JL, Valcárcel D, Martino R, et al. Encouraging results with inolimomab (anti-IL-2 receptor) as treatment for refractory acute graft-versus-host disease. *Biol Blood Marrow Transplant.* 2006;12:1135-1141.
115. van Groningen LF, Liefferink AM, de Haan AF, et al. Combination therapy with inolimomab and etanercept for severe steroid-refractory acute graft-versus-host disease. *Biol Blood Marrow Transplant.* 2016;22:179-182.
116. Lee SJ, Zahrieh D, Agura E, et al. Effect of up-front daclizumab when combined with steroids for the treatment of acute graft-versus-host disease: results of a randomized trial. *Blood.* 2004;104:1559-1564.
117. Levine JE, Paczesny S, Mineishi S, et al. Etanercept plus methylprednisolone as initial therapy for acute graft-versus-host disease. *Blood.* 2008;111:2470-2475.
118. Couriel DR, Saliba R, de Lima M, et al. A phase III study of infliximab and corticosteroids for the initial treatment of acute graft-versus-host disease. *Biol Blood Marrow Transplant.* 2009;15:1555-1562.
119. Alousi AM, Weisdorf DJ, Logan BR, et al. Etanercept, mycophenolate, denileukin, or pentostatin plus corticosteroids for acute graft-versus-host disease: a randomized phase 2 trial from the Blood and Marrow Transplant Clinical Trials Network. *Blood.* 2009;114:511-517.
120. Pidala J, Kim J, Anasetti C. Sirolimus as primary treatment of acute graft-versus-host disease following allogeneic hematopoietic cell transplantation. *Biol Blood Marrow Transplant.* 2009;15:881-885.
121. Introna M, Lucchini G, Dander E, et al. Treatment of graft versus host disease with mesenchymal stromal cells: a phase I study on 40 adult and pediatric patients. *Biol Blood Marrow Transplant.* 2014;20:375-381.
122. Abu-Dalle I, Reljic T, Nishihori T, et al. Extracorporeal photopheresis in steroid-refractory acute or chronic graft-versus-host disease: results of a systematic review of prospective studies. *Biol Blood Marrow Transplant.* 2014;20:1677-1686.
123. Alousi AM, Bassett R, Chen J, et al. A bayesian, phase II randomized trial of extracorporeal photopheresis (ECP) plus steroids versus steroids-alone in patients with newly diagnosed acute graft vs. host disease (GVHD): the addition of ECP improves GVHD response and the ability to taper steroids. *Blood.* 2015;126:854.
124. Schlaak M, Schwind S, Wetzig T, et al. UVA (UVA-1) therapy for the treatment of acute GVHD of the skin. *Bone Marrow Transplant.* 2010;45:1741-1748.
125. Furlong T, Leisenring W, Storb R, et al. Psoralen and ultraviolet A irradiation (PUVA) as therapy for steroid-resistant cutaneous acute graft-versus-host disease. *Biol Blood Marrow Transplant.* 2002;8:206-212.
126. Feldstein JV, Bolaños-Meade J, Anders VL, et al. Narrowband ultraviolet B phototherapy for the treatment of steroid-refractory and steroid-dependent acute graft-versus-host disease of the skin. *J Am Acad Dermatol.* 2011;65:733-738.
127. Garbutcheon-Singh KB, Fernández-Peñas P. Phototherapy for the treatment of cutaneous graft versus host disease. *Australas J Dermatol.* 2015;56: 93-99.
128. Le Blanc K, Frassoni F, Ball L, et al. Mesenchymal stem cells for treatment of steroid-resistant, severe, acute graft-versus-host disease: a phase II study. *Lancet.* 2008;371:1579-1586.
129. Wolff D, Gerbitz A, Ayuk F, et al. Consensus conference on clinical practice in chronic graft-versus-host disease (GVHD): first-line and topical treatment of chronic GVHD. *Biol Blood Marrow Transplant.* 2010;16: 1611-1628.
130. Choi CJ, Nghiem P. Tacrolimus ointment in the treatment of chronic cutaneous graft-vs-host disease: a case series of 18 patients. *Arch Dermatol.* 2001;137: 1202-1206.
131. Neuman DL, Farrar JE, Moresi JM, et al. Toxic absorption of tacrolimus [corrected] in a patient with severe acute graft-versus-host disease. *Bone Marrow Transplant.* 2005;36(10):919-920 [erratum in *Bone Marrow Transplant.* 2006;38:81].
132. Carpenter PA, Kitko CL, Elad S, et al. National Institutes of Health consensus development project on criteria for clinical trials in chronic graft-versus-host disease: V. The 2014 Ancillary Therapy and Supportive Care

Working Group Report. *Biol Blood Marrow Transplant.* 2015;21:1167-1187.
133. Connolly KL, Griffith JL, McEvoy M, et al. Ultraviolet A1 phototherapy beyond morphea: experience in 83 patients. *Photodermatol Photoimmunol Photomed.* 2015;31:289-295.
134. Wetzig T, Sticherling M, Simon JC, et al. Medium dose long-wavelength ultraviolet A (UVA1) phototherapy for the treatment of acute and chronic graft-versus-host disease of the skin. *Bone Marrow Transplant.* 2005;35:515-519.
135. Ständer H, Schiller M, Schwarz T. UVA1 therapy for sclerodermic graft-versus-host disease of the skin. *J Am Acad Dermatol.* 2002;46:799-800.
136. Calzavara Pinton P, Porta F, Izzi T, et al. Prospects for ultraviolet A1 phototherapy as a treatment for chronic cutaneous graft-versus-host disease. *Haematologica.* 2003;88:1169-1175.
137. Teske NM, Jacobe HT. Phototherapy for sclerosing skin conditions. *Clin Dermatol.* 2016;34:614-622.
138. Vogelsang GB, Wolff D, Altomonte V, et al. Treatment of chronic graft-versus-host disease with ultraviolet irradiation and psoralen (PUVA). *Bone Marrow Transplant.* 1996;17:1061-1067.
139. Ballester-Sánchez R, Navarro-Mira MÁ, de Unamuno-Bustos B, et al. The role of phototherapy in cutaneous chronic graft-vs-host disease: a retrospective study and review of the literature. *Actas Dermosifiliogr.* 2015;106:651-657.
140. Koc S, Leisenring W, Flowers ME, et al. Therapy for chronic graft-versus-host disease: a randomized trial comparing cyclosporine plus prednisone versus prednisone alone. *Blood.* 2002;100:48-51.
141. Lee SJ. Classification systems for chronic graft-versus-host disease. *Blood.* 2017;129(1):30-37.
142. Couriel DR, Hosing C, Saliba R, et al. Extracorporeal photochemotherapy for the treatment of steroid-resistant chronic GVHD. *Blood.* 2006;107:3074-3080.
143. Jagasia MH, Savani BN, Stricklin G, et al. Classic and overlap chronic graft-versus-host disease (cGVHD) is associated with superior outcome after extracorporeal photopheresis (ECP). *Biol Blood Marrow Transplant.* 2009;15:1288-1295.
144. Sbano P, Rubegni P, De Aloe GB, et al. Extracorporeal photochemotherapy for treatment of fasciitis in chronic graft-versus-host disease. *Bone Marrow Transplant.* 2004;33:869-870.
145. Baird K, Comis LE, Joe GO, et al. Imatinib mesylate for the treatment of steroid-refractory sclerotic-type cutaneous chronic graft-versus-host disease. *Biol Blood Marrow Transplant.* 2015;21:1083-1090.
146. de Masson A, Bouaziz JD, Peffault de Latour R, et al. Limited efficacy and tolerance of imatinib mesylate in steroid-refractory sclerodermatous chronic GVHD. *Blood.* 2012;120:5089-5090.
147. Olivieri A, Locatelli F, Zecca M, et al. Imatinib for refractory chronic graft-versus-host disease with fibrotic features. *Blood.* 2009;114:709-718.
148. Chen GL, Arai S, Flowers ME, et al. A phase 1 study of imatinib for corticosteroid-dependent/refractory chronic graft-versus-host disease: response does not correlate with anti-PDGFRA antibodies. *Blood.* 2011;118:4070-4078.
149. Magro L, Mohty M, Catteau B, et al. Imatinib mesylate as salvage therapy for refractory sclerotic chronic graft-versus-host disease. *Blood.* 2009;114:719-722.
150. Dubovsky JA, Flynn R, Du J, et al. Ibrutinib treatment ameliorates murine chronic graft-versus-host disease. *J Clin Invest.* 2014;124:4867-4876.
151. Schutt SD, Fu J, Nguyen H, et al. Inhibition of BTK and ITK with ibrutinib is effective in the prevention of chronic graft-versus-host disease in mice. *PLoS One.* 2015;10:e0137641.
152. Xu Y, Johnston HF, Forman SJ, et al. Oral administration of ibrutinib is ineffective at preventing scleroderma in chronic GVHD in two preclinical mouse models. *Blood.* 2014;124:3818-3818.
153. Zeiser R, Burchert A, Lengerke C, et al. Ruxolitinib in corticosteroid-refractory graft-versus-host disease after allogeneic stem cell transplantation: a multicenter survey. *Leukemia.* 2015;29:2062-2068.
154. Okiyama N, Furumoto Y, Villarroel VA, et al. Reversal of CD8 T-cell-mediated mucocutaneous graft-versus-host-like disease by the JAK inhibitor tofacitinib. *J Invest Dermatol.* 2014;134:992-1000.
155. Johnston LJ, Brown J, Shizuru JA, et al. Rapamycin (sirolimus) for treatment of chronic graft-versus-host disease. *Biol Blood Marrow Transplant.* 2005;11:47-55.
156. Pidala J, Kim J, Perkins J, et al. Mycophenolate mofetil for the management of steroid-refractory acute graft vs host disease. *Bone Marrow Transplant.* 2010;45:919-924.
157. Carnevale-Schianca F, Martin P, Sullivan K, et al. Changing from cyclosporine to tacrolimus as salvage therapy for chronic graft-versus-host disease. *Biol Blood Marrow Transplant.* 2000;6:613-620.
158. Vogelsang GB, Farmer ER, Hess AD, et al. Thalidomide for the treatment of chronic graft-versus-host disease. *N Engl J Med.* 1992;326:1055-1058.
159. Sullivan KM, Witherspoon RP, Storb R, et al. Prednisone and azathioprine compared with prednisone and placebo for treatment of chronic graft-v-host disease: prognostic influence of prolonged thrombocytopenia after allogeneic marrow transplantation. *Blood.* 1988;72:546-554.
160. de Lavallade H, Mohty M, Faucher C, et al. Low-dose methotrexate as salvage therapy for refractory graft-versus-host disease after reduced-intensity conditioning allogeneic stem cell transplantation. *Haematologica.* 2006;91:1438-1440.
161. Schmitt T, Luft T, Hegenbart U, et al. Pentostatin for treatment of steroid-refractory acute GVHD: a retrospective single-center analysis. *Bone Marrow Transplant.* 2011;46:580-585.
162. Mayer J, Krejcí M, Doubek M, et al. Pulse cyclophosphamide for corticosteroid-refractory graft-versus-host disease. *Bone Marrow Transplant.* 2005;35:699-705.
163. Lee SJ, Wegner SA, McGarigle CJ, et al. Treatment of chronic graft-versus-host disease with clofazimine. *Blood.* 1997;89:2298-2302.
164. Reddy P, Sun Y, Toubai T, et al. Histone deacetylase inhibition modulates indoleamine 2,3-dioxygenase-dependent DC functions and regulates experimental graft-versus-host disease in mice. *J Clin Invest.* 2008;118:2562-2573.
165. Morin F, Kavian N, Marut W, et al. Inhibition of EGFR tyrosine kinase by erlotinib prevents sclerodermatous graft-versus-host disease in a mouse model. *J Invest Dermatol.* 2015;135:2385-2393.
166. Busca A, Locatelli F, Marmont F, et al. Recombinant human soluble tumor necrosis factor receptor fusion protein as treatment for steroid refractory graft-versus-host disease following allogeneic hematopoietic stem cell transplantation. *Am J Hematol.*

2007;82:45-52.
167. Shapira MY, Abdul-Hai A, Resnick IB, et al. Alefacept treatment for refractory chronic extensive GVHD. *Bone Marrow Transplant*. 2009;43:339-343.
168. Koreth J, Kim HT, Jones KT, et al. Efficacy, durability, and response predictors of low-dose interleukin-2 therapy for chronic graft-versus-host disease. *Blood*. 2016;128:130-137.
169. Cohen JL, Trenado A, Vasey D, et al. CD4(+)CD25(+) immunoregulatory T cells: new therapeutics for graft-versus-host disease. *J Exp Med*. 2002;196:401-406.
170. Ringden O, Keating A. Mesenchymal stromal cells as treatment for chronic GVHD. *Bone Marrow Transplant*. 2011;46:163-164.
171. Hautmann AH, Wolff D, Hilgendorf I, et al. Total nodal irradiation in patients with severe treatment-refractory chronic graft-versus-host disease after allogeneic stem cell transplantation: response rates and immunomodulatory effects. *Radiother Oncol*. 2015;116:287-293.
172. Robin M, Guardiola P, Girinsky T, et al. Low-dose thoracoabdominal irradiation for the treatment of refractory chronic graft-versus-host disease. *Transplantation*. 2005;80:634-642.
173. Marcellus DC, Altomonte VL, Farmer ER, et al. Etretinate therapy for refractory sclerodermatous chronic graft-versus-host disease. *Blood*. 1999;93:66-70.
174. Sullivan KM, Storek J, Kopecky KJ, et al. A controlled trial of long-term administration of intravenous immunoglobulin to prevent late infection and chronic graft-vs.-host disease after marrow transplantation: clinical outcome and effect on subsequent immune recovery. *Biol Blood Marrow Transplant*. 1996;2:44-53.
175. Herrera AF, Kim HT, Bindra B, et al. A phase II study of bortezomib plus prednisone for initial therapy of chronic graft-versus-host disease. *Biol Blood Marrow Transplant*. 2014;20:1737-1743.
176. Zerr P, Palumbo-Zerr K, Distler A, et al. Inhibition of hedgehog signaling for the treatment of murine sclerodermatous chronic graft-versus-host disease. *Blood*. 2012;120:2909-2917.
177. Margaix-Muñoz M, Bagán JV, Jiménez Y, et al. Graft-versus-host disease affecting oral cavity. A review. *J Clin Exp Dent*. 2015;7:e138-e145.
178. Stratton P, Turner ML, Childs R, et al. Vulvovaginal chronic graft-versus-host disease with allogeneic hematopoietic stem cell transplantation. *Obstet Gynecol*. 2007;110:1041-1049.

Chapter 130 :: Hereditary Disorders of Genome Instability and DNA Repair
:: John J. DiGiovanna, Thomas M. Rünger, & Kenneth H. Kraemer

第一百三十章

基因组不稳定性和DNA修复障碍的遗传性疾病

中文导读

基因组对细胞功能起着控制作用，保持基因组的稳定对于细胞、组织和生物体的持续功能是很重要的。DNA是遗传信息的载体，它的结构经常受到破坏因素的威胁，包括氧化应激、紫外线（UV）和X射线辐射，以及化学试剂。本章介绍与基因组不稳定以及DNA修复或DNA维护的潜在缺陷机制相关的疾病，所有这些疾病都表现出明显的皮肤异常。分别介绍了DNA修复障碍的皮肤疾病中的着色性干皮病、着色性干皮病合并Cockayne综合征、毛发硫性营养不良（TTD）和基因组不稳定性相关皮肤病中的布鲁姆综合征、沃纳综合征、Rothmund-Thomson综合征、范可尼贫血、先天性角化不良的流行病学、临床表现、病因和发病机制、诊断与鉴别诊断、临床病程与预后、临床管理。

〔粟 娟〕

AT-A-GLANCE

- Genome instability characterizes a large group of inherited disorders with prominent cutaneous abnormalities; many have an increased cancer risk.
- Genome instability is caused by impaired repair and/or maintenance of DNA.
- Xeroderma pigmentosum is a prototype with impaired repair of environmentally induced DNA damage and a greatly increased frequency of sunlight-induced cancer.
- Although these disorders are rare, heterozygous carriers of affected genes, which may comprise several percent of the general population, may carry an increased cancer risk as well.

Because the genome exerts control of cellular function, maintaining genome stability is important for the continued function of cells, tissues, and organisms. DNA is the carrier of genetic information. Its structure is regularly threatened by damaging agents that include oxidative stress, ultraviolet (UV) and X radiation, and chemical agents. Although much damage is repaired, failure to maintain genomic integrity may lead to abnormal cell function or cell death. If the cell divides, progeny may accumulate additional damage and this progressive accumulation of damage can lead to malignancy.

This chapter describes the relevant skin disorders with genome instability and the underlying defective mechanisms of DNA repair or DNA maintenance (Tables 130-1 and 130-2). All of these disorders exhibit

TABLE 130-1
Clinical Features of Hereditary Disorders of Genome Instability and DNA Repair

DISORDER	CLINICAL FEATURES			INHERITANCE
	CUTANEOUS	NEOPLASIA	OTHER	
Disorders of Genome Instability With Defective DNA Repair				
Xeroderma pigmentosum (XP)	Photosensitivity (burning on minimal sun exposure in some patients); freckle-like (lentiginous) macules; poikiloderma (hyperpigmentation and hypopigmentation, atrophy, telangiectasia); skin cancer	Basal cell carcinoma (BCC), squamous cell carcinoma (SCC), melanoma, CNS tumors	Sensorineural deafness, progressive neurologic degeneration, primary loss of neurons (some patients)	Autosomal recessive
Cockayne syndrome (CS)	Photosensitivity (burning on sun exposure in some patients)	No increased incidence	Typical facial features (deep-set eyes; loss of subcutaneous fat); pigmentary retinal degeneration; postnatal growth failure; sensorineural deafness; progressive neurologic degeneration; primary dysmyelination; brain calcifications	Autosomal recessive
XP/CS complex	Photosensitivity (burning on sun exposure in some patients); freckle-like (lentiginous) macules; poikiloderma (hyperpigmentation and hypopigmentation, atrophy, telangiectasia); skin cancer	BCC, SCC	Neurologic changes of CS	Autosomal recessive
Trichothiodystrophy (TTD)	Brittle hair, photosensitivity (burning on minimal sun exposure in some patients); ichthyosis; collodion membrane; "tiger tail banding" of hair with polarized microscopy	No increased incidence	Congenital cataracts; short stature developmental delay; microcephaly; brain dysmyelination (failure to develop white matter); recurrent infections	Autosomal recessive (rare X-linked)
XP/TTD	Clinical features of both TTD and XP including skin cancer	BCC, SCC, melanoma	Clinical features of both TTD and XP	Autosomal recessive
Hereditary nonpolyposis colon cancer (HNPCC)/ Muir-Torre syndrome (MTS)	Sebaceous tumors (benign and malignant), keratoacanthomas	Low-grade cancer of the colon, endometrium, stomach, small intestine, hepatobiliary system, upper urethral tract, larynx, and ovary; sebaceous carcinoma; BCC with sebaceous differentiation		Autosomal dominant
Other Disorders of Genome Instability				
Bloom syndrome (BS)	Photosensitivity (burning on sun exposure); malar erythema; café-au-lait macules	Most cancer types, particularly leukemias, lymphomas, carcinomas of the breast and GI tract	Immune deficiency; growth retardation; unusual facies; male infertility and female subfertility; Type II diabetes	Autosomal recessive
Werner syndrome (WS)	Graying of hair; skin atrophy; leg ulcers; melanomas	Sarcomas; thyroid cancer; meningiomas; melanomas (acral lentiginous and mucous membrane melanomas)	Premature aging (atherosclerosis, diabetes mellitus, osteoporosis, cataracts)	Autosomal recessive

(Continued)

TABLE 130-1
Clinical Features of Hereditary Disorders of Genome Instability and DNA Repair (*Continued*)

	CLINICAL FEATURES			
DISORDER	**CUTANEOUS**	**NEOPLASIA**	**OTHER**	**INHERITANCE**
Rothmund-Thomson syndrome (RTS)	Photosensitivity (burning on sun exposure); poikiloderma; alopecia	Osteosarcomas; cutaneous SCC; and others	Skeletal abnormalities; growth deficiency; juvenile cataracts; osteoporosis	Autosomal recessive
Fanconi anemia (FA)	Café-au-lait macules	Myeloid leukemia; SCC of head and neck	Aplastic anemia; pancytopenia; growth retardation; thumb and other bone abnormalities	Autosomal recessive
Dyskeratosis congenita	Lacy, reticular pigmentation of neck and upper chest; nail dystrophy; premature gray hair; hyperhidrosis; skin cancer	Mucosal leukoplakia leading to cancer of anus or mouth; Hodgkin disease; pancreatic adenocarcinoma	Stenosis of lacrimal duct; anemia; pancytopenia; immunodeficiency; learning difficulties; deafness; brain calcifications; cerebellar hypoplasia; testicular atrophy; short stature; intrauterine growth retardation; retinopathy	X-linked recessive; autosomal dominant; autosomal recessive
Ataxia telangiectasia (AT)	Telangiectasias	T-cell leukemia, lymphomas	Progressive cerebellar ataxia; immune defects; hypogonadism; increased acute toxicity of therapeutic X-ray	Autosomal recessive
AT-like disorder (ATLD)	Similar to AT	Similar to AT	Similar to AT, but no ocular telangiectasias	Autosomal recessive
Nijmegen breakage syndrome (NBS)	Café-au-lait macule; vitiligo	B-cell and T-cell lymphomas; rhabdomyosarcoma; neuroblastoma	Immune defects; growth retardation; microcephaly; mental retardation; characteristic facies	Autosomal recessive
Seckel syndrome	Café-au-lait macules	Leukemia	Proportionate dwarfism; microcephaly; mental retardation; characteristic facies (receding forehead, narrow face, large, beaked nose, micrognathia); immune deficiency; pancytopenia	Autosomal recessive

prominent cutaneous abnormalities that involve dermatologists in their diagnosis and management. Most, but not all, are also characterized by an increased risk of malignancies. This demonstrates that the maintenance of genome integrity is important for the prevention of malignant transformation. Malignant transformation requires the accumulation of several mutations in specific genes of a single cell. Thus a mutator phenotype is often regarded a prerequisite for carcinogenesis, because without genome instability it would be exceedingly unlikely that all of those mutations would occur in a single cell.[1-4] The same genes that are affected in the hereditary genome instability disorders can also confer genome instability to individual cells when impaired through acquired mutations, thereby playing an important role early in spontaneous carcinogenesis.

In addition, although these heritable diseases are rare (1 in 100,000 to 1 in 1,000,000 people), heterozygous carriers of the affected genes (with 1 mutated allele and 1 normal allele) are more common, and may comprise several percent of the general population. These individuals are usually free of clinical symptoms, as most of these disorders are characterized by autosomal recessive inheritance. However, epidemiologic studies suggest that heterozygous carriers may have an increased risk of neoplasia as well.[5,6]

Spontaneous genome instability is present in Bloom syndrome (BS), ataxia telangiectasia, and Fanconi anemia (FA) as manifested by increased chromosome breakage in primary blood or skin cells. On the other hand, genome instability is present in cells from patients with xeroderma pigmentosum (XP) only after exposure to DNA-damaging agents such as UV radiation or other carcinogens such as benzo[*a*]pyrene, which is present in cigarette smoke. In some of the disorders discussed here, genome instability is caused by an impaired ability to repair damage to DNA introduced by certain physical or chemical agents. Cells are equipped with different DNA repair pathways that repair different types of DNA damage. The nucleotide excision repair (NER) pathway, which processes bulky

TABLE 130-2
Mechanisms of Hereditary Disorders of Genome Instability and DNA Repair

DISORDER	CELLULAR ABNORMALITIES	AFFECTED GENE(S)	IMPAIRED FUNCTION
Disorders of Genome Instability With Defective DNA Repair			
Xeroderma pigmentosum (XP)	Increased ultraviolet (UV)-induced cell killing and mutagenesis	XPA, XPB, XPC, XPD, XPE, XPF, XPG, or DNA polymerase η	Nucleotide excision repair: global genome and transcription-coupled DNA repair; translesional DNA synthesis (XP-variant)
Cockayne syndrome (CS)	Increased cell killing and mutagenesis after exposure to UV and ionizing radiation	CSA or CSB	Nucleotide excision repair: transcription-coupled DNA repair only
XP/CS complex	Increased UV-induced cell killing and mutagenesis	XPG, XPD, or XPB	Nucleotide excision repair: global genome and transcription-coupled DNA repair
Trichothiodystrophy (TTD)	Increased UV-induced cell killing	XPB, XPD, TTDA, or TTDN1, GTF2E2, RNF113A	Nucleotide excision repair: transcription-coupled pathway of nucleotide excision repair
XP/TTD	Same as XP	XPD	Nucleotide excision repair: global genome and transcription-coupled DNA repair
Hereditary nonpolyposis colon cancer (HNPCC)/Muir-Torre syndrome (MTS)	High level of microsatellite instability in tumors	hMSH2 (MTS, HNPCC1), hMLH1 (MTS, HNPCC2), PMS1 (HNPCC3), hPMS2 (HNPCC4), hMSH6 (HNPCC5), TGFBR2 (HNPCC6), or hMLH3 (HNPCC7)	Mismatch repair
Other Disorders of Genome Instability			
Bloom syndrome (BS)	Spontaneous chromosome breakage and rearrangements, increased sister chromatid exchanges, quadriradial chromosomes	BLM	A RecQ DNA helicase, recombination, replication
Werner syndrome (WS)	Chromosomal instability, accelerated telomere shortening	WRN	A RecQ DNA helicase, transcription, DNA repair (DSBR, SSBR, recombination), DNA replication, telomere maintenance
Rothmund-Thomson syndrome (RTS)	Chromosomal instability in response to ionizing radiation	RECQL4 (some patients)	A RecQ DNA helicase
Fanconi anemia (FA)	Increased sensitivity to DNA crosslinking agents	FANCA, FANCB, FANCC, FANCD1/BRCA2, FANCD2, FANCE, FANCF, FANCG/XRCC9, FANCI, FANCJ/BACH1/BRIP1, FANCL, FANCM, FANCN/PALB2	DNA damage signaling, recombination repair
Dyskeratosis congenita	Shortened telomeres	DKC1 X-linked; TERC, TERT, TINF2, autosomal dominant; TERT, NOLA3, NOLA2 autosomal recessive	Abnormal telomere biology
Ataxia telangiectasia (AT)	Increased spontaneous and X-ray–induced chromosome breakage; increased sensitivity to killing by ionizing radiation; impaired cell-cycle arrest and/or apoptosis in response to DNA damage	ATM	DNA damage signaling (control of cell cycle, apoptosis), repair of DNA double-strand breaks
AT-like disorder (ATLD)	Increased spontaneous and X-ray–induced chromosome breakage; increased sensitivity to killing by ionizing radiation; impaired DNA strand break repair	LIG4	DNA ligase 4, strand break repair
Nijmegen breakage syndrome (NBS)	Increased spontaneous and X-ray–induced chromosome breakage; increased sensitivity to killing by ionizing radiation	NBS1	Nibrin (p95), which is part of the MRE11–RAD50–NBS1 complex; DNA damage signaling; recombination; DNA double-strand break repair; cell-cycle checkpoint
Seckel syndrome	Spontaneous and mitomycin C– induced chromosome instability; sensitivity to killing by ultraviolet and DNA crosslinking agents	ATR	AT-related and RAD3-related protein; DNA damage response; cell-cycle checkpoints

DNA lesions, including UV-induced DNA photoproducts, is impaired in XP, Cockayne syndrome (CS), and trichothiodystrophy (TTD). Cells from patients with these conditions are characterized by increased cell death and mutagenesis. However, only XP patients have an increased cancer risk. The reason for this difference in cancer risk is not known.

Proteins encoded by some of the affected genes in XP, CS, and TTD are not only involved in DNA repair, but also in transcription and cellular DNA damage responses. Thus, mutations affecting different functions of the same gene (such as nervous system development or immune competence) appear to play a role in various phenotypes that are not directly linked to DNA repair functions and underlie several overlap syndromes between the 3 conditions (Table 130-3). The multisystem abnormalities of TTD may be a result of failure of the transcription function of the NER pathway proteins, or other proteins involved in transcription. Multiple clinical phenotypes of DNA repair diseases have been recognized and the relationship between the clinical phenotypes and their underlying molecular abnormalities is complex and depicted in Fig. 130-1. Mutations in different DNA repair genes can be associated with the same clinical phenotype. On the other hand, different mutations in one DNA repair gene can be associated with different clinical phenotypes. For example, mutations in the *XPD(ERCC2)* DNA repair/transcription gene have been associated with the following clinical phenotypes: XP, XP with neurologic abnormalities, the XP–CS complex, XP–TTD, COFS (cerebro-oculo-facio-skeletal) syndrome, or CS–TTD. In contrast to the defects in the NER pathway, XP variant, which is clinically indistinguishable from XP, is a disorder of DNA damage tolerance with mutations in the DNA polymerase eta *(POLH)*(pol η) gene. Although normal cells can bypass DNA damage during replication (translesional DNA synthesis), cells from XP-variant patients have a defect in this process. Defects in the DNA mismatch repair pathway result in hereditary nonpolyposis colon cancer (Lynch syndrome) and its subform, Muir-Torre syndrome (MTS). Muir-Torre syndrome has cutaneous features including sebaceous gland tumors.

Helicases are proteins that unwind DNA and are required for a multitude of metabolic processes involving DNA, such as transcription, replication, and repair. Two genes involved in NER are helicases that are also

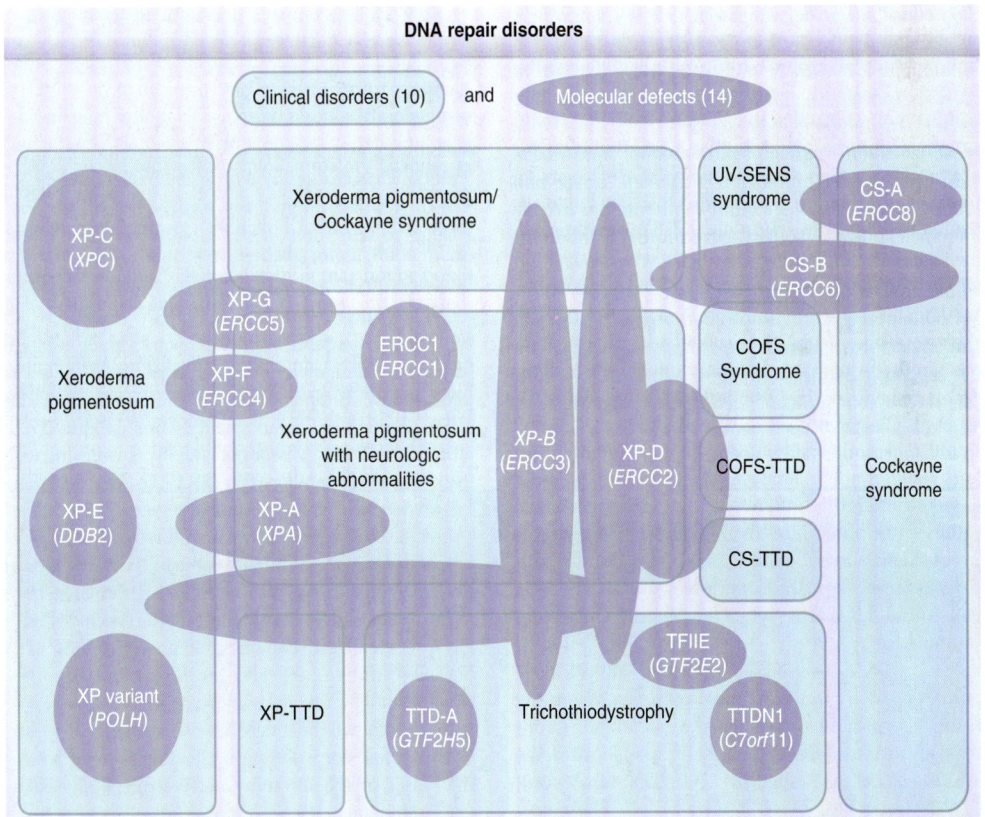

Figure 130-1 The relationship of clinical disorders (*light-blue rectangles*) to molecular defects (*dark-blue ovals*) in DNA repair disorders. A total of 10 clinical disorders and 14 molecular defects are represented. One disorder may be caused by mutations in several different genes. Conversely, different mutations in 1 gene may result in several different clinical diseases. Mutations in *RNF113A* (not shown) have been reported in 1 TTD family with X-linked inheritance. COFS syndrome, cerebro-oculo-facial-skeletal syndrome; CS, Cockayne syndrome; DDB2, double-strand DNA–binding protein 2; SENS, sensitive; TTD, trichothiodystrophy; UV, ultraviolet; XP, xeroderma pigmentosum. (Modified from DiGiovanna JJ and Kraemer KH.[13])

TABLE 130-3
DNA Repair Disorders and Molecular Defects

CLINICAL DISORDERS	MOLECULAR DEFECTS
Xeroderma pigmentosum	XP-C, XP variant, XP-D, XP-A, XP-F, XP-G, XP-E
Xeroderma pigmentosum with neurologic abnormalities	XP-A, XP-D, XP-B
Trichothiodystrophy	XP-D, TTD-A, XP-B, TTDN1, GTF2E2, RNF113A
Cockayne syndrome	CS-B, CS-A
Xeroderma pigmentosum–Cockayne syndrome complex	XP-G, XP-D, XP-B
Xeroderma pigmentosum–trichothiodystrophy complex	XP-D
Cerebro-ocular-facio-skeletal (COFS) syndrome	CS-B, XP-D

DISORDERS OF DNA REPAIR

XERODERMA PIGMENTOSUM

AT-A-GLANCE

- Xeroderma pigmentosum (XP) is an autosomal recessive disease characterized by sun sensitivity, with approximately 50% of patients having acute burning on minimal sun exposure.
- Onset of freckling (lentigines) on sun-exposed skin before age 2 years in most patients.
- Greatly increased risk of sunlight-induced cutaneous neoplasms (basal cell carcinoma, squamous cell carcinoma, melanoma) at an early age.
- Sunlight-induced ocular involvement (photophobia, keratitis, atrophy of lids, cancer).
- Progressive neurologic degeneration (progressive hearing loss and cognitive impairment) in approximately 25% of the patients.
- Cellular hypersensitivity to ultraviolet radiation and to certain chemicals in association with abnormal DNA repair.
- The most common causes of death are skin cancer, neurologic degeneration, and internal cancer. The median age at death of persons with XP with neurodegeneration (29 years) is younger than that of persons with XP without neurodegeneration (37 years).

part of the basal transcription factor, TFIIH. The *XPB* (*ERCC3*) gene product unwinds DNA in the 3′ to 5′ direction, whereas the *XPD* (*ERCC2*) gene product unwinds DNA in the opposite direction. Defects in these genes are associated with multiple clinical phenotypes (see above). The RecQ family of DNA helicases is highly conserved in evolution from bacteria to humans.[7,8] Of the 5 known human RecQ family members, 3 (BLM, which causes BS; WRN, which causes Werner syndrome [WS]; and RECQL4, which causes Rothmund-Thomson syndrome [RTS]) are mutated in distinct clinical disorders associated with chromosomal instability, cancer predisposition, and/or premature aging.[9]

Genetic instability can also result from abnormal telomere maintenance. Telomeres are long nucleotide (TTAGGG)n repeats that are important for the maintenance of chromosomal integrity.[10] Some telomeric repeats are lost at each cell division and shortened telomere lengths are a feature of aged cells. Accelerated telomere shortening is a hallmark of cells from patients with the cancer-prone disorder dyskeratosis congenita. In approximately half of dyskeratosis congenita patients, mutations have been found in 1 of 6 genes involved in telomere maintenance.[11]

BASC (*B*RCA1-*a*ssociated genome *s*urveillance *c*omplex) is a multienzyme complex centered around the BRCA1 protein in the nucleus.[12] It contains important DNA damage response proteins including ATM, ATR, the MRE11-RAD50-NBS1 complex, BRCA1, BLM, FANCD2, and MLH1. These proteins physically interact with each other. Genome instability may result from a defect in any of those and cause the genome instability disorders including ataxia-telangiectasia, Seckel syndrome, Nijmegen breakage syndrome, hereditary breast cancer, BS, FA, or hereditary colon cancer. BS and FA are reviewed here.

XP was first described in Vienna by Moriz Kaposi in the textbook of dermatology he published in 1870 with his father-in-law, Ferdinand Hebra. The disorder was first called xeroderma or parchment skin. Subsequently, the term *pigmentosum* was added for the greatly increased freckle-like pigmentation (Fig. 130-2A, B). See discussion in DiGiovanna and Kraemer[13] and Kraemer and colleagues.[14]

In 1968, hypersensitivity of cultured XP cells to UV damage was reported by Cleaver to be the result of defective DNA repair.[15] Most XP cells have a normal response to treatment with X-rays, indicating the specificity of the DNA repair defect. The defective genes for the 7 NER-defective forms of XP and the XP variant have been cloned and their functions are being investigated.[13]

In XP, many of the severe disease manifestations, such as cancer and corneal scarring leading to blindness, are the result of the interplay between genetic risk and environmental exposure. For example, XP patients who avoid UV radiation dramatically reduce or eliminate the probability of developing skin cancer and blindness.

EPIDEMIOLOGY

Patients have been reported worldwide in all races. XP occurs with a frequency of about 1 in 1 million persons in Europe and the United States.[16] The frequency is higher in certain populations. In Japan, prevalence is estimated at 1 in 22,000 persons.[17] It is relatively more common in areas such as the Middle East where marriage of close relatives is practiced. Founder mutations have been reported in Japan, India, Tunisia, North Africa, Israel, Spain, and Brazil. A review of 106 XP patients examined at the U.S. National Institutes of Health described observations between 1971 and 2009.[18] A report of 89 patients examined at the multidisciplinary XP service in the United Kingdom in a 5-year interval described heterogeneous clinical and laboratory features.[19]

CLINICAL FEATURES

Cutaneous Findings:

Skin: Approximately 50% of the patients with XP have a history of acute burning on minimal sun exposure.[18] The other 50% of patients tan normally without excessive burning of their skin (Fig. 130-3). In all patients, numerous freckle-like hyperpigmented macules (lentigines) appear predominately on sun-exposed skin. The median age of onset of the cutaneous symptoms in XP is between 1 and 2 years.[14] These generally spare sun-protected sites, such as the buttocks (see Fig. 130-2D). However, some severely sun-exposed patients may show pigmentary abnormalities in the axillae. Continued sun exposure causes the patient's skin to become dry and parchment-like with increased pigmentation, hence the name *xeroderma pigmentosum* ("dry pigmented skin"; see Fig. 130-2A). Premalignant actinic keratosis also develop at an early age. The appearance of sun-exposed skin in children with XP is similar to that occurring in farmers and sailors after many years of extreme sun exposure.

Cancer: Patients with XP who are younger than 20 years of age have a greater than 10,000-fold increased risk of cutaneous basal cell carcinoma, squamous cell carcinoma, or melanoma.[18] The median age of onset of nonmelanoma skin cancer reported in patients with XP is 8 years. Compared to the general population, XP patients have a greater than 50-year reduction in age of onset of first nonmelanoma skin cancer (and greater than 30-year reduction in first melanoma), which indicates the importance of DNA repair in protection from skin cancer in unaffected individuals (Fig. 130-4).

Noncutaneous Findings:

Eyes: Ocular abnormalities are almost as common as the cutaneous abnormalities and are an important feature of XP (see Fig. 130-2C).[20] The posterior portion of the eye (retina) is shielded from UV radiation by the anterior portion (lids, cornea, and conjunctiva). Clinical findings are strikingly limited to these anterior, UV-exposed structures. Photophobia is often present and may be associated with prominent conjunctival injection. Schirmer testing frequently reveals reduced tearing leading to dry eyes. Continued UV exposure of the eye may result in severe keratitis, leading to corneal opacification and vascularization. The lids develop increased pigmentation and loss of lashes. Atrophy of the skin of the lids results in ectropion, entropion, or, in severe cases, complete loss of the lids. Benign conjunctival inflammatory masses or papillomas of the lids may be present. Epithelioma, squamous cell carcinoma, and melanoma of UV-exposed portions of the eye are common. The ocular manifestations may be more severe in black patients.

Neurologic System: Neurologic abnormalities have been reported in approximately 25% of the patients.[18] The onset may be early in infancy or, in some patients, delayed until the second decade. The neurologic abnormalities may be mild (eg, isolated hyporeflexia) or severe, with progressive mental retardation, sensorineural deafness (beginning with high-frequency hearing loss), spasticity, or seizures. The most severe form, known as the *De Sanctis-Cacchione syndrome*, involves the cutaneous and ocular manifestations of classic XP plus additional neurologic and somatic abnormalities, including microcephaly, progressive mental deterioration, low intelligence, hyporeflexia or areflexia, choreoathetosis, ataxia, spasticity, Achilles tendon shortening leading to quadriparesis, dwarfism, and immature sexual development. The complete De Sanctis-Cacchione syndrome has been recognized in very few patients; however, many patients with XP have 1 or more of its neurologic features. In clinical practice, deep-tendon reflex testing and routine audiometry usually can serve as a screen for the presence of XP-associated neurologic abnormalities.[21] In cases where there is clinical evidence of early neurologic abnormalities, a brain MRI or CT scan may show enlarged ventricles.[22]

The predominant neuropathologic abnormality found at autopsy in patients with neurologic symptoms was loss (or absence) of neurons, particularly in the cerebrum and cerebellum.[23] There is evidence for a primary axonal degeneration in these patients. In a long-term followup study of 106 XP patients, those with neurodegeneration had a younger age at death (29 years) than those without neurodegeneration (37 years).[18]

Internal Cancers: Review of the world's literature on XP reveals a substantial number of cases of oral cavity neoplasms, particularly squamous cell carcinoma of the tip of the tongue, a presumed sun-exposed location.[14] Brain (sarcoma and medulloblastoma), CNS (astrocytoma of the spinal cord), lung, uterine, breast, pancreatic, gastric, renal, and testicular tumors, and leukemia have been reported in a few patients with XP. Overall, these reports suggest an approximate 10- to 20-fold increase in internal neoplasms in XP.[24,25]

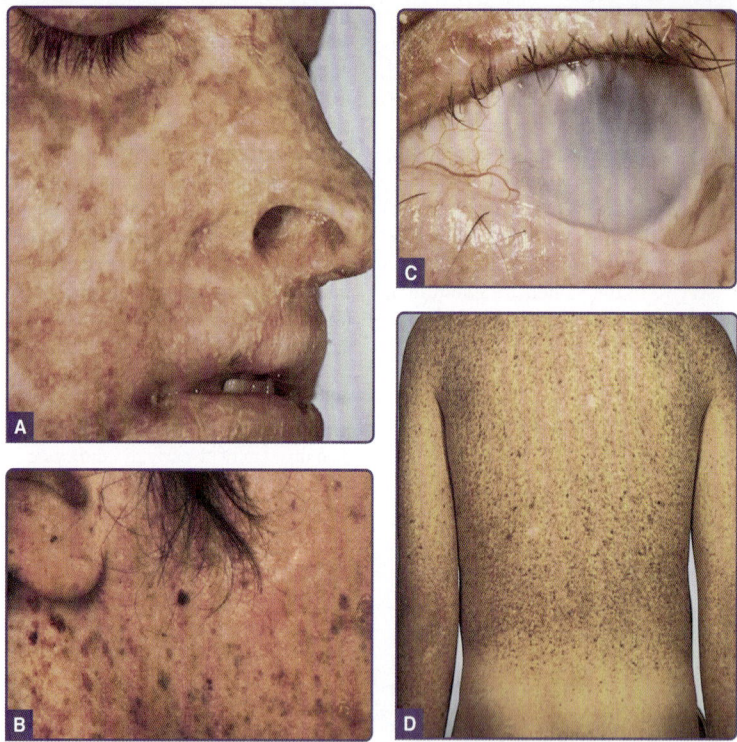

Figure 130-2 Xeroderma pigmentosum. **A,** Pigmentary changes, atrophy, dryness, and cheilitis in a 16-year-old patient. **B,** Cheek of a 14-year-old patient with pigmented macules of varying size and intensity, actinic keratosis, basal cell carcinoma, and a surgical scar. **C,** Corneal clouding, prominent conjunctival blood vasculature, and loss of lashes. **D,** Myriad pigmented macules of varying sizes and intensities and scattered hypopigmented areas on the back, with marked sparing of the sun-protected buttocks of a 14-year-old patient.

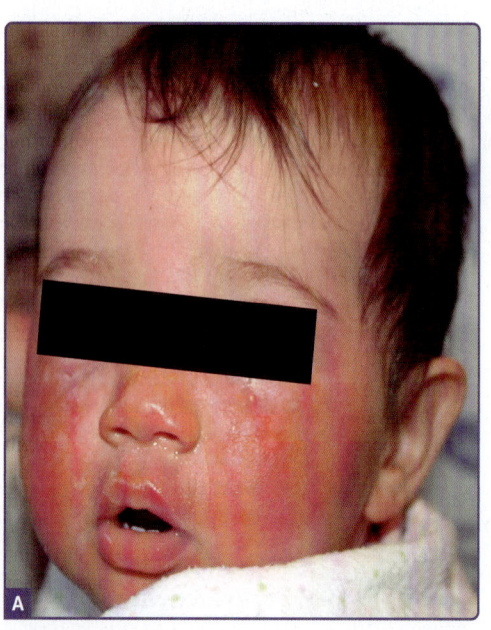
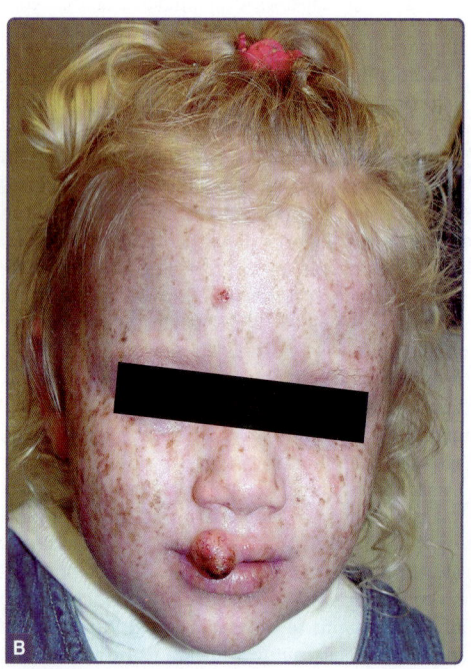

Figure 130-3 Xeroderma pigmentosum (XP): different sunburning clinical phenotypes. **A,** Complementation group XP-D patient at 9 months of age with severe blistering erythema of the malar area following minimal sun exposure. Note sparing of her forehead and eyes that were protected by a hat. **B,** Patient XP358BE (XP-C) at age 2 years did not sunburn easily but developed multiple hyperpigmented macules on her face. A rapidly growing squamous cell carcinoma or keratoacanthoma grew on her upper lip and a precancerous lesion appeared on her forehead.

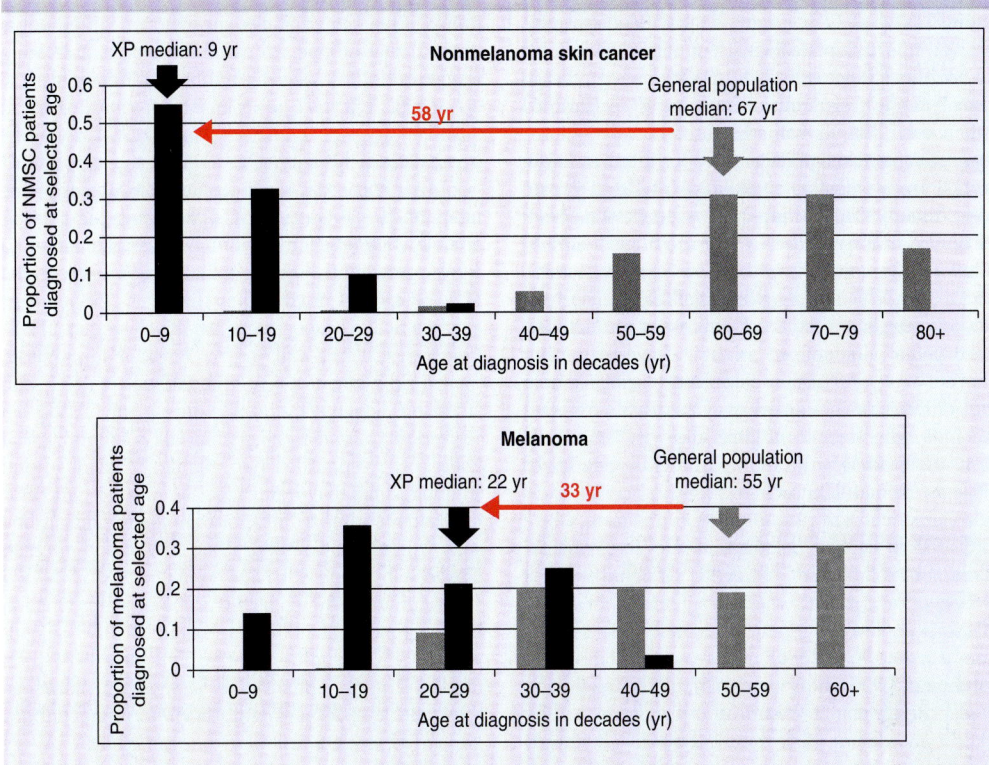

Figure 130-4 Xeroderma pigmentosum (XP) skin cancer by age at first skin cancer diagnosis and skin cancer type compared to U.S. general population. *Upper panel:* Proportion of nonmelanoma skin cancer (NMSC) patients diagnosed at selected ages. *Lower panel:* Proportion of melanoma patients diagnosed at selected ages. Compared to the U.S. general population, XP patients had a 58-year reduction in age of first NMSC, and a 33-year reduction in age of first melanoma. Individuals with both NMSC and melanoma were used for both analyses. (Adapted by permission from BMJ Publishing Group Ltd: Bradford PT, Goldstein AM, Tamura D, et al. Cancer and neurologic degeneration in xeroderma pigmentosum: long term follow-up characterises the role of DNA repair. *J Med Genet* 2011;48:168-76.[18])

ETIOLOGY AND PATHOGENESIS

Patients with XP are hypersensitive to UV radiation, as are their cultured cells. Cutaneous and ocular abnormalities are strikingly limited to UV-exposed areas and usually spare such UV-shielded locations as the axillae, buttocks, and retina. The fact that black patients with XP have an increased frequency of skin cancer suggests that a normally functioning DNA repair system provides greater protection against skin cancer than does the natural pigmentation of black skin.

Complementation Groups: Genetic heterogeneity among the XP DNA repair defects was found by fusing cultured fibroblasts from different patients and defining complementation groups. Seven such DNA excision repair-deficient complementation groups have been identified (named XP-A to XP-G) and the mutated genes have been identified (*DDB2, ERCC1, ERCC2, ERCC3, ERCC4, ERCC5, XPA*, and *XPC*; see Table 130-3).[13] Additional patients with clinical XP but normal NER are called *XP variants*. Studies of cellular hypersensitivity reveal a slightly increased sensitivity to UV-induced inhibition of cell growth that was potentiated by caffeine. Cells from XP-variant patients have a defect in an error-prone DNA polymerase *(POLH)*(pol η) that bypasses unrepaired DNA damage.[8]

There is a complex relationship among the DNA repair genes and clinical disease[13] (see Table 130-3 and Fig. 130-1; also see https://www.ncbi.nlm.nih.gov/books/NBK1397/ for review of XP). One clinical phenotype can be associated with defects in each of several genes. Conversely, mutations in one gene can be associated with several different clinical phenotypes.[18,19] These complex relationships and the roles of DNA repair genes in regulation of transcription and in immune functions are under intense investigation.

Complementation Group A: XP complementation group A (XP-A; see Table 130-3) contains patients with the most-severe neurologic and somatic abnormalities (the De Sanctis-Cacchione syndrome), as well as patients with minimal or no neurologic abnormalities. Long-term followup of these patients has revealed a relationship between the genotype and the phenotype.[18,19] Patients with the most-severe disease appear to have truncating mutations in both alleles of the *XPA* gene, leading to no detectible normal protein. In contrast, patients with minimal neurologic abnormalities have splice-site mutations that permit a small amount of normal messenger RNA (mRNA) to be made. Patients with *XPA* mutations have been reported in the United States, Europe, and the Middle East. It is the most common form of XP in Japan. Approximately 90% of Japanese XP-A patients have the same founder mutation, which is a single base substitution (see https://www.ncbi.nlm.nih.gov/books/NBK1397/). This finding has served as the basis for development of a rapid diagnostic assay for Japanese XP-A patients (including prenatal diagnosis) using polymerase chain reaction analysis of a small sample of DNA. Heterozygous carriers of this disease-causing mutation who have 1 mutated allele and 1 normal allele are estimated to comprise approximately 1% of the Japanese population.[17]

Complementation Group B: XP complementation group B (XP-B; Fig. 130-5) is composed of 5 patients in 4 kindreds who had the cutaneous abnormalities characteristic of XP (including neoplasms) in conjunction with neurologic and ocular abnormalities typical of CS. Another family had 2 adult sisters with XP but without CS who had ocular melanomas and were parents of normal children.[26] Surprisingly, a patient with TTD also was found to have a defect in the *XPB (ERCC3)* gene.

Complementation Group C: Patients in XP complementation group C (XP-C), with rare exceptions, have XP with skin and ocular involvement but without neurologic abnormalities.[13] This is the most common group in the United States, Europe, and Egypt, but is found rarely in Japan. Most patients have truncating mutations in both alleles leading to undetectable levels of *XPC* mRNA (the result of nonsense-mediated message decay).[19] However, a splice lariat branch-point mutation resulting in as little as 3% to 5% of normal mRNA resulted in milder clinical symptoms in 1 family in Turkey.[27] XP-C patients typically do not give a history of severe blistering sunburns on minimal sun exposure and at times are first diagnosed with the appearance of skin cancer in a child.[28]

Complementation Group D: Patients in XP complementation group D (XP-D) have been described with several different clinical phenotypes. They may have cutaneous XP with late onset of neurologic abnormalities in their second decade of life or XP with no neurologic abnormalities.[18,19] Two XP-D patients have been reported with clinical symptoms of both XP and CS. Cells from patients with a photosensitive form of TTD (without XP) also were assigned to the XP-D.[29] Two patients were reported with combined symptoms of both TTD and XP (1 patient had a skin cancer and the other died of metastatic melanoma) and mutations in the *XPD (ERCC2)* gene. Finally, a patient with COFS syndrome had a mutation in the *XPD* gene.

Complementation Group E: XP complementation group E (XP-E) was found in 1 kindred in Europe and in several kindreds in Japan. We studied adult patients from 3 kindreds from the United States and Germany

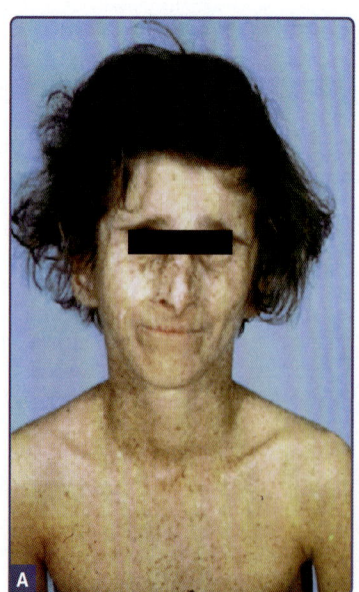 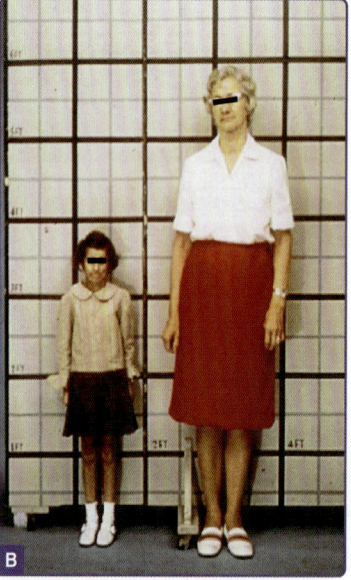

Figure 130-5 Xeroderma pigmentosum (XP)–Cockayne syndrome (CS) complex. **A,** A 28-year-old patient (XP11BE) in XP complementation group B with cutaneous changes of XP, including pigmentary changes and atrophy. She has a beak-like nose and loss of subcutaneous tissue, which are typical of Cockayne syndrome. **B,** The patient is of short stature (less than 4 ft. tall). Her mother, an obligate heterozygote, is clinically normal.

who had mutations in the *XPE (DDB2)* gene. These patients had no neurologic involvement.[30]

Complementation Group F: XP complementation group F (XP-F) patients are found mainly in Japan. Most of these patients have mild clinical symptoms without neurologic abnormalities or skin cancer.[18,19] However, we recently found 2 families with adult onset of severe neurodegeneration with mutations in the *XPF (ERCC4)* gene. The residual rate of DNA repair is very low (only 10% to 20% of normal).

Complementation Group G: Thirteen patients in XP complementation group G (XP-G) have been identified in the United States, Europe, and Japan (Fig. 130-6).[18,19] There is a large variation in clinical features among these patients. Several patients with mutations in the *XPG (ERCC5)* gene had clinical features of both XP and severe CS with cachexia and death in the first decade (see Fig. 130-5). Other patients with different mutations (missense mutations) in the same gene had no neurologic abnormalities, probably because of the low level of residual activity present in cells from these patients.[31]

Xeroderma Pigmentosum Variant: XP-variant cells have normal DNA NER and thus do not fall into any of the complementation groups of cells with

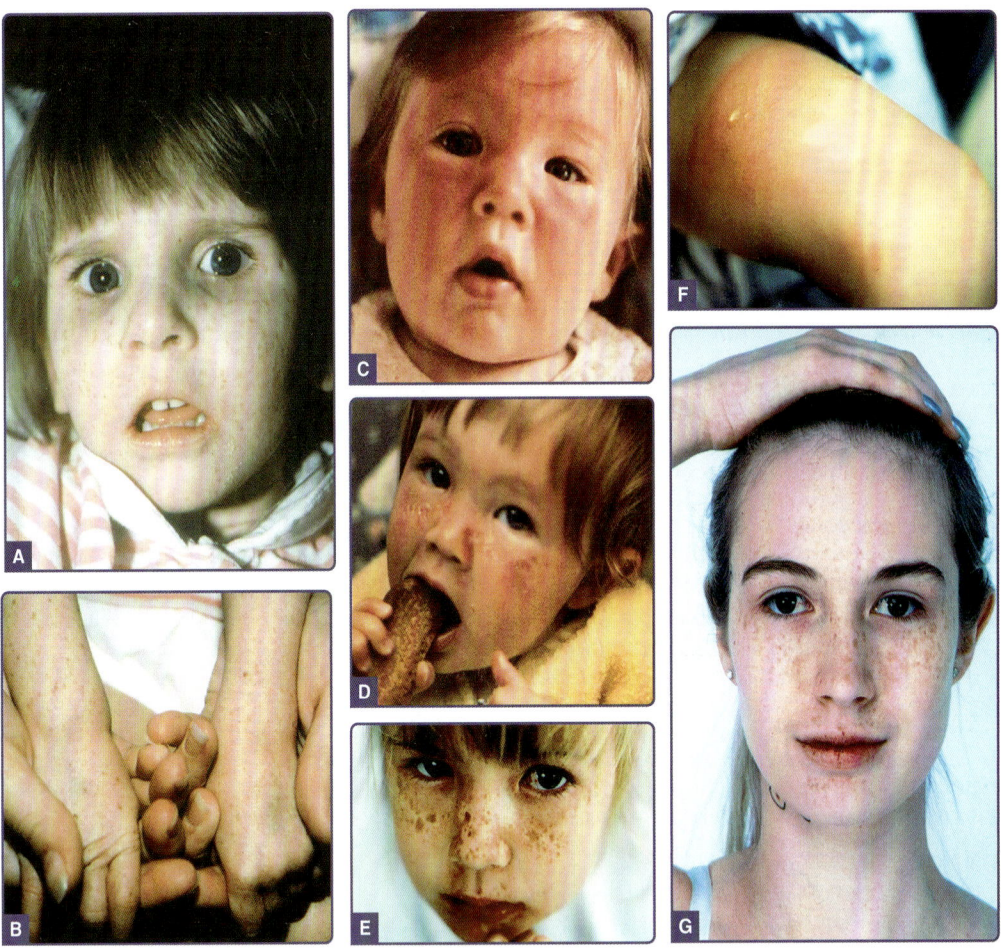

Figure 130-6 Severe and mild xeroderma pigmentosum complementation group G (XP-G) patients. **A** and **B,** XP82DC. **C** to **F,** XP65BE. **A,** Patient XP82DC at 3 years of age has deep-set eyes, which is characteristic of Cockayne syndrome (CS), and irregular lentiginous pigmentation on her face, which is characteristic of XP, indicating XP–CS complex. **B,** Patient XP82DC at 3 years of age has characteristic XP-pigmented lesions on her forearms and dorsa of hands along with thin, translucent skin with readily visible veins. The small size of her hands is apparent in comparison with the hands of her mother. **C,** Patient XP65BE at age 6 months experienced severe sunburn on her face with minimal sun exposure. Erythema and swelling are seen on skin of forehead, cheeks, and periorbital area. **D,** Patient XP65BE at age 9 months shows erythema and peeling of skin of malar area of face after sun exposure. **E,** Patient XP65BE at age 4.5 years shows pigmentary changes on her nose, malar area, and other portions of her face. **F,** Patient XP65BE at 4.5 years shows blistering sunburn on her upper thigh. Note spared area above knee where sunscreen was applied. **G,** Patient XP65BE shows minimal pigmentary changes on face and sparing of neck and hand. She used measures to protect her skin from sun exposure. (From Emmert S, Slor H, Busch DB, et al. Relationship of neurologic degeneration to genotype in three xeroderma pigmentosum group G patients. *J Invest Dermatol* 2002;118:972, with permission. Copyright © Society for Investigative Dermatology.)

defective DNA excision repair. However, there is a defect in an error-prone, translesional DNA damage bypass polymerase, *POLH* (pol η). Most XP-variant patients have clinical XP with no neurologic abnormalities.[18,19] The cutaneous and ocular abnormalities have been severe in some patients and mild in others.[32]

Parents: Both parents of XP patients are asymptomatic carriers of mutations in one of these genes. They are obligate heterozygotes with 1 mutated allele and 1 normal allele. There is a 1 in 4 chance that their offspring will have inherited a mutated allele from each parent and thus have symptomatic XP.

DIAGNOSIS (LABORATORY TESTING)

Cellular Hypersensitivity: Cultured cells from patients with XP generally grow normally when not exposed to damaging agents. However, the population growth rate or single-cell colony-forming ability is reduced to a greater extent than normal cells after exposure to UV radiation. A range of post-UV exposure colony-forming abilities has been found with fibroblasts from patients, some having extremely low post-UV exposure colony-forming ability and others having nearly normal survival.[13]

XP fibroblasts are deficient in their ability to repair some UV-damaged viruses or plasmids to a functionally active state. These host cell reactivation assays have detected an abnormality in every form of XP tested.

UV-irradiated XP fibroblasts are hypermutable compared to normal fibroblasts. This post-UV irradiation hypermutability is believed to be the basis of the increased frequency of sunlight-induced somatic mutations that lead to cancer in XP patients.[33]

Chromosome Abnormalities: XP cells generally are found to have a normal karyotype without excessive chromosome breakage or increased sister chromatid exchanges (as seen in BS). However, after exposure to UV radiation, abnormally large increases in chromosome breakage and in sister chromatid exchanges have been observed. The extent of this induced abnormality varies in different patients.

DNA Repair Testing: Incorporation of nucleotides into DNA following UV exposure of living, cultured cells (unscheduled DNA synthesis) is reduced in XP cells of complementation groups A to G. Unscheduled DNA synthesis is normal in cells from XP-variant patients.[13]

Drug and Chemical Hypersensitivity: A number of DNA-damaging agents other than UV radiation have been found to yield hypersensitive responses with XP cells. These agents include drugs (psoralens, chlorpromazine), cancer chemotherapeutic agents (cisplatin, carmustine), and chemical carcinogens (benzo[*a*]pyrene derivatives). Presumably, these agents induce DNA damage whose repair involves portions of the DNA repair pathways that are defective in XP.

DNA Sequence Analysis: Sequence analysis of DNA obtained from blood, cheek cells, or cultured cells is now available in CLIA (Clinical Laboratory Improvement Amendments)-certified laboratories. (See https://www.cms.gov/Regulations-and-Guidance/Legislation/CLIA/Laboratory_Registry.html for an updated listing of laboratories.)

Prenatal Diagnosis: In kindreds with an affected XP patient, prenatal diagnosis has been reported by measuring UV-induced unscheduled DNA synthesis in cultured amniotic fluid cells and by use of DNA diagnosis of trophoblast cells obtained early in pregnancy. DNA-based prenatal diagnoses also may be possible. (See https://www.cms.gov/Regulations-and-Guidance/Legislation/CLIA/Laboratory_Registry.html for an updated listing of laboratories.)

DIFFERENTIAL DIAGNOSIS

Other diseases with deficient NER and neurologic degeneration, such as CS (see below), may be considered. CS patients have abnormal myelin in the brain, retinal degeneration, and a low frequency of skin cancer. Other diseases with cutaneous photosensitivity, such as porphyria, RTS, and the allelic disorder Baller-Gerold syndrome, should be ruled out.

Hartnup disorder is a disorder of amino acid absorption resulting from biallelic pathogenic variants in *SLC6A19*, a nonpolar amino acid transporter. Affected individuals may have reduced levels of niacin with resulting pellagra-like symptoms of photosensitivity with dermatitis, diarrhea, and dementia. However, individuals with Hartnup disorder are not reported to have increased frequency of skin cancer.

The cutaneous findings of Carney complex may be confused with those of XP; however, Carney complex is characterized by lentigines without evidence of the usually associated signs of skin damage, such as atrophy and telangiectasia (ie, poikiloderma), and cutaneous findings are not limited to sun-exposed sites.[34]

CLINICAL COURSE AND PROGNOSIS

The most common causes of death are skin cancer, neurologic degeneration, and internal cancer. The median age at death of persons with XP with neurodegeneration (29 years) is younger than that of persons with XP without neurodegeneration (37 years).[18]

In a few families, patients who received an early diagnosis and used rigorous sun protection had fewer skin cancers and a longer life than did their affected siblings who did not use rigorous sun protection.[35]

MANAGEMENT

Management of patients with XP is based on early diagnosis, lifelong protection from UV radiation exposure, and early detection and treatment of neoplasms.[36] Diagnosis rests on recognition of the characteristic clinical features of XP and is confirmed by laboratory tests of cellular hypersensitivity to UV and defective DNA repair. Molecular determination of some of the XP disease-causing mutations is offered in a laboratory that is certified for clinical testing (see https://www.cms.gov/Regulations-and-Guidance/Legislation/CLIA/Laboratory_Registry.htmlgenetests.org for the most recent listing of CLIA-certified laboratories).

Interventions:

Sun Protection: Patients should be educated to protect all body surfaces from UV radiation by wearing protective clothing, UV-absorbing glasses, and long hair styles. They should adopt a lifestyle to minimize UV exposure and use sunscreens with high sun protective factor (SPF) ratings (minimum SPF 30) daily. Because the cells of individuals with XP are hypersensitive to UVA (found in sunlight), UVB (found in sunlight), and UVC (found in some artificial light sources), it is useful to measure UV light in an individual's home, school, or work environment with a light meter. The meter permits detection of high levels of environmental UV (such as halogen lamps) that can be eliminated. Although no standards exist for perfectly safe UV exposure in individuals with XP, the use of UV meters can alert individuals to unexpected sources of high levels of environmental UV.[36]

Patients should be examined frequently by a family member who has been instructed in recognition of cutaneous neoplasms. A set of color photographs of the entire skin surface with close-ups of lesions (including a ruler) is often extremely useful to both the patient and the physician in detecting new or changing lesions. A physician should examine patients at frequent intervals (approximately every 3 to 6 months depending on severity of skin disease). Premalignant lesions such as actinic keratoses may be treated by freezing with liquid nitrogen, or with topical 5-fluorouracil or imiquimod. Photodynamic therapy, using, for example, the topical photosensitizer 5-aminolevulinic acid followed by exposure to blue light, is an effective treatment modality for normal patients with multiple actinic keratoses. There are no data on the safety or efficacy of this treatment in XP patients. *Caution is recommended because an abnormal response to photodynamic therapy or other light-based or laser-based therapy cannot be excluded in XP cells.* Larger areas have been treated with therapeutic dermatome shaving or dermabrasion to remove the more damaged superficial epidermal layers. This procedure permits repopulation by cells from the follicles and glands, which are deeper and relatively UV-shielded.

Because cells from patients with XP are also hypersensitive to environmental mutagens such as benzo[a]pyrene found in cigarette smoke, prudence dictates that patients should be protected against these agents. One of our patients who smoked cigarettes for more than 10 years died of bronchogenic carcinoma of the lungs at age 37 years,[18] and another patient who smoked developed a lung cancer at age 48 years. Thus, we recommend that XP patients refrain from smoking cigarettes and that parents should protect children with XP from being exposed to secondhand smoke.

Cancer: Cutaneous neoplasms are treated in the same manner as in patients who do not have XP. However, special consideration should be given to the extent of actinic damage in the area surrounding the tumor and to the need for tissue conservation because of the very high risk of future tumors requiring surgical intervention. Typical procedures include electrodesiccation and curettage, surgical excision, or Mohs micrographic surgery. Although actinically damaged skin in non-XP patients is characterized by laxity and wrinkling, XP skin is atrophic and taut, complicating skin closure. Because multiple surgical procedures are often necessary, removal of undamaged skin should be minimized. Extremely severe cases have been treated by excision of large portions of the facial surface and grafting with uninvolved skin.

Most patients with XP are not abnormally sensitive to therapeutic X-rays, and XP patients have responded normally to full doses of therapeutic X-radiation for treatment of inoperable neoplasms such as an astrocytoma of the spinal cord, a frontal lobe astrocytoma, or recurrent squamous cell carcinoma in the orbit.[23]

Medications: In a controlled study, oral isotretinoin was effective in preventing new neoplasms in patients with multiple skin cancers.[37] Because of its toxicity (hepatic, hyperlipidemic, teratogenic, calcification of ligaments and tendons, premature closure of the epiphyses), oral isotretinoin should be reserved for patients with XP who are actively developing large numbers of new skin cancers. We found that the effective dose varies among patients and some patients may respond to doses of oral isotretinoin as low as 0.5 mg/kg/day.

One research study has reported that a bacterial DNA repair enzyme, denV T4 endonuclease, in a topical liposome-containing preparation, reduces the frequency of new actinic keratoses and basal cell carcinomas in XP patients.[38] As of 2018, this treatment has not been approved by the U.S. Food and Drug Administration (FDA).

A study treating multiple melanoma in situ lesions with intralesional interferon-α in 1 XP patient showed localized clearing only of lesions injected with the intralesional interferon-α but not with the control diluent.[39]

There are several case reports of XP patients responding to topical treatment with the immune modulator imiquimod. However, none of these reported long-term followup.

Oral vismodegib (Erivedge), an inhibitor of the hedgehog pathway, has been approved by the FDA for treatment of metastatic basal cell carcinoma or locally advanced basal cell carcinoma that has recurred following surgery. This drug also has been approved for use in individuals with basal cell carcinoma who are not candidates for surgery or for radiation therapy (see FDA package insert). Although this treatment may be appropriate for some individuals with XP, no studies on the efficacy of this drug in those with XP have been published. Oral vismodegib is also a teratogen, leading to embryo-fetal death, midline defects, missing digits, and other birth defects in an exposed embryo or fetus; effective contraception during and after vismodegib treatment is advised for both women and men. There is concern that vismodegib treatment of skin cancers having mixed basal cell carcinoma and squamous cell carcinoma histology might result in shrinking of the basal cell carcinoma component while permitting the squamous cell carcinoma component to proliferate.

Vitamin D is produced in the skin by a reaction involving exposure to UV radiation. Active adults with XP and skin cancers received sufficient vitamin D in their diet in the past to result in normal serum concentrations of the active form (1,25-dihydroxy vitamin D).[40] However, children protected from sunlight very early in life have had low serum concentration of 25-hydroxy vitamin D; one child became susceptible to bone fractures.[41] Dietary supplementation with oral vitamin D is recommended for persons with low serum concentration of serum vitamin D.[42]

Eyes: The eyes should be protected by wearing UV-absorbing glasses with side shields. Methylcellulose eye drops can be used to keep the cornea moist. Corneal transplantation has restored vision in patients with corneal opacity from severe keratitis. However, some of these suffered graft rejection as a result of neovascularization. Neoplasms of the lids, conjunctiva, and cornea are usually treated surgically. We are examining the possibility of using a swab to obtain cytologic specimens from the surface of the eye to determine if early neoplasms can be detected or excluded without the need for performing biopsies.[20]

Hearing Loss: Hearing aids can be of great help for individuals who have sensorineural hearing loss with learning difficulties in school.[21]

Heterozygotes: XP heterozygotes (parents and some other relatives) are carriers of the gene for XP but are clinically normal. There is limited epidemiologic evidence to indicate that such persons have an increased risk of developing skin cancer. Most tests of cell function or DNA repair yield normal responses with cells from XP heterozygotes.[43]

Patient Support Groups: The XP Family Support Group provides ongoing educational and community support to families and patients living with XP (XP Family Support Group, 10259 Atlantis Drive, Elk Grove, CA 95624; Phone: (916) 628-3814; Email: contact@xpfamilysupport.org). The XP Society has a summer camp with activities designed for light-sensitive individuals (https://www.xps.org; 437 Snydertown Road, Craryville, NY 12521-5224; Phone: 518-851-3466; Email: xps@xps.org).

COCKAYNE SYNDROME (INCLUDING XERODERMA PIGMENTOSUM–COCKAYNE SYNDROME OVERLAP)

AT-A-GLANCE

- Cockayne syndrome (CS) is an autosomal recessive disease with acute burning of the skin on minimal sun exposure.
- CS patients have developmental delay, microcephaly, progressive hearing loss, cataracts, and pigmentary retinal degeneration.
- A moderate type (CS Type I) has been distinguished from the an early-onset severe form (CS Type II) and a milder, late-onset form (CS Type III).
- Cells from CS patients have a defect in transcription coupled DNA repair with approximately two-thirds having mutations in the *CSB (ERCC6)* gene and one-third with mutations in the *CSA (ERCC8)* gene.

In 1936, E. A. Cockayne described a syndrome characterized by cachectic dwarfism, deafness, and pigmentary retinal degeneration with a characteristic "salt-and-pepper" appearance of the retina.[44]

EPIDEMIOLOGY

CS is a very rare, autosomal recessive degenerative disease with cutaneous, ocular, neurologic, and somatic abnormalities (see Table 130-1).[45] A review published in 1992 described 140 cases reported in the literature.[46] A nationwide survey of CS patients in Japan, published in 2015, reported 47 patients.[47] In 2015, the Cockayne Syndrome Natural History (CoSyNH) study described clinical findings in 102 patients from Europe, North Africa/Middle East, West Asia, and East Asia.[48] The incidence of CS has been estimated as 1.8 per million persons in native West European population and 2.7 per million live births overall.[16]

CLINICAL FEATURES

Cutaneous Findings: The skin has photosensitivity without the excessive pigmentary abnormalities seen in XP. There is marked loss of subcutaneous fat, resulting in a "wizened" appearance with typical deep-set eyes and prominent ears. A systematic dermatologic examination of 14 European CS patients and 2 COFS syndrome patients (ages 1 to 28 years) reported photosensitivity in 75% with sunburn after brief sun exposure.[49] Six patients had pigmented macules on sun-exposed skin but none developed skin neoplasms. Cyanotic acral edema of the extremities was present in 12 patients, 8 had nail dystrophy, and 7 had hair abnormalities.

Noncutaneous Findings: CS is a progressive disorder and most symptoms appear and worsen with time. The eyes are small (microphthalmia) and develop a characteristic sunken appearance over time because of loss of orbital fat. The ocular abnormalities include a progressive pigmentary retinal degeneration and optic atrophy leading to eventual blindness. Other manifestations include photophobia, early cataract, and diminished tearing leading to conjunctivitis, corneal infection, and scarring. The pupils are typically small with iris atrophy and poorly reactive to light. CS patients frequently have abnormal electroretinograms.[45,50]

Birth weight and early development are usually normal. Neurologic abnormalities, in addition to deafness, include peripheral neuropathy, normal pressure hydrocephalus, microcephaly, and segmental loss of myelin "tigroid leukodystrophy."[45]

The disease onset is usually in the second year of life with slowly progressive neurologic degeneration (CS Type I). Intellectual deterioration may be nonuniform, with some functions preserved better than others. A severe infantile form has been described (CS Type II) as well as a milder form with late onset (CS Type III). COFS syndrome with microcephaly and severe mental retardation and CAMFAK syndrome of congenital *c*ataracts, *m*icrocephaly, *f*ailure to thrive, and *k*yphoscoliosis have some similar features. A continuous spectrum of severity in CS has been proposed.[51] The most severe form is COFS syndrome, then CS Type II, CS Type I, and CS Type III. The mildest form is UVSS with photosensitivity without the systemic features of CS.

CS is not associated with an increased incidence of neoplasia.

ETIOLOGY AND PATHOGENESIS

CS is an autosomal recessive disorder caused by mutations in *CSB (ERCC6)* in approximately two-thirds of the patients, and in *CSA (ERCC8)* in approximately one-third.[51] Patients with mutations in these genes have similar clinical features. A survey in 2013 listed 78 different mutations in the *CSB* gene and 30 in the *CSA* gene from 120 genetically confirmed patients.[51] A patient with COFS syndrome was reported with a defect in *CSB* and another with a defect in *XPD*. These genes are part of the NER pathway and have a primary role in transcription coupled DNA repair.[13]

Parents: Both parents of CS patients are asymptomatic carriers of mutations in one of these genes. They are obligate heterozygotes with one mutated allele and one normal allele. There is a 1 in 4 chance that their offspring will have inherited a mutated allele from each parent and thus have symptomatic CS.

DIAGNOSIS

Diagnostic criteria for CS have been proposed[51] with mandatory major criteria of developmental delay, progressive growth failure, and progressive microcephaly. Minor criteria (3 out of 5) are cutaneous photosensitivity, pigmentary retinopathy and/or cataracts, progressive sensorineural hearing loss, tooth enamel hypoplasia, and enophthalmia (abnormally sunken eyes). In addition, brain imaging criteria include white matter hypomyelination, cerebellar atrophy or hypoplasia, and bilateral calcifications of the putamen.

COFS syndrome is an autosomal recessive disorder with microcephaly, cataracts, microphthalmia and arthrogryposis (congenital joint contractures usually associated with curtailed joint movement before birth).[51]

Laboratory Testing: Clinical laboratory testing often shows sensorineural deafness, neuropathic electromyogram, and slow motor nerve conduction velocity.[52] The electroencephalogram may be abnormal, and X-ray examination may show thickened skull and microcephaly. CT may be diagnostically useful in the detection of normal-pressure hydrocephalus and showing calcification of the basal ganglia and other structures (Fig. 130-7). MRI of the brain shows atrophy and dysmyelination of the cerebrum and cerebellum.[53] Bone age is usually normal. Height and weight are usually well below the third percentile for the age.[48]

Cellular Hypersensitivity: As with XP, cultured cells (fibroblasts or lymphocytes) from patients with CS are hypersensitive to UV-induced inhibition of growth and colony-forming ability. Host cell reactivation of UV-damaged adenovirus or plasmids is reduced, although generally to a lesser extent than in XP. Molecular determination of the CS-causing mutations is offered in a laboratory that is CLIA-certified for clinical testing (see https://www.cms.gov/Regulations-and-Guidance/Legislation/CLIA/Laboratory_Registry.htmlgenetests.org for a current list of laboratories that provide this service).

Prenatal Diagnosis: Prenatal diagnosis of CS has been performed based on the delay in recovery of post-UV radiation RNA synthesis and the increased cell killing by UV radiation. Molecular identification of the mutations is more commonly used currently for families with an affected child where the causative mutations are known (see https://www.cms.gov/Regulations-and-Guidance/Legislation/CLIA/Laboratory_Registry.htmlgenetests.org for a current list of laboratories that provide this service).

Clinical-Laboratory Correlation: Patients with defects in *CSA* or *CSB* have similar clinical features.[48,51]

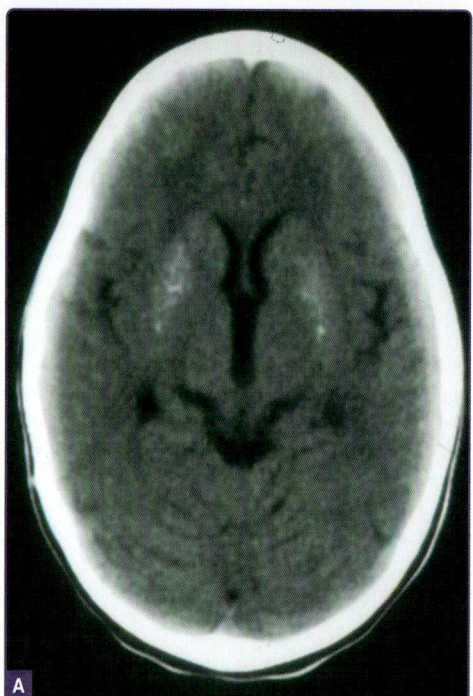 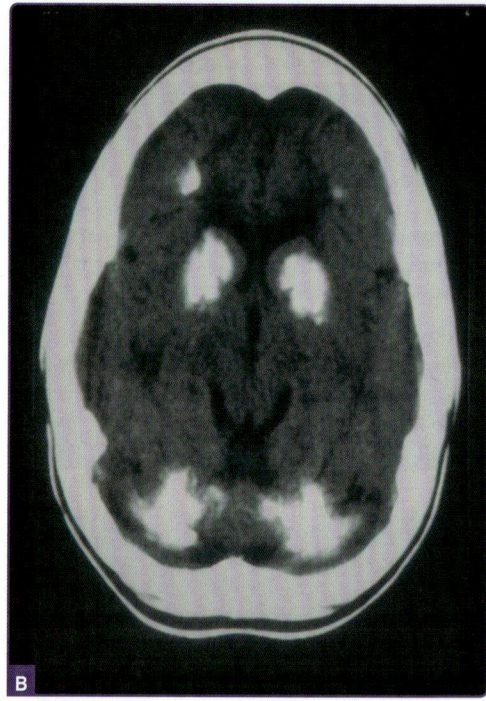

Figure 130-7 Cockayne syndrome. Calcification of brain visualized on CT scan. **A,** A 2-year-old patient with bilateral calcification of basal ganglia. **B,** A 15-year-old patient with extensive calcification involving basal ganglia, cerebellum, and cerebral hemispheres.

DIFFERENTIAL DIAGNOSIS

As CS patients have involvement of multiple organ systems with varying degrees of severity, some of the features may be present in other disorders (see discussion in Laugel[54]). Thus growth failure may be a common feature of many chromosomal, endocrine, or GI disorders. Calcifications in the brain are also seen in congenital infections such as rubella or toxoplasmosis, or in calcium or phosphate metabolism abnormalities. Cutaneous photosensitivity is also present in premature aging syndromes including XP (accompanied by early onset of freckle-like pigmentation and skin cancer), BS, progeria, WS, and RTS. Retinal pigmentary abnormalities and growth failure may be present in mitochondrial dystrophies. Other disorders with profound growth failure have characteristic physical appearance include Cornelia de Lange syndrome, Dubowitz syndrome, Hallermann-Streiff syndrome, Russell-Silver syndrome, and Seckel syndrome. Warburg MICRO syndrome has features of microcephaly, microcornea, congenital cataract, mental retardation, optic atrophy, and hypogenitalism,[55] but does not have rapidly progressive neurodegeneration or defective DNA repair.

CLINICAL COURSE AND PROGNOSIS

In the CoSyNH study of 102 patients from 81 families,[48] the mean age of the recruited individuals was 11.5 years (range: 3 months to 19 years). At the time of analysis, 28 individuals had died with a median age at death of 8.4 years (range: 17 months to 30 years). The presence of cataracts before 3 years of age was the single most important prognostic factor with a statistically significant association with reduced survival, earlier onset of hearing loss, and earlier onset of contractures.

MANAGEMENT

Recommendations for care of CS patients have been developed by the authors of the CoSyNH study of clinical findings in 102 patients.[48] These include molecular testing (*CSA [ERCC8]*, *CSB [ERCC6]* followed by *XPG [ERCC5]*, *XPD [ERCC2]* or *XPB [ERCC3]* if these are normal and features of XP–CS complex are present [see below]); multidisciplinary care (coordinating clinician, dietician, physiotherapist); annual surveillance (cataracts, retinal evaluation, hearing assessment, blood pressure monitoring); and laboratory testing (liver function tests, blood glucose). Supplementary feeding may be required, including use of a nasogastric tube or percutaneous gastrostomy. Hypertension, gastroesophageal reflux disease, and tremor may be treated with specific medications. Low temperature may reflect thyroid insufficiency and recurrent pneumonias may be related to swallowing difficulty.

Metronidazole for GI abnormalities was associated with acute liver failure in 8 CS patients (3 fatal within 11 days of treatment).[56] These authors state that metronidazole is contraindicated for CS patients.

Patient Support Group: The Share and Care Cockayne Syndrome Network (http://cockaynesyndrome.net or http://www.cockayne-syndrome.org) is an educational, advocacy, and support organization for CS patients and their families (Box 570618, Dallas, TX 75357).

XERODERMA PIGMENTOSUM–COCKAYNE SYNDROME COMPLEX

Approximately 12 patients with CS have been found to have, in addition to CS, clinical features of XP.[18,19,48] These features include freckle-like pigmentation on sun-exposed skin and cutaneous neoplasms (see Fig. 130-5). Cells from these XP–CS complex patients have reduced DNA excision repair, which is characteristic of XP. Clinically, these patients can be distinguished from XP patients with neurologic abnormalities by the presence of the CS features of pigmentary retinal degeneration, calcification of the basal ganglia, normal-pressure hydrocephalus, and hyperreflexia.[45,57,58] Cells from patients with this complex have been found to have mutations in 3 different XP genes: *XPG*, *XPD*, and *XPB* (see Table 130-3).

TRICHOTHIODYSTROPHY

AT-A-GLANCE

- Trichothiodystrophy is a rare genetic disorder characterized by sulfur-deficient brittle hair and a broad spectrum of clinical abnormalities.
- A diagnostic feature is tiger tail banding under polarizing microscopy with structural abnormalities of hair shafts.
- Typical clinical features include maternal pregnancy abnormalities, abnormal birth and development (collodion presentation, microcephaly, short stature, developmental delay), photosensitivity, and developmental abnormalities, such as the skin (hair and nails), brain, eyes, musculoskeletal system, and immune system (infections).

DEFINITIONS

TTD is a rare genetic disorder that is characterized by sulfur-deficient brittle hair and includes a broad spectrum of clinical abnormalities that may include photosensitivity, ichthyosis, intellectual impairment, short stature, microcephaly, characteristic facial features (protruding ears, micrognathia), recurrent infections, bilateral congenital cataracts, dystrophic nails, and other features (see Table 130-1; Fig. 130-8).[59-68] Although usually inherited as autosomal recessive, in one family an X-linked inheritance was described.[69] TTD encompasses patients who have been described as *Tay syndrome*, *Amish brittle hair syndrome*, *Sabinas brittle hair syndrome*, or *Pollitt syndrome*.

TTD is caused by different mutations in some of the same genes that cause XP. The functional defect in XP is abnormal DNA repair, whereas the abnormality in TTD is thought to be related to the transcription.

HISTORICAL PERSPECTIVE

In 1968, Pollitt reported a brother and sister with mental and physical growth retardation, trichorrhexis nodosa and other hair shaft defects, and identified that their hair had low cystine content, indicating deficiency of high sulfur hair proteins.[70] In 1971, Tay described 3 children of a Chinese family with an autosomal recessive disorder characterized by growth retardation, short stature, developmental delay, ichthyosis, and hair shaft defects.[59] In 1970, Brown described alternating hair shaft patterning in hair, and later, Baden and colleagues studied the hair from an Amish kindred, identifying reduced level of cystine and observed alternating light and dark bands in their hairs when viewed under polarizing microscopy.[71] Price proposed the term *trichothiodystrophy* (derived from Greek *tricho*: hair; *thio*: sulfur; *dys*: faulty; *trophe*: nourishment) recognizing the hair shaft sulfur deficiency as a marker for this symptom complex.[60]

EPIDEMIOLOGY

The disease is rare. A review attempting to capture all TTD cases reported up to the year 2005 only identified 112 cases worldwide. However, TTD is probably much more common and underdiagnosed because of failure to recognize the condition.

CLINICAL FEATURES

In addition to the diagnostic hair shaft features, TTD patients have a broad spectrum of multisystem abnormalities. Table 130-4 lists the clinical features seen in TTD as summarized from an extensive literature review.[66] Table 130-5 summarizes the findings in 1 patient.[72]

Cutaneous Findings: The newborn with TTD often has generalized redness or a mild collodion appearance, which typically clears over a few weeks. This may progress to ichthyosis, which is often mild and involves the trunk and scalp. Most TTD patients have short, broken hair (see Fig. 130-8A, B, and E), and some do not need to get haircuts. After an illness with fever, many have an episode of hair loss or "falling out." Under light microscopy with polarization, TTD hair shafts have a characteristic dark-and-light banding pattern that gives a "tiger tail" appearance (see Fig. 130-8F). Their hair shafts have multiple abnormalities, including undulating hair shaft surface (see

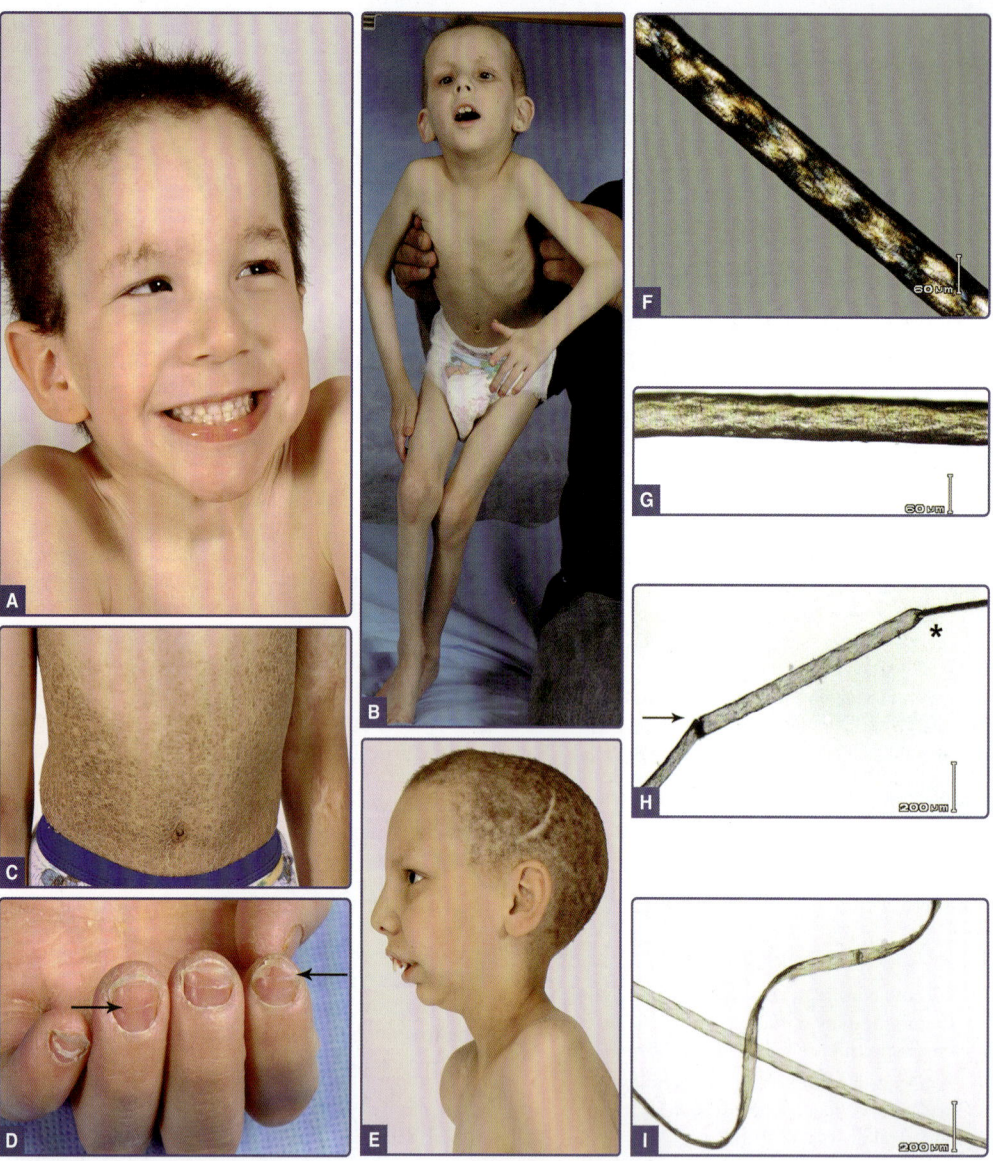

Figure 130-8 Trichothiodystrophy (TTD): clinical and microscopic hair findings. **A,** A 7-year-old boy with short, brittle scalp and eyebrow hair, and a smiling, outgoing demeanor. He had hip surgery at age 14 years, followed by a downward course and died approximately 7 months later of pneumonia. **B,** A 9-year-old girl with short stature, developmental delay, multiple infections, died 2 months after this picture of sepsis. **C, D,** and **E,** A 14-year-old boy with short brittle hair, dysmorphic facies, micrognathia, head elongation in the fronto-occipital plane (**E**). He also has ichthyosis (**C**), intellectual impairment, short stature, photosensitivity, osteosclerosis, neurologic abnormalities, recurrent infections, and nail abnormalities. **D,** Note the onychoschizias (distal nail plate split/layering at *arrows*). Light microscopy findings: **F,** TTD hair shafts displaying alternating light and dark "tiger tail" bands using polarizing microscopy. **G,** Irregular, undulating hair shaft with light microscopy **H,** Trichoschisis (*arrow*): clean, transverse cleavage fracture; marked narrowing of shaft diameter (*asterisk*). **I,** Ribboning. (Modified with permission from Liang C, Kraemer KH, Morris A, et al.[63])

Fig. 130-8G), trichoschisis (a clean transverse break through the hair; see Fig. 130-8H), trichorrhexis nodosa-like defects, and ribboning (see Fig. 130-8I).[63,64] Hair shafts are brittle because of a reduction of high-sulfur matrix proteins, and amino acid analysis of the hair demonstrates reduced levels of cysteine and cystine in hair shaft proteins. This is associated with a decrease in the ratio of strong to weak disulfide bonds within the hair shafts.[65] Approximately 50% of TTD patients have clinical photosensitivity that ranges from subtle to severe. However, in contrast to the typical clinical features of XP, patients with TTD do not develop poikilodermatous changes (hyperpigmentation, hypopigmentation, telangiectasias, and atrophy) nor skin cancer. Nails are brittle and may have onychoschizia, koilonychia (spooning) or other dystrophy. Rarely, patients may have an overlap syndrome with diluted features of both TTD and XP. They may have

TABLE 130-4
Most Frequent Clinical Manifestations of 112 Reported Patients with Trichothiodystrophy[a,66]

ABNORMALITY	# OF 112 PATIENTS	%
Short, brittle hair with shaft abnormalities	108	96
Developmental delay/intellectual impairment	96	86
Short stature	82	73
Facial dysmorphism (eg, microcephaly)	74	66
Ichthyosis	73	65
Ocular abnormality (eg, cataracts)	57	51
Infections	51	46
Photosensitivity	47	42

[a]Numbers may be artificially low because the presence of normal versus abnormal features are not always reported in case reports. Details of reported abnormal, reported normal, and unreported can be found in the "clinical array" in Faghri S, Tamura D, Kraemer KH, et al.[66]

TABLE 130-5
Clinical Features of a Patient with Trichothiodystrophy (TTD421BE), Showing the Broad Array of Abnormalities

- *Hair abnormalities:* tiger tail banding; brittle hair; sparse hair; other hair shaft abnormalities
- *Nail abnormalities:* brittle nails; koilonychias; soft nails
- *Skin abnormalities:* ichthyosis; photosensitivity; hypohidrosis
- *Oral abnormalities:* high-arched palate; abnormal teeth; frequent caries
- *Growth abnormalities:* short stature and poor weight gain (third percentile) and microcephaly (10th percentile)
- *Neonatal skin abnormalities:* collodion membrane; erythroderma
- *Neurologic abnormalities:* developmental delay; intellectual impairment; abnormal gait/ataxia; abnormal MRI results (diffuse dysmyelination)
- *Personality characteristics:* sociable/engaging/cheerful
- *Hematologic/immunologic abnormalities:* recurrent infections (particularly respiratory); neutropenia; elevated hemoglobin A_2; low serum immunoglobulin M
- *Maternal pregnancy and fetal abnormalities:* pregnancy-induced hypertension; spotting during pregnancy; abnormal prenatal screening (elevated maternal α-fetoprotein); premature birth; intrauterine growth restriction; birth weight low for gestational age; placental abnormalities

From Zhou X, Khan SG, Tamura D, et al.[72]

longer hair with some hair shaft features of TTD visible in only a portion of the hair shafts, and the pigmentary and skin cancers suggestive of XP.

Noncutaneous Findings: TTD children typically have a happy, friendly, and interactive personality but with a broad spectrum of abnormalities of growth and development. Extent of involvement varies from only hair and mild developmental impairment to severe multisystem abnormalities with a high mortality in childhood. Typical abnormalities (see Tables 130-4 and 130-5) include dysmorphic (eg, short stature, micrognathia, microcephaly), neurologic (developmental delay, intellectual impairment), ophthalmologic (congenital cataracts, nystagmus),[68] recurrent infections, musculoskeletal and bone (osteosclerosis of the axial skeleton with peripheral osteopenia, delayed bone age, contractures), and dental. Decreased red blood cell mean corpuscular volume and increased hemoglobin A_2 levels mimic β-thalassemia trait. Developmental delay may be associated with brain dysmyelination,[73] a feature similar to CS; however, patients do not have the retinal changes or brain calcifications of CS.

ETIOLOGY AND PATHOGENESIS

The majority of TTD patients have a defect in *XPD* (*ERCC2*). A few have mutations in *XPB* (*ERCC3*) or *TTDA* (*GTF2H5*) genes, which are components of TFIIH, a transcription factor that regulates both DNA repair and transcription. Mutations in the gene *GTF2E2*, which encodes the general transcription factor IIE (TF2E2), have recently been shown to cause TTD, supporting the theory that TTD is caused by impaired transcription.[74] Some TTD patients have mutations in the gene *TTDN1*,[75] and recently an X-linked form of TTD was associated with a mutation in the gene *RNF113A*,[69] but the molecular functions of these 2 genes are not yet known. It is believed that mutations that affect the repair function of the NER genes are associated with features of XP, whereas mutations affecting the transcription-related function results in features of TTD.[76] Most DNA repair disorders are inherited as autosomal recessive, requiring failure of the proteins encoded by each of 2 alleles, and different mutations in *XPD* can lead to a wide spectrum of clinical phenotypes. Some mutations in the *XPD* gene impair the repair function of the protein leading to clinical XP, while other mutations impair the transcription function leading to clinical TTD. Patients carrying mutations that impair both functions can have clinical overlap syndromes with features of both diseases.

DIAGNOSIS

The diagnosis of TTD is made on the basis of clinical features in association with characteristic hair shaft abnormalities. These include tiger tail banding under polarizing microscopy with hair shaft abnormalities and/or analysis of hair shafts for reduced sulfur content.[63] Identification of mutations known to cause TTD can confirm the diagnosis. However, because underlying genetic mutations have not been identified in all patients, failure to identify mutations does not diminish the clinical diagnosis.

A typical patient presentation in the newborn period is an infant with a preterm delivery, small for gestational age, short stature, micrognathia, congenital cataracts, and cryptorchidism, who may have erythroderma or a collodion membrane. These newborns are often in neonatal intensive care units and are at high risk for infection. Mothers frequently have a history of pregnancy difficulties, which can include hypertension, preeclampsia, or the more severe HELLP (hemolysis, elevated liver enzymes, low platelets) syndrome.[77,78]

A typical childhood presentation is a happy, outgoing child with short, brittle hair, developmental delay, short stature, microcephaly, micrognathia, abnormal myelination of the brain, recurrent infections, and feeding difficulties. Table 130-5 lists the clinical findings in 1 TTD patient, as an example of the diverse findings.[72]

Laboratory Testing: The diagnosis of TTD can be confirmed with examination of hair shafts (see Fig. 130-8F to I). TTD hair shafts display tiger tail banding under polarizing microscopy. In addition, they show a spectrum of typical hair shaft abnormalities, including trichoschisis, trichorrhexis nodosa–like fractures, surface irregularities, and ribboning.[63,64] Amino acid analysis of hair shafts can confirm reduced levels of cysteine and cystine.

Testing for mutations in the genes known to cause TTD (*XPD* [*ERCC2*]; *XPB* [*ERCC3*] or *TTDA* [*TFB5*]; *GTF2E2*; *TTDN*; *RNF113A*) can be performed. Patients with mutations in the *TTDN1* gene have a distinct TTD phenotype, are more likely to display autistic behaviors (compared to the usual socially interactive personality), and have delayed bone age and seizures; additionally, they are less likely to have low birth weight, collodion presentation, cataracts, and brain abnormal myelination.[79]

Imaging:

Brain Imaging: TTD patients fail to develop myelin in the brain and MRI can identify this dysmyelination. Rare patients can have overlap syndromes with features not only of TTD, but also of XP or CS. These patients may have features of brain atrophy (eg, dilated ventricles, loss of brain tissue volume). TTD–CS patients may have the deep-set eyes and pigmentary retinopathy of CS.

Bone Imaging: TTD patients have an unusual combination of osteosclerosis of the axial skeleton and osteopenia of the peripheral skeleton can be seen on radiographs or dual-energy x-ray absorptiometry (DEXA) scan.

Diagnostic Algorithm: Once the diagnosis is suspected because a patient has the characteristic newborn or childhood presentation described before (see "Diagnosis"), a lock of hair shafts can be cut for microscopic examination. The identification of hair shaft defects under regular light microscopy and tiger tail banding under polarizing lenses can confirm the diagnosis. Further confirmation can be obtained with amino acid analysis of hair shafts to identify low sulfur content. Mutation testing may identify a mutation in one of the associated genes, but mutations have not been identified in all patients, suggesting that there are other causative genes not yet identified.

CLINICAL COURSE AND PROGNOSIS

TTD children are prone to feeding difficulties, failure to thrive, and recurrent infections. In many children, relatively mild infections can quickly progress to systemic illness. A review of the literature identified a high mortality (>20%) in children younger than the age of 10 years, with most deaths caused by infection.[66]

MANAGEMENT

Management focuses on identification and support for individual clinical problems. Photosensitive patients should use sun-protective measures such as sunscreen, cover with clothing, and use sun-avoidance measures. Patients with developmental delay and intellectual impairment may benefit from neurologic and developmental assessment and support. Ophthalmologic consultation can identify developmental abnormalities such as congenital cataracts. Cataracts and refraction errors that impair vision can be treated.[68] In some patients, recurrent infections have been managed with prophylactic antibiotics or intravenous immunoglobulin. Patients generally have abnormal growth and difficulty maintaining weight. The reason for this is not known and may be a result of mitochondrial dysfunction. In some cases, gastrostomy tubes (G-tubes) may help maintain adequate nutrition.[80] Several of our TTD patients in their first or second decade of life have experienced progressive inability to walk from bilateral aseptic necrosis of their hips. Rehabilitation medicine and support can address musculoskeletal abnormalities and can help to maintain walking ability. In addition, a high frequency of complications occurs during pregnancies carrying an affected fetus. These can include intrauterine growth restriction, preeclampsia, preterm delivery, HELLP syndrome, and abnormal levels of maternal serum screening markers, highlighting the role of DNA repair in normal development.[78,81]

Patient Support Group: The Foundation for Ichthyosis and Related Skin Types (FIRST, http://www.firstskinfoundation.org/, 2616 N. Broad Street, Colmar, PA 18915) is an educational, advocacy and support organization for those affected by ichthyosis and related skin types.

DISORDERS OF GENOME INSTABILITY

BLOOM SYNDROME

BS is a rare, autosomal recessive disorder characterized by growth deficiency, unusual facies, sun-sensitive telangiectatic erythema, immunodeficiency, and predisposition to a variety of different cancers.[7,82]

AT-A-GLANCE

- Bloom Syndrome (BS) is a rare chromosome instability syndrome with a predisposition to a variety of cancers and multiple infections.
- BS is caused by a mutation in *BLM*, a RecQ helicase.
- Cells demonstrate impaired DNA recombination.
- Patients present with facial erythema and telangiectasia, an usual facies, and growth deficiency.
- No specific treatment is available.

EPIDEMIOLOGY

BS is most frequent among Ashkenazi Jews, who have a carrier frequency of 1%.[83] Approximately 250 patients have been recognized worldwide.

CLINICAL FEATURES

Cutaneous Findings: Facial erythema and telangiectasia superficially resembling lupus erythematosus (Fig. 130-9) are often present within the first few weeks after birth in the malar area, on the nose, and around the ears.[82] Sun exposure accentuates these abnormalities and may induce bullae, bleeding, and crusting of the lips and eyelids. Café-au-lait spots are common, at times accompanied by adjacent depigmented areas.

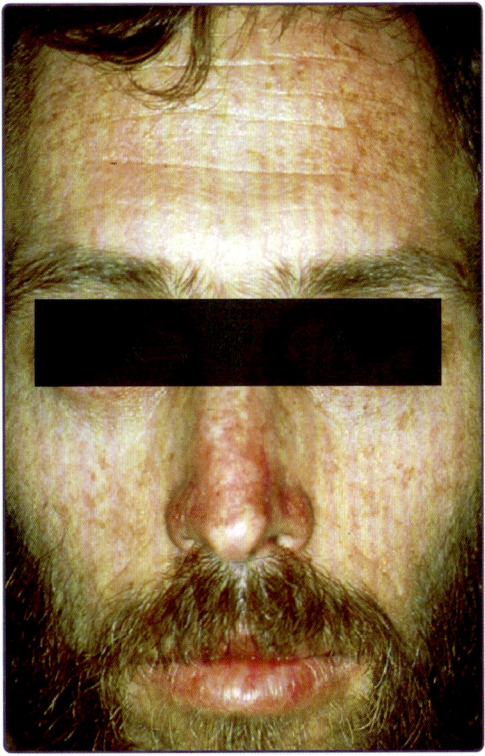

Figure 130-9 Bloom syndrome. Prominent telangiectasia in malar distribution.

Noncutaneous Findings: Patients are well proportioned but small. Adult height is usually less than 150 cm (5 feet). Patients have a long, narrow head with characteristic facies consisting of a narrow, prominent nose, relatively hypoplastic malar areas, and a receding chin.

Complications: Patients with BS are predisposed to multiple infections, as there is immune dysfunction. Fertility is decreased and diabetes mellitus is common. Approximately 20% of patients with BS develop malignancies, comprising a normal spectrum of cancer types, of which half occur before age 20 years.[82]

ETIOLOGY AND PATHOGENESIS

BS is caused by mutations in *BLM*, which encodes a RecQ helicase.[7,9,83-85] BS cells are characterized by an increase in the frequency of spontaneous sister chromatid exchanges and in exchanges between homologous chromosomes. The latter is often visualized by quadriradial chromosomes. These are 4-arm chromosomes most likely formed by recombination between 2 chromosomes (and almost never found in unaffected individuals). These observations demonstrate that BS cells are characterized by hyperrecombination. Although the exact mechanisms of how mutations in the BLM helicase lead to hyperrecombination are still not completely understood, it has been suggested that it interacts with the Fanconi anemia D2 protein (FANCD2; see below).[86] It also has been shown to participate in telomere replication and with that maintain telomere integrity.[87-89] Hyperrecombination may result in an increased frequency of loss of heterozygosity and through that mechanism, in conjunction with increased spontaneous mutation frequency, an increased frequency of malignant transformation. The immune deficiency, characterized by diminished immunoglobulin levels, reduced cellular proliferative response to mitogens, and decreased proliferation in the mixed leukocyte reaction, may be a result of impaired recombination of immunoglobulin and lymphocyte receptor genes, and probably further contributes to the increased cancer risk.

DIAGNOSIS

The observation of quadriradial chromosomes (observed in 0.5% to 14% of lymphocytes of BS patients) and the approximately 10-fold increased frequency of spontaneous sister chromatid exchanges are used to diagnose BS.[90] A founder deletion/insertion mutation in the *BLM* gene was identified in Ashkenazi Jews at a frequency of approximately 1% (BLM[Ash])[83,91] and can be used for DNA diagnosis of BS patients and carriers among Ashkenazi Jews.[92] Diagnostic testing for BS, including sequencing of *BLM* is offered in a number of laboratories that are CLIA-certified for clinical testing (see https://www.cms.gov/Regulations-and-Guidance/Legislation/CLIA/Laboratory_Registry.htmlgenetests.org for the most recent listing).

DIFFERENTIAL DIAGNOSIS

Table 130-1 outlines the clinical features of hereditary disorders of genome instability and DNA repair needed for the differential diagnosis. The differential diagnosis of BS includes other disorders, in that photosensitivity is seen in xeroderma pigmentosum and Rothmund-Thompson Syndrome, café-au-lait macules occur in neurofibromatosis, and early-onset telangiectasias are present in ataxia telangiectasia.

CLINICAL COURSE AND PROGNOSIS

Patients usually die before the age of 30 years from either cancer or infection.

MANAGEMENT

There is no specific treatment for BS. Early monitoring for the development of cancers is recommended.

WERNER SYNDROME (ADULT PROGERIA)

AT-A-GLANCE

- Werner syndrome (WS) is a rare disorder of premature aging (progeria) with an increased cancer risk.
- WS is caused by a mutation in WRN, a RecQ helicase.
- Cells demonstrate impaired DNA metabolism and a reduced replicative life span.
- Patients present with premature graying of hair, loss of subcutaneous fat, wrinkling of the skin, and cataracts starting in adolescence.
- Premature aging also affects other organs.
- No specific treatment is available.

WS is a rare, autosomal recessive disorder, characterized by several features of premature aging and an increased cancer risk.[93]

EPIDEMIOLOGY

More than 800 patients have been reported worldwide.[94] Most WS patients are Japanese.

CLINICAL FEATURES

Cutaneous Findings: Patients with WS are clinically normal until adolescence, when they do not show the usual growth spurt and start to prematurely develop features and diseases of aging, including graying and thinning of hair, loss of subcutaneous fat, and wrinkling of skin. Other features that are not part of the normal skin-aging process are scleroderma-like changes with subcutaneous atrophy, leg ulcers, and soft-tissue calcifications.

Noncutaneous Findings: Signs of premature aging also affect other organs and include Type 2 diabetes, osteoporosis, and cardiovascular disease secondary to atherosclerosis.[95] Often, ophthalmologists are the first to make the diagnosis of WS as cataracts develop early.[96] A feature that is not related to aging is a bird-like facies.

Complications: Although an increased incidence and early onset of cancer is related to aging, the 10:1 ratio between epithelial and mesenchymal cancer seen in a normally aging population is shifted to 1:1 in WS patients, with mostly thyroid epithelioid carcinomas, melanomas, meningiomas, soft-tissue sarcomas, hematologic neoplasias (mostly leukemias), and osteosarcomas.[97,98] As in the Japanese general population, most of the melanomas are of the acral-lentiginous type or arise from mucous membranes, and, consequently, are not considered to be related to UV exposure. Thyroid cancer occurs at a younger age in WS patients than in the Japanese general population.

ETIOLOGY AND PATHOGENESIS

WS is caused by a mutation in *WRN*, which encodes a RecQ helicase.[7,99,100] Most mutations of *WRN* result in truncation of the protein, sometimes by only a small amount, with loss of the nuclear targeting sequence. WRN is involved in many processes of DNA metabolism and *WRN* mutations cause various defects in DNA replication, recombination, base excision repair of oxidative DNA damage, repair of DNA strand breaks, DNA damage signaling, telomere maintenance, and transcription.[88] Cells from WS patients have a reduced replicative life span in culture[101] and show altered telomere structure and accelerated telomere attrition. Genome instability in WS cells is shown by an increased frequency of nonhomologous chromosome exchanges and of large chromosomal deletions.

Atypical Werner syndrome is a term used for patients in whom WS is suspected, but who do not carry *WRN* mutations. Several candidate genes have been identified.[93]

DIAGNOSIS

For the most recent listing of CLIA-certified laboratories offering diagnostic testing, including sequencing of the *WRN* gene, see https://www.cms.gov/Regulations-and-Guidance/Legislation/CLIA/Laboratory_Registry.htmlgenetests.org.

DIFFERENTIAL DIAGNOSIS

Table 130-1 outlines the clinical features of hereditary disorders of genome instability and DNA repair needed for the differential diagnosis. In addition, there are other hereditary conditions with premature aging, including, eg, Hutchinson-Gilford Progeria.

CLINICAL COURSE AND PROGNOSIS

Death from either myocardial infarction or cancer usually occurs before the age of 50 years.

MANAGEMENT

There is no specific treatment for WS. Early monitoring for the development of cancers, management of heart disease, and avoidance of risk factors for cardiovascular disease is recommended. Several pharmacologic interventions (mammalian target of rapamycin inhibitors, p38 mitogen-activated protein kinase inhibitors, and vitamin C) and stem cell-based treatments have been explored to alleviate the phenotypes of WS, but none of these have been studied in clinical applications.[93,102]

ROTHMUND-THOMSON SYNDROME

AT-A-GLANCE

- Rothmund-Thomson syndrome (RTS) is a rare chromosomal instability syndrome with an increased cancer risk and a typical poikiloderma that starts on the face during infancy.
- In two-thirds of patients, RTS is caused by a mutation in the DNA helicase RecQL4.
- Cells demonstrate impaired DNA metabolism and chromosomal instability.
- No specific treatment is available. Photoprotection is important.

RTS is a rare autosomal recessive disorder characterized by a hallmark poikiloderma, photosensitivity, short stature, bone abnormalities, and an increased risk for cancer.

EPIDEMIOLOGY

Approximately 400 patients worldwide have been described, but many may have been overlooked owing to the highly variable clinical presentations.

CLINICAL FEATURES

Cutaneous Findings: The hallmark of RTS is poikiloderma with variegated cutaneous pigmentation, atrophy, and telangiectasias beginning in infancy on the face, later spreading to the extremities and buttocks.[103-105,119] RTS patients are photosensitive and develop prominent erythema and facial swelling upon sun exposure early in life, which may be accompanied by blister formation. They also often have sparse scalp hair, eyebrows, and eyelashes, and abnormal nails.

Noncutaneous Findings: Other clinical features include juvenile cataracts, stunted growth, dental and skeletal abnormalities including radial bone defects and osteopenia.

Complications: RTS patients have a predisposition for cancer, in particular for osteosarcomas (32% of patients). Five percent of RTS patients also develop squamous cell carcinomas of the skin and 2% develop basal cell carcinomas.

ETIOLOGY AND PATHOGENESIS

Mutations in the helicase RecQL4 have been identified in approximately 67% of patients with RTS.[104,106,107] The gene defects of the other 33% of RTS patients remain unknown. RTS patients without *RECQL4* mutations (RTS Type 1) may not have an increased risk for osteosarcoma.[108] Two other syndromes that share many of the features of RTS, except the poikiloderma, Rapadilino syndrome and Baller-Gerold syndrome, are also caused by *RECQL4* mutations, but are now considered part of the spectrum of RecQL4 diseases.[104]

Cells from RTS patients are characterized by chromosomal instability with trisomy, aneuploidy, and chromosomal rearrangements, suggesting a role of RecQL4 in maintaining chromosome stability.[109,119] The exact function of the RecQL4 helicase remains unclear,[100,104,110,111] but likely, similar to the RecQ helicases mutated in BS and WS, includes a variety of functions involving DNA metabolism, including DNA replication, homologous recombination, DNA damage repair, and maintenance of mitochondrial and telomeric DNA integrity.

DIAGNOSIS

See https://www.cms.gov/Regulations-and-Guidance/Legislation/CLIA/Laboratory_Registry.htmlgenetests.org for the most recent listing of CLIA-certified laboratories offering diagnostic testing, including sequencing of the *RECQL4* gene.

DIFFERENTIAL DIAGNOSIS

Table 130-1 outlines the clinical features of hereditary disorders of genome instability and DNA repair needed for the differential diagnosis. Myeloblastic syndrome in childhood can also be seen in Fanconi anemia and dyskeratosis congenita.

CLINICAL COURSE AND PROGNOSIS

Life expectancy is limited by cancer, but is normal in RTS patients without cancer.[111]

MANAGEMENT

There is no specific treatment for RTS. Photoprotection and regular skin checks to screen for skin cancers are recommended. The telangiectatic component of the poikiloderma can be ameliorated by photocoagulation with a pulsed-dye laser. There are various yet inconsistent reports of cellular and clinical hypersensitivity to ionizing radiation and chemotherapeutic agents,[110] which must be considered when using radiation or chemotherapy for cancer treatment.

FANCONI ANEMIA

AT-A-GLANCE

- Fanconi anemia (FA) is a rare, genetically heterogeneous condition with an increased risk for aplastic anemia and cancer.
- Proteins encoded by the FA genes act in a common DNA damage-recognition-and-repair pathway that mediates DNA recombination.
- Cells are characterized by a hypersensitivity to DNA crosslinking agents.
- Cutaneous findings include diffuse hyperpigmentations and other pigment abnormalities.
- Growth retardation and abnormalities of the limbs, heart, kidney, and nervous system.
- No specific treatment is available. Allogeneic hematopoietic stem cell transplantation is the treatment of choice for aplastic anemia/myelodysplastic syndrome and leukemia.

FA is an autosomal recessive or in the case of Fanconi anemia complementation group B X-linked disease characterized by progressive pancytopenia, growth retardation, various congenital abnormalities of the heart, kidney, and limbs, and a predisposition to cancer.[112,113]

EPIDEMIOLOGY

More than 1200 patients have been reported to the International Fanconi Anemia Registry. The estimated incidence is 1 in 200,000 to 1 in 400,000 persons, but higher in Afrikaners (1 in 22,000) and Ashkenazi Jews (1 in 30,000).

CLINICAL FEATURES

Cutaneous Findings: Cutaneous abnormalities are present in almost 80% of patients (Figs. 130-10A to D).[112,113,116] Hyperpigmentation is present from birth or early childhood and is diffuse and accentuated over the neck, joints, and trunk. Café-au-lait spots and achromic lesions are also present.

Noncutaneous Findings: Hematopoietic manifestations usually have their onset before age 10 years and most commonly lead pediatricians to make the diagnosis of FA. These consist of a hypocellular bone marrow with progressive decrease in the number of circulating platelets, granulocytes, and erythrocytes. Skeletal malformations are common and often include aplasia or hypoplasia of the thumb, metacarpals, or radius.[112,113,115,116,117] Short stature, renal deformities, strabismus, microphthalmia, hypogonadism, and CNS abnormalities, including hyperreflexia and mild mental retardation, are also observed.

Complications: The frequency of acute myelogenous leukemia has been reported to be elevated 500-fold.[117,118,120,121] If patients survive aplastic anemia and/or leukemia (eg, as a result of bone marrow transplantation), they often develop solid tumors by the fifth decade of life, mostly squamous cell carcinomas of the head and neck and the anogenital area.

ETIOLOGY AND PATHOGENESIS

FA is genetically heterogeneous with 19 complementation groups (FANCA to FANCT). All 19 genes have been identified and all of the FA proteins have been shown to act in a common DNA damage recognition and repair pathway, which also involves *BRCA1* and *BRCA2* (These genes are mutated in hereditary breast cancer; *BRCA2* is identical to *FANCD1* and annotated as such) and multiple other proteins involved in cellular DNA damage responses.[122-135] Activation of this FA/BRCA pathway is thought to mediate DNA recombination to repair DNA strand breaks and DNA crosslinks, generated, for example, by ionizing radiation or DNA crosslinking agents, and to facilitate resolution of stalled replication forks.

DIAGNOSIS

Increased chromosome breakage after exposure to DNA crosslinking agents such as mitomycin C or diepoxybutane is a feature of FA. Central to the FA/BRCA pathway is the monoubiquitination of the FANCD2 protein. The inability of FA cells to ubiquitinate the FANCD2 protein, as shown in Western blots after, for example, exposure to DNA crosslinking agents, is currently used as a screening tool to confirm the diagnosis of FA. Diagnostic testing, including DNA sequencing for FA is offered in a number of laboratories that are CLIA-certified for clinical testing (see https://www.cms.gov/Regulations-and-Guidance/Legislation/CLIA/Laboratory_Registry.htmlgenetests.org for the most recent listing).

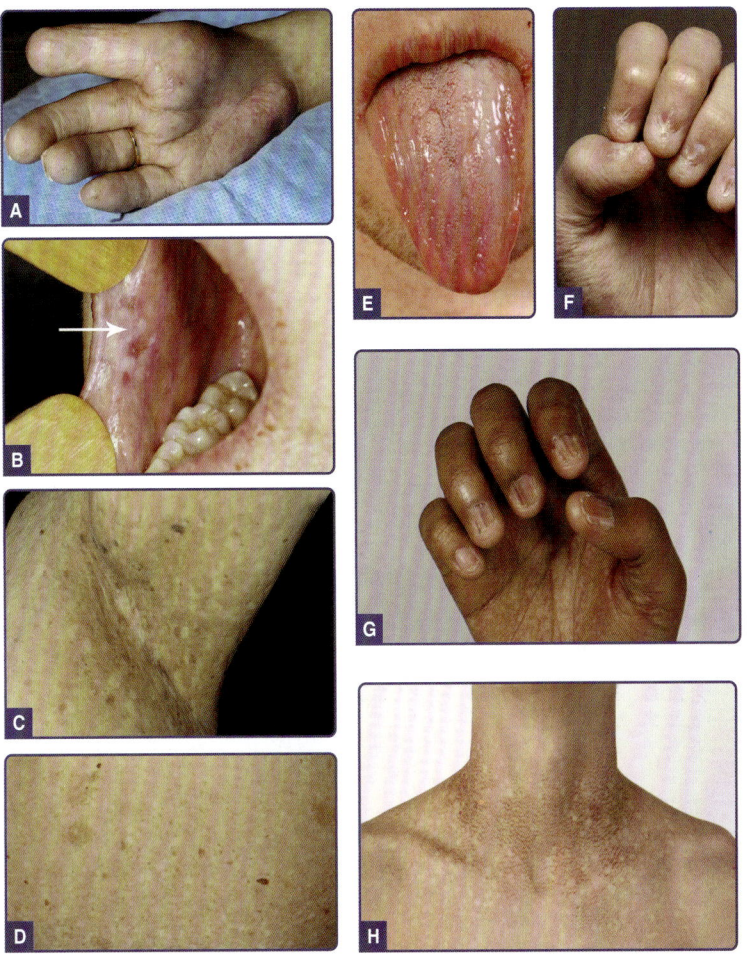

Figure 130-10 Skin and oral mucous membrane findings in Fanconi anemia (**A** to **D**) and dyskeratosis congenita (**E** to **H**). **A** to **D,** Fanconi anemia. **A,** Congenital absence of thumb. The second finger has been surgically altered to function as a thumb. Keratotic papules are present on the palm. **B,** Oral leukoplakia on right buccal mucosa (*arrow*). **C** and **D,** Dyspigmentation of Fanconi anemia. **C,** Hyperpigmentation of left axilla with discrete hyperpigmented and hypopigmented macules. **D,** Several irregular café-au-lait macules, smaller, fine, tanned, hyperpigmented macules, and dozens of guttate hypopigmented macules in the lower back. **E** to **H,** Dyskeratosis congenita. **E,** Oral leukoplakia involving the tongue. **F,** Severe atrophy of all fingernails and thickening of the palm. **G,** Longitudinal ridging and dystrophy of several fingernails with dyspigmentation and thickening of the palm. **H,** Poikiloderma showing reticular hypopigmentation and hyperpigmentation of the skin of the neck and chest. (Images **A-D,** Modified from Braun M, Giri N, Alter BP, et al. Thrombocytopenia, multiple mucosal squamous cell carcinomas, and dyspigmentation. *J Am Acad Dermatol* 2006;54:1056. Copyright © American Academy of Dermatology; Images **E-H,** Used with permission from Dr. Blanche Alter, NCI, Bethesda, MD.)

DIFFERENTIAL DIAGNOSIS

Table 130-1 outlines the clinical features of hereditary disorders of genome instability and DNA repair needed for the differential diagnosis.

CLINICAL COURSE AND PROGNOSIS

Life span is limited mostly by the associated malignancies.

MANAGEMENT

There is no specific treatment for FA, and patients should be followed by a multispecialty team of pediatricians, oncologists, dentists, and medical geneticists. Allogeneic hematopoietic stem cell transplantation is the treatment of choice for aplastic anemia/myelodysplastic syndrome and leukemia. Specific protocols have been developed to take into account the cellular hypersensitivities to DNA damaging chemotherapeutic agents in FA. Patients, physicians, and researchers may obtain information from the Fanconi Anemia

Research Fund, Inc. (http://www.fanconi.org) or from Fanconi Canada (http://www.fanconicanada.org).

DYSKERATOSIS CONGENITA

AT-A-GLANCE

- Dyskeratosis congenita is a rare telomere instability syndrome with an increased risk for pancytopenia, myelodysplasia, and acute myeloid leukemia.
- Dyskeratosis congenita is caused by a mutation in one of several telomere biology genes.
- Cells demonstrate shortened telomeres.
- Patients commonly present with a triad of reticulated hyperpigmentation, dystrophic nails, and mucosal leukoplakia.
- No specific treatment is available. Allogeneic hematopoietic stem cell transplantation is the treatment of choice for bone marrow failure and leukemia.

Dyskeratosis congenita, the Zinsser-Cole-Engman syndrome, is an X-linked multisystem disease with cutaneous, mucosal, ocular, GI, and hematologic abnormalities, and an increased incidence of cancer. There are also autosomal dominant and autosomal recessive forms. There is a broad phenotypic heterogeneity. Hoyeraal-Hreidarsson syndrome and Revesz syndrome are severe variants on the spectrum of telomere biology disorders. Less-severe variants with isolated manifestations, such as pulmonary fibrosis of myelodysplastic syndrome, also have been described.

EPIDEMIOLOGY

A registry at Hammersmith Hospital in London recruited 228 families having 354 affected patients from 40 countries.[136] More than 500 patients have been reported in the literature and the estimated incidence is 1 in 1 million persons.[137] Affected females may have either the autosomal dominant or autosomal recessive form.

CLINICAL FEATURES

Cutaneous Findings: The most common features are a triad of reticulated hyperpigmentation, dystrophic nails, and mucosal leukoplakia (see Fig. 130-10E to H).[138-141] During the first decade of life, patients develop reticulated poikiloderma in sun-exposed areas, with hyperpigmentation and, occasionally, bullae. Nail dystrophy is present in most patients beginning at approximately age 2 to 5 years. The nails initially split easily, then develop longitudinal ridging with irregular free edges. Eventually, the nails become smaller, resulting in only rudiments remaining. The fingernails are usually involved before the toenails. Other skin abnormalities include atrophic, wrinkled skin over the dorsum of hands and feet and hyperhidrosis and hyperkeratosis of palms and soles with disappearance of dermal ridges (absence of fingerprints).

Leukoplakia may be present in any mucosal site. The oral mucosa is the most frequent site, but leukoplakia is also found in the urethra, glans penis, vagina, and rectum. Lingual hyperkeratosis may be present.

Noncutaneous Findings: Approximately 50% of patients develop pancytopenia before the age of 10 years with a hematologic picture similar to FA. There is also a predisposition to both myelodysplasia and acute myeloid leukemia.[139,140]

Mucosal surfaces, such as the esophagus, urethra, and lacrimal duct, may become constricted and stenotic, resulting in dysphagia, dysuria, and epiphora. Multiple dental caries and early loss of teeth are common. Progressive pulmonary disease, including infections and fibrosis (and cirrhosis in some patients), was reported in 19% of affected males.[139] Approximately 20% of the patients had learning difficulties or mental retardation.[139] There are several reports of intracranial calcifications, especially of the basal ganglia,[142,143] similar to those seen in CS.

Complications: The majority (93%) of patients have been reported to develop bone marrow failure as the main cause (71%) of early death.[139,140] There is also an increased incidence of solid tumors, particularly squamous cell carcinoma of the mouth, rectum, cervix, vagina, esophagus, and skin. A large British kindred had Hodgkin disease and adenocarcinoma of the pancreas.[144]

ETIOLOGY AND PATHOGENESIS

Dyskeratosis congenita is caused by germline mutations in one of several telomere biology genes. *DKC1* is located on the q28 region of the X chromosome.[136,145-149] It encodes the protein dyskerin, which has a nucleolar function and a role in telomere maintenance and aging.[150-154] There is also evidence for an autosomal form with affected females[136,139,155,156] having mutations in the *TERC* gene, which is also involved in telomere function. Approximately 70% of the dyskeratosis congenita patients have a mutation in *DKC1*, *TERC*, or another gene involved in telomere biology (eg, *TERT*, *TINF2*, *NOLA2*, *NOLA3*, *NOP10*, *NHP2*, *WRAP53*, *CTC1*, *RTEL1*, *ACD*, and *PARN*). Many dyskeratosis congenita patients have very short telomeres and their telomere lengths decline with age. The shortest telomeres are associated with severe dyskeratosis congenita variants.[157]

DIAGNOSIS

Short telomere length is a typical finding in dyskeratosis congenita and used for diagnosis.[157] Testing for dyskeratosis congenita, including DNA sequencing, is offered in a number of laboratories that are CLIA-certified for clinical testing (see https://www.cms.gov/Regulations-and-Guidance/Legislation/CLIA/Laboratory_Registry.htmlgenetests.org for the most recent listing).

DIFFERENTIAL DIAGNOSIS

Table 130-1 outlines the clinical features of hereditary disorders of genome instability and DNA repair needed for the differential diagnosis.

CLINICAL COURSE AND PROGNOSIS

Life span is limited by bone marrow failure, myelodysplastic syndrome, and malignancies.

MANAGEMENT

There is no specific treatment of dyskeratosis congenita. Allogeneic hematopoietic stem cell transplantation is the treatment of choice for bone marrow failure and leukemia.[158] Lung transplantation may be considered for pulmonary fibrosis.

REFERENCES

1. Bielas JH, Loeb LA, Bielas JH, et al. Mutator phenotype in cancer: timing and perspectives. *Environ Mol Mutagen*. 2005;45:206-213.
2. Hoeijmakers JH. Genome maintenance mechanisms for preventing cancer. *Nature*. 2001;411:366-374.
3. Loeb LA. Cancer cells exhibit a mutator phenotype. *Adv Cancer Res*. 1998;72:25-56.
4. Mohrenweiser HW, Wilson DM 3rd, Jones IM,. Challenges and complexities in estimating both the functional impact and the disease risk associated with the extensive genetic variation in human DNA repair genes. *Mutat Res*. 2003;526:93-125.
5. Renwick A, Thompson D, Seal S, et al. ATM mutations that cause ataxia-telangiectasia are breast cancer susceptibility alleles. *Nat Genet*. 2006;38:873-875.
6. Su Y, Swift M. Mortality rates among carriers of ataxia-telangiectasia mutant alleles. *Ann Intern Med*. 2000;133:770-778.
7. Hickson ID. RecQ helicases: caretakers of the genome. *Nat Rev Cancer*. 2003;3:169-178.
8. Opresko PL, Cheng WH, Bohr VA. Junction of RecQ helicase biochemistry and human disease. *J Biol Chem*. 2004;279:18099-18102.
9. Harrigan JA, Bohr VA. Human diseases deficient in RecQ helicases. *Biochimie*. 2003;85:1185-1193.
10. Aubert G, Lansdorp PM. Telomeres and aging. *Physiol Rev*. 2008;88:557-579.
11. Savage SA, Alter BP. Dyskeratosis congenita. *Hematol Oncol Clin North Am*. 2009;23:215-231.
12. Wang Y, Cortez D, Yazdi P, et al. BASC, a super complex of BRCA1-associated proteins involved in the recognition and repair of aberrant DNA structures. *Genes Dev*. 2000;14:927-939.
13. DiGiovanna JJ, Kraemer KH. Shining a light on xeroderma pigmentosum. *J Invest Dermatol*. 2012;132:785-796.
14. Kraemer KH, Lee MM, Scotto J. Xeroderma pigmentosum. Cutaneous, ocular, and neurologic abnormalities in 830 published cases. *Arch Dermatol*. 1987;123:241-250.
15. Cleaver JE. Defective repair replication of DNA in xeroderma pigmentosum. *Nature*. 1968;218:652-656.
16. Kleijer WJ, Laugel V, Berneburg M, et al. Incidence of DNA repair deficiency disorders in Western Europe: Xeroderma pigmentosum, Cockayne syndrome and trichothiodystrophy. *DNA Repair (Amst)*. 2008;7:744-750.
17. Hirai Y, Kodama Y, Moriwaki S, et al. Heterozygous individuals bearing a founder mutation in the XPA DNA repair gene comprise nearly 1% of the Japanese population. *Mutat Res*. 2006;601:171-178.
18. Bradford PT, Goldstein AM, Tamura D, et al. Cancer and neurologic degeneration in xeroderma pigmentosum: long term follow-up characterises the role of DNA repair. *J Med Genet*. 2011;48:168-176.
19. Fassihi H, Sethi M, Fawcett H, et al. Deep phenotyping of 89 xeroderma pigmentosum patients reveals unexpected heterogeneity dependent on the precise molecular defect. *Proc Natl Acad Sci U S A*. 2016;113:E1236-E1245.
20. Brooks BP, Thompson AH, Bishop RJ, et al. Ocular manifestations of xeroderma pigmentosum: long-term follow-up highlights the role of DNA repair in protection from sun damage. *Ophthalmology*. 2013;120:1324-1336.
21. Totonchy MB, Tamura D, Pantell MS, et al. Auditory analysis of xeroderma pigmentosum 1971-2012: hearing function, sun sensitivity and DNA repair predict neurological degeneration. *Brain*. 2013;136:194-208.
22. Kraemer KH, Patronas NJ, Schiffmann R, et al. Xeroderma pigmentosum, trichothiodystrophy and Cockayne syndrome: a complex genotype-phenotype relationship. *Neuroscience*. 2007;145:1388-1396.
23. Lai JP, Liu YC, Alimchandani M, et al. The influence of DNA repair on neurological degeneration, cachexia, skin cancer and internal neoplasms: autopsy report of four xeroderma pigmentosum patients (XP-A, XP-C and XP-D). *Acta Neuropathol Commun*. 2013;1:4.
24. Kraemer KH, Lee MM, Scotto J. DNA repair protects against cutaneous and internal neoplasia: evidence from xeroderma pigmentosum. *Carcinogenesis*. 1984;5:511-514.
25. Kraemer KH, Lee MM, Andrews AD, et al. The role of sunlight and DNA repair in melanoma and nonmelanoma skin cancer. The xeroderma pigmentosum paradigm. *Arch Dermatol*. 1994;130:1018-1021.
26. Oh KS, Khan SG, Jaspers NG, et al. Phenotypic heterogeneity in the XPB DNA helicase gene (ERCC3): xeroderma pigmentosum without and with Cockayne syndrome. *Hum Mutat*. 2006;27:1092-1103.
27. Khan SG, Metin A, Gozukara E, et al. Two essential splice lariat branchpoint sequences in one intron in a xeroderma pigmentosum DNA repair gene: mutations result in reduced XPC mRNA levels that correlate with cancer risk. *Hum Mol Genet*. 2004;13:343-352.

28. Khan SG, Oh KS, Emmert S, et al. XPC initiation codon mutation in xeroderma pigmentosum patients with and without neurological symptoms. *DNA Repair (Amst)*. 2009;8:114-125.
29. Boyle J, Ueda T, Oh KS, et al. Persistence of repair proteins at unrepaired DNA damage distinguishes diseases with ERCC2 (XPD) mutations: cancer-prone xeroderma pigmentosum vs. non-cancer-prone trichothiodystrophy. *Hum Mutat*. 2008;29:1194-1208.
30. Oh KS, Emmert S, Tamura D, et al. Multiple skin cancers in adults with mutations in the XP-E (DDB2) DNA repair gene. *J Invest Dermatol*. 2011;131:785-788.
31. Emmert S, Slor H, Busch DB, et al. Relationship of neurologic degeneration to genotype in three xeroderma pigmentosum group G patients. *J Invest Dermatol*. 2002;118:972-982.
32. Inui H, Oh KS, Nadem C, et al. Xeroderma pigmentosum-variant patients from America, Europe, and Asia. *J Invest Dermatol*. 2008;128:2055-2068.
33. Reid-Bayliss KS, Arron ST, Loeb LA, et al. Why Cockayne syndrome patients do not get cancer despite their DNA repair deficiency. *Proc Natl Acad Sci U S A*. 2016;113:10151-10156.
34. Correa R, Salpea P, Stratakis CA. Carney complex: an update. *Eur J Endocrinol*. 2015;173:M85-M97.
35. Slor H, Batko S, Khan SG, et al. Clinical, cellular, and molecular features of an Israeli xeroderma pigmentosum family with a frameshift mutation in the XPC gene: sun protection prolongs life. *J Invest Dermatol*. 2000;115:974-980.
36. Tamura D, DiGiovanna JJ, Khan SG, et al. Living with xeroderma pigmentosum: comprehensive photoprotection for highly photosensitive patients. *Photodermatol Photoimmunol Photomed*. 2014;30:146-152.
37. Kraemer KH, DiGiovanna JJ, Moshell AN, et al. Prevention of skin cancer in xeroderma pigmentosum with the use of oral isotretinoin. *N Engl J Med*. 1988;318:1633-1637.
38. Yarosh D, Klein J, O'Conner A, et al. Effect of topically applied T4 endonuclease V in liposomes on skin cancer in xeroderma pigmentosum: a randomized study. *Lancet*. 2001;357:926-929.
39. Turner ML, Moshell AN, Corbett DW, et al. Clearing of melanoma in situ with intralesional interferon alfa in a patient with xeroderma pigmentosum. *Arch Dermatol*. 1994;130:1491-1494.
40. Sollitto RB, Kraemer KH, DiGiovanna JJ. Normal vitamin D levels can be maintained despite rigorous photoprotection: six years' experience with xeroderma pigmentosum. *J Am Acad Dermatol*. 1997;37:942-947.
41. Ali JT, Mukasa Y, Coulson IH. Xeroderma pigmentosum: early diagnostic features and an adverse consequence of photoprotection. *Clin Exp Dermatol*. 2009;34:442-443.
42. Reichrath J. Sunlight, skin cancer and vitamin D: what are the conclusions of recent findings that protection against solar ultraviolet (UV) radiation causes 25-hydroxyvitamin D deficiency in solid organ-transplant recipients, xeroderma pigmentosum, and other risk groups? *J Steroid Biochem Mol Biol*. 2007;103:664-667.
43. Khan SG, Oh KS, Shahlavi T, et al. Reduced XPC DNA repair gene mRNA levels in clinically normal parents of xeroderma pigmentosum patients. *Carcinogenesis*. 2006;27:84-94.
44. Cockayne EA. Dwarfism with retinal atrophy and deafness. *Arch Dis Child*. 1936;11:1-8.
45. Rapin I. Disorders of nucleotide excision repair. *Handb Clin Neurol*. 2013;113:1637-1650.
46. Nance MA, Berry SA. Cockayne syndrome: review of 140 cases. *Am J Med Genet*. 1992;42:68-84.
47. Kubota M, Ohta S, Ando A, et al. Nationwide survey of Cockayne syndrome in Japan: incidence, clinical course and prognosis. *Pediatr Int*. 2015;57:339-347.
48. Wilson BT, Stark Z, Sutton RE, et al. The Cockayne Syndrome Natural History (CoSyNH) study: clinical findings in 102 individuals and recommendations for care. *Genet Med*. 2016;18:483-493.
49. Frouin E, Laugel V, Durand M, et al. Dermatologic findings in 16 patients with Cockayne syndrome and cerebro-oculo-facial-skeletal syndrome. *JAMA Dermatol*. 2013;149:1414-1418.
50. Trese MG, Nudleman ED, Besirli CG. Peripheral retinal vasculopathy in Cockayne syndrome. *Retin Cases Brief Rep*. 2017;11(3):232-235.
51. Laugel V. Cockayne syndrome: the expanding clinical and mutational spectrum. *Mech Ageing Dev*. 2013;134:161-170.
52. Gitiaux C, Blin-Rochemaure N, Hully M, et al. Progressive demyelinating neuropathy correlates with clinical severity in Cockayne syndrome. *Clin Neurophysiol*. 2015;126:1435-1439.
53. Koob M, Rousseau F, Laugel V, et al. Cockayne syndrome: a diffusion tensor imaging and volumetric study. *Br J Radiol*. 2016;89:20151033.
54. Laugel V. Cockayne syndrome. In: Adam MP, Ardinger HH, Pagon RA, et al, eds. GeneReviews [Internet]. Seattle, WA: University of Washington; 1993-2018 [December 28, 2000; updated June 14, 2012]. https://www.ncbi.nlm.nih.gov/books/NBK1342/#cockayne.Summary
55. Graham JM Jr, Hennekam R, Dobyns WB, et al. MICRO syndrome: an entity distinct from COFS syndrome. *Am J Med Genet A*. 2004;128A:235-245.
56. Wilson BT, Strong A, O'Kelly S, et al. Metronidazole toxicity in Cockayne syndrome: a case series. *Pediatrics*. 2015;136:e706-e708.
57. Lindenbaum Y, Dickson D, Rosenbaum P, et al. Xeroderma pigmentosum/Cockayne syndrome complex: first neuropathological study and review of eight other cases. *Eur J Paediatr Neurol*. 2001;5:225-242.
58. Rapin I, Lindenbaum Y, Dickson DW, et al. Cockayne syndrome and xeroderma pigmentosum. *Neurology*. 2000;55:1442-1449.
59. Tay CH. Ichthyosiform erythroderma, hair shaft abnormalities, and mental and growth retardation. A new recessive disorder. *Arch Dermatol*. 1971;104:4-13.
60. Price VH, Odom RB, Ward WH, et al. Trichothiodystrophy: sulfur-deficient brittle hair as a marker for a neuroectodermal symptom complex. *Arch Dermatol*. 1980;116:1375-1384.
61. Lehmann AR, Francis AJ, Giannelli F. Prenatal diagnosis of Cockayne's syndrome. *Lancet*. 1985;1:486-488.
62. Itin PH, Sarasin A, Pittelkow MR. Trichothiodystrophy: update on the sulfur-deficient brittle hair syndromes. *J Am Acad Dermatol*. 2001;44:891-920; quiz 921-924.
63. Liang C, Kraemer KH, Morris A, et al. Characterization of tiger-tail banding and hair shaft abnormalities in trichothiodystrophy. *J Am Acad Dermatol*. 2005;52:224-232.
64. Liang C, Morris A, Schlucker S, et al. Structural and molecular hair abnormalities in trichothiodystrophy. *J Invest Dermatol*. 2006;126:2210-2216.
65. Schlucker S, Liang C, Strehle KR, et al. Conformational differences in protein disulfide linkages between

normal hair and hair from subjects with trichothiodystrophy: a quantitative analysis by Raman microspectroscopy. *Biopolymers*. 2006;82:615-622.
66. Faghri S, Tamura D, Kraemer KH, et al. Trichothiodystrophy: a systematic review of 112 published cases characterises a wide spectrum of clinical manifestations. *J Med Genet*. 2008;45:609-621.
67. Laugel V, Dalloz C, Durand M, et al. Mutation update for the CSB/ERCC6 and CSA/ERCC8 genes involved in Cockayne syndrome. *Hum Mutat*. 2010;31:113-126.
68. Brooks BP, Thompson AH, Clayton JA, et al. Ocular manifestations of trichothiodystrophy. *Ophthalmology*. 2011;118:2335-2342.
69. Corbett MA, Dudding-Byth T, Crock PA, et al. A novel X-linked trichothiodystrophy associated with a nonsense mutation in RNF113A. *J Med Genet*. 2015;52:269-274.
70. Pollitt RJ, Jenner FA, Davies M. Sibs with mental and physical retardation and trichorrhexis nodosa with abnormal amino acid composition of the hair. *Arch Dis Child*. 1968;43:211-216.
71. Baden HP, Jackson CE, Weiss L, et al. The physicochemical properties of hair in the BIDS syndrome. *Am J Hum Genet*. 1976;28:514-521.
72. Zhou X, Khan SG, Tamura D, et al. Brittle hair, developmental delay, neurologic abnormalities, and photosensitivity in a 4-year-old girl. *J Am Acad Dermatol*. 2010;63:323-328.
73. Ostergaard JR, Christensen T. The central nervous system in Tay syndrome. *Neuropediatrics*. 1996;27:326-330.
74. Kuschal C, Botta E, Orioli D, et al. GTF2E2 mutations destabilize the general transcription factor complex TFIIE in individuals with DNA repair-proficient trichothiodystrophy. *Am J Hum Genet*. 2016;98:627-642.
75. Nakabayashi K, Amann D, Ren Y, et al. Identification of C7orf11 (TTDN1) gene mutations and genetic heterogeneity in nonphotosensitive trichothiodystrophy. *Am J Hum Genet*. 2005;76:510-516.
76. Dubaele S, Proietti De Santis L, Bienstock RJ, et al. Basal transcription defect discriminates between xeroderma pigmentosum and trichothiodystrophy in XPD patients. *Mol Cell*. 2003;11:1635-1646.
77. Moslehi R, Signore C, Tamura D, et al. Adverse effects of trichothiodystrophy DNA repair and transcription gene disorder on human fetal development. *Clin Genet*. 2010;77:365-373.
78. Tamura D, Merideth M, DiGiovanna JJ, et al. High-risk pregnancy and neonatal complications in the DNA repair and transcription disorder trichothiodystrophy: report of 27 affected pregnancies. *Prenat Diagn*. 2011;31:1046-1053.
79. Heller ER, Khan SG, Kuschal C, et al. Mutations in the TTDN1 gene are associated with a distinct trichothiodystrophy phenotype. *J Invest Dermatol*. 2015;135:734-741.
80. Atkinson EC, Thiara D, Tamura D, et al. Growth and nutrition in children with trichothiodystrophy. *J Pediatr Gastroenterol Nutr*. 2014;59:458-464.
81. Tamura D, Khan SG, Merideth M, et al. Effect of mutations in XPD(ERCC2) on pregnancy and prenatal development in mothers of patients with trichothiodystrophy or xeroderma pigmentosum. *Eur J Hum Genet*. 2012;20:1308-1310.
82. German J. Bloom's syndrome. XX. The first 100 cancers. *Cancer Genet Cytogenet*. 1997;93:100-106.
83. Shahrabani-Gargir L, Shomrat R, Yaron Y, et al. High frequency of a common Bloom syndrome Ashkenazi mutation among Jews of Polish origin. *Genet Test*. 1998;2:293-296.
84. Singh DK, Ahn B, Bohr VA. Roles of RECQ helicases in recombination based DNA repair, genomic stability and aging. *Biogerontology*. 2009;10:235-252.
85. Thompson LH, Schild D. Recombinational DNA repair and human disease. *Mutat Res*. 2002;509:49-78.
86. Panneerselvam J, Wang H, Zhang J, et al. BLM promotes the activation of Fanconi anemia signaling pathway. *Oncotarget*. 2016;7:32351-32361.
87. Drosopoulos WC, Kosiyatrakul ST, Schildkraut CL. BLM helicase facilitates telomere replication during leading strand synthesis of telomeres. *J Cell Biol*. 2015;210:191-208.
88. Kong CM, Lee XW, Wang X. Telomere shortening in human diseases. *FEBS J*. 2013;280:3180-3193.
89. Zimmermann M, Kibe T, Kabir S, et al. TRF1 negotiates TTAGGG repeat-associated replication problems by recruiting the BLM helicase and the TPP1/POT1 repressor of ATR signaling. *Genes Dev*. 2014;28:2477-2491.
90. Chaganti RS, Schonberg S, German J. A manyfold increase in sister chromatid exchanges in Bloom's syndrome lymphocytes. *Proc Natl Acad Sci U S A*. 1974;7:4508-4512.
91. Peleg L, Pesso R, Goldman B, et al. Bloom syndrome and Fanconi's anemia: rate and ethnic origin of mutation carriers in Israel. *Isr Med Assoc J*. 2002;4:95-97.
92. Khan SG, Levy HL, Legerski R, et al. Xeroderma pigmentosum group C splice mutation associated with autism and hypoglycinemia. *J Invest Dermatol*. 1998;115:791-796.
93. Oshima J, Sidorova JM, Monnat RJ Jr. Werner syndrome: clinical features, pathogenesis and potential therapeutic interventions. *Ageing Res Rev*. 2017;33:105-114.
94. Ishikawa Y, Sugano H, Matsumoto T, et al. Unusual features of thyroid carcinomas in Japanese patients with Werner syndrome and possible genotype-phenotype relations to cell type and race. *Cancer*. 1999;85:1345-1352.
95. Epstein CE, Martin GM, Schultz AL, et al. Werner syndrome. A review of its symptomatology, natural history, pathologic features, genetics and relationship to the natural aging process. *Medicine (Baltimore)*. 1966;45:177-221.
96. Ruprecht KW. Ophthalmological aspects in patients with Werner's syndrome. *Arch Gerontol Geriatr*. 1989;9:263-270.
97. Goto M, Miller RW, Ishikawa Y, et al. Excess of rare cancers in Werner syndrome (adult progeria). *Cancer Epidemiol Biomarkers Prev*. 1996;5:239-246.
98. Monnat RJ Jr. "...Rewritten in the skin": clues to skin biology and aging from inherited disease. *J Invest Dermatol*. 2015;135:1484-1490.
99. Chen L, Huang S, Lee L, et al. WRN, the protein deficient in Werner syndrome, plays a critical structural role in optimizing DNA repair. *Aging Cell*. 2003;2:191-199.
100. Opresko PL, Cheng WH, von KC, et al. Werner syndrome and the function of the Werner protein; what they can teach us about the molecular aging process. *Carcinogenesis*. 2003;24:791-802.
101. Morita K, Nishigori C, Sasaki MS, et al. Werner's syndrome—chromosome analyses of cultured fibroblasts and mitogen-stimulated lymphocytes. *Br J Dermatol*. 1997;136:620-623.
102. Li Y, Zhang W, Chang L, et al. Vitamin C alleviates aging defects in a stem cell model for Werner syndrome.

Protein Cell. 2016;7:478-488.
103. Larizza L, Roversi G, Volpi L. Rothmund-Thomson syndrome. *Orphanet J Rare Dis.* 2010;5:2.
104. Lu L, Jin W, Wang LL. Aging in Rothmund-Thomson syndrome and related RECQL4 genetic disorders. *Ageing Res Rev.* 2017;33:30-35.
105. Wang LL, Levy ML, Lewis RA, et al. Clinical manifestations in a cohort of 41 Rothmund-Thomson syndrome patients. *Am J Med Genet.* 2001;102:11-17.
106. Kitao S, Shimamoto A, Goto M, et al. Mutations in RECQL4 cause a subset of cases of Rothmund-Thomson syndrome. *Nat Genet.* 1999;22:82-84.
107. Suter AA, Itin P, Heinimann K, et al. Rothmund-Thomson Syndrome: novel pathogenic mutations and frequencies of variants in the RECQL4 and USB1 (C16orf57) gene. *Mol Genet Genomic Med.* 2016;4:359-366.
108. Wang LL, Gannavarapu A, Kozinetz CA, et al. Association between osteosarcoma and deleterious mutations in the RECQL4 gene in Rothmund-Thomson syndrome. *J Natl Cancer Inst.* 2003;95:669-674.
109. Smith PJ, Paterson MC. Enhanced radiosensitivity and defective DNA repair in cultured fibroblasts derived from Rothmund Thomson syndrome patients. *Mutat Res.* 1982;94:213-228.
110. Yin J, Kwon YT, Varshavsky A, et al. RECQL4, mutated in the Rothmund-Thomson and RAPADILINO syndromes, interacts with ubiquitin ligases UBR1 and UBR2 of the N-end rule pathway. *Hum Mol Genet.* 2004;13:2421-2430.
111. Croteau DL, Popuri V, Opresko PL, et al. Human RecQ helicases in DNA repair, recombination, and replication. *Annu Rev Biochem.* 2014;83:519-552.
112. Kutler DI, Singh B, Satagopan J, et al. A 20-year perspective on the International Fanconi Anemia Registry (IFAR). *Blood.* 2003;101:1249-1256.
113. Auerbach AD. Fanconi anemia. *Dermatol Clin.* 1995;13:41-49.
114. Saftig P, Hunziker E, Wehmeyer O, et al. Impaired osteoclastic bone resorption leads to osteopetrosis in cathepsin-K-deficient mice. *Proc Natl Acad Sci U S A.* 1998;95:13453-13458.
115. Shimamura A, Alter BP. Pathophysiology and management of inherited bone marrow failure syndromes. *Blood Rev.* 2010;24:101-122.
116. De Kerviler E, Guermazi A, Zagdanski AM, et al. The clinical and radiological features of Fanconi's anaemia. *Clin Radiol.* 2000;55:340-345.
117. Gmyrek D, Syllm-Rapoport I. On Fanconi's anemia. Analysis of 129 cases [in German]. *Z Kinderheilkd.* 1964;91:297-337.
118. Alter BP. Cancer in Fanconi anemia, 1927-2001 [see comment]. *Cancer.* 2003;97:425-440.
119. Kerr B, Ashcroft GS, Scott D, et al. Rothmund-Thomson syndrome: two case reports show heterogeneous cutaneous abnormalities, an association with genetically programmed ageing changes, and increased chromosomal radiosensitivity. *J Med Genet.* 1996;33:928-934.
120. Auerbach AD, Allen RG. Leukemia and preleukemia in Fanconi anemia patients. A review of the literature and report of the International Fanconi Anemia Registry. *Cancer Genet Cytogenet.* 1991;51:1-12.
121. Rosenberg PS, Greene MH, Alter BP. Cancer incidence in persons with Fanconi anemia [see comment]. *Blood.* 2003;101:822-826.
122. Bogliolo M, Cabre O, Callen E, et al. The Fanconi anaemia genome stability and tumour suppressor network. *Mutagenesis.* 2002;17:529-538.
123. Ceccaldi R, Sarangi P, D'Andrea AD. The Fanconi anaemia pathway: new players and new functions. *Nat Rev Mol Cell Biol.* 2016;17:337-349.
124. D'Andrea AD, Grompe M. The Fanconi anemia/BRCA pathway. *Nat Rev Cancer.* 2003;3:23-34.
125. Dong H, Nebert DW, Bruford EA, et al. Update of the human and mouse Fanconi anemia genes. *Hum Genomics.* 2015;9:32.
126. Dunn J, Potter M, Rees A, et al. Activation of the Fanconi anemia/BRCA pathway and recombination repair in the cellular response to solar UV. *Cancer Res.* 2006;66(23):11140-11147.
127. Garcia-Higuera I, Taniguchi T, Ganesan S, et al. Interaction of the Fanconi anemia proteins and BRCA1 in a common pathway. *Mol Cell.* 2001;7:249-262.
128. Howlett NG, Taniguchi T, Durkin SG, et al. The Fanconi anemia pathway is required for the DNA replication stress response and for the regulation of common fragile site stability. *Hum Mol Genet.* 2005;14:693-701.
129. Joenje H, Patel KJ. The emerging genetic and molecular basis of Fanconi anemia. *Nat Rev Genet.* 2001;2:446-457.
130. Lomonosov M, Anand S, Sangrithi M, et al. Stabilization of stalled DNA replication forks by the BRCA2 breast cancer susceptibility protein. *Genes Dev.* 2003;17:3017-3022.
131. Osborn AJ, Elledge SJ, Zou L. Checking on the fork: the DNA-replication stress-response pathway. *Trends Cell Biol.* 2002;12:509-516.
132. Taniguchi T, D'Andrea AD. Molecular pathogenesis of Fanconi anemia: recent progress. *Blood.* 2006;107:4223-4233.
133. Taniguchi T, Garcia-Higuera I, Xu B, et al. Convergence of the Fanconi anemia and ataxia telangiectasia signaling pathways. *Cell.* 2002;109:459-472.
134. Thompson LH, Hinz JM, Yamada NA, et al. How Fanconi anemia proteins promote the four Rs: replication, recombination, repair, and recovery. *Environ Mol Mutagen.* 2005;45:128-142.
135. Wang W. Emergence of a DNA-damage response network consisting of Fanconi anaemia and BRCA proteins. *Nat Rev Genet.* 2007;8:735-748.
136. Vulliamy TJ, Marrone A, Knight SW, et al. Mutations in dyskeratosis congenita: their impact on telomere length and the diversity of clinical presentation. *Blood.* 2006;107:2680-2685.
137. Alter BP, Giri N, Savage SA, et al. Cancer in dyskeratosis congenita. *Blood.* 2009;113:6549-6557.
138. Dokal I. Dyskeratosis congenita in all its forms. *Br J Haematol.* 2000;110:768-779.
139. Knight S, Vulliamy T, Copplestone A, et al. Dyskeratosis congenita (DC) registry: identification of new features of DC. *Br J Haematol.* 1998;103:990-996.
140. Savage SA. Dyskeratosis congenita. In: Adam MP, Ardinger HH, Pagon RA, et al, eds. GeneReviews [Internet]. Seattle, WA: University of Washington; 1993-2018 [November 12, 2009; updated May 26, 2016]. https://www.ncbi.nlm.nih.gov/books/NBK22301/#dkc.Summary
141. Sirinavin C, Trowbridge AA. Dyskeratosis congenita: clinical features and genetic aspects. Report of a family and review of the literature. *J Med Genet.* 1975;12:339-354.
142. Kelly TE, Stelling CB. Dyskeratosis congenita: radiologic features. *Pediatr Radiol.* 1982;12:31-36.
143. Mills SE, Cooper PH, Beacham BE, et al. Intracranial

calcifications and dyskeratosis congenita. *Arch Dermatol*. 1979;115:1437-1439.
144. Connor JM, Teague RH. Dyskeratosis congenita. Report of a large kindred. *Br J Dermatol*. 1981;105:321-325.
145. Hassock S, Vetrie D, Giannelli F. Mapping and characterization of the X-linked dyskeratosis congenita (DKC) gene. *Genomics*. 1999;55:21-27.
146. Dokal I, Bungey J, Williamson P, et al. Dyskeratosis congenita fibroblasts are abnormal and have unbalanced chromosomal rearrangements. *Blood*. 1992;80:3090-3096.
147. Heiss NS, Knight SW, Vulliamy TJ, et al. X-linked dyskeratosis congenita is caused by mutations in a highly conserved gene with putative nucleolar functions. *Nat Genet*. 1998;19:32-38.
148. Knight SW, Heiss NS, Vulliamy TJ, et al. X-linked dyskeratosis congenita is predominantly caused by missense mutations in the DKC1 gene. *Am J Hum Genet*. 1999;65:50-58.
149. Vulliamy TJ, Knight SW, Heiss NS, et al. Dyskeratosis congenita caused by a 3′ deletion: germline and somatic mosaicism in a female carrier. *Blood*. 1999;94:1254-1260.
150. Mitchell JR, Wood E, Collins K. A telomerase component is defective in the human disease dyskeratosis congenita. *Nature*. 1999;402:551-555.
151. Marciniak RA, Johnson FB, Guarente L. Dyskeratosis congenita, telomeres and human ageing. *Trends Genet*. 2000;16:193-195.
152. Vulliamy TJ, Knight SW, Mason PJ, et al. Very short telomeres in the peripheral blood of patients with X-linked and autosomal dyskeratosis congenita. *Blood Cells Mol Dis*. 2001;27:353-357.
153. Dokal I. Dyskeratosis congenita. A disease of premature ageing. *Lancet*. 2001;358(suppl):S27.
154. Collins K, Mitchell JR. Telomerase in the human organism. *Oncogene*. 2002;21:564-579.
155. Elliott AM, Graham GE, Bernstein M, et al. Dyskeratosis congenita: an autosomal recessive variant. *Am J Med Genet*. 1999;83:178-182.
156. Vulliamy T, Marrone A, Goldman F, et al. The RNA component of telomerase is mutated in autosomal dominant dyskeratosis congenita. *Nature*. 2001;413:432-435.
157. Alter BP, Rosenberg PS, Giri N, et al. Telomere length is associated with disease severity and declines with age in dyskeratosis congenita. *Haematologica*. 2012;97:353-359.
158. Ghavamzadeh A, Alimoghadam K, Nasseri P, et al. Correction of bone marrow failure in dyskeratosis congenita by bone marrow transplantation. *Bone Marrow Transplant*. 1999;23:299-301.

Chapter 131 :: Ectodermal Dysplasias
:: Elizabeth L. Nieman & Dorothy Katherine Grange

第一百三十一章
外胚层发育不良

中文导读

外胚层发育不良（EDS）是一组复杂的异质性的遗传性疾病，具有共同的发育缺陷，其共同的发育缺陷涉及至少2种典型的胚胎外胚层结构：头发、牙齿、指甲、汗液和其他外分泌腺和皮脂腺。

〔粟　娟〕

AT-A-GLANCE

- A group of inherited disorders characterized by developmental abnormalities in 2 or more ectodermal structures.
- These include hair, teeth, nails, and sebaceous and sweat glands.
- There may be abnormalities in nonectodermal structures and functions.
- Distinction is based on clinical features, mode of inheritance, and molecular/genetic findings.
- Clinically distinct disorders may be due to different mutations in the same gene (allelic heterogeneity), and clinically similar conditions may be due to mutations in different genes (locus heterogeneity).

INTRODUCTION

The ectodermal dysplasias (EDs) are a complex and heterogenous group of inherited disorders that share developmental defects involving at least 2 of the major structures classically known to derive from the embryonic ectoderm: hair, teeth, nails, and sweat and other eccrine and sebaceous glands. Developmental disorders involving only one type of ectodermal structure, even if associated with other congenital malformations, are not classified as EDs. There are almost 200 conditions classified as EDs, and given the varied clinical presentations and clinical overlap, it can be difficult to diagnose them precisely.[1]

Various classification schemes have been proposed over the past several decades to help in ordering and thinking about these disorders. Freire-Maia and Pinheiro published an exhaustive review and classification system, with later updates, for these disorders using a numeric system.[2] Although this system developed a rational approach to a previously chaotic field, it has little use in clinical practice and does not account for the pathogenesis or genetics of specific conditions. Over the past few decades, many of the genes responsible for these disorders have been identified, leading to several attempts to reclassify the EDs based on molecular and developmental biopsy. In 2008, an international ED classification conference consisting of health care providers, researchers, patient advocate representatives, and administrators convened in an attempt to move toward a more useful and unified system. In 2009, a conference report was released outlining the goal of creating an integrated ED classification system based on the most recent clinical and molecular information available.[3] Given the rate of discovery of new molecular information, this has been challenging. Thus, in 2012, a second international conference was held resulting in the development of a multi-axis model approach to EDs.[4] This model will be based on a clinical/phenotype axis, a gene-based axis, and a functional/pathways axis and is still in the process of creation.

This chapter will only cover the EDs that are more common and most likely to present to a dermatologist for diagnosis and medical attention. As much as possible, it will be organized in concordance with the ED international classification conference, limited by the complexities discussed above. Given the evolving landscape of EDs, the reader is directed to the following resources for the most current information on EDs: https://omim.org (Online Catalog of Mendelian Inheritance in Man) and http://www.ncbi.nlm.nih.gov/gtr/ (an up-to-date listing of laboratories offering molecular testing).

Figure 131-1 is an algorithm showing the clinical approach to the diagnosis of EDs. The first step in the algorithm for making a specific diagnosis of an ED is to determine the presence of sweating (hidrotic) or absence of sweating (hypohidrotic/anhidrotic). The involvement of other ectodermal structures and of non–ectodermal derived tissues provides further branching points in a diagnostic hierarchy. Mode of inheritance may differ within a seemingly uniform diagnostic group, and care must be taken in evaluating family members before providing genetic counseling.

The National Foundation for Ectodermal Dysplasias (NFED; http://www.nfed.org) is a lay support group that has numerous informative pamphlets for families and physicians, as well as a strong advocacy program for dental care, insurance coverage, and research. With the knowledge gained from studies on the molecular pathways leading to EDs, there is hope that molecular-based therapies will be able to treat or replace defective or missing teeth, hair follicles, or eccrine sweat glands.[5-7]

HYPOHIDROTIC ECTODERMAL DYSPLASIA: XLHED, ADHED, ARHED, HED-ID

INTRODUCTION

One of the earliest descriptions of hypohidrotic ectodermal dysplasia (HED) was in 1848, and involved male first cousins and their grandmother with sparse hair, missing teeth, and dry skin.[8] HED is the most common ED,[9] specifically the X-linked recessive (XLHED) form of HED, and accounts for 80% of the families registered with NFED. There are several forms of HED, including XLHED (also known as Christ–Siemens–Touraine

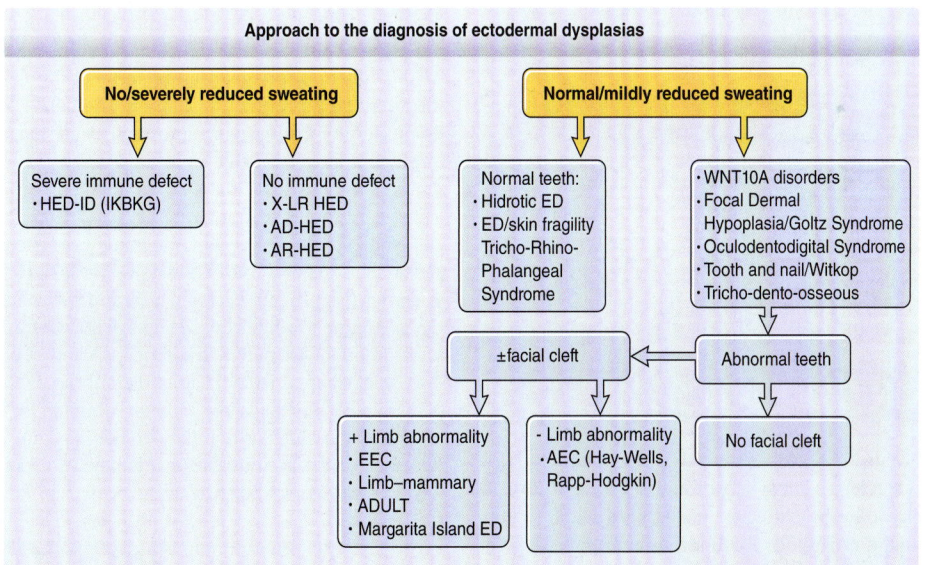

Figure 131-1 Approach to the diagnosis of ectodermal dysplasias. AD = autosomal dominant; ADULT = *a*cro-*d*ermato-*u*ngual-*l*acrimal-*t*ooth syndrome; AEC = *a*nkyloblepharon filiforme adnatum–*e*ctodermal dysplasia–*c*left palate syndrome; AR = autosomal recessive; ED = ectodermal dysplasia; EEC = ectrodactyly–ED–cleft lip/palate syndrome; HED = hypohidrotic ectodermal dysplasia; IM = immune defects; X-LR = X-linked recessive.

syndrome), autosomal dominant HED (ADHED), autosomal recessive HED (ARHED), and HED with immunodeficiency (HED-ID). The autosomal dominant and autosomal recessive forms of HED are similar to XLHED, although the autosomal dominant form may be milder.[10] HED-ID should be considered in a male with HED and recurrent or significant infections.[11,12]

AT-A-GLANCE

- Variants:
  - XLHED (OMIM 305100): XLR mutation of *EDA1* on Xq12-q13.1 encoding the triggering ligand molecule ectodysplasin-A
  - ADHED (OMIM 129490): AD mutation of *EDARADD/EDAR* on 1q42.2-q43/2q11-q13; the intracellular molecule adaptor of EDAR death domain/transmembrane receptor of EDA
  - ARHED (OMIM 224900): AR mutation of *EDARADD/EDAR* on 1q42.2-q43/2q11-q13; the intracellular molecule adaptor of EDAR death domain/transmembrane receptor of EDA
  - HED with immune deficiency (HED-ID; OMIM 300291): XLR mutation of *IKBKG* on Xq28 encoding NF-κB cytoplasmic inhibitor (also referred to as NF-κB essential modulator/NEMO)
- Ectodermal features: characterized by hypotrichosis, hypohidrosis, and hypodontia.
- Systemic features: characteristic facial features with frontal bossing and depressed midface. Often associated with atopic dermatitis, asthma, upper respiratory tract infections, pneumonias

EPIDEMIOLOGY

XLHED occurs in all racial groups and is thought to have an incidence at birth of anywhere from 1 in 5,000 to 100,000 births.[10,13,14] Accurate prevalence and incidence data are not available for the other forms of HED.

CLINICAL FEATURES

Clinical features across the variants are similar. HED is characterized by hypotrichosis, hypohidrosis, and hypodontia. Affected males with XLHED may present at birth with a collodion membrane or with marked scaling of the skin,[15] similar to congenital ichthyosis.

Scalp hair is usually sparse, fine, and blonde. It may thicken and darken at puberty, and secondary sexual hair is typically normal. Other body hair is usually sparse or absent.

The ability to sweat is significantly compromised, and most affected males with XLHED have marked heat intolerance.[16] The inability to sweat adequately in response to environmental heat results in an elevation of core temperature and bouts of unexplained high fevers, usually leading to an extensive workup for infectious disease, malignancy, or autoimmune disease before the correct diagnosis is recognized. In an older series of patients, intellectual disability was reported as a feature of XLHED. Currently, this is believed to have been due to damage from prolonged high fevers and seizures and not to be an intrinsic feature of the disorder.[17] Individuals with ADHED appear to have a milder defect in the ability to sweat.

The nails are usually normal, although there are reports of thin, fragile nails.[18] Fingerprint ridges are effaced. Periorbital wrinkling and hyperpigmentation are typical and often present at birth (Fig. 131-2). Eczema affects more than two-thirds of affected males and almost half of affected females.[19] Hyperplasia of sebaceous glands, particularly on the face, can develop over time and appear as small, pearly, skin-colored to white papules that may resemble milia.

Hypodontia, oligodontia, or anodontia are invariable features of XLHED in affected males. Hypoplastic alveolar ridges in an affected infant can be an early clue to the diagnosis of the disorder. Teeth that do erupt are usually peg-shaped and small (Fig. 131-2B).

The facial features of the disorder are characterized by frontal bossing and a depressed midface with a saddle nose and full, everted lips. Otolaryngologic and pulmonary manifestations include thick nasal secretions and impaction, ozena (atrophic rhinitis), sinusitis, recurrent upper respiratory tract infections and pneumonias, decreased saliva production, hoarse voice, and an increased frequency of asthma. The increased frequency of respiratory tract infections has been attributed to hypoplastic or absent mucus-secreting glands in the bronchial tree.[20] Gastroesophageal reflux and feeding difficulties may be a problem in infancy. The basis for this is unknown. Preliminary studies suggest that there may be failure to thrive in infancy and early childhood in as many as 20% to 40% of affected boys, with catch-up growth seen later.[21]

Female carriers for XLHED may be affected as severely as males or may show few, if any, signs of the disorder (Fig. 131-3). Between 60% and 80% of carrier females express some clinical signs of the disorder; the most frequent are patchy hypotrichosis and hypodontia or peg-shaped teeth. Heat intolerance, if present, is usually mild. Adult carrier women comment that they do not sweat much or that they do not like very warm weather, but it is unusual for a female to experience fever because of inability to sweat.[22]

ETIOLOGY AND PATHOGENESIS

HED is genetically heterogenous, with several forms related to different genes involved in the tumor necrosis factor α (TNF-α) signaling pathway.[9] Mutations in this pathway lead to interruption of the

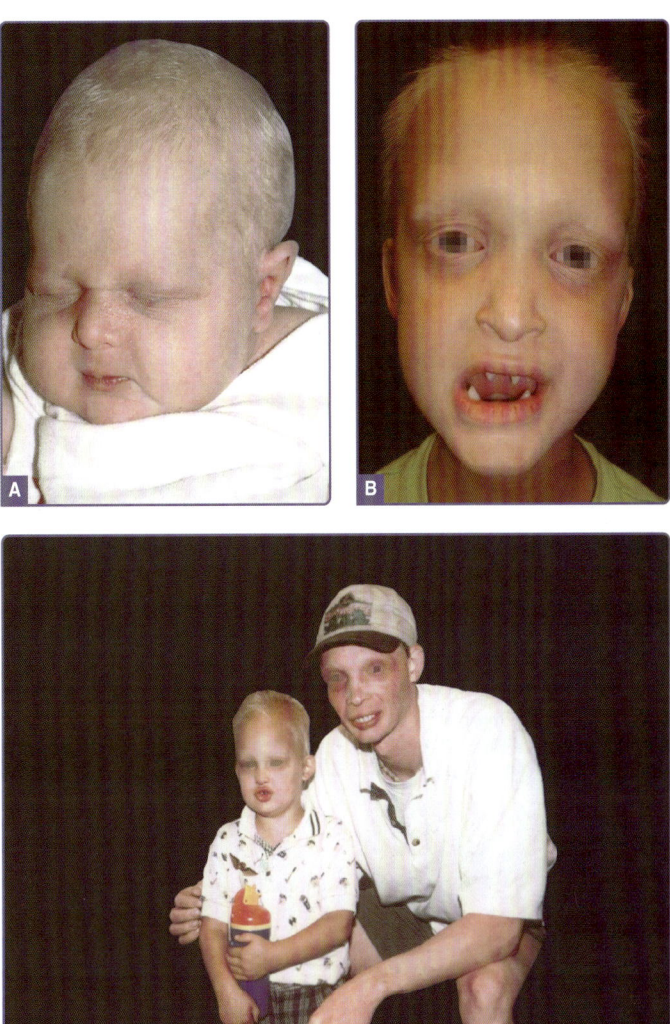

Figure 131-2 Hypohidrotic ectodermal dysplasia. **A,** Newborn with periorbital wrinkling, beaked nose. Diagnosis would not be suspected unless there was a positive family history. **B,** Peg-shaped teeth; fine periorbital wrinkling can be appreciated. **C,** Two unrelated males with X-linked hypohidrotic ectodermal dysplasia; adult is wearing dentures; periorbital wrinkling and hyperpigmentation are evident. (Used with permission from the National Foundation for Ectodermal Dysplasias.)

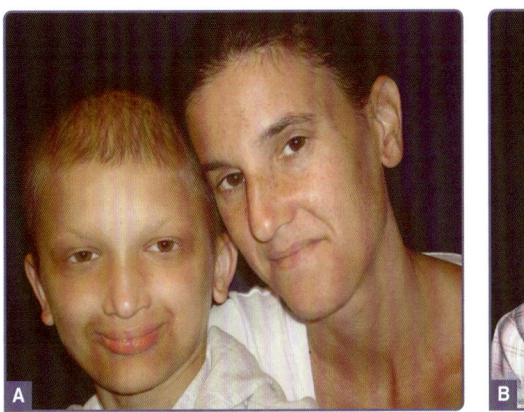
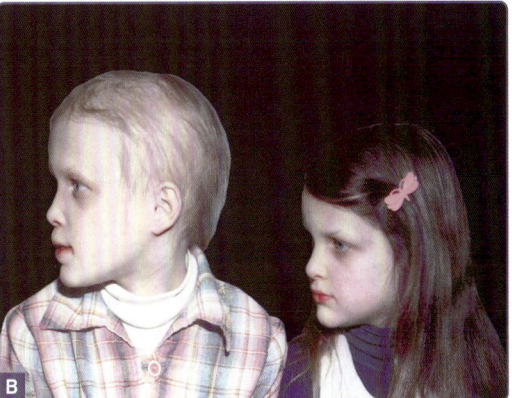

Figure 131-3 Hypohidrotic ectodermal dysplasia. **A,** Female carrier of X-linked hypohidrotic ectodermal dysplasia with her affected son. **B,** Two sisters with X-linked hypohidrotic ectodermal dysplasia manifesting to different degrees. Note periorbital hyperpigmentation, full everted lips, and sculpted noses. (Reproduced from Sybert V. Hypohidrotic ectodermal dysplasia: Argument against an autosomal recessive form clinically indistinguishable from X-linked hypohidrotic ectodermal dysplasia (Christ-Siemens-Touraine syndrome). *Pediatr Dermatol.* 1989;6:76-81; with permission. Copyright © 1989 John Wiley & Sons.)

interaction between epithelial cells and underlying mesenchyme, leading to the clinically observed features that are similar between the different forms of HED. Figure 131-4 demonstrates the ectodysplasin signal transduction pathway and how it relates to each form of HED.

XLHED results from alterations in the gene *EDA1* encoding ectodysplasin-A located at Xq12-13.1.[10] Approximately 70% of affected males inherited the mutation from a carrier mother. *EDA1* codes for a transmembrane protein, ectodysplasin, which plays a role in regulation of the formation of ectodermal structures. It forms trimers and is expressed in keratinocytes, the outer root sheath of hair follicles, and sweat glands. It localizes to the lateral and apical surfaces of cells. A multitude of mutations in this gene causing XLHED have been identified. Interfamilial and intrafamilial variation occurs, but there are reports of genotype-phenotype correlation of skin and hair findings.[23]

Mutations in the autosomal genes, *EDAR*, located at 2q11-q13 and *EDARADD*, located at 1q42.2-q43, have been implicated in both an autosomal dominant form of hypohidrotic ectodermal dysplasia (ADHED; OMIM 129490) and in an autosomal recessive form (ARHED; OMIM 224900). As discussed above, these entities are clinically similar to XLHED, but are rarer. EDAR acts as a receptor for ectodysplasin and EDARADD acts as an intracellular adaptor protein that assists in transmitting the signal from the activated EDA receptor to the nucleus of the cell.[10]

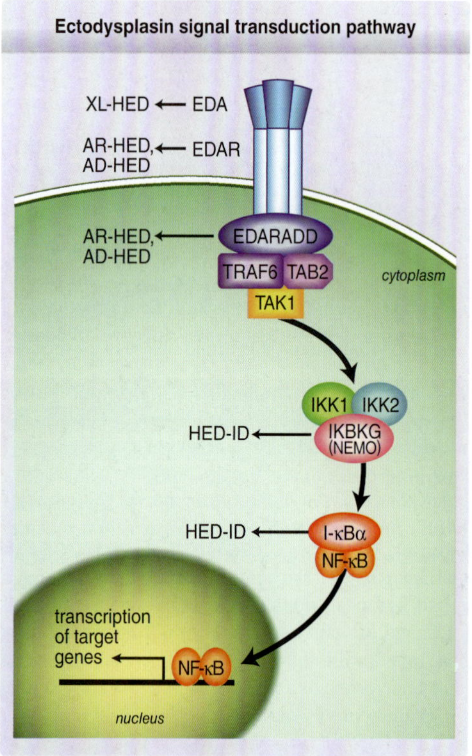

Certain mutations in the X-linked *IKBKG* gene, which causes incontinentia pigmenti (IP) in females have been shown to result in HED-ID in males. There are 2 similar OMIM defined syndromes, HED-ID (OMIM#300291) and ectodermal dysplasia, anhidrotic with immunodeficiency, osteopetrosis, and lymphedema (OLEDAID; OMIM#300301) that describe males with ED and immune deficiency with mutations in *IKBKG*.[11,12] These patients demonstrate ED along with dysgammaglobulinemia and significant early morbidity and mortality. The complexity of the NFKB signaling pathway accounts for the diverse genotypes of HED-ID and immunologic phenotypes.

DIAGNOSIS

The diagnosis of HED is recognized readily when expected, such as when a child is born into a family with a known history of HED. However, without advance knowledge, the diagnosis can initially be clinically challenging. As the patient ages, the characteristic features of hypotrichosis, hypohidrosis, and hypodontia become more evident.[22] Hypoplastic alveolar ridges, indicating lack of teeth, can be an early diagnostic clue. A Panorex view of the jaw can assist in making the correct diagnosis. Although rarely necessary, evaluation of sweating by examination for sweat pores with iodine solution, quantification of pilocarpine-induced sweating,[23] or skin biopsy to assess for the absence of eccrine structures in the scalp and/or palmar region may help confirm a diagnosis.[24] In an isolated, fully expressing female, the autosomal dominant and recessive forms of HED need to be considered. Family history review is necessary, and mothers always should be examined fully to detect mild manifestations of the X-linked form. With the recent expansion and development of molecular genetic testing, definitive genetic diagnosis is becoming more readily available. Referral to a pediatric dermatologist or geneticist can assist in diagnosis.

On histopathology, the epidermis is thinned and flattened. There is a reduction in the number of sebaceous glands and hair follicles. Eccrine glands are absent or incompletely developed. Histologic evaluation of the skin is usually not necessary.

DIFFERENTIAL DIAGNOSIS

Table 131-1 reviews the differential diagnoses for many of the ectodermal dysplasias discussed in this chapter.

The scaling skin at birth may result in a misdiagnosis of congenital ichthyosis. Recurrent fever may be thought to have an infectious source or underlying autoinflammatory disorder.

Figure 131-4 Ectodysplasin signal transduction pathway. (Image **B**, Reproduced from Rimoin D, Pyeritz R, Korf B, eds. *Emery and Rimoin's Principles and Practice of Medical Genetics*, 6th ed. Oxford, UK: Academic Press; 2013; Fig. 148-5; with permission. Copyright © Elsevier.)

TABLE 131-1
Differential Diagnosis of Some Diagnostic Features of Ectodermal Dysplasias

- Collodion membrane
  - Self-healing collodion baby
  - Neutral lipid storage disease
  - Autosomal recessive congenital ichthyosis
    - Nonbullous congenital ichthyosiform erythroderma
    - Lamellar ichthyosis
  - Trichothiodystrophy
  - Storage diseases (eg, Gaucher)
  - Chondrodysplasia punctata
- Ankyloblepharon filiforme adnatum (AFA)
  - Lethal popliteal pterygium syndrome
  - Popliteal pterygium syndrome
  - Isolated AFA
  - AFA and cleft palate
- Hypodontia
  - Isolated hypodontia
  - Incontinentia pigmenti
- Skin fragility/erosions
  - Epidermolysis bullosa (all subtypes)
  - Incontinentia pigmenti
  - Acrodermatitis enteropathica
  - Congenital erythropoietic porphyria
- Atrophic streaks
  - Incontinentia pigmenti—stage 4
  - MIDAS (microphthalmia, dermal aplasia, and sclerocornea)
  - Focal dermal hypoplasia

CLINICAL COURSE, PROGNOSIS, AND MANAGEMENT

Maintenance of cool ambient temperatures is vital to prevent hyperpyrexia. Most children do well with simple measures, such as wet T-shirts and headbands, air conditioning in home and school, etc. Occasionally, cooling vests allow a broader range of participation in sports and vigorous physical activity in warm climates.

Dental restoration is of primary importance, and early implementation of dentures and ultimate use of dental implants are mainstays of treatment.

Management of otolaryngologic complications, asthma, and recurrent infections needs to be individualized. The eczema may be quite refractory to care and difficult to manage.

Infants with HED are at increased risk of death due to hyperthermia and potentially other features of the disorder, such as infection.[25,26] In a survey of the Ectodermal Dysplasia International Registry (EDIR), 21% of XLHED reported a family history of infant or childhood death.[19]

Although infancy and childhood are complicated by many problems, most individuals with HED lead adult lives that allow them to function successfully in society. Heat intolerance seems to decrease because of the development of some ability to sweat in adolescence or to the development adaptation of lifestyle, or both.

Recombinant ectodysplasin protein injections of pregnant affected mice led to permanent rescue of the phenotypic features in the offspring.[27] Further, early postnatal injections were also shown to ameliorate the developmental defects. Similar results have been noted in affected canine models who were infused with recombinant ectodysplasin protein in the postnatal period, with resultant normalization of teeth, lacrimation, and sweating ability, as well as decreased eye and respiratory infections.[28,29] These developments in animal models have been encouraging. There are currently human trials under way.

HIDROTIC ECTODERMAL DYSPLASIA (CLOUSTON)

AT-A-GLANCE

- OMIM 129500, AD mutation of *GJB6* on 13q12 which encodes connexin 30, a connexin protein of the intercellular junction
- Sparse, wiry pale hair with progressive alopecia; variable onychodystrophy; progressive palmoplantar hyperkeratosis
- Normal sweating and teeth

EPIDEMIOLOGY

Hidrotic ED was first described in a French–Canadian kindred.[30] It has been reported in other ethnic groups, but the majority of affected individuals can trace their ancestry back to an original French–Canadian settler.

CLINICAL FEATURES

The scalp hair is wiry, brittle, and pale, and there is often patchy alopecia (Fig. 131-5). This progresses in adult life and may lead to total alopecia. Body and facial hair are affected. The nails may be milky white in infancy and early childhood, gradually thickening and becoming dystrophic. The nail plates in adults are thick, short, and slow growing. They separate distally from the nail bed (Fig. 131-5C), and may cause pain. Anonychia has been reported. Not all the nails are necessarily affected to the same degree. Progressive palmar/plantar hyperkeratosis is common (Fig. 131-5B). In contrast to HED, sweating is normal, as are the teeth. Oral leukoplakia has been reported. Conjunctivitis and blepharitis, possibly due to poor function of sparse eyelashes, are common.[31]

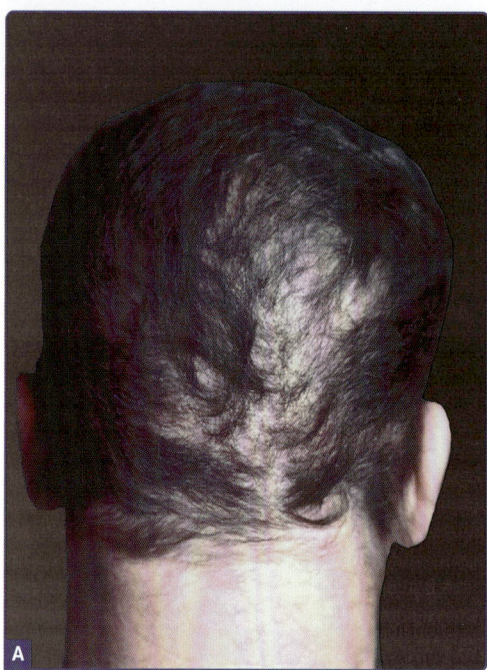
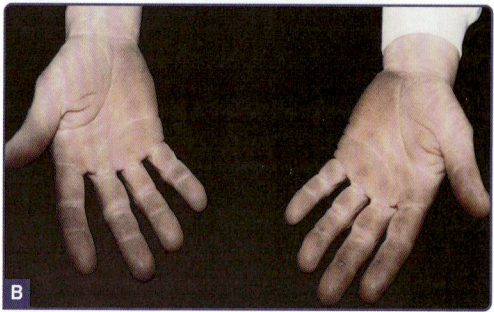
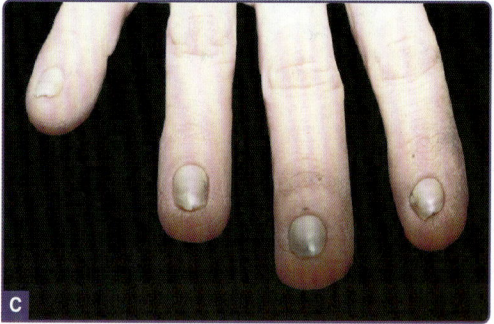

Figure 131-5 Hidrotic ectodermal dysplasia (Clouston syndrome). **A,** Patchy alopecia in adult. Coarseness of hair can be appreciated. **B,** Palmar hyperkeratosis. **C,** Nail dystrophy.

ETIOLOGY AND PATHOGENESIS

Hidrotic ED is autosomal dominant with variable expression, and the degree of severity can vary within and between families. Males and females are affected in equal numbers and to equal degree.

The disorder is caused by mutations in a connexin gene, *GJB6*, which encodes the intercellular junction protein connexin 30.[32] Different mutations in the same gene are responsible for a form of nonsyndromic autosomal dominant deafness. Connexin mutations are involved in several other genodermatoses, such as keratitis-ichthyosis-deafness (KID) syndrome (Chaps. 47 and 48).

DIAGNOSIS

The diagnosis is straightforward with time. The involvement of nails and hair and palmar/plantar thickening, in the absence of other signs of ED, are reasonably specific. Again, genetic testing can be confirmatory.[31]

On histopathology, the thickened palms and soles show orthohyperkeratosis with a normal granular layer.

On electron microscopy, an increase in the number of desmosomes in the cells of the stratum corneum is found. The hair shows nonspecific changes.

DIFFERENTIAL DIAGNOSIS

Other palmar/plantar hyperkeratoses do not have similar hair changes. Orofacial clefting differentiates other forms of autosomal dominant hidrotic EDs, such as ankyloblepharon–ED–cleft palate (AEC) syndrome. Although the nail changes are similar to those of pachyonychia congenita, the hair changes are distinctive.

CLINICAL COURSE, PROGNOSIS, AND MANAGEMENT

Occasionally, ablation of the nail matrix is necessary for relief of pain. Wigs may provide cosmetic benefit. Treatment of the palmoplantar keratoderma is not specific and minimally successful.

ID SYNDROMES:
AEC (HAY–WELLS/RAPP–
HODGKIN); EEC; LIMB–
MAMMARY SYNDROME;
ACRO-DERMATO-UNGUAL–
LACRIMAL–TOOTH (ADULT)
SYNDROME; ISOLATED
SPLIT HAND–SPLIT FOOT
MALFORMATION

> **AT-A-GLANCE**
>
> - Variants: all of the conditions below are AD with a mutation of *TP63* on 3q27, which encodes the p63 transcription protein
>   - Ankyloblepharon-ectodermal defects-clefting (AEC)/Hay–Wells/Rapp–Hodgkin syndrome (AEC/Hay–Wells OMIM 106260; Rapp–Hodgkin syndrome OMIM 129400)
>   - Limb–mammary syndrome (OMIM 603543)
>   - Acro-dermato-ungual-lacrimal-tooth (ADULT) syndrome (OMIM 103285)
>   - Ectrodactyly-ED-cleft lip/palate syndrome 3 (EEC3; OMIM 604292)
> - Ectodermal features: collodion membrane at birth, dry thin skin, erosive scalp dermatitis, patchy alopecia, coarse light hair, dyspigmentation, variable nail dystrophy.
> - Systemic features: Ankyloblepharon filiforme adnatum, lacrimal duct atresia, cleft lip/palate, hypodontia, syndactyly, ectopic breast tissue and hypospadias.

INTRODUCTION

Mutations in *p63*, a tumor-suppressor gene mapped to 3q27, have been found in most, but not all, individuals with ankyloblepharon-ectodermal defects-clefting (AEC; Hay–Wells; Rapp–Hodgkin) syndrome.[33] The gene is expressed widely, including in the basal cells of proliferating epithelial tissues. Mutations in the same gene cause some cases of isolated split hand–split foot malformation, limb–mammary syndrome, and acro-dermato-ungual-lacrimal-tooth (ADULT) syndrome. There appear to be some genotype–phenotype correlations.[34]

AEC (HAY–WELLS/RAPP–HODGKIN) SYNDROME

EPIDEMIOLOGY

Hay–Wells syndrome was first described in 1976,[35] and has been found in ethnically and geographically disparate families. Rapp–Hodgkin syndrome was first described in 1968,[36] and although it had many clinical similarities to Hay–Wells syndrome, it was once thought to be a distinct clinical entity. More recently, it has become evident that Rapp–Hodgkin syndrome and Hay–Wells syndrome are allelic and should be considered variants of the same disorder, AEC syndrome.[37,38]

CLINICAL FEATURES

Eighty to 90% of affected infants present at birth with shiny red, cracking, peeling skin, and superficial erosions, similar to the appearance of a collodion membrane (Fig. 131-6A).[18] This sheds within a few weeks, and the skin underneath is dry and thin.

The scalp is almost invariably affected. Many individuals have chronic erosive dermatitis with abnormal granulation tissue on the scalp and recurrent bacterial infections (Fig. 131-6B).[39] There is alopecia of the scalp of variable extent along with hair that is often wiry, coarse, and light in color with an uncombable appearance. Sparseness to absence of body hair is typical.

Cutaneous dyspigmentation, both hypo- and hyperpigmentation, can be quite striking and is seen universally in affected patients.[40,41] The nails may be normal, hyperconvex and thickened, absent, or partially dystrophic, and all changes can be found in a single individual and can worsen with age. Effaced dermatoglyphics and palmoplantar erosive changes are also quite common. Sweating may be normal to slightly decreased. Although most affected individuals describe subjective heat intolerance, frank hyperpyrexia is uncommon.

Ankyloblepharon filiforme adnatum (AFA), the term for strands of skin between the eyelids, is seen in approximately 70% of affected infants (Fig. 131-6C). These may tear spontaneously prior to birth, and minimally involve the lateral eyelids or require surgical lysis. Lacrimal duct atresia or obstruction is common.

Supernumerary nipples and ectopic breast tissue are seen occasionally, as is mild cutaneous syndactyly of the second and third toes. More prominent limb defects, including ectrodactyly (abnormal development of the median rays of the hands and feet), have been observed.[42]

Historically, the main clinical differences between Hay–Wells and Rapp–Hodgkin syndrome included characteristic facial features with a short nasal columella and maxillary hypoplasia, thin upper lip, and full lower lip associated with Rapp–Hodgkin syndrome (Fig. 131-7A,B). Also, with Rapp–Hodgkin syndrome, the teeth may be conical and prone to caries (Fig. 131-7D), lacrimal puncta are aplastic in almost one-third of affected individuals, but AFA is rare, and

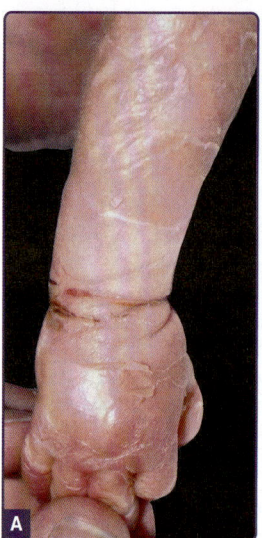
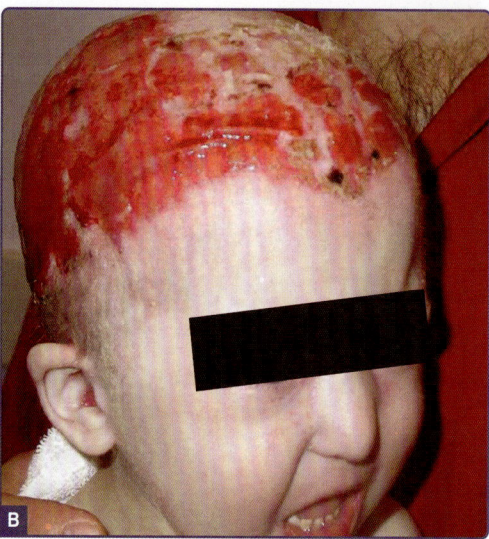
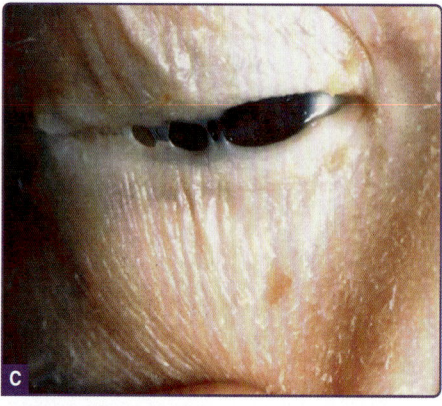

Figure 131-6 Ankyloblepharon filiforme adnatum–ectodermal dysplasia–cleft palate (Hay–Wells) syndrome. **A,** Newborn with peeling collodion membrane. **B,** Scalp erosions. **C,** Fine strands of tissue (ankyloblepharon filiforme adnatum) between eyelids.

scalp involvement with breakdown and granulation tissue formation is far less common.

Cleft palate, with or without cleft lip, occurs in 80% to 100% of reported cases, with some cases displaying submucosal cleft palate alone.[43] There is typically hypodontia with missing or misshapen teeth, and maxillary hypoplasia is also common.[44] Malformed auricles have been described in some. Recurrent otitis media and secondary conductive hearing loss are common and may be consequences of the cleft palate. Hypospadias has been described in affected males, and labial hypoplasia with absence of the opening of the vagina has been reported in a single female. These features are also reminiscent of the EEC syndrome.

DIAGNOSIS

See discussion of etiology and pathogenesis for information on genetic testing.

On histopathology, consistent changes include mild epidermal atrophy, focal orthokeratosis, prominent superficial vascular plexus, and pigment incontinence with melanophages.[45] Electron microscopy of hairs shows a defective cuticular structure, atrophy and loss of melanin, along with structural abnormalities including pili torti and pili trianguli et canaliculi. There is a decrease in the keratins of the basal and suprabasal layers of the epidermis and disorganized keratin filaments in the stratum corneum.

DIFFERENTIAL DIAGNOSIS

Among the autosomal dominant EDs associated with clefting, EEC syndrome is characterized by bony hand and foot abnormalities not typically seen in AEC and also lacks the ankyloblepharon. The peeling, eroded skin of the newborn can lead to misdiagnosis of epidermolysis bullosa or congenital ichthyosis. AFA can occur in the absence of syndromic associations, and strands of tissue between the eyelids have been seen in several forms of arthrogryposis and in CHANDS (*c*urly *h*air, *a*nkyloblepharon, and *n*ail *d*ysplasia syndrome), an autosomal recessive form of ED.

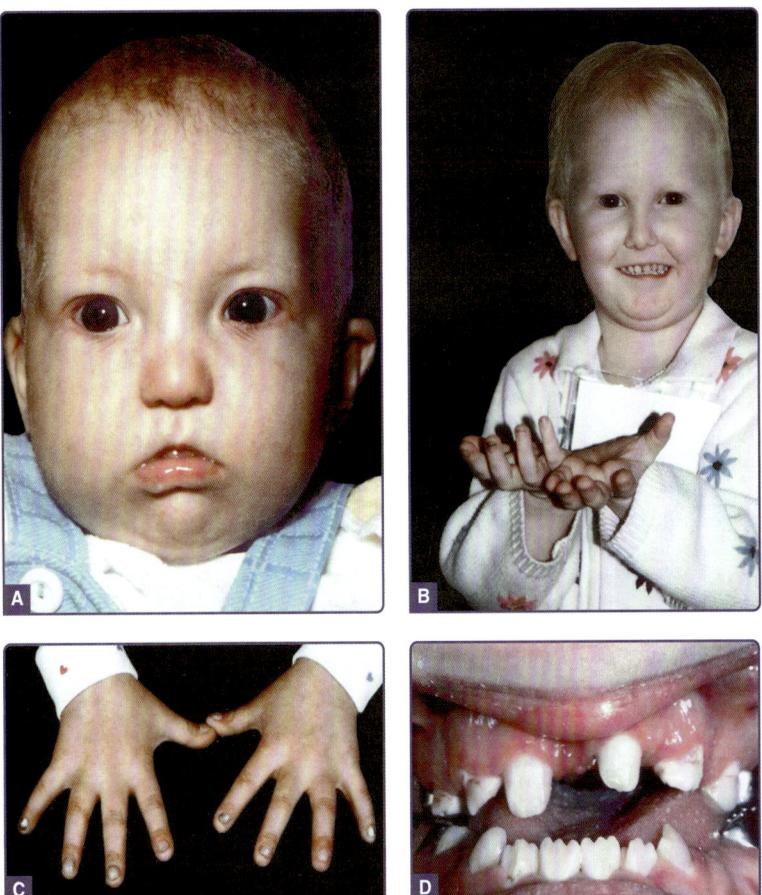

Figure 131-7 Rapp–Hodgkin syndrome. **A,** Affected infant at 5 months. **B,** Fine, blond, sparse hair; beginnings of nail changes on middle finger of right hand. **C,** Abnormal nails in same patient as (**A**), at age 4½ years with thickened and friable nail plates. **D,** Abnormal dentition, missing teeth, and peg teeth. (Images A and C, From Schroeder HW Jr, Sybert VP. Rapp-Hodgkin ectodermal dysplasia. *J Pediatr*. 1987;110(1):72-75; with permission. Copyright © Elsevier. Image **B**, Used with permission from the National Foundation for Ectodermal Dysplasias.)

CLINICAL COURSE, PROGNOSIS, AND MANAGEMENT

Light emollients should be used until the collodion membrane sheds. Ankyloblepharon may require surgical lysis. Ongoing ocular hygiene is important. The skin erosions, especially of the scalp, are difficult to manage and prone to excessive granulation tissue and secondary infection. They should be managed with gentle wound care, dilute bleach or other antimicrobial soaks. Occlusive dressings should be avoided.[40] Grafting of skin to the scalp has not proven successful in most instances. Clefting requires a team approach for repair and followup for secondary issues, such as feeding difficulties, speech defects, orthodontia, and ear infections.

EEC SYNDROME (OMIM 129900, 604292)

EEC syndrome is an ED classified as a multiple congenital anomaly syndrome because it has major involvement of structures other than those derived from the ectoderm. There are 3 variants of EEC syndrome, EEC1 (OMIM 129900), EEC2 (no OMIM number) and EEC3 (OMIM 604292). EEC1 and EEC2 have unknown gene product mutations, but EEC1 has been linked to a mutation on chromosome 7. EEC3 is caused by an autosomal dominant mutation in the tumor-suppressor gene *TP63*, designating the EECs as p63-related EDs. EEC syndrome has occurred in all racial groups worldwide, and all 3 forms share clinical manifestations.

CLINICAL FEATURES

The ectodermal dysplasia manifestations may be quite mild. The hair is usually blonde, coarse, and dry. It may be sparse and slow growing. Axillary and pubic hair also may be affected. The nails are dystrophic in approximately four-fifths of individuals with transverse ridging, pitting, and slow growth. Dry skin and thickening of the palms and soles can occur. Sweating is usually normal.[46]

The major distinguishing feature of EEC syndrome is ectrodactyly (Figs. 131-8A-C). The feet are involved more frequently than the hands, and there may be asymmetry of involvement.

Cleft palate, with or without cleft lip, occurs in 70% to 100% of affected individuals.[46,47] Hypodontia and premature loss of secondary teeth and the dental abnormalities associated with clefting are found in most affected individuals. Lacrimal gland abnormalities and secondary conductive hearing loss are common. Genitourinary abnormalities that include hydronephrosis and structural renal or genital malformations affect one-third or more of persons with EEC syndrome. Although intellectual disability has been reported, it is not believed to be an inherent feature of the disorder.

DIFFERENTIAL DIAGNOSIS

Disorders with limb defects that need to be considered in the differential diagnosis of EEC syndrome are odontotrichomelic syndrome (OMIM 273400), in which there are severe absence deformities of the limbs, and aplasia cutis congenita with limb defects (Adams–Oliver syndrome, OMIM 100300), which does not have clefting or ectodermal defects other than absence of skin. Cutis marmorata telangiectatica congenita (Chap. 103) has been described in some individuals with Adams–Oliver syndrome. Other EDs with clefting include AEC and limb–mammary syndrome, all of which are allelic to EEC syndrome. Ectrodactyly with cleft palate without ED (OMIM 129830) may be a distinct entity. There appear to be some families with EEC in whom linkage studies have suggested other causal genes located at different chromosomal loci. Prenatal diagnosis by ultrasound for detection of limb abnormalities is unreliable; genetic testing may prove useful in some families.

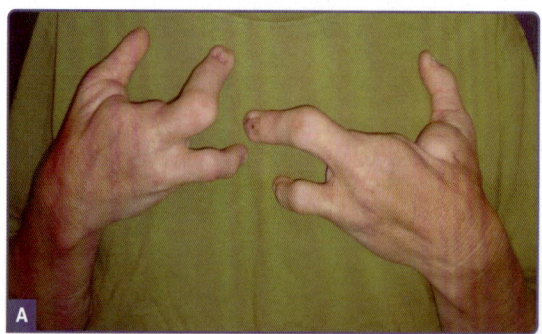
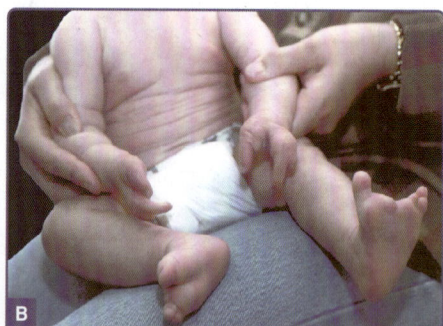
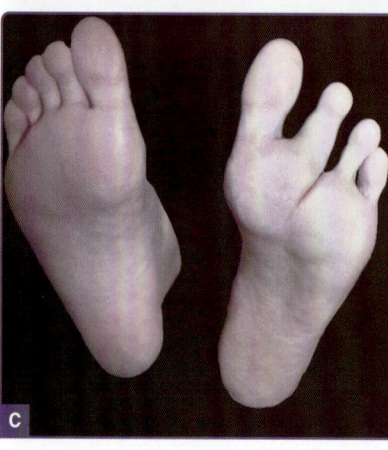
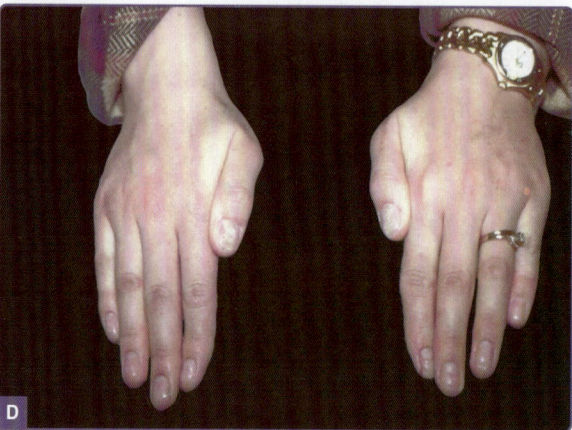

Figure 131-8 Ectrodactyly–ectodermal dysplasia–clefting syndrome. **A**, Hands of an affected adult. **B**, Hands and feet of affected infant. **C** and **D**, Feet and hands of parent of infant in (**B**) demonstrating variability of expression both among limbs and between family members. Note the nail dystrophy in the mildly affected mother, especially evident on the thumbs.

CLINICAL COURSE, PROGNOSIS, AND MANAGEMENT

As for other EDs with orofacial clefting and ophthalmologic involvement, management requires a team approach. Similarly, treatment for the limb defects must be individualized. Renal ultrasonography and a high index of suspicion for urinary tract problems are appropriate and warranted.

P63-RELATED ECTODERMAL DYSPLASIA SYNDROMES

ETIOLOGY AND PATHOGENESIS

AEC, EEC, split hand–split foot malformation, limb–mammary syndrome, and ADULT syndrome are caused by mutations in the tumor-suppressor gene *TP63* mapped to 3q27. Different mutations within this gene have been implicated in the pathogenesis of these syndromes.[34,48] *TP63* is expressed widely, including in the basal cells of proliferating epithelial tissues.

AEC syndrome is an autosomal dominant disorder with complete penetrance and variable expression. The majority of alterations identified thus far in AEC syndrome have been missense mutations in the sterile α motif (SAM) domain of p63.

EEC syndrome is an autosomal dominant disorder with variable expression and reduced penetrance. Mutations in *TP63* have been found in most, but not all, individuals with EEC syndrome. The majority of mutations result in single–amino acid substitutions in the DNA-binding domain of p63.[33]

Similar to EEC, mutations in the DNA-binding domain of *TP63* are also found in split hand–split foot malformation.[49] Frameshift mutations in *TP63* cause limb–mammary syndrome, in which ectodermal structures other than the mammary gland often, but not always, appear normal. Among 3 unrelated families with ADULT syndrome, all shared the same point mutation in *p63*.[50]

WNT10A DISORDERS: ODONTO-ONYCHO-DERMAL DYSPLASIA (OODD), SCHOPF–SCHULZ–PASSARGE SYNDROME (SSPS)

AT-A-GLANCE

- Variants: all of the below are AR with a mutation of *WNT10A* (wingless-type MMTV integration site family, member 10A) on 2q35, which mediates β catenin–mediated specific intracellular signaling
    - Odonto-onycho-dermal dysplasia (OODD; OMIM 257980)
    - Schopf–Schulz–Passarge Syndrome (SSPS; OMIM 224750)
- Both OODD and SSPS demonstrate variable degrees of hypodontia, dystrophic nails, hypotrichosis, palmar plantar hyperkeratosis with hyperhidrosis, hypohidrosis on rest of body.
- SSPS is also characterized by eyelid hidrocystomas

INTRODUCTION

Odonto-onycho-dermal dysplasia (OODD) and Schopf–Schulz–Passarge Syndrome (SSPS) are both forms of ED caused by mutations in the *WNT10A* gene.

EPIDEMIOLOGY

Mutations in *WNT10A* have been reported in about 9% of EDs and in 25% of hypohidrotic ED (HED) patients who do not have mutations in *EDA*.[51,52] With recent advances in molecular genetic testing, *WNT10A* mutations have been found in about 16% of suspected cases of HED.[9]

CLINICAL FEATURES

OODD has a broad spectrum of clinical features. The most consistent finding is severe hypodontia to anodontia of the permanent teeth. Primary teeth are almost always normal in number but may be small and widely spaced (Fig. 131-9A).[53-55] The tongue may be smooth, with decreased fungiform and filiform papillae. The nails are dystrophic, and there can be congenital anonychia. Hair is absent at birth, progressing to dry, thin hair in older individuals. Eyebrows may be sparse. Skin changes include palmar erythema, palmar plantar hyperkeratosis (Fig. 131-9B),[56] and keratosis pilaris. The palms and soles commonly have hyperhidrosis, although there is hypohidrosis elsewhere on the body.

SSPS is characterized by eyelid hidrocystomas; in addition, the findings described above in OODD.[57]

ETIOLOGY AND PATHOGENESIS

OODD and SSPS are caused by mutations in *WNT10A* (wingless-type MMTV integrations site family, member 10A) gene.[57] Most cases are autosomal recessive, but up to 50% of heterozygotes may display clinical features.

DIAGNOSIS

On histopathology, the skin shows orthokeratosis, hyperkeratosis, hypergranulosis, and mild acanthosis. When

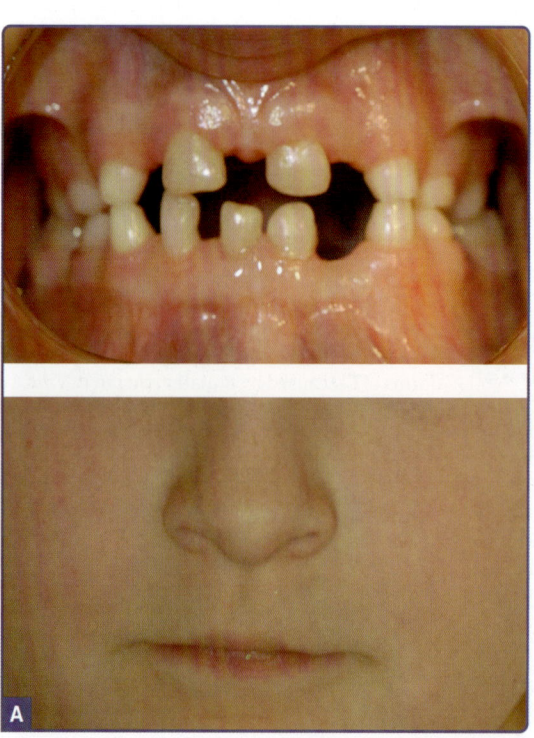
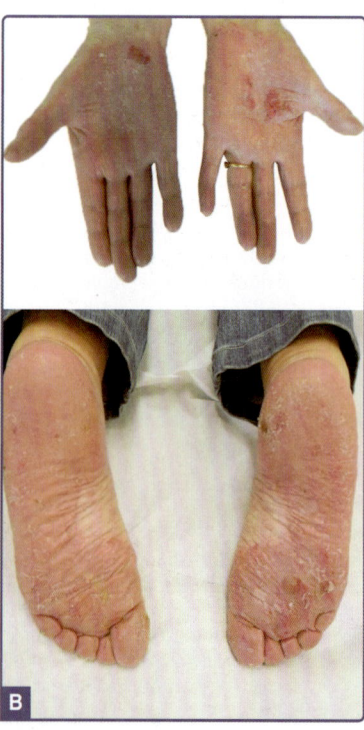

Figure 131-9 WNT10A disorders. **A,** Note the widely spaced and scattered missing deciduous teeth with the characteristic thin upper lip. (Image reused from Bergendal B, Norderyd J, Zhou X, et al. Abnormal primary and permanent dentitions with ectodermal symptoms predict WNT10A deficiency. BMC Med Genet. 2016;17(1):88 with permission from BioMed Central.) **B,** Erythematous hyperkeratosis with erosions and fissures of the palmar hands and the plantar feet. (Images reused from Krøigård AB, Clemmensen O, Gjørup H, et al. Odonto-onycho-dermal dysplasia in a patient homozygous for a WNT10A nonsense mutation and mild manifestations of ectodermal dysplasia in carriers of the mutation. BMC Dermatol. 2016;16:3, with permission from BioMed Central.)

examined by EM, the hairs of OODD have longitudinal depressions. Again, genetic testing can be helpful.

CLINICAL COURSE, PROGNOSIS, AND MANAGEMENT

Restorative dentistry is important. Hyperkeratosis management is nonspecific and the nails usually require no treatment. There is potential increased risk of nonmelanoma skin cancer in SSP, and patients should be monitored appropriately.

FOCAL DERMAL HYPOPLASIA (GOLTZ SYNDROME; GOLTZ-GORLIN SYNDROME)

AT-A-GLANCE

- OMIM 305600
- XLD, *PORCN*, Xp11.23, involved in membrane targeting and secretion of Wnt proteins necessary for embryonic tissue development
- Cutaneous features: Blaschkoid dermal atrophy with fat herniations; progressive papillomas; patchy alopecia
- Extracutaneous features: microphthalmia and colobomas; oligodontia and enamel defects; numerous skeletal anomalies including syndactyly and osteopathia striata; developmental delays in 15%

INTRODUCTION

Focal dermal hypoplasia (FDH) is a rare ectodermal dysplasia with multisystem involvement, including skin, teeth, bones, and eyes with variable clinical manifestations.[58]

EPIDEMIOLOGY

FDH was first described in 1934.[59] Subsequently, there have been more than 200 case reports published.

CLINICAL FEATURES

The skin changes of FDH are the primary diagnostic features with considerable variability because of both postzygotic somatic mosaicism in both males and females and random X-chromosome inactivation in females. There is linear, punctate, streaky cribriform atrophy (Fig. 131-10), with telangiectasia distributed along the lines of Blaschko. The cribriform atrophy is marked by tiny ice pick–like depressions in the skin. Areas of thinned to absent dermis are irregularly distributed and the resultant herniations of fat appear as yellow–pink excrescences that are easily depressed on the skin surface (Fig. 131-10). Papillomas that may be raspberry-like or vascular develop throughout life and favor the perigenital, perioral, intertriginous, and mucosal surfaces. Other dermatologic features include pigmentary changes, patchy alopecia, brittle or sparse hair, and palmar and plantar hyperkeratoses. Some individuals have had hyperhidrosis and some have had aplasia cutis congenita.

The other organ systems most frequently involved in FDH are the skeleton, CNS, teeth, and eyes. Microphthalmia and colobomas are common, and the diagnosis of FDH should prompt a full ophthalmologic evaluation. Oligodontia, tooth dysplasia, and enamel defects are common. The skeletal abnormalities are too numerous to list; the most common are vertical banding of the bones (osteopathia striata), syndactyly (both cutaneous and bony), ectrodactyly, asymmetry, oligodactyly, and short stature. Intellectual disability has been reported in approximately 15% of cases. Defects in other organ systems have been described in a minority of cases, including cardiac defects, abdominal wall defects, and renal malformations.

ETIOLOGY AND PATHOGENESIS

Focal dermal hypoplasia is an X-linked dominant disorder, usually lethal in males. Case reports of males with the condition are believed to be due to mosaicism for postzygotic somatic mutations (as is true for incontinentia pigmenti); the presence of some normal cells allows survival in the male. The mutated gene is *PORCN*, the human homolog of the porcupine gene in *Drosophila*. *PORCN* is thought to be important for palmitoylation and secretion of Wnt protein, a key regulator of the development of skin and bone.[60,61]

It is important to inquire about the family history of lost pregnancies and a skewed male–female ratio in offspring, as these are clues to the mother being a carrier. Both mothers and fathers should be examined

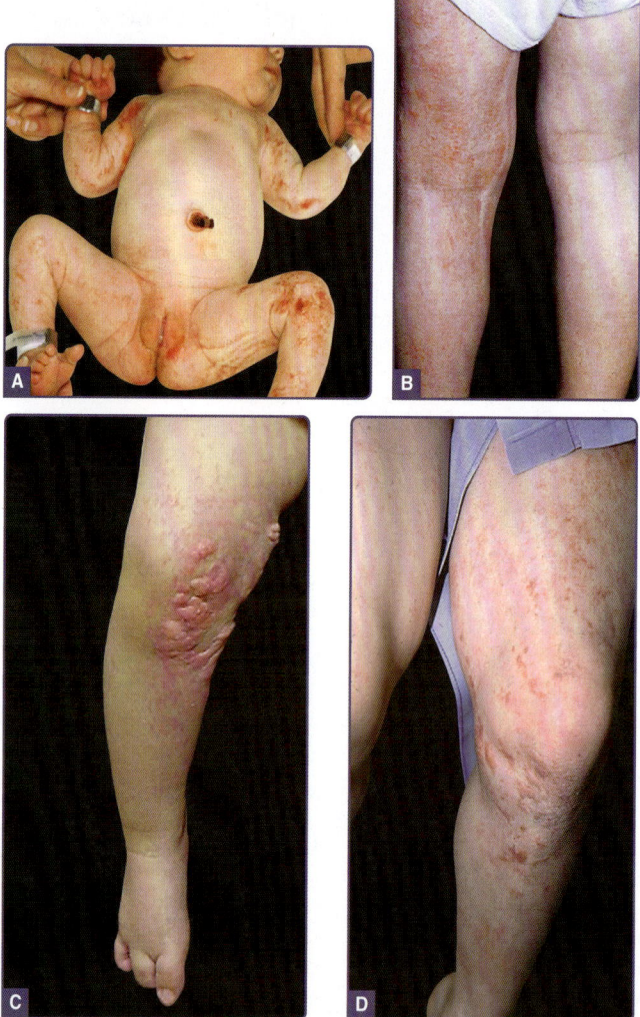

Figure 131-10 Focal dermal hypoplasia. **A,** Streaky and patchy involvement in the newborn. Note similarity to the distribution of lesions in incontinentia pigmenti. **B** and **C,** Same girl at age 2 showing atrophy and fat herniation. **D,** Now a young adult, erythema and atrophy, with dryness and scale, predominate. (Image **A,** From Sybert VP. *Genetic Skin Disorders*, 3rd ed. New York, NY: Oxford University Press; 2017; with permission.)

carefully; fathers may have subtle features and, presumably, represent individuals with postzygotic mutations for the *FDH* gene.

DIAGNOSIS

The diagnosis of FDH is challenging given the rarity of the syndrome. Biopsy can be helpful in demonstrating the dermal hypoplasia and increased capillaries in the papillary dermis.[58] Additionally, genetic testing is commercially available, but can be challenging in patients with postzygotic mutations.

DIFFERENTIAL DIAGNOSIS

Cribriform atrophy has been described in X-linked dominant Conradi–Hünermann syndrome (chondrodysplasia punctata), but ichthyosis is not a feature of FDH, and fat herniation is not part of Conradi–Hünermann. The Blaschkoid distribution of the atrophic lesions of IP is similar, but the blistering and hyperkeratosis of IP are not found in FDH. In microphthalmia and linear skin defects/microphthalmia, dermal aplasia, sclerocornea (MIDAS; OMIM 309801), the skin defects are limited to the head and neck; there is atrophy and scarring of the skin more similar to aplasia cutis congenita and not dermal atrophy alone. The disorders do share similar ocular abnormalities.

CLINICAL COURSE, PROGNOSIS, AND MANAGEMENT

There is no specific treatment for the dermatologic and systemic features of FDH. Areas of atrophy may be prone to infection or become erosive. Papillomas can be excised if they interfere with function. Referral to otolaryngology may be necessary for management of papillomas of the larynx or trachea and preoperative evaluation for these lesions should be considered.[62] Use of vascular lasers to decrease the erythema of telangiectatic areas may have cosmetic benefit. As with most X-linked dominant disorders, clinical involvement varies considerably, and the range in severity is marked. This makes prognostic counseling difficult early in infancy, and usually it is wise to counsel patience and reassurance until the extent to which there is systemic involvement becomes clear.

INCONTINENTIA PIGMENTI

AT-A-GLANCE

- OMIM 308300
- XLD, *IKBKG* (also called NEMO), Xp28, encodes the I-kappa-B kinase gamma subunit protein involved in cell protection from apoptosis
- Cutaneous features: 4 characteristic stages involving (1) vesicobullous lesions; (2) verrucous lesions; (3) hyperpigmentation; and (4) hypopigmentation and atrophy. May also see hypotrichosis, cicatricial alopecia, and tooth defects.
- Extracutaneous features: ophthalmologic complications, CNS manifestations (seizures, developmental delay)

INTRODUCTION

Incontinentia pigmenti (IP), also known as male-lethal type Bloch–Sulzberger syndrome, was first described in 1906 by Garrod.[63] IP is an ectodermal dysplasia with highly variable involvement of skin, teeth, hair, nails, eyes, and the CNS.[64] The skin findings are the first clinical manifestation.[65]

EPIDEMIOLOGY

IP occurs in 1 in 50,000 to 150,000 newborns.[65] It is X-linked dominant and usually lethal in male fetuses; however, similar to FDH, there are reports of male cases in the setting of late postzygotic mutations, seg- mental involvement, or XXY genotype.

CLINICAL FEATURES

There are 4 characteristic stages of skin lesions, all of which occur along the lines of Blaschko. Not every stage may occur, and some stages may overlap.

- Stage I: Perinatal inflammatory stage with erythema, vesicles, and pustules with individual lesions lasting for several days to weeks (Fig. 131-11A). Present at birth in 50% and by 2 weeks of age in 90%. Typically resolves by 4 to 6 months, but may have recurrences with illnesses.[66]
- Stage II: Verrucous and hyperkeratotic papules persistent for several weeks to months, with reports of it lasting up to years (Fig. 131-11B).
- Stage III: Hyperpigmentation that usually presents around 6 months of age and persists for several years, with reports of persistence into adulthood. Highly variable extent, often unrelated to the distribution in the previous stages. Most frequently involves the groin and axillae.[64]
- Stage IV: Hypopigmentation and atrophy in previously affected areas. Starts with the resolution of the previous stages and lasting into adulthood.

Many of the cutaneous features resolve or become very subtle by the 20 years of age. Cicatricial and patchy alopecia are common and tend to be persistent. In adult females, areas of hypotrichosis on the legs and whorled alopecia of the scalp can be helpful clinically.[67]

Nail dystrophy is common during the second stage, but often mild.[64] There is a wide range of teeth findings, including hypodontia, microdontia, adontia, and conical teeth.

Ophthalmological involvement is present in 20% to 77%[64,65] of affected individuals and includes retinal neovascularization, strabismus, cataracts, optic atrophy, and retinal pigmentary abnormalities. It is important to screen for eye findings at the time of diagnosis because retinal neovascularization can result in retinal detachment, with the highest risk in the neonatal period and up to the first 6 years of life.[64] Given the risk of decreased visual acuity, repeat eye examinations are necessary.

CNS involvement is estimated at 10% to 30%, although it may be lower.[64,65] CNS abnormalities range from a single seizure to encephalopathy, ischemic stroke, and significant developmental delay. Symptoms most often present in the first year of life, which is consistent with the hypothesis that neurologic manifestations are a result of inflammation and vasculopathy/ischemia.[68] CNS manifestations highly impact morbidity and mortality, and predictive features, such as retinal neovascularization and male gender, are helpful for assessing risk.[68]

Unilateral breast aplasia is uncommon, but should be alert one to the possible diagnosis of IP.[69]

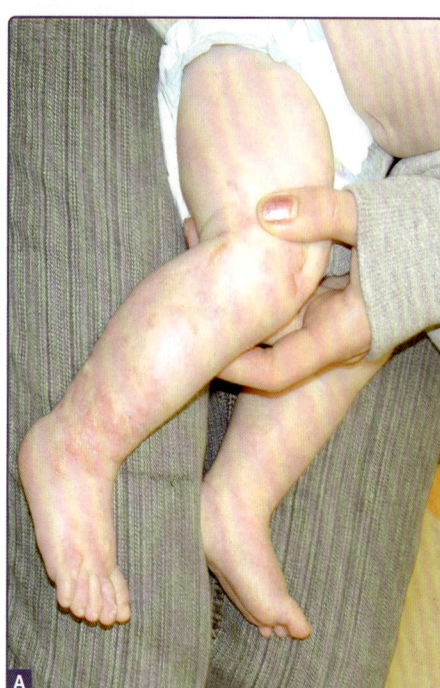 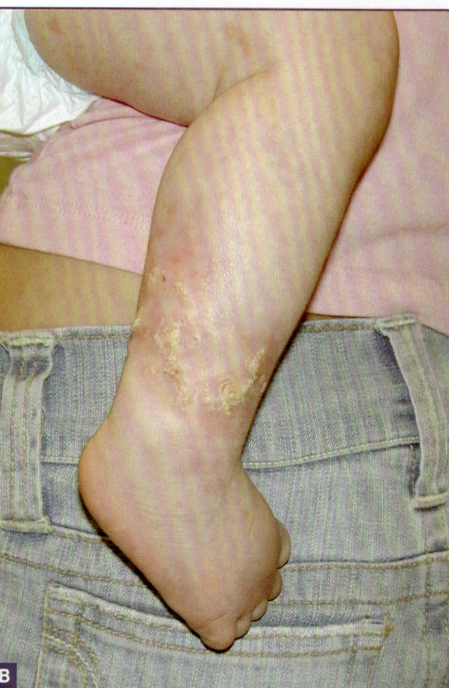

Figure 131-11 Incontinentia pigmenti. **A,** Stage I. Edematous erythematous papules and vesicles following the lines of Blaschko on the lower leg. Note the early stage II verrucous papules on the toes. **B,** Stage II. Hyperkeratotic papules and papules and plaques with surrounding erythema. (Reproduced from Rimoin D, Pyeritz R, Korf B, eds. *Emery and Rimoin's Principles and Practice of Medical Genetics*, 6th ed. Oxford, UK: Academic Press; 2013; Figure 148-15; with permission. Copyright © Elsevier.)

ETIOLOGY AND PATHOGENESIS

IP is an X-linked dominant disorder, typically lethal in males (see discussion regarding mosaicism for postzygotic mutations above in FDH). About 80% of IP are due to mutations in the *IKBKG* gene, which encodes the I-kappa-B kinase gamma subunit protein (IKK-gamma). More than 50 distinct postzygotic somatic mutation variants in the *IKBKG* gene have been reported.

The IKK-gamma protein is widely expressed and binds to the IKK-alpha and IKK-beta proteins to activate the KF-kappa-B complex. This complex protects cells from TNF-induced apoptosis. The different stages of IP represent cell death of affected cells that are unable to activate this protective complex. It is proposed that after cells with the *IKBKG* mutation undergo apoptosis, they are replaced by unaffected cells. Late recurrences may be due to persistence of affected keratinocytes in the sites of previous lesions.[65]

DIAGNOSIS

In 2014, Minic et al updated the diagnostic criteria. Major criteria include any of the 4 stages of skin lesions. Minor criteria include dental, ocular, CNS, hair, nail, palate, breast, and nipple anomalies; family history; multiple male miscarriages; and histopathologic skin findings.[64,69]

Skin biopsy greatly aids in diagnosis, especially in suspected males, and histopathology is stage specific. Biopsy of vesiculobullous lesions reveals a spongiotic epidermis with eosinophilic infiltrates and microabscesses, and dyskeratosis. Verrucous lesions demonstrate hyperkeratosis, papillomatosis, and dyskeratosis.

Genetic testing is commercially available for *IKBKG* common deletion/duplication and gene sequencing, which identifies IP and HED-ID. About 75% of affected patients have the common 11.7kb deletion of exons 4 to 10.[65] Testing can confirm a clinical diagnosis, detect female carriers, and evaluate at-risk pregnancies in families carrying the IKBKG mutation. Without family history, prenatal diagnosis is difficult as there are no characteristic ultrasound features other than intrauterine growth retardation.[64]

DIFFERENTIAL DIAGNOSIS

The differential for IP depends on what point in the time course the patient is presenting. In the neonatal period, vesiculobullous disorders, including HSV,

VZV, bullous impetigo, bullous mastocytosis, and epidermolysis bullosa, and other mosaic disorders, such as focal dermal hypoplasia and epidermal nevus syndrome, may be considered. Later on, linear epidermal nevus, ILVEN, and pigmentary mosaicism, can appear similar.

CLINICAL COURSE, PROGNOSIS, AND MANAGEMENT

Most affected individuals without significant complications in infancy do well with a normal life expectancy. Treatment is symptom directed. The skin changes do not require specific treatment other than wound care of blisters to prevent secondary infection.[64] There are reports of topical corticosteroids minimizing inflammation and accelerating healing in the first stage.[66] As with other EDs, dental evaluation and restoration is important.

A baseline eye examination at diagnosis and following the recommended guidelines for repeat examinations during the first 3 years of life is critical. Peripheral retinal photocoagulation can reduce the risk of retinal detachment. Referral to neurology at time of diagnosis for a comprehensive examination and anticipatory guidance should be considered and is imperative for the management of seizures, spasticity, or other deficits if needed.[64] If neurologic symptoms are present, MRI and EEG should be performed. MRI can be considered in affected individuals with retinal neovascularization.[64]

TOOTH AND NAIL SYNDROME (WITKOP SYNDROME)

AT-A-GLANCE

- OMIM 189500, AD mutation of *MSX1* on 4p16.1, which encodes the transcription factor Msx1
- Characterized by small, friable nails at birth that may improve over time; may have fine, sparse hair. Primary teeth are usually unaffected, but secondary teeth fail to erupt or have partial absence

EPIDEMIOLOGY

The earliest case was reported by Witkop in 1965, when he described a pedigree demonstrating autosomal dominant inheritance. Along with Hudson, he later went on to describe 23 cases in 6 families in 1975.[70] All demonstrated hypoplastic nails and hypodontia; the latter manifested as failure of permanent teeth to erupt.

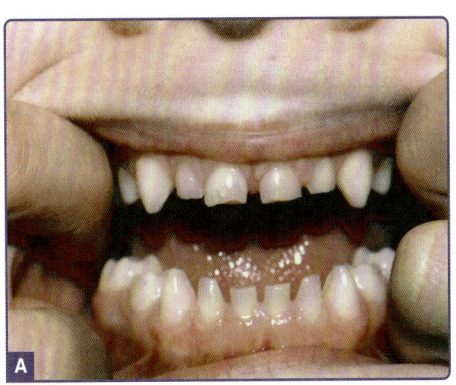
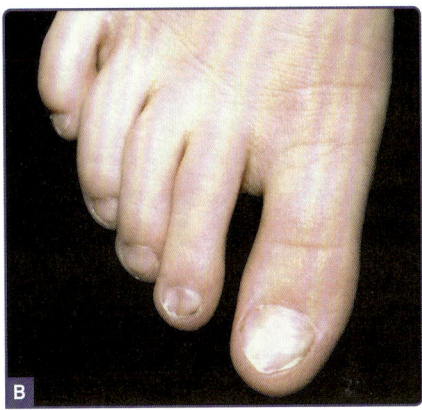

Figure 131-12 Tooth–nail syndrome. **A,** Primary teeth still in place; failure of adult teeth to erupt. **B,** Dystrophic toenails with flattening of nail plates.

CLINICAL FEATURES

In tooth and nail syndrome, the nails are thin, small, and friable and may show koilonychia at birth. Toenails are usually more severely involved than fingernails (Fig. 131-12). Nail changes improve with age and may be unappreciated in affected adults. A few individuals have reported thin, fine hair.[71]

The primary teeth usually are unaffected, although they may be small. The secondary teeth may fail to erupt, and there can be partial or total absence (Fig. 131-12A). The mandibular incisors, second molars, and maxillary canines are missing most often.[70] No other ectodermal structures are affected.

ETIOLOGY AND PATHOGENESIS

A nonsense mutation in *MSX1*, a gene expressed in the developing teeth and nail beds, was first identified in 2001 in a 3-generation family.[72] In 2013, an unrelated patient was found to have an *MSX1* mutation as well.[73] Other mutations in *MSX1* have been associated with isolated tooth agenesis or tooth agenesis with cleft palate, and mouse models have demonstrated the role of *MSX1* in tooth and nail development.[72] Tooth and nail syndrome is autosomal dominant, with variable expression and intrafamilial variability.

DIAGNOSIS

This is an easy condition to miss. The nail changes may be subtle. The tooth abnormalities may be mild enough to escape detection by a physician. The lack of associated features, either dermatologic or systemic, readily distinguish Witkop syndrome from other EDs. Genetic testing is available.

DIFFERENTIAL DIAGNOSIS

There is a presumed autosomal recessive disorder termed taurodontia, absent teeth, and sparse hair (OMIM 272980) that appears similar.[74] Taurodontia refers to teeth with an elongated body and pulp chamber and short roots.

CLINICAL COURSE, PROGNOSIS, AND MANAGEMENT

The nails usually require no treatment. Restorative dentistry is important.

TRICHO-DENTO-OSSEOUS (TDO) SYNDROME

AT-A-GLANCE

- OMIM 190320, AD mutation of *DLX3* on 17q21.3-q22, which encodes the transcription factor homeobox protein DLX-3
- Ectodermal features: teeth, nail, and hair changes in the setting of normal sweating and skin
- Systemic features: increased bone density

INTRODUCTION

Tricho-dento-osseous (TDO) syndrome is a rare autosomal dominant ED that involves the teeth, hair, nails, and bone.[75] It has been described in several families, although exact epidemiologic information is lacking.

CLINICAL FEATURES

TDO involves the hair, teeth, and nails. Hair is kinky or extremely curly, especially during the neonatal period. Dental findings include enamel hypoplasia, hypocalcification, and taurodontism (enlargement of the body of the tooth and pulp chamber) in both primary and secondary teeth. Nails are often thickened with splitting in the superficial layers. Sweat gland function and skin are unaffected.

Skeletal findings included increased bone density of the long bones and skull. There can be craniosynostosis resulting in dolichocephaly.[76]

ETIOLOGY AND PATHOGENESIS

TDO is an autosomal dominant disorder caused by mutations in *DLX3*, which encodes the human distal-less homeobox. Depending on the mutation, there are different severities in phenotype, but penetrance is usually complete.[77] The DLX3 protein is a transcriptional activator in the development and differentiation of epithelial tissue and has been shown to regulate hair follicles.[78,79]

DIAGNOSIS

Clinical molecular genetic testing is available through several labs.

DIFFERENTIAL DIAGNOSIS

TDO has the same dental findings as amelogenesis imperfecta (hypomaturation-hypoplasia type) with taurodontism (AIHHT), but AIHHT lacks hair and nail findings.

CLINICAL COURSE, PROGNOSIS, AND MANAGEMENT

Management includes dental care for the enamel hypoplasia. Given its autosomal dominant nature, genetic counseling should be provided.

OCULO-DENTO-DIGITAL DYSPLASIA (ODDD)

AT A GLANCE

- OMIM 164200
- AD mutation of *GJA1* on 6p21-23.2, which encodes connexin 43, a connexin protein of the intercellular junction
- Characterized by sparse hair, enamel hypoplasia, camptodactyly, and small eyes

INTRODUCTION

Oculo-dento-digital dysplasia (ODDD) is an autosomal dominant ED with variable expression.

CLINICAL FEATURES

ODDD patients have sparse, dry, slow-growing scalp hair with absent or sparse eyelashes. Both the primary and secondary teeth have enamel hypoplasia, resulting in small, yellow, and friable teeth prone to decay. Sweat glands and skin are normal.

Although vision is normal, the eyes have short palpebral fissures with microcornea and/or microphthalmia. Digital changes include camptodactyly of the fourth and fifth fingers in more than 80% of cases, with possible syndactyly of the fourth and fifth digits. Other skeletal anomalies include hyperostosis of the skull, broad ribs and clavicles, and abnormal trabeculation of the long bones.[80]

ETIOLOGY AND PATHOGENESIS

ODDD is autosomal dominant and caused by mutations in the gene for connexin-43 (*GJA1*).[81] Clinical molecular genetic testing is available.

CLINICAL COURSE, PROGNOSIS, AND MANAGEMENT

Management includes dental care of the enamel hypoplasia. Although vision is normal, patients should be followed by ophthalmology as 10% to 15% develop glaucoma.[82]

TRICHO-RHINO-PHALANGEAL SYNDROME

AT-A-GLANCE

- Variants:
  - TRPS I (OMIM 190350): AD mutation of *TRPS1* on 8q23.2; mutation in the same gene causes TRPS III (OMIM 190351)
  - TRPS II (Langer–Giedion Syndrome; OMIM 150230): AD, contiguous gene syndrome involving TRPS1 and EXT1, 8q24.11-q24.13
- Characterized by sparse hair, prominent nose, receding chin, and cone-shaped epiphyses leading to deviation of the middle phalanges

INTRODUCTION

Tricho-rhino-phalangeal (TRP) syndrome is an AD malformation syndrome characterized by distinctive craniofacial and skeletal anomalies. Although it is not considered a typical ED given the involvement of hair alone without involvement of the teeth, nails, or sweat/sebaceous glands, this chapter best encompasses its other features.

CLINICAL FEATURES

TRPS I patients have sparse, brittle, slow-growing scalp hair. On light microscopy, pili torti can be appreciated. They have a prominent, pear-shaped nose with a broad high nasal bridge and bulbous tip. The philtrum is long and flat with a thin upper lip and receding chin (Fig. 131-13).[83]

Digital changes may not appear until several years of age and include cone-shaped epiphyses and deviation of the middle phalanges giving the appearance of crooked fingers. Other skeletal abnormalities include hip malformations and short stature.[84]

TRPS III has the features above in addition to the presence of severe brachydactyly and more pronounced short stature.[85] TRPSII combines the features of TRPS1 and multiple exostoses type 1. Additionally, these patients often have intellectual disabilities.[86]

ETIOLOGY AND PATHOGENESIS

TRPS I and TRPS III are autosomal dominant and caused by a mutation in *TRPS1*, a transcription factor

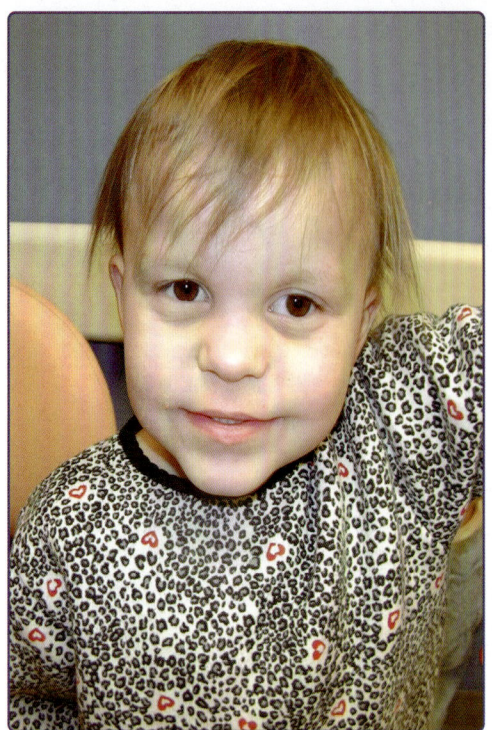

Figure 131-13 Tricho-rhino-phalangeal syndrome. Note the sparse hair and eyebrows, bulbous nose and thin upper lip.

zinc finger protein.[83] TRPS II is caused by a deletion that includes both *TRPS1* and *EXT1*. Genetic testing is available to assist with diagnosis.

CLINICAL COURSE, PROGNOSIS, AND MANAGEMENT

For short stature, consideration should be given to growth hormone treatment on an individual basis.[87] The skeletal changes should be monitored and managed appropriately for pain if needed. Otoplasty and rhinoplasty can provide aesthetic correction.[88]

ACKNOWLEDGMENTS

The authors acknowledge the contributions of Alanna F. Bree, Nnenna Agim, and Virginia P. Sybert, authors of prior versions of this chapter.

REFERENCES

1. Visinoni AF, Lisboa-Costa T, Pagnan NA, et al. Ectodermal dysplasias: clinical and molecular review. *Am J Med Genet A*. 2009;149a(9):1980-2002.
2. Pinheiro M, Freire-Maia N. Ectodermal dysplasias: a clinical classification and a causal review. *Am J Med Genet*. 1994;53(2):153-162.
3. Salinas CF, Jorgenson RJ, Wright JT, et al. 2008 International Conference on Ectodermal Dysplasias Classification: conference report. *Am J Med Genet A*. 2009;149a(9):1958-1969.
4. Salinas CF, Irvine AD, Itin PH, et al. Second International Conference on a classification of ectodermal dysplasias: development of a multiaxis model. *Am J Med Genet A*. 2014;164a(10):2482-2489.
5. Modino SA, Sharpe PT. Tissue engineering of teeth using adult stem cells. *Arch Oral Biol*. 2005;50(2):255-258.
6. Del Rio M, Gache Y, Jorcano JL, et al. Current approaches and perspectives in human keratinocyte-based gene therapies. *Gene Ther*. 2004;11(suppl 1):S57-S63.
7. Ohyama M, Vogel JC. Gene delivery to the hair follicle. *J Investig Dermatol Symp Proc*. 2003;8(2):204-206.
8. Thurnam J. Two cases in which the skin, hair and teeth were very imperfectly developed. *Med Chir Trans*. 1848;31:71-82.
9. Cluzeau C, Hadj-Rabia S, Jambou M, et al. Only four genes (*EDA1*, *EDAR*, *EDARADD*, and *WNT10A*) account for 90% of hypohidrotic/anhidrotic ectodermal dysplasia cases. *Hum Mutat*. 2011;32(1):70-72.
10. Trzeciak WH, Koczorowski R. Molecular basis of hypohidrotic ectodermal dysplasia: an update. *J Appl Genet*. 2016;57(1):51-61.
11. Zonana J, Elder ME, Schneider LC, et al. A novel X-linked disorder of immune deficiency and hypohidrotic ectodermal dysplasia is allelic to incontinentia pigmenti and due to mutations in IKK-gamma (NEMO). *Am J Hum Genet*. 2000;67(6):1555-1562.
12. Doffinger R, Smahi A, Bessia C, et al. X-linked anhidrotic ectodermal dysplasia with immunodeficiency is caused by impaired NF-kappaB signaling. *Nat Genet*. 2001;27(3):277-285.
13. Stevenson AC, Kerr CB. On the distribution of frequencies of mutation to genes determining harmful traits in man. *Mutat Res*. 1967;4(3):339-352.
14. Kishore M, Panat SR, Aggarwal A, et al. Hypohidrotic ectodermal dysplasia (ED): a case series. *J Clin Diagn Res*. 2014;8(1):273-275.
15. Scaling skin in the neonate: a clue to the early diagnosis of X-linked hypohidrotic ectodermal dysplasia (Christ-Siemens-Touraine syndrome). The Executive and Scientific Advisory Boards of the National Foundation for Ectodermal Dysplasias, Mascoutah, Illinois. *J Pediatr*. 1989;114(4, pt 1):600-602.
16. Basu S, Mitra M, Ghosh A. Evaluation of sweat production by pilocarpine iontophoresis: a noninvasive screening tool for hypohidrosis in ectodermal dysplasia. *Indian J Clin Biochem*. 2013;28(4):433-435.
17. Clarke A, Phillips DI, Brown R, et al. Clinical aspects of X-linked hypohidrotic ectodermal dysplasia. *Arch Dis Child*. 1987;62(10):989-996.
18. Sybert VP. *Genetic Skin Disorders*. New York: Oxford University Press; 1997.
19. Fete M, Hermann J, Behrens J, et al. X-linked hypohidrotic ectodermal dysplasia (XLHED): clinical and diagnostic insights from an international patient registry. *Am J Med Genet A*. 2014;164a(10):2437-2442.
20. Zankl A, Addor MC, Cousin P, et al. Fatal outcome in a female monozygotic twin with X-linked hypohidrotic ectodermal dysplasia (XLHED) due to a de novo t(X;9) translocation with probable disruption of the EDA gene. *Eur J Pediatr*. 2001;160(5):296-299.

21. Motil KJ, Fete TJ, Fraley JK, et al. Growth characteristics of children with ectodermal dysplasia syndromes. *Pediatrics.* 2005;116(2):e229-234.
22. Wright JT, Grange DK, Richter MK. Hypohidrotic ectodermal dysplasia. In: Pagon RA, Adam MP, Ardinger HH, et al, eds. *GeneReviews(R).* Seattle (WA): University of Washington, Seattle, 1993.
23. Burger K, Schneider AT, Wohlfart S, et al. Genotype-phenotype correlation in boys with X-linked hypohidrotic ectodermal dysplasia. *Am J Med Genet A.* 2014;164a(10):2424-2432.
24. Rouse C, Siegfried E, Breer W, et al. Hair and sweat glands in families with hypohidrotic ectodermal dysplasia: further characterization. *Arch Dermatol.* 2004;140(7):850-855.
25. Bernstein R, Hatchuel I, Jenkins T. Hypohidrotic ectodermal dysplasia and sudden infant death syndrome. *Lancet.* 1980;2(8202):1024.
26. Ogden E, Schandl C, Tormos LM. Death due to complications of anhidrotic ectodermal dysplasia. *J Forensic Sci.* 2014;59(6):1672-1674.
27. Gaide O, Schneider P. Permanent correction of an inherited ectodermal dysplasia with recombinant EDA. *Nat Med.* 2003;9(5):614-618.
28. Casal ML, Lewis JR, Mauldin EA, et al. Significant correction of disease after postnatal administration of recombinant ectodysplasin A in canine X-linked ectodermal dysplasia. *Am J Hum Genet.* 2007;81(5):1050-1056.
29. Mauldin EA, Gaide O, Schneider P, et al. Neonatal treatment with recombinant ectodysplasin prevents respiratory disease in dogs with X-linked ectodermal dysplasia. *Am J Med Genet A.* 2009;149a(9):2045-2049.
30. Clouston HR. The major forms of hereditary ectodermal dysplasia: (with an autopsy and biopsies on the anhydrotic type). *CMAJ.* 1939;40(1):1-7.
31. Der Kaloustian VM. Hidrotic ectodermal dysplasia 2. In: Pagon RA, Adam MP, Ardinger HH, et al, eds. *GeneReviews(R).* Seattle, WA: University of Washington, Seattle, 1993.
32. Lamartine J, Munhoz Essenfelder G, Kibar Z, et al. Mutations in GJB6 cause hidrotic ectodermal dysplasia. *Nat Genet.* 2000;26(2):142-144.
33. Celli J, Duijf P, Hamel BC, et al. Heterozygous germline mutations in the p53 homolog p63 are the cause of EEC syndrome. *Cell.* 1999;99(2):143-153.
34. van Bokhoven H, Hamel BC, Bamshad M, et al. p63 Gene mutations in EEC syndrome, limb-mammary syndrome, and isolated split hand-split foot malformation suggest a genotype-phenotype correlation. *Am J Hum Genet.* 2001;69(3):481-492.
35. Hay RJ, Wells RS. The syndrome of ankyloblepharon, ectodermal defects and cleft lip and palate: an autosomal dominant condition. *Br J Dermatol.* 1976;94(3):277-289.
36. Rapp RS, Hodgkin WE. Anhidrotic ectodermal dysplasia: autosomal dominant inheritance with palate and lip anomalies. *J Med Genet.* 1968;5(4):269-272.
37. Kannu P, Savarirayan R, Ozoemena L, et al. Rapp-Hodgkin ectodermal dysplasia syndrome: the clinical and molecular overlap with Hay-Wells syndrome. *Am J Med Genet A.* 2006;140(8):887-891.
38. Clements SE, Techanukul T, Holden ST, et al. Rapp-Hodgkin and Hay-Wells ectodermal dysplasia syndromes represent a variable spectrum of the same genetic disorder. *Br J Dermatol.* 2010;163(3):624-629.
39. Vanderhooft SL, Stephan MJ, Sybert VP. Severe skin erosions and scalp infections in AEC syndrome. *Pediatr Dermatol.* 1993;10(4):334-340.
40. Julapalli MR, Scher RK, Sybert VP, et al. Dermatologic findings of ankyloblepharon-ectodermal defects-cleft lip/palate (AEC) syndrome. *Am J Med Genet A.* 2009;149a(9):1900-1906.
41. Berk DR, Crone K, Bayliss SJ. AEC syndrome caused by a novel p63 mutation and demonstrating erythroderma followed by extensive depigmentation. *Pediatr Dermatol.* 2009;26(5):617-618.
42. Sutton VR, Plunkett K, Dang DX, et al. Craniofacial and anthropometric phenotype in ankyloblepharon-ectodermal defects-cleft lip/palate syndrome (Hay-Wells syndrome) in a cohort of 17 patients. *Am J Med Genet A.* 2009;149a(9):1916-1921.
43. Cole P, Hatef DA, Kaufman Y, et al. Facial clefting and oro-auditory pathway manifestations in ankyloblepharon-ectodermal defects-cleft lip/palate (AEC) syndrome. *Am J Med Genet A.* 2009;149a(9):1910-1915.
44. Farrington F, Lausten L. Oral findings in ankyloblepharon-ectodermal dysplasia-cleft lip/palate (AEC) syndrome. *Am J Med Genet A.* 2009;149a(9):1907-1909.
45. Dishop MK, Bree AF, Hicks MJ. Pathologic changes of skin and hair in ankyloblepharon-ectodermal defects-cleft lip/palate (AEC) syndrome. *Am J Med Genet A.* 2009;149a(9):1935-1941.
46. Buss PW, Hughes HE, Clarke A. Twenty-four cases of the EEC syndrome: clinical presentation and management. *J Med Genet.* 1995;32(9):716-723.
47. Roelfsema NM, Cobben JM. The EEC syndrome: a literature study. *Clin Dysmorphol.* 1996;5(2):115-127.
48. McGrath JA, Duijf PH, Doetsch V, et al. Hay-Wells syndrome is caused by heterozygous missense mutations in the SAM domain of p63. *Hum Mol Genet.* 2001;10(3):221-229.
49. Ianakiev P, Kilpatrick MW, Toudjarska I, et al. Split-hand/split-foot malformation is caused by mutations in the p63 gene on 3q27. *Am J Hum Genet.* 2000;67(1):59-66.
50. Rinne T, Spadoni E, Kjaer KW, et al. Delineation of the ADULT syndrome phenotype due to arginine 298 mutations of the p63 gene. *Eur J Hum Genet.* 2006;14(8):904-910.
51. Bohring A, Stamm T, Spaich C, et al. WNT10A mutations are a frequent cause of a broad spectrum of ectodermal dysplasias with sex-biased manifestation pattern in heterozygotes. *Am J Hum Genet.* 2009;85(1):97-105.
52. Nawaz S, Klar J, Wajid M, et al. WNT10A missense mutation associated with a complete odonto-onychodermal dysplasia syndrome. *Eur J Hum Genet.* 2009;17(12):1600-1605.
53. Megarbane H, Haddad M, Delague V, et al. Further delineation of the odonto-onycho-dermal dysplasia syndrome. *Am J Med Genet A.* 2004;129a(2):193-197.
54. Arzoo PS, Klar J, Bergendal B, et al. WNT10A mutations account for (1/4) of population-based isolated oligodontia and show phenotypic correlations. *Am J Med Genet A.* 2014;164a(2):353-359.
55. Bergendal B, Norderyd J, Zhou X, et al. Abnormal primary and permanent dentitions with ectodermal symptoms predict WNT10A deficiency. *BMC Med Genet.* 2016;17(1):88.
56. Kroigard AB, Clemmensen O, Gjorup H, et al. Odonto-onycho-dermal dysplasia in a patient homozygous for a WNT10A nonsense mutation and mild manifestations of ectodermal dysplasia in carriers of the mutation. *BMC Dermatol.* 2016;16:3.

57. Castori M, Ruggieri S, Giannetti L, et al. Schopf-Schulz-Passarge syndrome: further delineation of the phenotype and genetic considerations. *Acta Derm Venereol.* 2008;88(6):607-612.
58. Ko CJ, Antaya RJ, Zubek A, et al. Revisiting histopathologic findings in Goltz syndrome. *J Cutan Pathol.* 2016;43(5):418-421.
59. Goltz RW. Focal dermal hypoplasia syndrome. An update. *Arch Dermatol.* 1992;128(8):1108-1111.
60. Grzeschik KH, Bornholdt D, Oeffner F, et al. Deficiency of PORCN, a regulator of Wnt signaling, is associated with focal dermal hypoplasia. *Nat Genet.* 2007;39(7):833-835.
61. Wang X, Reid Sutton V, Omar Peraza-Llanes J, et al. Mutations in X-linked PORCN, a putative regulator of Wnt signaling, cause focal dermal hypoplasia. *Nat Genet.* 2007;39(7):836-838.
62. Bostwick B, Van den Veyver IB, Sutton VR. Focal dermal hypoplasia. In: Pagon RA, Adam MP, Ardinger HH, et al, eds. *GeneReviews(R).* Seattle, WA: University of Washington, Seattle, 1993.
63. Arenas-Sordo Mde L, Vallejo-Vega B, Hernandez-Zamora E, et al. Incontinentia pigmenti (IP2): familiar case report with affected men. Literature review. *Med Oral Patol Oral Cir Bucal.* 2005;10(suppl 2):E122-E129.
64. Scheuerle AE, Ursini MV. Incontinentia Pigmenti. In: Adam MP, Ardinger HH, Pagon RA, et al, eds. *GeneReviews((R)).* Seattle, WA: University of Washington, Seattle, 1993.
65. Fusco F, Paciolla M, Conte MI, et al. Incontinentia pigmenti: report on data from 2000 to 2013. *Orphanet J Rare Dis.* 2014;9:93.
66. Darne S, Carmichael AJ. Isolated recurrence of vesicobullous incontinentia pigmenti in a schoolgirl. *Br J Dermatol.* 2007;156(3):600-602.
67. Popli U, Yesudian PD. Whorled scarring alopecia—the only adult marker of incontinentia pigmenti. *Int J Trichology.* 2018;10(1):24-25.
68. Meuwissen ME, Mancini GM. Neurological findings in incontinentia pigmenti; a review. *Eur J Hum Genet.* 2012;55(5):323-331.
69. Minic S, Trpinac D, Obradovic M. Incontinentia pigmenti diagnostic criteria update. *Clin Genet.* 2014;85(6):536-542.
70. Hudson CD, Witkop CJ. Autosomal dominant hypodontia with nail dysgenesis. Report of twenty-nine cases in six families. *Oral Surg Oral Med Oral Pathol.* 1975;39(3):409-423.
71. Garzon MC, Paller AS. What syndrome is this? Witkop tooth and nail syndrome. *Pediatr Dermatol.* 1996;13(1):63-64.
72. Jumlongras D, Bei M, Stimson JM, et al. A nonsense mutation in MSX1 causes Witkop syndrome. *Am J Hum Genet.* 2001;69(1):67-74.
73. Ghaderi F, Hekmat S, Ghaderi R, et al. MSX1 mutation in witkop syndrome; a case report. *Iran J Med Sci.* 2013;38(2)(suppl):191-194.
74. Moller KT, Gorlin RJ, Wedge B. Oligodontia, taurodontia, and sparse hair growth—a syndrome. *J Speech Hear Disord.* 1973;38(2):268-271.
75. Islam M, Lurie AG, Reichenberger E. Clinical features of tricho-dento-osseous syndrome and presentation of three new cases: an addition to clinical heterogeneity. *Oral Surg Oral Med Oral Pathol Oral Radiol Endod.* 2005;100(6):736-742.
76. Haldeman RJ, Cooper LF, Hart TC, et al. Increased bone density associated with DLX3 mutation in the tricho-dento-osseous syndrome. *Bone.* 2004;35(4):988-997.
77. Wright JT, Hong SP, Simmons D, et al. DLX3 c.561_562delCT mutation causes attenuated phenotype of tricho-dento-osseous syndrome. *Am J Med Genet A.* 2008;146a(3):343-349.
78. Bryan JT, Morasso MI. The Dlx3 protein harbors basic residues required for nuclear localization, transcriptional activity and binding to Msx1. *J Cell Sci.* 2000;113(pt 22):4013-4023.
79. Hwang J, Mehrani T, Millar SE, et al. Dlx3 is a crucial regulator of hair follicle differentiation and cycling. *Development (Cambridge, England).* 2008;135(18):3149-3159.
80. Judisch GF, Martin-Casals A, Hanson JW, et al. Oculodentodigital dysplasia. Four new reports and a literature review. *Arch Ophthalmol.* 1979;97(5):878-884.
81. Paznekas WA, Karczeski B, Vermeer S, et al. GJA1 mutations, variants, and connexin 43 dysfunction as it relates to the oculodentodigital dysplasia phenotype. *Hum Mutat.* 2009;30(5):724-733.
82. Mosaed S, Jacobsen BH, Lin KY. Case report: imaging and treatment of ophthalmic manifestations in oculodentodigital dysplasia. *BMC Ophthalmol.* 2016;16:5.
83. Momeni P, Glockner G, Schmidt O, et al. Mutations in a new gene, encoding a zinc-finger protein, cause tricho-rhino-phalangeal syndrome type I. *Nat Genet.* 2000;24(1):71-74.
84. Izumi K, Takagi M, Parikh AS, et al. Late manifestations of tricho-rhino-pharyngeal syndrome in a patient: Expanded skeletal phenotype in adulthood. *Am J Med Genet A.* 2010;152a(8):2115-2119.
85. Ludecke HJ, Schaper J, Meinecke P, et al. Genotypic and phenotypic spectrum in tricho-rhino-phalangeal syndrome types I and III. *Am J Hum Genet.* 2001;68(1):81-91.
86. Ludecke HJ, Wagner MJ, Nardmann J, et al. Molecular dissection of a contiguous gene syndrome: localization of the genes involved in the Langer-Giedion syndrome. *Hum Mol Genet.* 1995;4(1):31-36.
87. Merjaneh L, Parks JS, Muir AB, et al. A novel TRPS1 gene mutation causing trichorhinophalangeal syndrome with growth hormone responsive short stature: a case report and review of the literature. *Int J Pediatr Endocrinol.* 2014;2014(1):16.
88. Morioka D, Hosaka Y. Aesthetic and plastic surgery for trichorhinophalangeal syndrome. *Aesthetic Plast Surg.* 2000;24(1):39-45.

Chapter 132 :: Genetic Immunodeficiency Diseases
:: Ramsay L. Fuleihan & Amy S. Paller

第一百三十二章
遗传性免疫缺陷病

中文导读

原发性免疫缺陷病是一种遗传性免疫系统疾病，导致感染易感性增加，发病率和死亡率增加。许多遗传性免疫缺陷疾病与各种皮肤异常有关，识别这些临床特征可能有助于早期诊断原发性免疫缺陷。皮肤异常可能包括皮肤感染、特应性或脂溢性皮炎、黄斑红斑、脱发、伤口愈合不良、紫癜、瘀斑、毛细血管扩张、色素稀释、皮肤肉芽肿、广泛疣、血管性水肿和狼疮样改变。其他临床特征通常包括发育不良、内脏感染、自身免疫性疾病、结缔组织/风湿病、过敏反应和肿瘤。

遗传性免疫缺陷疾病分为五类：抗体缺陷、细胞缺陷、抗体和细胞联合缺陷、吞噬和细胞杀伤障碍及补体缺陷。细胞缺陷容易引起慢性皮肤黏膜念珠菌病。抗体和细胞联合缺陷可表现为Wiskott-Aldrich综合征、外胚层发育不良伴免疫缺陷、共济失调毛细血管扩张等。吞噬和细胞杀伤功能紊乱可引起慢性肉芽肿性疾病、高免疫球蛋白E综合征、Ché Diak-Higashi综合征等。补体缺陷可引起遗传性血管性水肿。本章分别介绍了这五类疾病的临床特点、病因和发病机制、诊断、临床病程、预后和处理。

OVERVIEW OF GENETIC IMMUNODEFICIENCY DISEASES

Primary immunodeficiency diseases are inherited disorders of the immune system that result in an increased susceptibility to infection and an increased morbidity and mortality.[1] Many of these genetic immunodeficiency diseases are associated with a variety of cutaneous abnormalities, and recognition of these clinical features may allow an early diagnosis of primary immunodeficiency. Cutaneous abnormalities may include cutaneous infections, atopic-like or seborrheic-like dermatitis, macular erythemas, alopecia, poor wound healing, purpura, petechiae, telangiectasias, pigmentary dilution, cutaneous granulomas, extensive warts, angioedema, and lupus-like changes (Table 132-1). Other clinical features often include failure to thrive, visceral infection, autoimmune disorders, connective tissue/rheumatologic diseases, allergic reactions, and neoplasias.

CLINICAL FEATURES

Immunodeficiency should be suspected when patients have recurrent infections of increased duration or severity, particularly with unusual organisms. Incomplete clearing of infections, unexpected or severe complications of infection, or poor response to antibiotics may be associated.[2] Affected infants often grow poorly

TABLE 132-1
Manifestations of Genetic Immunodeficiencies

CUTANEOUS MANIFESTATIONS	ASSOCIATED IMMUNODEFICIENCY	CUTANEOUS MANIFESTATIONS	ASSOCIATED IMMUNODEFICIENCY
Angioedema	Hereditary angioedema	Lupus-like cutaneous change	IgA deficiency Chronic granulomatous disease, autosomal recessive Chronic granulomatous disease, X-linked carrier Common variable immunodeficiency Complement deficiency, early components Elevated IgM with hypogammaglobulinemia
Atopic-like dermatitis	IgA deficiency/IgM deficiency Chronic granulomatous disease Common variable immunodeficiency Elevated IgM with hypogammaglobulinemia Ectodermal dysplasia with immunodeficiency Hyperimmunoglobulinemia E syndrome Severe combined immunodeficiency Wiskott-Aldrich syndrome X-linked agammaglobulinemia	Mucocutaneous telangiectasias	Ataxia-telangiectasia
		Petechiae and/or purpura	Chédiak-Higashi syndrome
		Pigmentary dilution/silvery hair	Griscelli syndrome
		Pyoderma gangrenosum-like ulcerations	Wiskott-Aldrich syndrome Chédiak-Higashi syndrome Griscelli syndrome IgA deficiency Chédiak-Higashi syndrome Chronic granulomatous disease Hyperimmunoglobulinemia E syndrome Leukocyte adhesion deficiency
Cutaneous abscesses	Chronic granulomatous disease Hyperimmunoglobulinemia E syndrome Leukocyte adhesion deficiency	Seborrheic-like or exfoliative dermatitis	X-linked hypogammaglobulinemia Ataxia-telangiectasia "Leiner" phenotype: complement deficiency or dysfunction
Cutaneous granulomas	Ataxia-telangiectasia Chronic granulomatous disease Chronic mucocutaneous candidiasis Common variable immunodeficiency Severe combined immunodeficiency, especially *TAP2* deficiency X-linked hypogammaglobulinemia	Warts, extensive	Severe combined immunodeficiency X-linked agammaglobulinemia Common variable immunodeficiency Elevated IgM with hypogammaglobulinemia Epidermodysplasia verruciformis (see Chap. 166) IgM deficiency Severe combined immunodeficiency after transplantation (mutations in *IL2RG* or *JAK3*) WHIM syndrome
Cutaneous candidal infection	Chronic mucocutaneous candidiasis DiGeorge syndrome Hyperimmunoglobulinemia E syndrome Severe combined immunodeficiency especially TAP2 deficiency		
Eosinophilic folliculitis, infantile	Hyperimmunoglobulinemia E syndrome		
Graft-versus-host disease	DiGeorge syndrome Severe combined immunodeficiency		

Ig, immunoglobulin; TAP, transporter associated with antigen processing or transporter, ATP-binding cassette; WHIM, warts, hypogammaglobulinemia, infections, myelokathexis.

(failure to thrive). The most common noncutaneous abnormalities are infections, diarrhea, vomiting, hepatosplenomegaly, arthritis, adenopathy or paucity of lymph nodes/tonsils, and hematologic abnormalities.

The classification of genetic immunodeficiency disorders includes: (a) antibody deficiencies, (b) cellular deficiencies, (c) combined antibody and cellular deficiencies, (d) disorders of phagocytosis and cell killing, and (e) complement defects. The characteristic clinical signs of each group suggest that proper classification and laboratory tests may be used to confirm the diagnosis. The laboratory testing and clinical patterns of illness associated with each group of immunodeficiency disorders that allow their differential diagnosis are outlined in Table 132-2 and Fig. 132-1. The most important disorder in the differential diagnosis of all genetic immunodeficiency disorders is HIV infection. In addition to the lack of HIV antigen as detected by polymerase chain reaction in patients with genetic immunodeficiency, other features help to differentiate the disorders. Patients with HIV infection tend to show an inverted CD4-to-CD8 ratio and hypergammaglobulinemia, in contrast to the hypogammaglobulinemia of many patients with genetic immunodeficiency.

ANTIBODY DEFICIENCY DISORDERS

AGAMMAGLOBULINEMIA

AT-A-GLANCE

- Synonym: Bruton disease.
- Early-onset, recurrent bacterial infections.
- Absent or barely detectable tonsillar and cervical lymph node tissue.
- Profound hypogammaglobulinemia and decreased or absent peripheral B cells.

CLINICAL FEATURES

Agammaglobulinemia is characterized by recurrent pyogenic infections that often begin after 6 months of age, concurrent with the waning of maternal immunoglobulins. These patients have absent or barely detectable tonsils and cervical lymph nodes.[3] Skin infections, especially furunculosis and impetigo, are common and often surround body orifices. An atopic-like eczematous eruption that fails to improve with immunoglobulin (Ig) therapy has been described in many affected children. Pyoderma gangrenosum and noninfectious cutaneous granulomas have been reported. Childhood exanthematous disorders are handled appropriately, but the infections may recur, owing to a failure to develop specific antibodies.

Recurrent otitis media, sinusitis, bronchitis, and pneumonia are the earliest infectious manifestations and usually are caused by pneumococci, staphylococci, or *Haemophilus*. Untreated pulmonary infections may lead to progressive bronchiectasis and chronic pulmonary disease.[4] Patients can also suffer from chronic enteroviral infections and hearing loss from repeated otitis and sinusitis infections. Other common bacterial infections include conjunctivitis, osteomyelitis, septic arthritis, and meningitis. Protracted diarrhea may be caused by infection, particularly with *Giardia*, *Salmonella*, *Campylobacter*, or *Cryptosporidium* spp. Three virus groups cause problems: enterovirus, hepatitis B virus, and rotavirus. Patients have developed paralysis after administration of the live polio vaccine. A rheumatoid-like arthritis, characterized by chronic inflammation and swelling of the large joints, may develop in as many as one-third to one-half of boys with X-linked agammaglobulinemia (XLA) and is often caused by mycoplasmal infection (*Ureaplasma urealyticum*). Disseminated echovirus infection has caused meningoencephalitis and a dermatomyositis-like disorder with brawny edema, induration of the muscles with accompanying weakness, muscle contractures, and poikiloderma.

TABLE 132-2
Patterns Associated with Primary Immune Deficiency

DISORDER	INFECTION	OTHER
Antibody	Sinopulmonary (pyogenic bacteria)	Autoimmune disease (autoantibodies, inflammatory bowel disease)
	GI (enterovirus, *Giardia*)	Minimal growth retardation
	Normal handling of fungal and viral infections (exception is enterovirus)	Paucity of lymphoid tissue
Cellular	Low-grade or opportunistic infections	Growth retardation
	Pneumonia (pyogenic bacteria, *Pneumocystis*, viruses)	Graft-versus-host disease
	GI (viruses)	Fatal infections from live vaccines
	Skin, mucous membranes (fungi)	Malignancy
Phagocytosis and cell killing	Skin, reticuloendothelial system (*Staphylococcus*, enteric bacteria, *Aspergillus*, *Mycobacteria*)	Ulcerative stomatitis
Complement	Alternative, late components	Early components
	Sepsis/blood-borne (streptococci, pneumococci, *Neisseria*)	Autoimmune disease (systemic lupus erythematosus, glomerulonephritis)
		C1 esterase inhibitor deficiency
		Angioedema

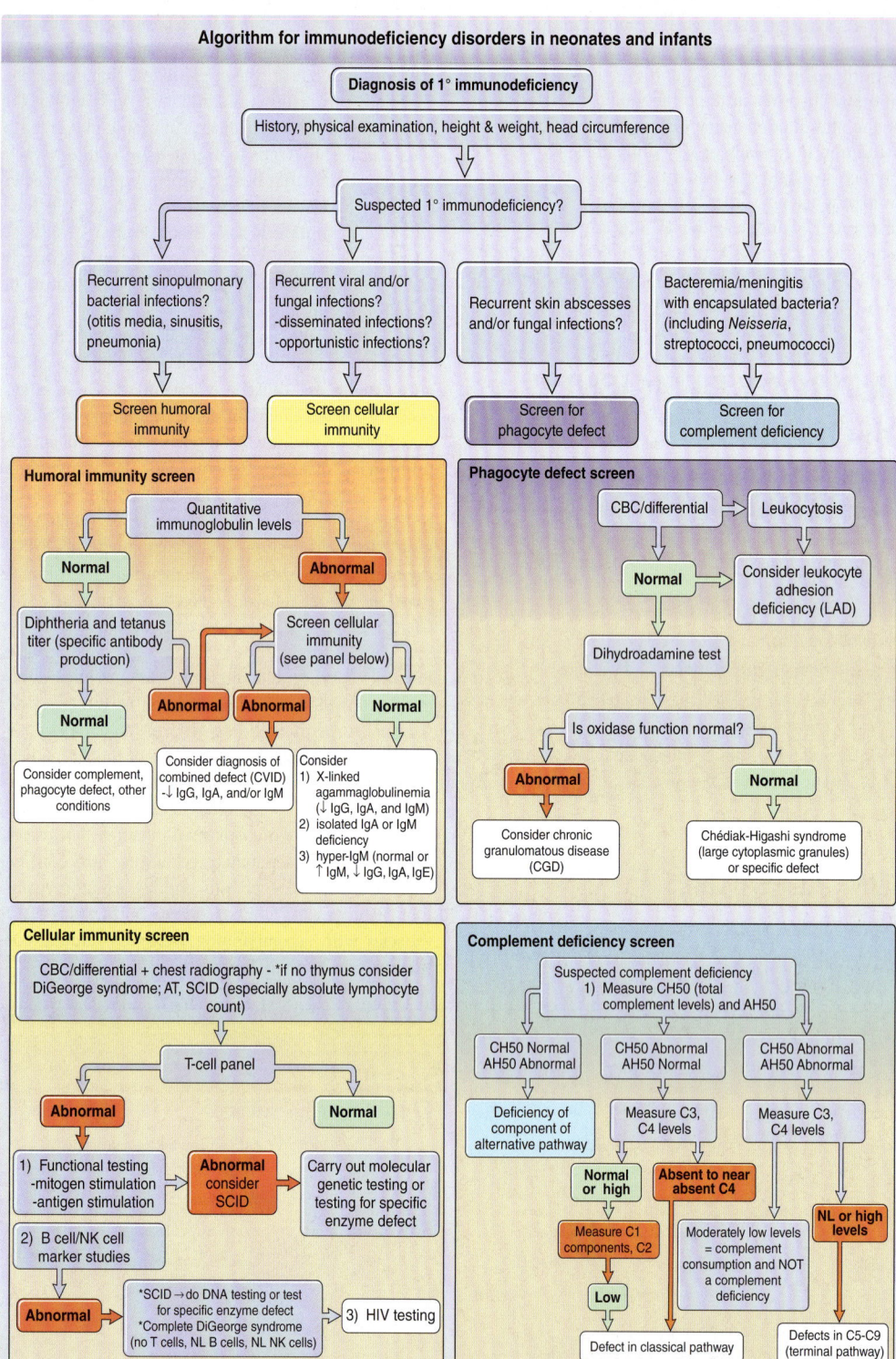

Figure 132-1 Algorithm for immunodeficiency disorders in neonates and infants. If the clinical presentation is concerning for severe combined immunodeficiency (SCID), this is a medical emergency and the patient needs immediate referral to an immunologist. AH50, alternative pathway 50% hemolytic activity; AT, ataxia-telangiectasia; CBC, complete blood cell count; CH50, 50% hemolytic complement; CVID, common variable immunodeficiency; Ig, immunoglobulin; NK cell, natural killer cell; NL, normal; ↓, decreased; ↑, increased.

ETIOLOGY AND PATHOGENESIS

Agammaglobulinemia results from failure of development of B cells, most commonly from gene defects that prevent the assembly of a full B-cell antigen receptor. XLA is the most common cause of agammaglobulinemia and results from defects in a cytoplasmic tyrosine kinase, Bruton tyrosine kinase. XLA is inherited in an X-linked fashion, and approximately 50% of affected boys have a family history of the disorder.[5] Autosomal recessive agammaglobulinemia affects males and females equally and results from defects in the genes that encode for components of the pre–B-cell and B-cell receptors or in BLNK (B-cell linker), a scaffold protein that assembles signaling molecules associated with the pre–B-cell and B-cell receptor.

DIAGNOSIS

The diagnosis of agammaglobulinemia is made by serum concentrations of IgG, IgA, and IgM that are far below the 95% confidence limits for appropriate controls (usually less than 100 mg/dL total Ig) and by the virtual absence of B cells in the peripheral circulation (<1% of normal). The absence of the Bruton tyrosine kinase protein in patients with XLA can be detected by flow cytometry. Identification of a defect in one of the known genetic causes of agammaglobulinemia confirms the diagnosis and allows for genetic counseling and prenatal diagnosis.

CLINICAL COURSE, PROGNOSIS, AND MANAGEMENT

Early Ig replacement, intravenously or subcutaneously, and antibiotic use markedly reduces the risk of infections, although it may not be helpful in diminishing the risk and morbidity of chronic lung disease or chronic enterovirus infection.

COMMON VARIABLE IMMUNODEFICIENCY

AT-A-GLANCE

- Heterogeneous group of disorders in which both antibody deficiency and abnormalities of T cells may be found.
- Most common underlying gene defect is in the transmembrane activator and calcium-modulating cyclophilin ligand interactor (TACI) gene.
- May manifest during childhood, with peak onset in the second and third decades of life.

(Continued)

AT-A-GLANCE (Continued)

- Diagnosis requires the presence of low levels of serum immunoglobulin (Ig) G with either low IgM and/or low IgA, defective antibody response to immunization, especially with pneumococcal antigens, with recurrent infections and/or typical autoimmune complications.
- Variable severity of autoimmune and infectious complications.

CLINICAL FEATURES

Common variable immunodeficiency (CVID) usually presents in young adults, but approximately 20% of cases are diagnosed before the age of 21 years.[6] Patients have infections similar to those in patients with XLA, particularly sinopulmonary infections, but are less susceptible to enteroviral infections and more susceptible to *Giardia* infections. Many patients with CVID have liver disease and GI disease, causing malabsorption syndromes. Noncaseating granulomas of skin (Fig. 132-2), lungs, liver, and spleen have been reported. Caseating granulomas of the skin and viscera, although rare, also have been described.[7,8] Extensive warts can be a major problem in individuals with CVID (Fig. 132-3). A comparison of skin manifestations in patients with CVID compared to IgA deficiency found that there was an increased incidence of atopic dermatitis without an elevated IgE level in patients with IgA deficiency, while there

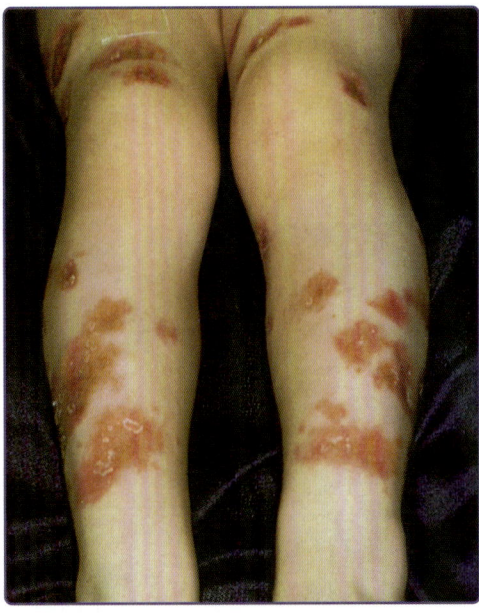

Figure 132-2 Noncaseating granulomas on the legs of a child with common variable immunodeficiency. Cultures and special stains showed no organisms.

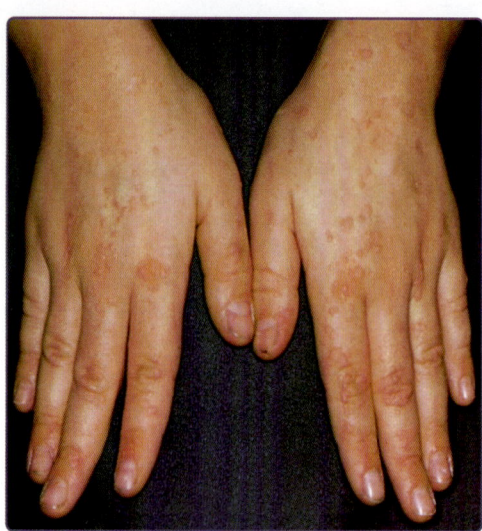

Figure 132-3 The dorsal aspect of the hands were covered with recalcitrant verrucae vulgaris in this girl with common variable immunodeficiency.

was an increased prevalence of psoriasis, skin infections, acne, alopecia, vitiligo, and aphthous ulcers in patients with CVID.[9] Lymphoid tissues often are enlarged, and splenomegaly with hypersplenism is also found, with 8.2% of CVID patients undergoing splenectomy.[6] Autoimmune disorders are especially frequent (28.6%), particularly autoimmune thrombocytopenia, autoimmune hemolytic anemia, rheumatoid arthritis, sicca syndrome, and pernicious anemia. Alopecia areata and lupus also have been described. In 10% to 20% of CVID patients, at least 1 family member is also immunodeficient, particularly with CVID or IgA deficiency.[10] The incidence of lymphoreticular malignancy and gastric carcinoma are markedly increased, particularly in the fifth and sixth decades of life.

SELECTIVE IMMUNOGLOBULIN DISORDERS

AT-A-GLANCE

- Immunoglobulin A deficiency is usually asymptomatic; only 10% to 15% of affected individuals demonstrate clinical manifestations, including bacterial sinopulmonary infections and autoimmune disorders.

CELLULAR DEFICIENCIES

CHRONIC MUCOCUTANEOUS CANDIDIASIS

AT-A-GLANCE

- Heterogeneous group of disorders with altered immune responses selective to *Candida*.
- Recurrent, progressive candidal infections of the skin, nails, and mucous membranes.
- May be associated with the later development of endocrinopathy (APECED [*a*utoimmune *p*oly*e*ndocrinopathy, *c*andidiasis, and *e*ctodermal *d*ystrophy]).

Several clinical subtypes of chronic mucocutaneous candidiasis (CMC) have been defined (Table 132-3). They have varied clinical manifestations, variable immunodeficiency, and different forms of genetic inheritance. Patients with CMC may have childhood or mature onset, and familial or sporadic occurrence. In addition, CMC may be present with or without endocrinopathy. Patients with autoimmune polyendocrinopathy, candidiasis, and ectodermal dystrophy (APECED or autoimmune polyendocrine syndrome, Type 1) often have affected siblings. APECED and other familial forms of CMC are autosomal recessive. Autosomal dominant inheritance is seen in patients with associated keratitis.

CLINICAL FEATURES

Patients with CMC have recurrent, progressive infections of the skin, nails, and mucous membranes most commonly caused by *Candida albicans*. Depending on the subtype, the clinical presentation ranges from recurrent, recalcitrant thrush (Fig. 132-4) to mild erythematous scaling plaques (Fig. 132-5) with a few dystrophic nails to severe generalized, crusted granulomatous plaques (Fig. 132-6). The cutaneous plaques occur most commonly in intertriginous areas, periorificial sites, and the scalp, but they may be generalized. The nails are thickened, brittle, and discolored, and the paronychial areas are often erythematous, swollen, and tender. Scalp infections may lead to scarring and alopecia. Although the oral mucosa is the most frequent site of mucosal alteration, esophageal, genital, and laryngeal mucosae may be affected. Strictures may be formed by candidal infection at these mucosal sites. Scrapings and cultures from cutaneous or mucosal lesions demonstrate candidal organisms.

TABLE 132-3
Subgroups of Chronic Mucocutaneous Candidiasis

CHRONIC MUCOCUTANEOUS CANDIDIASIS TYPE	INHERITANCE/GENE DEFECT	CLINICAL FEATURES	ASSOCIATED FEATURES
Familial chronic mucocutaneous candidiasis	Autosomal dominant gain-of-function mutations in *STAT1*	Candidiasis of the oral mucosa, nails and skin often begin in infancy; occasionally dermatophyte infections; squamous cell carcinoma, dental enamel defects, arterial aneurysms have been described	Most common are thyroid disease, vitiligo and alopecia areata, but other immune-mediated disorders occur with increased frequency May have bacterial (especially skin and lungs), and viral infections; invasive fungal and mycobacterial infections are uncommon
Autoimmune polyendocrinopathy, candidiasis, and ectodermal dystrophy (APECED) syndrome	Autosomal recessive Mutations in the *AIRE* (autoimmune regulator) gene More common in the Finnish population, Iranian Jews, and Sardinians	Oral and diaper area candidiasis > skin and nail begin before 5 years of age; up to 60% have urticarial eruptions	Often does not develop until adolescence or adulthood Hypoparathyroidism (90%) Hypoadrenalism (80%) Chronic diarrhea (up to 80%) Dental enamel hypoplasia (70%) Hypogonadism (up to 50%) Hepatitis (up to 40%) Pneumonitis (up to 40%) Sjögren syndrome (up to 40%) Alopecia areata (30%) Vitiligo (20%) Thyroid disease (20%) Diabetes (Type 1) (20%) Pernicious anemia (20%) Keratoconjunctivitis (20%) Hypopituitarism (15%) Hyposplenism (15%) Hypertension (15%) Nephritis (10%) Mucosal squamous cell carcinoma (10% of adults) Almost 100% have anti-Type I interferon antibodies Other autoantibodies common
Others	Autosomal recessive IL-17RA, IL-17RC (interleukin-17 receptors A and C) TRAF3IP2 (TRAF3-interacting protein 2) RORC (RAR-related orphan receptor C) CARD9 deficiency (caspase recruitment domain family member 9) Dectin-1 deficiency	All with mucosal candidiasis, dermatophytes	 Mycobacterial infections (RORC) Invasive fungal infections (especially of brain) (CARD9)

Other genetic disorders with increased risk of chronic candida infections:
- Acrodermatitis enteropathica
- DiGeorge syndrome
- Ectodermal dysplasia-ectrodactyly-clefting
- Hypohidrotic ectodermal dysplasia with immunodeficiency (NFκB [nuclear factor kappa B] IA)
- Hyper-IgE syndrome
- Interleukin-12B/ IL-12RB1 deficiency
- Multiple carboxylase deficiency
- Severe combined immunodeficiency

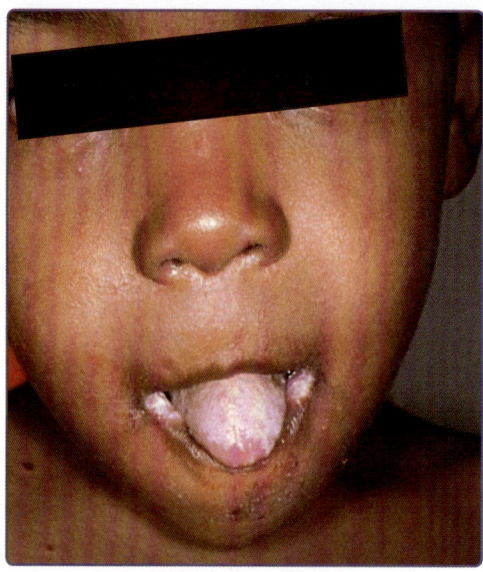

Figure 132-4 Recurrent thrush and candidal cheilitis in a boy with mucocutaneous candidiasis.

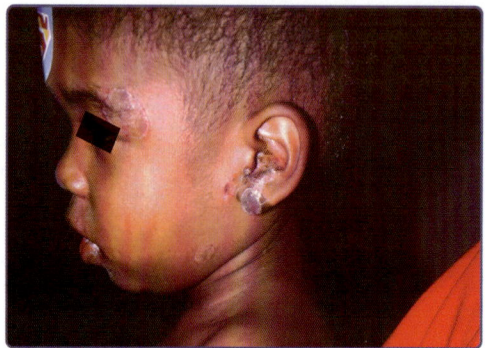

Figure 132-5 Cutaneous candidal infections with hyperkeratotic candidal granulomas. The child responded to oral azole antifungal medications, but not to topical medications.

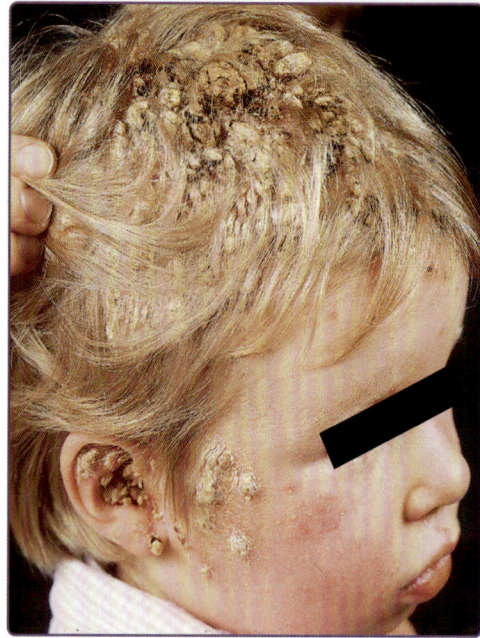

Figure 132-6 This 3-year-old child with hypothyroidism had oral thrush, intertriginous candidiasis, verrucous crusting on the scalp and face, and candidal onychomycosis. The warty growths shown in the photograph consisted of dried pus and serum, and grew only *Candida albicans*.

Patients with CMC rarely develop systemic candidiasis, but 50% may develop recurrent or severe infections caused by other organisms. In one study, 81% of patients with early-onset CMC also had infections with bacteria, fungi, and parasites, including bacterial septicemia.[11] Concomitant dermatophyte infections may occur.

In patients with APECED, the candidal infections tend to begin by 5 years of age, although the endocrinologic dysfunction may not be apparent until 12 to 13 years of age (see Fig. 132-6). The most commonly associated endocrinopathies are hypoparathyroidism (88%) and hypoadrenocorticism (60%). One-third of patients have candidiasis, hypoparathyroidism, and defective adrenal function. Other associated endocrinopathies or autoimmune disorders include gonadal insufficiency (45%), alopecia areata (20%), pernicious anemia (16%), thyroid abnormalities (12%), chronic active hepatitis or juvenile cirrhosis (9%), vitiligo, diabetes mellitus, and hypopituitarism. Chronic diarrhea and malabsorption have been reported in 25% of patients and usually are associated with hypoparathyroidism. Some affected patients also have pulmonary fibrosis, dental enamel hypoplasia, and keratoconjunctivitis. The "ectodermal dysplasia" features are likely to be secondary to the candidal infections or autoimmunity. Patients with APECED often have autoimmune antibodies, including antithyroglobulin, antimicrosomal, antiadrenal, and antimelanocyte antibodies, and rheumatoid factor. Autoantibodies also have been found in patients with CMC who do not have clinical endocrinologic disease.

ETIOLOGY AND PATHOGENESIS

T-helper 17 (Th17) cells play a critical role in immune defense against *Candida* and are impaired in their responsiveness in both APECED and non-APECED CMC patients.[12] Heterozygous mutations that activate the signal transducer and activator of transcription 1 gene (*STAT1*) are the most common cause,[13,14] and repress expression of interleukin (IL)-17 while promoting interferon signaling (see Table 132-3).[15-18] Mutations in isoforms of IL-17, IL-17 receptors, or *TRAF3IP2*, which regulates responses to IL-17, also have been described. APECED, an autosomal recessive form, results from loss-of-function mutations in the autoimmune regulator gene (*AIRE*). *AIRE* regulates the expression of self-antigens in thymic medullary epithelial cells, promoting immune tolerance through negative selection of autoreactive T cells and generation of antigen-specific regulatory T cells.[19] The retention of peripheral tissue-specific autoreactive T cells in APECED leads to the production of neutralizing autoantibodies, including against Th17-associated cytokines, leading to *Candida* infections and autoimmune disease.[20,21] Predisposition to *Candida* and dermatophyte infections is also a feature of mutations in the caspase recruitment domain family member-9 gene (*CARD9*)[22] and in the gene encoding dectin-1.[23]

DIAGNOSIS

Scrapings and cultures from lesions show candidal organisms. If a biopsy is done, the *C. albicans* are seen only in the stratum corneum. Evidence of an immunologic defect, including skin test anergy and deficient in vitro lymphoproliferation or cytokine release in response to *Candida* antigens, is found in 75% of CMC patients. However, the variability reflects the underlying heterogeneity of CMC. Autoantibodies against Type I interferons are a sensitive and specific marker for APECED.[24]

DIFFERENTIAL DIAGNOSIS

Frequent *Candida* infections in infants, especially thrush, commonly accompany recurrent use of antibiotics, such as for otitis; without a reason for the recurrent *Candida* infections, HIV infection and CMC should be considered. Autoimmune disorders and endocrinopathies are a feature of IPEX (*i*mmune dysregulation, *p*olyendocrinopathy, *e*nteropathy, *X*-linked) syndrome,[25] but infections tend to be bacterial. However, fungal, bacterial, and viral infections may accompany autoimmune endocrinopathies in IL-2 receptor α chain (CD25) deficiency.[26]

CLINICAL COURSE, PROGNOSIS, AND TREATMENT

Candidal lesions in patients with CMC generally respond to long-term systemically administered azole antifungal agents (itraconazole, fluconazole) or terbinafine.[27] Patients who are resistant usually respond to voriconazole (with its risk of phototoxicity), posaconazole, echinocandins, and/or amphotericin B with or without flucytosine. Cutaneous granulomas often are less responsive despite clearance of infection. Other therapies are granulocyte colony-stimulating factor (may increase IL-17 production),[28] nail avulsion, drainage of abscesses, and debridement of thick-crusted cutaneous plaques.

All patients with CMC should have an annual endocrine evaluation and patients with documented endocrinopathy or a family history of APECED should be monitored more closely. Patients who have a history of infections other than candidal should have further evaluation of their immune status.

CARTILAGE–HAIR HYPOPLASIA SYNDROME

AT-A-GLANCE

- Synonym: metaphyseal chondrodysplasia McKusick type.
- Autosomal recessive disorder, common in Amish and Finnish populations.
- Mutations in the RNA component of a ribonucleoprotein endoribonuclease, leading to defective cell-mediated and humoral immunity.
- Characterized by fine, sparse, hypopigmented hair, and short-limbed dwarfism.
- Supportive treatment with appropriate antibiotic use; bone marrow transplantation corrects immune deficiency but not dermis or cartilage.

COMBINED ANTIBODY AND T-CELL DEFICIENCY

HYPERIMMUNOGLOBULIN M SYNDROME

AT-A-GLANCE

- Most cases of hyperimmunoglobulin M syndrome have the X-linked recessive form with deficiency of CD40 ligand; common clinical features are recurrent sinopulmonary and GI tract infections, oral ulcerations, and verrucae.
- Autosomal recessive hyperimmunoglobulin M syndrome, except CD40 deficiency, does not have a susceptibility to opportunistic infections and lymphoid hyperplasia.

WISKOTT–ALDRICH SYNDROME

AT-A-GLANCE

- X-linked recessive.
- Mutations in WASP (Wiskott-Aldrich syndrome protein).

- Recalcitrant dermatitis.
- Recurrent pyogenic infections.
- Hemorrhage caused by thrombocytopenia and platelet dysfunction.
- Therapy: bone marrow stem cell transplantation.

CLINICAL FEATURES

Wiskott-Aldrich syndrome (WAS) is an X-linked recessive disorder with an incidence of approximately 4 per 1 million male births.[29,30] The classic triad of WAS is (a) hemorrhage caused by thrombocytopenia and platelet dysfunction, (b) recurrent pyogenic infections, and (c) recalcitrant dermatitis, but this triad appears in only 25% of patients. The bleeding diathesis, which is the most common manifestation of mutations in WAS, being present in 84% of patients, often manifests initially during the first weeks or months of life with bloody diarrhea. Epistaxis, hematemesis, hematuria, mucocutaneous petechiae, and intracranial hemorrhage also may occur. Recurrent bacterial infections begin in infancy as levels of placentally transmitted maternal antibodies diminish. These infections include furunculosis, conjunctivitis, otitis media and otitis externa, pansinusitis, pneumonia, meningitis, and septicemia. Infections with encapsulated bacteria such as *Pneumococcus*, *Haemophilus influenzae*, and *Neisseria meningitidis* predominate. Patients are also susceptible to infections caused by herpes and other viruses and to *Pneumocystis jiroveci*.

The atopic dermatitis associated with WAS, which occurs in approximately 80% of patients, usually develops during the first few months of life and may be quite severe. The face, scalp, and flexural areas are the most severely involved, although patients commonly have widespread involvement with progressive lichenification. The eruption may be more exfoliative than that of atopic dermatitis in individuals without WAS, and excoriated areas frequently have serosanguineous crusts (Fig. 132-7). Secondary bacterial infection of eczematous lesions is common, as are eczema herpeticum (Fig. 132-8) and molluscum contagiosum. IgE-mediated allergic problems, such as urticaria, food allergies, and asthma, are seen in addition to the atopic dermatitis.

Up to 40% of patients with WAS develop an autoimmune disorder.[31] The most common are vasculitis (particularly involving the skin, GI tract, brain, and heart) in 20% of patients, autoimmune hemolytic anemia in 14% of patients, and IgA nephropathy in up to 10% of patients.[32] Other immune-mediated cutaneous manifestations are angioedema, dermatomyositis, pyoderma gangrenosum, and erythema nodosum. Hepatosplenomegaly is common, and lymphadenopathy, transient arthritis, and joint effusions are present occasionally.

ETIOLOGY AND PATHOGENESIS

The defective gene is *WASP*, mapped to Xp11.22-11.23, which encodes WASP, a hematopoietic specific

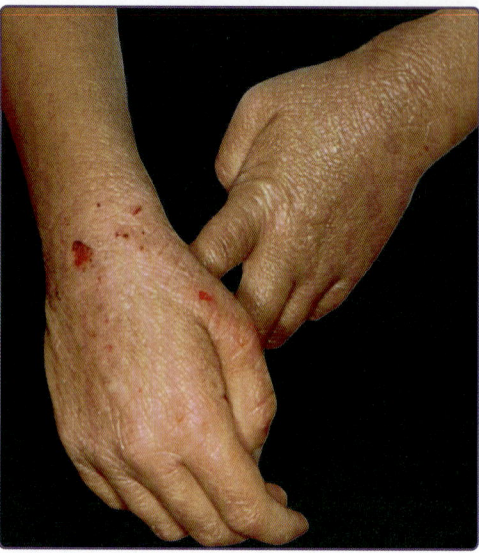

Figure 132-7 Severe atopic dermatitis in a boy with Wiskott-Aldrich syndrome. Note the serosanguineous crusting.

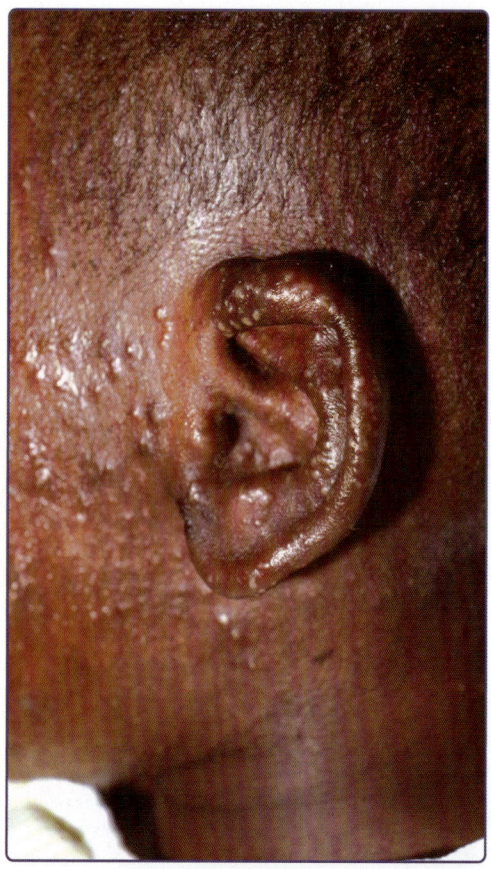

Figure 132-8 Herpetic infection with pustules on the ear of a teenager with Wiskott-Aldrich syndrome. The patient was blind in this left eye owing to a previous ocular infection. After the pictured infection, the patient was administered prophylactic acyclovir and had no subsequent herpetic infections for a decade. Eventually, he became resistant to acyclovir and succumbed to his immunodeficiency.

cytoplasmic protein that functions in signaling and cytoskeletal organization. WASP couples the signals arising at the cell membrane with reorganization of the cellular cytoskeleton, resulting in cellular activation and promotion of cell motility.[33] Mutations in WASP affect organization of the immunologic synapse and T-cell activation, T-lymphocyte and B-lymphocyte migration, and initiation of the primary antibody response. There is a strong phenotype–genotype correlation; classic WAS occurs when WASP is absent or truncated, whereas X-linked thrombocytopenia occurs when mutated WASP is expressed. The atopic dermatitis is likely associated with the observed skewing of CD4+ T-cell differentiation toward Th2 cells with suppression of Th1 and regulatory T cells differentiation.[34] Alteration in homeostasis of peripheral B cells and reduced activation of regulatory T cells is thought to promote the development of the autoimmune manifestations of WAS.[35-37] Given the expression of WASP on epidermal Langerhans cells, abnormal interactions of Langerhans cells with T cells and the ability of Langerhans cells to move to the lymph node after antigen stimulation may be involved as well.

WAS patients have decreased function and number of both T and B lymphocytes, beginning in the first years of life. The lymphocytes of patients with WAS lack microvilli formed by actin bundles, resulting in defective chemotaxis and, in some patients, there is decreased expression of sialoglycoproteins (eg, CD43 and others) on lymphocytes and platelets. Defects in humoral immunity include abnormal serum Ig and decreased antibody response to polysaccharide antigens. WAS patients also have defects in natural killer (NK) cell cytotoxicity, dendritic cell migration, and activation, and impaired macrophage chemotaxis.

DIAGNOSIS

The diagnosis is suspected on the basis of the platelet abnormalities and associated atopic dermatitis, and confirmed by laboratory testing, particularly genotyping to identify the *WASP* mutation. The thrombocytopenia of WAS is persistent, and platelet counts may range from 1000 to 80,000 platelets/μL. A platelet count of <70,000/μL is required for formal diagnostic criteria. The platelets are small, and platelet aggregation is defective. Levels of IgM and, sometimes, IgG are low, and isohemagglutinins are absent. IgA, IgE, and IgD levels usually are elevated. Eosinophilia, leukopenia, and lymphopenia are also seen. Delayed hypersensitivity skin-test reactivity is diminished, and patients fail to respond to polysaccharide antigens. WASP can be detected by flow cytometry using intracellular staining with an antibody to WASP and sequencing of the *WASP* gene can confirm the diagnosis of WAS or X-linked thrombocytopenia, which results also from mutations in the *WASP* gene that do not affect immune function. Mutation analysis allows for prenatal diagnosis. Female carriers of WAS can be detected by their selective inactivation of the abnormal X chromosome in lymphocytes and platelets.[38]

DIFFERENTIAL DIAGNOSIS

Other immunodeficiencies are characterized by eczematous dermatitis and increased susceptibility to infections, but WAS can usually be distinguished by the bleeding tendency and laboratory evidence of microthrombocytopenia.

CLINICAL COURSE, PROGNOSIS, AND TREATMENT

Therapeutic interventions allow some patients with WAS to survive into adulthood; however, a significant proportion die before the age of 10 years from infections secondary to hemorrhage, malignancies, or the complications of transplantation.[29,39]

Thirteen percent of patients with WAS develop lymphoreticular malignancies, especially non-Hodgkin lymphoma (especially diffuse large B-cell lymphomas), with a predominance of extranodal and brain involvement. Development of autoimmune hemolytic anemia is a poor prognostic factor and associated with the development of lymphoid malignancies; overall, 25% of patients with autoimmunity develop a malignancy.[32] 10% of patients die from these malignancies, usually as adolescents or young adults.

Appropriate antibiotics, immunizations, and transfusions of platelets and plasma decrease the risk of fatal infections and hemorrhage. Immunoglobulin replacement therapy is useful in some patients. Splenectomy has been advocated to ameliorate the bleeding abnormality in patients with recurrent severe hemorrhage, but this procedure increases the risk of infection from encapsulated bacterial organisms. Topical glucocorticoid preparations and Ig replacement may improve the dermatitis, and chronic administration of oral acyclovir is appropriate for patients with recurrent eczema herpeticum.

Bone marrow or stem cell transplantation is the treatment of choice for patients with recurrent problems, especially significant autoimmunity.[29,39] Full engraftment results in normal platelet number and function, normal immunologic status, and clearance of the dermatitis (T-lymphocyte engraftment). The 5-year survival rate for children younger than 5 years of age with human leukocyte antigen (HLA)-matched sibling donors is 87%; older patients and those with mismatched donors have survival rates of approximately 50%. Lentivirally transduced, WAS-reconstituted, autologous CD34+ cells have been administered in gene therapy trials, resulting in sustained clinical benefit in the majority of treated patients; dermatitis is improved or cleared and the risk of infection and autoimmune manifestations is reduced.[37,40,41] To avoid the risk of insertional oncogenesis from viral vectors, ongoing trials use self-inactivating lentiviral vectors and, more recently, zinc finger nucleases as a nonviral approach to the correction of WAS cells.[42]

SEVERE COMBINED IMMUNODEFICIENCY

AT-A-GLANCE

- Heterogeneous group of X-linked and autosomal recessive disorders with deficient cell-mediated and humoral immunity.
- Failure to thrive in early infancy; diarrhea; recurrent mucocutaneous candidiasis, bacterial, and viral infections; risk of graft-versus-host disease.
- Hematopoietic stem cell transplantation may provide a long-term cure.

Table 132-4 outlines the subtypes of severe combined immunodeficiency.

CLINICAL FEATURES

Infants with severe combined immunodeficiency (SCID) usually fail to gain weight by 3 to 6 months of age, following the onset of recurrent sinopulmonary and skin infections.[43,44] Persistent mucocutaneous candidiasis is often present at the time of diagnosis, and systemic candidal infections occur occasionally. Patients with SCID also may have chronic diarrhea and malabsorption caused by viral infections. *P. jiroveci* (*carinii*) pneumonia is often a presenting feature. Although bacterial infections usually respond to systemic antibiotics, viral infections tend to be fatal. Infants with SCID lack palpable lymphoid tissue despite recurrent infections.

In addition to cutaneous bacterial and candidal infections, the most common cutaneous eruptions are morbilliform or resemble seborrheic dermatitis. In some infants with SCID, biopsy sections show graft-versus-host disease (GVHD) (see Chap. 129). GVHD may result from in utero exposure to maternal lymphocytes, which is usually nonfatal, from transfusion with nonirradiated blood products, which is usually fatal, or may follow stem cell transplantation. Patients with GVHD most commonly present acutely with morbilliform erythema, papular dermatitis, or diffuse erythroderma. The face, neck, palms, and soles are usually affected initially, before the eruption becomes generalized. Severe cases are complicated by diffuse bullae or toxic epidermal necrolysis. The clinical presentation of GVHD from maternal engraftment (without transplantation) is indistinguishable from the clinical presentation of GVHD from transplantation, but histopathologic features differ.[45] Biopsy sections from GVHD secondary to maternal engraftment show psoriasiform hyperplasia with parakeratosis and variable spongiosis in contrast to the vacuolar interface pattern observed in conventional GVHD. Overall, 83% of SCID patients with maternal engraftment develop skin manifestations. Oral and genital ulcerations are also seen in SCID, particularly in Athabascan-speaking Native American children with a defect in the *Artemis* gene.[46] Patients with Omenn syndrome show erythroderma, hepatosplenomegaly and lymphadenopathy with eosinophilia and increased IgE production.[47] B cells tend to be undetectable, and T cells, although often increased in number, are nonfunctional. Omenn syndrome has been shown to be a phenotype with several underlying genetic bases. Most patients have RAG1/RAG2 mutations, but the phenotype of Omenn syndrome has been described in patients with mutations in *Artemis* and IL-7R. Two individuals with cartilage-hair hypoplasia and another with complete DiGeorge syndrome also showed features of Omenn syndrome.

The natural history of SCID is changing with the introduction of newborn screening for SCID and other T-cell lymphopenia.[48] Except for a few causes of SCID that may not present with T-cell lymphopenia at birth, patients are identified by newborn screening soon after birth and the diagnosis is established before serious infections develop. Early stem cell transplantation provides an excellent outcome irrespective of the source of the stem cells or the preparation regimen.[49]

ECTODERMAL DYSPLASIA WITH IMMUNODEFICIENCY

AT-A-GLANCE

- Mutations in nuclear factor κB (NF-κB) essential modulator, leading to abnormal NF-κB signaling.
- Characteristic facies of hypohidrotic ectodermal dysplasia.
- Often severe immunodeficiency; bacterial, atypical mycobacterial, and viral infections are common.
- Therapy: stem cell transplantation can correct the immunodeficiency but not the other features of the disease.

EPIDEMIOLOGY

X-linked recessive transmission is most common with an estimated incidence of 1:250,000 live male births.[50] An autosomal dominant form of ectodermal dysplasia with immunodeficiency also has been described.[51]

TABLE 132-4
Subtypes of Severe Combined Immunodeficiency

LYMPHOCYTE PROFILE	DISORDER	GENE	GENE PRODUCT FUNCTION
T–/B–/NK–	ADA deficiency[a,b]	ADA	Enzyme necessary for detoxification of metabolic products of the purine salvage pathway that cause lymphocytes to undergo apoptosis
	PNP deficiency	PNP	Enzyme necessary for detoxification of metabolic products of the purine salvage pathway that cause lymphocytes to undergo apoptosis: located downstream from ADA
T–/B–/NK+	RAG 1 or 2[c]	RAG1/RAG2	Required for somatic V, D, and J rearrangements during B and T-cell development
	Artemis deficiency[d,e]	Artemis	Required for DNA repair during somatic V, D, and J rearrangements during B-cell and T-cell development
	LIG4 syndrome[e,93]	LIG4	Ligase required for ATP-dependent repair of double-stranded DNA
T–/B+/NK–	X-linked severe combined immunodeficiency[a]	IL2RG	Common γ chain of IL-2, IL-4, IL-7, IL-9, IL-15, and IL-21
	Janus protein kinase deficiency	JAK3	Tyrosine kinase; primary signal transducer from common γ chain
T–/B+/NK+	IL-7 receptor (IL-7R) deficiency	IL7R	α Chain of IL-7 receptor
	T-cell receptor/CD3 complex deficiency	CD3δ and CD3ε	Facilitates expression of T-cell receptor/CD3 complex; block at pre–T-cell receptor stage of development
	CD45 deficiency[92]	PTPRC	Phosphatase that regulates immune cell signaling
	Winged helix nude deficiency	WHN	Defect in thymic development. Human homolog of nude mouse with total alopecia and onychodystrophy; critical transcription factor for thymic development
Other Defects in T-Cell Development			
CD4+ CD8– /B+/NK+	CD8 deficiency[94]	CD8A	Promotes survival and differentiation of activated T cells to memory CD8+ T cells
	ZAP-70 deficiency	ZAP-70	Signaling tyrosine kinase
	MHC class I deficiency/TAP deficiency (bare lymphocyte syndrome I)	TAP1 TAP2	Transporter associated with antigen processing, transports peptides to assemble the class I molecule, dysregulated NK cells
CD4[low] CD8+/B+/NK+	MHC class II deficiency (bare lymphocyte syndrome II)	CIITA RFXB RFX5 RFXAP	Defects in the transactivating factors of MHC II molecules, nonfunctional CD4 T cells if present
T+/B+/NK+	T-cell receptor/CD3 complex deficiency	CD3γ	Chain facilitates expression of T-cell receptor/CD3 complex

[a]Most common severe combined immunodeficiency defects. X-linked severe combined immunodeficiency accounts for approximately 50% of patients. Adenosine deaminase deficiency accounts for approximately 20% of patients.

[b]Eighty-five percent to 90% of patients present in infancy with severe immunodeficiency; one-half have skeletal deformities, neurologic symptoms, behavior problems, and decreased IQ.

[c]Deletions/frameshift mutations of RAG1/RAG2 genes result in severe combined immunodeficiency phenotype. Less-severe mutations result in Omenn syndrome, which is clinically distinct from other forms of severe combined immunodeficiency. Mutations in other genes may lead to the Omenn phenotype and immunodeficiency.

[d]Common genetic defect seen in Athabascan-speaking Native Americans, the defect is called SCIDA in this population. Gene frequency may be as high as 2%. These patients have a higher incidence of oral/genital ulcers.

[e]Both Artemis and LIG4 mutations lead to hypersensitivity to irradiation.

ADA, adenosine deaminase; ATP, adenosine triphosphate; IL, interleukin; MHC, major histocompatibility complex; NK, natural killer cell; PNP, purine nucleoside phosphorylase; RAG, recombination activating gene; TAP, transporter associated with antigen processing.

ETIOLOGY AND PATHOGENESIS

Several genetic disorders result from gene mutations in the nuclear factor κB (NF-κB) essential modulator (NEMO) and lead to abnormal NF-κB signaling (see Chaps. 75 and 131). One of these, hypohidrotic ectodermal dysplasia with immunodeficiency, results from hypomorphic mutations in the NEMO gene (also called *ectodermal dysplasia, anhidrotic, with immunodeficiency* or *Hyperimmunoglobulinemia M, immunodeficiency, X-linked with ectodermal dysplasia*). NF-κB is a DNA-binding transcription factor, and its ability to transcribe genes is regulated by a cytoplasmic inhibitor, IKB (inhibitor of nuclear factor κB). NF-κB signaling affects inflammation, apoptosis, development, and immunity. NF-κB activation requires phosphorylation of IKB by IKB kinase (IKK). IKK is composed of 2 catalytic components (IKKα and IKKβ) and a regulatory subunit, IKKγ or NEMO. NEMO has no catalytic function, but is the structural scaffold that supports the IKK complex. When NEMO is absent or defective, no functional IKK complex is formed and, as a result, NF-κB cannot translocate to the nucleus and activate gene transcription.

The hypomorphic mutations that cause anhidrotic ectodermal dysplasia with immunodeficiency allow early survival in males, in contrast to the large deletions in *NEMO* (usually of exons 4 to 10) that lead to incontinentia pigmenti in carrier females and fetal death in affected males (see Chap. 75). Female carriers of hypomorphic *NEMO* mutations often show mild features of incontinentia pigmenti, but may also express an incontinentia pigmenti phenotype with transient immunodeficiency.[52] In boys with hypomorphic mutations of *NEMO*, the ectodermal dysplasia phenotype results from impaired NF-κB signaling.[53] Immunodeficiency results from impaired NF-κB activation in response to signaling via antigen receptors, Toll-like receptors, IL-1 receptor, and the tumor necrosis factor (TNF) receptor family.[54] Gain-of-function mutations in IKBα, the component of the inhibitor of NF-κB that is phosphorylated by IKK, lead to an autosomal dominant form of ectodermal dysplasia with a distinct immunologic phenotype, characterized by a profound T-cell deficiency, but normal NK cytotoxicity and responses to *Mycobacteria*. Mutations in *NEMO* that cause immunodeficiency without the ectodermal dysplasia phenotype also have been reported.

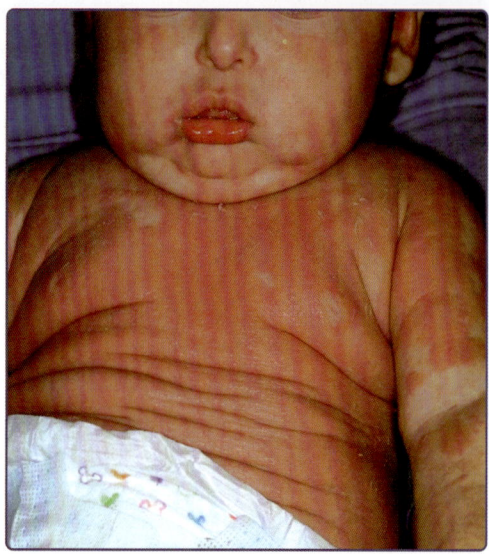

Figure 132-9 Ectodermal dysplasia with immunodeficiency gene mutation. This boy with a hypomorphic mutation in *NEMO* (nuclear factor κB essential modulator) showed failure to thrive, slightly exfoliative dermatitis, and the typical facial features of hypohidrotic ectodermal dysplasia. Note the small chin, the "pouty" lower lip, thin upper lip, and small, pinched nose with malar hypoplasia. His mother had a pigmented streak following a line of Blaschko, typical of that seen in incontinentia pigmenti. (Used with permission from Dr. Anthony Mancini.)

CLINICAL FEATURES

Affected patients present with classic characteristics of hypohidrotic ectodermal dysplasia (Fig. 132-9). These include the characteristic facies, hypotrichosis or atrichia, hypohidrosis (leading to heat intolerance), hypodontia or anodontia with conical incisors, and associated dermatitis (see Chap. 131). A subset of patients has associated osteopetrosis and lymphedema in association with severe immunodeficiency. Boys with immunodeficiency from *NEMO* mutations without the features of hypohidrotic ectodermal dysplasia also have been described. In an analysis of 72 patients with *NEMO* mutations, only 77% had ectodermal dysplasia.[50] Bacterial infections early in infancy are common, particularly sepsis, pneumonia, otitis, sinusitis, and lymphadenitis. Recurrent pneumonias may lead to bronchiectasis. Common pathogens include *Streptococcus pneumoniae*, *H. influenzae*, *Klebsiella*, *Salmonella*, and *Pseudomonas*. Infections with atypical *Mycobacteria* and viruses, including cytomegalovirus (systemic and GI involvement), herpes simplex virus, molluscum contagiosum, human papillomavirus, and *Pneumocystis carinii*, are also reported.

The immunodeficiency is often severe, but its characteristics are variable with an apparent genotype–phenotype correlation that can be further identified by in vitro reconstitution of the mutations. Immune dysfunction includes impaired B-cell Ig class switching with hypogammaglobulinemia (and often increased levels of IgM and/or IgA), impaired specific antibody production (particularly to polysaccharide antigens), deficient NK cell cytotoxicity, poor cytokine production in response to CD40 signaling, and autoinflammation, especially of the gut. Biopsy of skin may show evidence of keratinocyte apoptosis, reflecting the dysfunction in NF-κB signaling, and must be differentiated from GVHD.

TREATMENT AND PROGNOSIS

There is an increased mortality, with 36% of patients dying at a mean age of 6.4 years.[50] Therapy is guided by the patient's clinical and immunologic phenotype. Ectodermal dysplasia is treated supportively (see Chap. 131). Patients with impaired antibody production may benefit from Ig replacement. All infections (bacterial and viral) should be treated aggressively with the appropriate antibiotics/antivirals. Prophylaxis for both *P. jiroveci* and *Mycobacterium avium-intracellulare* should be considered. Stem cell transplantation may lead to immune reconstitution but may not correct the other manifestations of the disease.[55] The mothers and sisters of these patients should be offered genetic testing for the *NEMO* mutation and counseling.

ATAXIA-TELANGIECTASIA

AT-A-GLANCE

- Autosomal recessive disorder with mutations in *ataxia-telangiectasia mutated (ATM)*.
- Early onset of ataxia with progressive neurologic deterioration; conjunctival telangiectasia first appears in preschool years in most patients.
- Sinopulmonary infections, lymphoreticular neoplasia.
- Deficiency of IgA, IgE, IgG_2, IgG_4; variable manifestations of T-cell deficiency; high levels α-fetoprotein; chromosomal breaks; sensitive to irradiation.

EPIDEMIOLOGY

Ataxia-telangiectasia (AT; Online Mendelian Inheritance in Man [OMIM] #208900), also called *Louis-Bar syndrome*, is an autosomal recessive disorder with an estimated incidence of up to 1:40,000 and a carrier rate of up to 1%. Carriers have an increased risk of breast cancer, hematologic malignancies,[56,57] and ischemic heart disease, with a reduced life expectancy of approximately 8 years.[58] These heterozygotes show an increased risk of chromosomal breaks after exposure to irradiation in vitro, suggesting that mammograms in known carriers of AT are contraindicated.

CLINICAL FEATURES

Characteristic oculocutaneous telangiectasias begin near the ocular canthi and progress across the bulbar conjunctivae (Fig. 132-10). These telangiectasias usually appear when patients are 3 to 6 years of age; rarely have they been described at earlier ages. Cutaneous telangiectasias subsequently may develop on the malar prominences, ears, eyelids, anterior chest, and popliteal and antecubital fossae, and the dorsal aspects of the hands and feet (Fig. 132-11). The telangiectasias may be subtle and resemble fine petechiae, especially in the flexural areas. The development of telangiectasias may be related to sun exposure, because ocular, but not cutaneous, telangiectasias develop in affected dark-skinned children. The development of telangiectasias may relate, at least in part, to the sensitivity of some AT strains to ultraviolet light.[59]

Progeric changes of the skin, including xerosis and gray hair, occur in 90% of patients.[60] During adolescence, the facial skin may become progressively more atrophic and sclerotic, causing a mask-like appearance. Occasionally, the ears, arms, and hands also become sclerodermatous. The hair may be diffusely gray by adolescence, and subcutaneous fat is generally lost in childhood. Recurrent severe impetigo often develops. Seborrheic dermatitis occurs in many patients, and the associated blepharitis may lead to a diagnosis of blepharoconjunctivitis rather than ocular telangiectasia. Mottled hyperpigmentation and hypopigmentation commonly occur and, together with the telangiectasias and atrophy, can resemble the poikiloderma of radiodermatitis, actinic damage, or scleroderma. Other pigmentary changes include café-au-lait spots that may be found in a dermatomal distribution, multiple ephelides, and vitiligo. Hypertrichosis of the arms and legs, alopecia areata, multiple warts, atopic dermatitis, keratosis pilaris, nummular eczema, and acanthosis nigricans also have been described in association with AT. Among the most common cutaneous manifestations are noninfectious cutaneous granulomas (Fig. 132-12).[61] These persistent, atrophic, and often ulcerative lesions are often mistaken for other granulomatous processes, including sarcoidosis, necrobiosis lipoidica diabeticorum, granuloma annulare, and granulomatous dermatitis.

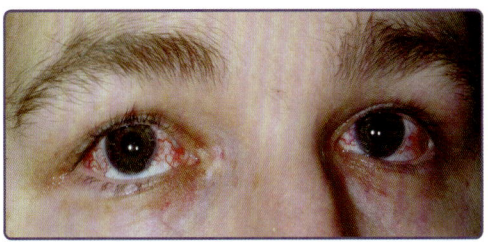

Figure 132-10 Bulbar conjunctival telangiectasias in a patient with ataxia-telangiectasia.

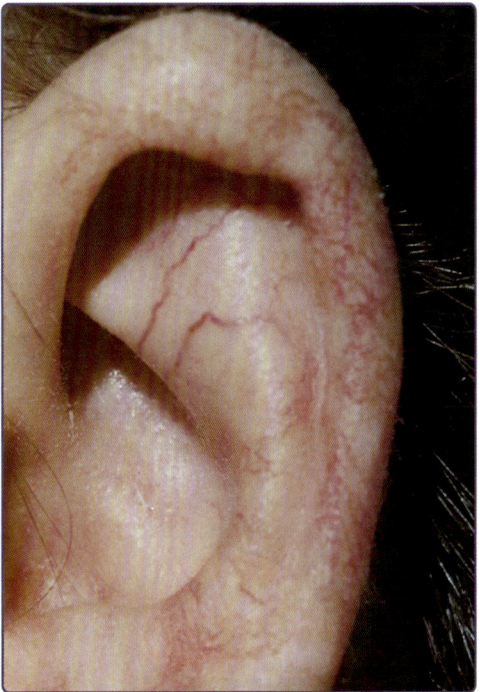

Figure 132-11 Ataxia-telangiectasia. Telangiectasias inside and on the helix.

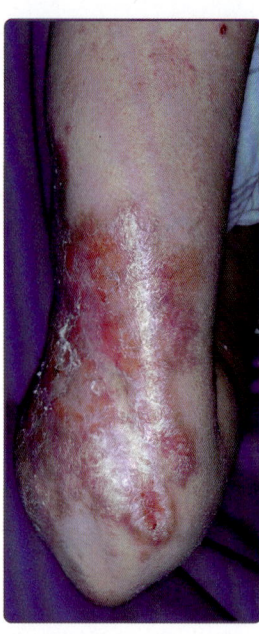

Figure 132-12 Noninfectious granulomatous dermatitis of a patient with ataxia-telangiectasia. These persistent lesions tend to ulcerate, but often respond to injections of triamcinolone acetonide.

Usually, the progressive cerebellar ataxia first becomes apparent during infancy (median age: 1.2 years) with swaying of the head and trunk and apraxia of eye movements, often years before skin or conjunctival abnormalities develop. In childhood, dysarthric speech, drooling, choreoathetosis, and myoclonic jerks become prominent. The diagnosis of AT is usually made at a median age of 7 years, after appearance of the mucocutaneous telangiectasia. Patients usually require a wheelchair by their teenage years.

Recurrent bacterial and viral sinopulmonary infections occur in up to 80% of patients; these are the most common cause of death, which is usually from bronchiectasis and respiratory failure. Approximately 75% of patients with AT may have growth retardation and endocrine disorders, especially ovarian agenesis or testicular hypoplasia and insulin-resistant diabetes.

Neoplasia occurs in 40% of surviving adolescents or young adults, although lymphoid malignancy has been described as the presenting sign during infancy. Most common are lymphomas (especially B-cell lymphoma; 200-fold increased risk) and leukemia (especially T-cell chronic lymphocytic leukemia; 70-fold increased risk). Basal cell carcinomas have been reported in young adults.

Patients with AT tend to have both humoral and cellular immunologic abnormalities. Serum IgA and IgE are absent or deficient in 70% and up to 80% of patients, respectively. Circulating anti-IgA antibodies are common in AT patients with IgA deficiency. Approximately 60% of patients have selective IgG_2 and IgG_4 deficiencies. Defective cell-mediated immunity is found in 70% of patients, particularly lymphopenia and deficient in vitro responses to antigens and mitogens; T cells bearing γ/δ receptors are increased in number, while CD4+ T cells tend to be reduced.

Virtually all patients have elevated levels of α-fetoprotein (which is particularly significant after 2 years of age), and many have detectable carcinoembryonic antigen. Patients with AT often have elevated hepatic transaminases (40% to 50%), and glucose intolerance. DNA is exquisitely sensitive to X-irradiation, and patients also show an increased rate of telomere shortening. Spontaneous chromosomal abnormalities (fragments, breaks, gaps, and translocations) occur 2 to 18 times more frequently in patients with AT than in normal individuals and mainly involve chromosomes 2, 7, and 14. Rearrangements of chromosomes 7 and 14, and especially 14:14 translocations, seem to predict the development of lymphoreticular malignancy, including leukemia. The thymus is absent or hypoplastic, and the spleen may be reduced in size.

Among techniques to confirm diagnosis are an elevated serum α-fetoprotein level in children older than 8 months of age, analysis of radioresistant DNA synthesis (which demonstrates an abnormal S-phase checkpoint), radiosensitivity testing with the colony survival assay, immunoblotting for the ATM (ataxia-telangiectasia mutated) protein, assessment of ATM kinase activity, and molecular genetic testing.

PROGNOSIS, CLINICAL COURSE, AND TREATMENT

Therapy for AT is supportive and includes administration of antibiotics for infection, physiotherapy for pulmonary bronchiectasis, physical therapy to prevent contractures in patients with neurologic dysfunction, and sunscreens and sun avoidance to diminish actinic-like changes. Patients should be aggressively screened for malignancy, especially after the first decade of life. Intralesional injections of triamcinolone have helped promote healing of the painful, associated ulcerations, although the lesions do not clear completely with treatment. Autopsy findings indicate that approximately 50% of the patients die from pulmonary disease, the most common cause of death. Lymphoreticular malignancies, including lymphoid leukemia, are the second most common cause of death (15% of patients with AT). The remaining patients tend to die of both pulmonary disease and malignancy. Therapeutic radiation and radiomimetic chemotherapeutic agents, especially bleomycin, may lead to extensive tissue necrosis. The administration of small doses of other chemotherapeutic drugs and low-dose, fractionated radiation is the least-harmful means of managing these malignancies. In a small subset of patients with milder AT, treatment with aminoglycosides increased ATM gene function.[62] Death usually occurs by late childhood or early adolescence; the oldest surviving patient died at the age of 50 years. Prenatal diagnosis is currently best achieved by DNA analysis.

DISORDERS OF PHAGOCYTOSIS AND CELL KILLING

Patients with defects in phagocyte function or cell killing typically present during infancy or childhood with recurrent, unusual, and/or difficult-to-clear bacterial infections. Infections commonly seen include those of skin or mucosa, lung, lymph nodes, deep-tissue abscesses, or childhood periodontitis. The most distinctive disorders of phagocytosis and cell killing are chronic granulomatous disease (CGD), leukocyte adhesion deficiencies, Hyperimmunoglobulinemia E syndrome (HIES), and the silvery hair syndromes with immunodeficiency.[63] However, several disorders with neutropenia, neutrophil dysfunction, or cytokine dysfunction also lead to a decreased ability to engulf and/or kill organisms. These are reviewed in Table 132-5.

CHRONIC GRANULOMATOUS DISEASE

AT-A-GLANCE

- Group of disorders in which defective production of reactive oxygen intermediates impairs intracellular killing of microorganisms.
- X-linked or autosomal recessive.
- Mutations in genes that encode components of nicotinamide adenine dinucleotide phosphate oxidase system.
- Pneumonias, lymphadenopathy, hepatosplenomegaly, and skin infections.
- Granulomas, most commonly of lungs and liver.
- Lupus-like inflammation in carriers (X-linked) and patients.

CGD is a heterogeneous group of X-linked and autosomal recessive disorders.[64,65] Ninety percent of patients with the disorder are male, and the overall incidence is 1 in 200,000 to 250,000 persons. X-linked disease with deficiency of gp91^{phox} occurs in 70% of affected individuals with signs and symptoms manifesting in the first year of life. Individuals with autosomal recessive disease are more likely to have some nicotinamide adenine dinucleotide phosphate (NADPH) oxidase activity, tend to present later in life (mean age of onset: 8 years), have milder signs and symptoms, and have longer survival.[66,67]

CLINICAL FEATURES

Pyodermas with associated regional lymphadenopathy/adenitis and dermatitis tend to affect body sites that are exposed to organisms, especially on the skin and lungs. Staphylococcal abscesses are found in 40% of patients, particularly of the perianal area, nares, and ears. Purulent inflammatory reactions may develop at sites of lymph node drainage or minor cutaneous trauma and heal slowly with scarring. Ecthyma gangrenosum may be the presentation in a neonate.[68] Staphylococcal infections are the most common, but other bacterial and fungal organisms that are killed by generation of reactive oxygen species may cause infection (*Aspergillus* spp., *Burkholderia cepacia*, *Candida* spp., *Klebsiella* spp., mycobacteria (including severe/disseminated bacille Calmette-Guérin infection),[69] *Nocardia* spp., and *Serratia marcescens* (especially abscesses with ulceration and osteomyelitis).[70]

Patients with CGD often develop chronic inflammatory granulomas, most commonly of the lungs and liver. Cutaneous granulomas are nodular and often necrotic. Granulomas can occlude vital structures, especially of the GI and genitourinary systems. Intraoral ulcerations resembling aphthous stomatitis, chronic gingivitis, perioral ulcers, scalp folliculitis, and seborrheic dermatitis also have been described in many patients. Female carriers for X-linked CGD do not have the increased risk of infections but may have cutaneous lesions of discoid or systemic lupus erythematosus, Jessner lymphocytic infiltration of the skin, aphthous stomatitis, granulomatous cheilitis, photosensitivity, and/or Raynaud phenomenon.[71,72]

The lymph nodes, lungs, liver, spleen, and GI tract are the most frequent areas of noncutaneous involvement. Suppurative lymphadenitis with abscess and fistula formation usually affects cervical nodes. Pneumonia occurs in almost all affected children and may lead to abscess formation, cavitation, and empyema. Hepatosplenomegaly has been reported in 80% to 90% of patients; more than 30% of patients develop hepatic abscesses, and staphylococcal liver abscesses are almost pathognomonic to CGD. Other excessive inflammatory responses can include hemophagocytic lymphohistiocytosis[73] or features that resemble inflammatory bowel disease (anal fistulae, diarrhea), IgA nephropathy, sarcoidosis, and rheumatoid arthritis.[74,75]

Patients with bacterial and *Nocardia* spp. infections tend to be symptomatic and frequently have leukocytosis, anemia, and elevated sedimentation rate. In contrast, lack of fever, normal erythrocyte sedimentation rate, and few symptoms are more common in *Aspergillus* spp. infections. Thus, laboratory values within normal limits do not rule out infection in a CGD patient. Patients show an increased erythrocyte sedimentation rate, hypergammaglobulinemia, leukocytosis, and mild anemia; other immune function tests are otherwise usually normal.

TABLE 132-5
Other Disorders of Phagocytosis or Cell Killing

DISORDER	GENETICS	GENE	FUNCTIONAL CONSEQUENCE	CLINICAL FINDINGS
Neutropenia				
Cyclic neutropenia	AD	ELA2	Defects in neutrophil elastase	Cycles of neutropenia and monocytopenia, approximately every 3 weeks; oral ulcers and fever when low
Severe congenital neutropenia	AD	ELA1	Defects in neutrophil elastase lead to abnormal neutrophil trafficking	Neutropenia, myelodysplastic syndrome, and acute myelogenous leukemia; neutropenia and lymphopenia; myeloid progenitors in circulation
	AD	GF11	Repressor of elastase transcription leads to accumulation of elastase	
Shwachman-Diamond syndrome (SBDS)	AR	SBDS	SBDS protein participates in metabolism of ribosomal RNA	Pancytopenia with myelodysplastic syndrome and acute myelogenous leukemia; pancreatic insufficiency; chondrodysplasia
WHIM[128]	AD	CXCR4	Receptor regulates development and migration of neutrophils; affects viral entry into cells	Chronic cutaneous and cervical warts, antibiotic-responsive bacterial sinopulmonary infections; often low Ig levels, peripheral neutropenia in the face of bone marrow hypercellularity (myelokathexis), and distinctive neutrophil morphology
Cytokine Defects				
	AR	IL12B	Absence of component of IL-12 and IL-23 that stimulates IFN-γ production	Severe mycobacterial infections. Disseminated bacille Calmette-Guérin after vaccination; severe *Salmonella* infections
	AR	IL12RB1	β_1-Chain of IL-12 and IL-23 receptors	
	AR, AD	IFNGR1	Affects ligand binding to IFN-γ receptor	
	AR	IFNR2	Affects IFN-γ receptor signaling	
	AR, AD	STAT1	Affects transcription in IFN receptor signaling	Also severe viral infections
	AR	STAT5B	As in Stat1, but also growth hormone receptor signaling	Also growth hormone insensitivity
Defects of Killing				
Myeloperoxidase deficiency	AR	MPO	Myeloperoxidase required for bacterial killing	Especially *Staphylococcus aureus* and candidal infections; may be asymptomatic
Specific granule deficiency	AR	C/EBPE	C/EBPε transcription factor required for granulocyte differentiation	Recurrent bacterial infections; neutrophils with 2 lobes

AD, autosomal dominant; AR, autosomal recessive; IFN, interferon; IL, interleukin; WHIM, warts, hypoimmunoglobulinemia, infections, and myelokathexis.

ETIOLOGY AND PATHOGENESIS

CGD is caused by defects in the reduced NADPH oxidase, the enzyme complex responsible for the generation of superoxide. Normal bactericidal activity after phagocytosis requires the NADPH oxidase system, which consists of NADPH, an unusual phagocyte cytochrome b (b_{558}), and cytosolic proteins. In patients with CGD, this membrane-associated NADPH oxidase system fails to produce superoxide and other toxic oxygen metabolites. The oxidative molecules have direct microbicidal activity, but also act as intracellular signaling molecules, activating the release of primary granule proteins neutrophil elastase and cathepsin G inside the phagocytic vacuole that, in turn, are necessary to kill microbes. Mouse models of CGD show decreased regulatory T-cell activity, unrestrained γ/δ T-cell activity, and increased production of IL-1β, IL-8, and IL-17.[76] NADPH oxidase also modulates major histocompatibility complex Class II antigen presentation by B cells.[77]

In X-linked kindreds (approximately 70%), the *CYBB* gene encoding the gp91[phox] (phagocyte oxidase) subunit of cytochrome b_{558} is mutated. Patients with autosomal recessive CGD are deficient in NADPH oxidase cytosolic factors (p47[phox]—encoded by *NCF1*—in approximately 20% of patients; p67[phox]—encoded by *NCF2*—in ≤5%; and p40[phox]—encoded by *NCF4*—very rare); occasionally, the p22[phox] (γ subunit of cytochrome b_{558}), which contains a docking site for p47[phox], is deficient (mutation in *CYBA*; ≤5% of patients). It is thought that cytochrome b_{558} is the membrane attachment site for these cytosolic factors that translocate from the cytosol to the plasma membrane, assembling oxidase components to allow activation of the NADPH oxidase.

The types of microbial organisms that cause infections in patients with CGD require intracellular killing and are usually catalase-positive. Only 5 organisms are responsible for the overwhelming majority of infections in CGD in North America and Europe: *Staphylococcus aureus*, *S. marcescens*, *B. cepacia*, *Nocardia* spp., and *Aspergillus* spp. The intense humoral and granulomatous responses of CGD are thought to be compensatory in the robust but ineffectual response to organisms.

DIAGNOSIS

The diagnosis of CGD is made on the basis of assays that rely on superoxide production. The dihydrorhodamine flow cytometry-based test (DHR 123 assay) is currently favored and can readily identify patients or carriers of X-linked disease[78]; the ferricytochrome c reduction assay is another quantitative measure of the respiratory burst. The screening test for CGD is the nitroblue tetrazolium (NBT) reduction assay, in which the yellow NBT becomes insoluble, oxidized form (blue formazan) when precipitated with normal oxidative metabolism. Quantitative NBT tests and chemiluminescence assays also may be performed. Immunoblot analysis confirms the absence of the glycoprotein 91^{phox} (gp91^{phox}) component; because deficiency of one component of cytochrome b$_{558}$ leads to absence of the other, sequencing of the *gp91*^{phox} or *p22*^{phox} gene is necessary if absence is noted by immunoblot analysis. Immunoblots that show the absence of p47^{phox} or p67^{phox} can be diagnostic.

Biopsy of cutaneous granulomas shows histiocytic infiltrates associated with foreign-body giant cells and accumulation of neutrophils with necrosis. Although the histopathologic features of lupus erythematosus-like skin lesions in CGD patients and carriers may resemble those of lupus patients, immunofluorescence examination of lesional skin is usually negative.

DIFFERENTIAL DIAGNOSIS

Although the tests to measure respiratory burst are an easy screening test, other disorders of phagocytosis may be confused with CGD. Among these are the leukocyte adhesion defects (see section "Leukocyte Adhesion Deficiencies"), Shwachman-Diamond syndrome, myeloperoxidase deficiency, and defects in Toll receptor, interferon, or IL-12 signaling.

CLINICAL COURSE, PROGNOSIS, AND TREATMENT

Patients with X-linked CGD, p22^{phox} CGD, and p67^{phox} CGD tend to have a more-severe clinical course compared to patients with p47^{phox} CGD. The mean age of diagnosis of X-linked CGD is 3 years of age, and of autosomal recessive forms, 8 years of age. More than 90% of patients with non-p47^{phox} CGD have undetectable levels of superoxide production. Some patients develop severe infections as early as infancy whereas others unexpectedly develop a serious infection typical of CGD later during childhood.

Small foci of localized inflammation may not be associated with fever and may be difficult to detect without vigorous investigation of the lungs, liver, and bones by routine screening radiographs, scans, or ultrasonography. Cultures should be performed to identify the infectious agent, and invasive procedures may be necessary to obtain adequate tissue samples.

Patients with evidence of infection should be treated empirically with broad-spectrum parenteral antibiotics that cover *S. aureus* as well as Gram-negative organisms.[79] Intravenous therapy should be continued for at least 10 to 14 days, followed by a several-week course of oral antibiotics. Surgical interventions (drainage, debridement) may be required for deeper infections (Table 132-6). Trimethoprim-sulfamethoxazole therapy decreases the incidence of bacterial infection without increasing the incidence of fungal infection. Itraconazole is an effective agent for prophylaxis for

TABLE 132-6
Treatment of Chronic Granulomatous Disease

TREATMENT	INDICATION	DOSE
Trimethoprim-sulfamethoxazole[a] (dicloxacillin if allergic)	Bacterial infections	5 mg/kg/day divided twice daily
Itraconazole[a]	Fungal infections	100 mg/day if patient weighs <50 kg; 200 mg/day if patient weighs >50 kg
Interferon-γ[a]	Infections	50 mcg/m^2 subcutaneously 3 × /week
Leukocyte transfusion	Life-threatening infections	
Bone marrow transplantation	Life-threatening infections	
Systemic glucocorticoids	Granulomas, particularly if obstructive	
Debridement/drainage/surgical intervention	Abscesses (particularly liver)	

[a]Regardless of genetic subgroup, the current recommendation is to use prophylaxis with trimethoprim-sulfamethoxazole, itraconazole, and interferon-γ.[136]

fungal infections.[80] Prophylactic interferon (IFN)-γ decreases the number and severity of infections without increasing the incidence of chronic inflammatory complications in both X-linked and autosomal recessive CGD.[81] Use of IFN-γ is not accompanied by any measurable improvement in NADPH oxidase activity; its clinical benefit is related to enhanced phagocyte function and killing by nonoxidative mechanisms. Granulocyte transfusions have been used for rapidly progressive, life-threatening infections. The prophylactic administration of antibiotics and IFN-γ has reduced the mortality of CGD to approximately 2% per patient-year for autosomal CGD and 5% per year for X-linked CGD.[65] The most common causes of death are pneumonia and/or sepsis caused by *Aspergillus* or *B. cepacia*. Systemic glucocorticoids have been helpful for patients with obstructive visceral granulomas. Other therapies that may be of benefit for the inflammatory manifestations include anakinra, azathioprine, hydroxychloroquine, pioglitazone,[82] sirolimus, and thalidomide[83]; TNF inhibitors improve the colitis, but increase the risk of infection.

Stem cell transplantation may cure CGD and its use has increased.[84] Younger patients without infection at transplantation have the best outcome (survival >95%), but reduced-intensity conditioning regimens have been used for older individuals (including adults) and patients with recalcitrant infections or inflammation,[85] and should be considered if recurrent serious infections or corticosteroid-dependent inflammatory disease before irreversible organ damage occurs.[86]

Gene therapy has been performed for the p47^{phox}-deficient and X-linked forms of CGD. The use of retroviruses, however, may lead to insertional oncogenesis and myelodysplasia, necessitating safer approaches such as self-inactivating lentiviral vectors or nonviral techniques.[86-90]

LEUKOCYTE ADHESION DEFICIENCIES

AT-A-GLANCE

- Group of 4 disorders: 3 autosomal recessive (mutations in *ITGB2*, *SLC35C1*, or *FERMT3*) and 1 autosomal dominant (mutations in *Rac2*).
- Gingivitis and periodontitis.
- Poor wound healing; delayed separation of the umbilical stump and development of pyoderma gangrenosum-like necrotic ulcerations after wounding.
- Life-threatening bacterial and fungal infections.

HYPERIMMUNOGLOBU-LINEMIA E SYNDROME

AT-A-GLANCE

- Synonyms: Job syndrome, Buckley syndrome, hyperimmunoglobulin E recurrent infection syndrome.
- Most cases are autosomal dominant, but recessive forms with some different features have been described.
- Classic triad: (a) recurrent staphylococcal skin abscesses, (b) pneumonia with pneumatocele formation, and (c) high serum levels of IgE.
- Atopic dermatitis is a common manifestation.
- Scoliosis, fractures, and dental abnormalities are uniquely features of the more prevalent, autosomal dominant form.
- Autosomal recessive cases have severe viral infections and can develop severe neurologic complications.

HIES is rare (incidence 1 in 10^6).[91] It is found equally in males and females. Most cases are sporadic or consistent with an autosomal dominant inheritance. Autosomal recessive inheritance also has been described, but patients show different associated features.

CLINICAL FEATURES

The clinical presentation of individual patients with HIES may vary greatly.[91-93] Table 132-7 summarizes the most common clinical features and laboratory values of patients with sporadic or autosomal dominant HIES. The neonatal or infantile rash of HIES is often a papulopustular eruption with prominent crusting distributed on the scalp, face, neck, axillae, and diaper area.[94,95] The most consistent finding on skin biopsy is an eosinophilic spongiotic dermatitis, sometimes centered in the dermal follicles.[94] Early candidal infections of the skin, mucosae, and nails and/or infantile atopic dermatitis are other presentations; in patients with the eosinophilic papulopustules, the atopic dermatitis commonly follows later in infancy. Superinfection of the dermatitis with *S. aureus* is very common,[95] and patients show high levels of antistaphylococcal IgE antibodies. Staphylococcal skin infections include impetigo, furunculosis, paronychia, cellulitis, and characteristic "cold" abscesses (Fig. 132-13) that do not demonstrate the anticipated degree of erythema, warmth, and purulence. The abscesses occur most commonly on the head and neck and in intertriginous areas. Recurrent streptococcal pyoderma may also develop.

Pulmonary bacterial pneumonia, abscesses, and empyema are the most frequent systemic infections and may result in pneumatoceles that serve as the nidus for bacterial (often *Pseudomonas aeruginosa*) or fungal

TABLE 132-7
Characteristics of Hyperimmunoglobulinemia E Syndrome[131]

	INCIDENCE (%)
Immune System	
▪ Dermatitis	100
▪ Skin abscesses	87
▪ Recurrent pneumonia (3 or more, proved by radiography)	87
▪ Pneumatoceles	77
▪ Mucocutaneous candidiasis	83
Skeletal System	
▪ Characteristic fades	83
▪ Wide nose	65
▪ Failure of dental exfoliation (>3 teeth)	72
▪ Hyperextensibility	68
▪ Recurrent pathologic fractures	57
▪ Scoliosis (>10°)	63
Laboratory Values	
▪ Immunoglobulin E >2000 IU/mL or >10 times the age-specific norm	97
▪ Eosinophilia (>2 SD above the norm)	93

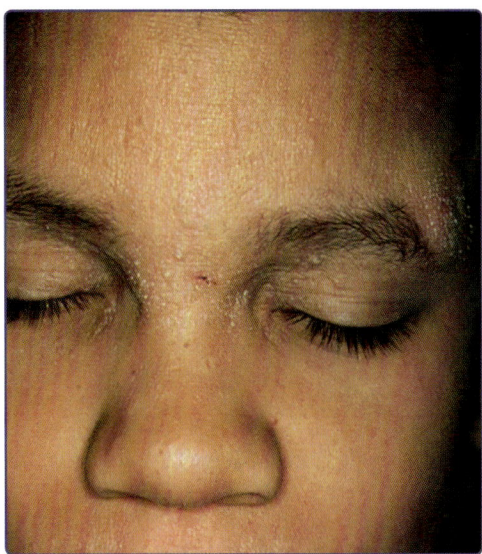

Figure 132-13 Coarse facial features, atopic dermatitis furuncles, and a cold abscess at the glabella in a boy with Hyperimmunoglobulinemia E syndrome.

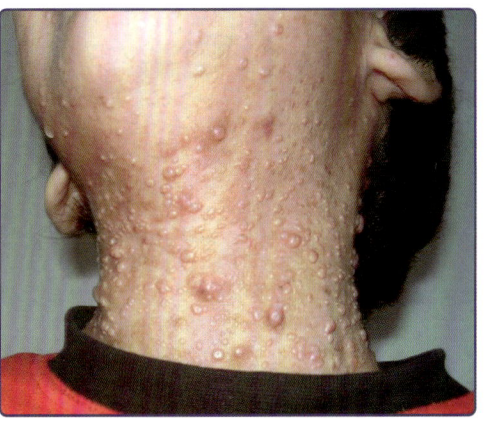

Figure 132-14 This boy with autosomal recessive HIES caused by a *DOCK8* (dedicator of cytokinesis 8) mutation shows extensive molluscum contagiosum infection on the neck. (Used with permission from Dr. I. Barlan.)

(especially *Aspergillus*) infection. The most common infecting organisms are *S. aureus* and *H. influenzae*. Other than pneumonias, deep-seated infections, bacteremia, and sepsis are rare.[96]

Facial and skeletal abnormalities are common. Patients develop progressive coarsening of facial features (see Fig. 132-13), probably reflecting the skeletal defects, but the recurrent facial pustulation and lichenification from dermatitis may contribute. Distinctive facial features, including prominent forehead, a broad nasal bridge, and wide nasal tip are universally present by the age of 16 years. Dental anomalies include retention of primary teeth and lack of eruption of secondary teeth.[97] Osteopenia is common, and 57% of patients have had at least 3 pathologic fractures, especially of the long bones, ribs, and pelvis.[98,99] Scoliosis occurs in 63% of adult patients and hyperextensibility of joints in 68% of patients.[96] Milder phenotypes may reflect mosaicism.[100]

Autosomal recessive disease shares with autosomal recessive HIES the high serum IgE levels, peripheral eosinophilia, chronic eczematous dermatitis, and recurrent skin (including cold abscesses) and respiratory tract staphylococcal infections. However, patients with autosomal recessive HIES show no tendency to form pneumatoceles and have no skeletal or dental abnormalities.[101] Instead, autosomal recessive HIES is characterized by recurrent viral infections (eg, molluscum contagiosum, warts, herpes simplex and varicella-zoster), opportunistic infections, autoimmunity and devastating neurologic complications (especially vasculitis) that are often fatal in childhood (Fig. 132-14).[102-107] Of patients with autosomal recessive HIES, up to 24% may have the neonatal the neonatal papulopustular eruption and food allergies/asthma are more common than in autosomal dominant HIES. Patients with autosomal recessive HIES have an increased risk of mucocutaneous squamous cell carcinoma and lymphomas.

ETIOLOGY AND PATHOGENESIS

Three different gene defects have been identified in HIES. The most common is a dominant negative mutation in signal transducer and activator of transcription 3 (STAT3),[108,109] and is associated with a severe reduction of Th17 cells.[110] STAT3 signals downstream of IL-6, which, together with transforming growth factor–β, is important for the development of Th17 cells. The Th17 cell deficiency accounts for the increased susceptibility to *Candida* infection and, as Th17 activation is key, for innate immunity at epithelial surfaces through the development of antimicrobial peptides. The decreased cytokine signaling may account for the "cold" abscesses and destructive inflammation from increased expression of other proinflammatory cytokines. The osteopenia of HIES is thought to result from loss of STAT3-dependent downregulation of osteoclast differentiation.

Autosomal recessive HIES most often results from biallelic mutations in the dedicator of cytokinesis 8 (*DOCK8*), which encodes for a protein that is implicated in the regulation of the actin cytoskeleton that is critical for T-cell expansion and antibody responses.[102,103]

Mutations in *TYK2* have been found in a single patient with HIES,[111] although other patients with *TYK2* deficiency have increased viral and mycobacterial infections, but not HIES, suggesting that HIES may not be an important feature. Biallelic mutations in phosphoglucomutase 3, a glycosylation enzyme, also have been found to underlie an HIES-like autosomal recessive disorder with elevated IgE levels, atopy, autoimmunity, and neurocognitive abnormalities.[112-114]

DIAGNOSIS

By definition, serum IgE levels must be elevated, but normal levels of IgE increase markedly during childhood. Diagnostic criteria for autosomal dominant HIES have been established that include IgE levels greater than 1000 IU/mL and a weighted score of 5 clinical features (typical newborn rash, recurrent pneumonia, pathologic bone fractures, characteristic facies, and a high palate)[115]; these features and Th17 cell deficiency lead to a "probably" diagnosis, but are definitive with a heterozygous *STAT3* mutation. It should be recognized, however, that normal levels of IgE are age-dependent. Levels greater than 2000 IU/mL are seen in adolescents and adults; considerably lower levels are seen during infancy, given that the upper limit of normal in infants younger than age 1 year is 12.7 IU/mL and by 5 years of age is 47.1 IU/mL; an IgE level 10-fold above the 95th percentile for age is required for diagnosis. Eosinophilia of at least 2 SD above normal (usually above 700 cells/μL) is also a clinical manifestation. The total white blood cell count is typically normal and often fails to elevate in the setting of acute infection.

In the autosomal recessive forms, eosinophilia tends to be more severe (eg, 17,500/μL).[116] These patients have a global defect in T-cell activation (CD4>CD8 cells), which may explain their susceptibility to viral infections (including herpes and molluscum) in addition to bacterial and fungal infections. In contrast to autosomal dominant HIES, autosomal recessive HIES is associated with Th2 cell skewing. Deficiency of DOCK8 expression can be detected by flow cytometry.[117]

DIFFERENTIAL DIAGNOSIS

HIES is often considered in young pediatric patients with atopic dermatitis or WAS because of the high levels of IgE, eosinophilia, dermatitis, and recurrent staphylococcal infections. The coarse facial features, osteopenia, recurrent pneumonia, and cold abscesses of autosomal dominant HIES help to distinguish it; the presence of platelet abnormalities also helps to distinguish WAS. In a study of 70 pediatric patients with a serum IgE level higher than 2000 IU/mL, 54 (77%) had atopic dermatitis and only 6 (8%) had HIES; the IgE level did not correlate with the diagnosis of HIES.[118] Other immunodeficiency syndromes can be confused with HIES (eg, Omenn, DiGeorge, IPEX, and IRAK-4 [IL-1R–associated kinase 4] deficiency), as well as Netherton syndrome and GVHD. Early candidal infections may lead to consideration of mucocutaneous candidiasis (and with mosaic STAT3 mutations, candida infections may be present without detectable Th17 cell deficiency.[100]

CLINICAL COURSE, PROGNOSIS, AND TREATMENT

Given the lack of correlation between serum levels of IgE, eosinophilia, and the susceptibility to severe infections, the clinical course is difficult to predict. Patients with autosomal recessive HIES have a more severe course related to the neurologic complications.

Antistaphylococcal antibiotics are effective for most cutaneous infections in patients with HIES, and oral triazole antifungals treat the mucocutaneous candidiasis. The prophylactic use of antistaphylococcal antibiotics markedly reduces the incidence of skin abscesses and pneumonia. The cutaneous and pulmonary abscesses often require incision and drainage and may require partial lung resections. Intravenous immunoglobulin therapy has been used successfully. Intravenous immunoglobulin may influence IgE levels as a consequence of an increased Ig catabolism or neutralization of the IgE. Ascorbic acid and cimetidine have decreased the number of infections and the chemotactic defect in some patients. Isotretinoin has been reported to eliminate the recurrent staphylococcal abscesses in an isolated patient without any change in immunologic status. Cyclosporine also has been used with good clinical and laboratory response. IFN-γ has shown inconsistent effects on IgE levels and infection susceptibility. Alendronate has been administered for the osteopenia.[99] There are anecdotal reports of improvement of the eczematous dermatitis of HIES with use of omalizumab, a monoclonal antibody directed against IgE.[119] INF-α has effectively treated the numerous warts[120] and severe herpetic infections[121,122] in DOCK8-deficient HIES. Stem cell transplantation is generally reserved for DOCK8-deficient HIES,[123-125] but has been successful in severe cases of STAT3-deficient HIES.[126]

WHIM SYNDROME

WHIM (*w*arts, *h*ypogammaglobulinemia, *i*nfections, and *m*yelokathexis) syndrome is an immunodeficiency that is characterized by neutropenia, hypogammaglobulinemia, and a susceptibility to infection by human papillomavirus. The disorder results from defects in the chemokine receptor gene *CXCR4*,[127,128] and thus mature neutrophils are not able to exit the bone marrow (myelokathexis). The susceptibility to human papillomavirus infections suggests an important role for CXCR4 in immunity to this virus. Plerixafor, a CXCR4 antagonist, increases circulating leukocytes, reduces infections and, in combination with imiquimod, markedly reduces associated warts that had previously been resistant to treatment.[129]

SILVERY HAIR SYNDROMES: CHÉDIAK-HIGASHI AND GRISCELLI SYNDROMES

The silvery hair syndromes comprise a group of autosomal recessive disorders in which a peculiar metallic sheen to hair, and often to skin, is noted (see also Chap. 75). Of these, Chédiak-Higashi and Griscelli (Type 2) syndromes have associated immunodeficiency (Table 132-8). Another syndrome with silvery hair, Elejalde syndrome, does not have associated immunodeficiency and may be allelic with the myosin 5a-deficient form of Griscelli syndrome (GS), with severe associated CNS dysfunction.

CHÉDIAK-HIGASHI SYNDROME

AT-A-GLANCE

- Autosomal recessive disorder of vesicle trafficking that results in giant organelles, including melanosomes, leukocyte granules, and platelet-dense granules.
- Mutations in *LYST*.
- Silvery hair; pigment speckling and often hyperpigmentation on nose and ears.
- Variable degree of photophobia and nystagmus.
- Diagnosis can be confirmed by pigment clumping in hair shaft and leukocyte granules in blood smears.
- Recurrent pyogenic infections and a mild bleeding diathesis.
- Life-threatening "accelerated phase" with pancytopenia and organomegaly as a result of lymphohistiocytic infiltration.
- Progressive neurologic deterioration.
- Therapy: transplantation.

EPIDEMIOLOGY

Chédiak-Higashi syndrome (CHS) is a rare autosomal recessive disorder.[130,131] Parental consanguinity is often reported, and there are approximately 300 reported cases worldwide.

CLINICAL FINDINGS

Patients usually first show manifestations during infancy or early childhood. Pigment abnormalities occur in 75% of patients, particularly the silver sheen to the hair (Fig. 132-15A). Ocular hypopigmentation may cause photophobia, and strabismus and nystagmus are common. Visual acuity does not tend to be reduced. The skin is typically fair compared to other family members, but dark, slate-colored areas of pigmentation and diffuse, speckled hypopigmentation may be seen in the sun-exposed skin of dark-skinned individuals.[132-134]

Infections can be observed in the newborn period and continue throughout the lifetime of the patient. Infections most commonly involve the skin, lungs, and respiratory tract where microbes such as *S. aureus*, *Streptococcus pyogenes*, and *Pneumococcus* are prevalent. Deep ulcerations resembling pyoderma gangrenosum have been described.

Neurologic manifestations include muscle weakness, cranial and peripheral neuropathy, and progressive neurologic deterioration. CHS patients also exhibit a mild coagulation defect. Patients bruise easily, manifest petechiae, and have some mucosal bleeding, although platelet numbers remain normal.

ETIOLOGY AND PATHOGENESIS

CHS is caused by mutations in the *LYST* gene, located on chromosome 1q42, which encodes a protein required for the final steps of vesicle trafficking and secretion.[135] The *LYST* gene is expressed in lysosomes and other secretory organelles (melanosomes, cytolytic granules, and platelet dense granules). Characteristic giant granules are thought to result from altered granule maturation and fusion. Enlarged melanosomes are unable to be transferred to keratinocytes. NK cells and cytotoxic T lymphocytes do not release proteolytic enzymes necessary for target cell killing. Cytotoxic T-lymphocyte–associated antigen is trapped in abnormally large vesicles rather than on the cell surface and thus may be unable to regulate T-cell activation, increasing the risk of lymphoproliferative disease. Platelet-dense granules are delayed in secretion of storage pools required for normal coagulation. Diminished chemotaxis of neutrophils and monocytes and delayed intracellular microorganism killing are often associated.

DIAGNOSIS

Diagnosis is usually suspected clinically because of the silvery sheen to the hair. The finding of large cytoplasmic granules in blood leukocytes is highly

TABLE 132-8
Characteristics of Griscelli and Chédiak-Higashi Syndromes

	GRISCELLI (GS1)	GRISCELLI (GS2)	GRISCELLI (GS3)	CHÉDIAK-HIGASHI
Gene defect/protein	*MYO5A*/myosin5a	*RAB27A*/Rab27a	a. Slac2-a/mlph b. *MYO5A* F-exon deletion	LYST/lysosomal transport protein
Functional consequence	Intracellular organelle transport and neurotransmitter secretion; interacts with Slac2-a/mlph	GTPase for organelle movement and transfer. Essential for T- and NK-lymphocyte cytotoxic granule release and target cell death; interacts with Slac2-a/mlph	Interacts with both myosin 5a and Rab27 to form a protein complex essential for melanosome movement to melanocytes	Protein required for final steps of membrane fusion and vesicle trafficking
Tissue expression	Brain; not in cytotoxic cells	Cytotoxic cells; not in brain	Slac2-a/mlph is not in cytotoxic cells	
Clinical features	Silvery metallic hair; mild skin pigment dilution; onset of neurologic disorder in infancy	Silvery metallic hair; mild skin pigment dilution; severe immune disorder with hemophagocytic syndrome; neurologic symptoms are associated with hemophagocytic syndrome and CNS infiltration	Silvery metallic hair	Silvery metallic hair and skin; recurrent infections; bleeding tendencies; progressive neurologic defects; immune disorder with hemophagocytic syndrome
Immune defects	None	T- and NK-cell function; hypogammaglobulinemia	None	T- and NK-cell function, diminished neutrophil chemotaxis and bactericidal activity
Hair mount	Large, uneven clusters of pigment	Same as GS1	Same as GS1	Granular, evenly distributed pigment
Skin in light microscopy	Pigmentary dilution in keratinocytes, accumulation of melanosomes in melanocytes	Same as GS1	Same as GS1	Pigmentary dilution in both keratinocytes and melanocytes
Skin in electron microscopy	Mature melanosomes filling epidermal melanocytes	Same as GS1	Same as GS1	Reduced numbers of giant melanosomes
Leukocyte granules	None	None	None	Large, cytoplasmic

GTPase, guanosine triphosphatase; mlph, melanophilin; NK, natural killer.

diagnostic. Hair shafts have evenly distributed small pigment granules (see Fig. 132-15B), in contrast to the irregular, large pigmentary clumping of GS (see Fig. 132-15C). Although not performed for diagnostic purposes, skin biopsy shows pigmentary dilution in both melanocytes and keratinocytes, and electron microscopy reveals giant melanosomes.

DIFFERENTIAL DIAGNOSIS

The silvery hair sheen is also seen in GS, but an unusual metallic hair sheen and skin hypopigmentation is a component as well of Hermansky-Pudlak syndrome (see Chap. 75). Silvery hair also has been described in a neonate with hypoproteinemia from congenital hydrops fetalis; the hair spontaneously repigmented[136] with clinical improvement. Pseudo-CHS granules are seen on smears in some cases of acute leukemia.[137]

The hemophagocytic syndrome associated with lymphohistiocytic proliferation of silvery hair syndromes needs to be distinguished from massive lymphoproliferation in other immunodeficiency disorders, particularly X-linked lymphoproliferative disorder (see "Antibody Deficiency Disorders" above), familial hemophagocytic lymphohistiocytosis, autoimmune lymphoproliferative syndrome, and immunodeficiency caused by mutations in the IL-2R. *Familial hemophagocytic lymphohistiocytosis* is a group of autosomal recessive disorders with hemophagocytosis and absence of NK-cell cytotoxicity that tends to be fatal without early stem cell transplantation.[138,139] The condition can result from mutations in either *PRF1*, which encodes perforin; *UNC13D*, which encodes Munc 13-4[140]; *STX11*, encoding syntaxin 11; or *STXBP2*, encoding Munc 18-2. All of these proteins are involved in the exocytosis and function of cytotoxic intracellular granules NK cells and cytotoxic T lymphocytes.

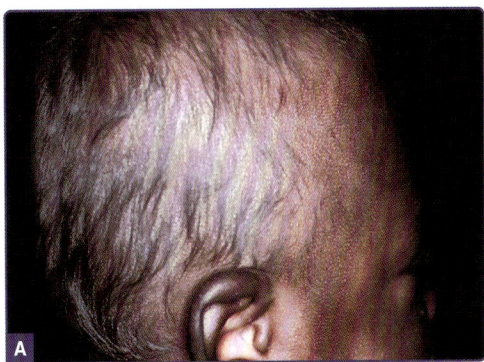
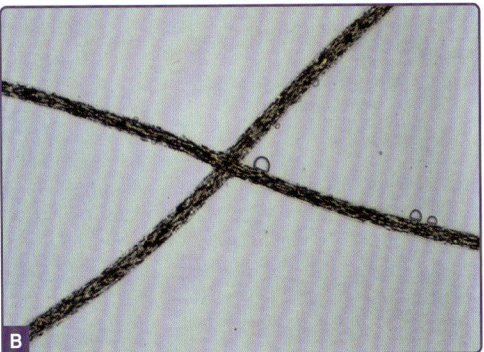
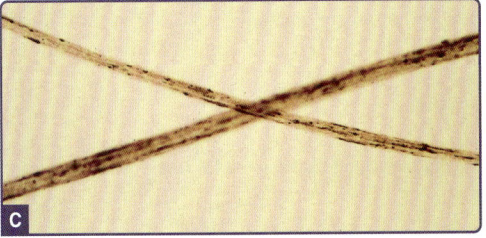

Figure 132-15 Silvery hair syndromes. **A,** Silvery sheen to the hair in a black infant; the patient had darkly pigmented eyes and skin. Note the accentuation of pigmentation on the ear helix. **B,** Small, evenly clumped pigment granules in the hairs of Chédiak-Higashi syndrome. **C,** Larger aggregates of irregularly spaced pigmentation in the hairs of a patient with Griscelli syndrome.

Patients demonstrate bacterial, viral, and fungal infections because of early apoptosis of the developing thymic T lymphocytes.

PROGNOSIS, CLINICAL COURSE, AND TREATMENT

The "accelerated phase" of hemophagocytic lymphohistiocytosis occurs in 85% of CHS patients and is usually triggered by Epstein-Barr virus infection. Viscera become infiltrated with lymphoid and histiocytic cells, which are sometimes atypical in appearance. Hepatosplenomegaly with jaundice, lymphadenopathy, pancytopenia, and a leukemia-like gingivitis with pseudomembranous sloughing of the buccal mucosa are associated. In this phase, petechiae, bruising and gingival bleeding are commonly seen, resulting from the thrombocytopenia and decreased hepatic synthesis of coagulation factors. Overwhelming infection or hemorrhage during the accelerated phase often lead to death. CHS may present with the accelerated phase.[144]

The mean age of death for untransplanted patients with CHS is 6 years, usually from overwhelming infection or hemorrhage during the lymphoma-like accelerated phase. Prenatal diagnosis has been achieved by examination of hair from fetal scalp biopsies and of leukocytes from fetal blood samples.

The treatment of choice for patients with CHS is early transplantation,[145-148] which corrects the immunologic status but does not affect the pigment abnormality nor inhibit the development of neurologic disorders that grow increasingly worse with age. Reduced intensity conditioning has been used with success, especially in patients transplanted before the accelerated phase occurs. Absence of cytotoxic T-cell function has been touted as predictive of the later occurrence of hemophagocytic lymphohistiocytosis, and as a biomarker for early transplantation. Management of CHS is otherwise largely supportive, with use of prophylactic antibiotics to avoid recurrent infections. Acyclovir, high-dose intravenous γ-globulin, vincristine, cyclosporine, and prednisone have been used to control the accelerated phase, but the accelerated phase is usually fatal.

Mutations in several genes can lead to autosomal recessive or dominant autoimmune lymphoproliferative syndrome, also known as Canale-Smith syndrome.[141,142] These include the genes that encode Fas or CD95 (*TNFRSF6*), the cell-surface apoptosis receptor, and its ligand (*TNFSF6*), and the caspase proteins 8 and 10, proteases in the cascade leading to apoptosis. This group of disorders features autoimmune disorders (cytopenias, leukocytoclastic vasculitis, lupus erythematosus) and an increased risk of lymphoma, and is associated with increased numbers of circulating CD4−/CD8− α/β T cells. Immunodeficiency with extensive lymphocytic infiltration of viscera is also a manifestation of autosomal recessive mutations in the α chain of the IL-2 receptor.[143]

GRISCELLI SYNDROME

AT-A-GLANCE

- Autosomal recessive group of disorders.
- Mutations in *MYO5A* (more neurologic), *RAB27A* (hemophagocytosis), or *Slac-2a*.
- Silvery hair is a hallmark.

- Diagnosis can be confirmed by pigment clumping in hair shaft, but smears show no leukocyte granules.
- Hemophagocytosis often precipitated by Epstein-Barr virus infection.
- Treatment: transplantation.

EPIDEMIOLOGY

The majority of affected patients with this autosomal recessive disorder are of Mediterranean or Middle Eastern origin and born into consanguineous families.

CLINICAL FINDINGS

The pigmentary dilution of GS is often limited to the hair, characterized by a silver-gray sheen with a few cases of skin involvement. The hair shaft shows large uneven clusters of pigment (see Fig. 132-15C) and the skin shows pigmentary dilution in keratinocytes but accumulation of melanosomes in melanocytes. Electron microscopy reveals numerous stage IV melanosomes in epidermal melanocytes. In contrast to CHS, smears of leukocytes do not show giant granules. The additional clinical features present in each subtype are dependent on the function and tissue expression of the defective protein. Patients with GS1 have a primary neurologic disorder that presents in infancy with hypotonia and developmental delay. Severe immune disorder characterized by hemophagocytic syndrome or an "accelerated phase of the disease" is seen in GS2. Hemophagocytic syndrome is characterized by infiltration of various organ systems by activated lymphocytes and macrophages. It develops at mean age of 36 months, and often is precipitated by a virus, particularly Epstein-Barr virus. Patients have fever, hepatosplenomegaly, neurologic impairment, coagulopathy, and pancytopenia. Patients with GS3 present solely with the pigmentary abnormalities.[149,150]

ETIOLOGY AND PATHOGENESIS

Mutations in 3 genes may underlie GS. GS1 is caused by a mutation in the *MYO5A* gene that encodes myosin-5a, a motor protein responsible for intracellular organelle transport. *MYO5A* is abundantly expressed in brain tissue and is important for neurotransmitter secretion. It is not expressed in cytotoxic cells. GS2 is caused by a mutation in the *RAB27A* gene, which encodes Rab27a, a guanosine triphosphatase protein involved in the function of the intracellular-regulated secretory pathway. It is essential for T-lymphocyte and NK-lymphocyte cytotoxic granule release and cell death. This defective cytotoxic activity most likely leads to the uncontrolled activation of lymphocytes and macrophages in the hemophagocytic syndrome.

Both *MYO5A* and *RAB27A* have been mapped to chromosome 15q21.1. The third type, GS3, is the result of a homozygous missense mutation in *Slac2-a/melanophilin* or a deletion of the *MYO5A* F-exon.[151] Melanophilin (also not expressed in cytotoxic cells) encodes a member of the Rab effector family and interacts with both myosin-5a (through the F-exon) and *RAB27A* to form a triprotein complex essential for the capture and local transport of melanosomes to the melanocytes (Fig. 132-16). All 3 genetic subtypes share the inability to construct this complex for melanosome transport, thus leading to the characteristic pigmentary abnormality of GS.

PROGNOSIS, CLINICAL COURSE, AND TREATMENT

GS has been uniformly fatal but now can be reversed by successful hematopoietic stem cell transplantation. Of patients with GS2, 85% have mutations in the *RAB27A* gene that lead to early protein truncation. They have the most-severe form of the disease, with early development of hemophagocytic syndrome and rapid progression. The median survival from the onset of the accelerated phase to death in these patients is 5 months. Most patients die by 5 years of age secondary to progressive CNS disease or recurrent infections. Missense mutations in the *RAB27A* gene show a milder phenotype

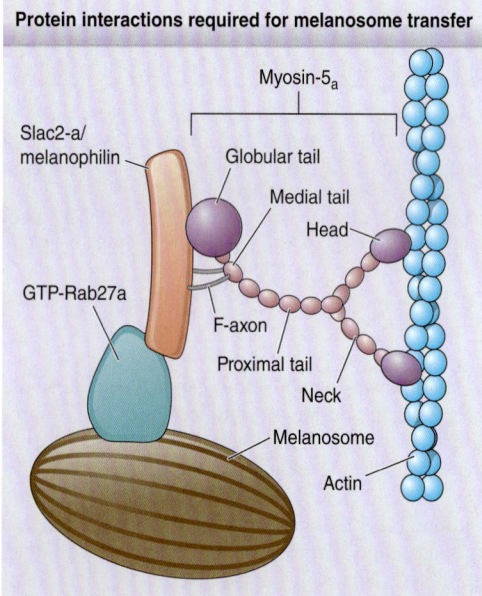

Figure 132-16 Protein interactions required for melanosome transfer. GTP, guanosine triphosphate. (Adapted with permission of ASCI: Ménasché G, Ho CH, Sanal O, et al. Griscelli syndrome restricted to hypopigmentation results from a melanophilin defect (GS3) or a MYO5A F-exon deletion (GS1). *J Clin Invest*. 2003;112:450-456. Permission conveyed through Copyright Clearance Center, Inc.)

with later age of hemophagocytic syndrome onset and a good response to chemotherapy treatment. Patients with GS1 do not develop hemophagocytic syndrome. Prenatal diagnosis has been achieved by examination of hair from fetal scalp biopsies and DNA analysis.

COMPLEMENT DEFICIENCY DISORDERS

AT-A-GLANCE

- Deficiency or dysfunction of early complement components is associated with autoimmune disorders, particularly systemic lupus erythematosus.
- Deficiency or dysfunction of early complement components leads to risk of infections caused by encapsulated bacteria.
- Deficiency of late complement components markedly increases susceptibility to neisserial infections.

Table 132-9 outlines the clinical manifestations of hereditary deficiency or dysfunction of complement components.

HEREDITARY ANGIOEDEMA

Hereditary angioedema (HAE) is almost always inherited in an autosomal dominant fashion with a spontaneous mutation rate of 25% (for clinical features and management, see Chap. 41).[152] It occurs in 1 in 150,000 persons and has no racial or ethnic predilection. Seventy-five percent of patients report a positive family history. There are 3 types of HAE. Type I is characterized by low antigenic levels of C1 inhibitor (C1 INH) and affects 85% of patients, whereas the remainder of patients have Type II, with low functional levels but normal/high antigenic levels of C1 INH. A third type of HAE does not show a deficiency of C1 INH. This type of HAE was previously thought to only affect women, although eventually, a family was described in which three male family members were affected.[153] One family in which the disease is transmitted as an autosomal recessive trait because of a mutation in the promoter region of the gene has been identified.[154]

HAE causes significant morbidity, especially if attacks are frequent and laryngeal edema is a

TABLE 132-9
Clinical Manifestations of Hereditary Deficiency or Dysfunction of Complement Components

MANIFESTATION	COMPONENT	PATHWAY	ASSOCIATIONS
Infection	C1q, C1r, C1s, C4, C2, C3	Classical	Autoimmune disorders, especially SLE
			Increased encapsulated bacterial infections
	Mannan-binding lectin	Lectin	Pyogenic infections in neonates and children (SLE)
	Factors H, I	Inhibitors, alternative	Recurrent pyogenic infections (C3 depletion)
	Properdin	Stabilizer, alternative	Fulminant neisserial infections
	CR3	Receptor for iC3b	LAD (see LAD Type 1)
	C5 to C9	Terminal (membrane attack complex)	Recurrent neisserial infections; milder with C9 deficiency
Autoimmune disorders	C1, C4, C2	Classical	Autoimmune disorders, especially SLE
			Increased encapsulated bacterial infections
			SLE
Exfoliative erythroderma	C3, C5	Shared, terminal	Failure to thrive, diarrhea, infections
Angioedema	C1 esterase inhibitor	Inhibitor, classical	Angioedema
Renal disease and/or hemolysis	Factor H	Inhibitor, alternative	Glomerulonephritis, atypical hemolytic uremic syndrome
	Decay accelerating factor (CD59)	Inhibitor, alternative	Hemolysis, thrombosis
	Membrane cofactor protein (CD46)	Inhibitor, alternative	Atypical hemolytic uremic syndrome
	C3	Shared	Membranoproliferative glomerulonephritis, severe bacterial infections

LAD, leukocyte adhesion deficiency; SLE, systemic lupus erythematosus.

significant risk for mortality. There are several treatment modalities available including the use of attenuated androgens, antifibrinolytic agents, plasma-derived C1 INH, a kallikrein inhibitor and a bradykinin receptor antagonist.[152] Plasma-derived C1 INH can be used acutely to treat angioedema attacks or preventatively if attacks are frequent or before known procedures.

REFERENCES

1. Picard C, Al-Herz W, Bousfiha A, et al. Primary immunodeficiency diseases: an update on the classification from the International Union of Immunological Societies Expert Committee for Primary Immunodeficiency 2015. *J Clin Immunol*. 2015;35(8):696-726.
2. Ochs HD, Hagin D. Primary immunodeficiency disorders: general classification, new molecular insights, and practical approach to diagnosis and treatment. *Ann Allergy Asthma Immunol*. 2014;112(6):489-495.
3. Smith CIE, Berglöf A. X-Linked Agammaglobulinemia. In: Adam MP, Ardinger HH, Pagon RA, et al., eds. *GeneReviews* [Internet]. Seattle, WA: University of Washington; 1993-2016. 2001 [updated August 4, 2016]. https://www.ncbi.nlm.nih.gov/books/NBK1453/.
4. Winkelstein JA, Marino MC, Lederman HM, et al. X-linked agammaglobulinemia: report on a United States registry of 201 patients. *Medicine (Baltimore)*. 2006;85(4):193-202.
5. Berglof A, Turunen JJ, Gissberg O, et al. Agammaglobulinemia: causative mutations and their implications for novel therapies. *Expert Rev Clin Immunol*. 2013;9(12):1205-1221.
6. Resnick ES, Moshier EL, Godbold JH, et al. Morbidity and mortality in common variable immune deficiency over 4 decades. *Blood*. 2012;119(7):1650-1657.
7. Pierson JC, Camisa C, Lawlor KB, et al. Cutaneous and visceral granulomas in common variable immunodeficiency. *Cutis*. 1993;52:221.
8. Torrelo A, Mediero IG, Zambrano A. Caseating cutaneous granulomas in a child with common variable immunodeficiency. *Pediatr Dermatol*. 1995;12:170.
9. Gualdi G, Lougaris V, Baronio M, et al. Burden of skin disease in selective IgA deficiency and common variable immunodeficiency. *J Investig Allergol Clin Immunol*. 2015;25(5):369-371.
10. Cunningham-Rundles C, Bodian C. Common variable immunodeficiency: clinical and immunological features of 248 patients. *Clin Immunol*. 1999;92:34.
11. Herrod HG. Chronic mucocutaneous candidiasis in childhood and complications of non-*Candida* infection: a report of the Pediatric Immunodeficiency Collaborative Study Group. *J Pediatr*. 1990;116:377-382.
12. Soltész B, Tóth B, Sarkadi AK, et al. The evolving view of IL-17-mediated immunity in defense against mucocutaneous candidiasis in humans. *Int Rev Immunol*. 2015;34:348-363.
13. van de Veerdonk FL, Plantinga TS, Hoischen A, et al. STAT1 mutations in autosomal dominant chronic mucocutaneous candidiasis. *N Engl J Med*. 2011;365:54-61.
14. Depner M, Fuchs S, Raabe J, et al. The extended clinical phenotype of 26 patients with chronic mucocutaneous candidiasis due to gain-of-function mutations in STAT1. *J Clin Immunol*. 2016;36:73-84.
15. Toubiana J, Okada S, Hiller J, et al. Heterozygous STAT1 gain-of-function mutations underlie an unexpectedly broad clinical phenotype. *Blood*. 2016;127:3154-3164.
16. Puel A, Cypowyj S, Bustamante J, et al. Chronic mucocutaneous candidiasis in humans with inborn errors of interleukin-17 immunity. *Science*. 2011;332:65-68.
17. Boisson B, Wang C, Pedergnana V, et al. An ACT1 mutation selectively abolishes interleukin-17 responses in humans with chronic mucocutaneous candidiasis. *Immunity*. 2013;39:676-686.
18. Ling Y, Cypowyj S, Aytekin C, et al. Inherited IL-17RC deficiency in patients with chronic mucocutaneous candidiasis. *J Exp Med*. 2015;212:619-631.
19. Anderson MS, Su MA. AIRE expands: new roles in immune tolerance and beyond. *Nat Rev Immunol*. 2016;16:247-258.
20. Ferre EM, Rose SR, Rosenzweig SD, et al. Redefined clinical features and diagnostic criteria in autoimmune polyendocrinopathy-candidiasis-ectodermal dystrophy. *JCI Insight*. 2016;1:13.
21. Wolff AS, Sarkadi AK, Maródi L, et al. Anti-cytokine autoantibodies preceding onset of autoimmune polyendocrine syndrome type I features in early childhood. *J Clin Immunol*. 2013;33:1341-1348.
22. Glocker EO, Hennigs A, Nabavi M, et al. A homozygous CARD9 mutation in a family with susceptibility to fungal infections. *N Engl J Med*. 2009;361:1727-1735.
23. Ferwerda B, Ferwerda G, Plantinga TS, et al. Human dectin-1 deficiency and mucocutaneous fungal infections. *N Engl J Med*. 2009;361:1760-1767.
24. Meloni A, Furcas M, Cetani F, et al. Autoantibodies against type I interferons as an additional diagnostic criterion for autoimmune polyendocrine syndrome type 1. *J Clin Endocrinol Metab*. 2008;93:4389-4397.
25. Halabi-Tawil M, Ruemmele FM, Fraitag S, et al. Cutaneous manifestations of immune dysregulation, polyendocrinopathy, enteropathy, X-linked (IPEX) syndrome. *Br J Dermatol*. 2009;160:645-651.
26. Caudy AA, Reddy ST, Chatila T, et al. CD25 deficiency causes an immune dysregulation, polyendocrinopathy, enteropathy, X-linked-like syndrome, and defective IL-10 expression from CD4 lymphocytes. *J Allergy Clin Immunol*. 2007;119:482-487.
27. van de Veerdonk FL, Netea MG. Treatment options for chronic mucocutaneous candidiasis. *J Infect*. 2016;72(suppl):S56-S60.
28. Wildbaum G, Shahar E, Katz R, et al. Continuous G-CSF therapy for isolated chronic mucocutaneous candidiasis: complete clinical remission with restoration of IL-17 secretion. *J Allergy Clin Immunol*. 2013;132:761-764.
29. Buchbinder D, Nugent DJ, Fillipovich AH, et al. Wiskott-Aldrich syndrome: diagnosis, current management, and emerging treatments. *Appl Clin Genet*. 2014;7:55-66.
30. Massaad MJ, Ramesh N, Geha RS, et al. Wiskott-Aldrich syndrome: a comprehensive review. *Ann N Y Acad Sci*. 2013;1285:26-43.
31. Dupuis-Girod S, Medioni J, Haddad E, et al. Autoimmunity in Wiskott-Aldrich syndrome: risk factors, clinical features, and outcome in a single-center cohort of 55 patients. *Pediatrics*. 2003;111:e622-e627.
32. Sullivan KE, Mullen CA, Blaese RM, et al. A multiinstitutional survey of the Wiskott-Aldrich syndrome. *J Pediatr*. 1994;125(6, pt 1):876-885.
33. Cotta-de-Almeida V, Dupré L, Guipouy D, et al. Signal

33. integration during T lymphocyte activation and function: Lessons from the Wiskott-Aldrich syndrome. *Front Immunol.* 2015;6:47.
34. Bosticardo M, Marangoni F, Aiuti A, et al. Recent advances in understanding the pathophysiology of Wiskott-Aldrich syndrome. *Blood.* 2009;113(25):6288-6295.
35. Dosanjh A. Autoimmunity and immunodeficiency. *Pediatr Rev.* 2015;36:489-494.
36. Volpi S, Santori E, Abernethy K, et al. N-WASP is required for B-cell-mediated autoimmunity in Wiskott-Aldrich syndrome. *Blood.* 2016;127:216-220.
37. Pala F, Morbach H, Castiello MC, et al. Lentiviral-mediated gene therapy restores B cell tolerance in Wiskott-Aldrich syndrome patients. *J Clin Invest.* 2015;125:3941-3951.
38. Winkelstein JA, Fearon E. Carrier detection of the X-linked primary immunodeficiency diseases using X-chromosome inactivation analysis. *J Allergy Clin Immunol.* 1990;85:1090-1097.
39. Worth AJ, Thrasher AJ. Current and emerging treatment options for Wiskott-Aldrich syndrome. *Expert Rev Clin Immunol.* 2015;11:1015-1032.
40. Braun CJ, Boztug K, Paruzynski A, et al. Gene therapy for Wiskott-Aldrich syndrome—long-term efficacy and genotoxicity. *Sci Transl Med.* 2014;6(227):227ra33.
41. Aiuti A, Biasco L, Scaramuzza S, et al. Lentiviral hematopoietic stem cell gene therapy in patients with Wiskott-Aldrich syndrome. *Science.* 2013;341:1233151.
42. Laskowski TJ, Van Caeneghem Y, Pourebrahim R, et al. Gene correction of iPSCs from a Wiskott-Aldrich syndrome patient normalizes the lymphoid developmental and functional defects. *Stem Cell Reports.* 2016;7:139-148.
43. Chinn IK, Shearer WT. Severe combined immunodeficiency disorders. *Immunol Allergy Clin North Am.* 2015;35(4):671-694.
44. Rivers L, Gaspar HB. Severe combined immunodeficiency: recent developments and guidance on clinical management. *Arch Dis Child.* 2015;100(7):667-672.
45. Denianke KS, Frieden IJ, Cowan MJ, et al. Cutaneous manifestations of maternal engraftment in patients with severe combined immunodeficiency: a clinicopathologic study. *Bone Marrow Transplant.* 2001;28(3):227-233.
46. Kwong PC, O'Marcaigh AS, Howard R, et al. Oral and genital ulceration: a unique presentation of immunodeficiency in Athabascan-speaking American Indian children with severe combined immunodeficiency. *Arch Dermatol.* 1999;135(8):927-931.
47. Marrella V, Maina V, Villa A. Omenn syndrome does not live by V(D)J recombination alone. *Curr Opin Allergy Clin Immunol.* 2011;11(6):525-531.
48. Kwan A, Abraham RS, Currier R, et al. Newborn screening for severe combined immunodeficiency in 11 screening programs in the United States. *JAMA.* 2014;312(7):729-738.
49. Pai SY, Logan BR, Griffith LM, et al. Transplantation outcomes for severe combined immunodeficiency, 2000-2009. *N Engl J Med.* 2014;371(5):434-446.
50. Hanson EP, Monaco-Shawver L, Solt LA, et al. Hypomorphic nuclear factor-kappaB essential modulator mutation database and reconstitution system identifies phenotypic and immunologic diversity. *J Allergy Clin Immunol.* 2008;122(6):1169-1177.e16.
51. Courtois G, Smahi A, Reichenbach J, et al. A hypermorphic IkappaBalpha mutation is associated with autosomal dominant anhidrotic ectodermal dysplasia and T cell immunodeficiency. *J Clin Invest.* 2003;112(7):1108-1115.
52. Martinez-Pomar N, Munoz-Saa I, Heine-Suner D, et al. A new mutation in exon 7 of NEMO gene: late skewed X-chromosome inactivation in an incontinentia pigmenti female patient with immunodeficiency. *Hum Genet.* 2005;118(3-4):458-465.
53. Orange JS, Geha RS. Finding NEMO: genetic disorders of NF-[kappa]B activation. *J Clin Invest.* 2003;112:983.
54. Uzel G. The range of defects associated with nuclear factor kappaB essential modulator. *Curr Opin Allergy Clin Immunol.* 2005;5:513.
55. Fish JD, Duerst RE, Gelfand EW, et al. Challenges in the use of allogeneic hematopoietic SCT for ectodermal dysplasia with immune deficiency. *Bone Marrow Transplant.* 2009;43(3):217-221.
56. Scott SP, Bendix R, Chen P, et al. Missense mutations but not allelic variants alter the function of ATM by dominant interference in patients with breast cancer. *Proc Natl Acad Sci U S A.* 2002;99(2):925-930.
57. Rothblum-Oviatt C, Wright J, Lefton-Greif MA, et al. Ataxia telangiectasia: a review. *Orphanet J Rare Dis.* 2016;11(1):159.
58. Swift M, Morrell D, Massey RB, et al. Incidence of cancer in 161 families affected by ataxia-telangiectasia. *N Engl J Med.* 1991;325(26):1831-1836.
59. Hannan MA, Hellani A, Al-Khodairy FM, et al. Deficiency in the repair of UV-induced DNA damage in human skin fibroblasts compromised for the ATM gene. *Carcinogenesis.* 2002;23(10):1617-1624.
60. Cohen LE, Tanner DJ, Schaefer HG, et al. Common and uncommon cutaneous findings in patients with ataxia-telangiectasia. *J Am Acad Dermatol.* 1984;10(3):431-438.
61. Paller AS, Massey RB, Curtis MA, et al. Cutaneous granulomatous lesions in patients with ataxia-telangiectasia. *J Pediatr.* 1991;119(6):917-922.
62. Lai CH, Chun HH, Nahas SA, et al. Correction of ATM gene function by aminoglycoside-induced read-through of premature termination codons. *Proc Natl Acad Sci U S A.* 2004;101(44):15676-15681.
63. Dinauer MC. Disorders of neutrophil function: an overview. *Methods Mol Biol.* 2007;412:489.
64. Chiriaco M, Salfa I, Di Matteo G, et al. Chronic granulomatous disease: clinical, molecular, and therapeutic aspects. *Pediatr Allergy Immunol.* 2016;27:242-253.
65. Winkelstein JA, Marino MC, Johnston RB Jr, et al. Chronic granulomatous disease. Report on a national registry of 368 patients. *Medicine (Baltimore).* 2000;79(3):155-169.
66. Köker MY, Camcioğlu Y, van Leeuwen K, et al. Clinical, functional, and genetic characterization of chronic granulomatous disease in 89 Turkish patients. *J Allergy Clin Immunol.* 2013;132:1156-1163.
67. Kuhns DB, Alvord WG, Heller T, et al. Residual NADPH oxidase and survival in chronic granulomatous disease. *N Engl J Med.* 2010;363:2600-2610.
68. Prendiville B, Nopper AJ, Lawrence H, et al. Chronic granulomatous disease presenting with ecthyma gangrenosum in a neonate. *J Am Acad Dermatol.* 2014;71:e44-e45.
69. Marciano BE, Spalding C, Fitzgerald A, et al. Common severe infections in chronic granulomatous disease. *Clin Infect Dis.* 2015;60:1176-1183.
70. Friend JC, Hilligoss DM, Marquesen M, et al. Skin ulcers and disseminated abscesses are characteristic of *Serratia marcescens* infection in older patients with chronic granulomatous disease. *J Allergy Clin Immunol.*

2009;124:164-166.
71. Foti C, Cassano N, Martire B, et al. Lupus erythematosus-like lesions in a carrier of X-linked chronic granulomatous disease: a case report and personal considerations. *Int J Dermatol*. 2004;43(11):840-842.
72. Cale CM, Morton L, Goldblatt D. Cutaneous and other lupus-like symptoms in carriers of X-linked chronic granulomatous disease: incidence and autoimmune serology. *Clin Exp Immunol*. 2007;148:79-84.
73. Valentine G, Thomas TA, Nguyen T, et al. Chronic granulomatous disease presenting as hemophagocytic lymphohistiocytosis: a case report. *Pediatrics*. 2014;134:e1727-e1730.
74. De Ravin SS, Naumann N, Cowen EW, et al. Chronic granulomatous disease as a risk factor for autoimmune disease. *J Allergy Clin Immunol*. 2008;122:1097-1103.
75. Magnani A, Brosselin P, Beauté J, et al. Inflammatory manifestations in a single-center cohort of patients with chronic granulomatous disease. *J Allergy Clin Immunol*. 2014;134:655-662.
76. Lekstrom-Himes JA, Kuhns DB, Alvord WG, et al. Inhibition of human neutrophil IL-8 production by hydrogen peroxide and dysregulation in chronic granulomatous disease. *J Immunol*. 2005;174:411-417.
77. Crotzer VL, Matute JD, Arias AA, et al. Cutting edge: NADPH oxidase modulates MHC class II antigen presentation by B cells. *J Immunol*. 2012;189:3800-3804.
78. Jirapongsananuruk O, Malech HL, Kuhns DB, et al. Diagnostic paradigm for evaluation of male patients with chronic granulomatous disease, based on the dihydrorhodamine 123 assay. *J Allergy Clin Immunol*. 2003;111:374-379.
79. Kang EM, Malech HL. Advances in treatment for chronic granulomatous disease. *Immunol Res*. 2009;43:77-84.
80. Gallin JI, Alling DW, Malech HL, et al. Itraconazole to prevent fungal infections in chronic granulomatous disease. *N Engl J Med*. 2003;348(24):2416-2422.
81. A controlled trial of interferon gamma to prevent infection in chronic granulomatous disease. The International Chronic Granulomatous Disease Cooperative Study Group. *N Engl J Med*. 1991;324(8):509-516.
82. Migliavacca M, Assanelli A, Ferrua F, et al. Pioglitazone as a novel therapeutic approach in chronic granulomatous disease. *J Allergy Clin Immunol*. 2016;137:1913-1915.
83. Noel N, Mahlaoui N, Blanche S, et al. Efficacy and safety of thalidomide in patients with inflammatory manifestations of chronic granulomatous disease: a retrospective case series. *J Allergy Clin Immunol*. 2013;132:997-1000.
84. Martinez CA, Shah S, Shearer WT, et al. Excellent survival after sibling or unrelated donor stem cell transplantation for chronic granulomatous disease. *J Allergy Clin Immunol*. 2012;129:176-183.
85. Güngör T, Teira P, Slatter M, et al. Reduced-intensity conditioning and HLA-matched haemopoietic stem-cell transplantation in patients with chronic granulomatous disease: a prospective multicentre study. *Lancet*. 2014;383:436-448.
86. Cole T, Pearce MS, Cant AJ, et al. Clinical outcome in children with chronic granulomatous disease managed conservatively or with hematopoietic stem cell transplantation. *J Allergy Clin Immunol*. 2013;132:1150-1155.
87. Malech HL, Mapels PB, Whiting-Theoblad N, et al. Prolonged production of NADPH oxidase-corrected granulocytes after gene therapy of chronic granulomatous disease. *Proc Natl Acad Sci U S A*. 1997;94:12133-12138.
88. Stein S, Ott MG, Schultze-Strasser S, et al. Genomic instability and myelodysplasia with monosomy 7 consequent to EVI1 activation after gene therapy for chronic granulomatous disease. *Nat Med*. 2010;16:198-204.
89. Kaufmann KB, Chiriaco M, Siler U, et al. Gene therapy for chronic granulomatous disease: current status and future perspectives. *Curr Gene Ther*. 2014;14:447-460.
90. De Ravin SS, Reik A, Liu PQ, et al. Targeted gene addition in human CD34(+) hematopoietic cells for correction of X-linked chronic granulomatous disease. *Nat Biotechnol*. 2016;34:424-429.
91. Grimbacher B, Holland SM, Gallin JI, et al. Hyper-IgE syndrome with recurrent infections: an autosomal dominant multisystem disorder. *N Engl J Med*. 1999;340:692-702.
92. Farmand S, Sundin M. Hyper-IgE syndromes: recent advances in pathogenesis, diagnostics and clinical care. *Curr Opin Hematol*. 2015;22(1):12-22.
93. Chandesris MO, Melki I, Natividad A, et al. Autosomal dominant STAT3 deficiency and hyper-IgE syndrome: molecular, cellular, and clinical features from a French national survey. *Medicine (Baltimore)*. 2012;91:e1-e19.
94. Chamlin SL, McCalmont TH, Cunningham BB, et al. Cutaneous manifestations of hyper-IgE syndrome in infants and children. *J Pediatr*. 2002;141:572-575.
95. Eberting CL, Davis J, Puck JM, et al. Dermatitis and the newborn rash of hyper-IgE syndrome. *Arch Dermatol*. 2004;140:1119-1125.
96. Grimbacher B, Holland SM, Puck JM. Hyper-IgE syndromes. *Immunol Rev*. 2005;203:244.
97. Esposito L, Poletti L, Maspero C, et al. Hyper-IgE syndrome: dental implications. *Oral Surg Oral Med Oral Pathol Oral Radiol*. 2012;114(2):147-153.
98. Sowerwine KJ, Shaw PA, Gu W, et al. Bone density and fractures in autosomal dominant hyper IgE syndrome. *J Clin Immunol*. 2014;34(2):260-264.
99. Scheuerman O, Hoffer V, Cohen AH, et al. Reduced bone density in patients with autosomal dominant hyper-IgE syndrome. *J Clin Immunol*. 2013;33(5):903-908.
100. Hsu AP, Sowerwine KJ, Lawrence MG, et al. Intermediate phenotypes in patients with autosomal dominant hyper-IgE syndrome caused by somatic mosaicism. *J Allergy Clin Immunol*. 2013;131(6):1586-1593.
101. Renner ED, Puck JM, Holland SM, et al. Autosomal recessive hyperimmunoglobulin E syndrome: A distinct disease entity. *J Pediatr*. 2004;144(1):93-99.
102. Zhang Q, Davis JC, Lamborn IT, et al. Combined immunodeficiency associated with DOCK8 mutations. *N Engl J Med*. 2009;361:2046-2055.
103. Engelhardt KR, Gertz ME, Keles S, et al. The extended clinical phenotype of 64 patients with dedicator of cytokinesis 8 deficiency. *J Allergy Clin Immunol*. 2015;136:402-412.
104. Aydin SE, Kilic SS, Aytekin C, et al. DOCK8 deficiency: clinical and immunological phenotype and treatment options—a review of 136 patients. *J Clin Immunol*. 2015;35(2):189-198.
105. Chu EY, Freeman AF, Jing H, et al. Cutaneous manifestations of DOCK8 deficiency syndrome. *Arch Dermatol*. 2012;148:79-84.
106. Boos AC, Hagl B, Schlesinger A, et al. Atopic der-

matitis, STAT3- and DOCK8-hyper-IgE syndromes differ in IgE-based sensitization pattern. *Allergy*. 2014;69:943-953.
107. Alsum Z, Hawwari A, Alsmadi O, et al. Clinical, immunological and molecular characterization of DOCK8 and DOCK8-like deficient patients: single center experience of twenty-five patients. *J Clin Immunol*. 2013;33:55-67.
108. Minegishi Y, Saito M, Tsuchiya S, et al. Dominant-negative mutations in the DNA-binding domain of STAT3 cause hyper-IgE syndrome. *Nature*. 2007;448(7157):1058-1062.
109. Holland SM, DeLeo FR, Elloumi HZ, et al. STAT3 mutations in the hyper-IgE syndrome. *N Engl J Med*. 2007;357(16):1608-1619.
110. Renner ED, Rylaarsdam S, Anover-Sombke S, et al. Novel signal transducer and activator of transcription 3 (STAT3) mutations, reduced T(H)17 cell numbers, and variably defective STAT3 phosphorylation in hyper-IgE syndrome. *J Allergy Clin Immunol*. 2008;122(1):181-187.
111. Minegishi Y, Saito M, Morio T, et al. Human tyrosine kinase 2 deficiency reveals its requisite roles in multiple cytokine signals involved in innate and acquired immunity. *Immunity*. 2006;25:745-755.
112. Sassi A, Lazaroski S, Wu G, et al. Hypomorphic homozygous mutations in phosphoglucomutase 3 (PGM3) impair immunity and increase serum IgE levels. *J Allergy Clin Immunol*. 2014;133:1410-1419.
113. Zhang Y, Yu X, Ichikawa M, et al. Autosomal recessive phosphoglucomutase 3 (PGM3) mutations link glycosylation defects to atopy, immune deficiency, autoimmunity, and neurocognitive impairment. *J Allergy Clin Immunol*. 2014;133:1400-1409.
114. Yang L, Fliegauf M, Grimbacher B, et al. Hyper-IgE syndromes: reviewing PGM3 deficiency. *Curr Opin Pediatr*. 2014;26:697-703.
115. Woellner C, Gertz EM, Schäffer AA, et al. Mutations in STAT3 and diagnostic guidelines for hyper-IgE syndrome. *J Allergy Clin Immunol*. 2010;125:424-432.
116. Boos AC, Hagl B, Schlesinger A, et al. Atopic dermatitis, STAT3- and DOCK8-hyper-IgE syndromes differ in IgE-based sensitization pattern. *Allergy*. 2014;69:943-953.
117. Pai SY, de Boer H, Massaad MJ, et al. Flow cytometry diagnosis of dedicator of cytokinesis 8 (DOCK8) deficiency. *J Allergy Clin Immunol*. 2014;134(1):221-223.
118. Joshi AY, Iyer VN, Boyce TG, et al. Elevated serum immunoglobulin E (IgE): when to suspect hyper-IgE syndrome: a 10-year pediatric tertiary care center experience. *Allergy Asthma Proc*. 2009;30:23-27.
119. Bard S, Paravisini A, Avilés-Izquierdo JA, et al. Eczematous dermatitis in the setting of hyper-IgE syndrome successfully treated with omalizumab. *Arch Dermatol*. 2008;144:1662-1663.
120. Al-Zahrani D, Raddadi A, Massaad M, et al. Successful interferon-alpha 2b therapy for unremitting warts in a patient with DOCK8 deficiency. *Clin Immunol*. 2014;153:104-108.
121. Keles S, Jabara HH, Reisli I, et al. Plasmacytoid dendritic cell depletion in DOCK8 deficiency: rescue of severe herpetic infections with IFN-alpha 2b therapy. *J Allergy Clin Immunol*. 2014;133:1753-1755.e3.
122. Papan C, Hagl B, Heinz V, et al. Beneficial IFN-alpha treatment of tumorous herpes simplex blepharoconjunctivitis in dedicator of cytokinesis 8 deficiency. *J Allergy Clin Immunol*. 2014;133:1456-1458.
123. Cuellar-Rodriguez J, Freeman AF, Grossman J, et al. Matched related and unrelated donor hematopoietic stem cell transplantation for DOCK8 deficiency. *Biol Blood Marrow Transplant*. 2015;21:1037-1045.
124. Gatz SA, Benninghoff U, Schutz C, et al. Curative treatment of autosomal-recessive hyper-IgE syndrome by hematopoietic cell transplantation. *Bone Marrow Transplant*. 2011;46:552-556.
125. Boztug H, Karitnig-Weiss C, Ausserer B, et al. Clinical and immunological correction of DOCK8 deficiency by allogeneic hematopoietic stem cell transplantation following a reduced toxicity conditioning regimen. *Pediatr Hematol Oncol*. 2012;29:585-594.
126. Patel NC, Gallagher JL, Torgerson TR, et al. Successful haploidentical donor hematopoietic stem cell transplant and restoration of STAT3 function in an adolescent with autosomal dominant hyper-IgE syndrome. *J Clin Immunol*. 2015;35:479-485.
127. Wolach B, Eliakim A, Pomeranz A, et al. Cyclosporin treatment of hyperimmunoglobulin E syndrome. *Lancet*. 1996;347(8993):67.
128. Al Ustwani O, Kurzrock R, Wetzler M. Genetics on a WHIM. *Br J Haematol*. 2014;164(1):15-23.
129. McDermott DH, Liu Q, Velez D, et al. A phase 1 clinical trial of long-term, low-dose treatment of WHIM syndrome with the CXCR4 antagonist plerixafor. *Blood*. 2014;123(15):2308-2316.
130. Nagai K, Ochi F, Terui K, et al. Clinical characteristics and outcomes of Chédiak-Higashi syndrome: a nationwide survey of Japan. *Pediatr Blood Cancer*. 2013;60(10):1582-1586.
131. Introne WJ, Westbroek W, Golas GA, et al. Chediak-Higashi syndrome. In: Adam MP, Ardinger HH, Pagon RA, et al., eds. *GeneReviews* [Internet]. Seattle, WA: University of Washington; 1993-2018. 2009 [updated January 15, 2015]. https://www.ncbi.nlm.nih.gov/books/NBK5188/.
132. Anderson LL, Paller AS, Malpass D, et al. Chediak-Higashi syndrome in a black child. *Pediatr Dermatol*. 1992;9:31-36.
133. Al-Khenaizan S. Hyperpigmentation in Chediak-Higashi syndrome. *J Am Acad Dermatol*. 2003;49:S244-S246.
134. Raghuveer C, Murthy SC, Mithuna MN, et al. Silvery hair with speckled dyspigmentation: Chediak-Higashi syndrome in three Indian siblings. *Int J Trichology*. 2015;7:133-135.
135. Huizing M, Helip-Wooley A, Westbroek W, et al. Disorders of lysosome-related organelle biogenesis: Clinical and molecular genetics. *Annu Rev Genomics Hum Genet*. 2008;9:359-386.
136. Galve J, Martín-Santiago A, Clavero C, et al. Spontaneous repigmentation of silvery hair in an infant with congenital hydrops fetalis and hypoproteinemia. *Cutis*. 2016;97:E1-E5.
137. Vargas MT, Escamilla V, Morales-Camacho RM, et al. Multiple pseudo-Chediak-Higashi inclusions associated with MYC deletion in a patient with acute myeloid leukemia. *Acta Haematol*. 2015;133(4):321-323.
138. Cetica V, Sieni E, Pende D, et al. Genetic predisposition to hemophagocytic lymphohistiocytosis: report on 500 patients from the Italian registry. *J Allergy Clin Immunol*. 2016;137(1):188-196.
139. Degar B. Familial hemophagocytic lymphohistiocytosis. *Hematol Oncol Clin North Am*. 2015;29(5):903-913.
140. Giri PP, Biswas N, Chakravarty S. Familial hemophagocytic lymphohistiocytosis due to mutation

of UNC13D gene. *Indian J Hematol Blood Transfus.* 2016;32(suppl 1):344-346.
141. Straus SE, Jaffe ES, Puck JM, et al. The development of lymphomas in families with autoimmune lymphoproliferative syndrome with germline Fas mutations and defective lymphocyte apoptosis. *Blood.* 2001;98(1):194-200.
142. George LA, Teachey DT. Optimal management of autoimmune lymphoproliferative syndrome in children. *Paediatr Drugs.* 2016;18(4):261-272.
143. Sharfe N, Dadi HK, Shahar M, et al. Human immune disorder arising from mutation of the alpha chain of the interleukin-2 receptor. *Proc Natl Acad Sci U S A.* 1997;94(7):3168-3171.
144. Maaloul I, Talmoudi J, Chabchoub I, et al. Chediak-Higashi syndrome presenting in accelerated phase: a case report and literature review. *Hematol Oncol Stem Cell Ther.* 2016;9(2):71-75.
145. Umeda K, Adachi S, Horikoshi Y, et al. Allogeneic hematopoietic stem cell transplantation for Chediak-Higashi syndrome. *Pediatr Transplant.* 2016;20:271-275.
146. Hamidieh AA, Pourpak Z, Yari K, et al. Hematopoietic stem cell transplantation with a reduced-intensity conditioning regimen in pediatric patients with Griscelli syndrome type 2. *Pediatr Transplant.* 2013;17:487-491.
147. Trottestam H, Beutel K, Meeths M, et al. Treatment of the X-linked lymphoproliferative, Griscelli and Chédiak-Higashi syndromes by HLH directed therapy. *Pediatr Blood Cancer.* 2009;52:268-272.
148. Lozano ML, Rivera J, Sánchez-Guiu I, et al. Towards the targeted management of Chediak-Higashi syndrome. *Orphanet J Rare Dis.* 2014;9:132.
149. Westbroek W, Klar A, Cullinane AR, et al. Cellular and clinical report of new Griscelli syndrome type III cases. *Pigment Cell Melanoma Res.* 2012;25:47-56.
150. Nouriel A, Zisquit J, Helfand AM, et al. Griscelli syndrome type 3: two new cases and review of the literature. *Pediatr Dermatol.* 2015;32:e245-e248.
151. Ménasché G, Ho CH, Sanal O, et al. Griscelli syndrome restricted to hypopigmentation results from a melanophilin defect (GS3) or a MYO5A F-exon deletion (GS1). *J Clin Invest.* 2003;112(3):450-456.
152. Cicardi M, Aberer W, Banerji A, et al. Classification, diagnosis, and approach to treatment for angioedema: consensus report from the Hereditary Angioedema International Working Group. *Allergy.* 2014;69(5):602-616.
153. Bork K, Gül D, Dewald G. Hereditary angio-oedema with normal C1 inhibitor in a family with affected women and men. *Br J Dermatol.* 2006;154(3):542-545.
154. Verpy E, Biasotto M, Brai M, et al. Exhaustive mutation scanning by fluorescence-assisted mismatch analysis discloses new genotype-phenotype correlations in angioedema. *Am J Hum Genet.* 1996;59(2):308-319.

Chapter 133 :: Skin Manifestations of Internal Organ Disorders
:: Amy K. Forrestel & Robert G. Micheletti

第一百三十三章

内脏疾病的皮肤表现

中文导读

皮肤表现与患者的整体健康有关。本章重点关注心血管、肺、肝、胃肠道和肾脏疾病的皮肤表现。

首先心血管系统疾病可出现的皮肤改变包括耳垂弗兰克征、银屑病、遗传性结缔组织病、自身免疫性结缔组织病及红皮病等。

呼吸系统疾病的一般皮肤表现包括发绀和杵状指。此外,结节病、抗中性粒细胞抗体相关性小血管炎、自身免疫性结缔组织病、黄甲综合征、水源性掌跖角皮病、呼吸道的感染性疾病等都与呼吸系统及皮肤改变有关。

肝脏疾病中肝豆状核变性、病毒性肝炎和原发性胆汁性肝硬化等可能会有特征性的皮肤变化或与某些皮肤病相关。可能出现血管病变(包括毛细血管扩张、蜘蛛痣和手掌红斑等)、指甲改变、黄疸、色素变化、淤胆性瘙痒症及激素引起的皮肤变化等。

胃肠系统中同时影响皮肤的疾病有消化道出血、吸收不良/腹泻和腹痛。消化道出血可合并小血管炎、免疫球蛋白A血管炎、结节性多动脉炎和Behcet综合征等。吸收不良的皮肤可表现为干燥症、湿疹性皮炎、唇炎、脱发或毛发质地改变、指甲改变和色素沉着。食管受累的常见皮肤病因包括水疱性皮肤病(大疱性表皮松解症、瘢痕性类天疱疮)、扁平苔藓、风湿病(Behcet综合征,SSC)、中毒性表皮坏死松解症、Darier病和念珠菌、单纯疱疹病毒感染。并特别提到了疱疹样皮炎、炎症性肠病、息肉病综合征等。

肾脏疾病患者出现各种与代谢异常相关的皮肤表现,包括贫血、钙磷调节失调和糖耐量减低。皮肤表现包括面色发黄、瘙痒、干燥、获得性穿孔性皮肤病、假性卟啉症、钙缺乏和尿毒症。

甲状腺疾病的皮肤改变在表133-7中进行了概述。

〔粟 娟〕

Frequently, cutaneous findings are relevant to the overall health of a patient. Even though some findings on the skin are the result of multisystem disease processes that affect the whole organism, primary skin diseases may also impact other organs and overall health, particularly when severe or longstanding.

A comprehensive chapter on cutaneous manifestations of systemic disease could encompass much of dermatology. This chapter's goal is to provide general information and principles, highlight key diseases that may not be discussed elsewhere, and group disorders into quick-reference charts organized by organ system. This chapter specifically focuses on cutaneous manifestations of cardiovascular, pulmonary, hepatic, GI, and renal disease.

CARDIOVASCULAR SYSTEM

Disturbances in the cardiovascular system causing decreased cardiac output can produce marked skin changes. Cyanosis is a purple-blue discoloration of the skin caused by an increase in the absolute amount of desaturated hemoglobin. It can be classified as "central," in which low arterial oxygen saturation is caused by lung disease or shunt physiology, or "peripheral," in which arterial oxygen saturation is normal but flow is reduced because of low-output cardiac failure or vasoconstriction. Central cyanosis is usually visible in warm areas of the skin, like the tongue, oral mucosa, and conjunctivae. Peripheral cyanosis is seen in cooler areas such as the nose, lips, earlobes, and fingertips.

In the acute setting (shock), the extremities can become cool and clammy with associated peripheral cyanosis, livedo, and mottling. If severe, this can progress into gangrene of the digits. Vasopressor medications used to support the blood pressure can exacerbate this problem by causing peripheral vasoconstriction. Chronic poor peripheral blood flow from heart failure or peripheral vascular disease can produce chronic edema, venous stasis, decreased hair, and ulceration of the lower legs.

Nail changes associated with cardiovascular disease include clubbing and the Quincke pulsation, which is flushing of the nail beds synchronous with the heartbeat, indicative of aortic regurgitation.

SELECT CONDITIONS

Table 133-1 outlines select conditions with cardiovascular and cutaneous manifestations.

ENDOCARDITIS

Cutaneous signs of endocarditis include Osler nodes, Janeway lesions, subungual splinter hemorrhages, purpura, and petechiae. Osler nodes and Janeway lesions may both present as erythematous or hemorrhagic macules, papules, or nodules. Whereas Osler nodes result from immune complex deposition and are painful, tender, and located distally on the digital tufts, Janeway lesions are nontender and located proximally on the palms and soles. Histologically, Osler nodes are a perivasculitis or necrotizing vasculitis *without* microabscess formation, whereas Janeway lesions exhibit vasculitis *with* microabscess formation. Both also may be found in patients with other conditions, namely systemic lupus erythematosus, gonococcemia, hemolytic anemia, and typhoid fever.

EARLOBE CREASE

The cutaneous finding of a diagonal earlobe crease (Frank sign) has been (controversially) associated with an increased risk of coronary artery disease. The finding is more common with older age and theorized to be a result of age-related loss of dermal and vascular elastic fibers.[1]

PSORIASIS

Psoriasis is recognized as a multisystem inflammatory disease associated with a number of important comorbidities. These include metabolic syndrome, obesity, nonalcoholic fatty liver disease, Type 2 diabetes mellitus, and cardiovascular disease (including increased myocardial infarction, stroke, and peripheral vascular disease).[2] Investigation into the impact of psoriasis treatment on these comorbid conditions is ongoing, but there have been reports of decreased rates of myocardial infarction after treatment with tumor necrosis factor inhibitors and methotrexate.[3]

INHERITED CONNECTIVE TISSUE DISEASE

Mutations causing defects in the structure and function of connective tissue (eg, collagen, elastic fibers) can lead to significant cutaneous and cardiovascular pathology. Diseases in this category include Ehlers-Danlos syndrome, Marfan syndrome, cutis laxa, progeria, and pseudoxanthoma elasticum. Loss of the supportive tissue results in skin that is hyperelastic, fragile, lax, and heals poorly. Vessel walls are similarly weakened. Patients can have aneurysms, dissections, and rupture of major arteries, as well as valvular prolapse and insufficiency. Progeria and progeroid conditions (such as Werner syndrome) have atrophic, tight skin with signs of premature aging like gray hair, accelerated atherosclerosis, and myocardial infarction.

AUTOIMMUNE CONNECTIVE TISSUE DISEASE

Systemic Lupus Erythematosus: Systemic lupus erythematosus (SLE) can affect all aspects of the heart and pericardium. Pericarditis is the most

TABLE 133-1
Conditions with Cardiovascular and Cutaneous Manifestations

DISEASE	CARDIAC FINDINGS	CUTANEOUS FINDINGS
Genetic		
Cardiofaciocutaneous syndrome	Structural heart defects, hypertrophic CMO	Ichthyosis, keratosis pilaris, sparse curly hair, coarse facies
Costello syndrome	Arrhythmias, structural heart defects, hypertrophic CMO	Loose skin, large mouth, acanthosis nigricans, periorificial papillomas
Carvajal syndrome	Dilated left ventricular CMO	Woolly hair, palmoplantar keratoderma
Cutis laxa	Aortic dilation and rupture, pulmonary artery stenosis, right-sided heart failure	Loose skin
Ehlers-Danlos syndrome	Aortic dilation and dissection, MV prolapse	Skin hyperelastic and fragile, delayed wound healing, atrophic scars
Fabry disease	Hypertrophic CMO, atherosclerosis, conduction abnormalities	Angiokeratoma corporis diffusum
Hemochromatosis	Dilated CMO, electrical disturbances	Diffuse skin hyperpigmentation
Homocystinuria	MV and TV prolapse, atherosclerosis	Livedo reticularis, malar rash, diffuse hypopigmentation, tissue-paper scars
LEOPARD syndrome	Conduction abnormalities, PV stenosis, hypertrophic CMO	Lentigines, café-au-lait macules
Marfan syndrome	Aortic dilation and dissection, MV and TV prolapse and regurgitation	Striae, arachnodactyly, elastosis perforans serpiginosa
Naxos disease	Dilated left ventricular CMO	Palmoplantar striate keratoderma, woolly scalp hair
NAME/LAMB/Carney complex	Atrial myxoma	Lentigines, coarse facies, blue nevi, cutaneous myxomas
Noonan syndrome	PV stenosis, hypertrophic CMO	Webbed neck, keratosis pilaris atrophicans, keloids, lymphedema
Progeria	Accelerated atherosclerosis	Graying and loss of hair; thin, hardened skin; mottled hyperpigmentation
Pseudoxanthoma elasticum	Accelerated atherosclerosis, MI, renovascular hypertension	Yellow papules and plaques, lax skin
Tuberous sclerosis	Cardiac rhabdomyomas, arrhythmias	Facial angiofibromas, periungual fibromas, ash-leaf macules, shagreen patch
Werner syndrome	Accelerated atherosclerosis	Graying and loss of hair; thin, hardened skin; ankle ulcerations
Neoplastic/Paraneoplastic		
Atrial myxoma	CHF, mitral regurgitation, constrictive pericarditis, arrhythmia	Embolic phenomena, peripheral cyanosis
Multicentric reticulohistiocytosis	Pericarditis, myocarditis, cardiomegaly, CHF	Erythematous nodules of the hands, extremities
Infectious		
Trichinosis	Eosinophilic infiltrate causing myocarditis, arrhythmias	Periorbital edema, splinter hemorrhages
Autoimmune/Rheumatologic		
Behçet syndrome	Pancarditis, coronary arteritis/aneurysm, arrhythmias, valvulopathy, thrombosis	Oral and genital ulcers, pustular eruptions, pyoderma gangrenosum-like lesions
Dermatomyositis	Myocarditis, conduction abnormalities, CHF. Increased risk of MI	Gottron papules, heliotrope rash, shawl sign, mechanic's hands
Polyarteritis nodosa	Coronary artery involvement, MI	Palpable purpura, livedo racemosa, subcutaneous nodules, ulcerations
Reactive arthritis	Valvulopathy, pericarditis	Keratoderma blenorrhagicum
Relapsing polychondritis	Valvulopathy, aneurysm, pericarditis, heart block, coronary arteritis	Red, edematous ears (sparing ear lobes), nasal tip
Rheumatoid arthritis	Pericarditis, myocarditis. Increased risk of CAD, CHF, atrial fibrillation	Rheumatoid nodules, ulcers, neutrophilic dermatosis
Rheumatic fever	Acute: pancarditis; Late: valvulopathy	Erythema marginatum, subcutaneous nodules

(Continued)

TABLE 133-1
Conditions with Cardiovascular and Cutaneous Manifestations (Continued)

DISEASE	CARDIAC FINDINGS	CUTANEOUS FINDINGS
Systemic lupus erythematosus	Pericarditis, myocarditis, conduction abnormalities, valvulopathy (Libman-Sacks), complete heart block (neonatal)	Malar rash, photosensitivity, oral ulcers, discoid, subacute, and other skin lesions
Systemic sclerosis	Pericarditis, myocarditis arrhythmias, pulmonary artery hypertension	Raynaud phenomenon, sclerosis, dyspigmentation, microstomia
Inflammatory		
DRESS	Eosinophilic myocarditis, pericarditis, conduction abnormalities	Diffuse morbilliform eruption with facial erythema and edema
Psoriasis	Increased cardiovascular disease, atherosclerosis	Well-demarcated erythematous plaques with micaceous scale
Kawasaki	Coronary artery aneurysm	Polymorphous exanthema, desquamation of palms and soles, lips
Erythroderma	Risk for high-output cardiac failure	Diffuse exfoliative erythema
Other		
Amyloidosis	CHF, conduction abnormalities, syncope, sudden death, restrictive CMO	Purpura, periorbital ecchymosis, waxy papules and plaques
Cholesterol emboli	Atherosclerotic vessels; embolization of cholesterol crystals	Livedo reticularis, ulcers, digital cyanosis
Erythromelalgia	Atherosclerosis, hypertension	Recurrent episodes of burning pain, erythema, and warmth in hands/feet
PHACES syndrome	Aortic coarctation, aortic arch abnormalities, structural abnormalities	Segmental infantile hemangioma
Sarcoidosis	Conduction abnormalities, arrhythmias, CMO, CHF, sudden cardiac death	Papules, nodules, plaques—predilection for scars and tattoos

CAD, coronary artery disease; CHF, congestive heart failure; CMO, cardiomyopathy; DRESS, drug rash with eosinophilia and systemic symptoms; LAMB, lentigines, atrial myxoma, mucocutaneous myxoma, and blue nevi; LEOPARD, lentigines, electrocardiographic abnormalities, ocular hypertelorism, pulmonary stenosis, abnormalities of genitalia, retardation of growth, and deafness; MI, myocardial infarction; MV, mitral valve; NAME, nevi, atrial myxoma, myxoid neurofibromas, and ephelides; PHACES, posterior fossa malformations, facial hemangiomas, arterial anomalies, cardiac anomalies and aortic coarctation, eye anomalies, and sternal clefting and/or supraumbilical raphe; PV, pulmonic valve; TV, tricuspid valve.

common manifestation, occurring in approximately 25% of patients during the course of their disease.[4] Pericarditis may be more common in patients with drug-induced lupus or photosensitive discoid lesions. Myocarditis is uncommon but can cause severe cardiomyopathy and arrhythmias. In Libman-Sacks endocarditis, deposits of immune complexes, fibrin, platelet thrombi, and mononuclear cells can build up on heart valves. This condition can cause significant mitral or aortic insufficiency as well as serve as a source of emboli resulting in purpuric macules at acral sites. It is often associated with the presence of antiphospholipid antibodies.[5] Patients with SLE also have an increased risk of coronary artery disease. Neonatal lupus occurs from transplacental transfer of maternal antibodies (most often anti-Ro/SSA).[6] It can cause an annular rash similar to subacute cutaneous lupus and, in some newborns, complete heart block.

Systemic Sclerosis: Pericarditis is common in systemic sclerosis (SSc) and may result in effusions and tamponade with significant associated morbidity. Small vessel disease of the myocardium causing patchy fibrosis is a hallmark of SSc and can cause systolic or diastolic heart failure as well as arrhythmias and sudden death.[7] Patients are also at increased risk of myocardial infarction.

ERYTHRODERMA

As a consequence of extensive peripheral vasodilation, erythrodermic patients, particularly those with preexisting cardiomyopathy, are at risk for high-output cardiac failure with secondary end-organ damage, such as liver and renal insufficiency.

PULMONARY SYSTEM

General cutaneous findings in pulmonary disease include cyanosis and clubbing. Digital clubbing is characterized by increased distal fingertip mass and longitudinal and transverse nail plate curvature. The Lovibond angle (ie, the angle between the nail plate and the proximal nailfold) is greater than 180 degrees in clubbed nails and typically less than 160 degrees in normal nails. Although digital clubbing can be hereditary, it is much more frequently seen in association with pulmonary or cardiovascular diseases, including lung cancer, interstitial pulmonary fibrosis, pulmonary tuberculosis, congestive heart failure, and cyanotic congenital heart disease. It occurs less frequently in extrathoracic disease such as inflammatory bowel disease and cirrhosis.

SELECT CONDITIONS

Table 133-2 outlines select conditions with pulmonary and cutaneous manifestations.

SARCOIDOSIS

Sarcoidosis is a multisystem granulomatous disease of unknown etiology most commonly affecting the respiratory tract (90%), skin (25%), and eyes. The skin manifestations are protean and consist of noncaseating granulomas that classically appear as smooth papules, plaques, or nodules, but can be psoriasiform, ulcerative, verrucous, or photodistributed. Lesions frequently appear around the mouth and nose and form within scars and tattoos. Many other nonspecific cutaneous findings can occur, including ichthyosis, erythema nodosum, and alopecia. Bilateral hilar adenopathy is the most common intrathoracic manifestation, but patients can develop severe parenchymal disease. Patients are often asymptomatic but may have dyspnea, chronic nonproductive cough, or severe respiratory failure.[8] Lupus pernio and angiolupoid sarcoidosis (extensive telangiectatic lesions) are often associated with chronic sarcoidosis and persistent pulmonary involvement. Additionally, patients with a high burden of lesions around the nose have higher rates of pulmonary fibrosis and sarcoidosis involving the upper respiratory tract.[9]

ANTINEUTROPHILIC CYTOPLASMIC ANTIBODY–ASSOCIATED VASCULITIS

The antineutrophilic cytoplasmic antibody–associated vasculitides are characterized by pauci-immune necrotizing vasculitis of small to medium-sized vessels, which can affect multiple organs, including the lungs and skin.

Granulomatosis with polyangiitis (formerly Wegener granulomatosis) classically presents with granulomatous inflammation of the upper and lower respiratory tract resulting in rhinorrhea, sinusitis, epistaxis, nasal septal perforation, dyspnea, cough, and hemoptysis. Chest imaging shows irregular infiltrates and nodules. Skin findings include palpable purpura, oral ulcers, friable gingiva, pyoderma gangrenosum-like lesions, and papulonecrotic lesions on the extensor surfaces. In eosinophilic granulomatosis with polyangiitis (formerly Churg-Strauss syndrome), allergic rhinitis, nasal polyps, and asthma are followed by eosinophilic granulomatous infiltration with pulmonary infiltrates, pleural effusion, and nodules. Skin findings include palpable purpura, livedo reticularis, and urticarial lesions. Pulmonary involvement in microscopic polyangiitis, including dyspnea and pulmonary infiltrates without significant upper airway involvement, is the result of vasculitis without granulomatous inflammation. Skin findings include purpura, erythematous patches, livedo reticularis, urticarial papules, and ulcers.

TABLE 133-2
Conditions with Pulmonary and Cutaneous Manifestations

DISEASE	PULMONARY FINDINGS	CUTANEOUS FINDINGS
Genetic		
Birt-Hogg-Dube syndrome	Lung cysts, spontaneous pneumothorax	Fibrofolliculomas, trichodiscomas, acrochordons
Hereditary hemorrhagic telangiectasia	Pulmonary vascular malformations, pulmonary hypertension	Mucosal, facial, and acral mat telangiectasias
Lipoid proteinosis	Weak cry or hoarseness from infiltration of laryngeal mucosa	Beaded papules on eyelid margin; verrucous keratotic plaques on the elbows, knees, hands
Marfan syndrome	Emphysematous changes, spontaneous pneumothorax	Striae, decreased subcutaneous fat, arachnodactyly, elastosis perforans serpiginosa
Yellow nail syndrome	Sinusitis, bronchiectasis, pleural effusions, respiratory tract infections	Nails thick, yellow/green color, increased curvature, onycholysis, absent lunulae
Neoplastic/Paraneoplastic		
Kaposi sarcoma	Asymptomatic or cough, hemoptysis; more common in AIDS-associated KS	Red/purple macules, papules, plaques, or nodules on skin and mucosa
Lymphomatoid granulomatosis	Pulmonary infiltrates, cavitary nodules, hemoptysis	Morbilliform exanthem, erythema, nodules, ulcers
Paraneoplastic pemphigus	Bronchiolitis obliterans	Mucocutaneous erosions and ulcerations
Multicentric reticulohistiocytosis	Pleural effusions, infiltrates	Erythematous nodules on hands, extremities

(Continued)

TABLE 133-2
Conditions with Pulmonary and Cutaneous Manifestations (Continued)

DISEASE	PULMONARY FINDINGS	CUTANEOUS FINDINGS
Infectious		
Invasive aspergillosis	Nodules, patchy infiltrates; cough, hemoptysis	Necrotic violaceous papules and plaques
Blastomycosis	Asymptomatic vs chronic > acute pneumonia. ARDS rare	Papulopustules and verrucous, crusted plaques
Cryptococcosis	Range from asymptomatic infection to severe pneumonia and ARDS	Protean; umbilicated or acneiform papules, nodules, plaques, ulceration
Larva migrans	Rare; persistent dry cough; eosinophilic, migratory infiltrates	Erythematous papule at site of larva penetration, serpiginous migratory tracks
Strongyloidiasis	Dry cough, dyspnea, wheezing, hemoptysis, ARDS	Ground itch at site of contact, urticarial eruption, periumbilical purpura
Tuberculosis	Hilar lymphadenopathy, nodules, cavitary lesions with cough, hemoptysis	Lupus vulgaris, scrofuloderma, orificial TB, miliary TB, tuberculids
Varicella	Pneumonia with patchy infiltrates, tachypnea, dry cough, hemoptysis	Papulovesicles, pustules, hemorrhagic crusts at different stages of development
Autoimmune/Rheumatologic		
Behçet syndrome	Pulmonary vascular lesions, infarction, hemoptysis, pleural effusions	Oral/genital ulcers, pustular eruptions, pyoderma gangrenosum-like lesions
Eosinophilic granulomatosis with polyangiitis (Churg-Strauss syndrome)	Allergic rhinitis, nasal polyps, asthma; later patchy infiltrates, nodules, pleural effusions	Palpable purpura, urticarial lesions, livedo reticularis, nonspecific dermatitis
Dermatomyositis	Interstitial lung disease	Gottron papules, heliotrope rash, shawl sign, mechanic's hands
Granulomatosis with polyangiitis (Wegener syndrome)	Sinusitis, epistaxis, nasal septal perforation, cough, hemoptysis	Palpable purpura, friable gingiva, ulcers, papulonecrotic lesions
Microscopic polyangiitis	Capillaritis, pulmonary infiltrates; no upper airway involvement	Palpable purpura, livedo reticularis, ulcers
Relapsing polychondritis	Hoarseness, structural insufficiency and airway collapse	Red, edematous ears (sparing ear lobes), nasal tip
Rheumatoid arthritis	ILD, rheumatoid nodules, bronchiolitis obliterans	Rheumatoid nodules, palpable purpura, ulcers, neutrophilic dermatoses
Systemic lupus erythematosus	Pleuritis, pneumonitis, diffuse alveolar hemorrhage, pulmonary hypertension	Malar rash, photosensitivity, oral ulcers, discoid, subacute, and other skin lesions
Systemic sclerosis	ILD, pulmonary hypertension	Raynaud phenomenon, sclerosis, dyspigmentation, microstomia
Urticarial vasculitis	Cough, dyspnea, hemoptysis, COPD, pleuritis, pleural effusions	Urticarial papules and plaques, often with purpuric component
Inflammatory		
Drug reaction with eosinophilia and systemic symptoms	Interstitial pneumonitis, pleural effusions	Diffuse morbilliform eruption with facial erythema and edema
Sweet syndrome	Neutrophilic alveolitis, pleural effusions, ARDS	Pink-purple edematous papules, nodules, plaques; pathergy
Other		
Amyloidosis	Pleural effusions, hoarseness, airway obstruction	Purpura, periorbital ecchymosis, waxy papules and plaques
Graft-versus-host disease	Bronchiolitis obliterans	*Acute:* morbilliform exanthem; *Chronic:* poikiloderma, lichen planus-like, scleroderma-like
Sarcoidosis	Hilar lymphadenopathy, parenchymal opacities. Cough, dyspnea, chest pain	Papules, nodules, plaques–predilection for scars and tattoos
Fat embolism syndrome	Hypoxemia, dyspnea	Petechial rash

ARDS, acute respiratory distress syndrome; COPD, chronic obstructive pulmonary disease; ILD, interstitial lung disease; KS, Kaposi sarcoma; TB, tuberculosis.

AUTOIMMUNE CONNECTIVE TISSUE DISEASE

Rheumatoid Arthritis: Interstitial lung disease (ILD) is the most common pulmonary manifestation of rheumatoid arthritis and appears to correlate with high levels of rheumatoid factor.[10] Rheumatoid nodules in the lungs are often asymptomatic and occur more frequently in patients with concurrent subcutaneous nodules. Upper airway obstruction and bronchiolitis obliterans can also be seen.

Systemic Lupus Erythematosus: Pleuritis with or without pleural effusions occurs in half of patients with SLE. Primary lung involvement in SLE is varied and can include diffuse interstitial pneumonitis, acute pneumonitis, diffuse alveolar hemorrhage, diaphragm dysfunction with decreased lung volume, pulmonary hypertension with cor pulmonale, and fibrosing alveolitis.[11]

Systemic Sclerosis: Pulmonary involvement is seen in more than 70% of patients with SSc. The 2 main presentations are ILD and pulmonary arterial hypertension caused by pulmonary vascular disease, which can progress to cor pulmonale and right-sided heart failure. Symptoms usually consist of dyspnea on exertion and a nonproductive cough. There is also an increased risk of malignant lung neoplasms.

Dermatomyositis: ILD is seen in at least 10% of dermatomyositis cases, including both classic and amyopathic disease. Patients with antibodies to MDA-5 or to aminoacyl-transfer RNA synthetase enzymes such as Jo-1 have a much higher risk of ILD (up to 70%), and the disease in this context can be rapidly progressive and fatal.[12] Antisynthetase syndrome is a constellation of fever, myositis, inflammatory polyarthritis, ILD, Raynaud phenomenon, and mechanic's hands in a patient with anti–transfer RNA antibodies.

YELLOW NAIL SYNDROME

Yellow nail syndrome is an idiopathic phenomenon in which all 20 nails become thickened and yellow or yellow-green and overcurved. The cuticle disappears, and onycholysis and nail plate shedding are common. The nail abnormalities are associated with lymphedema and respiratory tract involvement, including pleural effusions, chronic bronchitis, bronchiectasis, and sinusitis.[13]

AQUAGENIC WRINKLING OF THE PALMS

Aquagenic wrinkling of the palms, also known as aquagenic palmoplantar keratoderma, is a rare condition with transient formation of edematous, translucent papules and plaques on the palms and digital pads within minutes of water exposure. Aquagenic wrinkling of the palms is associated with cystic fibrosis. The mechanism is unknown, but it is hypothesized that increased tonicity of sweat and increased aquaporins in eccrine sweat glands in patients with cystic fibrosis cause an osmotic shift of water across the epidermis.[14,15]

INFECTIOUS DISEASES

Various infectious diseases that primarily affect the respiratory tract may present with characteristic cutaneous findings that can aid in diagnosis. These include tuberculosis, endemic mycoses (eg, coccidiomycosis, blastomycosis), and angioinvasive fungi (eg, aspergillosis, mucormycosis).

HEPATOBILIARY SYSTEM

The stigmata of hepatobiliary disease and cirrhosis are well recognized but nonspecific.[16] Diseases such as hemochromatosis, Wilson disease, viral hepatitis, and primary biliary cirrhosis can have characteristic skin changes or be associated with certain dermatologic disorders, as discussed below.

VASCULAR LESIONS

Vascular lesions are common and include telangiectasias, spider angiomas, and palmar erythema. Spider angiomas are so named because of their structure with a central arteriole from which several small, twisted vessels radiate. Pressure over the central arteriole causes blanching of the whole lesion. Size ranges from that of a pinhead to 2 cm. Lesions are predominately located on the face, neck, and upper chest. In alcoholic cirrhosis, they are associated with the presence of esophageal varicosities and may be a predictive marker of future risk of esophageal bleeding.[17] Spider angiomas are also seen in healthy children. Other telangiectasias can be confluent in sun-exposed areas, giving the impression of almost exanthematous redness. This is known as "dollar paper markings," after the small threads visible in paper money held up to the light. It is thought that vascular lesions are related to estrogen levels, as they can be associated with pregnancy, oral contraceptive pills, and men receiving estrogen therapy for prostate cancer. Portal hypertension causes development of porto-systemic collaterals, which appear as dilated abdominal wall veins (caput medusa).

NAIL CHANGES

In liver disease, nails can show a variety of changes such as clubbing, koilonychia (spoon shape), thickening, transverse white lines (Muehrcke nails), and brittleness. "Terry nails" are opaque and white except for a distal horizontal band that retains its normal pink color. Blue discoloration of the lunulae can be seen in Wilson disease. Koilonychia is associated with hemochromatosis as well as iron deficiency anemia.

JAUNDICE

Hyperbilirubinemia causes jaundice when bilirubin and its metabolites are bound by cells and connective tissue, producing a generalized yellow discoloration of the skin, mucous membranes, sclerae (ie, icterus), and other body tissues. This becomes evident when total serum bilirubin levels are above 3. Involvement of the sclerae differentiates jaundice from other causes of skin pigmentation, including carotenemia, quinacrine and busulfan dyspigmentation, and lycopenemia as a result of the ingestion of tomato juice. In addition to hepatobiliary disease, the hyperbilirubinemia may result from hemolysis, premature birth, and hereditary disorders such as Crigler-Najjar and Gilbert syndromes.

PIGMENTARY CHANGES

In addition to jaundice, liver disease is associated with other pigmentary changes. Patients with longstanding cirrhosis may develop guttate hypomelanosis or a diffuse muddy gray color.[18] In primary biliary cirrhosis (PBC), hyperpigmentation is common and can be generalized or in photodistributed areas, in linear palmar creases, or chloasma-like around the mouth and eyes. Accentuation of normal freckling and areolar pigmentation can also occur. In hemochromatosis, the skin can have a striking generalized metallic gray or bronze-brown color. There is accentuation in sun-exposed and traumatized skin, and occasionally there is buccal and conjunctival pigmentation.[19] The mechanism of hyperpigmentation varies. The pigmentation in PBC or longstanding cirrhosis is predominantly due to excess melanin with no stainable iron, whereas in hemochromatosis, both hemosiderin and excess melanin are present in the skin.

CHOLESTATIC PRURITUS

Pruritus can be severe and refractory in hepatobiliary disease. It is more common in primary biliary sclerosis, sclerosing cholangitis, and biliary obstruction compared to intrahepatic cholestasis. It is usually most severe on the extremities and only rarely involves the neck, face, and genitalia. Retained cutaneous bile acids are implicated, and bile salt-chelating resins typically provide some relief. However, there is poor correlation between plasma bilirubin and the severity of pruritus.

HORMONE-INDUCED SKIN CHANGES

Both sexes can experience striae distensae and loss of forearm, axillary, and pubic hair. Men may have a decreased rate of growth of facial hair, gynecomastia, and testicular atrophy.

OTHER SIGNS

Ascites may cause marked abdominal distension. Poor synthetic hepatic function causes hypoalbuminemia, which can result in edema and subsequent stasis dermatitis. Low fibrinogen and clotting factors, vitamin K deficiency, and decreased and dysfunctional platelets may result in purpura, epistaxis, and gingival bleeding.

SPECIFIC CONDITIONS

Table 133-3 outlines select conditions with hepatobiliary and cutaneous manifestations.

HEMOCHROMATOSIS

In hemochromatosis, a mutation in the *HFE* gene leads to increased intestinal iron absorption and subsequent iron overload. Iron deposition in the liver causes hepatomegaly, transaminitis, and eventual cirrhosis. There is an increased risk of hepatocellular carcinoma. Diffuse bronze hyperpigmentation is visible in approximately 70% of patients at presentation and is a result of both iron deposition and increased melanin.[20]

GRAFT-VERSUS-HOST DISEASE

Graft-versus-host disease (GVHD) is a common complication of allogeneic hematopoietic stem cell transplant when transplanted immune cells (the graft) recognize cells of the transplant recipient (the host) as foreign and initiate an immune response against host cells. The most commonly affected organs are the skin, liver, and GI tract. Liver disease usually occurs in patients with skin and gut involvement and is characterized by cholestatic injury. GVHD of the lower GI tract manifests with abdominal pain and diarrhea. Upper GI tract involvement can include xerostomia, mucositis, dysphagia, esophageal stricture, nausea, and vomiting. In the skin, acute GVHD most commonly presents with a nonspecific morbilliform eruption. In chronic GVHD, dermatologic findings are protean and include poikiloderma, lichen planus-like, and lichen sclerosis, morphea, or scleroderma-like lesions. The eyes and oral mucosa are commonly involved. GVHD severity staging includes serum bilirubin levels, quantity of diarrhea, and extent of skin involvement.

TABLE 133-3
Conditions with Hepatobiliary and Cutaneous Manifestations

DISEASE	HEPATOBILIARY FINDINGS	CUTANEOUS FINDINGS
Genetic		
Hereditary hemorrhagic telangiectasia	Vascular malformations, high-output heart failure, biliary disease	Mucosal, facial, and acral mat telangiectasias
Erythropoietic porphyria	Protoporphyric hepatopathy	Sun sensitivity (burning, erythema, papulovesicles), lichenification dorsal hands
Hemochromatosis	Hepatomegaly, fibrosis, cirrhosis, increased risk for hepatocellular carcinoma	Bronze hyperpigmentation
Hereditary coproporphyria	Hepatocellular injury	Similar to porphyria cutanea tarda
Porphyria cutanea tarda	Hepatocellular injury	Photosensitivity with bullae, fragility, dyspigmentation
Variegate porphyria	Hepatocellular injury, increased risk hepatocellular carcinoma	Fragility, bullae, milia
Neoplastic/Paraneoplastic		
Langerhans cell histiocytosis	Cystic lesions, hepatocellular injury, sclerosing cholangitis	Erythematous to brown papules, plaques and nodules with scale, crusting
Mastocytosis	Hepatomegaly, hepatocellular injury, mast cell infiltration	Red-brown papules (urticaria pigmentosa), diffuse telangiectatic (TMEP [telangiectasia macularis eruptiva perstans]), skin thickening (diffuse cutaneous)
Infectious		
Schistosomiasis	Periportal fibrosis, portal hypertension, normal hepatocellular function	Cercarial dermatitis, Katayama fever, granulomatous genital and perianal lesions
Syphilis	Syphilitic hepatitis	Papulosquamous eruption involving palmoplantar surfaces, chancre, alopecia
Toxocariasis	Hepatic granulomas, hepatomegaly	Urticaria, cutaneous nodules
Tuberculosis	Hepatocellular or cholestatic injury, hepatic granulomas	Lupus vulgaris, scrofuloderma, orificial TB (tuberculosis), miliary TB, tuberculids
Varicella	Immunocompromised hosts–hepatitis	Vesiculopapules
Autoimmune/Rheumatologic		
Primary biliary cirrhosis	Biliary duct destruction, fibrosis	Pruritus, hyperpigmentation, lichen planus
Systemic lupus erythematosus	Hepatitis, thrombosis caused by antiphospholipid antibodies (Budd-Chiari, hepatic venoocclusive disease)	Malar rash, photosensitivity, oral ulcers, discoid, subacute, and other skin lesions
Inflammatory		
DRESS (drug rash with eosinophilia and systemic symptoms)	Most common organ involved; hepatitis	Diffuse morbilliform eruption with facial erythema and edema
Graft-versus-host disease	Cholestatic injury	*Acute:* morbilliform exanthem; *Chronic:* poikiloderma, lichen planus-like, scleroderma-like
Kawasaki	Transaminitis	Polymorphous exanthema, edema or desquamation of palms/soles, lips
Other		
Sarcoidosis	Most asymptomatic; granulomatous infiltration; cirrhosis rare	Papules, nodules, plaques—predilection for scars and tattoos
Amyloidosis	Hepatomegaly, cirrhosis	Purpura, periorbital ecchymosis, waxy papules and plaques

WILSON DISEASE

Wilson disease is a hereditary condition in which defective cellular copper transport leads to accumulation of copper in several organs—most commonly the liver, brain, and cornea. Corneal deposition is visible in the form of Kayser-Fleischer rings, which are brown or gray-green rings that can be seen with slit-lamp examination or occasionally are grossly visible.

PRIMARY BILIARY CIRRHOSIS

PBC is an autoimmune disease associated with antimitochondrial antibodies typically affecting women 40 to 60 years of age in which intrahepatic bile ducts are destroyed, resulting in hyperbilirubinemia and cirrhosis. It is notable because of the constellation of pruritus, jaundice, diffuse hyperpigmentation, and xanthomas seen in the disease. The xanthomas are typically eruptive, planar, or occasionally tuberous. Pruritus is common and often severe, and it precedes the development of jaundice. Hyperpigmentation occurs in 25% to 50% of patients and is caused by melanin deposition.[16] Lichen planus has a well-recognized association with PBC and may occur in either the presence or absence of penicillamine. The skin lesions can resolve following liver transplantation.[21] Occasionally, PBC occurs in conjunction with limited SSc (CREST [calcinosis cutis, Raynaud phenomenon, esophageal motility disorder, sclerodactyly, and telangiectasia] syndrome), a phenotype that is referred to as Reynolds syndrome. Patients with PBC also have a higher incidence of anticentromere antibodies (especially the antiprotein C isotype) and Sjögren syndrome.[22]

HEPATITIS

In any of the viral hepatitides, acute infection may result in a transient morbilliform, urticarial, or petechial rash. Hepatitis B (HBV) and hepatitis C virus (HCV) infection have some overlapping and unique cutaneous features (Table 133-4). Both HBV and HCV are associated with cryoglobulinemia, although it is more common in HCV infection. Mixed cryoglobulinemia in HCV infection is usually Type III, and it may indicate the presence of active viral replication.[23] Patients may develop recurrent palpable and retiform purpura, acrocyanosis, arthritis, mononeuritis, glomerulonephritis, and other complications.

Polyarteritis nodosa can be associated with HBV infection. In this setting, medium-vessel vasculitis is thought to result from the formation of immune complexes containing hepatitis B surface antigen and immunoglobulin.

Gianotti-Crosti syndrome (papular acrodermatitis) is an eruption of monomorphic, flat-topped, erythematous papules on the face and limbs. It is most often seen in children as a result of Epstein-Barr virus, but can be associated with HBV and, less often, HCV. This eruption is usually self-limited and asymptomatic and is occasionally accompanied by lymphadenopathy. Other infectious agents and immunizations have been implicated in papular acrodermatitis.[24]

GASTROINTESTINAL SYSTEM

Diseases affecting both the skin and GI tract can cause GI bleeding, malabsorption/diarrhea, and abdominal pain.

GASTROINTESTINAL BLEEDING

Several diseases associated with GI bleeding also have cutaneous findings. These include diseases with vascular malformations such as hereditary hemorrhagic telangiectasia; defects in connective tissue such as pseudoxanthoma elasticum and Ehlers-Danlos, vascular type; neoplasms such as Kaposi sarcoma and mastocytosis; inflammatory bowel disease; and polyposis syndromes. Many vasculitides can affect the vessels of the gut and cause bleeding, including small vessel vasculitis, immunoglobulin A vasculitis (Henoch-Schönlein purpura), polyarteritis nodosa, and Behçet syndrome.

MALABSORPTION

Diseases causing dysmotility, GI infections, pancreatitis or pancreatic insufficiency, chronic inflammation, and short gut can all cause malabsorption and malnutrition.

Cutaneous manifestations of malnutrition are detailed elsewhere (see Chap. 123) but may include xerosis, eczematous dermatitis, cheilitis, alopecia or changes in hair texture, nail changes, and hyperpigmentation.

ABDOMINAL PAIN

This category is wide and encompasses many of the conditions listed above. In addition to these, neuropathic pain from herpes zoster can mimic an acute abdomen (particularly when pain precedes skin findings). Some porphyrias cause flares of abdominal

TABLE 133-4
Cutaneous Findings Associated with Hepatitis B and Hepatitis C

HEPATITIS B	HEPATITIS C
Small vessel vasculitis	Small vessel vasculitis
Urticaria, urticarial vasculitis	Urticaria, urticarial vasculitis
Serum sickness–like reaction	Serum sickness–like reaction
Pruritus	Pruritus
Erythema multiforme	Erythema multiforme
Cryoglobulinemia (C>B)	Cryoglobulinemia (C>B)
Porphyria cutanea tarda (C>B)	Porphyria cutanea tarda (C>B)
Sarcoidosis after interferon/ribavirin (C>B)	Sarcoidosis after interferon/ribavirin (C>B)
Erythema nodosum (B>C)	Erythema nodosum (B>C)
Gianotti-Crosti syndrome (B>C)	Gianotti-Crosti syndrome (B>C)
Polyarteritis nodosa	Lichen planus–erosive oral disease
	Necrolytic acral erythema

pain, and acute allergic reactions and anaphylaxis often have prominent abdominal discomfort. Bruising of the skin around the umbilicus (Cullen sign) or the flanks (Grey Turner sign) are well-known features of acute pancreatitis but occur in less than 3% of cases.[24] Chronic pancreatitis may cause tender, subcutaneous nodular areas of fat necrosis (pancreatic panniculitis) that may ulcerate.

ESOPHAGEAL INVOLVEMENT

Extension of dermatologic disease into the pharynx and esophagus can cause significant dysphagia. Common etiologies include blistering dermatoses (epidermolysis bullosa, cicatricial pemphigoid), lichen planus, rheumatologic disorders (Behçet syndrome, SSc), toxic epidermal necrolysis, Darier disease, and infection (*Candida*, herpes simplex virus).

SPECIFIC CONDITIONS

Table 133-5 outlines select conditions with GI and cutaneous manifestations.

KAPOSI SARCOMA

Visceral involvement is more common in AIDS-related Kaposi sarcoma than in classic Kaposi sarcoma. The most common organs involved are the GI tract and lungs. Prior to antiretroviral therapy, the GI tract was involved in 40% of patients with Kaposi sarcoma at initial diagnosis and in up to 80% at autopsy. GI Kaposi sarcoma can occur in the absence of cutaneous lesions and can be asymptomatic, or it may cause abdominal pain, weight loss, or bleeding.

DERMATITIS HERPETIFORMIS

Dermatitis herpetiformis is a cutaneous finding that occurs in celiac disease when antitransglutaminase antibodies bind to keratinocytes. It is intensely pruritic and presents with grouped excoriated papules and vesicles over the buttocks and extensor surfaces.

INFLAMMATORY BOWEL DISEASE

Inflammatory bowel disease (IBD) manifests with recurrent episodes of abdominal pain, GI bleeding, and diarrhea. Ulcerative colitis involves the rectum and colon, whereas Crohn disease can involve any area of the intestinal tract and is often discontinuous. There are multiple cutaneous findings associated with IBD.

Oral lesions, including aphthae, are common and appear to be related to active bowel inflammation. Aphthae are nonspecific and can be seen in healthy patients. Crohn disease is associated with granulomatous cheilitis and granulomatous nodules in the oral mucosa, which can coalesce to give a "cobblestone" appearance.

Granulomas may also occur in the perineum, at colostomy and ileostomy sites, and in association with

TABLE 133-5
Conditions with Gastrointestinal and Cutaneous Manifestations

DISEASE	GI FINDINGS	CUTANEOUS FINDINGS
Genetic		
Blue rubber bleb nevus syndrome	GI bleeding from venous malformations in gut; chronic anemia > acute hemorrhage	Dark blue papules, nodules
Cowden disease	Esophageal acanthosis; stomach, small intestine, colon polyps; colorectal cancer	Facial trichilemmomas, oral papillomas with cobblestoning, acral keratoses
Cronkhite-Canada syndrome	Polyposis stomach and bowel; abdominal pain, severe protein-losing enteropathy	Patchy alopecia, nail changes, hyperpigmentation
Ehlers-Danlos syndrome, vascular	Diverticula, hernias, bowel perforation (sigmoid colon)	Thin translucent skin, characteristic facies, acrogeria
Fabry disease	Abdominal pain, diarrhea	Angiokeratoma corporis diffusum
Hereditary hemorrhagic telangiectasia	GI bleeding, most commonly stomach or duodenum	Mat telangiectasias (arteriovenous malformations)
Gardner syndrome	Adenomatous polyposis	Epidermoid cysts, fibromas, lipomas, pilomatricomas, facial osteomas
Muir-Torre syndrome	Colorectal cancer	Sebaceous neoplasms, keratoacanthomas
Neurofibromatosis I	GI stromal tumors	Café-au-lait macules, axillary freckling, neurofibromas, Lisch nodules
Peutz-Jeghers	Hamartomatous polyposis, mainly in small intestine, recurrent intussusception; increased risk adenocarcinoma	Pigmented macules around mouth, lips, buccal mucosa, digits
Porphyria-variegate	Abdominal pain	Fragility, blisters in sun-exposed skin
Pseudoxanthoma elasticum	GI bleeding	Yellow-orange papules and plaques, lax skin

(Continued)

TABLE 133-5
Conditions with Gastrointestinal and Cutaneous Manifestations (Continued)

DISEASE	GI FINDINGS	CUTANEOUS FINDINGS
Neoplastic/Paraneoplastic		
Carcinoid syndrome	Small bowel tumors cause 75%; abdominal cramps, diarrhea	Flushing, pellagra, facial edema and induration
Glucagonoma	Chronic diarrhea, abdominal pain, glucose intolerance, diabetes mellitus	Necrolytic migratory erythema
Mastocytosis	Of patients with abdominal symptoms, one-third experience pain, vomiting, diarrhea, bleeding	Red-brown papules (urticaria pigmentosa), diffuse telangiectatic (TMEP [telangiectasia macularis eruptiva perstans]), skin thickening (diffuse cutaneous)
Kaposi sarcoma	GI bleeding	Red/purple macules, papules, plaques, or nodules on skin and mucosa
Infectious		
Herpes zoster	Abdominal pain may mimic acute abdomen and precede cutaneous signs	Grouped vesicles in a dermatomal distribution
Strongyloidiasis	Abdominal pain, vomiting, diarrhea	Ground itch at site of contact, perianal urticarial eruption, periumbilical purpura
Tuberculosis	Enteritis, peritonitis	Lupus vulgaris, scrofuloderma, orificial tuberculosis (TB), miliary TB, tuberculids
Typhoid fever	Abdominal pain, diarrhea, constipation, intestinal perforation	Rose spots–salmon-colored macules on trunk
Autoimmune/Rheumatologic		
Behçet syndrome	Abdominal pain, diarrhea, bleeding, ulceration	Oral/genital ulcers, pustular eruptions, pyoderma gangrenosum-like lesions
Henoch-Schönlein purpura	Abdominal pain, vomiting, bloody diarrhea, intussusception	Palpable purpura of legs and buttocks
Malignant atrophic papulosis	GI bleeding, abdominal pain, diarrhea, bowel perforation	Crops of porcelain-white atrophic papules with telangiectatic border
Polyarteritis nodosa	Abdominal pain, nausea, melena, diarrhea; mesenteric arteritis, bowel ischemia	Subcutaneous nodules, livedo reticularis, ulcers
Systemic lupus erythematosus	Esophagitis, intestinal pseudoobstruction, protein-losing enteropathy, pancreatitis, mesenteric vasculitis, peritonitis	Malar rash, photosensitivity, oral ulcers, discoid, subacute, and other skin lesions
Systemic sclerosis	Dysphagia, reflux, gastroparesis, malabsorption, pseudoobstruction	Raynaud phenomenon, sclerosis, sclerodactyly, dyspigmentation, microstomia
Inflammatory		
Angioedema	Abdominal pain	Urticaria, edema
Crohn disease	Granulomatous inflammation of the bowel, often with skip lesions	Aphthae, granulomatous cheilitis, oral cobblestoning, erythema nodosum, vasculitis, pyoderma gangrenosum, perianal fistulae, ulcers
Pancreatitis	Abdominal pain, nausea, vomiting, diarrhea	Cullen sign, Grey Turner sign, panniculitis
Ulcerative colitis	Continuous inflammation of the rectum and large bowel; risk of toxic megacolon	Aphthae, pyoderma gangrenosum, vasculitis, erythema nodosum, fissures
Other		
Amyloidosis	GI bleeding, gastroparesis, constipation, intestinal pseudoobstruction	Purpura, periorbital ecchymosis, waxy papules and plaques
Scurvy	Gingivitis, gradual GI blood loss resulting in anemia	Perifollicular purpura, corkscrew hairs, conjunctival hemorrhage

scars, sinuses, and fistulas. Rarely, granulomas occur at sites not contiguous with the bowel, such as the trunk and limbs, a finding termed *metastatic* Crohn disease.

Neutrophilic dermatoses are associated with both ulcerative colitis and Crohn disease. Pyoderma gangrenosum is classic, seen in 1% to 10% of patients.[25] IBD is the most common cause of pyoderma gangrenosum, responsible for 25% to 50% of cases. Pyoderma gangrenosum ulcers characteristically present with a violaceous or metallic gray undermined border and can preferentially involve the peristomal area, as well as sites of trauma. The activity of pyoderma gangrenosum does not necessarily parallel the activity of the IBD. Other IBD-associated neutrophilic dermatoses include Sweet syndrome, acneiform lesions, and panniculitis.

Other reactive dermatoses associated with IBD include small vessel vasculitis, polyarteritis nodosa, erythema multiforme, and epidermolysis bullosa acquisita. Additionally, IBD is associated with an increased frequency of alopecia areata, vitiligo, digital clubbing, and cutaneous signs of malnutrition.

POLYPOSIS SYNDROMES

There are 2 groups of hereditary polyposis: adenomatous syndromes (eg, familial adenomatous polyposis, Gardner syndrome) and hamartomatous syndromes (eg, Peutz-Jeghers and Cronkhite-Canada syndromes). Adenomas have proven malignant potential. Hamartomatous polyps represent proliferation and malformation of connective tissue of the intestinal mucosa and have less risk of malignancy. True adenomatous polyps are rare except in the colon and rectum, whereas hamartomatous lesions occur in all parts of the gut.

Familial adenomatous polyposis is an autosomal dominant condition consisting of many adenomatous polyps without extracolonic manifestations. It leads to colorectal cancer with nearly 100% certainty starting at age 20 to 30 years.

Gardner syndrome is a variant of familial adenomatous polyposis with the addition of epidermoid cysts, fibromas, lipomas, desmoid tumors, pilomatricomas, and osteomas of the facial bones and skull. The cutaneous lesions frequently predate GI manifestations.[26]

Peutz-Jeghers syndrome is characterized by small darkly pigmented macules on the lips, buccal mucosa, and digits. A histologically unique type of hamartomatous polyp occurs, mainly in the small intestine, which predisposes to recurrent intussusception. Bleeding is relatively rare, but up to 2% of patients develop adenocarcinoma of the stomach, duodenum, and colon. There is also an increased risk of malignancy in general.[27]

Cronkhite-Canada syndrome manifests on the skin with patchy alopecia and characteristic nail changes. Inflammatory polyps are present in the stomach and bowel, and abdominal pain with a severe protein-losing enteropathy is common.[28]

BOWEL-ASSOCIATED DERMATOSIS-ARTHRITIS SYNDROME

Following any surgery that results in formation of blind bowel loops (eg, jejunoileal bypass, biliopancreatic diversion, bowel resection), patients may present with a constellation of findings called bowel-associated dermatosis-arthritis syndrome.[29] Bowel-associated dermatosis-arthritis syndrome consists of a serum sickness-like syndrome with fever, malaise, arthritis, and myalgia followed by a skin eruption. The polyarthritis is nonerosive, asymmetric, episodic, and affects both small and large joints. Typical skin lesions include erythematous macules with central vesicle or pustule formation; however, erythema nodosum and panniculitis also have been described. The pathogenesis is uncertain, but the disease may be related to bacterial overgrowth and immune complex formation.

RENAL SYSTEM

Patients with end-stage renal disease (ESRD) develop a variety of cutaneous findings related to metabolic abnormalities, including anemia, calcium-phosphate dysregulation, and glucose intolerance. Skin manifestations include a sallow appearance, pruritus, xerosis, acquired perforating dermatosis, pseudoporphyria, calciphylaxis, and uremic frost.

The skin can be pale as a consequence of anemia and often exhibits a distinctive muddy hue, partly from accumulation of carotenoid and nitrogenous pigments (urochromes) in the dermis.[30] Uremic frost results from eccrine deposition of urea crystals on the skin surface of individuals with severe uremia.

RENAL PRURITUS

Renal pruritus is a major problem and may be seen in as many as 90% of those undergoing hemodialysis.[31-33] The etiology is thought to be multifactorial, including xerosis, peripheral neuropathy, mast cell hyperplasia, and increased serum histamine, vitamin A, parathyroid hormone, and inflammatory factors.[34-36] Clinically, the skin may appear normal or demonstrate secondary changes such as lichenification, excoriation, and hyperpigmentation.

NAIL CHANGES

Lindsay nails (half-and-half nails) are seen frequently in patients on dialysis and resolve with renal transplantation. They are characterized by a dull-white color proximally and a nonblanching red, pink, or brown color distally. Other abnormalities include Beau lines, onycholysis, and nailfold capillary abnormalities.

SPECIFIC CONDITIONS

Table 133-6 outlines select conditions with renal and cutaneous manifestations.

CALCIPHYLAXIS

Metastatic calcification in ESRD results from dysfunction of calcium and phosphate homeostasis. Calcification of vessels is common in ESRD and is seldom symptomatic. Occasionally, however, deposition of calcium phosphate in the media of cutaneous vessels results in downstream ischemia and infarct known as calciphylaxis. Painful violaceous mottling and fixed livedo reticularis progress to firm plaques of retiform

TABLE 133-6
Conditions with Renal and Cutaneous Manifestations

DISEASE	RENAL FINDINGS	CUTANEOUS FINDINGS
Genetic		
Birt-Hogg-Dube	Renal tumors	Fibrofolliculomas, trichodiscomas, acrochordons, connective tissue nevi
Fabry disease	Proteinuria, renal cysts, renal failure	Angiokeratoma corporis diffusum
Familial cutaneous leiomyomatosis	Renal cell carcinoma	Cutaneous leiomyomas
Nail-patella syndrome	Glomerulonephritis, proteinuria, renal tubular defects	Triangular lunulae, nail hypoplasia
Tuberous sclerosis	Renal angiomyolipomas, polycystic kidney disease, renal cell carcinoma	Facial angiofibromas, periungual fibromas, ash leaf macules, shagreen patch, connective tissue nevi
Von Hippel-Lindau disease	Renal cysts, clear-cell renal cell carcinomas	Nonspecific; hemangiomas and café-au-lait spots[a]
Infectious		
Loiasis	Hematuria, proteinuria	Transient edema (Calabar swelling) in areas of migrating worms, conjunctivitis
Autoimmune/Rheumatologic		
Behçet syndrome	Glomerulonephritis, interstitial nephritis	Oral and genital ulcers, acneiform pustules, pyoderma gangrenosum-like lesions
Henoch-Schönlein purpura	Glomerulonephritis (immunoglobulin A nephropathy)	Palpable purpura
Granulomatosis with polyangiitis (Wegener)	Glomerulonephritis	Palpable purpura, friable gingiva, ulcers, papulonecrotic lesions
Microscopic polyangiitis	Glomerulonephritis	Palpable purpura, erythematous patches, livedo reticularis, ulcers
Polyarteritis nodosa	Renal artery aneurysms, glomerulonephritis, hypertension	Subcutaneous nodules, livedo reticularis, ulcers
Rheumatoid arthritis	Glomerulonephritis, rheumatoid vasculitis	Rheumatoid nodules, ulcers, neutrophilic dermatoses
Systemic lupus erythematosus	Glomerulonephritis	Malar rash, photosensitivity, oral ulcers, discoid, subacute, and other skin lesions
Systemic sclerosis	Malignant hypertension, rapidly progressive renal failure	Sclerosis, sclerodactyly, poikiloderma, telangiectasia
Inflammatory		
DRESS (drug rash with eosinophilia and systemic symptoms)	Nephritis, hematuria, proteinuria	Diffuse morbilliform eruption with facial erythema and edema
Other		
Amyloidosis	Proteinuria, renal insufficiency	Purpura, periorbital ecchymoses, subcutaneous nodules or waxy plaques
Cholesterol emboli	Hematuria, eosinophiluria	Distal cyanosis, cutaneous necrosis, retiform purpura, splinter hemorrhages
Graft-versus-host disease	Nephritis or nephrotic syndrome	Acute: morbilliform exanthem; Chronic: poikiloderma, lichen planus-like, scleroderma-like
Nephrogenic fibrosing dermopathy	Renal insufficiency	Sclerosis of the extremities
Sarcoidosis	Hypercalciuria, nephrolithiasis, interstitial nephritis, granulomas	Papules, nodules, plaques–predilection for scars and tattoos

[a]Amin A, Burgess E. Skin manifestations associated with kidney cancer. *Semin Oncol.* 2016;43(3):408-412.

purpura, followed by black eschar, and ulceration. Mortality is high—roughly 50% at 1 year—most often from sepsis. Parathyroid hormone is usually elevated, while the calcium-phosphate product is often normal when checked. Treatment of calciphylaxis is multimodal and includes sodium thiosulfate, low calcium bath dialysis, non–calcium phosphate binders, bisphosphonates, calcimimetics, debridement of necrotic tissue, and aggressive wound care.

BULLOUS DISEASES OF HEMODIALYSIS

Porphyria cutanea tarda may occur in patients with ESRD on dialysis. Although the etiology of this phenomenon is unclear, inadequate clearance of plasma-bound porphyrins by the kidneys or hemodialysis may lead to porphyrin deposition in the skin, with resulting skin fragility and blister formation in sun-exposed areas.[37,38] Patients on hemodialysis may also produce or be exposed to compounds that alter normal heme synthesis.

Bullous dermatosis of dialysis or pseudoporphyria may occur in up to one-fifth of patients on hemodialysis. This condition is often clinically indistinguishable from porphyria cutanea tarda. Hypertrichosis is less common, and plasma porphyrin levels are typically normal.

When treating porphyria cutanea tarda or pseudoporphyria, phlebotomy can reduce iron levels in the liver, allowing new hepatic uroporphyrinogen decarboxylase to be formed.[39] However, patients with ESRD often have significant anemia and cannot tolerate phlebotomy. Erythropoietin may both lower total body iron stores and support phlebotomy as needed.[40,41] Low-dose hydroxychloroquine or chloroquine effectively clear porphyrins from the liver, but these may not be eliminated in the setting of poor renal function. Deferoxamine may lower serum porphyrin levels in some patients. Renal transplantation is an option in refractory disease.[42]

ACQUIRED PERFORATING DERMATOSES (KYRLE DISEASE)

Acquired perforating dermatoses are a spectrum of disorders associated with ESRD and diabetes that involve transepidermal elimination of collagen or elastic fibers. They occur in up to 10% of patients undergoing hemodialysis.[43] Clinically, patients develop hyperkeratotic papules or nodules with a central crust-filled plug on the trunk and extensor surfaces, often in a linear distribution.

Proposed mechanisms include diabetic microangiopathy, dysregulation of vitamin A or vitamin D metabolism, abnormality of collagen or elastic fibers, and inflammation and connective tissue degradation by dermal deposition of substances such as uric acid and calcium pyrophosphate.[44] Many authorities regard this entity as a response to trauma caused by scratching in chronic renal pruritus. Successful treatment depends on addressing the underlying etiology of pruritus. Topical and intralesional glucocorticoids, topical and systemic retinoids, cryotherapy, and ultraviolet light may be useful.

THYROID DISORDERS

Table 133-7 outlines the manifestations of thyroid disorders (see also Chap. 137, "Diabetes and Other Endocrine Diseases").

REFERENCES

1. Agouridis AP, Elisaf MS, Nair DR, et al. Ear lobe crease: a marker of coronary artery disease? *Arch Med Sci*. 2015;11(6):1145-1155.
2. Gelfand JM, Neimann AL, Shin DB, et al. Risk of myocardial infarction in patients with psoriasis. *JAMA*. 2006;296(14):1735.
3. Hugh J, Van Voorhees AS, Nijhawan RI, et al. From the Medical Board of the National Psoriasis Foundation: the risk of cardiovascular disease in individuals with psoriasis and the potential impact of current therapies. *J Am Acad Dermatol*. 2014;70(1):168.
4. Miner JJ, Kim AH. Cardiac manifestations of systemic lupus erythematosus. *Rheum Dis Clin North Am*. 2014; 40(1):51-60.
5. Moder KG, Miller TD, Tazelaar HD. Cardiac involvement in systemic lupus erythematosus. *Mayo Clin Proc*. 1999;74(3):275-284.
6. Friedman DM, Rupel A, Buyon JP. Epidemiology, etiology, detection, and treatment of autoantibody-associated congenital heart block in neonatal lupus. *Curr Rheumatol Rep*. 2007;9(2):101-108.
7. Steen V. Targeted therapy for systemic sclerosis. *Autoimmun Rev*. 2006;5(2):122-124.
8. Baydur A, Alsalek M, Louie SG, et al. Respiratory muscle strength, lung function, and dyspnea in patients with sarcoidosis. *Chest*. 2001;120(1):102-108.
9. Rosenbach MA, English JC, Callen JP. Sarcoidosis. In: Callen J, Jorizzo J, eds. *Dermatological Signs of Systemic Disease*. St. Louis, MO: Elsevier; 2017:305-314.
10. Tanoue LT. Pulmonary manifestations of rheumatoid arthritis. *Clin Chest Med*. 1998;19(4):667.
11. Keane MP, Lynch JP III. Pleuropulmonary manifestations of systemic lupus erythematosus. *Thorax*. 2000;55(2):159-166.
12. Marie I, Hachulla E, Cherin P, et al. Interstitial lung disease in dermatomyositis and polymyositis. *Arthritis Rheum*. 2002;47(6):614.
13. Bull RH, Fenton DA, Mortimer PS. Lymphatic function in the yellow nail syndrome. *Br J Dermatol*. 1996;134(2): 307-312.
14. Arkin LM, Flory JH, Shin DB, et al. High prevalence of aquagenic wrinkling of the palms in patients with cystic fibrosis and association with measurable increases in transepidermal water loss. *Pediatr Dermatol*. 2012;29(5): 560-566.
15. Johns MK. Skin wrinkling in cystic fibrosis. *Med Biol Illus*. 1975;25(4):205-210.
16. Koulentaki M, Ioannidou D, Stefanidou M, et al. Dermatological manifestations in primary biliary

TABLE 133-7
Thyroid Disorders

DISEASE	THYROID FINDINGS	CUTANEOUS FINDINGS
Genetic		
Birt-Hogg-Dube syndrome	Medullary thyroid cancer	Fibrofolliculomas, trichodiscomas, fibrous papules, acrochordons, connective tissue nevi
Cowden syndrome	Follicular and papillary thyroid cancer; thyroid adenomas	Trichilemmomas
Werner syndrome	Thyroid cancer	Scleroderma-like changes with subcutaneous atrophy, leg ulcers, soft tissue calcifications, bird-like facies
Multiple endocrine neoplasia (MEN) 2A	Medullary thyroid cancer	Lichen amyloidosis
MEN 2B	Medullary thyroid cancer	Neuromas (which may involve all mucosal surfaces: oral mucosa, lips, tongue, conjunctivae); café-au-lait spots, facial lentigines, hyperpigmentation of the hands and feet
Drug reaction with eosinophilia and systemic symptoms (DRESS)	Thyroiditis	Exanthem, exfoliative dermatitis, pustular eruptions, Stevens-Johnson syndrome/toxic epidermal necrolysis
Autoimmune/Rheumatologic		
Grave disease	Autoimmune thyroid disease	Thyroid dermopathy (pretibial myxedema): painless nonpitting nodules and plaques with a waxy, indurated texture; thyroid acropachy (digital clubbing, soft-tissue swelling of the hands and feet); hyperpigmentation
Toxic multinodular goiter	Hyperthyroidism	Soft, warm, velvety skin texture; pruritus; diffuse nonscarring alopecia; soft, shiny brittle nails with increased rate of growth; Plummer nails; patient may also have vitiligo
Hashimoto thyroiditis	Hypothyroidism	Associated with alopecia areata, connective tissue disease (lupus and dermatomyositis), bullous pemphigoid, dermatitis herpetiformis, and chronic mucocutaneous candidiasis
Hypothyroidism	Hypothyroidism	Myxedema; atopic dermatitis, keratosis pilaris, fine wrinkling, impaired wound healing; absence of hair on lateral third of eyebrow (Hertoghe sign); slow-growing, brittle nails with hoarseness

cirrhosis patients: a case control study. *Am J Gastroenterol.* 2006;101(3):541.

17. Foutch PG, Sullivan JA, Gaines JA, et al. Cutaneous vascular spiders in cirrhotic patients: correlation with hemorrhage from esophageal varices. *Am J Gastroenterol.* 1988;83(7):723-726.
18. Viraben R, Couret B, Gorguet B. Disseminated reticulate hypomelanosis developing during primary biliary cirrhosis. *Dermatology.* 1997;195(4):382-383.
19. Smith KE, Fenske NA. Cutaneous manifestations of alcohol abuse. *J Am Acad Dermatol.* 2000;43:1-16; quiz 16-18.
20. Niederau C, Strohmeyer G, Stremmel W. Epidemiology, clinical spectrum and prognosis of hemochromatosis. *Adv Exp Med Biol.* 1994;356:293.
21. Oleaga JM, Gardeazabal J, Sanz de Galdeano C, et al. Generalized lichen planus associated with primary biliary cirrhosis which resolved after liver transplantation. *Acta Derm Venereol.* 1995;75(1):87.
22. Graham-Brown RA, Sarkany I, Sherlock S. Lichen planus and primary biliary cirrhosis. *Br J Dermatol.* 1982;106(6):699-703.
23. Nan DN, Fernandez-Ayala M, Garcia-Palomo D, et al. Atypical skin lesions associated with mixed cryoglobulinaemia and hepatitis C virus infection in a cocaine-consuming patient. *Br J Dermatol.* 2000;143(6):1330-1331.
24. Tay YK. Gianotti-Crosti syndrome following immunization. *Pediatr Dermatol.* 2110;18(3):262.
25. Bem J, Bradley EL III. Subcutaneous manifestations of severe acute pancreatitis. *Pancreas.* 1999;16(4):551-555.
26. Friedman S, Marion JF, Scheri E, et al. Intravenous cyclosporine in refractory pyoderma gangrenosum complicating inflammatory bowel disease. *Inflamm Bowel Dis.* 2001;7(1):1-7.
27. Tsao H. Update on familial cancer syndromes and the skin. *J Am Acad Dermatol.* 2000;42(6):939-969.
28. Doxey BW, Kuwada SK, Burt RW. Inherited polyposis syndromes: Molecular mechanisms, clinicopathology, and genetic testing. *Clin Gastroenterol Hepatol.* 2005;3(7):633-641.
29. Harned RK, Buck JL, Sobin LH. The hamartomatous polyposis syndromes: clinical and radiologic features. *AJR Am J Roentgenol.* 1995;164(3):565-571.
30. Kemp DR, Gin D. Bowel-associated dermatosis-arthritis syndrome. *Med J Aust.* 1990;152(1):43-45.
31. Murakami K, Nakanishi Y, Wakamatsu K, et al. Serum levels of 5-s-cysteinyldopa are correlated with skin colors in hemodialysis patients but not in peritoneal dialysis patients. *Blood Purif.* 2009;28(3):209-215.
32. Gilchrest BA, Stern RS, Steinman TI, et al. Clinical features of pruritus among patients undergoing maintenance hemodialysis. *Arch Dermatol.* 1982;118(3):154-156.
33. Stahle-Backdahl M. Uremic pruritus. *Semin Dermatol.* 1995;14(4):297-301.

34. Szepietowski JC, Sikora M, Kusztal M, et al. Uremic pruritus: a clinical study of maintenance hemodialysis patients. *J Dermatol*. 2002;29(10):621-627.
35. Mettang M, Weisshaar E. Pruritus: control of itch in patients undergoing dialysis. *Skin Therapy Lett*. 2010;15(2):1-5.
36. Vahlquist A, Stenstrom E, Torma H. Vitamin A and beta-carotene concentrations at different depths of the epidermis: a preliminary study in the cow snout. *Ups J Med Sci*. 1987;92(3):253-257.
37. Murtagh FE, Addington-Hall JM, Edmonds PM, et al. Symptoms in advanced renal disease: a cross-sectional survey of symptom prevalence in stage 5 chronic kidney disease managed without dialysis. *J Palliat Med*. 2007;10(6):1266-1276.
38. Poh-Fitzpatrick MB, Masullo AS, Grossman ME. Porphyria cutanea tarda associated with chronic renal disease and hemodialysis. *Arch Dermatol*. 1980;116(2):191-195.
39. Poh-Fitzpatrick MB, Sosin AE, Bemis J. Porphyrin levels in plasma and erythrocytes of chronic hemodialysis patients. *J Am Acad Dermatol*. 1982;7(1):100-104.
40. Kelly MA, O'Rourke KD: Treatment of porphyria cutanea tarda with phlebotomy in a patient on peritoneal dialysis. *J Am Acad Dermatol*. 2001;44(2)(suppl):336-338.
41. Anderson KE, Goeger DE, Carson RW, et al. Erythropoietin for the treatment of porphyria cutanea tarda in a patient on long-term hemodialysis. *N Engl J Med*. 1990;322(5):315-317.
42. Sarkell B, Patterson JW. Treatment of porphyria cutanea tarda of end-stage renal disease with erythropoietin. *J Am Acad Dermatol*. 1993;29(3):499-500.
43. Stevens BR, Fleischer AB, Piering F, et al. Porphyria cutanea tarda in the setting of renal failure. Response to renal transplantation. *Arch Dermatol*. 1993;129(3):337-339.
44. Farrell AM. Acquired perforating dermatosis in renal and diabetic patients. *Lancet*. 1997;349(9056):895-866.
45. Haftek M, Euvrard S, Kanitakis J, et al. Acquired perforating dermatosis of diabetes mellitus and renal failure: further ultrastructural clues to its pathogenesis. *J Cutan Pathol*. 1993;20(4):350-355.

Chapter 134 :: Cutaneous Paraneoplastic Syndromes :: Manasmon Chairatchaneeboon & Ellen J. Kim

第一百三十四章
皮肤副肿瘤综合征

中文导读

皮肤副肿瘤综合征包含多种皮肤疾病，提示存在远处恶性肿瘤。在某些情况下，它们可能出现在癌症诊断之前，有助于发现一种隐匿性癌症，或者它们也可能预示着先前癌症缓解患者的复发。因此，及时识别皮肤副肿瘤综合征可能可以在可治疗的阶段发现潜在的恶性肿瘤。本章除介绍了经典的副肿瘤性皮肤病外，还讨论了肿瘤直接累及皮肤和具有恶性潜在性的遗传性皮肤病。

主要介绍了：①角化过度性皮肤病，包括黑棘皮病、获得性鱼鳞病、牛肚掌、Leser-Trélat征、巴泽斯副肿瘤性肢端角化症；②胶原血管病，包括皮肌炎、进行性系统性硬化症；③反应性红斑，如匍行性回状红斑、坏死松解性游走性红斑；④中性粒细胞皮肤疾病，包括Sweet综合征、坏疽性脓皮病；⑤皮肤增生性疾病，包括多中心网状组织细胞增多症、坏死性黄色肉芽肿；⑥真皮沉积，如硬化性黏液水肿、系统性淀粉样变性；⑦大疱性疾病，包括副肿瘤性天疱疮、大疱性类天疱疮、疱疹样皮炎；⑧其他疾病，如获得性多毛症、特鲁索综合征；⑨直接累及皮肤的肿瘤等疾病的相关内容。

〔粟 娟〕

CUTANEOUS PARANEOPLASTIC SYNDROMES

Paraneoplastic syndromes refer to the remote effects of underlying neoplastic diseases. The clinical syndromes can occur in various organ systems, including endocrine, neuromuscular, cardiovascular, cutaneous, hematologic, GI, and renal. The symptoms are not the direct effect of metastases or tumor invasion, but may result from substances produced by the tumor (eg. hormones, peptides, or cytokines) or from immunologic or inflammatory reactions between malignant and normal tissues.

Cutaneous paraneoplastic syndromes (Table 134-1) are diverse dermatologic entities that suggest the presence of a remote malignancy. In some instances, they may appear before a cancer diagnosis and contribute to the discovery of an occult cancer, or they may also indicate recurrence in a patient with prior remission of cancer. Consequently, prompt recognition of the cutaneous paraneoplastic syndromes may lead to the detection of an underlying malignancy at an early and highly-treatable stage. However, the paraneoplastic manifestations may predate the diagnosis of the related neoplasm by many months or years. If an underlying cancer is not detectible, careful followup should continue for several years.

In addition to classic paraneoplastic dermatoses, this chapter also discusses direct tumor involvement of the skin and genodermatoses with malignant potential (Table 134-2). Although paraneoplastic dermatoses are not frequently seen in the clinical setting, recognition of these cancer-associated skin lesions is very important. The dermatologist may play a significant role in diagnosing an occult malignancy at earlier stages of disease.

HYPERKERATOTIC DERMATOSES

ACANTHOSIS NIGRICANS

Chap. 137, "Diabetes and Other Endocrine Diseases," provides additional information on benign acanthosis nigricans.

The term *acanthosis nigricans* was originally proposed by Unna, although the first cases were malignancy associated and described independently by Pollitzer and by Janovsky in 1890. Curth clinically classified acanthosis nigricans into malignant, benign, or syndromic acanthosis nigricans, or pseudoacanthosis nigricans (obesity related). Today acanthosis nigricans is classified into 2 broad categories: benign (familial, obesity related, hyperinsulinemic states, autoimmune disease associated) or malignant (malignancy associated). Malignant acanthosis nigricans typically occurs in older patients and frequently coexists with other paraneoplastic dermatoses such as tripe palms and the sign of Leser-Trélat.[1]

EPIDEMIOLOGY

The majority (80%) of acanthosis nigricans occurs idiopathically or in benign conditions such as endocrinopathies, heritable diseases, or drug use. Malignancy-associated acanthosis nigricans is rare, with approximately 1000 cases reported in the literature. It usually occurs in individuals older than 40 years of age, without gender, racial, or genetic predilection.[1]

AT-A-GLANCE

- Acanthosis nigricans is a cutaneous marker, most commonly of insulin resistance and less frequently of genetic disorders and malignancy.
- Characterized by symmetric hyperpigmented, hyperkeratotic, verrucous plaques with a velvety texture on intertriginous skin and occasionally mucocutaneous areas.
- Darker skin pigmentation, insulin resistance, and obesity are more commonly associated with benign acanthosis nigricans.
- Malignant acanthosis nigricans often appears rapidly in older individuals and can involve atypical areas such as mucosal surfaces.

CLINICAL FEATURES

The skin lesions first appear as a symmetric hyperpigmentation or a dirty appearance of the skin, followed by thickening and increased skin markings, resulting in hyperpigmented velvety plaques. The colors may vary and include yellow, brown, gray, and black. Although the skin lesions of acanthosis nigricans can occur almost anywhere on the body, they tend to affect the skinfold, flexural, and intertriginous areas. The most commonly involved locations are the axillae, neck, external genitalia, groin, face, inner thighs, antecubital and popliteal fossae, umbilicus, and perianal area. Acrochordons may develop, superimposed on the acanthosis nigricans or on other locations (Fig. 134-1). Hyperkeratosis of the nipple and areola also has been noted. Mucosal involvement tends to occur in the malignant form, but can also be seen in acanthosis nigricans without malignancy and is characterized by papillomatosis and thickening of mucosa with or without hyperpigmentation involving the oral cavity (lips, tongue, buccal mucosa, and palate) (Fig. 134-2), and, rarely, the esophagus, eyes, larynx, and anal and genital mucosae. Typically, patients with acanthosis nigricans are asymptomatic, but pruritus can be a problem in some patients. Oral and esophageal papillomatosis can cause sore mouth and dysphagia.[1]

The lesions of malignant and benign acanthosis nigricans are indistinguishable. However, malignancy-associated acanthosis nigricans usually appears abruptly and extensively. Mucosal involvement and generalized pruritus are more common. The co-occurrence with florid cutaneous papillomatosis and other paraneoplastic skin lesions, such as tripe palms (see "Tripe Palms" section) and Leser-Trélat sign (see "Leser-Trélat Sign" section), suggests the malignancy-associated form of acanthosis nigricans. Many types of malignancies have been reported in association with malignant acanthosis nigricans. A literature review shows that up to 90% of patients have an associated intraabdominal adenocarcinoma, of which approximately 60% are gastric cancer. Cancers of the uterus, liver, intestinal, ovary, kidney, breast, lung, pancreas, bladder, thyroid, and gallbladder have been reported, as have lymphoma and mycosis fungoides.[1]

ETIOLOGY AND PATHOGENESIS

The pathogenesis of acanthosis nigricans is poorly understood. In benign acanthosis nigricans, there is evidence that insulin plays a significant role through insulin-like growth factor-1 receptor signaling pathway (see Chap. 137). In acanthosis nigricans associated with inherited syndromes, insulin-like growth factor-1 receptor and fibroblast growth factor receptors may be implicated. In addition, genetic studies also demonstrate activation mutations of fibroblast growth factor receptors.[2]

In malignancy-associated acanthosis nigricans, it is proposed that the tumor produces transforming growth factor-α that is similar in structure to

TABLE 134-1
Classic Paraneoplastic Dermatoses

PARANEOPLASTIC DERMATOSIS	MAJOR INTERNAL MALIGNANCY	PERCENT WITH CANCER	UNIQUE FEATURES
Hyperkeratotic Diseases			
Acanthosis nigricans	Adenocarcinomas: intraabdominal; gastric cancer (CA) (60%)	Unknown	Older age, rapid course, extensive, and oral involvement indicate malignancy associations; more common in benign condition with insulin resistance and metabolic syndromes
Acquired ichthyosis	Hodgkin lymphoma most common	Unknown	Spares flexures, palms, soles; can occur in several benign conditions
Pityriasis rotunda	GI and hematologic malignancies; hepatocellular CA most common	30% of Type I	Type I: African/Asian; <30 lesions, high rate of malignancy. Type II: whites, familial; >30 lesions, cancer rare
Tripe palms	Lung CA most common; gastric CA second	>90%	Coexists with acanthosis nigricans in 70%
Leser-Trélat sign	Adenocarcinomas: GI (32%); lymphoproliferative disorders (20%)	Unknown	Seborrheic keratoses (SKs) with early onset, eruptive nature, pruritus; coexistence with acanthosis nigricans and/or tripe palms suggests paraneoplastic type
Bazex syndrome	Squamous cell carcinoma (SCC) of upper aerodigestive tract	Nearly 100%	Acral papulosquamous lesions (ears, nose), paronychia, onychodystrophy
Collagen–Vascular Diseases			
Dermatomyositis	Women: ovarian and breast CA. Men: GI, respiratory tract CA. Asians: nasopharyngeal CA	18%-25%	Older age, males predominate; refractory or flaring of previously well-controlled disease may signal malignancy
Progressive systemic sclerosis	Lung CA	3%-11%	Older age of onset, diffuse cutaneous disease, and RNA polymerase III autoantibodies
Reactive Erythemas			
Erythema gyratum repens	Lung CA	70%	Migratory "wood-grain" pattern; erythema
Necrolytic migratory erythema	Glucagonoma (pancreatic α cell tumor)	Nearly 100%	Can be first sign of glucagonoma syndrome; early recognition is important; most have metastatic tumors at the time of diagnosis
Neutrophilic Dermatoses			
Sweet syndrome	Acute myeloid leukemia (AML) most common	20%	Bullous and ulcerated skin lesions, subcutaneous nodules, oral mucosal involvement, anemia, and abnormal platelet count are more common with malignancy
Pyoderma gangrenosum	AML most common	4%-20%	Atypical presentation more common with malignancy; may be on a continuum with Sweet syndrome; immunoglobulin (Ig) A paraproteinemia is the most frequent associated gammopathy
Dermal Proliferative Diseases			
Multicentric reticulohistiocytosis	No specific cancer type or location	25%	Not parallel to malignancy
Necrobiotic xanthogranuloma	Monoclonal gammopathy of undetermined significance (MGUS) most common	80% (gammopathy)	Either IgG κ or λ light-chain monoclonal gammopathy; periorbital involvement, especially with necrosis; may develop multiple myeloma, recommend lifelong followup
Disorders of Dermal Deposition			
Scleromyxedema	MGUS most common; multiple myeloma rare	80% (gammopathy)	Most have IgG λ light-chain monoclonal gammopathy; only rarely convert to multiple myeloma, but poor prognosis if conversion occurs
Systemic amyloidosis	Multiple myeloma	20%	Macroglossia, pinch purpura, carpal tunnel clues to systemic amyloidosis; amyloid light chain (AL) amyloidosis is the most common form associated with malignancy; 1-year mean survival time

(Continued)

TABLE 134-1
Classic Paraneoplastic Dermatoses (*Continued*)

PARANEOPLASTIC DERMATOSIS	MAJOR INTERNAL MALIGNANCY	PERCENT WITH CANCER	UNIQUE FEATURES
Bullous Disorders			
Paraneoplastic pemphigus	Lymphoproliferative disorders; non-Hodgkin lymphoma most common; chronic lymphocytic leukemia (CLL) second most common	Nearly 100%	Can occur in Castleman disease and thymoma; parallels benign, but not malignant, tumors
Dermatitis herpetiformis	Non-Hodgkin lymphoma most common	4%	Occurs significantly more often in patients who do not follow a gluten-free diet
Other Changes			
Hypertrichosis lanuginosa acquisita	Men: lung, colorectal CA Women: colorectal, lung, or breast CA	Nearly 100%	Excessive downy hair initially concentrated on face, spreading caudally; usually appears in advanced or metastatic carcinomas
Trousseau syndrome	Pancreatic, brain, lung CA	20%-30%	Deep vein thrombosis (DVT) of unusual sites (eg. upper limbs), thrombosis of visceral organs and brain, and arterial thromboembolism suggest cancer association

epidermal growth factor and binds to epidermal growth factor receptors and stimulates keratinocyte proliferation, which leads to development of acanthosis nigricans. This theory was based on observations in which the skin disorders improved or resolved following treatment of the underlying malignancy. For example, elevated urinary transforming growth factor-α and increased expression of epidermal growth factor receptor in lesional skin were noted in a patient with acanthosis nigricans, acrochordons, Leser-Trélat sign, and melanoma. The enhanced expression of this cytokine and its receptor normalized after removal of the melanoma, and the accompanying skin lesions improved postoperatively. In addition, some authors suggest that fibroblast growth factor and insulin-like growth factor-1 also may play a role in the pathogenesis of malignancy-associated acanthosis nigricans.[2,3]

DIAGNOSIS

Diagnosis of acanthosis nigricans is based on clinical features and distribution of the lesions. Histopathologic study is needed only to confirm diagnosis

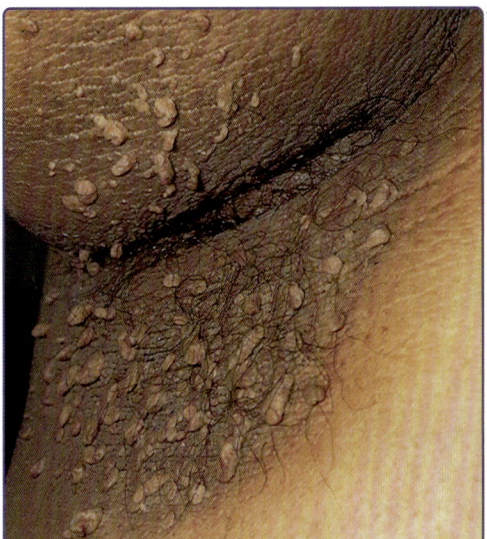

Figure 134-1 Acanthosis nigricans involving the axilla with numerous acrochordons.

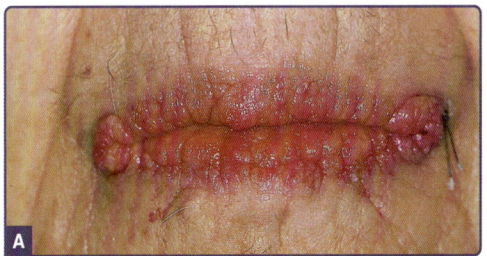

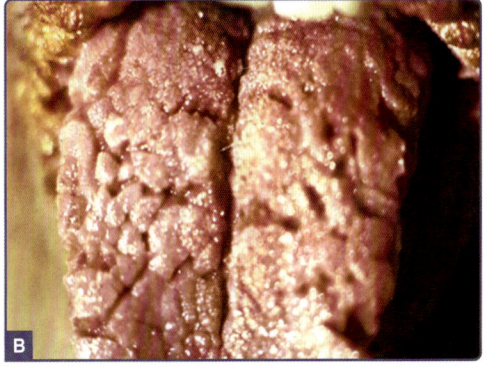

Figure 134-2 Acanthosis nigricans. **A,** Verrucous and papillomatous growths of the vermilion border of the lip. **B,** Velvety thickening of the tongue. (**A** and **B** are not the same patient.) (**A** and **B,** From Wolff K, Johnson RA. *Fitzpatrick's Color Atlas and Synopsis of Clinical Dermatology*, 6th ed. New York, NY: McGraw-Hill; 2009, with permission.)

TABLE 134-2
Genetic Syndromes Involving Skin and/or Mucous Membranes and Associated with Malignancy

SYNDROME	GENE/PROTEIN DEFECT	CUTANEOUS FINDINGS	OTHER CHARACTERISTIC FEATURES	MAJOR ASSOCIATED INTERNAL MALIGNANCY	MINOR ASSOCIATED INTERNAL MALIGNANCY
Autosomal Dominant					
Birt-Hogg-Dubé syndrome[41]	FLCN	Fibrofolliculomas, trichodiscomas, acrochordons	Lung cysts, emphysema, recurrent spontaneous pneumothoraces	Renal carcinoma	Lipoma, parathyroid adenoma
Carney complex[42,43]	PRKAR1A	Mucocutaneous myxomas, nevi, lentigines, blue nevi	Adrenocortical disease	Myxomas (cardiac, skin), Sertoli cell testicular cancer	Other testicular cancers, breast cancer, thyroid neoplasms, pituitary adenoma, psammomatous melanotic schwannomas, ovarian tumors, osteochondromyxoma
Cowden disease[41,43,44]	PTEN (phosphatase and tensin homolog)	Trichilemmomas, acral papules and keratoses, oral papillomas, sclerotic fibromas	Macrocephaly, cerebellar dysfunction	Breast cancer, thyroid cancer, endometrial cancer, hamartomatous intestinal polyps	Colorectal cancer, kidney cancer, liposarcoma, malignant melanoma
Gardner disease[41,45]	APC	Epidermoid cysts, fibromas, pilomatricomas	Congenital hypertrophy of retinal pigment epithelium (CHRPE), supernumerary teeth, osteomas, desmoid tumors	Intestinal polyposis and colorectal adenocarcinoma (near 100%)	Thyroid cancer, bone and CNS tumors, pancreatic and hepatic carcinomas, hepatoblastomas, adrenal adenomas
Gorlin syndrome/nevoid basal cell carcinoma (BCC) syndrome[44,46]	PTCH1, PTCH2, SUFU	Multiple BCCs, epidermoid cysts, milia, palmoplantar pits	Calcified falx cerebri, bifid ribs, odontogenic cysts, macrocephaly, frontal bossing, hypertelorism	BCC, medulloblastoma	Meningiomas, ovarian fibromas and fibrosarcomas, ovarian desmoids, cardiac fibromas, rhabdomyosarcomas, ameloblastoma
Howel-Evans syndrome[43]	TOC	Palmoplantar keratoderma (non-transgrediens), oral leukoplakia	Esophageal papillomas	Esophageal carcinoma (up to 90%)	
Multiple endocrine neoplasia (MEN) I syndrome[42,44]	MEN1	Angiofibromas, collagenomas, lipomas	Various endocrine sequelae based on underlying tumor	Parathyroid adenomas, pancreatic islet cell tumors, gastrinomas, anterior pituitary tumors	Carcinoid tumors, adrenal cortical tumors, thyroid adenomas
MEN IIa syndrome[44]	RET	Scapular macular or lichen amyloidosis	Hirschsprung disease; no mucosal neuromas or marfanoid habitus	Medullary thyroid carcinoma (95%), pheochromocytomas, parathyroid tumors	
MEN IIb/III syndrome[43]	RET	Mucosal neuromas, thickened eyelids and lips, circumoral lentigines, diffuse pigmentation of the hands and feet, café-au-lait macules (CALMs)	Marfanoid habitus	Medullary thyroid carcinoma (95%), pheochromocytoma; no parathyroid tumors	Conjunctival neuromas, intestinal ganglioneuromas
Muir-Torre syndrome[41,46]	MLH1, MSH2, MSH6	Sebaceous tumors (epitheliomas, hyperplasias, adenomas, carcinomas), keratoacanthomas		Colorectal carcinomas, genitourinary cancers	Breast, lung, head and neck, small intestine carcinomas, hematologic malignancies

TABLE 134-2
Genetic Syndromes Involving Skin and/or Mucous Membranes and Associated with Malignancy (Continued)

Syndrome	Gene	Skin/Mucous Membrane Findings	Other Findings	Associated Malignancies
Neurofibromatosis (NF) I[44,45]	NF1	CALMs, NF, plexiform NF, axillary/inguinal freckling	Lisch nodules, glaucoma, sphenoid wing dysplasia, pseudoarthrosis of tibia, learning difficulties, seizures	Optic gliomas, neurofibrosarcoma, juvenile myelomonocytic leukemia	Astrocytomas, ependymoma, meningioma, peripheral nerve sheath tumor, pheochromocytoma, hematologic malignancies
Neurofibromatosis II[43,45]	NF2	Schwannomas, NF, CALMs, plexiform NF	Juvenile posterior subcapsular cataracts, deafness	Bilateral vestibular schwannomas (near 100%), spinal tumors, meningiomas	Gliomas, astrocytomas, intramedullary ependymomas
Peutz-Jeghers syndrome[43,44]	STK11	Perioral and mucosal lentigines	Intussusception, bowel obstruction	Multiple GI hamartomatous polyps (near 100%), GI carcinoma	Pancreatic, esophageal, breast cancer, ovarian cancer, lung cancer
Reed syndrome[41] (hereditary leiomyomatosis and renal cell carcinoma)	FH	Cutaneous leiomyomas (piloleiomyomas)	Uterine leiomyoma	Renal carcinoma	
Tuberous sclerosis[42,43]	TSC1, TSC2	Ash-leaf macules, shagreen patches, CALMs, facial angiofibromas, periungual fibromas, dental enamel pits	Tonic–clonic seizures, paraventricular calcification, subependymal nodules, retinal hamartomas, learning disabilities, autism	Intracranial cortical/subcortical tubers (near 100%), cardiac rhabdomyomas, renal angiomyolipomas, lung lymphangiomyomatosis	
Autosomal Recessive					
Ataxia-telangiectasia[43,44]	ATM	Telangiectasias (skin and conjunctiva), mask-like progeric facies, CALMs, poikiloderma	Ataxia, nystagmus, choreoathetosis, immunodeficiency, CNS degeneration, growth deficiency, radiosensitivity	Leukemia/lymphomas	Various solid tumors
Bloom syndrome[44,46]	BLM/RECQL3	Cheilitis, CALMs, malar poikiloderma	Immunodeficiency, short stature, hypogonadism, high-pitched voice	Leukemia/lymphoma; GI adenocarcinoma	Other solid tumors of various organs
Chédiak-Higashi syndrome[43]	LYST	Partial oculocutaneous albinism, silver hair, slate-gray skin, ecchymoses	Immunodeficiency, pyogenic infections (Staphylococcus), photophobia, neurodegeneration, mild coagulation defect	Lymphoma-like accelerated phase (85%)	
Fanconi anemia[43,44]	FANC	Short stature, CALMs microcephaly, thumb and/or radial anomalies thenar hypoplasia	Short stature, multiple birth anomalies, microcephaly, bone marrow failure, infection, radial anomalies	Acute myeloid leukemia/myelodysplastic syndrome, SCC	Gynecologic tumors, brain tumors, Wilms tumor, neuroblastoma
Griscelli syndrome[43]	RAB27A, MYO5A	Silver hair, partial albinism	Immunodeficiency, pancytopenia, neurodegeneration (MYO5A), hemophagocytic syndrome (RAB27A)	Lymphoma-like accelerated phase	
Rothmund-Thomson syndrome[46]	RecQL4	Poikiloderma, nail dystrophy, acral keratoses, photosensitivity, hypotrichosis	Short stature, radial anomalies, juvenile cataracts, hypogonadism	Osteogenic sarcomas	Nonmelanoma skin cancers, fibrosarcoma, non-Hodgkin lymphoma, thyroid adenoma, gastric carcinoma

TABLE 134-2
Genetic Syndromes Involving Skin and/or Mucous Membranes and Associated with Malignancy (Continued)

SYNDROME	GENE/PROTEIN DEFECT	CUTANEOUS FINDINGS	OTHER CHARACTERISTIC FEATURES	MAJOR ASSOCIATED INTERNAL MALIGNANCY	MINOR ASSOCIATED INTERNAL MALIGNANCY
Werner syndrome[43,46]	RecQL2	Premature aging, bird-like facies, sclerodermoid changes, ulcers	Short stature, cataracts, diabetes, osteoporosis, abnormal voice, hypogonadism, muscular atrophy	Thyroid carcinomas	Meningiomas, malignant melanoma, sarcomas, hematologic malignancies
Xeroderma pigmentosum (XP)[43,44]	XP (multiple proteins that form DNA repair complex), XPA to XPG, and XPV	Photosensitivity, actinic keratoses, lentigines, poikiloderma	Photophobia, multiple ocular complications, neurodegeneration (XPA, XPD)	Cutaneous cancers (BCC, SCC, and melanoma 100%), ocular cancers	Sarcomas, leukemia, lung cancer, breast cancer, gastric cancer, brain tumors
X-Linked Recessive					
Dyskeratosis congenita[43,44]	DKC1 (XLR); TERT/TERD (AD); NOP10 (AR)	Leukoplakia, nail dystrophy, reticulate pigmentation, poikilodermatous skin changes, alopecia, premature graying of the hair, palmoplantar hyperkeratosis, adermatoglyphia, hyperhidrosis	Pancytopenia, various ocular complications, mental retardation, pulmonary complications, esophageal stricture, microcephaly	Cutaneous and mucosal SCC, acute myeloid leukemia/myelodysplastic syndrome	Hodgkin lymphoma, GI carcinoma
Wiskott-Aldrich syndrome (WAS)[43]	WASP	Eczema, petechiae/purpura	Immunodeficiency (decreased IgM), recurrent infections, thrombocytopenia	Lymphomas/leukemia	Kaposi sarcoma, smooth muscle tumors, cerebellar astrocytoma
X-linked ichthyosis	STS	Adherent brown scales that spares face, palms, soles and flexural creases	Failure of maternal labor, comma-shaped corneal opacities, cryptorchidism	Testicular cancer	
Sporadic					
Beckwith-Wiedemann syndrome[43,44]	p57, H19, LIT1, ICR1, CDKN1C, NSD1	Capillary malformation, macroglossia, linear indentations on earlobes creases, helical pits	Omphalocele, mental retardation, hemihypertrophy, neonatal hypoglycemia	Wilms tumor, hepatoblastoma	Adrenocortical tumors, rhabdomyosarcoma, glioblastoma, neuroblastoma
Familial atypical multiple mole melanoma syndrome (dysplastic nevus syndrome)[43,44]	CDKN2A	Multiple dysplastic nevi, melanomas		Melanomas, pancreatic cancer	Lung, laryngeal, and breast carcinomas, SCC of the oropharynx
Maffucci syndrome	IDH1, IDH2	Venous malformations	Enchondromas, secondary fractures	Chondrosarcoma	Angiosarcoma and lymphangiosarcoma, fibrosarcoma, osteosarcoma

in problematic cases. Histopathology of acanthosis nigricans classically shows hyperkeratosis and epidermal papillomatosis. There is only slight acanthosis and usually no hyperpigmentation. Horn pseudocyst formation and increased melanin pigmentation can be observed in some cases. The brown color of the lesion is caused by hyperkeratosis rather than melanin. The histopathologic findings cannot be distinguished from confluent and reticulated papillomatosis of Gougerot and Carteaud, seborrheic keratosis, or epidermal nevus.

DIFFERENTIAL DIAGNOSIS

The clinical differential diagnoses of malignant acanthosis nigricans include the conditions that present hyperpigmentation and patches or plaques in either flexural areas or a generalized distribution. Psoriasiform dermatitis, atopic dermatitis, pellagra, resolving pemphigus vegetans, parapsoriasis, cutaneous T-cell lymphoma, infections (eg. candidiasis, erythrasma, tinea corporis/cruris), pigmentary disorders (eg. hemochromatosis, Addison disease, Dowling-Degos disease), and others (eg, confluent and reticulated papillomatosis of Gougerot and Carteaud, Becker melanosis, epidermal nevus, and terra firma-forme dermatosis) are included in the differential diagnoses.

CLINICAL COURSE AND PROGNOSIS

Malignant acanthosis nigricans can occur before, during, or after the detection of cancer. It tends to parallel the course of the underlying malignancy. Skin lesions may regress after treatment of the underlying cancers, and recur following relapse or metastasis of the malignancies. Unfortunately, most associated malignancies present at an advanced stage, and thus the prognosis is usually poor.[2,4]

MANAGEMENT

Evaluation and studies are recommended in suspicious cases to identify the underlying endocrinopathy or malignancy. Older patients presenting with unintentional weight loss, rapid and extensive acanthosis nigricans with mucosal involvement, and have concomitant paraneoplastic skin lesions, should be investigated for underlying malignancy, especially of the GI tract.

Cosmetic appearance is often the patient's primary concern. Management of any co-occurring disease or malignancy often improves and may even resolve the acanthosis nigricans. Topical keratolytics, including the retinoids, and oral retinoids can reduce the appearance of acanthosis nigricans. Other oral medications reported to show improvement include dietary fish oil, metformin, and cyproheptadine, possibly by inhibition of tumor-secreted growth factors in the case of cyproheptadine. Other therapies found beneficial in case reports include calcipotriol, trichloroacetic acid peeling, and long-pulsed alexandrite laser.[3]

ACQUIRED ICHTHYOSIS

Chapter 47, "The Ichthyoses," provides additional information on acquired ichthyosis.

Acquired ichthyosis occurs in adulthood and may be associated with malignancies, endocrine and metabolic diseases, HIV and other infections, autoimmune diseases, nutritional deficiency, and drug reactions. Clinical manifestations include diffuse, symmetrical, plate-like scaling on trunk and extensor extremities, which usually spares flexures, palms, and soles. Malignancies associated with acquired ichthyosis include CD30+ lymphoproliferative disorders, mycosis fungoides, leiomyosarcoma, Kaposi sarcoma, multiple myeloma, and carcinomas of the ovary, breast, lung, and cervix. Hodgkin disease is the most common neoplasm; the ichthyosis usually occurs simultaneously with or after the diagnosis of lymphoma. As a sudden onset of ichthyosis in an adult may be a presenting sign of underlying malignancy, a careful malignancy screening, especially for lymphoma, is important. In lymphomas, acquired ichthyosis can be a cutaneous sign of the disease or a paraneoplastic phenomenon. However, this may be very difficult to identify in some cases, such as in mycosis fungoides, in which clinical and histopathologic findings can be indistinguishable between ichthyosiform mycosis fungoides and acquired ichthyosis related to mycosis fungoides.[5]

PITYRIASIS ROTUNDA

Pityriasis rotunda, a rare cutaneous disorder, is considered by some as a variant of acquired ichthyosis. It has been observed in association with chronic diseases, infections, and malignancies. GI (most commonly hepatocellular carcinoma) and hematologic malignancies are frequently reported among the various types of associated malignancies. However, pityriasis rotunda can occur in healthy people as well. Skin manifestations are characteristic, consisting of perfectly round or oval, asymptomatic, well-defined, hypopigmented or hyperpigmented ichthyosiform scaly patches that appear on the trunk and proximal extremities.[5] Type 1 pityriasis rotunda is associated with underlying malignant or systemic disease and presents with <30 skin lesions. It is more common in black and East Asian patients. Type 2 or familial pityriasis rotunda occurs in white patients and presents with more than 30 lesions (usually hypopigmented), and is not associated with any underlying disease.[5] Treatment of underlying disease may lead to resolution of skin lesions in Type 1 patients. In Type 2 patients, spontaneous improvement may be seen by adulthood. Topical treatments, such as retinoids, salicyclic acid, and lactic acid are useful treatments for the dryness and scaling associated with this condition.[5]

TRIPE PALMS

The term *tripe* refers to a rugose surface of the edible lining of a bovine foregut. It was first implicated in a clinical diagnosis of the keratoderma with ridging pattern of the palms and fingers in 1963, when a patient reported to his doctor that his hands looked similar to tripe. Tripe palms was first described in the literature by Clarke in 1977. He reported a patient with squamous cell carcinoma of the lung accompanied by malignant acanthosis nigricans and thickening of the palms in tripe pattern. Tripe palms has been recognized as a cutaneous sign of internal malignancy since then.[6]

EPIDEMIOLOGY

Tripe palms is a rare paraneoplastic dermatosis with approximately 100 cases reported in the literature. The association with malignancy is high, with a greater than 90% occurrence. It is found almost exclusively in adults, and is more common in men than in women.[6]

CLINICAL FEATURES

The palms are rough, thickened, and velvety with exaggerated dermatoglyphics. The texture of the ventral surface of hand and fingers may be moss-like, cobbled, or honeycombed (Fig. 134-3). Tripe palms usually coexists with malignant acanthosis nigricans, observed in approximately 70% of the patients. Several authors suggest that tripe palms may be a form of palmar acanthosis nigricans. The co-occurrence with other paraneoplastic skin lesions, such as florid cutaneous papillomatosis, pruritus, clubbing of the digits, and the sign of Leser-Trélat, can be also seen.[6]

Pulmonary and gastric carcinoma account for more than 50% of neoplasms associated with tripe palms. In patients with only tripe palms, pulmonary carcinoma is the most frequently associated malignancy, especially the squamous cell type. In patients with both tripe palms and acanthosis nigricans, gastric carcinoma is the most common carcinoma, followed by lung carcinoma. Other malignancies less often associated with tripe palms include those of the genitourinary tract, breast, head, and neck.[6,7]

ETIOLOGY AND PATHOGENESIS

Specific mechanisms of development have not been fully elucidated. Similar to acanthosis nigricans (see "Acanthosis Nigricans" section), there is limited evidence for the role of transforming growth factor-α released by tumor cells, inducing cellular proliferation in the pathogenesis of tripe palms. It is believed that tripe palms can be a variant of malignant acanthosis nigricans.[7]

DIAGNOSIS

Histopathology of tripe palms includes hyperkeratosis, acanthosis, and papillomatosis. These features closely resemble those pathologic findings observed in acanthosis nigricans and seborrheic keratoses. Additional findings can include dermal mucin and mast cells in approximately 20% of specimens.

DIFFERENTIAL DIAGNOSIS

The clinical differential diagnosis of tripe palms includes pachydermoperiostosis, hypertrophic pulmonary osteoarthropathy, acromegaly, thyroid acropachy, palmoplantar keratoderma, and acanthosis nigricans.

CLINICAL COURSE AND PROGNOSIS

Paraneoplastic tripe palms can occur before (48%), concurrently (21%), or after (31%) the diagnosis of malignancy. In one-third of patients, tripe palms parallels the course of the associated malignancy. The appearance of tripe palms in a known case of malignancy may be a sign of recurrence or metastasis of the tumor.[6]

MANAGEMENT

A complete malignancy workup, especially to rule out lung and stomach carcinoma, should be performed in all patients with tripe palms because of the high percentage of associated malignancy. A minimum workup should include a medical history, a complete physical examination, routine laboratory studies, a chest roentgenogram, and either a radiographic or an endoscopic evaluation of the upper GI tract. Additional

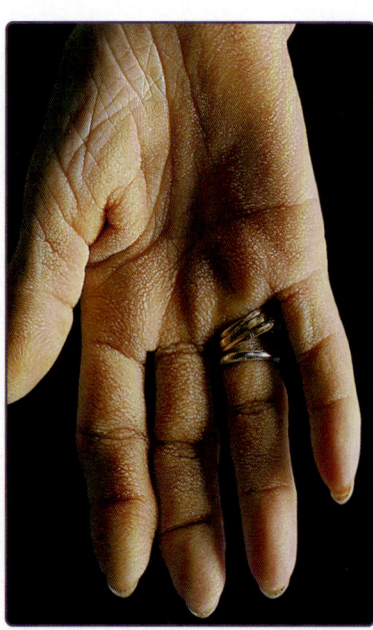

Figure 134-3 Tripe palm. The palmar ridges show maximal accentuation, thus mimicking the mucosa of the stomach of a ruminant.

investigations should be indicated by the findings of the initial workup.

Treatment of tripe palms is difficult and primarily aimed at the underlying malignancy. There is no specific therapy for tripe palms. Similar to acanthosis nigricans, there are anecdotal reports of improvement with oral retinoids alone and in combination with metformin. Approximately 30% of cases of tripe palms will resolve with treatment of the underlying tumor. However, there are many cases where remission of the cancer had no effect.

LESER-TRÉLAT SIGN

AT-A-GLANCE

- Rapid and eruptive increase in number and size of seborrheic keratoses.
- Pruritus is common.
- Often occurs with malignant acanthosis nigricans.
- Adenocarcinomas of the GI tract are the most common associated cancer, followed by lymphoproliferative malignancies.
- Rarely seen in benign conditions, such as pregnancy, HIV, heart transplantation, acromegaly, erythroderma, and drug reaction.

The sign of Leser-Trélat is characterized by the sudden increase in size and number of seborrheic keratoses (SKs) related to internal malignancy. This phenomenon is attributed to Edmund Leser and Ulysse Trélat, two European surgeons, who observed cherry hemangiomas (but not SKs) in patients with cancer in 1890. In 1900, Hollander was the first person who associated the appearance of numerous SKs with internal malignancy.[7,8]

EPIDEMIOLOGY

The sign of Leser-Trélat is a rare paraneoplastic dermatosis that occurs with equal frequency between men and women and among different races. Similar to the occurrence of malignancy, this sign is more common in older individuals.

This entity has remained controversial because the prevalence of both SKs and cancer is increased in the older population. Moreover, the identification of eruptive SKs is often based on the patient's self-reporting which is subjective. In a large population-based study of 1752 consecutive cases of SKs, there was no statistical evidence of an increased incidence of internal malignancy compared to the general population. Subanalysis of those presenting with eruptive SKs also failed to demonstrate an increased risk of internal malignancy. In other large studies of patients with SKs and a recent solid tumor, a comparison with age- and sex-matched controls has not demonstrated a difference in either the clinical features or numbers of SKs.[9] As such, large epidemiologic studies have not provided the evidence needed to conclusively define this sign as a true paraneoplastic dermatosis.

Although large studies have not shown a statistical difference, anecdotal evidence exists demonstrating that this sign may signify an internal malignancy. First, there are reports of eruptive SKs in patients in their 20s with internal malignancies. Clinically, Leser-Trélat sign often coexists with malignant acanthosis nigricans, a more established paraneoplastic phenomenon. Additionally, alterations in growth factor expression differ from control patients. Together, this suggests that the Leser-Trélat sign is a legitimate, but extremely uncommon, paraneoplastic dermatosis.[7,8]

CLINICAL FEATURES

Clinical features signifying a paraneoplastic phenomenon include numerous, widespread, eruptive SKs, predominantly on trunk and extremities. However, quantification of eruptive SKs in terms of length of the eruptive period and number and size of SKs required for the diagnosis is lacking. Individual SKs found in the sign of Leser-Trélat are similar to normal SKs, both clinically and histologically. Pruritus is a significant feature occurring in approximately half of patients. Cooccurrence with other hyperkeratotic paraneoplastic dermatoses is common, with approximately one-third having acanthosis nigricans. There are some case reports of Leser-Trélat sign coexisting with tripe palms as well.[8] The rapid occurrence of pruritic, eruptive SKs, especially in the setting of acanthosis nigricans should alert the clinician to a potential internal malignancy (Fig. 134-4).

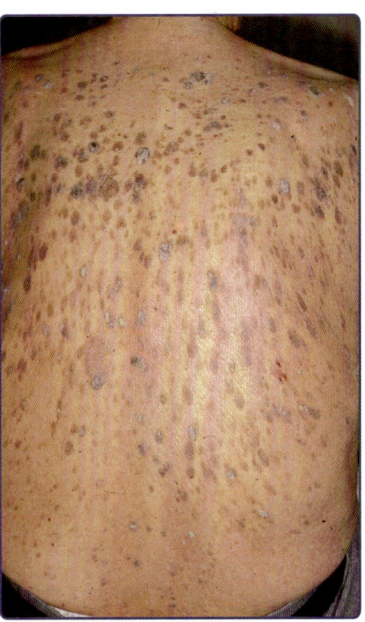

Figure 134-4 Leser-Trélat sign consisting of multiple pruritic eruptive seborrheic keratoses.

Adenocarcinomas account for the majority of malignancies described with the sign of Leser-Trélat, in 32% of which the Leser-Trélat sign is associated with GI tract malignancies, particularly gastric cancer. Lymphoproliferative disorders, including Sézary syndrome, mycosis fungoides, other lymphomas, and leukemia, are the second most common associated malignancies, occurring in approximately 20% of patients. Other tumors, such as lung, bladder, kidney, and ovarian cancers, and melanoma, also have been reported.[7]

A Leser-Trélat–like eruption or eruptive SKs have been rarely reported in the setting of benign conditions, such as pregnancy, HIV, heart transplantation, acromegaly, and erythroderma, and in association with drugs, such as cytarabine and tumor necrosis factor-α inhibitors.[7,10] The term pseudosign of Leser-Trélat has been used to designate nonmalignancy-associated eruptive SKs. Unfortunately, these examples do not help to further define an already confusing and controversial clinical entity.

ETIOLOGY AND PATHOGENESIS

An exact pathogenesis has yet to be elucidated. However, similar to acanthosis nigricans and tripe palms, evidence also exists with the Leser-Trélat sign that an alteration in growth factor homeostasis is contributory. In several instances, a state of increased growth factor expression has been observed, with increased urinary levels of epidermal growth factors and transforming growth factor-α detected in patients with an underlying malignancy and eruptive SKs. Subsequently, growth factor levels decreased following primary tumor resection.[7]

In addition to increased levels of growth factor expression, lesional skin in paraneoplastic acanthosis nigricans and SKs has alterations in the extracellular matrix. It is unknown what the direct impact of growth factor signaling has on the skin. Proposed ideas include either inducing a hyperproliferative state primarily or by altering the surrounding environment such as via the extracellular matrix. These similar mechanisms further support the idea of a continuum between acanthosis nigricans and the Leser-Trélat sign.

DIAGNOSIS

A skin biopsy may be done to confirm the diagnosis. Histopathologic findings of SK in this syndrome are the same as the common SK and include epidermal hyperkeratosis, papillomatosis, and acanthosis with cystic inclusion of keratinous material (horn pseudocysts).

DIFFERENTIAL DIAGNOSIS

Differential diagnosis of the individual skin lesion in this syndrome is the same as for SKs, consisting of fibroepithelial polyp, epidermal nevus, melanocytic nevus, pigmented basal cell carcinoma, squamous cell carcinoma, malignant melanoma, warty dyskeratoma, verruca vulgaris, and condyloma acuminatum. In extensive and generalized SKs, which can appear in older healthy individuals, it is important to distinguish the benign presentation from the signs of Leser-Trélat.

CLINICAL COURSE AND PROGNOSIS

Leser-Trélat sign can develop from approximately 5 months prior to 10 months after the diagnosis of malignancy. More than half of the patients have metastatic tumors at the time of diagnosis. The prognosis is poor, with an estimated survival time of 1 year after diagnosis. This eruption parallels the course of the underlying malignancy in some cases, but not as a general rule.

MANAGEMENT

Treatment should be directed toward the underlying tumor. If the lesions are symptomatic or cosmetically concerning to the patient, local treatment of SK, such as α-hydroxy acids, retinoids, trichloroacetic acid, cryosurgery with or without curettage, dermabrasion, laser, and shave removal, can be performed.

ACROKERATOSIS PARANEOPLASTICA OF BAZEX

AT-A-GLANCE

- Characteristic cutaneous lesions and distribution symmetrically involving the helices, nose, cheeks, digits, and nails.
- Lesions evolve from nonspecific dermatitis and paronychia to inflammatory plaques, acral keratoderma, and nail plate changes.
- Skin lesions often predate detection of internal malignancy.
- Upper aerodigestive tract malignancy is the most common.

Acrokeratosis paraneoplastica of Bazex was first presented in 1965 at the French Dermatological Society. Bazex and his colleagues described a patient with scaly erythematous lesions of the extremities who had a carcinoma of the pyriform fossa, whose skin lesions cleared after treatment of the carcinoma. The lesions were proposed as a cutaneous marker of internal malignancy.[11]

This condition is also known as Bazex syndrome, which is an eponym used to describe 2 different clinical entities. The first refers to *acrokeratosis paraneoplastica of Bazex*, which is discussed in this chapter, and the second is Bazex-Dupré-Christol syndrome, a very rare genodermatosis, characterized by congenital hypotrichosis, follicular atrophoderma, and basal cell carcinomas arising at an early age.

EPIDEMIOLOGY

More than 100 cases of Bazex syndrome have been reported in the medical literature. This condition is highly associated with underlying malignancy. It occurs almost exclusively in males older than age 40 years. Approximately 60% of the associated malignancies are squamous cell carcinomas of the upper aerodigestive tract. The second most common is lung cancer. Other less-common tumor locations are genitourinary and lower GI tract.[12]

CLINICAL FEATURES

The characteristic cutaneous findings are symmetrical erythematous to violaceous scaly patches or plaques over the acral extremities, ears, and bridge of the nose. Hyperpigmentation tends to appear in dark-skinned individuals. Vesicles and bullae are occasionally observed on the hands and feet. A bulbous enlargement of the distal phalanges has been described. The most common sites of involvement are the nails (77%), ears (76%), fingers (65%), nose (62%), palms (56%)/hands (51%), and soles (49%)/feet (44%). Several patients have an additional cutaneous paraneoplastic syndrome, which includes acquired ichthyosis, Leser-Trélat sign, and clubbing.[12] Bazex and Griffiths described 3 stages of skin lesions that parallel the growth and dissemination of the underlying tumor.

In the first stage, the neoplasm is frequently undetected. The helices, nose, fingers, and toes are usually affected in a symmetrical fashion. Early lesions are ill-defined scaly papules, simulating a nonspecific dermatitis. The eruption is classically asymptomatic, but pruritus may be a problem. Paronychia is the first sign of nail involvement (Fig. 134-5) and may be tender. Nail dystrophy, subungual hyperkeratosis, and onycholysis progressing to complete destruction of the nail plate have been reported.

During the second stage, the tumor exhibits symptoms, resulting from local extension or metastatic spread, and the skin eruption becomes more extensive. The typical red-to-purple scaly plaques may involve the whole pinna, cheeks, or upper lip. The palms and soles develop a keratoderma that often spares the central volar surfaces, but may lead to painful fissures (Fig. 134-6). Nail plate changes include yellowing, thickening, onycholysis, and ridging, both horizontal and vertical.

The final stage is observed when the tumor goes untreated or fails to respond to treatment. All of the above signs and symptoms persist as the papulosquamous lesions begin to appear on other sites, such as trunk, elbows, knees, scalp, and dorsal hands and feet. Rarely, vesicles and bullae may be present, most commonly on the fingers, hands, and feet. Nail changes can be quite variable, ranging from the typical thickening to nail atrophy and loss of the nail plate.

ETIOLOGY AND PATHOGENESIS

The pathophysiology of acrokeratosis paraneoplastica remains unclear. Many authors propose an immunologic mechanism in which the antibodies against the tumor crossreact with keratinocyte and basement membrane antigen, or a T cell-mediated immune response to tumor-like antigens in the epidermis. The findings of immunoglobulins (IgG, IgA, IgM) and complement (C3) along the basement membrane zone in some patients have been observed. Some authors also suggest that epidermal growth factor secreted by the tumor may play a role in epidermal hyperplasia

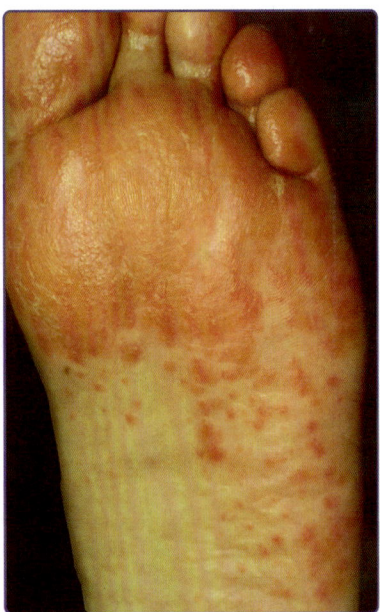

Figure 134-6 Keratoderma characteristically spares central aspects of plantar (and palmar) surfaces in acrokeratosis paraneoplastica.

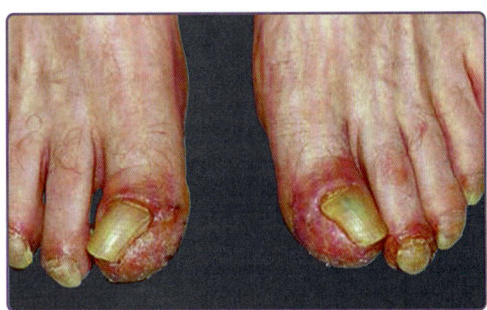

Figure 134-5 Distal edema of toes, painful generalized paronychia, and distal subungual hyperkeratosis in early acrokeratosis paraneoplastica.

and hyperkeratosis, as mentioned in other hyperkeratotic dermatoses in this chapter. Other hypotheses include low serum levels of vitamin A and zinc.[12]

DIAGNOSIS

Histopathology is somewhat nonspecific. Psoriasiform dermatitis is the most common pattern. Hyperkeratosis, parakeratosis, and a superficial lymphohistiocytic infiltrate are the main histopathologic features. The interface changes, including vacuolar degeneration, dyskeratotic keratinocytes, lichenoid infiltrate, and melanin-containing macrophages in the dermis, are reported less frequently.[12]

In the context of histopathologic and characteristic cutaneous findings, acrokeratosis paraneoplastica of Bazex could be a possible diagnosis. If the patients have no history of malignancy, appropriate investigations should be promptly performed.

DIFFERENTIAL DIAGNOSIS

The differential diagnoses include psoriasis, pityriasis rubra pilaris, seborrheic or contact dermatitis, eczematous drug eruption, infections (eg. dermatophytosis, onychomycosis), lupus erythematosus, palmoplantar keratodermas, and mycosis fungoides. The distinguishing clinical feature, which is nearly always present in acrokeratosis paraneoplastica, is involvement of the helices of the ears (Fig. 134-7) and the tip of the nose. Typically, Bazex syndrome is resistant to conventional treatment.

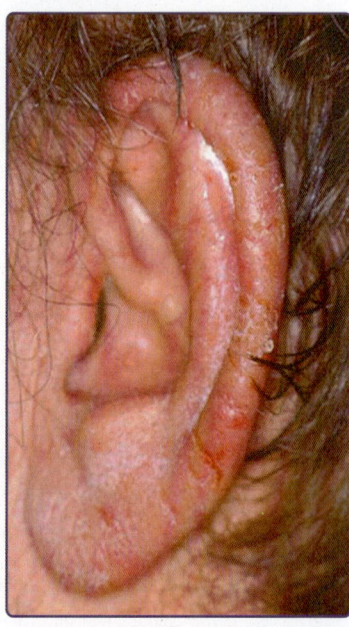

Figure 134-7 Characteristic helical inflammation with scale in acrokeratosis paraneoplastica.

CLINICAL COURSE AND PROGNOSIS

The skin eruption can occur before (67%), simultaneously (18%), or after (15%) the diagnosis of the neoplasm. The cutaneous lesions precede the diagnosis of the tumor by an average of 12 months. Acrokeratosis paraneoplastica is expected to resolve after successful treatment of the underlying malignancy and can reappear with tumor recurrence. However, nail dystrophy and pigmentary skin changes may persist despite significant improvement in the underlying malignancy and other skin lesions.[12]

MANAGEMENT

Treatment of the primary neoplasm is the most effective therapy. The skin lesions are typically resistant to standard therapies for hyperkeratotic conditions and few treatments specific for the cutaneous component of acrokeratosis paraneoplastica have been reported. Systemic retinoids have been used with variable success. Isolated reports suggest benefit from oral psoralen and ultraviolet A phototherapy, topical salicylic acid, and corticosteroids.

COLLAGEN–VASCULAR DISEASE

DERMATOMYOSITIS

Chapter 62, "Dermatomyositis," provides additional information on dermatomyositis.

Adult-onset dermatomyositis (DM) is significantly associated with malignancy. The risk of cancer is higher in DM than in polymyositis alone. Approximately 18% to 25% of patients with adult-onset DM may have malignancy, which is associated with decreased survival. The malignancy may occur before, simultaneously, or after the diagnosis of DM. The course of DM does not always follow the course of the malignancy. In contrast, juvenile-onset DM does not have a strongly increased risk of malignancy.

The clinical manifestations of DM with or without associated malignancy are similar. Previous studies reported predictive signs of accompanying malignancy, such as cutaneous necrosis, cutaneous vasculitis, lack of interstitial lung disease, dysphagia, male gender, elevated erythrocyte sedimentation rate, and an older age at onset. However, some of these findings are inconsistent and remain controversial. Recently, anti-p155 antibodies have been reported as a promising cancer marker in adult patients with DM.

Types of associated malignancies vary among studies and may reflect differences in malignancy risk across different populations. Lung, breast, ovarian, cervical, pancreatic, gastric, colorectal, and prostate malignancies are frequently reported; hematologic malignancies may also occur in association with DM. It has been noted that nasopharyngeal carcinoma is more common in the Asian population.[13]

In adult patients with DM, the risk of malignancy is highest in the first year after diagnosis, then steadily declines and remains slightly elevated even after 5 years. Therefore, all adult patients with DM should be evaluated for malignancy at the time of diagnosis, followed by long-term surveillance. There is no definitive guidelines for cancer screening in patients with DM. Most authors recommend an initial screening that includes a comprehensive history and physical examination (including a pelvic examination in women), standard laboratory tests (complete blood count, complete metabolic panel, urinalysis, stool occult blood testing), and chest radiography. Further investigation is directed by any abnormal findings. Some clinicians also recommend a colonoscopy and CT scans of the chest, abdomen, and pelvis. Additional age-, gender-, and ethnicity-appropriate malignancy screening, including a transvaginal pelvic sonography, Papanicolaou smear, and mammography for female patients, or an evaluation by an ear-nose-throat physician to exclude nasopharyngeal carcinoma for patients of Asian descent, should be considered.[13]

PROGRESSIVE SYSTEMIC SCLEROSIS

Chapter 63, "Systemic Sclerosis," provides additional information on progressive systemic sclerosis.

The majority of epidemiologic studies reveal an increased risk of cancer in patients with progressive systemic sclerosis (PSS) compared with general population, and demonstrated that men are at higher risk than women. The frequency of malignancy is approximately 3% to 11%.[14] The risk of cancer is higher within the first 12 months after a PSS diagnosis, and may be a paraneoplastic phenomenon. However, other studies included in a newer metaanalysis did not demonstrate an increase in the risk of cancer.[15]

Lung, bladder, breast, liver, esophageal, and oropharyngeal carcinoma, nonmelanoma skin cancer, and hematologic malignancies have been frequently reported in association with PSS. Lung cancer is the most frequent type of cancer in most studies, and may be associated with the presence of interstitial lung disease, as well as with history of smoking. Interestingly, there is a 25-fold increased incidence of tongue cancer in one U.S. study.[14,16]

This increased risk of cancer could be the result of damage from chronic inflammation and fibrosis, immunosuppressive therapies for PSS, an environmental exposure, and/or a genetic susceptibility to the development of both cancer and autoimmunity. Although the data are controversial, some studies suggest that the risk of cancer may be greater in patients with diffuse cutaneous disease. Several newer studies confirm an increased risk of cancer-associated PSS in patients with RNA polymerase III autoantibodies or an older age of PSS onset. These groups of patients may benefit from aggressive malignancy screening at diagnosis and long-term cancer surveillance.[16]

REACTIVE ERYTHEMAS

ERYTHEMA GYRATUM REPENS

Chapter 46, "Erythema Annulare Centrifugum and Other Figurate Erythemas," provides additional information on erythema gyratum repens.

This particular annular (*gyratum* is Latin for circle) erythema was thought to be one of the most specific dermatoses associated with underlying neoplasia. However, newer data demonstrate a higher proportion of associated benign conditions than previously reported. Erythema gyratum repens is a rare disease that presents with dramatic appearance and evolution. Nearly 100 cases are reported in the literature. It mostly affects adults in their 60s, men more than women (ratio: 2:1).

Numerous serpiginous bands are arranged in a parallel configuration of concentric red swirls over most of the body. This presentation is occasionally referred to as a "wood-grain" appearance (Fig. 134-8). Even more striking is the relatively rapid rate at which lesions migrate (*repens* is Latin for creeping), estimated at 1 cm per day. A fine scale may be found along the trailing edge of erythema (Fig. 134-9). The hands, feet, and face are commonly spared, except for occasional volar hyperkeratosis. Ichthyosis is

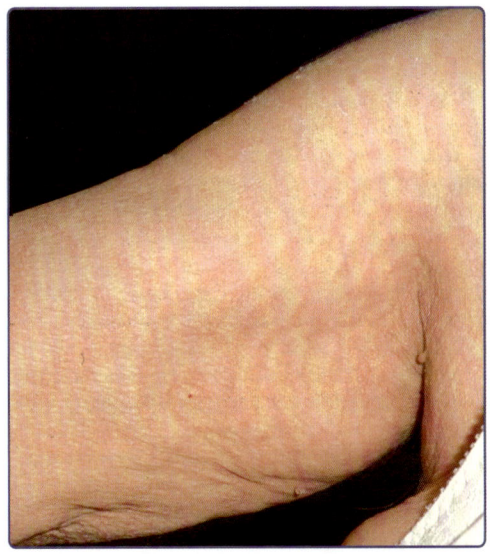

Figure 134-8 Erythema gyratum repens. Serpiginous parallel bands on axilla and arm. (Used with permission from Michael Adler.)

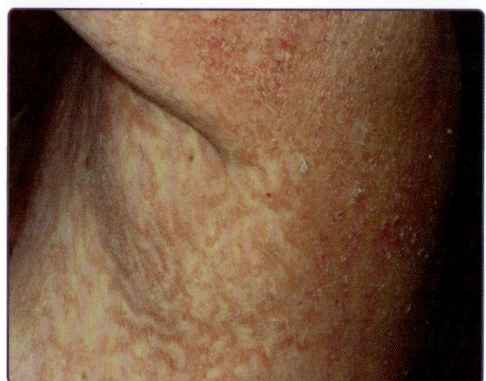

Figure 134-9 Erythema gyratum repens. Characteristic "wood-grain" pattern of erythema and slight scale in a woman with breast cancer. (Used with permission from Jill McKenzie, MD.)

present in many cases. Pruritus is universal and may be severe.[17]

An underlying malignancy is associated with erythema gyratum repens approximately 70% of the time. In more than 80% of cases, the cutaneous eruption appears before the diagnosis of malignancy with a mean period of 7 months (range: 1 to 72 months), but it can occur simultaneously or after the diagnosis of malignancy. Among patients with associated carcinoma, almost half of cases have lung cancer, whereas 8% have stomach cancer, 7% have esophageal cancer, and 5% have breast cancer. Individual case reports of many other types of associated tumors are published, as well as 5% of cases with an unknown primary. In those individuals with erythema gyratum repens who did not have a detectible underlying malignancy; some cases were idiopathic; some presented with concurrent conditions including concomitant skin disease (pityriasis rubra pilaris, psoriasis, ichthyosis), connective tissue disease (CREST [calcinosis cutis, Raynaud phenomenon, esophageal motility disorder, sclerodactyly, and telangiectasia] syndrome, rheumatoid arthritis), infection (tuberculosis), hypereosinophilic syndrome, or drug reaction (azathioprine).[18]

The exact etiology of erythema gyratum repens is unknown, but it has been suggested that the tumor may induce a chemical alteration of the normal components of the surrounding tissue. Molecular mimicry ensues as the inflammatory response directed against the tumor crossreacts with benign cutaneous proteins. This theory is supported by documentation of IgG and C3 deposition at the basement membrane of affected skin and bronchial basement membrane in one case associated with lung cancer. Migration characterizes all of the figurate erythemas, but is notably rapid in erythema gyratum repens. The mechanism for this is not clear, although some studies have focused on fibroblast activity. Inflammatory cells and/or fibroblasts may mediate ground substance alterations, which may localize the inflammation that orchestrates the movement of the infiltrate in a patterned mode.[17]

Treatment of erythema gyratum repens involves locating and treating the primary malignancy. With adequate control of the cancer the rash usually abates, but this may not be possible in cases that are widely metastatic at the time of diagnosis. Otherwise, the eruption is often treatment resistant, although variable results occur with systemic steroids. Topical steroids, vitamin A, and azathioprine have not been beneficial. The eruption has been known to resolve immediately before death, possibly because of generalized ante mortem immunosuppression.[17]

NECROLYTIC MIGRATORY ERYTHEMA

AT-A-GLANCE

- Painful, eroded, crusted intertriginous, and facial skin eruption.
- Highly suggestive of pancreatic malignancy (glucagonoma).
- Half of tumors are metastatic at the time of diagnosis.
- Pseudoglucagonoma syndrome occurs in absence of glucagonoma.
- Skin improves with treatment of underlying nutritional aberrations.

In 1942, Becker first described a patient with cutaneous eruptions in association with α-cell pancreatic tumor. In 1966, McGavran found another patient with similar clinical presentation and had hyperglucagonemia. Later, necrolytic migratory erythema (NME) was coined by Wilkinson in 1973 to describe the distinctive rash in patients with pancreatic cancer.[19]

EPIDEMIOLOGY

NME is a very rare paraneoplastic skin disorder that is considered a hallmark of glucagonoma and is present in more than two-thirds of patients at the time of tumor diagnosis.[19] Glucagonoma is an extremely rare, slow-growing neuroendocrine tumor of the α cells of the pancreas. The global incidence is approximately 1 in every 20 million people. It typically presents with glucagonoma syndrome.[2] There is no gender or race predilection, and it most commonly affects people in their sixth decade.

CLINICAL FEATURES

The skin lesions of NME are polymorphous, but erosions and crusts are usually apparent. Primary lesions are erythematous patches that evolve into plaques and develop central bullae. The blisters erode rapidly, form crusts, and eventually resolve. The erythematous and eroded annular patches and plaques coalesce into large geographic areas. They are typically painful and pruritic. The eruption disappears and reappears spontaneously over the course of weeks. The distribution of NME is characteristic and includes intertriginous areas (eg. groin, perineum, buttocks, and lower abdomen), the central face (especially perioral), and distal extremities (Fig. 134-10). Mucosal involvement manifests as angular cheilitis, atrophic glossitis, and stomatitis. Dystrophic nails may accompany the syndrome.[19,20]

Glucagonoma syndrome is characterized by NME, weight loss, sore mouth, diarrhea, diabetes mellitus, deep vein thrombosis, normochromic normocytic anemia, and neuropsychiatric disorders. Weight loss is the most common presenting sign. The glucagonoma tends to grow slowly. Metastasis to the liver, regional lymph nodes, and bone is common, but appears in late stage of the disease. Pseudoglucagonoma syndrome presents identically, but the α cell pancreatic tumor is not present, which may explain why the serum glucagon levels are not elevated. Underlying diseases identified in patients with the pseudosyndrome include liver disease, pancreatitis, celiac sprue, inflammatory bowel disease, acrodermatitis enteropathica, pellagra, and nonpancreatic malignancies.[19,20]

Because NME can be the first manifestation of the syndromes, early recognition is important and may provide a better outcome.

ETIOLOGY AND PATHOGENESIS

The exact cause of NME remains unclear. The skin rash can be attributed to the metabolic effects of excess glucagon, as resolution of the rash can occur after surgical removal of the glucagonoma or normalizing the glucagon level with medication. Hyperglucagonemia stimulates hepatic gluconeogenesis leading to an increase in blood glucose level. The amino acid consumption in gluconeogenesis pathway contributes to a decrease in serum amino acid. Hypoaminoacidemia resulting in epidermal protein deficiency (histidine and tryptophan) may provoke epidermal necrosis. Glucagon also increases cutaneous levels of arachidonic acid, prostaglandins, and leukotrienes, which may induce a cutaneous inflammatory reaction. However, NME cannot be completely attributed to hyperglucagonemia, because it may appear without elevated levels of glucagon or a pancreatic tumor, as reported in pseudoglucagonoma syndrome. Deficiency of zinc, protein, essential fatty acid, and vitamin B may also play a role in NME development.[20]

DIAGNOSIS

The histopathology of NME is characteristic, but not pathognomonic. Acute lesions exhibit a striking degree of epidermal necrosis in the upper layers of the stratum spinosum and may detach from the viable epidermis underneath. Neutrophiic infiltrates in the necrotic layer resulting in subcorneal pustules can be observed. Chronic lesions show a psoriasiform dermatitis. Parakeratosis, loss of granular layers, basal vacuolization, and scattered necrotic keratinocytes may be demonstrated. These findings can be also seen in other nutritional deficiencies, graft-versus-host disease, connective tissue disorders, and phototoxic drug eruptions.[19,20]

Laboratory abnormalities include a dramatically elevated serum glucagon, usually greater than 1000 pg/mL (reference range: 50 to 150 pg/mL). Most patients have hyperglycemia and a normochromic normocytic anemia. Abnormal liver function is present and serum levels of amino acids, total protein, albumin, and cholesterol are low. Occasionally, zinc levels are also decreased. Imaging studies should be performed to detect the pancreatic tumor. Various methods, such as angiography, ultrasonography, CT, MRI, positron emission tomography, octreotide scintigraphy, and somatostatin receptor scintigraphy, have been used to identify the pancreatic tumor.[20]

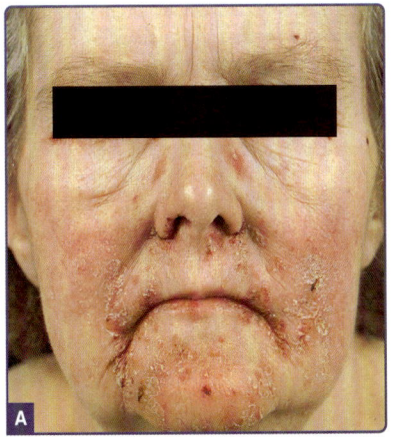
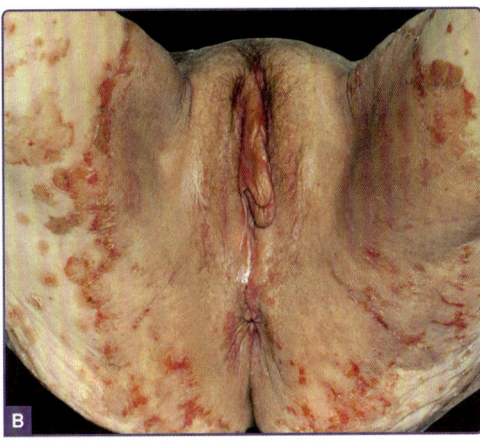

Figure 134-10 The glucagonoma syndrome, necrolytic migratory erythema. Flaccid and papulovesicular lesions (**A**) with erosions, crusting, and fissures around the orifices, and (**B**) appearing as geographic, circinate "necrolytic migratory erythema" in the groin. (**A** and **B** are not the same patient.)

DIFFERENTIAL DIAGNOSIS

Other disorders with cutaneous manifestations similar to NME include acrodermatitis enteropathica, nutritional deficiencies, psoriasis, eczema, seborrheic dermatitis, candidiasis, superficial pemphigus, and side effects of certain chemotherapies.

CLINICAL COURSE AND PROGNOSIS

In NME associated with glucagonoma syndrome, the course of the disease varies according to the stage at which the tumor is diagnosed. If the glucagonoma is not metastatic and can be completely resected, symptoms of the syndrome will resolve. Unfortunately, by the time of diagnosis, tumors are frequently large and metastatic in most cases. Fortunately, the tumors are slow growing and patients may experience symptom improvement by surgically reducing the tumor burden, although survival may not be affected by the procedure.

MANAGEMENT

The underlying cause for hyperglucagonemia must be addressed to eradicate the painful skin disease. For patients with glucagonoma, resection of the tumor is important for symptom relief. Complete surgical removal can be curative if the tumor is confined to the pancreas. This tumor is often resistant to chemotherapy. Somatostatin analog (octreotide, pasireotide, and lanreotide) improves the cutaneous symptoms and may delay tumor progression. Other therapeutic modalities, such as interferon, everolimus (mammalian target of rapamycin inhibitor), sunitinib (tyrosine kinase inhibitor), and peptide receptor radionuclide therapy, have been reported with favorable results. Supplementation to correct zinc, amino acid, or fatty acid deficiencies improves skin lesions in some cases.[19]

NEUTROPHILIC DERMATOSES

SWEET SYNDROME

Chapter 36, "Sweet Syndrome," provides additional information on Sweet syndrome.

Sweet syndrome, also known as acute febrile neutrophilic dermatosis, is characterized by fever, leukocytosis, and skin papules or plaques caused by dermal neutrophils. Malignancy is reported in approximately 21% of patients diagnosed with Sweet syndrome, either hematologic (15%) or solid (6%) malignancy. The most commonly-associated hematologic malignancy is acute myeloblastic leukemia. Other hematologic neoplasms include myeloproliferative neoplasms, diffuse large B-cell lymphoma, Hodgkin lymphoma, myelodysplastic syndrome, and myelofibrosis. The most common solid malignancies associated with Sweet syndrome are carcinomas of the genitourinary organs, breast, and GI tract, most frequently adenocarcinomas (57%).[21] Several authors proposed the features to distinguish malignancy-associated Sweet syndrome from the classical form of the disease. Malignancy-associated Sweet syndrome is less-often preceded by upper respiratory tract infection, and the onset is temporally associated with the new discovery or relapse of cancer. In addition, there is no sex preponderance, whereas female sex is predominant in the classical form.[22]

Clinically, bullous and ulcerated skin lesions, subcutaneous nodules, and oral mucosal involvement may be more frequently observed in malignancy-associated than in classical Sweet syndrome. Laboratory abnormalities, including anemia (82% to 83%) and abnormal platelet count (68%), are reported in malignancy-associated Sweet syndrome. Although peripheral leukocytosis is one of the diagnostic criteria of Sweet syndrome, neutropenia can be observed in some patients with malignancy-associated Sweet syndrome. A small number of patients with hematologic malignancy demonstrate leukemia cutis concurrently with Sweet syndrome in lesional skin biopsy.[21,22]

The onset of Sweet syndrome can precede, follow, or appear concurrently with the diagnosis of a patient's neoplasm. The duration of Sweet syndrome is variable. Recurrence of lesions can occur not only in malignancy-affected patients, but also in individuals with either idiopathic or disease-associated Sweet syndrome. There are no specific guidelines for the treatment of malignancy-associated Sweet syndrome. Systemic corticosteroid and other standard treatments that are used in classical or idiopathic sweet syndrome are the mainstay of therapy. Successful treatment of underlying malignancy may result in complete resolution of malignancy-associated Sweet syndrome, and the reappearance of dermatologic findings may signify relapse of cancer.[21,22]

PYODERMA GANGRENOSUM

Chapter 37, "Pyoderma Gangrenosum," provides additional information on pyoderma gangrenosum.

Pyoderma gangrenosum (PG) is a rare, painful, ulcerating neutrophilic dermatosis associated with various internal diseases. The incidence of malignancy in patients with PG varies among studies, occurring in approximately 4% to 20% of PG patients.[23]

Hematologic malignancy is the most common associated neoplasm; other associated malignancies include acute and chronic myelogenous leukemia, chronic lymphocytic leukemia, multiple myeloma, myelodysplastic syndrome, polycythemia vera, Hodgkin lymphoma, and cutaneous T-cell lymphoma. Atypical features of PG, such as abrupt onset, superficial lesions, hemorrhagic bullae, and involvement of the upper extremities have been described in 27% of PG patients with underlying hematologic disease or malignancy.[24] Improvement of bullous PG with treatment of the underlying malignancy has been documented.

Monoclonal gammopathy of undetermined significance has been described by several authors as an associated condition with PG, with IgA as the most frequently associated paraproteinemia.[23] These gammopathies are clinically benign, but they occasionally progress to myeloma. Therefore, long-term monitoring is recommended.

Underlying solid tumors can also occur in patients with PG. Cancers of various organs, such as breast, prostate, lung, bladder, colon, liver, ovary, larynx, glioblastoma multiforme, and melanoma, have been occasionally reported.[23]

DERMAL PROLIFERATIVE DISORDERS

MULTICENTRIC RETICULOHISTIOCYTOSIS

Chapter 117, "Histiocytosis," provides additional information on multicentric reticulohistiocytosis.

Multicentric reticulohistiocytosis (MRH) is a rare, systemic disease presenting with destructive polyarthritis and typical cutaneous lesions. The isolated or grouped reddish brown to skin-colored papules and nodules are seen predominantly on the face and hands with a characteristic "coral bead" appearance of periungual papules. Up to 25% of patients have associated malignancies, and in some cases the diagnosis of multicentric reticulohistiocytosis precedes the diagnosis of cancer.[25]

There is no predominant type of associated cancer in this disease. Various neoplasms, including breast, lung, thyroid, GI, urogenital, sarcoma, lymphoma, leukemia, and melanoma, have been reported. The course of the disease may be self limtied without joint deformity; waxing and waning; or aggressive with mutilating arthritis. Spontaneous remission usually occurs after many years. It does not run a parallel course with the associated malignancy in the majority of patients. Treatment of the accompanying cancer will resolve joint and skin disease only in some reported cases. It is still debated among several authors whether to label multicentric reticulohistiocytosis as a paraneoplastic disorder. Regardless, a complete workup for underlying malignancy should be performed in every patient diagnosed with multicentric reticulohistiocytosis.[26]

NECROBIOTIC XANTHOGRANULOMA

Chapter 57, "Intercellular IgA Dermatosis (IgA Pemphigus)," provides additional information on necrobiotic xanthogranuloma.

Necrobiotic xanthogranuloma is a rare, non–Langerhans cell histiocytosis with a strong association with hematologic disorders. The skin is the most common site of involvement and more than 80% of patients have periorbital lesions. Extracutaneous involvement is rare. The lesions appear as yellowish to red-orange or violaceous papules, plaques, or nodules, with areas of ulceration, telangiectasia, or atrophy. Most of the cases are asymptomatic with an indolent course.

Up to 80% of patients have monoclonal gammopathy of IgG type with either a κ or λ light chain.[27] The most common associated plasma cell dyscrasias are monoclonal gammopathies of undetermined significance, smoldering multiple myeloma, and multiple myeloma. Other hematologic abnormalities, including non-Hodgkin lymphoma, chronic lymphocytic leukemia, Hodgkin lymphoma, and lymphoplasmacytic lymphoma, may occur in association with necrobiotic xanthogranuloma.[27]

Patients with necrobiotic xanthogranuloma associated with monoclonal gammopathy are at risk of conversion to multiple myeloma. Consequently, careful monitoring should be continued for early detection of disease progression.[27]

DERMAL DEPOSITION

SCLEROMYXEDEMA

Chapter 67, "Scleredema and Scleromyxedema," provides additional information on scleromyxedema.

Scleromyxedema, the generalized form of papular mucinosis (lichen myxedematosus), is an uncommon disease associated with monoclonal gammopathy and systemic organ involvement. The typical cutaneous manifestations have a predilection for the face, arms, and hands. Cardiopulmonary, rheumatologic, GI, and neurologic involvement is common. The majority (80%) of patients with scleromyxedema has an IgGλ light chain monoclonal gammopathy of undetermined significance. Serum protein electrophoresis should be performed in conjunction with thyroid studies to rule out thyroid dysfunction and myxedema. Fortunately, the paraproteinemia only rarely converts to multiple myeloma, but when it occurs, it portends a poor prognosis. There are several case reports of other hematologic and nonhematologic malignancies among patients with scleromyxedema, including leukemia, Hodgkin or non-Hodgkin lymphoma, and some solid tumors. However, it is uncertain if some of the associated malignancies are incidental or associated with the treatment of scleromyxedema with agents, such as melphalan as a secondary malignancy.[28] The course of the disease is usually progressive and major systemic organ involvement may contribute to poor outcome.

SYSTEMIC AMYLOIDOSIS

Chapter 124, "The Porphyrias," provides additional information on systemic amyloidosis.

Primary systemic amyloidosis is referred to as AL

amyloidosis, in which there is extracellular deposition of fibrils of monoclonal immunoglobulin light chain typically produced by a small plasma cell clone. Secondary (AA) amyloidosis occurs with autoimmune or inflammatory diseases, malignancies, and chronic infections. Skin manifestations of systemic amyloidosis include "pinch purpura" (periorbital bruising), macroglossia, and, less commonly, waxy skin thickening and subcutaneous nodules.

AL amyloidosis is the most common form associated with malignancy. The prognosis is generally poor, with median survival time if left untreated of 12 months. In AL amyloidosis, multiple organs and tissues (kidney, heart, liver, peripheral/autonomic nerve, soft tissue) are generally involved. It is important to distinguish the skin lesions in systemic AL amyloidosis from the less-common, localized, cutaneous variant, which does not progress to multisystem involvement.

Multiple myeloma is the most common associated malignancy, and is seen in approximately 20% of patients with AL amyloidosis.[29] Other neoplasms, such as non-Hodgkin lymphoma, mucosa-associated lymphoid tissue lymphoma, lymphoplasmacytic lymphoma, and other single case reports of solid-organ tumors, have been rarely reported. For all patients with suspected AL amyloidosis, serum and urine protein electrophoresis/immunofixation electrophoresis, serum free light chain assay, bone marrow biopsy, and skeletal imaging should be performed at baseline to rule out the presence of multiple myeloma.[30]

Some investigators have described an increased risk of non-Hodgkin lymphoma in transthyretin amyloidosis (ATTR).[31] In addition, certain neoplasms, such as hepatocellular carcinoma, renal cell carcinoma, Castleman disease, Hodgkin disease, and adult hairy cell leukemia, can cause reactive or secondary (AA) amyloidosis.[30]

BULLOUS DISORDERS

PARANEOPLASTIC PEMPHIGUS

Chapter 53, "Paraneoplastic Pemphigus," provides additional information on paraneoplastic pemphigus.

Paraneoplastic pemphigus is a life-threatening condition with a high mortality rate. Painful, hemorrhagic oral erosions are the earliest characteristic clinical finding. The polymorphous skin eruption, composed of pemphigus-like, bullous pemphigoid–like, erythema multiforme–like, graft-versus-host disease–like and lichen planus–like skin lesions, may involve any site. Multiorgan involvement, such as of the lung, thyroid, kidney, smooth muscle, and GI tract, is documented. The pathogenesis of paraneoplastic pemphigus involves both cellular and humoral immunity. Nearly all patients have an underlying neoplasm, most frequently a lymphoproliferative disease. The most commonly reported associated neoplasms are non-Hodgkin lymphoma, chronic lymphocytic leukemia, Castleman disease, and thymoma. The prognosis is poor in patients with malignancy-associated paraneoplastic pemphigus but may be better in patients with benign tumors.[32]

DERMATITIS HERPETIFORMIS

Chapter 59, "Dermatitis Herpetiformis," provides additional information on dermatitis herpetiformis.

Dermatitis herpetiformis is an autoimmune skin condition that presents as a severely pruritic skin eruption with polymorphous lesions and is associated with gluten sensitivity. The majority of studies have demonstrated a significantly increased risk of non-Hodgkin lymphoma in patients with dermatitis herpetiformis, even though the risk of malignancy overall is similar to general population.[33,34] It has been noticed that patients with longstanding dermatitis herpetiformis are at particular risk. The reported frequency of associated malignancy in patients with dermatitis herpetiformis is up to 4.3%, predominantly in males.[33] However, patients with dermatitis herpetiformis do not appear to have an increased mortality rate despite this association with non-Hodgkin lymphoma.[33,34]

The lymphomas associated with dermatitis herpetiformis can be either B-cell or T-cell lymphomas, and may occur both in and outside the GI tract as nodal or extranodal disease. In addition, the enteropathy-associated T-cell lymphoma, typically associated with celiac disease, has been reported in dermatitis herpetiformis patients.[34] A gluten-free diet may protect against the development of cancer, but more studies are needed to confirm this finding.[33,34]

BULLOUS PEMPHIGOID

Chapter 54, "Bullous Pemphigoid," provides additional information on bullous pemphigoid.

Bullous pemphigoid (BP) is an autoimmune blistering disorder that presents in elderly patients with intact skin blisters and pruritus. It remains debated whether there is an increased risk of malignancy in bullous pemphigoid, other than the risk related to the age of the patient. Several studies, including newer large epidemiologic studies, have not found an association between bullous pemphigoid and cancer. Other studies, however, especially from Japan, demonstrated a higher risk of malignancy in bullous pemphigoid patients, compared to the normal population. Many authors discourage a routine cancer screening in bullous pemphigoid patients, except in early-onset pemphigoid, history of malignancy, or standard treatment failure.[35]

MISCELLANEOUS

HYPERTRICHOSIS LANUGINOSA ACQUISITA

Acquired hypertrichosis lanuginosa ("malignant down") is a rare condition characterized by the relatively-sudden appearance of long, fine, nonpigmented lanugo (Latin for *down*) hairs. The lanugo hairs most frequently appear on the face and ears early in the course (Fig. 134-11). The hairs may grow to an impressive length; eyebrows and eyelashes may grow to inches long. The long fine hairs also may be seen on the trunk and limbs, including the axillae, but the palms, soles, suprapubic, and genital areas are usually spared. Acquired hypertrichosis lanuginosa often develops in a cephalocaudal direction and may be accompanied by glossitis, hypertrophy of tongue papillae, oral hyperpigmentation, disturbances of taste and smell, acanthosis nigricans, diarrhea, adenopathy, and weight loss.[36]

This condition is frequently paraneoplastic and can be a marker of an underlying malignancy. It usually appears in advanced or metastasized carcinomas, and thus has a poor prognosis. The most commonly associated malignancies are lung and colorectal cancer in men, and colorectal cancer followed by lung and breast cancer in women. Ovary, uterus, and urinary bladder carcinoma, lymphoma, and leukemia also have been found in patients with acquired hypertrichosis lanuginosa, as have other malignancies.[37]

Acquired hypertrichosis lanuginosa must be distinguished from hirsutism and hypertrichosis associated with nonmalignant causes, including metabolic and endocrine diseases, such as anorexia nervosa, thyrotoxicosis, and porphyria cutanea tarda (see Chap. 124), or medications such as cyclosporine, phenytoin, penicillamine, spironolactone, psoralens, corticosteroids, interferon, diazoxide, or minoxidil.[36,37]

Patients presenting with acquired hypertrichosis lanuginosa without history of drug administration or underlying metabolic and endocrine or malignant diseases, should be suspected of an underlying cancer. Appropriate diagnostic evaluations for the occult malignancy, especially of the lung, colon, rectum areas, and breast, should be considered.

TROUSSEAU SYNDROME

The definition of Trousseau syndrome has evolved over time. It originally described the occurrence of migratory thrombophlebitis associated with underlying gastric cancer. Later, it was expanded by several authors to include cancer-associated hypercoagulability with a wide range of clinical manifestations, including abnormal coagulation tests without clinical symptoms, superficial migratory thrombophlebitis, deep vein thrombosis, marantic endocarditis, pulmonary embolism, and massive thromboembolic phenomenon associated with disseminated intravascular coagulation. Venous thromboembolism (VTE) seems to be the most frequent clinical manifestation.[38]

Clinically, VTE in patients with malignancy can be more severe and more extensive than in patients without malignancy. Deep vein thrombosis of unusual sites, such as upper limbs, thrombosis of visceral organs and brain, and arterial thromboembolism have been reported to occur in cancer-associated cases. Trousseau syndrome composes approximately 20% to 30% of all VTE patients, and occurs in 1% to 8% of patients with underlying malignancy. The incidence has increased, possibly as a result of the more frequent use of newer thrombogenic chemotherapeutic and immunomodulatory agents (eg, thalidomide or lenalidomide) and the longer survival period in cancer patients. Unfortunately, VTE is the second most common cause of death in patients with cancer. Patients with active cancer have a 4 to 7 times higher risk of thrombosis than the normal population, and the risk is highest in certain cancers, such as pancreatic, brain, lung, stomach, and ovarian cancers.[38-40]

Although the pathogenesis of Trousseau syndrome in cancer patients is unclear, multiple factors are likely to be involved in the thrombogenic process. The combination of abnormal blood flow or stasis, vessel wall injury, and blood hypercoagulability, referred to as the *Virchow triad*, contributes to thrombus formation. Several studies have described the overexpression of tissue factor by tumor cells and the increase of plasma microparticles, which are involved in the coagulation pathway. Chemotherapy and tumor necrosis may induce inflammatory cytokines resulting in endothelial cell injury. Neutrophil extracellular traps (NETs), released as a result of neutrophil programmed cell

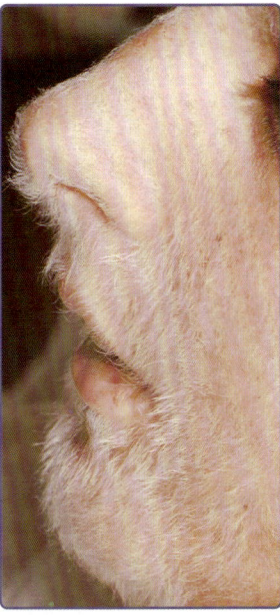

Figure 134-11 Hypertrichosis lanuginosa acquisita in a 19-year-old woman with pancreatic carcinoma.

death (NETosis), have effects on the intrinsic coagulation pathway. Moreover, several investigators have documented specific signaling pathways that contribute to the procoagulant phenotype of cancer cells, resulting from mutations in oncogenes (eg, K-*ras*, EGFR, PML/RAR-α, MET) and tumor suppressor genes (eg, *p53*, *PTEN*).[38,40]

As Trousseau syndrome can be a presenting manifestation of an occult cancer, several authors suggest an age-specific and sex-specific malignancy screening test in patients with idiopathic VTE. Treatment of the underlying malignancy along with anticoagulant therapy is recommended. Low-molecular-weight heparin is the first-line treatment.

GENETIC SYNDROMES INVOLVING SKIN AND/OR MUCOUS MEMBRANES AND ASSOCIATED WITH MALIGNANCY

It is important for clinicians to recognize cutaneous features of genetic conditions that predispose to internal malignancy. In several cases, cutaneous features predate the development of malignancy and increased surveillance may improve overall survival in these patients. For malignancies associated with a genodermatosis, there may be an increased risk for family members to develop cancer and appropriate genetic counseling and testing should be considered.

Table 134-2 outlines the characteristic cutaneous findings and the major associated internal malignancies for the genodermatoses with cancer susceptibility.[41-46]

DIRECT TUMOR INVOLVEMENT OF THE SKIN

CUTANEOUS METASTASES

Cutaneous metastases represent involvement of the skin by metastatic spread of a distant primary tumor. The overall incidence of cutaneous involvement is approximately 5%. The most common malignancies to metastasize to the skin in women are breast cancer, followed by colon cancer and melanoma. In men, the most common are lung cancer, followed by colon cancer and melanoma.[47]

Cutaneous metastases most commonly appear as a rapid onset of solitary or multiple, asymptomatic, skin-colored, mobile, firm, round or oval nodule(s). Metastatic breast cancer can present with various forms of skin lesions. For example, carcinoma erysipelatoides, presents with warm, tender erythematous patches or plaques resembling erysipelas or cellulitis (Fig. 134-12A), but without fever or leukocytosis. Another clinical variant is the leather-like skin changes of sclerosing metastatic breast cancer, known as carcinoma en cuirasse, which may later present as nodules and ulceration (Fig. 134-12B, C). Although carcinoma en cuirasse has been reported as the presenting sign of breast cancer, it more commonly occurs as a local recurrence after treatment of an underlying breast cancer. Both carcinoma erysipelatoides and carcinoma en cuirasse are not restricted to breast cancer; they also can be seen in lung, kidney, GI tract, and other metastasizing malignancies.[48] Metastases from malignant melanoma are usually pigmented (Fig. 134-13). Often there is a bluish tint to the lesion, even if it is deep in the skin. However, even if the primary tumor was pigmented, the metastases may be amelanotic and vice versa.

The thorax is the most common site for cutaneous metastasis, as a result of the high frequency of metastatic breast and lung cancers. The scalp is another common site, for metastases from lung (Fig. 134-14), kidney, and breast tumors. On the scalp, the metastatic tumors typically present as single or multiple firm nodules, but scarring alopecia, known as *alopecia neoplastica*, can be occasionally seen, especially from

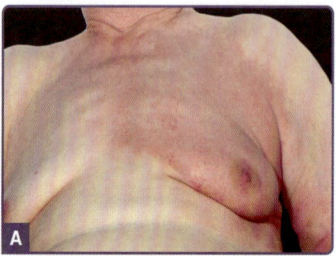

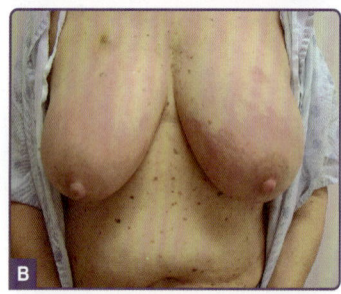

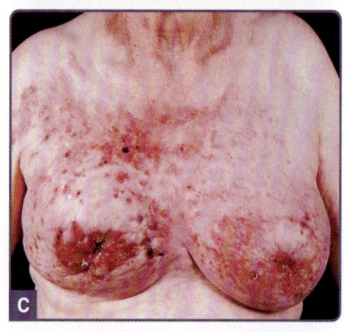

Figure 134-12 **A,** Carcinoma erysipelatoides. Intralymphatic spread of mammary carcinoma that manifests as erysipelas-like erythema. **B,** Bilateral cutaneous metastases from underlying breast carcinoma. **C,** Carcinoma en cuirasse involving both breasts and thoracic wall.

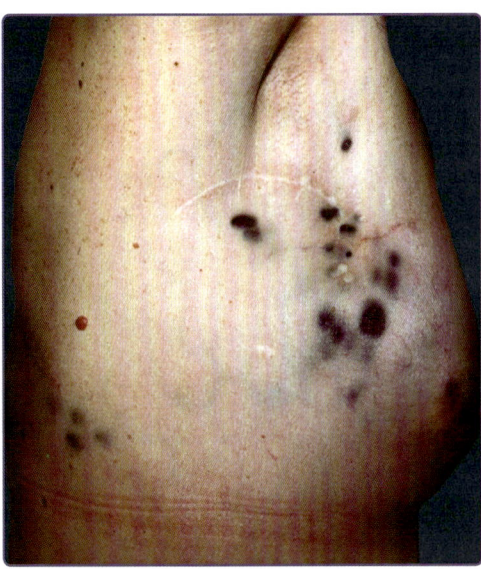

Figure 134-13 Deeply pigmented cutaneous metastases from melanoma.

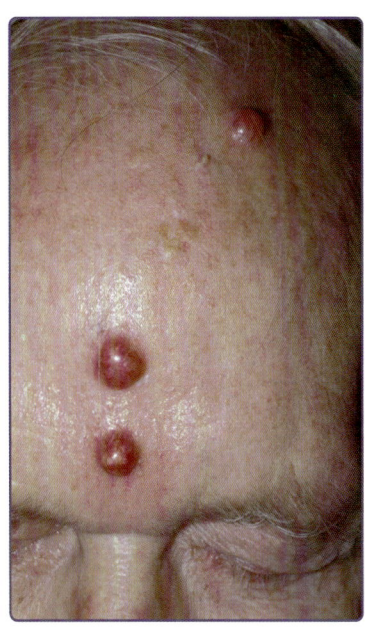

Figure 134-14 Metastatic lung cancer presenting as forehead nodules.

metastatic breast cancer. The face and neck may be involved by metastases from oropharyngeal carcinomas. Metastases from renal and thyroid carcinoma may be pulsatile and may have a bruit.[48]

Several histopathologic features may help identify the source of the primary tumor. Microscopically, the collection of neoplastic cells, which usually resemble their malignancy of origin, is generally seen in the dermis and/or subcutaneous tissue. Additional features, such as tumor cells in an "Indian filing" pattern, lymphovascular invasion, necrosis, and a tumor-free "grenz zone," are also helpful for the diagnosis of metastatic skin lesions. In some types of cancers or poorly differentiated tumors, immunohistochemical staining is often required to achieve the correct diagnosis. For example, the immunohistochemical panel of CK7, CK20, and S-100 is a helpful tool in the diagnoses of breast, lung, and GI cancers and melanoma. Additional recommended markers include TTF-1 (thyroid transcription factor-1; lung), HMB-45 (homatropine methylbromide; melanoma), PSA (prostate-specific antigen; prostate), estrogen/progesterone receptors (breast), and chromogranin (neuroendocrine tumors).[47,48]

Cutaneous metastases may indicate advanced disease and a poor prognosis. The estimated mean survival after the diagnosis of cutaneous metastases is 50% at 6 months. However, according to recent studies, patients with breast cancer may have a better prognosis than those with other cancers.[48]

LEUKEMIA AND LYMPHOMA CUTIS

Chapter 119, "Cutaneous Lymphoma," provides additional information on leukemia and lymphoma cutis.

Cutaneous metastases from leukemia and lymphoma are referred to as leukemia cutis and lymphoma cutis, respectively. Skin manifestations may have similar appearances in both diseases. The lesions generally appear as pink, red, and/or brown-to-purple macules, papules, plaques, and nodules, and are usually firm and painless.

Leukemia cutis is an extramedullary manifestation of leukemia, characterized by an invasion of leukemic cells into the epidermis, dermis, or subcutis. The skin eruptions can appear on the trunk, extremities, and head without sites of predilection. Occasionally, erythema, macules, blisters, ulcers, and erythroderma may be seen. Mucosal involvement, especially gum hypertrophy, is common. Nodular or plaque-like infiltration of the face can lead to the development of leonine facies. Rapid and generalized eruption of cutaneous lesions may suggest an acute form of leukemia. Leukemia cutis most frequently develops in patients with acute myeloid leukemia, particularly monocytic (M5) and myelomonocytic (M4) subtypes, but it can also occur in patients with other leukemia subtypes, such as chronic lymphocytic leukemia, chronic myeloid leukemia, chronic myelomonocytic leukemia, and acute lymphocytic leukemia. Most patients with leukemia cutis develop it after a known diagnosis of leukemia, but in rare cases, "aleukemic" leukemia cutis or leukemia cutis without systemic involvement can appear as a presenting manifestation months or years before developing systemic involvement. A skin biopsy is essential to confirm the diagnosis. Immunohistochemical and molecular genetic methods are essential for determining the subtype of leukemia. Treatment is targeted to the specific type of underlying leukemia. Some authors suggest that the appearance of leukemia cutis may indicate aggressive disease and a poor prognosis.[49]

Lymphoma cutis occurs when systemic lymphoma spreads secondarily to the skin. At times, it may be difficult to distinguish the primary cutaneous lymphoma from lymphoma cutis. Further staging evaluation is needed to document the origins of cutaneous lymphomas. Cutaneous dissemination can occur in both T-cell and B-cell lymphomas. Systemic anaplastic large-cell lymphoma is a T-cell lymphoma in which skin involvement occurs more commonly in the anaplastic lymphoma kinase–negative subtype. In adult T-cell leukemia-lymphoma, more than half of patients present with skin lesions at the time of diagnosis with chronic and smoldering subtypes resembling mycosis fungoides skin lesions. Cutaneous dissemination in Hodgkin lymphoma is much less frequent than in non-Hodgkin lymphoma.

Many types of systemic B-cell lymphomas can also have extranodal spread to the skin (systemic follicular lymphoma, marginal zone lymphoma, or diffuse large B-cell lymphoma), although primary cutaneous B-cell lymphomas may be more common than secondary skin involvement by systemic B-cell lymphomas. In lymphomatoid granulomatosis, skin is the most common extrapulmonary site, with lymphomatoid granulomatosis occurring in a progressive pattern in 50% of cases. Other rare types of B-cell lymphomas with cutaneous involvement include intravascular B-cell lymphoma and precursor B-cell lymphoblastic lymphoma.[50]

PAGET AND EXTRAMAMMARY PAGET DISEASES

Chapter 114, "Paget Disease," provides additional information on Paget and extramammary Paget diseases.

Paget disease of the nipple is a chronic erythematous scaling eruption of the nipple and areola indicating ductal carcinoma of the underlying breast. Extramammary Paget disease most commonly occurs in the anogenital skin, followed by the axillae and penis. It is classified into 3 types. The most common type appears as a primary intraepidermal adenocarcinoma. The second type (25%) is associated with visceral malignancy, most commonly of GI or genitourinary systems. The third type, the least common, is associated with an adjacent sweat gland carcinoma.

REFERENCES

1. Shah A, Jack A, Liu H, et al. Neoplastic/paraneoplastic dermatitis, fasciitis, and panniculitis. *Rheum Dis Clin North Am*. 2011;37(4):573-592.
2. Torley D, Bellus GA, Munro CS. Genes, growth factors and acanthosis nigricans. *Br J Dermatol*. 2002;147(6):1096-1101.
3. Higgins SP, Freemark M, Prose NS. Acanthosis nigricans: a practical approach to evaluation and management. *Dermatol Online J*. 2008;14(9):2.
4. Zur RL, Shapero J, Shapero H. Pityriasis rotunda diagnosed in Canada: case presentation and review of the literature. *J Cutan Med Surg*. 2013;17(6):426-428.
5. Patel N, Spencer LA, English JC 3rd, et al. Acquired ichthyosis. *J Am Acad Dermatol*. 2006;55(4):647-656.
6. Cohen PR, Grossman ME, Silvers DN, et al. Tripe palms and cancer. *Clin Dermatol*. 1993;11(1):165-173.
7. Silva JA, Mesquita Kde C, Igreja AC, et al. Paraneoplastic cutaneous manifestations: concepts and updates. *An Bras Dermatol*. 2013;88(1):9-22.
8. Nanda A, Mamon HJ, Fuchs CS. Sign of Leser-Trélat in newly diagnosed advanced gastric adenocarcinoma. *J Clin Oncol*. 20 2008;26(30):4992-4993.
9. Fink AM, Filz D, Krajnik G, et al. Seborrhoeic keratoses in patients with internal malignancies: a case-control study with prospective accrual of patients. *J Eur Acad Dermatol Venereol*. 2009;23(11):1316-1319.
10. Eastman KL, Knezevich SR, Raugi GJ. Eruptive seborrheic keratoses associated with adalimumab use. *J Dermatol Case Rep*. 30 2013;7(2):60-63.
11. Bazex A, Dupre A, Christol B, et al. Paraneoplastic acrokeratosis [in French]. *Bull Soc Fr Dermatol Syphiligr*. 1969;76(4):537-538.
12. Bolognia JL. Bazex syndrome: acrokeratosis paraneoplastica. *Semin Dermatol*. 1995;14(2):84-89.
13. Femia AN, Vleugels RA, Callen JP. Cutaneous dermatomyositis: an updated review of treatment options and internal associations. *Am J Clin Dermatol*. 2013;14(4):291-313.
14. Szekanecz E, Szamosi S, Horvath A, et al. Malignancies associated with systemic sclerosis. *Autoimmun Rev*. 2012;11(12):852-855.
15. Onishi A, Sugiyama D, Kumagai S, et al. Cancer incidence in systemic sclerosis: meta-analysis of population-based cohort studies. *Arthritis Rheum*. 2013;65(7):1913-1921.
16. Shah AA, Casciola-Rosen L. Cancer and scleroderma: a paraneoplastic disease with implications for malignancy screening. *Curr Opin Rheumatol*. 2015;27(6):563-570.
17. Boyd AS, Neldner KH, Menter A. Erythema gyratum repens: a paraneoplastic eruption. *J Am Acad Dermatol*. 1992;26(5, pt 1):757-762.
18. Rongioletti F, Fausti V, Parodi A. Erythema gyratum repens induced by pegylated interferon alfa for chronic hepatitis C. *Arch Dermatol*. 2012;148(10):1213-1214.
19. John AM, Schwartz RA. Glucagonoma syndrome: a review and update on treatment. *J Eur Acad Dermatol*

Venereol. 2016;30(12):2016-2022.
20. Grewal P, Salopek TG. Is necrolytic migratory erythema due to glucagonoma a misnomer? A more apt name might be mucosal and intertriginous erosive dermatitis. *J Cutan Med Surg.* 2012;16(2):76-82.
21. Raza S, Kirkland RS, Patel AA, et al. Insight into Sweet's syndrome and associated-malignancy: a review of the current literature. *Int J Oncol.* 2013;42(5):1516-1522.
22. Cohen PR. Sweet's syndrome—a comprehensive review of an acute febrile neutrophilic dermatosis. *Orphanet J Rare Dis.* 2007;2:34.
23. Al Ghazal P, Herberger K, Schaller J, et al. Associated factors and comorbidities in patients with pyoderma gangrenosum in Germany: a retrospective multicentric analysis in 259 patients. *Orphanet J Rare Dis.* 2013;8:136.
24. Bennett ML, Jackson JM, Jorizzo JL, et al. Pyoderma gangrenosum. A comparison of typical and atypical forms with an emphasis on time to remission. Case review of 86 patients from 2 institutions. *Medicine (Baltimore).* 2000;79(1):37-46.
25. El-Haddad B, Hammoud D, Shaver T, et al. Malignancy-associated multicentric reticulohistiocytosis. *Rheumatol Int.* 2011;31(9):1235-1238.
26. Islam AD, Naguwa SM, Cheema GS, et al. Multicentric reticulohistiocytosis: a rare yet challenging disease. *Clin Rev Allergy Immunol.* 2013;45(2):281-289.
27. Higgins LS, Go RS, Dingli D, et al. Clinical features and treatment outcomes of patients with necrobiotic xanthogranuloma associated with monoclonal gammopathies. *Clin Lymphoma Myeloma Leuk.* 2016;16(8):447-452.
28. Hummers LK. Scleromyxedema. *Curr Opin Rheumatol.* 2014;26(6):658-662.
29. Elsaman AM, Radwan AR, Akmatov MK, et al. Amyloid arthropathy associated with multiple myeloma: a systematic analysis of 101 reported cases. *Semin Arthritis Rheum.* 2013;43(3):405-412.
30. Merlini G, Seldin DC, Gertz MA. Amyloidosis: pathogenesis and new therapeutic options. *J Clin Oncol.* 2011;29(14):1924-1933.
31. Hemminki K, Li X, Forsti A, et al. Cancer risk in amyloidosis patients in Sweden with novel findings on non-Hodgkin lymphoma and skin cancer. *Ann Oncol.* 2014;25(2):511-518.
32. Frew JW, Murrell DF. Paraneoplastic pemphigus (paraneoplastic autoimmune multiorgan syndrome): clinical presentations and pathogenesis. *Dermatol Clin.* 2011;29(3):419-425, viii.
33. Collin P, Pukkala E, Reunala T. Malignancy and survival in dermatitis herpetiformis: a comparison with coeliac disease. *Gut.* 1996;38(4):528-530.
34. Viljamaa M, Kaukinen K, Pukkala E, et al. Malignancies and mortality in patients with coeliac disease and dermatitis herpetiformis: 30-year population-based study. *Dig Liver Dis.* 2006;38(6):374-380.
35. Balestri R, Magnano M, La Placa M, et al. Malignancies in bullous pemphigoid: a controversial association. *J Dermatol.* 2016;43(2):125-133.
36. Hovenden AL. Hypertrichosis lanuginosa acquisita associated with malignancy. *Clin Dermatol.* 1993;11(1):99-106.
37. Slee PH, van der Waal RI, Schagen van Leeuwen JH, et al. Paraneoplastic hypertrichosis lanuginosa acquisita: uncommon or overlooked? *Br J Dermatol.* 2007;157(6):1087-1092.
38. Dicke C, Langer F. Pathophysiology of Trousseau's syndrome. *Hamostaseologie.* 2015;35(1):52-59.
39. Timp JF, Braekkan SK, Versteeg HH, et al. Epidemiology of cancer-associated venous thrombosis. *Blood.* 2013;122(10):1712-1723.
40. Key NS, Khorana AA, Mackman N, et al. Thrombosis in cancer: research priorities identified by a National Cancer Institute/National Heart, Lung, and Blood Institute Strategic Working Group. *Cancer Res.* 2016;76(13):3671-3675.
41. Ponti G, Pellacani G, Seidenari S, et al. Cancer-associated genodermatoses: skin neoplasms as clues to hereditary tumor syndromes. *Crit Rev Oncol Hematol.* 2013;85(3):239-256.
42. Shen Z, Hoffman JD, Hao F, et al. More than just skin deep: fasciocutaneous clues to genetic syndromes with malignancies. *Oncologist.* 2012;17(7):930-936.
43. Reyes MA, Eisen DB. Inherited syndromes. *Dermatol Ther.* 2010;23(6):606-642.
44. Kuhlen M, Borkhardt A. Cancer susceptibility syndromes in children in the area of broad clinical use of massive parallel sequencing. *Eur J Pediatr.* 2015;174(8):987-997.
45. Somoano B, Tsao H. Genodermatoses with cutaneous tumors and internal malignancies. *Dermatol Clin.* 2008;26(1):69-87, viii.
46. Jaju PD, Ransohoff KJ, Tang JY, et al. Familial skin cancer syndromes: increased risk of nonmelanotic skin cancers and extracutaneous tumors. *J Am Acad Dermatol.* 2016;74(3):437-451; quiz 452-434.
47. El Khoury J, Khalifeh I, Kibbi AG, et al. Cutaneous metastasis: clinicopathological study of 72 patients from a tertiary care center in Lebanon. *Int J Dermatol.* 2014;53(2):147-158.
48. Fernandez-Anton Martinez MC, Parra-Blanco V, Aviles Izquierdo JA, et al. Cutaneous metastases of internal tumors. *Actas Dermosifiliogr.* 2013;104(10):841-853.
49. Wagner G, Fenchel K, Back W, et al. Leukemia cutis-epidemiology, clinical presentation, and differential diagnoses. *J Dtsch Dermatol Ges.* 2012;10(1):27-36.
50. Oluwole OO, Zic JA, Douds JJ, et al. Cutaneous manifestations and management of hematologic neoplasms. *Semin Oncol.* 2016;43(3):370-383.

Chapter 135 :: The Neurofibromatoses
:: Robert Listernick & Joel Charrow

第一百三十五章

神经纤维瘤病

中文导读

神经纤维瘤病是一种染色体显性疾病，发病率为1/3000。本章介绍了该病的：①临床特点，包括咖啡斑、三叉神经性雀斑、离散神经纤维瘤、丛状神经纤维瘤、视路肿瘤、明显的骨性病变；②病因和发病机制，介绍了1型和2型神经纤维瘤病均是常染色体显性方式遗传；③临床病程、预后和处理，建议使用全身磁共振检查，注意骨骼并发症，关注恶性肿瘤的风险，以及可能出现的血管病变、智力和学习障碍，并提到了1型神经纤维瘤病需要进行多学科的治疗，包括眼科、皮肤科等。

〔粟 娟〕

AT-A-GLANCE

- Autosomal dominant condition with incidence of 1 in 3000 live births.
- Diagnosed clinically if 2 major features are present (see Table 135-1).
- Cutaneous neurofibromas:
  - Softer than the surrounding connective tissue and protrude just above the skin surface or lie just under the skin with an overlying violaceous hue.
- Subcutaneous neurofibromas:
  - Arise from peripheral nerves, both under the skin and deep in the viscera.
  - Generally much harder.
- Plexiform neurofibromas:
  - Generally present at birth or apparent during the first several years of life.
  - May lead to disfigurement, blindness (secondary to amblyopia, glaucoma, or proptosis), loss of limb function, or organ dysfunction by compression of vital structures.
- Mosaic neurofibromatosis Type 1 (segmental NF-1):
  - Manifestations of NF-1, usually limited to one area of the body.
  - Occurs as result of a postconceptional mutation in the *NF1* gene, leading to somatic mosaicism.

CLINICAL FEATURES

A consensus development conference was held by the National Institutes of Health in 1987 to establish diagnostic criteria to promote better clinical research and care of patients with neurofibromatosis Type 1 (NF-1).[1] The 7 diagnostic features recognized at this conference (Table 135-1), and the recommendation that 2 or more of these 7 features be present before a diagnosis of NF-1 is established, have proven extremely useful and continue to be used without modification more than 30 years later. Perhaps the one caveat is the identification of a separate autosomal dominant syndrome caused by an inactivating mutation of the gene encoding sprouty-related EVH1 domain-containing protein 1 (*SPRED1*), which leads to the development of café-au-lait spots, intertriginous freckling, and macrocephaly,

TABLE 135-1
Diagnostic Criteria for Neurofibromatosis Type 1[a]

- Six or more café-au-lait macules larger than 5 mm in greatest diameter in prepubertal individuals, and larger than 15 mm in greatest diameter in postpubertal individuals.
- Two or more neurofibromas of any type *or* 1 plexiform neurofibroma.
- Freckling in the axillary or inguinal regions.
- Optic glioma.
- Two or more iris Lisch nodules.
- A distinctive osseous lesion such as sphenoid dysplasia or thinning of long bone cortex with or without pseudarthrosis.
- A first-degree relative (parent, sibling, or offspring) with neurofibromatosis Type 1 by the above criteria.

[a]Patient must meet 2 or more of the listed criteria for diagnosis.

but none of the other manifestations of NF-1 (Legius syndrome).[2]

CAFÉ-AU-LAIT SPOTS

Café-au-lait spots, which are flat, pigmented macules, are often the first manifestation of NF-1 to appear (Fig. 135-1). Frequently present at birth, they become more numerous as the infant grows; new ones may continue to appear throughout the first decade of life. Once noticed, they tend to grow in size in proportion to the overall growth of the child. Although infrequently found on the face, they may be noted anywhere on the body. The size, shape, and contour of café-au-lait spots are of no diagnostic significance, and the oft-quoted adage about smooth-edged café-au-lait spots being more typical of NF-1 rather than McCune-Albright syndrome is incorrect. When café-au-lait spots overlap each other, the area of overlap may be darker than either individual spot. When found within slate grey macules, they are typically surrounded by a more lightly pigmented halo. Individuals with large numbers of café-au-lait spots do not have "more-severe" NF-1, and the location of the macules in no way predicts the location of subsequent neurofibromas.

Café-au-lait spots represent collections of heavily pigmented melanocytes of neural crest origin in the epidermis. Although the cells may contain increased numbers of "giant" melanosomes, or melanin macroglobules, these are not unique to NF-1, and their presence or absence in biopsies is not helpful diagnostically.

INTERTRIGINOUS FRECKLING

Café-au-lait spots smaller than 5 mm are referred to as freckles, and are commonly present in the axillae, inguinal region, and under the breasts (Fig. 135-2). Unlike ordinary freckles in these locations, these lesions are not related to sun exposure, and are considered virtually pathognomonic of NF-1 (Crowe sign). Of all children ultimately diagnosed with NF-1, 81% will have intertriginous freckling by age 6 years.[3]

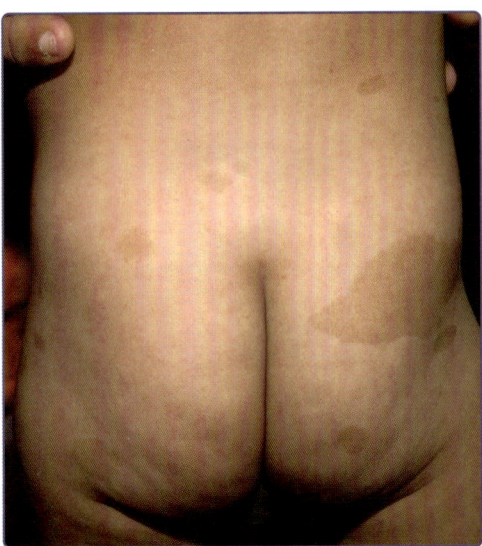

Figure 135-1 Café-au-lait spots.

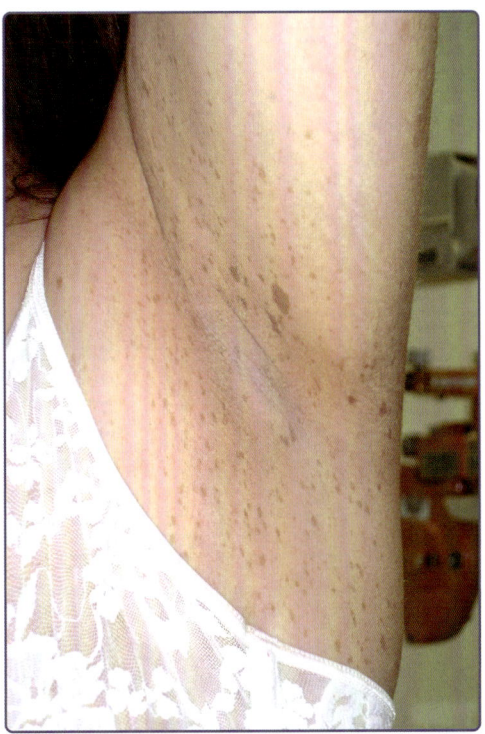

Figure 135-2 Axillary freckling.

DISCRETE NEUROFIBROMAS

Neurofibromas, which consist of Schwann cells, mast cells, fibroblasts, and perineural cells, are benign nerve sheath tumors that appear as discrete masses arising from peripheral nerves.[4] Cutaneous neurofibromas protrude just above the skin surface or lie just under the skin with an overlying violaceous hue (Fig. 135-3). They are softer than the surrounding connective tissue, often creating a "buttonholing" sensation when a finger is rubbed gently over the surface (Fig. 135-4). Subcutaneous neurofibromas that arise from peripheral nerves, both under the skin and deep in the viscera, are generally much harder (Fig. 135-5). If they arise from the dorsal root ganglia, they may grow through neural foramina, compressing the spinal cord, creating a "dumbbell" appearance. Subcutaneous neurofibromas in the neck may feel like a "beaded necklace," often being confused with lymph nodes. While fewer than 20% of children younger than 10 years of age have cutaneous neurofibromas, neurofibromas generally start appearing after puberty and increase in number as the patient grows older. Women who have NF-1 often comment on the appearance of cutaneous neurofibromas during pregnancy. The majority of adult patients with NF-1 probably have numerous asymptomatic deep neurofibromas involving the dorsal roots and other larger nerves. On occasion, neurofibroma-associated pruritus may be severe enough to require treatment with antihistamines.

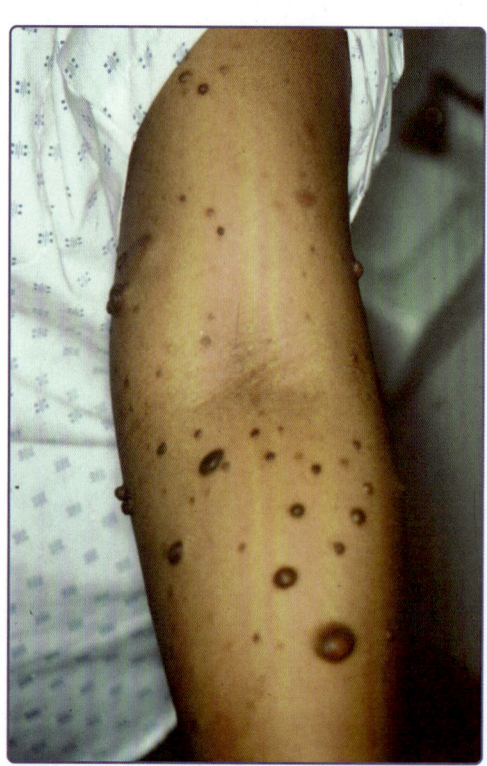

Figure 135-3 Cutaneous neurofibromas with overlying hyperpigmentation.

PLEXIFORM NEUROFIBROMAS

Plexiform neurofibromas, histologically similar to discrete neurofibromas, are benign peripheral nerve sheath tumors that involve single or multiple nerve fascicles, often arising from branches of major nerves.[5] They may elicit a "wormy" sensation on palpation, as a person feels multiple thickened nerve fascicles. Often there is overlying hyperpigmentation ("giant café-au-lait spot") or hypertrichosis (Fig. 135-6). Most plexiform neurofibromas are present at birth or become apparent during the first several years of life. Externally visible plexiform neurofibromas are easily identified and may lead to disfigurement, blindness (secondary to amblyopia, glaucoma, or proptosis), or loss of limb function (Figs. 135-7

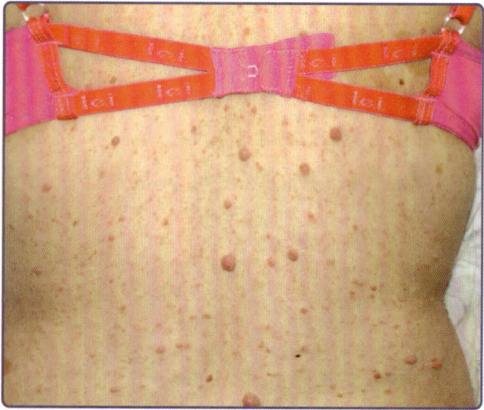

Figure 135-4 Multiple cutaneous neurofibromas.

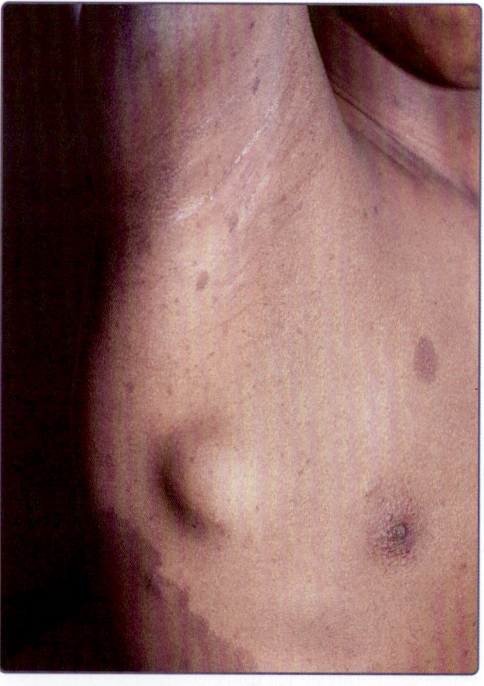

Figure 135-5 Subcutaneous neurofibroma.

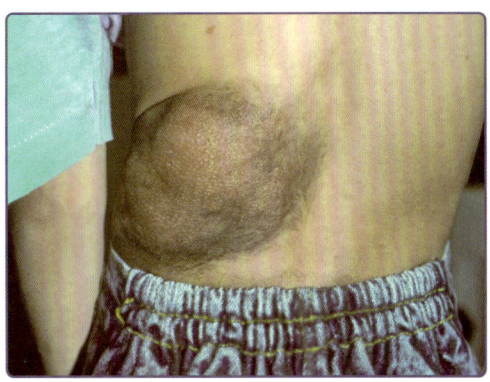

Figure 135-6 Plexiform neurofibroma with overlying hyperpigmentation and hypertrichosis.

to 135-9). In contrast, thoracic or abdominal plexiform neurofibromas may have no external manifestations but may have equally devastating consequences as a consequence of invasion or compression of vital structures (eg, ureters, bowel, spinal cord).

The growth rate of plexiform neurofibromas is highly variable. Periods of rapid growth alternating with long periods of quiescence are common. Malignant peripheral nerve sheath tumors, which generally arise from plexiform neurofibromas, may develop silently in deep plexiform neurofibromas and not give rise to symptoms until distant metastases have occurred. Even though loss of heterozygosity of *NF1* may lead to the formation of benign neurofibromas, the generation of malignant transformation of a benign plexiform neurofibroma may be caused by cell-cycle regulators beyond the *RAS* oncogene. For example, mice that have null mutations in both the *Nf1* and *p53* genes uniformly develop malignant tumors.[6] Physicians caring for individuals with NF-1 should be alert to development of a malignancy; plexiform neurofibromas should be biopsied if they exhibit rapid growth or cause significant pain or focal neurologic dysfunction. Positron emission tomography with 2-deoxy-2-[fluorine-18]fluoro-D-glucose integrated with computed tomography (^{18}F-FDG PET/CT) can be extremely useful in identifying the development of malignant peripheral nerve sheath tumor within a preexisting plexiform neurofibroma.[7,8]

OPTIC PATHWAY TUMORS

Approximately 15% of children with NF-1 will develop optic pathway tumors (OPTs); however, less than half of these patients will ever develop symptoms, giving an overall incidence of *symptomatic* OPT of 7%.[9,10] Recent series of NF-1–associated OPTs have identified an approximately 2:1 female predominance of patients, as well as a lower incidence in African American children. These observations suggest the possibility that either hormonal factors or modifying genes may influence the development and prognosis of OPTs.[11,12]

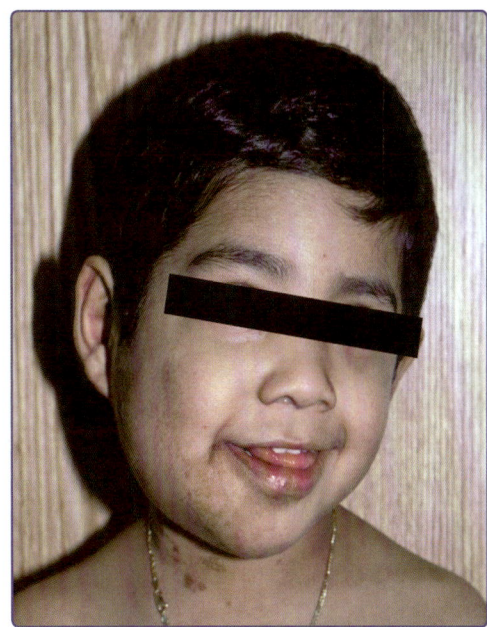

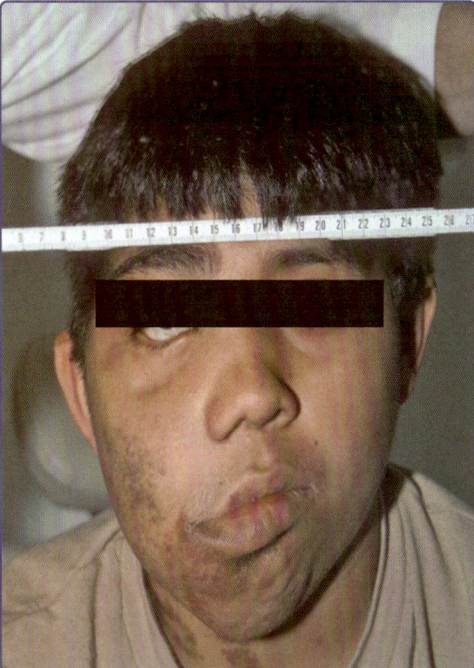

Figure 135-7 Progressive growth of facial plexiform neurofibroma.

The period of greatest risk for the development of symptomatic OPTs in NF-1 is during the first 6 years of life; the development of a symptomatic tumor after age 6 years is extremely unusual.[13,14] Thus, physicians caring for children with NF-1 should be sensitive to the signs and symptoms of OPTs in this young age group. Approximately 30% of children with symptomatic OPTs will present with the rapid onset of proptosis, with moderate to severe visual loss in the affected eye (Fig. 135-10). Another 30% of children who have

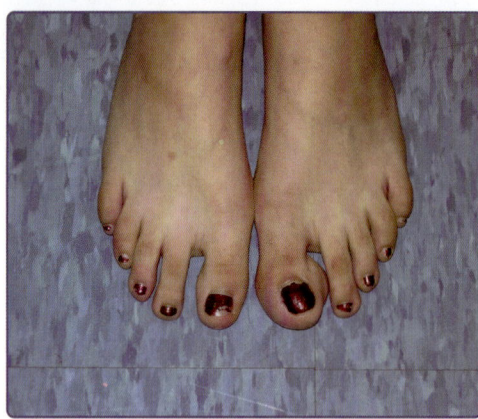

Figure 135-8 Plexiform neurofibroma of left first toe leading to isolated macrodactyly.

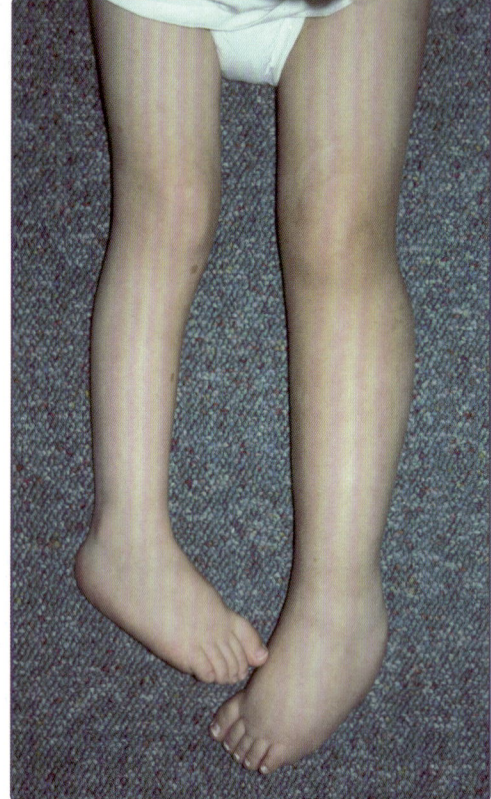

Figure 135-9 Plexiform neurofibroma of left lower extremity leading to leg-length discrepancy.

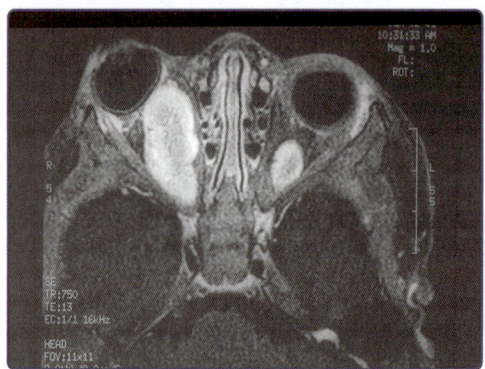

Figure 135-10 Intraorbital optic nerve tumor causing proptosis.

symptomatic OPTs will have abnormal ophthalmologic examinations, without any visual symptoms, leading to discovery of the tumors. As young children rarely complain of visual loss, even when severe, thorough annual eye examinations are imperative in all young children with NF-1. When present, ophthalmologic signs may include an afferent papillary defect, optic nerve atrophy, papilledema, strabismus, or defects in color vision. Finally, as many as 40% of children who have chiasmal tumors develop precocious puberty.[15] Accelerated linear growth will be the first sign of precocious puberty, underscoring the need for all children with NF-1 to have annual assessments of growth using standard growth charts. Children with chiasmal tumors often have no ophthalmologic symptoms or signs. Early detection of precocious puberty is important as both the accelerated linear growth and the development of secondary sexual characteristics can be can be aborted with the use of a long-acting luteinizing hormone-releasing hormone agonist.

LISCH NODULES

Lisch nodules are slightly raised, well-circumscribed melanocytic hamartomas of the iris thought to be virtually pathognomonic of NF-1 (Fig. 135-11). They are best seen using a slitlamp, which is necessary to distinguish them from the more commonly seen flat iris nevi, which are not associated with NF-1. They do not cause any functional impairment of vision. The frequency with which they are found increases with age; although Lisch nodules are found in more than 90% of adults with NF-1, only 30% of children with NF-1 who are younger than 6 years of age have them.[3]

DISTINCTIVE OSSEOUS LESIONS

There are 2 bony lesions distinctive enough to be included in the diagnostic criteria for NF-1. The first, dysplasia of the wing of the sphenoid bone, results in poor formation of the wall and/or floor of the orbit (Fig. 135-12). This congenital mesodermal dysplasia may be, but is not always, clinically apparent, leading to proptosis (from herniation of meninges or brain into the orbit) or enophthalmos.

Dysplasia of a long bone, characterized by congenital thinning and bowing, affects approximately 2% of children with NF-1 (Fig. 135-13). Although the tibia is

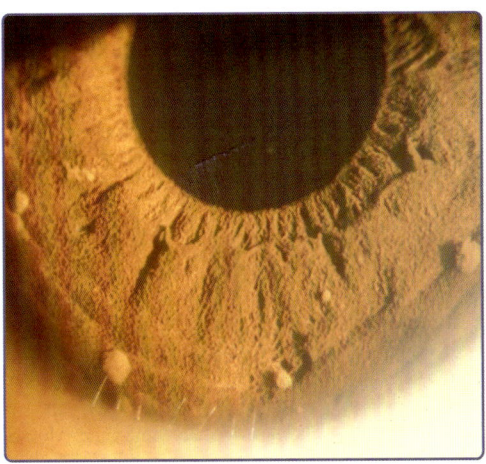

Figure 135-11 Lisch nodules.

most commonly affected, the femur, humerus and other long bones also may be involved. Even when the bone is intact, thinning and bowing produce a visible deformity, and the weakened mechanical properties of the bone predispose to fracture, particularly in the weight-bearing bones. Failure of primary union following a fracture results in a "false joint," or pseudarthrosis.[16]

ETIOLOGY AND PATHOGENESIS

EPIDEMIOLOGY

The "modern age" of neurofibromatosis began in 1981, with Riccardi's detailed clinical descriptions of the features and natural history of von Recklinghausen disease and the subsequent description of "central neurofibromatosis with bilateral acoustic neuroma."[17] With the availability of gene-based diagnosis, several distinct clinical syndromes have been identified: (a) NF-1, also known as von Recklinghausen disease; (b) NF-2, whose cardinal feature is the development of bilateral vestibular schwannomas; (c) segmental or mosaic NF-1; (d) Legius syndrome (*SPRED1* mutation) leading to autosomal dominant transmission of café-au-lait spots, intertriginous freckling, and macrocephaly; and (e) schwannomatosis. Both NF-1 and NF-2 occur equally in all ethnic groups. NF-1 occurs at an incidence of 1 in 3000 live births, whereas NF-2 is much less common with an estimated incidence of 1 in 40,000 live births.

GENETICS

NF-1 is inherited in an autosomal dominant fashion. Although the expressivity of NF-1 varies considerably, even among individuals in the same family who are genotypically identical, the disorder is considered to

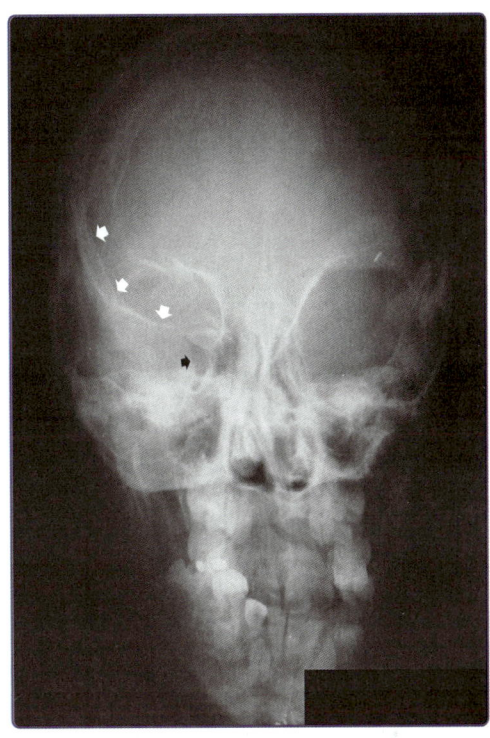

Figure 135-12 Sphenoid wing dysplasia. Arrows outline normal sphenoid wing in wall of right orbit. Contralateral sphenoid wing is dysplastic.

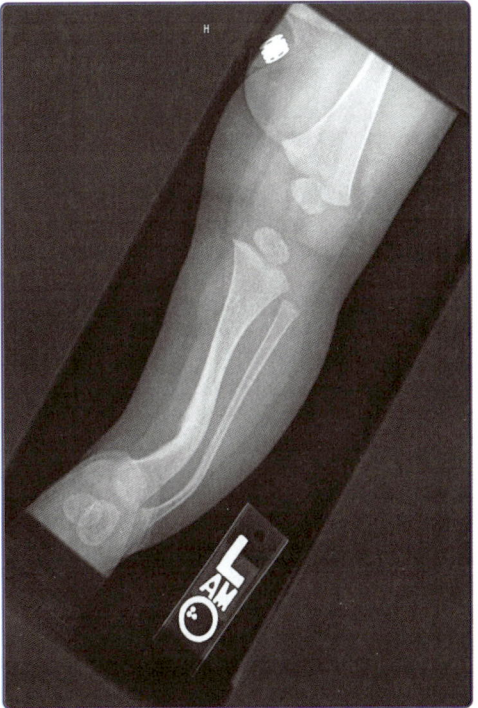

Figure 135-13 Tibial and fibular dysplasia.

be 100% penetrant. Thus, apparent skipping of NF-1 between generations may be the result of misdiagnosis, nonpaternity, or the occurrence of a new mutation in the grandchild. Although a large number of *NF1* mutations have been described, only 2 genotype–phenotype correlations have been noted. Individuals who have deletions of the entire gene have an increased risk of facial dysmorphism, intellectual disability, early appearance of neurofibromas, and the presence of plexiform neurofibromas.[18] In addition, individuals who have a specific 3 base pair in-frame deletion in exon 17 of *NF1* may have café-au-lait spots, intertriginous freckling and Lisch nodules, but do not develop cutaneous, subcutaneous, or plexiform neurofibromas.[19] There is evidence that NF-1 is more severe when inherited from the mother rather than from the father.

NF1 is located on the long arm of chromosome 17, and encodes a protein called *neurofibromin*. Homozygosity for mutant *NF1* alleles has not been reported, probably because it is a lethal condition. *NF1* has an unusually high mutation rate, estimated at 2.4×10^{-5} to 10^{-4} gametes per generation, one of the highest of known inherited disorders. This may reflect the large size of the gene, which spans 350 kb of genomic DNA, and contains 59 exons that encode a peptide containing more than 2800 amino acids.[20] An alternative hypothesis is that there is some structural property of the gene that renders it particularly susceptible to mutation. New mutations account for approximately 50% of cases, and are usually on the paternally inherited allele. In contrast to many other dominant disorders, the frequency of new mutations does not appear to increase with advancing paternal age.[11]

MOLECULAR BIOLOGY

Most *NF1* mutations result in reduced intracellular levels of the *NF1* gene product, neurofibromin; this appears to be sufficient to cause many of the clinical manifestations of the disease. Tumorigenesis, including the development of benign dermal neurofibromas, appears to be dependent on inactivation of the normal *NF1* allele in somatic cells, a process referred to as loss of heterozygosity.[21] Loss of heterozygosity is a critical step in tumorigenesis in many inherited cancer predisposition syndromes (eg, retinoblastoma, Li-Fraumeni syndrome), and the genes involved are called *tumor-suppressor genes*. Tumorigenesis is initiated when both copies of the gene cease functioning normally—the first as a result of an inherited mutation, and the second as the result of a second somatic "hit" interfering with the function of the previously normal allele.

Neurofibromin is found in a variety of cell types, including neurons, oligodendrocytes, and nonmyelinating Schwann cells. Considerable evidence has been developed for the role of neurofibromin as a negative regulator of Ras.[20] The *RAS* gene family encodes membrane-associated, guanine nucleotide-binding proteins that are involved in the regulation of cellular proliferation, differentiation, and learning. Ras exists in an active (Ras-GTP [guanosine triphosphate]) and inactive (Ras-GDP [guanosine diphosphate]) state. By favoring conversion of Ras from its active state to its inactive state, neurofibromin downregulates the downstream effects of Ras, which include promoting learning, memory, synaptic plasticity, and cell growth and proliferation. Mediators of the downstream effects of Ras include mitogen-activated protein kinase (MAPK), phosphatidylinositol 3'-kinase, protein kinase B, and mammalian target of rapamycin kinase.[22] *SPRED1* also inhibits activation of the MAPK pathway.[22]

In the brain, there are 3 major isoforms of Ras; K-*ras* is the primary target of neurofibromin activity.[23] Activation of Ras by neurofibromin stimulates G-protein activity, resulting in activation of adenylyl cyclase. Cyclic adenosine monophosphate and other downstream intermediates appear to play a role in cell growth, learning, and memory. Neurofibromin also associates with microtubules and plays a role in regulating γ-aminobutyric acid-ergic inhibitory neuronal activity in the hippocampus.[24]

Ras is a membrane-bound protein, and requires farnesylation (addition of a C15 isoprenoid to a cysteine residue near the C-terminus) for activity, a process that is catalyzed by farnesyltransferase. Agents that inhibit farnesyltransferase cause general inhibition of the Ras pathway, much as neurofibromin does. Farnesyltransferase inhibitors reverse the proliferative phenotype in *Nf1*-deficient mouse cells, and can reverse spatial learning impairments in a mouse model of NF-1, by decreasing Ras levels.[25] Inhibitors of downstream kinases of the MAPK pathway, such as MAPK kinase (MEK), have been shown to shrink plexiform neurofibromas in mouse models, leading the way for clinical trials that are ongoing.[26]

Loss of heterozygosity of *NF1* in Schwann cells has been shown to be a necessary event for the development of both discrete and plexiform neurofibromas.[27] Plexiform neurofibromas are comprised of Schwann cells, macrophages, mast cells, neurons and fibroblasts. Interestingly, neurofibromin-deficient Schwann cells secrete a substance that stimulates mast cell migration, which, in turn, stimulates production of extracellular matrix and angiogenesis.[5] Astrocytes lacking *NF1* expression cannot form optic nerve gliomas on their own; a brain environment heterozygous for *NF1* is necessary for the development of these tumors. Microglia, CNS immune surveillance cells, are involved in both optic nerve glioma formation and maintenance.[28]

DIAGNOSIS

Despite the identification of the *NF1* gene and its complete sequencing, the diagnosis of NF-1 remains primarily a clinical one. Although laboratory confirmation of the diagnosis is extremely useful in specific circumstances, in most cases it is unnecessary. As no common mutations have been identified, molecular diagnosis can only be based on strategies that screen the entire gene for mutations. This testing is available for both presymptomatic individuals and can be applied to prenatal diagnosis of NF-1 when a mutation has been identified in an affected parent.

Inexperienced clinicians often biopsy cutaneous masses in an effort to confirm the diagnosis of NF-1 in an individual with multiple café-au-lait spots or other stigmata of NF-1. Such procedures are invariably unnecessary as the clinical diagnosis of NF-1 is usually quite straightforward. Biopsy of a plexiform neurofibroma should be reserved for those situations in which the physician wishes to exclude the possibility of a malignancy.

DIFFERENTIAL DIAGNOSIS

There are numerous syndromes in which café-au-lait spots may be seen (Table 135-2). However, there are several syndromes that have overlapping phenotypes with NF-1 that have caused confusion in the past.

NEUROFIBROMATOSIS TYPE 2

AT-A-GLANCE

- Autosomal dominant disorder with incidence of 1 in 40,000 live births.
- Hallmark is the presence of bilateral vestibular schwannomas.
- At risk for development of multiple meningiomas, schwannomas, gliomas, and neurofibromas throughout neural axis.

TABLE 135-2
Differential Diagnosis of Syndromes Associated with Multiple Café-au-Lait Spots

Most Likely
- Neurofibromatosis Type 1
- Neurofibromatosis Type 2
- Familial café-au-lait spots (consider Legius syndrome)
- LEOPARD (lentigines, electrocardiographic abnormalities, ocular hypertelorism, pulmonary stenosis, abnormalities of genitalia, retardation of growth, and deafness) syndrome

Less Likely
- Tuberous sclerosis
- Fanconi anemia
- Multiple endocrine neoplasia Type 2B
- Bannayan-Riley-Ruvalcaba syndrome
- McCune-Albright syndrome (polyostotic fibrous dysplasia)
- Bloom syndrome
- Ataxia-telangiectasia

NF-2 is an autosomal dominant condition characterized by bilateral vestibular schwannomas, meningiomas (intracranial, intraspinal, and optic nerve sheath), schwannomas (dorsal roots of the spinal cord, peripheral nerves, and cranial nerves), ependymomas and gliomas of the CNS, and juvenile posterior subcapsular cataracts.[29] The estimated birth incidence is 1 in 40,000 live births. Even though it is much less common than NF-1, its morbidity is much greater, with patients frequently becoming paralyzed and deaf. The most recent clinical diagnostic criteria have led to increased sensitivity in establishing the diagnosis, particularly in those cases without a positive family history (Table 135-3). Approximately 60% of patients present in adulthood with hearing loss, tinnitus, or loss of balance. The younger the age at presentation, the greater the ultimate severity of the disease. Children are more apt to present with a non–eighth nerve tumor, such as an optic nerve sheath meningioma. Ophthalmologic findings include juvenile posterior subcapsular cataracts (60% to 80% of patients), retinal hamartomas, combined hamartomas of the retina and retinal pigment epithelium, and optic nerve sheath meningiomas.[30,31]

Individuals with NF-2 may have several café-au-lait spots, but rarely have more than 6; intertriginous freckling is not seen. The characteristic cutaneous lesion of NF-2 is the cutaneous schwannoma (Fig. 135-14). It is a plaque-like, slightly raised lesion with a faint violaceous hue, occasionally with hair. Less commonly, cutaneous neurofibromas, indistinguishable from those seen in NF-1, may be found.

NF-2 is caused by mutations in a gene on chromosome 22 which encodes the membrane-related protein merlin. As in NF-1, the *NF2* gene is a tumor-suppressor gene that downregulates cellular growth. The exact cellular pathways by which this control is exerted have yet to be delineated.

MOSAIC NEUROFIBROMATOSIS TYPE 1

The term *segmental neurofibromatosis* or *mosaic NF-1* refers to individuals who have manifestations of NF-1,

TABLE 135-3
Diagnostic Criteria for Neurofibromatosis Type 2

1. Bilateral vestibular schwannomas **or**
2. A first-degree relative with neurofibromatosis Type 2 (NF-2) **and**
   - Unilateral vestibular schwannoma **or**
   - Any 2 of: meningioma, schwannoma, glioma, neurofibroma, posterior subcapsular lenticular opacities
3. Unilateral vestibular schwannoma **and**
   - Any 2 of: meningioma, schwannoma, glioma, neurofibroma, posterior subcapsular lenticular opacities
4. Multiple meningiomas **and**
   - Unilateral vestibular schwannoma **or**
   - Any two of: schwannoma, glioma, neurofibroma, cataract

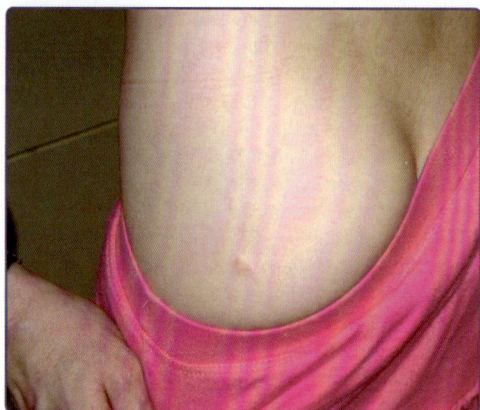

Figure 135-14 Cutaneous schwannoma.

usually café-au-lait macules and neurofibromas, limited to one area of the body.[32] Ruggieri and Huson have proposed use of the term *mosaic localized NF-1* for these individuals, as an acknowledgment that the pathogenesis of this condition is a postconceptional mutation in *NF1* leading to somatic mosaicism.[33] Somatic mosaicism was confirmed in a patient in whom the mutant *NF1* allele was present in a mosaic pattern in cultured fibroblasts from a café-au-lait macule and absent in fibroblasts from normal skin.[34]

The vast majority of patients with segmental NF-1 have café-au-lait macules or intertriginous freckling

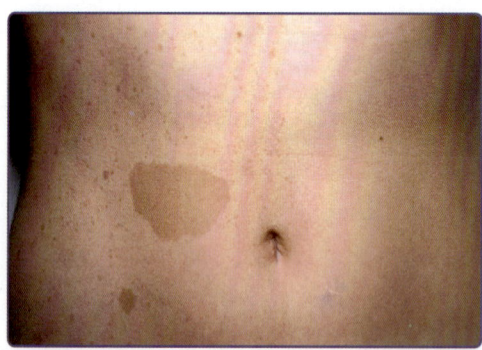

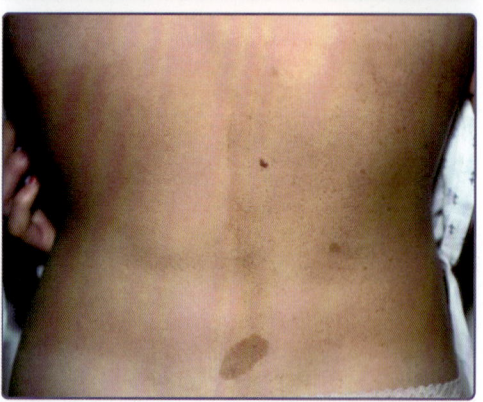

Figure 135-15 Mosaic neurofibromatosis Type 1. Note that the café-au-lait spots and freckling are limited to one side of body.

limited to one area of the body (Fig. 135-15). These individuals are at risk for developing complications of NF-1 in the affected area, most commonly neurofibromas. Localized manifestations of NF-1 other than café-au-lait macules, freckling, or cutaneous neurofibromas may also represent examples of somatic mosaicism. There have been numerous reports of isolated plexiform neurofibromas, including 1 case in which loss of heterozygosity of *NF1* in Schwann cells from the tumor was demonstrated. As only 50% of cases of tibial pseudarthrosis occur in the context of NF-1, the others may actually represent cases of mosaic NF-1. Other examples of mosaic NF-1 include a child who had a unilateral optic pathway glioma that acted that acted biologically like an NF-1–associated tumor and individuals with isolated sphenoid bone dysplasia.

Genetic counseling of patients with segmental NF-1 is problematic. Many of these patients are misdiagnosed as having NF-1, leading to unnecessary anxiety and inappropriate genetic counseling. In addition, gonadal mosaicism for NF-1 has been demonstrated; patients with segmental NF-1 have had offspring with complete NF-1.

NEUROFIBROMATOSIS TYPE 1–NOONAN SYNDROME

It has been recognized that there are individuals who meet the diagnostic criteria for NF-1, yet have many features of Noonan syndrome, which is characterized by hypertelorism, ptosis, downslanting palpebral fissures, low-set, posteriorly rotated ears, webbed neck, pectus deformities, and short stature. More than 50% of children with Noonan syndrome have cardiovascular disease, most commonly pulmonary valve stenosis. Noonan syndrome is caused by mutations in the gene *PTPN11* in 50% of cases. Mutations in multiple other genes (*KRAS*, *SOS1*, *BRAF*, *MEK1*, *MEK2*, *RIT1*, *HRAS*, and *RAF1*) also are associated with this phenotype. Genetic testing shows that most individuals with LEOPARD (lentigines, electrocardiographic abnormalities, ocular hypertelorism, pulmonary stenosis, abnormalities of genitalia, retardation of growth, and deafness) syndrome also have mutations in *PTPN11*.[35] Studies have documented mutations in the *NF1* gene in 16 of 17 unrelated subjects who clinically had the NF-1–Noonan phenotype; no mutations in *PTPN11* were found.[36] Thus, it appears that the vast majority of cases of NF-1–Noonan syndrome are caused by mutations in *NF1*.

LEGIUS SYNDROME

Families have been identified who have autosomal dominant transmission of café-au-lait spots, intertriginous freckling, and macrocephaly without any other manifestations of NF-1, including neurofibromas, in whom no *NF1* mutation was detected. Further genetic studies of these individuals revealed mutations in

SPRED1, a gene that negatively regulates the MAPK pathway.[2] None of these individuals has discrete neurofibromas, plexiform neurofibromas, Lisch nodules, OPTs, or NF-1–specific bony abnormalities. A study of 15 families with Legius syndrome documented a normal full scale IQ in affected individuals but a significantly lower performance IQ when compared to unaffected family members.[37] Genetic testing for *SPRED1* mutations is available in individuals suspected of having Legius syndrome in whom sequencing of *NF1* has failed to detect a mutation.

SCHWANNOMATOSIS

It had been noted for some time that there are patients who develop multiple schwannomas but who fail to develop other manifestations of NF-2, particularly vestibular schwannomas. Patients with this condition, now called *schwannomatosis*, develop multiple, painful schwannomas within peripheral nerves and paraspinal nerve roots.[38] The tumors most often start appearing during the second and third decades of life. Surgery of individual lesions is often necessary to treat intractable pain. In contrast to NF-2, individuals with schwannomatosis have a normal life span. Before making a diagnosis of schwannomatosis, it is extremely important to exclude the possibility of NF-2 by both genetic testing and performing an MRI scan to look for vestibular schwannomas. Current diagnostic criteria for a *definite* diagnosis of schwannomatosis in individuals 30 years of age or older include: (a) 2 or more nonintradermal schwannomas, at least 1 with histologic confirmation, and (b) diagnostic criteria for NF-2 not fulfilled, and (c) no evidence of vestibular schwannoma on MRI, and (d) no first-degree relative with NF-2, and (e) no germline *NF2* mutation.[39] Germline mutations in the tumor-suppressor genes *SMARCB1/INI1*, previously implicated in the development of rhabdoid tumors in infants and young children, as well as mutations in *LTZR1* have been identified as the cause of a large number of the familial cases of schwannomatosis. However, most cases are sporadic and caused by mutations in as-yet unidentified genes.[40]

CLINICAL COURSE, PROGNOSIS, AND MANAGEMENT

RADIOGRAPHIC EVALUATION

There is debate as to whether patients with NF-1 should be "screened" for the presence of hidden, internal plexiform neurofibromas; newer studies using whole-body MRI have demonstrated an incidence as high as 55%.[41,42] If current chemotherapeutic trials prove successful in the treatment of rapidly growing tumors, their identification at an early age may become more important using this technique.

SKELETAL COMPLICATIONS

All children with NF-1 should be regularly screened for scoliosis, beginning in early childhood. Scoliosis is the most common skeletal manifestation of NF-1, affecting 10% to 30% of patients. Scoliosis is divided into dystrophic and nondystrophic types. Dystrophic scoliosis is the result of primary bone dysplasia, and may present very early in childhood, typically resulting in a sharply angulated curve spanning relatively few vertebral bodies (Fig. 135-16). It is often accompanied by extreme rotation, scalloping of the posterior margins of the vertebral bodies, vertebral wedging, defective pedicles, and enlargement of the neural foramina and spinal canal. The curvature may progress rapidly, necessitating surgery that may be particularly complicated because of the complex, multiplanar curves, poor quality of bone, potential for nerve root and spinal cord injury, and the presence of intraspinal and extraspinal neurofibromas. The nondystrophic type of scoliosis is more common, and is similar to idiopathic scoliosis in adolescents. Many children can be managed expectantly or with bracing.[43]

Localized regions of bony overgrowth may also occur in children with NF-1 and are often in areas free of neurofibromas. The overgrowth may affect only a single digit or a larger region such as a hand or an extremity, but true hemihypertrophy is unusual. Bony overgrowth may also occur in a region affected by a plexiform neurofibroma.

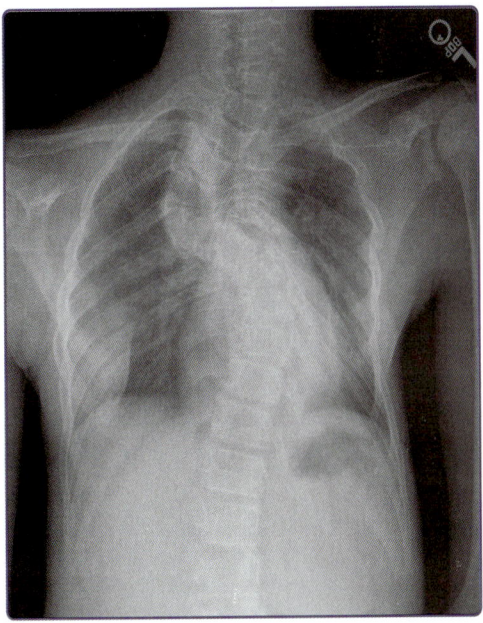

Figure 135-16 Dystrophic scoliosis.

CANCER

There is little doubt that NF-1 predisposes an individual to an increased risk for certain cancers. In a population-based Finnish study, an estimated lifetime cancer risk was 59.6%. Individuals with NF-1 were found to be at increased risk for cancers not traditionally thought to be part of the NF-1 spectrum of disease, most notably breast cancer which had a standardized incidence ratio of 11.1 for NF-1 women younger than 40 years of age when compared to women in the general population.[44]

MALIGNANT PERIPHERAL NERVE SHEATH TUMORS

Malignant peripheral nerve sheath tumors almost exclusively arise from preexisting plexiform neurofibromas. Estimates of the lifetime risk for the development of this tumor vary but may be as high as 13%.[45] As the outcome of therapy is poor, physicians should be diligently aware of the early symptoms referable to these tumors, including a rapidly growing mass or unexplained pain or dysfunction. Although conventional imaging cannot identify malignant tissue within a benign plexiform neurofibroma, newer modalities, such as ^{18}F-FDG PET coupled with either CT or MRI, have been shown to have excellent sensitivity and specificity.[7,8]

PHEOCHROMOCYTOMA

Pheochromocytoma clearly is associated with NF-1, with an incidence potentially as high as 1.4%. In a comprehensive review, the mean age at presentation was 42 years; 84% had solitary adrenal tumors, 10% had bilateral adrenal tumors, and 6% had ectopic tumors in the abdominal sympathetic chain, organ of Zuckerkandl, and the bladder.[46] Catecholamine-associated symptoms and hypertension each were present in 61% of the patients; 22% of the patients had neither of these findings. Malignant pheochromocytomas were found in 11.5% of patients, often with distant metastases at presentation. Loss of heterozygosity of the *NF1* has been demonstrated both in NF-1–associated and sporadic pheochromocytomas.[47]

LEUKEMIA

There is an increased risk of juvenile chronic myelomonocytic leukemia and acute lymphoblastic leukemia in children with NF-1. Homozygous inactivation of *NF1* in the bone marrow cells children with NF-1 and malignant myeloid disorders has been identified, suggesting that neurofibromin plays a role in down-regulating the growth of immature myeloid cells.[48] In addition, a population-based study in the United Kingdom identified that NF-1 individuals had a relative risk of developing acute lymphoblastic leukemia of 5.4 times the general population.[49]

OTHER TUMORS

Children with NF-1 may develop juvenile xanthogranulomas, which are yellowish papules less than 1 cm in diameter that are usually found on the head or trunk and may be multiple (Fig. 135-17). An unusual association between juvenile xanthogranulomas, NF-1, and the development of myeloid leukemias has been reported.[50] Although the pathogenesis is obscure, this association also has been observed independent of NF-1. Some authors have recommended "screening" blood counts for individuals who have juvenile xanthogranulomas and NF-1. Given that the precise magnitude of the risk is unknown, but certainly extremely small, this recommendation only serves to increase parental anxiety without providing any useful information and is not endorsed by the authors.

Rhabdomyosarcoma also occurs more frequently in individuals with NF-1.[51] Other tumors that appear to occur more frequently in adults with NF-1 are somatostatinomas of the duodenum and the ampulla of Vater, and GI stromal tumors. Compared to those tumors seen in non–NF-1 individuals, GI stromal tumors in NF-1 rarely arise in the pancreas, are smaller, and generally are not associated with hormonal symptoms (ie, diabetes, steatorrhea, and gallbladder disease).[52]

VASCULOPATHY

Patients with NF-1 may have a vasculopathy affecting essentially any arterial vessel. Clinical manifestations may include renal artery stenosis with hypertension, cerebral infarcts, bleeding aneurysms, and intermittent claudication of an extremity. This vasculopathy is a developmental problem not related to compression

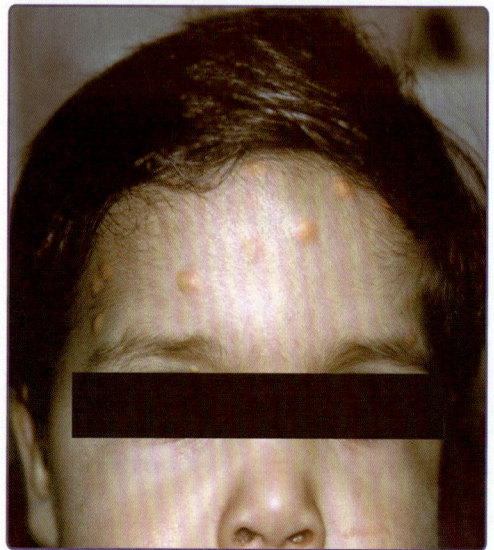

Figure 135-17 Multiple juvenile xanthogranulomas on the forehead.

of an arteriole by a neurofibroma, and appears to be acquired after birth, as the appearance of new lesions and the progression of preexisting ones have been described. Characteristic pathologic changes have been described in all layers of the vascular wall which ultimately leads to narrowing of the arterial lumen.

The most commonly identified vascular lesion in patients with NF-1 is in the renal artery, leading to renovascular hypertension.[53] Renal artery vasculopathy should be considered in any adult NF-1 patient with hypertension that is not easily controlled with a single antihypertensive medication; all NF-1 children should be evaluated for this complication. Aortography with selective angiography of the renal arteries should be used to confirm the diagnosis. If the blood pressure is uncontrollable using oral antihypertensives, percutaneous transluminal angioplasty can be performed and repeated if initially unsuccessful. Cerebral artery vasculopathy may lead to poststenotic proliferation of small capillaries, termed, *moyamoya*, which can recurrently bleed leading to strokes.

UNIDENTIFIED BRIGHT OBJECTS

Brain MRI of children with NF-1 frequently demonstrates regions of increased signal intensity on T2-weighted images, referred to as "unidentified bright objects" or UBOs (Fig. 135-18). UBOs may be found in the internal capsule, basal ganglia, cortex, cerebellar hemispheres, optic tract, or brainstem. They do not enhance and are not associated with compression of surrounding tissue, which distinguish them from neoplasms. UBOs are present in approximately 60% of children with NF-1, but disappear with age and are uncommon in adults. They are not associated with focal neurologic signs and are of uncertain significance. Past histopathologic studies have shown that the UBOs corresponded to areas of myelin vacuolization with increased water content. In addition, a recent study using diffusion tensor imaging provided further evidence that UBOs were caused by changes in the intramyelin water pool without demyelination or axonal damage.[54]

INTELLIGENCE AND LEARNING DISABILITIES

Contrary to gross misstatements in the older literature, the mean IQ of patients with NF-1 is only 5 to 10 points lower than the general population and unaffected siblings. However, learning disabilities, defined as discrepancies between ability (intellect) and performance, are quite common with an estimated prevalence of 30% to 60%.[55] Although earlier reports suggested there might be a specific "cognitive phenotype" in NF-1 characterized by an excess of visual/perceptual disabilities, newer studies demonstrate that verbal deficits (eg, reading) are at least as common as nonverbal disabilities in individuals with NF-1. These learning disabilities are lifelong and can affect adult functioning. Many children with NF-1 also have poor attention and impulse control, and may be diagnosed with attention deficit hyperactivity disorder, significantly interfering with school performance and learning. Stimulant medications may have a profound beneficial effect on the ability of these individuals to succeed academically and professionally.[56,57]

MANAGEMENT OF NEUROFIBROMATOSIS TYPE 1

Individuals with NF-1 are best cared for within a multidisciplinary clinic that has access to a wide range

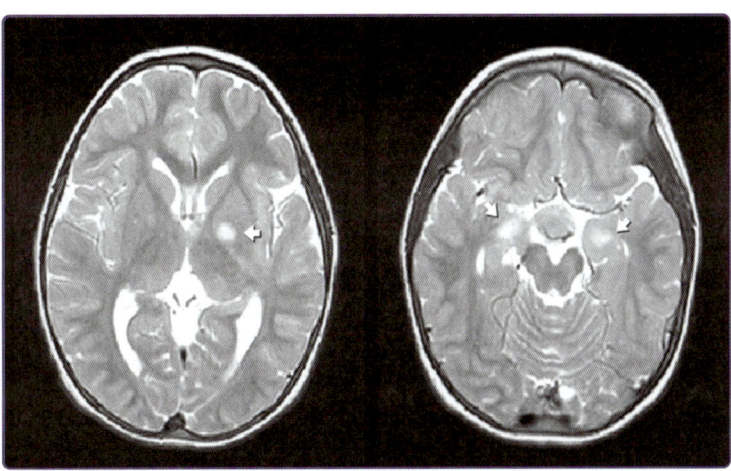

Figure 135-18 T2-weighted MRI hyperintensity, termed "unidentified bright object."

of subspecialists. The exact physician composition of the clinic is less important than the ability to obtain expeditious subspecialty consultation. All first-degree relatives should be examined for the cutaneous manifestations of NF-1 and should undergo slitlamp examination at the first visit to ascertain the presence of Lisch nodules. Yearly visits allow the physician to identify NF-1 complications early, while providing counseling and dissemination of information regarding NF-1. Individuals and families can obtain further information from the websites of the 2 national support groups: the Children's Tumor Foundation (www.ctf.org) and the Neurofibromatosis Network (www.nfnetwork.org).

All children with NF-1 who are 10 years old or younger should have yearly complete ophthalmologic examinations looking for signs of an OPT. These should include assessment of visual acuity, color vision, visual fields, funduscopy, and slitlamp examination. As almost all OPTs arise in children in this age group, the frequency of ophthalmologic examinations can be reduced in children older than 10 years of age. Yearly measurements of weight and height should be plotted on standardized growth charts, as the earliest indication of precocious puberty may be accelerated linear growth. Blood pressure measurements should be obtained at each visit to look for signs of renovascular hypertension. In addition, the spine should be examined each year for early signs of scoliosis.

CAFÉ-AU-LAIT SPOTS

Café-au-lait spots on the face are unusual in individuals with NF-1. On occasion, they do occur and affected individuals may seek to improve cosmesis. Attempts at removing café-au-lait spots with laser therapy have provided very mixed results. Copper vapor laser therapy provided good to excellent results in 15 of 16 treated patients.[58] Use of the Q-switched 755-nm alexandrite laser produced good to excellent results in 56% of treated patients and poor results in 17%.[59] Use of low-fluence 1064-nm Q-switched neodymium:yttrium-aluminum-garnet (Nd:YAG) laser therapy induced greater than 50% clearance in 75% of the café-au-lait spots treated.[60]

DISCRETE CUTANEOUS NEUROFIBROMAS

Discrete cutaneous neurofibromas may be removed surgically to improve cosmesis or to prevent local irritation, for example, in the hairline while brushing or on the foot rubbing against the shoe. Deeper neurofibromas may require surgical removal when pushing on vital structures, such as a dorsal root neurofibroma that infiltrates the neural foramen and compresses the spinal cord. Complications of surgery include regrowth of the original tumor and nerve damage. In individuals who have severe pruritus from a large burden of cutaneous neurofibromas, antihistamines may provide symptomatic relief. Uncontrolled anecdotal case reports suggest that ketotifen, an antihistamine and mast cell stabilizer, has provided relief from pruritus and pain and prevented the rapid growth of new neurofibromas.[61] Use of the carbon dioxide laser under general anesthesia to remove hundreds of cutaneous neurofibromas has resulted in markedly increased quality of life and decreased pain and pruritus for patients.[62] The residua of a flat smooth depigmented scar was not thought to be an impediment to such surgery by most patients. In another study, when compared to electrosurgery and carbon dioxide laser ablation, erbium:yttrium aluminium garnet (Er:YAG) laser ablation was superior.[63]

PLEXIFORM NEUROFIBROMAS

Until recently, the treatment of plexiform neurofibromas was limited to surgical debulking either to improve cosmesis or to prevent loss of function (eg, upper airway obstruction, blindness). Such surgery was highly limited in its efficacy; complete resection was impossible given the highly infiltrative nature of these tumors and tumor regrowth was common. Thus, there has been considerable interest in the development of nontraditional chemotherapy for use against these tumors. Unsurprisingly, the design of studies to test the efficacy of such agents was initially fraught with complications. Plexiform neurofibromas are quite different biologically from more conventional solid neoplasms. Lack of growth following treatment may be part of the natural history of the tumor rather than a true therapeutic response. In addition, tumor burden may be difficult to quantify radiographically; plexiform neurofibromas may "spread" along nerve roots sending out multiple finger-like projections, quite different than a single, solid tumor mass.

These difficulties largely have been overcome by data collected at the National Cancer Institute. Volumetric MRI has enabled researchers to accurately measure changes in growth of complex tumors in 3 dimensions and to show that tumor volume was a meaningful end point to use in clinical trials.[64] They demonstrated that younger patients had the most rapid growth of plexiform tumors that that new plexiform tumors were extremely unlikely to appear after the first few years of life.[65] Finally, the hormonal changes in puberty did not seem to accelerate the growth of these tumors.[66]

Armed with this information, several studies were performed to assess the impact of biologics on the growth of plexiform neurofibromas. Studies using pirfenidone, an antifibrotic agent that decreases proliferation of fibroblasts and collagen matrix synthesis, and a farnesyltransferase inhibitor that downregulates *Ras*, did not yield promising results.[67,68] Sirolimus, an inhibitor of the mammalian target of rapamycin, prolonged the time to progression by only 4 months in patients with progressive plexiform neurofibromas.[69] Based on in vitro studies of the important role of mast cell c-Kit receptor signaling, administration of imatinib to a 3-year-old with an unresectable airway plexiform neurofibroma led to 70% diminution in size during 3 months of therapy.[70] In addition, in a subsequent study, 17% of patients receiving imatinib had a 20% or more decrease in tumor volume.[71] If future studies demonstrate potential efficacy, the role of screening imaging to detect "hidden" plexiform neurofibromas will need to be readdressed.

OPTIC PATHWAY TUMORS

There has been considerable debate regarding the role of screening neuroimaging in the care of asymptomatic children with NF-1. Routine "screening" would be important if it led to early detection of OPTs and early initiation of therapy that prevented visual deterioration. A longitudinal study of children with NF-1 failed to identify any tumors in which early detection altered the patient's clinical course.[9] Moreover, targeted screening of very young children with NF-1, the high-risk group for the development of OPTs, failed, as 3 children developed symptomatic tumors shortly after having had normal MRI scans.[72] Brainstem tumors in both children and adults with NF-1 are generally more indolent than their counterparts in non–NF-1 individuals, suggesting that routine screening would not be beneficial.[73] Thus, the National Neurofibromatosis Foundation Optic Pathway Task Force has recommended against routine screening neuroimaging of all children with NF-1.[14] Although there are no comparable longitudinal data for adults regarding the performance of "routine" MRI scans of the head and spinal cord, it seems reasonable to perform such testing only in individuals who have symptoms or signs suggestive of CNS pathology.

Once identified, OPT should be followed by serial MRI and ophthalmologic examinations. Traditionally, treatment had been initiated only after demonstration of clear radiographic progression or deterioration of vision. However, a recent multicenter retrospective study from 10 institutions of 115 children treated for OPTs demonstrated that radiographic outcomes did not predict visual acuity outcomes.[74] Because the goal of treatment should be preservation of vision with minimization of side effects of therapy, tumor growth without visual decline might not be a priori an acceptable reason to institute therapy. When necessary, treatment with carboplatin and vincristine has proven effective in the management of these tumors.[75] Radiation therapy, while a mainstay of treatment of progressive CNS neoplasms not associated with NF-1, is not appropriate for NF-1–associated OPTs because of the risk of vasculopathy, second malignancies, and detrimental neurocognitive and endocrinologic side effects in very young children.

REFERENCES

1. Neurofibromatosis. Conference statement. National Institutes of Health Consensus Development Conference. *Arch Neurol*. 1988;45(5):575-578.
2. Denayer E, Chmara M, Brems H, et al. Legius syndrome in fourteen families. *Hum Mutat*. 2011;32(1):E1985-E1998.
3. Obringer AC, Meadows AT, Zackai EH. The diagnosis of neurofibromatosis-1 in the child under the age of 6 years. *Am J Dis Child*. 1989;143(6):717-719.
4. Carroll SL, Ratner N. How does the Schwann cell lineage form tumors in NF1? *Glia*. 2008;56(14):1590-1605.
5. Staser K, Yang FC, Clapp DW. Pathogenesis of plexiform neurofibroma: tumor-stromal/hematopoietic interactions in tumor progression. *Annu Rev Pathol*. 2012;7:469-495.
6. Brossier NM, Carroll SL. Genetically engineered mouse models shed new light on the pathogenesis of neurofibromatosis type I-related neoplasms of the peripheral nervous system. *Brain Res Bull*. 2012;88(1):58-71.
7. Ferner RE, Golding JF, Smith M, et al. [18F]2-fluoro-2-deoxy-D-glucose positron emission tomography (FDG PET) as a diagnostic tool for neurofibromatosis 1 (NF1) associated malignant peripheral nerve sheath tumours (MPNSTs): a long-term clinical study. *Ann Oncol*. 2008;19(2):390-394.
8. Combemale P, Valeyrie-Allanore L, Giammarile F, et al. Utility of 18F-FDG PET with a semi-quantitative index in the detection of sarcomatous transformation in patients with neurofibromatosis type 1. *PLoS One*. 2014;9(2):e85954.
9. Listernick R, Charrow J, Greenwald M, et al. Natural history of optic pathway tumors in children with neurofibromatosis type 1: a longitudinal study. *J Pediatr*. 1994;125(1):63-66.
10. Listernick R, Charrow J, Greenwald MJ, et al. Optic gliomas in children with neurofibromatosis type 1. *J Pediatr*. 1989;114(5):788-792.
11. Johnson KJ, Fisher MJ, Listernick RL, et al. Parent-of-origin in individuals with familial neurofibromatosis type 1 and optic pathway gliomas. *Fam Cancer*. 2012;11(4):653-656.
12. Diggs-Andrews KA, Brown JA, Gianino SM, et al. Sex is a major determinant of neuronal dysfunction in neurofibromatosis type 1. *Ann Neurol*. 2014;75(2):309-316.
13. Listernick R, Ferner RE, Liu GT, et al. Optic pathway gliomas in neurofibromatosis-1: controversies and recommendations. *Ann Neurol*. 2007;61(3):189-198.
14. Listernick R, Louis DN, Packer RJ, et al. Optic pathway gliomas in children with neurofibromatosis 1: consensus statement from the NF1 Optic Pathway Glioma Task Force. *Ann Neurol*. 1997;41(2):143-149.
15. Habiby R, Silverman B, Listernick R, et al. Precocious puberty in children with neurofibromatosis type 1. *J Pediatr*. 1995;126(3):364-367.
16. Stevenson DA, Little D, Armstrong L, et al. Approaches to treating NF1 tibial pseudarthrosis: consensus from the Children's Tumor Foundation NF1 Bone Abnormalities Consortium. *J Pediatr Orthop*. 2013;33(3):269-275.
17. Riccardi VM. Von Recklinghausen neurofibromatosis. *N Engl J Med*. 1981;305(27):1617-1627.
18. Kluwe L, Nguyen R, Vogt J, et al. Internal tumor burden in neurofibromatosis type I patients with large NF1 deletions. *Genes Chromosomes Cancer*. 2012;51(5):447-451.
19. Upadhyaya M, Huson SM, Davies M, et al. An absence of cutaneous neurofibromas associated with a 3-bp inframe deletion in exon 17 of the NF1 gene (c.2970-2972 delAAT): evidence of a clinically significant NF1 genotype-phenotype correlation. *Am J Hum Genet*. 2007;80(1):140-151.
20. Ratner N, Miller SJ. A RASopathy gene commonly mutated in cancer: the neurofibromatosis type 1 tumour suppressor. *Nat Rev Cancer*. 2015;15(5):290-301.
21. Spurlock G, Knight SJ, Thomas N, et al. Molecular evolution of a neurofibroma to malignant peripheral nerve sheath tumor (MPNST) in an NF1 patient: correlation between histopathological, clinical and

molecular findings. *J Cancer Res Clin Oncol*. 2010;136(12):1869-1880.
22. Hirata Y, Brems H, Suzuki M, et al. Interaction between a domain of the negative regulator of the Ras-ERK pathway, SPRED1 protein, and the GTPase-activating protein-related domain of neurofibromin is implicated in Legius syndrome and neurofibromatosis type 1. *J Biol Chem*. 2016;291(7):3124-3134.
23. Dasgupta B, Li W, Perry A, et al. Glioma formation in neurofibromatosis 1 reflects preferential activation of K-RAS in astrocytes. *Cancer Res*. 2005;65(1):236-245.
24. Li C, Cheng Y, Gutmann DA, et al. Differential localization of the neurofibromatosis 1 (NF1) gene product, neurofibromin, with the F-actin or microtubule cytoskeleton during differentiation of telencephalic neurons. *Brain Res Dev Brain Res*. 2001;130(2):231-248.
25. Costa RM, Federov NB, Kogan JH, et al. Mechanism for the learning deficits in a mouse model of neurofibromatosis type 1. *Nature*. 2002;415(6871):526-530.
26. Jessen WJ, Miller SJ, Jousma E, et al. MEK inhibition exhibits efficacy in human and mouse neurofibromatosis tumors. *J Clin Invest*. 2013;123(1):340-347.
27. Steinmann K, Kluwe L, Friedrich RE, et al. Mechanisms of loss of heterozygosity in neurofibromatosis type 1-associated plexiform neurofibromas. *J Invest Dermatol*. 2009;129(3):615-621.
28. Gutmann DH. Microglia in the tumor microenvironment: taking their TOLL on glioma biology. *Neuro Oncol*. 2015;17(2):171-173.
29. Slattery WH. Neurofibromatosis type 2. *Otolaryngol Clin North Am*. 2015;48(3):443-460.
30. Firestone BK, Arias JD, Shields CL, et al. Bilateral combined hamartomas of the retina and retinal pigment epithelium as the presenting feature of neurofibromatosis type 2 (Wishart type). *J Pediatr Ophthalmol Strabismus*. 2014;51:e33-e36.
31. McLaughlin ME, Pepin SM, Maccollin M, et al. Ocular pathologic findings of neurofibromatosis type 2. *Arch Ophthalmol*. 2007;125(3):389-394.
32. Tanito K, Ota A, Kamide R, et al. Clinical features of 58 Japanese patients with mosaic neurofibromatosis 1. *J Dermatol*. 2014;41(8):724-728.
33. Ruggieri M, Huson SM. The clinical and diagnostic implications of mosaicism in the neurofibromatoses. *Neurology*. 2001;56(11):1433-1443.
34. Tinschert S, Naumann I, Stegmann E, et al. Segmental neurofibromatosis is caused by somatic mutation of the neurofibromatosis type 1 (NF1) gene. *Eur J Hum Genet*. 2000;8(6):455-459.
35. Tartaglia M, Gelb BD, Zenker M. Noonan syndrome and clinically related disorders. *Baillieres Best Pract Res Clin Endocrinol Metab*. 2011;25(1):161-179.
36. De Luca A, Bottillo I, Sarkozy A, et al. NF1 gene mutations represent the major molecular event underlying neurofibromatosis-Noonan syndrome. *Am J Hum Genet*. 2005;77(6):1092-1101.
37. Denayer E, Descheemaeker MJ, Stewart DR, et al. Observations on intelligence and behavior in 15 patients with Legius syndrome. *Am J Med Genet C Semin Med Genet*. 2011;157C(2):123-128.
38. Lu-Emerson C, Plotkin SR. The neurofibromatoses. Part 2: NF2 and schwannomatosis. *Rev Neurol Dis*. 2009;6(3):E81-E86.
39. Baser ME, Friedman JM, Evans DG. Increasing the specificity of diagnostic criteria for schwannomatosis. *Neurology*. 2006;66(5):730-732.
40. Smith MJ, Isidor B, Beetz C, et al. Mutations in LZTR1 add to the complex heterogeneity of schwannomatosis. *Neurology*. 2015;84(2):141-147.
41. Jett K, Nguyen R, Arman D, et al. Quantitative associations of scalp and body subcutaneous neurofibromas with internal plexiform tumors in neurofibromatosis 1. *Am J Med Genet A*. 2015;167(7):1518-1524.
42. Plotkin SR, Bredella MA, Cai W, et al. Quantitative assessment of whole-body tumor burden in adult patients with neurofibromatosis. *PLoS One*. 2012;7(4):e35711.
43. Crawford AH, Herrera-Soto J. Scoliosis associated with neurofibromatosis. *Orthop Clin North Am*. 2007;38(4):553-562.
44. Uusitalo E, Leppavirta J, Koffert A, et al. Incidence and mortality of neurofibromatosis: a total population study in Finland. *J Invest Dermatol*. 2015;135(3):904-906.
45. Evans DG, Baser ME, McGaughran J, et al. Malignant peripheral nerve sheath tumours in neurofibromatosis 1. *J Med Genet*. 2002;39(5):311-314.
46. Walther MM, Herring J, Enquist E, et al. von Recklinghausen's disease and pheochromocytomas. *J Urol*. 1999;162(5):1582-1586.
47. Bausch B, Borozdin W, Mautner VF, et al. Germline NF1 mutational spectra and loss-of-heterozygosity analyses in patients with pheochromocytoma and neurofibromatosis type 1. *J Clin Endocrinol Metab*. 2007;92(7):2784-2792.
48. Staser K, Park SJ, Rhodes SD, et al. Normal hematopoiesis and neurofibromin-deficient myeloproliferative disease require Erk. *J Clin Invest*. 2013;123(1):329-334.
49. Stiller CA, Chessells JM, Fitchett M. Neurofibromatosis and childhood leukaemia/lymphoma: a population-based UKCCSG study. *Br J Cancer*. 1994;70(5):969-972.
50. Jans SR, Schomerus E, Bygum A. Neurofibromatosis type 1 diagnosed in a child based on multiple juvenile xanthogranulomas and juvenile myelomonocytic leukemia. *Pediatr Dermatol*. 2015;32(1):e29-e32.
51. Crucis A, Richer W, Brugieres L, et al. Rhabdomyosarcomas in children with neurofibromatosis type I: a national historical cohort. *Pediatr Blood Cancer*. 2015;62(10):1733-1738.
52. Takazawa Y, Sakurai S, Sakuma Y, et al. Gastrointestinal stromal tumors of neurofibromatosis type I (von Recklinghausen's disease). *Am J Surg Pathol*. 2005;29(6):755-763.
53. Srinivasan A, Krishnamurthy G, Fontalvo-Herazo L, et al. Spectrum of renal findings in pediatric fibromuscular dysplasia and neurofibromatosis type 1. *Pediatr Radiol*. 2011;41(3):308-316.
54. Billiet T, Madler B, D'Arco F, et al. Characterizing the microstructural basis of "unidentified bright objects" in neurofibromatosis type 1: a combined in vivo multi-component T2 relaxation and multi-shell diffusion MRI analysis. *Neuroimage Clin*. 2014;4:649-658.
55. Sangster J, Shores EA, Watt S, et al. The cognitive profile of preschool-aged children with neurofibromatosis type 1. *Child Neuropsychol*. 2011;17(1):1-16.
56. Lidzba K, Granstroem S, Leark RA, et al. Pharmacotherapy of attention deficit in neurofibromatosis type 1: effects on cognition. *Neuropediatrics*. 2014;45(4):240-246.
57. Lion-Francois L, Gueyffier F, Mercier C, et al. The effect of methylphenidate on neurofibromatosis type 1: a randomised, double-blind, placebo-controlled, crossover trial. *Orphanet J Rare Dis*. 2014;9:142.
58. Somyos K, Boonchu K, Somsak K, et al. Copper vapour laser treatment of cafe-au-lait macules. *Br J Dermatol*. 1996;135(6):964-968.
59. Wang Y, Qian H, Lu Z. Treatment of cafe au lait macules in Chinese patients with a Q-switched 755-nm alexandrite laser. *J Dermatolog Treat*. 2012;23(6):431-436.

60. Kim HR, Ha JM, Park MS, et al. A low-fluence 1064-nm Q-switched neodymium-doped yttrium aluminium garnet laser for the treatment of cafe-au-lait macules. *J Am Acad Dermatol*. 2015;73(3):477-483.
61. Riccardi VM. Ketotifen suppression of NF1 neurofibroma growth over 30 years. *Am J Med Genet A*. 2015;167(7):1570-1577.
62. Meni C, Sbidian E, Moreno JC, et al. Treatment of neurofibromas with a carbon dioxide laser: a retrospective cross-sectional study of 106 patients. *Dermatology*. 2015;230(3):263-268.
63. Kriechbaumer LK, Susani M, Kircher SG, et al. Comparative study of CO2- and Er:YAG laser ablation of multiple cutaneous neurofibromas in von Recklinghausen's disease. *Lasers Med Sci*. 2014;29(3):1083-1091.
64. Dombi E, Solomon J, Gillespie AJ, et al. NF1 plexiform neurofibroma growth rate by volumetric MRI: relationship to age and body weight. *Neurology*. 2007;68(9):643-647.
65. Nguyen R, Dombi E, Widemann BC, et al. Growth dynamics of plexiform neurofibromas: a retrospective cohort study of 201 patients with neurofibromatosis 1. *Orphanet J Rare Dis*. 2012;7:75.
66. Dagalakis U, Lodish M, Dombi E, et al. Puberty and plexiform neurofibroma tumor growth in patients with neurofibromatosis type I. *J Pediatr*. 2014;164(3):620-624.
67. Widemann BC, Babovic-Vuksanovic D, Dombi E, et al. Phase II trial of pirfenidone in children and young adults with neurofibromatosis type 1 and progressive plexiform neurofibromas. *Pediatr Blood Cancer*. 2014;61(9):1598-1602.
68. Widemann BC, Dombi E, Gillespie A, et al. Phase 2 randomized, flexible crossover, double-blinded, placebo-controlled trial of the farnesyltransferase inhibitor tipifarnib in children and young adults with neurofibromatosis type 1 and progressive plexiform neurofibromas. *Neuro Oncol*. 2014;16(5):707-718.
69. Weiss B, Widemann BC, Wolters P, et al. Sirolimus for non-progressive NF1-associated plexiform neurofibromas: an NF clinical trials consortium phase II study. *Pediatr Blood Cancer*. 2014;61(6):982-986.
70. Yang FC, Ingram DA, Chen S, et al. Nf1-dependent tumors require a microenvironment containing Nf1+/− and c-kit-dependent bone marrow. *Cell*. 2008;135(3):437-448.
71. Robertson KA, Nalepa G, Yang FC, et al. Imatinib mesylate for plexiform neurofibromas in patients with neurofibromatosis type 1: a phase 2 trial. *Lancet Oncol*. 2012;13(12):1218-1224.
72. Listernick R, Charrow J, Greenwald M. Emergence of optic pathway gliomas in children with neurofibromatosis type 1 after normal neuroimaging results. *J Pediatr*. 1992;121(4):584-587.
73. Ullrich NJ, Raja AI, Irons MB, et al. Brainstem lesions in neurofibromatosis type 1. *Neurosurgery*. 2007;61(4):762-766; discussion 766-767.
74. Fisher MJ, Loguidice M, Gutmann DH, et al. Visual outcomes in children with neurofibromatosis type 1-associated optic pathway glioma following chemotherapy: a multicenter retrospective analysis. *Neuro Oncol*. 2012;14(6):790-797.
75. Brossier NM, Gutmann DH. Improving outcomes for neurofibromatosis 1-associated brain tumors. *Expert Rev Anticancer Ther*. 2015;15(4):415-423.

Chapter 136 :: Tuberous Sclerosis Complex
:: Thomas N. Darling

第一百三十六章

结节性硬化症

中文导读

结节性硬化症（TSC）是一种遗传性疾病，影响多个器官，通常是大脑、心脏、肾脏、肺和皮肤。TSC通常在婴儿期表现为癫痫发作，有部分患者直到成年才被诊断出来。大多数人将经历与广泛的认知、行为和精神障碍相关的困难，这些障碍被统称为TSC相关的神经精神障碍。皮肤损害对生活质量有不利影响，皮肤科医生经常参与诊断或治疗TSC的皮肤表现。其皮肤临床表现包括色素沉着斑片、面部血管纤维瘤、鲨革斑、前额斑块和甲周纤维瘤，以及少见的牙齿坑蚀和口内纤维瘤。其病因主要是由肿瘤抑制基因TSC1或TSC2突变引起的，其诊断是基于遗传或临床特征，同时可行组织病理学检查。相关影像学检查及分子诊断等可以用来辅助诊断。结节性硬化症患者的总体存活率较正常人降低，但一部分患者寿命正常，几乎没有并发症。药物治疗上主要是mTOR抑制药的使用，同时需要注意该病的监测和筛查。

〔粟 娟〕

AT-A-GLANCE

- Autosomal dominant syndrome with variable expressivity.
- Manifested by hamartomatous tumors in multiple organs, including brain (causing seizures), eyes, heart, kidneys, lungs, and skin.
- Skin lesions occur in nearly all individuals and are important for diagnosis.
- Skin lesions include hypomelanotic macules, "confetti" lesions, facial angiofibromas, fibrous cephalic plaques, shagreen patches, and ungual fibromas.
- Hypomelanotic macules appear at birth or shortly thereafter and are most useful in early diagnosis.
- Although the skin lesions are benign, they may require treatment because of symptoms or disfigurement.
- Skin lesions can be treated with surgery or topical sirolimus.

Tuberous sclerosis complex (TSC) is a genetic disease caused by mutations in a tumor-suppressor gene, either *TSC1* or *TSC2*, which affects multiple organs, typically the brain, heart, kidneys, lungs, and skin.[1] TSC commonly presents with seizures during infancy but some individuals remain undiagnosed until adulthood.[2] Most individuals will experience difficulties related to a wide range of cognitive, behavioral, and psychiatric disorders encompassed by the umbrella term TSC-associated neuropsychiatric disorders (TAND).[3] Skin lesions adversely affect quality of life[4] and dermatologists are frequently called upon to diagnose or treat the skin manifestations of TSC.

EPIDEMIOLOGY

The incidence of TSC is as high as 1 in 6000 live births with a prevalence of approximately 1 in 25,000.[5,6] It occurs with equal frequency in males and females and in different races and ethnicities. Hereditary transmission is evident in approximately one-third of patients. Sporadic disease occurs in about two-thirds of patients, caused by de novo mutations.[7]

CLINICAL FEATURES

CUTANEOUS FINDINGS

Individuals with TSC may develop multiple different types of skin findings, including hypomelanotic macules, facial angiofibromas, fibrous cephalic plaques, shagreen patches, and ungual fibromas.[8] Some skin findings, such as hypomelanotic macules, may appear at birth, whereas others, such as ungual fibromas, may not appear until adulthood. Most individuals eventually manifest at least 1 skin finding, but there is variability in severity between individuals.[9] The ability to recognize TSC-related skin findings is important for diagnosis as skin lesions constitute several of the major and minor features for clinical diagnosis (see section "Diagnosis").[10,11]

HYPOMELANOTIC MACULES

Hypomelanotic macules (Fig. 136-1) are observed in more than 90% of children with TSC.[12,13] The macules are often present at birth or appear within the first few years of life and may fade or disappear in adulthood.[9] The ultraviolet light of a Wood lamp may improve detection, especially in lightly pigmented individuals (Fig. 136-2).[8]

Hypomelanotic macules typically measure 0.5 to 3.0 cm in diameter. They are off-white and incompletely depigmented as in vitiligo. Some are oval at one end and taper to a point at the other. Such lesions are called *ash-leaf spots* because of their resemblance to the leaf of the European mountain ash.[14] They number from 1 to more than 20. They can be located anywhere on the body, but tend to occur most often on the trunk and buttocks. When located on the scalp, they cause poliosis.[12]

Three or more hypopigmented macules measuring 5 mm or greater in longest dimension constitutes a major feature for the diagnosis of tuberous sclerosis.[10] One or 2, and in rare individuals up to 3, hypomelanotic macules occur in 4.7% of the general population.[15] A less-common type of hypopigmentation is the "confetti" skin lesion (Fig. 136-3), which is considered a minor feature for diagnosis.[10] It typically occurs on the legs below the knees or on the forearms, and consists of multiple hypopigmented macules 2 to 3 mm in diameter.[12,14]

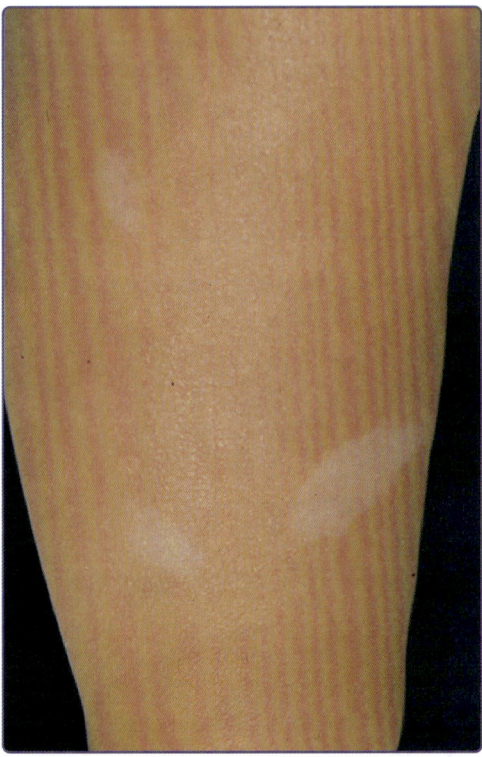

Figure 136-1 Hypomelanotic ash-leaf macules on the lower leg of a child with tuberous sclerosis complex.

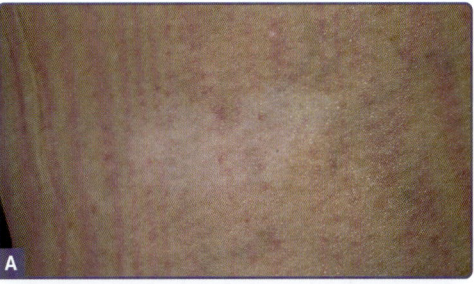

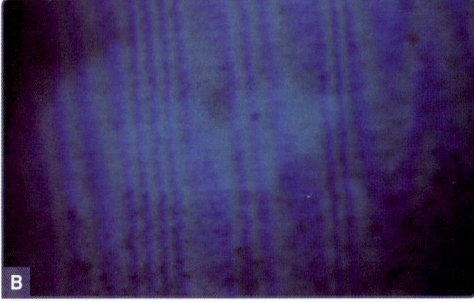

Figure 136-2 **A,** Hypomelanotic macules on the lateral chest of an adult with tuberous sclerosis complex. The macules may be easily overlooked. **B,** Wood lamp accentuates the macules.

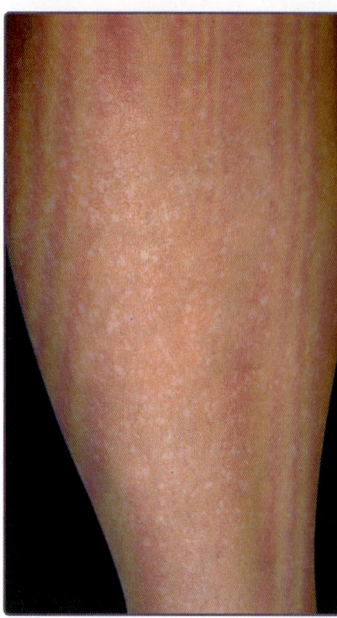

Figure 136-3 Confetti-like hypopigmented macules on the lower leg of an adult with tuberous sclerosis complex.

darker pigmentation. They occur on the central face and are often concentrated in the alar grooves (Fig. 136-5), extending symmetrically onto the cheeks and to the nose, nasal opening, and chin, with relative sparing of the upper lip and lateral face. They may number from 1 to more than 100. Lesions may coalesce to form large nodules, especially in the alar grooves.[12,13] Sometimes lesions occur on the forehead, scalp, or eyelids. Adults may develop angiofibromas on the nipples.[16] Angiofibromas may be unilateral in rare cases. Unilateral angiofibromas may indicate a segmental or mosaic defects.[17]

The development of papules may be preceded by mild erythema that is intensified by emotion or heat. During puberty, angiofibromas may grow in size and number. During adulthood they tend to be stable in size, but redness may gradually diminish.[8]

Three or more angiofibromas comprise a major feature.[10] A solitary angiofibroma is clinically and histologically indistinguishable from the fibrous papule that occurs sporadically as a single lesion in the general population. The development of multiple angiofibromas with onset later in adolescence or early adulthood is not specific for TSC and may, instead, indicate multiple endocrine neoplasia Type 1 or Birt-Hogg-Dubé syndrome.[11]

FACIAL ANGIOFIBROMAS

Angiofibromas generally appear between 2 and 5 years of age and eventually affect 75% to 90% of patients.[9,12,13] These 1 to 3 mm in diameter, pink to red papules have a smooth surface (Fig. 136-4). They may be hyperpigmented, especially in individuals with

FIBROUS CEPHALIC PLAQUE

The fibrous cephalic plaque, previously called forehead plaque, may be congenital or show gradual development over years.[12] It is present in approximately 40% of patients.[9,12,13] It is an irregular, soft to firm, connective tissue nevus with the color of the normal surrounding skin, red, or hyperpigmented in darkly pigmented individuals (Fig. 136-6). The plaque classically develops on the forehead, but can occur on the scalp, cheeks, and elsewhere on the face. The fibrous cephalic plaque and/or multiple angiofibromas is a major feature for diagnosis.[10]

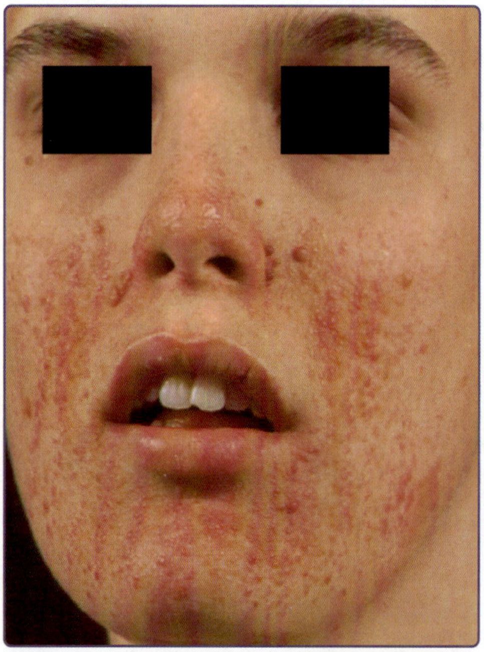

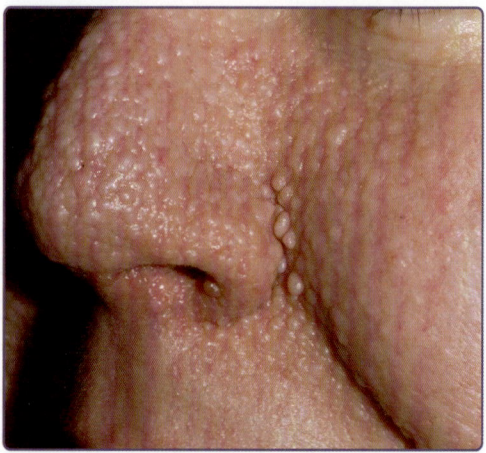

Figure 136-4 Multiple facial angiofibromas on the nose, cheeks, and chin, with relative sparing of the upper lip is commonly observed in tuberous sclerosis complex.

Figure 136-5 Angiofibromas are often larger in the alar grooves and may become less erythematous over time, as in this adult with tuberous sclerosis complex.

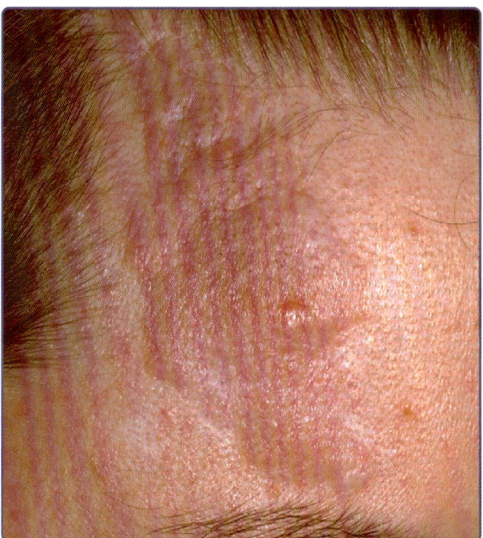

Figure 136-6 The forehead fibrous plaque in tuberous sclerosis complex is often pink-red and has a bumpy surface and irregular outline.

SHAGREEN PATCH

The shagreen patch is observed in approximately 50% of patients.[9,12,13] It may be present in infancy, but usually becomes apparent later. It is a firm or rubbery irregular plaque ranging in size from 1 to 10 cm (Fig. 136-7). The surface may appear bumpy with coalescing papules and nodules, or the patch may have the surface appearance of an orange peel. The color may be that of the surrounding skin, or it may be slightly pink or brown. There may be scattered smaller oval papules with or without a larger plaque (Fig. 136-8). The most common location is on the lower back to sacral region; less commonly, the patch is on the mid or upper back, buttocks, or thighs.[8]

UNGUAL FIBROMAS

Ungual fibromas, also known as *Koenen tumors*, usually appear after the first decade and eventually affect more than 85% of adults with TSC.[9,13] They are more common on the toes than on the fingers.[18]

Ungual fibromas measure 1 mm to 1 cm in diameter. They arise from under the proximal nailfold (periungual fibromas) and under the nail plate (subungual fibromas). Periungual fibromas are red papules and nodules that are firm, pointed, and hyperkeratotic, or soft and rounded (Fig. 136-9). They press on the nail matrix and cause a longitudinal groove, and sometimes a groove forms without an evident papule (Fig. 136-10).[18] Subungual fibromas are visible through the nail plate as red or white oval lesions or as red papules emerging from the distal nail plate, causing distal subungual onycholysis (Fig. 136-11). In addition to ungual fibromas, individuals with TSC may develop "red comets" (subungual red streaks), splinter hemorrhages, and longitudinal leukonychia.[18]

The presence of 2 or more ungual fibromas is a major feature for diagnosis of TSC.[10] Solitary lesions (also termed *acral* or *acquired digital fibrokeratomas*) are also observed in the general population, especially after nail trauma.[19]

OTHER SKIN LESIONS

Folliculocystic and collagen hamartomas are large plaques with follicular comedo-like openings and cysts observed in association with TSC.[20] Molluscum fibrosum pendulum (skin tags) is the name given to multiple fibroepithelial polyps in TSC (Fig. 136-12).[12] Skin tags are common in the general population, so these are not useful for diagnosis. Miliary fibromas are patches of multiple minute papules, usually on the neck or trunk that appear like "gooseflesh."[8] Pachydermodactyly is a benign thickening of the proximal fingers that has been observed in a few patients with TSC.[18]

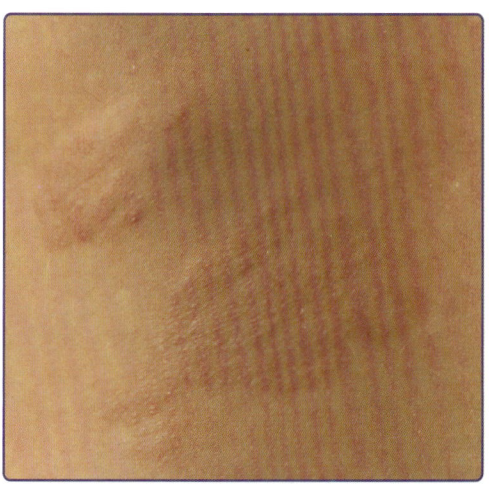

Figure 136-7 The shagreen patch in tuberous sclerosis complex is a firm, bumpy plaque that is usually located on the lower back.

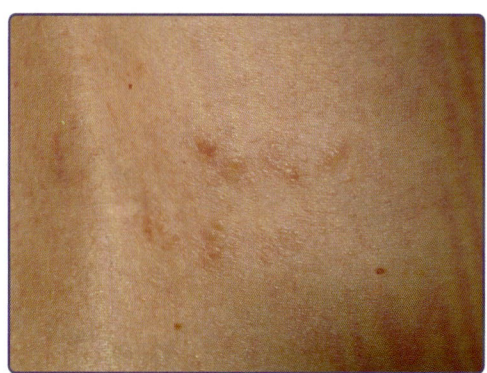

Figure 136-8 The shagreen patch may consist of grouped, dermal papules that are minimally elevated above the skin.

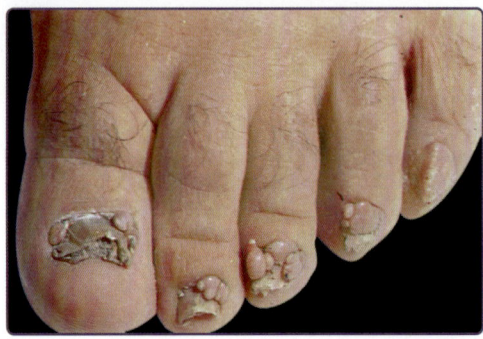

Figure 136-9 Multiple periungual and subungual fibromas on the toes in a patient with tuberous sclerosis complex.

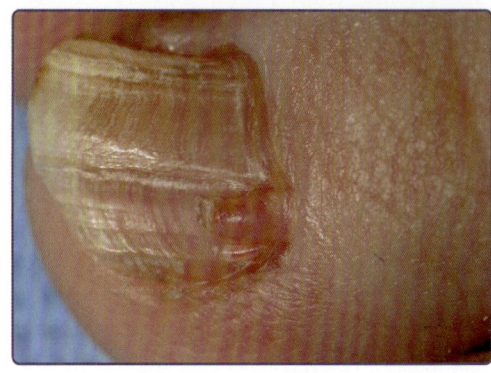

Figure 136-10 Periungual fibromas emanating from the proximal nailfold in tuberous sclerosis complex causes a longitudinal groove in the nail.

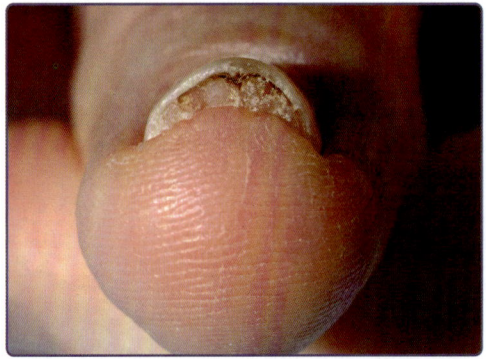

Figure 136-11 Subungual fibromas may disrupt the normal nail anatomy in tuberous sclerosis complex, causing distal onycholysis.

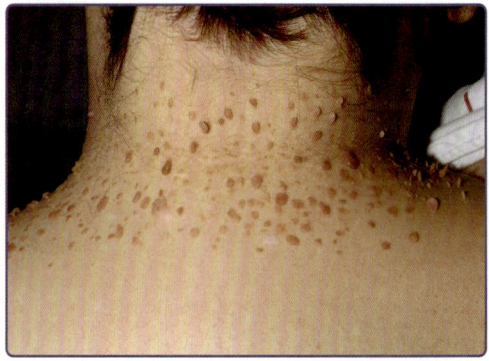

Figure 136-12 Molluscum fibrosum pendulum, another name for multiple skin tags in tuberous sclerosis complex, is observed on the neck in this patient.

DENTAL PITTING

Multiple pits of the dental enamel are observed in up to 100% of TSC patients.[21] These pits can be tiny pinpoint lesions or larger crater-like lesions (Fig. 136-13). They occur on both deciduous and permanent teeth. The identification of these lesions is enhanced by using a dental plaque stain. Dental pits can also be seen in the general population, albeit with lower prevalence and at lower numbers than in TSC.[21] The presence of more than 3 dental pits is a minor feature for diagnosis.[10]

INTRAORAL FIBROMAS

Approximately 50% of TSC patients have intraoral fibromas (Fig. 136-14).[13] These sometimes occur in the

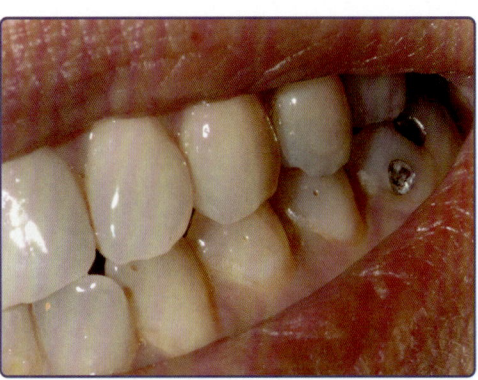

Figure 136-13 Multiple dental enamel pits are seen in nearly all patients with tuberous sclerosis complex.

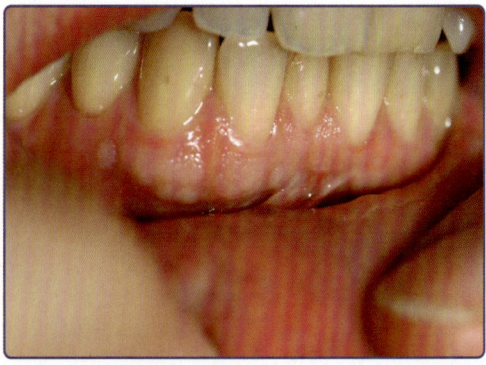

Figure 136-14 Multiple gingival fibromas in an adult with tuberous sclerosis complex.

first decade but are more common in adulthood. They are most common on the gingivae, but also occur on the buccal and labial mucosa, hard palate, and tongue. Some patients have diffuse gingival overgrowth. Gingival overgrowth is a common side effect of anticonvulsants, especially phenytoin and cyclosporine, but gingival overgrowth can be observed in TSC even in patients not treated with anticonvulsants or immunosuppressive agents.[21] Two or more intraoral fibromas are a minor feature for diagnosis.[10] Oral fibromas in the general population are typically single and form at sites of trauma, usually on the tongue or buccal mucosa.[21]

NONCUTANEOUS FINDINGS

BRAIN

Cerebral lesions include cortical dysplasia (tubers and white matter migration lines), subependymal nodules, and subependymal giant cell astrocytomas. Seizures occur in approximately 80% of patients, with onset in most patients in the first 3 years of life. Epilepsy is most likely infantile spasms or focal seizures, but may be tonic, atonic, or tonic–clonic seizures.[22] The first-line treatment of infantile spasms is vigabatrin.[23] Seizures are treated with anticonvulsant drugs as used in other forms of epilepsy. Epilepsy surgery may be required for seizures intractable to anticonvulsant therapy.[23] Other approaches used to reduce seizures include ketogenic diet, vagus nerve stimulation, and possibly mammalian target of rapamycin (mTOR) inhibitors.[22]

TAND encompasses a range of behavioral, intellectual, and psychosocial difficulties.[3] Approximately half of individuals with TSC will have intellectual disability, ranging from mild to profound. Even those with normal intellectual abilities may have deficits in recall memory, attention, or executive function. Nearly half of individuals with TSC have autism spectrum disorder or attention deficit hyperactivity disorder. Aggressive behavior, impulsivity, and sleep disorders are also common, and adolescents and adults may have anxiety and depressive disorders. TSC affects self-esteem and family and peer relationships.[22]

Subependymal nodules occur in approximately 80% of individuals with TSC, and subependymal giant cell astrocytomas develop in approximately 5% to 15% of individuals with TSC. Subependymal giant cell astrocytomas may be treated using an mTOR inhibitor or acute obstructive hydrocephalus may require surgical resection and possibly shunting.[22,23]

HEART

Cardiac rhabdomyomas occur in approximately 80% of infants with TSC and nearly 100% of fetuses with multiple cardiac rhabdomyomas have TSC.[24] These neoplasms are often asymptomatic and spontaneously regress, but they may cause fetal hydrops and stillbirth or heart failure shortly after birth. Treatment of cardiac rhabdomyomas with mTOR inhibitors may speed regression. Cardiac arrhythmias are common in TSC, including slow, fast, and irregular rhythms.[24]

KIDNEYS

Angiomyolipomas are observed in up to 80% of TSC patients and are usually renal but may be hepatic.[10,25] Additional renal lesions include renal cysts in approximately 30% and renal cell carcinoma in 2% to 3% of TSC patients. Polycystic kidney disease from contiguous *TSC2-PKD1* deletion is present in approximately 1 in 20 patients.[25] Renal lesions can cause renal insufficiency, hypertension, and potentially fatal retroperitoneal hemorrhage. Patients may require selective embolization followed by corticosteroids as first-line therapy for angiomyolipomas with acute hemorrhage. Treatment with an mTOR inhibitor is first-line therapy for asymptomatic growing angiomyolipomas.[23,25]

LUNGS

Lung involvement in TSC includes lymphangioleiomyomatosis (LAM), multifocal micronodular pneumocyte hyperplasia, and clear cell tumors of the lung.[10] LAM develops in females with TSC during the third or fourth decade of life and the risk of disease increases with age. Radiographic evidence of LAM was observed in up to 80% of adult females with TSC older than age 40 years.[26] It may cause spontaneous pneumothorax, chylothorax, dyspnea, cough, and hemoptysis.[27] mTOR inhibitors may be used to treat LAM patients with moderate to severe lung disease or rapid progression.[23]

EYES

Retinal hamartomas are observed in 30% to 50% of TSC patients.[10] The most common type is flat and translucent. Also common are elevated, opaque, and sometimes calcified multinodular "mulberry" lesions.[28] Retinal hamartomas are usually stable in size but enucleation has been required for enlarging retinal astrocytomas. Retinal hamartomas can be similar to retinal lesions in neurofibromatosis Type 1 and may appear similar to retinoblastomas.[28] TSC patients may also have retinal achromic patches that appear as hypopigmented patches in the retina.[10]

OTHER ORGANS

Hamartomatous polyps have been observed in the colon and rectum of TSC patients.[29] Benign tumors sometimes occur in the spleen, thymus, and thyroid. TSC also may be associated with pituitary, parathyroid, and islet cell tumors.[30] Arterial stenotic-occlusive disease and arterial aneurysms including aortic and intracranial aneurysms have been observed.[31] Bone lesions in TSC are usually asymptomatic and may be sclerotic (calvaria, pelvis, vertebrae, ribs, and long bones) or cystic (phalanges).[32,33]

COMPLICATIONS

None of the skin lesions in TSC is prone to malignant degeneration, but the lesions can be a major cosmetic concern for the patient, causing social isolation and difficulties with self-esteem.[34] Angiofibromas, facial plaques, and ungual fibromas can be painful or bleed spontaneously or in response to minor trauma. Ungual fibromas can cause nail dystrophy and eventual loss of the nail. Large facial lesions may obstruct vision or occlude the nasal passages.[35]

ETIOLOGY AND PATHOGENESIS

TSC is caused by mutations in a tumor-suppressor gene, either *TSC1* or *TSC2*. The *TSC1* gene maps to chromosome band 9q34 and consists of 23 exons that encodes a 130-kDa protein called *hamartin* or TSC1. The *TSC2* gene maps to chromosome band 16p13.3 and includes 42 exons that encodes a 200-kDa protein called *tuberin* or TSC2.[7] The mutations observed in patients with TSC are inactivating mutations located anywhere along the sequence of *TSC1* or *TSC2*.[7] Consistent with Knudson's 2-hit hypothesis, most TSC tumors, including skin tumors, show a second somatic mutation that inactivates the wild-type allele.[36] TSC1 and TSC2 form a complex that inhibits signaling through the mechanistic target of rapamycin complex 1 (mTORC1) pathway (Fig. 136-15). Loss of TSC1/TSC2 function leads to increased mTORC1 signaling and increased cell growth.[37] Sirolimus (rapamycin) inhibits mTORC1 activity and treats TSC tumors. A xenograft mouse model of TSC demonstrated that TSC2-null fibroblast-like cells are the inciting cells in angiofibromas, inducing angiogenesis and hair

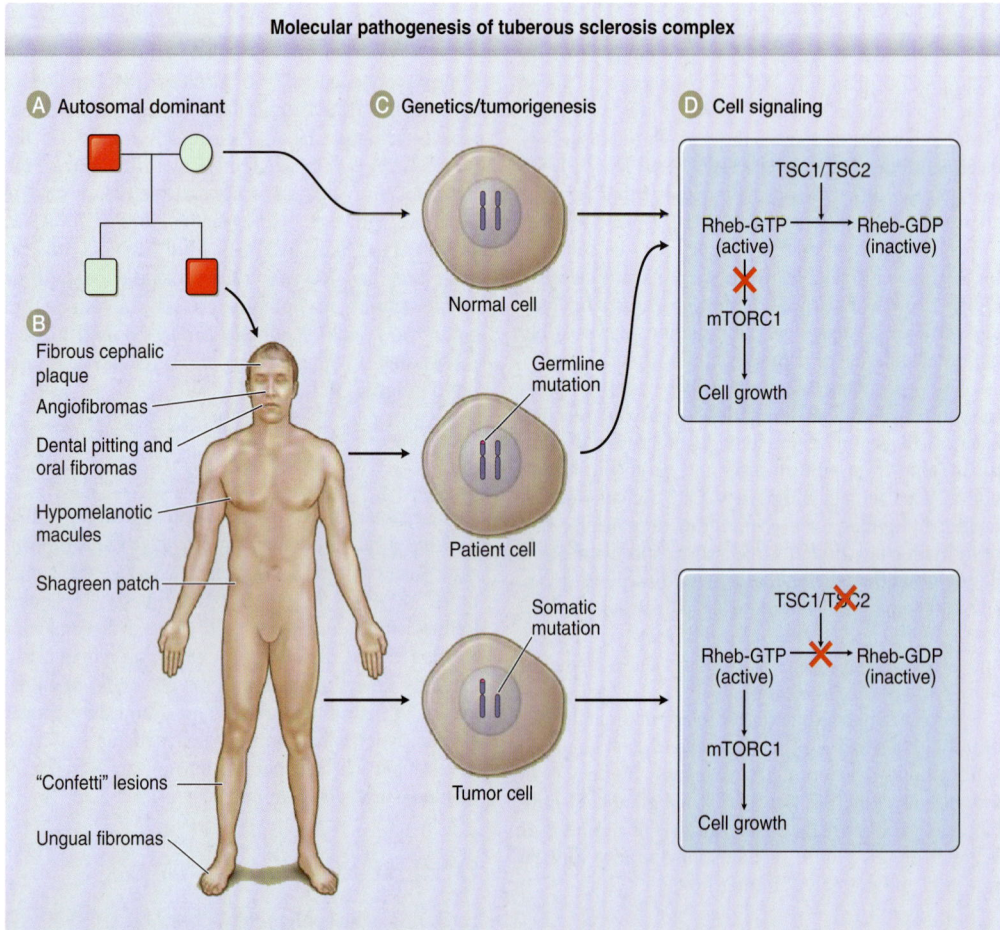

Figure 136-15 Molecular pathogenesis of tuberous sclerosis complex (TSC). **A,** An example is shown in which a mutation in *TSC2* is passed from the father (*red square*) to the son (*red square*), whereas the mother (*white circle*) and another son (*white square*) are unaffected. **B,** Skin lesions are observed in the son at the indicated locations. **C,** A cell from the mother shows 2 normal alleles for *TSC2* on chromosome band 16p13.3. A cell from the son shows the *TSC2* mutation inherited from his father. A tumor from the son has this germline mutation and a "second-hit" mutation, detectable as loss of heterozygosity at this locus, that inactivates the other allele. **D,** TSC2, in a complex with TSC1, is a guanosine triphosphatase–activating protein, converting active Ras-homolog enriched in brain (Rheb) guanosine triphosphate (GTP) to inactive Rheb guanosine diphosphate (GDP). Rheb-GTP activates mammalian target of rapamycin complex 1 (mTORC1), a kinase that increases protein translation and cell growth, so TSC2 normally acts to inhibit cell growth. Loss of TSC2 function in tumors results in increased levels of Rheb-GTP, activation of mTORC1, and increased cell growth.

follicle neogenesis. Treatment with rapamycin normalized the pathologic changes but failed to eradicate the TSC2-null cells.[38]

RISK FACTORS

Patients with mutations in *TSC2* tend to exhibit a more-severe phenotype than those with mutations in *TSC1*. Immediately adjacent to *TSC2* on chromosome 16 is *PKD1*, the gene mutated in polycystic kidney disease. Some patients with TSC have severe, early-onset renal cystic disease, and most of these patients have a contiguous deletion of *TSC2* and *PKD1*.[7] Tuber count and early onset epilepsy is associated with impairment of intellectual abilities.[39] Skin manifestations have been reported in association with epilepsy, including higher likelihood of epilepsy in those with angiofibromas or shagreen patch,[40] and fibrous forehead plaque with ipsilateral cerebral abnormalities and contralateral seizures.[41] Analysis of somatic second-hit mutations in angiofibromas has shown the presence of ultraviolet-signature mutations, suggesting that sun exposure may worsen TSC skin findings.[36]

DIAGNOSIS

The diagnosis of TSC is based on either genetic or clinical criteria (Table 136-1).[10] The genetic criterion requires the identification of a mutation in *TSC1* or *TSC2* that clearly inactivates the function of the TSC1 or TSC2 proteins in DNA from normal tissue. The demonstration of a pathogenic mutation is sufficient to make a definite diagnosis of TSC. Using standard approaches for DNA analysis, approximately 10% to 25% of individuals with TSC will have no mutation identified. Therefore, a normal result does not exclude the possibility of TSC and clinical criteria are still important. The clinical criteria are categorized as major or minor features, with cutaneous and oral lesions comprising 4 of 11 major features and 3 of 6 minor features. Using clinical criteria, a definite diagnosis of TSC requires the presence of 2 or more major features or 1 major feature with 2 or more minor features. A possible diagnosis of TSC is made based on the presence of either 1 major feature or 2 or more minor features.[10]

SUPPORTIVE STUDIES

PATHOLOGY

A skin biopsy may be useful when internal manifestations of TSC are lacking or if the diagnosis of TSC hinges on skin lesions for satisfying clinical criteria.[11] Hypomelanotic macules have normal numbers of melanocytes, in contrast to the lesions of vitiligo, in which melanocytes are absent. The melanocytes in hypomelanotic macules have poorly developed dendritic processes, and melanosomes are decreased in numbers, size, and melanization.[42] Angiofibromas contain plump, spindle-shaped, or stellate fibroblastic cells in the dermis among increased numbers of dilated vessels (Fig. 136-16). Collagen fibers are oriented in an onionskin pattern around follicles and vessels. The epidermis shows melanocytic hyperplasia

TABLE 136-1
Diagnostic Criteria for Tuberous Sclerosis Complex (Updated at 2012 Conference)

Genetic Criterion
Pathogenic mutation in *TSC1* or *TSC2* in DNA from normal tissue

Major Features
1. Hypomelanotic macules (≥3, at least 5 mm diameter)
2. Angiofibromas (≥3) or fibrous cephalic plaque
3. Ungual fibromas (≥2)
4. Shagreen patch
5. Multiple retinal hamartomas
6. Cortical dysplasias[a]
7. Subependymal nodules
8. Subependymal giant cell astrocytoma
9. Cardiac rhabdomyoma
10. Lymphangioleiomyomatosis[b]
11. Angiomyolipomas (≥2)[b]

Minor Features
1. "Confetti" skin lesions
2. Dental enamel pits (≥3)
3. Intraoral fibromas (≥2)
4. Retinal achromic patch
5. Multiple renal cysts
6. Nonrenal hamartomas

[a]Includes tubers and cerebral white matter radial migration lines.
[b]A combination of the 2 major clinical features (lymphangioleiomyomatosis and angiomyolipomas) without other features does not meet criteria for a definite diagnosis.
Definite diagnosis: Pathogenic mutation *or* 2 major features *or* 1 major feature with ≥2 minor features.
Possible diagnosis: One major feature *or* ≥2 minor features.

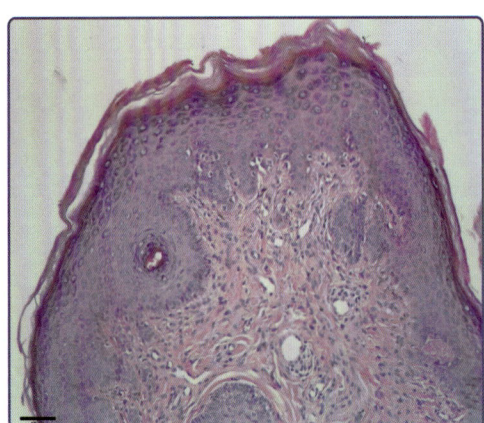

Figure 136-16 Angiofibromas are composed of ectatic vessels and fibroblastic cells that can be large, stellate, and sometimes multinucleated. There is fibrosis that may form concentric rings around vessels and adnexal structures.

and flattening of rete ridges. Periungual fibromas are similar, but with more extensive hyperkeratosis and a variable increase in vascularity (Fig. 136-17). The shagreen patch has sclerotic bundles of collagen in the reticular dermis, often with reduced elastic fibers (Fig. 136-18).[8]

IMAGING AND LABORATORY TESTING

Besides dermatologic and ophthalmologic examination, the initial evaluation of a patient suspected to have TSC includes MRI of the brain and abdomen.[23] MRI of the brain, with and without gadolinium, evaluates for tubers, subependymal nodules, migrational defects, and subependymal giant cell astrocytoma. MRI of the abdomen assesses for renal angiomyolipomas and cysts, as well as extrarenal hamartomas and aortic aneurysms. These imaging studies and additional studies described next are used to confirm the diagnosis of TSC and to determine the extent of disease in those known to have TSC. Additional studies include (a) a baseline routine electroencephalogram even without reported seizures; (b) evaluation for TAND; (c) blood pressure and renal glomerular filtration rate; (d) high-resolution chest computed tomography (HRCT) and pulmonary function testing if symptomatic or as baseline in asymptomatic females 18 years of age or older; (e) an echocardiogram and electrocardiogram to evaluate for rhabdomyomas and arrhythmia in pediatric patients, especially if younger than 3 years of age; and (f) a baseline electrocardiogram at any age.[23]

MOLECULAR DIAGNOSIS

The identification of a pathogenic mutation in *TSC1* or *TSC2* is now sufficient for the diagnosis of TSC even without diagnostic clinical findings.[10] Genetic testing may yield false-negative or inconclusive results in approximately 10% to 25% of TSC patients.[1] Most of these cases are caused by intronic mutations or somatic mosaicism.[43] Molecular genetic testing can provide additional information for genetic counseling, and it can be used in prenatal diagnosis. When a pathogenic mutation has been identified, it may be used to screen at-risk family members.[1]

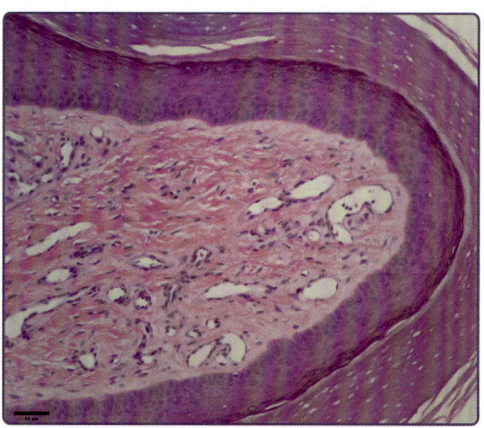

Figure 136-17 Periungual fibromas may exhibit dense collagen bundles and ectatic vessels, sparse to increased fibroblastic cells, and acanthosis and hyperkeratosis.

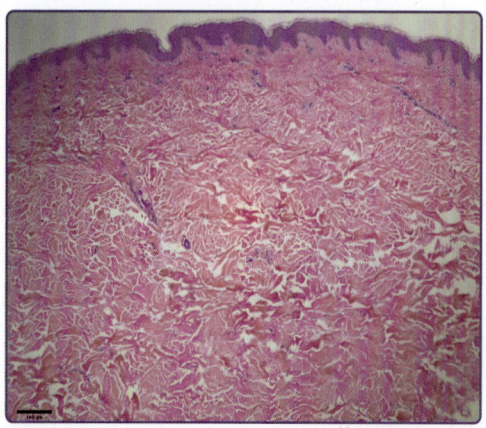

Figure 136-18 The shagreen patch shows thickened collagen bundles that appear disordered. Elastic fibers are decreased in amount compared to normal skin.

DIAGNOSTIC ALGORITHM

Individuals with skin findings suggestive of 1 cutaneous major feature of TSC should be queried for TSC-associated symptoms and family history. A thorough skin and oral examination should be performed. Those manifesting at least 1 additional major feature or 2 minor features should undergo TSC diagnostic evaluation to determine baseline disease extent.[23] In absence of additional skin or oral lesions, skin biopsy may be performed to confirm the clinical diagnosis (Fig. 136-19). Individuals with skin lesions characteristic of TSC should proceed to complete diagnostic evaluation. Those with skin lesions nonspecific or atypical of TSC should be first considered for other conditions to avoid unnecessary TSC workup.[44] Some patients will not meet criteria for a definitive diagnosis. These patients should receive a diagnosis of possible TSC and consideration given to performing a future reevaluation.

DIFFERENTIAL DIAGNOSIS

Tables 136-2, 136-3, 136-4, and 136-5 summarize differential diagnoses for several major features of TSC.

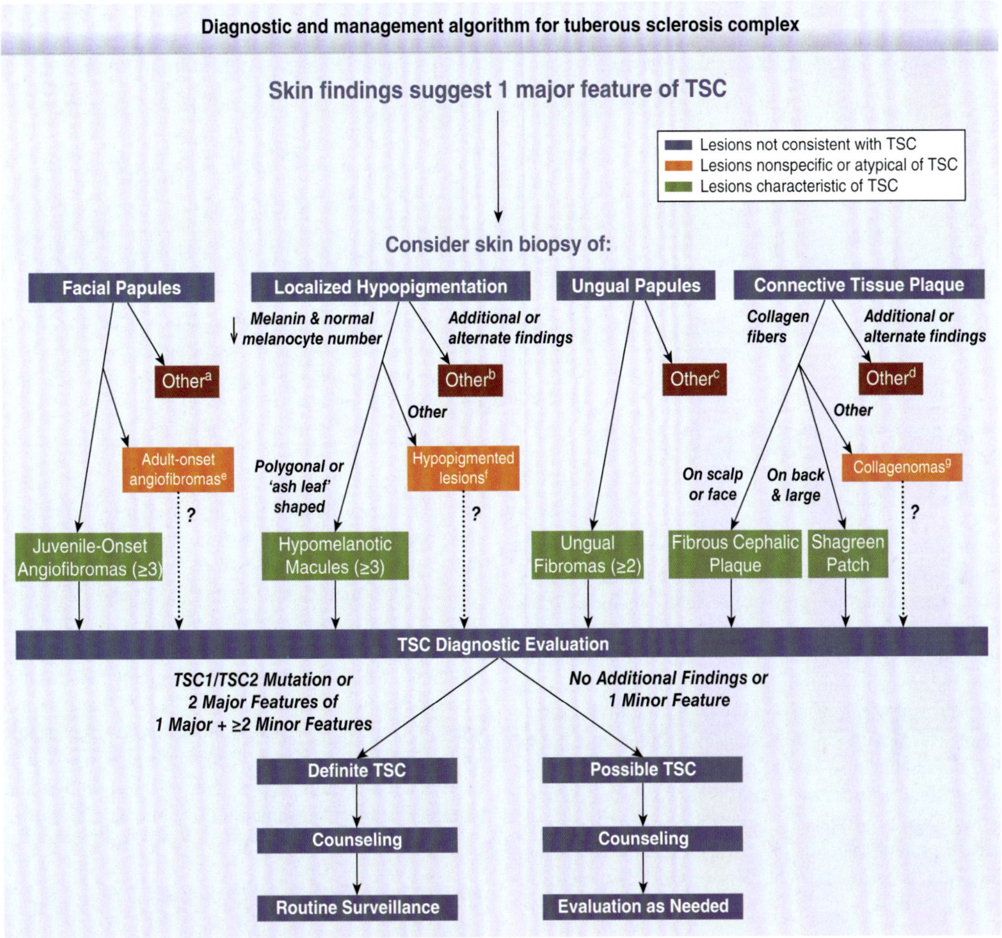

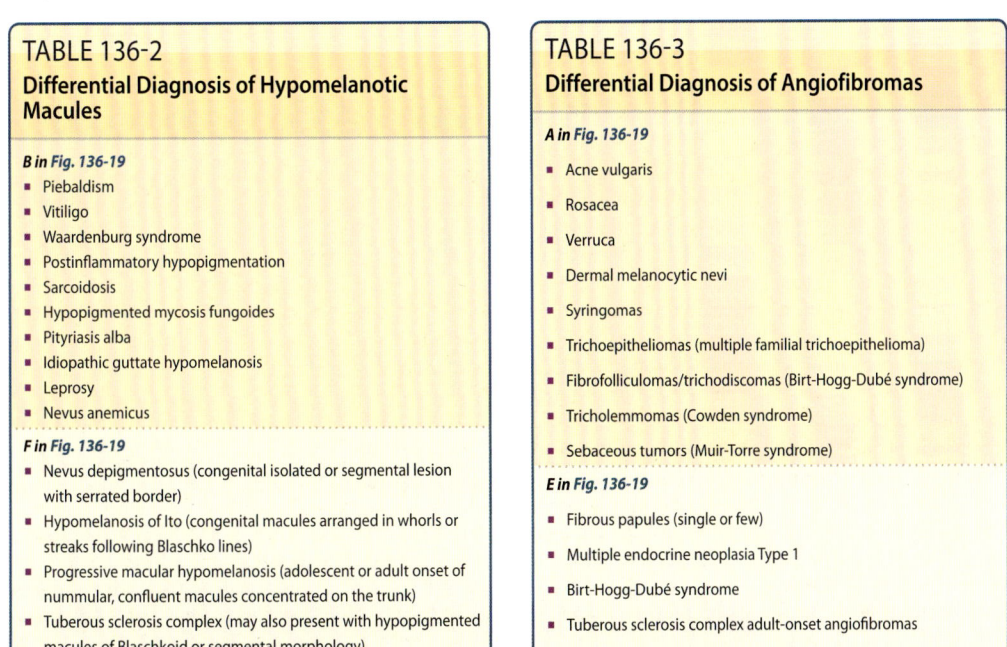

Figure 136-19 Diagnostic and management algorithm for tuberous sclerosis complex (TSC). Skin lesions may be categorized as not consistent (*red*), nonspecific or atypical (*orange*), or characteristic (*green*) of TSC. **A** and **E**, see Table 136-3; **B** and **F**, see Table 136-2; **C**, see Table 136-4; **D** and **G**, see Table 136-5. (Adapted from Nathan N, Burke K, Moss J, et al. A diagnostic and management algorithm for individuals with an isolated skin finding suggestive of tuberous sclerosis complex. *Br J Dermatol*. 2017;176(1):220-223.)

TABLE 136-2
Differential Diagnosis of Hypomelanotic Macules

B in Fig. 136-19
- Piebaldism
- Vitiligo
- Waardenburg syndrome
- Postinflammatory hypopigmentation
- Sarcoidosis
- Hypopigmented mycosis fungoides
- Pityriasis alba
- Idiopathic guttate hypomelanosis
- Leprosy
- Nevus anemicus

F in Fig. 136-19
- Nevus depigmentosus (congenital isolated or segmental lesion with serrated border)
- Hypomelanosis of Ito (congenital macules arranged in whorls or streaks following Blaschko lines)
- Progressive macular hypomelanosis (adolescent or adult onset of nummular, confluent macules concentrated on the trunk)
- Tuberous sclerosis complex (may also present with hypopigmented macules of Blaschkoid or segmental morphology)

TABLE 136-3
Differential Diagnosis of Angiofibromas

A in Fig. 136-19
- Acne vulgaris
- Rosacea
- Verruca
- Dermal melanocytic nevi
- Syringomas
- Trichoepitheliomas (multiple familial trichoepithelioma)
- Fibrofolliculomas/trichodiscomas (Birt-Hogg-Dubé syndrome)
- Tricholemmomas (Cowden syndrome)
- Sebaceous tumors (Muir-Torre syndrome)

E in Fig. 136-19
- Fibrous papules (single or few)
- Multiple endocrine neoplasia Type 1
- Birt-Hogg-Dubé syndrome
- Tuberous sclerosis complex adult-onset angiofibromas

TABLE 136-4
Differential Diagnosis of Ungual Fibroma

C in Fig. 136-19
- Digital mucous cyst
- Subungual exostosis
- Subungual corn (heloma)
- Wart
- Pyogenic granuloma
- Squamous cell carcinoma
- Onychomycosis
- Psoriasis

TABLE 136-5
Differential Diagnosis of Shagreen Patch

D in Fig. 136-19
- Nonfamilial elastoma or familial elastoma
- Dermatofibrosis lenticularis disseminata (in Buschke-Ollendorf syndrome)
- Dermal nevi
- Xanthomas
- Granulomatous disease

G in Fig. 136-19
- Familial cutaneous collagenomas or eruptive collagenoma
- Multiple endocrine neoplasia Type 1 collagenomas
- Sclerotic fibroma (Cowden syndrome)
- Isolated connective tissue nevus
- Tuberous sclerosis complex collagenomas

CLINICAL COURSE AND PROGNOSIS

Individuals with tuberous sclerosis exhibit decreased overall survival compared with the general population. The causes of premature death include renal failure, intractable seizures, obstructive hydrocephalus, cardiac outflow obstruction, arrhythmia, respiratory failure, pneumothorax, and hemorrhage from an aneurysm or a tumor, especially angiomyolipomas.[45,46] Fatal events may occur at any age. Brain and heart tumors may cause death in infancy, whereas lung and kidney tumors are more likely to cause premature death in adulthood. The prognosis for the individual patient depends on disease expressivity. Some individuals have a normal life span with few medical complications.

MANAGEMENT

MEDICATIONS

The management of TSC skin tumors has changed with the use of mTOR inhibitors. The U.S. Food and Drug Administration has approved oral mTOR inhibitors for treating several TSC-associated tumors, such as everolimus for subependymal giant cell astrocytomas and renal angiomyolipomas, and sirolimus for LAM.[47] Most patients treated with an oral mTOR inhibitor for internal tumors will show improvement in their skin lesions.[48,49] Therefore, appropriate management may involve monitoring for skin improvement in those on systemic therapy. Oral mTOR inhibitors may delay wound healing, but surgical intervention may be indicated for lesions failing to respond to oral therapy or for urgent clinical situations such as bleeding or functional impairment.[11]

Systemic treatment with mTOR inhibitors is associated with a variety of adverse effects, such as stomatitis, mouth ulceration, acne-like skin lesions, infections, hypertriglyceridemia, hypercholesterolemia, bone marrow suppression, proteinuria, joint pain, and noninfectious pneumonitis. The potential for these adverse effects limits the use of systemic mTOR inhibitors in the treatment of skin lesions alone.[11] To reduce the potential for adverse effects, several investigators have used mTOR inhibitors applied topically. Angiofibromas in most patients became flatter and decreased in redness.[50] Hypomelanotic macules increased in pigmentation.[51] Adverse effects were minimal and systemic levels were mostly undetectable.[50] A double-blind, placebo-controlled, phase 2 randomized clinical trial showed that topical sirolimus 0.2% gel was safe and effective for treating TSC angiofibromas.[52] It is expected that long-term treatment will be required and skin lesions may worsen after discontinuing therapy.

PROCEDURES

Indications for treatment of TSC-related skin lesions may include pain, bleeding, functional interference, or disruption of social interactions.[11] Angiofibromas have been treated by excision, curettage, chemical peel, cryosurgery, dermabrasion, electrosurgery, and different types of laser procedures.[8,11,35,53] Multiple sessions using several approaches may be required for optimal results. Potential complications of surgical treatments include infection, hypertrophic scarring, postinflammatory hyperpigmentation, and hypopigmentation. Treated angiofibromas tend to recur over a couple of years, and new lesions may form.[35] Ungual fibromas are usually treated by excision, but these lesions also have a high recurrence rate. Hypomelanotic macules may be temporarily concealed using self-tanning lotions or makeup matched to the person's skin color. The shagreen patch is usually left untreated, but it can be excised.[8,35]

COUNSELING

Upon diagnosing an infant with TSC, a major aspect of care is answering questions and addressing the concerns of the family. Unfortunately, many parents report negative experiences because of physician insensitivity and the provision of inaccurate information and inadequate support.[54] Parents should be educated about possible evolution or development of skin lesions and available treatments. Parents should be advised to maintain good sun protection for their children as this may lessen the future severity of angiofibromas.[11] Other important educational aspects include informing parents to recognize infantile spasms, discussing the potential need for an individual educational program, and counseling adolescent and adult females about the risks of smoking or estrogen use in oral contraceptives because of their potential to worsen LAM.[23] Patients should be promptly referred to other specialists, social services, and genetic counseling as indicated. Inform individuals and families about organizations dedicated to TSC, such as the Tuberous Sclerosis Alliance (http://www.tsalliance.org).

SURVEILLANCE

After diagnosis, the patient should have periodic surveillance for the development of new lesions or changes in existing lesions.[23] MRI of the brain is recommended every 1 to 3 years in asymptomatic TSC patients younger than age 25 years to monitor for development of subependymal giant cell astrocytoma and, more frequently, for positive findings. MRI of the abdomen should be performed every 1 to 3 years to evaluate for progression of angiomyolipomas and renal cystic disease. Additional recommendations include: (a) annual screening for TAND throughout childhood and as needed; (b) annual tests of blood pressure and renal glomerular filtration rate; (c) clinical screening for LAM symptoms and HRCT every 5 to 10 years for asymptomatic at-risk individuals, or, for those with LAM, annual pulmonary function testing and HRCT every 2 to 3 years; (d) electrocardiogram every 3 to 5 years in asymptomatic patients of all ages and, for pediatric patients with asymptomatic cardiac rhabdomyomas, echocardiogram every 1 to 3 years until resolved; (e) annual skin examination; (f) dental examination every 6 months with panoramic radiographs by age 7 years; and (g) annual ophthalmologic evaluation in patients with previously identified ophthalmologic lesions or vision symptoms.[23]

SCREENING

A child with TSC may be born to parents who do not carry the diagnosis of TSC. This may represent a de novo mutation, parental mosaicism, or it may indicate that 1 parent has a very mild form of TSC that has escaped detection. Both parents should be carefully screened for clinical manifestations or for the pathogenic mutation, if known. Screening begins with examination of the skin, oral mucosa, teeth, and retina. Most affected family members will show TSC lesions with this approach, but additional imaging studies are recommended in their absence.[1] If 1 parent has TSC, there is a 50% chance that subsequent children will inherit the mutation. To identify additional family members at risk of TSC, obtain a 3-generation family history.[23]

If neither parent has TSC, it is possible that there is alternate paternity or undisclosed adoption. Another possibility is that 1 parent is mosaic for a mutation in *TSC1* or *TSC2*.[43] This has profound implications for genetic counseling. Whereas it would be extremely unlikely for parents of a child with a de novo mutation to have another affected child, germline mosaicism in 1 parent increases the risk of having another child with TSC. An estimate of the overall risk that apparently unaffected parents will have a second child with TSC is approximately 1% to 2%.[1]

REFERENCES

1. Northrup H, Koenig MK, Pearson DA, et al. Tuberous sclerosis complex. In: Adam MP, Ardinger HH, Pagon RA, et al, eds. *GeneReviews*. Seattle, WA: University of Washington; 1993-2018 [updated September 3, 2015].
2. Seibert D, Hong CH, Takeuchi F, et al. Recognition of tuberous sclerosis in adult women: delayed presentation with life-threatening consequences. *Ann Intern Med*. 2011;154(12):806-813, W-294.
3. de Vries PJ, Whittemore VH, Leclezio L, et al. Tuberous sclerosis associated neuropsychiatric disorders (TAND) and the TAND Checklist. *Pediatr Neurol*. 2015;52(1):25-35.
4. Crall C, Valle M, Kapur K, et al. Effect of angiofibromas on quality of life and access to care in tuberous sclerosis patients and their caregivers. *Pediatr Dermatol*. 2016;33(5):518-525.
5. Devlin LA, Shepherd CH, Crawford H, et al. Tuberous sclerosis complex: clinical features, diagnosis, and prevalence within Northern Ireland. *Dev Med Child Neurol*. 2006;48(6):495-499.
6. Osborne JP, Fryer A, Webb D. Epidemiology of tuberous sclerosis. *Ann N Y Acad Sci*. 1991;615:125-127.
7. Curatolo P, Moavero R, Roberto D, et al. Genotype/phenotype correlations in tuberous sclerosis complex. *Semin Pediatr Neurol*. 2015;22(4):259-273.
8. Darling TN, Moss J, Mausner M. Dermatologic manifestations of tuberous sclerosis complex. In: Kwiatkowski DJ, Whittemore VH, Thiele EA, eds. *Tuberous Sclerosis Complex: Genes, Clinical Features, and Therapeutics*. Weinheim, Germany: Wiley-VCH Verlag; 2010:285-309.
9. Wataya-Kaneda M, Tanaka M, Hamasaki T, et al. Trends in the prevalence of tuberous sclerosis complex manifestations: an epidemiological study of 166 Japanese patients. *PLoS One*. 2013;8(5):e63910.
10. Northrup H, Krueger DA. Tuberous sclerosis complex diagnostic criteria update: recommendations of the 2012 International Tuberous Sclerosis Complex Consensus Conference. *Pediatr Neurol*. 2013;49(4):243-254.
11. Teng JM, Cowen EW, Wataya-Kaneda M, et al. Dermatologic and dental aspects of the 2012 International Tuberous Sclerosis Complex Consensus Statements. *JAMA Dermatol*. 2014;150(10):1095-1101.
12. Jozwiak S, Schwartz RA, Janniger CK, et al. Skin lesions in children with tuberous sclerosis complex: their prevalence, natural course, and diagnostic significance. *Int J*

13. Webb DW, Clarke A, Fryer A, et al. The cutaneous features of tuberous sclerosis: a population study. *Br J Dermatol*. 1996;135(1):1-5.
14. Fitzpatrick TB. History and significance of white macules, earliest visible sign of tuberous sclerosis. *Ann N Y Acad Sci*. 1991;615:26-35.
15. Vanderhooft SL, Francis JS, Pagon RA, et al. Prevalence of hypopigmented macules in a healthy population. *J Pediatr*. 1996;129(3):355-361.
16. Nathan N, Tyburczy ME, Hamieh L, et al. Nipple Angiofibromas with loss of TSC2 are associated with tuberous sclerosis complex. *J Invest Dermatol*. 2016;136(2):535-538.
17. Hall MR, Kovach BT, Miller JL. Unilateral facial angiofibromas without other evidence of tuberous sclerosis: case report and review of the literature. *Cutis*. 2007;80(4):284-288.
18. Aldrich CS, Hong CH, Groves L, et al. Acral lesions in tuberous sclerosis complex: insights into pathogenesis. *J Am Acad Dermatol*. 2010;63(2):244-251.
19. Zeller J, Friedmann D, Clerici T, et al. The significance of a single periungual fibroma: report of seven cases. *Arch Dermatol*. 1995;131(12):1465-1466.
20. Torrelo A, Hadj-Rabia S, Colmenero I, et al. Folliculocystic and collagen hamartoma of tuberous sclerosis complex. *J Am Acad Dermatol*. 2012;66(4): 617-621.
21. Sparling JD, Hong CH, Brahim JS, et al. Oral findings in 58 adults with tuberous sclerosis complex. *J Am Acad Dermatol*. 2007;56(5):786-790.
22. Curatolo P, Moavero R, de Vries PJ. Neurological and neuropsychiatric aspects of tuberous sclerosis complex. *Lancet Neurol*. 2015;14(7):733-745.
23. Krueger DA, Northrup H. Tuberous sclerosis complex surveillance and management: recommendations of the 2012 International Tuberous Sclerosis Complex Consensus Conference. *Pediatr Neurol*. 2013;49(4): 255-265.
24. Hinton RB, Prakash A, Romp RL, et al. Cardiovascular manifestations of tuberous sclerosis complex and summary of the revised diagnostic criteria and surveillance and management recommendations from the International Tuberous Sclerosis Consensus Group. *J Am Heart Assoc*. 2014;3(6):e001493.
25. Kingswood JC, Bissler JJ, Budde K, et al. Review of the tuberous sclerosis renal guidelines from the 2012 Consensus Conference: Current Data and Future Study. *Nephron*. 2016;134(2):51-58.
26. Cudzilo CJ, Szczesniak RD, Brody AS, et al. Lymphangioleiomyomatosis screening in women with tuberous sclerosis. *Chest*. 2013;144(2):578-585.
27. Johnson SR, Taveira-DaSilva AM, Moss J. Lymphangioleiomyomatosis. *Clin Chest Med*. 2016;37(3):389-403.
28. Hodgson N, Kinori M, Goldbaum MH, et al. Ophthalmic manifestations of tuberous sclerosis: a review. *Clin Exp Ophthalmol*. 2017;45(1):81-86.
29. Santos L, Brcic I, Unterweger G, et al. Hamartomatous polyposis in tuberous sclerosis complex: case report and review of the literature. *Pathol Res Pract*. 2015;211(12):1025-1029.
30. Dworakowska D, Grossman AB. Are neuroendocrine tumours a feature of tuberous sclerosis? A systematic review. *Endocr Relat Cancer*. 2009;16(1):45-58.
31. Salerno AE, Marsenic O, Meyers KE, et al. Vascular involvement in tuberous sclerosis. *Pediatr Nephrol*. 2010;25(8):1555-1561.
32. Avila NA, Dwyer AJ, Rabel A, et al. CT of sclerotic bone lesions: imaging features differentiating tuberous sclerosis complex with lymphangioleiomyomatosis from sporadic lymphangioleiomyomatosis. *Radiology*. 2010;254(3):851-857.
33. Manoukian SB, Kowal DJ. Comprehensive imaging manifestations of tuberous sclerosis. *AJR Am J Roentgenol*. 2015;204(5):933-943.
34. Kane Y. The "bumps" on my face. *J Am Acad Dermatol*. 2004;51(1)(suppl):S11-S12.
35. Sweeney SM. Pediatric dermatologic surgery: a surgical approach to the cutaneous features of tuberous sclerosis complex. *Adv Dermatol*. 2004;20:117-135.
36. Tyburczy ME, Wang JA, Li S, et al. Sun exposure causes somatic second-hit mutations and angiofibroma development in tuberous sclerosis complex. *Hum Mol Genet*. 2014;23(8):2023-2029.
37. Laplante M, Sabatini DM. mTOR signaling in growth control and disease. *Cell*. 2012;149(2):274-293.
38. Li S, Thangapazham RL, Wang JA, et al. Human TSC2-null fibroblast-like cells induce hair follicle neogenesis and hamartoma morphogenesis. *Nat Commun*. 2011;2:235.
39. Bolton PF, Clifford M, Tye C, et al. Intellectual abilities in tuberous sclerosis complex: risk factors and correlates from the Tuberous Sclerosis 2000 Study. *Psychol Med*. 2015;45(11):2321-2331.
40. Jeong A, Wong M. Systemic disease manifestations associated with epilepsy in tuberous sclerosis complex. *Epilepsia*. 2016;57(9):1443-1449.
41. Galahitiyawa J, Wanigasinghe J, Seneviratne J, et al. Cutaneous markers of systemic manifestations of tuberous sclerosis complex. *Int J Dermatol*. 2015;54(1): e52-e55.
42. Jimbow K. Tuberous sclerosis and guttate leukodermas. *Semin Cutan Med Surg*. 1997;16(1):30-35.
43. Tyburczy ME, Dies KA, Glass J, et al. Mosaic and intronic mutations in TSC1/TSC2 explain the majority of TSC patients with no mutation identified by conventional testing. *PLoS Genet*. 2015;11(11):e1005637.
44. Nathan N, Burke K, Moss J, et al. A diagnostic and management algorithm for individuals with an isolated skin finding suggestive of tuberous sclerosis complex. *Br J Dermatol*. 2017;176(1):220-223.
45. Shepherd CW, Gomez MR, Lie JT, et al. Causes of death in patients with tuberous sclerosis. *Mayo Clin Proc*. 1991;66(8):792-796.
46. Byard RW, Blumbergs PC, James RA. Mechanisms of unexpected death in tuberous sclerosis. *J Forensic Sci*. 2003;48(1):172-176.
47. Capal JK, Franz DN. Profile of everolimus in the treatment of tuberous sclerosis complex: an evidence-based review of its place in therapy. *Neuropsychiatr Dis Treat*. 2016;12:2165-2172.
48. Nathan N, Wang JA, Li S, et al. Improvement of tuberous sclerosis complex (TSC) skin tumors during long-term treatment with oral sirolimus. *J Am Acad Dermatol*. 2015;73(5):802-808.
49. Sasongko TH, Ismail NF, Zabidi-Hussin Z. Rapamycin and rapalogs for tuberous sclerosis complex. *Cochrane Database Syst Rev*. 2016;7:CD011272.
50. Jozwiak S, Sadowski K, Kotulska K, et al. Topical use of mammalian target of rapamycin (mTOR) Inhibitors in tuberous sclerosis complex—a comprehensive review of the literature. *Pediatr Neurol*. 2016;61:21-27.
51. Wataya-Kaneda M, Tanaka M, Yang L, et al. Clinical and histologic analysis of the efficacy of topical rapamycin therapy against hypomelanotic macules in tuberous sclerosis complex. *JAMA Dermatol*. 2015;151(7): 722-730.

Dermatol. 1998;37(12):911-917.

52. Wataya-Kaneda M, Nakamura A, Tanaka M, et al. Efficacy and Safety of Topical Sirolimus Therapy for Facial Angiofibromas in the Tuberous Sclerosis Complex: A Randomized Clinical Trial. *JAMA Dermatol*. 2017;153(1):39-48.
53. Ali FR, Mallipeddi R, Craythorne EE, et al. Our experience of carbon dioxide laser ablation of angiofibromas: case series and literature review. *J Cosmet Laser Ther*. 2016;18(7):372-375.
54. Whitehead LC, Gosling V. Parent's perceptions of interactions with health professionals in the pathway to gaining a diagnosis of tuberous sclerosis (TS) and beyond. *Res Dev Disabil*. 2003;24(2):109-119.

Chapter 137 :: Diabetes and Other Endocrine Diseases
April Schachtel & Andrea Kalus

第一百三十七章
糖尿病和其他内分泌疾病

中文导读

几乎所有的糖尿病患者都有与病情相关的皮肤表现，部分皮肤状况是相关代谢变化的直接结果，如高血糖和高脂血症。血管、神经或免疫系统的进行性损害也是导致皮肤症状的重要原因。但仍有其他糖尿病相关皮肤病的机制仍不清楚。

本章首先介绍了与代谢、血管、神经或免疫异常相关的糖尿病皮肤病变，如黑棘皮病、糖尿病性皮肤增厚、关节活动受限（LJM）与硬皮病样综合征、糖尿病性硬肿症、发疹性黄色瘤、皮肤感染、糖尿病溃疡；接下来介绍了与糖尿病相关但发病机制不明的皮肤疾病如类脂渐进性坏死、化脓性肉芽肿、糖尿病皮肤病、获得性穿孔性疾病、糖尿病性水疱病。

同时介绍了其他内分泌疾病如肥胖与代谢综合征可引起表皮屏障功能的改变，皮肤皱褶的增大而出汗增加，淋巴引流不良，伤口愈合不良，以及微血管的反应性受损等；甲状腺功能亢进症可出现皮肤弥漫性瘙痒、柔软、有光泽和易碎的指甲、Plummer指甲、白癜风、胫前粘液水肿、甲状腺肢端肥厚、色素沉着、荨麻疹等。在甲状腺功能减退症中，皮肤凉爽苍白干燥、皮肤黄橙色改变、黏液水肿、头发粗糙干燥、指甲生长缓慢增厚可能与斑秃、白癜风、结缔组织病（包括狼疮和皮肌炎）、大疱性类天疱疮、疱疹性皮炎和慢性黏膜皮肤念珠菌病（CMC）等相关。甲状旁腺功能亢进症患者可出现皮肤钙质沉着症或者罕见但危及生命的钙质疏松症，而甲状旁腺功能减退症与鳞屑、角化过度和水肿性浮肿的皮肤有关。肾上腺疾病包括库欣综合征的常见皮肤症状有容易擦伤和皮肤变薄、轻度多毛症等，Addison病最常见的皮肤表现是皮肤和黏膜色素沉着。

本章最后提到了雌激素、黄体酮、雄激素以及生长激素紊乱都可以出现相应的皮肤改变。

〔粟　娟〕

DIABETES MELLITUS

AT-A-GLANCE

- The incidence of diabetes in America is increasing steadily with the epidemic of obesity.
- Fourteen percent of health care expenditures in America are diabetes related.
- Metabolic abnormalities in glucose and insulin relate directly to diabetic thick skin, limited joint mobility, eruptive xanthomas, and acanthosis nigricans.
- Neuropathy, vasculopathy, and immune dysfunction associated with diabetes contribute directly to lower-extremity ulcers and certain cutaneous infections.
- Diabetes-associated skin conditions without a known pathogenesis include: necrobiosis lipoidica, granuloma annulare, diabetic dermopathy, acquired perforating dermatosis, and bullosis diabeticorum.

EPIDEMIOLOGY

Diabetes mellitus (DM) is a major cause of morbidity and mortality in the United States; 2017 estimates suggest 23.4 million Americans have known diabetes.[1] Approximately 14% of all health care expenditures in the United States are directly attributable to the medical care of diabetes. Men and women diagnosed with diabetes at age 40 years are expected to lose 12 and 14 life-years, respectively.[2] Major studies show that tight glycemic control decreases microvascular disease (ie, retinopathy, neuropathy, nephropathy), but that coronary vascular disease, the major contributor to morbidity and mortality in patients with diabetes, receives no benefit from intensive glycemic control in patients with longstanding diabetes. In one large, randomized, controlled trial with approximately a third of patients having known coronary artery disease, intensive glycemic control was, in fact, associated with an increase in mortality. Newly diagnosed Type 2 diabetes appears to have long-term benefit from similar degrees of tight control.[3] New guidelines for glycemic control (glycosylated hemoglobin [HbA_{1c}] <7%) attempt to balance this body of evidence.[4] Tight glycemic control may have a beneficial effect on a subset of skin-related, diabetes-associated disorders, but evidence is generally lacking.

Diabetes is characterized by a state of relative or complete insulin deficiency, leading to defects in glucose, fat, and protein metabolism. In Type 1 diabetes (formerly insulin-dependent DM), an insufficiency of insulin occurs through a gradual, immune-mediated destruction of β islet cells in the pancreas, marked by autoantibodies. In Type 2 diabetes (formerly noninsulin-dependent DM), chronic hyperglycemia occurs mainly through end-organ insulin resistance followed by a progressive decrease in pancreatic insulin release associated with aging. Diabetes can be diagnosed by a fasting blood glucose level of 126 mg/dL or higher, a random value of 200 mg/dL or higher, or an HbA_{1c} level of 6.5% or above. A genetic predisposition and a strong association with obesity exist in Type 2 diabetes. In both types of diabetes, abnormalities of insulin and elevated blood glucose levels lead to metabolic, vascular, neuropathic, and immunologic abnormalities. Affected organs include the cardiovascular, renal, and nervous systems, the eyes, and the skin.

CLINICAL FEATURES

Nearly all patients with diabetes have cutaneous findings related to their condition, including those listed in Table 137-1. Some diabetes-associated skin conditions are a direct result of the related metabolic changes such as hyperglycemia and hyperlipidemia. Progressive damage to the vascular, neurologic, or immune systems also contributes significantly to skin manifestations. The mechanisms for other diabetes-associated

TABLE 137-1
Approach to the Patient with Diabetes

Cutaneous Findings in Diabetes
- Acanthosis nigricans
- Limited joint mobility and scleroderma-like syndrome
- Scleredema diabeticorum
- Eruptive xanthomas
- Bacterial infections (streptococcal, malignant external otitis, necrotizing fasciitis)
- Fungal infections (candidal, onychomycosis, mucormycosis)
- Foot ulcers
- Necrobiosis lipoidica
- Granuloma annulare
- Diabetic dermopathy
- Acquired perforating disorders
- Bullosis diabeticorum

Related Features in Diabetes
- Retinopathy
- Nephropathy
- Neuropathy
- Cardiovascular disease
- Peripheral vascular disease
- Hyperlipidemia
- Hypertension

Diagnosis
- Diabetes can be diagnosed by a fasting blood glucose level of 126 mg/dL or higher, a random value of 200 mg/dL or higher, or an HbA_{1c} level of 6.5% or above.

Management
- Diet and exercise
- Referral to primary care provider or endocrinologist for medical management with either oral hypoglycemic agents or insulin
- Always perform a foot examination
- Address modifiable risk factors

skin conditions remain unknown. The cutaneous disorders associated with DM are characterized in the following section by disorders with evidence for metabolic, vascular, neurologic, or immunologic pathogenesis induced by glucose and insulin abnormalities and by disorders associated with diabetes, but without a clear pathogenesis.

ETIOLOGY AND PATHOGENESIS

Hyperglycemia leads to nonenzymatic glycosylation of structural and regulatory proteins, including collagen. Although nonenzymatic glycosylation occurs normally with aging, the process is greatly accelerated in diabetes.[5,6] Nonenzymatic glycosylation leads to the formation of advanced glycation end products (AGEs) that are responsible for decreases in both acid solubility and enzymatic digestion of cutaneous collagen. Disorders such as diabetic thick skin and limited joint mobility (LJM) are thought to result directly from accumulation of AGEs.[7] Studies show that the degree of cutaneous AGEs correlates strongly with retinopathy, nephropathy, and other microvascular complications of diabetes.[8] There is increased interest in noninvasive measurement of AGEs in the skin and correlation with diabetes micro and macro vascular risks.[9]

Derangements of immunoregulatory mechanisms also occur in diabetes. Hyperglycemia and ketoacidosis diminish chemotaxis, phagocytosis, and bactericidal ability of white blood cells.[10] Historically, infections were a major cause of death in the diabetic patient. This has changed dramatically with improved glucose control and antibiotic use. Despite these improvements, certain infections, such as malignant external otitis, necrotizing soft-tissue infections, and the devastating disease of mucormycosis, occur more frequently in patients with diabetes.[11]

Metabolic abnormalities, including hyperinsulinemia, as is seen in early insulin-resistant Type 2 diabetes, contribute to cutaneous manifestations. The action of insulin on the insulin-like growth factor-1 (IGF1) receptor appears to mediate the abnormal epidermal proliferation and resulting phenotype of acanthosis nigricans.[12] Dysregulated lipid metabolism occurs with diabetes-associated insulin deficiency. Defective lipid processing can lead to massive hypertriglyceridemia, manifesting in the skin as eruptive xanthomas. Naturally, disorders of lipid processing also play an integral role in the vasculopathies of diabetes.

Macroangiopathy and microangiopathy contribute significantly to the cutaneous complications of diabetes. In patients with diabetes, there is increased "leakiness" or vessel wall permeability, decreased vascular responsiveness to sympathetic innervation, and less ability to respond to thermal and hypoxemic stress.[10] Combined with arteriosclerosis of large vessels, these microvascular abnormalities contribute to the formation of diabetic ulcers. In addition, a loss of cutaneous sensory innervation occurs with diabetes, predisposing patients to infection and injury. The loss of neuroinflammatory cell signaling plays a causal role in nonhealing, lower-extremity ulcers.[13] Patients with diabetes who lack lower-extremity vibratory perception have a 15.5-fold increased probability of leg amputation.[14]

CUTANEOUS DISORDERS OF DIABETES MELLITUS ASSOCIATED WITH METABOLIC, VASCULAR, NEUROLOGIC OR IMMUNOLOGIC ABNORMALITIES

ACANTHOSIS NIGRICANS

Epidemiology: Acanthosis nigricans is probably the most readily recognized skin manifestation of diabetes. Acanthosis nigricans is common in the general population, and most cases are linked to obesity and insulin resistance. In some cases, increased androgen production is also identified.[15,16] Drug-related and idiopathic acanthosis nigricans or familial acanthosis nigricans are additional causes.[17] In general, though, acanthosis nigricans should be considered a prognostic indicator for developing Type 2 diabetes.[18] The prevalence of acanthosis nigricans varies among different ethnic groups. In one study, despite similar obesity rates, the prevalence was lower in whites (0.5%) and Hispanics (5%) than in African American children (13%).[16] This finding suggests a possible genetic predisposition or increased sensitivity of the skin to hyperinsulinemia among certain populations.[18] Although historical data emphasizes the relationship between acanthosis nigricans and malignancy, a true association is rare.[19] Only when the onset is particularly rapid, the clinical findings are florid, or in the nonobese or nondiabetic adult with acanthosis nigricans is an evaluation for malignancy beyond routine age-appropriate screening warranted.

Clinical Features: Acanthosis nigricans presents as brown to gray-black papillomatous cutaneous thickening in the flexural areas, including the posterolateral neck, axillae, groin, and abdominal folds. The distribution is usually symmetric. The affected skin has a dirty, velvety texture. In some cases, oral, esophageal, pharyngeal, laryngeal, conjunctival, and anogenital mucosal surfaces may be involved. In general, however, the back of the neck is the most consistently and severely affected area (Fig. 137-1).[18] The development of superimposed acrochordons in involved areas is well described (Fig. 137-2). In particularly florid

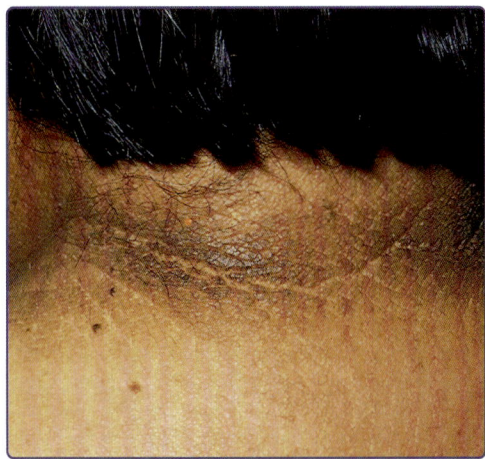

Figure 137-1 Acanthosis nigricans involving the neck.

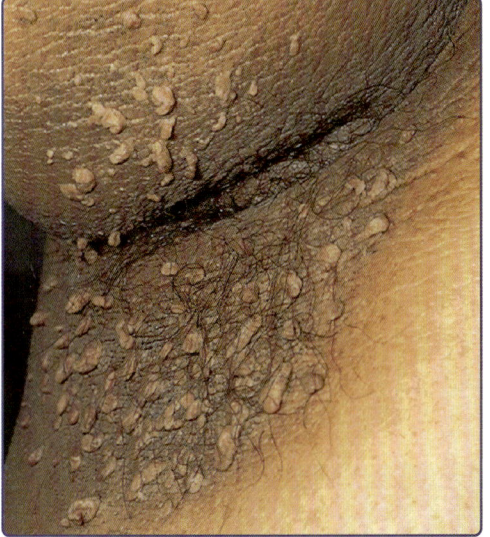

Figure 137-2 Acanthosis nigricans involving the axilla with numerous acrochordons.

cases, involvement on the back of the hands over the knuckles and even on the palms can be seen. When the palms are involved, the rugated appearance of the palmar surface has been called *tripe palms* and is usually associated with acanthosis nigricans seen in the setting of malignancy. In the majority of cases, the most important factor in diagnosing acanthosis nigricans is recognizing the usually associated hyperinsulinemia, which is a known risk factor for Type 2 diabetes and the metabolic syndrome.

The histopathology of clinical lesions demonstrates papillomatosis and hyperkeratosis but minimal acanthosis. Hyperpigmentation of the basal layer has been variably demonstrated, and the brown color of the lesions is attributed to the hyperkeratosis by most.[20,21]

Etiology and Pathogenesis: Insulin clearly plays a central role in the presentation of acanthosis nigricans. In a subset of women with hyperandrogenism and insulin resistance with acanthosis nigricans, loss-of-function mutations in the insulin receptor or anti–insulin-receptor antibodies can be found (Type A and Type B syndrome).[22] It is postulated that excess growth factor stimulation in the skin causes the aberrant proliferation of keratinocytes and fibroblasts that results in the phenotype of acanthosis nigricans.[15] In states of insulin resistance and hyperinsulinemia, acanthosis nigricans may result from excess insulin binding to IGF1 receptors on keratinocytes and fibroblasts.[12] IGF1 receptors are expressed on basal keratinocytes and are upregulated in proliferative conditions.[23] Studies show that high concentrations of insulin stimulate fibroblast proliferation through IGF1 receptors in vitro.[24] Other members of the tyrosine kinase receptor family, including the epidermal growth factor receptor and the fibroblast growth factor receptor, have been implicated in acanthosis nigricans. Several genetic syndromes (Crouzon and SADDAN [severe achondroplasia with developmental delay and acanthosis nigricans]) with mutations in fibroblast growth factor receptor 3 result in acanthosis nigricans in the absence of hyperinsulinemia or obesity, implicating this growth factor receptor in the pathogenesis of acanthosis nigricans.[23] In several reports of acanthosis nigricans associated with malignancy, evidence suggests that transforming growth factor-β released from the tumor cells may stimulate keratinocyte proliferation via the epidermal growth factor receptors.[25,26] Support for the role of different growth factors in the pathogenesis of acanthosis nigricans continues to accrue.

In addition to the direct effects of hyperinsulinemia on keratinocytes, insulin also appears to augment androgen levels in women. High insulin levels stimulate the production of ovarian androgens and ovarian hypertrophy with cystic changes.[22] Although associated with elevated androgen levels, the acanthosis nigricans in women with polycystic ovarian syndrome (PCOS) does not respond reliably to antiandrogen therapy, implicating the relative importance of hyperinsulinemia over hyperandrogenism in acanthosis nigricans. Several drugs also have been reported to cause acanthosis nigricans, including systemic glucocorticoids, nicotinic acid, and estrogens such as diethylstilbestrol.[15]

Management: Treatment of acanthosis nigricans is generally ineffective. Topical treatment with calcipotriol,[27] salicylic acid, glycolic acid peels, urea, systemic, and topical retinoids have all been used with anecdotal success.[28] Long-pulsed alexandrite laser was effective in 1 patient.[29] When identifiable, treatment of the underlying cause may be beneficial. Improvement or resolution does occur with weight loss in some obese patients.[12,15] Medications that improve insulin sensitivity, such as metformin, have a theoretic benefit. Removal of an offending medication generally results in clearance of the skin.[30] In patients with acanthosis nigricans in association with malignancy, there is usually improvement following treatment of the underlying malignancy. The skin finding may present before or after the diagnosis of malignancy is made. When it is associated with malignancy, a tumor of intraabdominal origin, usually gastric, is seen in the majority of cases.[31] It has been repeatedly described that patients' skin improves with chemotherapy and remits with recurrences.

DIABETIC THICK SKIN

Several specific syndromes are associated with localized thickening of the skin in diabetes. The common underlying pathogenesis involves biochemical alterations in dermal collagen and mucopolysaccharides. The clinical syndromes are a result of increased deposition and improper degradation of these constituents, likely related to the formation of AGEs.

LIMITED JOINT MOBILITY AND SCLERODERMA-LIKE SYNDROME

Diabetic LJM, or cheiroarthropathy, presents as tightness and thickening of the skin and periarticular connective tissue of the fingers, resulting in a painless loss of joint mobility. Initial involvement of the distal interphalangeal joints of the fifth digit usually progresses proximally to involve all fingers. Larger joints of the elbow, knee, and foot may be affected. The actual joint space, however, remains uninvolved, as LJM is not a true arthropathy. This disorder is characterized by the "prayer sign," which is an inability to approximate the palmar surfaces and interphalangeal joint spaces with the hands pressed together and fingers separated (Fig. 137-3). In addition to joint contractures, the skin may appear thickened, waxy, and smooth with apparent loss of adnexa, resembling skin changes in scleroderma.

Of adult patients with Type 1 diabetes, 30% to 50% have LJM, and it is common in Type 2 diabetes as well. LJM is associated with increased duration of diabetes and poor glucose control.[32,33] One longitudinal prospective study showed a 2.5-fold increase in the risk of LJM for every unit increase in the HbA_{1c}.[33] In addition, it appears that LJM may be correlated with the presence of microvascular disease.[34]

Most important, the evidence indicates that intensive insulin therapy is central in prevention and, possibly, treatment of LJM and scleroderma-like syndrome. Long-term tight glycemic control leads to decreased skin AGEs,[8] and tight glycemic control is associated with delayed onset and severity of LJM.[33] On the basis of improvements in diabetes management, a fourfold reduction in the frequency of LJM has been reported.[35] Treatment of LJM is difficult and should focus on tight control of blood glucose as well as physical therapy to preserve active range of motion.

Although the scleroderma-like skin changes can occur independently, they often occur together with LJM in patients with diabetes. The scleroderma-like syndrome is not associated with systemic sclerosis but does correlate with the duration of diabetes, the severity of joint contractures, and retinopathy.[36] It appears that the historical description of "diabetic hand syndrome" represents a combination of LJM and the scleroderma-like syndrome.

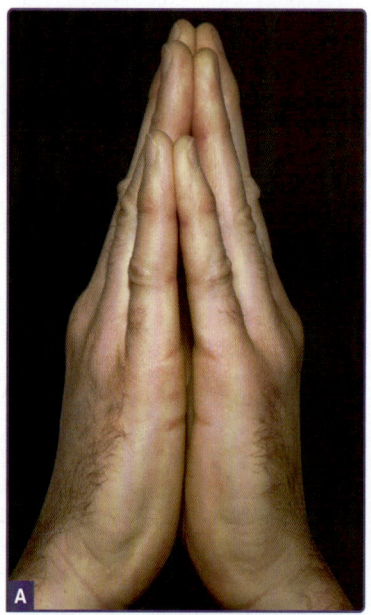 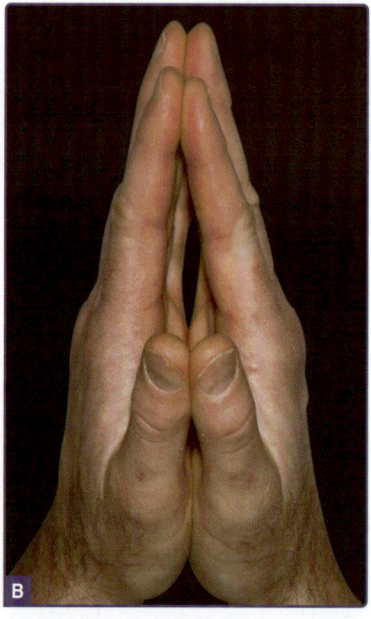

Figure 137-3 Limited joint mobility in a 31-year-old male patient with Type 1 diabetes mellitus. The patient is unable to approximate the palmar surface of the proximal and distal interphalangeal joints with palms pressed together (known as the "prayer sign"). **A,** Ulnar view; only fingertips are approximated. **B,** Radial view; straining to press palms together.

SCLEREDEMA DIABETICORUM (SEE CHAP. 67)

Scleredema of diabetes (scleredema diabeticorum) presents with the insidious onset of painless, symmetric induration and thickening of the skin on the upper back and neck. Spreading to the face, shoulders, and anterior torso also may occur. The skin retains a nonpitting, woody, *peau d'orange* quality. Identical changes occur with postinfectious scleredema, usually associated with streptococcal pharyngitis. In scleredema associated with infection, however, the onset is often sudden, and the symptoms usually remit over time. Scleredema diabeticorum affects 2.5% to 14% of patients with diabetes.[37,38] Scleredema diabeticorum is a disease of longstanding diabetes associated with obesity. Most patients have Type 2 diabetes. This disorder has not been reported in children.

The pathogenesis of scleredema diabeticorum is postulated to be unregulated production of extracellular matrix molecules by fibroblasts, leading to thickened collagen bundles and increased deposition of glycosaminoglycans (mainly hyaluronic acid). Studies using in vitro fibroblast analysis from involved skin have variably demonstrated increased synthesis of glycosaminoglycans and Type 1 collagen.[39] However, most of these reports involved nondiabetic patients with paraproteinemia and are based on small numbers of cases.

Patients with scleredema diabeticorum may experience decreased sensation to pain and light touch over the affected areas and difficulties with upper-extremity and neck range of motion. Extreme cases may result in full loss of range of motion. Unlike in LJM and scleroderma-like syndrome, the presence of scleredema does not correlate with retinopathy, nephropathy, neuropathy, or principal vascular disease.[37] However, no large-scale prospective study has been done. Most patients with scleredema diabeticorum become insulin dependent, are difficult to treat, and have multiple complications of diabetes.[39] Treatment of scleredema diabeticorum is usually unsuccessful. Case reports describe treatment with radiotherapy, low-dose methotrexate, bath psoralen and ultraviolet A light (PUVA), extracorporeal photopheresis, factor XIII, and prostaglandin E_1.[40-42] Weight reduction and physical therapy to preserve range of motion may be useful.

ERUPTIVE XANTHOMAS (SEE CHAP. 126)

Eruptive xanthomas present clinically as 1-mm to 4-mm, reddish-yellow papules on the buttocks and extensor surfaces of the extremities (Fig. 137-4). The lesions occur in crops and may coalesce into plaques over time. Although eruptive xanthomas are generally asymptomatic, there is often underlying severe hypertriglyceridemia (>1000 mg/dL) and potentially undiagnosed diabetes. Uncontrolled diabetes is a common cause of massive hypertriglyceridemia. Histologic and biochemical studies show that lipoproteins (mainly chylomicrons) in the blood permeate cutaneous vessel walls and accumulate in macrophages in the dermis.[43] Initially, triglycerides predominate in the skin lesions but, because triglycerides are mobilized more easily than cholesterol, the lesions contain progressively more cholesterol as they resolve.[43]

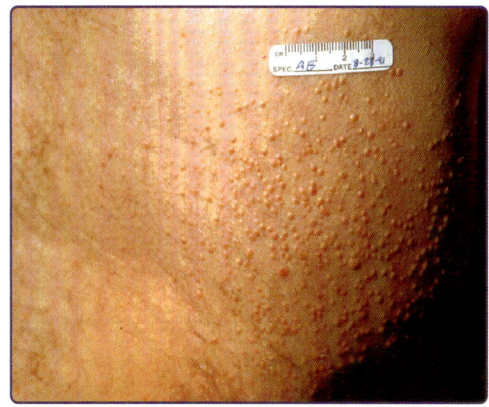

Figure 137-4 Eruptive xanthomas appear as yellow-orange papules and plaques on a male patient with Type 2 diabetes mellitus. (Used with permission from Greg Raugi, MD.)

In addition to eruptive xanthomas, triglyceride levels above 4000 mg/dL may cause lipemia retinalis. On funduscopic examination, lipemia retinalis appears as pale pink to white retinal arterioles and venules. The fundus may have a milky hue. Untreated, severe hypertriglyceridemia may also present clinically with abdominal pain, hepatosplenomegaly, pancreatitis, or dyspnea from decreased pulmonary diffusing capacity and abnormal hemoglobin oxygen affinity.[44] Treatment of hypertriglyceridemia involves lifestyle modification and control of the underlying diabetes. The eruptive xanthomas respond rapidly and usually resolve completely in 6 to 8 weeks.[45]

CUTANEOUS INFECTIONS

In diabetic patients, there is not strong evidence for an increased susceptibility to infections in general, but several skin infections do occur more commonly, with greater severity, or with a greater risk for complications in patients with DM. Joshi and colleagues have reviewed this subject.[11]

There is extensive research on the pathogenesis of immune dysfunction in diabetes. Although some studies could not detect defects at the cellular level,[46] other studies show that leukocyte chemotaxis, adherence, and phagocytosis are impaired in patients with diabetes, especially during hyperglycemia and diabetic acidosis.[47] Further studies show that cutaneous T-cell function and response to antigen challenge are also decreased in diabetes.[11] Table 137-2 outlines some of the skin infections that occur more commonly or more severely in diabetic patients.

TABLE 137-2
Infections More Common or More Severe in Diabetic Patients

BACTERIA	FUNGAL AND YEAST
▪ Invasive group B *Streptococcus*	▪ Candida
▪ Invasive group A *Streptococcus*	▪ Dermatophyte
▪ Malignant external otitis	▪ Rhinocerebral mucormycosis
▪ Necrotizing fasciitis	

DIABETIC ULCERS

Epidemiology: Foot ulcers are a significant problem for patients with diabetes, occurring in 15% to 25% of diabetic patients.[48] Patients with diabetes have an estimated increased risk of lower-extremity amputation that is 10 to 30 times greater than that of the general population. Lower-extremity ulcers account for 25% of all hospital stays for patients with diabetes and are the proximal cause of amputation in 84% of patients.[49] Of diabetic patients with foot ulcers, 14% to 24% will eventually undergo amputation.[50]

Clinical Features: Callus formation precedes necrosis and breakdown of tissue over bony prominences of feet, usually on great toe and sole, over first and/or second metacarpophalangeal joints. Ulcers are surrounded by a ring of callus and may extend to underlying joint and bone (Fig. 137-5). Complications are soft-tissue infection and osteomyelitis.

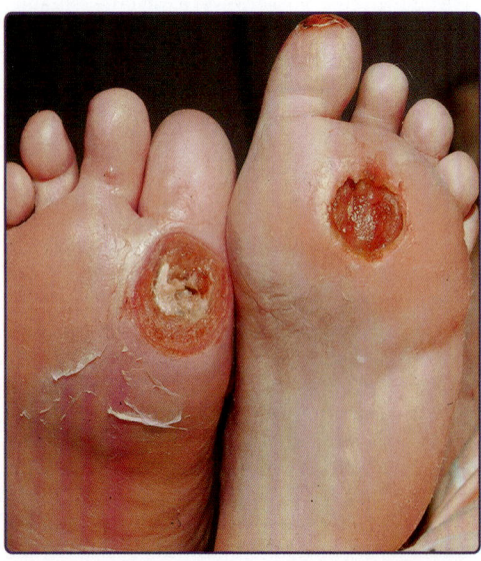

Figure 137-5 "Diabetic foot." Two larger ulcers overlying the first right and second left metacarpophalangeal joints in a 56-year-old man with diabetes of 20 years' duration. There is significant sensory neuropathy and peripheral vascular disease.

Etiology and Pathogenesis: Many of the factors previously described in this chapter contribute to the pathogenesis of diabetic ulcers. Peripheral neuropathy, pressure, and trauma are thought to play prominent roles in the development of diabetic ulcers. Neuropathy (associated with uncontrolled hyperglycemia) is one of the major predictors of diabetic ulcers.[14] Patients with diabetes also suffer the loss of cutaneous sensory nerves.[51] The subsequent diminished neuroinflammatory signaling via neuropeptides to keratinocytes, fibroblasts, endothelial cells, and inflammatory cells may adversely affect wound healing.[52] Excessive plantar pressure develops from foot deformities (Charcot arthropathy). In a study of 314 diabetic patients with ulcers, ill-fitting shoes and socks were the most common reasons for foot ulcers.[53] Callus formation is a sign of excess friction and often precedes foot ulcers. Wearing running shoes demonstrates a measurable reduction of calluses.[54] Once an ulcer develops, peripheral vascular disease and intrinsic wound healing disturbances contribute to adverse outcomes. Known factors associated with foot ulceration in the setting of diabetes include previous foot ulceration, prior lower-extremity amputation, long duration of diabetes (>10 years), impaired visual acuity, onychomycosis, and poor glycemic control.[55]

Management: Treatment of diabetic ulcers requires modification of factors that contribute to ulcer formation, including, stasis dermatitis, leg edema, and skin infection. Standard therapy for neuropathic diabetic ulcers includes debridement, off-loading (often non–weight-bearing), moist wound care, and protective dressings (Fig. 137-6).

There has been substantial interest in developing adjunctive therapies for diabetic ulcers, including growth factors and skin-replacement products, but data have not supported their use as a replacement for standard wound care. Recombinant platelet-derived growth factor for the topical treatment of diabetic foot ulcers demonstrates a modest benefit if used with adequate off-loading, debridement, and control of infection.[56] A large multicenter, clinical trial of a bilayered living skin equivalent[57] showed 56% healing at 12 weeks as compared with 38% healing at 12 weeks for standard care. The most favorable published results for a monolayered living skin equivalent and platelet-derived growth factor show roughly comparable improvement in healing to that reported for bilayered living skin equivalents when each is compared with standard care or placebo.[57] These technologies await definitive analysis of cost-effectiveness compared with standard older approaches. Even though the studies available do not support the routine use of these biologic approaches, these approaches may have a role in the treatment of large ulcers (>2 cm) or of ulcers that are poorly responsive to standard therapy. A recent meta-analysis makes the point that, typically, a higher percentage of ulcers heal during a 12-week study period with biologic products than with standard therapy, but analysis of cost-effectiveness is made difficult by differences in study designs, short duration of studies,

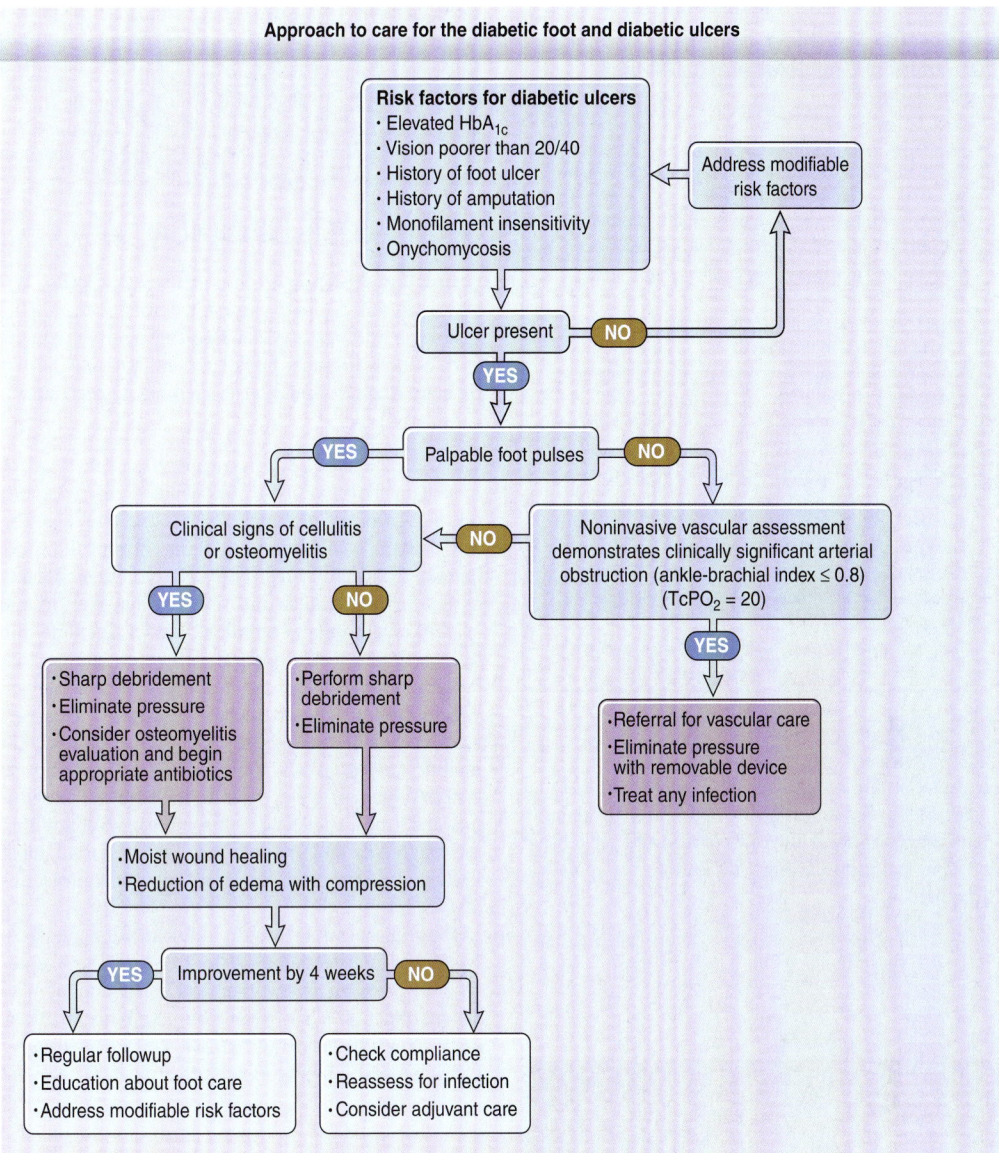

Figure 137-6 Approach to the care of the diabetic foot and diabetic ulcers. HbA_{1c}, hemoglobin A_{1c}; $TcPO_2$, transcutaneous oxygen tension.

different cost structures, the absence of quality-of-life measures, and pharmaceutical funding of the primary studies and analysis.[58]

Prevention: Ulcer prevention is the most important intervention physicians and other health care professionals can provide for diabetic patients. An excellent review of ulcer prevention was published by Singh and colleagues.[48] Optimizing glycemic control is well supported to prevent the neuropathy that is so intimately associated with foot ulceration. The risk of a foot ulcer increases in nearly direct proportion to every 1% increase in HbA_{1c}.[55] Foot examination should be part of every patient visit if diabetes is on the problem list. Failure to perceive touch of a Semmes-Weinstein 10-g monofilament means a patient lacks protective sensation in the foot tested. If tinea pedis is present, it should be treated to prevent the associated skin barrier disruption. Smoking cessation should be encouraged. Patients should be counseled about the importance of daily foot care (Table 137-3).

Specialized ulcer care teams have published impressive results on the prevention and healing of ulcers.[59] This multidisciplinary team approach is becoming more important in the treatment of diabetic ulcers in large population centers. Patients with a history

TABLE 137-3
General Foot Care Guidelines for Patients with Diabetes

- Examine feet every day, including areas between the toes.
- Regular washing of feet with careful drying, especially between the toes.
- Water temperature should always be less than 37°C (98.6°F) and checked first with the hand rather than the foot.
- Barefoot walking indoors or outdoors and wearing of shoes without socks is discouraged.
- Daily inspection and palpation of the inside of the shoes for irregular surfaces or foreign objects.
- If vision is impaired, patients should not try to treat their feet (eg, nails) by themselves.
- Emollients should be used for dry skin, but not between the toes.
- Change stockings daily.
- Stockings should be worn with seams inside out or, preferably, without any seams at all.
- Nails should be cut straight across.
- Corns and calluses should not be cut by patients but by a health care provider.
- The patient must ensure that the feet are examined regularly by a health care provider.
- The patient should seek early health care attention for any blister, cut, scratch, sore, ingrown toenail, or dermatitis.

of ulceration are at high risk for reulceration (34% at 1 year, 61% at 3 years, and 70% at 5 years).[60] Intensifying education (formal foot care classes) and prevention efforts in this group, along with lifelong surveillance, is required.

DISORDERS ASSOCIATED WITH DIABETES MELLITUS BUT OF UNKNOWN PATHOGENESIS

NECROBIOSIS LIPOIDICA

Coined by Urbach in 1932 as *necrobiosis lipoidica diabeticorum*, this disorder was named after characteristic histologic findings and was first described in patients with diabetes. Because not all patients have concurrent diabetes, the shortened term, *necrobiosis lipoidica* (NL) is preferred.

Clinical Features: Classically, NL presents with 1 to several sharply demarcated yellow-brown plaques on the anterior pretibial region (Fig. 137-7). The lesions have a violaceous, irregular border that may be raised and indurated. Early on, NL often presents as red-brown papules and nodules that may mimic sarcoid or granuloma annulare (GA). Over time, the lesions flatten, and a central yellow or orange area becomes atrophic, and, commonly, telangiectasias are visible, taking on the characteristic "glazed-porcelain" sheen. Aside from the shins, other sites of predilection include ankles, calves, thighs, and feet. Fifteen percent of patients develop lesions on the upper extremities and trunk that tend to be more papulonodular. Although pain and pruritus have been reported, most lesions are asymptomatic. Anesthesia of the plaques does occur.[61]

The clinical course is often indolent, with spontaneous remission in less than 20% of cases.[10] The plaques tend to stabilize over time, and formation of new lesions tapers off. However, the possibility of ulceration, a poor spontaneous remission rate, and cosmetic concerns lead patients to seek treatment. Ulceration,

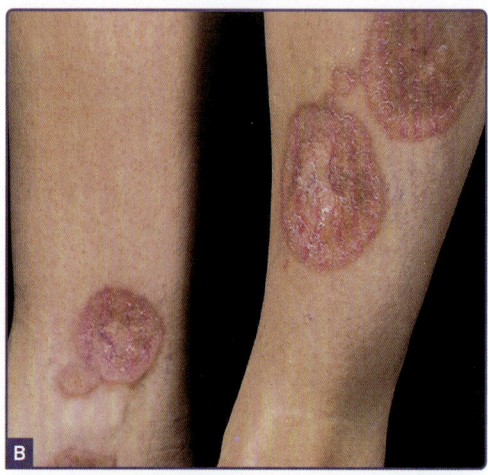

Figure 137-7 Necrobiosis lipoidica. **A,** A single orange plaque with atrophy of the overlying epidermis and arborizing telangiectasias is seen on the lower leg of a patient with diabetes mellitus; the crust marks an area of early ulceration. **B,** Older lesions with striking central atrophy involving both the dermis and epidermis.

the most serious complication, occurs in approximately 13% to 35% of cases on the legs.[62,63] A few cases of squamous cell carcinoma arising in chronic ulcerative lesions of NL have been reported.[64] Multiple reports document the association of NL with GA and sarcoidosis.[65]

Epidemiology and Pathogenesis: Epidemiologic data show that the mean age of onset is around 30 years, with women representing 3 times more cases than men.[62] The most often quoted statistics concerning the association of NL with diabetes are from a 1966 retrospective study at the Mayo Clinic. Of 171 patients with NL, 67% had diabetes at diagnosis, and another 5% to 10% had glucose tolerance abnormalities.[62] However, in a 1999-study of 65 patients with NL, only 11% had diabetes after 15 years of followup.[66] Conversely, the prevalence of NL has been found to be only 0.3% to 3% in patients with diabetes.[62] Although lacking full concordance, NL definitely has a strong association with diabetes and remains a valid marker of the disease. The pathogenesis of this skin disease is unclear.[63] The degree of hyperglycemia and diabetic control does not appear to correlate with the presence of NL.[67]

Management: Treatment of NL is disappointing. Case reports and small, uncontrolled trials provide the basis for treatment decisions. Early application of potent topical glucocorticoids might slow progression.[63] Although improvement can be seen with intralesional injection of glucocorticoids to the active border, the risk of ulceration with this treatment modality should be considered. A few case reports and 1 series of 6 patients[68] showed benefit with short-term systemic glucocorticoids. Aspirin and dipyridamole have produced variable results.[63] Anecdotal reports exist that support the use of tumor necrosis factor-α inhibitors, topical retinoids, and topical PUVA. Treatment with fumaric acid esters in 18 patients was reported to improve lesions clinically and histologically.[69]

Given the generally benign nature of the lesions, physicians should consider the adage "do no harm." Focus should be on prevention of ulcers. When ulceration occurs in patients with NL, the same wound care principles apply as for all diabetic ulcers. Healing of ulcerated lesions with cyclosporine has been demonstrated in several patients.[70] Surgical excision down to fascia and split-thickness skin grafting remain as the last resort for recalcitrant ulcers in NL.[71]

GRANULOMA ANNULARE (SEE CHAP. 34)

The association of GA with diabetes is weaker than that of NL. Although most patients with GA are in good health, without underlying systemic illness, an association with diabetes is supported in the literature. Dabski and Winklemann[72] found diabetes in 9.7% of patients with localized GA and 21% of patients with generalized GA. An additional small retrospective case-control study showed an increased prevalence of diabetes among patients with GA (18%) as compared with the prevalence in age-matched controls (8%).[73] Furthermore, there is an impression that diabetes is found more frequently in patients with adult-onset GA and in those with generalized or perforating GA, and that these patients tend to experience a more chronic, relapsing course of GA. The pathogenesis is unclear. Clinical findings and treatment of GA are discussed in Chap. 34.

DIABETIC DERMOPATHY

Clinical Features: Atrophic skin lesions of the lower extremity, or shin spots, were first characterized and proposed as a cutaneous marker for diabetes in 1964.[74] Shortly after, Binkley coined the term *diabetic dermopathy* to correlate the pathologic changes with those of retinopathy, nephropathy, and neuropathy.[75] Diabetic dermopathy presents as small (<1 cm), atrophic, pink to brown, scar-like macules on the pretibial areas (Fig. 137-8). The lesions are asymptomatic and clear within 1 to 2 years with slight residual atrophy or hypopigmentation.[75] The appearance of new lesions gives the sense that the pigmentation and atrophy are persistent.

An association seems to exist between diabetic dermopathy and the more serious complications of diabetes. In a study of 173 patients with diabetes, the incidence of shin spots correlated with the duration of diabetes and the presence of retinopathy, nephropathy, and neuropathy.[76] Diabetic dermopathy does not, however, correlate with obesity or hypertension in patients with diabetes.[77] No treatment is necessary for the individual atrophic tibial lesions. They are asymptomatic and are not directly associated with an increase in morbidity.

Etiology and Pathogenesis: Controversy has existed about the disorder's etiology, specificity for diabetes, and association with other microangiopathic complications of diabetes.

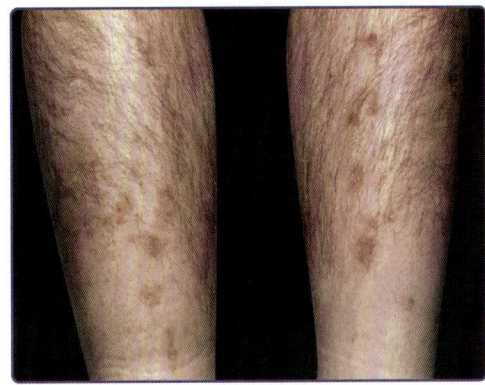

Figure 137-8 Diabetic dermopathy with hyperpigmented macules on the anterior lower legs.

The prevalence of shin spots in ambulatory patients with diabetes varies. In a population-based study from Sweden, diabetic dermopathy was found in 33% of patients with Type 1 diabetes and in 39% of patients with Type 2 diabetes, compared with 2% of controls.[78] In other studies, the prevalence rate for individuals without diabetes ranges from 1.5% for healthy medical students to 20% for a group of nondiabetic endocrine patients.[77] Diabetic dermopathy occurs more often in patients with an increased duration of diabetes and is more frequent in men.[77]

It is likely that the lesions are related to antecedent trauma. Lithner[79] induced diabetic dermopathy on the legs of diabetic patients with heat and cold injury, whereas nondiabetic control subjects healed without residual change. When questioned, most patients attribute the changes to injury, but are often unable to recall preceding trauma.

ACQUIRED PERFORATING DISORDERS (SEE CHAP. 71)

The acquired perforating disorders comprise an overlapping group of disorders characterized by transepidermal elimination or "spitting" of altered dermal constituents. Included in this group are Kyrle disease, reactive perforating collagenosis, perforating folliculitis, and elastosis perforans serpiginosa.[80] These disorders and their treatment[81] are fully described in Chap. 71.

Clinically, these lesions appear as pruritic, keratotic papules mainly on the extensor surfaces of the extremities. Papules and nodules with a perforating component may also occur on the trunk and face. Many are follicular and contain a prominent central keratotic plug. The papules may be grouped, or coalesce to form verrucous plaques. Treatment of the perforating disorders is usually unsuccessful. Retinoic acid, topical glucocorticoids, and PUVA are partially successful.[81]

BULLOSIS DIABETICORUM

Clinical Features: The abrupt, spontaneous development of blisters on the lower extremities without other demonstrable cause is a rare characteristic skin manifestation of diabetes. Bullosis diabeticorum is characterized by bullae on the lower extremities, usually the toes, feet, and shins, arising in normal skin. Occasionally, the distal upper extremities are involved. The blisters are usually painless and not pruritic. Healing occurs within 2 to 5 weeks and rarely leaves scarring. The condition may recur as successive crops of bullae over many years. Studies of affected individuals excluded other blistering skin disorders, and revealed no abnormalities of porphyrin metabolism.[82] Histopathologic examination of the bullae shows an inconsistent level of separation varying from intraepidermal to subepidermal.[83] No immunopathologic features are consistently observed (Table 137-4).

TABLE 137-4
Differential Diagnosis and Evaluation of Bullosis Diabeticorum

Differential Diagnosis
- Bullous impetigo
- Bullous pemphigoid
- Epidermolysis bullosa acquisita
- Porphyria cutanea tarda
- Bullous erythema multiforme
- Insect bite reaction

Laboratory Tests
- Skin biopsy for histology and immunofluorescence
- Bacterial cultures
- Screening for porphyrins

Bullosis diabeticorum runs a benign course without involvement of large body surface areas. The only serious complication is that of secondary infection, which should be managed with culture and appropriate antibiotics if suspected. Otherwise, therapy is supportive. The real importance of this disorder is that of correct diagnosis because several of the blistering skin diseases have a high rate of morbidity and require potentially toxic systemic treatments. Exclusion of these entities is important. The patient should be educated, reassured, and wound care implemented.

Etiology and Pathogenesis: The pathogenesis of diabetic bullae is unknown. Patients with bullosis diabeticorum do not have a history of antecedent trauma or infection. One study found a decreased threshold to suction-induced blister formation in patients with diabetes.[82] Reduced suction blister time is also observed with increasing age in nondiabetic subjects.[83] Although a history of antecedent trauma is not elicited, this finding suggests a role of increased skin fragility in diabetic bullae. Perhaps the formation of AGEs leads to increased fragility.

OBESITY AND THE METABOLIC SYNDROME

EPIDEMIOLOGY

Obesity is characterized by excess fat mass and defined according to the body mass index (BMI [kg/m^2]), a calculation based on weight and height (BMI = body weight [in kg] ÷ square of stature [height in meters]). BMI is correlated with body fat and the World Health Organization defines overweight as a BMI greater than 25 and obesity as greater than 30 kg/m^2. For Americans, the risk of becoming overweight or obese in adulthood is high. As part of the National Health and Nutrition Examination Survey (NHANES) in 2012, 35% of adults were obese.[84]

CLINICAL FEATURES

Physiologic changes in the skin related to obesity include alterations in epidermal barrier function,[85,86] increased sweating along with larger skin folds, increased skin surface pH in intertriginous areas,[87] poor lymphatic drainage, impaired wound healing in animal models,[88] and impaired responsiveness of the microvasculature.[89] Several reviews regarding obesity and dermatology have been published.[90,91] Table 137-5 lists the cutaneous disorders seen in obesity. Detailed discussion of findings and treatments for these disorders are found in the appropriate sections of the text.

It is now well recognized that the presence of abdominal—central rather than subcutaneous—obesity (more than just increased BMI) is associated with insulin resistance, hyperlipidemia, hypertension, and vascular inflammation (Table 137-6). The coexistence of these disorders increases the risk for diabetes and cardiovascular disease and has been called the metabolic syndrome. It is not clear that the metabolic syndrome confers risk beyond that of the individual components, but because the traits cooccur, those with 1 trait are likely to have others. The most important therapy is weight reduction and exercise along with adequate control of cardiac risk factors.

ETIOLOGY AND PATHOGENESIS

Contributing factors to obesity are nutritional choices, activity and exercise, medications, and, rarely, one of several endocrine disorders. In the setting of nutrient excess and weight gain, numerous comorbid factors occur that may contribute to further weight gain by increasing energy intake or decreasing energy expenditure. These include inflammation and insulin resistance, depression and emotional eating, degenerative joint disease, obstructive sleep apnea, gonadal dysfunction, vitamin D deficiency. Familial studies suggest a strong genetic basis for human obesity. The genetics of obesity are complex, although most human obesity is likely polygenic, multiple single genes have been identified as key regulators of body adiposity. Three of these genes (leptin, proopiomelanocortin [POMC], and agouti-related protein [AgRP]) with dermatologic relevance are discussed in detail below.

The hormone leptin is secreted by adipose tissue in proportion to total body fat. Leptin regulates energy homeostasis, neuroendocrine function, and metabolism.[92] Rare cases in humans have shown that leptin deficiency causes extreme obesity, hyperphagia, diabetes, neuroendocrine abnormalities, and infertility, all of which can be reversed by administration of exogenous leptin. However, most obese humans are leptin resistant, have high circulating levels of leptin, and pharmacologic leptin administration has not proven to be a successful weight-loss strategy. Leptin resistance appears to be at the hypothalamic leptin receptor or downstream.[92] Congenital and acquired forms of lipoatrophy (HIV or highly active antiretroviral therapy associated) are characterized by low leptin levels and metabolic abnormalities, including insulin resistance, hyperlipidemia, and fatty liver. Leptin treatment in these patients can improve insulin resistance, lipid abnormalities, and fat distribution.[93,94]

Leptin stimulates the hypothalamic melanocortin pathway including hypothalamic neurons expressing POMC. Cleavage of POMC results in peptide agonists for all 5 homologous melanocortin receptors. The melanocortin 1 receptor (MC1R) is expressed on melanocytes and mutations in MC1R are known to cause red hair and fair skin.[95] Inactivating mutations in MC4R and to a lesser degree MC3R are associated with obesity. Studies estimate that inactivating mutations in MC4R account for up to 6% of all severe cases of early-onset obesity. Further emphasizing the importance of the POMC pathway is the finding that homozygous loss of function of POMC (complete

TABLE 137-6
Definition of the Metabolic Syndrome (Any 3 of 5 Traits)

1. Abdominal Obesity
2. Serum triglycerides ≥150 mg/dL (or drug treatment of elevated triglycerides)
3. Serum high-density lipoprotein cholesterol (HDL-C) <40 mg/dL in men and <50 mg/dL in women (or drug treatment of low HDL-C)
4. Blood pressure ≥130/85 mm Hg (or drug treatment of elevated blood pressure)
5. Fasting plasma glucose ≥100 mg/dL (or drug treatment of elevated blood glucose)

TABLE 137-5
Cutaneous Disorders Associated with Obesity

Metabolic
- Acanthosis nigricans
- Acrochordons
- Keratosis pilaris
- Hyperandrogenism
- Hirsutism
- Tophaceous gout

Infectious
- Candidiasis
- Dermatophytosis
- Intertrigo
- Cellulitis
- Erysipelas
- Necrotizing fasciitis

Mechanical
- Plantar hyperkeratosis
- Striae distensae
- Lymphedema
- Elephantiasis nostras verrucosa
- Venous stasis
- Cellulite

Miscellaneous
- Hidradenitis suppurativa
- Adiposis dolorosa
- Psoriasis

POMC deficiency) produces obesity, pale skin, and red hair.[96]

AgRP is an endogenous hypothalamic melanocortin receptor antagonist, which causes obesity when overexpressed. Although studies have found high serum AgRP levels in obese men,[97] the role of AgRP in common obesity is unclear. The gene is closely related to *agouti,* a skin pigmentation gene, which causes yellow coat color and obesity when overexpressed in mice.

The hormonal regulation of obesity is similarly complex and several gut hormones are likely involved in the regulation of food intake. The gastric-derived, appetite-stimulating hormone ghrelin impacts obesity and diabetes by modulating body weight, insulin secretion, and gastric motility.[98] Serum ghrelin levels rise before meals and are thought to promote food intake. Sharp rises are seen in states of starvation and after weight loss in obesity. This likely contributes to weight regain. Interestingly, postgastric bypass surgery patients have altered ghrelin secretion and this may be one of the reasons for the long-term success of this surgical treatment of obesity.[99] Ghrelin receptors are located in the pituitary and hypothalamus and stimulate growth hormone (GH1) release and regulate energy expenditure (see Fig. 137-15).[93] Ghrelin antagonists have been considered as a treatment of obesity, metabolic syndrome, and diabetes.

MANAGEMENT

The cornerstones of treatment of overweight and obesity are dietary changes, increased physical activity, and behavioral modification. In high-risk patients with comorbid conditions, pharmacologic therapy (orlistat or lorcaserin, among others) can be considered as an additional intervention. In clinically severe obesity, surgical therapies may be appropriate. All successful patients will require long-term nutritional adjustments that reduce caloric intake. The role of liposuction in weight loss has been studied and despite the removal of a large volume of subcutaneous adipose tissue there was no improvement seen in the metabolic risk factors associated with obesity.[100,101]

THYROID DISEASE

> ### AT-A-GLANCE
>
> - The most common cause of hyperthyroidism is Graves disease, characterized by the triad of autoimmune thyroid disease, eye disease, and thyroid dermopathy (pretibial myxedema).
> - Toxic multinodular goiter is another cause of hyperthyroidism that should be considered, particularly in elderly individuals.
> - Serious signs of thyrotoxicosis include atrial fibrillation and fever.
> - Hashimoto thyroiditis and thyroid ablation for treatment of hyperthyroidism are the 2 most common causes of hypothyroidism.
> - The best screening test for thyroid disease is thyrotropin (thyroid-stimulating hormone), which is elevated in hypothyroidism and depressed or absent in hyperthyroidism.

EPIDEMIOLOGY

Thyroid disease is very common worldwide. Enlargement of the thyroid gland, known as goiter, is estimated to affect around 700 million people worldwide.[102] The majority of these worldwide cases are secondary to iodine deficiency. However, hypothyroidism and hyperthyroidism are very prevalent even in industrialized countries. The overall incidence of hyperthyroidism in the U.S. population is estimated at 1%, but may be 4 to 5 times higher in older women.[103] As salt is routinely iodized in these countries, the major causes of goiter are Hashimoto thyroiditis, multinodular goiter, and Graves disease. Graves disease accounts for 60% to 80% of all cases of hyperthyroidism and was first described as an association between goiter, palpitations, and exophthalmos.[104] Although the incidence of Graves disease is similar between whites and Asians, it appears to be lower in blacks.[104] After Graves disease, the next most common cause of hyperthyroidism is *toxic multinodular goiter.*[105] *Toxic adenoma* and *toxic multinodular goiter* refer to the hyperplastic growth of thyroid tissue that functions independently of thyroid-stimulating hormone (TSH) regulation, resulting in inappropriately elevated levels of thyroid hormone. Toxic multinodular goiter is more common in areas of low iodine intake, particularly in patients older than age 50 years.[106]

Population-based screening with laboratory testing found hypothyroidism in 4.6% of the U.S. population, and more than 90% of individuals identified with hypothyroidism were asymptomatic.[103]

The majority of thyroid disease is acquired, but thyroid disease also can be congenital. Congenital hypothyroidism is the most common treatable cause of intellectual disability, and occurs in up to 1 in 3000 neonates worldwide. Causes are an absent or anatomically defective gland, inborn errors of thyroid metabolism, or iodine deficiency.[107] Congenital hyperthyroidism is much less common, and although 0.2% of pregnant women have Graves disease, only approximately 1% of the resultant neonates will have hyperthyroidism, with most cases resulting from the transfer of maternal thyroid-activating autoantibodies.[108]

CLINICAL FEATURES

CUTANEOUS MANIFESTATIONS OF HYPERTHYROIDISM

Table 137-7 describes an approach to the patient with hyperthyroidism.

The cutaneous changes of hyperthyroidism have been likened to infant's skin and described as soft, warm, and velvety in texture. Pruritus can be a manifestation of thyroid disease, and laboratory screening for thyroid disease is often included when working up patients experiencing diffuse pruritus without obvious rash. Scalp hair in patients with hyperthyroidism is often soft and fine, and in certain cases may be accompanied by a diffuse nonscarring alopecia analogous to telogen effluvium. Patients with hyperthyroidism frequently have soft, shiny, and brittle nails with an increased rate of growth. A small percentage of patients with hyperthyroidism will have Plummer nails, which exhibit a concave shape with distal onycholysis (see Chap. 91). Plummer nails also can be found in a variety of other conditions and are not pathognomonic for hyperthyroidism. Vitiligo appears to be overrepresented in patients with Graves disease, but not in patients with other forms of hyperthyroidism. Vitiligo often predates the diagnosis of thyroid disease and does not improve with the treatment of the hyperthyroidism (see Chap. 76).

Thyroid dermopathy (in the past referred to as *pretibial myxedema*) is a classic manifestation of Graves disease (see Fig. 137-11). The term *thyroid dermopathy* is used in this chapter because the lesions can occur at any site on the body, are not limited to the pretibial region, and the name does not suggest myxedema as a cause.[109] It is most commonly seen with Graves disease, but has been reported in patients with Hashimoto thyroiditis as well. Although there are reports of patients who have presented with thyroid dermopathy as their initial finding, thyroid dermopathy is usually a late manifestation of thyroid disease. Almost all patients with thyroid dermopathy also have thyroid ophthalmopathy, another manifestation of Graves disease.[110] The presence of thyroid dermopathy and acropachy are markers of the severity of the autoimmune disease process and signal a risk for severe ophthalmopathy.[111] The clinical appearance of thyroid dermopathy can be quite varied. Classically, thyroid dermopathy occurs bilaterally as painless nonpitting nodules and plaques with variable coloring and a waxy, indurated texture (Fig. 137-9). The distribution can range from localized to diffuse, but by far the most common location is on the extensor surfaces of the legs.[110] In some cases the skin has a peau d'orange appearance. An extreme form of diffuse thyroid dermopathy has been termed the *elephantiasic* variant, which occurs in less than

TABLE 137-7
Approach to the Patient with Hyperthyroidism

Cutaneous Findings in Hyperthyroidism
- Soft, velvety, infant-like skin
- Thyroid dermopathy (in Graves disease)
- Soft, fine hair with diffuse nonscarring alopecia
- Facial flushing
- Palmar erythema
- Hyperpigmentation
- Plummer nails
- Thyroid acropachy (in Graves disease)
- Hyperpigmentation

Related Features
- Hyperhidrosis
- Atrial fibrillation
- Ophthalmopathy (in Graves disease)
- Goiter
- High-output heart failure
- "Thyroid storm"

Diagnosis
- Best initial test is serum thyroid-stimulating hormone (low in hyperthyroidism)
- Other tests include serum free thyroxine (T_4), total triiodothyronine (T_3), and thyrotropin receptor antibodies
- Radioactive iodine uptake and imaging

Management
- Appropriate surgical and endocrine consultation
- Propranolol for symptomatic treatment of tremor, tachycardia, and sweating, if no contraindications are present
- Propylthiouracil to inhibit thyroid hormone metabolism and conversion of T_4 to T_3
- Methimazole to inhibit thyroid hormone synthesis
- Radioiodine ablation of the thyroid gland

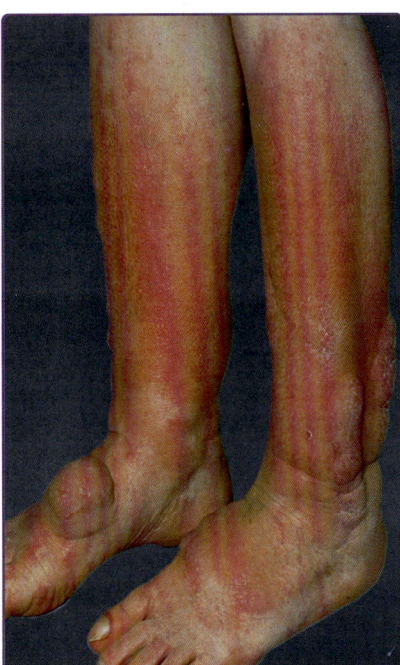

Figure 137-9 Hyperthyroidism with thyroid dermopathy in a classic location on the anterior shins. Note that infiltrated plaques extend to the calf and are partially hyperkeratotic. An isolated nodule is also present on the dorsum of the foot.

1% of patients with Graves disease and is characterized by progressive thickening and gray-black hyperpigmentation of the pretibial skin accompanied by a woody, firm edema with nodule formation.[109] Biopsies of thyroid dermopathy reveal a thickened dermis with splayed collagen fibrils and abundant mucin, usually hyaluronic acid, in the interstitial space.

The exact pathophysiology underlying thyroid dermopathy is still unclear. Autoantibodies that bind the TSH receptor (TSHR) on fibroblasts are seen and may trigger synthesis of glycosaminoglycans. However, antibodies that bind TSHR on fibroblasts are present in patients without thyroid dermopathy, indicating there are likely other factors involved. The presence of dependent edema in the lower extremities may contribute to either fibroblast stimulation or hyaluronic acid accumulation, and thus account for the tendency of thyroid dermopathy to occur in this anatomic site.[109]

Thyroid acropachy refers to digital clubbing, soft-tissue swelling of the hands and feet, and the presence of characteristic periosteal reactions.[109] This very rare clinical finding is almost always associated with thyroid dermopathy and exophthalmos, and typically presents after the diagnosis and treatment of hyperthyroidism. Like thyroid dermopathy, thyroid acropachy also has been reported in patients with hypothyroidism or euthyroidism. Clubbing occurs most frequently on the first, second, and fifth metacarpals, the proximal phalanges of the hand, and the first metatarsal and proximal phalanges of the feet.[109] The radiographic findings are characterized by a lamellar periosteal reaction of the hands or wrists, with long bones only rarely involved. Because increased osteoblastic activity has been observed in the diaphyseal parts of small bones, the use of bone scan has been suggested as a sensitive way to aid in diagnosis.[112] The mechanisms underlying thyroid acropachy remain unknown, although interestingly, a large case series identified a disproportionately high percentage of smokers (80%) in patients with thyroid acropachy.[113]

Systemic signs and symptoms of hyperthyroidism and hypothyroidism are variably present and are summarized in Table 137-8. The effects of excess thyroid hormone on other organ systems can also result in cutaneous findings. Hyperpigmentation similar to that seen in Addison disease has been seen with patients with hyperthyroidism, with increased pigment in the palmar creases, gingiva, and buccal mucosa that is usually more prominent in individuals with darker skin. It has been postulated that the hyperpigmentation may be the result of increased corticotropin (ACTH) resulting from accelerated cortisol metabolism.[109] The cardiovascular effects of thyroid hormone excess include atrial fibrillation, increased cardiac output, and decreased peripheral vascular resistance, resulting in increased blood flow to the skin which manifests as facial flushing and palmar erythema. The increase in metabolism, along with increased peripheral blood flow and temperature dysregulation, can also result in a generalized hyperhidrosis as well as high-output cardiac failure.

TABLE 137-8
Symptoms, Clinical Findings, and Complications of Thyroid Disease

HYPERTHYROIDISM	HYPOTHYROIDISM
Symptoms	**Symptoms**
▪ Unintentional weight loss	▪ Unexplained weight gain
▪ Heat intolerance/sweating	▪ Fatigue
▪ Palpitations	▪ Cold intolerance
▪ Agitation/emotional lability	▪ Constipation
▪ Multiple daily loose stools	▪ Dry skin
▪ Pruritus	▪ Muscle weakness
▪ Weakness	▪ Carpal tunnel syndrome
▪ Oligomenorrhea in women	▪ Hoarseness
	▪ Decreased body temperature
	▪ Facial swelling
	▪ Menorrhagia in women
Clinical Findings and Complications	**Clinical Findings and Complications**
▪ Goiter	▪ Goiter
▪ Tachycardia	▪ Cold, doughy skin
▪ Atrial fibrillation	▪ Bradycardia
▪ High-output cardiac failure	▪ Facial and finger swelling
▪ Fine tremor	▪ Slowed relaxation of deep tendon reflexes
▪ Hot sweaty extremities	▪ Hair loss/lateral eyebrow loss
▪ Ophthalmopathy	▪ Pericardial effusion
▪ Agitation/confusion	▪ Myocardial infarction or congestive heart failure with aggressive thyroid hormone replacement
▪ Muscle weakness/wasting	▪ Coma and death without treatment
▪ "Thyroid storm" with fever, confusion, dehydration, and eventual death, if untreated	

There is extensive literature regarding the association between thyroid disease and urticaria (see Chap. 41).[114] Several studies have found a much higher incidence of thyroid disease in patients with chronic urticaria compared with control populations, although the mechanism behind this association remains unclear. Treatment with levothyroxine has been reported to improve the urticaria in some patients with thyroid disease, particularly Hashimoto thyroiditis, but strong evidence is lacking.[115,116] Other dermatologic conditions that have been reported in association with Graves disease include dermatitis herpetiformis, Sweet syndrome, pemphigoid gestationis, vitiligo, pemphigus vulgaris, anetoderma, and middermal elastolysis.[109]

CUTANEOUS MANIFESTATIONS OF HYPOTHYROIDISM

Table 137-9 outlines an approach to the patient with hypothyroidism.

In hypothyroidism, decreased core temperature and increased peripheral vasoconstriction cause the skin to be cool and pale. The skin is also xerotic, and the stratum corneum is poorly hydrated. The xerosis can mimic acquired ichthyosis. Histologically, the epidermis is thin, and there is hyperkeratosis with follicular plugging. The generalized distribution of these findings can help distinguish these changes from those of atopic dermatitis and keratosis pilaris, which tend to be more prominent on the extremities. A fine wrinkling of the skin also can be seen. Yellow-orange discoloration of the skin can be seen secondary to the accumulation of beta-carotene in the stratum corneum, which is thought to be the result of increased circulating carotene from diminished hepatic conversion of beta-carotene to vitamin A. This "pseudojaundice" can be distinguished from true jaundice because it spares the sclerae.[117] Hypothyroidism is also a rare cause of acquired palmoplantar keratoderma, which responds well to treatment with thyroxine.[118]

Myxedema is the most classic finding associated with hypothyroidism and is distinct from the thyroid dermopathy seen with Graves disease. Myxedema occurs as a result of dermal accumulation of mucopolysaccharides, namely, hyaluronic acid and chondroitin sulfate, and tends to resolve with treatment of the hypothyroidism. The myxedema tends to be generalized but can appear more striking in the extremities. Characteristic facial changes can be seen, including a broadened nose, thickened lips, puffy eyelids, and macroglossia with a smooth and clumsy tongue. The skin can be doughy, swollen, and waxy, but without pitting. Wound healing is impaired.

The hair in patients with hypothyroidism is coarse, dry, and brittle with slowed growth. The alopecia seen in hypothyroidism can be either diffuse or patchy. Hypothyroidism can result in increased numbers of hair follicles in telogen, as well as telogen effluvium when the onset of hypothyroidism is abrupt. There can be a characteristic pattern of eyebrow loss involving the outer third of the eyebrows. Although body hair can be diminished, hypothyroidism can also result in increased lanugo hair on the back, shoulders, and extremities. The nails in hypothyroidism grow slowly and can be thickened and brittle with longitudinal and transverse striations.

Hypothyroidism caused by iodine deficiency or Hashimoto thyroiditis can be associated with goiter. In patients with a goiter, compression of the recurrent laryngeal nerve can result in hoarseness. Large goiters can cause tracheal or esophageal displacement. In extreme cases, large retrosternal goiters can cause the Pemberton sign, which consists of facial plethora when patients raise their arms above their head owing to compression of the jugular veins.[119] Hashimoto thyroiditis also is associated with several other dermatologic disorders, including alopecia areata, vitiligo, connective tissue disease (including lupus and dermatomyositis), bullous pemphigoid, dermatitis herpetiformis, and chronic mucocutaneous candidiasis (CMC).[120-124]

ETIOLOGY AND PATHOGENESIS

Thyroid hormone is synthesized in the thyroid gland and plays an important role in regulating the body's metabolism. Hyperthyroidism is the result of excess levels of thyroid hormone, whereas hypothyroidism is characterized by hypometabolism secondary to inappropriately low levels of thyroid hormone. Thyroid hormone synthesis is heavily dependent on iodine and consequently changes in iodine intake can result in both hyperthyroidism and hypothyroidism.

Synthesis of thyroid hormone is regulated by the pituitary gland via the release of TSH in response to hypothalamic production of thyrotropin-releasing hormone. TSH acts on the thyroid gland by binding to the TSHR, a G-protein–coupled receptor, triggering thyroid hormone synthesis and release. Levels of TSH and thyrotropin-releasing hormone are both tightly controlled by circulating levels of thyroxine (T_4) and triiodothyronine (T_3), which provide feedback regulation. Inappropriate activation of TSHR is thought to cause the hyperthyroidism seen in Graves disease, in which almost all patients have long-acting thyroid-stimulating autoantibodies that bind and activate TSHR.[125]

Most thyroid hormone in the blood is bound by plasma proteins. These include thyroid-binding globulin, which is the major determinant of protein binding.

TABLE 137-9
Approach to the Patient with Hypothyroidism

Cutaneous Findings
- Myxedema
- Cool temperature
- Doughy, dry skin with fine wrinkling
- Yellow-orange carotenemia
- Dry, brittle hair
- Slow growth of hair and nails

Related Features
- Macroglossia
- Broadened nose, thickened lips, puffy eyelids
- Impaired wound healing
- Cretinism in patients with congenital hypothyroidism
- "Myxedema coma"

Diagnosis
- Best initial test is serum thyroid-stimulating hormone (elevated in hypothyroidism)
- Other useful tests include serum free thyroxine (T_4), total triiodothyronine (T_3), antithyroperoxidase (anti-TPO) antibodies, and lipid panel

Management
- Appropriate endocrine consultation
- Oral thyroxine replacement (usually in the range of 75 to 150 μg/day)
- Careful followup for heart, lung, and adrenal disease

TABLE 137-10
Medical Conditions That Can Affect Thyroid Hormone Levels

Increased Thyroid-Binding Globulin
- Pregnancy
- Infectious/chronic active hepatitis
- Cirrhosis
- Acute intermittent porphyria

Decreased Thyroid-Binding Globulin
- Hereditary thyroid-binding globulin deficiency
- Severe systemic illness
- Active acromegaly
- Cushing syndrome
- Nephrotic syndrome

Decreased Peripheral Conversion of Thyroxine (T_4) to Triiodothyronine (T_3)
- Fasting/malnutrition
- Systemic illness
- Physical trauma
- Postoperative state

A variety of medical conditions (Table 137-10) and medications (Table 137-11) can alter levels of thyroid hormone-binding proteins and/or peripheral conversion of T_4 to T_3 (which is responsible for most of thyroid hormone's effects).[126]

TABLE 137-11
Medications Affecting Thyroid Hormone Levels

Drugs That Affect Thyroid Hormone Secretion
- Lithium (decreases secretion)
- Iodide (can increase or decrease secretion)
- Amiodarone (contains iodine, can increase or decrease secretion)

Drugs That Increase Serum Thyroid-Binding Globulin Concentrations
- Estrogens/tamoxifen
- Heroin/methadone
- 5-Fluorouracil

Drugs That Decrease Serum Thyroid-Binding Globulin Concentrations
- Androgens
- Anabolic steroids
- Slow-release nicotinic acid
- Glucocorticoids

Drugs That Increase Metabolism of Thyroid Hormone
- Phenobarbital
- Rifampin
- Phenytoin
- Carbamazepine
- Tyrosine kinase inhibitors (imatinib, sorafenib, etc.)[131]

Drugs That Decrease Deiodination of Thyroxine to Triiodothyronine
- Propylthiouracil (used to treat hyperthyroidism)
- Amiodarone
- β-Blockers
- Glucocorticoids
- Certain radiographic contrast dyes

Drugs That Decrease Thyroid-Stimulating Hormone
- Bexarotene

Adapted from Surks MI, Sievert R. Drugs and thyroid function. *N Engl J Med*. 1995;333:1688.

Hyperthyroidism can be broadly classified into 2 categories: (a) high radioiodine (radioactive iodine) uptake and (b) low radioiodine uptake. The presence of high radioiodine uptake indicates increased synthesis of thyroid hormone, whereas diminished or absent radioiodine uptake suggests either an exogenous source of thyroid hormone or the thyroid inflammation with release of preformed thyroid hormone into the circulation. Evidence suggests that genetic predisposition as well as environmental factors, including infection, may play a role in the pathogenesis of autoimmune thyroid disease.[127] In the case of toxic adenoma, molecular studies have identified a high prevalence of TSHR mutations, resulting in a receptor that triggers thyroid hormone synthesis in the absence of bound TSH.[128]

Although some of the cutaneous findings seen in hyperthyroidism are indirect consequences of thyroid hormone's actions on other tissues, most of the skin manifestations of thyroid disease result from the direct effects of thyroid hormones on the keratinized epithelium of the epidermis, hair, and nails as well as effects on stromal cells in the dermis. Thyroid hormone is essential for optimal epidermal proliferation both in vitro and in vivo.[129] Thyroid hormone regulates genes involved in keratinocyte proliferation, stimulates the expression of certain keratins, and plays an important role in hair growth and hair cycling by acting on the stem cells in the hair follicle bulge.[129,130]

Ironically, the most common cause of hypothyroidism without a goiter is the surgical or radioiodine-induced ablation of the thyroid gland for the treatment of Graves disease. The most common cause of hypothyroidism with a goiter in North America is Hashimoto thyroiditis. Less common causes of hypothyroidism include inherited defects in hormone synthesis or drugs that affect hormone synthesis or metabolism (see Table 137-11). Bexarotene, a selective retinoid-X–receptor agonist (see Chap. 119) used to treat cutaneous T-cell lymphoma, causes a central hypothyroidism by suppressing the production and release of TSH, which leads to decreased levels of T_3 and T_4.[131,132] Hypopituitarism is another rare cause of hypothyroidism.

DIAGNOSIS AND LABORATORY TESTS

The diagnosis of thyroid-related cutaneous disease is often suspected clinically, although in certain instances a skin biopsy may prove helpful in confirming the diagnosis. The clinical diagnosis of thyroid disease is confirmed by abnormal thyroid function tests. Serum TSH is recommended as an initial screen, and any abnormalities in TSH should be followed up with measurements of serum free T_4 to confirm whether the abnormal TSH truly reflects a thyroid disorder. Other tests that can be useful include measurement of serum total T_3 and antithyroid antibodies. This combination of tests will diagnose the vast majority of patients with suspected thyroid disease.

MANAGEMENT

The mainstay of treatment of the cutaneous findings of thyroid disease is normalization of thyroid function, either through replacement of thyroid hormone for hypothyroidism or through the use of medications, radioiodine ablation, or surgery for hyperthyroidism. Complete or partial remission of cutaneous findings can be seen even in the absence of any localized topical treatment.[113] However, thyroid dermopathy and thyroid acropachy can persist even in patients who are effectively treated for their thyroid disease, and the current treatment options for thyroid dermopathy can be classified as either experimental or palliative at best. Topical glucocorticoids with adjuvant compression have been used with some success for many years.[117] Other reported treatments for thyroid dermopathy include systemic corticosteroids, intralesional corticosteroids, octreotide, intravenous immunoglobulin, plasmapheresis, pentoxifylline, complete decongestive physiotherapy, and even surgical excision (not recommended given the high rate of recurrence after surgery).[113,133,134] The success of these therapies is still controversial and based on small, uncontrolled case series and anecdotal reports. No specific treatment for thyroid acropachy is available. It is typically less symptomatic than thyroid dermopathy, although pain management is sometimes required. Tobacco use is thought to be a risk factor for severe manifestations of Graves disease and patients who use tobacco should be strongly urged to quit.[113]

PARATHYROID DISEASE

AT-A-GLANCE

- The most common cause of hypercalcemia in outpatients is hyperparathyroidism, whereas the most common cause of hypercalcemia in hospitalized patients is malignancy.
- The most common causes of hypocalcemia are vitamin D deficiency and surgically induced hypoparathyroidism.
- Calciphylaxis is most commonly seen in the setting of secondary hyperparathyroidism related to renal failure.

EPIDEMIOLOGY

The annual incidence of primary hyperparathyroidism has decreased since 1992 to about 20 cases per 100,000 person-years, potentially reflecting a decrease in the use of ionizing radiation to the neck, which is a known risk factor for developing primary hyperparathyroidism.[135] The majority of cases occur in individuals older than 45 years of age, with an approximate 2:1 female-to-male predominance.

CLINICAL FEATURES

Parathyroid disease most often presents with abnormal serum calcium levels. Table 137-12 outlines the physical findings and symptoms associated with hypercalcemia and hypocalcemia. Skin manifestations are rare in patients with hyperparathyroidism and hypercalcemia but can be impressive. Table 137-13 outlines the suggested approach to a patient with suspected hyperparathyroidism. Cutaneous calcinosis (sometimes referred to as *calcinosis cutis* or *metastatic calcinosis*) is thought to be partly caused by the combination of elevated calcium and phosphate (see Chap. 128).[136] Subcutaneous calcifications are typically found in a symmetric distribution, often overlying large joints or in linearly arrayed papules and plaques that are skin-colored and firm to palpation (Fig. 137-10). These lesions can be pruritic and can exert pressure on surrounding tissues. Chronic urticaria also is associated with hyperparathyroidism.[137] Signs or symptoms of hyperparathyroidism in combination with certain cutaneous tumors, such as angiofibromas, collagenomas, café-au-lait macules, and lipomas, should prompt a workup for multiple endocrine neoplasia Type 1 (MEN1). MEN1 is caused by mutations in the *MEN1* gene and characterized by tumors of the anterior pituitary, pancreas, and parathyroid glands. Table 137-14 shows the differential diagnosis of hypercalcemia.

Calciphylaxis (also called calcific uremic arteriolopathy) is a rare, but life-threatening, cutaneous condition associated with hyperparathyroidism. Calciphylaxis occurs most often in the setting of chronic renal failure and secondary hyperparathyroidism, although there are reports of calciphylaxis associated with primary hyperparathyroidism and normal renal function. Other risk factors include obesity, diabetes, protein C

TABLE 137-12

Physical Findings Associated with Hypercalcemia and Hypocalcemia

Hypercalcemia
- Anorexia
- Nausea and vomiting
- Constipation
- Muscle weakness and bone pain
- Lethargy and coma
- Anxiety and depression
- Polyuria and polydipsia
- Nephrolithiasis

Hypocalcemia
- Increased neuromuscular irritability and tetany
- Chvostek sign: induced tetany of the facial muscles induced by tapping the facial nerve just anterior to the ear
- Trousseau sign of hypocalcemia: carpal spasm with inflation of blood pressure cuff
- Peripheral and perioral paresthesias
- Seizures
- Bronchospasm/laryngospasm
- Lengthening of QT interval on electrocardiogram

TABLE 137-13
Approach to the Patient with Suspected Hyperparathyroidism

Cutaneous Findings
- Cutaneous (metastatic) calcinosis
- Calciphylaxis

Related Disorders
- Renal disease
- Multiple endocrine neoplasia Type 1 (MEN1) with angiofibromas, collagenomas, café-au-lait macules, and lipomas
- History of head/neck irradiation

Diagnosis
- Best initial tests are serum calcium and serum parathyroid hormone levels
- If malignancy is suspected, serum parathyroid hormone–related peptide

Management
- Identify underlying cause of hyperparathyroidism
- Appropriate endocrine, surgery, and nephrology consultation
- Hospitalization for acute cases with severe hypercalcemia
- Aggressive fluid resuscitation to treat severe hypercalcemia
- Phosphate replacement as warranted
- Dialysis as needed for acute renal failure
- Calciphylaxis warrants aggressive wound care and management of infections
- Surgical parathyroidectomy

or protein S deficiency, and warfarin administration. Calciphylaxis is caused by calcium deposition in the walls of small- to medium-sized vessels, resulting in vascular occlusion and overlying skin necrosis. Clinically, patients present initially with tender violaceous patches that may exhibit a mottled or reticular pattern. Subsequently, involved areas become indurated and exquisitely painful, with eventual ulceration and eschar formation that can lead to tissue gangrene (Fig. 137-11). Both the trunk and extremities can be involved, and the most common locations are the thighs, buttocks, and breasts. Most patients with calciphylaxis have a normal calcium-phosphate product (serum calcium × serum phosphate), although a calcium-phosphate product of greater than 70 mg/dL has often been cited as a predisposing risk factor. The histologic finding of calcium deposits in vessel walls coupled with compatible clinical findings is diagnostic. Calciphylaxis has a very poor prognosis, with reported mortality rates up to 80%, usually from infection. Excellent wound care and management of infections is critical. An accumulating number of case reports using the calcium-sequestering compound sodium thiosulfate in an intravenous infusion have demonstrated considerable efficacy, particularly in patients with renal disease.[138] Even though large clinical trials are lacking, the lack of any serious short-term side effects reported with sodium thiosulfate suggests serious consideration of this therapy for patients with calciphylaxis. Parathyroidectomy has been effective in the treatment of some, but not all, patients with calciphylaxis and hyperparathyroidism, and firm evidence that supports this practice is lacking. The calcimimetic agent cinacalcet has shown promise in some case reports in the treatment of calciphylaxis in patients with hyperparathyroidism.[139] There are also small case series reporting successful treatment of calciphylaxis using hyperbaric oxygen.[140]

Hypoparathyroidism is associated with scaly, hyperkeratotic, and edematous puffy skin (Table 137-15).[141] Patients may complain of paresthesias secondary to

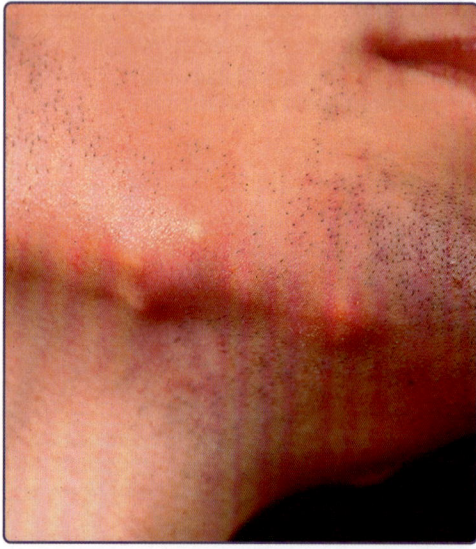

Figure 137-10 Papules of cutaneous calcinosis are arranged in a linear array in the skin overlying the mandible.

TABLE 137-14
Differential Diagnosis of Hypercalcemia

Increased Parathyroid Hormone
- Solitary adenoma
- Multiple adenomas (ie, multiple endocrine neoplasia Type 1 [MEN1])
- Tertiary hyperparathyroidism with renal failure

Increased Parathyroid Hormone-Related Peptide
- Squamous cell carcinoma
- Renal carcinoma
- Bladder carcinoma
- Human T-cell leukemia virus Type 1
- Breast cancer
- Lymphoma

Increased Serum 1,25-OH Vitamin D
- Sarcoidosis
- Excess ingestion

Increased Bone Resorption of Calcium
- Myeloma
- Lymphoma
- Breast cancer

Renal Failure
- Secondary hyperparathyroidism
- Tertiary hyperparathyroidism
- Vitamin D intoxication

Milk-Alkali Syndrome (Hypercalcemia Associated with Ingestion of Calcium-Based Antacids and Milk)

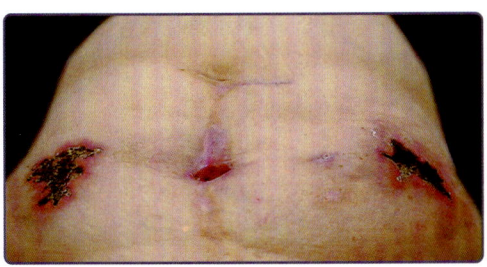

Figure 137-11 Calciphylaxis in a patient with chronic renal failure. Note the stellate-shaped necrotic plaques on the abdomen and the scars from peritoneal dialysis. The thighs and buttocks are often involved. A deep biopsy that includes subcutaneous fat can help make the diagnosis if it demonstrates the characteristic findings of calcification in the media of small- and medium-sized vessels. Histologically, subcutaneous calcium deposits and fat necrosis also can be seen.

hypocalcemia. Patchy alopecia and generalized thinning of the hair have been reported. Nails can be brittle with transverse ridging. Hypoparathyroidism with hypocalcemia is associated with flares of psoriasis, which is interesting in light of the response of psoriasis to the Vitamin D analog calcipotriene.[142] These skin abnormalities often resolve with normalization of serum calcium levels, suggesting that they are the result of changes in calcium homeostasis rather than parathyroid hormone (PTH) deficiency.

Hypoparathyroidism in the setting of familial autoimmune polyglandular syndrome Type 1 is associated with CMC and adrenal failure.[143] The CMC can precede the diagnosis of hypoparathyroidism, although the CMC does not improve significantly with treatment of the hypoparathyroidism with calcium and vitamin D. Other findings in these patients include dental enamel hypoplasia, vitiligo, and the cutaneous manifestations of adrenal failure (see section "Addison Disease").

Pseudohypoparathyroidism is the term for end-organ lack of responsiveness to PTH. The hypocalcemia and hyperphosphatemia of hypoparathyroidism is present, but serum PTH is elevated. Although several variants of pseudohypoparathyroidism have been described, perhaps the best characterized is Albright hereditary osteodystrophy.[144] These patients present with a constellation of findings that include short stature, developmental delay, obesity, rounded facies, dental hypoplasia, and shortened bones of the hands and feet. Characteristic shortening of the fourth metacarpal leads to a dimpling of the fourth knuckle, known as the *Albright sign*. These patients can also have subcutaneous ossifications and calcifications.

ETIOLOGY AND PATHOGENESIS

PTH is synthesized and secreted by the parathyroid glands in response to low levels of serum calcium and acts as one of the main regulators of calcium in the body. Elevations in serum PTH (hyperparathyroidism) increase serum calcium, whereas decreased levels of PTH (hypoparathyroidism) can lead to hypocalcemia. PTH acts through varying mechanisms that include the stimulation of vitamin D production, stimulation of calcium absorption in the GI tract, regulation of renal reabsorption of calcium and phosphate, and direct regulation of calcium mobilization from bone. Circulating free calcium acts on the parathyroid glands to control the release of PTH. Serum PTH then acts on target tissues by binding the PTH/PTH-related peptide (PTHrP) receptor, which is mainly expressed in the kidneys and bones, resulting in changes in calcium metabolism and an increase in serum calcium. Because abnormal levels of PTH primarily alter levels of serum calcium, it is not surprising that the skin manifestations of parathyroid disease are primarily the result of calcium dysregulation. The skin is likely a site of PTH action, although the exact effects of PTH on skin are not well understood. Keratinocytes produce a PTH-related peptide (PTHrP) that has been implicated in regulating keratinocyte growth and differentiation and uses the same receptors as PTH.[145-148] PTHrP-receptor interactions are thought to play in important role in the regulation of the hair cycle.[149] Elevated PTHrP also can be seen in the setting of squamous cell carcinomas and other malignancies and can result in malignancy-related hypercalcemia in these patients.[150]

Primary hyperparathyroidism results from abnormal function of the parathyroid gland, resulting in inappropriately elevated levels of PTH. In 80% of diagnosed cases, the cause of hyperparathyroidism is parathyroid hyperplasia, parathyroid carcinoma, or a parathyroid adenoma.

Secondary hyperparathyroidism occurs most often in the setting of renal disease. Altered metabolism of calcium, vitamin D, and phosphorous leads to elevated

TABLE 137-15
Approach to the Patient with Suspected Hypoparathyroidism

Cutaneous Findings
- Scaly, hyperkeratotic, puffy skin
- Patchy alopecia with thinning hair
- Brittle nails with transverse ridging

Related Findings
- Paresthesias
- Neuromuscular irritability
- Bronchospasm or laryngospasm
- Electrocardiogram changes

Diagnosis
- Serum calcium, phosphorous, and intact parathyroid hormone levels
- Serum magnesium levels to rule out hypomagnesemia
- Electrocardiogram to rule out QT elongation

Management
- Vitamin D or vitamin D metabolites (eg, calcitriol at 0.2 to 1 μg/day)
- Calcium supplementation at 2 to 3 g of elemental calcium per day
- Magnesium supplementation when appropriate
- Endocrinology and nephrology consultation

PTH. Hypersecretion of PTH results in hyperphosphatemia, and because of end-organ resistance to PTH there is persistent hypocalcemia despite the elevated PTH. In patients with renal failure and longstanding secondary hyperparathyroidism, hyperplastic parathyroid tissue can become autoactivated, resulting in tertiary hyperparathyroidism. This condition is characterized by persistent hypersecretion of PTH despite hypercalcemia.

Primary hypoparathyroidism is most often iatrogenic as a result of the removal of the parathyroid glands during a thyroidectomy. There are also several genetic and nongenetic congenital causes of primary hypoparathyroidism, although these are much less common. Secondary hypoparathyroidism refers to decreased PTH secretion secondary to a primary process that causes hypercalcemia.

DIAGNOSIS AND LABORATORY TESTS

The diagnosis of parathyroid disease can be made with measurements of serum calcium, phosphorous, and intact PTH. Total calcium levels may need to be corrected for low albumin. In the case of hypercalcemia related to malignancy, measurement of PTHrP also may be useful in the workup.

MANAGEMENT

The main treatment for hyperparathyroidism is partial or total parathyroidectomy (see Table 137-13). For hypoparathyroidism, treatment focuses on correction of serum calcium and phosphate (see Table 137-13). In the setting of acute hypercalcemia, aggressive fluid and electrolyte management are essential.

DISORDERS OF THE ADRENAL GLANDS

AT-A-GLANCE

- Excessive production of cortisol manifests as Cushing syndrome and results from pituitary oversecretion of corticotropin or excess production of cortisol by the adrenal glands.
- Destruction of the adrenal gland with resulting loss of glucocorticoids, mineralocorticoids, and adrenal androgens is known as Addison disease.
- Although many etiologies of Addison disease are described, the most common cause is autoimmune destruction with detectable circulating autoantibodies.

CUSHING SYNDROME

Cushing syndrome describes chronic exposure to excess corticosteroids. The most common cause is exogenous corticosteroid administration, but there are endogenous causes as well. In the normal physiology of the hypothalamic–pituitary–adrenal axis, corticotropin-releasing hormone is secreted from the hypothalamus and stimulates the production of corticotropin, also known as ACTH, by the anterior pituitary. ACTH is synthesized as part of a larger precursor molecule, POMC. The relationship of POMC to ACTH is important in diseases of the adrenal gland and the resulting skin manifestations. POMC is processed into several peptides, including melanocyte-stimulating hormone and ACTH, which stimulate the production of cortisol from the adrenal cortex. In a classic negative feedback manner, cortisol inhibits corticotropin-releasing hormone and ACTH production.

CLINICAL FEATURES

The clinical presentation of Cushing syndrome may be subtle (Table 137-16). Skin findings may be present, and if careful attention is paid to the relationship of skin findings and systemic complaints, the diagnosis can be made early in the clinical course. Common skin complaints are easy bruisability and skin thinning. Mild hypertrichosis often of the lanugo type and acne may occur. Frank hirsutism and severe acne raise the possibility of a tumor that also secretes androgens. The development of multiple violaceous striae wider than 1 cm on the abdomen or proximal extremities is highly suggestive of Cushing

TABLE 137-16
Approach to the Patient with Cushing Syndrome

Cutaneous Findings in Cushing Syndrome
- Increased central adiposity (moon facies and buffalo hump) with thinning of the extremities
- Skin thinning and easy bruisability
- Violaceous striae
- Acanthosis nigricans
- Increased dermatophyte and candidal skin and nail infections
- Hyperpigmentation (rare)

Related Features
- Diabetes
- Hypertension
- Osteoporosis
- Irregular menses

Diagnosis
- Measurement of 24-hour urinary free cortisol and late-night salivary cortisol
- Failure to suppress cortisol production with a low-dose dexamethasone suppression test

Management
- Appropriate endocrine and surgical consultation
- Surgical removal of pituitary or adrenal tumor
- Adrenal enzyme inhibitors
- Radiation therapy

syndrome. The width and color of these striae differentiate them from the striae commonly seen in pregnancy and weight gain. Relatively dramatic changes in fat distribution often occur along with a generalized gain in weight. Central obesity develops, along with concurrent thinning of the arms and legs with loss of muscle mass. Increased facial fat results in a rounded appearance of the face, often with increased redness and telangiectasias. This appearance has been referred to as a *moon facies*. In addition to truncal obesity, there is an increase in the size of the dorsocervical fat pad, known as a *buffalo hump* and there is increased fat in the supraclavicular fossae. Men may experience gynecomastia.

Although unusual, hyperpigmentation can occur in cases of Cushing syndrome caused by a massive increase in ACTH production either from the pituitary or, more commonly, an ectopic source.[151] ACTH itself, in addition to melanocyte-stimulating hormone derived from POMC, can stimulate increased melanin synthesis. This is similar to the hyperpigmentation more commonly associated with Addison disease. Acanthosis nigricans also may be seen because Cushing syndrome contributes to insulin resistance, and patients often develop diabetes. The immunosuppressive effects of glucocorticoids result in increased dermatophyte and candidal nail and skin infections. Women may experience irregular menses or amenorrhea. Additional extracutaneous signs and symptoms of Cushing syndrome include hypertension, osteoporosis, and decreased muscle mass and strength.[151]

EPIDEMIOLOGY, ETIOLOGY, AND PATHOGENESIS

The overall incidence of endogenous Cushing syndrome is about 10 persons per 1 million persons per year, with a female predominance.[152] It can be divided into 2 categories. The first category is caused by inappropriately high secretion of ACTH, usually from a pituitary microadenoma. It is given the unique name of *Cushing disease*. The excess ACTH drives glucocorticoid production in the adrenals. Rarely, ectopic (nonpituitary) production of ACTH results in Cushing syndrome. This clinical presentation is most often associated with a pulmonary carcinoid tumor or small cell lung carcinoma, although numerous other tumor types have been reported.[153] The second category of endogenous Cushing syndrome results from excess cortisol produced by the adrenal cortex independent of regulation by ACTH. This is usually caused by an adrenal adenoma, which may be benign or malignant, or is the result of generalized hyperplasia of the adrenal gland. Cushing syndrome can be seen in the McCune-Albright syndrome and in association with primary pigmented nodular adrenocortical disease in the Carney complex.[154,155]

DIAGNOSIS AND LABORATORY TESTS

Diagnostic confirmation of Cushing syndrome requires demonstration of excess cortisol production. The Endocrine Society recommends testing with a 24-hour urine free cortisol (repeated at least twice), late night salivary cortisol (repeated twice), or a low-dose dexamethasone suppression test.[156] Additional testing, including a high-dose dexamethasone suppression test, can be useful to determine if the source of the excess cortisol production is from the pituitary or elsewhere. Hypercortisolism may be present in patients without true Cushing syndrome. This is known as *pseudo-Cushing syndrome* and can be caused by obesity, major depressive disorders, and chronic alcohol abuse. It resolves with treatment of the underlying condition.

MANAGEMENT

The primary treatment of Cushing syndrome is surgical removal of the ectopic focus of ACTH production. Cure is achieved in the majority of patients, but resistant disease requires radiation in the case of pituitary disease or medical therapy with adrenal enzyme inhibitors such as ketoconazole or the adrenolytic agent mitotane.[151] Historically, Cushing syndrome was treated with bilateral adrenalectomy. This frequently resulted in Nelson syndrome, which is characterized by unchecked ACTH production from an enlarging pituitary adenoma with resulting hyperpigmentation. Neurosurgical resection of the tumor is considered first-line therapy.[157]

ADDISON DISEASE

CLINICAL FEATURES

Table 137-17 outlines an approach to the patient with Addison disease.

Destruction of the adrenal glands and the resulting life-threatening deficiency of glucocorticoids and

TABLE 137-17
Approach to the Patient with Addison Disease

Cutaneous Findings in Addison Disease
- Hyperpigmentation of skin and mucous membranes
- Longitudinal pigmented bands in the nails
- Vitiligo
- Decreased axillary and pubic hair in women
- Calcification of auricular cartilage in men

Related Features
- Abdominal pain
- Electrolyte abnormalities (hyponatremia and hyperkalemia)
- Postural hypotension
- Anorexia and weight loss
- Fatigue
- Shock, coma, and death, if untreated

Diagnosis
- Failure to respond adequately to corticotropin stimulation test

Management
- Lifelong replacement therapy of glucocorticoids and mineralocorticoids

mineralocorticoids is known as *Addison disease*. The estimated prevalence is 120 per million persons in Western countries.[158,159] It is suspected that many more cases remain undiagnosed. The most recognized cutaneous manifestation of Addison disease is hyperpigmentation of skin and mucous membranes. This occurs after longstanding adrenal insufficiency and would not be present in a patient with acute adrenal crisis unless the patient also had a history of chronic adrenal insufficiency. The hyperpigmentation is accentuated in sun-exposed areas, flexural folds, and skin creases, including the creases on the palms (Fig. 137-12). Pigment may develop in scars and longitudinal pigmented bands may appear in the nails. These pigment changes develop because persistently low cortisol levels do not provide negative regulatory feedback to the hypothalamus and pituitary. This results in unchecked production of POMC, ACTH, and melanocyte-stimulating hormone, which increase melanogenesis. Interestingly, vitiligo can be also seen in 10% to 20% of these patients.[160] Axillary and pubic hair may be sparse in women because of the loss of adrenal androgens. This does not occur in men because the testes maintain adequate androgen levels. Adrenal insufficiency can also cause calcification of auricular cartilage, known as "petrified ears."[161] Extracutaneous symptoms include weakness, anorexia, weight loss, abdominal pain, postural hypotension, and electrolyte abnormalities.

ETIOLOGY AND PATHOGENESIS

Historically, the most common cause of Addison disease was tuberculosis infection, but now autoimmune disease as part of the autoimmune polyglandular syndromes 1 and 2 is the most common etiology. In autoimmune cases, circulating autoantibodies can be detected to enzymes of the adrenal cortex, including 21-hydroxylase and 17-hydroxylase. There is lymphocytic infiltration of the adrenal glands with damage and scarring as a result.

Infectious causes of adrenal insufficiency remain the next most common etiology; tuberculosis is still a major problem in many areas of the world. Addison disease is increasingly recognized in patients with AIDS and, in these patients, infection with cytomegalovirus and *Mycobacterium avium-intracellulare* are common causes.[162,163] Fungal infections, including histoplasmosis, blastomycosis, paracoccidioidomycosis, coccidioidomycosis, and cryptococcosis, also are reported to cause Addison disease.[163] Bilateral adrenal hemorrhage in the setting of an acute severe bacterial infection is known as the *Waterhouse-Friderichsen syndrome*. Classically, this is a result of meningococcal infection, although other infectious causes have been reported.[163] Other rare causes of Addison disease include medications, congenital adrenal hypoplasia, and infiltrative disorders such as amyloidosis, sarcoidosis, and metastatic carcinomas. The surgical treatment of Cushing syndrome can be an additional cause of adrenal insufficiency.

DIAGNOSIS AND LABORATORY TESTS

Acute adrenal crisis can develop in the setting of chronic adrenal insufficiency and may be life-threatening. In an acute crisis, a blood sample should be obtained for measurement of cortisol, but therapy with intravenous hydrocortisone should be instituted immediately. In chronic adrenal insufficiency, the diagnosis is confirmed using the cosyntropin stimulation test. This involves the IV administration of synthetic ACTH and the measurement of serum cortisol 30 and 60 minutes later. Inability to produce adequate cortisol is diagnostic. Chronic replacement therapy is necessary and may require dose adjustments for illness or

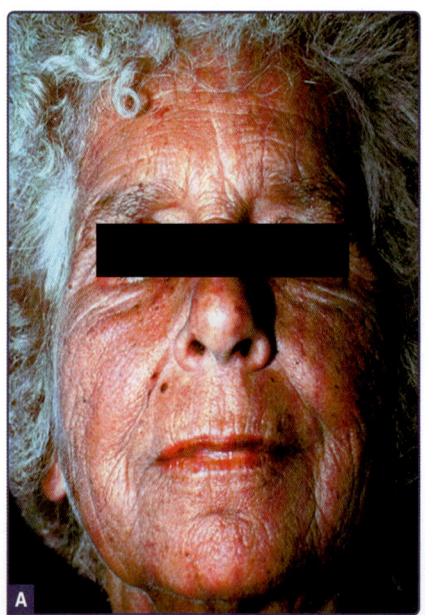

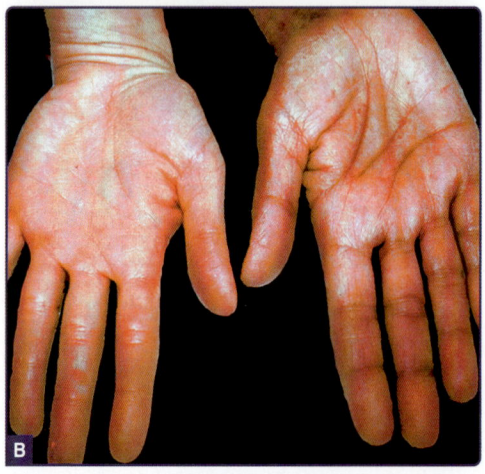

Figure 137-12 **A,** This patient with Addison disease demonstrates the characteristic hyperpigmentation of the skin with accentuation in sun-exposed areas. **B,** Palmar creases are also hyperpigmented compared to a normal hand.

severe stress. The cutaneous findings improve gradually with treatment, with the exception of auricular calcification.

ESTROGEN AND PROGESTERONE

AT-A-GLANCE

- Exogenous estrogen, either through oral contraceptives or hormone replacement, is the most common cause of estrogen excess.
- Wrinkling, xerosis, and atrophy are signs of estrogen deficiency.
- Triple-ingredient preparations are first-line therapy for treating melasma if patients are not content with covering cosmetics.

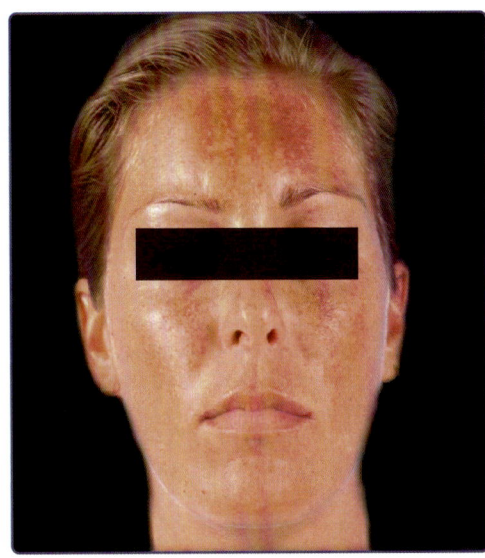

Figure 137-13 Melasma is demonstrated in a symmetric pattern on the face of a young woman. The upper lip is also a common site of involvement.

EPIDEMIOLOGY

The most commonly encountered cause of estrogen excess is the pharmacologic use of estrogens for birth control, treatment of dysfunctional uterine bleeding, or postmenopausal hormone replacement. Approximately 25% of women of child-bearing age in the United States use oral contraceptives.[164] Ovarian, testicular, or hypothalamic tumors can also cause estrogen excess. Estrogen deficiency occurs most commonly as a result of menopause, which occurs around 50 years of age on average. Other, less common causes of estrogen deficiency include pituitary or gonadal failure and exercise-induced amenorrhea.

CLINICAL FEATURES: CUTANEOUS MANIFESTATIONS OF ESTROGEN EXCESS AND DEFICIENCY

Estrogen can have both desired and undesired effects on the skin. Estrogen replacement therapy in postmenopausal women can reverse epidermal atrophy and restore cutaneous collagen. The inhibitory actions of estrogen on sebum production can lead to improvement of acne with oral contraceptive therapy, particularly with the use of estrogen-dominant preparations. Despite high circulating estriol during pregnancy, the relative androgen excess due to elevated progesterone can exacerbate acne in some patients. Telogen effluvium characterized by diffuse loss of scalp or body hair can occur after delivery or discontinuation of oral contraceptives. Both pregnant women and patients taking synthetic estrogens can be more prone to certain side effects of estrogen, including telangiectasias, palmar erythema, spider angiomas, and pigmentary changes.

Melanocytic lesions, including preexisting nevi and malignant melanoma, can darken during pregnancy. Hyperpigmentation of the nipples, linea nigra, and genitalia also can be seen. Melasma, sometimes referred to as the *mask of pregnancy*, presents as irregularly shaped, hyperpigmented patches on the forehead, cheeks, nose, upper lip, chin, and neck (Fig. 137-13). It is associated with pregnancy and oral contraceptive use, among other factors. Although melasma may improve after delivery, it can persist or reoccur with subsequent pregnancies. Melasma may persist even after discontinuation of the oral contraceptives. In the very rare cases of men with melasma, the etiology is thought to be sun exposure or familial susceptibility rather than estrogen excess, but the clinicopathologic features are similar to those seen in female patients.[165]

In clinical states characterized by elevated estrogen levels, including pregnancy and the use of oral contraceptives, increased hair growth over the face, breasts, and extremities can be seen. This phenomenon may be a result of the complex interplay of estrogens and androgenic hormones rather than a direct effect of increased estrogen levels on the hair follicles themselves. Autoimmune progesterone dermatitis and estrogen dermatitis have been described in the literature and are characterized by a polymorphous eruption marked by cyclical premenstrual flares that may include pruritus, eczematous dermatitis, and urticaria. The diagnosis may be made by separate subcutaneous injection of both estrogen and progesterone in the skin of the forearm. Persistence of a papule for more than 24 hours is considered a positive test, as is the presence of an immediate urticarial wheal that fades over hours in the case of urticaria.[166] Oral contraceptives have been implicated as a cause of erythema nodosum. Pregnancy and high estrogen levels also are associated with hyperkeratosis of the nipples.[167]

Estrogen deficiency from either menopause or pituitary failure can result in hot flashes, epithelial atrophy of the genitalia, and decreased breast size. Certain medications, such as danazol, leuprolide, and clomiphene citrate, can induce a pharmacologic menopause that presents with flushing. Flushing episodes accompanied by uncomfortable heat lasting several minutes can occur in younger women immediately before or during their period when estrogen levels are at their lowest.

ETIOLOGY AND PATHOGENESIS

Estrogen receptors are found throughout the skin, including on keratinocytes, sebaceous glands, eccrine and apocrine glands, in hair follicles, on dermal fibroblasts, and on melanocytes. In women of reproductive age, reported variations in dermatologic responses seen throughout the menstrual cycle suggest that estrogens and progesterone have important effects on the clinical presentation of numerous disease states of the skin.[168] Estrogen receptors are found in greater numbers in women compared with men. The main observations regarding the effects of estrogen on skin come from studies of postmenopausal women, in whom estrogen deprivation leads to skin wrinkling, xerosis, and atrophy. Increased epidermal and dermal thickness, increased water-holding capacity, changes in lipid composition of the stratum corneum, and improvement in skin laxity all occur with estrogen replacement, highlighting the important effects of this hormone throughout the skin.[169] Estrogen deficiency also has been reported to hinder wound healing, which subsequently improves with estrogen replacement. Estrogens also are reported to suppress sebaceous gland function and tend to inhibit hair growth.

The most potent naturally occurring estrogen is estradiol, which is the principal estrogen secreted by the ovaries. Estrone, another estrogen secreted by the ovaries, is synthesized primarily in peripheral tissues. During pregnancy, the main estrogen is estriol, which is synthesized by the placenta. Progesterone is the main hormone secreted by the corpus luteum, and peak levels are seen after ovulation. Gonadal hormones are not entirely specific, and progesterone is able to crossreact by binding to androgen receptors to exert androgenic or antiandrogenic effects.

MANAGEMENT

The Pigmentary Disorders Academy generated a consensus statement on the treatment of melasma and recommended the use of fixed "triple-ingredient" combinations as first-line therapy.[170] Topical retinoids, corticosteroids, azelaic acid, and hydroquinone-based bleaching creams have been used in various combinations to treat melasma for many years. Kligman's formula, first developed in 1975, is the classic triple-ingredient melasma preparation, consisting of 5% hydroquinone, 0.1% tretinoin, and 0.1% dexamethasone in a hydrophilic ointment. Dual-ingredient combinations or single agents are reasonable alternatives. For refractory cases, chemical peels (ie, glycolic acid or trichloroacetic acid) in combination with topical therapy can be tried, but postinflammatory hyperpigmentation is a concern. Lasers also can be considered but have shown variable results. Given the exacerbation of hyperpigmentation with sun exposure, sun avoidance and the consistent use of broad-spectrum sunscreens is very important in the treatment of all patients with melasma.

ANDROGENIC HORMONES

AT-A-GLANCE

- The peripheral conversion of testosterone to 5α-dihydrotestosterone is important in the pathophysiology of androgenetic alopecia.
- Hirsutism secondary to androgen excess has a characteristic distribution that includes the beard area, chest, back, and suprapubic region.

EPIDEMIOLOGY

In males, cutaneous manifestations of androgen excess occur most commonly with either the onset of sexual maturation or with androgen replacement therapy. Androgen-secreting tumors are a much less common cause of androgen excess. In women, androgen excess can occur from congenital adrenal hyperplasia (CAH). CAH is the result of a deficiency of enzymes in adrenal enzymes such as 21-hydroxylase (encoded by the gene *CYP21A2*), which accounts for more than 90% of cases of CAH.[171] Deficiency of CYP21 is inherited as an autosomal recessive trait and results in accumulation of 17-hydroxyprogesterone. Although the progestins in oral contraceptives are listed as potential causes of hirsutism because of their chemical similarity to testosterone, they likely do not cause androgenic effects at clinically used doses based on data from animal studies. PCOS occurs in approximately 5% of premenopausal women in the United States, and is characterized by insulin resistance, polycystic ovaries, and the presence of androgenic cutaneous findings such as acne, hirsutism, and androgenetic alopecia. PCOS is also associated with the metabolic syndrome, which is characterized by obesity, hypertension, lipid abnormalities, diabetes, and heart disease. Androgenetic alopecia affects approximately 50% of men older than age 40 years, and potentially as many women as well, with most patients showing signs of alopecia by age 30 years (see Chap. 85).

CLINICAL FEATURES: CUTANEOUS MANIFESTATIONS OF ANDROGEN EXCESS

Androgen-related skin conditions are commonly seen in dermatology practice. Although our knowledge regarding acne pathogenesis is still incomplete, at least part of acne's pathophysiology involves the response of sebaceous glands to androgens. In most males and females, acne tends to subside after adolescence (see Chap. 78). Cases of severe persistent acne should elicit a differential diagnosis that includes causes of persistent androgen excess, including CAH, PCOS in women, or an androgen-secreting tumor (Fig. 137-14), in addition to rosacea and chemically-induced acne. In the appropriate clinical setting, laboratory studies may be helpful in determining the source of androgen excess (Table 137-18). Performance-enhancing anabolic steroids are derivatives of testosterone, and the resulting androgen excess can manifest as acne.

There is some genetic variation underlying the response of hair follicles to androgens as evidenced by the varying degrees of hirsutism seen among women with different ethnic backgrounds but similar serum androgen levels. Hirsutism secondary to androgen excess occurs in a characteristic distribution involving the beard region of the face, the chest, the upper back, and the suprapubic area.

Paradoxically, although androgens can cause excess hair, they are also responsible for male-pattern (androgenetic) alopecia. Scalp hairs are converted first to indeterminate hairs and then to vellus hairs. In men, the pattern is characteristic and consists of symmetric recession of the hairline on the frontal and frontoparietal scalp along with hair loss on the vertex. In women, the frontal hairline is usually preserved, and the pattern is mostly diffuse thinning of the crown of the scalp without areas of frank alopecia. Although androgenetic alopecia can be acquired in patients with androgen excess, it is most commonly an incompletely characterized genetic disorder that appears to be inherited in an autosomal dominant manner (see Chap. 85).

TABLE 137-18
Approach to the Female Patient with Suspected Hyperandrogenism

History and Physical Findings Concerning for Hyperandrogenism
- Sudden onset of acne
- Severe acne refractory to conventional treatments
- Irregular menstrual periods
- Hirsutism

Laboratory Evaluation[a]
- Dehydroepiandrosterone sulfate (DHEA-S): screens for adrenal androgen source
  - Elevated in adrenal tumors and congenital adrenal hyperplasia
- Testosterone: screens for ovarian source
  - Elevated in polycystic ovarian syndrome
  - Some adrenal tumors can also secrete testosterone
- Luteinizing hormone–follicle stimulating hormone ratio
  - Ratio >2 to 3 can be consistent with polycystic ovarian syndrome

[a]Laboratory evaluation is most accurate when patient is off oral contraceptives for 4 to 6 weeks and if tests are drawn before menses.
Adapted from Thiboutot D. Acne: hormonal concepts and therapy. *Clin Dermatol*. 2004;22:419.

ETIOLOGY AND PATHOGENESIS

Like estrogen receptors, androgen receptors are also present throughout the skin. In men, androgens are synthesized in the testes and adrenal glands, whereas in women androgens are secreted by the ovaries and adrenal glands. In addition to testosterone, progesterone, dehydroepiandrosterone (DHEA), and DHEA sulfate (DHEA-S) are all natural androgens that can

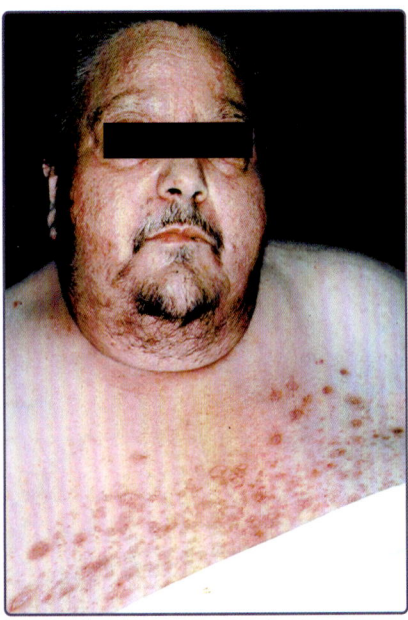

Figure 137-14 Hyperandrogenism manifests clinically in this woman with an androgen-secreting adrenal tumor. Note the characteristic facial hair, the receding hairline, and the acneiform eruption on the chest.

lead to cutaneous findings when they are present in excess.[172] Testosterone is subsequently converted in peripheral target tissues to the active metabolite 5α-dihydrotestosterone (5α-DHT) by the enzyme 5α-reductase. 5α-DHT binds the androgen receptor with greater affinity than testosterone.

Androgens are significant regulators of hair growth and sebaceous gland function. Androgens also play a role in the control of wound healing, epidermal differentiation, and the regulation of dermal fibroblasts. Androgen receptors have a trophic distribution throughout the body that is most evident with the appearance of "male pattern" hair growth on the face, chest, and back, as well as areas of hair loss on the scalp. Both estrogens and androgens bind to sex hormone–binding globulin. Sex hormone–binding globulin levels are decreased by the synthetic progestins found in oral contraceptives (eg, norgestrel, norethindrone, norgestimate, and desogestrel), as well as in obesity, acromegaly, hypothyroidism, and insulin resistance. The decreased sex hormone–binding globulin results in higher levels of circulating androgens and accounts, in part, for why androgenic findings can be associated with these conditions.

MANAGEMENT

In women whose acne appears to be hormonally driven, the use of antiandrogens, including the diuretic spironolactone, or oral contraceptive pills containing progestins with low androgenic or antiandrogenic activity, may prove more effective than conventional topical and oral acne medications. These drugs act as competitive inhibitors of dihydrotestosterone binding to androgen receptors. Specific 5α-reductase inhibitors, such as finasteride, can be used to treat androgenetic alopecia, although this medication is contraindicated in women of child-bearing age because of possible effects on development of genitalia and gonads in the male fetus. The use of finasteride has been linked to an increased risk of high-grade prostate cancer but without an increase in the absolute risk of prostate cancer in men, although similar data on men using finasteride for hair loss has not been reported.[173] Other side effects of finasteride therapy in men include depression, decreased libido, and erectile dysfunction.[174] These sexual adverse effects are persistent despite stopping finasteride in some patients. Finasteride treatment in postmenopausal women has not demonstrated significant benefit in a large placebo-controlled trial.[175]

Cyproterone acetate is an antiandrogen and progestin that is not available in the United States, although it has shown promise in the treatment of acne when used in other countries in oral contraceptive preparations. Flutamide is an androgen receptor antagonist that is rarely used due to the risk of fatal hepatitis as well as concerns about effects on fetal development in women of child-bearing age.[176]

DISORDERS OF GROWTH HORMONE

AT-A-GLANCE

- Growth hormone plays a central role in longitudinal growth.
- In children, growth hormone deficiency manifests as short stature, while gigantism occurs from oversecretion of growth hormone before puberty, when the growth plates in long bones are still open.
- The disease acromegaly occurs in adults after the growth plates have closed.
- Acromegaly results from oversecretion of growth hormone, usually from a pituitary adenoma.

ACROMEGALY

Growth hormone (GH) is secreted by the pituitary in a pulsatile fashion and reaches its maximum rate of secretion during puberty and then declines over time. Secretion of GH is primarily regulated by GH-releasing hormone (GHRH), somatostatin, and the natural GH secretagogue ghrelin.[177] GHRH and ghrelin stimulate the release of GH, whereas somatostatin has an inhibitory effect. The peripheral effects of GH are largely indirectly mediated through production of IGF1 in the liver. GH contributes significantly to linear growth in children, increases protein synthesis, mobilizes stored triglycerides, and antagonizes the action of insulin (Fig. 137-15).

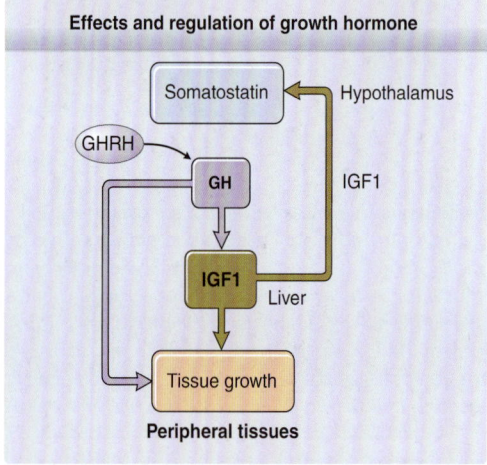

Figure 137-15 Effects and regulation of growth hormone (GH). GHRH, growth hormone–releasing hormone; IGF1, insulin-like growth factor-1.

CLINICAL FEATURES

Table 137-19 outlines an approach to the patient with acromegaly.

The clinical manifestations of acromegaly include the overgrowth of bone and connective tissue, metabolic effects, and localized tumor mass effects. The onset is insidious, and the average age at the time of diagnosis is 40 to 45 years, although the condition has often been present for many years before the diagnosis.[178] The metabolic effects include diabetes, hypertension, and hyperlipidemia. There is a gradual coarsening of facial features with frontal bone bossing and increasing shoe, ring, glove, and hat size (Fig. 137-16B).[179] Macroglossia and prognathism of the jaw may be seen. The skin becomes thickened, almost doughy, with deep prominent grooves on the forehead and around the nasolabial folds (Fig. 137-16A). Cutis verticis gyrata may develop on the scalp. Heel pads and the pads of the digits become thickened. Nails are thickened and brittle, and some patients develop hirsutism. Hyperhidrosis and malodor are common. Many patients develop acanthosis nigricans and multiple acrochordons with or without frank diabetes. Retinal angioid streaks can be seen in acromegaly (as well as in osteogenesis imperfecta and pseudoxanthoma elasticum). Histologically, there is dense deposition of glycosaminoglycans in the papillary and superficial reticular dermis. Often, coarse collagen bundles with normal elastin and increased numbers of fibroblasts are seen in the dermis.

TABLE 137-19
Approach to the Patient with Acromegaly

Cutaneous Findings in Acromegaly
- Enlargement of hands and feet with a doughy texture
- Increased ring, glove, shoe, and hat size
- Jaw enlargement with separation of teeth (prognathism)
- Frontal bossing
- Macroglossia
- Cutis verticis gyrata
- Acanthosis nigricans
- Hirsutism
- Hyperhidrosis
- Thick brittle nails

Related Features
- Diabetes
- Hypertension
- Hyperlipidemia

Diagnosis
- Elevated serum insulin-like growth factor-1 levels
- Failure to suppress growth hormone levels by oral glucose-tolerance test

Management
- Appropriate endocrine and surgical consultation
- Surgical removal of adenoma by transsphenoidal resection
- Somatostatin analogs or growth hormone receptor antagonists for residual disease
- Radiation therapy is an option for resistant cases

ETIOLOGY AND PATHOGENESIS

Excessive production of GH is almost always caused by a pituitary adenoma. In children, this results in pituitary gigantism, whereas in adults, excessive GH manifests as the clinical syndrome acromegaly. This syndrome is diagnosed in approximately 11 people per 1 million every year in the United States.[180] Very rarely, acromegaly is caused by a GH-producing tumor in the hypothalamus or by an ectopic tumor such as small cell lung cancer or carcinoid tumor.[179] The incidence of acromegaly caused by pituitary tumors is approximately 10% to 12% in patients with Carney complex, a genetic syndrome characterized by pigmented lesions, myxomas, and multiple endocrine tumors.[181] It is also present in approximately 20% of patients with McCune-Albright syndrome.[182]

DIAGNOSIS AND LABORATORY TESTS

Measurement of serum GH is highly variable and diagnostically unreliable because of the pulsatile pattern of secretion. Plasma IGF1 levels are dependent on GH and are fairly stable throughout a 24-hour period. Therefore, serum IGF1 levels can be used as a surrogate measurement of GH, and are elevated in acromegaly. Further workup with assistance from a consulting endocrinologist may include an oral glucose tolerance test. In the proper clinical setting, failure to suppress the GH level to less than 1 ng/mL 1 to 2 hours after 75 g of oral glucose is diagnostic for acromegaly.[179]

MANAGEMENT

Because most cases of GH excess are caused by a pituitary adenoma, the primary therapy is surgical removal. This is most commonly accomplished through a selective transsphenoidal resection.[179] Residual disease after surgery is more common in larger adenomas. Somatostatin analogs such as octreotide inhibit GH secretion and are used for the medical treatment of residual disease after surgery. They are increasingly being considered as potential primary therapy in select cases. In resistant cases, radiation therapy can be considered.

GROWTH HORMONE DEFICIENCY AND PANHYPOPITUITARISM

GH deficiency occurs in both children and adults and can be inherited or acquired. The primary clinical manifestation of this deficiency in children is

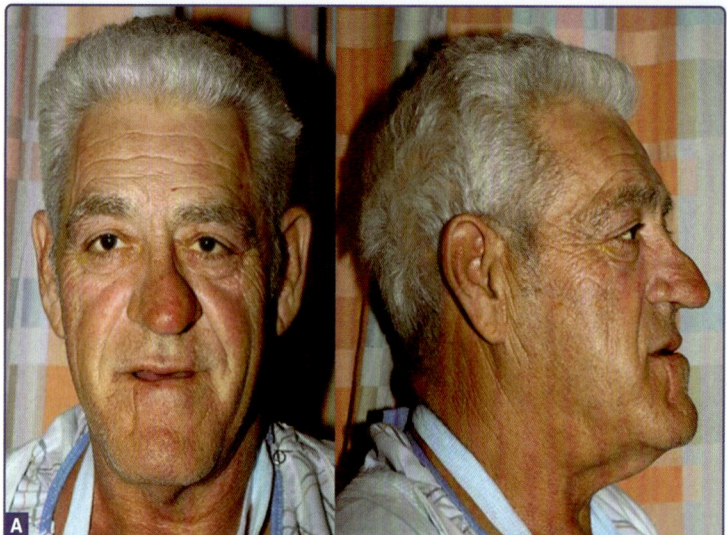

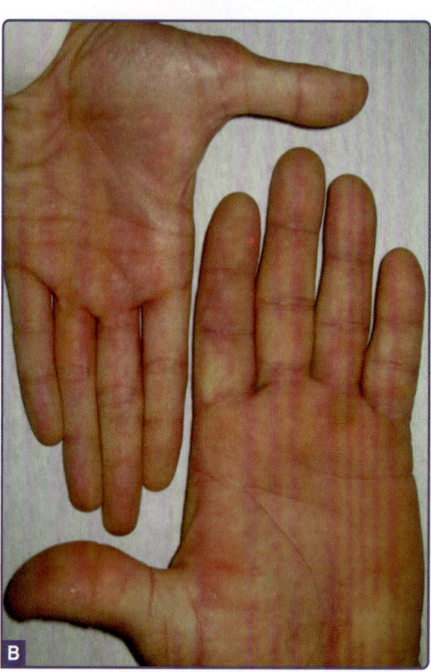

Figure 137-16 **A,** The facial changes in acromegaly include temporal wasting, broadening of the nose, deep grooves on the forehead and around the nasolabial folds, as well as jaw enlargement. **B,** Acral enlargement is a prominent feature of acromegaly and is easily demonstrated in comparison with a normal hand. (Used with permission from Brad Anawalt, MD.)

abnormally short stature. This can be corrected by the administration of GH. The clinical presentation of GH deficiency in adults includes decreased lean body mass, decreased strength and exercise capacity (partly the result of decreased sweating) and a loss of general vitality. GH replacement therapy in adults is a complex discussion that is beyond the scope of this chapter. Practice guidelines have been established by the Endocrine Society for the assessment and treatment of GH deficiency in adults.[183] In patients with panhypopituitarism, there is total loss of all pituitary function, including GH secretion (Table 137-20). These patients typically present with symptoms from either a space-occupying lesion in the pituitary or hormone dysregulation. These

TABLE 137-20
Causes of Hypopituitarism

- Mass lesions: nonfunctioning pituitary adenoma, cyst, craniopharyngioma, metastasis
- Infectious causes: tuberculosis, histoplasmosis
- Pituitary infarction: known as Sheehan syndrome when occurs in the setting of childbirth
- Pituitary apoplexy: sudden hemorrhage into the pituitary
- Lymphocytic hypophysitis
- Infiltrative disorders: hemochromatosis, sarcoidosis, Langerhans cell histiocytosis
- Head trauma
- Surgery or radiation

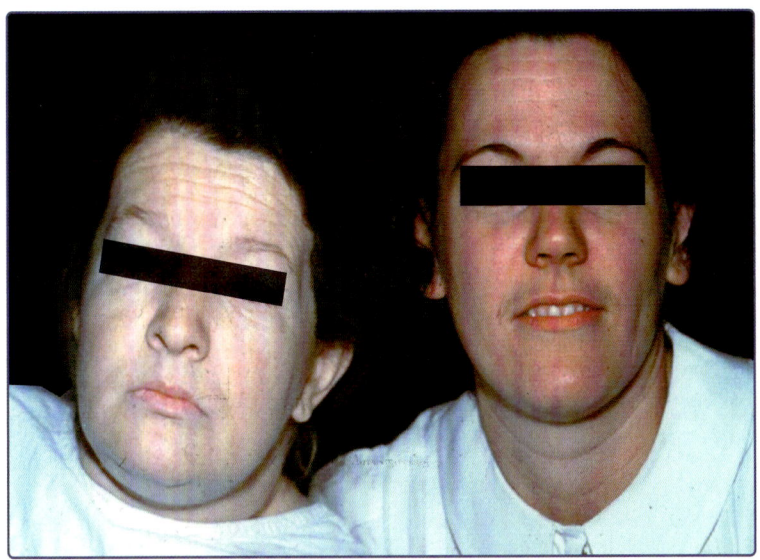

Figure 137-17 In this patient with panhypopituitarism, fine wrinkling and pale skin can be seen as well as other features suggestive of hypothyroidism. Her decreased pigmentation is contrasted by that of her nurse on the right. Patients with panhypopituitarism often present with findings of multiple endocrine disorders.

symptoms may be a manifestation of imbalance in any number of endocrine systems that are regulated at the level of the pituitary including features of hypothyroidism. Skin findings that have been described in these patients include fine wrinkling of the skin, decreased pigmentation, and decreased to absent pubic and axillary hair (Fig. 137-17).

ACKNOWLEDGMENTS

We acknowledge and sincerely appreciate the contributions to this chapter from the authors of previous editions, Dr. John Olerud and Dr. Andy Chien.

REFERENCES

1. Economic Costs of Diabetes in the U.S. in 2017. *Diabetes Care*. 2018;41(5):917-928.
2. Narayan KM, Boyle JP, Thompson TJ, et al. Lifetime risk for diabetes mellitus in the United States. *JAMA*. 2003;290(14):1884-1890.
3. Holman RR, Paul SK, Bethel MA, et al. 10-year follow-up of intensive glucose control in type 2 diabetes. *N Engl J Med*. 2008;359(15):1577-1589.
4. Skyler JS, Bergenstal R, Bonow RO, et al. Intensive glycemic control and the prevention of cardiovascular events: implications of the ACCORD, ADVANCE, and VA diabetes trials: a position statement of the American Diabetes Association and a scientific statement of the American College of Cardiology Foundation and the American Heart Association. *Diabetes Care*. 2009;32(1):187-192.
5. Beisswenger PJ, Moore LL, Curphey TJ. Relationship between glycemic control and collagen-linked advanced glycosylation end products in type I diabetes. *Diabetes Care*. 1993;16(5):689-694.
6. Dyer DG, Dunn JA, Thorpe SR, et al. Accumulation of Maillard reaction products in skin collagen in diabetes and aging. *J Clin Invest*. 1993;91(6):2463-2469.
7. Buckingham BA, Uitto J, Sandborg C, et al. Scleroderma-like changes in insulin-dependent diabetes mellitus: clinical and biochemical studies. *Diabetes Care*. 1984;7(2):163-169.
8. Monnier VM, Bautista O, Kenny D, et al. Skin collagen glycation, glycoxidation, and crosslinking are lower in subjects with long-term intensive versus conventional therapy of type 1 diabetes: relevance of glycated collagen products versus HbA1c as markers of diabetic complications. DCCT Skin Collagen Ancillary Study Group. Diabetes Control and Complications Trial. *Diabetes*. 1999;48(4):870-880.
9. Noordzij MJ, Mulder DJ, Oomen PH, et al. Skin autofluorescence and risk of micro- and macro-vascular complications in patients with Type 2 diabetes mellitus—a multi-centre study. *Diabet Med*. 2012;29(12):1556-1561.
10. Olerud JE. *Ellenburg & Rifkin's Diabetes Mellitus*. 6th ed. New York, NY: McGraw-Hill; 2003.
11. Joshi N, Caputo GM, Weitekamp MR, et al. Infections in patients with diabetes mellitus. *N Engl J Med*. 1999;341(25):1906-1912.
12. Cruz PD Jr, Hud JA Jr. Excess insulin binding to insulin-like growth factor receptors: proposed mechanism for acanthosis nigricans. *J Invest Dermatol*. 1992;98(6)(suppl):82S-85S.
13. Ansel JC, Armstrong CA, Song I, et al. Interactions of the skin and nervous system. *J Investig Dermatol Symp Proc*. 1997;2(1):23-26.
14. Reiber GE, Pecoraro RE, Koepsell TD. Risk factors for amputation in patients with diabetes mellitus. A case-control study. *Ann Intern Med*. 1992;117(2):97-105.
15. Schwartz RA. Acanthosis nigricans. *J Am Acad Dermatol*. 1994;31(1):1-19; quiz 20-22.
16. Stuart CA, Pate CJ, Peters EJ. Prevalence of acanthosis nigricans in an unselected population. *Am J Med*. 1989;87(3):269-272.

17. Tasjian D, Jarratt M. Familial acanthosis nigricans. *Arch Dermatol*. 1984;120(10):1351-1354.
18. Stuart CA, Gilkison CR, Smith MM, et al. Acanthosis nigricans as a risk factor for non-insulin dependent diabetes mellitus. *Clin Pediatr (Phila)*. 1998;37(2):73-79.
19. Andreev V. Malignant acanthosis nigricans. *Semin Dermatol*. 1984;3(4):265.
20. Brown J, Winkelmann RK. Acanthosis nigricans: a study of 90 cases. *Medicine (Baltimore)*. 1968;47(1):33-51.
21. Elder D, Elenitsas R, Jaworsky C, et al, eds. *Lever's Histopathology of the Skin*. 8th ed. Philadelphia, PA: Lippincott Williams and Wilkins; 1997.
22. Dunaif A. Insulin resistance and the polycystic ovary syndrome: mechanism and implications for pathogenesis. *Endocr Rev*. 1997;18(6):774-800.
23. Torley D, Bellus GA, Munro CS. Genes, growth factors and acanthosis nigricans. *Br J Dermatol*. 2002;147(6):1096-1101.
24. Flier JS, Usher P, Moses AC. Monoclonal antibody to the type I insulin-like growth factor (IGF-I) receptor blocks IGF-I receptor-mediated DNA synthesis: clarification of the mitogenic mechanisms of IGF-I and insulin in human skin fibroblasts. *Proc Natl Acad Sci U S A*. 1986;83(3):664-668.
25. Ellis DL, Kafka SP, Chow JC, et al. Melanoma, growth factors, acanthosis nigricans, the sign of Leser-Trelat, and multiple acrochordons. A possible role for alpha-transforming growth factor in cutaneous paraneoplastic syndromes. *N Engl J Med*. 1987;317(25):1582-1587.
26. Koyama S, Ikeda K, Sato M, et al. Transforming growth factor-alpha (TGF alpha)-producing gastric carcinoma with acanthosis nigricans: an endocrine effect of TGF alpha in the pathogenesis of cutaneous paraneoplastic syndrome and epithelial hyperplasia of the esophagus. *J Gastroenterol*. 1997;32(1):71-77.
27. Bohm M, Luger TA, Metze D. Treatment of mixed-type acanthosis nigricans with topical calcipotriol. *Br J Dermatol*. 1998;139(5):932-934.
28. Blobstein SH. Topical therapy with tretinoin and ammonium lactate for acanthosis nigricans associated with obesity. *Cutis*. 2003;71(1):33-34.
29. Rosenbach A, Ram R. Treatment of acanthosis nigricans of the axillae using a long-pulsed (5-msec) alexandrite laser. *Dermatol Surg*. 2004;30(8):1158-1160.
30. Coates P, Shuttleworth D, Rees A. Resolution of nicotinic acid-induced acanthosis nigricans by substitution of an analogue (acipimox) in a patient with type V hyperlipidaemia. *Br J Dermatol*. 1992;126(4):412-414.
31. Kebria MM, Belinson J, Kim R, et al. Malignant acanthosis nigricans, tripe palms and the sign of Leser-Tre'lat, a hint to the diagnosis of early stage ovarian cancer: a case report and review of the literature. *Gynecol Oncol*. 2006;101(2):353-355.
32. Frost D, Beischer W. Limited joint mobility in type 1 diabetic patients: associations with microangiopathy and subclinical macroangiopathy are different in men and women. *Diabetes Care*. 2001;24(1):95-99.
33. Silverstein JH, Gordon G, Pollock BH, et al. Long-term glycemic control influences the onset of limited joint mobility in type 1 diabetes. *J Pediatr*. 1998;132(6):944-947.
34. Rosenbloom AL, Silverstein JH, Lezotte DC, et al. Limited joint mobility in childhood diabetes mellitus indicates increased risk for microvascular disease. *N Engl J Med*. 1981;305(4):191-194.
35. Infante JR, Rosenbloom AL, Silverstein JH, et al. Changes in frequency and severity of limited joint mobility in children with type 1 diabetes mellitus between 1976-78 and 1998. *J Pediatr*. 2001;138(1):33-37.
36. Buckingham B, Perejda AJ, Sandborg C, et al. Skin, joint, and pulmonary changes in type I diabetes mellitus. *Am J Dis Child*. 1986;140(5):420-423.
37. Cole GW, Headley J, Skowsky R. Scleredema diabeticorum: a common and distinct cutaneous manifestation of diabetes mellitus. *Diabetes Care*. 1983;6(2):189-192.
38. Sattar MA, Diab S, Sugathan TN, et al. Scleroedema diabeticorum: a minor but often unrecognized complication of diabetes mellitus. *Diabet Med*. 1988;5(5):465-468.
39. Varga J, Gotta S, Li L, et al. Scleredema adultorum: case report and demonstration of abnormal expression of extracellular matrix genes in skin fibroblasts in vivo and in vitro. *Br J Dermatol*. 1995;132(6):992-999.
40. Cohn BA, Wheeler CE Jr, Briggaman RA. Scleredema adultorum of Buschke and diabetes mellitus. *Arch Dermatol*. 1970;101(1):27-35.
41. Seyger MM, van den Hoogen FH, de Mare S, et al. A patient with a severe scleroedema diabeticorum, partially responding to low-dose methotrexate. *Dermatology*. 1999;198(2):177-179.
42. Lee MW, Choi JH, Sung KJ, et al. Electron beam therapy in patients with scleredema. *Acta Derm Venereol*. 2000;80(4):307-308.
43. Parker F, Bagdade JD, Odland GF, et al. Evidence for the chylomicron origin of lipids accumulating in diabetic eruptive xanthomas: a correlative lipid biochemical, histochemical, and electron microscopic study. *J Clin Invest*. 1970;49(12):2172-2187.
44. Chait A, Robertson HT, Brunzell JD. Chylomicronemia syndrome in diabetes mellitus. *Diabetes Care*. 1981;4(3):343-348.
45. Parker F. Xanthomas and hyperlipidemias. *J Am Acad Dermatol*. 1985;13(1):1-30.
46. Valerius NH, Eff C, Hansen NE, et al. Neutrophil and lymphocyte function in patients with diabetes mellitus. *Acta Med Scand*. 1982;211(6):463-467.
47. Gallacher SJ, Thomson G, Fraser WD, et al. Neutrophil bactericidal function in diabetes mellitus: evidence for association with blood glucose control. *Diabet Med*. 1995;12(10):916-920.
48. Singh N, Armstrong DG, Lipsky BA. Preventing foot ulcers in patients with diabetes. *JAMA*. 2005;293(2):217-228.
49. Pecoraro RE, Reiber GE, Burgess EM. Pathways to diabetic limb amputation. Basis for prevention. *Diabetes Care*. 1990;13(5):513-521.
50. American Diabetes Association. Consensus Development Conference on Diabetic Foot Wound Care: 7-8 April 1999, Boston, Massachusetts. American Diabetes Association. *Diabetes Care*. 1999;22(8):1354-1360.
51. Levy DM, Karanth SS, Springall DR, et al. Depletion of cutaneous nerves and neuropeptides in diabetes mellitus: an immunocytochemical study. *Diabetologia*. 1989;32(7):427-433.
52. Antezana M, Sullivan S, Usui M, et al. Neutral endopeptidase activity is increased in the skin of subjects with diabetic ulcers. *J Invest Dermatol*. 2002;119(6):1400-1404.
53. Apelqvist J, Larsson J, Agardh CD. The influence of external precipitating factors and peripheral neuropathy on

53. the development and outcome of diabetic foot ulcers. *J Diabet Complications*. 1990;4(1):21-25.
54. Soulier SM. The use of running shoes in the prevention of plantar diabetic ulcers. *J Am Podiatr Med Assoc*. 1986;76(7):395-400.
55. Boyko EJ, Ahroni JH, Cohen V, et al. Prediction of diabetic foot ulcer occurrence using commonly available clinical information: the Seattle Diabetic Foot Study. *Diabetes Care*. 2006;29(6):1202-1207.
56. Wieman TJ, Smiell JM, Su Y. Efficacy and safety of a topical gel formulation of recombinant human platelet-derived growth factor-BB (becaplermin) in patients with chronic neuropathic diabetic ulcers. A phase III randomized placebo-controlled double-blind study. *Diabetes Care*. 1998;21(5):822-827.
57. Edmonds M, Bates M, Doxford M, et al. New treatments in ulcer healing and wound infection. *Diabetes Metab Res Rev*. 2000;16(suppl 1):S51-S54.
58. Langer A, Rogowski W. Systematic review of economic evaluations of human cell-derived wound care products for the treatment of venous leg and diabetic foot ulcers. *BMC Health Serv Res*. 2009;9:115.
59. Van Gils CC, Wheeler LA, Mellstrom M, et al. Amputation prevention by vascular surgery and podiatry collaboration in high-risk diabetic and nondiabetic patients. The Operation Desert Foot experience. *Diabetes Care*. 1999;22(5):678-683.
60. Apelqvist J, Larsson J, Agardh CD. Long-term prognosis for diabetic patients with foot ulcers. *J Intern Med*. 1993;233(6):485-491.
61. Mann RJ, Harman RR. Cutaneous anaesthesia in necrobiosis lipoidica. *Br J Dermatol*. 1984;110(3):323-325.
62. Muller SA, Winkelmann RK. Necrobiosis lipoidica diabeticorum. A clinical and pathological investigation of 171 cases. *Arch Dermatol*. 1966;93(3):272-281.
63. Lowitt MH, Dover JS. Necrobiosis lipoidica. *J Am Acad Dermatol*. 1991;25(5, pt 1):735-748.
64. Imtiaz KE, Khaleeli AA. Squamous cell carcinoma developing in necrobiosis lipoidica. *Diabet Med*. 2001;18(4):325-328.
65. Crosby DL, Woodley DT, Leonard DD. Concomitant granuloma annulare and necrobiosis lipoidica. Report of a case and review of the literature. *Dermatologica*. 1991;183(3):225-229.
66. O'Toole EA, Kennedy U, Nolan JJ, et al. Necrobiosis lipoidica: only a minority of patients have diabetes mellitus. *Br J Dermatol*. 1999;140(2):283-286.
67. Dandona P, Freedman D, Barter S, et al. Glycosylated haemoglobin in patients with necrobiosis lipoidica and granuloma annulare. *Clin Exp Dermatol*. 1981;6(3):299-302.
68. Petzelbauer P, Wolff K, Tappeiner G. Necrobiosis lipoidica: treatment with systemic corticosteroids. *Br J Dermatol*. 1992;126(6):542-545.
69. Kreuter A, Knierim C, Stucker M, et al. Fumaric acid esters in necrobiosis lipoidica: results of a prospective noncontrolled study. *Br J Dermatol*. 2005;153(4):802-807.
70. Darvay A, Acland KM, Russell-Jones R. Persistent ulcerated necrobiosis lipoidica responding to treatment with cyclosporin. *Br J Dermatol*. 1999;141(4):725-727.
71. Dubin BJ, Kaplan EN. The surgical treatment of necrobiosis lipoidica diabeticorum. *Plast Reconstr Surg*. 1977;60(3):421-428.
72. Dabski K, Winkelmann RK. Generalized granuloma annulare: clinical and laboratory findings in 100 patients. *J Am Acad Dermatol*. 1989;20(1):39-47.
73. Veraldi S, Bencini PL, Drudi E, et al. Laboratory abnormalities in granuloma annulare: a case-control study. *Br J Dermatol*. 1997;136(4):652-653.
74. Melin H. An atrophic circumscribed skin lesion in the lower extremities of diabetics. *Acta Med Scand*. 1964;176(suppl 423):1-75.
75. Binkley GW. Dermopathy in diabetes mellitus. *Arch Dermatol*. 1965;92(1):106-107.
76. Shemer A, Bergman R, Linn S, et al. Diabetic dermopathy and internal complications in diabetes mellitus. *Int J Dermatol*. 1998;37(2):113-115.
77. Danowski TS, Sabeh G, Sarver ME, et al. Shin spots and diabetes mellitus. *Am J Med Sci*. 1966;251(5):570-575.
78. Borssen B, Bergenheim T, Lithner F. The epidemiology of foot lesions in diabetic patients aged 15-50 years. *Diabet Med*. 1990;7(5):438-444.
79. Lithner F. Cutaneous reactions of the extremities of diabetics to local thermal trauma. *Acta Med Scand*. 1975;198(4):319-325.
80. Rapini RP, Herbert AA, Drucker CR. Acquired perforating dermatosis. Evidence for combined transepidermal elimination of both collagen and elastic fibers. *Arch Dermatol*. 1989;125(8):1074-1078.
81. Faver IR, Daoud MS, Su WP. Acquired reactive perforating collagenosis. Report of six cases and review of the literature. *J Am Acad Dermatol*. 1994;30(4):575-580.
82. Bernstein JE, Levine LE, Medenica MM, et al. Reduced threshold to suction-induced blister formation in insulin-dependent diabetics. *J Am Acad Dermatol*. 1983;8(6):790-791.
83. Toonstra J. Bullosis diabeticorum. Report of a case with a review of the literature. *J Am Acad Dermatol*. 1985;13(5, pt 1):799-805.
84. Ogden CL, Carroll MD, Kit BK, et al. Prevalence of childhood and adult obesity in the United States, 2011-2012. *JAMA*. 2014;311(8):806-814.
85. Loffler H, Aramaki JU, Effendy I. The influence of body mass index on skin susceptibility to sodium lauryl sulphate. *Skin Res Technol*. 2002;8(1):19-22.
86. Guida B, Nino M, Perrino NR, et al. The impact of obesity on skin disease and epidermal permeability barrier status. *J Eur Acad Dermatol Venereol*. 2010;24(2):191-195.
87. Yosipovitch G, Tur E, Cohen O, et al. Skin surface pH in intertriginous areas in NIDDM patients. Possible correlation to candidal intertrigo. *Diabetes Care*. 1993;16(4):560-563.
88. Enser M, Avery NC. Mechanical and chemical properties of the skin and its collagen from lean and obese-hyperglycaemic (ob/ob) mice. *Diabetologia*. 1984;27(1):44-49.
89. de Jongh RT, Serné EH, IJzerman RG, et al. Impaired local microvascular vasodilatory effects of insulin and reduced skin microvascular vasomotion in obese women. *Microvasc Res*. 2008;75(2):256-262.
90. Yosipovitch G, DeVore A, Dawn A. Obesity and the skin: skin physiology and skin manifestations of obesity. *J Am Acad Dermatol*. 2007;56(6):901-916; quiz 917-920.
91. Scheinfeld NS. Obesity and dermatology. *Clin Dermatol*. 2004;22(4):303-309.
92. Kelesidis T, Kelesidis I, Chou S, et al. Narrative review: the role of leptin in human physiology: emerging clinical applications. *Ann Intern Med*. 2010;152(2):93-100.
93. Oral EA, Simha V, Ruiz E, et al. Leptin-replacement therapy for lipodystrophy. *N Engl J Med*. 2002;346(8):570-578.

94. Lee JH, Chan JL, Sourlas E, et al. Recombinant methionyl human leptin therapy in replacement doses improves insulin resistance and metabolic profile in patients with lipoatrophy and metabolic syndrome induced by the highly active antiretroviral therapy. *J Clin Endocrinol Metab*. 2006;91(7):2605-2611.
95. Schaffer JV, Bolognia JL. The melanocortin-1 receptor: red hair and beyond. *Arch Dermatol*. 2001;137(11): 1477-1485.
96. Krude H, Biebermann H, Luck W, et al. Severe early-onset obesity, adrenal insufficiency and red hair pigmentation caused by POMC mutations in humans. *Nat Genet*. 1998;19(2):155-157.
97. Katsuki A, Sumida Y, Gabazza EC, et al. Plasma levels of agouti-related protein are increased in obese men. *J Clin Endocrinol Metab*. 2001;86(5):1921-1924.
98. Sonnett TE, Levien TL, Gates BJ, et al. Diabetes mellitus, inflammation, obesity: proposed treatment pathways for current and future therapies. *Ann Pharmacother*. 2010;44(4):701-711.
99. Inui A, Asakawa A, Bowers CY, et al. Ghrelin, appetite, and gastric motility: the emerging role of the stomach as an endocrine organ. *FASEB J*. 2004;18(3):439-456.
100. Klein S, Fontana L, Young VL, et al. Absence of an effect of liposuction on insulin action and risk factors for coronary heart disease. *N Engl J Med*. 2004;350(25): 2549-2557.
101. Mohammed BS, Cohen S, Reeds D, et al. Long-term effects of large-volume liposuction on metabolic risk factors for coronary heart disease. *Obesity (Silver Spring)*. 2008;16(12):2648-2651.
102. Andersson M, Takkouche B, Egli I, et al. Current global iodine status and progress over the last decade towards the elimination of iodine deficiency. *Bull World Health Organ*. 2005;83(7):518-525.
103. Hollowell JG, Staehling NW, Flanders WD, et al. Serum TSH, T(4), and thyroid antibodies in the United States population (1988 to 1994): National Health and Nutrition Examination Survey (NHANES III). *J Clin Endocrinol Metab*. 2002;87(2):489-499.
104. Weetman AP. Graves' disease. *N Engl J Med*. 2000;343(17):1236-1248.
105. De Leo S, Lee SY, Braverman LE. Hyperthyroidism. *Lancet*. 2016;388(10047):906-918.
106. Laurberg P, Cerqueira C, Ovesen L, et al. Iodine intake as a determinant of thyroid disorders in populations. *Best Pract Res Clin Endocrinol Metab*. 2010;24(1):13-27.
107. Buyukgebiz A. Congenital hypothyroidism clinical aspects and late consequences. *Pediatr Endocrinol Rev*. 2003;1(suppl 2):185-190; discussion 190.
108. Polak M. Hyperthyroidism in early infancy: pathogenesis, clinical features and diagnosis with a focus on neonatal hyperthyroidism. *Thyroid*. 1998;8(12): 1171-1177.
109. Ai J, Leonhardt JM, Heymann WR. Autoimmune thyroid diseases: etiology, pathogenesis, and dermatologic manifestations. *J Am Acad Dermatol*. 2003;48(5):641-659; quiz 660-662.
110. Fatourechi V, Pajouhi M, Fransway AF. Dermopathy of Graves disease (pretibial myxedema). Review of 150 cases. *Medicine (Baltimore)*. 1994;73(1):1-7.
111. Fatourechi V, Bartley GB, Eghbali-Fatourechi GZ, et al. Graves' dermopathy and acropachy are markers of severe Graves' ophthalmopathy. *Thyroid*. 2003;13(12): 1141-1144.
112. Parker LN, Wu SY, Lai MK, et al. The early diagnosis of atypical thyroid acropachy. *Arch Intern Med*. 1982;142(9):1749-1751.
113. Fatourechi V, Ahmed DD, Schwartz KM. Thyroid acropachy: report of 40 patients treated at a single institution in a 26-year period. *J Clin Endocrinol Metab*. 2002;87(12):5435-5441.
114. Dreskin SC, Andrews KY. The thyroid and urticaria. *Curr Opin Allergy Clin Immunol*. 2005;5(5):408-412.
115. Kim DH, Sung NH, Lee AY. Effect of levothyroxine treatment on clinical symptoms in hypothyroid patients with chronic urticaria and thyroid autoimmunity. *Ann Dermatol*. 2016;28(2):199-204.
116. Bagnasco M, Minciullo PL, Saraceno GS, et al. Urticaria and thyroid autoimmunity. *Thyroid*. 2011;21(4): 401-410.
117. Doshi DN, Blyumin ML, Kimball AB. Cutaneous manifestations of thyroid disease. *Clin Dermatol*. 2008;26(3):283-287.
118. Miller JJ, Roling D, Spiers E, et al. Palmoplantar keratoderma associated with hypothyroidism. *Br J Dermatol*. 1998;139(4):741-742.
119. Basaria S, Salvatori R. Images in clinical medicine. Pemberton's sign. *N Engl J Med*. 2004;350(13):1338.
120. Biro E, Szekanecz Z, Czirjak L, et al. Association of systemic and thyroid autoimmune diseases. *Clin Rheumatol*. 2006;25(2):240-245.
121. Callen JP, McCall MW. Bullous pemphigoid and Hashimoto's thyroiditis. *J Am Acad Dermatol*. 1981;5(5): 558-560.
122. Coleman R, Hay RJ. Chronic mucocutaneous candidosis associated with hypothyroidism: a distinct syndrome? *Br J Dermatol*. 1997;136(1):24-29.
123. Puavilai S, Puavilai G, Charuwichitratana S, et al. Prevalence of thyroid diseases in patients with alopecia areata. *Int J Dermatol*. 1994;33(9):632-633.
124. Zettinig G, Weissel M, Flores J, et al. Dermatitis herpetiformis is associated with atrophic but not with goitrous variant of Hashimoto's thyroiditis. *Eur J Clin Invest*. 2000;30(1):53-57.
125. Rees Smith B, McLachlan SM, Furmaniak J. Autoantibodies to the thyrotropin receptor. *Endocr Rev*. 1988;9(1):106-121.
126. Surks MI, Sievert R. Drugs and thyroid function. *N Engl J Med*. 1995;333(25):1688-1694.
127. Prabhakar BS, Bahn RS, Smith TJ. Current perspective on the pathogenesis of Graves' disease and ophthalmopathy. *Endocr Rev*. 2003;24(6):802-835.
128. Derwahl M, Manole D, Sobke A, et al. Pathogenesis of toxic thyroid adenomas and nodules: relevance of activating mutations in the TSH-receptor and Gs-alpha gene, the possible role of iodine deficiency and secondary and TSH-independent molecular mechanisms. *Exp Clin Endocrinol Diabetes*. 1998;106(suppl 4): S6-S9.
129. Safer JD, Crawford TM, Holick MF. Topical thyroid hormone accelerates wound healing in mice. *Endocrinology*. 2005;146(10):4425-4430.
130. Contreras-Jurado C, Lorz C, Garcia-Serrano L, et al. Thyroid hormone signaling controls hair follicle stem cell function. *Mol Biol Cell*. 2015;26(7):1263-1272.
131. Hamnvik OP, Larsen PR, Marqusee E. Thyroid dysfunction from antineoplastic agents. *J Natl Cancer Inst*. 2011;103(21):1572-1587.
132. Sherman SI, Gopal J, Haugen BR, et al. Central hypothyroidism associated with retinoid X receptor-selective ligands. *N Engl J Med*. 1999;340(14):1075-1079.

133. Pingsmann A, Ockenfels HM, Patsalis T. Surgical excision of pseudotumorous pretibial myxedema. *Foot Ankle Int.* 1996;17(2):107-110.
134. Susser WS, Heermans AG, Chapman MS, et al. Elephantiasic pretibial myxedema: a novel treatment for an uncommon disorder. *J Am Acad Dermatol.* 2002;46(5):723-726.
135. Wermers RA, Khosla S, Atkinson EJ, et al. Incidence of primary hyperparathyroidism in Rochester, Minnesota, 1993-2001: an update on the changing epidemiology of the disease. *J Bone Miner Res.* 2006;21(1):171-177.
136. Walsh JS, Fairley JA. Calcifying disorders of the skin. *J Am Acad Dermatol.* 1995;33(5, pt 1):693-706; quiz 707-710.
137. Dagher HN, Aboujaoude ZC, Jabbour SA. Chronic urticaria: an unusual initial manifestation of primary hyperparathyroidism. *Endocr Pract.* 2002;8(1):47-49.
138. Schlieper G, Brandenburg V, Ketteler M, et al. Sodium thiosulfate in the treatment of calcific uremic arteriolopathy. *Nat Rev Nephrol.* 2009;5(9):539-543.
139. Vedvyas C, Winterfield LS, Vleugels RA. Calciphylaxis: a systematic review of existing and emerging therapies. *J Am Acad Dermatol.* 2012;67(6):e253-e260.
140. An J, Devaney B, Ooi KY, et al. Hyperbaric oxygen in the treatment of calciphylaxis: a case series and literature review. *Nephrology (Carlton).* 2015;20(7):444-450.
141. Jabbour SA. Cutaneous manifestations of endocrine disorders: a guide for dermatologists. *Am J Clin Dermatol.* 2003;4(5):315-331.
142. Lee Y, Nam YH, Lee JH, et al. Hypocalcaemia-induced pustular psoriasis-like skin eruption. *Br J Dermatol.* 2005;152(3):591-593.
143. Makitie O, Sochett EB, Bondestam S, et al. Bone health in autoimmune polyendocrinopathy-candidiasis-ectodermal dystrophy (APECED): findings in 25 adults. *Clin Endocrinol (Oxf).* 2006;64(5):489-494.
144. Wilson LC, Hall CM. Albright's hereditary osteodystrophy and pseudohypoparathyroidism. *Semin Musculoskelet Radiol.* 2002;6(4):273-283.
145. Foley J, Longely BJ, Wysolmerski JJ, et al. PTHrP regulates epidermal differentiation in adult mice. *J Invest Dermatol.* 1998;111(6):1122-1128.
146. Sharpe GR, Dillon JP, Durham B, et al. Human keratinocytes express transcripts for three isoforms of parathyroid hormone-related protein (PTHrP), but not for the parathyroid hormone/PTHrP receptor: effects of 1,25(OH)2 vitamin D3. *Br J Dermatol.* 1998;138(6):944-951.
147. Lowik CW, Hoekman K, Offringa R, et al. Regulation of parathyroid hormonelike protein production in cultured normal and malignant keratinocytes. *J Invest Dermatol.* 1992;98(2):198-203.
148. Atillasoy EJ, Burtis WJ, Milstone LM. Immunohistochemical localization of parathyroid hormone-related protein (PTHRP) in normal human skin. *J Invest Dermatol.* 1991;96(2):277-280.
149. Diamond AG, Gonterman RM, Anderson AL, et al. Parathyroid hormone hormone-related protein and the PTH receptor regulate angiogenesis of the skin. *J Invest Dermatol.* 2006;126(9):2127-2134.
150. Donovan PJ, Achong N, Griffin K, et al. PTHrP-mediated hypercalcemia: causes and survival in 138 patients. *J Clin Endocrinol Metab.* 2015;100(5):2024-2029.
151. Orth DN. Cushing's syndrome. *N Engl J Med.* 1995;332(12):791-803.
152. Beauregard C, Dickstein G, Lacroix A. Classic and recent etiologies of Cushing's syndrome: diagnosis and therapy. *Treat Endocrinol.* 2002;1(2):79-94.
153. Ilias I, Torpy DJ, Pacak K, et al. Cushing's syndrome due to ectopic corticotropin secretion: twenty years' experience at the National Institutes of Health. *J Clin Endocrinol Metab.* 2005;90(8):4955-4962.
154. Jabbour SA. Skin manifestations of hormone-secreting tumors. *Dermatol Ther.* 2010;23(6):643-650.
155. Stratakis CA. Cushing syndrome caused by adrenocortical tumors and hyperplasias (corticotropin-independent Cushing syndrome). *Endocr Dev.* 2008;13:117-132.
156. Nieman LK, Biller BM, Findling JW, et al. The diagnosis of Cushing's syndrome: an Endocrine Society clinical practice guideline. *J Clin Endocrinol Metab.* 2008;93(5):1526-1540.
157. Palermo NE, Ananthakrishnan S. Re-examining Nelson's syndrome. *Curr Opin Endocrinol Diabetes Obes.* 2015;22(4):313-318.
158. Ten S, New M, Maclaren N. Clinical review 130: Addison's disease 2001. *J Clin Endocrinol Metab.* 2001;86(7):2909-2922.
159. Laureti S, Vecchi L, Santeusanio F, et al. Is the prevalence of Addison's disease underestimated? *J Clin Endocrinol Metab.* 1999;84(5):1762.
160. Zelissen PM, Bast EJ, Croughs RJ. Associated autoimmunity in Addison's disease. *J Autoimmun.* 1995;8(1):121-130.
161. Barkan A, Glantz I. Calcification of auricular cartilages in patients with hypopituitarism. *J Clin Endocrinol Metab.* 1982;55(2):354-357.
162. Jameson JL, De Groot LJ. *Endocrinology: Adult and Pediatric.* Philadelphia, PA: Elsevier Health Sciences; 2010.
163. Alevritis EM, Sarubbi FA, Jordan RM, et al. Infectious causes of adrenal insufficiency. *South Med J.* 2003;96(9):888-890.
164. Daniels K, Daugherty J, Jones J, et al. Current contraceptive use and variation by selected characteristics among women aged 15-44: United States, 2011-2013. *Natl Health Stat Report.* 2015(86):1-14.
165. Sarkar R, Puri P, Jain RK, et al. Melasma in men: a clinical, aetiological and histological study. *J Eur Acad Dermatol Venereol.* 2010;24(7):768-772.
166. Shelley WB, Shelley ED, Talanin NY, et al. Estrogen dermatitis. *J Am Acad Dermatol.* 1995;32(1):25-31.
167. Higgins HW, Jenkins J, Horn TD, et al. Pregnancy-associated hyperkeratosis of the nipple: a report of 25 cases. *JAMA Dermatol.* 2013;149(6):722-726.
168. Farage MA, Berardesca E, Maibach H. The possible relevance of sex hormones on irritant and allergic responses: their importance for skin testing. *Contact Dermatitis.* 2010;62(2):67-74.
169. Hall G, Phillips TJ. Estrogen and skin: the effects of estrogen, menopause, and hormone replacement therapy on the skin. *J Am Acad Dermatol.* 2005;53(4):555-568; quiz 569-572.
170. Rendon M, Berneburg M, Arellano I, et al. Treatment of melasma. *J Am Acad Dermatol.* 2006;54(5)(suppl 2):S272-S281.
171. Forest MG. Recent advances in the diagnosis and management of congenital adrenal hyperplasia due to 21-hydroxylase deficiency. *Hum Reprod Update.* 2004;10(6):469-485.
172. Chen W, Thiboutot D, Zouboulis CC. Cutaneous androgen metabolism: basic research and clinical perspectives. *J Invest Dermatol.* 2002;119(5):992-1007.
173. Wilt TJ, MacDonald R, Hagerty K, et al. Five-alpha-reductase Inhibitors for prostate cancer prevention. *Cochrane Database Syst Rev.* 2008(2):Cd007091.

174. Traish AM, Melcangi RC, Bortolato M, et al. Adverse effects of 5α-reductase inhibitors: what do we know, don't know, and need to know? *Rev Endocr Metab Disord*. 2015;16(3):177-198.
175. van Zuuren EJ, Fedorowicz Z, Schoones J. Interventions for female pattern hair loss. *Cochrane Database Syst Rev*. 2016;(5):Cd007628.
176. Thiboutot D. Acne: hormonal concepts and therapy. *Clin Dermatol*. 2004;22(5):419-428.
177. Khatib N, Gaidhane S, Gaidhane AM, et al. Ghrelin: ghrelin as a regulatory peptide in growth hormone secretion. *J Clin Diagn Res*. 2014;8(8):MC13-MC17.
178. Rajasoorya C, Holdaway IM, Wrightson P, et al. Determinants of clinical outcome and survival in acromegaly. *Clin Endocrinol (Oxf)*. 1994;41(1):95-102.
179. Melmed S. Acromegaly. *N Engl J Med*. 2006;355(24):2558-2573.
180. Burton T, Le Nestour E, Neary M, et al. Incidence and prevalence of acromegaly in a large US health plan database. *Pituitary*. 2016;19:262-267.
181. Correa R, Salpea P, Stratakis C. Carney complex: an update. *Eur J Endocrinol*. 2015;173(4):M85-M97.
182. Salenave S, Boyce AM, Collins MT, et al. Acromegaly and McCune-Albright syndrome. *J Clin Endocrinol Metab*. 2014;99(6):1955-1969.
183. Molitch ME, Clemmons DR, Malozowski S, et al. Evaluation and treatment of adult growth hormone deficiency: an Endocrine Society clinical practice guideline. *J Clin Endocrinol Metab*. 2011;96(6):1587-1609.

图书在版编目（CIP）数据

菲兹帕里克皮肤病学：第9版：双语版：汉、英文. 中册 /[美] 康斯文（Sewon Kang）等主编；陈翔，粟娟等编译.—长沙：湖南科学技术出版社，2020.10
（西医经典名著集成）
ISBN 978-7-5710-0760-7

Ⅰ.①菲… Ⅱ.①康… ②陈… ③粟…Ⅲ.①皮肤病学—汉、英文 Ⅳ.①R751

中国版本图书馆 CIP 数据核字(2020)第 189071 号

Sewon Kang, Masayuki Amagai, Anna L. Brucker, Alexander H. Enk, David J. Margolis, Amy J. McMichael, Jeffrey S. Orringer
Fitzpatrick's Dermatology, Ninth Edition, 2-Volume Set
ISBN 9780071837795
Copyright ©2019 by McGraw-Hill Education.

All Rights reserved. No part of this publication may be reproduced or transmitted in any form or by any means, electronic or mechanical, including without limitation photocopying, recording, taping, or any database, information or retrieval system, without the prior written permission of the publisher.

This authorized Bilingual edition is jointly published by McGraw-Hill Education and Hunan Science & Technology Press. This edition is authorized for sale in the People's Republic of China only, excluding Hong Kong, Macao SAR and Taiwan.

Translation Copyright © 2020 by McGraw-Hill Education and Hunan Science & Technology Press.

版权所有。未经出版人事先书面许可，对本出版物的任何部分不得以任何方式或途径复制或传播，包括但不限于复印、录制、录音，或通过任何数据库、信息或可检索的系统。

本授权双语版由麦格劳-希尔教育出版公司和湖南科学技术出版社合作出版。此版本经授权仅限在中华人民共和国境内（不包括香港特别行政区、澳门特别行政区和台湾省）销售。

翻译版权©2020 由麦格劳-希尔教育出版公司与湖南科学技术出版社所有。

本书封面贴有 McGraw-Hill Education 公司防伪标签，无标签者不得销售。
著作权合同登记号 18-2020-188

西医经典名著集成
FEIZIPALIKE PIFUBINGXUE

菲兹帕里克皮肤病学　第 9 版（双语版）中册

主　　编：	[美]康斯文（Sewon Kang），[日]天谷正之（Masayuki Amagai），[美]安娜 L. 布鲁克纳（Anna L. Brucker），[德]亚历山大 H. 恩（Alexander H. Enk），[美]大卫 J. 马戈利斯（David J. Margolis），[美]艾美 J. 麦克迈克尔（Amy J. McMichael），[美]杰弗里 S. 奥林格（Jeffrey S. Orringer）
编 译 者：	陈翔，粟娟等
责任编辑：	李　忠　杨　颖
出版发行：	湖南科学技术出版社
社　　址：	长沙市湘雅路 276 号
	http://www.hnstp.com
印　　刷：	湖南凌宇纸品有限公司
厂　　址：	长沙市长沙县黄花镇黄花工业园
邮　　编：	410137
版　　次：	2020 年 10 月第 1 版
印　　次：	2020 年 10 月第 1 次印刷
开　　本：	787mm×1092mm　1/16
印　　张：	81
字　　数：	4210 千字
书　　号：	ISBN 978-7-5710-0760-7
定　　价：	1050.00 元（上、中、下册）

（版权所有·翻印必究）